GENETIC DISORDERS AND THE FETUS

GENETIC DISORDERS AND THE FETUS

DIAGNOSIS, PREVENTION, AND TREATMENT

Fifth Edition

Edited by
AUBREY MILUNSKY, MB.B.Ch., D.Sc., F.R.C.P., F.A.C.M.G., D.C.H.
Professor of Human Genetics, Pediatrics,
Obstetrics and Gynecology, and Pathology
and Director, Center for Human Genetics
Boston University School of Medicine
Boston, Massachusettts

THE JOHNS HOPKINS UNIVERSITY PRESS
Baltimore and London

The Johns Hopkins University Press
2715 North Charles Street
Baltimore, Maryland 21218-4363
www.press.jhu.edu

Library of Congress Cataloging-in-Publication Data

Genetic disorders and the fetus: diagnosis, prevention, and treatment / edited by Aubrey Milunsky.
   —5th ed.
      p.   cm.
   Includes bibliographical references and index.
   ISBN 0-8018-7928-0 (hardcover : alk. paper)
   1. Prenatal diagnosis.   2. Fetus—Diseases—Genetic aspects.   3. Fetus—Abnormalities—
Genetic aspects.
   [DNLM: 1. Genetic Diseases, Inborn.   2. Prenatal Diagnosis.   3. Fetal Diseases—genetics.
QZ 50 G3244   2004]   I. Milunsky, Aubrey.
RG628.G46   2004
618.3′2042—dc22   2003018312

A catalog record for this book is available from the British Library.

Dedicated to

Laura
for her love, understanding, and support

and to

my grandchildren,
Julie, Miranda, and Cody,
who endow life with joy and meaning

Contents

Preface to the Fifth Edition

In this electronic age, it takes but a moment to reach the medical literature and to begin to explore a subject, no matter how small or vast. With such access, then, a justifiable question could be why a major reference text like this one is at all necessary. This in turn begets the question about the purpose and utility of any such text. As an inveterate life-long reader and frequent consulter of leading medical texts, my response might resonate with the experience of others.

Most, I think, would seek an up-to-date text that is a major repository of facts and knowledge with accurate information and reliable recommendations. It should be easy to read and contain valuable tabulated data, good illustrations, and concepts presented with clarity. The authors, preferably drawn internationally, should be experts, and their authoritative contributions and perspectives should reflect critical analysis, synthesis, and the wisdom of their experience. Facts should be easily accessed via a comprehensive index, and the text should be thoroughly referenced. Such a text should serve as a stimulus to research and be an important source of guidance in the care of patients. Mindful of these quintessential elements and with the collaboration of outstanding experts, this fifth edition, reflecting the current and future state-of-the-art in prenatal genetic diagnosis, has come to fruition.

A comprehensive discussion of the principles and practice of genetic counseling sets the stage for this volume and focuses on preconception, perinatal, and postnatal counseling. Particular attention is given to predictive prenatal diagnosis, more especially because the prenatal detection of adult-onset serious to lethal genetic disorders will increasingly demand attention. Malignancies, neurodegenerative disorders, and potentially fatal cardiovascular disorders have already become prime considerations. The complexities of the necessary communications, the expertise and knowledge necessary, coupled with the time required, make peremptory genetic counseling by a busy practitioner effectively taboo.

A discussion of the fundamentals of amniocentesis, with special reference to their application and risks, focuses on the issues raised by early amniocentesis, the discussion being informed by new data on this subject. An extensive compilation of data on amniotic fluid and its constituents as well as on cell culture techniques precedes the remarkable personal distillation of an enormous experience with chorionic villus sampling. The authors provide extremely valuable insights, guidance, and lessons from their vast experience. Invaluable to every prenatal diagnostic facility and associated geneticists and counselors is the extensive compilation of facts and details concerning the prenatal detection of chromosome abnormalities. The depth and breadth of the information provided will serve as a unique resource to those engaged daily in prenatal genetic diagnosis. The incidental prenatal detection of fetal sex chromosome abnormality invokes considerable patient anxiety and necessitates in-depth knowledge by the counselor of future developmental prognosis in such cases. Continuing the life-long tradition of the late Arthur Robinson, the most up-to date information is provided to assist the unprepared parents who must grapple with very difficult decisions. Further refinements in the use of fluorescent in situ hybridization for prenatal diagnosis is reflected in an analysis of the major published series with a critical appraisal of the cumulative experience now recast into standard guidelines. Complicating counseling for the fragile X syndrome is the recent recognition of the late-onset tremor/ataxia syndrome among premutation (especially male) carriers. Completion of the Human Genome Project has resulted in rapid gene discovery, resulting in an extensive list of disorders now amenable to molecular prenatal diagnosis. The indications, limitations, pitfalls, and guidelines in the use of the now widely available molecular tools for prenatal diagnosis established the basis for a wide-ranging key chapter on this subject. Nongeneticists are now cautioned to first determine precise information before assuming that DNA analysis is not available for definitive diagnosis, carrier detection, prenatal, or predictive diagnosis.

Authoritative, up-to-date reviews, analyses, synthesis, and guidance in sequential chapters cover the prenatal diagnosis for disorders of lipid, mucopolysaccharide, amino acid, and carbohydrate disorders of metabolism, as well as those disorders involving folate and cobalamin metabolism. Detailed attention to the prenatal diagnosis and carrier detection of cystic fibrosis constitutes a section made more important through guidelines published by the American College of Obstetricians and Gynecologists. New advances for prenatal diagnosis are presented in depth for congenital adrenal hyperplasia and the immunodeficiency disorders.

Once again, a superlative discourse is provided on the prenatal detection of the hemoglobinopathies. Given the enormous advances in molecular analysis of the collagen and related genes, new opportunities for the prenatal detection of connective tissue disorders have now arisen.

Multianalyte second-trimester maternal serum screening for neural tube and chromosomal defects is among the most important advances in prenatal diagnosis and is fully integrated into routine antenatal care. First-trimester maternal serum screening coupled with fetal ultrasound study is now rapidly gaining ground as an earlier and valuable diagnostic modality. Integration of first- and second-trimester maternal serum results coupled with ultrasound analysis has reached a highly impressive rate of detection of pregnancies requiring definitive prenatal diagnosis. The wide-ranging considerations, implications, pitfalls, policies, and guidelines for maternal serum screening constitute the substance of two extensive discussions.

The art and complementary experience of fetal anomaly detection by ultrasound in early and late pregnancy are captured in two chapters that reflect the unique and extensive experience of the authors. Expansion of the authoritative chapter on fetal magnetic resonance imaging continues to add remarkable advances in the detection of complex fetal malformations.

A comprehensive chapter focuses on the various techniques, indications, limitations, complications, and guidelines concerning pregnancy termination. Experience with preimplantation genetic diagnosis, while still limited to a relatively small number of centers, has grown remarkably in the number of disorders now successfully detected. Advantages even beyond direct genetic diagnosis have become apparent and are detailed in this authoritative chapter. While fetal cell sampling from the maternal circulation has yet to gain a foothold in noninvasive prenatal diagnosis, new and exciting advances have dawned from the analysis of fetal DNA and RNA in the maternal circulation.

While fetal gene therapy remains more hope than reality, surgical interventions have steadily made inroads and chalked up some successes in this very challenging territory. The reintroduction of a chapter on the prenatal detection of infectious diseases that may lead to fetal malformations reflects the now-standard use of molecular methods for precise prenatal detection. Even so, the authors caution about both indications and interpretations.

The profound ethical and legal dilemmas and quandaries that arise in the context of genetic testing and prenatal diagnosis receive in-depth consideration by very experienced analysts. This discussion rounds off the fifth edition, which is a veritable repository of information on prenatal genetic diagnosis and is very heavily referenced, full of guidance, and, we hope, reflective of the enormous cumulative experience and wisdom of the many authors. Indeed, this edition encompasses 173 tables, 104 figures, 6 color plates, and 7286 references. The valuable and comprehensive index should facilitate both study and easy reference.

I hope this edition will bring into sharper focus the need for preconception risk determination, voluntary genetic testing, and genetic counseling, and replace the anachronistic habit of attending to all these issues in the late first or early second trimester of pregnancy. In addition, the emerging reality demands recognition that indications for prenatal genetic diagnosis have moved far beyond maternal age-related risks to pre-emptive maternal serum screening and molecular analyses of parents and fetus. Once again, the goal of this text is to provide a major source of guidance and reference on prenatal genetic diagnosis, stimulate research, and in particular, help physicians provide prospective reassurance to parents, so that they may avoid either conceiving offspring with a serious/lethal genetic disorder or having affected offspring that could have been detected prenatally.

Acknowledgments

More than 30 years ago, with prenatal diagnosis still in its infancy, a single author was able to write an entire book on this subject. That monograph, *The Prenatal Diagnosis of Hereditary Disorders*, spawned five subsequent editions. These accomplishments were achieved only by the invaluable and authoritative contributions, wisdom, and sheer excellence of the contributing authors. I am extremely grateful to all of these remarkable physicians and scientists who have been willing to share their expertise and precious time in contributing to these volumes.

I am also most grateful for all the work of my senior executive secretary, Mrs. Marilyn McPhail, who, in the face of heavy adversity and despite a heavy workload, maintained her outstanding dedication to perfection. My thanks and appreciation are also extended to Ms. Wendy Harris, the medical editor at the Johns Hopkins University Press, who has guided this edition yet again to a very efficient conclusion (witness the late 2003 references).

List of Contributors

Leena Ala-Kokko, M.D., Ph.D., Professor of Medicine, Center for Gene Therapy, Tulane University Health Sciences Center, New Orleans, Louisiana

Svetlana Arbuzova, M.D., Ph.D., D.Med.Sc., Professor of Obstetrics and Gynecology, Donetsk Medical University; and Head, Donetsk Interregional Medico-Genetics Center, Dunetsk, Ukraine

Gideon Bach, Ph.D., Professor and Chair, Department of Human Genetics, Hadassah University Hospital, Jerusalem, Israel

Peter A. Benn, Ph.D., Professor, Departments of Genetics and Developmental Biology, Pediatrics, and Laboratory Medicine; and Director, Human Genetics Laboratories, University of Connecticut Health Center, Farmington, Connecticut

Diana W. Bianchi, M.D., Natalie V. Zucker Professor of Pediatrics, Obstetrics and Gynecology and Vice-Chair for Research and Academic Affairs, Department of Pediatrics, Tufts University School of Medicine; Chief, Division of Genetics, Department of Pediatrics, Tufts-New England Medical Center, Boston, Massachusetts

Bruno Brambati, M.D., Director, Prenatal Diagnosis Center, Milan, Italy

W. Ted Brown, M.D., Ph.D., F.A.C.M.G., Chair, Department of Human Genetics, and Director of the Jervis Clinic, New York State Institute for Basic Research in Developmental Disabilities, Staten Island, New York

Stuart Campbell, M.B.B.S., F.R.C.O.G., Professor and Chair, Department of Obstetrics and Gynaecology, St. George's Hospital, London, United Kingdom

Jacob A. Canick, Ph.D., F.A.C.B., Professor, Department of Pathology and Laboratory Medicine, Brown Medical School; and Director, Division of Prenatal and Special Testing, Women and Infants Hospital, Providence, Rhode Island

Yuan-Tsong Chen, M.D., Ph.D., Professor and Chief, Division of Medical Genetics, Department of Pediatrics, Duke University Medical Center, Durham, North Carolina

Frank A. Chervenak, M.D., Given Foundation Professor and Chair, Department of Obstetrics and Gynecology and Gynecologist-in-Chief, New York-Presbyterian Hospital; and Weill Medical College of Cornell University, New York, New York

Howard S. Cuckle, B.A., M.Sc., D.Phil., Professor of Reproductive Epidemiology, Center for Reproduction, Growth and Development, School of Medicine, University of Leeds, Leeds, United Kingdom

Fernand Daffos, M.D., Head, Department of Fetal Medicine, Institut de Puériculture et de Périnatalogie, Paris, France

Louis Dallaire, M.D., Ph.D., F.R.C.P.(C), F.A.C.M.G., F.C.C.M.G., Professor Emeritus, School of Medicine, University of Montreal; Service of Medical Genetics and Research Center, Sainte-Justine Hospital, Montrèal, Quèbec, Canada.

Sherman Elias, M.D., F.A.C.O.G., F.A.C.M.G., F.A.C.S., John J. Sciarra Professor and Chair, Department of Obstetrics and Gynecology, Feinberg School of Medicine, Northwestern University, Chicago, Illinois

Diana L. Farmer, M.D., Professor of Surgery, Pediatrics, and Obstetrics, Gynecology and Reproductive Sciences, University of California, San Francisco; and Chief, Division of Pediatric Surgery, UCSF Children's Hospital, San Francisco, California

Gerald L. Feldman, M.D., Ph.D., Associate Professor, Center for Molecular Medicine and Genetics and Departments of Pediatrics and Pathology, Wayne State University School of Medicine; Director, Clinical Genetics Services, and Director, Molecular Genetics Diagnostic Laboratory, Detroit Medical Center-University Laboratories, Detroit, Michigan

Michael R. Harrison, M.D., Professor of Surgery, Pediatrics, and Obstetrics, Gynecology and Reproductive Sciences; and Director, Fetal Treatment Center, University of California, San Francisco, San Francisco, California

Lillian Y. F. Hsu, M.D., Professor of Pediatrics and of Obstetrics and Gynecology, New York University School of Medicine, New York, New York; Director Emeritus, Prenatal Diagnosis Laboratory of New York City, New York

Anne M. Hubbard, M.D., Associate Professor, Department of Radiology, University of Pennsylvania School of Medicine; and Associate Professor of Radiology, The Children's Hospital of Philadelphia, Philadelphia, Pennsylvania

James C. Hyland, M.D., Ph.D., Assistant Professor of Pathology and Director, DNA Diagnostics, Center for Gene Therapy, Tulane University Health Sciences Center, New Orleans, Louisiana

François Jacquemard, M.D., Assistant, Department of Fetal Medicine, Institut de Puériculture de Paris, Paris, France

Edmund C. Jenkins, Ph.D., F.A.C.M.G., Adjunct Professor, Graduate Program, City University of New York, New York; and Chair, Department of Cytogenetics, and Director, Specialty Clinical Laboratories, New York State Institute for Basic Research in Developmental Disabilities, Staten Island, New York

Anver Kuliev, M.D., Ph.D., Director of Research, Reproductive Genetics Institute, Chicago, Illinois

Hanmin Lee, M.D., Assistant Professor of Surgery, Pediatrics, and Obstetrics, Gynecology and Reproductive Sciences, University of California, San Francisco, San Francisco, California

Roseann Mandell, B.A., Lab Supervisor, Clinical Neurochemistry Laboratory, Department of Pathology; and Lab Manager, Amino Acid Disorders Laboratory, Department of Neurology, Massachusetts General Hospital, Boston, Massachusetts

Laurence B. McCullough, Ph.D., Professor of Medicine and Medical Ethics, Center for Medical Ethics and Health Policy, Baylor College of Medicine, Houston, Texas

Jeff M. Milunsky, M.D., F.A.C.M.G., Associate Professor of Pediatrics, Genetics and Genomics; Associate Director, Center for Human Genetics, and Director, Clinical Genetics, Center for Human Genetics, Boston University School of Medicine, Boston, Massachusetts

Véronique Mirlesse, M.D., Assistant, Department of Fetal Medicine, Institut de Puériculture de Paris, Paris, France

Kristin G. Monaghan, Ph.D., Director, DNA Diagnostics Laboratory, Department of Medical Genetics, Henry Ford Medical System; and Assistant Professor, Center for Molecular Medicine and Genetics, Wayne State University School of Medicine, Detroit, Michigan

Kypros H. Nicolaides, M.B.B.S., M.R.C.O.G., Professor and Director, Harris Birthright Research Center for Fetal Medicine, King's College School of Medicine, London, United Kingdom

Kerilyn K. Nobuhara, M.D., Assistant Professor of Surgery and Pediatrics, University of California, San Francisco, San Francisco, California

John M. Old, Ph.D., F.R.C.Path., Consultant Clinical Scientist and Reader in Haematology, National Haemoglobinopathy Reference Laboratory, Oxford Haemophilia Centre, Churchill Hospital, Oxford, United Kingdom

Mary Z. Pelias, Ph.D., J.D., Professor, Department of Genetics, Louisiana State University Health Sciences Center, New Orleans, Louisiana

John A. Phillips III, M.D., David T. Karzon Professor of Pediatrics and Professor of Biochemistry, Medicine and Pathology, Harvie Branscomb Distinguished Professor, Director, Division of Medical Genetics, Department of Pediatrics, Vanderbilt University School of Medicine, Nashville, Tennessee

Thomas W. Prior, Ph.D., Professor of Pathology and Neurology and Director of Molecular Pathology, Ohio State University, Columbus, Ohio

Jennifer M. Puck, M.D., Chief, Genetics and Molecular Biology Branch, National Human Genome Research Institute, and Senior Staff Physician, Warren Magnussen Clinical Center, National Institutes of Health, Bethesda, Maryland

Stéphane Romand, M.D., Assistant, Laboratoire d'Immunoanalyses et Recherche sur la Toxoplasmose, Institut de Puériculture de Paris, Paris, France

David S. Rosenblatt, M.D., Professor and Chair, Department of Human Genetics, and Professor, Departments of Medicine, Pediatrics, and Biology, McGill University; Director, Division of Medical Genetics, Department of Medicine, McGill University Health Center, Montreal, Quebec, Canada

Stuart Schwartz, Ph.D., Associate Professor and Director, Center for Human Genetics Laboratory, Department of Genetics, Case Western Reserve University School of Medicine, Cleveland, Ohio

Vivian E. Shih, M.D., Professor, Department of Neurology, Harvard Medical School; and Pediatrician, Associate Neurologist, and Director, Clinical Neurochemistry and Amino Acid Disorders Laboratory, Massachusetts General Hospital, Boston, Massachusetts

Lee P. Shulman, M.D., Professor and Head, Section of Reproductive Genetics, Department of Obstetrics and Gynecology, Feinberg School of Medicine, Northwestern University, Evanston, Illinois

Joe Leigh Simpson, M.D., F.A.C.O.G., F.A.C.M.G., F.R.C.O.G., Ernst W. Bertner Chairman and Professor, Department of Obstetrics and Gynecology; and Professor, Department of Human and Molecular Genetics, Baylor College of Medicine, Houston, Texas

Phyllis W. Speiser, M.D., Professor, Department of Pediatrics, New York University School of Medicine, New York, New York; and Director, Division of Pediatric Endocrinology, Schneider Children's Hospital, North Shore–LIJ Health System, New Hyde Park, New York, New York

Philippe Thulliez, M.D., Head of Department, Laboratoire d'Immunoanalyses et Recherche sur la Toxoplasmose, Institut de Puériculture de Paris, Paris, France

Lucia Tului, Ph.D., M.D., Senior Scientist, Prenatal Diagnosis Center, Milan, Italy

Daniel L. Van Dyke, Ph.D., Mayo Clinic Cytogenetics Laboratory, Rochester, Minnesota

Yury Verlinsky, Ph.D., Director, Reproductive Genetics Institute, Chicago, Illinois

Yves G. Ville, M.D., Senior Lecturer and Director, Fetal Medicine Unit, St. George's Hospital Medical School, London, United Kingdom

Cindy L. Vnencak-Jones, Ph.D., Associate Professor of Pathology and Pediatrics, Vanderbilt University School of Medicine, Nashville, Tennessee

Bryan G. Winchester, M.A., Ph.D., Professor of Biochemistry and Head, Biochemistry, Endocrinology and Metabolism Unit, Institute of Child Health, London, United Kingdom

J. W. Wladimiroff, M.D., Ph.D., F.R.C.O.G., Professor, Department of Obstetrics and Gynaecology, University Hospital Rotterdam-Dijkzigt, Rotterdam, The Netherlands

Elisabeth P. Young, B.Sc., Department of Chemical Pathology, Great Ormond Street Hospital, London, United Kingdom

GENETIC DISORDERS AND THE FETUS

"Make assurance double sure."
Shakespeare, *Macbeth*

Aubrey Milunsky, MB.B.Ch., D.Sc., F.R.C.P., F.A.C.M.G., D.C.H., and Jeff M. Milunsky, M.D., F.A.C.M.G.

1

Genetic Counseling: Preconception, Prenatal, and Perinatal

Sequencing of the human genome has spawned much hope in the hearts and minds of millions affected by genetic disorders and their loved ones. While hope might spring eternal, reality is more daunting, and gene therapy has remained largely elusive. Early and continuing experience with advances in molecular genetics has translated into additional and more precise diagnostic tests. The widening scope of molecular diagnostics has increased opportunities for predictive, preconception, preimplantation, and prenatal diagnosis. Consequently, genetic counseling for prenatal diagnosis can be expected increasingly to involve early adult-onset malignancies, neurodegenerative, cardiovascular, and other fatal genetic disorders, as well as those with significant morbidity.

Against this background, physicians in all specialties are expected to be cognizant of new developments in genetics that facilitate the prevention or avoidance of genetic or acquired defects. In context, women at risk for having progeny with defects expect to be informed about their odds and options, preferably during preconception counseling. Their concerns are serious, given the significant contribution of genetic disorders to morbidity and mortality in children and adults.

THE BURDEN OF GENETIC DISORDERS AND CONGENITAL MALFORMATIONS

Various measures reflect the population burden of genetic disease and congenital anomalies. Common assessments include the incidence or prevalence of the disorder/defect, the associated morbidity and mortality, the degree of disability and suffering, life expectancy, and economic burden. Indeed, many factors influence efforts to accurately determine the incidence or prevalence of congenital anomalies or genetic disorders. Table 1.1 encompasses the majority of known etiologic categories, discussed below, which help explain sometimes striking differences among major studies. It is almost impossible to account for all these potentially confounding factors in a study, and rarely has any one study come close.

The availability of prenatal diagnosis and more recently the advent of maternal serum screening for neural tube defects (NTDs) and Down syndrome (DS) have also affected

Table 1.1. Factors that influence estimates of the incidence or prevalence in the newborn
of a congenital malformation (CM) or genetic disorder

Maternal age
Use of maternal serum screening for Down syndrome
Use of maternal serum screening for neural tube defects
Frequency, inclusion, and exclusion of stillbirths, fetal deaths, and elective pregnancy termination
Maternal diabetes and gestational diabetes
Previous affected child
Availability and use of expertise in prenatal diagnostic ultrasound
History of recurrent spontaneous abortion
Multiple pregnancy rate
Maternal epilepsy, lupus erythematosus, and other illnesses
Maternal alcohol abuse
Maternal obesity
Family history
Consanguinity
Maternal fever or use of hot tub in the first 6 weeks of pregnancy
Incidence and severity of prematurity
Use of folic acid supplementation
Economic level in developed or developing world
Later manifestation or onset of disorder
Previous maternal immunization/vaccination
Frequency of certain infectious diseases
Maternal use of medication
Case selection, bias and ascertainment
Definitions of major and minor congenital anomalies
Use of perinatal necropsy
Use of registry data
Use of death certificates
Training and expertise in examination of newborns
In vitro fertilization
Intracytoplasmic sperm injection
Season of the year
Paternal age

---

the birth frequency of these two most common congenital defects. A French study of the
impact of prenatal diagnosis over a 21-year period (1979–1999) in a well-defined population showed a drop of 80 percent in the birth prevalence of DS.[1] A study from Newcastle, England, based on ascertainment of all cases of NTDs revealed a twofold reduction
in the birth prevalence between 1984–1990 and 1991–1996.[2] A Scottish study aimed at
assessing the impact of prenatal diagnosis on the prevalence of DS from 1980 to 1996.
Both births and pregnancy terminations were included. Pregnancy terminations for DS
rose from 29 percent to about 60 percent.[3]

The effect of folic acid supplementation, via tablet or food fortification, on the prevalence of NTDs, now well known to reduce the frequency of NTDs by up to 70 percent,[4–6]
has only recently been assessed in this context. A Canadian study focused on the effect
of supplementation on the prevalence of open NTDs among 336,963 women. The authors
reported that the prevalence of open NTDs declined from 1.13 in 1,000 pregnancies before fortification to 0.58 in 1,000 pregnancies thereafter.[7]

In a population-based cohort study by the Metropolitan Atlanta Congenital Defects
Program, the risk of congenital malformations was assessed among 264,392 infants with

known gestational ages born between 1989 and 1995. Premature infants (<37 weeks of gestation) were found to be more than twice as likely to have been born with congenital malformations than infants at term.[8]

Incidence/prevalence rates of congenital defects are directly influenced by when and how diagnoses are made. Highlighting the importance of how early a diagnosis is made after birth, the use of echocardiography and the stratification of severity of congenital heart defects, Hoffman and Kaplan[9] clarified how different studies reported the incidence of congenital heart defects varying from 4 in 1,000 to 50 in 1,000 livebirths. They reported an incidence of moderate and severe forms of congenital heart disease in about 6 in 1,000 livebirths, a figure that would rise to 19 in 1,000 livebirths if the potentially serious bi-cuspid aortic valve is included. They noted that if all forms of congenital heart disease (including tiny muscular ventricular septal defects) were considered, the incidence increases to 75 in 1,000 livebirths.

The frequency of congenital defects is also influenced by the presence or absence of such defects in at least one parent. A Norwegian Medical Birth Registry Population-Based Cohort Study of 486,207 males recorded that 12,292 (2.53 percent) had been born with a congenital defect.[10] Among the offspring of these affected males, 5.1 percent had a congenital defect, compared with 2.1 percent of offspring of males without such defects (relative risk, 2.4).

The prevalence of maternal obesity also has the potential for influencing the rate of congenital anomalies. Watkins et al.,[11] in a population-based case controlled study excluding women with preexisting diabetes, compared the risks of selected congenital defects among obese women with those of average-weight women. They noted significant odds ratios for spina bifida (3.5), omphalocele (3.3), heart defects (2.0), and multiple anomalies (2.0). Others[12] found a 2.2-fold increased risk of spina bifida in the offspring of obese women. Our studies[13,14] have pointed in the direction of a prediabetic state or gestational diabetes as the biologic mechanism accounting for the increased rate of congenital anomalies in the offspring of obese women. In contrast, markedly underweight women reportedly have a 3.2-fold increased risk of having offspring with gastroschisis.[15]

The frequency of congenital hypothyroidism, now known to be associated with up to a fourfold increased risk of additional congenital malformations, represents yet another factor that may influence incidence/prevalence rates of congenital anomalies. A French study of 129 infants with congenital hypothyroidism noted that 15.5 percent had associated congenital anomalies.[16] Nine of the infants had congenital heart defects (6.9 percent).

Women with epilepsy who are taking anticonvulsant medications have an increased risk of having offspring with congenital malformations, noted in a recent study as 2.7-fold greater than those without epilepsy.[17]

Congenital Malformations and Infant Morbidity and Mortality

The leading cause of infant death in the United States in 2000 was congenital malformations, deformations, and chromosomal abnormalities, accounting for 20.5 percent of all infant deaths.[18] Congenital malformations, deformations, and chromosomal abnormalities accounted for 17.3 percent of all infant deaths occurring between 28 days and 11 months of life. The rank order of leading causes of infant death varied substantially by race and if the mother was Hispanic. Congenital malformations ranked first as the cause of infant death except in black and Puerto Rican mothers, for whom low birth weight was the leading cause.[19]

Survival is clearly dependent on the severity or lethality of the congenital defect. The Centers for Disease Control and Prevention assessed mortality rates for infants born with trisomy 13 and trisomy 18. Using death certificates and other source data, the authors identified 5,515 infants born with trisomy 13 and 8,750 born with trisomy 18. The median age at death for both trisomy 13 and trisomy 18 was 10 days. Survival to at least 1 year occurred in 5.6 percent of those born with trisomy 13 or trisomy 18.[20] A regional study in the Netherlands noted lethal congenital malformations in 51 percent of stillbirths and 70 percent among those who died during the neonatal period.[21] A Glasgow, Scotland, study focused on the survival of infants with congenital anomalies up to the age of 5 years. They used a population-based and systematically validated registry of congenital anomalies containing 6,153 anomalous livebirths. Survival rates for these infants to the age of 5 was: chromosomal anomalies (48 percent), neural tube defects (72 percent), respiratory system anomalies (74 percent), congenital heart disease (75 percent), nervous system anomalies (77 percent), and Down syndrome (84 percent).[22] Survival rates among males with congenital defects was 84 percent, compared with 97 percent in those born unaffected.[10] Liu et al.[23] examined temporal changes in fetal and infant deaths caused by congenital malformations in Canada, England, Wales, and the United States. They concluded that the major factor responsible for the accelerated decline in infant deaths was prenatal diagnosis and elective abortion of fetuses with abnormalities. Given the frequency of DS, a more detailed discussion follows. NTDs are discussed in chapter 21.

Down Syndrome

The special problems and associated defects in DS are well known, as is the increasing life expectancy. Studies from Japan,[24] Denmark,[25] England,[26] Australia,[27] and Canada[28,29] highlight the increased life expectancy with DS. Baird and Sadovnick[28] reported a large study of 1,610 individuals with DS identified in more than 1,500,000 consecutive livebirths in British Columbia from 1908 to 1981. They constructed survival curves (Figure 1.1) and a life table (Table 1.2) for DS and for the general population.[30] Their estimates show that 44.4 percent and 13.6 percent of liveborn individuals with DS will survive to 60 and 68 years, respectively, compared with 86.4 percent and 78.4 percent of the general population. In another report,[31] these authors have analyzed the causes of death in DS, highlighting congenital defects and cardiovascular and respiratory illnesses as the most important.

Additional studies of mortality rates in individuals with DS revealed that those up to about 35 years of age were little different from others who were mentally retarded. Subsequently, however, mortality rates in DS doubled every 6.4 years, compared with 9.6 years for other mentally retarded individuals.[31] Life tables constructed by these authors indicated a life expectancy of 55 years for a 1-year-old patient with DS and mild/moderate retardation and a life expectancy of 43 years for a 1-year-old patient with DS and profound mental retardation.

More recently, a study from the Centers for Disease Control and Prevention focused on a death certificate study of 17,897 individuals with DS born between 1983 and 1997.[32] These authors reported that the median age at death for those with DS increased from 25 years in 1983 to 49 years in 1997 (Figure 1.2). They also observed that the median age at death was significantly lower among blacks and people of other races when compared with whites with DS. The authors acknowledge the limitations of their study given the known problems with the epidemiologic use of death certificates.

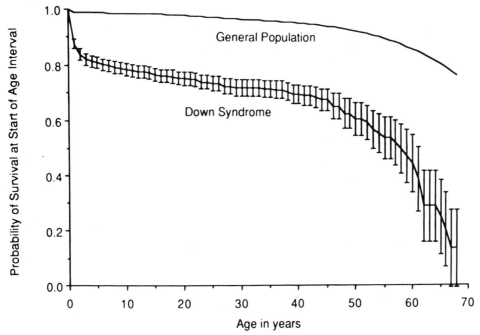

Fig. 1.1. Survival curves for Down syndrome and for the general population of British Columbia. *Source*: Baird and Sadovnik, 1987.[28]

An Australian cohort study of 1,332 people with DS who had registered for intellectual disability services between 1953 and 2000 calculated a life expectancy of 58.6 years, with 25 percent expected to live to 62.9 years. The oldest person with DS was alive at 73 years of age. Their calculations concluded that 75 percent of people with DS would survive to 50 years, 50 percent to 58.6, and 25 percent to 62.9.[33] The authors cautioned that this study was not a birth cohort and also omitted some deaths that occurred in infancy or early childhood. Nevertheless, they found that life expectancy of those with DS is approaching that of the general population of Australia, now approximating 76 years for males and 81.7 years for females.

Table 1.3 reflects the common associated defects that occur in DS and the more common complications that can be anticipated, monitored, prevented and treated.

Incidence and Prevalence

Estimates of aneuploidy in oocytes and sperm reach 18–19 percent and 3–4 percent, respectively.[34] Not surprisingly, then, about 1 in 13 conceptions results in a chromosomally defective conceptus,[35] while about 50 percent of first-trimester spontaneous abortions are associated with chromosomal anomalies.[36] Clinically significant chromosomal defects occur in 0.65 percent of all births; an additional 0.2 percent of babies are born with balanced structural chromosome rearrangements (see also chapter 6) that have implications for reproduction later in life. Between 5.6 and 11.5 percent of stillbirths and neonatal deaths have chromosomal defects.[37]

Table 1.2. Life expectancy with Down syndrome, to age 68 years

Age	Total	Deaths	Withdrawals	Survival at Start of Age Interval (%)
0	1,337	164	0	100.00
1	1,173	51	0	87.73
2	1,122	23	0	83.92
3	1,099	10	29	82.20
4	1,060	5	35	81.44
5	1,020	10	33	81.05
6	977	5	37	80.24
7	935	6	20	79.82
8	909	3	30	79.31
9	876	7	28	79.04
10	841	2	27	78.40
11	812	4	28	78.21
12	780	2	34	77.82
13	744	3	21	77.61
14	720	6	35	77.30
15	679	3	41	76.64
16	635	1	34	76.29
17	600	1	26	76.16
18	573	4	36	76.03
19	533	1	35	75.48
20	497	1	46	75.34
21	450	1	26	75.18
22	423	5	40	75.01
23	378	0	38	74.08
24	340	2	50	74.08
25	288	0	46	73.61
26	242	3	38	73.61
27	201	0	36	72.62
28	165	1	36	72.62
29	128	0	37	72.12
30	91	0	35	72.12
31	56	0	30	72.12
32	26	0	26	72.12
33	255	1	19	72.12
34	235	0	27	71.83
35	208	1	7	71.83
36	200	0	12	71.48
37	188	2	21	71.48
38	165	2	12	70.67
39	151	0	15	69.78
40	136	1	8	69.78
41	127	0	11	69.25
42	116	1	17	69.25
43	98	1	5	68.61
44	92	0	6	67.89
45	86	3	4	67.89
46	79	0	5	65.47
47	74	3	4	65.47
48	67	0	4	62.74
49	63	2	4	62.74
50	57	0	1	60.68
51	56	1	7	60.68

Table 1.2. Life expectancy with Down syndrome, to age 68 years (continued)

Age	Total	Deaths	Withdrawals	Survival at Start of Age Interval (%)
52	48	2	5	59.53
53	41	1	2	56.91
54	38	1	6	55.49
55	31	0	2	53.96
56	29	1	3	53.90
57	25	1	4	51.94
58	20	1	1	49.68
59	18	1	1	47.14
60	16	2	1	44.44
61	13	3	2	38.71
62	8	0	0	29.03
63	8	0	1	29.03
64	7	1	0	29.03
65	6	1	1	24.88
66	4	1	2	20.36
67	1	0	0	13.57
68	1	0	1	13.57

Source: Baird and Sadovnick, 1989.[30]

Congenital malformations with obvious structural defects are found in about 2 percent of all births.[38] This was the figure in Spain among 710,815 livebirths,[39] with 2.25 percent in Liberia,[40] 2.03 percent in India,[41] and 2.53 percent among newborn males in Norway.[10] Factors that had an impact on the incidence/prevalence of congenital malformations were discussed above.

More than 9,000 monogenic disorders and traits have been catalogued.[42] Estimates based on 1 million consecutive livebirths in Canada suggested a monogenic disease in 3.6 in 1,000, consisting of autosomal dominant (1.4 in 1,000), autosomal recessive (1.7 in 1,000), and X-linked-recessive disorders (0.5 in 1,000).[43] Polygenic disorders occurred at a rate of 46.4 in 1,000 (Table 1.4).

At least 3–4 percent of all births are associated with a major congenital defect, mental retardation, or a genetic disorder, a rate that doubles by 7–8 years of age, given later-appearing and/or later-diagnosed genetic disorders.[44,45] If all congenital defects are considered, Baird et al.[43] estimated that 7.9 percent of liveborn individuals have some type of genetic disorder by about 25 years of age. These estimates are likely to be very low given, for example, the frequency of undetected defects such as bicuspid aortic valves (see below). These numbers lead to a significant genetic-disease burden and have accounted for 28–40 percent of hospital admissions in North America, Canada, and England.[46,47] Notwithstanding their frequency, the causes of up to 60 percent of congenital malformations remain obscure.[48]

THE GOAL AND PURPOSE OF PRENATAL DIAGNOSIS

The fundamental philosophy of prenatal genetic diagnosis is to provide reassurance to couples at risk that they may selectively have unaffected children even if their procreative risk for having defective offspring is unacceptably high.[49] Fetal defects serious enough to

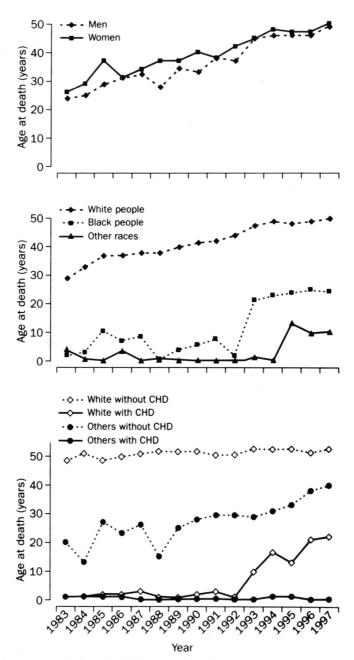

Fig. 1.2. Median age at death of people with Down syndrome by sex (upper), by racial group (middle), and with or without congenital heart defects (CHD) by racial group (lower). *Source*: Yang et al., 2002.[32]

warrant parental election of abortion are found in less than 5 percent of all cases studied, based on current indications for amniocentesis. When couples are at risk for having a seriously defective child, common experience shows that those with risks between 10 and 25 percent or even greater most often avoid pregnancies unless prenatal diagnosis is available. The advent of prenatal diagnosis has made it possible for such high-risk couples to

Table 1.3. Defects and complications associated with Down syndrome

	Percentage
Defect	
Congenital heart disease	±50
Mitral-valve prolapse	46
Aortic-valve regurgitation	17
Hearing impairment	38–78
Eye disorders[a]	80
Complication	
Obesity	Majority
Periodontal disease	±all
Orthodontic problems	±all
Hypothyroidism	15
Celiac disease	4.6–7.1
Juvenile rheumatoidlike arthritis	1.2
Atlantoaxial subluxation	
Diabetes mellitus	
Leukemia[b]	
Obstructive sleep apnea	Frequency greater than in general population
Epilepsy	
Testicular cancer[33c]	
Alzheimer disease and dementia [33c]	

[a]Includes cataracts, strabismus, nystagmus, refractive errors, keratoconus, glaucoma, and lens opacities.
[b]±20-fold excess.[33b]
Source: Data from Riozen and Patterson, 2003.[33a]

have children that they would otherwise never have conceived. As a consequence, the number of children born because of prenatal diagnosis is much higher than the very small number of pregnancies terminated because of the detection of grave fetal defects. Prenatal genetic studies are used in Western society virtually exclusively for the detection of defects generally characterized by irreparable mental retardation and/or irremediable, serious to fatal genetic disease. Sadly, at present, the ideal goal of prevention or treatment rather than abortion after prenatal detection of a fetal defect is achieved only rarely, with the exception of NTDs (see also chapter 21).

All couples or individuals concerned about the risks of genetic defects in their offspring should seek genetic counseling before conceiving. Such counseling is best provided in medical genetics departments of university medical centers with multiple-specialty clinical and laboratory teams. For the more common indications for amniocentesis (such as advanced maternal age), the well-informed obstetrician should be able to provide the necessary information. However, a salutary observation in one study revealed that 43.3 percent of patients referred for amniocentesis exclusively for advanced maternal age had additional genetic risks or significant concerns regarding one or more genetic or congenital disorders.[50] This group required more extensive genetic counseling.

PREREQUISITES FOR GENETIC COUNSELING

Genetic counseling is a communication process concerning the occurrence and the risk of recurrence of genetic disorders within a family. The aim of such counseling is to provide the counselee(s) with as complete an understanding of the disorder and/or problem as pos-

Table 1.4.　The frequencies of genetic disorders in 1,169,873 births, 1952–1983

Category	Rate per Million Livebirths	Percentage of Total Births
A.		
Dominant	1,395.4	0.14
Recessive	1,665.3	0.17
X-linked	532.4	0.05
Chromosomal	1,845.4	0.18
Multifactorial	46,582.6	4.64
Genetic unknown	1,164.2	0.12
Total	53,175.3	5.32[a]
B.		
All congenital anomalies 740–759[b]	52,808.2	5.28
Congenital anomalies with genetic etiology (included in section A)	26,584.2	2.66
C.		
Disorders in section A plus those congenital anomalies not already included	79,399.3	7.94

[a]Sum is not exact owing to rounding.
[b]International Classification of Disease numbers.
Source: Baird et al., 1988.[43]

sible and of all the options. The counseling process is also aimed at helping families cope with their problems and at assisting and supporting them in their decision making.

The personal right to found a family is considered inviolable. Such reproductive autonomy is enhanced by genetic counseling, a process that both emphasizes freedom of choice and reviews the available options in order to enrich the decision-making process. All couples have a right to know whether they have an increased risk of having children with genetic disease and to know which options pertain to their particular situation. The physician has a clear duty and obligation to communicate this information, to offer specific tests, or to refer couples for a second or more expert opinion. In the United States, at least, the full force of law supports the prospective parents' right to know (see also chapter 31).

As Kessler[51] stated so succinctly, "Because genetic counselors work with people filled with uncertainty, fear of the future, anguish, and a sense of personal failure," they have unusual challenges and opportunities "to understand clients, give them a sense of being understood, and help them feel more hopeful, more valued, and more capable of dealing with their life problems." The physician and genetic counselor providing genetic counseling should have a clear perception of the necessary prerequisites, guiding principles, and potential problems.

Knowledge of Disease

The need for a counselor to have extensive factual knowledge about disease in general, as well as about the disease for which counseling is being provided, hardly needs emphasis. Such knowledge should include how the diagnosis is made or confirmed, the recurrence risks, the mode of inheritance, the tests available to detect a carrier, the heterogeneity and pleiotropic nature of the disease, the quality of life associated with survival, prognosis, and the causes of death. When relevant, it is necessary to know about treatment and its efficacy.

The physician or genetic counselor who initiates genetic counseling for an apparently straightforward indication (e.g., advanced maternal age) may find one or more other familial conditions about which he or she has little or no familiarity. Such circumstances dictate referral for specialist consultation. A National Confidential Enquiry into counseling for genetic disorders by nongeneticists in the United Kingdom revealed that less than half of those with known high genetic risks were referred to medical geneticists.[52] This study focused on a review of 12,093 "genetic events" involving potentially avoidable cases of DS, NTDs, cystic fibrosis, β-thalassemia, and multiple endocrine neoplasia. Medical record reviews were frustrated by the poor quality of clinical notes, which lacked evidence of counseling. An urgent call was made for genetic management to be at least as well documented as surgical operations, drug records, and informed consent. A Dutch study evaluated the levels of knowledge, practical skills, and clinical genetic practices of 643 cardiologists. They noted low levels of self-reported knowledge and that only 38 percent had referred patients to clinical geneticists.[53]

After the prenatal diagnosis of a serious genetic disorder, the physician should be able to inform the family fully about the anticipated burden and to detail the effects of this burden on an affected child, the family, other siblings, the family economics, and the couple's sex life, along with any other pros and cons of continuing pregnancy. Exact details should also be known about the risks of elective abortion (see also chapter 26).

Expertise in Genetic Counseling

Genetic counseling is best provided by board-certified clinical geneticists and genetic counselors. In countries with this specialization, such service is provided by a team composed of clinical geneticists (physicians) and medical geneticists with doctorates, working in concert with clinical cytogeneticists, biochemical and molecular geneticists, and genetic counselors. Optional genetic counseling is attainable through this team approach. It is, however, impractical and not cost effective to provide such formal counseling for every woman before amniocentesis for advanced maternal age. It is necessary for the obstetrician to be fully informed about the indications for amniocentesis and to explain the techniques and requirements for obtaining the fluid, the limitations of the studies, the risks of chromosomal abnormality in the offspring of the patient being counseled, the risks of the procedure, and, when pertinent, all matters concerned with elective abortion of a defective fetus.

Gordis et al.[54] concluded that the way in which an obstetrician managed patients at risk regarding referral for genetic screening was closely related to that obstetrician's attitudes and education. Physicians in practice should be aware of the nuances and needs in the genetic-counseling process, including the key psychologic aspects.[55] Perhaps most important is the requirement that they recognize limitations in their knowledge of unusual or rare genetic disorders and be alert to situations requiring referral. Obstetricians or family practitioners are not expected to have an extensive knowledge of all diseases, but they should be able to recognize that a condition could be genetic. Concern about litigation should not act as a constant reminder to physicians of the need to consult or refer[56–58] (see also chapter 31).

Ability to Communicate

Many physicians are not born communicators, and most have not had formal teaching and training to hone their communication skills. Recognizing these deficiencies, the Royal

College of Physicians Working Party made specific recommendations for the teaching of communication skills to undergraduates and postgraduates.[59]

Simple language, an adequate allotment of time, and care and sensitivity are keys to successful genetic counseling. Technical jargon is avoided only through conscious effort. How an issue requiring a decision is framed,[60] and the nature of the language used,[61] may influence the patient's choice.[62] Counseling is facilitated when three key questions are asked: "Why did you come?" "What exactly do you hope to learn?" and "Have I answered all your questions and concerns?"

Although the explanation of exact statistical risks is important, patients often pay more attention to the actual burden or severity of the disease in question. A clear and accurate exposition of these aspects should be carefully provided. An essential ingredient of the counseling process is time. The busy practitioner can hardly expect to offer genetic counseling during a brief consultation. Distress and misunderstanding are invariable sequelae of such hastily delivered counseling.

Knowledge of Ancillary Needs

For the couple at high risk for having a child with a serious genetic disorder, prenatal diagnosis is not the sole option. Even in situations in which a particular disease is diagnosable prenatally, it is important to be certain that other avenues are explored. Prospective parents who are known, for example, to be carriers of an autosomal recessive disorder may be unaware of the possibility of sperm or ovum donation or may be unwilling to raise the question. This option may be viewed more favorably than amniocentesis and elective abortion. Physicians should be certain that their patients are familiar with all of the aforementioned important options, as well as with adoption, vasectomy, tubal ligation, treatments of the mother and/or fetus during pregnancy, and new methods of assisted reproduction (e.g., intracytoplasmic sperm injection,[63] epididymal sperm aspiration,[64] and preimplantation genetic diagnosis) (see also chapters 7 and 27).

Empathy

Much more than the communication of risk figures for a particular disorder is required in the genetic-counseling process. Warmth, care, sympathy, understanding, and insight into the human condition are necessary for effective communication. The difficulty of assimilating information and making rational decisions in the face of anxiety[65] should be recognized and vocalized. Empathy and sensitivity enable the counselor to anticipate and respond to unspoken fears and questions and are qualities that make the counseling experience most beneficial and valuable to the counselees.

For example, a couple may have been trying to conceive for 10 years and, having finally succeeded, may be confronted by a callous physician who is impatient about their concerns regarding amniocentesis and elective abortion. Another couple may have lost their only child to a metabolic genetic disease and may be seeking counseling to explore the possibilities for prenatal diagnosis in a subsequent pregnancy, or even treatment followed by prenatal diagnosis, as in the case of galactosemia. They may have in mind past problems encountered in prenatal diagnosis or may be aware of the uncertain outcome of treatment.

Sensitivity and awareness of the plight of prospective parents are critical prerequisites, and include the need to recognize and address the usually unspoken fears and anxieties.

Beyond the qualifications and factual knowledge of the counselor is the person, who is key to successful and effective counseling. Attitude, body language, warmth, manners, dress, tone of voice, and personality are facets that seriously influence the credibility and acceptance of the counseling offered. Curiously, counselors rarely realize during their counseling session that they are simultaneously being assessed. Patients assess the apparent knowledge and credibility of the counselor, seek and are encouraged by evidence of experience, and consider the information provided in light of the counselor's attitude, body language, and other nonverbal characteristics.

Quintessential prerequisites for the empathetic genetic counselor include:

1. Acknowledge the burden and empathize about the sadness or loss (e.g., a previous child; recurrent miscarriage; a deceased affected parent; a patient who has experienced mastectomy and chemotherapy for breast cancer with daughters at risk).
2. Vocalize the realization of the psychologic pain and distress the person or couple has experienced (e.g., recurrent pregnancy loss followed by multiple IVF efforts and subsequently a successful pregnancy with a fetal defect).
3. Compliment the coping that has been necessary, including the stress a couple might have to endure, despite sometimes conflicting feelings.
4. Recognize (and explain) psychologic difficulties in decision making when faced with a prenatal diagnosis of the same disorder affecting one parent (discussion of self-extinction, self-image, and issues of survival).
5. Fulfill the patient's need for hope and support and actively avoid any thoughtless comments[51] that may erode these fundamental prerequisites.

Sensitivity to Parental Guilt

Feelings of guilt invariably invade the genetic consultation; they should be anticipated, recognized, and dealt with directly. Assurance frequently does not suffice; witness the implacable guilt of the obligate maternal carrier of a serious X-linked disease. Explanations that we all carry harmful genes often helps. Mostly, however, encouragement to move anguish into action is important.

Guilt is not only the preserve of the obligate carrier. Affected parents inevitably also experience guilt on transmitting their defective genes.[66,67] Frequently, a parent expresses guilt about an occupation, medication, or illegal drug that they feel caused or contributed to their child's problem. Kessler et al.[67] advised that assuaging a parent's guilt may diminish the parents' power of effective prevention, in that guilt may serve as a defense from being powerless.

Guilt is often felt by healthy siblings of an affected child, who feel relatively neglected by their parents, and who also feel anger toward their parents and affected sibling. What is termed "survivor guilt" is increasingly recognized, as the new DNA technologies are exploited. Experience with Huntington disease and adult polycystic kidney disease[68–74] confirm not only survivor guilt with a new reality (a future) but also problems in relationships with close family members. Huggins et al.[71] found that about 10 percent of individuals receiving low-risk results experienced psychologic difficulties.

PRINCIPLES IN GENETIC COUNSELING

Ten key principles are discussed that guide genetic counseling in the preconception, prenatal, and perinatal periods. This section is in concert with consensus statements concerning ethical principles for genetics professionals.[75,76]

ACCURATE DIAGNOSIS

The clinical geneticist, obstetrician, or pediatrician is frequently confronted by a patient seeking guidance because of a certain genetic disease in the family. A previous child or a deceased sibling or parent may have had the disease in question. The genetic-counseling process cannot begin, however, without an accurate diagnosis. Information about the exact previous diagnosis is important not only for the communication of subsequent risks but also for precise future prenatal diagnosis. Hence, it is not sufficient to know that the previous child had a mucopolysaccharidosis; exactly which type and even subtype must be determined because each may have different enzymatic deficiencies (see also chapter 12). A history of limb girdle muscular dystrophy will also not facilitate prenatal diagnosis because there are two dominant types (1A and 1B) and six autosomal-recessive types (2A–2F).[77] Similarly, a history of epilepsy gives no clear indication which of at least eleven recognized genes[78,79] are involved.

Instead of simply accepting the patient's description of the disease—for example, muscular dystrophy or a mucopolysaccharidosis—the counselor must obtain confirmatory data. The unreliability of the maternal history, in this context, is remarkable, a positive predictive value of 47 percent having been documented.[80] Photographs of the deceased, autopsy reports, hospital records, results of carrier detection tests performed elsewhere, and other information may provide the crucial confirmation or negation of the diagnosis made previously. Important data after miscarriage may also influence counseling. In a study of ninety-one consecutive, spontaneously aborted fetuses, almost one-third had malformations, most associated with increased risks in subsequent pregnancies.[81]

Myotonic muscular dystrophy (DM), the most common adult muscular dystrophy, with an incidence of about 1 in 8,000,[82] serves as the paradigm for preconception, prenatal, and perinatal genetic counseling. Recognition of the pleomorphism of this disorder will, for example, alert the physician hearing a family history of one individual with DM, another with sudden death (cardiac conduction defect), and yet another relative with cataracts. Awareness of the autosomal dominant nature of this disorder and its genetic basis due to a dynamic mutation reflected in the number of trinucleotide (CTG) repeat units raises issues beyond the 50 percent risk of recurrence in the offspring of an affected parent. As the first disorder characterized with expanding trinucleotide repeats, the ob-

Table 1.5. Myotonic muscular dystrophy: potential pregnancy, neonatal, and other complications

Potential abortion
Fetal death
Polyhydramnios
Prolonged labor
Fetal distress
Uterine atony
Postpartum hemorrhage
Cardiac arrhythmias
Increased sensitivity to anesthetic and relaxant agents
Postoperative respiratory depression
Neonatal death
Arthrogryposis
Mental retardation

Source: Milunsky et al., 1995.[96]

servation linking the degree of disease severity to the number of triplet repeats was not long in coming.[82] In addition, the differences in severity when the mutation was passed via a maternal rather than a paternal gene focused attention on the fact that congenital DM was almost always a sign of the greatest severity and originating through maternal transmission. However, at least one exception has been noted.[83] There is about a 93–94 percent likelihood that the CTG repeat will expand on transmission. This process of genetic anticipation (increasing clinical severity over generations) is not inevitable. An estimated 6–7 percent of cases of DM are associated with a decrease in the number of triplet repeats or no change in number.[84] Rare cases also exist in which complete reversal of the mutation occurs with spontaneous correction to a normal range of triplet repeats.[85–88]

There are also reports of patients born with a decreased number of triplet repeats who nevertheless show no decrease in the severity of their DM.[89–92] It is unclear whether these cases in part reflect somatic or germ-line (either or both combined) mosaicism.[84] Somatic mosaicism is certainly well documented in DM with, for example, larger expansions being observed in skeletal muscle than in peripheral blood.[93] Another problem that complicates molecular diagnosis is that <2 percent of individuals without expanded triplet repeats nevertheless have DM.[84,94–97] Discussion about potential complications of pregnancy (Table 1.5) in the prospective affected mother is crucial.[98] (See discussion below on presymptomatic testing.)

The lack of CAG triplet expansion among individuals presenting with Huntington disease–like symptoms and a family history of neurodegenerative disease has focused attention on phenocopies of Huntington disease.[99,100] Estimates of such phenocopies range between 1 and 2.4 percent of patients manifesting Huntington disease–like symptoms even with a family history of a neurodegenerative disorder.[101] Among the reported phenocopies found thus far are a familial prion disease[99] and a triplet expansion (CAG/CTG) in the junctophilin-3 gene on chromosome 16 in patients presenting with Huntington disease–like manifestations.[100]

Nondirective Counseling

Physicians are accustomed to issuing therapeutic directives, and indeed, patients invariably depend on such instructions to improve their health status. Such directive approaches are not consonant with the overwhelming consensus of opinion that governs genetic counseling. Nondirective genetic counseling has been endorsed by medical geneticists,[78,102–106] as well as by the World Health Organization Expert Committee[106] on genetic counseling and in a multinational study focused on the attitudes of genetic counselors.[107,108] Kessler,[109] in an analysis of nondirective genetic counseling, proffered this definition: "Non-directiveness describes procedures aimed at promoting the autonomy and self-directedness of the client." The role of the physician and genetic counselor is to provide the most complete information available, remaining impartial and objective in this communication process albeit recognizing a tenet of medicine to prevent disease. This might not be an easy task. Hsia[110] validly observed that optimistic counselors may tell anxious individuals not to worry, whereas pessimistic ones might unwittingly exaggerate the significance of even small risks. Not unexpectedly, significant differences in counseling techniques mirror the divergent views of counselors on the goals, content, and process of genetic counseling.[111] Kessler,[109] on the other hand, believes that the difficulties counselors have with answering direct questions and being nondirective reveal a lack of skill and an incompetence, which he lays at the door of inadequate training. In calling for correction of the major inadequacies in counseling, training, and skill, he emphasized that nondirectiveness is an "active strategy" aimed at "evoking the client's competence and ability for self-direction."

Michie et al.[112] studied nondirectiveness in genetic counseling. They defined directiveness as advice and expressed views about or selective reinforcement of counselees' behavior, thoughts, or emotions. Not unexpectedly, they concluded that genetic counseling as currently practiced was not characterized, either by counselors, counselees, or a standardized rating scale they used, as uniformly nondirective.

Clarke[113] remarkably argued that nondirective genetic counseling in the context of prenatal diagnosis is "inevitably a sham," largely because of the "structure of the encounter between counselor and client." He further contended "that an offer of prenatal diagnosis implies a recommendation to accept that offer, which in turn entails a tacit recommendation to terminate a pregnancy" if the fetus is abnormal. Thirty years ago,[114] it was emphasized that the offer of prenatal diagnosis was not associated with any explicit or implicit commitment to abort. Clarke[113] further opined that "non-directive counseling was unattainable, despite the counselor's motives, since the offer and acceptance of genetic counseling has already set up a likely chain of events in everyone's mind." Experienced clinical geneticists were taken aback by his views,[115–117] and rightly so. He regarded reproductive choice as part of the "1980s consumerism model of clinical genetics."[118]

Clarke ignored a fundamental tenet of genetic counseling founded in a free society, where choice is not a fad but a right. His ideas suggest contempt for the views (and hence choices) of the public, maintaining that respect for the handicapped is not achievable in a society that "makes judgements about what types of people are worthy of life."[118] Others have reported that people's decision-making processes are more rational than they might appear to be.[119] Simms[120] noted that with hindsight, 80 percent of parents with handicapped children would have aborted their pregnancies. Later, in taking Clarke to task, she concluded that it was "his professional duty to advise parents to the best of his ability, not to make decisions for them. They will have to live with the consequences: he will not."[121]

The intrinsic danger of using a directive approach is the opportunity (even subconscious or inadvertent) for the physician to insinuate his or her own religious, racial, eugenic, or other beliefs or dictates of conscience into the counseling that is offered.[79] Some obstetricians, for example, are known to have specifically not offered or referred patients for prenatal genetic studies because of their antiabortion views, and have unconscionably exaggerated the specific risks of amniocentesis in order to discourage prenatal genetic studies. A Mexican study showed that physicians in specialties other than clinical genetics tend to counsel directively.[122]

The duty of the physician and genetic counselor is to communicate all the available information and then to assist a counselee to recognize his or her major priorities, beliefs, fears, and other concerns in order to make possible the counselee's rational decision making. To remain impartial is difficult and takes valuable time and conscious effort, but it is largely attainable. Time-pressed nongeneticists providing genetic counseling may easily experience slippage between choice and coercion.[123] The difficulty lies mainly in trying to remain impartial while aiming to prevent the occurrence of genetic disease. The insinuation of the physician's prejudices into the decision-making process of the counselee constitutes a moral affront to individual privacy and reproductive autonomy.[121]

In rare instances, family circumstances may challenge the need to adhere to personal autonomy and nondirective counseling. The right of one monozygous twin at 50 percent risk for Huntington disease not to know information after predictive testing should be respected. If there is possible harm to the co-twin, Chapman suggested that testing should "be denied in the absence of mutual consent."[124] She further argued that in the interest of beneficence, directive counseling is acceptable for individuals at 50 percent risk of Huntington disease, who suffer from depression, lack social support, and have a history of attempted suicide. For these patients, psychiatric evaluation and counseling, rather than predictive testing, have been recommended. Marteau et al.,[125] in a study of counseling following prenatal diagnosis of Klinefelter syndrome, found that pregnancy was almost two and a half times more likely to continue when counseling was provided by a geneticist.

Concern for the Individual

Many issues should be raised by the physician or genetic counselor during counseling. Communication should not depend on questions posed by the patient, who may not be cognizant of the subject's dimensions or the available options. For example, in the case of a couple who are at risk for having a profoundly retarded child, the physician should explore the consequences for the interrelationships of the couple, the effects on their other children, the suffering of the affected child, the possible social stigma, and the economic and other societal implications, as well as the need for contraception. Many feel that the economic burden of a defective offspring on society should at least be mentioned as part of a comprehensive view of all issues being considered. Although this may not be unreasonable, the major emphasis should focus on the concern for the individual, whose priorities, needs, and choices remain paramount. In the physician/counselor–patient relationship, concern for the individual should always override consideration of the needs of society. Many avenues exist for society to influence the actions of its citizens. In genetic counseling, the role of the physician is not that of an advocate for society.

A couple may elect to have an amniocentesis that is indeed indicated without making a commitment to pregnancy termination if the fetus is found to be defective. Some may deny such couples the opportunity for prenatal genetic studies. All couples have a right to have information about their fetus, and prenatal diagnosis is a fundamentally reassuring technique.[100] More than 95 percent of such couples do not need to consider elective abortion. The few who are initially ambivalent almost invariably move to terminate the pregnancy after the detection of a serious fetal defect. Nevertheless, abortion may be declined after the prenatal diagnosis of disorders such as trisomy 21, anencephaly, or trisomy 13. Concern for the individual includes providing ambivalent couples with the opportunity for reassurance or the choice to decline abortion with preparation for the consequences. Moreover, opportunities to save their offspring's life, or at least to improve the outcome, now exist in specific circumstances (e.g., for omphalocele).

Quite often, a patient declines an otherwise clearly indicated amniocentesis. Today, the standard of care dictates the need for an explanatory note in the patient's record. A brief letter to the patient noting the indication for prenatal study and that such study was declined is also helpful. Litigation has ensued in which patients have maintained that no amniocentesis had been offered, while obstetricians (without notes in the records) have taken an opposite view.

Truth in Counseling

Since the time of Hippocrates, physicians have often withheld the truth from their patients and, as Katz[126] emphasized in *The Silent World of Doctor and Patient*, defended the morality of this position. Sparing the patient emotional distress, removing hope and/or diminishing the physician's personal esteem may have been some of the quintessential reasons for the lack of truth-telling. Lantos,[127] while recognizing the modern change in moral sentiment, acknowledged that truth telling has become "morally obligatory." Notwithstanding his preference that he "would not want a doctor judging the morality of my decision," he remained uncertain about the value of the "comforting lie."

In a number of situations in genetic counseling, it is possible that the facts may be deliberately distorted, deemphasized, or even hidden. Obstetricians opposed to prenatal genetic studies and abortion of a defective fetus have been known to deny the genetic origin of a disorder, to describe it as a fluke occurrence, or to provide incorrect (much lower) recurrence figures.

The physician may be unable to establish an exact diagnosis, to be certain of the carrier status of an individual, or to predict accurately the outcome of pregnancy when faced with a very unusual fetal karyotype. Painful as it may be to both parties, the physician must ensure that patients understand the limitations completely. The unexpected finding, for example, of an XYY fetus should not be withheld from the parents, despite the inability to predict with certainty the ultimate development of an individual so affected.

In the course of a prenatal diagnostic study, blood samples from both parents may be called for to elucidate a potential diagnostic dilemma. On occasion, such studies unexpectedly reveal that the husband is not the biologic father of the fetus. Not sharing this information with the patient's husband may subsequently have legal implications. The management and resolution of such a problem will most often rest on the nature of the dilemma (for example, translocation, deletion) to be solved. Advising the mother of these findings, as well as the paternity issue, is necessary, as is documentation in the physician's notes.

The expanding use of prenatal diagnosis and the advent of molecular tools using recombinant-DNA techniques for carrier detection and prenatal diagnosis are likely to increase the frequency of detected nonpaternity. The warning that the rate of infidelity is higher than the rate of inborn errors of metabolism should not be reserved for medical students only. Management is invariably tricky, and medical, ethical, and legal issues abound. An important guiding principle is that the noncarrier male partner should not be misled.

Confidentiality and Trust

Action by the physician after the diagnosis of the carrier state for an X-linked disease demands more than simply offering prenatal studies in all subsequent pregnancies. There is an obligation to convey this information to the sisters of any such carrier female. The patient may, however, expressly forbid the physician to communicate this information, even to her sisters at risk. Certain legal pitfalls involving the transmission of privileged communications and breach of medical ethics[128] need to be considered by the conscientious physician faced with this rare but not unheard-of situation. The need for caution is clear when one realizes that in some states in the United States, the physician may lose his or her license to practice medicine after a breach of confidentiality.

Disclosure to third parties, other than relatives, also includes employers, insurance companies, and schools. It is hoped that the confidentiality of the physician-patient relationship and the patients' right to privacy and personal autonomy remain sacrosanct. The American Medical Association has affirmed the importance of keeping genetic information confidential.[128a] Established precedent for breaking this confidentiality relates to recognition by the physician of danger to a third party. Threats to kill a former girlfriend shared with a psychiatrist were recognized by the courts as knowledge that should have been communicated.[129,130] Certainly, the clinical notes and letters should reflect the geneticist's recommendation that the patient promptly contact the indicated close relatives who are at risk for a specific genetic disorder.

However, faced with an intractable patient, some guidance about disclosure is reflected in a statement issued by the American Society of Human Genetics in 1998.[131] When serious and foreseeable harm to at-risk relatives can be anticipated, when the disorder is preventable or treatable, or when reduction of risk through monitoring is achievable, disclosure is seen to be permissible. "The harm that may result from failure to disclose should outweigh the harm that may result from disclosure." In practice, few geneticists appear to have warned at-risk relatives without patient consent. The vast majority of medical geneticists who decided not to warn such relatives were concerned by patient confidentiality issues and legal liability.[132]

Timing of Genetic Counseling

Today, more than ever before, counseling before conception or marriage[133] may provide opportunities for carrier detection, prenatal diagnosis, or the presentation of other important options noted earlier. Therefore, the optimal time to initiate counseling is not during pregnancy. Counselees whose first antenatal visits occur after the second missed menstrual period miss the critical period of organogenesis, and patients referred well after conception have lost almost all their options except for selective abortion. Given the 70 percent protection afforded by periconceptional folic acid supplementation against the occurrence of an NTD[4–6] (see also chapter 21), there is a need to advise women about the importance of preconception care.

Confronted by a fatally malformed newborn, the physician may attempt to counsel a couple on the very day of the birth of such a defective child or before the mother's discharge from the hospital. Although communication and support are both vital during those fateful days, the physician needs to recognize the great difficulty that anguished patients would have in assimilating or comprehending even the essence of any counseling.[121,134,135] The physician/counselor should share with the couple his or her awareness that it is difficult to remember all the important information in the face of emotional upset and that it would be normal and expected for them to raise all the same questions some weeks later, when the entire subject could be fully covered. Support for the parents should continue to be available for many months.

Parental Counseling

Physicians/counselors have a duty to convey information about the known options, risks, benefits, and foreseeable consequences[56–58] to couples with increased risks of having children with genetic defects. Such a duty may be difficult, if not impossible, to fulfill if only one member of the couple attends genetic counseling. The issues are usually complex and are frequently compounded by feelings of guilt and by ignorance, family prejudices, religious obstacles, fear, and serious differences of opinion between spouses. Hence, when possible (at the time the appointment is made would seem to be best), the necessity that the couple attend together should be emphasized. Physicians/counselors have often seen an extremely anxious parent attend counseling alone and then have learned later of the counselee's incorrect interpretation to the spouse, lack of appreciation of the true risk figures, and unnecessary emotional chaos. Not even letters written to parents after the counseling session (a recommended procedure, to summarize the essence of the counseling provided) can safely substitute for face-to-face discussions with a couple, allowing for questions and interchange about the issues and an opportunity to examine the partner.

Genetic counselors should be cognizant of the complex interactive factors involved in parental reproductive decision making. Frets[136] confirmed the importance of the burden of the disease in question and found that the interpretation of risk (high or low) and the wish to have children were paramount factors. The absence of personal experience of the disease was also found to be a significant influence. Frets identified a number of factors that were independently and significantly associated with problems experienced by 43 percent of counseled couples. These included no postcounseling support, recognition of high risk, disapproval by relatives, the presence of an affected child, and decisions not to have a (or another) child.

Counselee Education

Hsia et al.[135] emphasized that genetic counseling is an educational process in which the counselee acquires a set of facts and options. Fraser's[101] essential message was that genetic counseling does not involve telling families what they *should* do but rather what they *can* do. We maintain that members of the health professions should adopt as a guiding principle the critical imperative that the concept of genetic counseling be introduced in high school and in continuing public education[110,137–139] about genetic disease. Children sensitized in school about the importance of the family history, elements of heredity, concepts of individual susceptibility and risk, and opportunities for anticipatory prevention of unnecessary catastrophes are likely to better comprehend pregnancy risks and options.

Genetic counseling and prenatal diagnostic services are of little avail if many women attend for their first antenatal visit after 16 weeks of gestation. Currently, this is the case in many urban hospitals in the Western world, where between 20 and 40 percent of obstetric patients arrive at this late time. Education beginning in high school and continued by public health authorities working in the public sector could effectively communicate the critical importance of preconception and prenatal care.

Duty to Recontact

The remarkable and rapid advances in medical genetics have introduced a "new" responsibility related to the well-established requirement to disclose risk information that materially bears on a patient's decision making.[140,141] Pelias[141] focused attention on the geneticist's continuing obligation to recontact patients when new information develops that would prove material to them, so far as personal health and childbearing are concerned (see also chapter 30). The implications raise serious ethical, legal, and policy issues.[131,141a,141b] Medical genetics consultations frequently involve only one encounter, and the requirement to contact that patient years later may be regarded as both irrational and unreasonable. Pelias pointed to a 1971 case[142] in which the University of Chicago failed to notify women who had been given diethylstilbestrol. The University had apparently become aware of the dangers of this drug but had delayed notification for 4–5 years. In yet another case, after a single visit to her gynecologist for insertion of an intrauterine device (a Dalkon Shield), a woman sued this physician for failing to notify her of the subsequently recognized risks of this device.[143] In that case, as Pelias noted, the court allowed the case to proceed because of the continuing status of the physician–patient relationship and because the physician had a "separate duty to act."[143]

In cases in which reasonable expectations for significant advances exist (e.g., tests for carrier detection or prenatal diagnosis), the authors recommend that the patient be in contact annually and/or before planned childbearing. Pelias[141] opined that this recommendation should be recorded in clinical notes and echoed in letters to referring physicians and patients alike. Ultimately, the responsibility to return for further counseling in the light of new advances must be vested with the patient's primary care physician and shared with the patient. To a variable extent, the patient's physician can be expected to remain cognizant of genetic risks family members may have and refer them for specific genetic counseling or testing when appropriate. However, given that tens of millions change their addresses annually and frequently seek other medical care, the patients themselves, once informed of potential advances and the need to remain in contact with a clinical geneticist, encumber personal responsibility.

Do No Harm

The classical exhortation *primum non nocere* (first do no harm) is as pertinent to clinical genetics as it is to medicine in all specialties. Attention to this principle arises particularly in the context of predictive genetic diagnosis, possible for a rapidly escalating number of neurodegenerative disorders (e.g., Huntington disease, Friedreich ataxia, the spinocerebellar ataxias) and certain potentially fatal conditions (e.g., multiple endocrine neoplasia type 2B). Published recommendations and guidelines[144] urge rigorous pretest and posttest genetic counseling and recommendations that testing of children younger than 18 years of age be proscribed, except in life-threatening disorders (e.g., multiple endocrine neoplasia type 2B). The inherent harm that could potentially be done by presymptomatic testing is the potential for demoralization and depression with possible suicidal consequences. Extreme caution is recommended in considering predictive testing for a disorder without curative, let alone meaningful, palliative treatment. Although for certain dominant disorders some 50 percent of individuals at risk may receive good news, the other 50 percent face, effectively, a death sentence. Given the remarkable pace of advances in human genetics, it may well be possible in the foreseeable future to develop a therapy that enhances the extant biologic mechanism already in place that delays the manifestations of later-onset disease for decades after birth. No life should be ruined by severe depression or suicide only to discover later that a critical palliative remedy has emerged.

Clearly, there are extraordinarily difficult circumstances related to planned childbearing in the face of 50 percent risks for a neurodegenerative disorder coupled with a wish not to know. In these special circumstances, predictive testing can be regarded as acceptable only if performed with extreme care, concern, and professionalism.

Preconception care should begin during visits to the family physician after menarche. Reiterated and expanding discussions on personal health habits that will affect both the adolescent herself and a future child provide a basis for promoting good health behavior, while a solid grounding in knowledge about the hazards of smoking, drugs, alcohol, sexually transmitted diseases, and nutrition is provided. Early adolescence is also a vital period during which to inculcate the importance of genes and the wisdom of assimilating and updating information on family history. Linkage of family history to the common experience of physical and mental handicap, outlined in the context of personal risk in childbearing, provides a compelling and cogent framework on which physicians, teachers, and parents can build.

This preparatory background may help educate all women about the importance of planning pregnancy. Over 50 percent of pregnancies in the United States are not planned and are often unintended.[145] Physicians also need to reorient their practices so that women of childbearing age understand that to optimize the chance of having a healthy child,[137] prenatal care is best initiated before conception and not after the second missed menstrual period, as is still anachronistically practiced so widely. Only genetic-related matters occupy the focus of the necessarily brief discussion that follows.

PRECONCEPTION GENETIC COUNSELING

Expectations at the first preconception visit include routine documentation of the medical, obstetric, and genetic history, including construction of a family pedigree. This activity includes a review of medical records, photographs (e.g., previous stillbirths), and pertinent autopsy reports, radiographs, brain scans, and chromosome or other special laboratory reports. Physical examination and needed special tests also focus on acquired and genetic disorders that could, during pregnancy, threaten maternal and/or fetal welfare. Previously undiagnosed/undetected disorders may be determined for the first time at this visit and may be important for planned childbearing and the selection of future prenatal diagnostic tests. There is a need to insist that the male partner attend the preconception visit (or absolutely the first prenatal visit), providing an opportunity to detect at least obvious genetic disorders and solidify information possibly provided earlier about his family history. The senior author recalls, over many years during prenatal diagnosis counseling for other issues, diagnosing various disorders in male partners who were wholly unaware of their conditions, including osteogenesis imperfecta, Treacher–Collins syndrome, tuberous sclerosis, neurofibromatosis, Charcot–Marie–Tooth (type 1A) disease, limb-girdle muscular dystrophy, facioscapulohumeral muscular dystrophy, blepharophimosis, mitral-valve prolapse, the XYY male, and spinocerebellar ataxia.

The first preconception visit also serves to instruct about the need for folic acid supplementation for the avoidance of NTDs and possibly other defects.[4–6] This counseling is particularly important given the remarkable observation in a Colorado study showing that 9 years after national folic acid recommendations were made, 53 percent of women who had had a pregnancy with offspring affected by a neural tube defect did not know about the need for additional folic acid supplementation to avoid recurrence.[146] Referral to other specialists (e.g., neurologists), for tailoring medication requirements to safer and possibly less teratogenic agents, is also recommended. This is also the time for specialists caring for the same patient to confer about the planned care of their patient through pregnancy and for documentation of that exchange to be made.

Indications for Preconception Genetic Counseling

The indications for preconception genetic counseling should be determined at the first visit and can be considered in a few clear categories.

Advanced Maternal Age

An arbitrary age of 35 years still functions in the United States as an expected standard of care, which requires that a prospective mother be informed of her risks of having a child with a chromosome defect, informed of the recommendation for prenatal diagnosis, and given an explanation of the risks of chorionic villus sampling (CVS) or amniocentesis, with the associated details related to any problems, pitfalls, or reservations. In some countries, largely for economic reasons, older ages have been used as an indication for prenatal study. Amniocentesis risks lower than 0.5 percent for fetal loss in some U.S. centers prompt the offer of such studies earlier than 35 years of age.

Excluding infants with chromosome abnormalities, a prospective analysis of 102,728 pregnancies (including abortions, stillbirths, and livebirths) in Texas found that the incidence of congenital malformations increased significantly and progressively in women after 25 years of age.[147] They found that an additional age-related risk of nonchromosome malformations was approximately 1 percent in women 35 years of age or older. The odds ratio for cardiac defects was 3.95 in infants of women 40 years of age or older when compared with women aged 20–24 years.

A Previous Fetus or Child with a Genetic Disorder

A genetic evaluation and counseling are usually indicated when a previous fetus or child has or had a genetic disorder, unless the matter is straightforward (e.g., previous trisomy 21) and the obstetrician is well informed. Careful inquiry should be made about the health status of a previous child. Failure or delay in the diagnosis of a monogenic disorder leaves the parents without the option of prenatal diagnosis in a subsequent pregnancy. Failure to make an early diagnosis of a genetic disorder during the first 5 years of life is not unusual. For example, the Rotterdam Clinical Genetics Group reported that 50 percent of children affected by neurofibromatosis had been treated for related symptoms before a specific diagnosis had been made.[148]

Not infrequently, distressed parents will select a different physician for a subsequent pregnancy and a new or more recent insight may shed light on the cause of the previous defect. For example, confined placental mosaicism (see also chapter 6) may now serve to explain the discrepancy between reported chromosomal findings at the time of CVS and fetal tissues obtained at elective abortion. Confined placental mosaicism may also serve to explain, through trisomic zygote rescue, the liveborn child with trisomy 15 evident in skin fibroblasts but not in peripheral blood.[149]

Given the heterogeneous nature of genetic disease, being alert to alternative mechanisms of causation will on occasion be rewarding. For example, during a consultation with a patient who had previously delivered a child with cystic fibrosis (CF), preparatory discussions about establishing the specific mutation from each parent could reveal that the father is not a carrier of the mutated CF gene. Although nonpaternity is more likely, a judicious approach would also include consideration of uniparental disomy.[150] This mode of inheritance in which an offspring can inherit two copies, part, or all of a chromosome from one parent and no copy from the other parent has been seen in a number of disorders, including Prader–Willi syndrome[151] and Angelman syndrome.[152,153] About 30 percent of cases of Prader–Willi syndrome are caused by maternal uniparental disomy.[151] These disorders then, represent situations in which one parent is the source of both gene mutations for a recessively inherited condition. Disorders involving chromosomes 11, 14, and 15 have been notable.[154] Uniparental disomy is caused primarily by meiotic nondisjunction events and followed by trisomy or monosomy "rescue."[155] Most cases described have been associated with advanced maternal age and have been detected primarily in the process of prenatal genetic studies.[155]

Recognition of the molecular basis of a disorder from which a previous child died may provide a couple an opportunity for prenatal diagnosis in a subsequent planned pregnancy. A caveat would be the availability of analyzable tissue from the deceased child. In the recent past this was mostly not done, but with the escalation of new discoveries in genetics, tissues are now being frozen for potential future DNA analysis. The establishment of the molecular basis of recognized syndromes, previously undetectable prenatally, now provides new opportunities for couples seeking prenatal diagnosis. Examples abound (see also chapter 10) and include some of the craniosynostosis syndromes, certain skeletal dysplasias, and many other disorders.

In one of our cases, a father with metaphyseal dysplasia of Schmid, troubled by the indignities and hurts of growing up with severe short stature, elected prenatal diagnosis at a preconception visit. Subsequent mutation analysis of conceived twins yielded a normal prenatal diagnosis result confirmed postnatally.[156]

Heterogeneity and pleiotropism also require consideration in the context of a previous child's disorder and anticipation of future prenatal diagnosis. For example, a child with sensorineural deafness and additional major features of Waardenburg syndrome (white forelock, heterochromia irides, and patchy skin hypopigmentation) may have a mutation in the *PAX3* gene[157] if dystopia canthorum and hypertelorism are present (Waardenburg syndrome type 1). The same features without hypertelorism constitute Waardenburg syndrome type 2 (WS-2). Since we cloned the gene for Waardenburg syndrome type 1,[157] sequencing has not yielded a mutation in a significant proportion of cases. For WS-2, mutations in the *MITF* gene and one report of a mutation in the *SLUG* gene, have been published.[158,159] The same team has reported *SLUG* gene deletions in piebaldism,[159a] apparently distinct from WS-2. Thus far, our experience indicates that <10 percent of WS-2 cases have a mutation in the *MITF* gene.

A Parent with a Genetic Disorder

Given the pace of advances in human genetics, physicians are advised to determine whether prenatal diagnosis has become available for the specific genetic disorder under discussion. Increasingly, these discussions may focus on a dominant genetic disorder affecting one parent and the concern vis-à-vis prenatal diagnosis and pregnancy termination is about personal existence and self-extinction. These consultations may invoke deep personal emotional conflict, especially when heterogeneity of the disorder is concerned, exemplified by the parent with normal intelligence and a definitive diagnosis of tuberous sclerosis facing uncertainty about the potential intellectual health of their offspring. Parental decisions are neither simple nor predictable. In a U.K. study[160] of 644 deaf individuals and 143 with hearing impairment, 2 percent opined that they would prefer to have deaf children and would consider an elective abortion if the fetus was found to be hearing. Certain genetic disorders may (1) threaten maternal health in pregnancy, (2) threaten fetal health and survival, or (3) be aggravated by pregnancy.

Genetic Disorders That Pregnancy May Aggravate. Dramatic advances in medical care have resulted in more women affected by genetic disorders surviving to childbearing age and becoming pregnant. There are several genetic disorders affecting the mother that can be aggravated and worsened during pregnancy. Awareness of these disorders facilitates better preconception anticipatory guidance and expectant management during pregnancy. Metabolic disorders that may worsen include ornithine transcarbamylase deficiency, homocystinuria, and lysinuric protein intolerance. Hyperammonemia during pregnancy/ delivery or postpartum coma may be the presenting signs of a female heterozygote with ornithine transcarbamylase deficiency.[161] Thrombophlebitis and other thromboembolic

events have been reported during pregnancy and operative delivery in women with homocystinuria.[162] Ehlers–Danlos syndrome and Marfan syndrome may have associated aor-
tic/vascular rupture and uterine rupture during pregnancy and delivery.[163] Sophisticated
care and counseling are necessary for women with Marfan syndrome who are considering pregnancy. Among the guidelines recommended by Lipscomb et al.[163] are:

1. Women with Marfan syndrome who are planning to have children should be encouraged to do so in their early twenties, given that the mean age for aortic dissection is 32 years.[164]
2. Women should be counseled that there is a significant likelihood of aortic dissection if the aortic root dimension exceeds 4.0 cm or if there has been a steady increase in this dimension over preceding visits.
3. Monthly echocardiography during pregnancy should begin as early as 6 weeks of
   gestation. They emphasize that aortic catastrophes are not confined to late pregnancy, labor, and the postnatal period.
4. Vaginal deliveries with epidural anesthesia are recommended for women with stable aortic measurements <4 cm during pregnancy.
5. Elective cesarean section with epidural anesthesia is recommended for women with
   changes in aortic root dimensions during pregnancy and for those with measurements exceeding 4 cm.
6. Hypertension must be treated aggressively, and ideally with beta blockers.[165]
7. Routine beta blocker treatment slows the rate of aortic dilatation and should be
   used at least after the first trimester.
8. Prophylactic antibiotics should be used because of the likely associated presence
   of mitral-valve prolapse.

First-trimester spontaneous abortion and gastrointestinal bleeding during pregnancy
have been described in women with pseudoxanthoma elasticum.[166] Worsening of the
mother's pulmonary status is seen with cystic fibrosis.[167] An increase in the size and number of neurofibromata during pregnancy in women affected with neurofibromatosis type
1 may occur (in 60 percent of 105 cases in one study[168]) and has resulted in both cos-
metic changes as well as significant morbidity (paraplegia with rapid growth of intraspinal
tumors).[169] Hypertension may be a problem for the pregnant patient with either neurofibromatosis type 1 or autosomal dominant polycystic kidney disease. As well as causing
potentially life-threatening events for both the fetus and mother affected by myotonic muscular dystrophy,[80,170] the condition itself may worsen during a pregnancy.[170] Hematologic
disorders may complicate pregnancy by altering normal physiology.

Carriers of hemophilia A are best cared for by a high-risk perinatal obstetric group.
Prenatal sex determination (whether or not prenatal diagnosis by mutation analysis is
elected) is important for the management of labor and delivery, with special reference to
the possible need for cesarean section. In addition, vacuum-assisted delivery with an affected male could result in a massive cephalohematoma requiring blood transfusion.[171]
Moreover, a high incidence of primary and secondary postpartum hemorrhage in hemophilia A (22 percent) and hemophilia B (11 percent)[171] carriers should further inform anticipatory care.

Maternal Genetic Disorders That May Threaten Fetal Health and Survival. Among the
more common examples in this category are diabetes (see discussion below), sickle cell
disease, epilepsy,[172] and lupus erythematosus. Fetal loss, stillbirth, and malformations are

the primary concerns. Lupus is associated with a significant frequency of congenital heart block,[173,174] and electronic fetal monitoring in the third trimester and during labor is important,[175] given available treatment options (see also chapter 29). As many as 60 percent of mothers of offspring with congenital heart block have lupus or other connective-tissue disorders. Maternal myotonic muscular dystrophy, which may be presymptomatic, is a key example in which both the life and health of the mother and fetus/child may be threatened.[96,176] In addition to the earlier discussion, serious-to-fatal fetal/neonatal complications can be anticipated.[96,176] One study showed that 12 percent of the offspring of affected women are stillborn or die as neonates, 9 percent survive although severely affected, and 29 percent are affected later.[177] Awareness of the obstetric-related risks facilitates optimal pregnancy care but does require in-depth preconception discussion.

Untreated maternal phenylketonuria represents a potentially unmitigated disaster for the fetus and child. Besides pregnancy loss, there is a >90 percent likelihood of mental retardation, cardiac, or other defects in the offspring of mothers who undertake pregnancy without being on strict preconception dietary therapy.[178]

Genetic Disorders That Pregnancy May Aggravate. Women who are severely affected by CF may jeopardize their survival by becoming pregnant and should be advised accordingly. Those with mild-to-moderate disease are likely to have a successful pregnancy. A French study in which the outcome was known for seventy-five patients noted a prematurity rate of 18 percent and one maternal death during pregnancy.[179] Later, some twelve deaths were recorded after pregnancy with only three in the year following the pregnancy. Four affected children were diagnosed after birth. Clearly, partners should be tested for their CF carrier status before the initiation of pregnancy in a woman with CF (see also chapter 15). A Norwegian study of pregnancy with CF noted preterm delivery in 24 percent of cases and the development of gestational diabetes in four of twenty-three patients.[180] Similar observations were made in a Swedish study, except that they noted an overall mortality rate of 19 percent among forty-eight patients.[181] If pregnancy is elected regardless of counseling, special care and attention will be necessary, and hospitalization is commonly needed at some time during the third trimester. Women with severe sickle cell disease may also become sicker during pregnancy and should be counseled accordingly. In some women, epilepsy is aggravated by pregnancy and could threaten the life of both mother and child. Given the potential teratogenic risks of anticonvulsants (in the 7–10 percent range),[182] change to the least teratogenic should be achieved in the preconception period and should be done under the direct guidance of a neurologist. Prospective mothers with insulin-dependent diabetes mellitus (IDDM) could find their disorder harder to control during pregnancy. Diabetes should be well controlled before pregnancy. The better the control, the lower the risk of having a child with congenital defects.[183–185] An Australian study noted that with good preconception care of type 1 IDDM, the major congenital malformation rate decreased from a high of 14 percent to 2.2 percent.[186] Notwithstanding extant knowledge about IDDM and pregnancy, a recent report of 273 women noted rates of stillbirth (1.85 percent), perinatal mortality (2.78 percent), and congenital anomalies (6 percent).[187] Maternal obesity clearly poses an increased risk of congenital malformations as noted in the discussion earlier, probably through a metabolic route involving prediabetes.[13]

Muscle weakness may increase during pregnancy in women with limb-girdle muscular dystrophy, leading to the need for assistance after delivery.[185] In women with congenital myopathies, including central core disease and cytoplasmic body myopathy, cesarean sections may occur more frequently and some deterioration in pregnancy and weakness after delivery may be experienced.[188] Anesthetic risks may be increased in women with central core disease in whom malignant hyperthermia may be a complication.[189]

A History of Infertility

About 10 percent of couples have infertility problems. A World Health Organization multicenter study concluded that the problem appeared predominantly in males in 20 percent of cases, predominantly in females in 38 percent, and in both partners in 27 percent. In the remaining 15 percent of cases, no definitive cause for the infertility was identified.[190] Care should be exercised in the preconception counseling of a couple with a history of infertility. In the absence of a recognizable cause, karyotyping of both should be considered. Unrecognized spontaneous abortions may have occurred without the patient's awareness, caused by structural chromosome defects. Recognized habitual abortion due to the same cause would also require cytogenetic analysis. Such studies may reveal that a parent (rarely both) may be found with a chromosomal rearrangement and have significant risks for bearing a child with mental retardation and/or malformations.

Other disorders characteristically associated with recurrent pregnancy loss include the X-linked disorders, steroid sulfatase deficiency,[191] and incontinentia pigmenti.[192]

Although the investigation to determine the cause of male or female infertility can be extensive, three observations are pertinent here. First, we recognized that congenital bilateral absence of the vas deferens (CBAVD),[136] which occurs in 1–2 percent of infertile males, is primarily a genital form of CF. Men with CBAVD should have CF gene mutation analysis. After analysis of 100 of the most common mutations we found that only 35.9 percent of men with CBAVD had two identifiable mutations, 31.5 percent had only one mutation recognized, and no CF mutation was found in the remainder.[193] Of interest is the observation of Traystman et al.[194] that CF carriers may be at higher risk for infertility than the population at large.

Some patients with CBAVD (21 percent in one study[195]) also had renal malformations. These patients may have a normal sweat test and thus far no recognizable mutations in the CF gene.[195] Renal ultrasound studies are recommended in all patients with CBAVD who have normal results on a sweat chloride test and no identified mutations.

The female partner of a male with CBAVD should routinely be tested for the common CF mutations. Such couples frequently consider epididymal sperm aspiration,[196,197] with pregnancy induced by in vitro fertilization. Precise prenatal diagnosis can be achieved only if specific mutations have been recognized.

Second, Y-chromosome microdeletions occur in 10–20 percent of men with "idiopathic" azoospermia or severe oligospermia.[198–200] Genes, including *DAZ* ("deleted in azoospermia"), *YRRM* (Y chromosome RNA recognition motif),[200,201] and others may be deleted singly or together in the region of Yq11.23.[202] Couples must be informed that male offspring of men with these interstitial deletions in the Y chromosome will have the same structural chromosome defect. The female partner of the male undergoing intractyoplasmic sperm injection (ICSI) needs explanations about procedures and medications for her that are not risk-free. Patients should realize that ICSI followed by in vitro fertilization is likely to achieve pregnancy rates between 20 and 24 percent,[203] a success rate not very different from the approximately 30 percent success rate in a single cycle after natural intercourse at the time of ovulation.[203] Pregnancy follow-up data from cases culled from thirty-five different programs reported in a European survey[204] and a major American study of 578 newborns showed no increased occurrence of congenital malformations.[63]

However, more recently, a statistically significant increase in sex chromosome defects has been observed[205] (see chapter 7). Prenatal diagnosis is recommended in all pregnancies following ICSI.

Third, even balanced reciprocal translocations in males may be associated with the arrest of spermatogenesis and resultant azoospermia.[206]

In one series of 150 infertile men with oligospermia or azoospermia, an abnormal karyotype was found in 10.6 percent of (16/180), 5.3 percent (8/150) had an AZF-c deletion, and 9.3 percent (14/150) had at least a single CF gene mutation.[207] This study revealed a genetic abnormality in 36/150 (24 percent) of men with oligospermia or azoospermia.

Parental Carrier of a Genetic Disorder

The first preconception visit should be the time to establish the carrier state for a chromosomal rearrangement or a gene mutation in prospective parents.

Physicians should be alerted to the possibility of chromosomal rearrangements or gene mutations that one or the other partner might carry relative to a history of previous recurrent spontaneous abortions, infertility, or previous offspring with a chromosomal or single gene defect. Referral for genetic counseling in these circumstances is appropriate given complex questions relative to risk, prognosis in a future pregnancy, and potential pitfalls/reservations concerning prenatal diagnosis (see also chapter 6).

Determination of single gene mutations in carriers may be prompted by the patient's ethnic group, a family history of a specific genetic disorder, or a previously affected offspring. In virtually all ethnic groups, particular recessive disorders occur more frequently than in the population at large (Table 1.6). Increasingly, carrier tests will become available for these various ethnic groups. Carrier testing for Tay–Sachs disease (Ashkenazi Jews), sickle cell disease (blacks), β-thalassemia (peoples of Mediterranean descent), and β-thalassemia (Asians) is regarded as standard, and indicated simply on the basis of ethnicity.

Individuals of French-Canadian ancestry living in New England were reported to have a maximum frequency of heterozygosity for Tay–Sachs disease or Sandhoff disease of 1 in 42.[209] Enzymatic analysis of hexosaminidase was confirmed by mutation analysis with exclusion of benign pseudodeficiency mutations. Notwithstanding these findings, which could reflect ascertainment bias, are the prior salutary observations of Palomaki et al.[210] These authors recorded no cases of Tay–Sachs disease in 41,000 births to couples who were *both* of French-Canadian ancestry. Further studies are necessary before formal recommendations can be made for carrier testing in this ethnic group.

A family history of CF is a direct indication for mutation analysis.[211] Moreover, given the ability to detect about 90 percent of CF carriers by routine testing of the most common mutations (see also chapter 15), all Caucasian couples should be offered these analyses at the preconception visit.[212] Unfortunately, even after DNA mutation analysis, couples may not be aware of the limitations of these results. In one study, over half of those having CF carrier tests were unaware of their residual risk after having received a negative test result,[213] while in another report only 62 percent correctly understood their results 6 months after testing.[214]

Among the many items to be considered during the preconception visit are the potential physical features indicative of sex-linked disorders that may manifest in female carriers (Table 1.7). With or without a family history of the disorder in question, referral to a clinical geneticist would be appropriate for final evaluation of possible implications.

Table 1.6. Common genetic disorders in various ethnic groups

Ethnic Group	Genetic Disorder
Africans (blacks)	Sickle-cell disease and other disorders of hemoglobin
	Alpha- and beta-thalassemia
	Glucose-6-phosphate dehydrogenase deficiency
	Benign familial leukopenia
	High blood pressure (in females)
Afrikaners (white South Africans)	Variegate porphyria
	Fanconi anemia
American Indians (of British Columbia)	Cleft lip or palate (or both)
Armenians	Familial Mediterranean fever
Ashkenazi Jews	A-beta-lipoproteinemia
	Bloom syndrome
	Breast cancer
	Colon cancer
	Congenital adrenal hyperplasia
	Dystonia musculorum deformans
	Factor XI (PTA) deficiency
	Familial dysautonomia
	Gaucher disease (adult form)
	Iminoglycinuria
	Meckel syndrome
	Niemann–Pick disease
	Pentosunria
	Spongy degeneration of the brain
	Stub thumbs
	Tay–Sachs disease
Chinese	Thalassemia (alpha)
	Glucose-6-phosphate dehydrogenase deficiency (Chinese type)
	Adult lactase deficiency
Eskimos	E_1 pseudocholinesterase deficiency
	Congenital adrenal hyperplasia
Finns	Aspartylglucosaminuria
	Congenital nephrosis
French Canadians	Neural tube defects
	Tay–Sachs disease
Irish	Neural tube defects
	Phenylketonuria
	Schizophrenia
Italians (northern)	Fucosidosis
Japanese and Koreans	Acatalasia
	Dyschromatosis universalis hereditaria
	Oguchi disease
Maori (Polynesians)	Clubfoot
Mediterranean peoples (Italians, Greeks, Sephardic Jews, Armenians, Turks, Spaniards, Cypriots)	Familial Mediterranean fever
	Glucose-6-phosphate dehydrogenase deficiency (Mediterranean type)
	Glycogen storage disease (type III)
	Thalassemia (mainly beta)
Norwegians	Cholestasis-lymphedema
	Phenylketonuria
Yugoslavs (of the Istrian Peninsula)	Schizophrenia

Source: Milunsky, 2001.[208]

Table 1.7. Signs in females who are carriers of X-linked-recessive disease

Selected Disorders	Key Feature(s) That May Occur	Selected References
Achromatopsia	Decreased visual acuity and myopia	215
Adrenoleukodystrophy	Neurologic and adrenal dysfunction	216,217
Alpha-thalassemia/mental retardation	Rare hemoglobin H inclusions in red blood cells	218
Alport syndrome	Microscopic hematuria and hearing impairment	219
Ameliogenesis imperfecta, hypomaturation type	Mottled enamel vertically arranged	220
Arthrogrypsos multiplex congenita	Club foot, contractures, hyperkyphosis	221
Borjeson syndrome	Tapered fingers, short widely spaced flexed toes, mild mental retardation	222
Choroideremia[a]	Choreoretinal dystrophy	223
Chronic granulomatous disease	Cutaneous and mucocutaneous lesions	224,225
Cleft palate	Bifid uvula	226
Conductive deafness with stapes fixation	Mild hearing loss	227
Congenital cataracts[b]	Posterior suture cataracts	228
Duchenne muscular dystrophy	Pseudohypertrophy, weakness, cardiomyopathy/ conduction defects	229–231
Dyskeratosis congenita	Retinal pigmentation	232
Emery–Dreifuss muscular dystrophy	Cardiomyopathy/conduction defects	233
Fabry disease	Angiokeratomas, corneal dystrophy, "burning hands and feet"	234
FG syndrome	Anterior displaced anus, facial dysmorphism	235
Fragile X syndrome	Mild-to-moderate mental retardation, behavioral aberrations, schizoaffective disorder, premature ovarian failure	236–238
G6PD deficiency	Hemolytic crises, neonatal hyperbilirubinemia	239,240
Hemophilia A and B	Bleeding tendency	241
Hypohydrotic ectodermal dysplasia	Sparse hair, decreased sweating	242
Lowe syndrome	Lenticular cataracts	243,244
Menkes disease	Patchy kinky hair, hypopigmentation	245,246
Myopia	Mild myopia	247
Nance–Horan syndrome[b]	Posterior Y-sutural cataracts and dental anomalies	248
Norrie disease	Retinal malformations	249
Ocular albinism type 1	Retinal/fundal pigmentary changes	250
Oligodontia	Hypodontia	251
Omithine transcarbamylase deficiency	Hyperammonemia, psychiatric/neurologic manifestations	252,253
Retinoschisis	Peripheral retinal changes	254
Retinitis pigmentosa	Night blindness, concentric reduction of visual field, pigmentary fundal degeneration, extinction of electroretinogram	255
Sideroblastic anemia	Minor red-cell abnormalities without anemia	256
Simpson–Golabi–Behmel syndrome	Extra lumbar/thoracic vertebrae, accessory nipples, facial dysmorphism	257
Split-hand/split-foot anomaly	Mild split-hand/split-foot anomaly	258
Spondyloepiphyseal dysplasia, late onset	Arthritis	259
Ulnar hypoplasia with lobster-claw deficiency of feet	Slight hypoplasia of ulnar side of hand and mild syndactyly of toes	260
Wiscott–Aldrich syndrome[a]	Abnormal platelets and lymphocytes	261,262
X-linked mental retardation	Short stature, hypertelorism	263,264
X-linked retinitis pigmentosa	Retinal changes	265

[a]Uncertain.

[b]May be same disorder.

Failure to recognize obvious features in a manifesting female may well result in a missed opportunity for prenatal genetic studies and an outcome characterized by a seriously affected male (or occasionally female) offspring. Of crucial additional importance in considering manifesting female carriers of sex-linked disorders is the realization that carrier females for Duchenne and Becker muscular dystrophy have preclinical or clinically evident myocardial involvement in up to a remarkable 84 percent of cases.[229] A study of 197 women and girls aged 5–60 years who were carriers of either Duchenne or Becker muscular dystrophy revealed progressive dilated cardiomyopathy, myocardial hypertrophy, and/or dysrhythmias. Careful and detailed annual evaluation of cardiac status is recommended for these carriers. Dilemmas may also occasionally arise in counseling, for example, for a mildly retarded female with fragile X syndrome, compounded in one report in which the partner was also retarded.[266] The involvement of close relatives is key to the counseling needs in this type of situation.

A Family History of a Genetic Disorder

The explicit naming of a specific genetic disorder when the family history is being discussed facilitates evaluation and any possible testing. Difficulties are introduced when neither family nor previous physicians have recognized a genetic disorder within the family. Such a disorder may not be uncommon (e.g., factor V Leiden deficiency) but nevertheless unrecognized. Clinical clues would include individuals in the family with deep-vein thrombosis, sudden death possibly due to a pulmonary embolus, and yet other individuals with recurrent pregnancy loss.[267,268] For some families, individuals with quite different apparent clinical features may in fact have the same disorder. For example, there may be two or more deceased family members who died from "kidney failure" and another one or two who died from a cerebral aneurysm or a sudden brain hemorrhage. Adult polycystic kidney disease (APKD) may be the diagnosis, which will require further investigation by both ultrasound and DNA analysis.[269] Moreover, two different genes for APKD have been cloned (about 85 percent of cases due to APKD1 and close to 15 percent due to APKD2)[270,271] and a rare third locus is known. In yet other families, a history of hearing impairment/deafness in some members and sudden death in others may translate to the autosomal recessive Jervell and Lange–Nielsen syndrome.[272] This disorder is characterized by severe congenital deafness, a prolonged QT interval, and large T waves, together with a tendency for syncope and sudden death due to ventricular fibrillation. Given that a number of genetic cardiac conduction defects have been recognized, a history of an unexplained sudden death in a family should lead to a routine electrocardiogram at or after the first preconception visit. Other disorders in which sudden death due to a conduction defect might have occurred, with or without a family history of cataract or muscle weakness, should raise the suspicion of myotonic muscular dystrophy.[82]

Rare named disorders in a pedigree should automatically raise the question of the need for genetic counseling. We have seen instances (e.g., pancreatitis) in which in view of its frequency the disorder was simply ascribed to alcohol or idiopathic categories. Hereditary pancreatitis, although rare, is an autosomal dominant disorder for which the gene has already been discovered.[273]

The pattern of inheritance of an unnamed disorder may signal a specific monogenic form of inheritance. For example, unexplained mental retardation on either side of the family calls for fragile X DNA carrier testing.[274] Moreover, unexpected segregation of a maternal premutation may have unpredicted consequences, including reversion of the triplet repeat number to the normal range.[275] Genetic counseling may be valuable, more especially because the phenomena of pleiotropism (several different effects from a single gene) and heterogeneity (a specific effect from several genes) may confound interpretation in any of these families.

Consanguinity

Consanguineous couples face increased risks of having children with autosomal recessive disorders—the closer the relationship the higher the risks. A study in the United Arab Emirates of 2,200 women ≥15 years of age (with a consanguinity rate of 50.5 percent) concluded that the occurrence of malignancies, congenital abnormalities, mental retardation, and physical handicap were significantly higher in the offspring of consanguineous couples.[276] The pooled incidence of all genetic defects regardless of the degree of consanguinity was 5.8 percent, in contrast with a nonconsanguineous rate of 1.2 percent, similar to an earlier study.[277] A Jordanian study also noted significantly higher rates of infant mortality, stillbirths, and congenital malformations among the offspring of consanguineous couples.[278] A Norwegian study of first-cousin Pakistani parents yielded a relative risk for birth defects of about twofold.[279] In that study, 28 percent of all birth defects were attributed to consanguinity.

The occurrence of rare, unusual, or unique syndromes invariably raises questions about potential consanguinity and common ancestral origins. Clinical geneticists will frequently be cautious in these situations, providing potential recurrence risks of 25 percent. Consanguineous couples may opt for the entire gamut of prenatal tests to diminish even their background risks, with special focus on their ethnic-specific risks.[139]

Environmental Exposures That Threaten Fetal Health

Concerns about normal fetal development after exposure to medications; illicit drugs; chemical, infectious, or physical agents; and/or maternal illness are among the most common reasons for genetic counseling *during* pregnancy. Many of these anxieties and frequently real risks could be avoided through preconception care. Public health authorities, vested with the care of the underprivileged in particular, need to focus their scarce resources on preconception and prenatal care and on the necessary public education regarding infectious diseases, immunization, nutrition, and genetic disorders.

In preconception planning, careful attention to broadly interpreted fetal "toxins" is necessary, and avoidance should be emphasized. Excessive alcohol drinking, smoking, illegal drug use, use of certain medications, and therapeutic X-rays may require discussion. An estimate of the incidence of the fetal alcohol syndrome is 1 in 1,000 births.[280] In another study, women who drank heavily during pregnancy were noted to have a 17 percent increased risk of major congenital defects.[281] There is a limited list of known and proven human drug teratogens.[139] Maternal use of specific teratogenic medications, such as isotretinoin, may be missed, unless the physician expressly inquires about them.

Preconception advice to avoid heat exposure in early pregnancy is now appropriate. Our observations (see also chapter 21) showed a 2.9 relative risk for having a child with a NTD in mothers who used a hot tub during the first 6 weeks of pregnancy.[282]

A report from the Spanish Collaborative Study of Congenital Malformations noted a 2.8-fold increased risk of DS in the offspring of women <35 years of age and who were taking oral contraceptives when they became pregnant.[283]

Identification of Preconception Options

The time to deal with unwanted risks is not during the second trimester of pregnancy, as is so often the case in practice. Preconception counseling will identify specific risks and attendant options, which include:

1. Decision not to have children (includes consideration of vasectomy or tubal ligation)
2. Adoption
3. In vitro fertilization
4. Gamete intrafallopian-tube transfer or allied techniques
5. Artificial insemination by donor
6. Ovum donation (includes surrogacy)
7. Intracytoplasmic sperm injection
8. carrier detection tests
9. Prenatal diagnosis (CVS, amniocentesis, cordocentesis, ultrasound)
10. Preimplantation genetic diagnosis
11. Fetal treatment for selected disorders
12. Folic acid supplementation in periconceptional period (see also chapter 21)
13. Selective abortion.

GENETIC COUNSELING AS A PRELUDE TO PRENATAL DIAGNOSIS

Prospective parents should understand their specific indication for prenatal tests and the limitations of such studies. Frequently, one or both members of a couple fail to appreciate how focused the prenatal diagnostic study will be. Either or both may have the idea that all causes of mental retardation or congenital defects will be detected or excluded. It is judicious for the physician to urge that both members of a couple come for the consultation before CVS or amniocentesis. Major advantages that flow from this arrangement include a clearer perception by the husband regarding risks and limitations, a more accurate insight into his family history, and an opportunity to detect an obvious (although unreported or undiagnosed) genetic disorder of importance (e.g., Treacher Collins syndrome, facioscapulohumeral dystrophy, or one of the orofacial–digital syndromes). Women making an appointment for genetic counseling should be informed about the importance of having their partner with them for the consultation, avoiding subsequent misunderstanding about risks, options, and limitations.

Before prenatal genetic studies are performed, a couple should understand the inherent limitations both of the laboratory studies and, when relevant, of ultrasound. For detection of chromosomal disorders, they should be aware of potential maternal cell admixture and mosaicism (see also chapter 6). When faced with potential X-linked hydrocephalus, microcephaly, or other serious X-linked disorders and the realization of less than 100 percent certainty of diagnosis, couples may elect fetal sex determination as the basis for their decision to keep or terminate a pregnancy at risk. For some biochemical assays and invariably for DNA linkage analyses, results may be less than 100 percent certain.

The time taken to determine the fetal karyotype or other biochemical parameters should be understood before amniocentesis. The known anxiety of this period can be appreciably aggravated by a long, unexpected wait for a result. The need for a second amniocentesis is rarer nowadays, but in some circumstances, fetal blood sampling remains an additional option that may need discussion. Despite the unlikely eventuality that no result may be obtained because of failed cell culture or contamination, this issue must be mentioned.

The potential possibility for false-positive or false-negative results should be carefully discussed when applicable. Any quandary stemming from the results of prenatal studies is best shared immediately with the couple. The role of the physician in these situations is not to cushion unexpected blows or to protect couples from information that may be difficult to interpret. All information available should be communicated, including the inability to accurately interpret the observations made.

Other key issues to be considered by the genetic counselor and discussed when appropriate with the consultant follow.

Informed Consent

Patients should be told that prenatal diagnosis is not error-free. Although the accuracy rate for prenatal diagnostic studies exceeds 99 percent, it is not 100 percent. Errors have occurred in all of the following ways, and most, at least in the United States, have been followed by frequently successful lawsuits[56–58,284,285] (see also chapter 31).

1. Failure to offer prenatal diagnosis.
2. Failure to provide accurate information regarding risks of occurrence or recurrence.
3. Failure to explain significantly abnormal results, with catastrophic consequences.
4. Failure to provide timely results of prenatal diagnosis, resulting in the birth of a child with trisomy 21.
5. Failure to communicate the recommendation from the laboratory to perform a second amniocentesis in view of failed cell culture, resulting in the birth of a child with a detectable chromosome defect.
6. Failure to determine the correct fetal sex or genetic disorder, due to maternal cell contamination.
7. Failure to diagnose a defect because of a sample or slide mix-up.
8. Failure to order indicated tests (e.g., karyotype of prospective mother when her sister, or sibling's child, had DS, chromosome type unknown).
9. Failure to analyze the fetal karyotype correctly.
10. Failure to recognize significant chromosomal mosaicism.
11. Incorrect performance or interpretation of a biochemical or DNA assay.
12. Incubator failure or infection of cell cultures, resulting in failure of cell growth, no time for a repeat study, and subsequent birth with a chromosomal (or detectable) anomaly.
13. Failure to offer maternal serum screening or to correctly interpret and act on results.
14. Failure to understand a laboratory report coupled with failure to clarify the results by contacting the laboratory.
15. Failure to detect obvious fetal defects on ultrasound.
16. Failure to recommend periconception folic acid supplementation (see also chapter 21) with subsequent birth of a child with a neural tube defect.
17. Failure to offer indicated carrier detection tests.
18. Failure to deliver a blood sample to the laboratory in a timely manner, with the subsequent birth of a child with spina bifida and hydrocephalus.
19. Failure to advise change or discontinuance of a teratogenic medication (e.g., valproic acid), resulting in the birth of a child with spina bifida.

20. Delay/failure in making a timely diagnosis of a serious genetic disorder in a previous child, thereby depriving parents of risk data and of the options for prenatal diagnosis (among others) in a subsequent pregnancy, resulting in a second affected child. Examples already litigated include phenylketonuria and Duchenne muscular dystrophy.

From a previous worldwide survey of prenatal diagnosis[285] and two formal amniocentesis studies,[286,287] an error rate between 0.1 and 0.6 percent seems likely. After communication of all the necessary information concerning amniocentesis and prenatal genetic studies pertinent to the couple and especially tailored to their particular situation, an informed consent form should be signed and witnessed. Consent forms used for minor surgery should suffice for amniocentesis. However, each laboratory should have a specific form covering all key eventualities.[285]

It is crucial to ensure not only that the language in the consent form is nontechnical and easily understandable, but also that the form is available in the language best understood by the couple. Although the medicolegal validity of such forms may still be questioned, the exercise ensures at least a basic discourse between doctor (or the doctor's staff) and patient. For patients who decline prenatal studies, maternal serum screening, or specific genetic tests, physicians are advised to document their discussion and the patient's refusal in the medical record. In successful litigation, some plaintiffs have claimed that prenatal diagnostic studies or maternal serum screening were neither discussed nor offered by their physicians.

Carrier Detection

Before any effort to make a prenatal diagnosis of an autosomal recessive or sex-linked biochemical disorder, the carrier state should be documented (see above). For autosomal recessive disorders, particular attention should be paid to the parents' ethnic origin (see Table 1.6). A previous birth of an affected child with an autosomal recessive disorder might alert the physician to consanguinity. DNA mutation analysis facilitates carrier detection for a host of disorders not previously detectable prenatally (see also chapter 10). Recognition of compound heterozygosity in a couple will influence discussions about prognosis and should also initiate tracking of carriers through the respective families.

Presymptomatic or Predictive Testing

Presymptomatic or predictive testing is available for a rapidly increasing number of disorders, especially neuromuscular and neurodegenerative (see also chapter 10). Huntington disease is the prototype, and predictive testing using guidelines promulgated by the World Federation of Neurology[144,288] and the International Huntington Association is well established. Various programs report that a majority of patients are able to cope when it is found that they are affected,[68–73,289–291] and at least after a 1-year follow-up, potential benefit has been shown even in those found to be at increased risk.[292] A European collaborative study evaluated 180 known carriers of the Huntington disease gene mutation and 271 noncarriers, all of whom received a predictive test result. Although the follow up was only 3 years for about half the group, pregnancies followed in 28 percent of noncarriers and only 14 percent of carriers.[293] Prenatal diagnosis was elected by about two-thirds of those who were carriers.

We, as others earlier,[294] remain very concerned about the use of a test that can generate a "no-hope" result and recommend long-term follow-up. Even in sophisticated programs offering Huntington disease tests, fewer than expected at-risk individuals requested testing.[295] A multicenter Canadian collaborative study evaluated the uptake, utilization, and outcome of 1,061 predictive tests, 15 prenatal tests, and 626 diagnostic tests from 1987 to 2000. The uptake for predictive testing was about 18 percent (range, 12.5 to 20.7 percent).[99] Of the 15 who had prenatal tests, 12 had an increased risk which led to pregnancy termination in all but 1.[99] The motivations leading to the very difficult decision to have or not to have a predictive test are being recognized as extremely complex.[296] In a Danish study before DNA tests were available, 1 in 20 individuals *at risk* for Huntington disease committed suicide, more than double the population rate,[297] highlighting earlier reports of high suicide rates,[298] and emphasizing the erosive effects of uncertainty. However, a worldwide assessment of suicide rates, suicide attempts, or psychiatric hospitalizations *after* predictive testing did not confirm a high rate of suicide.[299] In their worldwide questionnaire study sent to predictive-testing centers they noted that 44 individuals (0.97 percent) among 4,527 tested had 5 suicides, 21 suicide attempts, and 18 hospitalizations for psychiatric reasons. All those who committed suicide had signs of Huntington disease, while 11 (52.4 percent) of the 21 individuals who attempted suicide were symptomatic. Others have written about the psychologic burden created by knowledge of a disabling fatal disease decades before its onset.[300–306] Hayden[307] warned that it is inappropriate to introduce a predictive test that "has the potential for catastrophic reactions," without a support program, including pretest and posttest counseling and specified standards for laboratory analyses. In one study, 40 percent of individuals tested for Huntington disease and who received DNA results required psychotherapy.[308] A 5-year longitudinal study of psychologic distress after predictive testing for Huntington disease focused on twenty-four carriers and thirty-three tested noncarriers. Mean distress scores for both carriers and noncarriers were not significantly different, but carriers had less-positive feelings.[309] A subgroup of tested persons were found to have long-lasting psychologic distress.

On the other hand, an increasing number of examples already exist (see also chapter 10) in which presymptomatic testing is possible and important to either the patient or future offspring or both. Uptake has been high by individuals at risk, especially for various cancer syndromes.[310] Use of DNA linkage or mutation analysis for autosomal dominant polycystic kidney disease (ADPKD) [269–271,311] may lead to the diagnosis of an unsuspected associated intracranial aneurysm in 8 percent of cases (or 16 percent in those with a family history of intracranial aneurysm or subarachnoid hemorrhage[312]) and preemptive surgery, with avoidance of a life-threatening sudden cerebral hemorrhage. In a study of 141 affected individuals, 11 percent decided against bearing children on the basis of the risk.[313] These authors noted that only 4 percent of at-risk individuals between 18 and 40 years of age would seek elective abortion for an affected fetus. The importance of accurate presymptomatic tests for potential at-risk kidney donors has been emphasized.[314] Organ donation by a sibling of an individual with ADPKD, later found to be affected, has occurred more than once.

Individuals at 50 percent risk for familial polyposis coli (with inevitable malignancy for those with this mutated gene) who undergo at least annual colonoscopy could benefit from a massive reduction in risk (from 50 percent to <1 percent) after DNA analysis. Individuals in whom this mutation was found with greater than 99 percent certainty may elect more frequent colonoscopies and eventually elective colonic resections, thereby saving the lives of the vast majority. The need for involvement of clinical geneticists is especially evident in this and other disorders in which complex results may emerge.

Giardiello et al.[315] showed that physicians misinterpreted test results in almost one-third of cases.

Families with specific cancer syndromes, such as multiple endocrine neoplasia, Li–Fraumeni syndrome, or von Hippel–Lindau disease, may also benefit by the institution of appropriate surveillance for those shown to be affected by DNA haplotype or mutation analysis when they are still completely asymptomatic, once again—in all likelihood—saving their lives. For example, elective thyroidectomy is recommended for multiple endocrine neoplasia type 2B by 5 years of age in the child with this mutation, given the virtual 100 percent penetrance of this gene and the possible early appearance of cancer.[316] Predictive testing even of children at high genetic risk poses a host of complex issues.[317] Where life-threatening early-onset genetic disorders are concerned, testing in early childhood still requires the exercise of parental prerogatives. However, failure to test because of parental refusal may invite the reporting of child neglect.[318]

No longer hypothetical is the prenatal diagnosis request by a pregnant mother for fetal Huntington disease absent the knowledge of her partner at-risk who does not wish to know his genetic status. In preserving the partner's autonomy and recognizing maternal rights, we have in the past honored such requests. Mothers have in these circumstances, faced with an affected fetus, elected to terminate the pregnancy, invoking miscarriage as the reason to her unknowing partner. Distressing as it is to contemplate such a marital relationship, textured on the one hand by extreme care and by deceit born of sensitivity on the other hand, consider our report of symptomatic Huntington disease at 18 months of age and diagnosed at the age of 3 years.[319] These cases pose difficult ethical, moral, and legal questions, but at least in the United States, United Kingdom, and Australia,[320] a woman's request for prenatal diagnosis would be honored.

Homozygotes for Huntington disease are rare[321,322] and reported in 1 out of 1,007 patients (0.1 percent). Counseling a patient homozygous for Huntington disease about the 100 percent probability of transmitting the disorder to each child is equivalent to providing a nonrequested predictive test,[323] while failing to inform the patient of the risks would be regarded as the withholding of critical information. Pretest counseling in such cases would take into consideration a family history on both sides and therefore be able to anticipate the rare homozygous eventuality.

Identification of specific mutations in the breast/ovarian cancer susceptibility genes (*BRCA1* and *BRCA2*) have opened up difficult personal decision making as well as consideration concerning future prenatal diagnosis.[324] DudokdeWit et al. and his team laid out a detailed and systematic approach to counseling and testing in these families.[325] In their model approach, important themes and messages emerge, including:

1. Each person may have a different method of coping with threatening information and treatment options.
2. Predictive testing should not harm the family unit.
3. Special care and attention are necessary to obtain informed consent, protect privacy and confidentiality, and safeguard "divergent and conflicting intrafamilial and intergenerational interests."

A French study noted that 87.7 percent of women who were first-degree relatives of patients with breast cancer were in favor of predictive testing.[326] Two specific groups of women are especially involved. The first are those who, at a young age, have already had breast cancer, with or without a family history, and in whom a specific mutation has been identified. Recognizing their high risk for breast and/or ovarian cancer[327,327a] (about 65 percent [95 percent confidence interval, 44–78 percent] by age 70 for *BRCA1* mutation carriers for breast cancer and about 39 percent [95 percent confidence interval, 18–54 percent] for ovarian cancer and for BRCA2 carriers an estimated 45 percent (95 percent confidence interval, 31–56 percent) risk of breast cancer and an 11 percent (95 percent confidence interval, 2.4–19 percent) risk for ovarian cancer,[327b] These women have grappled with decisions about elective bilateral mastectomy and oophorectomy. This group of women may also consider prenatal diagnosis in view of their personal suffering and intent not to have a child subject to the same set of problems. They may well elect precise prenatal diagnosis based on specific mutation analysis.

The second group of women are of Ashkenazi Jewish ancestry. These Jewish women have a 2.5 percent risk of harboring two common mutations in *BRCA1* (185delAG and 5382insC) and 1 in *BRCA2* (6174delT) that account for the majority of breast cancers in this ethnic group.[328] Regardless of a family history of breast or ovarian cancer, the lifetime risk of breast cancer among Jewish female mutation carriers was 82 percent in a study of 1,008 index cases.[328a] Breast cancer risk by 50 years of age among mutation carriers born before 1940 was 24 percent, but 67 percent for those born after 1940.[328a] Lifetime ovarian cancer risks were 54 percent for *BRCA1* and 23 percent for *BRCA2* mutation carriers.[328a]

It can easily be anticipated that with identification of mutations for more and more serious/fatal monogenic genetic disorders (including cardiovascular, cerebrovascular, connective-tissue, and renal disorders, among others) that prospective parents may well elect prenatal diagnosis in an effort to avoid at least easily determinable genetic disorders. Discovery of the high frequency (28 percent) of a mutation (T to A at APC nucleotide 3920) in the familial adenomatous polyposis coli gene among Ashkenazi Jews with a family history of colorectal cancer[329] is also likely to be followed by thoughts of avoidance through prenatal diagnosis. This mutation has been found in 6 percent of Ashkenazi Jews.[329] Because the ability to determine whether a specific cancer will develop in the future, given identification of a particular mutation, much agonizing can be expected for many years. These quandaries will not and cannot be resolved in rushed visits to the physician's office as part of preconception or any other care. Moreover, developing knowledge about genotype/phenotype associations and many other aspects of genetic epidemiology will increasingly require referral to clinical geneticists.

Anticipation

In 1991 the first reports appeared of dynamic mutations resulting from the unstable expansion of trinucleotide repeats.[330] Thus far, seventeen such disorders with these unstable repeats have been described (Table 1.8). All disorders described thus far are autosomal dominant or X-linked, except for Friedreich ataxia, which is autosomal recessive and also unique in having intronic involvement.[331] Typically for these disorders (except for Friedreich ataxia), the carrier will have one normal allele and a second expanded allele.

These disorders (except for Friedreich ataxia) are also generally characterized by progressively earlier manifestations and/or more severe expression with succeeding generations. This genetic mechanism, called anticipation, is associated with further expansion of the specific triplet repeat, but there are also disorders with anticipation and no apparent dynamic mutations (Table 1.9). Indeed, these disorders characteristically have a direct relation between the number of repeats and the severity of disease and an inverse relation between the number of repeats and age of onset. These aspects of anticipation weigh heavily in preconception counseling when it becomes clear that the relatively mild-to-moderate status of a mother with myotonic muscular dystrophy, for example, is likely to be

Table 1.8. Dynamic mutations with triplet repeat expansion

Disease	Chromosome	Repeat Sequence	Size in Normal[a]	Size in Carrier[a]	Size in Affected[a]
Dentatorubral pallidoluysian atrophy	12p12–13	CAG	7–34	—	49–75
Fragile X syndrome[b]	Xq27.3	CGG	5–54	50–200	200 to >2000
Fragile XE	Xq27.3	GGC	6–25	116–133	200 to >850
Friedreich ataxia[b]	9q13	GAA	7–40	50–200	200 to >1200
Huntington disease	4p16.3	CAG	6–36	—	35–121
Kennedy disease (spinal bulbar muscular atrophy)	Xq11–12	CAG	12–34	—	40–62
Machado–Joseph disease	14q32.1	CAG	13–36	—	68–79
Myotonic dystrophy type 1	19q13.3	CTG	5–37	—	50 to >2000
Myotonic dystrophy type 2[c]	3q21.3	CCTG	<44	—	75–11,000
Spinocerebellar ataxia type 1	6p22–23	CAG	6–39	—	41–81
Spinocerebellar ataxia type 2	12q24.1	CAG	15–29	—	35–59
Spinocerebellar ataxia type 6	19p13	CAG	4–16	—	21–27
Spinocerebellar ataxia type 7	3p21.1	CAG	4–18	—	37–130
Spinocerebellar ataxia type 8	13q21	CTG	16–37	—	>90
Spinocerebellar ataxia type 10[d]	22q13-qter	ATTCT	10–22	—	>19,000
Spinocerebellar ataxia type 12	5q31–33	CAG	7–28	—	66–78
Spinocerebellar ataxia type 17	6q27	CAG	27–44	—	>45

[a]Variable ranges reported and overlapping sizes may occur.
[b]Mutation may not involve an expansion.
[c]Expansion involves four nucleotides.
[d]Expansion involves five nucleotides.

Table 1.9. Selected genetic disorders with anticipation

Disorders with anticipation
   See Table 1.8 of disorders with trinucleotide repeats (exception: Friedreich ataxia)
Disorders with suspected anticipation
   Adult-onset idiopathic dystonia
   Autosomal dominant acute myelogenous leukemia
   Autosomal dominant familial spastic paraplegia
   Autosomal dominant polycystic kidney disease (PKD1)
   Autosomal dominant rolandic epilepsy
   Behçet syndrome
   Bipolar affective disorder
   Crohn disease
   Facioscapulohumeral muscular dystrophy
   Familial adenomatous polyposis
   Familial amyloid polyneuropathy
   Familial breast cancer
   Familial paraganglioma
   Familial Parkinson disease
   Familial primary pulmonary hypertension
   Familial rheumatoid arthritis
   Hereditary nonpolyposis colorectal cancer
   Holt–Oram syndrome
   Meniere disease
   Oculodentodigital syndrome
   Restless legs syndrome
   Schizophrenia
   Total anomalous pulmonary venous return
   Unipolar affective disorder

Table 1.10. Examples of imprinting and human disease

Syndrome	Chromosomal Location	Parental Origin	Selected References
Angelman	15q11–q13	Maternal	335
Beckwith–Wiedemann	11p15.5	Paternal	336
Congenital hyperinsulinism	11p15	Maternal	337
Congenital myotonic muscular dystrophy	19q13.3	Maternal	338
Early embryonic failure	21	Maternal	339
Familial paraganglioma	11q23	Paternal	340
Hereditary myoclonus–dystonia	7q21	Maternal	341
Intrauterine and postnatal growth retardation	7	Maternal	342
Intrauterine growth retardation or miscarriage	16	Maternal	343
Mental retardation and dysmorphism	14	Paternal	344
Prader–Willi	15q11–q13	Paternal	345
Progressive osseous heteroplasia	20q13.3	Paternal	347
Pseudohypoparathyroidism	20q13.3	Paternal	346
Rett syndrome	Xq28	Paternal	351,352
Russell-Silver syndrome	7p11.2–p.13 7q31–qter	Maternal	348
Short stature	14	Maternal	349
Transient neonatal diabetes	6	Paternal	350

associated in the case of an affected child with severe disease manifesting as congenital myotonic muscular dystrophy.[80] More recent studies have shown that triplet size correlates significantly with muscular disability as well as mental and gonadal dysfunction.[332] These authors also noted that triplet repeat size did not correlate with the appearance of cataract, myotonia, gastrointestinal dysfunction, and cardiac abnormalities. They hypothesized that somatic mosaicism with different amplification rates in various tissues may be one possible explanation for the variable phenotypes.

This phenomenon of parent-of-origin difference in the expression of specific genes introduces genomic imprinting into the genetic counseling considerations. Some genes are genetically marked before fertilization so that they are transcriptionally silent at one of the parental loci in the offspring.[333] A number of disorders have been recognized in which genomic imprinting is especially important[334] (Table 1.10). One such example is Huntington disease. Paternal transmission of the gene is associated with earlier and more severe manifestations than would be the case after maternal transmission. Families at risk may not realize that Huntington disease may manifest in childhood, not only in the teens, but as early as 18 months of age.[319,353]

Genotype–Phenotype Associations

DNA mutation analysis has largely not clarified genotype–phenotype associations, with the exception of some key examples, such as cystic fibrosis (CF) and the ΔF508 mutation with severe disease. Notwithstanding this limitation, mutation analysis does provide precise prenatal diagnosis opportunities and detection of affected fetuses with compound heterozygosity.

Simple logic might have concluded that genotype at a single locus might predict phenotype. For monogenic disorders, this is frequently not the case. In the autosomal dominant Marfan syndrome (due to mutations in the chromosome 15 fibrillin gene), family members with the same mutation may have severe ocular, cardiovascular, and skeletal abnormalities, while siblings or other close affected relatives with the same mutation may have mild effects in only one of these systems.[354] In Gaucher disease with one of the common Ashkenazi Jewish mutations, only about one-third of homozygotes have significant clinical disease.[355] Apparently, at least two-thirds have mild or late-onset disease or remain asymptomatic. Compound heterozygotes for this disorder involving mutations L444P and N370S have included a patient with mild disease first diagnosed at 73 years of age, while another requiring enzyme-replacement therapy was diagnosed at the age of 4 years.[356] In CF, a strong correlation exists between genotype and pancreatic function, but only a weak association has been noted with the respiratory phenotype[357] (see discussion in chapter 15). Although individuals who are homozygous for the common CF mutation (ΔF508) can be anticipated to have classical CF, those with the less common mutation (R117H) are likely to have milder disease.[358] On occasion, an individual who is homozygous for the "severe" ΔF508 mutation might unexpectedly exhibit a mild pancreatic-sufficient phenotype. Illustrating the complexity of genotype–phenotype associations is the instance noted by Dork et al.[359] of a mildly affected ΔF508 homozygote whose one chromosome 7 carried both the common ΔF508 mutations and a cryptic R553Q mutation. Apparently, a second mutation in the same region may modify the effect of the common mutation, permitting some function of the chloride channel[360] and thereby ameliorating the severity of the disease.

The extensive mutational heterogeneity in hemophilia A[361] is related to not only variable clinical severity but also to the increased likelihood of anti-factor VIII antibodies (inhibitors) developing. Miller et al.[362] found about a fivefold higher risk of inhibitors developing in hemophiliac males with gene deletions compared with those without deletions.

Given the history of a previously affected offspring with a genetic disorder, the preconception visit serves as an ideal time to refocus on any putative diagnosis (or lack thereof) and to do newly available mutation analyses when applicable.

Mosaicism

Mosaicism is a common phenomenon (witness the normal process of X-inactivation and tissue differentiation) that results in functional mosaicism in females. Mosaicism might occur in somatic or germ-line cells. Its recognition is important, because a disorder may not be due to a new dominant mutation, despite healthy parents. Erroneous counseling could follow, with the provision of risks very much lower than would be the case if germline mosaicism existed. After the birth to healthy parents of a child with achondroplastic dwarfism, random risks of 1 in 10,000 might be given for recurrence. However, germ-line mosaicism has been described after the birth of a second affected child.[363] Similarly, the birth of a male with Duchenne muscular dystrophy (DMD), no family history, and no detectable mutation on DNA analysis of maternal peripheral leukocytes might lead to counseling based on spontaneous mutation rates. Once again, germ-line mosaicism is now well recognized in mothers of apparently sporadic sons with DMD, and the risk of recurrence in such cases approximates 7–14 percent if the at-risk X-haplotype is determined.[364] Germline mosaicism has also been documented for other disorders (Table 1.11) and undoubtedly occurs in some others yet to be discovered.

Somatic-cell mosaicism with mutations has been recognized in a number of distinctly different disorders, such as hypomelanosis of Ito, other syndromes with patchy pigmentary abnormalities of skin associated with mental retardation, and in some patients with

Table 1.11.   Selected monogenic disorders with established germ-line mosaicism

Disorder	Inheritance
Achondroplasia	AD
Adrenoleukodystrophy	X-L rec
Albright hereditary osteodystrophy	AD
α-Thalassemia mental retardation syndrome	X-L
Amyloid polyneuropathy	AD
Aniridia	AD
Apert syndrome	AD
Becker muscular dystrophy	X-L rec
Cantu syndrome	AD
Cerebellar ataxia with progressive macular dystrophy (SCA7)	AD
Charcot–Marie–Tooth disease type 1B	AD
Coffin–Lowry syndrome	X-L dom
Congenital contractural arachnodactyly	AD
Conradi–Hunnermann–Happle syndrome	X-L dom
Cowden disease	AD
Danon disease (lysosome-associated membrane protein-2 deficiency)	X-L rec
Dejerine–Sotas syndrome (HNSN III) with stomatocytosis	AD
Duchenne muscular dystrophy	X-L rec
Dyskeratosis congenita	X-L
EEC syndrome (ectrodactyly, ectodermal dysplasia, orofacial clefts)	AD
Epidermolysis bullosa simplex	AR
Facioscapulohumeral muscular dystrophy	AD
Factor X deficiency	AR
Familial hypertrophic cardiomyopathy	AD
Fibrodysplasia ossificans progressiva	AD
Fragile X syndrome (deletion-type)	X-L
Hemophilia B	X-L rec
Herlitz junctional epidermolysis bullosa	A rec
Holt–Oram syndrome	AD
Hunter syndrome	X-L rec
Incontinentia pigmenti	X-L dom
Karsch–Neugebauer syndrome	AD
Lissencephaly (males); "subcortical band heterotopia" (almost all females)	X-L rec
Multiple endocrine neoplasia I	AD
Myotubular myopathy	X-L rec
Neurofibromatosis type 1	AD
Neurofibromatosis type 2	AD
Oculocerebrorenal syndrome of Lowe	X-L
Ornithine transcarbamylase deficiency	X-L rec
Osteocraniostenosis	AD
Osteogenesis imperfecta	AD
Pseudoachondroplasia	AD
Severe combined immunodeficiency disease	X-L rec
Spondyloepimetaphyseal dysplasia	AD
Renal-coloboma syndrome	AD
Rett syndrome	X-L dom
Tuberous sclerosis	AD
Von Hippel–Lindau disease	AD
von Willebrand disease (type 2b)	X-L rec
Waardenburg syndrome	AD
Wiskott–Aldrich syndrome	X-L rec

AD = autosomal dominant; AR = autosomal recessive; X-L rec = X-linked recessive; X-L dom = X-linked dominant.

asymmetric growth retardation.[365,366] Germ-line mosaicism should be distinguished from somatic-cell mosaicism in which there is also gonadal involvement. In such cases, the patient with somatic-cell mosaicism is likely to have some signs, although possibly subtle, of the disorder in question, while those with germ-line mosaicism are not expected to show any signs of the disorder. Examples of somatic and gonadal mosaicism include autosomal dominant osteogenesis imperfecta,[367,368] Huntington disease,[369] and spinocerebellar ataxia type 2.[370] Lessons from these and the other examples quoted for germ-line mosaicism indicate a special need for caution in genetic counseling for disorders that appear to be sporadic.

Very careful examination of both parents for subtle indicators of the disorder in question is necessary, particularly in autosomal dominant and sex-linked recessive conditions. The autosomal dominant disorders are associated with 50 percent risks of recurrence, while the sex-linked disorders have 50 percent risk for males and 25 percent risk for recurrence in families. Pure germ-line mosaicism would likely yield risks considerably lower than these figures, such as 7–14 percent for females with gonadal mosaicism and X-linked Duchenne muscular dystrophy. A second caution relating to counseling such patients with an apparent sporadic disorder is the offer of prenatal diagnosis (possibly limited) despite the inability to demonstrate the affected status of the parent.

Chromosomal mosaicism is discussed in chapter 6, but note can be taken here of a possibly rare (and mostly undetected) autosomal trisomy. A history of subfertility with mostly mild dysmorphic features and normal intelligence have been reported in at least ten women with mosaic trisomy 18.[371]

GENETIC COUNSELING WHEN THE FETUS IS AFFECTED

The fateful day the anxious, waiting couple hears the grim news that their fetus has a malformation or genetic disorder will live on in their memories forever. Cognizance of this impact should inform the thoughts, actions, and communications of the physician called on to exercise consummate skill at such a poignant time. Couples may have traveled the road of hope and faith for many years, battling infertility only to be confronted by the devastating reality of a fetal anomaly. With hopes and dreams so suddenly dashed, doubt, anger, and denial surface rapidly. The compassionate physician will need to be fully armed with all the facts about the defect or be ready to obtain an immediate expert clinical genetics consultation for the couple.

Care should be taken in selecting a quiet, comfortable, private location that is safe from interruption. Ptacek and Eberhardt,[372] in reviewing the literature, noted consensus recommendations in breaking bad news that included the foregoing and sitting close enough for eye contact without physical barriers. Identifying a support person if the partner cannot/will not attend the consultation is important, and knowledge of available resources is valuable. All of the above points are preferences that have been vocalized by parents receiving bad news about their infants.[373]

Almost all patients would have reached this juncture through maternal serum screening, an ultrasound study, or amniocentesis/chorionic villus sampling for maternal age or for established known carriers, because of a previously affected child or a family history of a specified disorder. Not rarely, an anxious patient insists on an amniocentesis. On one such occasion, the patient stated, "My neighbor had a child with Down syndrome," only to discover from the requested amniocentesis study that her fetus also had a serious abnormality. Physicians are advised not to dissuade patients away from amniocentesis but rather to inform them about the risks of fetal loss balanced against the risk of fetal defects, distinctly different from recommendations for accepted indications.

Decision Making

The presence of both parents for the consultation concerning possible elective abortion for a fetal defect is critical in this situation. All the principles governing the delivery of genetic counseling and discussed earlier apply when parents face the need to decide to continue or terminate their pregnancy. A brief explanation of some of the key issues follow and are culled from over 35 years of experience in this very subject.

Doubt and disbelief crowd the parental senses in the face of such overwhelming anxiety. Was there a sample mix-up? How accurate is this diagnosis? How competent is the laboratory? Have they made errors in the past? How can we be certain that there has been no communication failure? Is there another couple with the same name? There are endless questions and endless doubts. Each and every one needs to be addressed carefully, slowly, and deliberately, with painstaking care to provide the necessary assurance and reassurance. Needless to say, the clinical geneticist must have thoroughly checked all the logistics and potential pitfalls before initiating this consultation. Errors have indeed occurred in the past.

The central portion of the communication will focus on the nature of the defect, and the physician or counselor providing the counseling should be fully informed about the disorder, its anticipated burden, the associated prognosis, life expectancy, and the possible need for lifetime care. A clear understanding of the potential for pain and suffering is necessary, and an exploration concerning the effect on both parents and their other children is second only to a discussion about the potential effects on the child who is born with the condition in question. Any uncertainties related to diagnosis, prognosis, pleiotropism, or heterogeneity should emerge promptly. Questions related to possible future pregnancies should be discussed, together with recurrence risks and options for prenatal diagnosis.

The question concerning a second amniocentesis is invariable, at least if not stated, certainly in the mind of the parents. There are occasions when a repeat test might be appropriate, especially if there is a failure to reconcile cytogenetic or molecular results with expected high-resolution ultrasound observations. Maternal cell contamination (see also chapter 6), while extremely unlikely in almost all circumstances, requires exclusion in some others. Certain prenatal diagnoses may not easily be interpretable, and a phenotype may not be predictable with certainty. A de novo supernumerary chromosome fragment in the prenatal cytogenetic analysis (see also chapter 6) is a key example. The sensitive counselor should offer second opinions in another center in such circumstances or when it is clear that the parents require additional perspectives. The compleat physician anticipates virtually all of the patient's questions, answers them before they are asked, and raises all the issues without waiting for either parent to vocalize them.

Occasionally, it is apparent that there are powerful disparate attitudes to abortion between the spouses. Such differences would best be considered during the preconception period, rather than for the first time when faced with a serious fetal defect. Resolution of this conflict is not the province of the physician or counselor, nor should either become arbitrator in this highly charged and very personal dispute, in which religious belief and matters of conscience may collide. The physician's or counselor's duty is to ensure that all facts are known and understood and that the pros and cons of various possible scenarios are identified in an impartial manner. A return appointment within days should be arranged. Questions of paternity have also suddenly emerged in this crisis period and can now be settled—sometimes with painful certainty.

Elective Abortion: Decision and Sequel

Among the greatest challenges clinical geneticists and genetic counselors face is the consultation in which the results of prenatal studies indicating a serious fetal defect is communicated to parents for the first time. The quintessential qualities a counselor will need to include maturity, experience, warmth and empathy, sensitivity, knowledge, communication skill, and insight into the psychology of human relationships, pregnancy, and grieving. Ample time (with follow-up visits) is critical. The principles and prerequisites for counseling discussed earlier apply fully in these circumstances, and the fact that this is a parental decision, not a medical "recommendation," should not need reiteration.

Anticipatory counseling in these consultations have been characterized by in-depth discussions of two areas: first, all medical and scientific aspects of the prenatal diagnosis made (and discussed earlier), and second, recognition and vocalization of emotional responses and reference to experiences (preferably published) of other couples in like circumstances when it was helpful. These sessions have then included explorations concerning guilt, a possible feeling of stigma (because of abortion), anger, upset, and how other couples have coped. All of this anticipatory counseling has been tinctured with support and hope when possible. Many couples have expressed their appreciation of this approach and indicated the benefits of having had these discussions before elective termination.

The importance of continuing follow-up visits with couples who have terminated pregnancy for fetal defects cannot be overemphasized. In an important study on the psychosocial sequelae in such cases, White-Van Mourik et al.[374] showed the long-range effects (Table 1.12). Display of emotional and somatic symptoms 1–2 years after abortion were not rare, and included partners. Although some couples grew closer in their relationships, separations, especially because of failed communication, increased irritability, and intolerance, were noted in 12 percent of the eighty-four patients studied.[374] Marital discord in these circumstances has been noted previously.[375,376] At least 50 percent of couples admitted to having problems in their sexual relationship. In addition, many couples indicated changed behavior toward their children, including overprotectiveness, anxiety, irritability, and consequent guilt and indifference.[374] White-Van Mourik et al.[374] noted that women with secondary infertility and those younger than 21 years of age (or immature women) had the most prolonged emotional, physical, and social difficulties.

Grief counseling becomes part of the consultations after elective termination, in which full recognition of bereavement is necessary. The psychology of mourning has been thoroughly explored by both Parkes[377] and Worden.[378] Worden emphasized how important it is for a bereaved individual to complete each of four stages in the mourning process:

1. Acceptance of the loss.
2. Resolving the pain of grieving.
3. Adjusting to life without the expected child.
4. Placing the loss in perspective.

The importance of allowing parents the option of holding the fetus (or later, the child) when appropriate is well recognized.[379,380] These authors have also called attention to the

Table 1.12. The frequency of emotions and somatic symptoms of 84 women and 68 men: overall and 24 months after terminating a pregnancy for fetal abnormality

	Women (%)	Men (%)	Women after 24 Months (%)	Men after 24 Months (%)
Feeling				
Sadness	95	85	60	47
Depression	79	47	12	6
Anger	78	33	27	7
Fear	77	37	46	17
Guilt	68	22	33	7
Failure	61	26	24	14
Shame	40	9	18	4
Vulnerability	35	0	18	0
Relief	30	32	16	16
Isolation	27	20	11	6
Numbness	23	0	0	0
Panic spells	20	0	5	0
Withdrawal	0	32	0	13
Left out	0	12	0	0
Somatic symptom				
Crying	82	50	22	5
Irritable	67	38	19	3
No concentration	57	41	7	1
Listlessness	56	17	2	0
Sleeplessness	47	19	2	1
Tiredness	42	21	6	3
Loss of appetite	31	10	0	0
Nightmares	24	7	5	0
Palpitations	17	—	6	0
Headaches	9	8	2	0

Source: White-Van Mourik et al., 1992.[374]

complex tasks of mourning for a woman who is faced with one defective twin when pregnancy reduction or birth might occur.

Notwithstanding anticipated loss and grief, Seller et al.,[380] reflecting our own experience as well, emphasized that many couples recover from the trauma of fetal loss "surprisingly quickly." Insinuation of this reality is helpful to couples in consultations both before and after elective termination. Moreover, couples' orientation toward the grieving process achieves an important balance when they gain sufficient insight into the long-term emotional, physical, economic, and social consequences they might have needed to contemplate if prenatal diagnosis had not been available.

Testing the Other Children

Invariably, parents faced with the news of their affected fetus question the need to test their other children. Answers in the affirmative are appropriate when diagnosis of a disorder is possible. Carrier-detection tests, however, need careful consideration and are most appropriately postponed until the late teens, when genetic counseling should be offered. Given the complex dilemmas and far-reaching implications of testing asymptomatic children for disorders that may manifest many years later, parents would best be advised to delay consideration of such decisions while in the midst of dealing with an existing fetal defect. In later consultations, the thorny territory of predictive genetic testing of children can be reviewed at length.[381–385] Fanos[381] emphasized that testing adolescents "may alter the achievement of developmental tasks, including seeking freedom from parental figures, establishment of personal identity, handling of sexual energies, and remodeling of former idealizations of self and others." Fanos also emphasized that parental bonding may be compromised by genetic testing when the child's genetic health is questionable. Parents may react to the possible loss or impairment of a child by developing an emotional distance, recognized as the vulnerable child syndrome.[386] Other aspects, including interference with the normal development of a child's self-concept, introduce issues of survivor guilt, or increase levels of anxiety already initiated by family illnesses or loss.[386] Predictive testing of children for later-manifesting neurodegenerative or other disorders would rarely be recommended, except in circumstances in which early diagnosis could offer preventive or therapeutic benefit.

PERINATAL GENETIC COUNSELING

A similar spectrum of issues and concerns are faced after the detection and delivery of a child with a genetic disorder or an anomaly. Pregnancy with a defective fetus may have been continued from the first or second trimester of pregnancy, or a diagnosis may be made in the third trimester or at the delivery of a living or stillborn child. The principles and prerequisites for genetic counseling discussed earlier apply equally in all these circumstances.[387] Special attention should be focused on assuaging aspects of guilt and shame. Difficult as it may be for some physicians,[388,389] close rapport, patient visitation, and sincerity are necessary at these times, even when faced with commonly experienced anger. A misstep by the physician in these circumstances in failing to continue (it is to be hoped) the rapport already established during pregnancy care provides the spark that fuels litigation in relevant cases.

Despite anger, grief, and the gamut of expected emotions, the attending physician (not the resident and not the nurse!) should take care to urge an autopsy when appropriate. Diagnosis of certain disorders (e.g., congenital nephrosis) can be made by promptly collected and appropriately prepared renal tissue for electron microscopy, if mutation analysis (see chapter 10) is unavailable. In circumstances in which parents steadfastly withhold permission for autopsy (which is optimal), magnetic resonance imaging could provide some useful acceptable alternative when fetal anomalies are expected.[390] The autopsy is the last opportunity parents will have to determine causation, which may ultimately be critical in their future childbearing plans and also for their previous children. A formal protocol for evaluating the cause of stillbirth or perinatal death is important (Table 1.13) to secure a definitive diagnosis, thereby laying the foundation for providing accurate recurrence risks and future precise prenatal diagnosis. In addition, care should be taken in the face of known or suspected genetic disorders in which mutation analysis now or in the future may be critical, to obtain tissue for DNA banking or for establishing a cell line. Later, parents may return and seriously question the failure of the physician to secure tissues or DNA that would have been so meaningful in future planning (e.g., congenital nephrosis, spinal muscular atrophy).

Psychologic support is important for couples who have lost an offspring from any cause, a situation compounded by fetal or congenital abnormality.[391] The birth (or prenatal detection) of twins discordant for a chromosomal disorder is not rare, given the increased frequency of multiple pregnancy associated with advanced maternal age.

Table 1.13.   Protocol for evaluating the cause of stillbirth or perinatal death

1. Review genetic, medical, and obstetric history.
2. Determine possible consanguinity.
3. Gently and persistently recommend that parents permit a complete autopsy.
4. Obtain photographs, including full face and profile, whole body, and, when applicable, detailed pictures of any specific abnormality (e.g., of digits).
5. Obtain full body skeletal radiographs.
6. Consider full-body magnetic resonance imaging,[390] if autopsy is not permitted.
7. Carefully document any dysmorphic features.
8. Obtain heparinized cord or fetal blood sample for chromosomal or DNA analysis.
9. Obtain fetal serum for infectious disease studies (e.g., parvovirus, cytomegalovirus, toxoplasmosis).
10. Obtain fetal tissue sample (sterile fascia best) for cell culture aimed at chromosome analysis or biochemical or DNA studies.
11. Obtain parental blood samples for chromosome analysis, when indicated.
12. Communicate final autopsy results and conclusions of special analyses.
13. Provide follow-up counseling, including a summary letter.

Pregnancy reduction (see also chapter 26) or the death of one twin or delivery of both evokes severely conflicting emotions that may well affect the mother's care for the surviving child.[392] Considerable psychologic skill must be marshaled by physicians if meaningful care and support are to be provided.[393]

Supporting telephone calls from doctor and staff and encouragement to attend appointments every 6 weeks, or more frequently when appropriate, are often appreciated by patients. Review of the autopsy report and discussion with reiterative counseling should be expected of all physicians. Frequently, parents receive an autopsy report by mail without further opportunity for explanation and discussion. In one study, 27 percent failed to received autopsy results.[394] Providing contacts with groups whose focus is the disorder in question is also valuable. In the United States, the vast majority of these groups have combined to form the Alliance of Genetic Support Groups, which acts as a central clearinghouse and referral center.

Family Matters

Beyond all the "medical" steps taken in the wake of stillbirth or perinatal death due to fetal defects are critical matters important to the family and its future. Active, mature, and informed management is necessary in these difficult and frequently poignant situations. Regardless of the cause of the child's defect(s), maternal guilt is almost invariable and sometimes profound. Recognition of a definitive cause unrelated to a maternal origin should be explained in early discussions and reiterated later. For autosomal recessive disorders or with even more problematic X-linked disorders, maternal culpability is real and not easily assuaged. The fact that we all carry harmful genes, some of which we may have directly inherited, while others may have undergone mutation, may need in-depth discussion. Mostly, it is possible and important to reassure mothers that the outcome was not due to something they did wrong. Where the obverse is true, much effort will be needed for management of guilt[395] and shame and for planning actions that promise a better future with ways to avert another adverse outcome.

Attention to details that have a very important role in the mourning process include ensuring that the child be given a name and, in the case of the death of a defective fetus in the third trimester, that the parents' wishes for a marked grave be determined. As noted earlier, most caretakers feel that parents are helped by both seeing and holding the baby.[379,380,396] Although some may experience initial revulsion when the subject is mentioned, gentle coaxing and explanations about experience of other couples may help grieving parents. Even with badly disfigured offspring, it is possible for parents to cradle a mostly covered baby whose normal parts, such as hands and feet, can be held. Important mementos that parents should be offered are photographs, a lock of hair, the baby's name band, or clothing.[392,393] Ultimately, these concrete emblems of the baby's existence assist parents in the mourning process, although the desperate emptiness that mothers especially feel is not easily remedied. Photos may also be helpful in providing comfort for other children and for grandparents. Parents will also vary in their choice of traditional or small, private funerals. Physicians should ensure that parents have the time to make these various decisions and assist by keeping the child in the ward for some hours when necessary.

Both parents should be encouraged to return for continuing consultations during the mourning period.[397] Mourning may run its course for 6–24 months. These consultations will serve to explore aspects of depression, guilt, anger, denial, possible marital discord, and physical symptoms such as frigidity or impotence. Impulsive decisions for sterilization should be discouraged in the face of overwhelming grief. Advice should be given about safe, reliable, and relatively long-term contraception.[398] Similarly, parents should be fully informed about the consequences of having a "replacement child" very soon after their loss.[399,400] That child may well become a continuing vehicle of grief for the parents, who may then become overanxious and overprotective. Subsequently, they may bedevil the future of the replacement child with constant references to the lost baby, creating a fantasy image of perfection that the replacement child could never fulfill. Such a child may well have trouble establishing his or her own identity.

The Surviving Children

Distraught parents frequently seek advice about how to tell their other children. Responses should be tailored to the age of the child in question, to the child's level of understanding, and against a background of the religious and cultural beliefs of the family. A key principle to appreciate is that having reached the stage of cognizance regarding the loss, a child needs and seeks personal security. Hence, the parents' attention should be focused on love, warmth, and repetitive reassurance, especially about (possibly) unstated feelings of previous wrongdoing and personal culpability. Advice about grieving together instead of being and feeling overwhelmed in front of their children is also helpful advice. Focusing on the children's thoughts and activities is beneficial rather than lapsing into a state of emotional paralysis, which can only serve to aggravate the family's psychodynamics adversely.

THE EFFICACY OF GENETIC COUNSELING

The essential goal of the communication process in genetic counseling is to achieve as complete an understanding by the counselee(s) as possible, thereby enabling the most rational decision making. Parental decisions to have additional affected progeny should not be viewed as a failure of genetic counseling. Although the physician's goal is the prevention of genetic disease, the orientation of the prospective parents may be quite different. A fully informed couple, both of whom had achondroplasia, requested prenatal diagnosis with the expressed goal of aborting a normal unaffected fetus so as to be able to raise a child like themselves. Would anyone construe this as a failure in genetic counseling?

Clarke et al.[401] considered three prime facets that could possibly evaluate the efficacy of genetic counseling: (1) recall of risk figures and other relevant information by the counselee(s); (2) the effect on reproductive planning; and (3) actual reproductive behavior. Their conclusions, reflecting a Western consensus, were that there are too many subjective and variable factors involved in the recall of risk figures and other genetic counseling information to provide any adequate measure of efficacy. Further, assessing reproductive intentions may prejudge the service the counselee wishes as well as the fact that there are too many confounding factors that have an impact on reproductive planning. Moreover, how many years after counseling would be required to assess the impact on reproductive planning? They regarded evaluation of reproductive plans as "a poor proxy for reproductive behavior." In dispensing with assessments of actual reproductive behavior in the face of counseling about such risks, they pointed to the complex set of social and other factors that confound the use of this item as an outcome measure. They did, however, recommend that efficacy be assessed against the background goals of genetic counseling aimed at evaluation of the understanding of the counselee(s) of their own particular risks and options.

Evaluation of the efficacy of genetic counseling[44,135] should therefore concentrate on the degree of knowledge acquired (including the retention of the counselee(s) with regard to the indicated probabilities) and the rationality of decision making (especially concerning further reproduction). Frequent contraceptive failures in high-risk families highlight the need for very explicit counseling.[402]

Important points made by Emery et al.[403] in their prospective study of 200 counselors included the demonstrated need for follow-up after counseling, especially when it is suspected that the comprehension of the counselee(s) is not good. This seemed particularly important in chromosomal and X-linked recessive disorders. They noted that the proportion deterred from having children increased with time and that more than one-third of their patients opted for sterilization within 2 years of counseling.

A number of studies[403–406] document the failure of comprehension by the counselee(s). The reports do not reflect objective measures of the skill or adequacy of genetic counseling and the possible value of a summary letter to the patient of the information provided after the counseling visit. Sorenson et al.[407] prospectively studied 2,220 counselees who were seen by 205 professionals in 47 clinics located in 25 states and the District of Columbia. They gathered information not only on the counselees but also on the counselors and the clinics in which genetic counseling was provided. They, too, documented that 53 percent of counselees did not comprehend their risks later, while 40 percent of the counselees given a specific diagnosis did not appear to know it after their counseling. They thoroughly explored the multiple and complex issues that potentially contributed to the obvious educational failure that they (and others) have observed. In another study of parents with a Down syndrome child, Swerts[408] noted that of those who had genetic counseling, 45 percent recalled recurrence risks accurately, 21 percent were incorrect, and 34 percent did not remember their risks.

Genetic counseling can be considered successful when counselees, shown to be well informed, make careful, rational decisions regardless of whether their physicians consider their position to be ill advised. Notwithstanding obvious benefits of counseling, Wertz et al.[409] found that reproductive uncertainty is often not eliminated because it is related to factors beyond the scope of counseling.

In considering the effectiveness of genetic counseling, Sorenson et al.[407] summarized the essence of their conclusion:

In many respects, an overall assessment of the effectiveness of counseling, at least the counseling we assessed in this study, is confronted with the problem of whether the glass is half full or half empty. That is, about half of the clients who could have learned their risk did, but about half did not. And, over half of the clients who could have learned their diagnosis did, but the remainder did not. In a similar vein, clients report that just over half of their genetic medical questions and concerns were discussed, but about half were not. The picture for sociomedical concerns and questions was markedly worse however. And, reproductively, just over half of those coming to counseling to obtain information to use in making their reproductive plans reported counseling influenced these plans, but about half did not. Any overall assessment must point to the fact that counseling has been effective for many clients, but ineffective for an almost equal number.

A critical analysis of the literature by Kessler[410] concluded that published studies on reproductive outcome after genetic counseling reveal no major impact of counseling. Moreover, decisions made before counseling largely determined reproduction after counseling.

In a study of patients' expectations of genetic counseling, it was revealed that the majority had their expectations fulfilled. When patients' expectations for reassurance and advice were met, they were subsequently less concerned and had less anxiety compared with when such expectations were not fulfilled.

The limited efficacy of genetic counseling revealed in the study by Sorenson et al.[407] reflects the consequences of multiple factors, not the least of which are poor lay understanding of science and a lack or inadequacy of formal training of counselors in clinical genetics,[108] as discussed earlier. Efficacy, of course, is not solely related to counselee satisfaction. Efforts to educate the public about the importance of genetics in their personal lives have been made by one of us in a series of books (translated into nine languages) over a quarter of a century.[132,134,139,208] In addition to public education, and its concomitant effect of educating physicians generally, formal specialist certification in the United States, Canada, and the United Kingdom and acceptance of clinical genetics as a specialty approved by the American Medical Association will undoubtedly improve the efficacy of genetic counseling.

REFERENCES

1. Stoll C, Alembik Y, Dott B, et al. Impact of prenatal diagnosis on livebirth prevalence of children with congenital anomalies. Ann Genet 2002;45;115.
2. Rankin J, Glinianaia S, Brown R, Renwick M. The changing prevalence of neural tube defects: a population-based study in the north of England, 1984–96. Northern Congenital Abnormality Survey Steering Group. Paediatr Perinat Epidemiol 2000;14:104.
3. Iliyasu Z, Gilmour WH, Stone DH. Prevalence of Down syndrome in Glasgow, 1980–96: the growing impact of prenatal diagnosis on younger mothers. Health Bull (Edinb) 2002;60:20.
4. Milunsky A, Jick H, Jick SS, et al. Multivitamin/folic acid supplementation in the earliest weeks of pregnancy reduces the prevalence of neural tube defects. JAMA 1989;262:2847.
5. MRC Vitamin Study Research Group. Prevention of neural tube defects: results of the Medical Research Council Vitamin Study. Lancet 1991;338:131.
6. Czeizel AE, Dudas I. Prevention of the first occurrence of neural-tube defects by periconceptional vitamin supplementation. N Engl J Med 1992;327:1832.
7. Ray JG, Meier C, Vermeulen MJ, et al. Association of neural tube defects and folic acid food fortification in Canada. Lancet 2002;360:2047.
8. Rasmussen SA, Moore CA, Paulozzi LJ, et al. Risk for birth defects among premature infants: a population-based study. J Pediatr 2001;138:668.
9. Hoffman JI, Kaplan S. The incidence of congenital heart disease. J Am Coll Cardiol 2002;39:1890.

10. Lie RT, Wilcox AJ, Skjaerven R. Survival and reproduction among males with birth defects and risk of recurrence in their children. JAMA 2001;285:755.

11. Watkins ML, Rasmussen SA, Honein MA, et al. Maternal obesity and risk for birth defects. Pediatrics 2003;111:1152.

12. Shaw GM, Todoroff K, Finnell RH, et al. Spina bifida phenotypes in infants or fetuses of obese mothers. Teratology 2000;61:376.

13. Moore LL, Singer MR, Bradlee ML, et al. A prospective study of the risk of congenital defects associated with maternal obesity and diabetes mellitus. Epidemiology 2000;11:689.

14. Moore LL, Bradlee ML, Singer MR, et al. Chromosomal anomalies among the offspring of women with gestational diabetes. Am J Epidemiol 2002;155:719.

15. Lam PK, Torfs C, Brand RJ. A low pregnancy body mass index is a risk factor for an offspring with gastroschisis.

16. Stoll C, Dott B, Alembik Y, et al. Congenital anomalies associated with congenital hypothyroidism. Ann Genet 1999;42:17.

17. Olafsson E, Hallgrimsson JT, Hauser WA, et al. Pregnancies of women with epilepsy: a population-based study in Ireland. Epilepsia 1998;39:887.

18. Deaths, percent of total deaths, and death rates for the 10 leading causes of death in selected age groups, by race and sex: United States, 2000. Natl Vital Stat Rep 2002;50,13.

19. Infant deaths and mortality rates for the five leading causes of infant death by race and Hispanic origin of mother: United States, 2000. Natl Vital Stat Rep 2002;50:21.

20. Rasmussen SA, Wong LY, Yang Q, et al. Population-based analyses of mortality in trisomy 13 and trisomy 18. Pediatrics 2003;111:777.

21. DeGalan-Roosen AE, Kuijpers JC, Meershoek AP, et al. Contribution of congenital malformations to perinatal mortality: a 10 years prospective regional study in The Netherlands. Eur J Obstet Gynecol Reprod Biol 1998;80:55.

22. Dastgiri S, Gilmour WH, Stone DH. Survival of children born with congenital anomalies. Arch Dis Child 2003;88:391.

23. Liu S, Joseph KS, Wen SW. Trends in fetal and infant deaths caused by congenital anomalies. Semin Perinatol 2002;26:268.

24. Masaki M, Higurashi M, Iijima K, et al. Mortality and survival for Down syndrome in Japan. Am J Hum Genet 1981;33:629.

25. Dupont A, Vaeth M, Videbech P. Mortality and life expectancy of Down's syndrome in Denmark. J Ment Defic Res 1986;30:111.

26. Fryers T. Survival in Down's syndrome. J Ment Defic Res 1986;30:101.

27. Malone Q. Mortality and survival of the Down's syndrome population in Western Australia. J Ment Defic Res 1988;32:59.

28. Baird PA, Sadovnick AD. Life expectancy in Down syndrome adults. Lancet 1988;2:1354.

29. Baird PA, Sadovnick AD. Life expectancy in Down syndrome. J Pediatr 1987;110:849.

30. Baird PA, Sadovnick AD. Life tables for Down syndrome. Hum Genet 1989;82:291.

31. Strauss D, Eyman RK. Mortality of people with mental retardation in California with and without Down syndrome, 1986–1991. Am J Ment Retard 1996;100:643.

32. Yang Q, Rasmussen SA, Friedman JM. Mortality associated with Down's syndrome in the USA from 1983 to 1997: a population-based study. Lancet 2002;359:1019.

33. Glasson EJ, Sullivan SG, Hussain R, et al. The changing survival profile of people with Down's syndrome: implications for genetic counseling. Clin Genet 2002;62:390.

33a. Riozen NJ, Patterson D. Down's syndrome. Lancet 2003;361:1281.

33b. Hasle H, Clemmensen IH, Mikkelsen M. Risks of leukemia and solid tumours in individuals with Down's syndrome. Lancet 2000;355:165.

33c. Hill DA, Gridley G, Cnattingius S, et al. Mortality and cancer incidence among individuals with Down syndrome. Arch Intern Med 2003;163:705.

34. Martin RH, Ko E, Rademaker A. Distribution of aneuploidy in human gametes: comparison between human sperm and oocytes. Am J Med Genet 1991;39:321.

35. Plachot M. Chromosome analysis of oocytes and embryos. In: Verlinsky Y, Kuliev A, eds. Preimplantation genetics. New York: Plenum Press, 1991:103.

36. Boué J, Boué A, Lazar P. Retrospective and prospective epidemiological studies of 1500 karyotyped spontaneous human abortions. Teratology 1975;12:11.

37. Alberman ED, Creasy MR. Frequency of chromosomal abnormalities in miscarriages and perinatal deaths. J Med Genet 1977;14:313.

38. Holmes-Seidle M, Ryyvanen M, Lindenbaum RH. Parental decisions regarding termination of pregnancy following prenatal detection of sex chromosome abnormality. Prenat Diagn 1987;7:239.

39. Martinez-Frias ML, Bermejo E, Cereijo A, et al. Epidemiological aspects of Mendelian syndromes in a Spanish population sample. II. Autosomal recessive malformation syndromes. Am J Med Genet 1991; 38:626.

40. Njoh J, Chellaram R, Ramas L. Congenital abnormalities in Liberian neonates. West Afr J Med 1991;10:439.

41. Verma IC. Burden of genetic disorders in India. Indian J Pediatr 2001;67:893.

42. McKusick VA. Mendelian inheritance in man, 12th ed. Baltimore: Johns Hopkins University Press, 1998.

43. Baird PA, Anderson TW, Newcombe HB, et al. Genetic disorders in children and young adults: a population study. Am J Hum Genet 1988;42:677.

44. Milunsky A. The prevention of genetic disease and mental retardation. Philadelphia: WB Saunders, 1975.

45. Myrianthopoulos NC. Malformations in children from one to seven years. New York: Alan R. Liss, 1985.

46. Galjaard H. Genetic metabolic diseases: early diagnosis and prenatal analysis. Amsterdam: Elsevier/North-Holland, 1980.

47. Scriver CR, Neal JL, Saginur R, et al. The frequency of genetic disease and congenital malformation among patients in a pediatric hospital. Can Med Assoc J 1973;108:1111.

48. Brent RL. The magnitude of the problem of congenital malformations. In: Marois M, ed. Prevention of physical and mental congenital defects. Part A: The scope of the problem. New York: Alan R. Liss, 1985:55.

49. Milunsky A. The prenatal diagnosis of hereditary disorders. Springfield, IL: Charles C Thomas, 1973.

50. Rubin SP, Malin J, Maidman J. Genetic counseling before prenatal diagnosis for advanced maternal age: an important medical safeguard. Obstet Gynecol 1983;62:155.

51. Kessler S. Psychological aspects of genetic counseling. XIII. Empathy and decency. J Genet Couns 1999;8:333.

52. Harris R, Lane B, Harris H, et al. National Confidential Enquiry into counseling for genetic disorders by non-geneticists: general recommendations and specific standards for improving care. Br J Obstet Gynaecol 1999;106:658.

53. van Langen IM, Birnie E, Leschot NJ, et al. Genetic knowledge and counseling skills of Dutch cardiologists: sufficient for the genomics era? Eur Heart J 2003;24:560.

54. Gordis L, Childs B, Roseman MG. Obstetricians' attitudes toward genetic screening. Am J Public Health 1977;67:469.

55. Kessler S. Psychological aspects of genetic counseling. XII. More on counseling skills. J Genet Couns 1998;7:263.

56. Milunsky A, Annas GJ. Genetics and the law. New York: Plenum Press, 1976.

57. Milunsky A, Annas GJ. Genetics and the law II. New York: Plenum Press, 1980.

58. Milunsky A, Annas GJ. Genetics and the law III. New York: Plenum Press, 1985.

59. Working Party of the Royal College of Physicians. Improving communication between doctors and patients. J R Coll Physicians Lond 1997;31:258.

60. Welkenhuysen M, Evers-Kiebooms G, d'Ydewalle G. The language of uncertainty in genetic risk communication: framing and verbal versus numerical information. Patient Educ Couns 2001;43:179.

61. Benkendorf JL, Prince MB, Rose MA, et al. Does indirect speech promote nondirective genetic counseling? Results of a sociolinguistic investigation. Am J Med Genet 2001;106:199.

62. Abramsky L, Fletcher O. Interpreting information: what is said, what is heard: a questionnaire study of health professionals and members of the public. Prenat Diagn 2002;22:1188.

63. Palermo GD, Colombero LT, Schattman GL, et al. Evolution of pregnancies and initial follow-up of newborns delivered after intracytoplasmic sperm injection. JAMA 1996;276:1893.

64. Girardi SK, Schlegel PN. Microsurgical epididymal sperm aspiration: review of techniques, preoperative considerations, and results. J Androl 1996;17:5.

65. Eden OB, Black I, MacKinlay GA, et al. Communication with parents of children with cancer. Palliat Med 1994;8:105.

66. Targum SD. Psychotherapeutic considerations in genetic counseling. Am J Med Genet 1981;8:281.

67. Kessler S, Kessler H, Ward P. Psychological aspects of genetic counseling. III. Management of guilt and shame. Am J Med Genet 1984;17:673.

68. Hayden MR, Canadian Collaborative Study of Predictive Testing for HD. Predictive medicine for late onset disorders: the experience for Huntington disease. Am J Hum Genet 1991;49:50.

69. Tibben A, Vegter-van der Vlis M, Skraastad MI, et al. Presymptomatic DNA-testing for Huntington disease in the Netherlands. Am J Hum Genet 1991;49:316.

70. Craufurd D, Dodge A, Kerzin-Storrar L, et al. Psychosocial impact of presymptomatic predictive testing for Huntington's disease. Am J Hum Genet 1991;49:311.

71. Huggins M, Bloch M, Kanani S, et al. Ethical and legal dilemmas arising during predictive testing for adult-onset disease: the experience of Huntington disease. Am J Hum Genet 1990;47:4.

72. Folstein SE. Presymptomatic testing for Huntington's disease: outcome of 136 at-risk persons who requested testing. Am J Hum Genet 1991;49:62.

73. Wiggins S, Whyte P, Hayden M, et al. No harm, potential benefit: the one year follow-up of participants in the Canadian Collaborative Study of Predictive Testing for Huntington's Disease. Am J Hum Genet 1991;49:317.

74. Ravine D, Walker RG, Sheffield JL, et al. Experience of family screening for autosomal dominant polycystic kidney disease. Am J Hum Genet 1991;49:50.

75. Baumiller RC, Comley S, Cunningham G, et al. Code of ethical principles for genetics professionals. Am J Med Genet 1996;65:177.

76. Baumiller RC, Cunningham G, Fisher N, et al. Code of ethical principles for genetics professionals: an explication. Am J Med Genet 1996:65:179.

77. Brown RH Jr. Dystrophin-associated proteins and the muscular dystrophies. Annu Rev Med 1997;48;457.

78. Guerrini R, Casari G, Marini C. The genetic and molecular basis of epilepsy. Trends Mol Med 2003;9:300.

79. Chang BS, Lowenstein DH. Epilepsy. N Engl J Med 2003;349:1257.

80. Rasmussen SA, Mulinare J, Khoury MJ, et al. Evaluation of birth defect histories obtained through maternal interviews. Am J Hum Genet 1990;46:478.

81. Haxton MJ, Bell J. Fetal anatomical abnormalities and other associated factors in middle-trimester abortion and their relevance to patient counseling. Br J Obstet Gynaecol 1983;90:501.

82. Harper PS. Myotonic dystrophy, 2nd ed. London: WB Saunders, 1989.

83. Bergoffen J, Kant J, Sladky J, et al. Paternal transmission of congenital myotonic dystrophy. J Med Genet 1994;31:518.

84. Wieringa B. Myotonic dystrophy reviewed: Back to the future? Hum Mol Genet 1994;3:1.

85. Shelbourne P, Winqvist R, Kunert E, et al. Unstable DNA may be responsible for the incomplete penetrance of the myotonic dystrophy phenotype. Hum Mol Genet 1992;1:467.

86. Brunner HG, Jansen G, Nillesen W, et al. Reverse mutation in myotonic dystrophy. N Engl J Med 1993;328:476.

87. O'Hoy KL, Tsilfidis C, Mahadevan MS, et al. Reduction in size of the myotonic dystrophy trinucleotide repeat mutation during transmission. Science 1993;259:809.

88. Brook JD. Retreat of the triplet repeat? Nat Genet 1993;3:279.

89. Cobo AM, Baiget M, Lopez de Munain A, et al. Sex-related difference in intergenerational expansion of myotonic dystrophy gene. Lancet 1993;341:1159.

90. Hunter AG, Jacob P, O'Hoy K, et al. Decrease in the size of the myotonic dystrophy CTG repeat during transmission from parent to child: implications for genetic counseling and genetic anticipation. Am J Med Genet 1993;45:401.

91. Ashizawa T, Anvret M, Baiget M, et al. Characteristics of intergenerational contractions of the CTG repeat in myotonic dystrophy. Am J Hum Genet 1994;54:414.

92. Abeliovich D, Lerer I, Pashut-Lavon I, et al. Negative expansion of the myotonic dystrophy unstable sequence. Am J Hum Genet 1993;52:1175.

93. Ashizawa T, Dunne PW, Ward PA, et al. Effects of the sex of myotonic dystrophy patients on the unstable triplet repeat in their affected offspring. Neurol 1994;44:120.

94. Anvret M, Ahlberg G, Grandell U, et al. Larger expansions of the CTG repeat in muscle compared to lymphocytes from patients with myotonic dystrophy. Hum Mol Genet 1993;2:1397.

95. Abbruzzese C, Krahe R, Liguori M, et al. Myotonic dystrophy phenotype without expansion of (CTGn) repeat: an entity distinct from proximal myotonic myopathy? J Neurol 1996;243:715.

96. Ricker K, Koch MC, Lehmann-Horn F, et al. Proximal myotonic myopathy: clinical features of a multisystem disorder similar to myotonic dystrophy. Arch Neurol 1995;52:25.

97. Thornton CA, Griggs R, Moxley RT. Myotonic dystrophy with no trinucleotide repeat expansion. Ann Neurol 1994;35:269.

98. Milunsky A, Skare JC, Milunsky JM, et al. Prenatal diagnosis of myotonic muscular dystrophy with DNA probes. Am J Obstet Gynecol 1991;164:751.

99. Moore RC, Xiang F, Monaghan J et al. Huntington disease phenocopy is a familial prion disease. Am J Hum Genet 2001;69:1385.

100. Stevanin G, Camuzat A, Holmes SE et al. CAG/CTG repeat expansions at the Huntington's disease-like 2 locus are rare in Huntington's disease patients. Neurology 2002;58:965.

101. Creighton S, Almqvist EW, MacGregor D, et al. Predictive, pre-natal and diagnostic genetic testing for Huntington's disease: the experience in Canada from 1987 to 2000. Clin Genet 2003;63:462.

102. Fraser FC. Genetic counseling. Am J Hum Genet 1974;26:636.

103. Clow CL, Fraser C, Laberge C, et al. On the application of knowledge to the patient with genetic disease. In: Steinberg AG, Bearn AG, eds. Progress in medical genetics, vol. 9. New York: Grune & Stratton, 1979:159.

104. Shaw MW. Genetic counseling. Science 1974;184:751.

105. Emery AEH. Genetic counseling. BMJ 1975;3:219.

106. World Health Organization Expert Committee. Genetic counseling. WHO Tech Rep 1969;416:1.

107. Wertz DC, Fletcher JC. Attitudes of genetic counselors: a multinational survey. Am J Hum Genet 1988;42:592.

108. Wertz DC, Fletcher JC, Mulvihill JJ. Medical geneticists confront ethical dilemmas: cross-cultural comparisons among 18 nations. Am J Hum Genet 1990;46:1200.

109. Kessler S. Psychological aspects of genetic counseling. XI. Nondirectiveness revisited. Am J Med Genet 1997;72:164.

110. Hsia YE. Choosing my children's genes: genetic counseling. In: Lipkin M, Rowley PT, eds. Genetic responsibility. New York: Plenum Press, 1974:43.

111. Sorenson JR, Culbert AF. Counselors and counseling orientations: unexamined topics in evaluation. In: Lubs HA, de la Cruz F, eds. Genetic counseling. New York: Raven Press, 1977:131.

112. Michie S, Bron F, Bobrow M, et al. Nondirectiveness in genetic counseling: an empirical study. Am J Hum Genet 1997;60:40.

113. Clarke A. Is non-directive genetic counseling possible? Lancet 1991;338:998.

114. Milunsky A, Littlefield JW, Kanfer JN, et al. Prenatal genetic diagnosis. N Engl J Med 1970;283:1370, 1441, 1498.

115. Super M. Non-directive genetic counseling. Lancet 1991;338:1266.

116. Pembrey M. Non-directive genetic counseling. Lancet 1991;338:1267.

117. Harris R, Hopkins A. Non-directive genetic counseling. Lancet 1991;338:1268.

118. Clarke A. Non-directive genetic counseling. Lancet 1991;338:1524.

119. Einhorn HJ, Hogarth RM. Behavioral decision theory: processes of judgment and choice. Annu Rev Psychol 1981;32:53.

120. Simms M. Informed dissent: The view of some mothers of severely mentally handicapped young adults. J Med Ethics 1986;12:72.

121. Simms M. Non-directive genetic counseling. Lancet 1991;338:1268.

122. Carnevale A, Lisker R, Villa AR, et al. Counseling following diagnosis of a fetal abnormality: comparison of different clinical specialists in Mexico. Am J Med Genet 1997;69:23.

123. Williams C, Alderson P, Farsides B. Is nondirectiveness possible within the context of antenatal screening and testing? Soc Sci Med 2002;54:339.

124. Chapman MA. Predictive testing for adult-onset genetic disease: ethical and legal implications of the use of linkage analysis for Huntington disease. Am J Hum Genet 1990;47:1.

125. Marteau TM, Nippert I, Hall S, et al. Outcomes of pregnancies diagnosed with Klinefelter syndrome: the possible influence of health professionals. Prenat Diagn 2002;22:562.

126. Katz J. The silent world of doctor and patient. New York: Free Press, 1984.

127. Lantos JD. Should we always tell children the truth? Perspect Biol Med 1996;40:78.

128. Capron AM. Autonomy, confidentiality and quality care in genetic counseling. In: Capron AM, Lappe M, Murray RF, et al., eds. Genetic counseling: facts, values and norms. New York: Alan R. Liss, 1979:307.

128a. AMA Policy H-140.899. Disclosure of familial risk in genetic testing. In Code of Medical Ethics. Chicago: American Medical Association, 2003.

129. Tarasoff v. Regents of Univ. of Cal., 17 Cal.3d 425,131 Cal.Rptr 14,551 P.2d 334 (1976).

130. Davis v. Lhim, 124 Mich.App.291, 335 N.W.2d 481 (1983).

131. ASHG statement. Professional disclosure of familial genetic information. The American Society of Human Genetics Social Issues Subcommittee on Familial Disclosure. Am J Hum Genet 1998;62:474.

132. Falk MJ, Dugan RB, O'Riordan MA, et al. Medical geneticists' duty to warn at-risk relatives for genetic disease. Am J Med Genet 2003;120A:374.

133. Milunsky A. Genetic disorders and the fetus: diagnosis, prevention and treatment, 2nd ed. New York: Plenum Press, 1986.

134. Milunsky A. Know your genes. Boston: Houghton-Mifflin, 1977.

135. Hsia YE, Hirschhorn K, Silverberg RL, et al. Counseling in genetics. New York: Alan R. Liss, 1979.

136. Frets PG. The reproductive decision after genetic counseling. Ph.D. thesis. Rotterdam: Erasmus University, 1990.

137. Milunsky A. How to have the healthiest baby you can. New York: Simon & Schuster, 1987.

138. Milunsky A. Choices, not chances: an essential guide to your heredity and health. Boston: Little, Brown, 1989.

139. Milunsky A. Heredity and your family's health. Baltimore: Johns Hopkins University Press, 1992.

140. Cantebury v. Spence, 464 F.2d 772 (D.C. Cir. 1972).

141. Pelias MZ. Duty to disclose in medical genetics: a legal perspective. Am J Med Genet 1991;39:347.

141a. Hirschhorn K, Fleischer LD, Godmilow L, et al. Duty to re-contact. Genet Med 1999;1:171.

141b. Hunter AG, Sharpe N, Mullen M, et al. Ethical, legal, and practical concerns about recontacting patient to inform them of new information: the case in medical genetics. Am J Med Genet 2001;103:265.

142. Mink v. University of Chicago, 460F.Supp.713 (N.D.Ill.1978).

143. Tresemer v. Barke, 86 Cal.App.3d 656, 150 Cal.Rptr 384 (1978).

144. Committee of the International Huntington Association and the World Federation of Neurology. Guidelines for the molecular genetics predictive test in Huntington's disease. J Med Genet 1994;31:555.

145. Jones EF, Forrest JD, Henshaw SK, et al. Unintended pregnancy, contraceptive practice and family planning services in developed countries. Fam Plann Perspect 1988;20:53.

146. Rinsky-Eng J, Miller L. Knowledge, use, and education regarding folic acid supplementation: continuation study of women in Colorado who had a pregnancy affected by a neural tube defect. Teratology 2002;66:S29.

147. Hollier LM, Leveno KJ, Kelly MA, et al. Maternal age and malformations in singleton births. Obstet Gynecol 2000;96:701.

148. Cnossen MH, Smit FJ, deGoede-Bolder A, et al. Diagnostic delay in neurofibromatosis type 1. Eur J Pediatr 1997;156:482.

149. Milunsky JM, Wyandt HE, Huang X-L, et al. Trisomy 15 mosaicism and uniparental disomy (UPD) in a liveborn infant. Am J Med Genet 1996;61:269.

150. Spence JE, Perciaccante RG, Greig GM, et al. Uniparental disomy as a mechanism for human genetic disease. Am J Hum Genet 1988;42:217.

151. Nicholls RD, Knoll JHM, Butler MG, et al. Genetic imprinting suggested by maternal uniparental heterodisomy in nondeletion Prader–Willi syndrome. Nature 1989;342:281.

152. Malcolm S, Clayton-Smith J, Nichols M, et al. Uniparental paternal disomy in Angelman's syndrome. Lancet 1991;337:694.

153. Brzustowicz LM, Alitto BA, Matseoane D, et al. Paternal isodisomy for chromosome 5 in a child with spinal muscular atrophy. Am J Hum Genet 54:1994;54:482.

154. Kalousek DK, Barrett I. Genomic imprinting related to prenatal diagnosis. Prenat Diagn 1994;14:1191.

155. Ledbetter DH, Engel E. Uniparental disomy in humans: development of an imprinting map and its implications for prenatal diagnosis. Hum Mol Genet 1995;4:1757.

156. Milunsky JM, Maher T, Lebo R, et al. Prenatal diagnosis for Schmid metaphyseal chondrodysplasia in twins. Fetal Diagn Ther 1998;13:167.

157. Baldwin CT, Hoth CF, Amos JA, et al. An exonic mutation in the HuP2 paired domain gene causes Waardenburg's syndrome. Nature 1992;355:637.

158. Bondurand N, Pingault V, Goerich DE, et al. Interaction among SOX10, PAX3 and MITF, three genes altered in Waardenburg syndrome. Hum Mol Genet 2000;9:1907.

159. Sanchez-Martin M, Rodriguez-Garcia A, Perez-Losada J, et al. SLUG (SNAI2) deletions in patients with Waardenburg disease. Hum Mol Genet 2002;11:3231.

159a. Sanchez-Martin M, Perez-Losada J, Rodriguez-Garcia A, et al. Deletion of the SLUG (SNAI2) gene results in human piebaldism. Am J Med Genet 2003;122A:125.

160. Middleton A, Hewison J, Mueller R. Prenatal diagnosis for inherited deafness: what is the potential demand? J Genet Couns 2001;10:121.

161. Horwich AL, Fenton WA. Precarious balance of nitrogen metabolism in women with a urea-cycle defect. N Engl J Med 1990;322:1668.

162. Parris WCV, Quimby CW. Anesthetic considerations for the patient with homocystinuria. Anesth Analg 1982;61:708.

163. Lipscomb KJ, Smith JC, Clarke B, et al. Outcome of pregnancy in women with Marfan's syndrome. Br J Obstet Gynaecol 1997;104:201.

164. Murdoch JL, Walker BA, Halpern BL, et al. Life expectancy and causes of death in the Marfan syndrome. N Engl J Med 1972;286:804.

165. Shores J, Berger K, Murphy E, et al. Progression of aortic dilatation and the benefit of long-term beta-adrenergic blockade in Marfan's syndrome. N Engl J Med 1994;330:1335.

166. Viljoen D. Pseudoxanthoma elasticum. In: Beighton P, ed. McKusick's heritable disorders of connective tissue, 5th ed. St. Louis: Mosby, 1993:347.

167. Clinton MJ, Nierderman MS, Matthay RA. Maternal pulmonary disorders complicating pregnancy. In Reece EA, Hobbins JC, Mahoney MJ, et al., eds. Medicine of the fetus and mother. Philadelphia: JB Lippincott, 1992:955.

168. Dugoff L, Sujansky E. Neurofibromatosis type 1 and pregnancy. Am J Med Genet 1996;66:7.

169. Riccardi VM, Mulvihill JJ. Advances in neurology: neurofibromatosis (von Recklinghausen disease). New York: Raven Press, 1981:95.

170. Jaffe R, Mock M, Abramowicz J. Myotonic dystrophy and pregnancy: a review. Obstet Gynecol Surv 1986;31:272.

171. Kadir RA, Economides DL, Braithwaite J, et al. The obstetric experience of carriers of haemophilia. Br J Obstet Gynaecol 1997;104:7:803.

172. Pennell PB. Pregnancy in the woman with epilepsy: maternal and fetal outcomes. Semin Neurol 2002;22:299.

173. McCue CM, Mantakas ME, Tingelstad JB, et al. Congenital heart block in newborns of mothers with connective tissue disease. Circulation 1977;56:82.

174. Chamcides L, Truex RC, Vetter V, et al. Association of maternal systemic lupus erythematosus and congenital complete heart block. N Engl J Med 1977;297:1204.

175. Walsh EP, Keane JF, Sanders SP. Fetal cardiac dysrhythmias: detection and management. In: Milunsky A, Friedman EA, Gluck L, eds. Advances in perinatal medicine, vol. 4. New York: Plenum Press, 1985:63.

176. Milunsky JM, Skare JC, Milunsky A. Presymptomatic diagnosis of myotonic muscular dystrophy with linked DNA probes. Am J Med Sci 1991;301:231.

177. Harper PS. Practical genetic counseling, 2nd ed. Bristol: John Wright, 1984.

178. Lenke RR, Levy HL. Maternal phenylketonuria and hyperphenylalaninemia. N Engl J Med 1980;303:1202.

179. Gillet D, de Braekeleer M, Bellis G, et al. Cystic fibrosis and pregnancy: report from French data (1980–1999). BJOG 2002;109:912.

180. Odegaard I, Stray-Pedersen B, Hallberg K, et al. Maternal and fetal morbidity in pregnancies of Norwegian and Swedish women with cystic fibrosis. Acta Obstet Gynecol Scand 2002;81:698.

181. Gilljam M, Antoniou M, Shin J, et al. Pregnancy in cystic fibrosis: fetal and maternal outcome. Chest 2000;118:85.

182. Kelly TE, Edwards P, Rein M, et al. Teratogenicity of anticonvulsant drugs. II. A prospective study. Am J Med Genet 1984;19:435.

183. Chung CS, Myrianthopoulos NC. Factors affecting risks of congenital malformations. II. Effect of maternal diabetes. New York: Grune & Stratton, 1975.

184. Milunsky A, Alpert E, Kitzmiller JL, et al. Prenatal diagnosis of neural tube defects. VIII. The importance of serum alpha-fetoprotein screening in diabetic pregnant women. Am J Obstet Gynecol 1982;142:1030.

185. Miller E, Hare JW, Cloherty JP, et al. Elevated maternal HbA1c in early pregnancy and major congenital anomalies in infants of diabetic mothers. N Engl J Med 1981;304:1331.

186. McElvy SS, Miodovnik M, Rosenn B, et al. A focused preconceptional and early pregnancy program in women with type 1 diabetes reduces perinatal mortality and malformation rates to general population levels. J Matern Fetal Med 2000;9:14.

187. Penney GC, Mair G, Pearson DW, et al. Outcomes of pregnancies in women with type 1 diabetes in Scotland: a national population-based study. BJOG 2003;110:315.

188. Rudnik-Schöneborn S, Glauner B, Röhrig D, et al. Obstetric aspects in women with facioscapulohumeral muscular dystrophy, limb-girdle muscular dystrophy, and congenital myopathies. Arch Neurol 1997;54:888.

189. Frank JP, Harati Y, Butler IJ, et al. Central core disease and malignant hyperthermia syndrome. Ann Neurol 1980;7:11.

190. World Health Organization. Towards more objectivity in diagnosis and management of male infertility. Int J Androl 1987;7:1.

191. Scriver CR, Beaudet AL, Sly WS, et al. The metabolic and molecular bases of inherited disease, 7th ed., vol. II. New York: McGraw-Hill, 1995:B3008.

192. Turnpenny PD, Gunasegaran R, Smith NC, et al. Recurrent miscarriage, cystic hygroma and incontinentia pigmenti. Br J Obstet Gynaecol 1992;99:920.

193. Anguiano A, Oates RD, Amos JA, et al. Congenital bilateral absence of the vas deferens: a primarily genital form of cystic fibrosis. JAMA 1992;267:1794.

194. Traystman MD, Schulte NA, MacDonald M, et al. Mutation analysis for cystic fibrosis to determine carrier status in 167 sperm donors from the Nebraska Genetic Semen Bank. Hum Mutat 1994;4:271.

195. Augarten A, Yahav Y, Kerem BS, et al. Congenital bilateral absence of vas deferens in the absence of cystic fibrosis. Lancet 1994;344:1473.

196. Temple-Smith PD, Southwick GJ, Yates CA, et al. Human pregnancy by IVF using sperm aspirated from the epididymis. J In Vitro Fertil Embryo Transfer 1985;2:119.

197. Silber SJ, Ord T, Balmaceda J, et al. Congenital absence of the vas deferens: the fertilizing capacity of human epididymal sperm. N Engl J Med 1990;7:147.

198. Vogt P, Chandley AC, Hargrave TV, et al. Microdeletions in interval 6 of the Y-chromosome of males with idiopathic sterility point to disruption of AZF, a human spermatogenesis gene. Hum Genet 1992;89:491.

199. Reijo R, Lee TY, Salo P, et al. Diverse spermatogenic effects in humans caused by Y chromosome deletions encompassing a novel RNA-binding protein gene. Nat Genet 1995;10:383.

200. Najmabadi H, Huang V, Yen P, et al. Substantial prevalence of microdeletions of the Y chromosome in infertile men with idiopathic azoospermia and oligospermia detected using a sequence-tagged site-based mapping strategy. J Clin Endocrinol Metab 1996;71:1347.

201. Ma K, Inglis JD, Sharkey A, et al. A Y chromosome gene family with RNA-binding protein homology; candidates for the azoospermia factor AZF controlling human spermatogenesis. Cell 1993;73:1287.

202. Reijo R, Alagappan RK, Patrizio P, et al. Severe oligozoospermia resulting from deletions of azoospermia factor gene on Y chromosome. Lancet 1996;347:1290.

203. deKretser DM. Male infertility. Lancet 1997;349:787.

204. Bonduelle M, Hamberger L, Joris H, et al. Assisted reproduction by intracytoplasmic sperm injection: an ESHRE survey of clinical experiences until December 1993. Hum Reprod Update 1995;1:3.

205. Meschede D, Horst J. Sex chromosomal anomalies in pregnancies conceived through intracytoplasmic sperm injection: a case for genetic counseling. Hum Reprod 1997:12:1125.

206. Chandley AC. Meiotic studies and fertility in human translocation carriers. In: Daniel A, ed. The cytogenetics of mammalian autosomal rearrangements. New York: Alan R. Liss, 1988:370.

207. Dohle GR, Halley DJ, Van Hemel JO, et al. Genetic risk factors in infertile men with severe oligozoospermia and azoospermia. Hum Reprod 2002;17:13.

208. Milunsky A. Your genetic destiny: know your genes, secure your health, save your life. Cambridge, UK: Perseus Books, 2001.

209. Prence EM, Jerome CA, Triggs-Raine BL, et al. Heterozygosity for Tay-Sachs and Sandhoff diseases among Massachusetts residents with French Canadian background. J Med Screen 1997;4:133.

210. Palomaki GE, Williams J, Haddow JE, et al. Tay–Sachs disease in persons of French-Canadian heritage in northern New England. Am J Med Genet 1995;56:409.

211. American Society of Human Genetics. Statement of the American Society of Human Genetics on cystic fibrosis carrier screening. Am J Hum Genet 1992;51:1443.

212. National Institutes of Health Consensus Development Conference Statement. Bethesda, MD: National Institutes of Health, 1997.

213. Denayer L, Welkenhuysen M, Evers-Kiebooms G, et al. Risk perception after CF carrier testing and impact of the test result on reproductive decision making. Am J Med Genet 1997;69:422.

214. Henneman L, Bramsen I, Van Der Ploeg HM, et al. Preconception cystic fibrosis carrier couple screening: impact, understanding, and satisfaction. Genet Test 2003;6:195.

215. Pinckers A. X-linked progressive cone dystrophy. Doc Ophthalmol Proc Ser 1982;33:399.

216. el-Deiry SS, Naidu S, Blevins LS, et al. Assessment of adrenal function in women heterozygous for adrenoleukodystrophy. J Clin Endocrinol Metab 1997;82:856.

217. Menage P, Carreau V, Tourbah A, et al. Les adrenoleucodystrophies heterozygotes symptomatiques de l'adulte: 10 cas. Rev Neurol 1993;149:445.

218. Gibbons RJ, Suthers GK, Wilkie AOM, et al. X-linked alpha-thalassemia/mental retardation (ATR-X) syndrome: location to Xq12–q21.31 by X inactivation and linkage analysis. Am J Hum Genet 1992;51:1136.

219. Hasstedt SJ, Atkin CL, San Juan AC Jr. Genetic heterogeneity among kindreds with Alport syndrome. Am J Hum Genet 1986;38:940.

220. Patel RR, Hovijitra S, Kafrawy AH, et al. X-linked (recessive) hypomaturation amelogenesis imperfecta: a prosthodontic, genetic, and histopathologic report. J Prosthet Dent 1991;66:398.

221. Hennekam RCM, Barth PG, Van Lookeren Campagne W, et al. A family with severe X-linked arthrogryposis. Eur J Pediatr 1991;150:656.

222. Mathews KD, Ardinger HH, Nishimura DY, et al. Linkage localization of Borjeson–Forssman–Lehmann syndrome. Am J Med Genet 1989;34:470.

223. Karna J. Choroideremia: a clinical and genetic study of 84 Finnish patients and 126 female carriers. Acta Ophthalmol Suppl 1986;176:1.

224. Romera MG, Martin MM, Gonzalez E. Chronic granulomatous disease: a case study of a symptomatic carrier. J Invest Allerg Clin Immunol 1997;7:57.

225. Lovas JG, Issekutz A, Walsh N, et al. Lupus erythematosus-like oral mucosal and skin lesions in a carrier of chronic granulomatous disease: chronic granulomatous disease carrier genodermatosis. Oral Surg Oral Med Oral Pathol Oral Rad Endod 1995;80:78.

226. Rollnick BR, Kaye CI. Mendelian inheritance of isolated nonsyndromic cleft palate. Am J Med Genet 1986;24:465.

227. Cremers CWRJ, Huygen PLM. Clinical features of female heterozygotes in the X-linked mixed deafness syndrome (with perilymphatic gusher during stapes surgery). Int J Pediatr Otorhinolaryngol 1983;6:179.

228. Walsh FB, Wegman ME. Pedigree of hereditary cataract, illustrating sex-limited type. Bull Johns Hopkins Hosp 1937;61:125.

229. Politano L, Nigro V, Nigro G, et al. Development of cardiomyopathy in female carriers of Duchenne and Becker muscular dystrophies. JAMA 1996;275:1335.

230. Matthews PM, Benjamin D, Van Bakel I, et al. Muscle X-inactivation patterns and dystrophin expression in Duchenne muscular dystrophy carriers. Neuromuscul Disord 1995;5:209.

231. Azofeifa J, Voit T, Hubner C, et al. X-chromosome methylation in manifesting and healthy carriers of dystrophinopathies: concordance of activation ratios among first degree female relatives and skewed inactivation as cause of the affected phenotypes. Hum Genet 1995;96:167.

232. Schnur RE, Heymann WR. Reticulate hyperpigmentation. Semin Cutan Med Surg 1997;16:72.

233. Emery AEH. Emery–Dreifuss syndrome. J Med Genet 1989;26:637.

234. Ropers HH, Wienker TF, Grimm T, et al. Evidence for preferential X-chromosome inactivation in a family with Fabry disease. Am J Hum Genet 1977;29:361.

235. Thompson EM, Baraitser M, Lindenbaum RH, et al. The FG syndrome: seven new cases. Clin Genet 1985;27:582.

236. Vianna-Morgante AM, Costa SS, Pares AS, et al. FRAXA premutation associated with premature ovarian failure. Am J Med Genet 1996;64:373.

237. Sobesky WE, Taylor AK, Pennington BF, et al. Molecular/clinical correlations in females with fragile X. Am J Med Genet 1996;64:340.

238. Franke P, Maier W, Hautzinger M, et al. Fragile-X carrier females: evidence for a distinct psychopathological phenotype? Am J Med Genet 1996;64:334.

239. Russo G, Mollica F, Pavone L, et al. Hemolytic crises of favism in Sicilian females heterozygous for G-6-PD deficiency. Pediatrics 1972;49:854.

240. Meloni T, Forteleoni G, Dore A, et al. Neonatal hyperbilirubinaemia in heterozygous glucose-6-phosphate dehydrogenase deficient females. Br J Haematol 1983;53:241.

241. Mauser Bunchoten EP, van Houwelingen JC, Sjamsoedin Visser EJ, et al. Bleeding symptoms in carriers of hemophilia A and B. Thromb Haemost 1988;59:349.

242. Vabres P, Larregu M. X-linked genodermatoses. Ann Dermatol Venereol 1995;122:154.

243. Holmes LB, McGowan BL, Efron ML. Lowe's syndrome: a search for the carrier state. Pediatrics 1969;44:359.

244. Endres W. Inherited metabolic diseases affecting the carrier. J Inherit Metab Dis 1997;20:9.

245. Lorette G, Toutain A, Barthes M, et al. Menkes syndrome: an unusual pigmentation anomaly in a mother and three sisters. Ann Pediatr 1992;39:453.

246. Collie WR, Moore CM, Goka TJ, et al. Pili torti as marker for carriers of Menkes disease. Lancet 1978;1:607.

247. Bartsocas CS, Kastrantas AD. X-linked form of myopia. Hum Hered 1981;31:199.

248. Nance WE, Warburg M, Bixler D, et al. Congenital X-linked cataract, dental anomalies and brachymetacarpalia. Birth Defects Orig Artic Ser 1974;10:285.

249. Kellner U, Fuchs S, Bornfeld N, et al. Ocular phenotypes associated with two mutations (R121W, C126X) in the Norrie disease gene. Ophthalmol Genet 1996;17:67.

250. Charles SJ, Moore AT, Zhang Y, et al. Carrier detection in X linked ocular albinism using linked DNA polymorphisms. Br J Ophthalmol 1994;78:539.

251. Erpenstein H, Pfeiffer RA. Geschlechsgebunden-dominant erbliche Zahnunterzahl. Humangenetik 1967;4:280.

252. Herinklake S, Boker K, Manns M. Fatal clinical course of ornithine transcarbamylase deficiency in an adult heterozygous female patient. Digestion 1977;58:83.

253. Fries MH, Kuller JA, Jurecki E, et al. Prenatal counseling in heterozygotes for ornithine transcarbamylase deficiency in an adult heterozygous female patient. Digestion 1997;58:83.

254. Kaplan J, Pelet A, Hentari H, et al. Contribution to carrier detection and genetic counseling in X linked retinoschisis. J Med Genet 1991;28:383.

255. Souied E, Segues B, Ghazi I, et al. Severe manifestations in carrier females in X linked retinitis pigmentosa. J Med Genet 1997;34:793.

256. Harris JW, Danish EH, Brittenham GM, et al. Pyridoxine responsive hereditary sideroblastic erythropoiesis and iron overload: two microcytic subpopulations in the affected male, one normocytic and one microcytic subpopulation in the obligate female carrier. Am J Hematol 1993;42:400.

257. McKusick VA. Mendelian inheritance in man, 11th ed. Baltimore: Johns Hopkins University Press, 1994:2530.

258. Ahmad M, Abbas H, Haque S, et al. X-chromosomally inherited split-hand/split foot anomaly in a Pakistani kindred. Hum Genet 1987;75:169.

259. McKusick VA. Mendelian inheritance in man, 11th ed. Baltimore: Johns Hopkins University Press, 1994:2535.

260. van den Berghe H, Dequeker J, Fryns JP, et al. Familial occurrence of severe ulnar aplasia and lobster claw feet: a new syndrome. Hum Genet 1978;42:109.

261. Wengler G, Gorlin JB, Williamson JM, et al. Nonrandom inactivation of the X chromosome in early lineage hematopoietic cells in carriers of Wiskott–Aldrich syndrome. Blood 1995;85:2471.

262. Peacocke M, Siminovitch KA. The Wiskott–Aldrich syndrome. Semin Dermatol 1993;12:247.

263. Stoll C, Geraudel A, Chauvin A. New X-linked syndrome of mental retardation, short stature, and hypertelorism. Am J Med Genet 1991;39:474.

264. Atkin JF, Flaitz K, Patil S, et al. A new X-linked mental retardation syndrome. Am J Med Genet 1985;21:697.

265. Nowakowski R. Ocular manifestations in female carriers of X-linked disorders. J Am Optom Assoc 1995;66:352.

266. de Vries BB, van den Boer-van den Berg HM, Niermeijer MF, et al. Dilemmas in counseling females with the fragile X syndrome. J Med Genet 1999;36:167.

267. Simioni P, Prandoni P, Lensing AW, et al. The risk of recurrent venous thromboembolism in patients with an Arg5066Gln mutation in the gene for factor V (factor V Leiden). N Engl J Med 1997;336:399.

268. Brenner B, Blumenfeld Z. Thrombophilia and fetal loss. Blood Rev 1997;11:72.

269. Bear JC, Parfrey PS, Morgan JM, et al. Autosomal dominant polycystic kidney disease: new information for genetic counseling. Am J Med Genet 1992;43:539.

270. Reeders ST, Breuning MH, Davies KE, et al. A highly polymorphic DNA marker linked to adult polycystic kidney disease on chromosome 16. Nature 1985;317:542.

271. Veldhuisen B, Saris JJ, deHaij S, et al. A spectrum of mutations in the second gene for autosomal dominant polycystic kidney disease (PKD2). Am J Hum Genet 1997;61:547.

272. Neyroud N, Tesson F, Denjoy I, et al. A novel mutation in the potassium channel gene KVLQT1 causes the Jervell and Lange–Nielsen cardioauditory syndrome. Nat Genet 1997;15:186.

273. Gorry MC, Gabbaizedeh D, Furey W, et al. Mutations in the cationic trypsinogen gene are associated with recurrent acute and chronic pancreatitis. Gastroenterology 1997;113:1063.

274. Ryynänen Markku, Kirkinen P, Mannermaa A, et al. Carrier diagnosis of the fragile X syndrome: a challenge in antenatal clinics. Am J Obstet Gynecol 1995;172:1236.

275. Mornet E, Chateau C, Taillandier A, et al. Recurrent and unexpected segregation of the FMR1 CGG repeat in a family with fragile X syndrome. Hum Genet 1996;97:512.

276. Abdulrazzaq YM, Bener A, Al-Gazali LI, et al. A study of possible deleterious effects of consanguinity. Clin Genet 1997;51:167.

277. Bundey S, Alam H, Kaur A, et al. Race, consanguinity and social features in Birmingham babies: a basis for prospective study. J Epidemiol Commun Health 1990;44:130.

278. Khoury SA, Massad DF. Consanguinity, fertility, reproductive wastage, infant mortality and congenital malformations in Jordan. Saudi Med J 2000;21:150.

279. Stoltenberg C, Magnus P, Lie RT, et al. Birth defects and parental consanguinity in Norway. Am J Epidemiol 1997;145:439.

280. Jones KL. Smith's recognizable patterns of human malformation, 5th ed. Philadelphia: WB Saunders, 1997:555.

281. Ouellette EM, Rosett HL, Rosman NP, et al. Adverse effects on offspring of maternal alcohol abuse during pregnancy. N Engl J Med 1977;297:527.

282. Milunsky A, Ulcickas M, Rothman KJ, et al. Maternal heat exposure and neural tube defects. JAMA 1992;268:882.

283. Martinez-Frias ML, Bermejo E, Rodriguez-Pinilla E, et al. Periconceptional exposure to contraceptive pills and risk for Down syndrome. J Perinatol 2001;21:288.

284. Reilly PR, Milunsky A. Medicolegal aspects of prenatal diagnosis. In: Milunsky A, ed. Genetic disorders and the fetus: diagnosis, prevention and treatment. New York: Plenum Press, 1979:603.

285. Milunsky A. Genetic disorders and the fetus: diagnosis, prevention and treatment. New York: Plenum Press, 1979.

286. NICHD National Registry for Amniocentesis Study Group. Midtrimester amniocentesis for prenatal diagnosis: safety and accuracy. JAMA 1976;236:1471.

287. Simpson NE, Dallaire L, Miller JR, et al. Prenatal diagnosis of genetic disease in Canada: report of a collaborative study. Can Med Assoc J 1976;115:739.

288. International Huntington Association and World Federation of Neurology. Guidelines for the molecular genetics predictive test in Huntington's disease. Neurology 1994;44:1533.

289. Tibben A, Duivenvoorden J, Niermeijer MF, et al. Psychological effects of presymptomatic DNA testing for Huntington's disease in the Dutch program. Psychosom Med 1994;56:526.

290. Lawson K, Wiggins S, Green T, et al. Adverse psychological events occurring in the first year after predictive testing for Huntington's disease. J Med Genet 1996;33:856.

291. Tibben A, Frets PG, Van de Kamp JJP, et al. On attitudes and appreciation six months after predictive DNA testing for Huntington's disease in the Dutch program. Am J Med Genet 1993;48:103.

292. Wiggins S, Whyte P, Huggins M, et al. The psychological consequences of predictive testing for Huntington's disease. N Engl J Med 1992;327:1401.

293. Evers-Kiebooms G, Nys K, Harper P, et al. Predictive DNA-testing for Huntington's disease and reproductive decision making: a European collaborative study. Eur J Hum Genet 2002;10:167.

294. Perry TL. Some ethical problems in Huntington's chorea. Can Med Assoc J 1981;125:1098.

295. Quaid KA, Brandt J, Faden RR, et al. Knowledge, attitude, and the decision to be tested for Huntington's disease. Clin Genet 1989;36:431.

296. Evers-Kiebooms G, Swerts A, Cassimann JJ, et al. The motivation of at-risk individuals and their partners in deciding for or against predictive testing for Huntington's disease. Clin Genet 1989;35:29.

297. Sorenson SA, Fenger K. Suicide in patients with Huntington's disease and their sibs. Am J Hum Genet 1991;49:316.

298. Schoenfeld M, Myers RH, Cupples LA, et al. Increased rate of suicide among patients with Huntington's disease. J Neurol Neurosurg Psychiatry 1984;47:1283.

299. Almqvist EW, Bloch M, Brinkman R, et al, on behalf of an International Huntington Disease Collaborative Group. A worldwide assessment of the frequency of suicide, suicide attempts or psychiatric hospitalization after predictive testing for Huntington disease. Am J Hum Genet 1999;64:1293.

300. Kessler S, Field T, Worth L, et al. Attitudes of persons at risk for Huntington's disease toward predictive testing. Am J Med Genet 1987;26:259.

301. Meissen GJ, Myers RH, Mastromauro CA, et al. Predictive testing for Huntington's disease with use of a linked DNA marker. N Engl J Med 1988;318:535.

302. Evers-Kiebooms G, Cassiman JJ, van den Berghe. Attitudes towards predictive testing in Huntington's chorea: a recent survey in Belgium. J Med Genet 1987;24:275.

303. Markel DS, Young AB, Penney JB. At-risk persons' attitudes toward presymptomatic and prenatal testing of Huntington's disease in Michigan. Am J Med Genet 1987;26:295.

304. Lamport AN. Presymptomatic testing for Huntington's chorea: ethical and legal issues. Am J Med Genet 1987;26:307.

305. Bloch M, Fahy M, Fox S, et al. Predictive testing for Huntington's disease. II. Demographic characteristics, life-style patterns, attitudes, and psychosocial assessments of the first fifty-one test candidates. Am J Med Genet 1989;32:217.

306. Taylor CA, Myers RH. Long-term impact of Huntington disease linkage testing. Am J Med Genet 1997:70:365.

307. Hayden MR. Predictive testing for Huntington disease: are we ready for widespread community implementation? Am J Med Genet 1991;40:515.

308. Nance MA, Leroy BS, Orr HT, et al. Protocol for genetic testing in Huntington disease: three years of experience in Minnesota. Am J Med Genet 1991;40:518.

309. Decruyenaere M, Evers-Kiebooms G, Cloostermans T, et al. Psychological distress in the 5-year period after predictive testing for Huntington's disease. Eur J Hum Genet 2003;11:30.

310. Evans DGR, Maher EF, Macleod R, et al. Uptake of genetic testing for cancer predisposition. J Med Genet 1997;34:746.
311. Deltas CC, Christodoulou K, Tjakouri C, et al. Presymptomatic molecular diagnosis of autosomal dominant polycystic kidney disease using PKD1- and PKD2-linked markers in Cypriot families. Clin Genet 1996;50:10.
312. Pirson Y, Chaveau D. Intracranial aneurysms in autosomal dominant polycystic kidney disease. In: Watson ML, Torres VE, eds. Polycystic kidney disease. Oxford: Oxford University Press, 1996:530.
313. Sujansky E, Kreutzer SB, Johnson AM, et al. Attitudes of at-risk and affected individuals regarding presymptomatic testing for autosomal dominant polycystic kidney disease. Am J Med Genet 1990;35:510.
314. Hannig VL, Hopkins JR, Johnson HK, et al. Presymptomatic testing for adult onset polycystic kidney disease in at-risk kidney transplant donors. Am J Med Genet 1991;40:425.
315. Giardiello FM, Brensinger JD, Petersen GM, et al. The use and interpretation of commercial APC gene testing for familial adenomatous polyposis. N Engl J Med 1997;336:823.
316. Telander RL, Zimmerman D, Sizemore GW, et al. Medullary carcinoma in children: results of early detection and surgery. Arch Surg 1989;124:841.
317. Ross LF. Predictive genetic testing for conditions that present in childhood. Kennedy Inst Ethics J 2002;12:225.
318. Wertz DC, Fanos JH, Reilly PR. Genetic testing for children and adolescents: who decides? JAMA 1994;272:875.
319. Milunsky JM, Maher TA, Loose BA, et al. XL PCR for the detection of large trinucleotide expansions in juvenile Huntington's disease. Clin Genet 2003;64:70.
320. Tassicker R, Savulescu J, Skene L, et al. Prenatal diagnosis requests for Huntington's disease when the father is at risk and does not want to know his genetic status: clinical, legal, and ethical viewpoints. BMJ 2003;326:331.
321. Gusella JF, McNeil S, Persichetti F, et al. Huntington's disease. Cold Spring Harb Symp Quant Biol 1996;61:615.
322. Kremer B, Goldberg P, Andrew SE, A worldwide study of the Huntington's disease mutation: the sensitivity and specificity of measuring CAG repeats. N Engl J Med 1994;330:1401.
323. Alonso ME, Yescas P, Rasmussen A, et al. Homozygosity in Huntington's disease: new ethical dilemma caused by molecular diagnosis. Clin Genet 2002;61:437.
324. Lancaster JM, Wiseman RW, Berchuck A. An inevitable dilemma: prenatal testing for mutations in the BRCA1 breast-ovarian cancer susceptibility gene. Obstet Gynecol 1996;87:306.
325. DudokdeWit AC, Tibben A, Frets PG, et al. BRCA1 in the family: a case description of the psychological implications. Am J Med Genet 1997;71:63.
326. Julian-Reynier C, Eisinger F, Vennin P, et al. Attitudes towards cancer predictive testing and transmission of information to the family. J Med Genet 1996;33:731.
327. Lancaster JM, Wiseman RW, Berchuck A. An inevitable dilemma: prenatal testing for mutations in the BRCA1 breast-ovarian cancer susceptibility gene. Obstet Gynecol 1996;87:306.
327a. Wooster R, Weber BL. Breast and ovarian cancer. N Eng J Med 2003;348:2339.
327b. Antoniou A, Pharoah PD, Narod S, et al. Average risks of breast and ovarian cancer associated with BRCA1 or BRCA2 mutations detected in case series unselected for family history: a combined analysis of 22 studies. Am J Hum Genet 2003;72:1117.
328. Burke W, Daly M, Garber J, et al. Recommendations for follow-up care of individuals with an inherited predisposition to cancer. II. BRCA1 and BRCA2. Cancer Genetics Studies Consortium. JAMA 1997;277:997.
328a. King M-C, Marks JH, Mandell JB. Breast and ovarian cancer risks due to inherited mutations in BRCA1 and BRCA2. Science 2003:302;643.
329. Laken SJ, Petersen GM, Gruber SB, et al. Familial colorectal cancer in Ashkenazim due to a hypermutable tract in APC. Nat Genet 1997;17:79.
330. Warburton D, Kline J, Stein Z, et al. Does the karyotype of a spontaneous abortion predict the karyotype of a subsequent abortion? Evidence from 273 women with two karyotyped spontaneous abortions. Am J Hum Genet 1987;41:465.
331. Campuzano V, Montermini L, Molot MD, et al. Friedreich's ataxia: autosomal recessive disease caused by an intronic GA triplet repeat expansion. Science 1996;271:1423.
332. Jaspert A, Fahsold R, Grehl H, et al. Myotonic dystrophy: correlation of clinical symptoms with the size of the CTG trinucleotide repeat. J Neurol 1995;242:99.
333. Kalousek DK, Barrett I. Genomic imprinting related to prenatal diagnosis. Prenat Diagn 1994;14:1191.
334. Deal CL. Parental genomic imprinting. Curr Opin Pediatr 1995;7:445.

335. Clayton-Smith J, Laan L. Angelman syndrome: a review of the clinical and genetic aspects. J Med Genet 2003;40:87.

336. Walter J, Paulsen M. Imprinting and disease. Semin Cell Dev Biol 2003;14:101.

337. Fournet JC, Mayaud C, de Lonlay P, et al. Loss of imprinted genes and paternal SUR1 mutations lead to focal form of congenital hyperinsulinism. Horm Res 2000;53:2.

338. Passos-Bueno MR, Cerqueira A, Vainzof M, et al. Myotonic dystrophy: genetic, clinical, and molecular analysis of patients from 41 Brazilian families. J Med Genet 1995;32:14.

339. Judson H, Hayward BE, Sheridan E, et al. A global disorder of imprinting in the human female germ line. Nature 2002;416:539.

340. van Schothorst EM, Jansen JC, Bardoel AF, et al. Confinement of PGL, an imprinted gene causing hereditary paragangliomas, to a 2-cM interval on 11q22–q23 and exclusion of DRD2 and NCAM as candidate genes. Eur J Hum Genet 1996;4:267.

341. Muller B, Hedrich K, Kock N, et al. Evidence that paternal expression of the epsilon-sarcoglycan gene accounts for reduced penetrance in myoclonus-dystonia. Am J Hum Genet 2002;71:1303.

342. Fokstuen S, Ginsburg C, Zachmann M, et al. Maternal uniparental disomy 14 as a cause of intrauterine growth retardation and early onset of puberty. J Pediatr 1999;134:689.

343. Eggermann T, Zerres K, Eggermann K, et al. Uniparental disomy: clinical indications for testing in growth retardation. Eur J Pediatr 2002;161:305.

344. Davies W, Isles AR, Wilkinson LS. Imprinted genes and mental dysfunction. Ann Med 2001;33:428.

345. Perk J, Makedonski K, Lande L, et al. The imprinting mechanism of the Prader–Willi/Angelman regional control center. EMBO J 2002;21:5807.

346. Bastepe M, Juppner H. Pseudohypoparathyroidism: new insights into an old disease. Endocrinol Metab Clin North Am 2000;29:569.

347. Shore EM, Ahn J, Jan de Beur S, et al. Paternally inherited inactivating mutations of the GNAS1 gene in progressive osseous heteroplasia. N Engl J Med 2002;346:99.

348. Hitchins MP, Stanier P, Preece MA, et al. Silver-Russell syndrome: a dissection of the genetic aetiology and candidate chromosomal regions. J Med Genet 2001;38:810.

349. Hannula K, Lipsanen-Nyman M, Kristo P, et al. Genetic screening for maternal uniparental disomy of chromosome 7 in prenatal and postnatal growth retardation of unknown cause. Pediatrics 2002;109:441.

350. Temple IK, Shield JP. Transient neonatal diabetes, a disorder of imprinting. J Med Genet 2002;39:872.

351. Balmer D, Arredondo J, Samaco RC, et al. MECP2 mutations in Rett syndrome adversely affect lymphocyte growth, but do not affect imprinted gene expression in blood or brain. Hum Genet 2002;110:545.

352. Girard M, Couvert P, Carrie A, et al. Parental origin of de novo MECP2 mutations in Rett syndrome. Eur J Hum Genet 2001;9:231.

353. Turpin JC. Huntington chorea in children. Arch Fr Pediatr 1993;50:119.

354. Pyeritz RE, McKusick VA. The Marfan syndrome: diagnosis and management. N Engl J Med 1979;300:772.

355. Beutler E, Nguyen NJ, Henneberger MW, et al. Gaucher disease: gene frequencies in the Ashkenazi Jewish population. Am J Hum Genet 1993;53:85.

356. Lewis BD, Nelson PV, Robertson EF, et al. Mutation analysis of 28 Gaucher disease patients: the Australasian experience. Am J Med Genet 1994;49:218.

357. Kerem E, Corey M, Kerem B, et al. The relationship between genotype and phenotype in cystic fibrosis: analysis of the most common mutation. N Engl J Med 1990;323:1517.

358. Cystic Fibrosis Genotype-Phenotype Consortium. Correlation between genotype and phenotype in patients with cystic fibrosis. N Engl J Med 1993;329:1308.

359. Dork T, Wulbrand U, Richter T, et al. Cystic fibrosis with three mutations in the cystic fibrosis transmembrane regulator gene. Hum Genet 1991;87:441.

360. Le C, Ramjeesingh M, Reys E, et al. The cystic fibrosis mutation (F508) does not influence the chloride channel activity of CFTR. Nat Genet 1993;3:311.

361. Tuddenham EGD. Factor VIII and haemophilia A. Baillieres Clin Haematol 1989;2:849.

362. Miller DS, Steinbrecher RA, Wieland K, et al. The molecular genetic analysis of haemophilia A: characterization of six partial deletions in the factor VIII gene. Hum Genet 1990;86:219.

363. Hoo JJ. Alternative explanations for recurrent achondroplasia in siblings with normal parents. Clin Genet 1984;25:553.

364. Bakker E, Veenema H, Den Dunnen JT, et al. Germinal mosaicism increases the recurrence risk for "new" Duchenne muscular dystrophy mutations. J Med Genet 1989;26:553.

365. Donnai D, Read AP, McKeown C, et al. Hypomelanosis of Ito-A manifestation of mosaicism or chimerism. J Med Genet 1988;25:809.

366. Thomas IT, Frias JL, Cantu ES, et al. Association of pigmentary anomalies with chromosomal and genetic mosaicism and chimerism. Am J Hum Genet 1989;45:193.

367. Raghunath M, Mackay K, Dalgleish R, et al. Genetic counseling on brittle grounds: recurring osteogenesis imperfecta due to parental mosaicism for a dominant mutation. Eur J Pediatr 1995;154:123.

368. Lund AM, Nicholls AC, Schwartz M, et al. Parental mosaicism and autosomal dominant mutations causing structural abnormalities of collagen I are frequent in families with osteogenesis imperfecta type III/IV. Acta Paediatr 1997;86:711.

369. Telenius H, Kremer B, Goldberg YP, et al. Somatic and gonadal mosaicism of the Huntington disease gene CAG repeat in brain and sperm. Nat Genet 1994;6:409.

370. Cancel G, Durr A, Didierjean O, et al. Molecular and clinical correlations in spinocerebellar ataxia 2: a study of 32 families. Hum Mol Genet 1997;6:709.

371. Satge D, Geneix A, Goburdhun J, et al. A history of miscarriages and mild prognathism as possible mode of presentation of mosaic trisomy 18 in women. Clin Genet 1996;50:470.

372. Ptacek JT, Eberhardt TL. Breaking bad news. JAMA 1996;276:496.

373. Bond CF, Anderson EL. The reluctance to transmit bad news: private discomfort or public display? J Eur Soc Psychol 1987;23:176.

374. White-Van Mourik MCA, Connor JM, Ferguson-Smith MA. The psychosocial sequelae of a second-trimester termination of pregnancy for fetal abnormality. Prenat Diagn 1992;12:189.

375. Blumberg BD, Golbus MC, Hanson K. The psychological sequelae of abortion performed for a genetic indication. Am J Obstet Gynecol 1975;122:799.

376. Blumberg BD. The emotional implications of prenatal diagnosis. In: Emery, AEH, Pullen IM, eds. Psychological aspects of genetic counseling. London: Academic Press, 1984:202.

377. Parkes CM. Bereavement. Studies of grief in adult life. London: Tavistock Publications, 1972.

378. Worden JW. Grief counseling and grief therapy, 2nd ed. New York: Springer, 1991.

379. Appleton R, Gibson B, Hey E. The loss of a baby at birth: the role of the bereavement officer. Br J Obstet Gynaecol 1993;100:51.

380. Seller M, Barnes C, Ross S, et al. Grief and mid-trimester fetal loss. Prenat Diagn 1993;13:341.

381. Fanos JH. Developmental tasks of childhood and adolescence: implications for genetic testing. Am J Med Genet 1997;71:22.

382. Andrews LB, Fullarton JE, Holtzman NA, et al. Assessing genetic risks: implications for health and social policy. Washington, DC: National Academy Press, 1994:297.

383. Wertz DC, Fanos JH, Reilly PR. Genetic testing for children and adolescents: who decides? JAMA 1994;272:875.

384. Clinical Genetics Society (UK). Report of a Working Party: the genetic testing of children. J Med Genet 1994;31:785.

385. American Society of Human Genetics and American College of Medical Genetics. Points to consider: ethical, legal and psychosocial implications of genetic testing in children and adolescents. Am J Hum Genet 1995;57:1233.

386. Green M, Solnit AJ. Reactions to the threatened loss of a child: a vulnerable child syndrome. Pediatrics 1964;34:58.

387. McIntosh N, Eldrige C. Neonatal death: the neglected side of neonatal care? Arch Dis Child 1984;59:585.

388. Bourne S. The psychological effects of a stillbirth on women and their doctors. J R Coll Gen Pract 1968:16:103.

389. Crowther ME. Communication following a stillbirth or neonatal death: room for improvement. Br J Obstet Gynaecol 1995;102:952.

390. Brookes JAS, Hall-Craggs MA, Sams VR, et al. Non-invasive perinatal necropsy by magnetic resonance imaging. Lancet 1996;348:1139.

391. Nicholas AM, Lewin TJ. Grief reactions of parental couples: congenital handicap and cot death. Med J Aust 1986;144:292.

392. Lewis E, Bryan E. Management of perinatal loss of a twin. BMJ 1988;297:1321.

393. Lewis E. Stillbirth: psychological consequences and strategies of management. In: Milunsky A, ed. Advances in perinatal medicine, vol. 3. New York: Plenum, 1983:205.

394. McPhee SJ, Bottles K, Lo B, et al. To redeem them from death: reactions of family members to autopsy. Am J Med 1986;80:665.

395. Irvin NA, Kennell JH, Klaus MH. Caring for the parents of an infant with a congenital malformation. In: Warkany J, ed. Congenital malformations: notes and comments. Chicago: Year Book Medical Publishers, 1971.

396. Klaus MH, Kennell JH. Caring for parents of an infant who dies: Maternal infant bonding. St. Louis: CV Mosby, 1976.

397. Furlong RM, Hobbins JC. Grief in the perinatal period. Obstet Gynecol 1983;61:497.

398. Shulman LP, Grevengood C, Phillips OP, et al. Family planning decisions after prenatal detection of fetal abnormalities. Am J Obstet Gynecol 1994;171:1373.

399. Rowe J, Clyman R, Green C, et al. Follow-up of families who experience a perinatal death. Pediatrics 1978;62:166.

400. Forrest GC, Standish E, Baum JD. Support after perinatal death: a study of support and counseling after bereavement. BMJ 1982;285:1475.

401. Clarke A, Parsons E, Williams A. Outcomes and process in genetic counseling. Clin Genet 1996;50:462.

402. Antley RM. Variables in the outcome of genetic counseling. Soc Biol 1976;23:108.

403. Emery AEH, Raeburn JA, Skinner R. Prospective study of genetic counseling. BMJ 1979;1:253.

404. Taylor K, Merill RE. Progress in the delivery of health care: genetic counseling. Am J Dis Child 1970:119:209.

405. Sibinga MS, Friedman CG. Complexities of parental understanding for phenylketonuria. Pediatrics 1971;48:216.

406. Reynolds BD, Puck MH, Robinson A. Genetic counseling: an appraisal. Clin Genet 1974;5:177.

407. Sorenson JR, Swazey JP, Scotch NA. Effective genetic counseling: more informed clients. In: Reproductive pasts, reproductive futures: Genetic counseling and its effectiveness. New York: Alan R. Liss, 1981:79.

408. Swerts A. Impact of genetic counseling and prenatal diagnosis for Down syndrome and neural tube defects. Birth Defects Orig Artic Ser 1987;23(2):61.

409. Wertz DC, Sorenson JR, Heeren TC. Clients' interpretation of risks provided in genetic counseling. Am J Hum Genet 1986;39:253.

410. Kessler S. Psychological aspects of genetic counseling. VI. A critical review of the literature dealing with education and reproduction. Am J Med Genet 1989;34:340.

Sherman Elias, M.D., F.A.C.O.G., F.A.C.M.G., F.A.C.S., and Joe Leigh Simpson, M.D., F.A.C.O.G., F.A.C.M.G., F.R.C.O.G.

2

Amniocentesis and Fetal Blood Sampling

Amniocentesis was first used in Germany in the early 1880s to treat hydramnios.[1,2] In 1930, Menees et al.[3] used amniocentesis to inject contrast media into the amniotic sac, to evaluate the fetus, and to localize the placenta. The procedure of using amniocentesis to introduce hypertonic saline into the amniotic sac to terminate pregnancy was first used in 1937.[4] In 1950 Alvarez of Uruguay performed amniocentesis to assess fetal well-being.[5] The use of amniocentesis increased rapidly in the 1950s, when spectrophotometric analysis of bilirubin proved valuable in monitoring fetuses with Rh isoimmunization.[5,6]

Amniocentesis for exclusively genetic indications evolved in the mid-1950s. Several investigators demonstrated that fetal sex could be determined by X-chromatin analysis of amniotic fluid cells (AFCs).[7–9] In 1966, Steele and Breg[10] reported the feasibility of performing chromosomal analysis of AFCs, thereby formally introducing the prenatal diagnosis of genetic disorders. The next year, Jacobson and Barter[11] reported the first prenatal diagnosis of a chromosomal abnormality (a balanced D/D translocation). In 1968, Valenti et al.[12] and Nadler[13] reported the in utero detection of Down syndrome, with confirmation after elective abortion. That same year, Nadler[13] diagnosed galactosemia in fetal AFCs, the first detection of a mendelian disorder. Within the next few years, numerous investigators reported successful prenatal diagnosis of a wide variety of chromosomal and metabolic disorders.[14] In 1970, Nadler and Gerbie[15] summarized their initial experience in performing genetic amniocentesis in 142 patients during 155 pregnancies. By demonstrating both diagnostic accuracy and a relatively low risk, their landmark report helped establish prenatal diagnosis through amniocentesis as an integral part of modern obstetric care.[16]

In this chapter, we consider the current technique and the safety of genetic amniocentesis. We also consider fetal blood sampling, the second most commonly employed invasive prenatal diagnostic procedure in the second and third trimesters. Indications and methods of prenatal diagnosis are considered in detail throughout this text, as well as elsewhere by us.[17–22]

AMNIOCENTESIS

Prerequisites

Consistently reliable and safe diagnosis can be achieved only by a team that provides the necessary expertise. Ideally, couples should have the opportunity to discuss their genetic risks and available antenatal studies before pregnancy.[17,21,23] The counselor should elicit an accurate history, confirm the diagnosis of any abnormality in question, be aware of diagnostic capabilities, and be cognizant of psychological defenses (e.g., denial, guilt reactions, and blame) engendered during genetic counseling. Couples must understand the risks of amniocentesis itself, the accuracy and limitations of antenatal diagnosis, the time required before results become available, technical problems potentially necessitating a second amniocentesis, and the rare possibility of an inability to make a diagnosis.

Amniocentesis should be performed only by an obstetrician who (1) is experienced in this procedure, (2) has the availability of high-quality ultrasonography, and (3) has access to a laboratory with experience in performing prenatal diagnostic studies.[20,24,25] We believe that only obstetricians should perform the procedure, not because of technical difficulty but because the operator must always be prepared to deal with the potential complications of the procedure. If an abnormality is detected and the couple elects to terminate the pregnancy, the obstetrician must either perform the abortion or refer the family to an obstetrician who will act on their request.

Technique of Amniocentesis

Timing

Traditionally, amniocentesis has been performed at about the fifteenth and sixteenth weeks of gestation (menstrual weeks). At this time, the ratio of viable to nonviable cells is greatest compared with procedures performed later in gestation.[26] In addition, the uterus is accessible by an abdominal approach and contains sufficient amniotic fluid (AF) (200–250 mL) to permit 20–30 mL to be aspirated safely. Amniocentesis earlier in gestation (i.e., <14 weeks) is discussed below. Transvaginal amniocentesis has historically not been recommended, because of its technical difficulty and because of associated infection and spontaneous abortion.[27] Whether the proscription is still appropriate in this era of sophisticated ultrasonography is untested.

Surgical Aspects

Amniocentesis for genetic diagnosis is performed in an outpatient facility. In preparation for the procedure, the patient empties her bladder so that inadvertent aspiration of urine does not occur. A careful ultrasonographic examination is performed and a needle-insertion site is selected. The needle is inserted, preferably in the midline fundal area of the uterus, employing concurrent ultrasound guidance; however, this site does not always correspond to the location of the optimal pocket of amniotic fluid. Not infrequently, a lower uterine segment or a lateral approach is required. Tabor et al.[28] found that transplacental needle insertion increased the risk of the procedure, but Tharmaratnam, et al.[29] did not. Nonetheless, the placenta should logically be avoided when possible. If reaching the optimal pocket of AF requires traversing the placenta, it is desirable to select the thinnest possible part of the placenta through which the needle can be directed. Usually, this site is at the periphery of the placenta. The umbilical cord and its insertion site should be especially identified and avoided. The risk for fetal complications has not been proved to be increased when transplacental amniocentesis is performed by experienced operators, compared with nontransplacental procedures.[30] The maternal bowel and bladder should also be located, because these structures should also be avoided; it is essential to avoid the former, whereas the latter is painful to traverse. A local anesthetic (e.g., 2–3 mL of 1 percent xylocaine) may or may not be used; however, local anesthesia does not appear to affect the level of pain of the procedure.[31] Counseling before amniocentesis should emphasize that the actual pain and anxiety experienced during the procedure is significantly lower than expected.[32] After the maternal skin has been cleansed with an iodine-based solution and/or alcohol-based solution, sterile drapes are placed around the needle-insertion site to help maintain an aseptic field. A disposable 22-gauge spinal needle with stylet is most frequently used (and is recommended by us).

During the entire procedure, ultrasonographic monitoring with continuous visualization of the needle should be performed. Ultrasound gel is applied adjacent to the insertion site, and a real-time transducer is held in position by an assistant such that the ultrasound beam is directed at a 15–20° angle from the parallel of the planned needle track (see Figure 2.1). Simultaneous ultrasound produces some distortion of the angle of the needle entering the uterus. If the obstetrician is standing on the patient's right side and inserts the needle perpendicular to the horizontal plane, the needle can be observed coming from the side of the screen. That is, a needle directed perpendicular (12 o'clock) appears to enter at a 15–20° angle (2 o'clock). On insertion, the entire length of the needle should be observed on the screen, with the tip being identified by a "flare" produced by the beveled end. The tactile perception by the operator of the needle passing through the various tissues is important for proper needle placement. In nulliparous patients especially, the operator appreciates the needle passing through the rectus fascia. Tactile sensation is greatest if one places his/her index finger on the top of the needle stylet, pushing down. The patient may respond to peritoneal entry with a transient sensation of pain. The operator next appreciates a firm sensation as the uterus is traversed, and sometimes a "popping" sensation when the amniotic membranes are pierced. Distinguishing chorion from amnion is not usually possible after the first trimester, but it may be possible early in gestation.

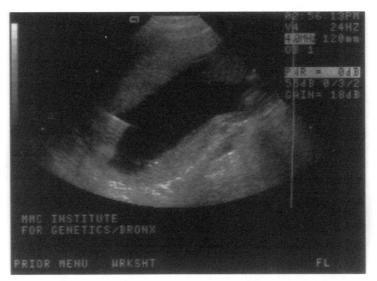

Fig. 2.1. Amniocentesis being performed under direct, continuous ultrasound scanning (sector transducer, 3.5 MHz). Although the needle is being introduced perpendicular to the skin, the angle of the ultrasound beam in relation to the needle causes an illusion, so the needle appears to be entering the amniotic cavity at the 10 o'clock position.

After assurance that the needle is in its proper location, the stylet is moved and a 10- or 20-cc syringe attached. The tip is typically more easily identified on removal of the stylet. If freely flowing AF is not obtained on aspiration, the needle must be repositioned with stylet in place. One should not "search" for AF by applying suction on the syringe plunger while redirecting the needle. Sometimes, only minimal repositioning is necessary, such as rotating the needle to redirect the bevel. After the needle tip has been satisfactorily positioned in the amniotic cavity, the stylet is removed permanently. The first several milliliters are theoretically most likely to contain maternal cells from blood vessels, the abdominal wall, or the myometrium; therefore, this initial sample is usually discarded or set aside for AF α-fetoprotein (AF-AFP) assay. However, this fluid may be used to differentiate AF from inadvertently obtained maternal urine (discussed later). Twenty to 30 mL of AF are aspirated into sterile, disposable plastic syringes, although as little as 3 to 5 mL AF has been shown to suffice for reliable prenatal cytogenetic results.[33] It is preferable to use 10- or 20-mL syringes because only gentle traction on the barrel of the syringe is desirable or necessary. Overly vigorous traction in search of fluid, especially with a 30- to 50-mL syringe, can result in the amniotic membranes being drawn into the needle. After the AF has been obtained, it is either left in the labeled syringes or transferred into labeled flasks, which are transported at ambient temperature directly to the laboratory.

Any given attempt at amniocentesis may be unsuccessful. In the 1972–1975 U.S. collaborative study,[34] which did not use ultrasound, no AF was aspirated in 5.9 percent of cases. In the Canadian collaborative study[35] the frequency of failure was 10.6 percent with the same technique. At present, it is unusual for experienced operators to fail to obtain a specimen. Because concurrent ultrasound has become routine, failure to obtain AF occurs far less often. Some failures may be due to uterine contractions, which may obliterate or alter the AF space beneath the needle. Other failures may be due to improper placement of the needle or "tenting" of the membranes (i.e., impingement of the membranes without piercing them) such that the needle does not penetrate into the amniotic cavity.[36,37] This is much more problematic with early amniocentesis (i.e., before the fourteenth week, as discussed below). The ability to obtain AF is related to the experience of the operator, the use of ultrasonography, and the gestational age at which the procedure is performed. If performed at 15–16 weeks of gestation by experienced prenatal diagnosticians, failure to obtain AF should be far less than 1 percent,[24,38–41] in fact very unusual. After a failed amniocentesis, a second procedure may be attempted on the same day. However, another failure probably dictates postponement for 3–7 days. Even if not appreciated, a second failure may indicate overestimated gestational age or oligohydramnios.

Often, AF and urine are indistinguishable in appearance. Analysis of cells derived from maternal urine obviously could lead to erroneous interpretations of fetal status. Inadvertent aspiration of maternal urine is a particular risk if a suprapubic needle insertion is chosen. If the origin of aspirated fluid is in doubt, tests should be performed to determine its origin. Pirani et al.[42] recommend use of reagent strips for albumin to differentiate AF from urine. The AF contains albumin and glucose, whereas urine does not. However, this test may be unreliable if the pregnancy is complicated by diabetes mellitus, renal disease, or hydramnios. Guibaud et al.[43] advocate analyzing fluid for urea and potassium. Both show much higher levels in urine than in AF. Urea and potassium levels indeed differentiate AF from urine, but in most institutions these tests cannot be performed quickly. Elias et al.[44] found that the crystalline arborization pattern characteristic of AF is observed if the fluid is allowed to dry on an acid-cleansed slide and examined under low-power

(3×100) magnification. This test differentiated AF from urine with a high degree of accuracy; however, only rarely are any tests necessary.

After amniocentesis, intact fetal heart motions should be documented by ultrasonographic visualization. The patient should be observed briefly after the procedure and should be instructed to report any vaginal fluid loss or bleeding, severe uterine cramping (mild cramping for several hours after the procedure is not uncommon), or fever. Reasonably normal activities may be resumed after the procedure; however, we recommend that strenuous exercise (e.g., jogging or aerobic exercises) and coitus be avoided for a day.

Technical skills in performing amniocentesis have traditionally been taught by trainees observing experienced operators followed by the trainees performing the procedure under the direct supervision of the mentors. Pittini et al.[45] developed a high-fidelity simulator-based curriculum for teaching amniocentesis that showed that students' performance improved with experience on the simulator. Whether the skills acquired on a simulator are transferable to the clinical setting remains to be seen.

Ultrasound Concurrent with Amniocentesis

Almost all investigators regard it as mandatory that amniocentesis be performed under continuous ultrasound guidance. That is, a real-time transducer is placed on the abdomen in such a way that the needle tip can be continuously monitored throughout its entry.[39,46–50] Our own technique has already been described above.

In 1983, Benacerraf and Frigoletto[51] evaluated this approach in 232 of 235 consecutive amniocenteses (184 for prenatal diagnosis, 52 for monitoring pulmonary maturity in cases of Rh incompatibility). Among the 232 procedures in which direct ultrasonographic guidance was attempted, 7 were bloody taps, of which 6 cleared after the first milliliter was withdrawn. Six unsuccessful ("dry") taps necessitated a second attempt, which yielded clear AF in all except one case. In the one case, no AF was obtained after two attempts, and the patient declined a third attempt. The authors stated that "a significant number of patients were saved second attempts" and that "the rate of dry taps was 2.6 percent and the initial bloody tap rate was 2.9 percent, both substantially lower than those previously reported in the literature." However, Benacerraf and Frigoletto[51] acknowledge that their experience was probably similar to that of other experienced obstetricians. Thus, their data cannot be considered definitive.

Romero et al.[39] compared 688 patients undergoing genetic amniocentesis immediately after ultrasound (i.e., scanning followed immediately by skin asepsis and needle insertion) to 612 patients undergoing "sonographically monitored" amniocentesis (i.e., continuous monitoring of the needle throughout the procedure). The former group was studied from 1980 to 1981, the latter from 1981 to 1982. Amniocentesis results were also correlated with the operator's experience. In the sonographically monitored group, there was a statistically significant decrease in the frequencies of bloody taps and dry taps ($p < 0.0001$) and also in the number of patients requiring multiple needle insertions ($p < 0.0001$). Continuous ultrasound monitoring was most advantageous for operators who had experienced a relatively higher intraoperative complication rate when ultrasound was used only before the procedure. That is, the monitored technique allowed an inexperienced operator to acquire a satisfactory level of performance in a relatively short time (e.g., after only twenty amniocenteses). After this short interval, the least experienced operator (a Fellow in Maternal–Fetal Medicine) had frequencies of bloody and dry taps similar to those of the most experienced obstetrician of the unit. However, the authors acknowledge that increasing experience of all operators could have accounted for some of the ostensible improvement. A further limitation is that the study was not a prospective randomized clinical trial but rather a comparison using a historical control group.

Among 918 singleton amniocenteses performed under continuous ultrasound guidance (during 1981–1983), Williamson et al.[52] reported a fetal death rate (<28 weeks) after the procedure of only 0.89 percent, and no deaths occurred within 2 weeks of the procedure. This rate was compared with a retrospective analysis of an equivalent number of procedures performed during 1977–1980, in which the loss rate was 1.9 percent. In the latter interval, many amniocenteses were performed hours after the ultrasound examination.[53] As with similar reports, a concurrent control group was not available. Thus, although added safety using their newer technique is again suggested, a definitive statement could not be made.

Andreasen and Kristoffersen[54] prospectively sought to correlate placental localization with the performance of amniocentesis, particularly as assessed by spontaneous abortion. The study group consisted of 1,289 women undergoing amniocentesis and 256 control women who did not undergo the procedure "because there were no indications for it." Localization of the placenta per se had no influence on the frequency of abortion: 2.2 percent in the study group versus 0.8 percent in controls ($p = 5.14$). In patients in whom the placenta was traversed during the amniocentesis, the spontaneous abortion rate was significantly increased to 6.3 percent ($p < 0.002$). The mean age of women undergoing amniocentesis was 34.1 years, whereas among the controls the mean age was 30.1 years ($p < 0.001$). Thus, the background spontaneous abortion rates between the study group and the control group cannot be considered comparable.

Published data as well as our own clinical experience led us to conclude that all genetic amniocenteses must be preceded immediately by a careful ultrasonographic evaluation. We also believe that continuous ultrasonographic monitoring of the needle tip throughout the amniocentesis is mandatory. This is particularly beneficial for the relatively inexperienced operator or in potentially difficult amniocenteses (e.g., multiple gestation, leiomyomata of the uterus, or obesity).

Leiomyomata may complicate performance of amniocentesis. Realize, however, that some uterine contractions may mimic leiomyomata. Salvador et al.[55] reported a retrospective analysis of 128 women with leiomyomata uteri who underwent amniocentesis, matched with 218 women without leiomyomas undergoing amniocentesis and 128 women with leiomyomas not undergoing amniocentesis. The incidence of spontaneous abortion was 6.3 percent among the cases, 0.8 percent in the amniocentesis-only controls, and 7.0 percent in the leiomyoma-only controls. The authors concluded that women with leiomyomas are at increased risk, but second-trimester amniocentesis does not appear to further increase the risk.

Frequency of Multiple Gestations

The rate of monozygous (MZ) twins appears to be relatively constant in all populations at 3–4 per 1,000 births. The rate is largely independent of race, parity, age, and ovulation-induction factors. By contrast, such variables play an important role in the rate of dizygous (DZ) twinning, which varies between 7 and 11 per 1,000 births.[56] Ovulation-inducing agents alter this rate dramatically. For example, March[57] reported a 9.1 percent multiple pregnancy rate in 143 women treated with human menopausal–human chorionic gonadotropin for 661 cycles. Moreover, in pregnancies after in vitro fertilization, in which it is common practice to transfer three or four embryos, the frequency of multiple gestations is about 30 percent.[58–60] Of particular importance to prenatal diagnosis is the increase of DZ twinning with advancing maternal age and increasing parity.[59,61–63] The frequency of twinning increases with any increase in age up to 40 years or for any parity up to seven. Twin pregnancies are less than one-third as common in women under 20 years of age with no previous children as in women 35–40 years of age with four or more previous children.

Dizygotic twins are almost invariably discordant for Down syndrome.[64,65] By contrast, MZ twins are invariably concordant for Down syndrome. Discordance for cytogenetic abnormalities other than trisomy 21 is presumed for DZ twins.[66] Meyers et al.[67] calculated maternal age-specific risks for chromosomal abnormalities in twin gestations, based on existing tables of chromosomal abnormalities in singleton gestations. Figures are provided for the risks of one or both twins being affected with Down syndrome or any chromosomal abnormality, either at the time of midtrimester amniocentesis or as live-births. However, a caveat is that these otherwise useful figures fail to take into account the age-related increase in DZ twins, compared with age-independent rates in MZ twins.

Diagnosis of Multiple Gestations

By the early second trimester, multiple gestations are readily detectable by ultrasonography.[68] Uterine size larger than expected on the basis of the last menstrual period is another common sign of possible multiple gestation, as is increased maternal serum α-fetoprotein (MSAFP). If multiple gestations are detected, the patient can still be offered antenatal diagnosis. In fact, genetic amniocentesis can be performed successfully in more than 95 percent in twin pregnancies with ostensibly no increased risk over patients undergoing amniocentesis in singleton pregnancies.[46]

Amniocentesis Technique with Multiple Gestations

In most centers, separate amniocentesis of each sac is employed to assess the status of each fetus (see Figures 2.2 and 2.3). Each amniotic sac may be identified if the clinician injects a dye (i.e., 2–3 mL of the blue dye indigo carmine diluted 1:10 in bacteriostatic water) immediately after aspiration of the first AF sample but before withdrawal of the needle. Methylene blue dye is proscribed because it has been associated with high risk of small-intestine atresia and fetal death.[70] After completion of the first amniocentesis, a second amniocentesis is performed in the ultrasonographically located area of the other fetus. Visualization of the membranes separating the sacs is generally possible (see Figure 2.3). Aspiration of clear AF indicates that the second sac was successfully entered; aspiration of blue-tinged AF indicates that the original sac was re-entered.[68]

Single-needle insertion under ultrasound guidance to sample both sacs in twins has been reported,[47,48] but we still prefer the dye technique described above. In particular, we worry that single-puncture techniques could lead to cross-contamination between sacs, resulting in diagnostic inaccuracies. The technique of Jeanty et al.[49] employs a single myometrial needle puncture into the first amniotic sac and then through the membranous septum into the second sac. We believe that this technique does not necessarily facilitate amniocentesis of a twin gestation and that it could potentially result in inaccurate cytogenetic analyses from incidental admixture of AF occurring when the needle is introduced into the second from the first amniotic cavity. In addition, a single puncture could potentially result in higher rates of fetal morbidity and mortality, specifically from fetal injury, membrane shearing, or amniotic band syndrome.

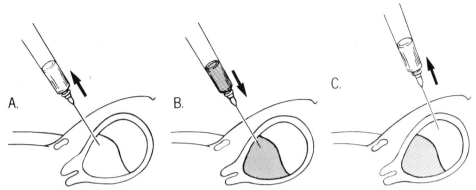

Fig. 2.2. The technique for amniocentesis in twin gestations. *A,* Fluid is aspirated from the first amniotic sac. *B,* Blue indigo carmine dye is instilled into the first amniotic sac. *C,* Clear fluid is aspirated from the ultrasonographically determined location of the second fetus. Clear fluid confirms that the second amniotic sac was successfully sampled. *Source:* Elias et al., 1980.[69]

Using the regimen we prefer or a slight variation thereof, experienced investigators have long been successful in obtaining information regarding both fetuses in more than 90–95 percent of cases.[50,69,71–82] In 1991, Anderson et al.[46] reported their experience with amniocentesis in 339 multiple gestations (330 twins, 9 triplets). The loss rate (to 28 weeks) in this group was 3.57 percent, compared with their singleton spontaneous abortion rate of 0.60 percent. They opined that this increased abortion rate after amniocentesis may represent only the increased natural loss rate in multiple gestations and did not indicate any increased risk added by the procedure. Yukobowich and coworkers[83] retrospectively compared 476 twin gestations undergoing amniocentesis at 17 to 18 weeks, 489 singleton gestations undergoing amniocentesis at 17 to 18 weeks, and 477 twin gestations not undergoing amniocentesis at 17 to 18 weeks. Loss rates up to 4 weeks after the procedure were 2.7 percent, 0.6 percent, and 0.6 percent, respectively. One problem with this and

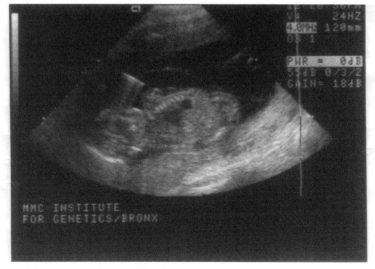

Fig. 2.3. Amniocentesis being performed under direct, continuous ultrasound scanning (sector transducer, 3.5 MHz) in a twin gestation.

other studies is that maternal age was not taken into account by logistic regression, nor were indications and other variables. Although there appears to be no greater frequency of amniocentesis-related complications of twin gestations as compared with singleton pregnancies, a formal clinical trial would be required for a definitive statement.

In our combined prenatal diagnosis programs, we have performed genetic amniocentesis in more than 500 twin pregnancies. Our overall success rate over several decades in sampling both amniotic sacs is well over 95 percent, and virtually 100 percent since the universal application of concurrent high-quality ultrasound that allows visualization of fetal membranes. In the few unsuccessful cases, there was a reason to suspect that there was relatively little AF in one twin's sac. Triplets (and presumably gestations of greater multiplicity) can be managed by sequentially injecting dye into successive sacs after the withdrawal of clear AF in each case. The number of aspirations of clear AF should equal the number of fetuses. As long as clear fluid can be aspirated, one can be reassured that a new amniotic sac has been entered. We have also performed amniocentesis in several triplet pregnancies, successfully aspirating fluid from all three gestational sacs. Others have reported similar experience.[78,81,82] Still, data are insufficient to make any statements regarding risks of amniocentesis in triplet gestations.

Rh Isoimmunization in Amniocentesis

The propriety of administering Rh(D) immunoglobulin (RhIG) to prevent Rh immunization in unsensitized women with Rh-positive fetuses remains controversial. Fetomaternal transfusion by disruption of the fetoplacental circulation logically might have an immunizing effect; however, the magnitude of this putative risk has not been determined. The task is difficult because one must consider variables such as ABO compatibility, number of needle insertions, placental location, and amount of fetal blood transfused into the maternal circulation. Nonetheless, Rh sensitization after second-trimester amniocentesis has clearly been observed.[84–86]

Postpartum administration of RhIG to Rh-negative unsensitized women delivered of Rh-positive infants is known to prevent Rh hemolytic disease of the newborn in subsequent pregnancies.[87] Thus, the efficacy of administering RhIG after genetic amniocentesis can be assumed. Indeed, Khalil et al.[88] reported only one sensitization among 300 (0.3 percent) at-risk women who received 300 μg of RhIG after amniocentesis. By contrast, among 615 Rh-negative women at risk for sensitization who did not receive RhIG after amniocentesis, Golbus et al.[86] reported that 12 (2.1 percent) became sensitized. These two data sets were actually not statistically different, but they suggested a trend toward decreasing sensitization when RhIG was given after genetic amniocentesis. Similarly, in the U.K. collaborative study,[84] sensitization of Rh-negative women who underwent amniocentesis was more common in the subjects not given RhIG (3 of 58; 5.2 percent) than in those given RhIG (0 of 59; 0 percent) or in women not undergoing amniocentesis (controls) (1 of 65; 0.6 percent). Although these differences were also not statistically significant, pooling data from several studies yields the estimate that amniocentesis increases the risk of Rh sensitization by about 1 percent over the background risk of 1.5 percent. Murray et al. calculated that 2.5 percent of Rh-negative women who undergo amniocentesis and who are carrying Rh-positive fetuses will be sensitized.[89] On the other hand, Tabor et al. reported a series of 655 Rh-negative women who had no anti-D antibody in their serum at genetic amniocentesis, 361 of whom were delivered of Rh-positive infants.[90] Prophylactic treatment with anti-D immunoglobulin was not given at amniocentesis, yet few were immunized. Tabor et al. concluded that the immunization rate after genetic amniocentesis was no higher than the spontaneous immunization rate during pregnancy.[90]

The only reason that we could imagine for not administering RhIG relates to the theoretical concerns that remain regarding the safety of its administration. As a 7S immunoglobulin, RhIG is known to cross the placenta and, in theory, could adversely affect the fetus by hemolyzing fetal red blood cells. However, this does not appear to be an issue, at least with the dose administered.[91] A second potentially deleterious outcome might be chronic toxicity related to exposing the immunologically "naïve" immune system of a 16- to 18-week fetus to pooled human serum globulins.[92] Finally, inappropriately small amounts of RhIG may actually augment the immune response. Based on both theoretical concerns and some limited experimental evidence, augmentation is a phenomenon in which very low circulating levels of an antibody may paradoxically enhance rather than deter antibody production; in the present context, this might occur when a new challenge with Rh-positive cells is introduced.[89,93]

Data implicating RhIG with adverse pregnancy outcome can indeed be cited. In 1979, Miles and Kaback surveyed ten large antenatal diagnostic centers in the United States to determine the effects of RhIG administration. Fetal losses were 60 percent higher in RhIG-treated pregnancies, suggesting a possible detrimental effect of such administration before 20 weeks of gestation. Other data revealed six fetal deaths in seventy-eight RhIG-treated, Rh-negative pregnancies.[94] Although not statistically significant (probably because of small sample size), this study raised the possibility that midtrimester administration of RhIG may be associated with fetal risk. In 1982 Golbus et al. concluded that prophylactic RhIG should not be administered after genetic amniocentesis.[86] However, in the 1984 retrospective study of Khalil et al.,[88] no significant differences were seen in the frequency of pregnancy wastage, intrauterine growth restriction, preterm delivery, lowered mean birth weight, and congenital defects between the RhIG and the control groups. Similar conclusions were reached by Crane et al.,[95] who in 1984 studied 147 Rh-negative women who received RhIG and 150 matched controls who did not.

What is the current recommendation? Virtually all operators advocate routine use of RhIG. However, the dose to be administered remains controversial. The American College of Obstetricians and Gynecologists[96] currently recommends a 300-μg dose of RhIG after second-trimester amniocentesis. However, Khalil et al.[88] administered a lower dose if Kleihauer–Betke stain or MSAFP after amniocentesis suggests a small fetomaternal hemorrhage. They administer 10 μg of RhIG for every 1 mL of fetal blood in the maternal circulation. In the United Kingdom, the recommended dose of RhIG is 50 μg before 20 weeks of gestation and 100 μg thereafter.[97] We routinely administer 300 μg of RhIG after genetic amniocentesis.

Discolored Amniotic Fluid

Occasionally, brown or green AF is observed in second-trimester amniocenteses.[34,38,82,98,99] Using spectrophotometric absorbance at 440–408 nm and measurements of free hemoglobin, Hankins et al.[99] demonstrated that the brown- or green-stained AF indicated intra-amniotic hemorrhage before amniocentesis, the discoloration specifically resulting from breakdown of blood products.

In the 1972–1975 U.S. collaborative study,[34] brown AF was associated with unfavorable pregnancy outcome; five of twenty such AF specimens were associated with fetal loss. Among 2,000 genetic amniocenteses performed in a subsequent decade, Dacus et al.[82] encountered 42 (2.1 percent) brown AF specimens. The prevalence of brown AF was 12.5 percent in women who later had a spontaneous abortion, compared with only 1.5 percent in their entire series. Among 923 amniocentesis reported by Cruikshank et al. in 1983,[53] seventeen fluids were discolored: nine green and eight "mahogany"-colored. Five of these seventeen patients (29.4 percent) had spontaneous abortions. In 1979 Golbus et al.[38] reported thirty-six (1.2 percent) discolored AF samples among 3,000 samples. Seven of the discolored fluid samples had an elevated AFP concentration, and all thirty-six discolored fluid samples were associated with fetal death. Among the thirty-six discolored fluid samples, there were six in which culture failure occurred. Among the thirty successful cultures, there were three chromosomal abnormalities: one trisomy 21, one trisomy 13, and one apparently balanced de novo translocation 46,XX,rcp(2;8)(q11;q24). Hankins et al.[99] found eighty-three discolored AF samples (seventy-seven green, six brown) among 1,227 amniocenteses. When compared with case-matched control subjects, patients with discolored AF showed no differences in the frequency of spontaneous abortions, cytogenetic abnormalities, infant abnormalities, preterm labor, or cesarean section deliveries. The only statistically significant difference between control and test patients was bleeding before amniocentesis (one of eighty-three control; thirty-two of eighty-three discolored) ($p <$ 0.001). Finally in 1986, Zorn et al.[100] reported 110 discolored AF samples among 3,349 amniocenteses. A significantly increased pregnancy loss rate (9 percent) was observed with discolored AF, in comparison with the entire group of pregnancies in which amniocentesis was performed at the same institution during the same period of time (1.6 percent). Using spectrophotometry, electrophoresis, isoelectric focusing, and chromatography, it was determined that in most cases the discoloring pigment was blood rather than meconium.

One caveat in interpreting the above studies is that all were conducted in the era before routine ultrasound. With ultrasound now ubiquitous, almost certainly many cases of fetal death would have been identified and managed earlier in pregnancy (i.e., before when traditional amniocentesis would have been performed [15–16 weeks]).

Safety of Genetic Amniocentesis

Potential risks of midtrimester amniocentesis are divided into those affecting the mother and those affecting the fetus.

Maternal Risks

Life-threatening maternal risks are almost nonexistent. Amnionitis occurs in approximately 1 per 1,000 women who undergo amniocentesis.[101] This may lead to fetal loss, but only the extraordinary case seems to be life threatening to the mother. A 1979 workshop identified one maternal death caused by complications of amniocentesis, apparently culled from more than 20,000 procedures.[102] Further details have never been published. We are unaware of any other claims of maternal deaths attributable to genetic amniocentesis. Additional potential complications include hemorrhage, injury to an intra-abdominal viscus, and blood-group sensitization.

Minor maternal problems, however, are not rare. In the 1972–1975 National Institute of Child Health and Development (NICHD) National Registry for Amniocentesis Study Group,[34] 2–3 percent of women experienced transient spotting or vaginal leakage of AF after amniocentesis. Although almost always limited in amount and duration, AF leakage could persist and lead to pregnancy loss. Oligohydramnios is a well-known cause of fetal deformation and pulmonary hypoplasia.[103] However, we have encountered several women who not only lost relatively large amounts of AF immediately after genetic amniocentesis but also continued to lose fluid for the remainder of the pregnancy. Surprisingly, all were delivered at term of normal infants.[104] We thus now recommend expectant obstetric management after persistent AF leakage, provided that couples are informed of the potential maternal and fetal risks. Appropriate surveillance should emphasize clinical indices of infection (e.g., increased leukocyte counts), ultrasonographic and clinical monitoring of fetal growth, and ultrasonographic assessment of AF volume. Such conservative management has been advocated by others as well.[105]

Uterine contractions (i.e., uterine cramping) immediately after amniocentesis are not rare. Again, expectant management and reassurance are generally all that is required. We have found that offering patients a single cup of coffee (nondecaffeinated), tea, or cocoa seems to decrease the occurrence of painful uterine contractions, presumably because of the β-sympathomimetic effects of the methyl xanthines in these liquids. Similarly, vaginal spotting is not rare but likewise is usually self-limited.

Direct Fetal Injury

Potential fetal risks include spontaneous abortion, injuries caused by needle puncture, placental separation, chorioamnionitis, premature labor, and injury caused by the withdrawal of AF (e.g., amniotic bands). Rare but reported direct needle injuries include ileocutaneous fistula, peritoneoparietal fistula, gangrene of an arm, ocular trauma, ileal atresia, porencephalic cysts, patellar disruption, brain injuries, peripheral nerve injury, and umbilical cord hematoma.[106–118] Some of these problems are more logically attributed to amniocentesis than others. Further, all except a few of these case reports occurred during the era before concurrent use of ultrasound.

In 1977, again before the routine use of ultrasound, Karp and Hayden[107] estimated the frequency of cutaneous scarring to be 1–3 percent if infants are carefully monitored for needle puncture scars. However, other studies have not observed nearly such a high frequency, and even if it was true in the mid-1970s, it seems no longer to be an issue. The U.K. collaborative amniocentesis study[84] indicated that genetic amniocentesis predisposes infants to severe orthopedic postural malformations (severe equinovarus or congenital hip dislocation). This proposition was supported by the view that such malformations can be caused by compression of the fetus as the result of decreased AF. However, this association was not seen either in the U.S. collaborative study[34] or in the Canadian collaborative study.[35,119] Furthermore, the claim was explicitly refuted in a case–control study comprising a total of 1,342 British infants.[120]

Mother-to-Fetus Transmission of HIV during Amniocentesis

Amniocentesis has been associated with an increase in the rate of vertical transmission of human immunodeficiency virus (HIV) type 1.[121–123] However, with the advent of zidovudine chemoprophylaxis, the risk of transmission as a result of amniocentesis has been markedly reduced. Bucceri and coworkers[122] reported nine HIV-infected women who underwent amniocentesis between 16 and 20 weeks of gestation. Six of these women were on chemoprophylaxis, and none of ten infants born to these women were infected. The International Perinatal HIV Group[124] reported that five of nine HIV-infected women not on chemoprophylaxis undergoing amniocentesis were delivered of infected infants, whereas none of five infants born to women taking zidovudine were infected. We conclude that HIV-infected women electing to have amniocentesis should be on chemoprophylaxis.

Pregnancy Losses

Although most spontaneous abortions occur during the first trimester, losses may also occur during the second trimester. Moreover, older women are relatively more likely to have a spontaneous abortion than are younger women.[125] Age-related phenomena could possibly influence frequencies of premature delivery and other adverse pregnancy outcomes. Thus, the only reports to which any real weight can be attached are those in which subjects undergoing amniocentesis are matched with controls not undergoing the procedure, after which the excess fetal loss in the subject group may thus be assessed. Three major national collaborative studies (U.S., U.K., and Canadian studies) of the risks of amniocentesis have now been published (see Table 2.1). A fourth major study, a randomized trial in Denmark, provides data appropriate for the 1990s. Again, most were conducted before routine use of concurrent ultrasound.

U.S. Collaborative Study

The first major prospective study, coordinated by the U.S. NICHD, 1972–1975, comprised 1,040 subjects and 992 matched controls.[34] The sample sizes were established on the basis of calculations indicating that a doubling in the risk of particular adverse occurrences (e.g., spontaneous abortion, prematurity) would be detected with high probability. Of the 1,040 women undergoing amniocentesis, 950 (91.3 percent) underwent the procedure performed

Table 2.1. Summary of collaborative amniocentesis studies

	U.S. Study (%)	U.S. Controls (%)	Canadian Study (%)	U.K. Study (%)	U.K. Controls (%)	U.K. Suppl. Study (%)	U.K. Suppl. Controls (%)
Patients	1,040	992	1,020	1,402	1,402	1,026	1,026
Fetal losses	36 (3.5)	32 (3.2)	33 (3.2)	38 (2.7)	20 (1.4)	27 (2.6)	11 (1.11)[a]
Maternal complications (within 72 hours or, in some cases, within 1 week of amniocentesis)	25 (2.4)	—	37 (3.6)	—	—	—	—
Amniocentesis needle injuries	1 (0.1)	—	—	4 (0.3)	3 (0.2)	—	—
Infants with respiratory distress syndrome	30 (3.1)	20 (2.1)	—	17 (1.2)	6 (0.4)	13 (1.3)	3 (0.3)
Infants with severe orthopedic postural injuries	—	—	20 (1.4)	0 (0.0)	4 (0.4)	4 (0.4)	—

Source: For U.S. study, data from NICHD Amniocentesis Registry 1976;[34] for Canadian study, data from Medical Research Council 1976;[35] for U.K. study, data from Working Party on Amniocentesis 1978.[84]

[a]Before 28 weeks of gestation.

for cytogenetic analysis and 90 (8.7 percent) underwent the procedure to evaluate the possible presence of an inborn error of metabolism.

The frequency of immediate complications (e.g., leaking of AF, bleeding) was 2.4 percent, as already noted. However, few of these complications proved serious. Of all women who underwent amniocentesis, 3.5 percent experienced fetal loss after the procedure; of pregnant controls, 3.2 percent experienced fetal loss. A fetal loss during a previous pregnancy did not increase the risk for another fetal loss in the amniocentesis group. Likewise, neither the volume of AF removed nor the number of amniocentesis procedures performed before obtaining fluid (i.e., on different days) correlated with the frequency of fetal loss. One statistically significant association was a direct relationship between the frequency of vaginal bleeding after the procedure and the number of needle insertions. Complications of labor and delivery were also infrequent and did not differ significantly between subjects and controls. A significant difference in cesarean section rates was probably unrelated to the amniocentesis procedure per se.

Evaluations of case and control infants showed similar birth weights and similar 5-minute Apgar scores. One infant in the amniocentesis group had a small mark on its back that resembled a dermal sinus, an anomaly that may or may not have been caused by the amniocentesis needle. In the U.S. collaborative study, no other injuries were found, nor were there differences in the overall frequency of anomalies. Physical examination at 1 year of age yielded a few additional abnormalities, some more common in one group than the other; however, overall anomaly rates were similar. There were no differences in neurologic findings or developmental status.

This study concluded that "midtrimester amniocentesis is an accurate and highly safe procedure that does not add significant risk to the pregnancy." A caveat is that the loss rate in the control group is considerably higher than expected for that stage of gestation; in the general population 3 percent is the loss rate expected from 9 weeks of gestation onward, and perhaps 1 percent from 16 weeks.[126] Rates would be expected to be higher in an older age cohort but to what extent is unclear. In retrospect, the possibility of unwitting selection bias in the control group cannot be excluded.

Canadian Collaborative Study

A Canadian collaborative group[35,119] conducted a similar prospective study in the 1970s, but without a concurrent control group. A total of 1,223 amniocenteses were performed during 1,020 pregnancies in 900 women. The frequency of pregnancy loss was 3.2 percent, a rate similar to that observed in the concurrently conducted U.S. collaborative study. The frequency of immediate amniocentesis complications (e.g., bleeding, AF leakage) was 3.6 percent, but most of these complicated pregnancies did not terminate in a spontaneous abortion. This study showed significantly greater fetal losses when more than two needle insertions were made on a single day and when needles of 19 gauge or larger were used. Newborns were not evaluated for needle injuries. The study concluded, "Amniocentesis for the diagnosis of certain classes of genetic disease can now be considered safe, accurate and reliable when carried out at about 16 weeks' gestation, monitored by ultrasound and performed by an obstetrician trained to carry out the procedure during the second trimester of pregnancy."

U.K. Collaborative Study

In contrast to the U.S. and Canadian studies, the U.K. collaborative study[84] reached several different conclusions. This study, published in 1978, comprised 2,428 amniocentesis subjects, an equal number of matched controls, and another 506 unmatched subjects. Matching criteria for controls and subjects were changed during the course of the study. Thus, results were reported in two parts: a main division (1,042 matched subjects) and a supplementary division (1,026 matched subjects).

In the overall study, there were 59 (2.4 percent) spontaneous abortions (less than 28 weeks) among subjects and 28 (1.2 percent) among controls. Stillbirth rates were 1.2 percent ($n = 528$) among the subjects and 0.8 percent ($n = 519$) among the controls. There were 27 (1.1 percent) neonatal deaths among subjects and 11 (0.5 percent) among controls. As published, the study suggested that amniocentesis was directly responsible for a fetal wastage rate of about 1.5 percent.[84] There was also a significant increase in severe unexplained respiratory difficulties in infants born to amniocentesis subjects (1.3 percent), compared with controls (0.4 percent). This increase was most marked among infants born between 34 and 37 gestational weeks: (8.2 percent amniocentesis subjects; 0.9 percent controls). Furthermore, orthopedic postural abnormalities (talipes equinovarus, congenital hip dislocation, and subluxation of the hip) were observed in 1 percent of subjects and 0.2 percent of controls.

Because the U.K. study is at odds with the North American studies, further comment is warranted. The U.K. subjects were significantly older than the controls (3 percent in North America vs. 4 percent in the U.K. study were older than 40 years of age) and thus not unexpectedly of significantly greater parity (19 percent North American vs. 85 percent U.K. subjects were parous). Age differences alone might account for some of the increased fetal losses and antepartum hemorrhage. Indeed, in comparison with the U.S. and Canadian studies, the British study showed an apparent deficit of fetal loss among the controls rather than excess among the subjects. On the other hand, longitudinal studies in the United Kingdom and North America of ultrasonographically monitored pregnancies revealed surprisingly few losses in pregnancies that were viable at 8–16 weeks.[126–128]

The most likely explanation for differences among studies is that the indications for prenatal diagnosis differed between the 1973–1975 U.S. study and the 1978 U.K. study. In the U.S. study, almost all procedures were performed because of either advanced maternal age or previous trisomic infants. In the U.K. study, 10 percent of subjects underwent amniocentesis because a previous child had a neural tube defect (NTD) and 30 percent underwent the procedure because of increased MSAFP. In particular, increased MSAFP is now known to presage abnormal obstetric outcome unrelated to underlying fetal anomalies (see also chapter 21). If one excludes the 40 percent of subjects who underwent amniocentesis because of potential risk for NTDs, no statistically significant differences in fetal loss exist between the amniocentesis and the control groups. However, risks remain absolutely higher in the amniocentesis group.

Danish Study

In 1986 Tabor et al. published results of a randomized, controlled study of amniocentesis performed in Denmark on 4,606 women aged 25–34 years who were without known risk factors for fetal genetic abnormalities.[40] Women with three or more previous spontaneous abortions, diabetes mellitus, multiple gestation, uterine anomalies, or intrauterine contraceptive devices were excluded. Maternal age, social group, smoking history, and number of previous induced and spontaneous abortions, stillbirths, livebirths, and low-birth-weight infants were comparable in the study and control groups, as was gestational age at the time of entry into the study. Amniocentesis was performed under real-time ultrasound guidance with an 18-gauge needle. Thus, this was the first collaborative study of amniocentesis safety that routinely required ultrasound. Follow-up information was available for all but three women. The spontaneous abortion rate after 16 weeks was 1.7 percent in patients who had undergone amniocentesis compared with 0.7 percent in controls ($p < 0.01$), with a 2.6-fold relative risk of spontaneously aborting if the placenta was traversed. The frequency of postural deformations in the infants did not differ between the two groups. However, respiratory distress syndrome was diagnosed more often (relative risk, 2.1) in the study group, and more infants were treated for pneumonia (relative risk, 2.5).

Thai Study

In 1998 Tongsong[129] and co-workers reported a large-scale cohort study from Thailand in which singleton pregnant women between 15 and 24 weeks of gestation undergoing amniocentesis were matched prospectively to controls on a one-to-one basis for maternal age, parity, and socioeconomic status. A total of 2,256 pairs were recruited. After excluding pairs lost to follow-up, those with fetal malformations, and those with major chromosomal abnormalities, 2,045 matched pairs were compared for pregnancy outcomes. There were no significant differences in fetal loss rates, premature deliveries, or placental abruptions between the two groups ($p > 0.5$). However, this study did not have sufficient statistical power to detect differences less than 1 percent.

Greek Study

The most recent comparative study is that of Papantoniou and coworkers,[130] who reported from Athens a retrospective analysis of 1,006 women undergoing amniocentesis with singleton pregnancies. Among these women, 708 had a history of first-trimester spontaneous abortions and/or a second-trimester spontaneous abortion or pregnancy termination. Controls consisted of 4,024 women undergoing amniocentesis and who had no risk factors. In both groups amniocentesis was performed between 16 and 18 weeks of gestation. When cases and controls were stratified according to maternal age, a statistically significant difference in the fetal loss rate was observed between women aged 20–34 years (2.54 percent) and women >40 years (5.1 percent). Women with a history of bleeding per vagina during the current pregnancy also had a higher fetal loss rate (6.5 percent) compared with controls (2.8 percent). Women with a history of previous spontaneous abortions/terminations had a fetal loss rate of 8 percent, compared with a 2.8 percent loss rate among controls.

Conclusions Regarding Pregnancy Loss

Likelihood of pregnancy loss reflects (a) the experience of the obstetrician performing the procedure, (b) characteristics of the amniotic fluid sample studied (e.g., presence or absence of increased AF-AFP), (c) adjunctive use of high-resolution ultrasound, and (d) indication for testing. Given potential confounding variables, it is not surprising that controversy persists on the exact risks.

Further contributing to the controversy is that the pathogenesis of fetal losses after amniocentesis remains surprisingly obscure. One can hypothesize various mechanisms: infection, premature labor, abruptio placentae or other placental damage, umbilical cord injury, direct fetal puncture, and rupture of the membranes. The most informative cases of fetal loss should be those occurring within the first week after the procedure. Even large centers encounter few such occurrences, and rarely are any potential causes identified.

Perhaps fetal arrhythmias or causes that would not produce anatomic changes are explanatory. In our collective experience, we recall about twelve fetal losses among perhaps 30,000 amniocenteses. In a few cases there was evidence of infection, but in most, there was no ostensible explanation (no infection; no trauma to fetus or placenta). Perhaps a vagal response led to fetal cardiac arrest.

Overall, we conclude that the conventionally stated pregnancy loss rate of 0.5 percent is no longer appropriate in experienced hands. Surely it is illogical to counsel the same 0.5 percent risk offered a quarter century ago when ultrasound was not available. In support, Armstrong et al.[131] followed the outcome after 28,613 procedures performed by obstetricians throughout the United States, mostly for advanced maternal age. The total loss rate (combined background plus procedure-related) was only 1:362. It seems likely that in experienced hands the procedure-related risk following traditional amniocentesis is no more than 0.2–0.3 percent. Most recently, Eddleman et al.[132a] aconcluded that the procedure related loss rate after midtrimester amniocentesis was 0.15 percent. This was based on 1,605 subjects undergoing midtrimester amniocentesis compared to 26,187 control subjects not undergoing midtrimester amniocentesis. Thus, we counsel patients that (1) the added risk of fetal loss attributable to amniocentesis has been stated to be about 0.5 percent, but a lower risk of 0.2–0.3 percent or less is far more likely in high-volume centers staffed by a limited number of experienced operators; (2) the risk of major fetal injury consistent with pregnancy continuation is very remote; (3) even needle scarring is rare; and (4) the maternal risk appears very minimal.

Early Amniocentesis

Amniocentesis at 15–18 menstrual weeks and chorionic villus sampling (CVS) at 10–12 weeks are both accepted as safe and accurate methods of prenatal diagnosis. With the advent of high-resolution ultrasound equipment, many physicians have opted to offer genetic amniocentesis before the customary minimum threshold of 15 weeks of gestation. Some programs not offering CVS have viewed early amniocentesis (EA) as an attractive alternative for patients who desire prenatal diagnosis before the stage of pregnancy when traditional amniocentesis is performed. In other medical centers, EA was explored to obviate the inconvenience for patients of having to be rescheduled if they presented for CVS but were determined to be beyond 12 weeks of gestation (yet still earlier than 15 weeks of gestation).

Technique

The technique for EA is essentially the same as for traditional amniocentesis, except that a smaller volume of AF is withdrawn. Most centers, including ours, use the guideline of 1 mL per week of gestation. Concurrent ultrasound-based guidance of the needle is particularly important, given the relatively small target area and the need to avoid the maternal bladder and bowel. It is necessary to be alert for tenting of the membranes by the needle, which in our experience is the most common cause of failing to obtain AF with the initial insertion. The earlier in gestation one attempts amniocentesis, the more problematic membrane tenting becomes, given incomplete fusion of the chorion and the amnion.[132] Although virtually always successful in obtaining an adequate specimen for cytogenetic and AF-AFP analysis, we observed tenting of the membranes in almost 10 percent of early amniocentesis procedures.

Early Amniocentesis: Initial Experience The use of EA appears to be gaining in popularity, as evidenced by the number of recent reports from centers describing their initial experiences. Many of these reports, however, remain in abstract form. Herein, we review only series that have been published in full. Most reports date from the early to mid-1990s, and only the most recent report from any given center is considered.

In 1987, Hanson et al.[133] reported 541 amniocenteses performed before the 15th week of gestation: 4 procedures during the 11th week of gestation, 36 during the 12th week, 149 during the 13th week, and 352 during the 14th week. In 479 (88.5 percent) procedures, AF was obtained with the first needle insertion; 41 cases (7.6 percent) required two needle insertions, and two (0.4 percent) required three needle insertions. In 19 (3.5 percent) cases, AF was not obtained during the first visit, and the patient had to be brought back for a second procedure. Follow-up data were obtained for 298 (96.8 percent) of 308 cases for which information was possible (i.e., patients who would have given birth by the completion date of this study). Normal fetal outcome was the result in 90.3 percent of deliveries; 4.7 percent of known fetal outcomes resulted in some kind of loss: 11 (3.6 percent) spontaneous abortions before 28 weeks, 2 (0.7 percent) stillbirths, and 1 (0.3 percent) neonatal death. There were no culture failures. A total of 13 (2.4 percent) chromosomal abnormalities were diagnosed among the 541 early amniocenteses.

Evans et al.[134] reported 227 EAs between 10 and 14 weeks of gestation; the number of procedures performed at a given week of gestation was not stated. Although tenting of the membranes was observed in 5 percent of cases, AF was obtained with a single needle insertion in every case. One pregnancy loss occurred within the first week after the procedure and another loss occurred before 24 weeks of gestation (exact week not specified). The number of pregnancies allowed to continue and the completeness of follow-up was also not stated. Six fetal chromosomal abnormalities were detected among 224 successful AF cultures; 3 (1.3 percent) cultures yielded no growth.

Among 615 amniocenteses performed between the 9th and 16th weeks of gestation (menstrual age), Elejalde et al.[135] reported 323 procedures performed before the 15th week of gestation. Three procedures were performed during the 9th week of gestation, 6 during the 10th week, 18 during the 11th week, 77 during the 12th week, 98 during the 13th week, and 121 during the 14th week. In 19 (5.9 percent) of the 323 EA cases, AF was not obtained at first needle insertion, thereby necessitating a second tap. None needed three insertions. In one additional case, AF was not obtained at 12 weeks, but amniocentesis was successful at 14 weeks. The number of fetal losses after amniocentesis at each week of gestation was 0 of 3 at 9 weeks, 0 of 6 at 10 weeks, 2 of 18 (11.0 percent) at 11 weeks, 3 of 77 (3.9 percent) at 12 weeks, 2 of 98 (2.0 percent) at 13 weeks, and 1 of 121 (0.8 percent) at 14 weeks. There was also one stillbirth (gestation at amniocentesis not given). In the overall series of 615 cases, 7 (1.1 percent) women had AF leakage within 24 hours of amniocentesis, with one subsequent fetal loss (week of procedure not stated); among the 323 women undergoing procedures before 15 weeks, five (1.6 percent) had leakage within 24 hours. Cytogenetic results from those amniocenteses were not specified, but two AF cultures failed.

In a similar study, Bombard and Rigdon[136] conducted a prospective pilot study in which 150 patients were offered either genetic amniocentesis at the traditional time ($n = 75$) or EA ($n = 75$) (11–14 weeks of gestation; mean gestational age, 12.7 weeks). The study and control groups were comparable with respect to maternal ages, indications for testing, race, obstetric history (specifically vaginal bleeding), and placental location. There were no significant differences between the study and control groups with respect to losses (one each), needle insertions (1.06 vs. 1.05), placental puncture (14 vs. 10), or the presence of discolored AF (0 vs. 4). There were seven cytogenetic abnormalities detected in the study group versus none in the control group, possibly reflecting the increased prevalence of chromosomal abnormalities early in gestation. In evaluating twenty-five of the study infants 3–5 years later, there was a tendency for increased risk of respiratory difficulties in the study group.[137] The number of affected patients did not exceed the general population risk for these disorders, but statistical power for meaningful conclusions was limited.

In 1990 Stripparo et al.[138] reported 505 amniocenteses from two centers in Italy; 395 of the procedures were performed before 15 weeks of gestation, based on ultrasonographic biometric measurements. Thirteen amniocenteses were performed during the 11th week of gestation, 42 during the 12th week, 158 during the 13th week, and 182 during the 14th week. Results were not stratified per week of gestation. Moreover, investigators were successful in obtaining AF in all cases, with only three cases requiring a second needle insertion. AF leakage occurred in six cases, all of which subsequently resulted in livebirths (albeit one delivered at 35 weeks, with mild respiratory distress syndrome). Among pregnancies allowed to continue, the fetal loss rates before 28 weeks of gestation, categorized according to week of gestation during which amniocentesis was performed, were 3 of 13 (23.1 percent) at 11 weeks, 5 of 41 (12.2 percent) at 12 weeks, 6 of 154 (3.9 percent) at 13 weeks, and 1 of 176 (0.6 percent) at 14 weeks. There were eight culture failures and ten (2.0 percent) chromosomal abnormalities in the 505 cases.

Penso et al.[139] reported 407 early amniocenteses, including one set of twins. These were performed at the following gestational ages: 9 at 11 weeks, 179 at 12 weeks, 177 at 13 weeks, and 42 at 14 weeks. There was no mention of needing to insert the needle more than once, nor was there mention of any failures in obtaining AF. Culture failure occurred in seven specimens (1.7 percent), and the frequency of chromosomal abnormalities was 3.8 percent. There were nine spontaneous abortions within 4 weeks of amniocentesis: one after a procedure performed during the 11th week of gestation, two after a 12th-week procedure, three after a 13th-week procedure, and three after a 14th-week procedure. There were six additional losses: three at <28 weeks and three at >28 weeks. Thus, the overall fetal loss rate was 25 of 389 (6.4 percent) in cases for which follow-up data were available. There were no neonatal deaths. The postprocedure incidence of AF leakage was 2.6 percent. Of particular interest, there were eight congenital orthopedic deformities, including four cases of clubbed feet and one case each of hyperextended knees, scoliosis, congenital dislocation of the knees, and congenital dislocation of the hips. Three of the eight postural deformities were associated with fluid leakage after amniocentesis.

Hackett et al.[140] reported 106 EAs between 11 and 14 weeks of gestation (ultrasound-based dating): Of these, five procedures were performed at 11 weeks, twenty-four at 12 weeks, forty-two at 13 weeks, and thirty-five at 14 weeks of gestation. There were also two "dry taps": in one of the two cases, a successful amniocentesis was performed 1 week later; in the other case, there were two additional unsuccessful attempts at 14 and 15 weeks, and finally, a successful transabdominal CVS (TA-CVS). All AF cultures grew successfully. Chromosome analysis revealed ninety-nine normal karyotypes, two balanced translocations, two tetraploids, and two cases of pseudomosaicism. There were two fetal losses: in one case, a spontaneous abortion occurred 1 week after an amniocentesis at 12 weeks of gestation; in the other case, a fetal death was diagnosed at 20 weeks of gestation, after an amniocentesis at 13 weeks of gestation. In both cases, the fetal chromosomal complements were normal. In two other cases, leakage of AF occurred: one case at 24 hours, after a 13th-week amniocentesis, and the other at 24 weeks gestation, after a 13th-week amniocentesis. Interpretation of these results is limited because 29 of the 103 continuing pregnancies were undelivered at the time of publication.

In contrast, the study of Bombard et al.,[141] which involved a single surgeon performing all procedures, was more reassuring. One hundred twenty-one patients underwent EA during these same gestational ages (i.e., 10–13 weeks). During the 24-month period, there was only one loss (0.8 percent), and there were no repeat procedures or culture failures. This compared favorably with results noted at later gestational ages (uncorrected fetal loss rate of 0.8 percent; 24 of 2,902). The only apparent methodologic difference was use of a thinner procedure needle (22-gauge) in the U.S. cohort.

Brumfield et al.[142] reported a retrospective, cohort study of 314 women undergoing EA (at 11–14 weeks of gestation) who were matched to 628 controls undergoing traditional genetic amniocentesis (16–19 weeks of gestation). Women who had an EA were significantly more likely to have postprocedural AF leakage (2.9 percent vs. 0.2 percent), postprocedure vaginal bleeding (1.9 percent vs. 0.2 percent), and a fetal loss within 30 days of the procedure (2.2 percent vs. 0.2 percent) than women undergoing traditional amniocentesis. However, as opined by Wilson et al.[143] several potential biases in the Brumfield report limit the validity of their conclusions. Selection biases included discrepancies of gestational age (i.e., cases and controls were not truly matched), limited use of continuous ultrasound guidance, and use of fetal abnormalities as an exclusion criterion.

The group at the University of Tennessee, Memphis, compared their first 250 EAs (14 weeks or less) to their first 250 cases of TA-CVS (9.5–12.9 weeks).[144] Culture failure rates for both procedures were 0.8 percent. Loss rates for EA and TA-CVS were 3.8 percent and 2.1 percent, respectively. Transplacental needle passage did not appear to increase the risk of pregnancy loss.[30,145] Included in this series were the results of EA in six twin gestations (mean, 11.9 weeks; range, 10.5–13.6 weeks), using a similar dye-injection technique as described for traditional amniocentesis (see above).[146] Both amniotic sacs were successfully sampled in each of six cases (five required two needle insertions, one required three needle insertions); all cultures yielded normal cytogenetic results; all six pregnancies resulted in the delivery of healthy infants.

In 1996 Diaz Vega and colleagues reported 181 ultrasound-guided genetic amniocenteses performed at 10–12 weeks of gestation, the most relevant time period to which EA would be offered as an alternative to CVS.[147] AF was obtained in 98.4 percent of the cases, on the first attempt in 167 of 181 patients. The culture success rate was 94.5 percent. There were three fetal losses (1.6 percent) at 12 days (ultrasound showed nuchal edema) and two fetal losses (1.1 percent) at 21 and 23 weeks of gestation. There was no control group, but the authors stated that the pregnancy outcome and perinatal results were similar to those in other centers in Spain.

Early Amniocentesis: Comparative Trials Except for some reports,[148] the early 1990s saw a tendency to conclude that EA was as safe as traditional amniocentesis. This may have been partly influenced by a desire to provide an alternative to first-trimester CVS. However, in the reports reviewed above, sample sizes were usually small, and the outcome measured was limited to fetal loss rates. Later and usually larger studies considered other outcomes and have arrived at less salutary conclusions.

In 1994 Nicolaides et al.[149] reported a prospective study comparing transabdominal CVS and EA at 10–13 weeks of gestation in a total of 1,492 singleton pregnancies. Patients were offered the option of having transabdominal CVS or EA or to be randomized into one of the two procedures, both being performed using a "freehand" technique with a 20-gauge needle. CVS was performed in 652 cases (375 by patient choice and 277 by randomization), and EA was performed in 840 cases (562 by patient choice and 278 by randomization). The two techniques were comparable at providing a sample (CVS, 99.3 percent; early amniocentesis, 100 percent) and the need for repeat testing (CVS, 2.5 percent; early amniocentesis, 2.1 percent). However, the main indications for repeat testing differed between the two groups. In the CVS group, the principal indication for repeat testing was chromosomal mosaicism (1.1 percent compared with 0.1 percent for early amniocentesis; $x^2 = 56.27$, $p < 0.01$), whereas in the early amniocentesis group, it was culture failure (2.0 percent compared with 0.6 percent for CVS; $x^2 = 55.26$, $p < .01$). The rate for culture failure in early amniocentesis was inversely related to gestational age: 7 of 168 (4.2 percent) at 10 weeks; 8 of 369 (2.2 percent) at 11 weeks; 2 of 192 (1.0 percent) at 12 weeks; and 0 of 111 at 13 weeks. Outcome was available in all but one case.

In the Nicolaides et al.[149] study spontaneous losses (intrauterine or neonatal death) after EA (total group, 4.9 percent; randomized subgroup, 5.8 percent) were significantly greater than after CVS (total group, 2.1 percent; randomized subgroup, 1.8 percent; difference, 2.8 percent, 95 percent confidence interval, 1.3–4.3 percent; and difference 4 percent, 95 percent confidence interval, 1.3–.7 percent). In the EA group, the incidence of talipes equinovarus (1.66 percent) was greater than in the CVS group, but this difference was not significantly different. The authors concluded that early amniocentesis at 10–11 weeks is associated with a significantly greater rate of fetal loss; at 12–13 weeks, the risk may also be greater.

Vandenbussche et al.[150] used an experimental design similar to that of Nicolaides et al.[149] Among 192 women, 102 consented to randomization and had a follow-up of at least 6 weeks after the procedure. Of the 102, 66 and 24 chose EA and CVS, respectively. There were 8 unintended fetal losses among 120 EAs, compared with none among 64 CVS procedures—a difference of 6.7 percent (95 percent confidence interval, 2.2–11.1 percent). These investigators believed that the risks of EA were so great that continuation of their trial could not be ethically justified.

Given these results, standard textbooks[151] began stating that EA "must be viewed with caution," being unlikely to be comparable in safety to either CVS or traditional amniocentesis. Further confirming concern was a Canadian collaborative study. In a preliminary study, in 1996 Johnson et al.[152] compared the safety of EA at (11–12 weeks, 6 days) to that of midtrimester amniocentesis (15–16 weeks, 6 days). Among 638 women randomized and followed to pregnancy completion, there were 27 of 344 (7.8 percent) spontaneous abortions and 25 of 399 (7.4 percent) induced abortions (difference: 0.4 percent; 95 percent confidence interval, 3.6–4.4 percent). There were no diagnostic errors. Johnson et al.[152] concluded that early amniocentesis appears to be as safe and accurate as midtrimester genetic amniocentesis. This led to the design of a larger presumably definitive study, called The Canadian Early and Mid-Trimester Amniocenteses Trial (CEMAT) Group.[153,154]

Unexpectedly, results of the full Canadian study were different from preliminary data of Johnson et al.[152] EAs ($n = 2,183$) were performed between 11 weeks, 0 days and 12 weeks, 6 days; midtrimester amniocenteses were performed between 15 weeks, 0 days, and 16 weeks, 6 days. In the EA ($n = 2,185$) cohort, 1,916 women (87.8 percent) underwent amniocentesis before 13 weeks of gestation. First, there was a significant difference in the total fetal losses for EA compared with midtrimester amniocenteses (7.6 percent vs. 5.9 percent); difference 1.7 percent, one-sided confidence interval, 2.98 percent, $p = 0.012$). A significant increase in talipes equinovarus was found in the EA group compared with the midtrimester amniocenteses group (1.3 percent vs. 0.1 percent, $p = 0.0001$). Even more disturbingly, there was a significant difference in postprocedural AF fluid leakage (EA 3.5 percent vs. midtrimester amniocenteses 1.7 percent, $p = 0.0007$). Failed procedures, multiple needle insertions and culture failures also occurred more frequently in the EA group.

In 1997 Sundberg et al.[155] reported a randomized cohort study encompassing 581 women undergoing 11th- to 13th-week EA and 579 undergoing 10th- to 12th-week transabdominal CVS. The most significant finding related to the striking difference in talipes equinovarus (TE): (1.7 percent EA vs. zero in CVS) and hip subluxation (0.8 percent EA vs. 0.2 percent CVS). The percentage of TE cases was almost identical to that observed by Nicolaides et al.[149] The greatest frequency of the anomaly was found when the gestational age at procedures was 80–88 days. AF leakage occurred in 4.4 percent of EA cases and in no CVS cases.

There was limited power to assess the fetal loss rate because the increased risk of anomalies necessitated cessation of the trial. However, despite CVS being performed earlier and being associated with more chromosomal abnormalities (1.6 percent vs. 0.7 percent), the total fetal loss rate was still the same or higher (5.4 percent) with EA compared with CVS (4.8 percent).

Conclusions virtually identical to those of the Canadian Early and Mid-Trimester Amniocentesis Trial (CEMAT)[153] and the Danish study of Sundberg et al.[155] were reached by a collaborative study funded by the National Institute of Child Health and Human Development that encompassed fourteen centers in the United States, Denmark, and Canada,[156] including ours. One important prerequisite was that in all participating centers, operators had to have performed at least twenty-five amniocentesis and twenty-five CVS procedures in the 11- to 14-week interval of gestation before the trial began. Subjects were then randomized between the two procedures, stratified by gestational week. Initially, gestational weeks 11–14 were to be studied, but following the report of Sundberg et al.[155] the study was confined first to 12–14 weeks and finally to only 13–14 weeks. On completion of the study, 3,698 cytogenetically normal subjects had been randomized. Unintended postprocedure losses <20 weeks (spontaneous plus therapeutic abortions related to procedure complications, such as amniotic band disruption or amniotic fluid leakage) were higher with EA than with late CVS. Overall, combined complications totaled 16 of 1878 in the CVS group versus 27 of 1820 EA group, nearing significance at 13 weeks ($p = 0.54$). With a larger sample significance would likely have reached $p < 0.05$ for fetal loss. Irrespective, the most significant finding of Philip and colleagues[156] was not procedure-related losses but rather increased talipes equinovarus (TE). Three cases followed CVS and 12 followed EA (relative risk, 4.13, 95 percent confidence interval, 1.17–14.6 percent; $p = 0.017$). No limb reduction defects were reported. TE was thus found by Nicolaides et al.,[149] CEMAT,[153] Sundberg et al.,[155] and Philip et al.[156]

Improving Culture Success in Early Amniocentesis

Because of relatively lower AF cell concentrations during the weeks when EA is performed (11–14 weeks), it has been suggested that filtration and recirculation of AF at EA might increase cell yield and reduce the culture time before karyotyping.[157–159] Such manipulations are probably unnecessary. In the series reported by Hanson et al.[160] 936 amniocenteses were performed at 12.8 weeks or less; mean culture time was 8.8 days (SD, 1.5 days), and only a single patient required a repeat procedure because of inadequate cell growth. Among 1,375 EA fluid samples (14 weeks or less), Lockwood and Neu[161] reported that 1,356 of 1,375 (98.6 percent) were successfully cultured and yielded cytogenetic results. Moreover, recent data suggest that the increased time required to perform filtration may increase the risk of AF leakage and fetal loss.[162]

A final unresolved concern is whether interpretation of AF-AFP and acetyl-cholinesterase carries the same sensitivity and specificity for detection of open NTDs compared with midtrimester analysis, especially when samples are obtained at 12 weeks of gestation or less.[163–165] (See also chapters 21 and 22.) Crandall and Chua identified 42 open NTDs among 7,440 amniocenteses performed between 11 and 15 weeks of gestation.[166] The detection rate was 100 percent each for anencephaly and spina bifida, and 78 percent for encephalocele using an AF-AFP threshold >2.0 MoM and positive acetyl-cholinesterase (AChE). Excluding fetal death and other obvious abnormalities, the false-positive rate using AF-AFP was 0.6 percent; for AChE, it was 0.1 percent. Among AF samples obtained before 13 weeks of gestation, the AChE false-positive rate was 6.3 percent. Nearly all samples showed two very faint bands that were easily distinguished from that which is noted in open NTD (i.e., true-positive results). However, the authors cautioned that there remain insufficient data to determine the sensitivity and specificity of these tests before 13 weeks of gestation. They recommended that MSAFP and ultrasound examination should be performed between 16 and 18 weeks of gestation for patients who have undergone EA.

Conclusions

It is not implausible that amniocentesis at 11–14 weeks of gestation should be a relatively safe and efficacious technique, as is the case for traditional amniocentesis (>15 weeks). However, available data are not supportive. In our opinion, EA cannot be recommended, especially before 14 gestational weeks.

1. Almost all reports of early amniocentesis describe relatively greater difficulty in obtaining AF, often due to membrane tenting and particularly if less than 13 weeks of gestation.
2. EA carries an increased risk of procedure-related loss, compared with both traditional amniocentesis as well as late CVS.
3. The prevalence of TE is unequivocally increased, and hip subluxation is probably as well.
4. Earlier favorable series often reached overarching conclusions. Most series define EA as a procedure performed between 10 and 14 weeks of gestation, yet the majority of these procedures were actually performed during the 13th and 14th weeks of gestation. Data concerning accuracy and safety must be stratified according to the week of gestation before generalizations are made.
5. Some data suggest increased risk for newborn respiratory distress after midtrimester amniocentesis.[40] Gestational weeks 12–14 (and earlier) are especially critical for fetal lung development, according to some authorities.[167] Thus, respiratory compromise after EA would also clearly be a concern. Indeed, Penso and colleagues[139] found pulmonary complications in 6.6 percent of infants born after EA; 1.6 percent of infants exhibit respiratory distress syndrome.
6. Concern has been raised about the interpretation of the presence of AChE before 13 weeks of gestation.[168] There are insufficient data to define the sensitivity and specificity of detecting open NTDs in AF obtained by early amniocentesis.[169]
7. The number of viable amniotic fluid cells increases with gestational age; therefore, not unexpectedly, the number of culture failures and the time required for

culture growth before harvesting might be increased at earlier gestational ages.[133,135] This has not, however, been the universal experience.

8. It is uncertain whether the AF cell types obtained by early amniocentesis are the same as those cultured from AF obtained from traditional amniocentesis. Such cells are derived from embryonic as well as extraembryonic tissues, and their composition in AF may differ at various gestational ages. Accordingly, rates of chromosomal mosaicism resulting from "confined placental mosaicism" could be higher in early amniocentesis compared with CVS or traditional amniocentesis.

FETAL BLOOD SAMPLING

For many years, fetal visualization and tissue sampling (e.g., blood, skin) within the gravid uterine cavity were accomplished by fetoscopy, a procedure in which a rigid endoscopic instrument was inserted percutaneously through the mother's abdomen and the target tissues (umbilical cord, fetus, and chorionic surface of the placenta) were directly evaluated.[170,171] This direct approach to fetal assessment has been replaced by a more indirect, potentially less morbid, ultrasonographically guided method. When fetal blood is withdrawn from the umbilical cord, the procedure may be referred to in several ways: fetal blood sampling, percutaneous umbilical blood sampling (PUBS), funicentesis, or cordocentesis. All terms are synonymous.

Fetal blood sampling for prenatal diagnosis is most often preferred for rapid fetal karyotyping, evaluation of fetal hematologic disorders, identification of fetal infection (by culture or molecular typing), drug therapy, and the treatment of fetal anemia by transfusion. PUBS for fetal blood chromosome analysis has been used to help clarify purported chromosomal mosaicism detected in cultured AF cells and/or chorionic villi.[172] Rapid assessment of fetal chromosome complement has been accomplished by "direct" cytogenetic analysis of uncultured nucleated blood cells.[173] Short-term fetal lymphocyte cultures usually can provide a cytogenetic result within 48–72 hours; direct analysis of spontaneously dividing cells can provide results within 24 hours. Such rapid sampling and evaluation become attractive in clinical scenarios in which patients present after the usual interval for prenatal diagnosis is past (e.g., 22–24 weeks of gestation), when the results from genetic amniocentesis would be completed only after elective pregnancy termination is no longer readily available in most locations.

In addition, many cases of fetal structural abnormalities such as intrauterine growth restriction (IUGR) do not become apparent until later in pregnancy—often the third trimester. In such instances, rapid results may prove useful for decision-making with regard to obstetric management and mode of delivery.[174,175] More recently, fluorescence in situ hybridization (FISH) and comparative genomic hybridization (CGH) technologies, employing chromosome-specific DNA probes have also been used for rapid prenatal diagnosis of aneuploidy using nucleated fetal erythrocytes from the umbilical cord as well as amniocytes.

FETAL HEMATOLOGIC DISORDERS

Fetal blood sampling was once used for the prenatal evaluation of many fetal hematologic abnormalities.[176] Normative hematologic and blood chemistry values have been reported and are applicable for second-trimester fetuses.[177–179] Furthermore, fetal hematocrit can be directly measured to assess fetal hemolysis resulting from Rh or other antigen incompatibility and isoimmunization states.[180] Previously, obstetricians had to rely on indirect evidence of fetal hemolysis such as maternal antibody titers, past obstetric history, abnormal ultrasound findings such as hydrops fetalis, and spectrophotometry of AF bilirubin. The need for subsequent fetal transfusions (which had theretofore been accomplished by the injection of compatible donor erythrocytes into the fetal peritoneal cavity) was based on somewhat arbitrary perinatal guidelines. Now, the decisions about which fetus, when in gestation, transfusion volume, and transfusion frequency can be made more rationally on the basis of actual fetal blood component analyses such as hemoglobin level, hematocrit level, blood group, direct antiglobulin titer, and reticulocyte count.[181,182] Fetal hemoglobin can be directly evaluated to diagnose sickle cell disease, α- or β-thalassemias, or other hemoglobinopathies,[171,183] although these disorders can now also be correctly identified employing DNA analysis of chorionic villi or AF cells. Fetal blood sampling can also be used to assess platelet quantity and quality of function.[184,185] PUBS is useful not only for the evaluation of maternal platelet antigen PLA2 in alloimmunization, but also, access to the fetal circulation allows for therapeutic alternatives including in utero platelet transfusion or maternal immunotherapy with γ-globulin or steroids.[186]

Fetal blood has also been used for the diagnosis of various coagulation factor abnormalities in the fetus, such as hemophilia A, hemophilia B, and von Willebrand disease.[179,187] In addition to hematologic studies, fetal blood samples have been used to diagnose autosomal recessive or X-linked immunologic deficiencies, including severe combined immunodeficiency (SCID), Chédiak–Higashi syndrome, Wiskott–Aldrich syndrome, and chronic granulomatous disease.[188–191]

Fetal Infection

Recovery of fetal blood permits assessment of viral, bacterial, and parasitic infections of the fetus (see chapter 30). Detection of fetal viral or parasitic infection is usually made on the basis of maternal antibody titers or ultrasound-detected fetal structural abnormalities (e.g., cranial microcalcifications). Serum fetal blood titers permit quantification of antibody titers.[192,193] In addition to antibody titers, PUBS can be used for direct analysis of viral, bacterial, and parasitic infections by culture of and/or molecular amplification of vector-specific DNA sequences in fetal blood.[193–198] Access to the fetal vasculature allows in utero transfusion for fetal anemia and hydrops caused by infections such as parvovirus B19.

Fetal Therapy

In addition to in utero vascular transfusion of blood products using PUBS, drug therapy is also possible. For example, fetal arrhythmias have been treated with the direct infusion of antiarrhythmic medications, and fetal paralysis may be induced to facilitate invasive procedures such as transfusions or for magnetic resonance imaging (MRI).[199] Fetal diagnosis and treatment of fetal goitrous hypothyroidism has also been reported.[200–202] (See also chapters 25 and 29.)

Technique of Fetal Blood Sampling

The technique now most commonly employed for fetal blood sampling is ultrasound-guided PUBS. Usually performed from 18 weeks of gestation onward, successful procedures have been reported as early as 12 weeks.[203–205]

PUBS can be performed as an outpatient procedure. Maternal sedation is usually unnecessary, but when a prolonged procedure is anticipated (such as with fetal transfusion), an oral benzodiazepine taken 1–2 hours before the procedure begins may be of benefit. Preliminary ultrasonographic examination of the fetus should be performed before PUBS to assess fetal viability, placental and umbilical cord location, fetal or placental abnormalities, and fetal position. A suitable site for needle insertion is then selected.

The skin over the needle insertion site is anesthetized with 0.5 mL of 1 percent xylocaine. A sterile field is established—we prefer cleansing the skin with an iodine-based solution and/or alcohol—and sterile drapes are applied. The ultrasound transducer is placed on the abdomen away from the sterile insertion site but at a location that permits visualization of the complete path of the needle from maternal skin to the target fetal blood vessel.

There are several potential sampling sites. Because of its fixed position, the umbilical cord root (site of placental attachment) is usually the site of choice whenever it is clearly visible and accessible. Alternatively, free loops of umbilical cord or the fetal hepatic vein are possibilities.[176,205,206] We prefer a 22-gauge, acute-angle, single end-port, echo-enhanced needle such as the "Ultra-Vue" procedure needle manufactured by Becton-Dickinson (Rutherford, NJ).

After percutaneous insertion of the spinal needle into the fetal blood vessel under direct ultrasound guidance, a small amount of blood is aspirated. The presence of fetal blood in this initial sample is confirmed using a model ZBI Coulter counter and channelizer to differentiate fetal or maternal blood on the basis of erythrocyte volume. An alternative "quick" bedside technique used in our institution is a modification of the Apt test. A drop of fetal blood is placed into a prepared KOH solution specifically set aside for PUBS testing. The amount of blood aspirated for diagnosis depends on the indication for diagnosis by PUBS but rarely exceeds 5 mL.

On completion of the fetal blood sampling procedure, the spinal needle is withdrawn and an ultrasound examination is performed to evaluate fetal status. At our centers, all women at risk for Rh isoimmunization receive 300 μg of Rh immune globulin after the procedure.

Safety of Fetal Blood Sampling

Fetal blood sampling appears to be a relatively safe procedure when performed by experienced surgeons, albeit carrying greater risk than either CVS or amniocentesis. However accurate statistical comparison of risk is difficult because fetuses undergoing PUBS are already at substantially increased risk—based on their indications for testing—compared with those undergoing CVS or amniocentesis. Genuine control groups are difficult to identify.

Maternal complications from PUBS are rare but include amnionitis and transplacental hemorrhage.[187,207] Data from large perinatal centers estimate that the fetal risks of death in utero or subsequent spontaneous abortion to be 3 percent or less after PUBS.[178,187,191,194,208–210] Collaborative data from fourteen North American centers, sampling 1,600 patients at varying gestational ages, revealed an uncorrected fetal loss rate of 1.6 percent.[211]

In 1993, Ghidini et al. used all the articles published in the English literature to estimate the incidence of complications related to PUBS, dividing losses according to when they occurred (before or after 28 weeks), concluding that the procedure carries a 1.4 percent risk of fetal loss before 28 weeks and a 1.4 percent risk of perinatal death after 28 weeks (total loss rate, 2.8 percent).[208] The authors used as a denominator the total number of patients on whom the procedure was performed before 28 weeks; this led to an underestimate of the loss rate before 24 weeks.

Buscaglia et al. reported their experience in performing 1,272 PUBS procedures.[210] Total procedure-related losses were 2.3 percent; 1.6 percent were intrauterine fetal deaths occurring within 48 hours of the procedure, and 0.7 percent were spontaneous abortions occurring within 2 weeks of the procedure.

In a 1996 review of 1,260 PUBS procedures performed at the University of Iowa ($n =$ 5,838) and the Tohoku University ($n =$ 5,422), Weiner and Okamura reported twelve procedure-related losses, yielding an overall perinatal loss rate of 0.9 percent.[211] For all diagnoses other than chromosomal abnormalities and severe intrauterine growth restriction, the procedure-related loss rate was 2 of 1,021 (0.2 percent).

Chinaiya et al.[205] performed fetal blood sampling on 382 women over a 7-year period from 13 weeks of gestation onward. In 292 of 382 (76.4 percent) cases, the intrahepatic part of the umbilical vein was targeted; in 70 of 382 (18.3 percent) cases, PUBS was performed; in 20 of 382 (5.2 percent) of cases, cardiocentesis was performed. Multivariate analysis showed an increased odds of fetal loss for PUBS and cardiocentesis compared with the intrahepatic vein (IHV) fetal blood sampling group. Fetal loss was significantly increased ($p > 0.01$) only in the cardiocentesis group for fetal loss, within 2 weeks of performing the procedure.

Baseline loss rates for patients undergoing PUBS or IHV sampling vary greatly with the indication for the procedure. Loss rates for fetuses with ultrasound-detected anomalies are far greater than for fetuses being evaluated for hemolytic diseases secondary to maternal blood-group sensitization. Studies directly comparing loss rates in control and treated groups have been published, none being randomized. The only cohort comparison study is by Tongsong et al.,[183] who followed 1,281 Thai women undergoing freehand cordocentesis between 16 and 24 weeks. Women with no overt fetal anomalies (and thus not requiring a procedure) served as controls. Indications for PUBS were increased risk for thalassemia (61 percent), rapid karyotyping (21 percent) or both (8.7 percent). Exclusion of some matched pairs left 1,029 pairs for comparisons. Loss rates were 3.2 percent (subjects) versus 1.8 percent (controls) with no differences in obstetric complications.

An overall confounder in all studies of this type is that baseline loss rates for patients undergoing PUBS or IHV fetal blood sampling vary greatly with the indication of the procedure.[212] Loss rates are far greater for fetuses with ultrasound-detected anomalies than for fetuses evaluated for hemolytic diseases secondary to maternal blood-group sensitization for late booking or for clarification of mosaicism at amniocentesis. Thus, data regarding loss rates in matched control and treated groups will be necessary to determine the true safety of PUBS and IHV fetal blood sampling. Overall, procedure-related loss rates of at least 1 percent, if not 1.5 percent, should be assumed.

The relationship between fetomaternal transfusion and pregnancy outcome was studied by Sikovanyecz et al.[213] Analyzing measurements of maternal serum α-fetoprotein levels before and after PUBS in 221 cases, maximum and mean amounts of fetomaternal transfusion were 1.067 mL and 0.061 mL, respectively. Positive correlation was found between fetomaternal transfusion and postprocedure bleeding time ($r = 0.174$, $p < 0.0129$) and duration of the procedure ($r = 0.165$, $p < 0.0171$). Comparing PUBS performed at the placental insertion site and at the free cord loop, a smaller amount of fetomaternal transfusion was observed in the latter ($p < 0.0123$). There was no association between the degree of maternofetal transfusion and pregnancy outcome. Potential fetal complications that may lead to fetal death or premature delivery included iatrogenic infection, premature rupture of the membranes, hemorrhage, severe fetal bradycardia, cord tamponade or thrombosis, and abruptio placenta.[176] Van Selm et al.[214] and Buscaglia et al.[210] also showed that PUBS is frequently associated with fetomaternal hemorrhage, which in turn was correlated with anterior position of the placenta, duration of the procedure, and number of needle insertions.

REFERENCES

1. Lambl D, Ein seltener fall von hydramnios. Zentralbl Gynaekol 1881;5:329.
2. Schatz F. Eine besondere art von ein seitiger polyhdramnic mit anderseitiger oligohydramnie bei zwillingen. Arch Gynecol 1882;19:392.
3. Menees TD, Miller JD, Holly LE. Amniography: preliminary report. AJR Am J Roentgenol 1930;24:363.
4. Aburel ME. Le declenchement du travail par injections intraamniotique de serum sale hypertonique. Gynecol Obstet 1937;36:398.
5. Gadow EC. Reaching the fetal environment: A tribute to Dr. Hermógenes Alvarez. Prenat Diagn 1998;18:870.
6. Bevis DCA. The antenatal prediction of haemolytic disease of the newborn. Lancet 1952;1:395.
7. Fuchs F, Riis P. Antenatal sex determination. Nature 1956;117:330.
8. Shettles LB. Nuclear morphology of cells in human amniotic fluid in relation to sex of infant. Am J Obstet Gynecol 1956;71:834.
9. Makowski EL, Prem K, Kaiser IH. Detection of sex of fetuses by the incidence of sex chromatin in nuclei of cells in amniotic fluid. Science 1945;123:542.
10. Steele MW, Breg WR Jr. Chromosome analysis of human amniotic fluid cells. Lancet 1966;1:383.
11. Jacobson CB, Barter RH. Intrauterine diagnosis and management of genetic defects. Am J Obstet Gynecol 1967;99:795.
12. Valenti C, Schutta EJ, Kehaty T. Prenatal diagnosis of Down's syndrome. Lancet 1968;2:220.
13. Nadler HL. Antenatal detection of hereditary disorders. Pediatrics 1968;42:912.
14. Milunsky A. The prenatal diagnosis of hereditary disorders. Springfield, IL: Charles C Thomas, 1973.
15. Nadler HL, Gerbie AB. Role of amniocentesis in the intrauterine detection of genetic disorders. N Engl J Med 1970;282:596.
16. Littlefield JW. The pregnancy at risk for a genetic disorder. N Engl J Med 1970;282:627.
17. Elias S, Annas GJ. Reproductive genetics and the law. Chicago: Year Book, 1987.
18. Simpson JL, Elias S. Prenatal diagnosis of genetic disorders. In: Creasy RK, Resnik R, eds. Maternal-fetal medicine: principles and practice, 2nd ed. Philadelphia: WB Saunders, 1989:78.
19. Verp MS, Simpson JL. Amniocentesis for prenatal genetic diagnosis. In: Filkins K, Russo JR, eds. Human prenatal diagnosis. New York: Marcel Decker, 1990:305.
20. Simpson JL, Elias S. Genetics in obstetrics and gynecology, 3rd ed. Philadelphia: WB Saunders, 2003.
21. Simpson JI. Genetic counseling and prenatal diagnosis. In: Gabbe SG, Niebyl JR, Simpson JL, eds. Obstetrics: normal and problem pregnancies, 4th ed. New York: Churchill Livingstone, 2003;187.
22. Shulman LP, Simpson JL, Elias S. Invasive prenatal genetic techniques. In: Sciarra JJ, ed. Gynecology and obstetrics, vol. 3. Philadelphia: JB Lippincott, 1992:1.
23. Elias S. Prenatal diagnosis of genetic disorders. In: Givens JR, ed. Endocrinology of pregnancy. Chicago: Year Book, 1980:327.
24. Gerbie AB, Elias S. Technique for midtrimester amniocentesis for prenatal diagnosis. Semin Perinatol 1980;4:159.
25. Gerbie AB, Elias S. Amniocentesis for antenatal diagnosis of genetic defects. Clin Obstet Gynecol 1989;7:5.
26. Emery AEH. Antenatal diagnosis of genetic disease. Mod Trends Hum Genet 1970; 1:267.
27. Scrimegeour JB. Amniocentesis: technique and complications. In: Emery AEH, ed. Antenatal diagnosis of genetic disease. Baltimore: Williams and Wilkins, 1973:11.
28. Tabor A, Philip J, Bang J, et al. Needle size and risk of miscarriage after amniocentesis. Lancet 1988;1:183.
29. Tharmaratnam S, Sadek S, Steele EK, et al. Transplacental early amniocentesis and pregnancy outcome. Br J Obstet Gynaecol 1998;105:228.
30. Bombard AT, Powers JF, Carter SM, et al. Procedure related fetal losses in transplacental versus nontransplacental genetic amniocentesis. Am J Obstet Gynecol 1995;172:868.
31. Van Schoubroeck D, Verhaeghe J. Does local anesthesia at mid-trimester amniocentesis decrease pain experience? A randomized trial in 220 patients. Ultrasound Obstet Gynecol 2000;16:536.
32. Ferber A, Onyeije CI, Zelop CM, et al. Maternal pain and anxiety in genetic amniocentesis: expectation versus reality. Ultrasound Obstet Gynecol 2002;19:13.

33. Sikkema-Raddatz B, van Echten J, van der Vlag J, et al. Minimal volume of amniotic fluid for reliable prenatal cytogenetic diagnosis. Prenat Diagn 2002;22:164.
34. NICHD National Registry for Amniocentesis Study Group. Midtrimester amniocentesis for prenatal diagnosis: safety and accuracy. JAMA 1976;236:1471.
35. Simpson NE, Dallaire L, Miller JR, et al. Prenatal diagnosis of genetic disease in Canada: report of a collaborative study. Can Med Assoc J 1976;15:739.
36. Finberg HJ, Frigoletto FD. Sonographic demonstration of uterine contraction during amniocentesis. Am J Obstet Gynecol 1981;139:740.
37. Platt LD, Devore GR, Gim OV, et al. Failed amniocentesis: the role of membrane tenting. Am J Obstet Gynecol 1982;144:479.
38. Golbus MS, Loughman WD, Epstein CJ, et al. Prenatal diagnosis in 3000 amniocenteses. N Engl J Med 1979;300:157.
39. Romero R, Jeanty P, Reece EA, et al. Sonographically monitored amniocentesis to decrease intraoperative complications. Obstet Gynecol 1985;65:426.
40. Tabor A, Philip J, Madsen MI, et al. Randomized controlled trial of genetic amniocentesis in 4606 low-risk women. Lancet 1986;1:1287.
41. Elias S, Simpson JL, unpublished data.
42. Pirani BBI, Doran TA, Benzie RJ. Amniotic fluid or maternal urine? Lancet 1976;1:303.
43. Guibaud S, Bonnet M, Dury A. Amniotic fluid or maternal uterine? Lancet 1976;1:746.
44. Elias S, Martin AO, Patel VA, et al. Analysis for amniotic fluid crystallization in second-trimester amniocentesis. Am J Obstet Gynecol 1979;133:401.
45. Pittini R, Oepkes D, Macrury K, et al. Teaching invasive perinatal procedures: assessment of a high fidelity simulator-based curriculum. Ultrasound Obstet Gynecol. 2002;19:478.
46. Anderson RL, Goldberg JD. Prenatal diagnosis in multiple gestations: 20 years' experience with amniocentesis. Prenat Diagn 1991;11:263.
47. Van Vugt JM, Nieuwint A, van Geijn HP. Single-needle insertion: an alternative technique for early second trimester genetic twin amniocentesis. Fetal Diagn Ther 1995;10:178.
48. Buscaglia M, Ghisoni L, Bellotti M, et al. Genetic amniocentesis in biamniotic twin pregnancies by a single insertion of the needle. Prenat Diagn 1995;15:17.
49. Jeanty P, Shah D, Roussis P. Single-needle insertion in twin gestations. Am J Obstet Gynecol 1980;138:169.
50. Henrion R, Papa F, Rouvillois JL, et al. L'amniocentese precoce en cas de grossesse gemellaire. Nouv Presse Med 1978;7:4119.
51. Benacerraf BR, Frigoletto FD. Amniocentesis under continuous ultrasound guidance: a series of 232 cases. Obstet Gynecol 1983;62:760.
52. Williamson RA, Vamer MW, Grant SS. Reduction in amniocentesis risks using a real-time needle guide procedure. Obstet Gynecol 1985;65:751.
53. Cruikshank DP, Vamer MW, Cruikshank JE, et al. Midtrimester amniocentesis: an analysis of 923 cases with neonatal follow-up. Am J Obstet Gynecol 1983;146:204.
54. Andreasen E, Kristoffersen K. Incidence of spontaneous abortion after amniocentesis: influence of placental localization and gynecologic history. Am J Perinatol 1989;6:268.
55. Salvador E, Bienstock J, Blakemore KJ, et al. Leiomyomata uteri, genetic amniocentesis, and the risk of second-trimester spontaneous abortion. Am J Obstet Gynecol. 2002;186:913.
56. MacGillivary I, Nylander POS, Corney G, et al. Human multiple reproduction. London: WB Saunders, 1975.
57. March CM. Improved pregnancy rate with monitoring of gonadotrophin therapy by three modalities. Am J Obstet Gynecol 1987;156:1473.
58. Dawson KJ, Rutherford AJ, Margara RA, et al. Reducing triplet pregnancies following in-vitro fertilisation. Lancet 1991;337:1543.
59. Society for Assisted Reproductive Technology. Assisted reproductive techniques in the United States and Canada: 1993 results generated from the American Society for Reproductive Medicine/Society for Reproductive Technology Registry. Fertil Steril 1995;64:13.
60. Jones HW Jr. Multiple births: how are we doing? Fertil Steril 2003;79:17.
61. Waterhouse JAH. Twinning in twin pedigrees. Br J Soc Med 1950;4:197.
62. Bulmer MG. Twinning rate in Europe during the war. BMJ 1959;1:29.
63. Myrianthopoulos N. An epidemiologic survey of twins in a large, prospectively studied population. Am J Hum Genet 1970;22:611.
64. Allen G, Baroff GS. Mongoloid twins and their siblings. Acta Genet 1955;5:294.
65. Zellweger H. Familial aggregates of the 21-trisomy syndrome. Ann NY Acad Sci 1968;155:784.

66. Rodis JF, Egan JRX, Craffey A, et al. Calculated risk of chromosomal abnormalities in twin gestations. Obstet Gynecol 1990;76:1037.

67. Meyers C, Adam R, Dungan J, et al. Aneuploidy in twin gestations: when is maternal age advanced? Obstet Gynecol 1997;89:248.

68. Elias S, Gerbie AB, Simpson JL, et al. Genetic amniocentesis in twin gestations. Am J Obstet Gynecol 1980;138:169.

69. Elias S, Gerbie A, Simpson JL. Genetic amniocentesis in twin gestations. Clin Genet 1980;17:300.

70. Kidd SA, Lancaster PAL, Anderson JC, et al. Fetal death after exposure to methylene blue dye during midtrimester amniocentesis in twin pregnancy. Prenat Diagn 1996;16:39.

71. Henry G, Robinson A. Genetic amniocentesis in twin pregnancies. Am J Hum Genet 1975;30:695.

72. Wolfe DA, Scheible FW, Young FE, et al. Genetic amniocentesis in multiple pregnancy. J Clin Ultrasound 1979;7:208.

73. Jassani MN, Merkatz IR, Brennan IN, et al. Twin pregnancy with discordance for Down's syndrome. Obstet Gynecol 1980;55 (suppl):455.

74. Bovicelli L, Michelacci L, Rizzo N, et al. Genetic amniocentesis in twin pregnancy. Prenat Diagn 1983;3:83.

75. Goldstein AI, Stills SM. Midtrimester amniocentesis in twin pregnancies. Am J Obstet Gynecol 1983;62:659.

76. Palle C, Anderson JW, Tobar A, et al. Increased risk of abortion after genetic amniocentesis in twin pregnancies. Prenat Diagn 1983;3:83.

77. Taylor MB, Anderson RL, Golbus MS. One hundred twin pregnancies in a prenatal diagnosis program. Am J Med Genet 1984;148:585.

78. Filkins K, Russo J. Genetic amniocentesis in multiple gestations. Prenat Diagn 1984;4:223.

79. Librach CL, Doran TA, Benzie RJ, et al. Genetic amniocentesis in seventy twin pregnancies. Am J Obstet Gynecol 1984;148:585.

80. Pijpers L, Jahoda MG, Vosters RP, et al. Genetic amniocentesis in twin pregnancies. Br J Obstet Gynaecol 1988;95:323.

81. Simpson JL. Procedures for prenatal diagnosis of genetic disorders. In: Golbus SG, Simpson JL, eds. Genetics in obstetrics and gynecology, 2nd ed. Philadelphia: WB Saunders, 1992:173.

82. Dacus JV, Wilroy RS, Summitt RL, et al. Genetic amniocentesis: a twelve years' experience. Am J Med Genet 1985;20:443.

83. Yukobowich E, Anteby EY, Cohen SM, et al. Risk of fetal loss in twin pregnancies undergoing second trimester amniocentesis (1). Obstet Gynecol. 2001;98:231.

84. Working Party on Amniocentesis: an assessment of hazards of amniocentesis. Br J Obstet Gynaecol 1978;85 (suppl 2):1.

85. Hill LM, Platt LD, Collage B. Rh-sensitization after genetic amniocentesis. Obstet Gynecol 1980;56:459.

86. Golbus MS, Stephens JD, Can HM, et al. Rh-isoimmunization following genetic amniocentesis. Prenat Diagn 1982;2:149.

87. Wyskowski DK, Flynt JW, Goldberg MF, et al. Rh hemolytic disease: epidemiologic surveillance in the United States, 1968 to 1975. JAMA 1979;242;1376.

88. Khalil MA, Tabsh MA, Lobherz TB, et al. Risks of prophylactic anti-D immunoglobulin after second-trimester amniocentesis. Am J Obstet Gynecol 1984;149:225.

89. Murray JC, Kasarp LE, Williamson RA, et al. Rh isoimmunization related to amniocentesis. Am J Med Genet 1983;16:527.

90. Tabor A, Jerne D, Bok JE. Incidence of rhesus immunization after genetic amniocentesis. BMJ 1986;293:533.

91. Gorman JG. New applications of Rh immune globulin: effect on protocols. In: Frigoletto FD Jr, Jewett JR, Konugres AA, eds. Rh hemolytic disease: new strategy for eradication. Boston: GK Hall, 1981:199.

92. Frigoletto FD Jr. Risk perspectives of Rh sensitization. In: Frigoletto FD Jr, Jewett JF, Konugres AA, eds. Rh hemolytic disease: new strategy for eradication. Boston: GK Hall, 1981:103.

93. Pollack, W, Gorman JG, Freda VI. Rh immune suppression: Past, present, and future. In: Frigoletto FD Jr, Jewett JF, Konugres AA, eds. Rh hemolytic disease: new strategy for eradications. Boston: GK Hall, 1981:9.

94. Miles JH, Kaback MD. Rh immune globulin after genetic amniocentesis. Clin Genet Res 1979;27:103A.

95. Crane JP, Rohland B, Larson D. Rh immune globulin after genetic amniocentesis: impact on pregnancy outcome. Am J Med Genet 1984;19:763.

96. ACOG Practice Bulletin, no. 4, 1999. Prevention of RhD isoimmunization. Washington DC: American College of Obstetricians and Gynecologists.

97. Turnbull AC, MacKenzie IZ. Second-trimester amniocentesis and termination of pregnancy. Br Med Bull 1983;39:315.

98. Karp LE, Schiller HS. Meconium staining of amniotic fluid at midtrimester amniocentesis. Obstet Gynecol 1977;50:475.

99. Hankins GD, Rowe J, Quirk JG, et al. Significance of brown and/or green amniotic fluid at the time of second trimester genetic amniocentesis. Obstet Gynecol 1984;64:353.

100. Zorn EM, Hanson FW, Greve LC, et al. Analysis of the significance of discolored amniotic fluid detected at mid-trimester amniocentesis. Am J Obstet Gynecol 1986;154:1234.

101. Murken JA, Stengel-Rutowski S, Schwinger E. Prenatal diagnosis. In: Proceedings of the third European Conference on Prenatal Diagnosis of Genetic Disorders. Stuttgart: Ferdinand Enke, 1979:132.

102. National Institute of Child Health and Human Development Consensus Conference on Antenatal Diagnosis December 1979, 1997. Washington, DC: Government Printing Office, 1979. NIH publication no. 80-1973.

103. Thomas IT, Smith DW. Oligohydramnios, cause of the nonrenal features of the Potter's syndrome, including pulmonary hypoplasia. J Pediatr 1974;84:811.

104. Simpson JL, Socol ML, Aladjem S, et al. Normal fetal growth despite persistent amniotic fluid leakage after genetic amniocentesis. Prenat Diagn 1981;1:277.

105. Crane JP, Rohland BM. Clinical significance of persistent amniotic fluid leakage after genetic amniocentesis. Prenat Diagn 1986;6:25.

106. Lamb MP. Gangrene of a fetal limb due to amniocentesis. Br J Obstet Gynaecol 1975;82:829.

107. Karp LE, Hayden PW. Fetal puncture during mid-trimester amniocentesis. Obstet Gynecol 1977;49:115.

108. Rickwood AMK. A case of ileal atresia and ileocutaneous fistula caused by amniocentesis. J Pediatr 1977;1:720.

109. Eply SL, Hanson JW, Cruickshank DP. Fetal injury with midtrimester diagnostic amniocentesis. Obstet Gynecol 1979;53:77.

110. Swift PFG, Driscoll IB, Vovles KDJ. Neonatal small bowel obstruction associated with amniocentesis. BMJ 1979;1:720.

111. Youroukos S, Papadelis F, Matsaniotis N. Porencephalic cysts after amniocentesis. Arch Dis Child 1980;55:814.

112. Merin S, Byth Y. Uniocular congenital blindness as a complication of midtrimester amniocentesis. Am J Ophthalmol 1980;80:299.

113. Isenberg SJ, Heckenlively JR. Traumatized eye with retinal damage from amniocentesis. J Pediatr Ophthalmol Strabismus 1988;25:196.

114. Adrnoni MM, BenEzra D. Ocular trauma following amniocentesis as the cause of leukocoria. J Pediatr Ophthalmol Strabismus 1988;25:196.

115. Gounot E, Cuzin B, Louis D, et al. Fistule peritoneo-parietale au decours d'une amniocentese precoce: a propos d'un cas. Chir Pediatr 1989;30:52.

116. Mancini J, Lethel V, Hugonenq C, et al. Brain injuries in early foetal life: consequences for brain development. Dev Med Child Neurol 2001;43:52.

117. Fines B, Ben-Ami TE, Yousefzadeh DK. Traumatic prenatal sigmoid perforation due to amniocentesis. Pediatr Radiol. 2001;31:440.

118. DeLong GR. Mid-gestation right basal ganglia lesion: clinical observations in two children. Neurology 2002; 59:54.

119. Medical Research Council. Diagnosis of genetic disease by amniocentesis during the second trimester of pregnancy. Ottawa, Canada: Medical Research Council, 1977.

120. Wald NJ, Terzian E, Vickers PA, et al. Congenital talipes and hip malformation in relation to amniocentesis: a case–control study. Lancet 1983;2:246.

121. Mandelbrot L, Mayaux MJ, Bongain A, et al. Obstetric factors and mother-to-child transmission of human immunodeficiency virus type 1: the French perinatal cohorts. SEROGEST French Pediatric HIV Infection Study Group. Am J Obstet Gynecol. 1996;175:661

122. Bucceri AM, Somigliana E, Vignali M. Early invasive diagnostic techniques during pregnancy in HIV-infected women. Acta Obstet Gynecol Scand 2001;80:82.

123. de Decker HP. Mother-to-fetus HIV transmission during amniocentesis—ethical concerns. S Afr Med J. 2002;92:124.

124. The International Perinatal HIV Group. The mode of delivery and the risk of vertical transmission of human immunodeficiency virus type 1. N Engl J Med 1999;179:590.

125. Stein Z, Kline J, Susser E, et al. Maternal age and spontaneous abortion. In: Porter IH, Hook EB, eds. Human embryonic and fetal death. New York: Academic Press, 1980:107.

126. Simpson JL. Incidence and timing of pregnancy losses: relevance to evaluating safety of early prenatal diagnosis. Am J Med Genet 1990;35:165.

127. Christiaens GCML, Stoutenbeek PH. Spontaneous abortion in proven intact pregnancies. Lancet 1984;2:572.

128. Wilson RD, Kendrick V, Wittman BK, et al. Risks of spontaneous abortion in ultrasonographically normal pregnancies. Lancet 1984;2:290.

129. Tongsong T, Wanapirak C, Sirivatanapa P, et al. Amniocentesis-related fetal loss: a cohort study. Obstet Gynecol 1998;92:64.

130. Papantoniou NE, Daskalakis GJ, Tziotis JG, et al. Risk factors predisposing to fetal loss following a second trimester amniocentesis. BJOG 2001;108:1053.

131. Armstrong J, Cohen AW, Bombard AT, et al. Comparison of amniocentesis-related loss rates between obstetrician-gynecologists and perinatologists. Obstet Gynecol 2002;99:65S.

132. Henry GP, Miller WA. Early amniocentesis. J Reprod Med 1992;37:396.

132a.Eddleman K, Berkowitz R, Kharbutli Y, et al. Pregnancy loss rates after midtrimester amniocentesis: The FASTER Trial. Am J Obstet Gynecol 2003;189:S111.

133. Hanson FW, Zorn EM, Tennant FR. Amniocentesis before 15 weeks' gestation: outcome, risks, and technical problems. Am J Obstet Gynecol 1987;156:1524.

134. Evans MI, Grogan A, Koppitch MS III, et al. Genetic diagnosis in the first trimester: the norm for the 1990s. Am J Obstet Gynecol 1989;160:1332.

135. Elejalde BR, de Elejalde MM, Acuna JM. Prospective study of amniocentesis performed between weeks 9 and 16 of gestation: its feasibility, risks, complications and use in early genetic prenatal diagnosis. Am J Med Genet 1990;35:188.

136. Bombard T, Rigdon DT. Prospective pilot evaluation of early (11–14 weeks' gestation) amniocentesis in 75 patients. Mil Med 1992;157:339.

137. Calhoun BC, Brehm W, Bombard AT. Early genetic amniocentesis and its relationship to respiratory difficulties in paediatric patients: a report of findings in patients and matched controls 3–5 years post-procedure. Prenat Diagn 1994;14:209.

138. Stripparo L, Buscaglia M, Longatti L. Genetic amniocentesis: 505 cases performed before the sixteenth week of gestation. Prenat Diagn 1990;10:359.

139. Penso CA, Sandstrom MM, Garber MF, et al. Early amniocentesis: report of 407 cases with neonatal follow-up. Obstet Gynecol 1990;76:1032.

140. Hackett GA, Smith ill, Rebello CTH, et al. Early amniocentesis at 11–14 weeks gestation for the diagnosis of fetal chromosomal abnormality: a clinical evaluation. Prenat Diagn 1991;11: 311.

141. Bombard AT, Carter SM, Nitowsky HM. Early amniocentesis versus chorionic villus sampling for fetal karyotyping. Lancet 1994;344:826.

142. Brumfield CG, Lin S, Conner W, et al. Pregnancy outcome following genetic amniocentesis at 11–14 versus 16–19 weeks' gestation. Obstet Gynecol 1996;88:114.

143. Wilson RD, Johnson J, Dansereau J. Pregnancy outcome following genetic amniocentesis at 11–14 versus 16–19 weeks' gestation. Obstet Gynecol 1996;88:638.

144. Shulman LP, Elias S, Phillips OP, et al. Amniocentesis performed at 14 weeks gestation or earlier: comparison with first- trimester chorionic villus sampling. Obstet Gynecol 1994;83:543.

145. Bravo RR, Shulman LP, Phillips OP, et al. Transplacental needle passage in early amniocentesis and pregnancy loss. Obstet Gynecol 1995;86:437.

146. Shulman LP, Elias S, Phillips OP, et al. Early twin amniocentesis prior to 14 weeks gestation. Prenat Diagn 1992;12:625.

147. Diaz Vega M, De La Cueva P, Leal C, et al. Early amniocentesis at 10–12 weeks' gestation. Prenat Diagn 1996;16:307.

148. Rao N, Pettenati M, Barry M, et al. Early amniocentesis: a cytogenetic evaluation of 1010 consecutive cases. Am J Hum Genet 1990;47:A283.

149. Nicolaides KH, Brizot ML, Patel F, et al. Comparison of chorionic villus sampling and amniocentesis for fetal karyotyping at 10–13 weeks gestation. Lancet 1994;344:435.

150. Vandenbussche FPHA, Kanhai HHH, Keirse MJNC. Safety of early amniocentesis. Lancet 1994;344:1032.

151. Simpson JL. Genetic counseling and prenatal diagnosis. In: Gabbe SG, Niebyl JR, Simpson JL, eds. Obstetrics: normal and problem pregnancies, 3rd ed. New York: Churchill Livingstone, 1996:215.

152. Johnson J, Wilson RD, Windsor EJT, et al. The Early Amniocentesis Study: a randomized clinical trial of early amniocentesis versus midtrimester amniocentesis. Fetal Diagn Ther 1996; 11:85.

153. The Canadian Early and Mid-Trimester Amniocentesis Trial Group. Randomized trial to assess safety and fetal outcome of early and midtrimester amniocentesis. Lancet 1998;351:242.

154. Johnson JM, Wilson RD, Singer J, et al. Technical factors in early amniocentesis predict adverse outcome: results of the Canadian Early (EA) versus Mid-trimester (MA) Amniocentesis Trial. Prenat Diagn 1999;19: 732.

155. Sundberg K, Bang J, Smidt-Jensen S, et al. Randomised study of risk of fetal loss related to early amniocentesis versus chorionic villus sampling. Lancet 1997;350:697.

156. Philip J, for the NICHD EATA Study Group. Greater risk associated with early amniocentesis compared to chorionic villus sampling: an international randomized trial. Am J Obstet Gynecol 2002;187:39A.

157. Kennerknecht I, Kramer S, Grab D, et al. Evaluation of amniotic fluid cell filtration: an experimental approach to early amniocentesis. Prenat Diagn 1993;13:247.

158. Sundberg K, Smidt-Jensen S, Lundsteen C, et al. Filtration and recirculation of early amniotic fluid: evaluation of cell cultures from 100 diagnostic cases. Prenat Diagn 1993;13:1101.

159. Byrne D, Marks K, Azar G, et al. Randomized study of early amniocentesis versus chorionic villus sampling: a technical and cytogenetic comparison of 650 patients. Ultrasound Obstet Gynecol 1991;1:235.

160. Hanson FW, Tennant F, Hune S, et al. Early amniocentesis: outcome, risks, and technical problems at 12.8 weeks. Am J Obstet Gynecol 1992;166:1707.

161. Lockwood DH, Neu RL. Cytogenetic analysis of 1,375 amniotic fluid specimens from pregnancies with gestational age less than 14 weeks. Prenat Diagn 1993;13:801.

162. Farran I, Sanchez MA, Mediano C, et al. Early amniocentesis with the filtration technique: neonatal outcome in 123 singleton pregnancies. Prenat Diagn 2002;22:859.

163. Watson JD, Craft P. Acetylcholinesterase determination in early amniocentesis. Am J Hum Genet 1989;70:664.

164. Crandall BF, Hanson FW, Tennant F. Acetylcholinesterase (AChE) electrophoresis and early amniocentesis. Am J Hum Genet 1989;45:A257.

165. Wathen NC, Campbell DJ, Kitau MJ, et al. Alpha-fetoprotein levels in amniotic fluid from 8 to 18 weeks of pregnancy. Br J Obstet Gynaecol 1993;100:380.

166. Crandall BF, Chua C. Detecting neural tube defects by amniocentesis between 11 and 15 weeks' gestation. Prenat Diagn 1995;15:339.

167. Hislop A, Fairweather D. Amniocentesis and lung growth: an animal experiment with clinical implications. Lancet 1982;2:271.

168. Burton BK, Nelson LH, Pettenati MJ. False-positive acetylcholinesterase with early amniocentesis. Obstet Gynecol 1989;74:607.

169. Jorgensen FS, Sundberg K, Loft AG, et al. Alpha-fetoprotein and acetylcholinesterase activity in first- and early second-trimester amniotic fluid. Prenat Diagn 1995;15:621.

170. Elias S. The role of fetoscopy in antenatal diagnosis. Clin Obstet Gynecol 1980;7:73.

171. Hobbins JC, Mahoney MJ. In utero diagnosis of hemoglobinopathies: technique for obtaining fetal blood. N Engl J Med 1974;290:1065.

172. Gosden C, Nicolaides KH, Rodeck CH. Fetal blood sampling in investigation of chromosome mosaicism in amniotic fluid culture. Lancet 1988;2:613.

173. Tipton RE, Therapel AT, Chang HT, et al. Rapid chromosome analysis using spontaneously dividing cells from umbilical cord blood (fetal and neonatal). Am J Obstet Gynecol 1990;161:1546.

174. Liou JD, Chen CP, Breg WR, et al. Fetal blood sampling and cytogenetic abnormalities. Prenat Diagn 1993;13:1.

175. Porreco RP, Harshbarger B, McGavran L. Rapid cytogenetic assessment of fetal blood samples. Obstet Gynecol 1993;82:242.

176. Ryan G, Rodeck CH. Fetal blood sampling. In: Simpson JL, Elias S eds. Essentials of prenatal diagnosis. New York: Churchill Livingstone, 1993:63.

177. Daffos F. Fetal blood sampling. Annu Rev Med 1989;40:319.

178. Forestier F, Daffos F, Rainau M, et al. Blood chemistry of normal human fetuses at midtrimester of pregnancy. Pediatr Res 1987;21:579.

179. Forestier F, Cox WL, Daffos F, et al. The assessment of fetal blood samples. Am J Obstet Gynecol 1988;158:1184.

180. Nicolaides KH, Clewel WH, Rodeck CH. Measurement of human fetoplacental blood volume in erythroblastosis fetalis. Am J Obstet Gynecol 1987;157:50.

181. Pardi G, Marconi M, Cetin I, et al. Fetal blood sampling during pregnancy: risks and diagnostic advantages. J Perinat Med 1994;22:513.

182. Bahado-Singh RO, Morotti R, Pirhonen J, et al. Invasive techniques for prenatal diagnosis: current concepts. J Assoc Acad Minority Phys 1995;6:28.

183. Tongsong T, Wanapirak C, Pkunavikatikul C, et al. Fetal loss rate associated with cordocentesis at midgestation. Am J Obstet Gynecol 2001;184:719.

184. Donnenfeld AE, Wiseman B, Lavi E, et al. Prenatal diagnosis of severe combined immunodeficiency. J Pediatr 1990;10:29.

185. Udom-Rice I, Bussel JB. Fetal and neonatal thrombocytopenia. Blood Rev 1995;9:57.
186. Bussel JB, Berkowitz RL, Mcfarland JG, et al. Antenatal treatment of neonatal alloimmune thrombocy-topenia. N Engl J Med 1988;319:1374.
187. Weiner CP. Cordocentesis for diagnostic indications: two years experience. Obstet Gynecol 1987;70:664.
188. Durandy A, Dumez Y, Guy-Grand D, et al. Prenatal diagnosis of severe combined immunodeficiency. J Pediatr 1982;101:995.
189. Holmberg L, Gustavii B, Jonsson A. A prenatal study of fetal platelet count and size with application to fetus at risk for Wiskott–Aldrich syndrome. J Pediatr 1983;102:773.
190. Diukman R, Tanigawa S, Cowan MJ, et al. Prenatal diagnosis of Chediak–Higashi syndrome. Prenat Diagn 1992; 12: 1877.
191. Rodeck CH, Nicolini U. Fetal blood sampling. Eur J Obstet Gynecol Reprod Biol 1988;28:85.
192. Daffos F, Forestier F, Capella-Pavlovsky M, et al. Prenatal management of 746 pregnancies at risk for con-genital toxoplasmosis. N Engl J Med 1988;318:271.
193. Peters MT, Nicolaides KH. Cordocentesis for the diagnosis and treatment of human fetal parvovirus in-fection. Obstet Gynecol 1990;75:501.
194. Hsieh PI, Ko TM, Chang FM, et al. Percutaneous ultrasound-guided fetal blood sampling: experience in the first 100 cases. Taiwan I Hsueh Hui Tsa Chi 1989;88:137.
195. Viscarello RR, Cullen MT, DeGennaro NJ, et al. Fetal blood sampling in human immunodeficiency virus seropositive women. Am J Obstet Gynecol 1992;167:1075.
196. Newton ER. Diagnosis of perinatal TORCH infections. Clin Obstet Gynecol 1999;42:59.
197. Azam AZ, Vial Y, Fawer CL, et al. Prenatal diagnosis of congenital cytomegalovirus infection. Obstet Gy-necol 2001;97:443.
198. Kailasam C, Brennand J, Cameron AD. Congenital parvovirus B19 infection: experience of a recent epi-demic. Fetal Diagn Ther 2001;16:18.
199. Moise KJ, Deter RL, Kirshon B, et al. Intravenous pancuronium bromide for fetal neuromuscular block-ade during intrauterine transfusion for red cell alloimmunization. Obstet Gynecol 1989;74:905.
200. Bellini P, Marinetti E, Arreghini A, et al. Treatment of maternal hyperthyroidism and fetal goiter. Minerva Ginecol 2000;52:25.
201. Gruner C, Kollert A, Wildt L, et al. Intrauterine treatment of fetal goitrous hypothyroidism controlled by determination of thyroid-stimulating hormone in fetal serum: a case report and review of the literature. Fetal Diagn Ther 2001;16:47.
202. Calderwood C, Williams H, Campbell IW, et al. Cordocentesis to predict fetal outcome after administra-tion of radioactive iodine for Graves' disease. J Obstet Gynaecol 2002;22:217.
203. Orlandi F, Damiani G, Jakil C, et al. Clinical results and fetal biochemical data on 140 early second trimester diagnostic cordocenteses. Acta Eur Fertil 1987;18:329.
204. Orlandi F, Damiani G, Jakil C, et al. The risks of early cordocentesis (12–21 weeks): analysis of 500 pro-cedures. Prenat Diagn 1990;10:425.
205. Chinaiya A, Venkat A, Dawn C, et al. Intrahepatic vein fetal blood sampling: current role in prenatal di-agnosis. J Obstet Gynaecol Res 1998;24:239.
206. Nicolini U, Nicolaides KH, Fisk NM, et al. Fetal blood sampling from the intrahepatic vein: analysis of safety and clinical experience with 214 procedures. Obstet Gynecol 1990;76:47.
207. Nicolini U, Kochenour NK, Greco P, et al. Consequences of fetomaternal hemorrhage after intrauterine transfusion. BMJ 1988;297:1379.
208. Ghidini A, Sepulveda W, Lockwood CJ, et al. Complications of fetal blood sampling. Am J Obstet Gy-necol 1993;168:1339.
209. Wilson RD, Farquarhson DF, Wittman BK, et al. Cordocentesis: overall pregnancy loss rate as important as procedure loss rate. Fetal Diagn Ther 1994;9:142.
210. Buscaglia M, Ghisoni L, Bellotti M, et al. Percutaneous umbilical blood sampling: indication, changes, and procedure loss rates in nine years' experience. Fetal Diagn Ther 1996;11:106.
211. Weiner CP, Okamura K. Diagnostic fetal blood sampling-technique related losses. Fetal Diagn Ther 1996;11:169.
212. Antsaklis A, Daskalakis G, Papantoniou N, et al. Fetal blood sampling—indication-related losses. Prenat Diagn 1998;18:934
213. Sikovanyecz J, Horvath E, Sallay E, et al. Fetomaternal transfusion and pregnancy outcome after cordo-centesis. Fetal Diagn Ther 2001;16:83.
214. Van Selm M, Kanhai HHH, Van Loon J. Detection of fetomaternal hemorrhage associated with cordo-centesis using serum alpha-fetoprotein and the Kleihauer technique. Prenat Diagn 1995;15:313.

Louis Dallaire, M.D., Ph.D., F.R.C.P.(C), F.A.C.M.G.,
F.C.C.M.G., and Aubrey Milunsky, MB.B.Ch., D.Sc.,
F.R.C.P., F.A.C.M.G., D.C.H.

3

Amniotic Fluid

Analysis of the chemical constituents of amniotic fluid (AF), which acts as a protective physical cushion for the fetus, has yielded valuable information for prenatal diagnosis, allowing assessment of fetal physiology and metabolism. Because the AF can be viewed as an extension of the fetal extracellular space,[1,2] an understanding of its origin, formation, and chemical constitution is crucial to prenatal diagnosis and fetal therapy. Early sampling of extracoelomic and amniotic fluids during the 8th to 12th weeks of pregnancy for the purpose of prenatal diagnosis has added valuable knowledge about the origin, formation, and content of AF. Cellular components are discussed in this chapter and in chapter 4.

AMNIOTIC FLUID DYNAMICS

Formation and Circulation

Knowledge remains incomplete regarding the anatomic pathways for the formation and circulation of AF.[3-6] Fluid exchange between the fetus and the mother occurs via a number of routes and through different mechanisms and may vary according to the stage of gestation. Large volumes of fluid are transferred across the fetal membranes, which are made up of five layers of amnion and four layers of chorion.[7] Electron microscopy of the amnion has revealed a complex system of tiny intracellular canals, which are connected to the intercellular canalicular system and the base of the cell.[8] The structure of the amniotic cavity is basically complete by about 10 weeks of gestation.[9] Studies in primates suggest that the AF is a transudate of the maternal plasma and becomes like other fetal fluids in the presence of the fetus, which contributes urine and other body secretions to the AF space.[10]

  Osmotic or diffusion permeability, hydrostatic pressure, chemical gradients, and other mechanisms are responsible for the fluid exchange between fetus and mother.[11] Intra-amniotic pressure measurements were obtained by Nicolini et al.[12] In normal pregnancies, this pressure at 16 weeks ranged between 1 and 14 mm Hg and increased with gestational age. Venous pressure obtained by the same technique was comparable to values reported previously. Fisk et al.[13] studied amniotic fluid pressure (AP) from 7 to 38 weeks of gestation) in 194 pregnancies. AP measured in mm Hg increased with gestational age and was not influenced by twin gestation, the deepest vertical pool, AF index, maternal age, parity, gravity, fetal sex, or time of delivery. They suggested that AP may be determined by anatomical and hormonal influences or gravid uterine musculature. The reference range given varied from a low of 1.1 to a high of 6.1 mm Hg at 8 weeks of gestation, compared with a low of 3.2 to a high of 13.1 mm Hg at 34 weeks of gestation. Barbera and co-workers[14] showed that intra-amniotic pressure does not vary much during amniocentesis performed between 13 and 18 weeks of gestation. The pressure was measured in mm Hg. Removing fluid samples, relative to the age of gestation, up to 12.6 percent of the total volume in early amniocentesis and 7.5 percent in a group of late genetic amniocenteses, did not change the AF pressure significantly. Studies by Tomoda et al.[15] in fetal sheep showed that artificially raising amniotic salt concentration or increasing amniotic osmolality with isotonic mannitol infusion reduced AF sodium concentration and elevated the fluid volume for more than 24 hr. As summarized by Brace,[16] there are three determinants of AF volume: (1) movements of water and solutes across the membranes; (2) the fetus's physiological regulation of flow rates, such as urine production and swallowing; and (3) maternal effects on transplacental fluid movement. In humans, the urine production per kg of body weight increases from 110 mL/kg/24 hr at 25 weeks to 190 mL/kg/24 hr at 35 weeks.[17]

During the second trimester of gestation, total AF turnover is complete within about 3 hr.[18–20] About 20 mL of AF/hr is swallowed by the fetus, that is approximately 500 mL/day.[21,22] At term, the exchange rate between fetus and mother may approach 500 mL/hr.[19,23] Active renal function is evident from the ability of the fetal kidney to concentrate radiopaque substances given intravenously to the mother, thereby allowing visualization of a fetal pyelogram.[24]

Several AF compounds reach a maximum or minimum level toward the end of the second trimester.[25] Understanding fetomaternal metabolism is of utmost importance in the evaluation of fetal development and particularly in the antenatal diagnosis of fetal demise.

Although the fetus depends largely on the placenta for the transport of nutrients, it is also protected from marked fluctuations in maternal metabolism. It was suggested[26] that the increase of creatinine, γ-glutamyl transferase, and β_2-microglobulin concentrations in AF after 10 weeks of gestation confirms the maturation of fetal glomerular function and reflects the fetal kidney development from the mesonephros to the metanephros. As stated by Clewell et al.,[27] "Since the fetal kidney cannot serve as a final excretory organ in utero, its function in fetal life has been obscure." It is generally accepted that AF is mainly produced by the fetal kidney as pregnancy progresses and that oligohydramnios may reflect renal structural anomalies or general growth retardation.[28]

Volume

The magnitude of fluid exchange also is uncertain. Interference with disposal in the routes of fluid production by a factor affecting only 1 percent of the volume may result in a significant increase or decrease in the total AF volume by as much as 1 L in 10 days.[18]

Various techniques have been used for the direct estimation of AF volume. Comparable results have been reported using dilution techniques, radioactive materials, or various dyes or chemicals.[4,5] Nelson[29] measured AF volumes in 46 cases before 20 weeks of gestation and summarized data culled from four other published series (see Table 3.1 and Figure 3.1). A highly variable although similar range of AF volumes was observed in other studies.[30–33] The mean volume seems to be about 207 mL at 16 weeks[29] and close to 400 mL at 20 weeks.[5] Queenan et al.[34] measured 115 AF volumes from 15 to 42 weeks of gestation by the p-aminohippurate method and found similar results with a wide normal

Table 3.1. The volume of AF recorded by different authors, by direct measurement

Duration of Gestation (weeks)	Number of Cases	Volume of Fluid (mL) Mean	SD
8	5	14.5	5.9
9	2	8.2	—
10	11	29.6	12.4
11	10	45.4	13.9
12	27	73.9	35.9
13	17	89.9	20.9
14	6	111.3	43.4
15	18	143.7	75.7
16	22	207.2	92.3
17	19	233.9	104.4
18	10	258.0	97.4
19	3	333.3	13.3
20	3	365.3	87.8

Source: Data from Wagner and Fuchs 1962,[30] Rhodes 1966,[31] Abramovich 1968,[32] Gillibrand 1969,[33] and Nelson 1972.[29]

range and no decrease at term. Later, Bhatt and co-workers[35] confirmed previously re-ported values for the second trimester. The accuracy of ultrasonic measurements of intra-amniotic volume using a parallel planimetric area method was assessed using a dye-dilution method during the second trimester and at term.[36] The parallel planimetric area method was found to carry acceptable table accuracy. As stressed by Moore[37] in a review of the clinical evaluation of AF volume, one criterion for acceptable volume assessment is the accuracy and reproducibility of measurements. In the ultrasonographic methods of as-sessing AF, the subjective assessment remains a good means of measuring AF volume. The vertical pocket measurement is simpler but remains a semiquantitative method with some limits in accuracy. The AF index is the result of the sum of the four maximum ver-tical pockets from each quadrant of the uterus. Percentiles are derived from the calcula-tion of the mean and standard deviation in each gestational week. This method probably is more reliable for assessing extremes of AF volume.

An incremental rise in volume of about 25 mL/week occurs from 11 to 15 weeks of gestation[31,32,38] and continues at a rate of approximately 50 mL/week from 15 to 28 weeks.[31,39,40] Total water accumulation in utero during pregnancy reaches about 4 L (fetus, 2,800 mL; placenta, 400 mL; AF, 800 mL).[11] AF turnover continues even after fetal death, but it is reduced by about 50 percent,[41] implying that membranes may be responsible for about half of the water exchange. This suggests that the membranes may have a larger role in water disposal than in production. Indeed, electron microscopic studies[42] correlate with an absorptive function of the membranes. According to Wintour and Shandley,[43] it is unlikely that excess AF production results solely from excess urine production or a fail-ure of the fetus to swallow amniotic fluid. The amnion must play a role in the mainte-nance of AF volume and composition. Earlier studies concluded that 25–50 percent of the fluid turnover takes place through the fetus in late pregnancy.[44]

Polyhydramnios is associated with fetal malformations in about 40 percent of cases.[45] Neural tube defects (NTDs) and disorders that impair deglutition or absorption of AF (esophageal and other intestinal atresias or obstructions) are the most common causes of polyhydramnios.[4,45–50] Among 41 patients with "idiopathic" polyhydramnios subject to polymerase chain reaction amplification and Southern blot analysis, 4 (9.7 percent) were

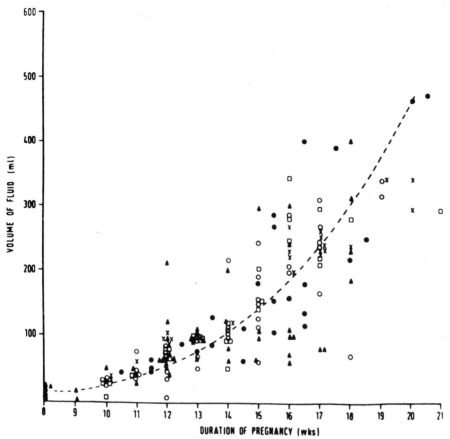

Fig. 3.1. The volume of AF at 8–21 weeks of gestation. Open circle = Wagner and Fuchs (1962);30N = 41. Open square = Rhodes (1966);31N = 26. Closed circle = Abramovich (1968)[32]; N = 28. X = Gillibrand (1969)[33]; N = 22. Closed triangle = Nelson (1972)[29]; N = 46. *Source*: Nelson 1972.[29]

found subsequently to have myotonic muscular dystrophy.[51] The development of polyhydramnios in anencephaly is believed to result from impaired swallowing by the fetus[47] or deficient antidiuretic hormone production by the defective fetus.[52] Polyhydramnios also occurs in maternal diabetes mellitus and may appear, especially early in pregnancy, in monozygotic twins.[47] Irrespective of the cause, there seems to be a risk of recurrence for polyhydramnios of between 0.06 and 8 percent.[45,46]

Ultrasonic assessment of fetal kidney function in normal and complicated pregnancies was undertaken by Kurjak et al.[53] The authors found that the hourly fetal urinary production rate was 2.2 mL/hr at 22 weeks of gestation, and it increased to 26.3 mL/hr at 40 weeks. This evaluation involved a combination of ultrasound and a furosemide test. They concluded that the regulation by the central nervous system does not play a large role in the control of fetal urination and that fetal polyuria does not explain polyhydramnios because the hourly output was normal in the patients studied. Weiner and Grose[54] indicated that umbilical venous pressure in humans was unrelated to gestational age and remained at 5.3 ± 2.3 mm Hg. Polyhydramnios was accompanied by elevated AF pressures.

Oligohydramnios, in contrast, is most often associated with disorders of the urinary tract that interfere with micturition, such as renal agenesis.[49,55,56] Placental insufficiency and ex-trauterine pregnancy also may cause oligohydramnios. However, a normal AF volume may occur even in the presence of urinary tract obstruction or bilateral renal agenesis.[4] A normal volume of AF has been found in 13 cases of hydronephrosis diagnosed by maternal sonography.[57] Only eight cases had confirmed urinary tract obstruction at birth, the other five were normal. Only one had long-term complications, but in that case, oligohydramnios had developed later during pregnancy. The authors suggest that fetal hydronephrosis associated with normal amounts of AF does not require intrauterine treatment. Appropriate intervention after birth should lead to normal renal function. Rarely, oligohydramnios may be extreme, even to the point at which there is virtually no AF. These extreme cases are frequently associated with amnion nodosum,[58,59] fetal defects, or placental problems.[47]

Abramovich[60] challenged the concept that swallowing and voiding are important factors in controlling the AF volume (AFV). He showed that some anencephalics may swallow considerable amounts of AF per day and that normal volumes were found in esophageal atresia and absence of fetal kidneys. Thus, other factors are involved in controlling the AFV. Chamberlain[61] has reviewed the studies done on abnormalities of AFV and altered perinatal outcome.

Gramellini and co-workers[62] constructed normal reference ranges of four ultrasound parameters for the evaluation of AFV during the second trimester and established normal curve limits suitable for use in clinical practice. Excluding cases of fetomaternal pathology from the 12th to the 24th week of gestation, the authors studied four parameters: the mean AF diameter, the two-diameter pocket, the largest vertical pocket, and the largest transverse pocket. The four parameters correlated well with the gestational week and with the biparietal diameter. All these parameters were found to have good intraoperative and interoperative reproducibility. The authors concluded that the use of an ultrasound semiquantitative method, based on the measurement of a single AF pocket and involving normal reference intervals according to gestational age, could improve the early diagnosis of AF variations during the second trimester.

Abnormal AFV is associated with increased maternal risk and perinatal morbidity and mortality, and it was stressed[63] that the invasive nature of AFV assessment limited its clinical utility. Refinements in quantifying the noninvasive sonographic assessment of AFV have improved the ability to identify at-risk pregnancies.

The sonographic evaluation of AF was reviewed by Schrimmer and Moore.[64] The practice of AF assessment has evolved from subjective observation to more sophisticated techniques for quantifying volume. The amniotic fluid index (AFI), introduced by Phelan et al. in 1987,[65] remains the most accepted and noninvasive method for assessing fluid status in singleton gestations, but oligohydramnios is more difficult to assess in multiple gestations, which are more frequent with advanced maternal age. The measurement of the single deepest AF pocket in each sac provides the most reproducible results. Hombo et al.[66] sonographically divided the intrauterine space into six segments and provided a regression equation to predict AFV. Sherer[67] cautioned that decreased AF volume is especially of concern when it occurs in conjunction with structural fetal anomalies, fetal growth restriction, and maternal disease, and others have noted an increased risk of fetal heart rate abnormalities.[68]

Origin

Much of the evidence that AF is derived largely (but not only) from maternal sources comes from the study of constituent proteins in the fluid[69–88] and was reviewed by Sutcliffe.[89] It is likely that the importance or relative contributions from maternal and fetal sources change as pregnancy progresses. Although urine is present in the fetal bladder at least as early as 12 weeks of gestation,[56] its contribution to AFV is likely to be significant only later in gestation.[29]

To some extent at least, the AF in early gestation is probably a dialysate of maternal serum, the total solute concentration being similar.[3] The bulk turnover of AF is completed in 1 day, but the diffusional exchange of some components such as water molecules is more active.[17] Experimental studies have shown that in sheep, large amounts of saliva and nasal secretions are produced late in gestation.[90] In his review on AFV, Brace[16] suggested that the human fetus may have a substantial volume of fluid of salivary origin. In contrast to previous reports,[91] it is now believed that there is a net outflow of fluid from the trachea. In humans, the phospholipids measured in AF, when lecithin/sphingomyelin (L/S) ratios are determined, are of pulmonary origin, and are not passed in significant quantities through the urine. Thus, a significant fraction of the secreted lung fluid in human fetuses seems to enter the AF.

Sutcliffe et al.[92] observed that the maternal serum protein group-specific component (Gc) is present in AF early in gestation. Their observations suggested that this protein enters the AF through the placenta or the fetal membranes. For this reason, they wisely cautioned against attempts at prenatal genetic diagnosis by examination of serum proteins or by linkage analysis using serum protein polymorphisms.

Brzezinski et al.[77] reported a fetal origin for the variant albumin in the rare bisalbuminemia. For various technical reasons, this claim, according to Sutcliffe,[89] was based on satisfactory evidence. Other studies concluded that most of the albumin in AF, at least near term, is of maternal origin.[93–95] Nevertheless, some AF albumin probably derives from the fetus because its concentration in fetal serum is greater than in maternal serum.[74,77,78] In addition, at least after 30 weeks of gestation, most of the AF antitrypsin, ceruloplasmin, Gc, orosomucoid, and transferrin are of maternal origin.[89]

Hemopexin, a β-glycoprotein, is found in AF[96] and is believed to be of maternal origin.[97] Another glycoprotein, β_2-microglobulin, has been noted to have concentrations in the AF in excess of those in maternal serum.[98] β_1-Glycoprotein (SP$_1$), produced by the syncytiotrophoblast, is elevated in AF in Meckel syndrome, but not in open NTDs and several other fetal disorders.[99,100] Indeed, at term, the concentration of β_2-microglobulin in AF is similar to that in cord serum and about twice that in maternal serum.[98] The inclination to conclude that this glycoprotein is of fetal origin may be quite incorrect, because the exact tissue(s) of origin is unknown. Because synthesis of β_2-microglobulin has been shown in lymphocytes,[100] and other glycoproteins are found on the surface of most cells, adjacent maternal tissues may be the most important source of AF β_2-microglobulin.

α_1-Fetoprotein (AFP) is clearly fetospecific, there being a steep gradient from fetal serum to AF. Acetylcholinesterase (AChE), which can be distinguished from nonspecific cholinesterases, is an extracellular component found in high concentration in the fetal brain (see chapter 21).

The D2-protein described by Jorgensen and Norgaard-Pedersen[101] in human AF is a neuronal membrane protein detectable in cerebrospinal fluid. Its presence in AF was proposed as an adjunct to the diagnosis of open NTDs. Sindic and co-workers[102] also found a protein called "S-100 protein" in the astrocytes of the nervous system. Neuron-specific enolase (NSE), a neuroendocrine tumor marker,[103] also has been assayed in AF. Neither the D2 and S-100 proteins nor NSE have proven more useful than AFP and AChE assays for NTDs (see chapter 21).

Gogiel et al.[104] studied the degradation products of collagen in AF. They suggested that nondialyzable collagenous polypeptides may be the products of the proteolytic conversion of procollagen into the monomeric form of this protein.

BIOCHEMICAL AND OTHER CHARACTERISTICS OF AF

One of the earliest of the physical and chemical properties of AF was reported from Japan in 1919.[105] Few studies were done over the next three decades,[106,107] mainly on samples obtained during the third trimester of pregnancy. Although AF frequently reflects the fetal status in many ways, providing opportunities both for prenatal diagnosis and for pregnancy management, its use may be confounded by maternal blood or tissue admixture. Campbell and co-workers[108] studied the composition of AF and extra-embryonic coelomic fluid (Figure 3.2) between 8 and 12 weeks of gestation. During that period, ultrasound-guided aspiration of amniotic and coelomic fluid was performed on 40 women before termination of pregnancy. Still unexplained, differences in electrolyte concentrations were statistically significant. Sodium, potassium, and bicarbonates were higher in AF, whereas chloride, urea, protein, bilirubin, albumin, glucose, creatinine, calcium, and phosphate were present in higher concentrations in extra-embryonic coelomic fluid. Those observations underline the significant difference in composition between the two embryonic fluids.

Proteins

The presence of a number of AF proteins, discussed previously herein, provides direct evidence as to their maternal or fetal origin.[69–88] Many maternal serum proteins gain access to the AF, thereby complicating the use of this fluid for prenatal diagnosis. Proteins of fetal origin probably derive from skin, amnion, chorion, umbilical cord, urine, and bronchial, buccal, and gastrointestinal secretions. Mapping of AF proteins by two-dimensional electrophoresis[109,110] showed the presence of more than 200 proteins. The proteins

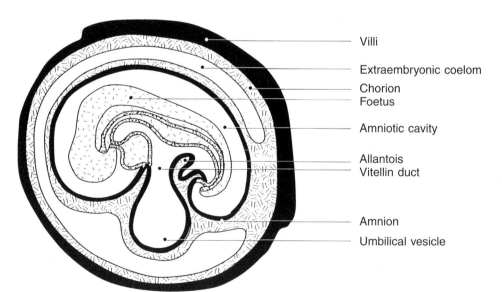

Fig. 3.2. The coelomic and amniotic fluid spaces during the first trimester of gestation.

in AF may be cellular,[111] free organelles,[112] or in solution. Protein constituents of basement membrane have been detected,[113] as has Tamm–Horsfall glycoprotein in human AF.[114] This glycoprotein originates from the kidney tubules, and its concentration increases from 0.9 mg/L at 16 weeks to 33 mg/L near term.

The glycosaminoglycan composition of human AF reveals[115] the major constituent to be hyaluronic acid (34 percent of total uronic acid) at 12–21 weeks of gestation; the rest is mostly chondroitins. Small amounts of heparan sulfate (6 percent) were also characterized.[115,116] The time in gestation when AF is sampled for chemical analysis is an important variable affecting glycosaminoglycan composition in both normal and pathological pregnancies.[115] The determination of glycosaminoglycan composition for prenatal diagnosis of the mucopolysaccharidoses is not recommended because both false-positive and false-negative results were obtained.

Decades ago, the mean protein concentration in AF at term was observed to be less than one-tenth that in maternal serum.[108] Subsequently, the ratios of albumin, transferrin, γ-globulin, ceruloplasmin, α_1-antitrypsin, and Gc[36,74] have been established. The prenatal detection of hemophilia B was attempted by the assay of factor IX and prothrombin in AF.[117]

Despite rapid processing of AF samples, the prothrombin was extensively cleaved, suggesting that it had been activated in vivo. On gel electrophoresis of AF samples, however, factor IX was only minimally cleaved. The prenatal diagnosis of hemophilia B is limited by assay sensitivity and reliability in fetal production or destruction of the gene product and a broadly distributed normal range. Today, carrier detection and prenatal diagnosis of hemophilia B is possible by direct analysis of DNA.[118]

The highest concentrations of albumin, α_1-antitrypsin, Gc, and transferrin have been noted between 20 and 30 weeks of gestation.[82] There is striking variability in the total protein concentration during pregnancy, increasing from a mean of about 3.5 mg/mL at 12 weeks to a maximum of about 8.0 mg/mL at approximately 25 weeks.[119–122] The concentration gradually falls to about 3 mg/mL between 25 and 35 weeks, with little change occurring thereafter.

Although most proteins in AF may be of maternal serum origin, nonserum proteins derived from the epithelial cells of the amnion[123–127] or from the maternal uterine decidua,[128] as well as other α_2-proteins and α_1-fetoprotein, have been described. It is likely that determinations of heretofore-unrecognized markers in AF will open up new horizons in the understanding and diagnosis of fetal defects. For example, Cornelia de Lange syndrome, so far recognized as a sporadic malformation syndrome, has been found to be associated with an absence or reduction in the maternal serum level of pregnancy-associated plasma protein-A (PAPP-A).[129,130] This finding may eventually shed some light on the etiology of this well-circumscribed but rare syndrome.[129] It is well known that a mixture of cells is found in AF samples obtained during the second trimester for prenatal diagnosis of genetic disease. Chitayat et al.[131] used a colon epithelial–specific monoclonal antibody (Mc-Ab) to determine the contribution of fetal colonic mucosal cells to the amniocyte population. The authors concluded that cell-specific Mc-Ab can be used to detect colon cells and that colonocytes are an important component of the AF cell (AFC) population.

Lipids

Lipids do not seem to be transported across the placenta from the mother to the fetus[132] and are not found in AF after maternal injection. In the first AF lipid study, Helmy and Hack[133] reported several compounds, including cholesterol and phosphatidylethanolamine. Biezenski et al.[134] described the lipid content of AF from the 26th week of gestation. Their determinations included monoglycerides, diglycerides, triglycerides, free fatty acids, free cholesterol, cholesterol esters, hydrocarbons, total nonpolar lipids, phospholipids, and estimated total lipid content of AF. The phospholipids measured included lysophosphatidylcholine, sphingomyelin, phosphatidylcholine, inositol, serine and ethanolamine, and phosphatidic acid and cardiolipin. They also established values for total fatty acids, including palmitic acid, palmitoleic acid, stearic acid, oleic acid, and linoleic acid. These workers concluded that total lipid was one-seventieth of that found in maternal plasma during pregnancy and about one-twentieth of that found in fetal plasma.

As far as the phospholipids are concerned, it seems that the phosphatidylserine normally found in AF and in the placenta is not present in maternal plasma.[135] The sphingomyelin content of AF seems to be much lower than in plasma.[134] Total cholesterol represents roughly one-third of the total lipids in AF. At least in the third trimester of pregnancy, Biezenski et al.[134] observed that the lipid profile remained essentially unchanged, despite the striking increase in AFV during this period. Near term, although the placenta prevents the transfer of maternal esterified fatty acids in the form of phospholipids, triglycerides, or cholesteryl esters, appreciable amounts of unesterified fatty acids and free cholesterol are transferred.[136] AF collected more than 2 weeks after fetal death show increased total lipid concentrations due mainly to increased free cholesterol, unesterified fatty acids, and hydrocarbons. Because the placenta and fetal membranes usually do not die with the fetus, continued function would allow the transfer of free fatty acids and free cholesterol, explaining the gradual elevation of the levels of these compounds in AF after fetal death.

Pomerance et al.[137] performed detailed lipid analyses of various complicated pregnancies, including hemolytic disease of the newborn, toxemia of pregnancy, diabetes, anencephaly, and hydramnios. They observed no specific diagnostic lipid pattern in any of these cases. Gardella et al.[138] found an association between lipopolysaccharide-binding protein and soluble CD-14 and preterm labor.

The Smith–Lemli–Opitz syndrome (SLOS)[139,140] is characterized by severe psychomotor retardation, genitourinary and skeletal anomalies. By measuring the sterol composition of plasma, erythrocytes, lens, cultured fibroblasts, and feces from five children with the syndrome, Tint et al.[141] demonstrated an elevation of 7-dehydrocholesterol and very low cholesterol values in the plasma and other tissues. The authors suggested that the deprivation of cholesterol was probably responsible for the abnormal fetal development.

In cholesterol biosynthesis, 7-dehydrocholesterol (7-DHC) is converted to cholesterol by sterol delta-7-reductase (7-DHC reductase). Dallaire et al.[142] and Tint et al.[143] were able to show that the abnormal sterol metabolism is present in utero: low cholesterol and elevated 7-DHC values were pathognomonic of the syndrome when observed in the AF of fetuses at risk. Wassif et al.[144] cloned a cDNA that encoded human sterol delta-7-reductase (DHCR7;60258) and identified mutant cDNAs in patients with SLOS. SLOS fibroblasts transfected with sterol DHCR7 cDNA showed a significant reduction in 7-DHC levels, compared with those in SLOS fibroblasts transfected with the vector alone. Four different mutant alleles were identified.[145–147] Attempts to treat infants affected with the syndrome opened the door to antenatal therapy.[148] Cholesterol supplementation with or without bile acids has been attempted in children with SLOS. There have been only modest improvements in photosensitivity, progressive polyneuropathy, and some growth and neurodevelopmental markers.[149–151] Treatment with a statin drug was considered as potentially harmful for some patients with SLOS.[152]

The fatty acid composition of AF[153,154] differs considerably from that found in maternal plasma. Fetal renal excretion seems to be the probable origin of part of the free fatty acids in AF, at least during the third trimester. The immunosuppressive activity of mouse and human AF has been studied by Rueda et al.,[155] who concluded that lipidlike factors may play a role as a nonspecific immunoregulatory mechanism that prevents the immune rejection of the conceptus by the mother.

Gluck et al.[156] pioneered the analysis of AF phospholipids for the assessment of fetal pulmonary maturity.[157,158] The surface-active phospholipids lecithin and sphingomyelin originate from the fetal lungs.[159] Lecithin apparently stabilizes the lining of the pulmonary villi, preventing their collapse at the end of expiration. A marked increase in the production of lecithin occurs at about 35 weeks of gestation.[160] As a consequence of the passage of the lecithin from the lung into the AF, an increase in the L/S ratio in AF occurs at about this time of gestation.[156] The correlation of the L/S ratio with the gestational age of the fetus has been demonstrated repeatedly.[161–172] Various disorders in pregnancy, including maternal, fetal, and placental complications, have been demonstrated to have a marked effect on the maturation of the fetal lung and hence the L/S ratio.

Any condition that affects the maturation of the fetal lung (either by accelerating or delaying the process), including maternal hypertension, placental insufficiency, and diabetes mellitus, renders the L/S ratio less valuable.[158] Moreover, the contamination by maternal blood of an AF sample may render the L/S test useless, with the direction of change incorrectly suggesting lung immaturity.[173]

Deleze et al.[174] and Heikkinen et al.[175] reported AF bile acid concentrations in normal and pathological pregnancy. Deleze et al.[176] found elevated bile acid concentrations in the AF of fetuses with intestinal obstructions. Such results are expected for all intestinal obstructions distal to the ampulla of Vater, where the fetal stomach content will be regurgitated into AF.[177] In general, the mean bile-acid concentrations in the AF were similar to those in the serum. However, in paired samples from individual patients, these two values did not correlate significantly.[175] High AF bile-acid concentrations might represent a threat to the fetus, but additional studies are needed to clarify this point.

Lamellar bodies, which are believed to be a form of pulmonary surfactant in AF, have been detected and have been characterized by electron microscopy,[178] as well as recently purified by gel chromatography.[179,180] They may allow better prediction of fetal lung maturity in the near future or could be used to predict and treat respiratory distress syndrome. A modified lamellar body phospholipid (LB-PL) assay exhibited better specificity than the L/S ratio or phosphatidylglycerol assay.[181]

Enzymes

Many enzymes have been found in the AF (see also chapters 11 and 12). Some have specific activities greater than those found in maternal serum, such as diamine oxidase[182] and phosphohexose isomerase,[183,184] whereas other enzymes have greater activity in maternal serum than in AF, such as histaminase[185,186] and creatine phosphokinase.[187] The activity of some enzymes in fetal serum exceeds that found in AF (e.g., glucose-6-phosphate dehydrogenase, malate dehydrogenase, glutamic-oxaloacetic transaminase, glutamic-pyruvate transaminase, and leucine aminopeptidase).[188,189] Some enzymes have been proposed as maturity indices: α-galactosidase,[190] pyruvate kinase,[191] alkaline phosphatase, γ-glutamyl transferase,[192] and prolidase.[193]

The lysosomal and microvillar enzymes in AF exhibit different activities as pregnancy progresses, as well as at the same stage in different pregnancies.[84,194] The exact reasons for fluctuating enzyme activities are not clearly understood. The most important factors influencing enzyme activity in the AF may be related to the state of the fetal skin. It is known that the fetal skin becomes impermeable to water[195] at about 20 weeks of gestation, when a number of enzymes change in their level of activity. At about the same time, fetal urine begins to contribute significantly to the AF.[196] Another important factor may be the recognized decrease in the activity of some specific placental lysosomal enzymes,[197] which also occurs at about 20 weeks of gestation. The developmental stage of the fetus may have some bearing on the AF content of lysosomal enzymes.[198] For example, the disappearance of α-glucosidase during the second trimester of pregnancy[198] may indicate that the fetal liver has assumed a major role in glucose homeostasis. Low activity of the placental form of AF alkaline phosphatase has been reported.[199,200]

The importance of knowing the developmental biology of enzymes of the AF is exemplified by observations made on lysosomal α-glucosidase. This enzyme is deficient in type II glycogenosis (Pompe disease) (see chapter 14) and the initial report indicated that there was no activity of this enzyme in AF from a fetus with Pompe disease.[201] Subsequent studies in another pregnancy, however, showed α-glucosidase activity in AF, whereas cultured AF cells showed no enzyme activity.[202] It turns out that the α-glucosidase in AF is caused by a maltase of fetal intestinal origin[203] that is different from the lysosomal α-glucosidase deficient in Pompe disease.[198] This enzyme shows considerable variation with gestation, being deficient in AF samples obtained after 22 weeks of gestation. Its determination in AF is of no value in the prenatal detection of this disorder.

At some stages of pregnancy, α-glucosidase has a specific activity in AF exceeding that found in both maternal or fetal serum.[84] This observation implies that there must be at least another source of these enzymes other than maternal–fetal serum. It is now known that this enzyme is of fetal intestinal origin.[203–205]

Lysosomal enzyme activities vary in relationship to gestational age.[78,206,207] Not unexpectedly, there is not total concurrence on the observations made about AF lysosomal enzyme activities. For example, the mean activities of β-galactosidase and N-acetyl-β-D-glucosaminidase reported by one group[208] differed by a factor of 2 from the mean activities observed by another group.[196] Technical aspects of the assays (especially the substrates used) and handling or storage of samples probably explain these reported differences.

Hexosaminidase seems to have the highest specific activity of the lysosomal enzymes in AF.[196] Except for α-glucosidase, α-arabinosidase, and β-glucosidase, lysosomal enzymes generally rise to their highest specific activities at term.[206] The specific activities of α-glucosidase and heat-labile alkaline phosphatase reach a peak of specific activity between 13 and 18 weeks of gestation. However, arylsulfatase A activity has not been demonstrated in AF.[200] However, Borresen and Van der Hagen[209] proposed that the prenatal detection of metachromatic leukodystrophy can be done on the basis of an arylsulfatase A deficiency in AF. Higher than normal activities of several lysosomal hydrolases were reported in the AF of a fetus affected with I-cell disease (mucolipidoses II).[211,212] All enzyme diagnostic tests based on cell-free AF should be used with care (see chapters 11 and 12).

In some specific inborn errors of metabolism, such as Tay–Sachs disease, the characteristic enzymatic deficiency (hexosaminidase A) may manifest in the AF.[213–215] Desnick et al.[216] found one fetus affected with Sandhoff disease (total hexosaminidase deficiency) that showed almost complete deficiency of this enzyme in the AF. This finding was confirmed in another Sandhoff-affected fetus in our laboratory.[217] Nevertheless, the varying rates of enzyme inactivation in AF and the possibilities of maternal or fetal serum contamination or maternal tissue admixture of different isozymes, in addition to points already made, suggest that total diagnostic reliance should not be placed on enzyme assays performed directly on cell-free AF. Whenever possible, correlation should be documented from the direct study of cultivated AF cells. Potier et al.[217] found that the AF samples with high total hexosaminidase activity also contained a high percentage of maternal serum hexosaminidase (form P).

Amino Acids

For a discussion of amino acid disorders, see chapter 13.

Studies[220,222,226] on amino acid concentrations in fetal tissues and AF were initiated when prenatal diagnosis was introduced to rule out genetic disorders in fetuses at risk. Dallaire et al.,[222] measured the concentration of amino acids and related compounds in 111 samples of AF and 89 maternal plasmas between the 10th and the 40th week of pregnancy. They found that the concentration of eight amino acids (Phe, Ser, Val, Leu, Ile, Lys, Ala, and His) decreased toward the end of the pregnancy. Thirteen amino acids (Gly, Ser, Thr, Asp, Asn, Glu, Arg, Met, Pro, Orn, Ans, Tau, and Cit) showed no significant change between 10 and 40 weeks of gestation, while ten were present in trace amounts (1-Mhis, 3-Mhis, Phser, Phethan, Asp, αAaa, αAba, $\frac{1}{2}$Cys, Cysth, Hypro). The great variation in lysine values between 10 and 20 weeks of pregnancy did not permit fetal age correlation studies. Hydroxyproline was found at a concentration of less than 0.04 mM at 10 weeks and 0.01 mM at 40 weeks. There was a marked elevation of amino acid concentrations in AF obtained from sacs containing two fetuses. Matched AF and maternal plasma samples, studied between 10 to 17 weeks of gestation, showed no significant correlation for that period, although amino acid concentration in AF tended to be higher near the end of the second trimester. Elevated levels of homocysteine have been noted in the second trimester independent of the methylenetetrahydrofolate reductase genotype.[223]

It had been postulated that the AF, being at first an isotonic transudate from the maternal plasma, may become hypotonic with the increase in fetal urine. A dilution factor could explain a general decrease in total amino acid concentration toward term, and the increase in urea and creatinine could come from the maturation of the urinary system. However, a change in fetal metabolism may explain the higher concentration of some amino acids during the end of pregnancy. The measure of amino acid concentration from the first urine samples obtained from normal newborn babies were, as expected, below AF levels. However Cockburn et al. had previously shown[228] a higher concentration of amino acids in urine samples collected during the 24-hr neonatal period.

The concentrations of amino acids were measured in samples of coelomic fluid obtained from normal pregnancies between 7 and 12 weeks of gestation.[224] The total molar concentration of the 18 amino acids measured was 2.3 times higher in coelomic fluid than in maternal serum, suggesting that levels of amino acids are influenced by placental synthesis and do not depend on maternal amino acid metabolism. Levels of amino acids were significantly higher in coelomic fluid than in AF. The authors concluded that amino acids in the coelomic fluid support the metabolism of the secondary yolk sac, the cavity being a nutrient reservoir for the fetus during the first trimester of pregnancy.

Jauniaux et al.[225] measured the distribution of amino acids between 7 and 11 weeks of gestation in homogenates of placental villi, in samples of coelomic and AF and maternal serum. They found a significant positive relation between maternal serum and placental tissue for 10 amino acids, indicating that active amino acid transport and accumulation by the human syncytiotrophoblast occurs as early as 7 weeks of gestation. The concentration distribution of individual amino acids in coelomic and AF were related, indicating a passive transfer through the amniotic membrane. Later, the authors[226] measured the concentration of 23 free amino acids in homogenates of fetal liver and samples of fetal plasma from 20 pregnancies between 12 and 17 weeks of gestation and compared those with matched samples of maternal plasma and AF. A fetomaternal plasma concentration gradient was observed for 21 amino acids, indicating that the fetomaternal amino acid gradient across the placenta is established from very early in pregnancy. The amino acid concentration pattern was similar in fetal plasma and AF but different in fetal liver, supporting the concept that it is essentially placental transport and metabolism that provides the fetus with these molecules.

Measurements of amino acids between the 13th and the 23rd week of gestation showed that the concentrations of Ala, Lys, Val, Glu, Pro, Thr, and Gly accounted for about 70 percent of the amino acids in amniotic fluids.[227] A negative correlation with gestational age (-0.34 to -0.24) was found for Leu, Val, Ile, Phe, Lys, Ala, Asp, Tyr, Glu, and Pro. The concentration of Gln increased slightly ($r = 0.18$), whereas the other amino acids did not change significantly during this period. Statistically significant positive correlations, at all gestational ages, were observed among Val, Leu, and Ile. These branched-chain amino acids also correlated positively with Phe, Lys, Asp, Thr, Ser, Glu, Pro, Gly, Ala, and Tyr, and the amino acids within this group correlated with each other. In addition, strong positive correlations were observed between Phe and Tyr and between Gly and Ser.

In humans,[229] AF amino acid levels are not influenced by normal variations in maternal amino acid concentrations. However, if the mother has an enzyme deficiency, a specific amino acid may be found in high concentration in the AF. Observation of a constant phenylalanine/tyrosine ratio in fetal AF supports the hypothesis that phenylalanine hydroxylase is present from the 9th week of pregnancy. Studies in *Ovis aries*[230] showed that if the animal was kept on a diet of 100 mg/kg phenylalanine per day, no change occurred in amniotic and allantoic fluids. However, intravenous injection of phenylalanine in the sheep is reflected by an increase in the fetal phenylalanine serum level. The prenatal diagnosis of phenylketonuria (PKU) is now based on a molecular study (see chapter 10) following the cloning of the human phenylalanine hydroxylase gene.[231,232] Malignant hyperphenylalaninemia can be diagnosed by measurement of dihydropteridine reductase, which is reported to be present in fetal cells at 16 weeks of gestation.[233] Although there is a high risk of fetal anomaly in the fetuses of untreated mothers with PKU,[234] there are situations in which the fetus shows defensive mechanisms probably related to the maternal phenylalanine serum level.

The increase of citrulline in the AF of a fetus affected with an argininosuccinate synthetase deficiency has been noted by Kamoun et al.[235] However, as stated by others,[236] measurement of the citrulline concentration in AF is an adjunct in the prenatal diagnosis of the severe neonatal form of citrullinemia. In two affected fetuses, the other amino acids were in the normal range, whereas citrulline showed a 10-fold increase. Chadefaux-Vekemans et al.[237] proposed the use of the citrulline/ornithine + arginine ratio, which is more discriminatory than citrulline concentration alone, when performing prenatal diagnosis of citrullinemia.

During the second trimester, there is accumulation of galactitol in the tissues of fetuses affected with galactosemia and also in AF. This could lead to an early prenatal diagnosis, although the enzymatic studies should be done to confirm the defect. It is interesting that galactitol accumulates in galactosemia and galactokinase-deficient patients.[239] Northrup et al.[240] reviewed studies on citrullinemia and compared the diagnostic techniques available for prenatal diagnosis. Although enzyme assay, quantitative determination of citrulline in AF, and ^{14}C citrulline incorporation by cultured fetal cells have been used, analysis of informative-restriction polymorphisms or precise mutation detection are the preferred methods of diagnosis (see chapters 10 and 13).

Coude and co-workers[241] studied organic acids in AF samples obtained by amniocentesis as early as 6–12 weeks of pregnancy. They state that methylmalonic and propionic acidemia could be diagnosed during the first trimester of pregnancy. Jakobs et al.[242] reviewed the usefulness of metabolite determinations in AF samples to diagnose amino and organic acidurias. Tyrosinemia type I and propionic acidemia have been diagnosed at the end of the first trimester via amniocentesis. One interesting finding related to amino acid metabolism has been the demonstration of succinylacetone in the AF of fetuses affected with hereditary tyrosinemia type I secondary to a deficiency of fumarylacetoacetate hydrolase in the liver.[218,219] Fumarylacetoacetate fumarylhydrolase, an enzyme involved in the tyrosine metabolic pathway,[221] is present in lymphocytes, fibroblasts, cultured amniocytes, and chorionic villi. Succinylacetone can be measured either by gas chromatography–mass spectrometry or by delta-aminolevulinate dehydratase inhibition assay. Prenatal diagnosis of tyrosinemia type I involving the measurement of succinylacetone in AF at 12 weeks of gestation has been offered to couples at risk since 1982.[219] However, affected fetuses and heterozygote carriers can now be identified by DNA analysis.

Fourteen metabolic disorders can be detected by a stable isotope dilution gas technique using chromatography and mass spectrometry with selected ion monitoring (GC-MS-SIM). Eleven other disorders are potential candidates for diagnosis by the same method. However, this has not been found to be useful for maple-syrup urine disease or lactic acidemia, which are caused by pyruvate carboxylase or pyruvate dehydrogenase deficiencies. The authors caution investigators against the use of this method for metabolic disorders in which metabolites are not specifically expressed in early pregnancy. A quantitative, rapid, sensitive and reproducible tandem mass spectrometry (MSMS) method for the one-step detection of amino acid and acylcarnitine concentrations is described[243] as most informative to measure low amino acid and acylcarnitine in AF.

MICROVILLAR ENZYMES

Intestinal microvillar enzyme activities (disaccharidases, alkaline phosphatase, and peptidases) in AF have been proposed as diagnostic markers for various pathological conditions, including cystic fibrosis (CF), chromosomal aberrations, intestinal obstruction, and fetal kidney dysfunction.

The Disaccharidases

AF disaccharidases have been used for the prenatal detection of intestinal obstruction, polycystic kidney disease, congenital nephrosis, and CF. The disaccharidases in AF were first noted by Antonowicz et al. in 1975.[244] Actual activity values were reported by Potier et al.[203] in the same year. In the human fetus, the disaccharidases are distributed in tissues such as intestine, kidney, and liver,[245] although they are more concentrated in the former two. They are localized in the brush-border membranes of the cells lining the villi of the fetal small intestine. Intestinal villi are well developed at 8–10 weeks of gestation, with the crypts approaching maturation at the time.[246] With the exception of lactase, which develops only a few weeks before term, disaccharidases are fully developed in the human fetal intestine as early as 10 weeks of gestation.[247–249] The fetal kidney contains only trehalase and some maltase activities in detectable quantities. The intestinal mucosa contains disaccharidases able to hydrolyze a variety of substrates, such as maltose, sucrose, trehalose, turanose, palatinose, lactose, cellobiose, isomaltose, and oligosaccharides. Few glycosidases are implicated in the hydrolysis of all these substrates: four α-glucosidases (glucoamylase, sucrase, isomaltase, and trehalase) and a β-glucosidase (lactase) (reviewed by Kenny and Maroux[250]). Their physiological function in the intestine is apparently to hydrolyze disaccharides and oligosaccharides, absorbed in the diet, into monosaccharides, which are transported through the mucosal surface into the bloodstream. The physiological function of trehalase and maltase in the kidney is not completely understood, but trehalase has been implicated in glucose transport mechanisms taking place in the kidney brush-border membranes.[251]

Origin of Amniotic Fluid Disaccharidases

In the AF, the disaccharidase activities apparently originate from both the fetal intestine and the kidney.[203–205] The disaccharidases are released into the amniotic cavity with the brush-border membranes, following desquamation of fetal enterocytes and kidney cells. The kidney disaccharidases (mainly trehalase) are detected in the AF at a later stage of gestation than the intestinal enzymes[201] and in fetuses affected with renal pathologies.[245,252]

The evidence in favor of the intestinal origin of most AF disaccharidases rests on the following observations: (a) the AF contains a full complement of disaccharidase activities similar to those of the fetal intestinal mucosa (maltase, sucrase, palatinase, trehalase, turanase, lactase, and cellobiase)[205–207]; (b) among the human fetal organs studied, disaccharidase activities are concentrated in the intestine, with the exception of trehalase and small amounts of maltase in the fetal kidney[197,245]; (c) AF disaccharidases have kinetic properties similar to those of intestinal disaccharidases, and they are bound to membrane debris in AF[203]; (d) there exists a close relationship between relative activities of disaccharidases in intestine and AF of individual fetuses[204]; (e) disaccharidase activities are deficient in the AF of fetuses with intestinal obstruction[252–254]; and finally, (f) fetal defecation was observed in utero by fetoscopy during the second trimester of gestation.[255] Claas et al.[256] provided immunologic and enzymologic evidence that the maltase activity of AF originates exclusively from the fetal intestine. Trehalase and lactase seem more sensitive to degradation of denaturation in the fetal intestinal lumen than maltase, sucrase, palatinase, and turanase. The amount of each disaccharidase released into the AF seems dictated by their relative sensitivities to proteolytic digestion in vivo.[256]

Intestinal microvilli of fetal origin have been characterized in AF after purification by CA^{2+}-precipitation of contaminating organelles followed by differential centrifugation of the microvillar membranes.[257,258] In the purified preparation, the specific activities of the intestinal microvillar marker enzymes maltase and sucrase increased about seventy-sevenfold over those in cell-free AF. AF microvilli contain typical enzymes of intestinal microvilli, including maltase, sucrase, trehalase, alkaline phosphatase, and γ-glutamyl transferase, and their morphology detected by electron microscopy resembles that of vesiculated intestinal microvilli. Jalanko et al.[259] also reported the presence of vesicles in AF, which they concluded originate in the fetal intestine. Prenatal detection of genetic diseases due to a deficiency of a protein expressed in these membranes or associated with abnormal morphology of microvilli seems feasible. Transport system activities expressed

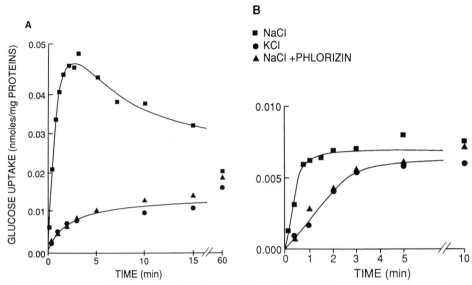

Fig. 3.3. The uptake of ^{3}H-glucose in microvilli prepared from fetal intestinal mucosa (A) and from amniotic fluid (B).

in these membranes can also be assayed by measuring the uptake of radioactive substrates. Na^+-dependent glucose transport, inhibitable by phlorizin, was demonstrated in microvilli purified from AF, suggesting that transporter systems can be assayed in these membranes (Figure 3.3). There is evidence that trehalase activity also could originate from the fetal kidney, at least in pathologic situations. First, it was noted that several fetuses with proven intestinal obstructions had normal trehalase activity, despite the fact that the other disaccharidases were almost completely deficient.[245,260,261] In addition, high trehalase activity (relative to the other disaccharidases) was found in the AF of fetuses with renal anomalies such as polycystic kidney disease[245] and congenital nephrotic syndrome.[261] In their study on the origin of α-glucosidase activity in human AF, Poenaru et al.[262] concluded, on the basis of both kinetic and immunologic evidence, that both renal and intestinal α-glucosidases were present.

Further biochemical characterization of trehalase from intestinal and kidney tissues revealed similar molecular size but a difference of isoelectric point between the two enzymes.[263] In the AF, isoelectric focusing revealed that the intestinal form (pI54.60) was present in samples collected before 21 weeks of gestation, whereas in samples obtained later in pregnancy, only the renal form (pI54.24) was present. In one fetus affected with polycystic kidney disease, the renal form of trehalase was markedly increased in the AF. In another fetus with intestinal obstruction, the intestinal form of trehalase, as well as other disaccharidase activities, were reduced in the AF. However, no systematic study on the clinical usefulness of AF trehalase for the detection of fetal renal anomalies has yet been conducted. Therefore, this test should be used with caution for diagnostic purposes.

Other Microvillar Enzyme Activities

Peptidases such as γ-glutamyl transpeptidase, leucine aminopeptidase, aminopeptidase M, and alkaline phosphatase are no longer used for the detection of CF (see chapter 15).

Development of AF Disaccharidases

On the basis of a comparison of specific activities (per mg of protein) of disaccharidases in the intestine and AF, it was concluded that during the second trimester, between 10 and 20 percent of the total proteins of AF could be of intestinal origin.[264] Developmental patterns of AF disaccharidases have been studied by Potier et al.[204] and Antonowicz et al.[205] All disaccharidase activities vary approximately in parallel during the course of gestation. They are present from 10 weeks of gestation, reach maximum values around 15–18 weeks, and drop rapidly to low values after 22 weeks. A comparison of the drop of disaccharidase activities as a function of the length of gestation is shown in Figure 3.4. All disaccharidases had a similar pattern, with the exception of trehalase activity, which increased after 22 weeks of gestation.

Potier et al.[204] suggested that the drop of disaccharidase activities at around 22 weeks of gestation is due to a combination of two physiologic mechanisms: (1) increasing fetal swallowing with age, and (2) accumulation of large quantities of meconium in the fetal intestine. It is known that the fetus swallows more and more with growth, which results in an increase in the reabsorption of AF proteins and disaccharidases. Gitlin et al.[265] reported that fetal swallowing is a major process by which proteins are cleared from the AF. In addition, as large quantities of meconium accumulate in the fetal intestine at around 22 weeks, the normal release of disaccharidases from the intestinal lumen to the amniotic cavity would be hampered. Mulivor et al.[266] observed a similar development pattern for intestinal alkaline phosphatase, and Pocknee and Abramovich[267] did so for AF trypsin activity. Such a pattern seems to be characteristic of the enzymes originating from, or transiting through, the fetal intestine.

To understand the mechanisms involved in the release and control of disaccharidase activities in AF, animal models suitable for studies have been investigated. Developmen-

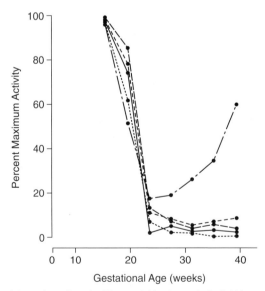

Fig. 3.4. A comparison of the various disaccharidase activities in amniotic fluid between 14 and 42 weeks of gestation, showing the different patterns of trehalase activity. All activities are expressed as a percentage of the mean activity at 14–17 weeks of gestation. – – = maltase, – – – – – = sucrase, – - – = trehalase, ———— = palatinase, ... = lactase.

tal patterns and properties of AF disaccharidase were studied in sheep[268] and rabbits.[269] The results of these studies on animal models support the conclusion that there is a relationship between meconium accumulation in the fetal intestine and the rapid fall of disaccharidase activities in the AF.[204]

Clinical Use of AF Disaccharidases

The AF disaccharidases have been used for the prenatal detection of fetal intestinal obstruction on the basis of low or absent activities in the AF.[245,254] In our laboratory, 16 fetuses between 16 and 20 weeks of gestation have been studied, who have different types of intestinal obstruction, with or without ventral wall defects and chromosomal syndromes, including imperforate anus, duodenal or jejunoileal atresia, and the autosomal recessive type of multiple intestinal atresia.[270] Van Diggelen et al.[254] reported on a fetus with anal atresia at 17 weeks of gestation. In all of these cases, disaccharidase activities were found to be below the normal range. Among the microvillar enzymes, the exclusively intestinal hydrolases maltase, sucrase, palatinase, and an intestinal form of alkaline phosphatase were the best markers to detect intestinal obstruction. Trehalase and γ-glutamyl transferase are distributed in other fetal organs and gave several false-negative results.[260]

Low or absent disaccharidase activities, as well as other microvillar enzyme activities (alkaline phosphatase and γ-glutamyl transferase),[254,271–273] have been reported in some fetuses affected with CF (see chapter 15). These fetuses seem to be unable to release their intestinal content normally into the amniotic cavity. It is important that the disaccharidase assay be performed no later than the 20th week of gestation, because after this period, some normal AF samples were found to have very low disaccharidase activities, which may be confounded with that of an affected fetus. In our hands, the disaccharidase test gave false-negative results in two fetuses with proven CF.[271] Six other fetuses with CF were deficient and were thus correctly identified retrospectively.[260]

The disaccharidase activities in AF are more specific to the fetal intestine and kidney than γ-glutamyl transferase.[274–277] However, both γ-glutamyl transferase and alkaline phosphatase show reduced activity levels in the AF of various pathologic pregnancies, such as trisomy 18[274] and trisomy 21.[275] Elevated activity of alkaline phosphatase has been observed in intrauterine fetal death, abdominal wall defect, Meckel syndrome, hydrops fetalis, and genital anomaly.[254] Elevated alkaline phosphatase activity in third-trimester AF is often associated with fetal disorders.

For the disaccharidase test to give valid results, the intestinal obstruction should hamper normal release of disaccharidases into the amniotic cavity. With multiple intestinal atresia, for instance, the intestinal obstruction is complete. In contrast, the situation is more complex with Hirschsprung disease, in which the intestinal obstruction may be incomplete. Our experience with two affected cases suggests that the disaccharidase test cannot be used for the prenatal detection of Hirschsprung disease because both fetuses had normal disaccharidase activities in the AF.[278]

Another intestinal malformation that possibly can be detected by a disaccharidase test in AF is the villus atrophy syndrome.[279] This is a recessively inherited condition characterized by an atrophy of intestinal villi and reduced disaccharidase activities in the intestinal mucosa. The disaccharidase activities would be expected to be low or deficient in the AF of an affected fetus. We had the opportunity to test such a pregnancy at risk and found normal disaccharidase activities in the AF. The newborn was subsequently found to be normal.[260]

Trehalase activity in AF has been used for the prenatal detection of fetal renal anomalies. Morin et al.[245] reported elevated trehalase/palatinase (or lactase) activity ratios in the AF of a fetus with polycystic kidney disease type II and of two fetuses with the congenital nephrotic syndrome of the Finnish type. These ratios were used as indices of the presence of renal trehalase in AF because palatinase and lactase are exclusively of intestinal origin.[245] All fetuses affected with renal congenital disease, in which a degeneration of kidney tissue is observed, can be expected to release higher than normal levels of renal trehalase activity in the amniotic cavity.

More recent studies confirmed the usefulness of trehalase determination in AF for the detection of polycystic kidney disease.[280] However, in our laboratory, two fetuses affected with congenital nephrosis gave false-negative levels of trehalase activity in the AF. Therefore, we believe that trehalase activity cannot be used as an index of congenital nephrosis, and prenatal detection must rely on an elevated AFP level and mutation analysis (chapters 10 and 21).

Low digestive enzyme activities in human AF can be observed[281] in normal and disease-affected pregnancies (CF, trisomy 21, and intestinal atresia). AFs were analyzed by proton nuclear magnetic resonance (NMR) spectroscopy in order to specify prenatally the etiology of low digestive enzyme activities observed at 17–18 weeks of amenorrhea. An unidentified resonance at 1.05 ppm was detected in seven of thirteen cases of CF-affected fetuses.

A simple method for the determination of the three isozymes of alkaline phosphatase (EC 3.1.3.1) contained in AF (fetal intestinal, placental, and liver-bone-kidney) is described by Sembaj et al.[282] Thus, the difference between total alkaline phosphatase activity and activity in the 100,000 g supernatant corresponds to fetal intestinal alkaline phosphatase. Mean percentages of the total alkaline phosphatase for each of the isozymes in AF were 81 percent for fetal intestinal alkaline phosphatase, 7.5 percent for placental alkaline phosphatase and 12.0 percent for liver–bone–kidney alkaline phosphatase.

During development,[283] the gastrointestinal tract undergoes marked changes in many physiologic and anatomic properties. The interactions between nutrition and intestinal development begin when fetuses start swallowing AF and extend past weaning. Hormonal control plays a major role in the ontogeny of the small intestine.

Karnak et al.[284] concluded in a study on esophageal ligation that AF ingestion has no significant effect on somatic growth but will affect the development of several organs and, in particular, gastric, small intestinal. and total gastrointestinal tract weights. Only the proximal portion of the small intestine lactase was decreased. The animal study involved the esophageal ligation of rabbit fetuses at 23 days of gestation. Sucrase and maltase activities were not measurable in both groups.

Recently, it has been shown[285] that, in human fetuses suffering from gastroschisis, there is an AF inflammatory response and that AF exchange, designed to disrupt the inflammatory loop, seems to have a favorable impact on outcome. The authors, therefore, designed in the fetal sheep a model of gastroschisis with and without esophageal ligation in which amnio-infusion significantly improved the deleterious process.

In conclusion, the disaccharidase test has a clinical utility for pregnancies presenting a risk of intestinal obstruction, such as the autosomal recessive type of multiple intestinal atresia,[270] polyhydramnios, or any other genetic indication of intestinal malformation compatible with reduced disaccharidase activities in the AF. Such test results would indicate the initiation of appropriate newborn care or provision of genetic counseling, including the option of elective abortion in families at risk for untreatable multiple intestinal obstructions. Results of low disaccharidase values are best followed by diagnostic ultrasound studies and, when necessary, the use of radiopaque substances for more certain delineation of the defect. Indications of renal degenerative diseases might also justify a disaccharidase test in conjunction with diagnostic ultrasound.

MISCELLANEOUS BIOCHEMICAL CONSTITUENTS AND OTHER CHARACTERISTICS OF AF

Various nonenzymatic constituents and characteristics of AF are listed in Table 3.2. Elevated values of biochemical constituents in AF may be nonspecific, such as 5-hydroxyindole-3-acetic acid in a fetus with Cornelia de Lange syndrome,[468] or acid-soluble glycoproteins in AF in CF.[377] Increased concentrations of amino acids (especially methionine, isoleucine, leucine, tyrosine, and phenylalanine) have been observed in the AF of fetuses with NTDs.[297] Two likely reasons are transudation across the defect and a nonspecific reflection of fetal distress with hypoxia. In contrast, a reduced amount of 5-hydroxyindole-3-acetic acid has been reported.[387,469] Certain other constituents of cell-free AF, such as 17-ketosteroids, are especially relevant to prenatal diagnosis (see chapter 16).

Starting from the principle that in several species studied, the D-amino nitrogen concentration is higher in the fetus than in the mother, Soltesz and co-workers[470] have studied venous and arterial blood amino acid levels in humans. Using fetoscopy between 18 and 21 weeks of gestation, in pretermination stages of pregnancy for social reasons, the authors have collected arterial and venous cord blood samples and measured amino acid concentrations. Values obtained were compared with maternal venous samples taken simultaneously. These results confirmed the existence of a fetomaternal gradient for amino acids during the second trimester of pregnancy: the total molar concentration of amino acids was at least twice as high in the fetal venous and arterial blood samples as in the maternal plasma. Keeping in mind that several manipulation factors may interfere with amino acid concentrations in fetal tissues, one can gain new insight from these experiments into fetomaternal exchange during pregnancy, and this should eventually allow determinations of amino acid and other nutrients during gestation.

A study of fetal insulin metabolism by Weiss et al.[400] confirmed that the insulin level increases in the AF of healthy, pregnant women from a value of 1.3 μU/mL at 13 weeks of gestation to a peak of 9.1 μU/mL at term. Similar values were noted by others,[471] with the added observation of a biphasic course of insulin concentration between 16 and 42 weeks of pregnancy and a zenith at the 30th week. In women receiving glucocorticoids or betamimetics or in fetuses with high glucose levels, the insulin levels may show a twofold increase, whereas very low levels are found in placental insufficiency and other conditions leading to fetal distress.

Hahn et al.[337] speculated that carnitine, which is involved in fatty acid metabolism, is retained by fetal tissues. Carnitine levels measured during pregnancy were found to be higher in cord than in maternal blood.

Thirteen major polypeptides, of which five had not been identified previously, were revealed by two different techniques. Their molecular weights ranged from 11 to 220 kDa. Prado et al.[437] suggest that those polypeptides might serve as useful references in molecular studies of fetal pathology. Maternal serum relaxin during pregnancy maintains the myometrial quiescence and facilitates uterine stroma remodeling during the uterine growth. In AF, this protein[445] rises from 58 ng/L at 10 weeks to 142 ng/L at 14 weeks and declines to 55 ng/l at 22 weeks. Relaxin may be derived from the decidualized endometrium

Table 3.2. Biochemical constituents and other characteristics of AF

Biochemical Constituent/Characteristic	Selected Reference(s): (See Text for Additional Sources)
Acetylcholine receptor	286
Acetylcholinesterase (AChE)	287,288
Acid–base	289,290
Adrenomedullin	291
α-fetoprotein	Chaper 21
Albumin	7,121,292
Alkaline phosphatase	266,272,293
α_1-Antitrypsin	292,294,295
α_1-Macroglobulin	292,296
Amino-acids	229,297,298–304
Amylase	305
Androgens	306
Angiogenin	307
Anticardiolipin antibodies	308
Antithrombin	296
Antiviral effect	309
Apolipoprotein	310
Apolipoprotein A	311
Arylsulfatase A	209
Atrial natriuretic factor	210
Bacteria	312
Bacterial growth, inhibitory effect	313–319
Basement membrane protein	113
β-Endorphin	320–323
β-Hydroxybutyrate	324
β_2-Microglobulin	98, 325–326
Bile pigments	265
Bilirubin	327–329
Bisphenol A	330
Blood group substances	331,332
Blood urea nitrogen	109
Cadmium	333
Candida albicans	334
Carcinoembryonic antigen	335
Calcium	336
Carnitine	337
Cathecolamine	338
Cerulopasmin	89,292
Cholesterol	121,137
Chorionic gonadotropin	306,339
Chorionic somatomammotropin	306
Citric acid	340
C-reactive protein	341,342
Clara cell protein	237
Complement	292
Copper	336,343
Cortisol	306,344–346
Creatine phosphokinase	187
Creatinine	120,122,347–352
Cystatin C	353,354
Cytokines	355–356
Cytomegalovirus	358
Decidua-associated protein	359

Table 3.2. Biochemical constituents and other characteristics of AF (continued)

Biochemical Constituent/Characteristic	Selected Reference(s): (See Text for Additional Sources)
Defensins	360,361
7-Dehydrocholesterol	233
Disaccharidases	203,204,362
Electrolytes	121,122,290,348
Estrogens	306,363–367
Factor IX	117
Fatty acids	137,368,368a
Ferritin	369
Fibronectin	370,371
Follicle-stimulating hormone (FSH)	339
Fractalkine	372
Free fatty acids	153
Fumarylacetoactetase	221
γ-Glutamyl transferase	373
Globulin	125,114,374
Globulin, cold-insoluble	375
Glucagon	376
Glucose	109,376
Glycoproteins	126,377
Glycosaminoglycans	112,115
Growth hormone	378–381
Growth-inhibiting property	382
Hemopexin	94
Homocysteine	223
Human leukocyte antigen G	383
Human leukocyte antigens (HLA)	384,385
Hydrocarbons	137
2-Hydroxybutyric acid	386
5-Hydroxindole-3-acetic acid	387
Hydroxyproline	388,389
Immunoglobulin	109,292,390–395
Inhibin (utero)	396–399
Insulin-like growth factor binding protein-1	357,357a,379
Insulin	376,400
Intercellular adhesion molecule	401
Interleukins	402–405
Iron	336
Isoferritin	406
Isomylases	407
Kallikrein	408
Lactoferrin	409
Lead	410
Lecithin/sphingomyelin (L/S) ratio	171,293,346,368,411–413
Lipids	134, 137
Lipopolysaccharide-binding protein	138
Luteinizing hormone (LH)	339
Lysosomal enzymes	205
Lysozyme	414, 415
Macroglobulin	296
Magnesium	336
Manganese	336
Meconium	416, 417
Metalloproteinase	418

Table 3.2. Biochemical constituents and other characteristics of AF (continued)

Biochemical Constituent/Characteristic	Selected Reference(s): (See Text for Additional Sources)
Metals	333
Muramidase (See Lysosyme)	
Mycoplasma	419
Neuraminic acid	420
Neurotrophins	421
Neuron-specific enolase	422
Nitric oxide	423
Nucleic acids	71
Nucleosome	72
Nicotine	424
Organic acids	70,425
Osmolality	121,426
Orosomucoid	131
Oxalate	427
Oygen tension	289
Oxytocin	428
Palmitic acid	171,293
PAPP-A	129
Peptidase activity	271,274
Peroxidase	415,429
Phospholipids	156,351,368,430–432
Phospholipase	433
Phytoestrogens	434
Plasminogen	296,435,436
Polypeptides	437
Procoagulant	438
Procollagen propeptides	439
Progesterone	306
Prolactin	306,440,441
Prostaglandin	306,442
Protein	77,89,121,122,292,443
Protein-bound iodine	444
Prothrombin	117
Pyruvate kinase	191
Relaxin	445
Renin	446
Rubella	447
Rubidium	410
Secretor typing	448
Selenium	333
Sialic acid	449
Sodium	18
Somatomedin	450–452
Spectrophotometry	453
Steroid hormones	306,454
Stromelysins	455
Succinylacetone	219
Surface-active material	378
Surface tension	456
Tamm–Horsfall glycoprotein	114
Testosterone	457–459
Thromboplastin	438,460
Thrombopoietin	461

Table 3.2. Biochemical constituents and other characteristics of AF (continued)

Biochemical Constituent/Characteristic	Selected Reference(s): (See Text for Additional Sources)
Trace elements	462
Transferrin	89,292
Triglyceride	121,137
3.3′,5′-Triiodothyronine	463
Trypsin	267
Ureaplasma urealyticum	419
Uric acid	121,348,348a
Urinary trypsin inhibitor	349
Vitamin A	464,465
Vitamin B$_{12}$	466
Vitamin D	467
Viral antibodies	395
Viruses	395
Volume of AF	4,5,7,29
Zinc	336,333

Note: For enzymes, see Table 11.1.

rather than the maternal circulation. In this study, there did not seem to be significant placental transfer or fetal synthesis of this peptide.

Trace Elements

AF copper and zinc are among the trace elements measured during pregnancy and found to have stable levels during the second and third trimesters.[343,472] No direct correlation has yet been made in AF studies between central nervous system development or enzymatic reactions and variations in trace element levels in humans. However, it is worth noting that studies in rats and mice showed that zinc deficiency in the diet potentiates the effects of alcohol on the progeny of pregnant mice.[473,474]

Furthermore, to those observations and another by Chez et al.[343] on copper and zinc, Hall et al.[462] combined proton-induced X-ray emission (PIXE) and direct plasma-atomic emission spectrometry (DCP-AES) for multi-element analysis. Their studies were done on AF samples obtained between 16 and 19 weeks of gestation (mean, 17.1 weeks) from women referred for advanced maternal age. Ninety samples were analyzed; the reported values are given here in an expanded table kindly provided by these authors (Table 3.3).

Copper, zinc, bromine, lead, and rubidium assays also were carried out,[410] using fluorescence X-spectrophotometry with dispersion of energy. The authors found no significant differences among groups of normal, hypotrophic, and trisomic fetuses. Using inductively coupled ICP-AES, Bussière et al.[336] studied calcium, copper, iron, magnesium, manganese, and zinc in normal second-trimester AF samples. The authors stressed that the wide dispersion of reported metal concentration values in AF may be secondary to sample variability, lack of technical uniformity, and the presence of contaminants. Nevertheless, results obtained for those trace elements are of the same order of magnitude as in previously published reports.[462,475,476] The values reported by Bussière et al.[336] were as follows: zinc, 27–81 ng mL^{-1}, calcium, 42–72 μg mL^{-1}; magnesium, 13.1–16.9 μg mL^{-1}; copper, 98–195 ng mL^{-1}; iron, −16–538 ng mL^{-1}; and manganese, 14–16 ng

Table 3.3. Trace elements in AF

Element (Z)	N	Mean	SD
B (5)	88	32.2	1.7
Mg (12)	200	16.0[a,b]	3.1
Al (13)	200	424.1	1.2
Si (14)	200	247.2	2.7
P (15)	200	28.3[a,b]	4.0
K (19)	200	148.4[b]	1.1
Ca (20)	200	73.2[a,b]	12.2
Ti (22)	200	13.2	2.0
V (23)	200	183.1	1.4
Cr (24)	200	4.9	1.9
Mn (25)	200	4.7	1.8
Fe (26)	200	3475.8	14.5
Co (27)	88	44.0	1.8
Ni (28)	200	24.0	2.2
Cu (29)	200	1437.0[b]	35.3
Zn (30)	88	216.5	15.1
Rb (37)	200	217.4	80.1
Sr (38)	200	21.2[a]	7.1
Ag (47)	88	15.1[a]	7.8
Sn (50)	88	95.6	1.5
Ba (56)	200	17.0	6.0
Pb (82)	88	116.7	1.4

[a]Concentration mg/mL.
[b]Arithmetic mean
Note: Mean gestational age, 17.1 weeks. All concentrations are ng/mL and except where noted.
Source: Hall et al., 1983[462] (see also Dawson et al., 1999[333]).

mL^{-1}. These results should be useful in prospective studies on fetal development and risk assessment of maternal exposure to toxic metals. Vitamin A levels had been measured by Parkinson et al.,[464] who later demonstrated that zinc levels were grossly elevated in mothers carrying a fetus with an NTD.[477] During the second trimester, the mean values of vitamin A were also raised in the presence of a fetal NTD. The concentration of vitamin A in the AF was 3.861.3 μg/100 mL, whereas in NTDs, the mean value was 5.761.6 μg/100 mL. Following this report, it was shown that the retinol AF values could not be used as a marker for the detection of fetal defects during the second trimester, as could have been expected in light of the knowledge of retinol binding protein and placental transfer.[465]

Tamura and co-workers[478] studied the relationships between AF and maternal blood nutrient concentrations. Zinc, copper and iron were measured by atomic absorption spectrophotometry. They found that the mean concentrations of plasma and red blood cell (RBC) folate, plasma and copper of the pregnant women were higher than those of healthy nonpregnant controls. Mean concentrations of plasma vitamin B_{12}, zinc, and iron levels and RBC zinc were similar to those of nonpregnant controls. AF folate, zinc, copper, and iron concentrations were significantly lower than plasma levels. However, this relationship was reversed for vitamin B_{12}. They found no correlation between AF and blood nutrient concentrations and pregnancy outcome. A number of studies have reported lower vitamin B_{12} concentrations in AF in the presence of fetal NTDs when compared with unaffected fetuses.[479–481]

Luglie and co-workers[482] studied the total concentration of mercury in AF and compared it with the number of occlusal extension of fillings using Ag amalgam. Women due to undergo amniocentesis were selected for the study. Mercury is one of the components of Ag amalgam that can pass into the organs and biologic fluids. The authors studied the possibility that mercury may pass through the placental barrier and reach the fetus. The aim of this study was "to evaluate the concentration of total mercury in human AF and compare it with the number and occlusal extension of fillings using Ag amalgam." Mercury levels in the AF were assayed using a spectrophotometer with atomic absorption and a FIAS-amalgam technique. No direct relationship was found with mercury levels. The occlusal extension of dental repairs was significantly correlated with metal concentrations. The authors recommend that silver amalgam should be used with considerable caution during pregnancy.

Milnerowicz et al.[483] suggested that smoking may have an impact on uterine blood vessels and may cause placental vascular insufficiency and changes in fetal membranes. In this study, the concentration of metals was determined by electrothermal atomic absorption spectrophotometry (ET-ASA). Zn and Cd were half the value and Pb ten times lower in AF from a small number of women as compared with a normal pregnancy. Cotinine and Cd were much higher in women with oligohydramnios who were also heavy smokers.

Creatinine/Cystatin C

In early pregnancy, the creatinine level in the AF is similar to that found in maternal serum, rising later in pregnancy to reach values twice those of maternal serum at term. In early gestation, it seems that creatinine moves from maternal to fetal serum and then to fetal urine and AF.[484] In late pregnancy, AF creatinine may originate from fetal muscle as well.

The accurate determination of fetal maturity is frequently of critical importance if the survival of the newborn is to be assured. Creatinine is one of the many indices used for the assessment of fetal maturity.[116,338,348,485,486] A number of authors have tried to improve on the maturity assessments provided by creatinine estimations alone, by combining the results of creatinine estimations, the percentage of lipid-positive cells,[487] and the L/S ratio for a more accurate assessment.[488] The simultaneous assessment of the three parameters correlates well with fetal maturity in normal pregnancy. However, in the very cases of abnormal pregnancy states (including diabetes, Rh isoimmunization, hypertensive disorders, intrauterine growth retardation, and hydramnios) in which guidance would be invaluable, these estimations, both singly and together, still leave the clinician with significant uncertainty.

As suggested by Muller et al.[353] prognosis on fetal outcome can rely only on sonography in cases of severe or mild uropathies, the most frequent being the obstructive anomalies. Serum creatinine cannot be used as a marker of glomerular filtration (GFR) because it crosses the placenta and is cleared by the mother. This is because during fetal life the mother supplies the fetus through the placenta with balanced nutrients, and fetal homeostasis is ensured without the intervention of the fetal kidneys. Therefore, the composition of the fetal urine depends only on renal function. Cystatin C has been shown to be an accurate marker of GFR in adults and infants, and can be considered as a marker of fetal renal tubular damage rather than a marker of GFR.

Mussap et al.[354] compared the diagnostic accuracy of cystatin C with that of creatinine in discriminating renal function in fetuses without ultrasonographic evidence of renal malformations from those with obstructive uropathies. Creatinine was measured by a kinetic Jaffe picric acid method and cystatin C by a nephelometric immunoassay. The maximum diagnostic accuracy of serum cystatin C in discriminating controls from fetal uropathies was 96 percent, whereas that of creatinine was 62 percent. The authors concluded that cystatin C may be considered a sensitive biochemical marker for the early identification of fetuses with obstructive uropathies.

Blood-Group Substances

The Lewis and soluble blood-group substances A, B, and H are known to be present in AF as early as 9–24 weeks of gestation.[221,332,489–492] The best evidence suggests that the AF Lewis substances and secretor types are of fetal origin. Because of their molecular weights (about 300,000),[493] the soluble blood-group substrates do not easily cross fetal membranes. Because the fetal ABH secretor and Lewis types can be determined from AF in early gestation, they may well be useful because of their linkage relationships to genetic disease. Examples include the linkage relationships of the ABO locus to the nail–patella syndrome[494] and the linkage of the secretor locus to the locus for myotonic muscular dystrophy.[495,496] Additional studies[448] confirmed the accuracy and reliability of AF secretor typing, using the semiquantitative hemagglutination inhibition procedure. The presence of some maternal blood contamination does not interfere with the reading, but maternal antibodies may be found in discolored fluids after maternal bleeding. Steinert disease or myotonic dystrophy is linked to the secretor locus, which is linked to the Lutheran blood group, Lu-Se-Dm, on chromosome 19. The prenatal diagnosis of myotonic muscular dystrophy is now accurately achieved by trinucleotide repeat analysis (chapter 10). Early on, Milunsky et al.[497] reported the prenatal diagnosis of six cases and stressed the risk of neurologic impairment when the mother herself is affected.

The development of fetoscopy facilitated the measurement of factor VIII coagulant antigen and factor VIII–related antigen. The ratio of factor VIII coagulant antigen to factor VIII–related antigen has a fairly constant value, and in three affected fetuses, a very low ratio was pathognomonic of classic hemophilia (see also chapter 2). This immunologic test does not apply to all families at risk, and has been replaced by molecular analysis (chapter 10).[498] Tersenov et al.[460] postulated that thromboplastin is the only blood-coagulating agent present in the AF.

Cell-free HLA-A and -B maternal and paternal antigens have been detected in AF samples obtained between 16 and 18 weeks of gestation. Deh et al.[385] reported this finding and stressed that paternal haplotypes or soluble HLA-A, -B, and -DR antigens have been found in the peripheral serum samples from pregnant women. HLA antigens can be detected in fetal tissues as early as the 6th week of pregnancy. The use of HLA antigens in the prenatal diagnosis of congenital adrenal hyperplasia is discussed in chapter 16.[384] Defective synthesis of HLA molecules is linked to the severe combined immunodeficiency syndrome.[499] Kleinbauer et al.[296] studied blood coagulation and fibrinolytic factor activities in the AF. Prothrombin rose during the last trimester, while factor X activity decreased. Plasminogen, α_1-antitrypsin, α_2-antiplasmin, antithrombin III, and α_2-macroglobulin levels did not change significantly during gestation.

Immunoglobulins

Immunoglobulins (IgA, IgA1, IgA2, and IgG) are measurable in AF samples tested between 11 and 40 weeks of gestation. Whereas IgG, IgD, and IgA levels increase from 11 to 25 weeks and then decrease until term, IgM levels have a tendency to remain constant until 35 weeks and then increase until term.[374] Davis et al.[500] found similar IgG levels in AF from the second trimester. Their study, however, dealt especially with antibodies to herpes simplex virus (HSV) type 1, which was found in 78 percent of AF samples tested. Antibodies to cytomegalovirus (CMV) were found in 84 percent of the same AF samples tested. During the course of this study, no viruses, bacteria, mycoplasma fungi, or chlamydiae were isolated from the samples. However, isolation of CMV has been successful in AF from two fetuses showing severe growth retardation and classical CMV infection.[502]

The immunologic activity of AF remains poorly understood,[503] and much remains to be learned about mechanisms involved in neonatal immune disease in babies born to mothers affected with systemic lupus erythematosus, idiopathic thrombocytopenic purpura, Graves disease, and myasthenia gravis. Auger et al.[334,504] studied the antibody response to *Candida albicans* during the second trimester. Specific IgG was detected in 94.7 percent of the samples and specific IgA in 98 percent. There was a predominance of IgA activity in the AF. There was no correlation between the IgG and IgA titers, suggesting a fetal origin for IgA, which would offer a functional advantage over maternally transmitted IgG. According to Jones et al.[109] "A major difference between AF and adult serum is the virtual absence of haptoglobin in the fluid. It is also absent from fetal serum and cord blood." Immunoglobulin C declines as pregnancy progresses toward term.[505]

ANTIBACTERIAL ACTIVITY OF AF

The rarity of infection following hundreds of thousands of amniocenteses during the second and third trimesters of pregnancy clearly suggests that some protective mechanism against bacterial infection is present in the AF. It is known that bacteria may occasionally be isolated from the AF of some patients who have no symptoms, suggesting an infectious process.[506–508] The implication always has been that AF has specific antibacterial activity: a substance bactericidal for *Bacillus subtilis* was found in about 17 percent of AF samples in one study.[509] Some investigators have concluded that AF has some antibacterial activity,[508,510] whereas others maintain that it has none or that it actually provides a good culture medium.[511,512]

Bacteriostatic Effect

A number of studies have supported the original contention of antibacterial activity by demonstrating that AF contains a substance that suppresses or inhibits bacterial growth.[313–315,501,513–515]

The exact nature of the bacteriostatic bactericidal substance within the AF has not been established. The first suggestion was lysozyme, an ubiquitous enzyme with lytic properties found in many tissues and secretions. Many studies have pointed to the bacteriostatic role of lysozyme.[414,515–519] However, subsequent studies have suggested that, among the wide variety of antibacterial compounds likely to be present in AF, zinc was one important component.[316,317] The antibacterial activity in zinc in AF seems to be dependent on the presence of a second organic component, which is heat stable and resists proteolytic digestion. This organic component may be a peptide with a molecular weight of less than 5,000 daltons.[377] Phosphate seems to reverse the AF inhibitory activity, possibly by interfering with the organic component rather than with the inorganic zinc.[297,377] The antimicrobial effect and bacteriolytic activity of AF have been studied on several strains.[319,520,521] Both lysozyme and β-lysin (a bactericidal substance) have been identified as early as the second trimester. Normal bacteriolytic activities have been found in pregnancies in which respiratory distress syndrome developed in the infants. On the other hand, lack of an antimicrobial effect of AF on anaerobic bacteria may be one explanation for the high incidence of spontaneous abortions in those conditions.

Other workers have concluded that AF inhibits *Staphylococcus aureus* throughout pregnancy, whereas clear inhibition of *Escherichia coli* and *Streptococcus agalactiae* appears during the third trimester.[382] It is important to note the ineffectiveness of AF against group B streptococci, the frequently documented cases of congenital infections, and the early deleterious effects of *Bacteroides fragilis*, especially in the first trimester.[522]

The effect of AF on bacterial growth also has been stressed by Ismail et al.[523] and Martius and Eschenbach[524] reviewed the literature on bacteria as a cause of the amnionitis that is often associated with premature labor. Bacterial proteases and lipases could play a role in weakening fetal membranes.

Isolation of Infectious Agents

Cerclage, an often-used surgical procedure, may be a cause of AF infections. Charles and Edwards[525] have isolated *Bacteroides bivius, Eubacterium lentum*, and *Staphylococcus epidermidis* from fluids obtained by amniocentesis after cervical cerclage during the second trimester. When performing prenatal diagnosis amniocentesis on patients who have had a cerclage in the preceding weeks, prophylactic antibiotic therapy may be indicated to prevent infectious complications. The isolation of *Mycoplasma hominis* and *Ureaplasma urealyticum* from AF during the second trimester has confirmed[419] previous reports suggesting that contamination of AF may be responsible more often than expected for prematurity, fetal loss, and amnionitis.

Uteroinhibin, a component isolated from AF during the second trimester, also can inhibit spontaneous contractions after the basal tone of the animal–intestinal–human–myometrium preparation. Pajor et al.[396] suggested that the inhibitory factor called "inhibin" might play a role in maintaining the resting state of the human uterus during pregnancy.

Auger et al.[334] demonstrated in vitro a stunted growth of *Candida albicans* in the presence of AF obtained during the second trimester. They suggested that the transferrin content is a factor in the growth-inhibiting activity. There is a high incidence of *C. albicans* genital infection during pregnancy, and problems caused by this should not be overlooked when chorionic villus sampling (CVS) is used for prenatal diagnosis. Other studies by the same group[504] revealed a specific fetal IgA response to *C. albicans* in AF, suggesting that this represents a more efficient defense mechanism than the maternally transmitted IgG.

The fetal origin of D-interferon has been suggested by Lebon et al.,[526] who detected small quantities of this substance in AF obtained between the 16th and 20th weeks of pregnancy. The absence of interferon in maternal serum and its presence in AF under physiologic conditions suggest that interferon may play a regulatory role during fetal development and also may possibly act as an antiviral agent.

The presence of specific IgM in fetal serum is not de facto evidence of fetal demise, nor is the recovery of rubella virus from placental tissue[447,527] evidence of fetal infection. However, an apparently unequivocal test for diagnosis of fetal rubella virus is provided by the polymerase chain reaction (see also chapter 30).[528] Bosma et al.[529] evaluated a reverse transcription–nested PCR assay (RT-PCR) for the diagnosis of congenitally acquired rubella in utero. The detection of rubella virus RNA by RT-PCR and the culture of tissues for the identification of the rubella virus was successful but not in all tissues tested, including the AF and chorionic villus samples.

Pons and co-workers[530] were the first to report a case of fetal varicella by AF viral culture and PCR analysis. (See also chapter 30.) The authors pointed to the need to obtain preventive vaccination for the nonimmunized group of women of childbearing age. To appreciate the risk of embryofetopathy in maternal varicella occurring before 20 weeks of gestation, Dufour et al.[531] studied seventeen cases before 20 weeks of gestation and noted no embryofetopathy.

The discovery of rare or as yet unknown infectious organisms may be revealed in AF from women who experience intrauterine fetal demise. A novel bacterium was isolated[532] and characterized from the AF of a woman who experienced intrauterine fetal demise in the second trimester of pregnancy. The bacterium was a slow-growing, gram-negative anaerobic coccobacillus belonging to the genus *Leptotrichia*. The isolate was characterized by sequencing and analyzing its 16S rRNA gene. The 1,493-pb 16S ribosomal DNA sequence had only 96 percent homology with *L. sangujinegens*. But *L. amnionii* is a distinct species and most closely related to *L. sanguegens*.[533,534]

AF inhibits the growth of aerobic and anaerobic bacteria and fungi, but the antimicrobial factors increase toward term and are not very active during the second trimester.[499] Furthermore, AF from patients with intra-amniotic infection is significantly less inhibitory to *E. coli*.[500] Cytomegalovirus can be isolated in culture from samples during the second trimester of pregnancy, and its presence is strongly indicative of a fetal infection.[535] Derouin and colleagues[536] suggested the use of tissue culture for the early prenatal diagnosis of toxoplasmosis. In one report, *Haemophilus influenzae* was ascertained as the cause of a postamniocentesis intra-amniotic infection[537] (see also chapter 30).

Studies have been made on the half-life and distribution of several antibiotics, particularly cephalosporin, in fetal tissues.[538,539] Among others, cefazolin has been studied and found to be absent from the fetus during the first trimester and present in fetal serum, urine, and AF in low concentrations during the second trimester. Because this study was performed after a single intramuscular injection to the mother, the authors warn that further investigations must be completed before one can claim that a specific antibiotic is nontoxic for the fetus.

HORMONES

Hormones and related metabolites have various origins and are present in measurable quantities in AF during the second trimester. Atkinson and co-workers[540] showed that coelomic fluid contains high concentrations of progesterone, 17β-estradiol and 17α-hydroxyprogesterone, which may be synthesized locally. Steroids other than progesterone are found in higher concentrations in coelomic fluid or maternal serum than in AF. The authors concluded that the free diffusion of steroids across the amnion is limited and that this may constitute a mechanism to protect the embryo from unwanted exposure to biologically active steroids. Abnormal findings may be related to placental dysfunction, renal or adrenal anomalies or insufficiency, or specific endocrine disorders of the reproductive organs; hormonal changes may also be linked to lipolysis or gluconeogenesis or thyroid, parathyroid, or pancreas malfunction. Several papers on hormone levels in AF from normal pregnancies have been published; a list of the major constituents is given in Table 3.4 for future reference in relation to studies of fetal malde-

Table 3.4. Hormones measured in AF during the second trimester

Hormone	AF Level	Approximate Time of Gestation (weeks)	Selected References
Androstenedione	Males: 658 ± 33 pg/mL	14–22	541
	Females: 360 ± 28 pg/mL	14–22	
Apolipoprotein A	2.1 ± 0.1 mg/L	16	311
	6.8 ± 1.6 mg/L	18	
Apolipoprotein A-I	2.3 ± 2.6 mg/dL	Second trimester	310
Apolipoprotein A-II	0.7 ± 0.08 mg/dL	Second trimester	
Apolipoprotein B	<2.0 mg/dL	Second trimester	
Apolipoprotein E	<0.5 mg/dL	Second trimester	
Cortisol	8.9 ng/mL	13–24	542
	13.8 ng/mL	37, 38	
Cortisol	2.89 μg/dL (age < 30 years)	17	381
	3.33 μg/dL (age > 30 years)	17	
Dopamine	880 pg/mL, SEM 98	Second trimester	366
Dopamine	1.19 ± 0.11 ng/mL	14, 16	441
β-Endorphin	65.3 ± 9.1 fmol/mL	16–21	543
β-Endorphin	228 ± 33.6 (SE) pg/mL	16–21	322
β-Endorphin	75.2 ± 14 fmol/mL	18–20	544
β-Endorphin	175 13 pg/mL	16–24	321
Epinephrine	449 pg/mL, SEM 52	Second trimester	338
Erythropoietin	1.20–6.53 U/L	Second and third trimesters	545,546
Estradiol	446.8 ± 73 pg/ml	16–20	547
Estradiol	Males: 85 ± 5.7 pg/mL	14–22	541
	Females: 162 ± 15 pg/mL	14–22	
Estrone	Males: 256 ± 18 pg/mL	14–22	548
	Females: 303 ± 30 pg/mL	14–22	
Estrone	234.1 ± ?.8 pg/mL	16–20	548
estriol-16-glucuronide	5 ng/mL	16	548
Follicle-stimulating hormone	Males: 1.36 ± 0.34 mIU/mL	14–22	541
	Females: 10.1 ± 1.6 mIU/mL	14–22	
β_1-Glycoprotein	110–7000 ng/mL	14–20	549
Gonadotropin LH	Males: 11–13 ng/mL	16–20	550
	Females: 18 ng/mL	16–20	
Gonadotropin hCG	2–5 IU/mL (both sexes)	16–20	550
Gonadotropin	5440 ± 570 mU/mL	15–16	549
Growth	9.32 ± 1.03 ng/mL (fasting)	17	381
17α-Hydroxypregnenolone	1.5 ± 0.3 ng/mL (unconjugated)	14–20	502,550a
Insulin	3.39 ± 0.54 mU/mL (fasting)	17	400
β-Lipoprotein	350 ± 15.8 fmol/mL	16–21	543
Progesterone	Males: 55 ± 3.4 pg/mL	14–22	541
	Females: 54 ± 4.5 pg/mL	14–22	
Progesterone	5200 ± 473 ng/dL 7	16–20	547
Prolactin	2633.5 ± 482.5 (SEM) ng/mL	16–20	547
Prolactin	1183.43 ng/L	15–16	551
Renin	130.2 ± 112.4 ng/mL	16–20	446
Testosterone	Males: 168.7 ± 95.4 pg/mL	10–20	552
	Females: 44.8 ± 26.3 pg/mL 10–20		
Testosterone	Males: 277 ± 16 pg/mL	14–22	541
	Females: 41 ± 3.7 pg/mL	14–22	
Testosterone	Males: 501.8 ± 185.8 pg/mL	12–15	553
	Females: 179 ± 50.5 pg/mL	12–15	
3.3′5′-Triiodothyronine	6.1 nmol/L	17–22	554
Thyroxine	6.5 nmol/L	17–22	554

velopment or endocrine dysfunction. It is not our aim to discuss the origin of the various proteins found in the AF, but it must be realized that fetal and maternal tissues produce hormones that have effects on enzyme synthesis, membrane transport systems, and, not the least, adenosine 3′,5′-cyclic phosphate (cyclic AMP). Measurement of steroid AF levels can be of some value in fetal sex determination and the evaluation of some pathologies, such as congenital adrenal hyperplasia and molar degeneration of the placenta.[555–558] On the other hand, steroid concentrations from fetuses with Klinefelter syndrome were found to be normal.[559,560] Robinson et al.[561] confirmed the value of AF testosterone measurement for sex determination between 14 and 20 weeks of gestation by finding no overlap among 48 male and 72 female fetuses. Although testosterone is elevated in the AF of male fetuses, there is no significant increase of dihydrotestosterone.[562] Testosterone glucuronide used in conjunction with unconjugated testosterone is found to be a good indicator for fetal sexing in AF[563] but replaced by Y-specific DNA (see chapter 8).

Levels of hepatocyte growth factor (HGF) are greater between 20 and 29 weeks of gestation than after 30 weeks. HFG was 300- to 400-fold higher in amnion during the second trimester than at term. Placenta and amnion produce and secrete HGF, which plays a role in fetal growth as well as the growth and differentiation of the placenta.[379]

An elevated insulinlike growth factor binding protein-1 level may be an early sign of intrauterine growth retardation. Studies[380] have shown an elevation of this protein at 15–16 weeks of gestation. With regard to fetal growth in the third trimester, 55 percent of all infants small for gestational age (birth weight lower than fifth percentile) were identified during this study.

Congenital adrenal hyperplasia can be diagnosed as early as 11 weeks of pregnancy by the determination of 17-hydroxyprogesterone in amniotic fluid. This diagnosis can be complemented by molecular studies using chorionic villi obtained at the same time.[564] Dodinval and Duvivier[565] caution against the use of AF steroids for sex determination or diagnosis of congenital adrenal hyperplasia; in both instances, an erroneous diagnosis is possible. Several early papers[566–569] summarized the status of prenatal diagnosis and treatment of congenital adrenal hyperplasia now updated in chapter 16.

Cortisol levels during the second trimester can be lowered by the administration of a synthetic glucocorticoid that crosses the placenta. This experiment was conducted as part of studies on the prevention of respiratory distress syndrome by stimulating lung maturation.[570]

The highest concentration of reverse triiodothyronine in AF occurs between 15 and 20 weeks of gestation.[571] Fetal thyroid function can be evaluated via amniocentesis, especially in families at risk, usually ascertained through newborn screening programs. Assay of thyroid-stimulating hormone (TSH) in AF may reveal fetal hypothyroidism. A fetal goiter was found on ultrasound examination and confirmed by thyroid function assays on AF. This led Perelman et al.[572] to administer levothyroxine sodium therapy in utero, and the authors reported the birth of a euthyroid infant. In pregnancies at high risk for fetal hypothyroidism, it may be advisable to consider prenatal investigation in view of in utero fetal therapy to prevent possible neurologic sequelae. Fetuses with primary pituitary dysgenesis have low levels of prolactin during the second trimester of pregnancy.[573]

Buscher et al.[545] measured the concentration of erythropoietin in AF from normal pregnancies and pregnancies with suspected hypoxia. Significantly elevated erythropoietin levels in AF were found in pregnancies complicated by maternal hypertension and low-birth-weight children. The authors suggest that elevated erythropoietin levels in AF may indicate chronic fetal hypoxia.[546]

Elevated levels of leptin in both AF and maternal serum of patients who had fetuses with a neural tube defect have been reported.[573,573a] The main source of leptin in AF when a fetal open neural tube defect was present was thought to be leakage from the cerebrospinal fluid.

Other components measured in AF include about 30 organic acids,[425] somatomedin,[450] surface-active material,[378] and β-endorphin.[320] The concentrations in AF at term of β-endorphin correlated with the degree of fetal distress. Pigmented AF seen at the time of amniocentesis at about 16 weeks of gestation usually reflect episodes of bleeding and transudation (see also chapters 2 and 21). In most cases, pregnancies progress to term normally. It is necessary to distinguish these cases from those in which meconium-stained fluid is found, which may arise from fetal distress with a higher risk of neonatal morbidity.[574–578]

DRUGS/TOXICANTS

Some drugs, such as meperidine, cross the placenta. This narcotic accumulates in AF, but the direct action of the drug on the fetus is not yet well understood. The amount of free methadone is four to five times that in the maternal plasma, but the active metabolite normeperidine is absent.[579]

Blocking factors in the fetus might alter the action of antibodies to acetylcholine receptor at the neuromuscular junction, thus preventing transient or neonatal myasthenia gravis until after birth.[286] Fetal hydantoin syndrome is observed in infants of epileptic mothers receiving some specific anticonvulsive drugs during pregnancy. Although the exact risk of fetal demise is unknown, it is believed that these mothers have a twofold increased risk of giving birth to a malformed infant, the main observations being mental deficiency, cleft lip and/or palate, heart defect, and minor skeletal anomalies. Buehler et al.[580] suggested that a deficiency of epoxide hydrolase would allow an elevation of oxidative metabolites. In their study of nineteen pregnancies at risk, four fetuses with low enzyme activity were found to have clinical features of the syndrome at birth (their mothers were on phenytoin monotherapy), whereas all fifteen other fetuses, with amniocyte enzyme activity about 30 percent of control values, were normal. Their results have yet to be confirmed. An accumulation of nicotine and its metabolites was reported[424] in AF samples obtained during the second trimester of self-reported smokers and in fetal arterial blood samples obtained at the time of delivery. Indeed, cotinine accumulation in the fetus was noted as early as 7 weeks of gestation in both active and passive smokers.[581] Even more troubling was the observation by Milunsky et al., who documented for the first time the presence of a tobacco-specific carcinogen in midtrimester AF of smoking mothers.[582]

An improved method for the determination of cocaine and norcocaine was developed by Sandberg and Olsen.[583] The detection limit for cocaine and norcocaine was 35 ng/mL, with a coefficient of variation of 7 percent for norcocaine. This method has been applied to human urine and guinea pig plasma, urine, and AF. A study on perinatal outcome and cocaine use[584] has shown a significant correlation between the presence of cocaine metabolites in neonates' urine and symptoms of acute cocaine intoxication. Multiple studies[585–587] of the infants of mothers who used cocaine during pregnancy showed no increase in teratogenicity. An increased risk of placental abruption and premature rupture of membranes was observed.[587]

In one report[588] on three women treated during pregnancy with fluvoxamine, sertraline, and venlafaxine, antidepressant concentrations were measured in AF, umbilical cord blood, and maternal blood using high-performance liquid chromatography with UV detection; antidepressant and metabolite concentrations were detectable in all amniotic fluid samples. No adverse effects of the medication were reported. The presence of these antidepressants in AF suggests that fetal exposure is continual and may occur via placental passage, fetal swallowing and fetal lung absorption.

Omtzigt et al.[589] report on three women with epilepsy who were taking long-term valproate. They measured the concentrations of the parent compound and thirteen of its metabolites by gas chromatography–mass spectrometry in AF, maternal serum, and 24-hr maternal urine samples. All metabolites of valproate present in the serum were detected in the AF at much lower concentrations. AF concentrations of valproate and several of its metabolites [(E) delta 2-valproate, (2E,3'E) delta 2,3'-valproate, and 3-keto-valproate] correlated with total valproate concentrations as well as with unbound valproate concentrations in maternal serum. The AF may act as a deep compartment, with slow appearance and disappearance of valproate and its main metabolites. The data also suggest that during the first and early second trimesters of pregnancy that the beta-oxidation of valproate decreases. In pregnancies associated with fetal neural tube defects ($n = 5$) significantly higher daily doses of valproate were used and higher levels of valproate were found in maternal serum. However, the metabolite patterns in maternal serum, 24-hr urine samples, and AF did not show any significant differences in pregnancies with neural tube defects. In-depth correlation studies of nonmedical drug metabolites in AF and of pregnancy outcome are warranted to evaluate the fetal exposure risk to maternal drug addiction or usage.

Bradman and co-workers[590] measured random amniotic fluid samples around 18 weeks of gestation for organophosphate, carbamate pesticides and metabolites synthetic pyrethoid metabolites, herbicides and chlorinated phenolic compounds. The authors suggest that amniotic fluid offers a unique opportunity to investigate fetal exposures to toxicants and pesticides. Previous studies by Whyatt and Barr[591] had shown an elevation of organophosphates in postpartum meconium samples. Wessels et al.[592] conclude that an appropriate use of markers of organophosphate pesticides can be a valuable tool in epidemiology of children's environmental health.

REFERENCES

1. Lind T, Parkin FM, Cheyne GA. Biochemical and cytological changes in liquor amnii with advancing gestation. J Obstet Gynaecol Br Commonw 1969;76:673.
2. Lind T, Hytten FE. Relation of amniotic fluid volume to fetal weight in the first half of pregnancy. Lancet 1970;1:1147.
3. Seeds AE Jr. Amniotic fluid and fetal water metabolism. In: Barnes AC, ed. Intrauterine development. Philadelphia: Lea & Febiger, 1968:129.
4. Ostergard DR. The physiology and clinical importance of amniotic fluid: a review. Obstet Gynecol Surv 1970;25:297.
5. Fuchs F. Volume of amniotic fluid at various stages of pregnancy. Clin Obstet Gynecol 1966;9:449.
6. Delecour M, Monnier JC, Codaccioni X. Connaissances actuelles sur la physiologie et la biochimie du liquide amniotique. Gynecol Obstet 1970;69:511.
7. Bourne GL. The anatomy of the human amnion and chorion. Proc R Soc Med 1966;59:1127.
8. Idem. The human amnion and chorion. London: Lloyd-Luke, 1962.
9. Hamilton WJ, Boyd JD, Mossman HW. Human embryology. Cambridge: Heffer, 1964.
10. Behrman RE, Parer JT, de Lannoy CW. Placental growth and the formation of amniotic fluid. Nature 1967;214:678.
11. Seeds AE Jr. Dynamics of amniotic fluid. In: Scommegna A, Epstein MB, eds. Amniotic fluid. New York: John Wiley, 1974:23.
12. Nicolini U, Fisk NM, Talbert DG, et al. Intrauterine manometry: technique and application to fetal pathology. Prenat Diagn 1989;9:243.

13. Fisk NM, Ronderos-Dumit D, Tannirandorn Y, et al. Normal amniotic fluid pressure throughout gestation. Br J Obstet Gynaecol 1992;99:18.

14. Barbera A, Buscaglia M, Ferrazzi E, et al. Intra-amniotic pressure is not affected by amniocentesis between 13 and 18 weeks of gestation. Eur J Obstet Gynecol Reprod Biol 1993;50:185.

15. Tomoda S, Brace RA, Longo LD. Amniotic fluid volume regulation: basal values and responses to fluid infusion and withdrawal in sheep. Am J Physiol 1987;252:380.

16. Brace RA. Amniotic fluid volume and its relationship to fetal fluid balance: review of experimental data. Semin Perinatol 1986;10:103.

17. Lotgering FK, Wallenburg HCS. Mechanisms of production and clearance of amniotic fluid. Semin Perinatol 1986;10:94.

18. Cox LW, Chalmers TA. The transfer of sodium to the amniotic fluid in normal and abnormal cases, determined by Na^{24} tracer methods. J Obstet Gynaecol Br Commonw 1953;60:222.

19. Hutchinson DL, Hunter CB, Neslen ED, et al. Exchange of water and electrolytes in the mechanism of amniotic fluid formation and the relationship of hydramnios. Surg Gynecol Obstet 1955;100:391.

20. Plentl AA, Hutchinson DL. Determination of deuterium exchange rates between maternal circulation and amniotic fluid. Proc Soc Exp Biol Med 1953;82:681.

21. Pritchard JA. Deglutition by normal and anencephalic fetuses. Obstet Gynecol 1965;25:289.

22. *Idem*. Fetal swallowing and amniotic fluid volume. Obstet Gynecol 1965;28:606.

23. Hutchinson DL, Gray MJ, Plentl AA, et al. The role of the fetus in the water exchange of the amniotic fluid of normal and hydroamniotic patients. J Clin Invest 1959;38:971.

24. Thomas CR, Lang EK, Lloyd FP. Fetal pyelography—a method for detecting fetal life: a preliminary report. Obstet Gynecol 1963;22:335.

25. Morgan DML, Hytten FE. Mid-trimester pregnancy: a time of tranquility of activity? Br J Obstet Gynaecol 1984;91:532.

26. Gulbis B, Jauniaux E, Jurkovic D, et al. Biochemical investigation of fetal renal maturation in early pregnancy. Pediatr Res 1996;39:731.

27. Clewell WH, Stys SJ, Battaglia FC. Fetal pathophysiology. Prenat Diagn 1984;7:181.

28. Hibbard BM. Polyhydramnios and oligohydramnios. Clin Obstet Gynecol 1972;5:1044.

29. Nelson MM. Amniotic fluid volumes in early pregnancy. J Obstet Gynaecol Br Commonw 1972;79:50.

30. Wagner G, Fuchs F. The volume of amniotic fluid in the first half of human pregnancy. J Obstet Gynaecol Br Commonw 1962;69:131.

31. Rhodes P. The volume of liquor amnii in early pregnancy. J Obstet Gynaecol Br Commonw 1966;73:23.

32. Abramovich DR. The volume of amniotic fluid in early pregnancy. J Obstet Gynaecol Br Commonw 1968;75:728.

33. Gillibrand PN. Changes in amniotic fluid volume with advancing pregnancy. J Obstet Gynaecol Br Commonw 1969;76:527.

34. Queenan JT, Thompson W, Whitfield CR, et al. Amniotic fluid volumes in normal pregnancies. Am J Obstet Gynecol 1972;114:34.

35. Bhatt RV, Acharya PT, Hazra MN, et al. Estimation of the volume of liquor in second trimester. Ind J Med Res 1978;67:767.

36. Geirsson RT, Patel NB, Christie AD. In-vivo accuracy of ultrasound measurements of intrauterine volume in pregnancy. Br J Obstet Gynaecol 1984;91:37.

37. Moore TR. Clinical evaluation of amniotic fluid volume. Semin Perinatol 1993;17:173.

38. Monie IW. The volume of the amniotic fluid in the early months of pregnancy. Am J Obstet Gynecol 1953;66:616.

39. Elliot PJ, Inman WHW. Volume of liquor amnii in normal and abnormal pregnancy. Lancet 1961;2:835.

40. Charles D, Jacoby HE, Burgess F. Amniotic fluid volumes in the second half of pregnancy. Am J Obstet Gynecol 1965;93:1042.

41. Tervila L. Transfer of water from maternal blood to amniotic fluid of live and dead fetuses in health and in some pathological conditions of the mother: a study with tritium-labelled water. Ann Chir Gynaecol Fenn Suppl 1964;53:131.

42. Bourne GL, Lacy D. Ultra-structure of human amnion and its possible relation to the circulation of amniotic fluid. Nature 1960;186:952.

43. Wintour EM, Shandley L. Effects of fetal fluid balance on amniotic fluid. Semin Perinatol 1993;17:158.

44. Gray MJ, Neslen ED, Plentl AA. Estimation of water transfer from amniotic fluid to fetus. Proc Soc Exp Biol Med 1956;92:463.

45. Stevenson AC, Davison BCC, Oakes MW. Genetic counseling. 2nd ed. Philadelphia: J.B. Lippincott, 1976.

46. Beischer N, Desmedt E, Ratten G, et al. The significance of recurrent polyhydramnios. Aust N Z J Obstet Gynaecol 1993;33:25.
47. Scott JS. The volume and circulation of the liquor amnii: Clinical observations. Proc R Soc Med 1966;59:1128.
48. Scott JS, Wilson JK. Hydramnios as an early sign of esophageal atresia. Lancet 1957;1:569.
49. Jeffcoate TNA, Scott JS. Polyhydramnios and oligohydramnios. Can Med Assoc J 1959;80:77.
50. Rivett LC. Hydramnios. Am J Obstet Gynecol 1946;52:890.
51. Esplin MS, Hallam S, Farrington PF, et al. Myotonic dystrophy is a significant cause of idiopathic polyhydramnios. Am J Obstet Gynecol 1998;179:974.
52. Benirschke K, McKay DC. The antidiuretic hormone in fetus and infant. Obstet Gynecol 1953;1:638.
53. Kurjak A, Kirkinen P, Latin V, et al. Ultrasonic assessment of fetal kidney function in normal and complicated pregnancies. Am J Obstet Gynecol 1981;141:266.
54. Weiner CP, Grose C. Prenatal diagnosis of congenital cytomegalovirus infection by virus isolation from amniotic fluid. Am J Obstet Gynecol 1990;163:1253.
55. Potter E. Bilateral absence of ureters and kidneys: a report of 50 cases. J Obstet Gynaecol Br Commonw 1965;25:3.
56. Green GH. Fetal renal hypoplasia and the origin of amniotic fluid. J Obstet Gynaecol Br Commonw 1955;62:592.
57. Hellstrom WJ, Kogan BA, Jeffrey RB Jr, et al. The natural history of prenatal hydronephrosis with normal amounts of amniotic fluid. Urology 1984;132:947.
58. Landing BH. Amnio nodosum: a lesion of the placenta apparently associated with deficient secretion of fetal urine. Am J Obstet Gynecol 1950;60:1339.
59. Scott JS, Bain AD. Amnion nodosum. Proc R Soc Med 1958;51:512.
60. Abramovich DR. Fetal factors influencing the volume and composition of liquor amnii. J Obstet Gynaecol Br Commonw 1970;77:865.
61. Chamberlain P. Amniotic fluid volume: ultrasound assessment and clinical significance. Semin Perinatol 1985;9:163.
62. Gramellini D, Chiaie D, Piantelli G, et al. Sonographic assessment of amniotic fluid volume between 11 and 24 weeks of gestation: construction of reference intervals related to gestational age. Ultrasound Obstet Gynecol. 2001; 17:410.
63. Larmon JE, Ross BS. Clinical utility of amniotic fluid volume assessment. Obstet Gynecol Clin North Am 1998;3:639.
64. Schrimmer DB, Moore TR. Sonographic evaluation of amniotic fluid volume. Clin Obstet Gynecol 2002;45:1026.
65. Phelan JP, Ahn MO Smith CV, et al. Amniotic fluid index measurements during pregnancy. J Reprod Med. 1987;32: 601.
66. Hombo Y, Ohshita M, Takamura S, et al. Direct prediction of amniotic fluid volume in the third trimester by 3-dimensional measurements of intrauterine pockets: a tool for routine clinical use. Am J Obstet Gynecol 2002;186:245.
67. Sherer DM. A review of amniotic fluid dynamics and the enigma of isolated oligohydramnios. Am J Perinatol 2002;19:253.
68. Voxman EG, Tran S, Wing DA. Low amniotic fluid index as a predictor of adverse perinatal outcome. J Perinatol 2002;22:282.
69. Barbani A. Il quadro proteico de liquido amniotico valutato electroforeticamenti e suoi rapporti col siero materno e quello fetale. Minerva Ginecol 1956;8:708.
70. Palliez R, Bisert G, Savary J, et al. Biochimie amniotique, complexes protéiques, acides organiques et cétoniques. Bull Soc R Belge Gynecol Obstet 1956;26:446.
71. Dawson EB, Harris WA, Evans DR, et al. Amniotic fluid amino and nucleic acid in normal and neural tube defect pregnancies: a comparison. J Reprod Med 1999;44:28.
72. Lu LC, Hsu CD. Elevated amniotic fluid nucleosome levels in women with intra-amniotic infection. Obstet Gynecol 1999;94:7.
73. Pahlman S, Esscher T, Bergvall P, et al. Purification and characterization of human neuron-specific enolase: radioimmunoassay development. Tumour Biol 1984;5:127.
74. Mentasti P. Il protidogramma del liquido amniotico valutazione con microelettroforesi libra. Minerva Ginecol 1959;2:547.
75. Strebel L. Immunoelectrophoretic studies of amniotic fluid: Comparison with umbilical cord blood and maternal venous blood. Biol Neonate 1960;2:55.
76. Abbas TM, Tovey JE. Proteins in liquor amnii. BMJ 1960;1:476.

77. Brzezinski A, Sadovsky E, Shafrir E. Electrophoretic distribution of proteins in amniotic fluid and in maternal and fetal serum. Am J Obstet Gynecol 1961;82:800.

78. *Idem.* Protein composition of early amniotic fluid and fetal serum with a case of bis-albuminaemia. Am J Obstet Gynecol 1964;89:488.

79. Derrington MM, Soothill JF. An immunochemical study of the proteins of amniotic fluid and maternal and fetal serum. J Obstet Gynaecol Br Commonw 1961;68:755.

80. Wild AE. The association between protein and bilirubin in liquor amnii. Clin Sci 1961;21:221.

81. Viergiver E, Stroup PE, Scheff MF, et al. Fractionation of amniotic fluid proteins by zone electrophoresis. Obstet Gynecol 1962;19:664.

82. Heron HJ. The electrophoresis of proteins of amniotic fluid. J Obstet Gynaecol Br Commonw 1966;73:91.

83. Usategui-Gomez M, Morgan DF. Maternal origin of the group specific (Gc) proteins in amniotic fluid. Nature 1966;212:1600.

84. Castelazo-Ayala L, Karchmer KS. Electrophoresis of proteins in normal and pathological pregnancies: correlation with maternal and fetal blood. J Int Fed Gynaecol Obstet 1968;6:67.

85. Kleist SV, Buff D, Burtin P. Relation entre les antigènes du liquide amniotique et du sérum foetal. Clin Chim Acta 1968;20:89.

86. Vernier J, Piquard M, Attarl B, et al. Etude électrophorétique et immunoélectrophorétique des protéines du liquide amniotique. C R Soc Biol 1969;163:1835.

87. Sutcliffe RG, Brock DJH. Immunological studies on the nature and origin of the major proteins in amniotic fluid. J Obstet Gynaecol Br Commonw 1973;80:721.

88. Fischbacher PH, Quinliyan WLC. Qualitative and quantitative analysis of the proteins in human amniotic fluid. Am J Obstet Gynecol 1970;108:1050.

89. Sutcliffe RG. The nature and origin of the soluble proteins in human amniotic fluid. Biol Rev 1975;50:1.

90. Harding R, Bocking AD, Sigger JN, et al. Composition and volume of fluid swallowed by fetal sheep. Q J Exp Physiol 1984;69:487.

91. Liley AW. Disorders of amniotic fluid. New York: Academic Press, 1972:157.

92. Sutcliffe RG, Brock DJH, Scrimgeour JB. Origin of amniotic fluid group-specific component. Nature 1972;238:400.

93. Dancis J, Lind J, Vara P. Transfer of proteins across the human placenta. In: Villee CA, ed. The placenta and fetal membranes. New York: Williams & Wilkins, 1960:185.

94. Dancis J, Lind J, Oratz M, et al. Placental transfer of proteins in human gestation. Am J Obstet Gynecol 1961;82:167.

95. Gitlin D, Kumante J, Urrusti J, et al. The selectivity of the human placenta in the transfer of plasma proteins from mother to fetus. J Clin Invest 1964;43:1938.

96. Muller-Eberhard U, Bashore R. Assessment of Rh disease by ratios of albumin and hemopexin to albumin in amniotic fluid. N Engl J Med 1970;282:1163.

97. Johnson AM, Umansky I, Alper AA, et al. Amniotic fluid proteins: maternal and fetal contributions. J Pediatr 1974;84:588.

98. Jonasson L-E, Ervin P-E, Wibell L. Content of beta$_2$-microglobulin and albumin in amniotic fluid. Acta Obstet Gynecol Scand 1974;53:63.

99. Heikinheimo M, Jalanko H, Leisti J, et al. Amniotic fluid pregnancy-specific beta$_1$-glycoprotein (SP$_1$) in fetal developmental disorders. Prenat Diagn 1984;4:147.

100. Bernier GM, Fanger MW. Synthesis of β_2-microglobulin by stimulated lymphocytes. J Immunol 1972;109:407.

101. Jorgensen OS, Norgaard-Pedersen B. The synaptic membrane D2-protein in amniotic fluid from pregnancies with fetal neural tube defects. Prenat Diagn 1981;1:3.

102. Sindic MF, Van Regemorter N, Verellen-Dumoulin C, et al. S-100 protein in amniotic fluid of anencephalic fetuses. Prenat Diagn 1984;4:297.

103. Anneren G, Esscher T, Larsson L, et al. S-100 protein and neuron-specific enolase in amniotic fluid as markers of abdominal wall and neural tube defects in the fetus. Prenat Diagn 1988;8:323.

104. Gogiel T, Bielecki DA, Bankowski E. Collagenous constituents of amniotic fluid. Acta Biochim Pol 1998;45:1037.

105. Uyeno D. The physical properties and chemical composition of human amniotic fluid. J Biol Chem 1919;37:77.

106. Flossner O, Kirstein F. Biochemische Untersuchungen über das menschliche Fruchtwasser. Z Biol (Munich) 1926;84:510.

107. Cantarow A, Stuckert H, Davies RC. Chemical composition of amniotic fluid: comparative study of human amniotic fluid and maternal blood. Surg Gynecol Obstet 1933;57:63.

108. Campbell J, Wathen N, Macintosh M, et al. Biochemical composition of amniotic fluid and extraembryonic coelomic fluid in the first trimester of pregnancy. Br J Obstet Gynaecol 1992;99:563.
109. Jones MI, Spragg SP, Webb T. Detection of proteins in human amniotic fluid using two-dimensional gel electrophoresis. Biol Neonate 1981;39:171.
110. Burdett P, Lizana J, Eneroth P, et al. Proteins of human amniotic fluid. II. Mapping by two-dimensional electrophoresis. Clin Chem 1982;28:935.
111. Nelson MM, Emery AEH. Amniotic fluid cells prenatal sex prediction and culture. BMJ 1970;1:523.
112. Salafsky IS, Nadler HL. Intracellular organelles and enzymes in cell-free amniotic fluid. Am J Obstet Gynecol 1971;111:1046.
113. Risteli L, Autic-Harmainen H, Von Koskull H, et al. Basement membrane proteins in human amniotic fluid. Clin Genet 1984;26:271.
114. Phimister GH, Marshall RD. Tamm–Horsfall glycoprotein in human amniotic fluid. Clin Chim Acta 1983;128:261.
115. Lee TY, Schafer IA. Glycosaminoglycan composition of human amniotic fluid. Biochim Biophys Acta 1974;354:264.
116. Duncan DM, Logan RW, Ferguson-Smith MA, et al. The measurement of acid mucopolysaccharides in amniotic fluid and urine. Clin Chim Acta 1973;45:73.
117. Thompson AR. Factor IX and prothrombin in amniotic fluid and fetal plasma: constraints on prenatal diagnosis of hemophilia B and evidence of proteolysis. Blood 1984;64:867.
118. Bottema CDK, Koeberl DD, Sommer SS. Direct carrier testing in 14 families with haemophilia B. Lancet 1989;2:526.
119. Queenan JT, Gadow EC, Bachner P, et al. Amniotic fluid proteins in normal and Rh-sensitized pregnancies. Am J Obstet Gynecol 1970;108:406.
120. Sutcliffe RG, Brock DJH. Observations on the origins of amniotic fluid enzymes. J Obstet Gynaecol Br Commonw 1972;79:902.
121. Benzie RJ, Doran TA, Harkins JL, et al. Composition of the amniotic fluid and maternal serum in pregnancy. Am J Obstet Gynecol 1974;119:798.
122. Jauniaux E, Gulbis B, Hyett J, et al. Biochemical analyses of mesenchymal fluid in early pregnancy. Am J Obstet Gynecol 1998;178:765.
123. Salmon J, Lambotte R, Sroliar V. Etude par immunofluorescence de la sécrétion du liquide amniotique humain. Arch Int Physiol Biochim Biophys 1962;70:731.
124. Lambotte R, Salmon J. Etude immunoélectrophorétique du liquide amniotique humain. C R Soc Biol 1962;156:530.
125. Lambotte R. Isolement et propriétés d'une alpha1–globuline spécifique du liquide amniotique humain. Arch Int Physiol Biochim Biophys 1966;74:284.
126. Lambotte R, Uhlenbruck G. Amniomucoids: a new class of hexosamine-rich glycoproteins. Nature 1966;212:290.
127. Lambotte R, Gosselin-Ray C. Analyse électrophorétique de la teneur en polysaccharides de l'alpha$_1$-globuline spécifique du liquide amniotique humain. Arch Int Physiol Biochim Biophys 1967;75:109.
128. Sutcliffe RG. Studies on the protein in amniotic fluid. Doctoral thesis. Edinburgh: Edinburgh University, 1972.
129. Westergard JG, Cheminitz J, Teisner B, et al. Pregnancy-associated plasma protein A: a possible marker in the classification and prenatal diagnosis of Cornelia de Lange syndrome. Prenat Diagn 1983;3:225.
130. Aitken DA, Ireland M, Berry E, et al. Second-trimester pregnancy associated plasma protein-A levels are reduced in Cornelia de Lange syndrome pregnancies. Prenat Diagn 1999;19:706.
131. Chitayat D, Marion RW, Squillante L, et al. Detection and enumeration of colonic mucosal cells in amniotic fluid using a colon epithelial–specific monoclonal antibody. Prenat Diagn 1990;10:725.
132. Biezenski JJ. Incorporation of 14C-1-palmitate into rabbits' fetal lipids in vivo. Am J Obstet Gynecol 1976;126:356.
133. Helmy FM, Hack MH. Comparison of the lipids in maternal and cord blood and of human amniotic fluid. Proc Soc Exp Biol Med 1962;110:91.
134. Biezenski JJ, Pomerance W, Goodman J. Studies on the origin of amniotic fluid lipids. Am J Obstet Gynecol 1968;102:853.
135. Vikrot O. Quantitative determination of plasma phospholipids in pregnant and non-pregnant women, with special reference to lysolecithin. Acta Med Scand 1964;175:443.
136. Robertson AF, Sprecher H. A review of human placental lipid metabolism and transport. Acta Paediatr Scand Suppl 1968;183:3.
137. Pomerance W, Biezenski JJ, Moltz A, et al. Origin of amniotic fluid lipids. II. Abnormal pregnancy. Obstet Gynecol 1971;38:379.

138. Gardella C, Hitti J, Martin TR, et al. Amniotic fluid lipopolysaccharide-binding protein and soluble CD14 as mediators of the inflammatory response in preterm labor. Am J Obstet Gynecol 2001;184:1241.

139. Smith DW, Lemli L, Opitz JM, et al. A newly recognized syndrome of multiple congenital anomalies. J Pediatr 1964;64:210.

140. Dallaire L. Syndrome of retardation with urogenital and skeletal anomalies (Smith–Lemli–Opitz syndrome): clinical features and mode of inheritance. J Med Genet 1969;6:113.

141. Tint GS, Irons M, Elias ER, et al. Defective cholesterol biosynthesis associated with the Smith–Lemli–Opitz syndrome. N Engl J Med 1994;330:107.

142. Dallaire L, Mitchell G, Giguere R, et al. Prenatal diagnosis of Smith–Lemli–Opitz syndrome is possible by measurement of 7-dehydrocholesterol in amniotic fluid. Prenat Diagn 1995;15:855.

143. Tint GS, Abuelo D, Till M, et al. Fetal Smith–Lemli–Opitz syndrome can be detected accurately and reliably by measuring amniotic fluid dehydrocholesterols. Prenat Diagn 1998;18:651.

144. Wassif CA, Maslen C, Kachilele-Linjewile S, et al. Mutations in the human sterol delta 7-reductase gene at 11q12–13 cause Smith–Lemli–Opitz syndrome. Am J Hum Genet 1998;63:55.

145. Fitzky B U, Witsch-Baumgartner M, Erdel M, et al. Mutations in the delta-7-sterol reductase gene in patients with the Smith–Lemli–Opitz syndrome. Proc Natl Acad Sci USA 1998;95:8181.

146. Yu H, Lee M-H, Starck L, et al. Spectrum of delta(7)-dehydrocholesterol reductase mutations in patients with the Smith–Lemli–Opitz (RSH) syndrome. Hum Mol Genet 2000;9:1385.

147. Yu H, Tint G S, Salen G, et al. Detection of a common mutation in the RSH or Smith–Lemli–Opitz syndrome by a PCR-RFLP assay: IVS8-1G-C is found in over sixty percent of US propositi. Am J Med Genet 2000;90:347.

148. Irons MB, Nores J, Stewart TL, et al. Antenatal therapy of Smith–Lemli–Opitz syndrome. Fetal Diagn Ther 1999;14:133.

149. Irons M, Elias ER, Abuelo D, et al. Treatment of Smith–Lemli–Opitz syndrome: results of a multicenter trial. Am J Med Genet 1997;68:311.

150. Starck L, Lovgren-Sandblom A, Bjorkhem I. Cholesterol treatment forever? The first Scandinavian trial of cholesterol supplementation in the cholesterol-synthesis defect Smith–Lemli–Opitz syndrome. J Intern Med 2002;252:314.

151. Azurdia RM, Anstey AV, Rhodes LE. Cholesterol supplementation objectively reduces photosensitivity in the Smith–Lemli–Opitz syndrome. Br J Dermatol 2001;144:143.

152. Starck L, Lovgren-Sandblom A, Bjorkhem I. Simvastatin treatment in the SLO syndrome: a safe approach? Am J Med Genet 2002;113:183.

153. Hagenfeldt L, Hagenfeldt K. Individual free fatty acids in amniotic fluid and in plasma of pregnant women. Br J Obstet Gynaecol 1976;83:383.

154. Lappin TRJ. The measurement of non-esterified fatty acids in icteric body fluids. Clin Chim Acta 1971;33:153.

155. Rueda R, Vargas ML, Garcia-Pacheco M, et al. Detection of immunoregulatory lipid-like factors in human amniotic fluid. Am J Reprod Immunol 1990;24:40.

156. Gluck L, Kulovich MV, Borer RC, et al. Diagnosis of the respiratory distress syndrome by amniocentesis. Am J Obstet Gynecol 1971;109:440.

157. Borer RC Jr, Gluck L, Freeman RK, et al. Prenatal prediction of the respiratory distress syndrome (RDS) (abstract). Pediatr Res 1971;5:655.

158. Gluck L, Kulovich MV. Lecithin/sphingomyelin ratios in amniotic fluid in normal and abnormal pregnancy. Am J Obstet Gynecol 1973;115:539.

159. Gluck L, Landowne RA, Kulovich MV. Biochemical development of surface activity in mammalian lung. Structural changes in lung lecithin during development of the rabbit fetus and newborn. Pediatr Res 1970;4:352.

160. Gluck L. Surfactant: 1972. Pediatr Clin North Am 1972;19:325.

161. Arvidson G, Ekelund H, Astedt B. Phospholipid composition of human amniotic fluid during gestation and at term. Acta Obstet Gynecol Scand 1972;51:71.

162. Biezenski JJ. Amniotic fluid phospholipids in early gestation. Obstet Gynecol 1973;41:825.

163. Donald IR, Freeman RK, Goebelsmann U, et al. Clinical experience with the amniotic fluid lecithin/sphingomyelin ratio. I. Antenatal prediction of pulmonary maturity. Am J Obstet Gynecol 1973;115:547.

164. Dewhurst CJ, Harvey DR, Dunham AM, et al. Prediction of respiratory-distress syndrome by estimation of surfactant in the amniotic fluid. Lancet 1973;1:1475.

165. Doran TA, Benzie RJ, Harkins JL, et al. Amniotic fluid tests for fetal maturity. Am J Obstet Gynecol 1974;119:829.

166. Freeman RK, Bateman BG, Goebelsmann U, et al. Clinical experience with the amniotic fluid lecithin/sphingomyelin ratio. II. The L/S ratio in "stressed pregnancies." Am J Obstet Gynecol 1974;119:239.
167. Caspi E, Schreyer I, Schreyer P, et al. Amniotic fluid volume, total phospholipids concentration and L/S ratio in term pregnancies. Obstet Gynecol 1975;46:584.
168. Caspi E, Schreyer P, Tamir I. The amniotic fluid foam test, L/S ratio, and total phospholipids in the evaluation of fetal lung maturity. Am J Obstet Gynecol 1975;122:323.
169. Caspi E, Schreyer P, Weinraub Z, et al. Changes in amniotic fluid lecithin phingomyelin ratio following maternal dexamethasone administration. Am J Obstet Gynecol 1975;122:327.
170. Frantz T, Lindback T, Skjaeraasen J, et al. Phospholipids in amniotic fluid. II. Lecithin fatty acid patterns related to gestation, maternal disease and fetal outcome. Acta Obstet Gynecol Scand 1975;54:33.
171. Ip MPC, Draisey TF, Thibert RJ, et al. Fetal lung maturity, as assessed by gas–liquid chromatographic determination of phospholipid palmitic acid in amniotic fluid. Clin Chem 1972;23:35.
172. Briand RL, Harold S, Blass KG. High-performance liquid chromatographic determination of the lecithin/sphingomyelin ratio in amniotic fluid. J Chromatogr 1981;223:277.
173. Gibbons JM, Huntley TE, Corral AG. Effect of maternal blood contamination on amniotic fluid analysis. Obstet Gynecol 1974;44:657.
174. Deleze G, Paumgartner G, Karlaganis G, et al. Bile acid pattern in human amniotic fluid. Eur J Clin Invest 1978;8:41.
175. Heikkinen J, Maentausta O, Tuimala R, et al. Amniotic fluid bile acids in normal and pathologic pregnancy. Obstet Gynecol 1980;56:60.
176. Deleze G, Sidiropoulos D, Paumgartner G. Determination of bile acid concentration in human amniotic fluid for the prenatal diagnosis of intestinal obstruction. Pediatrics 1977;59:647.
177. Shrand H. Vomiting in utero with intestinal atresia. Pediatrics 1972;49:767.
178. Hook GER, Gilmore LB, Tombopoulos EG, et al. Fetal lung lamellar bodies in human amniotic fluid. Am Rev Respir Dis 1978;117:541.
179. Oulton M, Martin TR, Faulkner GT. Developmental study of lamellar body fraction isolated from human amniotic fluid. Pediatr Res 1980;14:722.
180. Cavalieri RL, Woodling S. Purification of lamellar bodies from human amniotic fluid. Am J Obstet Gynecol 1984;150:409.
181. Ivie WM, Novy MJ, Reynolds JW, et al. Modified lamellar body phospholipid assay compared with L/S ratio and phosphatidylglycerol assay for assessment of fetal pulmonary status. Clin Chem J 1987;33:24.
182. Southern AL, Kobayashi Y, Brenner P, et al. Diamine oxidase activity in human maternal and fetal plasma and tissues at parturition. J Appl Physiol 1965;20:1048.
183. Lapan B, Friedman MM. Enzymes in the amniotic fluid and maternal serum. Am J Obstet Gynecol 1962;83:1337.
184. Usategui-Gomez M. Immunoglobulins and other proteins in amniotic fluid. In: Natelson S, Scommegno A, Epstein MB, eds. Amniotic fluid. New York: John Wiley, 1974:111.
185. Swanberg H. Histaminase in pregnancy. Acta Physiol Scand 1950;23:41.
186. Uuspaa VJ. High histaminase activity of human blood in pregnancy and in so-called placental haemochoriatis. Ann Med Exp Biol Fenn 1951;29:81.
187. Kerenyi T, Sarkozi L. Diagnosis of fetal death in utero by elevated amniotic fluid CPK levels. Obstet Gynecol 1974;44:215.
188. Geyer H, Schneider I. Enzyme in fruchtwasser. Z Klin Chem Klin Biochem 1970;8:141.
189. Geyer H. Zie Herkunft der Fruchtwasser-enzyme. Z Klin Chem Klin Biochem 1970;8:145.
190. Potier M, Dallaire L, Melançon SB. Amniotic fluid α-galactosidase activity: an indicator of gestational age. Gynecol Invest 1974;5:306.
191. Bacigalupo G, Meraner R. Pyruvate kinase in human amniotic fluid: a new indicator of fetal maturity in late pregnancy. J Perinat Med 1984;12:97.
192. Brocklehurst D, Wilde CE. Amniotic fluid alkaline phosphatase, γ-glutamyl transferase and 59-nucleotidase activity from 13–40 weeks' gestation as an index of fetal lung maturity. Clin Chem 1980;26:588.
193. Gurdol F, Genc S, Yalcin O, et al. The presence of prolidase activity in amniotic fluid and its evaluation as a maturity test. Biol Neonate 1995;67:34.
194. Butterworth J, Broadhead DM, Sutherland GR, et al. Lysosomal enzymes of amniotic fluid in relation to gestational age. Am J Obstet Gynecol 1974;119:821.
195. Parmley TH, Seeds AE. Fetal skin permeability to isotopic water (THO) in early pregnancy. Am J Obstet Gynecol 1970;108:128.

196. Lind T, Kendall A, Hytten FE. The role of the fetus in the formation of amniotic fluid. J Obstet Gynaecol Br Commonw 1972;79:289.

197. Wiederschain GY, Rosenfeld EL, Brusilovsky AI, et al. l-Fucosidase and other glycosidases in human placenta, fetus liver, and amniotic fluid at various stages of gestation. Clin Chim Acta 1971;35:99.

198. Fluharty AL, Scott ML, Porter MT, et al. Acid alpha-glucosidase in amniotic fluid. Biochem Med 1973;7:39.

199. Ind TE, Iles RK, Wathan NC, et al. Low levels of amniotic fluid placental alkaline phosphatase in Down's syndrome. Br J Obstet Gynaecol 1993;100:847.

200. Ind TE, Iles RK, Wathen NC, et al. Second trimester amniotic fluid placental alkaline phosphatase levels are low in Down's syndrome but not in other fetal abnormalities. Early Hum Dev 1994;37:39.

201. Nadler HL, Messina AM. In utero detection of type II glycogenosis (Pompe's disease). Lancet 1969;2:1277.

202. Nadler HL, Bigley RH, Hug G. Prenatal detection of Pompe's disease. Lancet 1970;2:369.

203. Potier M, Dallaire L, Melançon SB. Occurrence and properties of fetal intestinal glycosidases (disaccharidases) in human amniotic fluid. Biol Neonate 1975;27:141.

204. Potier M, Melançon SB, Dallaire L. Developmental patterns of intestinal disaccharidases in human amniotic fluid. Am J Obstet Gynecol 1978;131:73.

205. Antonowicz I, Milunsky A, Lebenthal E, et al. Disaccharidase and lysosomal enzyme activities in amniotic fluid, intestinal mucosa and meconium. Biol Neonate 1977;32:280.

206. Sutcliffe RG, Brock DJH, Robertson JG, et al. Enzymes, in amniotic fluid: a study of specific activity patterns during pregnancy. J Obstet Gynaecol Br Commonw 1972;79:895.

207. Butterworth J, Sutherland GR, Bain AD, et al. Lysosomal enzymes in amniotic fluid. Clin Chim Acta 1972;39:275.

208. Lowden JA, Cutz E, Conen PE, et al. Prenatal diagnosis of GM_1 gangliosidosis. N Engl J Med 1973;288:225.

209. Borresen AL, Van der Hagen CB. Metachromatic leukodystrophy. II. Direct determination of arylsulfatase A activity in amniotic fluid. Clin Genet 1973;4:442.

210. DiLieto A, Pollio F, Catalano D, et al. Atrial natriuretic factor in amniotic fluid and in maternal venous blood of pregnancies with fetal cardiac malformations and chromosomal abnormalities. J Matern Fetal Neonatal Med 2002;11:183.

211. Huijing F, Warren RJ, McLeod AGW. Elevated activity of lysosomal enzymes in amniotic fluid of a fetus with mucolipidosis II (I-cell disease). Clin Chim Acta 1973;44:453.

212. Poenaru L, Mezard C, Albi S, et al. Prenatal diagnosis of mucolipidosis type II on first trimester amniotic fluid. Prenat Diagn 1990;10:231.

213. Friedland J, Perle G, Saifer A, et al. Screening for Tay–Sachs disease in utero using amniotic fluid. Proc Soc Exp Biol Med 1971;136:1297.

214. O'Brien JS, Okada S, Fillerup DL, et al. Tay–Sachs disease: prenatal diagnosis. Science 1971;172:61.

215. Harzer K. Erste erfahrungen bei der pranatalen diagnose der Tay–Sachsschen Erkrankung durch isoelektrische fokussierung der hexosaminidase A aus amnion-flussigkeit. Klin Wochenschr 1974;52:145.

216. Desnick RJ, Krivit W, Sharp WL. In utero diagnosis of Sandhoff's disease. Biochem Biophys Res Commun 1973;51:20.

217. Potier M, Boire G, Dallaire L, et al. N-Acetyl-*b*-hexosaminidase isoenzymes of amniotic fluid and maternal serum: their relevance to prenatal diagnosis of the GM_2 gangliosidoses. Clin Chim Acta 1977;76:309.

218. Lindblad B, Lindstedt S, Steen G. On the enzymic defects in hereditary tyrosinemia. Proc Natl Acad Sci USA 1977;74:4641.

219. Gagné R, Lescault A, Grenier A, et al. Prenatal diagnosis of hereditary tyrosinaemia: measurement of succinylacetone in amniotic fluid. Prenat Diagn 1982;2:149.

220. Cockburn F, Robins SP, Forfar JO. Free amino-acid concentrations in fetal fluids. BMJ. 1970;3:747.

221. Kvittingen EA, Halvorsen S, Jellum E, et al. Deficient fumarylacetoacetate fumarylhydrolase activity in lymphocytes and fibroblasts from patients with hereditary tyrosinemia. Pediatr Res 1983;14:541.

222. Dallaire L, Gagnon M, Kinch RA. Fetal amino acid metabolism. Clin Res 1971;19:766.

223. Wenstrom KD, Johanning GL, Owen J, et al. Role of amniotic fluid homocysteine level and of fetal 5,10-methylenetetrahydrafolate reductase genotype in the etiology of neural tube defects. Am J Med Genet 2000;90:12.

224. Jauniaux E, Sherwood RA, Jurkovic D, et al. Amino acid concentrations in human embryological fluids. Hum Reprod 1994;9:1175.

225. Jauniaux E, Gulbis B, Gerlo E, et al. Free amino acid distribution inside the first trimester human gestational sac. Early Hum Dev 1998;51:159.

226. Jauniaux E, Gulbis B, Gerlo E. Free amino acids in human liver and fluids at 12–17 weeks of gestation. Hum Reprod 1999;14:1638.

227. Mesavage WC, Suchy SF, Weiner DL, et al. Amino acids in amniotic fluid in the second trimester of gestation. Prenat Diagn 2001;21:543.

228. Cockburn F, Giles M, Robins SP, Fonfar JO. Free amino acid composition of human amniotic fluid at term. J Obstet Gynaecol Br Commonw 1973;80:10

229. Dallaire L, Potier M, Melançon SB, et al. Fetomaternal amino acid metabolism. J Obstet Gynaecol Br Commonw 1974;81:761.

230. Dallaire L. La brebis: un modèle animal pour les recherches sur le diagnostic prénatal des maladies génétiques. Informations Vétérinaires 1975;18:41.

231. Woo SLC, Lidsky AS, Guttler F, et al. Cloned human phenylalanine hydroxylase gene allows prenatal diagnosis and carrier detection of classical phenylketonuria. Nature 1983;306:151.

232. Woo SLC. Collation of RFLP haplotypes at the human phenylalanine hydroxylase (PAH) locus. Am J Hum Genet 1988;43:781.

233. Firgaira FA, Cotton RGH, Danks DM, et al. Prenatal determination of dihydropteridine reductase in a normal fetus at risk for malignant hyperphenylalaninemia. Prenat Diagn 1983;3:7.

234. Levy HL, Waisbren SE. Effects of untreated maternal phenylketonuria and hyperphenylalaninemia on the fetus. N Engl J Med 1983;309:1269.

235. Kanoun P, Parvy DP, Dinh P, et al. Citrulline in amniotic fluid and the prenatal diagnosis of citrullinemia. Prenat Diagn 1983;3:53.

236. Kleijer WJ, Blom W, Huijmans JGM, et al. Prenatal diagnosis of citrullinemia: elevated levels of citrulline in the amniotic fluid in the three affected pregnancies. Prenat Diagn 1984;4:113.

237. Chadefaux-Vekemans B, Rabier D, Chabli A, et al. Improving the prenatal diagnosis of citrullinemia using citrulline/ornithine+arginine ratio in amniotic fluid. Prenat Diagn 2002;22:456.

238. De Jongh R, Vranken J, Kenis G, et al. Clara cell protein: concentrations in cerebrospinal fluid, serum and amniotic fluid. Cytokine 1998;10:441.

239. Pettit BR, Graham SK, Blau K. The analysis of hexitols in biological fluid by selected ion monitoring. Biomed Mass Spect 1980;7:309.

240. Northrup H, Beaudet AL, O'Brien WE. Prenatal diagnosis of citrullinaemia: review of a 10-year experience including recent use of DNA analysis. Br J Obstet Gynaecol 1990;98:162.

241. Coude M, Chadefaux B, Rabier D, et al. Early amniocentesis and amniotic fluid organic acid levels in the prenatal diagnosis of organic acidemias. Clin Chim Acta 1990;187:329.

242. Jakobs C, Ten Brink JH, Stellaard F. Prenatal diagnosis of inherited metabolic disorders by quantitation of characteristic metabolites in amniotic fluid: facts and future. Prenat Diagn 1990;10:265.

243. Braida L, Crovella S, Boniotto M, et al. A rapid and quantitative mass spectrometry method for determining the concentration of acylcarnitines and aminoacids in amniotic fluid. Prenat Diagn 2001;21:543.

244. Antonowicz I, Ishida S, Shwachman H. Studies in meconium from cystic fibrosis patients and controls. Pediatrics 1975;56:782.

245. Morin PR, Potier M, Dallaire L, et al. Prenatal detection of the autosomal recessive type of polycystic kidney disease by trehalase assay in amniotic fluid. Prenat Diagn 1981;1:75.

246. Arey LB. Developmental anatomy: a textbook and laboratory manual of embryology, 7th ed. Philadelphia: WB Saunders, 1965.

247. Dahlqvist A, Lindberg T. Development of the intestinal disaccharidase and alkaline phosphatase activities in the human fetus. Clin Sci 1966;30:517.

248. Auricchio S, Rubino A, Murset G. Intestinal glycosidase activities in the human embryo, fetus and newborn. Pediatrics 1965;35:944.

249. Antonowicz I, Chang SK, Grand RJ. Development and distribution of lysosomal enzymes and disaccharidases in human fetal intestine. Gastroenterology 1974;67:51.

250. Kenny AJ, Maroux S. Topology of microvillar membrane hydrolases of kidney and intestine. Physiol Rev 1982;62:91.

251. Grossman JW, Sacktor B. Histochemical localization of renal trehalase: demonstration of a tubular site. Science 1968;161:571.

252. Morin PR, Potier M, Dallaire L, et al. Prenatal detection of intestinal obstruction: deficient amniotic fluid disaccharidases in affected fetuses. Clin Genet 1980;18:217.

253. Potier M, Dallaire L, Melançon SB. Prenatal detection of intestinal obstruction by disaccharidase assay in amniotic fluid. Lancet 1977;2:982.

254. Van Diggelen OP, Janse HC, Kleijer WJ. Disaccharidases in amniotic fluid as a possible prenatal marker for cystic fibrosis. Lancet 1983;1:817.

255. Benzie RJ, Doran TA. The fetoscope: a new clinical tool for prenatal genetic diagnosis. Am J Obstet Gynecol 1975;121:460.

256. Claas AHW, Van Diggelen OP, Hauri HP, et al. Characteristics of maltase activity in amniotic fluid. Clin Chim Acta 1985;145:275.

257. Potier M, Morin PR, Melançon SB, et al. Differential stabilities of fetal intestinal disaccharidases determine their relative amounts released into amniotic fluid. Biol Neonate 1984;45:257.

258. Potier M, Cousineau J, Michaud L, et al. Fetal intestinal microvilli in human amniotic fluid. Prenat Diagn 1986;6:429.

259. Jalanko H, Rapola J, Lehtonen E. Particulate fraction in amniotic fluid at second trimester. J Clin Pathol 1985;38:1065.

260. Morin PR, Melançon SB, Dallaire L, et al. Prenatal detection of intestinal obstructions, aneuploidy syndromes, and cystic fibrosis by microvillar enzyme assays (disaccharidases, alkaline phosphatase, and glutamyl transferase) in amniotic fluid. Am J Med Genet 1987;26:405.

261. Morin PR, Potier M, Dallaire L, et al. Prenatal detection of the congenital nephrotic syndrome (Finnish type) by trehalase assay in amniotic fluid. Prenat Diagn 1984;4:257.

262. Poenaru L, Vinet MC, Dreyfus JC. Human amniotic fluid α-glucosidase. Clin Chim Acta 1981;117:53.

263. Elsliger MA, Dallaire L. Potier M. Fetal intestinal and renal origin of trehalase activity in human amniotic fluid. Clin Chim Acta 1993;216:91.

264. Potier M, Melançon SB, Dallaire L. Fetal intestinal disaccharidases in human amniotic fluid. Biomedicine 1976;25:167.

265. Gitlin D, Kumate J, Morales C, et al. The turnover of amniotic fluid protein in the human conceptus. Am J Obstet Gynecol 1972;113:632.

266. Mulivor RA, Mennuti MT, Harris H. Origin of the alkaline phosphatases in amniotic fluid. Am J Obstet Gynecol 1979;135:77.

267. Pocknee RC, Abramovich DR. Origin and levels of trypsin in amniotic fluid throughout pregnancy. Br J Obstet Gynecol 1982;89:142.

268. Potier M, Guay P, Lamothe P, et al. Origin and developmental patterns of lactase and other glycosidases in sheep amniotic and allantoic fluid. J Reprod Fertil 1979;57:49.

269. Morin PR. Etude d'un modèle expérimental pour le diagnostic prénatal de la fibrose kystique. Mémoire de Maîtrise. Montréal: Département de Sciences Cliniques, Université de Montréal, 1979.

270. Dallaire L, Perreault G. Hereditary multiple intestinal atresia. Birth Defects 1974;10:259.

271. Carbarns NJB, Gosden C, Brock DJH. Microvillar peptidase activity in amniotic fluid: possible use in the prenatal diagnosis of cystic fibrosis. Lancet 1983;1:329.

272. Brock DJH. Amniotic fluid alkaline phosphatase isoenzymes in early prenatal diagnosis of cystic fibrosis. Lancet 1983;2:941.

273. Morin PR, Potier M, Lasalle R, et al. Amniotic fluid disaccharidases in the prenatal detection of cystic fibrosis. Lancet 1983;2:621.

274. Jalanko H, Aula P. Decrease in gamma-glutamyl transpeptidase activity in early amniotic fluid in fetal trisomy 18 syndrome. BMJ 1982;284:1593.

275. Jalanko H. Developmental changes in gamma-glutamyl transpeptidase in human amniotic fluid. Oncodev Biol Med 198;4:252.

276. Moniz C, Nicolaides KH, Heys D, et al. Gamma-glutamyl transferase activity in fetal serum, maternal serum and amniotic fluid during gestation. J Clin Pathol 1984;37:700.

277. Brock DJH, Bedgood D, Hayward C. Amniotic fluid microvillar enzyme activities in the early detection of fetal abnormalities. Prenat Diagn 1984;4:261.

278. Jarmas AL, Weaver DD, Padilla LM, et al. Hirschsprung disease: etiologic implications of unsuccessful prenatal diagnosis. Am J Med Genet 1983;16:163.

279. Davidson GP, Cutz E, Hamilton JR, et al. Familial enteropathy: a syndrome of protracted diarrhea from birth, failure to thrive, and hypoplastic villi. Gastroenterology 1978;75:783.

280. Szabo M, Veress L, Teichmann F, et al. Amniotic fluid microvillar enzyme activity in fetal malformations. Clin Genet 1990;38:340.

281. Poloce F, Montegre M. Value of an assay of enzymatic activity in amniotic fluid for the detection of fetal anomalies. Rev Fr Gynecol Obstet. 1994;89:323

282. Sembaj A, Carriazo C, Sanz E, et al. Determination of alkaline phosphatase isozymes in amniotic fluid. Eur J Clin Chem Clin Biochem 1995;33: 281.

283. Perin NM, Thomson AB. Ontogeny of the small intestine. Arq Gastroenterol 1998;35:190.

284. Karnak I, Tanyel FC, Muftuoglu S, et al. Esophageal ligation: effects on the development of fetal organic systems. Eur J Pediatr Surg 1996;6:328.

285. de Lagausie P, Guibourdenche J, de Buis A, et al. Esophageal ligature in experimental gastroschisis. J Pediatr Surg 2002;37:1160.

286. Abramsky O, Brenner T, Lisak RP, et al. Significance in neonatal myasthenia gravis of inhibitory effect of amniotic fluid on binding of antibodies to acetylcholine receptor. Lancet 1979;2:1333.

287. Smith AD, Wald NJ, Cuckle HS, et al. Amniotic fluid acetylcholinesterase as a possible diagnostic test for neural tube defects in early pregnancy. Lancet 1979;1:685.

288. Brown CL, Colden KA, Hume RF, et al. Faint and positive amniotic fluid acetylcholinesterase with a normal sonogram. Am J Obstet Gynecol 1996;175:1000.

289. Johnell HE, Nilsson BA. Oxygen tension, acid–base status and electrolytes in human amniotic fluid. Acta Obstet Gynecol Scand 1971;50:183.

290. Symonds EM, Williams SS, Cellier KM. Maternal and fetal influences on the acid–base balance of human amniotic fluid. Obstet Gynecol 1971;37:742.

291. Yamashiro C, Kanenishi K, Akiyama M, et al. Adrenomedullin concentrations in early 2nd-trimester amniotic fluid: relation to preterm delivery and fetal growth at birth. Gyncecol Obstet Invest 2002;54:99.

292. Hulbis B, Jauniaux E, Cotton F, et al. Protein and enzyme patterns in the fluid cavities of the first trimester gestational sac: relevance to the absorptive role of secondary yolk sac. Mol Hum Reprod 1998;4:857.

293. Jalanko H, Heikinheimo M, Ryynanen M, et al. Alkaline phosphatase activity in amniotic fluid in pregnancies with fetal disorders. Prenat Diagn 1983;3:303.

294. Monaghan JM, Horn DB, Brock DJH. Alpha$_1$-antitrypsin in amniotic fluid. Lancet 1973;2:619.

295. Evans HE, Glass L, Mandl I. Alpha$_1$-antitrypsin concentration in amniotic fluid. Biol Neonate 1975;27:232.

296. Kleinbauer D, Klink F, Wagner T, et al. Blood coagulation and fibrinolytic factor activities in the amniotic fluid. Geburtshilfe Frauenheilkd 1988;48:397.

297. Emery AEH, Burt D, Scrimgeour JB. Aminoacid composition of amniotic fluid in central nervous system malformations. Lancet 1973;1:970.

298. Emery AEH, Burt D, Nelson MM, et al. Antenatal diagnosis and aminoacid composition of amniotic fluid. Lancet 1970;1:1307.

299. Reid DWJ, Campbell DJ, Yakymyshyn LY. Quantitative amino acids in amniotic fluid and maternal plasma in early and late pregnancy. Am J Obstet Gynecol 1971;111:251.

300. O'Neill RT, Morrow G III, Hammel D, et al. Diagnostic significance of amniotic fluid amino acids. Obstet Gynecol 1971;37:550.

301. Scott CR, Teng CC, Sagerson RN, et al. Amino acids in amniotic fluid: changes in concentrations during the first half of pregnancy. Pediatr Res 1972;6:659.

302. Cockburn F, Giles M, Robins SP, et al. Free amino acid composition of human amniotic fluid at term. J Obstet Gynaecol Br Commonw 1973;80:10.

303. Chadefaux B, Ceballos I, Rabier D. Prenatal diagnosis of argininosuccinic aciduria by assay or argininosuccinate in amniotic fluid at the 12th week of gestation. Am J Med Genet 1990;35:594.

304. Jauniaux E, Gulbis B, Gerlo E, et al. Free amino acid distribution inside the first trimester human gestational sac. Early Hum Dev 1998;51:159.

305. Fernandez de Castro A, Usategui-Gomez M, Spellacy WN. Amniotic fluid amylase. Am J Obstet Gynecol 1973;116:931.

306. Dawood MY. Hormones in amniotic fluid. Am J Obstet Gynecol 1977;128:576.

307. Madazli R, Atis A, Uzun H, Aksu F. Mid-trimester amniotic fluid angiogenin, lactate dehydrogenase and fibronectin in the prediction of preterm delivery. Eur J Obstet Gynecol Reprod Biol. 2003; 106:160.

308. Cohen SB, Goldenberg M, Rabinovici J, et al. Anti-cardiolipin antibodies in fetal blood and amniotic fluid derived from patients with the anti-phospholipid syndrome. Hum Reprod 2000;15:1170.

309. Pacsa AS, Pejtsik B. Impairment of immunity during pregnancy and antiviral effect of amniotic fluid. Lancet 1977;1:330.

310. Fainaru M, Deckelbaum R, Golbus MS. Apolipoproteins in human fetal blood and amniotic fluid in midtrimester pregnancy. Prenat Diagn 1981;1:125.

311. Ruelland A, Mention JE, Perrot Y, et al. The levels of apolipoprotein A in liquor in normal and pathological pregnancies. J Gynecol Obstet Biol Reprod 1982;11:241.

312. Lewis JF, Johnson P, Miller P. Evaluation of amniotic fluid for aerobic and anaerobic bacteria. Am J Clin Pathol 1976;65:58.

313. Bergman N, Bercovici B, Sacks T. Antibacterial activity of human amniotic fluid. Am J Obstet Gynecol 1972;114:520.

314. Kitzmiller JL, Highby S, Lucas WE. Retarded growth of *E. coli* in amniotic fluid. Obstet Gynecol 1973;41:38.

315. Larsen B, Snyder IS, Galask RP. Bacterial growth inhibition by amniotic fluid. I. In vitro evidence for bacterial growth-inhibiting activity. Am J Obstet Gynecol 1974;119:492.

316. Schlievert P, Johnson W, Galask RP. Bacterial growth inhibition by amniotic fluid. VI. Evidence for a zinc-peptide antibacterial system. Am J Obstet Gynecol 1976;125:906.

317. *Idem.* Bacterial growth inhibition by amniotic fluid. V. Phosphate-to-zinc ratio as a predictor of bacterial growth-inhibitory activity. Am J Obstet Gynecol 1976;125:899.

318. Prevedourakis C, Koumentakou E, Zolotas J, et al. *E. coli* growth inhibition by amniotic fluid. Acta Obstet Gynecol Scand 1976;55:245.

319. Ford LC, Delanse RJ, Lebherz TB. Identification of a bactericidal factor (B-lysin) in amniotic fluid at 14 and 40 weeks' gestation. Am J Obstet Gynecol 1977;127:788.

320. Gautray JP, Jolivet A, Vielh JP, et al. Presence of immunoassayable beta-endorphin in human amniotic fluid: elevation in cases of fetal distress. Am J Obstet Gynecol 1977;129:211.

321. Granat M, Sharf M, Weissman BA. Humoral endorphin in human body fluids during pregnancy. Gynecol Obstet Invest 1980;11:214.

322. Goebelsmann U, Abboud TK, Hoffman DI, et al. Beta-endorphin in pregnancy. Eur J Obstet Reprod Biol 1984;17:77.

323. Kofinas GD, Kofinas AD, Pyrgerou M, et al. Amniotic fluid beta-endorphin levels and labor. J Obstet Gynecol 1987;69:945.

324. Smith AL, Scanlon J. Amniotic fluid D(−)-beta-hydroxybutyrate and the dysmature newborn infant. Am J Obstet Gynecol 1973;115:569.

325. Hall PW III, Roux JF. Amniotic fluid beta-2-microglobulin concentration: an index of gestational age. Am J Obstet Gynecol 1974;120:56.

326. Gulbis B, Gervy C, Jauniaux E. Amniotic fluid biochemistry in second-trimester trisomic pregnancies: relationships to fetal organ maturation and dysfunction. Early Hum Dev 1998;52:211.

327. Perlman M. Golden liquor amnii. Lancet 1973;1:556.

328. Henneman CE, Anderson GV, Tejavej A, et al. Fetal maturation and amniotic fluid. Am J Obstet Gynecol 1970;108:302.

329. Ojala A. Studies on bilirubin in amniotic fluid with special reference to liver function tests. Oulu, Finland: Kirjapaino Osakeyhtio Kaleva, 1971.

330. Yamada H, Furuta I, Kato EH, et al. Maternal serum and amniotic fluid bisphenol A concentrations in the early second trimester. Reprod Toxicol 2002;16:735.

331. Arcilla MB, Sturgeon P. Lewis and ABH substances in amniotic fluid obtained by amniocentesis. Pediatr Res 1972;6:853.

332. Harper P, Bias WB, Hutchinson Jr, et al. ABH secretor status of the fetus: a genetic marker identifiable by amniocentesis. J Med Genet 1971;8:438.

333. Dawson EB, Evans DR, Nosovitch J. Third-trimester amniotic fluid metal levels associated with preeclampsia. Arch Environ Health 1999;54:412.

334. Auger P, Marquis G, Dallaire L, et al. Stunted growth of *Candida albicans* in human amniotic fluid in vitro. J Lab Clin Med 1980;95:272.

335. Tayyar M, Tutus A. The effect of maternal age, parity, and fetal sex on the amniotic fluid and maternal serum levels of CA 125, CA19.9, CA 15.3, and CEA. Int J Fertil Womens Med 1999;44:256.

336. Bussière L, Dumont J, Hubert J. Direct determination of calcium, copper, iron, magnesium, manganese and zinc in amniotic fluid samples using inductively coupled plasma–atomic mission spectrometry. Anal Chim Acta 1989;224:73.

337. Hahn P, Skala JP, Seccombe DW, et al. Carnitine content of blood and amniotic fluid. Pediatr Res 1977;11:878.

338. Divers WA Jr, Wilkes MM, Babaknia A, et al. An increase in catecholamines and metabolites in the amniotic fluid compartment from middle to late gestation. Am J Obstet Gynecol 1981;139:483.

339. Clements JA, Reyes FI, Winter JSD, et al. Studies on human sexual development. III. Fetal pituitary and serum, and amniotic fluid concentrations of LH, CG, and FSH. J Clin Endocrinol Metab 1976;42:9.

340. Anteby SC, Zukerman H, Gedelia I, et al. Citric acid in amniotic fluid. J Obstet Gynaecol Br Commonw 1973;80:27.

341. Ghezzi F, Franchi M, Raio L, et al. Elevated amniotic fluid C-reactive protein at the time of genetic amniocentesis is a marker for preterm delivery. Am J Obstet Gynecol 2002;186:268.

342. Raio L, Ghezzi F, Mueller MD, et al. Evidence of fetal C-reactive protein urinary excretion in early gestation. Obstet Gynecol 2003;101:1062.

343. Chez RA, Henkin RI, Fox R. Amniotic fluid copper and zinc concentrations in human pregnancy. Obstet Gynecol 1978;52:125.

344. Fencl MD, Tulchinsky D. Total cortisol in amniotic fluid and fetal lung maturation. N Engl J Med 1975;292:133.

345. Murphy BEP, Patrick J, Denton RL. Cortisol in amniotic fluid during human gestation. J Clin Endocrinol Metab 1975;40:164.

346. Sivakumaran T, Duncan ML, Effer SB, et al. Relationship between cortisol and lecithin/sphingomyelin ratios in human amniotic fluid. Am J Obstet Gynecol 1975;122:291.

347. Roopnarinesingh S. Amniotic fluid creatinine in normal and abnormal pregnancies. J Obstet Gynaecol Br Commonw 1970;77:785.

348. Doran TA, Bjerre S, Porter CJ. Creatinine, uric acid and electrolytes in amniotic fluid. Am J Obstet Gynecol 1970;106:325.

348a. Enlander D. Amniotic fluid indicators of fetal maturity. Obstet Gynecol 1972;40:605.

349. Kobayashi H, Suzuki K, Sugino Dl, et al. Urinary trypsin inhibitor levels in amniotic fluid of normal human pregnancy: decreased levels observed at parturition. Am J Obstet Gynecol 1999;180:141.

350. Moore WMO, Murphy PJ, David JA. Creatinine content of amniotic fluid in cases of retarded fetal growth. Am J Obstet Gynecol 1971;110:908.

351. Fex G, Holmberg N-G, Löfstrand T. Phospholipids and creatinine in amniotic fluid in relation to gestational age. I. Normal pregnancy. Acta Obstet Gynecol Scand 1975;54:425.

352. Cassady G, Hinkley C, Bailey P, et al. Amniotic fluid creatinine in pregnancies complicated by diabetes. Am J Obstet Gynecol 1975;122:13.

353. Muller F, Bernard MA, Benkirane A, et al. Fetal urine cystatin C as a predictor of postnatal renal function in bilateral uropathies. Clin Chem 1999;45:2292.

354. Mussap M, Fanos V, Pizzini C, et al. Predictive value of amniotic fluid cystatin C levels for the early identification of fetuses with obstructive uropathies. BJOG 2002;109:778.

355. Spong CY, Ghidini A, Ossandon M, et al. Are the cytokines interleukin-6 and angiogenin stable in frozen amniotic fluid? Am J Obstet Gynecol 1998;178:783.

356. Vesce F, Scapoli C, Giovannini G, et al. Cytokine imbalance in pregnancies with fetal chromosomal abnormalities. Hum Reprod 2002;17:803.

357. Verhaeghe J, Coopmans W, van Herck E, et al. IGF-I, IGF-II, IGF binding protein 1, and C-peptide in second trimester amniotic fluid are dependent on gestational age but do not predict weight at birth. Pediatr Res 1999;46:101.

357a. 307. Darj E, Lyrenas S. Insulin-like growth factor binding protein-1, a quick way to detect amniotic fluid. Acta Obstet Gynecol Scand 1998;77:295.

358. David LE, Tweed GV, Chin TDY, et al. Intrauterine diagnosis of cytomegalovirus infection: viral recovery from amniocentesis fluid. Am J Obstet Gynecol 1971;109:1217.

359. Halperin R, Halpern D, Hadas E, et al. Intrauterine levels of human decidua-associated protein (hDP) 200 in normal pregnancy and missed abortion. Gynecol Obstet Invest 1998;46:150.

360. Heine RP, Wiesenfeld H, Mortimer L, et al. Amniotic fluid defensins: potential markers of subclinical intrauterine infection. Clin Infect Dis 1998;27:513.

361. Espinoza J, Chaiworapongsa T, Romero R, et al. Antimicrobial peptides in amniotic fluid: defensins, calprotectin and bacterial/permeability-increasing protein in patients with microbial invasion of the amniotic cavity, intra-amniotic inflammation, preterm labor and premature rupture of membranes. J Matern Fetal Neonatal Med 2003;13:2.

362. Antonowicz I, Lebenthal E, Shwachman H. Disaccharidase activities in small intestinal mucosa in patients with cystic fibrosis. Pediatrics 1978;92:214.

363. Klopper A. Oestriol in amniotic fluid. Proc R Soc Med 1970;63:1090.

364. Pinkus GS, Pinkis JL. Fluorometric determination of total estrogens in amniotic fluid of normal and complicated pregnancies. Obstet Gynecol 1970;36:528.

365. Michie EA, Robertson JG. Amniotic and urinary oestriol assays in pregnancies complicated by rhesus immunization. J Obstet Gynaecol Br Commonw 1971;78:34.

366. Fencl M, Alonso C, Alba M. Estriol values in amniotic fluid in the course of normal pregnancy. Am J Obstet Gynecol 1972;113:367.

367. Sciarra JJ, Tagatz GE, Notation AD, et al. Estriol and estetrol in amniotic fluid. Am J Obstet Gynecol 1974;118:626.

368. Roux JF, Nakamura J, Frosolono M. Fatty acid composition and concentration of lecithin in the acetone fraction of amniotic fluid phospholipids. Am J Obstet Gynecol 1974;119:838.

368a. Das SK, Foster HW, Adhikary PK, et al. Gestational variation of fatty acid composition of human amniotic fluid lipids. Obstet Gynecol 1975;45:425.

369. Ramsey PS, Andrews WW, Goldenberg RL, et al. Elevated amniotic fluid ferritin levels are associated with inflammation-related pregnancy loss following mid-trimester amniocentesis. J Matern Fetal Neonatal Med 2002;11:302.

370. Robert JA, Romero R, Costigan K. Amniotic fluid concentrations of fibronectin and intra-amniotic infection. Am J Perinatol 1988;5:26.
371. Sakura M, Nakabayashi M, Takeda Y, et al. Elevated fetal fibronectin in midtrimester amniotic fluid is involved with the onset of preeclampsia. J Obstet Gynaecol Res 1998;24:73.
372. Shimoya K, Zhang Q, Tenma K, et al. Fractalkine (FRK) levels in amniotic fluid and its production during pregnancy. Mol Hum Reprod 2003;9:97.
373. Macek M, Annerén G, Gustavson KH, et al. Gamma-glutamyl transferase activity in the amniotic fluid of fetuses with chromosomal aberrations and inborn errors of metabolism. Clin Genet 1987;32:403.
374. Cederqvist LL, Ewool L, Bonsnes RW, et al. Detectability and pattern of immunoglobulins in normal amniotic fluid throughout gestation. Am J Obstet Gynecol 1978;130:220.
375. Chen AB, Mosesson MW, Solish GI. Identification of the cold-insoluble globulin of plasma in amniotic fluid. Am J Obstet Gynecol 1976;125:958.
376. Newman RI, Tutera G. The glucose–insulin ratio in amniotic fluid. Obstet Gynecol 1976;47:599.
377. Papp Z, Ember I, Juhasz E, et al. Acid-soluble glycoproteins in amniotic fluid and cystic fibrosis of the foetus. Clin Genet 1977;11:431.
378. Frosolono MF, Roux JR. Surface-active material in human amniotic fluid. Am J Obstet Gynecol 1978;130:562.
379. Hakala-Ala-Pietila TH, Koistinen RA, Salonen RK, et al. Elevated second-trimester amniotic fluid concentration of insulin-like growth factor binding protein-1 in fetal growth retardation. Am J Obstet Gynecol 1993;169:35.
380. Horibe N, Okamoto T, Itakura A, et al. Levels of hepatocyte growth factor in maternal serum and amniotic fluid. Am J Obstet Gynecol 1995;173:937.
381. Wisniewski L, Jezuita J, Bogoniowska Z, et al. II. Growth hormone in the amniotic fluid and blood serum of women in the 17th week of pregnancy. Ginekol Pol 1983;54:693.
382. Appelbaum PC, Shulman G, Chambers NL, et al. Studies on the growth-inhibiting property of amniotic fluids from two United States population groups. Am J Obstet Gynecol 1980;137:579.
383. Emmer PM, Steegers EA, van Lierop MJ, et al. Amniotic fluid soluble human leukocyte antigen G is markedly decreased in offspring with neural tube defects. Early Hum Dev 2002;66:101.
384. Couillin P, Nicolas H, Boué J, et al. HLA typing of amniotic fluid cells applied to prenatal diagnosis of congenital adrenal hyperplasia. Lancet 1979;1:1076.
385. Deh ME, Klouda PT, Levine M, et al. Detection, isolation and characterization of cell free HLA A and B antigens from human amniotic fluid. Tissue Antigens 1982;20:260.
386. Nicholls T, Hähnel R, Wilkinson S, et al. Identification of 2-hydroxybutyric acid in human amniotic fluid. Clin Chim Acta 1976;69:127.
387. Emery AEH, Brock DJH, Burt D, et al. Amniotic fluid composition in malformations of the fetal central nervous system. J Obstet Gynaecol Br Commonw 1974;81:512.
388. Shah SI, Alderman M, Queenan JT et al. Nondialyzable peptide-bound hydroxyproline in human amniotic fluid: an indicator of fetal growth. Am J Obstet Gynecol 1972;114:250.
389. Gogiel T, Bielecki DA, Bankowski E. Collagenous constituents of amniotic fluid. Acta Biochim Pol 1998;45:1037.
390. Monif GRG, Mendenhall HW. Immunoglobulin G levels and the titers of specific antiviral antibodies in amniotic fluid. Am J Obstet Gynecol 1970;108:651.
391. Curl CW. Immunoglobulin levels in amniotic fluid. Am J Obstet Gynecol 1971;109:408.
392. Rule AH, Lawrence D, Hager HJ, et al. IgA: Presence in meconium obtained from patients with cystic fibrosis. Pediatrics 1971;48:601.
393. Cederqvist LL, Queenan JT, Gadov EC, et al. The origin of gamma G globulins in human amniotic fluid. Am J Obstet Gynecol 1972;113:838.
394. Gadow EC, Floriani FA, Florin A. IgG levels in amniotic fluid. Am J Obstet Gynecol 1974;119:849.
395. Wilfert CM, Gradoville ML. In vitro viral studies of cells grown from human amniotic fluid samples. Am J Obstet Gynecol 1974;118:1073.
396. Pajor A, Grof J, Idel M, et al. Utero-inhibin: A new substance inhibiting uterine contraction, isolated from amniotic fluid. Acta Phys Acad Sci Hung 1982;59:325.
397. Wallace EM, D'Antona D, Shearing C, et al. Amniotic fluid levels of dimeric inhibins, pro-alpha C inhibin, activin A and follistatin in Down's syndrome. Clin Endocrinol 1999;50:669.
398. Thirunavukarasu PP, Lambert-Messerlian G, Robertson DM, et al. Molecular weight forms of inhibin A, inhibin B and pro-alphaC in maternal serum, amniotic fluid and placental extracts of normal and Down syndrome pregnancies. Prenat Diagn 2002;22:1086.

399. Wallace EM, Crossley JA, Riley SC, et al. Inhibin-B and pro-alphaC-containing inhibins in amniotic fluid from chromosomally normal and Down syndrome pregnancies. Prenat Diagn 1998;18:213.

400. Weiss PAM, Purstner P, Winter R, et al. Insulin levels in amniotic fluid of normal and abnormal pregnancies. Obstet Gynecol 1984;63:371.

401. Baviera G, D'Anna R, Corrado F, et al. ICAM-1 in maternal serum and amniotic fluid as an early marker of preeclampsia and IUGR. J Reprod Med 2002;47:191.

402. Hsu CD, Meaddough E, Aversa K, et al. The role of amniotic fluid L-selectin, GRO-alpha, and interleukin-8 in the pathogenesis of intraamniotic infection. Am J Obstet Gynecol 1998;178:428.

403. Nakabayashi M, Sakura MN, Takeda Y, et al. Elevated IL-6 in midtrimester amniotic fluid is involved with the onset of preeclampsia. Am J Reprod Immunol 1998;39:329.

404. Ghezzi F, Gomez R, Romero R, et al. Elevated interleukin-8 concentrations in amniotic fluid of mothers whose neonates subsequently develop bronchopulmonary dysplasia. Eur J Obstet Gynecol Reprod Biol 1998;78:5.

405. Fukuda H, Masuzaki H, Ishimaru T. Interleukin-6 and interleukin-1 receptor antagonist in amniotic fluid and cord blood in patients with pre-term, premature rupture of the membranes. Int J Gynaecol Obstet 2002;77:123.

406. Maymon R, Jauniaux E, Rodeck C, et al. Comparison of placental isoferritin levels in maternal serum and coelomic and amniotic fluids during first trimester human gestation. Hum Reprod 1998;13:1044.

407. Wolf RO, Taussig LM. Human amniotic fluid isoamylases: functional development of fetal pancreas and salivary glands. Obstet Gynecol 1973;41:337.

408. Magklara A, Scorilas A, Lopez-Otin C, et al. Human glandular kallikrein in breast milk, amniotic fluid, and breast cyst fluid. Clin Chem 1999;45:1774.

409. Otsuki K, Yoda A, Saito H, et al. Amniotic fluid lactoferrin in intrauterine infection. Placenta 1999;20:175.

410. Dott B, Maier EA, et al. Oligo-éléments du liquide amniotique des foetus normaux, hypotrophes et trisomiques 21. Rev Fr Gynecol Obstet 1990;85:45.

411. Blumenfeld TA, Driscoll JM, James LS. Lecithin/sphingomyelin ratios in tracheal and pharyngeal aspirates in respiratory distress syndrome. J Pediatr 1974;85:403.

412. Cowett RM, Unsworth EJ, Hakanson DO, et al. foam-stability test on gastric aspirate and the diagnosis of respiratory-distress syndrome. N Engl J Med 1975;293:413.

413. Mallikarjuneswara VR. Lecithin-sphingomyelin ratio in amniotic fluid, as assessed by a modified thin-layer chromatographic method in which a commercial pre-coated plate is used. Clin Chem 1975;21:260.

414. Cherry SH, Filler M, Harvey H. Lysozyme content of amniotic fluid. Am J Obstet Gynecol 1973;116:639.

415. Larsen B, Galask RP, Snyder IS. Muramidase and peroxidase activity of human amniotic fluid. Obstet Gynecol 1974;44:219.

416. Fujikura T, Klionsky B. The significance of meconium staining. Am J Obstet Gynecol 1975;121:45.

417. Mathews DM. Intestinal absorption of amino acids and peptides. Proc Nutr Soc 1972;31:171.

418. Moon JB, Kim JC, Yoon BH, et al. Amniotic fluid matrix metalloproteinase-8 and the development of cerebral palsy. J Perinat Med 2002;30:301.

419. Cassell GH, Davis RO, Waites KB, et al. Isolation of *Mycoplasma hominis* and *Ureaplasma urealyticum* from amniotic fluid at 16–20 weeks of gestation: potential effect on outcome of pregnancy. Sex Transm Dis 1983;10:294.

420. Kastner B, Schenk H, Weise W. The neuraminic acid/protein quotient in amniotic fluid: indicator for fetal maturity. Z Med Lab Diagn 1990;31:77.

421. Marx CE, Vance BJ,. Jarskog LF, et al. Nerve growth factor, brain-derived neurotrophic factor, and neurotrophin-3 levels in human amniotic fluid. Am J Obstet Gynecol 1999;181:1225.

422. Elimian A, Figueroa R, Patel K, et al. Reference values of amniotic fluid neuron-specific enolase. J Matern Fetal Med 2001;10:155.

423. Tranquilli AL, Bezzeccheri V, Scagnoli C, et al. Amniotic levels of vascular endothelial growth factor and nitric oxide at the second trimester in Down's syndrome. J Matern Fetal Neonatal Med 2003;13:28.

424. Ruhle W, Graf von Ballestrem CL, Pult HM, et al. Korrelation des Cotininspiegels in Fruchtwasser, Nabelarterienblut und mutterlichem Blut. Geburtshilfe Frauenheilkd 1995;55:156.

425. Nicholls TM, Hähnel R, Wilkinson SP. Organic acids in amniotic fluid. Clin Chim Acta 1978;84:11.

426. Mattison DR. Amniotic fluid osmolality. Obstet Gynecol 1970;36:420.

427. Wandzilak TR, Hanson FW, Williams HE, et al. The quantitation of oxalate in amniotic fluid by ion-chromatography. Clin Chim Acta 1989;185:131.

428. Seppala M, Aho I, Tissari A, et al. Radioimmunoassay of oxytocin in amniotic fluid, fetal urine, and meconium during late pregnancy and delivery. Am J Obstet Gynecol 1972;114:788.

429. Mihailovic M, Cvetkovic M, Ljubic A, et al. Selenium and malondialdehyde content and glutathione peroxidase activity in maternal and umbilical cord blood and amniotic fluid. Biol Trace Elem Res 2000;73:47.

430. Condorelli S, Cosmi EV, Scarpelli EM. Extrapulmonary source of amniotic fluid phospholipids. Am J
Obstet Gynecol 1974;118:842.

431. Lindback T, Frantz T. Effect of centrifugation on amniotic fluid phospholipid recovery. Acta Obstet Gynecol Scand 1975;54:101.

432. Neerhof MG, Dohnal JC, Ashwood ER, et al. Lamellar body counts: a consensus on protocol. Obstet Gynecol 2001;97:318.

433. Moon TC, Lee JH, Lee SH, et al. Detection and characterization of a type IIA secretory phospholipase
A2 inhibitory protein in human amniotic fluid. Biol Pharm Bull 2000;23:1163.

434. Foster WG, Chan S, Platt L, et al. Detection of phytoestrogens in samples of second trimester human amniotic fluid. Toxicol Lett 2002;129:199.

435. Vesce F, Scapoli C, Giovannini G, et al. Plasminogen activator system in serum and amniotic fluid of euploid and aneuploid pregnancies. Obstet Gynecol 2001;97:404.

436. Uszynski M, Klyszejko A, Zekanowska E. Plasminogen, alpha(2)-antiplasmin and complexes of plasmin-
alpha(2)-antiplasmin (PAP) in amniotic fluid and blood plasma of parturient women. Eur J Obstet Gynecol Reprod Biol 2000;93:167.

437. Prado VF, Reis DD, Pena SD. Biochemical and immunochemical identification of the fetal polypeptides
of human amniotic fluid during the second trimester of pregnancy. Braz J Med Biol Res 1990;23:121.

438. Phillips LL, Davidson EC. Procoagulant properties of amniotic fluid. J Obstet Gynecol 1972:113:911.

439. Kauppila S, Tekay A, Risteli L, et al. Type I and type III procollagen propeptides in amniotic fluid of
normal pregnancies and in a case of mild osteogenesis imperfecta. Eur J Clin Invest 1998;28:831.

440. Schenker JG, Ben-David M, Polishuk WZ. Prolactin in normal pregnancy: relationship of maternal, fetal,
and amniotic fluid levels. Am J Obstet Gynecol 1975;123:834.

441. Ben-Jonathan N, Munsick RA. Dopamine and prolactin in human pregnancy. J Clin Endocrinol Metab
1980;51:1019.

442. Singh EJ, Zuspan FP. content of amniotic fluid prostaglandins in normal, diabetic, and drug-abuse human
pregnancy. Am J Obstet Gynecol 1974;118:358.

443. Pitkin RM, Reynolds WA. Fetal ingestion and metabolism of amniotic fluid protein. Am J Obstet Gynecol 1975;23:356.

444. Kaufman S. Protein-bound iodine (PBI) in human amniotic fluid. J Pediatr 1966;68:990.

445. Johnson MR, Abbas A, Nicolaides KH, et al. Distribution of relaxin between human maternal and fetal
circulations and amniotic fluid. J Endocrinol 1992;134:313.

446. Franks RC, Hayashi RH. Maternal and fetal renin activity and renin and big renin concentrations in second-trimester pregnancy. Am J Obstet Gynecol 1979;134:20.

447. Cederqvist LL, Zervoudakis IA, Ewool L, et al. Prenatal diagnosis of congenital rubella. BMJ
1977;297:615.

448. Teichler D, Doherty RA. Amniotic fluid secretor typing: validation for use in prenatal prediction of myotonic dystrophy. Clin Genet 1980;18:257.

449. Renlung M, Aula P. Prenatal detection of Salla disease based upon increased free sialic acid in amniocytes. Am J Med Genet 1987;28:377.

450. Bala RM, Wright C, Bardai A, et al. Somatomedin bioactivity in serum and amniotic fluid during pregnancy. J Clin Endocrinol Metab 1978;46:649.

451. Chochinov RH, Mariz IK, Hajek AS, et al. Characterization of a protein in mid-term human amniotic
fluid which reacts in the somatomedin-C radioreceptor assay. J Clin Endocrinol Metab 1977;44:902.

452. Tham A, Wetterberg L, Sara VR. Immunoreactive somatomedin B in the human foetus and in women
during pregnancy. Acta Endocrinol 1987;115:218.

453. Niswander KR. Spectrophotometric analysis of amniotic fluid in early gestation. Am J Obstet Gynecol
1970;108:1296.

454. Schweitzer M, Giroud CJP. A comparison of the pattern of steroid glucuronides and sulfates in maternal
plasma, umbilical cord plasma, and amniotic fluid. II. J Clin Endocrinol Metab 1971;33:793.

455. Fortunato SJ, Menon R, Lombardi SJ. Stromelysins in placental membranes and amniotic fluid with premature rupture of membranes. Obstet Gynecol 1999;94:435.

456. Müller-Tyl E, Lempert J, Steinbereithner K, et al. Surface properties of the amniotic fluid in normal pregnancy. Am J Obstet Gynecol 1975;122:295.

457. Giles HR, Lox CD, Heine W, et al. Intrauterine fetal sex determination by radioimmunoassay of amniotic fluid testosterone. Gynecol Invest 1974;5:317.

458. Judd HL, Robinson JD, Young PE, et al. Amniotic fluid testosterone levels in midpregnancy. Obstet Gynecol 1976;48:690.

459. Belisle S, Fencl M deM, Tulchinsky E. Amniotic fluid testosterone and follicle-stimulating hormone in the determination of fetal sex. Am J Obstet Gynecol 1977;128:514.

460. Tersenov OA, Mikhaleva IV, Usol'tseva VA, et al. Coagulative activity of the amniotic fluid. Akush Ginekol (Mosk) 1989;1:43.

461. Sainio S, Javela K, Kekomaki R, et al. Thrombopoietin levels in cord blood plasma and amniotic fluid in fetuses with alloimmune thrombocytopenia and healthy controls. Br J Haematol 2000;109:330.

462. Hall, GS, Carr MJ, Cummins E, et al. Aluminum, barium, silicon, and strontium in amniotic fluid by emission spectrometry. Clin Chem 1983;29:1318.

463. Hüfner M, Grussendorf M, Lorenz U, et al. 3.39,59-Triiodothyronine (reverse T_3) in amniotic fluid and cord serum. Eur J Pediatr 1977;125:213.

464. Parkinson CE, Tan JC, Gal I. Vitamin A concentration in amniotic fluid and maternal serum related to neural-tube defects. Br J Obstet Gynaecol 1982;89:935.

465. Wallingford JC, Milunsky A, Underwood BA. Vitamin A and retinol-binding protein in amniotic fluid. Am J Clin Nutr 1983;38:377.

466. Gardiki-Kouidou P, Seller MJ. Amniotic fluid folate, vitamin B_{12} and transcobalamins in neural tube defects. Clin Genet 1988;33:441.

467. Weisman Y, Jaccard N, Legum C, et al. Prenatal diagnosis of vitamin D–dependent rickets, type II: response to 1,25-dihydroxyvitamin D in amniotic fluid cells and fetal tissues. J Clin Endocrinol Metab 1990;71:937.

468. Lacourt GC, Arendt J, Cox J, et al. Microcephalic dwarfism with associated low amniotic fluid 5-hydroxyindole-3-acetic acid (5HIAA): report of a case of Cornelia de Lange syndrome. Helv Paediatr Acta 1977;32:149.

469. Emery AEH, Eccleston D, Scrimgeour JB, et al. Amniotic fluid composition in malformations of the central nervous system. J Obstet Gynaecol Br Commonw 1972;79:154.

470. Soltesz G, Harris D, Mackenzie IZ, et al. The metabolic and endocrine milieu of the human fetus and mother at 18–21 weeks of gestation. I. Plasma amino acid concentrations. Pediatr Res 1985;19:91.

471. Weiss PA, Kainer F, Haeusler M, et al. Amniotic fluid insulin levels in nondiabetic pregnant women: an update. Arch Gynecol Obstet 1998;262:81.

472. Nusbaum MJ, Zettner A. The content of Ca, Mg Cu, Fe, Na and K in amniotic fluid from eleven to nineteen weeks' gestation. Am J Obstet Gynecol 1973;115:219.

473. Ruth RE, Goldsmith SK. Interaction between zinc deprivation and acute ethanol intoxication during pregnancy in rats. J Nutr 1981;111:2034.

474. Keppen LD, Pysher T, Rennert OM. Zinc deficiency acts as a co-teratogen with alcohol in fetal alcohol syndrome. Pediatr Res 1985;19:944.

475. Abdulla M, Lofberg L, Jagersted M, et al. Plasma and amniotic fluid chemical elements during pregnancy. In: Bratter P, Schramel P. Analytical chemistry in medicine and biology. Proceedings of the 2nd International Workshop. Berlin: Gruyter, 1983:517.

476. Ward N, Bryce-Smith DM, Minski M, et al. Multi element neutron activation analysis of amniotic fluid in relation to varying gestational membrane ruptures. In: Bratter P, Schramel P, eds. Analytical chemistry in medicine and biology. Proceedings of the 2nd International Workshops. Berlin: de Gruyter, 1983:483.

477. Parkinson CE, Tran JCY, Lewis PJ, et al. Amniotic fluid zinc and copper and neural tube defects. J Obstet Gynaecol 1981;1:207–12.

478. Tamura T, Weekes EW, Birch R, et al. Relationship between amniotic fluid and maternal blood nutrient levels. J Perinat Med 1994;22: 227.

479. Steen MT, Boddie AM, Fisher AJ, et al. Neural-tube defects are associated with low concentrations of cobalamin (vitamin B_{12}) in amniotic fluid. Prenat Diagn 1998;18:545.

480. Dawson EB, Evans DR, Van Hook JW. Amniotic fluid B_{12} and folate levels associated with neural tube defects. Am J Perinatol 1998;15:511.

481. Dawson EB, Evans DR, Harris WA, et al. Amniotic fluid B_{12}, calcium, and lead levels associated with neural tube defects. Am J Perinatol 1999;16:373.

482. Luglie PF, Frulio A, Campus G, et al. Mercury determination in human amniotic fluid: mercury determination in human amniotic fluid. Minerva Stomatol 2000;49:155.

483. Milnerowicz H, Zalewski J, Geneja R, et al. Levels of Cd, Pb in blood and Zn, Cu, Cd, Pb in amniotic fluid of tobacco smoking women during pregnancy complicated oligohydramnios or premature rupture of membranes. Ginekol Pol 2000;7:1311.

484. Hodari AA, Mariona FG, Houlihan RT, et al. Creatinine transport in the maternal–fetal complex. Obstet Gynecol 1973;41:47.

485. Pitkin RM, Swirek SJ. Amniotic fluid creatinine. Am J Obstet Gynecol 1967;98:1135.

486. Droegemueller W, Jackson C, Makowski EL, et al. Amniotic fluid examination as an aid in the assessment of gestational age. Am J Obstet Gynecol 1969;104:424.

487. Sharma SD, Trussell RR. The value of amniotic fluid examination in the assessment of fetal maturity. J Obstet Gynaecol Br Commonw 1970;77:215.

488. Doran TA, Malone RM, Benzie RJ, et al. Amniotic fluid tests for fetal maturity in normal and abnormal pregnancies. Am J Obstet Gynecol 1976;125:586.

489. Putkonen T. Ueber die gruppenspezifischen Eigenschaften verschiedener Korperflüssigkeiten. Acta Soc Med Fenn Duodecim Ser A 1930;14:113.

490. Freda JV. A-B-O (H) blood group substances in the human maternal–fetal barrier and amniotic fluid. Am J Obstet Gynecol 1958;76:407.

491. Prezestwor E. Distribution of ABH group substances in amniotic fluid. Poznan Tow Przyj Nauk 1964;29:197.

492. Turowska B, Bromboszca A. ABO group substances in the amniotic fluid. Przegl Lek 1967;23:731.

493. Giblett ER. Genetic markers in human blood. Oxford: Blackwell, 1969.

494. Renwick JH, Lawler SD. Genetical linkage between the ABO and nail–patella loci. Ann Hum Genet 1955;19:312.

495. Renwick JH, Bolling DR. An analysis procedure illustrated on a triple linkage of use for prenatal diagnosis of myotonic dystrophy. J Med Genet 1971;8:399.

496. Renwick JH, Bundey SE, Ferguson-Smith MA, et al. Confirmation of linkage of the loci for myotonic dystrophy and ABH selection. J Med Genet 1971;8:407.

497. Milunsky A, Skare JC, Milunsky JM, et al. Prenatal diagnosis of myotonic muscular dystrophy with linked deoxyribonucleic acid probes. Am J Obstet Gynecol 1991;164:751.

498. Firshein SL, Hoyer LW, Lazarchick J, et al. Prenatal diagnosis of classic hemophilia. N Engl J Med 1979;300:937.

499. Durandy A, Cerf-Bensussan N, Dumez Y, et al. Prenatal diagnosis of severe combined immunodeficiency with defective synthesis of HLA molecules. Prenat Diagn 1987;7:27.

500. Davis LE, McLaren LG, Stewart JA, et al. Immunological and microbiological studies of midtrimester amniotic fluid. Gynecol Obstet Invest 1983;16:261.

501. Altieri C, Maruotti G, Natale C, et al. In vitro survival of *Listeria monocytogenes* in human amniotic fluid. Zentralbl Hyg Umweltmed 1999;202:377.

502. Boulley AM, Vial M, Bessis R, et al. Antenatal diagnosis of 2 cases of cytomegalic inclusion disease. Arch Fr Pediatr 1984;41:123.

503. Gleicher N. Immunological influence of amniotic fluid. Lancet 1980;1:541.

504. Auger P, Marquis G, Dallaire L, et al. Natural occurrence of a humoral response to *Candida* in human amniotic fluid. Am J Obstet Gynecol 1980;136:1075.

505. Emelyanova AI, Mikheeva GA, Ermakova GG. Amniotic fluid immunoglobulins at different dates of pregnancy (in Russian). Akush Ginekol (Mosk) 1982;7:19.

506. Prevedourakis C, Stringou-Charlabis E, Kaskarelis D. Bacterial invasion of amniotic cavity during pregnancy and labor. Obstet Gynecol 1971;37:459.

507. Harwick HJ, Iuppa JB, Fekety FR. Microorganisms and amniotic fluid. Obstet Gynecol 1969;33:256.

508. Tafari N, Ross SM, Naeye RL, et al. Failure of bacterial growth inhibition by amniotic fluid. Am J Obstet Gynecol 1977;128:187.

509. Gusdon J. A bactericidin for *Bacillus subtilis* in pregnancy. J Immunol 1962;88:494.

510. Thadepalli H, Appleman MD, Maidman JE, et al. Antimicrobial effect of amniotic fluid against anaerobic bacteria. Am J Obstet Gynecol 1977;127:250.

511. Walsh H, Hildebrandt R, Prystowsky H. Growth inhibition factors in amniotic fluid. Am J Obstet Gynecol 1965;95:590.

512. Sarkany I, Gaylarde CC. The effect of amniotic fluid in bacterial growth. Br J Dermatol 1968;80:241.

513. Galask RP, Snyder IR. Bacterial inhibition by amniotic fluid. Am J Obstet Gynecol 1968;102:949.

514. Galask RP. Antimicrobial factors in amniotic fluid. Am J Obstet Gynecol 1970;106:59.

515. Florman A, Teubner D. Enhancement of bacterial growth in amniotic fluid by meconium. J Pediatr 1969;74:111.

516. Rozansky S, Persky B, Bercovici B. Antibacterial action of human cervical mucus. Proc Soc Exp Biol Med 1962;110:876.

517. Izaka K, Shirakawa H, Yamada M, et al. Method for isolation of human placental lysozyme. Anal Biochem 1971;42:299.

518. Schumacher GFB, Pearl MJ. Cyclic changes of muramidase (lysozyme in cervical mucus). J Reprod Med 1969;3:105.

519. Pokiodova NV, Babaian SS, Ermolieva ZV. Vydelenie lizotsima iz platsenty cheloveka. Antibiotiki 1971;16: 456.

520. Bratlid D, Lindback T. Bacteriolytic activity of amniotic fluid. Obstet Gynecol 1978;51:63.

521. Thadepalli H, Bach VT, Davidson EC Jr. Antimicrobial effect of amniotic fluid. Obstet Gynecol 1978;52:198.

522. Evaldson G, Nord CE. Amniotic fluid activity against *Bacteroides fragilis* and group B streptococci. Med Microbiol Immunol 1981;170:11.

523. Ismail MA, Salti GI, Moawad AH. Effect of amniotic fluid on bacterial recovery and growth: clinical implications. Obstet Gynecol Surv 1989;44:5711.

524. Martius J, Eschenbach DA. The role of bacterial vaginosis as a cause of amniotic fluid infection, chorioamnionitis and prematurity: a review. Arch Gynecol Obstet 1990;247:1.

525. Charles D, Edwards WR. Infectious complications of cervical cerclage. Am J Obstet Gynecol 1981; 141:1065.

526. Lebon P, Girard S, Thépot F, et al. Embryologie générale: présence constante d'interféron de type α dans les liquides amniotiques humains. C R Acad Sci Paris 1981;293:69.

527. Morgan-Capner P, Rodeck CH, Nicolaides KH. Prenatal detection of rubella-specific IgM in fetal sera. Prenat Diagn 1985;5:21.

528. Ho-Terrey L, Terrey GM, Londesborough P. Diagnosis of foetal rubella virus infection by polymerase chain reaction. J Gen Virol 1990;71:1607.

529. Bosma TJ, Corbett KM, Eckstein MB, et al. Use of PCR for prenatal and postnatal diagnosis of congenital rubella. J Clin Microbiol 1995;33:2881.

530. Pons JC, Vial P, Rozenberg F, et al. Prenatal diagnosis of fetal varicella in the second trimester of pregnancy J Gynecol Obstet Biol Reprod (Paris) 1995;24:829.

531. Dufour P, de Bievre P, Vinatier D, et al. Varicella and pregnancy. Eur J Obstet Gynecol Reprod Biol 1996;66:119.

532. Shukla SK, Meier PR, Mitchell PD, et al. *Leptotrichia amnionii* sp. *nov.*, a novel bacterium isolated. J Clin Microbiol 2002;40:3346.

533. Thadepalli H, Gangopadhyay PK, Maidman JE. Amniotic fluid analysis for antimicrobial factors. Int J Gynaecol Obstet 1982;20:65.

534. Blanco JD, Gibbs RS, Krebs LF, et al. The association between the absence of amniotic fluid bacterial inhibitory activity and intra-amniotic infection. Am J Obstet Gynecol 1982;143:749.

535. Grose C, Weiner CP. Prenatal diagnosis of congenital cytomegalovirus infection: two decades later. Am J Obstet Gynecol 1990;163:447.

536. Derouin F, Thulliez P, Candolfi E, et al. Early prenatal diagnosis of congenital toxoplasmosis using amniotic fluid samples and tissue culture. Eur J Clin Microb Infect Dis 1988;7:423.

537. Leiberman JR, Hagay ZJ, Dagan R. Intraamniotic *Haemophilus influenzae* infection. Arch Gynecol 1989;244:183.

538. Bernard B, Barton L, Abate M, et al. Maternal–fetal transfer of cefazolin in the first twenty weeks of pregnancy. J Infect Dis 1977;136:377.

539. Giamerellov H, Gazis J, Petrikkos G, et al. A study of cefoxitin, moxalactam, and ceftazidime kinetics in pregnancy. Am J Obstet Gynecol 1983;147:914.

540. Atkinson G, Campbell DJ, Cawood ML, et al. Steroids in human intrauterine fluids of early pregnancy. Clin Endocrinol 1996;44:435.

541. Mennuti MT, Wu CH, Mellman WJ. Amniotic fluid testosterone and follicle stimulating hormone levels as indicators of fetal sex during mid-pregnancy. Am J Med Genet 1977;1:211.

542. Peltonen J, Vinikka L, Laatikainen T. Amniotic fluid cortisol during gestation and its relation to fetal lung maturation. J Steroid Biochem 1977;8:1159.

543. Petrucha RA, Goebelsmann U, Hung TT, et al. Amniotic fluid β-endorphin and β-lipotropin concentrations during the second and third trimesters. Am J Obstet Gynecol 1983;146:644.

544. Genazzoni AR, Petraglia F, Parrini D, et al. Lack of correlation between amniotic fluid and maternal plasma contents of beta-endorphin, beta-lipotropin, and adrenocorticotropic hormone in normal and pathologic pregnancies. Am J Obstet Gynecol 1984;148:198.

545. Buscher U, Hertwig K, Dudenhausen JW. Detection of erythropoietin in amniotic fluid. Geburtshilfe Frauenheilkd 1996;56:243.

546. Kakuya F, Shirai M, Takase M, et al. Relationship between erythropoietin levels both in cord serum and amniotic fluid at birth and abnormal fetal heart rate records. Pediatr Int 2002;44:414.

547. Freeman R, Lev-Gur M, Koslowe R, et al. Maternal plasma and amniotic fluid levels of estradiol, estrone, progesterone and prolactin in early pregnancy. Obstet Gynecol 1984;63:507.

548. Sugar J, Dessy C, Alexander S, et al. Estriol-3-glucuronide and estriol-16-glucuronide in amniotic fluid during normal pregnancy. J Clin Endocrinol Metab 1980;50:137.

549. Heikinheimo M, Seppala M, Brock DJH. Pregnancy specific beta$_1$-glycoprotein and human chorionic gonadotrophin levels in amniotic fluid and maternal serum in the first half of pregnancy. Oncodev Biol Med 1980;1:71.

550. Dattatreyamurty B, Sheth AR, Purandare TV, et al. Gonadotropins during second trimester of pregnancy. I. LH and hCG levels in maternal serum and amniotic fluid and their relationship to the sex of the foetus. Acta Endocrinol 1979;91:692.

550a. Belisle S, Fencl M deM, Osathanondh R, et al. Sources of 17 alpha-hydroxypregnenolone and its sulfate in human pregnancy. J Clin Endocrinol Metab 1978;46:721.

551. Shi-hao Y. Prolactin in amniotic fluid and serum of women in early pregnancy. Jugosl Ginekol Opstet 1981;21:116.

552. Zondek T, Mansfield MD, Zondek LH. Amniotic fluid testosterone and fetal sex determination in the first half of pregnancy. Br J Obstet Gynaecol.1977;84:714.

553. Kunzig HJ, Meyer U, Schmitz-Roeckerath B, et al. Influence of fetal sex on the concentration of amniotic fluid testosterone: antenatal sex determination? Arch Gynakol 1977;223:75.

554. Cooper E, Anderson A, Bennett AH, et al. Radioimmunoassay of thyroxine and 3.39,59-triiodothyronine (reverse T$_3$) in human amniotic fluid. Clin Chim Acta 1982;118:57.

555. Dorner G, Stahl F, Rohde W, et al. Sex-specific testosterone and FSH concentrations in amniotic fluids of mid-pregnancy. Endokrinologie 1977;70:86.

556. Nazamani M, McDonough PG, Ellegood JO, et al. Maternal and amniotic fluid steroids throughout human pregnancy. Am J Obstet Gynecol 1979;134:674.

557. Wu CH, Mennuti MT, Mikhail G. Free and protein-bound steroids in amniotic fluid of midpregnancy. Am J Obstet Gynecol 1979;133:666.

558. Merger C, Blanc B, Ruf H, et al. The level of testosterone, delta 4-androstenedione, and S-DHA in liquor and fetal sex. J Gynecol Obstet Biol Reprod (Paris) 1983;10:567.

559. Carson DJ, Okuno A, Lee PA, et al. Amniotic fluid steroid levels. Am J Dis Child 1982;136:218.

560. Mean F, Pescia G, Vajda D, et al. Amniotic fluid testosterone in prenatal sex determination. J Genet Hum 1981;29:441.

561. Robinson JD, Judd HL, Young PE, et al. Amniotic fluid androgens and estrogens in midgestation. J Clin Endocrinol Metab 1977;45:755.

562. Abramovich DR, Herriot R, Stott J. Dihydrotestosterone levels at midpregnancy and term: a comparison with testosterone concentrations. J Obstet Gynaecol Br Commonw 1983;90:232.

563. Perera DM, McGarrigle HH, Lawrence DM, et al. Amniotic fluid testosterone and testosterone glucuronide levels in the determination of foetal sex. J Steroid Biochem 1987;26:273.

564. Raux-Demay M, Mornet E, et al. Early prenatal diagnosis of 21-hydroxylase deficiency using amniotic fluid 17-hydroxyprogesterone determination and DNA probes. Prenat Diagn 1989;9:457.

565. Dodinval P, Duvivier J. Diagnostic prénatal du sexe par dosage de la testostérone et de la F.S.H. amniotiques. J Genet Hum 1980;28:207.

566. Migeon CL. Comments about the need for prenatal treatment of congenital adrenal hyperplasia due to 21-hydroxylase deficiency. J Clin Endocrinol Metab 1990;70:836.

567. Speiser PW, Laforgia N, Kato J, et al. First trimester prenatal treatment and molecular genetic diagnosis of congenital adrenal hyperplasia (21-hydroxylase deficiency). J Clin Endocrinol Metab 1990;70:838.

568. Pang S, Pollack M, Marshall RN, et al. Prenatal treatment of congenital adrenal hyperplasia due to 21-hydroxylase deficiency. N Engl J Med 1990;322:111.

569. Loeuille GA, David M, Forest MG. Prenatal treatment of congenital adrenal hyperplasia: report of a new case. Eur J Pediatr 1990;149:237.

570. Blankstein J, Kraiem Z, Mashiah S, et al. Effect of dexamethasone administration at midgestation on cortisol levels in amniotic fluid. Isr J Med Sci 1979;15:945.

571. Friedrich E, Habedank M, Cooreman G, et al. Diagnostik der fötalen schilddrusenfunktion durch amniocentese. Z Geburtshilfe Perinatol 1981;185:96.

572. Perelman AH, Johnson RL, Clemons RD. Intrauterine diagnosis and treatment of fetal goitrous hypothyroidism. J Clin Endocrinol Metab 1990;71:618.

573. Stoll C, Willard D, Czernichow P, et al. Prenatal diagnosis of primary pituitary dysgenesis. Lancet 1978;1:932.

573a. Basbug M, Serin IS, Ozcelik B, et al. Correlation of elevated leptin levels in amniotic fluid and maternal serum in neural tube defects. Obstet Gynecol 2003;101:523.

574. Ledge M. Dark brown amniotic fluid: identification of contributing pigments. Br J Obstet Gynaecol 1981;88:632.

575. Svigos JM, Stewart-Rattray SF, Pridmore BR. Meconium-stained liquor at second trimester amniocentesis: is it significant? Aust NZ J Obstet Gynaecol 1981;21:5.

576. Immken L, Lee M, Stewart R, et al. Significance of meconium stained fluid in midtrimester amniocentesis. Birth Defects 1982;18:187.

577. Ron M, Cohen T, Yaffe H, et al. The clinical significance of blood-contaminated midtrimester amniocentesis. Acta Obstet Gynecol Scand 1982;61:43.

578. Hankins GDV, Rowe J, Quirk JG, et al. Significance of brown and/or green amniotic fluid at the time of second trimester genetic amniocentesis. Obstet Gynecol 1984;64:353.

579. Szeto HH, Zervoudakis IA, Cederqvist LL, et al. Amniotic fluid transfer of meperidine from maternal plasma in early pregnancy. Obstet Gynecol 1978;52:59.

580. Buehler BA, Delimont D, Van Waes M, et al. Prenatal prediction of risk of the fetal hydantoin syndrome. N Engl J Med 1990;31:322.

581. Jauniaux E, Gulbis B, Acharya G, et al. Maternal tobacco exposure and cotinine levels in fetal fluids in the first half of pregnancy. Obstet Gynecol 1999;93:25.

582. Milunsky A, Carmella SG, Ye M, et al. A tobacco-specific carcinogen in the fetus. Prenat Diagn 2000;20:307.

583. Sandberg JA, Olsen GD. Microassay for the simultaneous determination of cocaine, norcocaine, benzoylecgonine and benzoylnorecgonine by high-performance liquid chromatography. J Chromatogr 1990;525:113.

584. Mastrogiannis DS, Decavalas GO, Verma U, et al. Perinatal outcome after recent cocaine usage. Obstet Gynecol 1990;76:8.

585. Hadeed AJ, Siegel SR. Maternal cocaine use during pregnancy: effect on the newborn infant. Pediatrics. 1990;85:630.

586. Behnke M, Eyler FD, Garvan CW, et al. The search for congenital malformations in newborns with fetal cocaine exposure. Pediatrics 2001;107:E74.

587. Addis A, Moretti ME, Ahmed Syed F, et al. Fetal effects of cocaine: an updated meta-analysis. Reprod Toxicol 2001;15:341.

588. Hostetter A, Ritchie JC, Stowe ZN. Amniotic fluid and umbilical cord blood concentrations of antidepressants in three women. Biol Psychiatry 2000;48:1032.

589. Omtzigt JG, Nau H, Los FJ, et al. The disposition of valproate and its metabolites in the late first trimester and early second trimester of pregnancy in maternal serum, urine, and amniotic fluid: effect of dose, comedication, and the presence of spina bifida. Eur J Clin Pharmacol 1992;43:381.

590. Bradman A, Barr DB, Claus Henn BG, et al. Measurement of pesticides and other toxicants in amniotic fluid as a potential biomarker of prenatal exposure: a validation study. Environ Health Perspect. 2003;111:1779.

591. Whyatt RM, Barr DB. Measurement of organophosphate metabolites in postpartum meconium as a potential biomarker of prenatal exposure: a validation study. Environ Health Perspect. 2001;109:17

592. Wessels D, Barr DB, Mendola P. Use of Biomarkers to Indicate Exposure of Children to Organophosphate Pesticides: Implications for a Longitudinal Study of Children's Environmental Health. Environ Health Perspect. 2003;111:1939.

Daniel L. Van Dyke, Ph.D.

4

Amniotic Fluid Cell Culture

Amniotic fluid cell (AFC) culture is a well-established, routine procedure in prenatal diagnosis laboratories. The basic cell culture technology described by Milunsky in earlier versions of this chapter[1,2] has not changed and will remain worth consulting. What has changed are the improved speed to the final report, the success rate of cell culture, and the average quality of the chromosome banding. Because of optimized cell culture media, the use of growth factor supplements, high-quality plasticware, sophisticated incubators, and robotic cell harvest equipment, culture failures occur in less than 0.2 percent of all specimens processed by experienced laboratories. For the same reasons, the average reporting time has been reduced substantially.

ALTERNATIVES TO CELL CULTURE AND METAPHASE KARYOTYPE ANALYSIS

The prediction that AFC culture would largely be replaced by chorionic villus sampling (CVS) has not come true. The increasing acceptance and sophistication of maternal serum screening tests and high-resolution prenatal ultrasonography identified a greater number of at-risk pregnancies, especially in women under age 35. This resulted in an increase in the number of amniocentesis procedures. Now the number of amniocenteses for cell culture and karyotype studies is beginning to fall. This is primarily because women over age 35 are using screening-based risk figures to decide against prenatal diagnosis if their risks are deemed to be reduced based on triple, quadruple, or more complex screening tests that combine information from the first- and second-trimester serum assays and ultrasound examinations. With each additional chemical component of maternal serum screening has come a higher rate of detection and a lower false-positive rate—hence, fewer women are "screen positive" and many elect to forgo amniocentesis.[3] The use of early amniocentesis (9–14 gestational weeks) has been limited more by failure to obtain fluid and operator inexperience than by failing to grow cells from such early specimens.[4,5] Interphase fluorescence in situ hybridization (FISH) technology was also predicted to replace cell culture and metaphase karyotype analysis, at least outside the United States. This prediction has not been realized except for occasional cases of malformations identified by ultrasound examination and then diagnosed as aneuploid using FISH methods.[6,7] Most of these cases are still confirmed by cell culture and karyotype analysis, albeit after pregnancy termination. Interphase FISH analysis can identify 90–95 percent of the clinically relevant autosomal and sex chromosomal aneuploids, although up to 30 percent of all cytogenetic changes (e.g., mosaics and balanced translocations) are detected only by G-banded metaphase analysis.[8–15] Rapid and quantitative PCR methods have been employed to identify the common trisomies and sex chromosome aneuploid states,[16,17] and microarray technologies are also likely to be considered as alternatives to cell culture and metaphase karyotype analysis.[18]

ALTERNATIVES TO AMNIOTIC FLUID FOR PRENATAL DIAGNOSIS

Amniotic fluid may not be accessible in cases of severe cystic hygroma, pleural effusion, renal agenesis, or bladder outlet obstruction. In these situations, alternative sampling must be considered. Chorionic villus sampling is discussed elsewhere in this volume.[19] In cases of bladder outlet obstruction, it is possible to obtain fluid and cells for culture from the fetal bladder. In one study, fetal karyotype analysis was successful in 95 percent of 75 samples, with six chromosome abnormalities identified, and in fact cell culture was more successful than FISH studies.[20] Cases presenting with severe cystic hygroma, ascites, or pleural effusion are at significant risk for having a chromosomal abnormality, especially trisomy 21 or monosomy X.[21] Fluid drawn from any of these sources will contain cells that can be cultured like amniocytes and usually also include lymphocytes that can be cultured with phytohemagglutinin (PHA) and harvested very quickly.[22–24] Coelocentesis at 6 to 10 weeks of gestational has been proposed as an alternative to both CVS and amniocentesis, but has yet to garner wide acceptance.[25]

AMNIOTIC FLUID CELL TYPES

Cellular Contents of Native Fluids

The vast majority of nucleated cells in second-trimester amniocentesis fluids are incapable of in vitro attachment and growth, even though many of these cells may exclude trypan blue. These are cells with pale cytoplasm and small, densely staining nuclei. In their ultrastructural characteristics, they are reminiscent of fetal epidermal cells at 16 to 18 weeks of pregnancy[26,27]; exfoliation of such cells from the fetal epidermis has been directly observed.[28] It is not known why their number in a given fluid is so highly variable and whether this reflects the well-being of the fetus, for which other properties of the amniotic fluid (AF) may be more predictive.[29] Because the change of the fetal skin from a simple two-layered structure to the mature stratified epithelium takes place around the 16th week of gestation and occurs at different rates in different body zones, minor differences in gestational age might account for comparatively large differences in overall cornification and desquamation.[30] Classical cytology and transmission or scanning electron microscopy have attempted a subdivision of cells in midtrimester fluids.[31–34]

A variable number of cells attach to the culture substrate within 6 to 72 hours after incubation, but the number of colony-forming cells rarely amounts to more than 10 cells/mL fluid.[35,36] Cells that attach in less than 24 hours (rapidly adhering, or RA, cells), if present in clear fluids in large quantities, may indicate a neural tube defect (NTD).[29] Such cells often take on the characteristic elongated spindlelike appearance of neural crest cells in monolayer culture. In AFC cultures from NTD pregnancies, the rapidly adhering cells include at least two types: monocytic cells that have phagocytic activity, and cells of glial origin that lack phagocytic activity and stain positive for synaptophysin and neuron-specific enolase.[37,38] Rapidly adhering, phagocytic, esterase- and

Fc-receptor-positive cells are also found in AF from normal fetuses, albeit in more moderate quantities.[39]

In cases of abdominal wall defects, macrophagelike cells and even lymphocytelike cells responding to PHA have been described.[40] AF from distressed fetuses may likewise contain macrophagelike cells, which Gosden and Brock named fetal distress (FD) cells.[41] Such FD cells occur in spontaneous abortion, severe intrauterine growth retardation, and preeclampsia. They may originate from the placenta. Gosden published an excellent summary discussing the possible sources, characteristics, and gestation-related changes of the cellular constituents in midtrimester AF.[42]

Colony-Forming Cells: Morphology and Nomenclature

Multiple approaches have been used to characterize and classify colony-forming cell types. The ultimate goals of these efforts are the identification of specialized gene products and the elucidation of the in vivo sites of origin of clonable AFCs. The availability of specific antibodies to the intermediate filament components of the mammalian cell cytoskeleton has revolutionized histopathology.[43] These techniques provide the means for establishing tentative correlations between cell types in culture and their presumptive in vivo counterparts.[44] The impact of these methods on the understanding of the histiotype and possible origin of AFCs has been profound. In spite of this progress, many questions concerning the nature and in vivo origin of AFCs have not been entirely resolved.

Table 4.1 provides a synopsis of the current classification of human AFCs in culture. This table also summarizes some of the criteria used for classification and the various nomenclatures to which they have led (for a more extensive compilation of the properties of AFCs, see the review by Gosden[42]). Morphological criteria were applied first. They quickly led to the realization that a high degree of cytoplasmic and nuclear pleomorphism is the hallmark of cultured AFCs. In contrast to what is known from postnatally derived human skin fibroblast cultures, multinucleation is a frequent and distinctive feature of cultivated AFCs. One report describes 7 percent of AFCs having two nuclei and 1 percent showing three or more nuclei.[45] Within the clonal progeny of a single AF specimen, considerably more cells appear to be of epithelial than fibroblast origin. A cell type that looks very much like a prototype fibroblastlike cell at the individual cell level (Figure 4.1) was distinguished by Hoehn et al.[35] from classical fibroblasts on the basis of its "bull's-eye" colony pattern. Such a pattern is never observed with classical skin or embryonic lung fibroblasts. Figure 4.2 shows that the typical bull's-eye colony pattern is displayed by epithelioid (E) and by AF-type cells. The clonal pattern of F-type cells with whorl-like centers and parallel arrays of spindle-shaped cells is totally different. However, since shapes of individual cells and clonal units are influenced by culture conditions, these features are subject to change during long-term culture.[61] Any classification based solely on morphological criteria thus remains inadequate.

Biochemical Characterization

The distinctiveness of the AF type received support in a series of ultrastructural and cell secretion studies.[49–54] It was shown that hormones such as hCG, estrogen, and progesterone are produced by AF-type cells. From these observations, Priest et al. concluded that at least some AF-type cells must originate from (placental) trophoblast tissue.[51,52] In contrast, F-type AFCs failed to show hormone production, which is in keeping with their likely mesenchymal origin.[53,56,57] Human CVS cultures show even higher levels of hCG

Table 4.1. The classification of human second-trimester AFCs in culture (excluding RA cells)

Reference	Melancon et al.[30] Gerbie et al.[31]	Sutherland et al.[32]	Hoehn et al.[21,33]	Priest et al.[34-42]	Virtanen et al.[43]	Cremer et al.[44] Ochs et al.[45]
Criteria	Morphology, enzyme production	Morphology, growth behavior	Morphology, clone patterns, longevity, cytogenetics	Collagen and gonadotropin production, ultrastructure	IIF, intermediate filaments	Intermediate filaments, prokeratin peptides
Nomenclature	E (histidase)	EII	E	E	E2	E
		EI			E3	
					E4	ED
					E5	
	F (cystathionine synthetase)	EIII	AF	AF	E1	AF
		F	F	F	F	F

Note: AF = amniotic fluid-specific; E = epithelioid; ED = epithelial and densely packed;[45] F = fibroblastoid; IIF = indirect immunofluorescence microscopy. Dotted lines indicate correspondence between the various nomenclature (e.g., E3 corresponds to AF and E1). See also review by Gosden.[27]

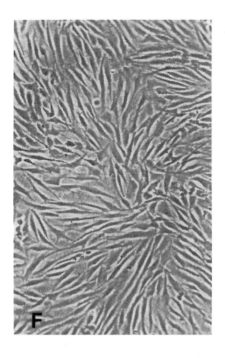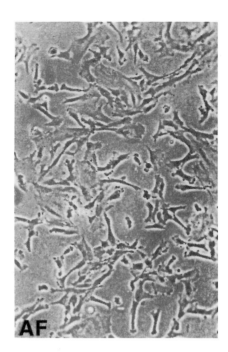

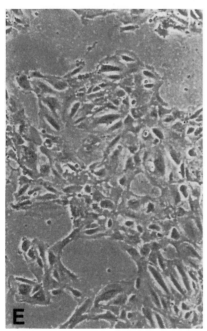

Fig. 4.1. Examples of living F, AF, and E morphotype cells observed by phase-contrast microscopy (3 × 6). Note the relative homogeneity of F-type, as opposed to the pleomorphism of AF- and E-type cells.

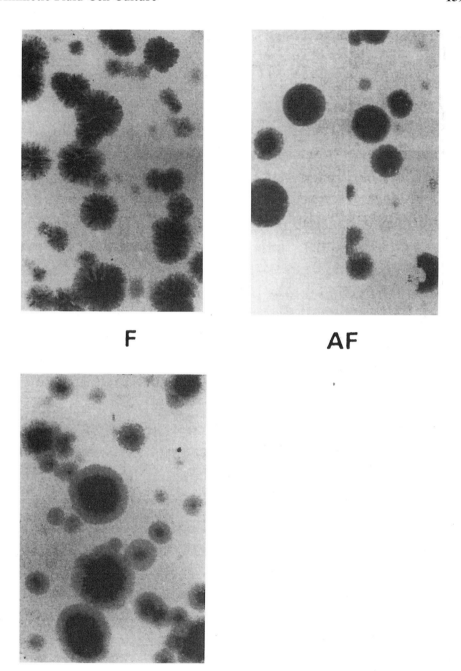

Fig. 4.2. Examples of fixed colonies of F, AF, and E clonal types at 2 weeks after plating. The AF- and E-type colonies display typical "bull's-eye" patterns. Compared to AF clones, the E-type clones display wider growth margins around the darkly stained central core. The examples of AF and E clones are from primary platings of uncentrifuged amniotic fluid at 17 weeks of gestational age. The F-clone examples are subclones derived from a single F-type primary clone isolated by a steel cloning cylinder and subsequent dilute plating on 2 x 3 inch glass slides. Crystal violet stain, four-fifths of actual size. Reproduced at 90 percent.

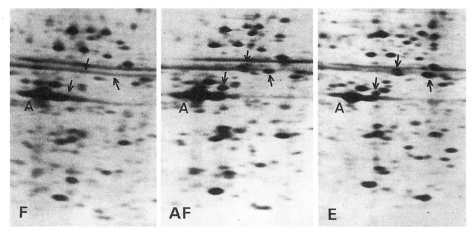

Fig. 4.3. Selected landscapes from two-dimensional (^{35}S)methionine-labeled polypeptide maps of F-, AF-, and E-type total-cell homogenates. Note that all three clone types are derived from a single amniotic fluid specimen, which rules out genotypic differences as a source of the apparent protein map differences. Horizontal dimension: isoelectric focusing; vertical dimension: polyacrylamide gradient gel electrophoresis. For technical details, see Johnston et al.[68] Arrows mark consistent differences of polypeptide spot patterns in the vicinity of the easily identifiable actin cluster (A).

secretion than AF-type AFC cultures.[62] The Priest laboratory also established that both AF- and F-type AFCs express human lymphocyte antigen (HLA) class I (HLA-ABC) but not class II (HLA-DR) surface antigens.[63]

Extracellular matrix studies by Crouch and Bornstein[64,65] and Crouch et al.[66] defined a number of qualitative differences between AF- and F-type AFCs. The differences in the types of procollagens produced were such that Bryant et al.[67] could use these as markers in fusion studies involving AF cells and postnatally derived skin fibroblasts. Examining whole-cell proteins by one- and two-parameter electrophoresis, Johnston et al.[68] provided additional evidence for the distinctiveness of the AF cell type (Figure 4.3). Several polypeptide spots were qualitatively different among F and AF clones (see arrows in Figure 4.3). Using a similar technique, Harrison et al.[69] demonstrated analogous differences. It furthermore provides convincing evidence for an apparent close ontogenetic relationship between E and AF cells, since their two-dimensional polypeptide patterns are nearly identical (Figure 4.3). For a more extensive discussion of the degrees of correlation between AFC morphotypes and their biochemical markers, see the review by Hoehn and Salk.[70]

Intermediate Filament System

The availability of antibodies to and the electrophoretic characterization of components of the cellular cytoskeleton were extended with great success to cultivated AFC types. For example, the close relationship between AF and E cells received overwhelming support from immunofluorescence studies using antibodies against epidermal keratins.[58,59] Such immunofluorescent staining of keratin filaments also confirmed the epithelioid nature of the vast majority of cells in AFC cultures.[71] However, it was soon noted that AF cells (labeled E1 by Virtanen; cf. Table 4.1) appeared to express intermediate-type filamentous structures that reacted with both prekeratin and vimentin antibodies. The conclusions from these early studies must be viewed in the context of the limited specificity (mostly to epidermal keratins) of the antibodies then available. This situation improved when Moll et al.[72] provided a comprehensive catalog of well-characterized prekeratin peptides. This new knowledge was rapidly applied to the identification of AFC clones. A landmark study by Ochs et al.[60] yielded two important findings: (1) not only AF but also F cells were shown to coexpress prekeratin and vimentin filaments; (2) the cytoplasmic margins of a singular cell type lit up strongly with desmoplakin-specific antibodies (Figure 4.4). These large, polygonal cells, labeled ED cells by Ochs et al. (Table 4.1), are only too familiar to pre-natal cell culturists because of their distinctive, cobblestone pattern, their low growth rate, and their resistance to trypsinization. They were pictured and referred to as sheathlike cells by Hoehn et al.[35] Coexpression of cytokeratin and vimentin filaments appears to be promoted by serial culture in many cell types of epithelioid origin. Ochs et al.[60] referred to the ED-cell as archetype E-cell, since it retains close cell-to-cell contacts by virtue of an abundant number of desmosomes. All other AFC E-cell types, and notably AF and F cells, have lost their desmosomes, together with a number of prokeratin peptides. They display only a remnant pattern of cytoskeletal structures (electrophoretically defined as cytokeratins 7, 8, 19, and 19).[60] The important point is that Ochs et al. viewed F-type AFCs as a distant but definite relative of an original E-cell lineage. This would fit with evidence for developmental epithelial-mesenchymal transitions.[73,74] F-type AFCs share many properties with classical fibroblastlike cells from postnatal skin or foreskin: shape, whorl clone pattern, production of collagenous matrixes, failure to produce hCG, ultra-structure, types of surface glycoproteins, and, last but not least, remarkable longevity. Fig-ure 4.5 shows that serially propagated derivative cultures of individual F, E, and AF clones show major differences in their longevities. In contrast to AF cells, genuine F cells can-not be cloned from every amniotic fluid sample.[48]

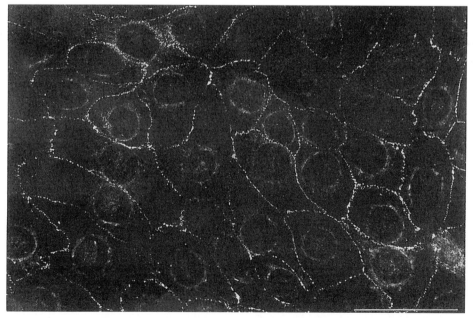

Fig. 4.4. Immunofluorescence staining of "ED"-type amniotic fluid cells using antibodies against desmo-plakin. The length of the bar is 0.05 mm. Note the exclusive reaction with cell boundaries (desmosomes). *Source*: Ochs et al., 1983.[60]

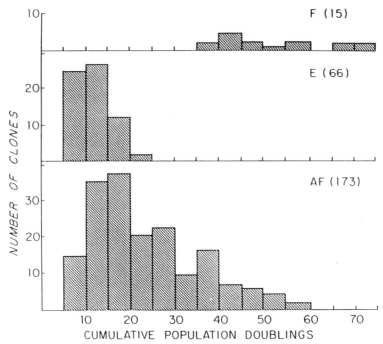

Fig. 4.5. Serial propagation and longevity of mass culture progeny of F-, E-, and AF-type amniotic fluid cell clones isolated individually from 20 consecutive amniotic fluid specimens (18 weeks of gestational age). The number of primary isolates of each clone type is given in parentheses. Note the relative paucity of F-type isolates from a total of 20 fluids. The progeny of F-type clones, however, reach the greatest number of cumulative population doublings. In contrast, all E-type isolates were short-lived, whereas AF-type isolates display a wide range of longevities.[35]

THE ORIGIN OF COLONY-FORMING CELL TYPES

Sites of origin of colony-forming amniotic fluid cells that are not at variance with either cytokeratin findings or anatomic considerations include fetal skin, the bronchopulmonary tract, and the collecting ducts of the kidney.[75] The latter site is of particular interest, since kidney tissue has been implicated as a source of trisomy 20 cells.[76] Cells staining with an antibody to glial fibrillary acidic protein (GFAP) occur in native fluids, even in the absence of neural tube defects, but they are not seen among colony-forming cells.[77]

Variation of enzyme expression[45,78,79] and morphological resemblance to either fetal urine[80] or amnion-derived cells[34] were the early clues to the possible sites of the in vivo origin of these cells. The Priest laboratory reported that human chorionic gonadotropin, normally produced by the placenta, appeared to be produced by AF-type, but not by F-type, cells in culture.[53,56,57,62,81] These studies suggest that the amniotic membranes contribute to the pool of proliferating AFCs.[82] Harris[83] arrived at a similar conclusion based on her comparative studies of glycoproteins secreted by AFCs.

Again, subsequent cytoskeleton studies contradicted these earlier findings. Regauer et al.[75] found that in situ and cultivated amniotic membrane cells display a much higher cytokeratin structural complexity than any of the AF-derived cell types. The authors therefore consider the amniotic membrane a rather unlikely source of clonable cells. Similarly, they failed to find any concordance between the cytokeratin pattern of urothelial cells and AFCs. Despite this powerful negative evidence, it does not seem all that unreasonable to believe that the fetal urine cells contribute to the AFC population. Several studies have shown that human fetal and postnatal urine contains cells that proliferate well in vitro.[20,76] Moreover, these urine-derived clones resemble AF-derived clones to an astonishing degree.[80,84] Using specific antibodies against urothelium, von Koskull et al.[85] provided results that tend to affirm the urinary origin of some types of AFCs. Although native AF at 16–18 weeks of gestation contains around 18 percent cells of colonic mucosal origin (as defined by a specific monoclonal antibody), none of the adherent cells appears to belong to this category.[86]

RESEARCH USE OF AMNIOTIC FLUID CELLS

In addition to their diagnostic value with respect to human chromosomal and metabolic disease, cultivated AFCs represent an important source of primary cell culture materials of human origin. Many of these cells can be grown in vitro for a considerable number of passages, and modern medium supplements facilitate their propagation. Except for human preputial epidermis, AF is the only source from which human epithelioid cells can be readily obtained without specialized culture techniques. AF-type AFCs are a readily accessible source of fibronectin and basement-membrane-type collagen. The uniqueness of AFCs is further highlighted by the fact that a single fluid specimen contains a variety of cell types, many of which presumably represent different cell lineages and various states of differentiation. Apparent differences in gene expression between such isogenic cultures can therefore safely be ascribed to developmental differentiation rather than genotypic variation. Laboratories handling AFCs for diagnostic purposes should be aware of the potential value of these materials for cell biologic investigations.[67, 87–91]

CELL CULTURE AND CELL HARVEST

Colony-Forming Cells

The total number of cells per milliliter of amniotic fluid increases with gestational age. Elejalde et al.[4] determined this number to be 9,000 cells/mL of fluid at 9 weeks, 100,000 cells/mL at 13 weeks, and more than 200,000 cells/mL of fluid at 16 weeks of gestation. Although the total number of nucleated cells per milliliter thus varies between 10^3 and more than 10^6, the number of colony-forming cells is much lower. Figure 4.6 shows that in platings of 16- to 18-week fluids, an average of 3.5 clones/mL are typically scored at day 12 after the initial plating. However, only 1.5 colonies/mL reach a clone size of at least 10^6 cells (corresponding to approximately 20 cumulative population doublings). Other laboratories report very similar values (e.g., Richkind and Risch[92]). In a series of 14- to 16-week amniocentesis specimens, Hoehn et al.[93] observed only 3.1 colonies/mL, but most were large colonies at day 12 after seeding. Kennerknecht et al.[94] reported surprisingly high clone counts in 7- to 9-week amniotic fluid (ranging from 7.9 to 12.2 colonies/mL), but the overall growth performance of these very early AFCs was not on a par with cells from later stages. Very late pregnancy fluids (weeks 24 to 32) show a significant decline in cloning efficiency, to less than 1.5 colonies/mL.

It is frequently asked how many cells should be placed in the standard 25 cm^2 flask and whether native fluids can be used without prior centrifugation. Because the cellular content of a given fluid sample is so highly variable, cell counts at the time of inoculation are not helpful. In a series of tests, Seguin and Palmer[95] determined that between 0.8 and 2.5 mL of uncentrifuged fluid per flask is optimal. Because human AF contains traces

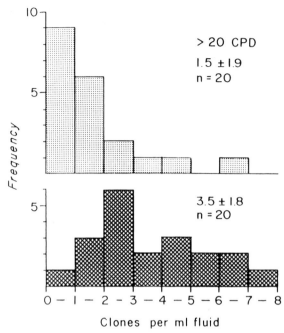

Fig. 4.6. Cloning efficiency of 20 consecutive amniotic fluid specimens (18 weeks of gestational age). Note that less than half of the colonies grow to more than 10^6 cells per clone (more than 20 cumulative population doublings).

of growth and attachment factors such as epidermal growth factor, interleukin-1, tumor necrosis factor alpha, fibronectin, and endothelin-1,[96] a 1:1 mixture of native fluid and growth medium has been recommended.[97] One should be aware, though, that cell growth inhibitors (e.g., IGFBP-1, an insulinlike growth factor binding protein) have also been found in human amniotic fluid.[98] The first feeding is recommended 3–4 days after the initiation of the culture. Although the proportion of erythrocytes may vary from 10^3 to 10^8 cells/mL, only the most severe blood contamination significantly retards or prevents cell growth. Such specimens can be treated with a brief exposure to 0.7 percent sodium citrate hypotonic solution before cell culture. For heavily blood-contaminated samples, a Ficoll–Hypaque fractionation procedure is an alternative to red blood cell lysis.[99,100]

Culture Techniques

The principle methodological difference between the flask and the in situ methods resides in the trypsinization step required for a suspension-type harvest. With the flask method, hypotonic and fixation steps are performed by repeated centrifugation and resuspension of the cell pellet in the appropriate solution. After two to three final changes of fixative (methanol:acetic acid, 3:1), aliquots of the cell pellet are taken up by the tip of a Pasteur pipette and dropped on precleaned glass slides. Regardless of whether primary cultures or subcultures are harvested by trypsinization, the resulting metaphase spreads can no longer be traced back to an individual parental colony. Some laboratories have used an intermediate form of cell harvest in which flask cultures are vigorously shaken or only briefly trypsinized to remove the loosely adherent mitotic cells. The remainder of the culture is then supplemented with fresh medium and can be reused for additional harvests.

When large numbers of cells are required for biochemical or molecular diagnostic studies, culture in T25 flasks remains the method of choice.

In Situ Procedure

Since the early 1980s, in situ culture and harvest has become the preferred method for cytogenetic studies (e.g., Chang et al.,[101] Schmid et al.,[102] Hoehn et al.,[103] Boue et al.,[104] Hecht et al.,[105] Tabor et al.[106]). The main advantages perceived by these laboratories are: (1) earlier culture harvest leading to a more speedy diagnosis (see below), (2) clonal (or, more correctly, colony) analysis leading to an easier distinction between genuine mosaicism and pseudomosaicism, and (3) recognition of maternal cell contamination on the basis of clonal morphology.

Maternal cell contamination (MCC) has been reported to occur in 0.15 to 0.54 percent of AFC cultures.[107–109] To minimize MCC, some laboratories prefer to discard the first 2 mL of amniotic fluid. PCR-detectable MCC of amniotic fluid samples has been reported to be common (4–17 percent of samples), and probably represents contamination by maternal blood. This contamination can be an important consideration for biochemical or molecular genetic studies.[110,111] However, our local experience is that none of 66 direct amniotic fluid samples has exhibited VNTR-detectable MCC (Monaghan K, Henry Ford Hospital, Detroit, MI, personal communication, May 16, 2003). This is consistent with the 0.5 percent rate of MCC in amniotic fluid cell cultures identified by PCR analysis by Smith et al.[112] This is also consistent with our local experience of finding MCC in 21 of 5108 (0.41 percent) consecutive amniotic fluid cell karyotype studies (i.e., one or two 46,XX colonies among 15 or more 46,XY colonies in the in situ harvests). Fortunately, MCC rarely confounds the interpretation of the laboratory results.

Guidelines and tables are now available concerning the number of metaphases to analyze by either suspension or in situ harvests to exclude mosaicism at a desired confidence level.[92,113–116] A deficit of these calculations is that they ignore the artifactual loss of chromosomes, which is more frequent with suspension than with in situ preparations. The influence of environmental conditions (e.g., relative humidity and temperature) during drying of chromosome spreads can influence chromosome spreading, and preparation aneuploidy has been well documented.[117,118] To search for mosaicism, the number of colonies sampled clearly is more informative than the number of metaphases analyzed,[119,120] but whether the gold standard should be a 15-colony analysis is the subject of some debate.[121,122]

Even though the in situ method has clear advantages over the flask method, it is more technically demanding. Laboratories using the in situ technique in conjunction with optimal culture media (e.g., Chang or AmnioMAX from Irvine Scientific or GIBCO, respectively) are able to karyotype most specimens in less than two weeks. Longer time intervals result from suboptimal cell growth conditions, adherence to a 5-day work week, or from other administrative rather than biological limitations. Many laboratories also employ a robotic harvesting system and an environmental control chamber to improve the number and quality of metaphase cells.[117,123,124]

Prototype Protocol

A prototype protocol[124] for in situ chromosome preparations employs Chang or AmnioMAX media and sterilized 22 mm^2 coverslips in sterile 35-mm Petri dishes. The laboratory is provided two or three transport tubes of amniotic fluid with patient identifiers, and if possible, numbered in sequence to indicate the first amniotic fluid aliquot, second, and so on. Complete media (2–3 mL) is mixed with AFCs suspended in 0.5 mL of amniotic fluid. This mixture is used to initiate two or three coverslip cultures, using surface tension to limit the cell suspension to the top of the coverslip. Each dish is labeled with patient identifiers and the number of the original amniotic fluid tube. Cultures are split among two or three incubators. After 12–24 hr of incubation, 1–1.5 mL of media are added to each culture, taking care not to disturb cells that have attached to the coverslip. The medium is replenished on day 3–5 of culture. When three or more light colonies have proliferated to 40–65 cells per colony, the culture is ready to harvest. Detailed records of the entire process are maintained.

Harvest methods including Colcemid and other pretreatments, slide-drying, and G-banding vary widely among laboratories and must be perfected locally. In our laboratory, preparation for harvest includes the addition of 50 μL ethidium bromide for 50 min and 10 μL Colcemid for an additional 30 min. Cells are gently exposed to hypotonic solution and then fixative. The coverslip is dried in a controlled way to optimize chromosome spreading, G-banded, and mounted on a microscope slide for karyotype analysis. Whenever possible, karyotype analysis includes metaphase cells from multiple culture vessels initiated from more than one original transport tube.

Automated harvesting for in situ chromosome analysis has been reported using a Tecan robotic sample processor. This instrument can process up to 104 Petri dishes with coverslips or 79 chamber slides in a single run.[125] The robotic harvesting equipment saves personnel time and improves consistency because the timing, rate, and quantity of aspiration and dispensing of media, hypotonic solution, and fixative are automated.

An environmental room or chamber that controls temperature, humidity, and airflow is helpful both to optimize the quality of the metaphase spreading and to reduce seasonal variations in harvest quality. The system must be optimized in each laboratory, but will probably provide high-quality preparations in the range of 50 percent relative humidity at 25°C.[117]

Cell Cycle Synchronization

Most indications for prenatal cytogenetic diagnosis do not call for high-resolution chromosome banding. If a high proportion of prometaphase spreads is required, the AFC cultures can be synchronized by adding either thymidine or 5-bromodeoxycytidine for 30 hr starting at 24 hr after the subcultivation of primary clones. After the removal of the blocking agent and addition of a low concentration of thymidine, the cultures are incubated for another 6.5–7 hr and then harvested without the use of Colcemid. This technique has been shown to yield a mitotic index between 3 and 4 percent, and at least half of the mitotic figures are in the desired prometaphase stage.[126] Other protocols recommend brief exposures to ethidium bromide or exposure to a mixture of agents including bromodeoxyuridine and Colcemid.[123,127–130]

ENHANCEMENT OF AMNIOTIC FLUID CELL GROWTH

Enrichment Techniques

Because so few cells in the fluid specimen are viable in the sense of cloning, it would be advantageous to increase the number of viable cells introduced into the cell cultures. Two studies have examined whether maternal activity and/or uterine agitation before amniocentesis affect the concentration of viable amniocytes in the fluid.[131,132] After correcting for gestational age, both studies were negative. Enrichment of the cell culture inoculums has been attempted via centrifugation of fluids through isopyknic gradients, both on microscale[133] and on macroscale.[100] With bloody specimens, these methods might be of some help, but they appear to be impractical for routine use. This limitation also holds for an enrichment technique by which the AF is returned to the fetus after aspiration, filtration, and reinjection of amniotic fluid as early as 12.5 gestational weeks.[134–137]

Growth on Extracellular Matrix Surface

The culture surface has a definite influence on the rate of attachment and proliferation. To attach to the culture surface, AFCs must create their own microenvironment, consisting of glycoproteins, collagen, laminin, and fibronectin, among others (extracellular matrix proteins). Fetal bovine serum contains fibronectin, and so does human AF at 15–18 weeks of gestation.[138] If serum concentrations of less than 10 percent are used (such as in Chang-type media supplements), the presence of AF in the culture setup might facilitate the coating of fibronectin on plastic surfaces. In a study by Chang and Jones,[97] optimal cloning and growth was observed when cultures were started with equal parts of AF and growth factor supplemented medium (including 4 percent fetal bovine serum). Two other studies have shown that the precoating of the usual plastic surfaces with extracellular matrix (ECM) improves both cloning and the rate of growth of AFCs.[139,140] In both laboratories, ECM-coated dishes were custom-made from bovine corneal endothelial cells. The use of such precoated surfaces may be advantageous for cell attachment and cloning if suboptimal media must be used. It appears impractical for routine use unless the laboratory is prepared to accept the extra expense involved in purchasing precoated dishes. A number of manufacturers offer such "biological" plasticware.

Reduction of Oxygen Supply

Other efforts directed at improving the cellular microenvironment take into account that the usual atmospheric oxygen conditions are not optimal for most mammalian cells in culture. Brackertz et al.[141] and Held and Soennichsen[142] provide convincing evidence for the improvement of AFC growth under hypoxic cell culture conditions. Because the effects of reduced oxygen are most distinctive among sparse cell populations, primary AFC cultures are likely to benefit most from hypoxia. A number of manufacturers now offer incubators that can be used with multiple gases. It is not very expensive to hook these up to a nitrogen tank to maintain a 3–5 percent (v/v) oxygen atmosphere. The cells do thrive. If such sophisticated incubators are opened frequently, however, their humidity tends to decrease, which might be a disadvantage for cells growing in open dishes.

Testing and Handling Fetal Bovine Serum

The single most important factor in determining the speed and success of prenatal cytogenetic diagnosis is the quality of the growth medium and its supplements.[36,97] Because the traditional medium supplement, fetal bovine serum, represents a complex mixture of growth-promoting substances, considerable effort has been directed toward formulating serum-free media in mammalian cell culture.[143] Human AFC culture has benefited greatly from the success of these efforts.[144,145] A milestone in AFC culture was the introduction of growth-factor-supplemented media by Chang and co-workers.[146,147]

Fetal bovine serum or Chang-type media, which includes serum, requires proper storage and handling to preserve its effectiveness. Freeze–thaw cycles and exposure to light are particular problems.[148] Proper handling includes:

1. Immediate transfer of serum to a $-20°C$ or colder freezer on delivery to the laboratory. Do not store serum in a frost-free freezer.
2. To thaw serum, place the bottle on a towel at room temperature for 30 min, then transfer to a 37°C water bath. As the serum thaws, agitate it periodically to mix the solutes. Once thawed, remove from the water bath.
3. Agitate the serum to mix the solutes well before heat inactivation or transferring to cell culture media.
4. Do not repeatedly freeze and thaw serum.
5. Shake and supercool serum so it refreezes rapidly.
6. Protect serum from exposure to light.

Defined Growth Factor Supplements

The commercial versions of the growth-factor-supplemented media are based on the formulation provided by Chang et al.[146,147] The classic "Chang medium" includes transferrin; selenium, insulin, triiodothyronine, glucagon, fibroblast growth factor, hydrocortisone, testosterone, estradiol, and progesterone. These factors are added to a 1:1 mixture of Dulbecco's modified Eagles' medium (DMEM) and Ham's F12 medium plus sodium bicarbonate, small amounts of HEPES buffer, and antibiotics. Chang et al. pointed out that their preferred basic medium mixture can be replaced by a number of other formulas (e.g., Ham's F10 or F12, Coon's modified Ham's F12, McCoy's 5A, RPMI 1640, DMEM, minimal essential medium, and TC 199) without detriment. Chang and AmnioMAX media, which differ in their buffering systems, are available for use in closed and open cell culture systems. As with other aspects of the cell culture art and science, local preferences vary with respect to choice of specialized media, fetal or newborn bovine serum, and whether to mix these media with less costly media.[101,123,124,147,149]

It is assumed that the various peptides, hormones, and trace elements act synergistically on the recruitment of cells into the cycle and keep them from reverting to the G0 stage after completed division. A greater number of cells within a colony will therefore stay in the proliferative pool. The cycle time of individual cells, with the possible exception of the duration of the G1 phase, is not likely to change. Unless Claussen's micropipette method[150] is used, a culture period of 5–7 days will thus remain the absolute minimum time requirement for prenatal cytogenetic diagnosis employing AFC cultures. In our laboratory, we have experimented with 12 hr Colcemid exposure and very early harvests. We obtained a small number of metaphase cells after 3 and even 2 days in cell culture, but the number of metaphases has not been sufficient for a complete analysis.

In view of the bothersome inconsistency of commercial Chang-type serum quality, most laboratories have switched to the routine use of culture medium supplements, with generally favorable results.[101,151] A typical early experience is that of Salk et al.,[152] who recorded growth failure for only 0.33 percent of 1,221 fluids set up in Chang media, whereas 1.53 percent of 4,758 cultures without growth supplements failed to grow. Average time from setup to signout was reduced from 20.3 to 12.8 days, and there was a significant improvement of the cloning efficiency in primary cultures. For most laboratories today, the growth failure rate ranges close to 0.2 percent, and probably 95 percent of reports are completed in 6–14 days, with a mean of 8–11 days to the final report.

Apart from the expense, a drawback noted by some users of Chang and AmnioMAX media is their limited shelf life. Lyophilized or other, more stable media supplements are offered by some manufacturers (e.g., Condimed, UltroSer), but cloning efficiency testing so far has failed to identify a commercial product that consistently yields higher cloning efficiencies than fresh lots of Chang media.[93] Use of Chang-type media may augment the incidence of chromosome breakage and chromosomal mosaicism in AFC cultures, but rarely to the extent that the cytogenetic interpretation is compromised.[152–155] This may result in part from the fact that Chang media can facilitate the growth of E-type colonies, and these colonies yield higher rates of (nonconstitutional) chromosome changes.[48,103] However, the advantages gained by the reduction of turnaround time and the substantial decrease of culture failures using Chang-type media appear to outweigh the potential drawbacks of increased chromosomal breakage and pseudomosaicism.

CULTURE FAILURE

In most laboratories, the rate of culture failure is below 1 percent, depending somewhat on the timing of the amniocentesis,[156] and in many laboratories it averages closer to 0.1 percent (Van Dyke D.L., unpublished data). There are multiple reasons for cell culture problems and outright failure.[157] With the increased experience of the obstetrician and the universal use of high-resolution ultrasonic equipment, maternal urine is now rarely received as a disguised amniotic fluid sample. Anecdotal evidence from some labs suggests that the risk of culture failure is higher in cases of fetal aneuploidy. In one published retrospective study, 56 (0.7 percent) of 7,872 amniotic fluid samples did not grow.[158] Twenty-four of these were judged technically inadequate and 10 were from women whose fetuses had died. Of the remaining 32 cases, 4 had proven (determined by repeat amniocentesis) and 4 had possible (extrapolated from fetal phenotype) aneuploidies. This 25 percent rate of growth failure associated with proven or likely chromosomal aberrations was not confirmed in a similar study comprising 6,369 cases and a growth failure rate of 1.2 percent.[159] A more recent study of 14,615 cases identified a higher incidence of culture failure in advanced pregnancies with abnormal ultrasound findings, but no association with aneuploidy.[160] In addition to a baseline level of less than 1 percent unexplained culture failure (the standard set by the American College of Medical Genetics is 2 percent),[115,116] a number of known hazards can interfere with cell growth.

Syringe Toxicity and Delayed Transportation

One serious hazard is the transmittal of fluid in toxic syringes or tubes.[161,162] Amniotic fluid samples should not be transported in syringes; rather, the fluid should always be promptly transferred and transported in conical centrifuge tubes with plastic caps, spinal tap tubes, or similar specimen transport containers. Rubber capped tubes and stoppered syringes should not be used as storage or transport containers for amniotic fluid. Recent problems reported in the United States prompted Becton, Dickinson to recommend minimizing both the residence time of amniotic fluid in the syringe and contact with the stopper attached to the plunger rod.[163]

Although it is advisable to deliver amniotic fluid samples to the laboratory without delay, in our experience with amniotic fluid specimens transported by courier and various delivery services, cell viability is maintained for at least five days assuming the sample is not exposed to extreme temperatures. There is one report of two successful cell cultures after unfortunate delays of 16 and 18 days.[164]

Contamination

Microbial contamination is a rare cause of culture failure in experienced laboratories and is by and large preventable.[165] (The AF itself has bactericidal properties, and there is no compelling reason for fluids to be pelleted before culturing.) The centrifugation step means additional hazard, and the protection provided by the supernatant is lost. If overwhelming microbial contamination is apparent within 24 hr after setup, it is probably caused by careless handling of the specimen between amniocentesis and delivery to the laboratory (e.g., leakage from loose screw caps or poorly packaged syringes).

Approximately 10–20 percent of all samples are cell-rich, and their turbidity creates considerable anxiety with regard to possible contamination. This also holds for brownish fluids containing cellular debris and granules in addition to erythrocytes. Seguin and Palmer[95] measured cell growth from clear, cloudy (cell-rich), bloody, and dark brown fluids. They showed that cloudy fluids yield better growth than clear ones. They confirm earlier observations[166] that very bloody fluids adversely affect the cloning efficiency. If bacterial or yeast contamination arises during the course of cell culture, it is by no means hopeless to attempt to salvage such cultures. Penicillin-, streptomycin-, or fungicide-supplemented media are used to feed cultures daily after initial frequent washings. Increased chromosomal breakage rates and elevated rates of pseudomosaicism may be observed in such salvaged cultures, but if the metaphase cells are analyzable, this rarely interferes with interpretation of the results.

Mycoplasma

Contrary to widespread belief, mycoplasma is not a significant problem in AFC culture. This is mainly due to better quality control by the serum manufacturers but also to the awareness of cell culturists that amniotic fluid cell cultures should never share incubator space with any established cell lines. Likewise, a shared water bath used for heating media and trypsin can be a source of mycoplasma contamination, since permanent cell lines, frequently shipped from laboratory to laboratory, remain the prevailing source of mycoplasma contamination. As additional protection, many laboratories heat-inactivate their sera before use (a 100-mL bottle thawed to room temperature is placed in a 56°C water bath for precisely 30 minutes). Commercial test kits are available for the detection of mycoplasma infections in cell cultures.[167]

Plasticware and Media Storage

There are occasional batches of cell-culture-grade plastic that do not, or barely, support cell attachment and growth. As with any component of the cell culture system, it is advisable to test new and old plasticware in parallel for toxicity and ability to support growth in vitro. It is important that there be immediate feedback to suppliers and manufacturers about such events. It seems prudent for a prenatal diagnosis laboratory to have at least two brands of culture containers on hand. Hoehn's laboratory has switched several times between Corning and Falcon and has tested additional brands because of considerable fluctuations in quality.[93] Single-chamber slides, which used to be plagued by leakage at 8–10 days of culture, have been improved and can be used for in situ harvests in lieu of flask or coverslip cultures.[106] They have remained expensive. With the advent of growth factor supplements, poor media or sera are rarely a cause of growth failure. The medium component most sensitive to degradation during storage (even at 4°C) is glutamine.

Incubator Failure

Incubator failure is not a trivial cause of culture loss. There are two main threats: one is breakdown of the gas supply or equipment. Values of pH close to or higher than 8 are not withstood by AFCs for more than 6–8 hr. On the other hand, a pH of less than 7.0 (for example, due to excess CO_2 in the incubator) causes cells to stop dividing. A second danger is the overheating of incubators caused by mechanical failure or human error. Connection of incubators to emergency power sources is important. Temperature- and gas-sensitive alarm systems are advisable.

Record Keeping and Quality Control

With the advent of highly standardized, commercially perfected cell culture technology, culture hazards have become a much rarer cause for concern in the prenatal diagnosis laboratory. Because of the greater number of specimens processed by the average laboratory, a variety of quality control measures need to be followed to avoid mistakes ranging from embarrassing culture mix-ups to catastrophic diagnostic errors. The most common and potentially serious laboratory errors are human errors in labeling and cross contamination of samples. Labeling errors can occur at any stage at which cells are transferred between vessels: in the amniocentesis procedure room, at culture initiation, during feeding and subculture, at harvest, during slide making, and even during microscope analysis. Cross contamination of cells between patient samples is most common at the time of cell culture harvest, especially for suspension harvests. For these reasons, quality control and quality assurance programs must include a nonpunitive recording system for all laboratory errors. In addition, a regular review of those errors should be performed to seek patterns of error that can be eliminated by the continuing education of laboratory staff or (often more effective) process improvement directed at reducing the opportunity for human error.

Laboratory directors and supervisors should be familiar with the College of American Pathologists Laboratory General and Cytogenetics checklists and the American College of Medical Genetics Standards and Guidelines.[115,116,168] Laboratories should also participate in a peer-review system such as the CAP Surveys for clinical cytogenetics and FISH.[169]

Safety in the Laboratory

It is the responsibility of the laboratory director and all of the laboratory staff to protect the rights, privacy, and health of employees, ancillary staff, and patients alike. In these times of acquired immunodeficiency syndrome (AIDS) and hepatitis C, amniotic fluid specimens and all cultures up to the stage of fixation should be treated as potentially hazardous. Universal precautions are essential. Available resources include the CAP Safety Checklist and excellent reviews of laboratory safety and management.[168,170–172]

ACKNOWLEDGMENT

I am indebted to Aubrey Milunsky, M.D., D.Sc., and Holger Hoehn, M.D., for having written this chapter in the previous editions of this book.

REFERENCES

1. Milunsky A. The prenatal diagnosis of hereditary disorders. Springfield: Thomas, 1973.
2. Milunsky A. Amniotic fluid cell culture. In: Milunsky A, ed. Genetic disorders and the fetus. New York: Plenum Press, 1979:75.

3. Wald NJ, Rodeck C, Hackshaw AK, et al. First and second trimester antenatal screening for Down's syndrome: the results of the serum, urine, and ultrasound screening study (SURUSS). Health Technol Assess 2003;7:1.
4. Elejalde BR, de Elejalde MM, Acuna JM, et al. Prospective study of amniocentesis performed between weeks 9 and 16 of gestation: its feasibility, risks, complications and use in early genetic prenatal diagnosis. Am J Med Genet 1990;35:188.
5. Daniel A, Ng A, Kuah KB, et al.. A study of early amniocentesis of prenatal cytogenetic diagnosis. Prenat Diagn 1998;18:21.
6. Lapidot-Lifson Y, Lebo RV, Flandermeyer MA, et al. Rapid aneuploid diagnosis of high-risk fetuses by fluorescence in situ hybridization. Am J Obstet Gynecol 1996;174:886.
7. D'Alton ME, Malone FD, Chelmow D, et al. Defining the role of fluorescence in situ hybridization on uncultured amniocytes for prenatal diagnosis of aneuploidies. Am J Obstet Gynecol 1997;176:769.
8. Kuo WL, Tenjin H, Segraves R, et al. Detection of aneuploidy involving chromosomes 13, 18 or 21 by fluorescence in situ hybridization (FISH) to interphase and metaphase amniocytes. Am J Hum Genet 1991;49:112.
9. Ried TH, Landes G, Dackowski W, et al. Multicolor fluorescence in situ hybridization for the simultaneous detection of probe sets for chromosomes 13, 18, 21, X and Y in uncultured amniotic fluid cells. Hum Mol Genet 1992;1:307.
10. Klinger K, Landes G, Shook D, et al. Rapid detection of chromosome aneuploidies in uncultured amniocytes by using fluorescence in situ hybridization (FISH). Am J Hum Genet 1992;51:55.
11. Ward BE, Gersen SL, Carelli MP, et al. Rapid prenatal diagnosis of chromosomal aneuploidies by fluorescence in situ hybridization: clinical experience with 4,500 specimens. Am J Hum Genet 1993;52:854.
12. Divane A, Carter NP, Spathas DH, et al. Rapid prenatal diagnosis of aneuploidy from uncultured amniotic fluid cells using five-colour fluorescence in situ hybridization. Prenat Diagn 1994;14:1061.
13. Gersen SL, Carelli MP, Klinger KW, et al. Rapid prenatal diagnosis of 14 cases of triploidy using FISH with multiple probes. Prenat Diagn 1995;15:1.
14. Evans MI, Henry GP, Miller WA, et al. International, collaborative assessment of 146,000 prenatal karyotypes: expected limitations if only chromosome-specific probes and fluorescent in-situ hybridization are used. Hum Reprod 1999;14:1213.
15. Feldman B, Ebrahim SA, Hazan SL, et al. Routine prenatal diagnosis of aneuploidy by FISH studies in high-risk pregnancies. Am J Med Genet 2000;90:233.
16. Verma L, Macdonald F, Leedham P, et al. Rapid and simple prenatal DNA diagnosis of Down's syndrome. Lancet 1998;352:9.
17. Pertl B, Kopp S, Kroisel PM, et al. Rapid detection of chromosome aneuploidies by quantitative fluorescence PCR: first application on 247 chorionic villus samples. J Med Genet 1999;36:300.
18. Veltman JA, Schoenmakers EFPM, Eussen BH, et al. High-throughput analysis of subtelomeric chromosome rearrangements by use of array-based comparative genomic hybridization. Am J Hum Genet 2002;70:1269.
19. Brambati B, Tului L. Prenatal genetic diagnosis through chorionic villus sampling. Chapter 5 in Milunsky A, ed., Genetic disorders and the fetus, 5th ed. Baltimore: Johns Hopkins University Press, 2004:179.
20. Donnenfeld AE, Lockwood D, Custer T, Lamb AN. Prenatal diagnosis from fetal urine in bladder outlet obstruction: success rates for traditional cytogenetic evaluation and interphase fluorescence in situ hybridization. Genet Med 2002;4:444.
21. Ville YG, Nicolaides KH, Campbell S. Prenatal diagnosis of fetal malformations by ultrasound. Chapter 23 in Milunsky A, ed., Genetic disorders and the fetus, 5th ed. Baltimore: Johns Hopkins University Press, 2004:900.
22. Golden WL, Schneider BF, Gustashaw KM, Jassani MN. Prenatal diagnosis of Turner syndrome using cells cultured from cystic hygromas in two pregnancies with normal maternal serum alpha-fetoprotein. Prenat Diagn 1989;9:683.
23. Wax JR, Blakemore KJ, Soloski MJ, et al. Fetal ascitic fluid: a new source of lymphocytes for rapid chromosomal analysis. Obstet Gynecol 1992;80:533.
24. Costa D, Borrell A, Margarit E, et al. Rapid fetal karyotype from cystic hygroma and pleural effusions. Prenat Diagn 1995;15:141.
25. Cruger DG, Bruun-Petersen G, Kolvraa D. Early prenatal diagnosis: standard cytogenetic analysis of coelomic cells obtained by coelocentesis. Prenat Diagn 1996;16:945.
26. Holbrook KA, Odland GF. The fine structure of developing epidermis: light, scanning, and transmission electron microscopy of the periderm. J Invest Dermatol 1975;65:16.
27. Holbrook KA, Odland GF. Regional development of the human epidermis in the first trimester embryo and

the second trimester fetus (ages related to the timing of amniocentesis and fetal biopsy). J Invest Dermatol 1980;80:161.

28. Tyden O, Bergstrom S, Nilsson BA. Origin of amniotic fluid cells in mid-trimester pregnancies. Br J Obstet Gynaecol 1981;88:278.

29. Gosden CM, Brock DJH. Morphology of rapidly adhering amniotic fluid cells as an aid to the diagnosis of neural tube defects. Lancet 1977;1:919.

30. Huisjes HJ. Cytology of the amniotic fluid and its clinical applications. In: Fairweather DVI, Eskes TKA, eds. Amniotic fluid research and clinical applications, 2nd ed. Amsterdam: Elsevier/North Holland, 1978:93.

31. Bergstrom S. Ultrastructure of cell detachment from the human fetus in early pregnancy. Acta Obstet Gynecol Scand 1980;59:169.

32. Tyden O, Bergstroem S, Nilsson BA. Origin of amniotic fluid cells in mid-trimester pregnancies. Br J Obstet Gynaecol 1981;88:278.

33. Schrage R, Buegelspacher HR, Wurster KG. Amniotic fluid cells in the second trimester of pregnancy. Acta Cytol 1982;26:407.

34. Agorastos T, Grussendorf EI, Weiss XX, et al. Zur Feinmorphologie der Fruchtwasserzellen. Z Gebursthilfe Perinatol 1982;186:41.

35. Hoehn H, Bryant EM, Karp LE, et al. Cultivated cells from diagnostic amniocentesis in second trimester pregnancies. I. Clonal morphology and growth potential. Pediatr Res 1974;8:746.

36. Felix JS, Doherty RA, Davis HT, et al. Amniotic fluid cell culture. I. Experimental design for evaluating cell culture variables: determination of optimal fetal calf serum concentration. Pediatr Res 1974;8:870.

37. Polgar K, Adnay R, Abel G, et al. Characterization of rapidly adhering amniotic fluid cells by combined immunofluorescence and phagocytosis assays. Am J Hum Genet 1989;45:786–792.

38. Greenebaum E, Mansukhani MM, Heller DS, et al. Open neural tube defects: immunocytochemical demonstration of neuro-epithelial cells in amniotic fluid. Diagn Cytopathol 1997;16:143.

39. Medina-Gomez P, McBride WH. Amniotic fluid macrophages from normal and malformed fetuses. Prenat Diagn 1986;6:195.

40. Roberts SH, Little E, Vaughan M, et al. Rapid prenatal diagnosis of Patau's syndrome in a fetus with an abdominal wall defect by 72 hour culture of cells from amniotic fluid. Prenat Diagn 1993;13:971.

41. Gosden CM, Brock DJH. Amniotic fluid cell morphology in early prenatal prediction of abortion and low birth weight. BMJ 1978;2:1186.

42. Gosden CM. Amniotic fluid cell types and culture. Br Med Bull 1983;39:348.

43. Osborn M, Weber K. Biology of disease: tumor diagnosis by intermediate filament typing: a novel tool for surgical pathology. Lab Invest 1983;48:372.

44. Franke WW, Appelhans B, Schmid E, et al. Identification and characterization of epithelial cells in mammalian tissues by immunofluorescence microscopy using antibodies to prekeratin. Differentiation 1979;15:7.

45. Melancon SB, Lee SY, Nadler HL. Histidase activity in cultivated human amniotic fluid cell cultures. Science 1971;173:627.

46. Gerbie AB, Melancon SB, Ryan C, et al. Cultivated epithelial-like cells and fibroblasts from amniotic fluid: their relationship to enzymatic and cytologic analysis. Am J Obstet Gynecol 1972;114:314.

47. Sutherland GR, Bauld R, Bain DJ. Observations on human amniotic fluid cell strains in serial culture. J Med Genet 1974;11:190.

48. Hoehn H, Bryant EM, Karp LE, et al. Cultivated cells from diagnostic amniocentesis in second trimester pregnancies. II. Cytogenetic parameters as functions of clonal type and preparative technique. Clin Genet 1975;7:29.

49. Priest RE, Priest JH, Laundon CH, et al. Multinucleate cells in cultures of human amniotic fluid form by fusion. Lab Invest 1980;43:140.

50. Megaw JW, Priest JH, Priest RE, et al. Differentiation in human amniotic fluid cell cultures. II. Secretion of epithelial basement membrane glycoprotein. J Med Genet 1977;14:163.

51. Priest RE, Priest JH, Moinuddin JF, et al. Differentiation in human amniotic fluid cell cultures. I. Collagen production. J Med Genet 1977;14:157.

52. Priest RE, Marimuthu KM, Priest JH. Origin of cells in amniotic fluid cultures: Ultrastructural features. Lab Invest 1978;39:106.

53. Priest RE, Priest JH, Moinhuddin JF, et al. Differentiation in human amniotic fluid cell cultures: Chorionic gonadotropin production. In Vitro 1979;15:142.

54. Thakar N, Priest RE, Priest JH. Estrogen production by cultured amniotic fluid cells. Clin Res 1982;30:888A.

55. O'Shannessy DJ, Priest RE, Priest JH. Metabolism of (4–14C) androstenedione by cells cultured from human amniotic fluid. J Steroid Biochem 1984;20:935.

56. Laundon CH, Priest JH, Priest RE. The characterization of hCG regulation in cultured human amniotic fluid cells. Prenat Diagn 1981;1:269.

57. Laundon CH, Priest JH, Priest RE. Characterization of hCG regulation in cultured human amniotic fluid cells. In Vitro 1983;19:911.

58. Virtanen I, von Koskull H, Lehto VP, et al. Cultured amniotic fluid cells characterized with antibodies against intermediate filaments in indirect immunofluorescence microscopy. J Clin Invest 1981;68:1348.

59. Cremer M, Treiss I, Cremer T, et al. Characterization of cells of amniotic fluids by immunological identification of intermediate-sized filaments: presence of cells of different tissue origins. Hum Genet 1981;59:373.

60. Ochs BA, Franke WW, Moll R, et al. Epithelial character and morphologic diversity of cell cultures from human amniotic fluids examined by immunofluorescence microscopy and gel electrophoresis of cytoskeletal proteins. Differentiation 1983;24:153.

61. Medina-Gomez P, Johnston TH. Cell morphology in long-term cultures of normal and abnormal amniotic fluids. Hum Genet 1982;60:310.

62. Chang HC, Jones OW. In vitro characteristics of human fetal cells obtained from chorionic villus sampling and amniocentesis. Prenat Diagn 1988;8:367.

63. Whitsett CF, Priest RE, Priest JH, et al. HLA typing of cultured amniotic fluid cells. Am J Clin Pathol 1983;79:186.

64. Crouch E, Bornstein P. Collagen synthesis by human amniotic fluid cells in culture: characterization of a procollagen with three identical pro alpha (I) chains. Biochemistry 1978;17:5495.

65. Crouch E, Bornstein P. Characterization of a type IV procollagen synthesized by human amniotic fluid cells in culture. J Biol Chem 1979;254:4197.

66. Crouch E, Balian G, Holbrook K, et al. Amniotic fluid fibronectin: characterization and synthesis by cells in culture. J Cell Biol 1978;78:701.

67. Bryant EM, Crouch E, Bornstein P, et al. Regulation of growth and gene activity in euploid hybrids between human neonatal fibroblasts and epithelioid amniotic fluid cells. Am J Hum Genet 1978;30:392.

68. Johnston P, Salk D, Martin GM, et al. Cultivated cells from mid-trimester amniotic fluids. IV. Cell type identification via one and two dimensional electrophoresis of clonal whole-cell homogenates. Prenat Diagn 1982;2:79.

69. Harrison H, Martin AO, Gemme MA, et al. Analysis of amniotic fluid supernatant and cellular proteins with high resolution two-dimensional electrophoresis. Am J Human Genet 1983;35:45A.

70. Hoehn H, Salk D. Morphological and biochemical heterogeneity of amniotic fluid cells in culture. Methods Cell Biol 1982;26:11.

71. Chen WW. Studies on the origin of human amniotic fluid cells by immunofluorescent staining of keratin filaments. J Med Genet 1982;19:433.

72. Moll R, Franke WW, Schiller DL, et al. The catalogue of human cytokeratins: patterns of expression in normal epithelia, tumors and cultured cells. Cell 1982;31:11.

73. Hay ED. Epithelial-mesenchymal transitions. Semin Dev Biol 1990;1:347.

74. Strutz F, Okada H, Lo CW, et al. Identification and characterization of a fibroblast marker: FSP1. J Cell Biol 1995;130:393.

75. Regauer S, Franke WW, Virtanen I. Intermediate filament cytoskeleton of amnion epithelium and cultured amnion epithelial cells: expression of epidermal cytokeratins in cells of a simple epithelium. J Cell Biol 1985;100:997.

76. Hsu LYF, Kaffe S, Perlis TE. A revisit of trisomy 20 mosaicism in prenatal diagnosis—an overview of 103 cases. Prenat Diagn 1991;11:7.

77. Bell JE, Barron L, Raab G. Antenatal detection of neural tube defects: comparison of biochemical and immunofluorescence methods. Prenat Diagn 1994;14:615.

78. Ven der Veer E, Kleijer WJ, de Josselin de Jong JE, et al. Lysosomal enzyme activities in different types of amniotic fluid cells measured by microchemical methods, combined with interference microscopy. Hum Genet 1978;40:285.

79. Burton BK, Gerbie AB, Nadler HL. Biochemical and biological problems and pitfalls of cell culture for prenatal diagnosis. In: Milunsky A, ed. Genetic disorders and the fetus. New York: Plenum Press, 1979:369.

80. Hoehn H, Bryant EM, Fantel AG, et al. Cultivated cells from diagnostic amniocentesis in second trimester pregnancies. III. The fetal urine as a potential source of clonable cells. Hum Genet 1975;29:285.

81. Chang HC, Jones OW. Amniocentesis: cell culture of human amniotic fluid in a hormone supplement. In:

Sato GH, Pardee AB, Sirbasku DA, eds. Growth of cells in hormonally defined media. Cold Spring Harbor, NY: Cold Spring Harbor Conferences on Cell Proliferation, 1982:1187.

82. Medina-Gomez P, Bard JBL. Analysis of normal and abnormal amniotic fluid cells in vitro by cinemicrography. Prenat Diagn 1983;3:311.

83. Harris A. Glycoproteins that distinguish different cell types in amniotic fluid. Hum Genet 1982;62:188.

84. Felix JS, Sun TT, Littlefield JW. Human epithelial cells cultured from urine: growth properties and keratin staining. In Vitro 1980;16:866.

85. Von Koskull H, Aula P, Trejdosiewicz LK, et al. Identification of cells from fetal bladder epithelium in human amniotic fluid. Hum Genet 1984;65:262.

86. Chitayat D, Marion RW, Squillante L, et al. Detection and enumeration of colonic mucosal cells in amniotic fluid using a colon epithelial-specific monoclonal antibody. Prenat Diagn 1990;10:725.

87. Darlington GJ. Applications of cell-fusion techniques to induce amniotic fluid cells to express special functions and for complementation analysis. Methods Cell Biol 1982;26:297.

88. Koch H, Bettecken T, Kubbies M, et al. Flow cytometric analysis of small DNA content differences in heterogeneous cell populations. Cytometry 1984;5:118.

89. Poot M, Esterbauer H, Rabinovitch PS, et al. Inhibition of cell proliferation by model compounds of lipid peroxidation contradicts causative role in cellular senescence. J Cell Physiol 1988;137:421.

90. Poot M, Kausch K, Koehler J, et al. The minor-groove binding DNA-ligands netropsin, distamycin A and berenil cause polyploidization via impairment of the G2 phase of the cell cycle. Cell Struct Funct 1990;15:151.

91. Eils R, Dietzel S, Bertin E, et al. Active and inactive X-chromosome territories in human female amniotic fluid cell nuclei can be differentiated by surface and shape but not by volume. J Cell Biol 1996;135:1427.

92. Richkind KE, Risch NJ. Sensitivity of chromosomal mosaicism detection by different tissue culture methods. Prenat Diagn 1990;10:519.

93. Hoehn HW. Fluid cell culture. In: Milunsky A, ed. Genetic disorders and the fetus, 4th ed. Baltimore: Johns Hopkins University Press, 1998;128.

94. Kennerknecht I, Baur-Aubele S, Grab D, et al. First trimester amniocentesis between the seventh and 13th weeks: evaluation of the earliest possible genetic diagnosis. Prenat Diagn 1992;12:595.

95. Seguin LR, Palmer CG. Variables influencing growth and morphology of colonies of cells from human amniotic fluid. Prenat Diagn 1983;3:107.

96. Casey ML, Word RA, MacDonald PC. Endothelin-I expression and regulation of endothelin mRNA and protein biosynthesis in vascular human amnion: potential source of amniotic fluid endothelin. J Biol Chem 1991;266:5762.

97. Chang HC, Jones OW. Reduction of sera requirements in amniotic fluid cell culture. Prenat Diagn 1985;5:305.

98. Liu L, Brinkman A, Blat C, et al. IGFBP-1, an insulin like growth factor binding protein, is a cell growth inhibitor. Biochem Biophys Res Commun 1991;174:673.

99. Gregson NM, Johnson M. Culture of bloody amniotic fluid for chromosome analysis: an improved method. J Med Genet 1980;17:388.

100. Chang HC, Jones OW, Bradshaw C, et al. Enhancement of human amniotic cell growth by Ficoll-paque gradient fractionation. In Vitro 1981;81.

101. Priest JH, Rao KW. Prenatal chromosome diagnosis. In: The AGT cytogenetics laboratory manual, 3rd ed. Philadelphia: Lippincott Williams & Wilkins, 1997:199.

102. Schmid W. A technique for in situ karyotyping of primary amniotic fluid cell cultures. Humangenetik 1975;30:325.

103. Hoehn H, Rodriguez ML, Norwood TH, et al. Mosaicism in amniotic fluid cell cultures: classification and significance. Am J Med Genet 1978;2:253.

104. Boue, J, Nicolas H, Barichard F, et al. Le clonage des cellules du liquide amniotique aide dans l'interpretation des mosaiques chromosomiques en diagnostic prenatal. Ann Genet 1979;22:3.

105. Hecht F, Peakman DC, Kaiser-McCaw B, et al. Amniocyte clones for prenatal cytogenetics. Am J Med Genet 1981;10:51.

106. Tabor A, Lind AM, Andersen AM, et al. A culture vessel for amniotic fluid cells allowing faster preparation of chromosome slides. Prenat Diagn 1984;4:451.

107. Benn PA, Hsu LYF. Maternal cell contamination of amniotic fluid cell cultures: results of a U.S. nationwide survey. Am J Med Genet 1983;15:297.

108. Bui TH, Iselius L, Lindsten J. European collaborative study on prenatal diagnosis: mosaicism, pseudomosaicism, and single abnormal cells in amniotic fluid cell cultures. Prenat Diagn 1984;4 (special issue):145.

109. Worton RG, Stern R. A Canadian collaborative study of mosaicism in amniotic fluid cell cultures. Prenat Diagn 1984;4 (special issue):131.
110. Batanian JR, Ledbetter DH, Fenwick RG. A simple VNTR-PCR method for detecting maternal cell contamination in prenatal diagnosis. Genet Test 1998;2:347.
111. Frederickson RM, Wang HS, Surh LC. Some caveats in PCR-based prenatal diagnosis on direct amniotic fluid versus cultured amniocytes. Prenat Diagn 1999;19:113.
112. Smith GW, Graham CA, Nevin J, Nevin NC. Detection of maternal cell contamination in amniotic fluid cell cultures using fluorescent labelled microsatellites. J Med Genet 1995;32:61.
113. Claussen U, Schäfer H, Trampisch H. Exclusion of chromosomal mosaicism in prenatal diagnosis. Hum Genet 1984;67:23.
114. Sikkema-Raddatz B, Castedo S, Te-Meerman GJ. Probability tables for exclusion of mosaicism in prenatal diagnosis. Prenat Diagn 1997;17:115.
115. Standards and guidelines for clinical genetics laboratories, 2nd ed. Bethesda, Md.: American College of Medical Genetics, 1999.
116. Standards and guidelines for clinical genetics laboratories, 3rd ed. http://www.acmg.net/Pages/ACMG_Activities/stds-2002/stdsmenu-n.htm (accessed on May 15, 2003).
117. Spurbeck JL, Zinsmeister AR, Meyer KJ, et al. Dynamics of chromosome spreading. Am J Med Genet 1996;61:387.
118. Henegariu O, Heerema NA, Wright LL, et al. Improvements in cytogenetic slide preparation: controlled chromosome spreading, chemical aging, and gradual denaturation. Cytometry 2001;43:101.
119. Cheung SW, Spitznagel E, Featherstone T, Crane JP. Exclusion of chromosomal mosaicism in amniotic fluid cultures: efficacy of in situ versus flask techniques. Prenat Diagn 1990;10:41.
120. Featherstone T, Cheung SW, Spitznagel E, et al. Exclusion of chromosomal mosaicism in amniotic fluid cultures: determination of number of colonies needed for accurate analysis. Prenat Diagn 1994;14:1009.
121. Cheng EY, Luthy DA, Dunne DF, et al. Is the 15-in situ clone protocol necessary to detect amniotic fluid mosaicism? Am J Obstet Gynecol 1995;173:1025.
122. Ing PS, Van Dyke DL, Caudill SP, et al. Detection of mosaicism in amniotic fluid cultures: a CYTO2000 collaborative study. Genet Med 1999;1:94.
123. Miron PM. Preparation, culture, and analysis of amniotic fluid samples. Curr Protocol Hum Genet 1994;8.4.1–8.4.17
124. Van Dyke DL, Roberson JR, Wiktor A. Prenatal Cytogenetic diagnosis. In: McClatchey KD, ed. Clinical laboratory medicine, 2nd ed. Philadelphia: Lippincott Williams & Wilkins, 2002:636.
125. Spurbeck JL, Carlson RO, Allen JE, et al. Culturing androbiotic harvesting of bone marrow, lymph nodes, peripheral blood, fibroblasts, and solid tumors with in situ techniques. Cancer Genet Cytogenet 1988;32:59.
126. Qu JY, Dallaire L, Lemieux N, et al. Synchronization of amniotic fluid cells for high resolution cytogenetics. Prenat Diagn 1989;9:49.
127. Hoo JJ, Jamro H, Schmutz S, et al. Preparation of high resolution chromosomes from amniotic fluid. Prenat Diagn 1983;3:265.
128. Shah JV, Verma RS, Rodriguez J, et al. Human chromosomes in prenatal diagnosis: a one step high resolution technique. Prenat Diagn 1983;3:253.
129. Cheung SW, Crane JP, Johnson A, et al. A simple method preparing prometaphase chromosomes from amniotic fluid cell cultures. Prenat Diagn 1987;7:383.
130. Spurbeck JL. Amniotic fluid harvest for high resolution: In situ using ethidium bromide. In: Burch M, ed. The ACT cytogenetics laboratory manual, 2nd ed. Houston: Raven Press, 1989:96–97.
131. Carlan SJ, Papenhausen P, O'Brien WF, et al. Effect of maternal–fetal movement on concentration of cells obtained at genetic amniocentesis. Am J Obstet Gynecol 1990;163:490.
132. Fisher RL, LaMotta J, McMorrow LE, et al. Effect of pre-amniocentesis uterine manipulation on amniocyte concentration and culture duration: a randomized, clinical trial. Prenat Diagn 1996;16:673.
133. Melnyk JH, Persinger G, Teplitz RLA. A micromethod for processing amniotic fluid cells. In Vitro 1979;15:200.
134. Byrne D, Marks K, Braude PR, et al. Amniofiltration in the first trimester feasibility, technical aspects and cytological outcome. Ultrasound Obstet Gynecol 1991;1:320.
135. Sundberg K, Smidt-Jensen S, Lundsteen C, et al. Filtration and recirculation of early amniotic fluid: Evaluation of cell cultures from 100 diagnostic cases. Prenat Diagn 1993;13:1101.
136. Sundberg K, Bang J, Brocks V, et al. Early sonographically guided amniocenteses with filtration technique: follow-up on 249 procedures. J Ultrasound Med 1995;14:585.

137. Sundberg K, Lundsteen C, Philip J. Early filtration amniocentesis for further investigation of mosaicism diagnosed by chorionic villus sampling. Prenat Diagn 1996;16:1121.
138. Kunsela P, Seppala M, Brock DJH, et al. Amniotic fluid fibronectin in normal pregnancy and in pregnancies with anencephalic fetus. Biomedicine 1978;29:296.
139. Vlodavsky I, Voss R, Yarkoni S, et al. Stimulation of human amniotic fluid cell proliferation and colony formation by cell plating on naturally produced extracellular matrix. Prenat Diagn 1982;2:13.
140. Crickard K, Golbus MS. Influence of extracellular matrix on the proliferation of human amniotic fluid cells in vitro. Prenat Diagn 1982;2:89.
141. Brackertz M, Kubbies M, Feige A, et al. Decreased oxygen supply enhances growth in culture of human mid-trimester amniotic fluid cells. Hum Genet 1983;64:334.
142. Held KR, Soennichsen S. The effect of oxygen tension on colony formation and cell proliferation of amniotic fluid cells. Prenat Diagn 1984;4:171.
143. Barnes D, Sato G. Serum free cell culture: a unifying approach. Cell 1980;8: 649.
144. Gospodarowicz D, Moran JS, Owashi ND. Effect of fibroblast growth factor and epidermal growth factor on the rate of growth of amniotic fluid-derived cells. J Clin Endocrinol Metab 1977;44:651.
145. Porreco RP, Bradshaw C, Sarkar S, et al. Enhanced growth of amniotic fluid cells in the presence of fibroblast growth factor. Obstet Gynecol 1980;55:55.
146. Chang HC, Jones OW. A new growth medium for human amniotic fluid cells. Karyogram 1981;7:54.
147. Chang HC, Jones OW, Masui H. Human amniotic fluid cells grown in a hormone-supplemented medium: Suitability for prenatal diagnosis. Proc Natl Acad Sci USA 1982;79:4795.
148. Freezing and thawing serum and other biological materials: optimal procedures minimize damage and maximize shelf-life. Art Sci Tissue Cult 1992;11:1–7. http://www.hyclone.com/pdf/ATSV11N2.PDF (accessed on May 15, 2003).
149. Biddle WC, Kuligowski S, Filby J, et al. AmnioMAX TM-C100: A new specialized cell culture medium for the propagation of human amniocytes. Focus 1992;14:3.
150. Claussen UJ. The pipette method: a new rapid technique for chromosome analysis in prenatal diagnosis. Hum Genet 1980;54:277.
151. Lawce H. Survey of amniotic fluid techniques. Karyogram 1986;12:47.
152. Salk D, Disteche C, Stenchever MR, et al. Routine use of Chang medium for prenatal diagnosis: improved growth and increased chromosomal breakage. Am J Hum Genet 1983;35:151A.
153. Masia A, Jenkins EC, Duncan C, et al. Chromosomal abnormalities in cultures with Chang medium. Am J Hum Genet 1986;39:260.
154. Krawczun MS, Jenkins EC, Masia A, et al. Chromosomal abnormalities in amniotic fluid cell cultures: a comparison of apparent pseudomosaicism in Chang and RPMI-1640 media. Clin Genet 1989;35:139.
155. Eiben B, Goebel R, Hansen S, et al. Early amniocentesis: a cytogenetic evaluation of over 1500 cases. Prenat Diagn 1994;14:497.
156. Assel BG, Lewis SM, Dickerman LH, et al. Single-operator comparison of early and mid-second trimester amniocentesis. Obstet Gynecol 1992;79:940.
157. Ryan J. Corning guide for identifying and correcting common cell growth problems. http://www.corning.com/lifesciences/ (accessed on May 19, 2003).
158. Persutte WH, Lenke RR. Failure of amniotic-fluid-cell growth: Is it related to fetal aneuploidy? Lancet 1995;345:96.
159. Elejalde BR, De Elejalde MM, Soto A. Amniotic-fluid cell growth and fetal aneuploidy. Lancet 1995;345:924.
160. Lam YH, Tang MHY, Sin SY, Ghosh A. Clinical significance of amniotic-fluid-cell culture failure. Prenat Diagn 1998;18:343.
161. Milunsky A, Bender CS. Failure of amniotic fluid cell growth with toxic tubes. N Engl J Med 1979;301:47.
162. Kohn G. Failure of amniotic fluid cell culture due to syringe toxicity. Prenat Diagn 1981;1:233.
163. Current information regarding BD™ syringes and amniocentesis. http://www.bd.com/injection/amnio/ (accessed on May 15, 2003).
164. Chiesa J, Bureau JP. Nothing ventured, nothing gained. Prenat Diagn 1999;19:894.
165. Ryan, J. Understanding and managing cell culture contamination. http://www.corning.com/lifesciences/ (accessed on May 19, 2003).
166. Felix JS, Doherty RA. Amniotic fluid cell culture. II. Evaluation of a red cell lysis procedure for culture of cells from blood-contaminated amniotic fluid. Clin Genet 1979;15:215.
167. Johansson KE, Bolske G. Evaluation and practical aspects of the use of a commercial DNA probe for detection of mycoplasma infections in cell cultures. J Biochem Biophys Methods 1989;19:185.

168. Sarewitz SJ, ed. Laboratory Accreditation Checklists. http://www.cap.org/html/ftpdirectory/checklistftp.html (accessed on May 19, 2003).
169. Laboratory Improvement Surveys/EXCEL. http://www.cap.org/html/lip/surveys.html (accessed on May 19, 2003).
170. Knutsen T. Laboratory safety, quality control, and regulations. In: The AGT cytogenetics laboratory manual, 3rd ed. Philadelphia: Lippincott Williams & Wilkins, 1997:597.
171. Holtge GA. Laboratory safety. In: McClatchey KD, ed. Clinical laboratory medicine, 2nd ed. Philadelphia: Lippincott Williams & Wilkins, 2002:78.
172. Travers EM, McClatchey KD. Basic laboratory management. In: McClatchey KD, ed. Clinical laboratory medicine, 2nd ed. Philadelphia: Lippincott Williams & Wilkins, 2002:3.

Bruno Brambati, M.D., and
Lucia Tului, Ph.D., M.D.

5

Prenatal Genetic Diagnosis through Chorionic Villus Sampling

Chorionic villus sampling (CVS) must be considered among the most important advances in obstetrics of the 1980s, and it is now an accepted method for the prenatal diagnosis of genetic disorders. In the past two decades, alternative sampling approaches have been evaluated and not found to be successful[1-9]; therefore, CVS is still the only established method for prenatal diagnosis in the first trimester and appears to be as safe and reliable as midtrimester amniocentesis (AC). Although AC remains the most common technique for prenatal diagnosis, since its inception CVS has gained popularity as a means of rapid prenatal diagnosis in early pregnancy.[10,11] The ability to achieve a first-trimester fetal diagnosis reduces the emotional and physical stress in couples at risk, maximizes patient privacy, and permits access to termination at a safer time in pregnancy. Studies on the acceptance of prenatal tests indicate that decisions are influenced by several individual and social factors: moral and religious objection, emotional reluctance, and legal barriers.[12] Prenatal diagnosis in the first trimester, when a physical awareness of the conceptus may not be present and pregnancy is not physically apparent, is expected to have less pronounced psychologic and behavioral effects on the mother. Reports comparing the emotional distress experienced by women undergoing AC and CVS have shown that the CVS approach evokes less anxiety, which lasts a shorter period of time, than does AC.[13] Moreover, women undergoing CVS reported significantly greater attachment to the fetus during the second trimester than did women undergoing amniocentesis.[14] Although the miscarriage rate was shown to be a determinant factor of the patient's attitude toward prenatal procedures, the great benefits of an early diagnosis prepared patients to accept a higher risk, up to five times that of midtrimester amniocentesis.[15-17] The acceptance rate of CVS in some places did not significantly change, even when the controversy regarding the possibility of an association between CVS and birth defects arose.[18] Furthermore, religion does not seem to be an insurmountable obstacle in the decision making for prenatal diagnosis and selective abortion during the first trimester, as was evident from a study on the acceptability of CVS in 180 pregnant women, the majority (73 percent) of whom had low genetic risk.[19] Of the 146 Roman Catholic patients, 86.6 percent proved to be well informed about the prohibition against abortion but were determined to undergo voluntary termination in the case of a severely affected fetus.

179

CVS for genetic indications was suggested in the late 1960s,[20] and a small but successful clinical experience was described in the 1970s by a Chinese group using a blind transcervical aspiration approach.[21] The second generation of ultrasound machines was the main determinant of the use of CVS in clinical practice, and Kazy et al.[22] in the early 1980s were the first to publish a successful transcervical experience using thin biopsy forceps under ultrasound guidance. However, only the publication of the initial experience by Old et al.[10] and by Brambati and Simoni[11] established genetic diagnosis in the first trimester as an integral part of the obstetrical armamentarium: hemoglobinopathies[10] and chromosome defects[11] were the first to be detected using chorionic tissue. In 1984, a World Health Organization (WHO) working group[23] recognized the great potential of CVS for increasing the acceptability of fetal diagnosis, raised questions about the risks of CVS, and emphasized the necessity for control studies before its extensive clinical use. Thereafter, the WHO Inherited Disease Program sponsored an international registry, to which more than 200,000 cases had been referred by the end of 1996 by 100 centers, 81 of which were listed as current reporters.[24]

REQUIREMENTS FOR A CVS PROGRAM

CVS, as well as other sampling techniques, should be performed only at medical centers that have a high level of expertise and experience, that are capable of applying the appropriate sampling approach, that intend to do a substantial number of such procedures, and that provide accurate follow-up of the cases. Obstetricians interested in CVS should be experienced in first-trimester ultrasonography, well versed in the pathophysiology and clinical aspects of early pregnancy, and well informed about human genetics and laboratory methods used in genetic analysis. Training can be suitably performed at 10–12 weeks of gestation either in cases of voluntary abortion or in diagnostic cases only under the direct supervision of a senior expert operator. Prior experience in amniocentesis and cordocentesis is an advantage in acquiring CVS skill. By this prerequisite, adequate skills can be acquired after about 200–300 cases (Table 5.1); thereafter, an annual practice of at least 300–400 CVS might be recommended to avoid any deterioration in the sampling performance (Table 5.2).[25,26] An efficient self-evaluation of the sampling expertise can be easily obtained by rating the number of double insertions (<5 percent), the too light tissue specimens (<5 to 10 percent), the mean sampled tissue value (between 20 and 40 mg), and the sampling failures (5 to 10 percent at the first and less than 1 percent at the second attempt) (Table 5.2).

Sonographic examination should precede sampling to confirm gestational age, to document fetal viability, to ascertain the number of fetuses and chorionicity, and to detect obvious fetal malformations and uterine wall abnormalities. When echo-free areas are observed, it is essential to differentiate between subchorionic hematoma and the so-called vanishing twin, thereby avoiding a potential diagnostic pitfall.[27] The placental site is generally easily recognized by the eighth gestational week as a characteristic hyperechogenic crescent area. Transabdominal scanning by a very-high-quality machine with a 3.5- to 5-MHz probe is a standard approach for acquiring fundamental information. In principle, sector and convex probes should be preferred to reliably guide the sampling device. Their small contact surface allows an optimal fit to the maternal abdomen and facilitates easy handling of the transducer in all the scanning sections, with a comprehensive visualization of the uterus still frequently situated near or below the pubis.

CVS is performed in an outpatient facility. No medical preparation is needed before transabdominal (TA) sampling, whereas vaginal infection should be searched for and eventually treated before transcervical aspiration (TC) sampling. A full bladder is not required;

Table 5.1. Learning curve for TC-CVS, using catheter aspiration, and TA-CVS freehand needling, observed in the first three years of experience (February 1983 to December 1985) by the same self-taught operator (B.B.) at the Mangiagalli Clinic, University of Milan

Series of Cases	TC-CVS					TA-CVS				
	No. of Attempts				Sampling Success (%)	No. of Attempts				Sampling Success (%)
	1	2	3	4		1	2	3	4	
1–100	71	18	3	4	96	94	6	—	—	100
101–200	89	9	1	—	99	93	6	—	—	99
201–300	87	12	—	—	99	95	5	—	—	100
301–400	95	5	—	—	100	95	5	—	—	100
401–500	94	6	—	—	100	97	3	—	—	100

Table 5.2. Efficiency and fetal loss risk of TA-CVS by a single operator (B.B.) in different year intervals and in relation to changes in sampling policy, Prenatal Diagnosis Center, Milan

	1986–1988	1992	1996
Number of consecutive cases	700	700	900
Weeks at CVS (% of cases)			
7–9	34	17	5
10–12	59	71	77
≥13	7	12	18
Feasibility of TA-CVS	98.6%	98.7%	98.4%
	(10 TA-CVS changed to TC-CVS)	(7 TA-CVS changed to TC-CVS) (1 TA-CVS postponed)	(15 TA-CVS postponed)
Success at the first attempt	98.4%	99.3%	99.2%
Sampling failure after two attempts	0.3%	0%	0.2%
Tissue weight (mg)			
Mean	28.3%	29.1%	29.3%
<10 mg	3.3%	2.5%	2.7%
Total fetal loss rate (<24 weeks)	1.48%	1.35%	0.84%

however, some filling may be advantageous to straighten the angle of a pronounced anteflexed uterus or to push intestinal loops away from the anterior uterine wall. Postoperative care includes some rest only for patients who experience spotting/bleeding or cramping. The operating room should contain a visiting table, facilities for scrubbing, ultrasound equipment, and an inverted microscope for a preliminary identification, weight evaluation, and selection of chorionic villi. It is generally advised to aspirate tissue with a syringe containing 2–3 ml of saline solution. If maternal blood is heavily present in the sample, it should be promptly removed to avoid villus inclusion in blood clots.

SAMPLING METHODS

Two main approaches are available for obtaining chorionic tissue: the placenta is reached, under continuous ultrasound monitoring, either through the maternal abdomen (TA-CVS),[28,29] by needling or through the cervical canal (TC-CVS), by the insertion of a catheter,[11,30] or a biopsy forceps (Figure 5.1).[31,32] Transvaginal needling guided by an intravaginal ultrasound probe has also been developed, but it is indicated only for patients in whom CVS by both conventional approaches (TA and TC) is impractical.[33] Although

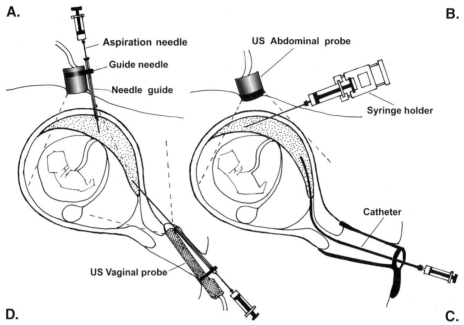

A.
- Aspiration needle
- Guide needle
- Needle guide

US Abdominal probe

Syringe holder

Catheter

US Vaginal probe

D.

C.

B.

Fig. 5.1. Diagrams of the four main CVS methods: *A,* double coaxial TA needle system with needle guide attached to the ultrasound probe; *B,* TA freehand spinal needle insertion, the syringe is mounted onto a holder; *C,* transcervical plastic catheter aspiration; and *D,* transvaginal needling by a needle guide attached to the ultrasound probe.

the published experiences have been performed mostly by TC sampling methods, the TA route has rapidly gained acceptance and at present is likely the most commonly used method in clinical practice.

Transcervical Aspiration Sampling

The most common instrument used[34] in TC sampling is a 26-cm-long, 1.5-mm-outer-diameter polyethylene cannula with a soft stainless steel blunt obturator.[35] The instrumentation for sampling also includes a speculum, a toothed tenaculum, a metal sound (hysterometer), and sponge forceps.

With the patient in the lithotomy position, and after antiseptic preparation of the external genitalia, the cervix is visualized and cleaned with a broad-spectrum antiseptic solution and may be grasped with a tenaculum to straighten the cervical canal. This maneuver has proven to be useful in the case of an anteflexed or retroflexed uterus, in which the placenta is anterior or posterior, respectively. However, this usually produces discomfort and sometimes may be very painful. Therefore, at least in the former condition, it is advantageous to obtain the same effect by filling the bladder. The hysterometer is introduced through the cervical canal to chart the path for the catheter on the ultrasound screen and to evaluate the curvature between the cervical canal and the placental site. The catheter is suitably curved and is slowly inserted through the cervical canal to enter into the placenta deeply, carefully avoiding any sac damage by membrane indentation. After the obturator has been removed, a 20-mL syringe containing nutrient medium or saline solution is attached, and the villi are aspirated by slowly moving the extremity of the catheter inside the placenta. The entire system is then withdrawn under negative pressure.

Transabdominal Aspiration Sampling

Two methodological approaches to TA sampling have been described.[28,29] A double coaxial needle system can be inserted percutaneously through a needle guide attached to the ultrasound probe.[29] The patient is placed in the supine position, the placental region is localized by a real-time sector scan, and the needle pathway is achieved by the needle guide. An 18-gauge, 15-cm guide needle is first introduced and then stopped at the edge of the placenta. Thereafter, a 22- or 20-gauge, 20-cm-long needle is passed through the outer needle, and the villi are aspirated into a syringe; the aspiration needle is repeatedly inserted until an adequate sample is obtained. The average time required to provide enough tissue is about 4 min.

As an alternative a single 20-gauge, 9- or 12-cm spinal needle can be used and inserted by a freehand ultrasound-guided approach (Figure 5.2). This approach is a three-step procedure: (1) the insertion point on the maternal abdominal surface and the sampling pathway are chosen in relation to the depth and the distance of the target as well as to the limited length of the needle; then (2) the needle is inserted through abdominal wall and stopped precisely next to the external uterine surface, with earlier confirmation of the correct direction the needle is pushed further into the placenta; and, finally, (3) the stylet is removed and a 30-mL syringe mounted onto a holder is attached (see Figure 5.1). Enough chorionic tissue is aspirated in about 20 sec by combining repeated suctions of about 20-mL depression and careful backward and forward movements of the needle along the placental axis. The sampling system is withdrawn by keeping a fully depressed syringe. After retrieval, confirmation of the amount and quality of chorionic tissue in a Petri dish through a dissecting microscope is advisable. Bladder filling might be very profitable for a safe

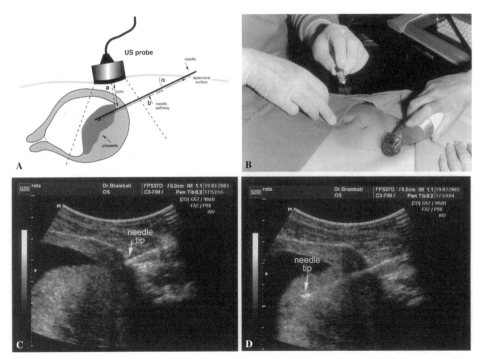

Fig. 5.2. Three-step TA freehand needling under continuous ultrasound control: *A* and *B*, the insertion point on maternal abdominal surface and the pathway (*α* angle) are chosen in relation to the depth (*a*) and the distance (*b*) of the target; *C*, the needle tip is stopped next to the uterine external surface; and finally, *D*, the needle is correctly pushed into the placenta.

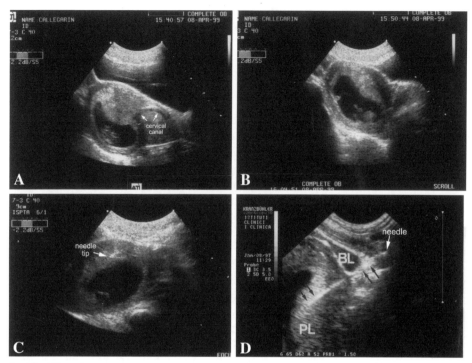

Fig. 5.3. Effect of bladder filling in retroflexed uteri: *A,* a full bladder makes impracticable TA needling in a 12-week pregnancy; *B* and *C,* however, after partial bladder emptying, needling becomes feasible and safe; *D,* a partially filled bladder indicates a safe pathway for a successful CVS (arrows show the needle) in a retroflexed uterus at 12 weeks of gestation. PL = placenta; BL = bladder.

and successful sampling in case the uterus is anteflexed or retroflexed (Figure 5.3). More than two sampling attempts either by TA-CVS or TC-CVS should be discouraged because a significant increase in fetal loss rate is expected.[36–38] Moreover, in case of failure or inadequate sample size at the first attempt, it is wise to evaluate any reason for the failure and to discuss with the patient/couple the opportunity for an additional attempt.

The freehand needle-insertion technique has some advantages when compared with the two-needle system. The needle is thinner and its direction can be easily adjusted when necessitated by abdominal wall or uterine displacements. Moreover, because the needle is not in direct contact with the transducer, neither a sterile ultrasound system nor a sterile contact gel are needed. In addition, the sampling procedure takes less time and the sampling devices are cheaper. However, the freehand technique is a two-person approach and demands the well-coordinated work of sonographer and operator; therefore, it may be more difficult to learn and run.

Efficiency of CVS

TA techniques appear to be more efficient between 8 and 12 weeks (Table 5.3): in the five published series, in which the failure rate after no more than three insertions of the sampling device was far more than 1 percent, TC-CVS was the only approach used. TA sampling provided an adequate amount of tissue at the first attempt in a significantly higher number of cases in the three randomized studies comparing TA- and TC-CVS (Table 5.4). However, the

Table 5.3. The major clinical experiences with first-trimester CVS

Study	CVS Technique	Cases (number)	Maternal Age	Gestation Weeks	Success Rate (%)	Fetal Losses (%) (<28 weeks)
Hogge et al.[39]	TC	950	NA	8–12	97	5.4
Brambati et al.[40]	TC	1,305	76% ≥ 35	7–12	99.2	3.9
Wade and Young[41]	TC	714	87% > 35	NA	NA	4.5
Jackson et al.[42]	TC	769	NA	NA	99.5	2.2
Green et al.[43]	TC	940	NA	9–12	99.4	2.5
Wass et al.[44]	TC	1,000	67.8% ≥ 37	9–12	99.3	4.1
Donner et al.[45]	TC	1,021	72% > 35	9–14	95	2.5
Jahoda et al.[46]	TC	1,449	65% > 36	8–11	97.8	5.1
Leschot et al.[47]	TC	947	NA	8–11	96.4	3.6
Miny et al.[48]	TC	1,173	80.9% > 35	NA	97.6	5.0
Evans et al.[49]	TC	1,055	NA	9–12	99.1	1.6[a]
Wass et al.[50]	TC	1,013	67.8% > 36	9–12	99.2	4.1
Bovicelli et al.[51]	TA	249	NA	9–13	99.7	3.6
Smidt-Jensen and Hahnemann[29]	TA	170	NA	8–11	99.4	3.6
Williams et al.[52]	TC	2,949	37 (mean)	9–12	99.7	1.9
Jackson and Wapner[53]	TC/TA	11,600	NA	NA	99.9	2.6
Palo et al.[54]	TA	821	91% ≥ 37	11.2 (mean)	99	1.9[a]
Chueh et al.[55]	TC	6,545	NA	9–12	NA	3.9
	TA	2,318	NA	9–12	NA	2.4
Lunshof et al.[32]	TC	1,936	90% ≥ 36	8–13	9.1	3.5[a]
Brambati et al.[56]	TC/TA	10,000	36 (median)	8–32	99.7	2.6
Brun et al.[57]	TA	10,741	36 (median)	8–38	99.9	1.7

[a]Losses up to 24 weeks.

NA = not available.

Table 5.4. Sampling performance and fetal loss in the three major randomized trials comparing TA-CVS and TC-CVS

Study	Number of Cases		Mean Tissue Weight (mg)		Success at the First Attempt (%)		Failure (%)		Deviation from the Allocated Procedure (%)		Total Losses (%)	
	TA	TC	TA	TC	TA	TC	TA	TC	TA	TC	TA	TC
Smidt-Jensen et al.[58]	1,027	1,010	29	31	98.1	96.0*	1.8	3.4	0.5	5.6	6.3	10.9[a]
Brambati et al.[59]	575	581	24	30.6*	96.7	89.7*	0.2	0.2	3.1	15.8*	16.5	15.5[b]
Jackson et al.[60]	1,944	1,929	20	25*	93.7	89.5*	1.4	2.4	3.5	3.3	2.6	2.6[a]

[a]All fetal losses before and after CVS (before 28 weeks).

[b]All fetal losses before and after CVS, including perinatal deaths.

[c]Only spontaneous fetal losses after CVS and before 28 weeks (elective abortions of chromosomally normal fetus are included).

*Statistically significant difference.

mean amount of villi obtained was higher by the TC route, although the range of weights was greater for TC than for TA.[58–60] The practicality of sampling was significantly higher for the TA technique in two of the randomized studies,[58,59] whereas no difference between techniques in the percentage of deviations from the allocated procedure was observed in the third

Table 5.5.   Late (>12 weeks) TA-CVS: Study characteristics, efficacy, and risk of fetal loss

Study	Number of Cases	Weeks at CVS	Tissue Weight (≥10 mg)	Sampling Failure	Fetal Loss (<28 weeks)	Indications
Monni et al.[61]	80	13–20	71.2%	None	None	thalassemia
Jahoda et al.[62]	567	12–17	90.3%	None	1.8%[a]	maternal age
Holzgreve et al.[63]	2,058	13–41	71.7%	None	10.4% (2.3%)[b]	30.5% SUF
Chieri and Aldini[64]	220	14–25	7.5%	9.1%	0.4%	maternal age, previous affected child, parental translocation
Podobaik et al.[65]	1,000	13–40	NA	None	0.3%	25% SUF
Camerun et al.[66]	551	18.2 ± 1.5 (mean ± SD)	NA	NA[c]	0.4%	Down syndrome screening risk ≥220
Brambati et al.[67]	871	13–14	91.6%[c]	None	0.8%[d]	76% maternal age, 19%
	924	15–20	91.6%[c]	None	0.4%[d]	Mendelian dis., 37% SUF

NA = not available   SUF = suspicious ultrasound findings
[a]undetermined number of cases at 12 weeks are included
[b]corrected rate excluding SUF cases
[c]>15 mg
[d]<24 weeks

study.[60] However, in this latter study, the very high number of cases excluded from the randomization because of specific contraindications seems to be the determining factor of the apparently identical feasibility rate. In our clinical experience, we found no association between sampling success rate and mean tissue size and placental location or timing of the first-trimester sampling.[56] The efficiency of the TA route does not apparently change after the 12th week of pregnancy, as all but one of the largest clinical experiences reported virtually 100 percent success rate with a low rate of repeated insertions (Table 5.5).

MULTIPLE PREGNANCIES

Multiple pregnancy poses a particular challenge to the obstetrician. Not only is at least one of the fetuses more likely to suffer from a genetic disorder or malformation, but the sampling approach may be more difficult, and discordance between fetuses for an anomaly may imply the need for a selective reduction. There was a steady decline in the incidence of multiple births in developed countries until the late 1970s. Since then, a slight increase in the number of twin pregnancies has been observed, whereas triplet and higher-order births have risen strikingly since the early 1980s.[68] Monozygotic twinning rates at birth are remarkably constant at about 3.5 per 1,000, whereas a fifteenfold variation in crude rates occurs for dizygotic twinning on a global scale, ranging from 2 to 7 per 1,000 to >20 per 1,000.[69] A twin pregnancy occurs more frequently than the number of twins observed at birth,[70] and high-resolution ultrasound has shown that at least one of two fetuses "vanishes" in 42–78 percent of cases.[71] Of particular interest to prenatal diagnosis is the increased rate of dizygotic twins with advancing maternal age and increasing parity. Fertility drugs and assisted conception techniques have contributed significantly to the increase of multiple pregnancies in the past 20 years,[72] and the rise in number can be expected to continue, at least in the short term.

    Using CVS for prenatal diagnosis in the first trimester has several technical advantages when compared with midtrimester amniocentesis: (a) the easier evaluation of the membranes and the accurate mapping of the uterus by ultrasound make both the prediction of chorionicity and amnionicity and the identification of the eventually affected fetus highly reliable[73–75]; (b) the use of rapid analytical methods (short-term culture karyotyping, enzymatic analysis on fresh tissue, and polymerase chain reaction amplification) make the result available in a few days, thereby avoiding substantial changes in the uterine topography; (c) if same-sex dichorionic twins are diagnosed, DNA polymorphism markers may be quickly checked to ensure retrieval of villi from the individual placentas[73,75]; (d) in case fetal reduction of an affected twin is requested, the intervention can still be done in the first trimester with lower emotional impact and lower medical risks.[76] Dichorionic twin pregnancy can easily be predicted when either two distinct placental sites are observed or, if the placentas are confluent, the septal thickness is at least 1.0 mm and the lambda sign is present[73–75] (Figure 5.4). In case of two distinct placental sites or monochorionic twins, the criteria for CVS are the same as for a singleton pregnancy. However, in dichorionic twins with fused placentas, no sonographic findings are available to distinguish monozygotic from dizygotic twins, and only sampling of both placentas can provide complete genetic information. The main criterion for a reliable sampling is to guide the extremity of the aspirating device close to the umbilical cord insertion, or next to the placental edge far from the confluence of the two placentas (Figure 5.4). A second rule is to avoid passing through the placenta of the second twin. This could, in some cases, be easily achieved by the combined use of TA-CVS and TC-CVS or, as an alternative, by using a double coaxial needle system. The double needle sampling system is made by a 19-gauge 9-cm-long guide needle and 21-gauge 15-cm-long sampling needle: the guide needle is first introduced through the co-twin placenta and stopped just after reaching the placenta to be sampled, thereafter sampling is performed by passing the thinner needle through the outer one[75] (Figure 5.4). If like-sex dichorionic twins are diagnosed from two different CVS specimens, and no chromosomal and DNA polymorphisms allow any differentiation between samples, later diagnostic confirmation by amniocentesis might be advisable.

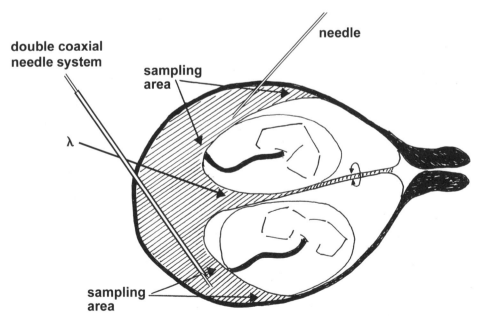

Fig. 5.4. Diagram of TA-CVS approach in dichorionic twin pregnancy with confluent placentas. If placenta can be reached only by going through the co-twin placenta, a double coaxial needle system allows a reliable and pure sampling.

Table 5.6. First trimester CVS in dichorionic twin pregnancies: fetal and neonatal loss rates compared to control population

	Brambati et al.[75]		De Catte et al.[79]**		Ayloz et al.[80]		Wapner et al.[78]	
	CVS	Controls	CVS	Controls	CVS	Controls	CVS	Controls***
No. of continuing pregnancies	147	63	102	101	110	175	158	70
Mean maternal age (± SD)	34.5 (4.4)	31.7* (4.0)	33.2 (3.7)	30.0 (4.3)	32 (NA)	31.5 (NA)	37 (median)	36 (median)
Mean GA at CVS (weeks)	10.4		10.9		11.1		10–12	16–18
No. of losses of TP at <20 weeks (%)	0	0	3 (2.9)	7 (6.9)	2 (1.8)	1 (0.6)	4 (2.5)	1 (1.4)
No. of losses of TP at ≥20 weeks (%)	0	0	3 (3.0)	1 (1.1)	0	0	1 (0.6)	3 (4.3)
Total alive newborns	289	126	193	185	216	339	309	140
Neonatal death (%)	6 (2.1)	8 (6.3)	4 (2.1)	7 (3.8)	NA	NA	7 (2.2)	3 (2.1)

GA = gestational age; TP = total pregnancy; NA = not available.
*$p < 0.0001$
**early (<22 weeks) and late (≥22 weeks) fetal loss
***mid-trimester amniocentesis

Genetic fetal investigation in twin pregnancy by first-trimester CVS is a safe and reliable approach.[75,77–80] In the major published experiences no statistical differences for fetal losses and perinatal complications have been observed between CVS and control populations[75,78–80] (Table 5.6). Diagnostic reliability was very high: the rate of wrong results due to erroneous sampling ranged between 0 percent and 0.9 percent.

TIMING OF CVS

CVS has been shown to be feasible as early as the sixth week of pregnancy. In the first and still largest study available, sampling was performed successfully in all of the 328 cases at high genetic risk[81] by TA freehand insertion of a 20- or 22-gauge spinal needle. No more than two needle insertions were carried out. In 20 percent of cases the embryo's crown-to-rump length (CRL) was 2–8 mm and in 80 percent it was 9–15 mm. Fetal karyotyping succeeded in 99.4 percent of cases, and no diagnostic failures were reported in enzymatic and DNA analyses.[81,82] However, the program was deliberately terminated because of the observation of an unusual number of fetal limb abnormalities, arousing suspicion of a causal relationship with the sampling procedure.[81] The methodological prerequisites of a safe TA-CVS are clear visualization of the uterine anatomy, precise definition of the placental limit, and absolute control of the needle path. Even in expert hands, these conditions are sometimes critical between 6 and 8 weeks of gestation, and chorionic plate vascular injury with fetal tissue damage may result from unsuitable technical approaches. More recently, a further experience of very early CVS has been published. CVS was offered to a population of Orthodox Jewish patients for whom abortion is permissible up to 40 days after conception. In 91 percent of cases, the TC catheter aspiration method was used for sampling (35 percent of cases at between 5 and 7 gestation weeks and 65 percent at 8 weeks), while only 9 percent of cases were sampled by TA needling, 85 percent of them at 8 weeks. In all cases, adequate tissue was obtained for diagnosis, and to provide an adequate amount of tissue in 6 percent of cases, three or more insertions were required.[83]

The recommended lowest limit of gestational age for sampling in clinical practice is between 9 and 10 weeks.[25,56] By this time, embryo viability is easily detectable, the placenta is clearly identifiable, and the conceptus is no longer in the embryonic development phase, during which most teratogenic effects occur. The upper limit for TC sampling has been suggested at 12–13 weeks. Indeed, as the pregnancy advances, the gestational sac increases in size, and by the end of the first trimester, the decidua capsularis generally fuses with the decidua parietalis. Thereafter, any attempt to insert the catheter between the uterine wall and the chorionic vesicle entails a higher risk of indenting and damaging the membranes. These difficulties can also be accentuated by the fact that the proximal placental edge may move far from the internal cervical os. However, transcervical sampling was recently successfully accomplished by thin biopsy forceps in 335 pregnancies at 12.1–15.0 weeks: diagnosis was obtained in 97.3 percent of cases, whereas the fetal loss rate up to 28 weeks was 3.1 percent, not significantly different from the values obtained by the authors in an earlier series between 8 and 12 weeks.[84] No procedural contraindications have been found for attempting CVS in the second and third trimesters via TA needling. The extension of TA-CVS beyond the first trimester has proven very convenient as an alternative to AC or cordocentesis (see Table 5.5) and is currently offered in three specific situations: (1) as an alternative to early second-trimester AC (before 15 weeks); (2) in late-booking cases to obtain fetal diagnosis in time for termination; and (3) at any time to acquire genetic information in cases at risk (e.g., suspicious ultrasound finding), especially if amniotic fluid or fetal blood sampling is confounded by technically unfavorable conditions (e.g., severe oligohydramnios).[56,61–65,67]

INDICATIONS FOR CVS

The indications for CVS are similar to those for AC, except when amniotic fluid studies are required (see discussion in chapters 1 and 6). Studies to detect chromosomal abnormalities are undoubtedly the most common reason for CVS. Banding of good quality can be obtained by culturing mesenchymal cells of chorionic villi; this process usually takes 10–15 days. Rapid karyotyping may be achieved by examining cytotrophoblastic cells arrested in metaphase, either immediately (within a few hours) after sampling or in a short-term (24–48 hr) culture. However, chromosome preparations obtained by the direct method are difficult to band and would not be suitable for detection of subtle chromosome anomalies. Therefore, a 12–14 day culture is suitable to provide the same standard of banding as usually achieved with amniotic fluid cell culture.

Chorionic tissue cells provide large amounts of metabolically active cytoplasm; therefore, direct assay is possible for many inherited metabolic diseases, yielding a diagnostic result within hours or days. In addition, the amount of DNA obtained from a conventional sampling allows reliable DNA analysis. This is not the case with amniotic fluid cells, in which the quantity and quality of DNA occasionally may be inadequate. Thus, chorionic tissue is at present the material of choice for prenatal diagnosis of mendelian diseases. The rapid progress of human genome research has broadened the range of gene defects directly detectable and facilitates prenatal diagnosis even in low-risk populations of the more frequent and severe conditions (e.g., cystic fibrosis, fragile X syndrome, nonsyndromic recessive deafness).[85–88]

At the individual level, the advantages of first-trimester CVS are evident when compared with AC. The preprocedure and postprocedure waiting periods are much shorter, no obvious complications threatening pregnancy (i.e., amniotic fluid leakage or amnionitis after amniocentesis) follow sampling, the decision to eventually end pregnancy is less stressful, and first-trimester abortion has a significantly lower rate of clinical complications, less profound emotional effect, and fewer legal limitations than a fifth month pregnancy interruption. Certain clinical conditions may also influence the choice of an early genetic diagnosis: namely, previous cesarean section, pending cerclage, and twin and higher multiple pregnancy in which selective fetal reduction is being considered.

CVS KARYOTYPING: PRINCIPLES AND PITFALLS

CVS is a well-established method for fetal karyotyping, and chorionic tissue informativeness has been based on the assumption that the chromosomal constitutions of fetus and chorionic tissue are identical. However, chromosomal mosaicism confined to the human placenta, first described by Kalousek and Dill in 1983,[89] was later confirmed by chorionic tissue karyotyping after first-trimester CVS.[90] By definition, confined placental mosaicism (CPM) is a dichotomy between the chromosomal constitution of placental tissues (both cytotrophoblast and chorionic stroma) and embryonic/fetal tissues, and it is usually detected in 1–2 percent of pregnancies studied by CVS.[56,91–93] CPM has been found less frequently after long-term culture (0.6 percent) than after direct or short-term incubation.[94] CPM can be explained by the fact that mitotic errors are expected to occur more frequently in the extraembryonic than in the embryonic lineage because the embryo proper is derived from only three progenitor cells in the sixty-four-celled blastocyst; the other cells give rise to extraembryonic structures.[95] Another explanation is that mitotic errors could involve true embryonic and extraembryonic cells equally, but the embryo has control mechanisms to limit the replication of cells with karyotypic abnormalities through mitotic loss of a supernumerary chromosome in subsequent cell division (trisomic zygote rescue), whereas in the placenta the abnormal cells may proliferate and be simply eliminated at delivery.[96] A positive correlation between maternal age and CPM has been preliminarily observed, although statistical significance has not been evaluated.[96]

Three types of CPM have been described.[97] In type I CPM, the most common, aneuploid cells are present only in direct or short-term cultured cytotrophoblast preparations. In the less common type II CPM, abnormal cells are observed only in cultured chorionic stromal cells. In the very rare type III CPM, abnormalities are present in both lineages. The European Collaborative Research on Mosaicism in CVS (EUCROMIC) is the largest study available; it is based on 92,246 CVS successfully karyotyped by seventy-nine laboratories. Mosaicism or nonmosaic fetoplacental discrepancy was found in 1,415 (1.5 percent) of the samples,[93] of which 192 were karyotyped after direct preparation or short-term incubation and long-term culture and further investigated by chromosome analysis of one or more types of fetal cells. Mosaicism involving trisomies 8, 9, 12, 15, and 20 was confirmed in all, although in a minority of cases, as mosaic trisomy in the fetus; trisomy 13 was confirmed as nonmosaic trisomy in two of fifteen fetuses; trisomy 18 in four of twenty-nine cases as mosaic, while trisomy 21 was the most frequently confirmed in the fetus (nine of twenty-two cases) as mosaic and nonmosaic trisomy. Trisomies 2, 3, 5, 7, 10, 11, 14, 16, and 22 were never confirmed in the fetus/neonate. Trisomies 15 and 16 were most often found in both cytotrophoblast and villus stroma. Mosaic trisomies 3, 7, and 20 were predominantly restricted to the cytotrophoblast, while mosaic trisomy 2 was restricted to the villus stroma. Three other major studies, totaling 49,500 CVS cases, show figures more or less in agreement for mosaic trisomy 21, 18, and 13 with the EUCROMIC study, and provide also information about mosaic trisomies XXX, XXY, XYY, and 45,X/46,XX and

Table 5.7. Confirmation rates of mosaic and non mosaic common aneuploidies in U.S. study,[91] U.K. study,[133] and our experience at Mangiagalli Clinic and Prenatal Diagnosis Center, Milan (unpublished data)

	U.S. Study		U.K. Study		Our Study	
Abnormality	Cases	Confirmed	Cases	Confirmed	Cases	Confirmed
47 +21	105	38/38	307	143/143	185	87/87
47 +18	31	8/8	146	59/59	67	23/23
47 +13	12	3/3	40	18/18	28	15/15
46/47 +21	12	2/6	15	5/11	16	7/15
46/47 +18	5	1/4	20	4/15	11	6/11
46/47 +13	5	0/3	10	3/8	12	4/12
47 XXX	4	2/2	20	8/8	10	7/7
47 XXY	13	6/6	21	8/8	20	15/15
47 XYY	7	3/3	11	7/7	6	4/4
46/47 XXX	2	0/1	3	2/3	4	1/4
46/47 XXY	1	0/1	4	1/2	3	1/3
46/47 XYY	0		1	—	2	0/2
45 X0	14	5/5	66	21/21	41	16/16
45/46 X0/XX	16	1/8	29	8/18	23	5/21
45/46 X0/XY	6	1/5	9	3/7	5	0/4
Total no. of CVS	11,473		20,527		17,500	

45,X /46,XY (Table 5.7): three of eight, two of six, zero of two, fourteen of forty-seven, and four of seventeen cases, respectively, were confirmed.

Uniparental Disomy (UPD)

If mosaicism or nonmosaic fetoplacental discrepancy involving a trisomy has originated through nondisjunction with subsequent reduction to disomy (embryo rescue), there is a theoretical risk of one in three for UPD in the fetus.[93] UPD is the abnormal inheritance of both homologous chromosomes from a single parent without representation from the other parent.[98] The phenotypic effect of UPD depends on which chromosome is involved, whether it contains imprinted genes or not, and on its parental origin. Fetal UPD has been described for chromosomes 2, 7, 9, 10, 11, 14, 15, 16, and 22, and in case of robertsonian translocations involving chromosome 14 and 15. However, there is evidence for imprinted genes with phenotypic effect linked to UPD only for chromosome 7 (Russell–Silver syndrome), 11 (Beckwith–Wiedemann syndrome), 14 (mental retardation and multiple anomalies), 15 (Prader–Willi and Angelman syndromes).

A further problem may arise from UPD when the uniparental chromosome pair is a duplicate of a same chromosome (isodisomy). The effect of this condition is to greatly increase the likelihood of inheriting a lethal or severe form of recessive disease. This occurred in two children with UPD for chromosome 7 from mothers who were carriers of a cystic fibrosis (CF) mutation, but whose fathers were not CF carriers.[99,100]

CPM and Intrauterine Growth Restriction (IUGR)

The association between CPM and IUGR was first suggested by Kalousek and Dill.[89] This report was followed by several others supporting an association between CPM for chromosomes 2, 7, 9, 14, 15, 16, 18, and 22, tetraploidy and growth restriction, fetal demise, and poor perinatal outcome.[101-111] The most likely mechanism to explain this associations could be a direct effect of the presence of a significant number of abnormal cells; this seems to be supported by the strong association observed between IUGR and higher levels of trisomic cells found by extensive cytogenetic investigation in the placenta after delivery.[112] In addition, the effect of the unbalanced parental imprinting in UPD eventually affecting the potentiality of fetal growth and viability should also be taken into account.[102]

However, there is no statistical evidence of the adverse effect of CPM on fetal outcome. In the retrospective collaborative study involving 21 UK laboratories, 73 cases of CPM were identified among 8,004 first-trimester referrals. The comparison with the control population failed to demonstrate a marked increase in adverse fetal outcome in the CPM group.[102] These results are in agreement with some other, less extensive CVS experiences.[104,113,114]

Some confounding factors have been suggested that may explain the conflicting evidence[102]: (a) the distribution of the trisomic cells in the placenta confining them to specific areas maybe heterogeneous[115]; (b) culture might select aberrant cells, or trisomic constitution could be an artifact of culture; (c) the abnormal karyotype might be the effect of the analysis of residual villi from an aneuploid twin that failed to develop[116,117]; (d) the effect might be mediated through abnormal growth factor expression from an imprinted gene in a specific involved chromosome; and (e) maternal origin of chromosomes in UPD might be a definite compounding factor in the pathogenesis of impaired fetal growth and adverse pregnancy outcome as observed with trisomy 16 CPM.[101,118,119]

Poor fetal outcome has been more frequently reported in CPM for chromosomes 16,[101,103,104,109,118–125] 7,[110] 22,[108,125] 2[104,126–129] 8,[130] and 9.[102,131]

Although in a number of CPM cases for trisomies 16, 22, and 2, placental chromosomal abnormality was associated with fetal/newborn malformations, the phenotypic effect of CPM on the fetus still remains to be demonstrated. Nevertheless, occasionally case reports raise serious concern given the placental chromosomal abnormality, the subsequent normal karyotype at amniocentesis and/or fetal blood sampling, and the later demonstration of the same abnormality in tissues of the abnormal newborn.[132]

Efficiency and Practical Recommendations

The accuracy of fetal karyotyping, on chorionic villi is very high and equivalent to that on amniocytes (Table 5.7). In the EUCROMIC study[134] on 62,865 karyotyped chorionic villi, true fetal mosaicism was diagnosed in 0.15 percent of samples, while CPM occurred in 1.0 percent. False-positive nonmosaic aberrations were observed in 0.15 percent and false-negative results in only 0.03 percent. False-negative results occurred, with only one exception (one of nineteen cases), after direct preparation alone. These figures give a sensitivity of CVS for fetal detection of chromosome aberrations of 98.9–99.6 percent (95 percent confidence interval [CI]) and a specificity of 98.5–98.8 percent (95 percent CI). It is expected that this high diagnostic accuracy in CVS karyotyping can be achieved only by performing the cytogenetic analysis after both direct and long-term culture preparations. Moreover, because all mosaic findings, including those with discordance between karyotyping techniques, are unreliable indicators of the fetal karyotype, further testing using AC, and rarely fetal blood sampling, are the most appropriate actions, providing more accurate means of differentiating between an abnormal fetal karyotype and CPM.[133] In case mosaic or nonmosaic autosomal trisomy is found in both cytotrophoblast and stroma, further examination by amniocentesis, ultrasound, and UPD testing might also be recommended in order to exclude fetal trisomy and UPD.[93]

CONTRAINDICATIONS TO CVS

Placental biopsy may be contraindicated for a number of reasons that apply either to both sampling routes or to only one of them. For TC approaches, vaginismus and cervical stenosis are absolute obstacles to the introduction of sampling devices, and a myoma of the lower uterine segment may seriously interfere with the passage of the catheter. Active vaginal infection is a contraindication for the TC approach, because specific treatment does not seem sufficient to remove any risk of ascending infection.[135] When the uterus is severely anteflexed or retroflexed, the placenta may not be accessible by the catheter through the cervical canal because of an overly pronounced curve of the sampling pathway: bladder filling and manipulation of the cervix by the speculum and/or the tenaculum are very helpful for safe and successful catheter placement. The retroflexed uterus may be a problem also for TA sampling; however, an accessible position of the placenta can generally be obtained by appropriate bladder filling or emptying (see Figure 5.3), otherwise sampling should be postponed waiting for a spontaneous rotation of the uterus.

History or evidence of vaginal bleeding is a very puzzling condition: the effect of CVS on pregnancy outcome is still unknown, but in these cases, the TA route is, in principle, preferable to avoid any potential risk of iatrogenic ascending infection. However, in our experience, CVS in patients with a history of sporadic bleeding and a normally developing conceptus on ultrasound showed no difference between the TA and TC route in the fetal loss rate.[35,136]

Fetomaternal hemorrhage may occur after CVS procedures, as documented by increased maternal serum-alpha-fetoprotein levels after sampling.[137-144] Therefore, there is a general consensus to administer anti-D immunoglobulin to Rhesus (Rh)-negative women at risk of isoimmunization. Previously sensitized Rh-negative women should be advised about the potential risk of an increased maternal antibody response from sampling, thereby worsening the outcome of erythroblastosis fetalis. CVS is not contraindicated in hemophilia carriers. However, it is advisable to treat the patient with less than 50 percent of factor VIII coagulant activity by 1-D-amino-8-D-arginine vasopressin intravenous infusion just before sampling. The significant increase of factor VIII serum levels rapidly conditioned by this antidiuretic hormone-like peptide minimizes any potential hemorrhagic consequence of the sampling.[145]

COMPLICATIONS OF CVS

Spotting/Bleeding

Vaginal spotting is the most frequent early complication after TC sampling and has been reported in up to 32.2 percent of patients.[60,146] Light to moderate bleeding occurs in a smaller percentage of cases (6.0–12.2 percent), and heavy transient hemorrhage is observed only occasionally.[36,52,59,60,146] As expected, hemorrhagic complications have been reported less frequently after TA-CVS, and the difference when compared with transcervical aspiration (1.3–1.9 percent versus 6.0 percent) was statistically significant in randomized studies.[59,60] Subchorionic hematoma, defined as an echo-free area between the uterine wall and the membranes, which is unusual after TA-CVS (0.3 percent),[40] has been reported in 3.1–4.0 percent of TC procedures[40,46] and generally is detected during the sonographic investigation, scheduled because of hemorrhage after sampling. No association between vaginal bleeding or subchorionic hematoma and the fetal loss rate was found,[35,60] although in single TC-CVS cases, these complications were the first clinical features of a sequence of events, including fluid leakage and chorioamnionitis, leading to fetal loss. In these cases, the retention of blood in the uterine cavity could have led to local subclinical infection or activation of thrombolysis, with subsequent membrane damage.[147]

Fluid Leakage/Oligohydramnios

Acute rupture of membranes is an uncommon complication: ovular sac perforation at the time of sampling occurred in 1–1.6 percent of cases undergoing blind TC aspiration[21,148,149] and has been reported in only one of the studies using ultrasound catheter guidance giving a rate as low as 0.2 percent.[39] However, severe oligohydramnios after an uncomplicated TC procedure and without a history of amniotic fluid (AF) leakage was reported by Wade and Young in 0.4 percent of 685 continuing pregnancies,[41] and an association between catheter aspiration and midtrimester membrane rupture and AF leakage was suspected by Jackson et al. in an unspecified number of oligohydramnios cases.[42] However, these complications are also observed in pregnancies not undergoing any sampling procedure. Therefore, reliable information on the true procedure-related incidence should be acquired only through controlled trials. In the U.S. trial for CVS risk evaluation,[146] no significant difference in AF leakage was observed within 4 days after TC-CVS or at a corresponding gestational age for the amniocentesis group. However, at the second ultrasound control, just before amniocentesis, leakage of AF was present only in CVS group (0.7 percent), probably as a persisting effect of membrane damage by the aspirating catheter.[146] The frequency of AF leakage after TC-CVS was confirmed in the U.S. randomized trial comparing TA and TC techniques[60]; the rate observed in the TC group was significantly higher than in the TA group (1.9 percent versus 0.5 percent). These figures were not confirmed by the Danish randomized study[58]: no statistical difference for postprocedural amniotic fluid leakage rate between TA-CVS (0.5 percent) and TC-CVS (0.6 percent) was observed, whereas the difference became highly significant when both CVS procedures were compared with AC (2.8 percent).

Infection

From the time the transcervical sampling route was suggested, introduction of bacteria into the uterine cavity with resulting microbial colonization and infection was a major concern. This potential risk was first demonstrated by Scialli et al.,[150] who isolated bacteria from 30 percent of catheters used for CVS. Brambati et al.[151] confirmed this finding in a study of 104 cases, in 50 percent of which the catheter was colonized, and culture revealed both aerobes and anaerobes, together with *Candida albicans*. However, no association between bacteria cultured from the catheter and pregnancy outcome could be demonstrated. So far, three cases of maternal septic shock have been reported 4–13 days after TC-CVS by repeated plastic catheter insertions[152–154]; their clinical evaluation clearly supports the probable causal relationship between TC-CVS and ascending infection. The incidence of post-TC-CVS chorioamnionitis is low, having been reported in 0.03–0.5 percent of cases,[35,43,52,53,78] and in some large series, no cases were observed.[36,46,50,58,155] However, there is some concern about the role of less serious infections in women who experience fetal loss after TC-CVS. In two studies, the evaluation of the clinical history of patients who underwent TC-CVS and spontaneously aborted revealed that infection was likely implicated in 13–41 percent of cases.[155,156] Therefore, despite the rarity of acute intrauterine infectious events, it seems wise to adhere strictly to aseptic procedures, to avoid multiple insertions of the sampling device through the cervical canal, to use a new sterile catheter for each insertion, and to choose the TA route whenever difficulties with a TC catheter are expected or have already arisen.

Intraperitoneal infection from using TA-CVS is a very rare event, but it may occur when the large intestine is punctured. In our experience, clinical symptoms of peritonitis were noted a few minutes after sampling in 3 of 8,479 cases (0.03 percent).[56] However, in only one case (0.01 percent), *Escherichia coli* was cultured in the cytogenetic culture medium, giving a strong suspicion of intestine perforation. In the other two cases, the medium was sterile, and symptoms were milder, suggesting that the peritoneal reaction resulted from bleeding at the external surface of the punctured uterine wall. Whatever the pathologic mechanism, following maternal rest, peritoneal irritation spontaneously resolved in all cases, within a few hours to a day, without any serious consequences for the mother or the fetus.

Fetomaternal Hemorrhage

Fetomaternal hemorrhage (FMH) may occur after first-trimester CVS. At the end of the fifth menstrual week, the intravillus vascular network connects with the umbilical–allantoic vessels and integrates into the general embryonic circulation. Thereafter, any disruption of villus integrity may cause fetal blood leakage. This has been demonstrated by a significant increase in the maternal serum α-fetoprotein (MSAFP) level reported in 40–70 percent of CVS cases.[137–144] FMH was also confirmed more recently by using techniques for detecting nucleated fetal red cells in maternal blood: the percentage of erythroblasts enriched from maternal blood that stained positive for ε- and γ-globin chains was significantly higher in the post-CVS samples compared with the pre-CVS samples, and this was supported by fluorescence in situ hybridization analysis for the Y chromosome.[157] In a randomized study between sampling techniques, the postprocedure MSAFP level increase was correlated with the biopsy method used; mean MSAFP values were significantly higher after TA than TC.[144] Moreover, a positive correlation was found between the magnitude of rise in MSAFP levels and the amount of chorionic tissue removed.[137–139,144,158] Attempts have been made to evaluate the extent of FMH, and in 5–18 percent of cases, fetal hemorrhage was calculated to exceed 0.1 mL[137,139,142,144]; a higher rate occurred after TA than after TC procedures.[144,159] This was explained by the fact that by TC sampling, the myometrium is not intentionally punctured, as is the case with TA sampling, thereby reducing the AFP leakage into the maternal blood.[144] The total fetal and placental blood volume calculated at 8–12 weeks of gestation ranged from 2.4 to 6.0 mL.[139] Therefore, fetal hemorrhage after CVS appears unlikely to harm fetal well-being by evoking a profound reaction and circulatory collapse.[160] However, an association between MSAFP increase and frequency of spontaneous abortion or fetal loss was found for the cases with the highest MSAFP level[138,144] or with a continuing rise in the first hour after CVS.[138] Fetal exsanguination was suspected after TA-CVS at 12 weeks in a case of fetal death after sampling with immediate postprocedural persisting fetal bradycardia, absent Doppler-flow in the umbilical cord, and a eighty-five-fold rise in the MSAFP level.[161]

FMH was also studied at 13–19 weeks in two small TA series[162,163]: MSAFP was elevated in virtually 100 percent of cases, and correlation was confirmed with the amount of villus tissue removed. Moreover, in 18 percent of cases, the volume of FMH approached or exceeded 21 percent of fetoplacental blood volume, but no fetomaternal exsanguination occurred. More recently, MSAFP was determined before and after TA-CVS in 300 patients between 13 and 16 weeks of gestation; Doppler recordings of the uterine artery, spiral artery, umbilical artery, and intraplacental arterioles were also performed before and after sampling. Maternal levels increased after sampling in only 6.7 percent of cases, and no correlation was found between AFP elevation, Doppler measurements, and spontaneous abortion.[65]

Therefore, it seems plausible that fetal blood released into the maternal circulation after CVS could result in maternal sensitization. Serologically, Rh antigen is fully expressed at an early stage of gestation and is shown to be capable of agglutinating megaloblasts of a 10-mm embryo.[164] Only a single case has been described in which CVS was suggested to have played a specific role in sensitizing an Rh-negative woman with a homozygous Rh-positive husband. She was correctly treated with anti-D immunoglobulin in previous pregnancies, but after CVS at 9 weeks, no anti-D immunoglobulin was administered, and anti-D antibodies were found in increasing amounts after the 27th week.[48] In view of the preceding considerations, anti-D prophylaxis in Rh-negative patients with an Rh-positive partner is recommended after CVS; a dose of 50 μg of anti-D immunoglobulin is fully protective. However, one should proceed with extreme caution when CVS is requested by previously sensitized women: even very small quantities of Rh-positive cells could enhance immunization in high responders.[165] The possibility of CVS aggravating preexisting Rh isoimmunization seems to be confirmed by sporadic cases in previously sensitized women in whom a sharp increase of antibody titers and/or severe erythroblastosis fetalis early in gestation were observed after first-trimester CVS.[35,166]

Another concern about first-trimester CVS is whether this procedure might alter the results of MSAFP screening for neural tube defects (NTDs) at 15–18 weeks of gestation; but no significant difference has been observed when the median of the post-CVS MSAFP values determined at 8–15 days after sampling was compared with the unsampled population.[139] Moreover, no significant difference in MSAFP concentrations was found at 15–18 weeks between post-CVS patients and controls.[43,139,144,167] Therefore, CVS in the first trimester does not appear to complicate the detection of NTDs in the second trimester, and MSAFP screening of open NTDs should be considered as useful and reliable for post-CVS patients as for the general population.[167] (See also chapter 21.)

Perinatal Complications

Data on preterm birth, small-for-date neonates, low birth weight, and perinatal mortality are available from only a small number of clinical CVS studies,[39,42,46,47,51,53,56,57,156] and thus far, no increased frequency has been found when CVS cases were compared with a control population.[56] Similar expectations were confirmed by the trials comparing CVS and AC,[36,57,58,146,155,168] in which no significant increase in these complications was observed in the CVS group. The Canadian study[155] drew attention to the increase in the crude perinatal mortality rate after CVS. However, the difference was not statistically significant and was not found in the other national control studies.[36,58,146] Moreover, no differences were found between TC and TA sampling approaches[58–60] except for a significantly lower birth weight in the TC group reported in the U.S. trial[36]; a similar, but not significant difference was also seen in the Italian trial.[59]

Pediatric Follow-up

Data on pediatric follow-up of infants resulting from CVS pregnancies are available only from the reports of the Ashan and Milan groups.[169,170] The Chinese[169] reported the clinical evaluation of 53 of 66 babies born after blind transcervical biopsy of chorionic villi by a 3-mm outer diameter metal cannula.[21] All of the children were normally developed, and at the time of the study, the youngest was 9 years of age and the oldest was 14. In the Italian experience, 274 children in our transcervical CVS group were evaluated at 3–5 years of age for somatic and psychomotor development.[170] Chorionic tissue was aspirated by a plastic cannula with a 1.5-mm outer diameter under continuous ultrasonic visualization.[40] Growth retardation ≤ third percentile) was present in four cases; three infants were underweight and the fourth was found to have a small head. Psychomotor delay was present in six cases (3.3 percent): in one infant with global delay, microcephaly was also present; one infant with gross motor delay had been born prematurely; one infant with cerebral palsy had a pathologic neonatal course.

More recently,[166] 1,509 women with singleton pregnancies who underwent TC-CVS by biopsy forceps at about 10 gestation weeks were matched by random electronic selection with 1,509 women with singleton pregnancies who had undergone AC. Long-term outcome was obtained by questionnaire, including pediatric morbidity and complications of motor development, speech, hearing, and visual function. No significant differences between infants after CVS and AC were reported. These findings appear to provide reassuring evidence with respect to invasive prenatal procedures and suggest that neither CVS nor midtrimester AC has a demonstrable impact on a child's health and development.

Fetal Loss

Evaluation of the risks of CVS has mostly focused on the issue of spontaneous abortion. The overall pregnancy loss rate after CVS was reported in a number of relatively large series in the first[29,32,39–57] as well as in the second trimester,[61,65,67,171] and the rates ranged from 1.6 to 5.4 percent (see Table 5.3) and from 0.3 to 2.3 percent (see Table 5.5), respectively; differences reflected not only the operator's skill and experience but also the week of gestation at which the procedures were performed and the maternal age distribution. Several variables, both technical and biologic, make it hazardous to evaluate the rate of fetal loss due to the procedure. These critical aspects are apparent in the data of the CVS registry sponsored by the World Health Organization's Inherited Disease Programme and the March of Dimes Birth Defects Foundation, revealing a marked difference in fetal loss rate between those centers with the greatest experience and those with the least, as well as among different sampling methods.[148]

Knowledge of the natural history of pregnancy failure is vitally important to interpret the procedure-related fetal loss correctly. Spontaneous fetal loss rate is dependent on maternal age and on the gestational period. The residual loss rate at 11 and 12 weeks (the gestational age usually recommended for CVS) is still notable, and the values reported in the two major studies providing life tables is 5.8 percent and 4.7 percent and 3.4 percent and 3.0 percent for 88.9 percent and 94.8 percent of pregnant women less than 35 years of age, respectively.[172,173] Although loss rates of chromosomally abnormal fetuses are strongly dependent on maternal age,[174,175] the incidence of chromosomally normal abortions rises with advancing maternal age, possibly as a result of anatomical and functional impairment of the uterus.[176] Therefore, the background spontaneous loss rate increases with maternal age. Two other factors, such as gestational age selection for sampling and the procedure's learning curve, may significantly affect fetal loss rates after CVS (see Tables 5.2 and 5.5). A sharp decrease in loss rates has been demonstrated throughout the first trimester: the rates fall dramatically from 9–11 percent by the end of the eighth week to 1.5–4.7 percent by the end of the third month.[172] It is difficult to quantify the impact of the operator's experience and skill on the fetal loss rate; nonetheless, higher spontaneous abortion rates were noted in the initial reports, followed by a decline as the teams gained experience.[35,37,47,52,156,177,178] A significant amount of training is required to develop the appropriate skill, the learning rate for TA-CVS being faster than that for TC-CVS (see Table 5.1).[40,136,179] The first-attempt sampling success rate has been suggested to be a more appropriate indicator of the operator's skill.[179] In fact, the number of times the sampling device has to be introduced before succeeding in adequate tissue aspiration has been found to be a factor directly influencing the frequency of the overall loss rate.[35,41,49,52,177,179] However, no difference was observed when repeated sampling was limited to two insertions,[52,56] and significance was achieved only when a comparison was made between one attempt and three or more.[52]

Given so many technical and biologic confounding variables, it was agreed that only controlled studies could adequately determine the short- and long-term risks of CVS through a longitudinal study of two comparable cohorts of offspring.[98] Because it was unrealistic to find a control group not undergoing any invasive procedure for genetic diagnosis, the comparison of CVS with AC was chosen.[180]

Canadian Study

The first major prospective study by the Medical Research Council involved 2,787 women, 35 years of age or older, who were assigned randomly to CVS at 9–12 weeks or to AC at 15–17 weeks[155] (Table 5.8). All eleven centers taking part in the trial used an ultrasound-guided sampling approach using a 1.5- to 1.7-mm-diameter plastic catheter. No more than three catheter insertions were allowed, and the operator had to perform at least thirty procedures and be successful in twenty-three of twenty-five consecutive cases before being admitted to the study. AC was performed by standard technique, and the size of the needle diameter varied between 20 and 22 gauge. The study was designed to detect a hypothesized difference of 3 percent in overall loss rate between groups. The observed difference in the total fetal losses (miscarriages, terminations, and stillbirths) between the two groups (0.6 percent) was not statistically significant. The excess of losses in the CVS group appeared as a consequence of a higher, although not significant, perinatal mortality rate.

Table 5.8. Controlled trials of CVS and AC: study characteristics, fetal and neonatal outcome

Study		Number of Centers	Cases Sampled (number)		CVS/Center (average number)	Total Fetal Losses (%)		LRDs (number)	
			CVS	AC		CVS	AC	CVS	AC
Canadian[155]		11	1,169	1,174	108	7.6	7.0	0	0
U.S.[146]		7	2,235	671	325	7.2	5.7	0	0
Danish[58]		2							
	TA-CVS		1,027		513	6.3		0	
				1,042			6.4		1
	TC-CVS		1,010		505	10.9[a]		0	
MRC-Europeans[36]		31	1,609	1,594	52	13.6[b]	9.0	1	0
Finnish[168]		1	400	400	400	7.8	8.3	0	0
Spanish[181]		1	318	363	318	2.2	2.8	0	0

LRDs = limb-reduction defects.
[a] = significant difference between TC-CVS and AC as well as TA-CVS.
[b] = significant difference between CVS and AC.

U.S. Study

A prospective multicenter study was coordinated by the National Institute of Child Health and Human Development (NICHD), but the control group undergoing AC could not be randomized[146] (see Table 5.8). Eleven university centers contributed a total of 2,235 CVS, performed at 10.6 ($\pm$0.84) weeks, and 671 AC, performed at 16.2 ($\pm$0.6) weeks. Each operator was requested to have completed at least 10 sampling procedures before enrolling in the study. However, on the basis of the total number of CVS procedures performed in the study period (about 20 months), it is very likely that the operators' experiences varied considerably; three of seven centers performed about 1,000 cases a year, compared with 100–300 procedures in the remaining four centers. CVS was performed by TC aspiration, using a plastic catheter, which usually had an outside diameter of 1.5 mm; amniocentesis was performed by conventional ultrasound-guided 20- or 22-gauge needle insertion. The study protocol fixed a maximum of three catheter insertions per patient in one session. However, a fourth insertion was carried out in 0.6 percent of cases, whereas second and third insertions were necessary in 14.3 percent and 4.4 percent of cases, respectively.

Among the common minor complications observed during the 3 weeks after sampling were cramping, spotting, and bleeding, which were reported more frequently in the CVS group, and no statistical difference was found between groups for fluid leakage and fever. The rate of combined losses due to spontaneous abortions, terminations, stillbirths, and neonatal deaths in the CVS group exceeded that for the AC group by only 0.8 percent, and the difference did not reach statistical significance. However, this difference did not persist after considering the reduction (1 percent) in fetal loss rate observed between CVS sampling and 28 weeks reported in the following NICHD randomized comparison of TA- and TC-CVS.[60] This finding suggests that the operators' skill may increase and that the inherent safety of CVS and AC in experienced hands may be equivalent.[60]

No positive association was found between the fetal loss rate and the amount of villus tissue recovered, whereas three or four attempts per procedure were associated with a significantly increased rate of loss when compared with a single attempt (10.8 percent versus 2.9 percent). The higher rate of perinatal losses in the CVS group found in the Canadian study[155] was not confirmed.

MRC-European Study

Since 1985, the British Medical Research Council has sponsored a multicenter randomized study for evaluating the safety and accuracy of CVS (see Table 5.8). The study lasted for 4 years, and 3,248 patients were randomized in thirty-one centers from seven European countries.[36] Two centers contributed 800 and 424 cases, respectively, whereas the number of cases recruited to the trial by the remaining centers ranged between 4 and 81 cases. A center was eligible to take part if each participating obstetrician had performed at least 30 procedures and had obtained a success rate of at least 92 percent in the most recent cases. The sampling techniques used were a catheter and a biopsy forceps introduced via the cervical canal in 64 percent and 8 percent of cases, respectively, whereas 28 percent of cases were sampled by TA needling. The characteristics of the sampling devices were not specified. The single centers were permitted to use more than one sampling technique, but the actual rate of each was not reported.

The success rate at the first insertion was 69 percent for CVS and 94 percent for AC, and more than one insertion was needed for 31 percent of CVS cases and 6 percent of

AC cases to attain 95.2 percent and 98.2 percent of success rate, respectively. Vaginal bleeding after sampling was more frequently observed in the TA-CVS and TC-CVS groups than in the AC group (2 percent and 7 percent, respectively, versus less than 1 percent). Amniotic fluid leakage was reported in both AC (0.5 percent) and TC-CVS (0.4 percent) groups, whereas no cases of leakage followed TA-CVS.

The fetal loss rate was higher after CVS, and the difference between techniques (4.6 percent) was statistically significant. This reflected a higher rate of fetal deaths before 28 weeks, selective termination for chromosomal anomalies, and neonatal death. The increased number of fetal deaths was due to a preponderance of very immature live born infants in the CVS group. No clear differences in the rate of late pregnancy complications (duration of gestation, birth weight, malformations) were found.

Finnish Study

This was a single-center trial[168] and the patients were recruited from the greater Helsinki area (see Table 5.8). The cases in this study were all included in the MRC-European trial[36] and comprised its largest single group. The patients were eligible if ultrasound revealed a singleton live fetus between 9 and 11 weeks; reasons for exclusion were blood discharge and vaginal infection or in situ contraceptive device. All CVS procedures were performed the same day of the trial entry by one of four operators, having performed at least thirty CVSs with a sample of 10 mg or more, by transcervical aspiration using a plastic cannula with an outer diameter of 1.45 mm. No more than three cannula insertions were allowed during one session. AC was performed at 16 gestational weeks under ultrasound guidance with a 22-gauge spinal needle. Sampling was successful at the first attempt in 69 percent of CVS and 99 percent of AC, and a second (24 percent) or third (5 percent) insertion was necessary to aspirate an adequate amount of chorionic villi, giving an overall success rate of 98.3 percent. The total fetal loss rates throughout pregnancy did not differ between sampling techniques. A total of 7.8 percent of all fetuses were lost (miscarriages, terminations, stillbirths, neonatal deaths) in the CVS group and 8.3 percent in the AC group.

Danish Study

The randomized project of the University Hospital in Copenhagen[58] has been more ambitious than the studies previously described (see Table 5.8). The study was designed as a three-way randomization of women at low risk (mother aged 35 years or older or father at least 50 years of age, family history of or anxiety about numerical chromosomal abnormalities, more than three spontaneous abortions) to evaluate sampling success and risk differences not only between CVS and AC, but also between TC-CVS and TA-CVS techniques. Women at high risk (history of translocation, late termination for any reason, fetus at risk of metabolic disease) were randomized only between TA-CVS and TC-CVS techniques. A total of 3,997 were recruited; 918 were at high risk. Two centers contributed to the study, with 86.4 percent and 13.6 percent of cases; moreover, participating obstetricians had to have performed at least twenty successful samplings of chorionic villi and amniotic fluid, and one of them sampled 71 percent of cases. TC-CVS was performed by 1.45-mm plastic catheter with a maximum of two cervical passages. TA-CVS was performed with the double-needle system.[29] AC was performed under ultrasound guidance using a needle guide and a 20-gauge needle.

In the low-risk group, the sampling success rate at the first attempt was 96.0 percent for TC-CVS, 98.1 percent for TA-CVS, and 99.7 percent for AC, with a statistically significant trend. No significant differences in total fetal losses were seen between the TA-CVS and AC groups (6.3 percent versus 6.4 percent), whereas the difference was significant when considering the TC-CVS group (10.9 percent). Within the TC-CVS group, the fetal loss rate was higher in the series of cases with 10 mg or less of chorionic tissue aspirated, but this was not so in the TA-CVS group. This fact was explained by a higher number of technically more complicated cases, in which more substantial manipulation of the uterus was probably necessary; the authors' preference is clearly expressed for the TA approach, giving better access to the placental site than TC sampling. After sampling, amniotic fluid leakage was reported in 0.6 percent, 0.5 percent, and 2.8 percent of cases ($p < 0.001$); spotting in 7.3 percent, 3.2 percent, and 1.9 percent of cases ($p < 0.001$); and bleeding in 8.6 percent, 4.7 percent, and 1.2 percent of cases ($p < 0.001$) for TC-CVS, TA-CVS, and AC, respectively. No differences between techniques were observed for stillbirths, neonatal deaths, and malformations.

Spanish Study

A 13-month-long trial comparing TA-CVS by a 1.9-mm-diameter forceps and AC by a 22-gauge spinal needle was more recently launched by the Prenatal Diagnosis Unit of the Hospital Clinic, University of Barcelona (see Table 5.8).[181] CVS was performed between 9 and 13 weeks of pregnancy, while AC ranged from 15 to 18 weeks. In both cases, continuous ultrasound visualization was used. Of the 1562 pregnant women requesting prenatal diagnosis, only 1011 were randomly allocated to one of the two sampling methods. However, withdrawal was recorded in about 28 percent in both groups, allowing randomized sampling in 318 and 363 cases in CVS and AC, respectively. The trial was discontinued when a second-trimester maternal serum biochemical Down syndrome screening policy was implemented in the same institution, precluding further randomization. The diagnostic success rate was 98 percent and 100 percent in the CVS and AC groups, respectively. No statistical difference was observed by comparing total spontaneous postprocedure fetal loss rates up to one week after birth: 2.2 percent in the CVS group and 2.8 percent in the AC group. Thus, the authors concluded that first-trimester TC-CVS by biopsy forceps should be considered as safe as AC.

CONTROVERSY OVER LIMB-REDUCTION DEFECTS

In early 1991, Firth et al.,[182] at the John Radcliffe Maternity Hospital, Oxford, U.K., reported an unusual cluster of four children with limb-reduction defects (LRDs) and oromandibular hypogenesis among 289 pregnancies in which TA-CVS was performed at 8.0–9.3 weeks of gestation. Samples were collected by way of an 18-gauge spinal needle under continuous ultrasound control. Three obstetricians did the CVS procedures (each had a case of limb abnormalities), and their sampling performance was based on an average of 60 CVSs per year. Subsequently, two other clusters of four LRD cases were reported.[81,183] In Milan, at Mangiagalli University Clinic, four severe LRDs, two of which were within the oromandibular-limb hypogenesis spectrum disorders, were detected early in the second trimester by ultrasound or observed at birth among 263 pregnancies intending to continue after the diagnosis of a fetus with a normal karyotype.[81] Sampling was performed at 6–7.6 weeks of gestation by freehand insertion of a 20- or a 22-gauge 9-cm-long spinal needle under continuous ultrasound surveillance.[28] LRD cases were reported only in cases sampled by a 20-gauge needle at 7 weeks of gestation. In Chicago, at Humana Hospital–Michael Reese, four transverse distal defects, including hypoplasia and absence of the fingers and toes, were observed among the 391 infants surviving after CVS was performed between 9 and 12 weeks. TC-CVS was performed in 58 percent of cases, in 39 percent by TA-CVS, and in the remaining cases both techniques were used.[183] In the three LRD cases, the TC procedure was performed using a catheter 19-mm in outer diameter, whereas the fourth case was observed after a TA-CVS performed using an 18-gauge (outer diameter, 1.24 mm) needle. In addition, in Taiwan, limb defects with and without CVS were surveyed by sending a questionnaire to 165 major obstetric units.[184] A total of 1,362 CVS procedures were performed in 1 year in the 67 hospitals, giving an average rate per unit and per year of 20 CVSs. The rate of LRD cases observed in the CVS population was significantly higher than in the general population (0.294 percent versus 0.032 percent). No information was made available on the sampling technique and precise weeks of pregnancy.

Recently, the Center for Genetics, Fetal, and Maternal Medicine at MCP Hahnemann University, Philadelphia, reported a case of total absence of lower limbs in one infant sampled at a CRL of 12 mm (7.3 weeks) by four attempts of TC catheter aspiration.[83] This case is one of the eighty-two CVSs performed in a 10-year program of very early genetic diagnosis offered to Orthodox Jewish patients. The mentioned reports on LRD clusters have some characteristics in common—early or very early gestation sampling,[81,83,182–184] poor operator expertise,[182–184] improper sampling device,[182–184] or wrong methodologic approach[81,83]—and each might have been a determinant factor of uncommon placental trauma. It is of some speculative relevance to remark that at the time of the four first reports[81,182–184] an unusual cluster of five severe LRDs was observed among approximately 300 live born infants at the University Hospital of Rotterdam, in the very short period of 44 days.[185] No single common cause was identified. A variety of factors were indicated as a potential teratogen in limb development, and in the only case undergoing CVS, sampling was performed at 12.2 weeks of gestation and the patient used a local nasal decongestant (xylometazoline). This agent, also used by one other patient, acts through vasoconstriction and probably passes through the placenta. This may imply that CVS may occasionally have systemic effects on the fetal circulation, resulting in teratogenic consequences.

When CVS is performed at a time (before 9–10 weeks) when the conceptus has the highest sensitivity to teratogenic agents, excessive trauma to the placenta and surrounding tissue could cause abnormalities during the phenocritical stage of embryologic development. Although no fetal hemodynamic changes have been observed after CVS,[65,186–188] direct hysteroscopic observations in pregnancies at 8–12 weeks being terminated immediately after intentionally vigorous placental trauma with a blunt instrument showed ecchymotic lesions on the head, face, and thorax of the fetus, and these findings were interpreted as the effects of placental trauma, supporting the view that extensive placental damage may be complicated by fetal lesions.[189] Several hypotheses regarding the pathogenesis of teratogenic effects of CVS have been proposed, the most probable concerning thromboembolism,[190] vasoconstriction,[191] and antibody-mediated reactions following maternofetal transfusion.[192,193] These hypotheses have the end-artery disruption theory in common: each developing limb has only one supporting artery before 10 gestational weeks; therefore, if end arteries are obstructed or constricted, or if immunologic factors damage the endothelium of end arteries, degeneration of the dependent tissues may follow.[194]

A burst of reports supporting or denying any association between LRDs and CVS followed.[195–206] Three case–control studies are available.[196,203,204] An investigation was made in seven European Registration of Congenital Anomalies and Twins (EUROCAT) registries, surveying a total of 607,996 births.[203] The exposure rate among cases of limb reduction was compared with the exposure rate among other anomalies and produced an odds ratio of 1.8, indicating that the risk was not significant. A population-based, multistate case–control study of limb deficiencies after CVS was developed in collaboration with the Centers for Disease Control, Atlanta.[205] One hundred thirty-one case–control pairs were drawn from a population of 421,489 births to women younger than 34 years of age. Information was obtained on 83 percent of subjects and 78 percent of control subjects. Seven of forty-six infants with transverse terminal deficiencies were exposed to CVS, and the defects were confined to the digits: five were missing only digital phalanges, whereas the only two cases of oromandibular-limb hypogenesis were exposed to amniocentesis. The overall risk for LRD after CVS was slightly but not significantly elevated, compared with the control population, whereas an association was found for all transverse digital deficiencies, giving a risk of 0.03 percent after CVS. However, difficulties of ascertainment and methodologic errors have raised criticism of this study, and it has also been suggested that a correct ascertainment might move findings of borderline significance into the nonsignificant range.[207] The same criticism is valuable for the case–control study performed in the Italian Multicentric Birth Defect Registry, which reported an elevenfold increase for TLDs in the cases exposed to CVS.[196] This strong association may be explained by the fact that half of the case subjects with LRDs underwent CVS before 8 complete weeks. Moreover, a major potential limitation of this study needs to be considered. The registry is hospital-based, and the unequal distribution of the contributing hospitals in the country may not be representative of the CVS cases.

A WHO statement based on the analysis of 76,476 cases with complete follow-up and referred to the WHO-CVS registry[25] did not find any evidence to suggest an increased risk of LRDs when CVS was performed after the eighth completed gestational week. These conclusions were confirmed by an updated analysis of the accumulated experience of 138,996 cases of the registry,[209] and more recently of 208,682 cases[24] (Table 5.9): the overall incidence of LRDs after CVS ranged between 5.7 and 5.08 per 10,000, compared with 5.2 and 6.2 in the general population[209–211] (see Table 5.9). In agreement with the

Table 5.9. Frequency of limb-reduction defects (LRDs) found in the major cohort CVS studies and congenital malformation registries

Source	Number of CVS Cases Intending to Continue	Number of Livebirths	Rate per 10,000
Thomas Jefferson University, Philadelphia[24]	13,629		4.4
Mangiagalli Clinic, University of Milan, and Prenatal Diagnosis Center*	16,597		3.0
Univ. of California, San Francisco[24]	10,386		6.7
Genetics and IVF Institute, Fairfax[24]	14,492		2.7
Pellegrin University Hospital, Bordeaux[57]	10,144		1.0
U.S. Collaborative Study[208]	76,476		4.3
WHO-CVS Registry[207]	138,996		5.7
WHO-CVS Registry[24]	208,682		5.08
Swedish Registry[209]		1,368,024	6.2
British Columbia Registry[210]		1,213,913	6.0
Italian Birth Defect Registry[211]		1,115,361	6.2
South America Registry[212]		2,917,074	5.2

*Including 10,900 previously reported cases, 1997.[56]

conclusions of the analysis of the WHO-CVS registry data, no increase in transverse LRD frequency was apparent in the five major single-center CVS experiences, four of which reported in the WHO-CVS registry[24] (see Table 5.9). Moreover, the overall rate of congenital anomalies in our study[56] was similar (1.96 percent versus 1.90 percent) to that reported in the Italian national hospital-based registry of malformations.[56,211] A special effort was made to apply to CVS cases the same classification criteria used by the Italian Birth Defects Registry (IPIMC); hospital or pediatrician reports were requested for pattern analysis of the major anomalies. When frequencies between our experience and that of the IPIMC were compared, no significant differences were observed, including LRDs (4.34/10,000 versus 6.16/10,000). These figures were confirmed in our experience until December 2001: the rate of LRDs observed on 16,597 consecutive CVS performed at 8 weeks or more was 3.01/10,000 (Table 5.10) (Brambati et al., unpublished data). The only significant differences with IPIMC were observed for polydactyly, diaphragmatic hernia, and vascular birthmarks (see Table 5.10). No explanations are available for the lower rate of polydactyly and diaphragmatic hernia in the CVS series. A slight but significantly higher frequency of congenital vascular birthmarks was found in the study group compared with the mean Italian population rate (0.152 percent versus 0.0702 percent, $p < 0.05$). However, the wide range of frequencies for the anomaly in different Italian regions (0.0114–0.1812 percent) would suggest that this finding may reflect the difficulty of discriminating between vascular malformations and hemangiomas, whenever the latter display a rapid postnatal proliferating phase. Our results cannot confirm the high rate in vascular birthmarks (21.1 percent) observed in a previous study,[212] in which unfortunately no distinction was made between malformations and vascular tumors (i.e., hemangiomas).[213]

Firth et al.[214] claimed a possible correlation between 75 LRDs and gestational age at CVS in an analysis of published data. Unfortunately, the diversity in the LRD classification between this study and the population-based registry used for comparison,[214] and the several erroneous duplications of LRD cases in the table listing details of the cases, make the conclusions of the study unreliable. In fact, the analysis by standardized methods of 77 infants or fetuses with limb defects from 138,996 pregnancies having CVS and reported to the WHO CVS registry was unable to confirm any correlation between gestational age at CVS and severity of defects.[215] Moreover, these results did not show any differences from the background population in the overall frequency or pattern distribution of limb deficiencies.

CONCLUSIONS

Important studies have been published and more are in progress aimed at understanding the pathophysiologic basis of hypothetical risks attributed to CVS. Notwithstanding these efforts, experienced centers have demonstrated that no significant adverse effects on the fetus should be expected from CVS when established methodologic prerequisites and timing of sampling are followed.

The transabdominal sampling technique, in our experience, has become the method of choice. Our preference for this approach has been based on a number of reasons: shorter learning time, lower rate of immediate complications, higher practicality and success rate at the first device insertion, no hazard of intrauterine infection, opportunity to extend sampling beyond the first trimester, and a wider range of diagnostic indications. However, it is plainly advisable that a complementary approach, namely transcervical or transvaginal sampling, should be mastered for appropriate chorion biopsy in any case. The high efficiency, the absence of complications after sampling, and the very low total abortion rate observed after 12

Table 5.10. Malformations detected in utero or at birth in 16,597 consecutive pregnancies intending to continue and undergoing CVS at Mangiagalli Clinic, University of Milan and Prenatal Diagnosis Center, Milan, compared to background incidence based on the Italian Birth Defects Registry (IPIMC) (144)*

Malformation	Cases (number)	This Study Rate/10,000	Rates IPIMC Rate/10,000	Rate Difference
Heart				
Total	58	34.94	27.28	N.S.
Ventral septal defect/atrial septal defect	33			
Pulmonary stenosis/atresia	5			
Cardiac malformation associated with other system malformations	3			
Others	17			
Gastrointestinal tract				
Total	7			
Esophageal atresia	5	4.21	2.86	N.S.
Hirschsprung diseases	2			
Neural tube defects				
Total	10			
Anencephaly	5	3.01	2.56	N.S.
Spina bifida	4	2.41	3.78	N.S.
Encephalocele	1	0.60	1.05	N.S.
Lungs				
Total	1			
Congenital cystic adenomatoid malformations	1			
Face/ear				
Total	27			
Cleft lip/palate	11	6.62	6.80	N.S.
Others	12			
Urogenital system				
Total	27			
Ureteropelvic junction defect	9			
Renal agenesis	3	1.81	1.60	N.S.
Cystic kidneys	5	3.01	2.52	N.S
Hypospadias	17	10.24	18.40	N.S
Others	9			
Abdominal defects				
Total	6			
Diaphragmatic hernia	3	1.81	2.66	($p < 0.25$)
Omphalocele	3	1.81	1.83	N.S.
Central nervous system				
Total	15			
Hydrocephalus	5	3.01	3.56	N.S.
Others	10			
Skin				
Total	31			
Vascular birthmarks	23	13.85	7.02	($p < .05$)
Others	8			
Miscellaneous				
Total	31			
Skeletal dysplasia				
Total	48			
Club foot	26	15.33	12.61	N.S.
Syndactyly[a]	4	2.41	3.17	N.S.
Polydactyly	4	2.41	8.61	($p < .01$)
Hip dysplasia	14			
Limb-reduction defects				
Total	5	3.01	6.16	N.S.
TLRDs	4	2.41	3.28[b]	N.S.

Note: CVS was performed by a single operator at eight or more gestational weeks.

N.S. = not significant. TLRDs = transverse limb-reduction defects.

[a]Between second and third toes excluded.

[b]Mastroiacovo et al., 1992.[128]

*These figures include previously published cases (15).

gestation weeks have made the use of CVS in the second trimester a valuable alternative to early and midtrimester amniocentesis, even in a population at low genetic risk.

Critical analysis of the literature demonstrates that where experience and skill are available, first-trimester CVS should be the gold standard for prenatal diagnosis. Given the promising developments (see also chapter 22) of biochemical markers in maternal blood[216,217,219] and fetal sonographic signs[218,219] for first-trimester screening for aneuploidies, the use of CVS for prompt and reliable diagnosis seems assured.

REFERENCES

1. Nicolaides K, Brizot Mde L, Patel F, et al. Comparison of chorionic villus sampling and amniocentesis for fetal karyotyping at 10–13 weeks' gestation. Lancet 1994;344:435.
2. Sundberg K, Bang J, Smidt-Jensen S, et al. Randomised study of risk of fetal loss related to early amniocentesis versus chorionic villus sampling. Lancet 1997;350:697.
3. Nagel HTC, Vandenbussche FPHA, Keirse MJNC, et al. Amniocentesis before 14 completed weeks as an alternative to transabdominal chorionic villus sampling: a controlled trial with infant follow-up. Prenat Diagn 1998;18:465.
4. The Canadian Early and Mid-Trimester Amniocentesis Trial (CEMAT) Group. Randomised trial to assess safety and fetal outcome of early and midtrimester amniocentesis. Lancet 1998;351:242.
5. Adinolfi M, Davics A, Sharif S, et al. Detection of trisomy 18 and Y-derived sequences in fetal nucleated cells obtained by transcervical flushing. Lancet 1993;342:403.
6. Adinolfi M, Sherlock J, Soothill P, et al. Molecular evidence of fetal-derived chromosome 21 markers (STRs) in transcervical samples. Prenat Diagn 1995;15:35.
7. Overton TG, Lighten AD, Fisk NM, et al. Prenatal diagnosis by minimally invasive first-trimester transcervical sampling is unreliable. Am J Obstet Gynecol 1996;175:382.
8. Bianchi DW, Simpson JL, Jackson LG, et al. Fetal gender and aneuploidy detection using fetal cells in maternal blood: analysis of NIFTY I data. Prenat Diagn 2002;22:609.
9. Bischoff FZ, Hahn S, Johnson KL, et al. Intact fetal cells in maternal plasma. are they really there? Lancet 2003;361:139.
10. Old JM, Ward RHT, Karagozlu F, et al. First-trimester fetal diagnosis for haemoglobinopathies: three cases. Lancet 1982;2:1414.
11. Brambati B, Simoni G. Fetal diagnosis of trisomy 21 in the first trimester of pregnancy. Lancet 1983;1:586.
12. Thomassen-Brepols LJ. Psychological aspects of prenatal diagnosis. In: Hicks EK, Berg JM, eds. The genetics of mental retardation. Boston: Kluwer Academic, 1988:45.
13. Spencer JW, Cox DN. Emotional responses of pregnant women to chorionic villi sampling or amniocentesis. Am J Obstet Gynecol 1987;157:1155.
14. Spencer JW, Cox DN. A comparison of chorionic villi sampling and amniocentesis: acceptability of procedure and maternal attachment to pregnancy. Obstet Gynecol 1988;72:714.
15. McCormack MJ, Rylance ME, Mackenzie WE, et al. Patients? attitudes following chorionic villus sampling. Prenat Diagn 1990;10:253.
16. Abramsky L, Rodeck CH. Women's choices for fetal chromosome analysis. Prenat Diagn 1991;11:23.
17. Cao A, Cossu P, Monni G, et al. Chorionic villus sampling and acceptance rate of prenatal diagnosis. Prenat Diagn 1987;7:531.
18. Cutillo DM, Hammond EA, Reeser SL, et al. Chorionic villus sampling utilization following reports of a possible association with fetal limb defects. Prenat Diagn 1994;14:327.
19. Tului L, Brambati B. Patient acceptability of first trimester prenatal diagnosis. Riv Ostet Ginecol 1990;2:129.
20. Mohr J. Foetal genetic diagnosis: development of techniques for early sampling of foetal cells. Acta Pathol Microbiol Scand 1968;73:73.
21. Ashan, Department of Obstetrics and Gynecology, Tietung Hospital of Ashan Iron and Steel Co., Ashan, China. Fetal sex prediction by sex chromatin of chorionic villi cells during early pregnancy. Chin Med J 1975;1:117.
22. Kazy Z, Rozovsky IS, Bakharev VA. Chorion biopsy in early pregnancy: a method of early prenatal diagnosis for inherited disorders. Prenat Diagn 1982;2:39.
23. WHO Working Group. Fetal diagnosis of hereditary diseases. Bull WHO 1984;62:345.
24. Jackson L. Personal communication, 1997.

25. Kuliev AM, Modell B, Jackson L, et al. Risk evaluation of CVS. Prenat Diagn 1993;13:197.

26. Lundsteen C, Vejerslev LO. Prenatal diagnosis in Denmark, Eur J Hum Genet 1997;5 (Suppl 1):14.

27. Tharapel AT, Elias S, Shulman LP, et al. Resorbed co-twin as an explanation for discrepant chorionic villus results: Non-mosaic 47,XX,+16 in villi (direct and culture) with normal (46,XX) amniotic fluid and neonatal blood. Prenat Diagn 1989;9:467.

28. Brambati B, Oldrini A, Lanzani A. Transabdominal chorionic villus sampling: a freehand ultrasound-guided technique. Am J Obstet Gynecol 1987;157:134.

29. Smidt-Jensen S, Hahnemann N. Danish experience. In: Liu DTW, Symonds EM, Golbus MS, eds. Chorion villus sampling. London: Chapman and Hall, 1987:145.

30. Ward RHT, Modell B, Petrou M, et al. A method for chorionic villus sampling in the first trimester of pregnancy under real time ultrasonic guidance. BMJ 1983;286:1542.

31. Dumez Y, Dommergues M. Chorionic villus sampling using rigid forceps under ultrasound control. In: Pescia G, Nguyen The H, eds. Chorionic villus sampling (CVS). Basel: Karger, 1986:22.

32. Lunshof S, Boer K, Leschot NJ, et al. Pregnancy outcome after transcervical CVS with flexible biopsy forceps: evaluation of risk factors. Prenat Diagn 1995;15:809.

33. Sidransky E, Black SH, Soenksen DM, et al. Transvaginal chorionic villus sampling. Prenat Diagn 1990;10:583.

34. Jackson L. CVS latest news. Philadelphia: WHO-CVS Registry, January 28, 1991.

35. Brambati B, Oldrini A, Ferrazzi E, et al. Chorionic villus sampling: an analysis of the obstetric experience of 1000 cases. Prenat Diagn 1987;7:157.

36. MRC Working Party on the Evaluation of Chorionic Villus Sampling. Medical Research Council European trial of chorionic villus sampling. Lancet 1991;337:1491.

37. Jackson LG, Wapner RJ. Risks of chorion villus sampling. Baillières Clin Obstet Gynaecol 1987;1:513.

38. Report of a WHO Consultation on first Trimester Fetal Diagnosis. Risk evaluation in chorionic villus sampling. Prenat Diagn 1986;6:451.

39. Hogge WA, Schonberg SA, Golbus MS. Chorion villus sampling: experience of the first 1000 cases. Am J Obstet Gynecol 1986;154:1249.

40. Brambati B, Lanzani A, Tului L. Transabdominal and transcervical chorionic villus sampling: efficiency and risk evaluation. Am J Med Genet 1990;35:160.

41. Wade RV, Young SR. Analysis of fetal loss after transcervical chorionic villus sampling: a review of 719 patients. Am J Obstet Gynecol 1989;161:513.

42. Jackson LG, Wapner RA, Barr MA. Safety of chorionic villus biopsy. Lancet 1986;1:674.

43. Green JE, Dorfmann A, Jones SL, et al. Chorionic villus sampling: experience with an initial 940 cases. Obstet Gynecol 1988;71:208.

44. Wass DM, Brown GA, Warren PS, et al. Completed follow-up of 1,000 consecutive transcervical chorionic villus samplings performed by a single operator. Aust NZ J Obstet Gynaecol 1991;31:240.

45. Donner C, Simon Ph, Karioun A, et al. Experience with 1251 transcervical chorionic villus samplings performed in the first trimester by a single team of operators. Eur J Obstet Gynecol Reprod Biol 1995;60:45.

46. Jahoda MGJ, Pijpers L, Reuss A, et al. Evaluation of transcervical chorionic villus sampling with a completed follow-up of 1550 consecutive pregnancies. Prenat Diagn 1989;9:621.

47. Leschot NJ, Wolf H, van Prooijen-Knegt, et al. Cytogenetic findings in 1250 chorionic villus samples obtained in the first trimester with clinical follow-up of the first 1000 pregnancies. Br J Obstet Gynaecol 1989;96:663.

48. Miny P, Basaran S, Pawlowitzki IH, et al. Validity of cytogenetic analysis from trophoblast tissue throughout gestation. Am J Med Genet 1989;33:136.

49. Evans M, Drugan A, Koppitch III FC, et al. Genetic diagnosis in the first trimester: the norm for the 1990s. Am J Obstet Gynecol 1989;160:1332.

50. Wass DM, Brown GA, Warren PS, et al. Complete follow-up of 1,000 consecutive chorionic villus samplings performed by a single operator. Aust NZ J Obstet Gynaecol 1991;31:240.

51. Bovicelli L, Rizzo N, Montacuti V, et al. Transabdominal villus sampling: analysis of 350 consecutive cases. Prenat Diagn 1988;8:495.

52. Williams III J, Wang BB, Rubin CH, et al. Chorionic villus sampling: experience with 3016 cases performed by a single operator. Obstet Gynecol 1992;80:1023.

53. Jackson L, Wapner RJ. Chorionic villus sampling. In: Simpson JL, Elias S, eds. Essentials of prenatal diagnosis. New York: Churchill Livingstone, 1993:45.

54. Palo P, Piiroinen O, Honkonen E, et al. Transabdominal chorionic villus sampling and amniocentesis for prenatal diagnosis: five years' experience at a university centre. Prenat Diagn 1994;14:157.

55. Chueh JT, Goldberg JM, Wohlferd MM, et al. Comparison of transcervical and transabdominal chorionic

villus sampling loss rates in nine thousand cases from a single center. Am J Obstet Gynecol 1995;173: 1277.

56. Brambati B, Tului L, Cislaghi C, et al. First 10,000 chorionic villus samplings performed on singleton pregnancies by a single operator. Prenat Diagn 1997;18:255.

57. Brun J-L, Mangione R, Gangho F, et al. Feasibility, accuracy and safety of chorionic villus sampling: a report of 10,741 cases. Prenat Diagn 2003;23:295.

58. Smidt-Jensen S, Permin M, Philip J, et al. Randomised comparison of amniocentesis and transabdominal and transcervical chorionic villus sampling. Lancet 1992;340:1237.

59. Brambati B, Terzian E, Tognoni G. Randomized clinical trial of transabdominal versus transcervical chorionic villus sampling methods. Prenat Diagn 1991;11:285.

60. Jackson LG, Zachary JM, Fowler SE, et al. A randomized comparison of transcervical and transabdominal chorionic villus sampling. N Engl J Med 1992;327:594.

61. Monni G, Ibba RM, Olla G, et al. Prenatal diagnosis of beta-thalassemia by second trimester chorionic villus sampling. Prenat Diagn 1988;8:495.

62. Jahoda MGJ, Pijpers L, Reuss A, et al. Transabdominal villus sampling in early second trimester: A safe sampling method for women of advanced age. Prenat Diagn 1990;10:307.

63. Holzgreve W, Miny P, Schloo R, et al. "Late CVS Registry": compilation of data from 24 centres. Prenat Diagn 1990;10:159.

64. Chieri PR, Aldini AJR. Feasibility of placental biopsy in the second trimester for fetal diagnosis. Am J Obstet Gynecol 1989;160:581.

65. Podobnik M, Ciglar S, Singer Z, et al. Transabdominal chorionic villus sampling in the second and third trimesters of high-risk pregnancies. Prenat Diagn 1997;17:125.

66. Camerun AD, Murphy KW, McNay MB, et al. Midtrimester chorionic villus sampling: An alternative approach? Am J Obstet Gynecol 1994;171:1035.

67. Brambati B, Tului L, Camurri L, et al. Early second trimester (13 to 20 weeks) transabdominal chorionic villus sampling (TA-CVS): a safe alternative method for both high and low risk populations. Prenat Diagn 2002;22:907.

68. Bryan EM. Twins and higher multiple births: a guide to their nature and nurture. London: Edward Arnold, 1992.

69. Little J, Thompson B. Descriptive epidemiology. In: MacGillivray I, Campbell DM, Thompson B, eds. Twinning and twins. Chichester: John Wiley, 1988:37.

70. Landy HJ, Keith L, Keith D. The vanishing twin. Acta Genet Med Gemellol 1982;31:179.

71. Blumenfeld Z, Dirnfeld M, Abramovici H, et al. Spontaneous fetal reduction in multiple gestations assessed by transvaginal ultrasound. Br J Obstet Gynaecol 1992;99:333.

72. Testart J, Plachot M, Mandelbaum J, et al. World collaborative report on IVF-ET and GIFT: 1989 results. Hum Reprod 1992;7:362.

73. Brambati B, Tului L, Lanzani A, et al. First-trimester diagnosis in multiple pregnancy: principles and potential pitfalls. Prenat Diagn 1991;11:767.

74. Sepulveda W, Sebire NJ, Hughes K, et al. The lambda sign at 10–14 weeks of gestation as a predictor of chronicity in twin pregnancies. Ultrasound Obstet Gynecol 1996;7:421.

75. Brambati B, Tului L, Guercilena S, et al. Outcome of first-trimester chorionic villus sampling for genetic investigation in multiple pregnancy. Ultrasound Obstet Gynecol 2001;17:209.

76. Evans MI, Goldberg JD, Dommergues M, et al. Efficacy of second-trimester selective termination for fetal abnormalities: international collaborative experience among the world's largest centers. Am J Obstet Gynecol 1994;171:90.

77. Pergament E, Schulman JD, Copeland K, et al. The risk and efficacy of chorionic villus sampling in multiple gestations. Prenat Diagn 1992;12:377.

78. Wapner RJ, Johnson A, Davis G, et al. Prenatal diagnosis in twin gestations: a comparison between second-trimester amniocentesis and first-trimester chorionic villus sampling. Obstet Gynecol 1993;82:49.

79. De Catte L, Liebaers I, Foulon W, et al. First trimester chorionic villus sampling in twin gestations. Am J Perinatol 1996;13:413.

80. Aytoz A, De Catte L, Camus M, et al. Obstetric outcome after prenatal diagnosis in pregnancies obtained after intracytoplasmic sperm injection. Hum Reprod 1998;13:2958.

81. Brambati B, Simoni G, Travi M, et al. Genetic diagnosis by chorionic villus sampling before 8 gestational weeks: efficiency, reliability, and risks in 317 completed pregnancies. Prenat Diagn 1992;12:789.

82. Minelli A, Piantanida M, Simoni G, et al. Prenatal diagnosis of metabolic diseases on chorionic villi obtained before the ninth week of pregnancy. Prenat Diagn 1992;12:959.

83. Wapner RJ, Evans MI, Davis G, et al. Procedural risks versus theology: chorionic villus sampling for Orthodox Jews at less than 8 weeks' gestation. Am J Obstet Gynecol 2002;186:1133.

84. Borrell A, Costa D, Delgado RD, et al. Transcervical chorionic villus sampling beyond 12 weeks of gestation. Ultrasound Obstet Gynecol 1996;7:416.

85. Brambati B, Anelli MC, Tului L. Prenatal cystic fibrosis screening in a low-risk population undergoing chorionic villus sampling for fetal karyotyping. Clin Genet 1996;50:23.

86. Di Cola G, Gallo P, Anelli MC, et al. PCR analysis of CGG trinucleotide repeat of FMR-1 gene in first trimester chorionic villi samples (abstract). Am J Hum Genet 1996;59(4 Suppl):A320.

87. Black SH, Bick DP, Maddalena A, et al. Pregnancy screening of cystic fibrosis in low-risk population. Lancet 1993;342:1112.

88. Schwartz M, Brandt NJ, Skovby F. Screening for carriers of cystic fibrosis among pregnant women: a pilot study. Eur J Hum Genet 1993;1:239.

89. Kalousek DK, Dill FJ. Chromosomal mosaicism confined to the placenta in human conceptions. Science 1983;221:665.

90. Simoni G, Gimelli G, Cuoco C, et al. Discordance between prenatal cytogenetic diagnosis after chorionic villus sampling and chromosomal constitution of the fetus. In: Fraccaro M, Simoni G, Brambati B, eds. First trimester fetal diagnosis, Berlin: Springer Verlag, 1985:137.

91. Ledbetter DH, Zachary JM, Simpson JL, et al. Cytogenetic results from the U.S. Collaborative Study on CVS. Prenat Diagn (special issue) 1992;12:317.

92. Association of Clinical Cytogeneticists Working Party on Chorionic Villi in Prenatal Diagnosis. Cytogenetic analysis of chorionic villi for prenatal diagnosis: an ACC collaborative study of U.K. data. Prenat Diagn 1994;14:363.

93. Hahnemann JM and Vejerslev LO. European Collaborative Research on Mosaicism in CVS (EUCROMIC): fetal and extrafetal cell lineages in 192 gestations with CVS mosaicism involving single autosomal trisomy. Am J Med Genet 1997;70:179.

94. Vejerslev LO, Mikkelsen M. The European collaborative study on mosaicism in chorionic villus sampling: data from 1986 to 1987. Prenat Diagn 1989;9:575.

95. Markert CL, Petters RM, Manufactured hexaparental mice show that adults are derived from three embryonic cells. Science 1978;202:56.

96. Simoni G, Sirchia M. Confined placental mosaicism. Prenat Diagn 1994;14:1185.

97. Kalousek DK. Confined placental mosaicism and intrauterine human development. Acta Med Auxol 1991;23:201.

98. Engel E, De Lozier-Blanchet CD. Uniparental disomy, isodisomy and imprinting: probable effects in man and strategies for their detection. Am J Med Genet 1991;40:432.

99. Spence EJ, Perciaccante RG, Greig GM, et al. Uniparental disomy as a mechanism for human genetic disease. Am J Hum Genet 1988;42:217.

100. Voss R, Ben-Simon E, Avital A, et al. Isodisomy of chromosome 7 in a patient with cystic fibrosis: could uniparental disomy be common in humans? Am J Hum Genet 1989;45:373.

101. Kalousek DK, Langlois S, Barrett I, et al. Uniparental disomy for chromosome 16 in humans. Am J Hum Genet 1993;52:8.

102. Wolstenholme J, Rooney DE and Davison EV. Confined placental mosaicism, IUGR, and adverse pregnancy outcome: a controlled retrospective U.K. collaborative survey. Prenat Diagn 1994;14:345.

103. Post JG, Nijhuis JG. Trisomy 16 confined to the placenta. Prenat Diagn 1992;12:1001.

104. Fryburg JS, Dimaio MS, Mahoney J. Post-natal placental confirmation of trisomy 2 and trisomy 16 detected at chorionic villus sampling: a possible association with intrauterine growth retardation and elevated maternal serum alpha-fetoprotein. Prenat Diagn 1992;12:157.

105. Johnson A, Wapner RJ, Davis GH, et al. Mosaicism in chorionic villus sampling: an association with poor perinatal outcome. Obstet Gynecol 1990;75:573.

106. Bryan J, Peters M, Pritchard G, et al. A second case of intrauterine growth retardation and primary hypospadias associated with trisomy 22 placenta but with biparental inheritance of chromosome 22 in the fetus. Prenat Diagn 2002;22:137.

107. Yeo L, Fisher A, Ranzini A, et al. Unique prenatal sonographic features of mosaic tetraploidy: 3 case histories. Am J Hum Genet 1977;61 (Suppl):A 166.

108. Stioui S, De Silvestris M, Molinari A, et al. Trisomic 22 placenta in a case of severe intrauterine growth retardation. Prenat Diagn 1989;9:673.

109. Wang BBT and Williams J III. Effect of confined placental mosaicism for trisomy 16 on fetal growth. Appl Cytogenet 1992;18:197.

110. Reddy KS, Blakemore KJ, Stetten G, et al. The significance of trisomy 7 mosaicism in chorionic villus culture. Prenat Diagn 1990;10:417.

111. Wapner RJ, Simpsom JL, Golbus MS, et al. Chorionic mosaicism: association with fetal loss but not with adverse perinatal outcome. Prenat Diagn 1992;12:347.

112. Kalousek DK, Howard-Peebles PN, Olson SB, et al. Confirmation of CVS mosaicism in term placentae and high frequency of intrauterine growth retardation association with confined placental mosaicism. Prenat Diagn 1991;11:743.

113. Schwinger E, Seidl E, Klink F, Rehder H. Chromosome mosaicism of the placenta: a cause of developmental failure of the fetus? Prenat Diagn 1989;9:639.

114. Roland B, Lynch L, Berkowitz G, et al. Confined placental mosaicism in CVS and pregnancy outcome. Prenat Diagn 1994;14:589.

115. Crane JP, Cheung SW. An embryonic model to explain cytogenetic inconsistencies observed in chorionic villus versus fetal tissue. Prenat Diagn 1988;8:119.

116. Tharapel AT, Elias S, Shulman LP, et al. Resorbed co-twin as an explanation for discrepant chorionic villus results: non-mosaic 47,XX,+16 in villi (direct and culture) with normal (46, XX) amniotic fluid and neonatal blood. Prenat Diagn 1989;9:467.

117. Callen DF, Fernandez H, Hull YJ, et al. A normal 46,XX infant with a 46,XX/69,XXY placenta: a major contribution to the placenta is from a resorbed twin. Prenat Diagn 1991;11:437.

118. Vaughan J, Ali Z, Bower S, et al. Human maternal uniparental disomy for chromosome 16 and fetal development. Prenat Diagn 1994;14:751.

119. Bennett P, Vaughan J, Henderson D, et al. Association between confined placental trisomy, fetal uniparental disomy, and early intrauterine growth retardation. Lancet 1992;340:1284.

120. Dworniczak B, Koppers B, Kurlemann G, et al. Uniparental disomy with normal phenotype. Lancet 1992;340:1285.

121. Kennerknecht I, Terinde R. Intrauterine growth retardation associated with chromosomal aneuploidy confined to the placenta: three observations: triple trisomy 6, 21, 22; trisomy 16; and trisomy 18. Prenat Diagn 1990;10:539.

122. Astner A, Schwinger E, Caliebe A, et al. Sonographically detected fetal and placental abnormalities associated with trisomy 16 confined to the placenta: a case report and review of the literature. Prenat Diagn 1998;18:1308.

123. Hashish AA, Monk N, Levell-Smith MP, et al. Trisomy 16 detected at chorionic villus sampling. Prenat Diagn 1989;9:427.

124. Simoni G, Brambati B, Maggi F, et al. Trisomy 16 confined to chorionic villi and unfavorable outcome of pregnancy. Ann Génét 1992;35:110.

125. Van Opstal D, Van Den Berg C, Deelen WH, et al. Prospective prenatal investigations on potential uniparental disomy in cases of confined placental trisomy. Prenat Diagn 1998;18:35.

126. Webb AL, Sturgiss S, Warwicker P, et al. Maternal uniparental disomy for chromosome 2 in association with confined placental mosaicism for trisomy 2 and severe intrauterine growth retardation. Prenat Diagn 1996;16:958.

127. Hansen WF, Bernard LE, Langlois S, et al. Maternal uniparental disomy of chromosome 2 and confined placental mosaicism for trisomy 2 in a fetus with intrauterine growth restriction, hypospadias, and oligohydramnios. Prenat Diagn 1997;17:443.

128. Harrison K, Eisenger K, Anyane-Yeboa K, et al. Maternal uniparental disomy of chromosome 2 in a baby with trisomy 2 mosaicism in amniotic fluid culture. Am J Med Genet 1995;58:147.

129. De Andreis C, Pariani S, Maggi F, et al. Trisomy 2 confined to the placenta in 2 cases with intrauterine growth delay. Acta Med Auxol 1992;24:21.

130. Saks E, McCoy MC, Damron J, et al. Confined placental mosaicism for trisomy 8 and intra-uterine growth retardation. Prenat Diagn 1998;18:1202.

131. Appelman Z, Rosensaft J, Chemke J, et al. Trisomy 9 confined to the placenta: prenatal diagnosis and neonatal follow-up. Am J Med Genet 1991;40:464.

132. Fryburg JS. Mosaicism in chorionic villus sampling. Obstet Gynecol Clin N Am 1993;20:523.

133. Smith K, Lowther G, Maher E, et al. The predictive value of findings of the common aneuploidies, trisomies 13, 18 and 21, and numerical sex chromosome abnormalities at CVS: experience from the ACC U.K. collaborative study. Prenat Diagn 1999;19:817.

134. Hahnemann JM, Vejerslev LO. Accuracy of cytogenetic findings on chorionic villus sampling (CVS): diagnostic consequences of CVS mosaicism and non-mosaic discrepancy in centres contributing to EUCROMIC 1986–1992. Prenat Diagn 1997;17:801.

135. Brambati B, Varotto F. Infection and chorionic villus sampling. Lancet 1985;2:609.

136. Brambati B, Lanzani A, Oldrini A. Transabdominal chorionic villus sampling: clinical experience of 1159 cases. Prenat Diagn 1988;8:609.

137. Blakemore KJ, Baumgarten A, Schoenfeld-Dimaio M, et al. Rise in maternal serum alpha-fetoprotein con-

centration after chorionic villus sampling and the possibility of isoimmunization. Am J Obstet Gynecol 1986;155:988.

138. Fuhrmann W, Atland K, Kohler A, et al. Feto-maternal transfusion after chorionic villus sampling. Hum Genet 1988;78:83.

139. Brambati B, Guercilena S, Bonacchi I, et al. Feto-maternal transfusion after chorionic villus sampling: clinical implications. Hum Reprod 1986;1:37.

140. Warren RC, Butler J, Morsman JM, et al. Does chorionic villus sampling cause fetomaternal haemorrhage? Lancet 1985;1:691.

141. Knott PD, Chan B, Ward RHT, et al. Changes in circulating alpha-fetoprotein and human chorionic gonadotrophin following chorionic villus sampling. Eur J Obstet Gynecol Reprod Biol 1988;27:277.

142. Mariona FG, Bhatia R, Syner FN, et al. Chorionic villi sampling changes maternal serum alpha-fetoprotein. Prenat Diagn 1986;6:69.

143. Perry TB, Vekemans MJJ, Lippman A, et al. Chorionic villus sampling: clinical experience, immediate complications and patients' attitudes. Am J Obstet Gynecol 1985;151:161.

144. Smidt-Jensen S, Philip J, Zachary JM, et al. Implications of maternal serum alpha-fetoprotein elevation caused by transabdominal and transcervical CVS. Prenat Diagn 1994;14:35.

145. Mannucci PM, Pareti FI, Ruggeri ZN, et al. 1-Deamino-8-D-arginine vasopressin: a new pharmacological approach to the management of haemophilia and Willebrand's disease. Lancet 1977;1:869.

146. Rhoads GG, Jackson LG, Schlesselman SA, et al. The safety and efficacy of chorionic villus sampling for early prenatal diagnosis of cytogenetic abnormalities. N Engl J Med 1989;320:610.

147. Jackson L. CVS latest news. Philadelphia: WHO-CVS Registry, May 28, 1987.

148. Horwell DH, Loeffler FE, Coleman DV. Assessment of a transcervical aspiration technique for chorionic villus biopsy in the first trimester of pregnancy. Br J Obstet Gynaecol 1983;90:196.

149. Brambati B, Oldrini A, Aladerun SA. Methods of chorionic villi sampling in the first trimester fetal diagnosis. In: Albertini A, Crosignani PG, eds. Progress in perinatal medicine. Amsterdam: Excerpta Medica, 1983:275.

150. Scialli AR, Neugebauer DL, Fabro S. Microbiology of the endocervix in patients undergoing chorionic villi sampling. In: Fraccaro M, Simoni G, Brambati B, eds. First trimester fetal diagnosis. Berlin: Springer Verlag, 1985:69.

151. Brambati B, Matarelli M, Varotto F. Septic complications after chorionic villus sampling. Lancet 1987;1:1212.

152. Leschot NJ, Wolf H, Verjaal M, et al. Chorionic villi sampling: cytogenetic and clinical findings in 500 pregnancies. BMJ 1987;295:407.

153. Barela AI, Kleinman GE, Golditch IM, et al. Septic shock with renal failure after chorionic villus sampling. Am J Obstet Gynecol 1986;154:1100.

154. Blakemore KJ, Mahoney MJ, Hobbins JC. Infection and chorionic villus sampling. Lancet 1985;2:339.

155. Canadian Collaborative CVS-Amniocentesis Clinical Trial Group. Multicentre randomized clinical trial of chorion villus sampling and amniocentesis. Lancet 1989;1:1.

156. Goldberg JD, Porter AE, Golbus MS. Current assessment of fetal losses as a direct consequence of chorionic villus sampling. Am J Med Genet 1990;35:174.

157. Al-Mufti R, Hambley H, Farzaneh F, Nicolaides KH. Distribution of fetal erythroblasts in maternal blood after chorionic villus sampling. Br J Obstet Gynaecol 2003;110:33.

158. Schulman LP, Meyers CM, Simpson JL, et al. Fetomaternal transfusion depends on the amount of villi aspirated but not on method of chorionic villus sampling. Am J Obstet Gynecol 1990;162:1185.

159. Rodeck CH, Sheldrake A, Beattie B, et al. Maternal serum alpha-fetoprotein after placental damage in chorionic villus sampling. Lancet 1993;341:500.

160. Linman JW. Physiologic and pathophysiologic effects of anemia. N Engl J Med 1968;279:812.

161. Los FJ, Jahoda MGJ, Wladimiroff JW, et al. Fetal exsanguination by chorionic villus sampling. Lancet 1993;342:1559.

162. Los FJ, Pijpers L, Jahoda MGJ, et al. Transabdominal villus sampling in the second trimester of pregnancy: feto-maternal transfusion in relation to fetal outcome. Prenat Diagn 1989;9:521.

163. Hogdall CK, Doran TA, Shime J, et al. Transabdominal villus sampling in the second trimester. Am J Obstet Gynecol 1988;158:345.

164. Bergstrom H, Nilsson LA, Nilsson L, et al. Demonstration of Rh antigen in a 38-day-old fetus. Am J Obstet Gynecol 1967;99:130.

165. Eklund J. Embryonic Rhesus-positive red cells stimulating a secondary response after early abortion. Lancet 1981;2:748.

166. Schaap AH, van der Pol HG, Boer K, et al. Long-term follow-up of infants after transcervical chorionic

villus sampling and after amniocentesis to compare congenital abnormalities and health status. Prenat Diagn 2002;22:598.

167. Sigler ME, Colyer CR, Pratt Rossiter J, et al. Maternal serum alpha-fetoprotein screening after chorionic villus sampling. Obstet Gynecol 1987;70:875.

168. Ammala P, Hiilesmaa VK, Liukkonen S, et al. Randomized trial comparing first-trimester transcervical chorionic villus sampling and second-trimester amniocentesis. Prenat Diagn 1993;13:919.

169. Anguo H, Bingru Z, Hong W. Long-term follow-up results after aspiration of chorionic villus during early pregnancy. In: Fraccaro M, Simoni G, Brambati B, eds. First trimester fetal diagnosis. Berlin: Springer Verlag, 1985:1.

170. Invernizzi L, Prina E, Alberti S, et al. Long-term follow-up of 274 children born from women who underwent first trimester CVS. In: Macek M, Ferguson-Smith MA, Spala M, eds. Early fetal diagnosis. Prague: Karolinum-Charles University Press, 1992:176.

171. Cameron AD, Murphy KW, McNay MB, et al. Midtrimester chorionic villus sampling: an alternative approach? Am J Obstet Gynecol 1994;171:1035.

172. Gustavii B. Chorionic biopsy and miscarriage in first trimester. Lancet 1984;1:562.

173. Hoesli IM, Walter-Goebel I, Tercanli S, et al. Percutaneous fetal loss rates in a non-selected population. Am J Med Genet 2001;100:106.

174. Hassold T. A cytogenetic study of repeated spontaneous abortions. Am J Hum Genet 1980;32:723.

175. Hook EB, Cross PK, Jackson L, et al. Maternal age-specific rates of 47,+21 and other cytogenetic abnormalities diagnosed in the first trimester of pregnancy in chorionic villus biopsy specimens: comparison with rates expected from observations at amniocentesis. Am J Hum Genet 1988;42:797.

176. Stein ZA. A woman's age: child bearing and child rearing. Am J Epidemiol 1985;121:327.

177. WHO Consultation on First Trimester Fetal Diagnosis. Risk evaluation in chorionic villus sampling. Prenat Diagn 1986;6:451.

178. Hunter AG, Muggah H, Ivey B, et al. Assessment of the early risks of chorionic villus sampling. Can Med Assoc J 1986;13:753.

179. Silver RK, MacGregor SN, Sholl JS, et al. An evaluation of the chorionic villus sampling learning curve. Am J Obstet Gynecol 1990;163:917.

180. Modell B. Chorionic villus sampling: evaluating safety and efficacy. Lancet 1985;1:737.

181. Borrell A, Fortuny A, Lazaro L, et al. First-trimester transcervical chorionic villus sampling by biopsy forceps versus mid-trimester amniocentesis: a randomized controlled trial project. Prenat Diagn 1999;19:1138.

182. Firth HV, Boyd PA, Chamberlain P, et al. Severe limb abnormalities after chorion villus sampling at 56–66 days' gestation. Lancet 1991;337:762.

183. Burton BK, Schulz CJ, Burd LI. Limb anomalies associated with chorionic villus sampling. Obstet Gynecol 1992;79:726.

184. Hsieh F-J, Shyu M-K, Sheu B-C, et al. Limb defects after chorionic villus sampling. Obstet Gynecol 1995;85:84.

185. van der Anker JN, van Vught EE, Zandwijken GRJ, et al. Severe limb abnormalities: analysis of a cluster of five cases born during a period of 45 days. Am J Med Genet 1993;45:659.

186. Zoppini C, Ludomirsky A, Godmilow L, et al. Acute hemodynamic effects induced by chorionic villus sampling: a preliminary investigation. Am J Obstet Gynecol 1993;169:902.

187. Jiang BY, Thorton JG, Griffith-Jones MD, et al. Utero-placental flow waveforms after CVS. Lancet 1992;339:147.

188. Ibba RM, Monni G, Olla G, et al. Umbilical artery velocity waveforms before and after chorionic villus sampling. Prenat Diagn 1994;14:199.

189. Quintero RA, Romero R, Mahoney MJ, et al. Embryoscopic demonstration of hemorrhagic lesions on the human embryo after placental trauma. Am J Obstet Gynecol 1993;168:756.

190. Scott R. Limb abnormalities after chorionic villus sampling. Lancet 1993;337:1038.

191. Firth HV, Boyd PA, Chamberlain PF, et al. Limb abnormalities and chorion villus sampling. Lancet 1991;338:51.

192. Los FJ, Noomen P, Vermeij-Keers Chr, et al. Chorionic villus sampling and materno-fetal transfusions: an immunological pathogenesis of vascular disruptive syndromes? Prenat Diagn 1996;16:193.

193. van der Zee DC, Bax KMA, Vermeij-Keers Chr. Maternoembryonic transfusion and congenital malformations. Prenat Diagn 1997;17:59.

194. Luijsterburg AJM, van der Zee DC, Gaillard JLJ, et al. Chorionic villus sampling and end-artery disruption of the fetus. Prenat Diagn 1997;17:71.

195. Miny P, Holzgreve W, Horst J, et al. Limb abnormalities and chorionic villus sampling. Lancet 1991;337:1423.

196. Mastroiacovo P, Botto LD, Cavalcanti PD, et al. Limb abnormalities following chorionic villus sampling: a registry based case–control study. Am J Med Genet 1992;44:856.

197. Monni G, Ibba RM, Olla G, et al. Limb reduction defects and chorionic villus sampling. Lancet 1991;337:1091.

198. Mahoney MJ. Limb abnormalities and chorionic villus sampling. Lancet 1991;337:1422.

199. Jackson LG, Wapner RJ, Brambati B. Limb abnormalities and chorionic villus sampling. Lancet 1991;337:1423.

200. Report of National Institute of Child Health and Human Development Workshop on chorionic villus sampling and limb and other defects, October 20, 1992. Am J Obstet Gynecol 1993;169:1.

201. Schloo R, Miny P, Holzgreve W, et al. Distal limb deficiency following chorionic villus sampling? Am J Med Genet 1992;42:404.

202. Blakemore K, Filkins K, Luthy DA, et al. Cook obstetrics and gynecology catheter multicenter chorionic villus sampling trial: comparison of birth defects with expected rates. Am J Obstet Gynecol 1993;169:1022.

203. Dolk H, Bertrand F, Lechat MF. Chorionic villus sampling and limb abnormalities. Lancet 1992;339:876.

204. Gruppo Italiano Diagnosi Embriofetali. Transverse limb reduction defects after chorion villus sampling: a retrospective cohort study. Prenat Diagn 1993;13:1051.

205. Olney RS, Khoury MJ, Alo CJ, et al. Increased risk for transverse digital deficiency after chorionic villus sampling (CVS): results of the US multistate case-control study, 1988–1992. Teratology 1994;49:376.

206. Silver RK, MacGregor SN, Muhlbach LH, et al. Congenital malformations subsequent to chorionic villus sampling: Outcome analysis of 1048 consecutive procedures. Prenat Diagn 1994;14:421.

207. Kuliev A, Jackson L, Froster U, et al. Chorionic villus sampling safety. Am J Obstet Gynecol 1996;174:807.

208. Jackson L. CVS latest news. Philadelphia: WHO-CVS Registry, March 31, 1993.

209. Kallen B, Rahmani TMC, Winberg J. Infants with congenital limb reduction registered in Swedish register of congenital malformations. Teratology 1984;29:73.

210. Froster-Iskenius UG, Baird AB. Limb reduction defects in over one million consecutive livebirths. Teratology 1989;39:127.

211. Indagine Policentrica Italiana sulle Malformazioni Congenite. 10 anni di sorveglianza sulle malformazioni congenite in Italia 1978B1987. Milan: CNM Edizioni Scientifiche, 1990.

212. Castilla EE, Cavalcanti DP, Dutra MG, et al. Limb reduction defects in South America. Br J Obstet Gynaecol 1995;102:393.

212. Burton BK, Schulz CJ, Angle B, et al. An increased incidence of haemangiomas in infants born following chorionic villus sampling (CVS). Prenat Diagn 1995;15:209.

213. Mulliken JB, Young AE. Vascular birthmarks: hemangiomas and malformations. Philadelphia: WB Saunders, 1990.

214. Firth HV, Boyd P, Chamberlain PF, et al. Analysis of limb reduction defects in babies exposed to chorionic villus sampling. Lancet 1994;343:1069.

215. Froster U, Jackson L. Limb defects and chorionic villus sampling: results from an international registry, 1992–94. Lancet 1996;347:489.

216. Brambati B, Tului L, Bonacchi I, et al. Serum PAPP-A and free β-hCG are first-trimester screening markers for Down syndrome. Prenat Diagn 1994;14:1043.

217. Krantz DA, Larsen JW, Buchanan PD, et al. First-trimester Down syndrome screening: free β-human chorionic gonadotropin and pregnancy-associated plasma protein A. Am J Obstet Gynecol 1996;174:612.

218. Snijders RJM, Johnson S, Sebire NJ, et al. First-trimester ultrasound screening for chromosomal defects. Ultrasound Obstet Gynecol 1996;7:216.

219. Nicolaides KH Screening for chromosomal defects. Untrasound Obstet Gynecol 1003;21:313.

Peter A. Benn, Ph.D., and Lillian Y. F. Hsu, M.D.

6

Prenatal Diagnosis of Chromosomal Abnormalities through Amniocentesis

In the mid-1950s, Serr et al.[1] and Fuchs and Riis[2] reported that fetal sex could be determined prenatally by examining the X-chromatin body in human amniotic fluid cells (AFC). A decade later, Steele and Breg[3] succeeded in culturing and karyotyping AFC. This important advance led to the widespread use of prenatal diagnosis by women at high risk of having chromosomally abnormal offspring. The development in the early 1980s of chorionic villus sampling (CVS) for first-trimester diagnosis[4,5] represented a further important advance in prenatal diagnosis (see chapter 5).

The trend among women to delay or continue childbearing into later ages, together with the use of maternal serum and fetal ultrasound screening to help identify high-risk pregnancies (chapters 22 and 23), have resulted in increased public awareness of genetic amniocentesis.[6–10] Evaluation of each woman's risk of having a child with a chromosomal abnormality is a standard component of contemporary obstetric care, and women who are considered to be at increased risk are routinely offered amniocentesis or CVS.

Prenatal cytogenetic diagnosis has been improved through the use of enriched culture media, adoption of in situ harvesting procedures, and significant reductions in test turnaround times. The development of molecular genetic technologies using fluorescence in situ hybridization (FISH) has added a new dimension to the diagnosis of chromosomal abnormalities (chapter 8). Notwithstanding these advances, cytogeneticists and medical geneticists still face considerable problems and pitfalls in diagnosis and counseling.

In addition to providing an overview of the incidence of chromosomal abnormalities and the indications for prenatal cytogenetic diagnosis, this chapter focuses on issues arising in the interpretation of prenatal cytogenetic diagnoses through amniocentesis.

THE INCIDENCE OF CHROMOSOMAL ABNORMALITIES

Data from Livebirths

Studies performed in the late 1960s and early 1970s (i.e., before the widespread use of prenatal diagnosis and pregnancy intervention) provide us with estimates for the frequencies of chromosomal abnormalities at birth. A combined survey of 68,159 livebirths[11–21] and a survey of 34,910 liveborns[22] found that 0.65–0.84 percent of newborns, or 1 in 119–154 livebirths, had a major chromosomal abnormality (Table 6.1). Trisomy

214

Table 6.1. Chromosomal abnormalities in liveborn babies

Type of Abnormality	Combined Surveys of 68,159 Liveborns[11-21]			Survey of 34,910 Newborns[22a]		
	Number of Cases	Rate per 1,000	Rate	Number of Cases	Rate per 1,000	Rate
Sex chromosomes, males						
47,XYY	45	1.03	1/969	21	1.18	1/851
47,XXY	45	1.03	1/969	28	1.57	1/638
Other	32	0.73	1/1,362	3	0.17	1/5,957
Sex chromosomes, females						
45,X	6	0.24	1/4,091	9[b]	0.53	1/1,893
47,XXX	27	1.09	1/909	18	1.06	1/947
Other	9	0.36	1/2,727	1	0.06	1/17,038
Sex chromosomes						
unknown phenotype	—	—	—	2	0.57	1/17,455
Autosomal trisomies						
47,+21	82	1.2	1/831	59	1.69	1/592
47,+18	9	0.13	1/7,573	10	0.29	1/3,491
47,+13	3	0.04	1/22,719	3	0.09	1/1,637
Other	2	0.02	1/34,079	1	0.03	1/34,910
Structural balanced rearrangements						
Robertsonian translocation						
rob(DqDq)	48	0.7	1/1,420	34[c]	0.97	1/1,027
rob(DqGq)	14	0.2	1/4,869	9[c]	0.26	1/3,879
Reciprocal and insertional						
translocation	64	0.93	1/1,065	49[c]	1.4	1/712
Inversion	13	0.19	1/5,243	12	0.34	1/2,909
Structural unbalanced						
Robertsonian	5	0.07	1/13,632	—	—	—
Reciprocal and insertional	9	0.13	1/7,573	—	—	—
Inversion	1	0.01	1/68,159	—	—	—
Deletion	5	0.07	1/13,632	4	0.11	1/8,728
Supernumerary marker	14	0.2	1/4,869	23	0.66	1/1,518
Other	9	0.13	1/7,573	8	0.23	1/4,364
Total abnormalities	442	6.48	1/154	294	8.42	1/119
Total number surveyed						
Males	43,612			17,872		
Females	24,547			17,038		

[a]Includes induced abortions after prenatal diagnosis. A proportion of the cases are also included in the combined surveys of 68,159 liveborns.

[b]Including all cases of 45,X mosaics.

[c]Including both balanced and unbalanced.

21 (Down syndrome) was shown to be the most frequent chromosomal anomaly, with an incidence of 1.2–1.7 per 1,000 liveborns or 1 in 592–831 liveborns. Sex chromosome aneuploidies were the next most common, with approximately one XYY and one XXY in every 900–1,000 male livebirths and one XXX in every 900–1,000 female livebirths. Excluding pericentric inversion of chromosome 9, structural balanced rearrangements had a frequency of approximately 2 per 1,000 livebirths.

These birth incidence rates underestimate the true rates that would be observed today in the absence of prenatal diagnosis and pregnancy intervention. The surveys of newborns from 1969 to 1975 used nonbanded, conventionally stained preparations. Based on the data derived from the prenatal cytogenetic diagnoses using moderate levels of banding, Jacobs et al.[23] estimated that the use of moderate levels of banding (400–500 bands) increased the detected frequency of unbalanced structural abnormalities from 0.052 to 0.061 percent. The incidence of balanced structural abnormalities was increased from 0.212 to 0.522 percent. Therefore, the total rate of chromosomal abnormalities detectable in the newborn should be increased from 0.60 percent in unbanded preparations to 0.92 percent in banded preparations. In addition, it is likely that the limited number of cells analyzed in some of the newborn studies resulted in an underestimation of mosaic aneuploidies.[24]

As well as these technical considerations, there are demographic factors that have altered the overall rates of chromosomal abnormality. In many countries, the proportion of pregnant women who are aged 35 or more has increased dramatically since the 1970s.[6] The frequency of trisomy 21, and many other chromosomal abnormalities, increases with maternal age. This maternal age effect is clearly illustrated in the data in Table 6.2. At a maternal age of 35 years, there is an approximately 0.3 percent risk of having a liveborn child with trisomy 21 and a 0.5 percent risk of having a child with any chromosomal abnormality. At 46 years of age, the risk rises to 5 percent for trisomy 21 and to 7.25 percent for any chromosomal abnormality.

Compilations of data from multiple sources have resulted in relatively well-defined maternal age-specific birth rate schedules for Down syndrome. [25,36–40] Rates for trisomy

Table 6.2. Maternal age-specific rates for Down syndrome and all chromosomal abnormalities

Maternal Age[a] (years)	Liveborn Statistics		At Amniocentesis		At CVS	
	Down Syndrome[b] (%)	All Chromosomal Abnormalities[c] (%)	Down Syndrome[d] (%)	All Chromosomal Abnormalities[e] (%)	Down Syndrome[f] (%)	All Chromosomal Abnormalities[g] (%)
35	0.30	0.52	0.33	0.77	0.39	1.02
36	0.37	0.63	0.43	0.94	0.52	1.29
37	0.47	0.77	0.55	1.15	0.70	1.63
38	0.61	0.96	0.72	1.40	0.95	2.06
39	0.78	1.21	0.93	1.72	1.27	2.60
40	1.02	1.55	1.21	2.10	1.71	3.29
41	1.32	1.98	1.58	2.56	2.30	4.15
42	1.73	2.56	2.05	3.13	3.10	5.25
43	2.27	3.31	2.66	3.82	4.17	6.63
44	2.97	4.29	3.45	4.67	5.62	8.38
45	3.89	5.57	4.48	5.71	7.56	10.58
46	5.08	7.24	5.83	6.97	10.17	13.37

Note: Excludes balanced translocations and inversions.

[a]Maternal age at delivery, with year truncation (i.e., 35 = 35–35.99 years, 36 = 36–36.99 years, etc.)

[b]Based on the eight study curve of Bray et al.[25]

[c]Conservative estimate based on trisomy 18 and 13 prevalences, 10% and 5%, respectively,[26] of the rate for Down syndrome; XYY 0.05% for all ages[24]; XXY and XXY same as the second trimester prevalence[27]; unbalanced Robertsonian translocations involving chromosome 13 imbalance, 0.04% for all ages[28]; Turner syndrome (including variants and mosaics), 0.01% for all ages[29]; and other abnormalities, 0.02–0.03% at all ages.[26]

[d]Based on regressed data for 108,868 women aged 35–46, with rates adjusted to reflect age at delivery.[27,30]

[e]Based on regressed data for 52,836 women aged 35–46, with rates adjusted to reflect age at delivery.[27]

[f]Based on regressed data for 22,775 women aged 35–46, with rates adjusted to reflect age at delivery.[31–35]

[g]Based on regressed data for 16,852 women aged 35–46, with rates adjusted to reflect age at delivery.[31–34] Excludes cases with trisomy 3, 7, 11, 14, 15, and 16 and diploid/tetraploid mosaicism. Overall rate is expected to be 1–2% higher when abnormalities considered to be confined to the placenta are included.

18 and trisomy 13 are approximately 10–15 percent and 5–10 percent, respectively, of those for Down syndrome.[26]

Data from Amniocentesis

The age-specific rates of Down syndrome, as well as that for all chromosomal abnormalities combined, are higher when diagnosed through amniocentesis than when diagnosed in livebirths (Table 6.2). These differences can be largely attributed to the increased spontaneous loss rates of fetuses with chromosomal abnormalities subsequent to the time of amniocentesis. Several approaches have been used to assess the rate of spontaneous loss between the time of prenatal diagnosis and full-term delivery. The first approach is based on follow-up data for women choosing to continue an affected pregnancy (Table 6.3).[41] Additional data for trisomy 21 suggested a somewhat higher loss rate, particularly early in the second trimester.[42] A second approach uses an actuarial survival analysis on all prenatally diagnosed cases, whether or not the affected pregnancy is terminated. This approach provides an estimated absolute loss rate of 24 percent for Down syndrome.[43] The third method compares the observed number of affected pregnancies with the expected number of chromosomally abnormal births.[44] This approach provides estimates for the loss rates that are strongly dependent on the precise birth rate curve chosen.[45,46]

A particularly useful database for evaluating the prevalence of second-trimester chromosomal abnormality is a European collaborative study involving 52,965 amniocenteses performed on women aged 35 or more (Table 6.4).[27] All chromosome aberrations present in this population were documented.

Based on amniocentesis data, it would appear that the frequency of structural chromosomal abnormalities is probably independent of maternal age.[27] Drawing on data from an analysis of 377,357 genetic amniocenteses, Warburton[47] reported that in every 10,000 amniocenteses, there would likely be 5 de novo reciprocal translocations, 1 de novo Robertsonian translocation, 1 de novo inversion, and 4 cases of de novo supernumerary small marker chromosomes, with close to a 1:1 ratio of satellited versus nonsatellited chromosomes (Table 6.5). The frequency of Robertsonian translocations appeared to be underestimated, probably because of underreporting.

Table 6.3. Excess and absolute fetal loss rates subsequent to amniocentesis

Abnormality	Total Cases	Fetal Deaths	Absolute Fetal Deaths (%)	Excess Fetal Deaths (%)
47,+21	110	32	29.1	25.6
47,+18	40	27	67.5	64.0
47,+13	10	4	40.0	36.5
47,XXX	65	0	0	(no excess)
47,XXY	67	3	4.5	(no excess)
47,XYY	56	2	3.6	(no excess)
45,X	16	11	68.8	65.3
46,XX/45,X	28	4	14.3	10.8
Balanced translocations and inversions	298	10	3.4	(no excess)
Markers, variants, fragments	38	0	0	(no excess)

Source: Data from Hook et al., 1989.[41]

Note: Absolute rates refer to the actual rate of losses observed and excess refers to the rate over and above that expected for fetuses with a normal karyotype (estimated in this study to be 3.5%).

Table 6.4. Crude maternal age-specific rates (%) for chromosomal abnormalities ascertained in women having amniocentesis because of advanced maternal age

Maternal Age (years)	No. of Pregnancies	Autosomal Aberrations								Sex Chromosome Aberrations							Total			All Aberrations
		+21	+18	+13	Extra Marker	Mosaic, etc.	Unbal.	Bal.	t(13q14q)	XXX	XXY	XYY	X0	Mosaic, etc.	Unbal.	Bal.	Abn.	Bal.	De novo	
35	5,409	0.35	0.07	0.05	0.04	0.04	0.02	0.26	0.07	0.07	0.09	0.05	0.05	—	0.05	0.05	0.91	0.39	0.02	1.29
36	6,103	0.57	0.08	0.03	0.03	—	0.05	0.21	0.08	0.08	0.08	0.02	0.10	0.05	—	0.02	1.09	0.31	0.03	1.41
37	6,956	0.68	0.09	0.03	0.07	0.07	0.04	0.18	0.03	0.07	0.04	0.03	0.06	0.06	—	0.03	1.24	0.26	0.04	1.50
38	7,926	0.81	0.15	0.04	0.02	0.02	0.04	0.19	0.08	0.08	0.08	0.02	0.08	0.04	0.02	—	1.39	0.26	0.04	1.65
39	7,682	1.09	0.19	0.06	0.05	0.03	0.05	0.16	0.03	0.12	0.16	0.04	0.03	0.04	0.01	0.04	1.87	0.22	0.05	2.10
40	7,174	1.23	0.25	0.12	0.08	0.03	0.07	0.17	0.06	0.06	0.15	0.03	0.04	0.04	0.03	—	2.13	0.22	0.01	2.36
41	4,763	1.47	0.36	0.17	0.06	0.04	0.02	0.17	0.02	0.15	0.29	0.04	—	0.04	—	—	2.64	0.19	0.02	2.83
42	3,156	2.19	0.63	0.19	0.06	0.13	—	0.19	0.06	0.28	0.35	0.03	0.03	0.03	—	—	3.77	0.24	0.03	4.01
43	1,912	3.24	0.78	0.05	0.10	0.10	0.05	—	0.05	0.31	0.31	—	—	—	—	—	5.02	0.05	—	5.07
44	1,015	2.95	0.49	—	—	—	0.05	—	0.10	0.49	0.39	—	—	—	0.05	—	4.33	0.10	—	4.43
45	508	4.53	0.39	0.20	0.39	0.20	—	—	—	0.39	0.98	0.20	—	—	—	—	7.28	—	0.2	7.28
46	232	8.19	0.43	—	—	—	—	—	—	0.43	1.29	—	—	—	—	—	10.30	—	—	10.34
>46	129	2.33	0.77	—	—	—	—	—	—	1.55	1.55	0.77	—	—	—	—	6.98	—	—	6.98
≥35	52,965	1.16	0.23	0.07	0.06	0.04	0.04	0.18	0.05	0.12	0.16	0.03	0.04	0.04	0.02	0.02	2.01	0.25	0.03	2.26

Source: Data from Ferguson-Smith and Yates, Table 2, 1984.[27] Reproduced by permission from John Wiley & Sons Ltd.

Abn. = all unbalanced abnormalities; Bal. = balanced structural abnormalities (excluding pericentic inversion 9); Unbal. = duplications, deficiencies arising from structural abnormalities.

Table 6.5. The incidence of de novo balanced structural rearrangements and supernumerary markers in 337,357 genetic amniocenteses

De Novo Rearrangement	Number of Cases	(%)
Reciprocal translocation	176	0.047
Robertsonian translocation	42	0.011
Inversion	33	0.009
Supernumerary small marker chromosome	162	0.04
Satellited marker	77	0.02
Nonsatellited marker	85	0.023
Total	413	0.109

Source: Data from Warburton, 1991.[47]

Data from Chorionic Villus Sampling

Published data are available for more than 16,000 chorionic villus specimens from women of advanced maternal age. These data show maternal age-specific prevalence for chromosomal abnormalities higher than that seen at amniocentesis (Table 6.2).

Data from Spontaneous Abortuses

Major chromosomal abnormalities have been found in 20–60 percent of first-trimester spontaneously aborted fetuses.[48–57] Of 8,841 spontaneous abortuses studied (Table 6.6), 3,613 (40.9 percent) were found to have chromosomal abnormalities. Of these, 52 percent were autosomal trisomies, 19 percent were 45,X, 22 percent were polyploidies, and 7 percent had other anomalies, such as a structural aberration, mosaicism, or monosomies other than 45,X. Warburton et al.[57] reported the largest series, which included 2,517 spontaneous abortions. In this series, trisomy was found for every autosome except chromosomes 1, 11, and 19. An extra chromosome 16 was the most commonly observed trisomy (30.2 percent of all trisomies). This study demonstrated once again that the frequency of all trisomies increases with maternal age. Monosomy X (45,X), however, was found to be associated with young maternal age: 32 percent of 45,X abortuses came from women with ages between 20 and 24 years. This association had also been noted in an earlier study.[58]

Table 6.6. The frequency of chromosomal abnormalities in unselected spontaneous abortions

	Number of Cases	(%)
Abortuses studied	8,841	
Abortuses with chromosomal aberrations	3,613	40.9
Types of chromosomal aberration		
Autosomal trisomy	1,890	52.3
45,X	689	19.1
Triploidy	586	16.2
Tetraploidy	119	5.5
Other	249	6.9

Source: Data from Hsu and Hirschhorn, 1977;[48] Boué et al., 1975;[49] Creasy et al., 1976;[50] Takahara et al., 1977;[51] Carr and Gedeon, 1978;[52] Geisler and Kleinebrecht, 1978;[53] Kajii et al., 1980;[54] Hassold et al., 1980;[55] Andrews et al., 1984;[56] Warburton et al., 1980.[57]

Data on Induced Abortuses

The largest series of cytogenetic studies of induced abortuses is to be found in the report of Kajii et al.[59] More than 7,000 induced abortuses were karyotyped. Chromosomal abnormalities were found in 5 percent of the 3,237 specimens that included both complete and incomplete tissues and in 1.1 percent of 3,816 specimens with complete tissue specimens alone. It is likely that the incomplete specimens contained a significant number of "blighted ova," either with no embryo or with a stunted embryo.

Data on Stillbirths and Neonatal Deaths

Stillbirth is defined as the birth of a dead fetus during the late second or the third trimester of pregnancy (gestational age, ≥ 28 weeks), whereas neonatal death refers to death occurring within the first 4 weeks after birth. To provide adequate counseling for parents, all cases of stillbirth and neonatal death must be properly investigated. Thus, cytogenetic evaluation has become an important component of perinatal autopsy.[60,61]

In a combined group of stillbirths and neonatal deaths, 52 (6.31 percent) of 823 karyotyped cases were found to have a major chromosomal abnormality[62–64] (Table 6.7). The average frequency of abnormal karyotypes was 11.9 percent for macerated stillbirths, 4.2 percent for nonmacerated stillbirths, and 6.0 percent for neonatal deaths. The most common abnormalities reported were trisomies 18, 13, and 21, as well as sex chromosome aneuploidies and unbalanced translocations. These frequencies of chromosomal abnormality in stillbirths and neonatal deaths were approximately 10 times higher than those in newborns (reviewed by Alberman and Creasy[65]). To increase the detection rate of chromosomal defects, it was suggested that all macerated fetuses and all perinatal deaths with multiple congenital malformations should be studied cytogenetically.[61]

INDICATIONS FOR PRENATAL CYTOGENETIC DIAGNOSIS

The President's Commission for the Study of Ethical Problems in Medicine and Biomedical and Behavioral Sciences[66] recommended that genetic amniocentesis for prenatal diagnosis should be available to all pregnant women. Today, with readily available genetics laboratories, any pregnant woman can choose to have a genetic amniocentesis, provided there is no financial barrier. However, such barriers do exist. Amniocentesis is considered an invasive procedure involving a risk of fetal loss (chapter 2). Therefore, amniocentesis is usually offered only to pregnant women with an increased risk of having an affected child. The indications for prenatal cytogenetic diagnosis are discussed below.

Table 6.7. The frequency of chromosomal abnormalities in stillbirths and neonatal deaths

		Abnormal	
	Number Karyotyped	Number	(%)
Macerated stillbirths	59	7	11.9
Nonmacerated stillbirths	215	9	4.2
Neonatal deaths	549	33	6.0
Total	823	52	6.3

Source: Data from Machin and Crolla, 1974;[62] Bauld et al., 1974;[63] and Kuleshov, 1976.[64]

Advanced Maternal Age

The data from livebirths,[26] genetic amniocenteses,[27,30] and spontaneous abortions[50,57] all demonstrate the close association between advanced maternal age and risk for fetal autosomal trisomies and trisomies involving sex chromosomes (except XYY). This association led to the advanced maternal age group (usually women aged 35 years or more) routinely being offered amniocentesis. The second-trimester risk for fetal Down syndrome for a 35-year-old woman is approximately 1:270, and this risk has been widely, but not universally, adopted as a criterion for offering amniocentesis in maternal serum screening programs (see Chapter 22). The decision to recommend amniocentesis at 35 years of age evolved as the risks of fetal chromosomal abnormality were balanced against possible procedural loss.

Serum and ultrasound screening tests can be used to alter the risk for fetal aneuploidy significantly in older women (see Chapters 22 and 23) and the use of these screening approaches as primary indicators for amniocentesis has been advocated.[7,67–70] However, current guidelines do still recommend that amniocentesis be offered to all women aged 35 or more.[71,72] Serum and ultrasound screening tests do not identify all age-associated aneuploidies. Moreover, the association between maternal age and fetal chromosomal abnormality can be a source of considerable anxiety, and a negative screening result is sometimes not sufficiently reassuring. It is not wise to deny prenatal cytogenetic diagnosis to any pregnant woman. It is likely that, even with further improvements in screening, maternal age alone will continue to be a reason for amniocentesis, at least for a proportion of women.

Carrier of a Balanced Structural Rearrangement

Although this indication represents only a small proportion (usually less than 5 percent) of prenatal diagnosis patients, the risk that these parents will bear offspring with an unbalanced chromosome complement is usually significantly higher than 1:270. The risk varies, depending on (a) which parent is the carrier, (b) the type of rearrangement, (c) the method of ascertainment, (d) the chromosome involved, and (e) the specific chromosome breakpoints.

Reciprocal Translocation

Reciprocal translocation is the result of chromosome breaks in two autosomal chromosomes and the subsequent exchange of chromosome segments. In an early report[73] of 609 prenatal diagnoses performed in cases in which one parent was a carrier of an apparently balanced reciprocal translocation, 71 fetuses (11.7 percent) had an unbalanced chromosome constitution. There was no apparent difference in rates for unbalanced offspring between cases with a carrier father versus those with a carrier mother. Daniel et al.[74] expanded the analysis to 1,157 amniocenteses, including the initial data from Boué and Gallano[73] (Table 6.8). Excluding the relatively commonly encountered t(11;22)(q23.3;q11.2), the overall risk for maternal carriers ($N = 557$) to have a fetus with an unbalanced chromosome rearrangement was 11.7 percent; it was 10.9 percent for paternal carriers ($N = 414$). Daniel et al.[74,75] showed that the frequency of fetuses with unbalanced chromosome constitutions was much higher when the family was ascertained through prior full-term unbalanced progeny compared with the frequency when ascertainment was through recurrent

Table 6.8. Segregation products at the time of prenatal diagnoses when a parent is a reciprocal translocation carrier (N = 1,010); frequencies (%) of balanced, normal, and unbalanced fetal chromosome complements by method of ascertainment

Ascertainment through	Maternal				Paternal				Grand Total
	Balanced	Normal	Unbalanced	Total	Balanced	Normal	Unbalanced	Total	
Term unbalanced progeny[a]	90 (38.6)	94 (40.3)	49 (21.0)	233	67 (39.0)	66 (38.4)	39 (22.7)	172	405
Recurrent miscarriages[a]	111 (53.9)	85 (41.3)	10 (4.9)	206	76 (55.5)	59 (43.1)	2 (1.5)	137	343
Other[a,b]	68 (57.6)	44 (37.3)	6 (5.1)	118	60 (57.1)	41 (39.1)	4 (3.8)	105	223
Overall[a]	269 (48.3)	223 (40.0)	65 (11.7)	557	203 (49.0)	166 (40.1)	45 (10.9)	414	971
t(11;22)(q23.3;q11.2)[c]	22 (73.3)	6 (20.0)	2 (6.7)	30	5 (55.6)	3 (33.3)	1 (11.1)	9	39

Source: Data from Daniel et al., 1989.[74]

Note: To avoid ascertainment bias, these data include only those cases in which the presence of the translocation in a parent was known before amniocentesis. Translocations with both 2:2 and 3:1 modes of segregation are considered together.

[a]Excludes t(11;22)(q23.3;q11.2).

[b]Reasons apparently unrelated to the presence of the rearrangement (e.g., advanced maternal age).

[c]All ascertainment modes. Unbalanced forms all arise through 3:1 segregation with +der(22) in these offspring.

miscarriage (21.0 percent versus 4.9 percent for maternal carriers; 22.7 percent versus 1.5 percent for paternal carriers).

Both the earlier data[73,75] and the updated data[74] showed that the risk rates for unbalanced segregants diagnosed through amniocentesis are inversely related to the size of the chromosome imbalance (measured as a percentage of the total haploid autosome length). Thus, a small imbalance is associated with a higher risk. It is likely that many larger imbalances are associated with lethality and early embryonic or fetal loss.

Daniel et al.[74] considered separately translocations that were known to show 3:1 segregation patterns. Excluding the common translocation t(11;22)(q23.3;q11.2), male carriers showed a much lower risk for chromosomally unbalanced progeny compared with female carriers. Male carriers of these translocations were far fewer than female carriers, suggesting an effect on male fertility. They also indicated that the risk for unbalanced segregants was higher for carriers of complex chromosome rearrangements with multiple breakpoints.

Regarding the question of whether a balanced structural chromosome rearrangement could predispose for an unrelated numerical chromosomal abnormality during meiosis—the so-called interchromosomal effect—the data of Daniel et al.[74] could not provide an answer. They indicated that a strong effect could not be established, but a weak effect also could not be excluded.

Robertsonian Translocation

Robertsonian translocation is also referred to as a centric fusion type of translocation. It is a fusion of the entire long arms of two acrocentric chromosomes (chromosomes 13, 14, and 15 of the D group and chromosomes 21 and 22 of the G group) after breakage in the short arms. In humans, an individual with what is called a "balanced Robertsonian" translocation shows only forty-five chromosomes, with the translocation chromosome containing the two complete long arms of the two acrocentric chromosomes involved. The short arm fragments of the two translocated chromosomes are lost.

Boué and Gallano[73] summarized the prenatal diagnosis results in 517 cases in which one parent was a carrier for a Robertsonian translocation involving nonhomologous chromosomes. An additional 406 cases were reported by Daniel et al.[74] After excluding cases in which the translocation was identified at the time of the prenatal diagnosis (and therefore biased toward balanced and unbalanced translocations), data were available for a total of 811 cases (Table 6.9).

There were 357 cases with rob(13q14q), of which 251 were maternal carriers and 106 were paternal carriers. Among these rob(13q14q) cases, only one prenatal diagnosis result showed an unbalanced translocation resulting in trisomy 13. The overall risk for this group of patients was therefore very low (0.3 percent). A relatively high proportion of the cases were ascertained through a history of recurrent miscarriages (30 percent in the study of Daniel et al.[74]). This translocation would thus appear to be associated with a high probability of early fetal loss.

The risk for unbalanced segregation products also appears to be low for other Robertsonian translocations *not* involving chromosome 21 (Table 6.9). Of the sixty such cases, only one unbalanced segregation product was observed. This case involved translocation trisomy 13 arising in a mother with a rob(13q22q).

In contrast, risks were much higher when the Robertsonian translocation involved chromosome 21. The excess risk was largely confined to a situation in which the mother was

Table 6.9. Segregation in Robertsonian translocations

Type of Translocation	Number of Diagnoses	Offspring		
		Normal	Balanced	Unbalanced (%)
rob(13q14q)	357	146	210	1 (0.3)
rob(13q15q)	24	6	18	0
rob(13q21q)	52	25	23	4 (7.7)
rob(13q22q)	8	2	5	1 (12.5)
rob(14q15q)	12	9	3	0
rob(14q21q)	282	106	144	32 (11.3)
rob(14q22q)	7	4	3	0
rob(15q21q)	29	16	12	1 (3.4)
rob(15q22q)	9	6	3	0
rob(21q22q)	31	14	14	4 (12.9)
Total	811	333[a]	435[a]	43 (5.3)

Source: Data from Boué and Gallano, 1984,[73] and Daniel et al., 1989.[74]

Note: To avoid ascertainment bias, these data include only those cases in which the presence of the translocation in a parent was known prior to amniocentesis.

[a]For all types of Robertsonian translocations combined, the excess of balanced segregation products over normal is statistically significant.

the carrier of the translocation (Table 6.10). The largest amount of data available was for rob(14q21q)mat. For these carrier women, the risk at amniocentesis of having a fetus affected with Down syndrome approached 15 percent. When the father was a carrier of the translocation, the corresponding risk was closer to 1 percent. Male carriers of this translocation were less common than female carriers, suggesting that these translocations may have an effect on male fertility.

Substantially fewer data were available for other Robertsonian translocations involving chromosome 21. Based on the data in Table 6.10, the risks assigned to rob(14q21q) would seem to be applicable to all Robertsonian translocations involving chromosome 21.

Balanced Robertsonian translocations can be associated with uniparental disomy (UPD), and for chromosomes 14 and 15 UPD is clinically significant.[76–78] The risks and management of Robertsonian translocations where a clinically significant UPD is theoretically possible are discussed below (see "Interpretation Issues: Chromosome Rearrangements" and "Uniparental Disomy in Familial and de novo Rearrangements"). As well as providing the risk for an unbalanced karyotype, pre-amniocentesis counseling for carrier parents should include information about the risk for UPD and the testing options available.

Table 6.10. Prenatal results for Robertsonian translocation involving a chromosome 21

Robertsonian Translocation	Maternal Carrier		Paternal Carrier	
	Total Cases	Unbalanced (%)	Total Cases	Unbalanced (%)
rob(13q21q)	32	4 (12.5)	20	0 (0)
rob(14q21q)	208	31 (14.9)	74	1 (1.4)
rob(15q21q)	18	1 (5.6)	9	0 (0)
rob(21q22q)	27	3 (11.1)	4	0 (0)
Total	285	39 (13.7)	107	1 (0.9)

Source: Data from Boué and Gallano, 1984,[73] and Daniel et al., 1989.[74]

Note: To avoid ascertainment bias, these data include only those cases in which the presence of the translocation in a parent was known prior to amniocentesis.

Chromosome Inversion

A chromosome inversion arises when there has been a double break in one chromosome, reversal of a segment, and repair of the inverted sequence. If the inversion includes the centromere, it is a pericentric inversion. If it is confined to a single arm of the chromosome, it is paracentric. When a germ cell with a pericentric inversion undergoes meiosis, the inverted chromosome must form a loop to line up all homologous segments for proper pairing. A crossover within the loop of the inversion may result in a gamete with an unbalanced chromosome constitution. This is sometimes called "aneusomy by recombination."[79]

In 118 prenatal diagnoses collected by Boué and Gallano[73] that were performed because of a balanced pericentric inversion in one parent (excluding inv(9)qh), 7 fetuses (5.9 percent) were found to have unbalanced karyotypes (carrier father, 4 percent; carrier mother, 7.5 percent).

The 1989 collection by Daniel et al.[74] ($N = 173$) (Table 6.11) showed an overall risk of 3.3 percent for maternal carriers ($N = 91$) and no increased risk for paternal carriers ($N = 82$). For pericentric inversions with small distal segments, the risks of unbalanced progeny are rather high (about 10–15 percent).[74]

The data set of Daniel et al.[74] included 46 parents with inv(2)(p11.2q13), 24 with inv(10)(p11.2q21.2), 9 with inv(1)(p13q21), and 5 with inv(5)(p13q13). No recombinants were observed for any of these common specific inversions. According to the study by Djalali et al.,[80] the risk for a carrier of inv(2)(p11.2q13) to have a spontaneous abortion or a stillborn child may be twice the basic risk in the general population. Isolated case reports have suggested that inv(2)(p11.2q13) could result in offspring with an unbalanced karyotype,[81,82] but these events appear to be very rare. We are unaware of any reports of recombinants involving inv(10)(p11.2q21.2)[83]; such events may be associated with early embryonic lethality. The commonly encountered inv(Y)(p11.2q11.2) and most other X- or Y-chromosome inversions should not result in recombinants because the X and Y chromosomes do not pair except in the pseudoautosomal regions. However, it cannot be concluded from these comments that all the commonly encountered inversions carry a minimal risk. The frequently seen inv(8)(p23q22) is associated with a 6.2 percent risk for a child with the recombinant 8 chromosome.[84] If the data of Daniel et al.[74] are confined to cases in which the inversion was known to be present in a parent before amniocentesis, and

Table 6.11. Prenatal results for pericentric inversions ($N = 173$)

Method of Ascertainment	Maternal Carrier				Paternal Carrier				Grand Total
	Balanced	Normal	Unbalanced	Total	Balanced	Normal	Unbalanced	Total	
Through term unbalanced progeny	6	1	1 (12.5%)	8	2	3	0	5	13
Through recurrent miscarriages	10	4	0	14	4	2	0	6	20
Other	63	4	2 (2.9%)	69	68	3	0	71	140
Total	79	9	3 (3.3%)	91	74	8	0	82	173

Source: Data from Daniel et al., 1989.[74]

Note: Includes all autosomal inversions and no sex chromosome inversions. Includes 120 cases in which the segregation of the inversion in a parent was not known before the amniocentesis. Results are therefore biased in favor of balanced and unbalanced karyotypes.

we also exclude sex chromosome inversions, the relatively well characterized inv(2)(p11.3q13), inv(8)(p23q22), and inv(10)(p11.2q21.2), there remain forty cases with only one recombinant (2.5 percent).

For carriers with a paracentric inversion, the overall risk of having an abnormal child is low. Prenatal cytogenetic diagnosis may not be warranted for those carriers because a crossover within the inverted loop during the meiotic pairing process would lead to the formation of an acentric fragment and a dicentric chromosome. Both of these are highly unstable and are frequently lost or further rearranged in subsequent cell divisions. Gametes with the resulting unbalanced chromosome constitutions (duplication/deletion), if fertilized, would result in zygotes with highly reduced viability. Most of these zygotes would be lost very early, probably before implantation.[85–88] Although the risk for live-born recombinants is therefore small, such births have occurred several times to female carriers.[85–87] The risk is increased if there is a history of repeated abortions, abnormal previous children, or both, for carrier members of the family. A recombinant is likely to be viable only when the distal breakpoint of the inversion is close to the telomere.[87] It is sometimes difficult to distinguish between paracentric inversion and intrachromosomal insertion,[89] and this has been the basis of some controversy regarding reproductive risks that should be used in counseling.[88–90]

Intrachromosomal Insertions and Interchromosomal Insertions

Intrachromosomal insertions are very rare and have been ascertained only through offspring with recombinant, unbalanced karyotypes.[91] For an individual with an intrachromosomal insertion, Madan and Menko have estimated the risk for a recombinant child to be about 15 percent.[91]

Interchromosomal insertions are also very rare and predominantly ascertained through offspring with unbalanced karyotypes. For carriers, the risk for unbalanced offspring has been assessed as 32 percent for male carriers and 36 percent for female carriers.[92]

Previous Child with a Chromosomal Abnormality

Trisomy

Arbuzova et al.[93] performed a meta-analysis on data from four sources that evaluated second-trimester risk for Down syndrome in women who had a previous child with trisomy 21 (Table 6.12). Based on 4,953 pregnancies, the overall risk for Down syndrome was 0.85 percent, which was 0.54 percent higher than that expected on the basis of maternal age alone. The analysis did not take into account the maternal age at which the initial affected birth occurred or the total number of prior births. Thus, recurrence was more likely to be due to maternal-age-associated factors in older women and more likely to be attributable to other predisposing factors in younger women. Women who had a previous Down syndrome child were also at increased risk for aneuploidy other than trisomy 21. The overall risk for aneuploidy, including trisomy 21, was 1.46 percent. The risk for Down syndrome (0.85 percent) and the risk for any aneuploidy (1.46 percent) are comparable to that of a 38- to 39-year-old with no prior history of Down syndrome (Table 6.2).

Fewer data are available to assess the recurrence risk when there has been a previous child or affected pregnancy with any other trisomy. In a multicenter study for the recurrence risk for trisomy 13 and 18,[98] a total of 1,259 prenatal diagnosis cases were collected, including 838 cases with a previous pregnancy with trisomy 18 and 421 cases with

Table 6.12. Excess rates of Down syndrome and other aneuploidy in women who have had a previous Down syndrome pregnancy

| Study Reference | Down Syndrome | | | | | | Other Aneuploidy[a] | Any Aneuploidy |
| | Maternal Age | | | | | Total | | |
	<25	25–29	30–34	35–39	40+			
MRC Canada[94]	0/51	0/96	1/64	0/24	1/7	2/242	2/242	4/242
Mikkelsen et al.[95]	2/199	1/452	1/418	3/244	0/75	7/1,388	10/1,388	17/1,388
Stene et al.[96]	3/331	7/826	2/734	6/343	1/119	19/2,353	13/2,353	32/2,353
Uehara et al.[97]	0/41	5/301	3/394	5/195	1/39	14/970	5/970	19/970
Total	5/622	13/1,675	7/1,610	14/806	3/240	42/4,953	30/4,953	72/4,943
Rate (%)	0.80	0.78	0.43	1.74	1.25	0.85	0.61	1.46
Expected (%)[b]	0.10	0.13	0.2	0.59	2.2	0.31	0.36	0.67
Excess (%)	0.70	0.65	0.23	1.15	−0.75	0.54	0.25	0.79

Source: Arbuzova et al., Table 1, 2001.[93] Reproduced by permission from Munksgaard International Publishers.

[a]Includes six cases of XXY, four cases of 45,X, four cases of +18, three cases of +13, three cases of XYY, two cases of XXX, two cases of markers, and five cases unspecified.

[b]Based on maternal-age-specific rate at birth with adjustment for fetal losses between amniocentesis and full term.

trisomy 13. The recurrence rate for trisomy was 1.9 percent for trisomy 18 (including two cases of trisomy 18; six cases of trisomy 21; five cases of trisomy 13; and one case each for trisomies 9, 12, and 15). For trisomy 13, the recurrence rate for trisomy was 0.7 percent (including two cases of trisomy 18 and one case of trisomy 21). There was an overall twofold increased risk compared with the age-specific risk.

An increased risk following the birth of a trisomic child may be attributable to (a) parental mosaicism, (b) a structural chromosome rearrangement (the interchromosomal effect), (c) Mendelian genes producing a higher risk of nondisjunction, (d) exogenous factors, (e) decreased rate of spontaneous loss of trisomic conceptions, or (f) reduced ovarian complement in women with an atypical advanced biologic age.[96,100] Parental trisomy 21 mosaicism was detected in 2.7 percent (based on a finding of two or more trisomy 21 cells) to 4.3 percent (based on the finding of a single trisomy 21 cell) in one study of 374 families[99] in which there was a child with Down syndrome. Mosaicism was found more frequently in the mother than in the father. Using DNA markers, Pangalos et al.[101] studied twenty-two families with recurrence of free trisomy 21 and observed parental mosaicism in five families. However, parental mosaicism does not explain the presence of an entirely different trisomy present in many of these families with recurrent aneuploidy.

De Novo Unbalanced Rearrangement

When an apparently de novo unbalanced translocation is identified, recurrence risk is generally considered to be low. However, there have been isolated case reports of recurrence following the birth of a Down syndrome child with an apparently de novo isochromosome 21q or rob(21q21q).[102] These cases can be explained by cryptic or germ-cell mosaicism involving the balanced form of the translocation in a parent. A survey of 112 families with apparently de novo unbalanced rob(21q21q) children failed to identify any additional examples of recurrence of rob(21q21q) among the 164 sibs of the affected children.[102] However, Steinberg et al.[102] suggest that prenatal diagnosis should still be available to these parents because the number of cases available in their study was insufficient to be entirely reassuring.

Presumably, recurrence risk would be even lower for germ-cell mosaicism involving a translocation in which normal segregation products were possible.

Previous Child with a Neural Tube Defect or Isolated Hydrocephalus

Barkai et al.[103] found an increased incidence of Down syndrome in families in which there was a history of a child with a neural tube defect or hydrocephalus. These observations might be explained by a common etiologic factor (such as mutation in a gene involved in folate metabolism), the identification of a subgroup of women with a greater probability for the in utero survival of fetuses with diverse abnormalities, or may simply be an as-certainment bias. Among the 744 pregnancies to women who had a prior neural tube de-fect or hydrocephalus affected pregnancy, there were 7 cases of Down syndrome (1 in 106). This would be approximately equivalent to the risk associated with a maternal age of approximately 39 and no known prior history (Table 6.2). The risk for a Down syn-drome pregnancy in a woman with a prior pregnancy with a child with a neural tube de-fect was estimated to be 0.8 percent higher than that expected on the basis of maternal age alone.[103] This preliminary study has serious limitations[103a] and will require a follow-up study with rigorous epidemiologic design to determine its accuracy.

Elevated Maternal Serum α-Fetoprotein

In a large study, Feuchtbaum et al.[104] reported a twofold increased prevalence of fetal chromosomal abnormalities in the pregnancies of women who had "unexplained" elevated maternal serum α-fetoprotein (MS-AFP) greater or equal to 2.5 MoM, relative to an un-matched population prevalence. In that study, "unexplained" MS-AFP referred to cases in which this serum protein was elevated and the result was not attributable to the presence of a ventral wall or neural tube defect. No significant excess was found when a cutoff of 2.0 MoM was used. The excess cases using the 2.5 MoM were mostly autosomal aneu-ploidies or triploidy and it is likely that many of these would have been associated with fetal anomalies identifiable by ultrasound. The excess risk for a serious chromosomal ab-normality in women with unexplained MS-AFP and normal ultrasound findings is there-fore likely to be minimal.

For cases in which an anomaly is identified by ultrasound, amniocentesis should be considered. See the section on "Abnormal Ultrasound Findings" (below) and chapter 21 for a fuller discussion.

Second-Trimester Maternal Serum Screening for Chromosomal Defects

Second-trimester maternal serum screening through MS-AFP, human chorionic go-nadotropin (hCG) unconjugated estriol (uE$_3$) and, recently, inhibin A, has become com-mon practice (see chapter 22 for a full discussion). We note, in passing, that this screening will identify not only pregnancies with fetal Down syndrome and trisomy 18 but also those complicated by 45,X, triploidy, and mosaic trisomy 16 and possibly other rare chromo-somal abnormalities.[105–107]

First-Trimester Screening for Chromosomal Defects

First-trimester screening through fetal biometric measurement of nuchal translucency and maternal serum biochemical tests can provide an effective protocol for detecting aneu-ploidy (see chapters 22 and 23 for a full discussion). Some patients who are positive on screening may elect to receive second-trimester amniocentesis instead of first-trimester CVS testing. In these patients, there is a greater likelihood that surviving fetuses with trisomies 21, 18, and 13 and triploidy and other cytogenetic abnormalities will be found.[108]

CVS Mosaicism

In 1–2 percent of CVS, a mosaic or nonmosaic abnormal chromosome complement is observed that is apparently not present in the fetus (see chapter 5). A follow-up amniocentesis has been recommended for all women who show a mosaic autosomal trisomy in CVS cultures (villus mesenchyme).[109] Amniocenteses may also be indicated for additional women with nonmosaic abnormalities, depending on the specific chromosomal abnormalities involved.

Abnormal Ultrasound Findings

A large number of studies have evaluated the risk for a chromosomal abnormality associated with the ultrasound identification of a fetal anomaly. Generally, the sonographic identification of anomalies is confined to a gestational age of 10–22 weeks, and the identification of some anomalies can be somewhat subjective in nature. Studies associating specific ultrasound findings with aneuploidy are often based on high-risk populations referred for ultrasound examinations because of maternal age, positive serum screening results, or other concerns. Therefore, the risk figures presented in Table 6.13 should be considered crude estimates. They do, however, provide some indication of the magnitude of risk together with a guide to the most common chromosomal abnormalities seen. In Table 6.14 the results from four large studies documenting the cytogenetic abnormalities in cases with abnormal ultrasound findings are presented. Additional information on the ultrasound detection of anomalies and their association with fetal aneuploidy can be found in chapter 23.

Very High Risk for Fetal Aneuploidy (>35 percent)

Some of the highest rates of cytogenetic abnormality are to be found in amniotic fluid specimens from pregnancies complicated by fetal cystic hygromas and nonimmune hydrops. Cystic hygromas are fluid accumulations in the lymphatics and are frequently associated with excess fluid in other tissues (nonimmune hydrops). Among second-trimester fetuses with cystic hygromas, only 37 percent show a normal karyotype.[121] A 45,X karyotype is observed in 43 percent of these cases; other abnormalities, including trisomies 21, 18, and 13, make up the remainder.

A distinction has been drawn between cystic hygroma (bilateral, septated, cystic structures) and nuchal edema (subcutaneous fluid accumulation).[142] Nuchal edema is visualized on first-trimester ultrasonography as an increased nuchal translucency, and this finding can also be associated with a very high risk for fetal chromosomal abnormality.[142] In the second trimester, distention of the nuchal skin fold also provides a marker for chromosomal abnormality.[134] For both first- and second-trimester nuchal measurements, the extent of the enlargement can be combined with serum screening results and some other ultrasound findings to revise the maternal age-specific risk for aneuploidy for individual patients.[143,144]

Cardiac defects are among the most commonly encountered congenital anomalies.[145,146] Approximately 19–48 percent of cases that would be apparent at birth might

Table 6.13. Frequency and types of chromosomal abnormalities in fetuses with ultrasound-detected fetal anomalies

Anomaly Identified by Ultrasound[a]	Risk (%)[b]	Common Chromosomal Abnormalities[c]	Reference
Abdominal wall defect			
Gastroschisis	Background	None	Hunter and Soothill[110]
Omphalocele	4.5–35	+18; +13; +21; 45,X; 3n; t(11p15.5)mat; dup(11p15.5)pat	Kilby et al.[111]
Agenesis of corpus callosum	10	+8; +13; +18; other	Gupta and Lilford[112]
Choroid plexus cyst, isolated	0.7	+18; +21	Gupta et al.[113]
Choroid plexus cyst, complex	10.5–12	+18; +21; 3n	Gupta et al.[113]
Cleft lip, with or without cleft palate	21.6	+13; +18; del; +21; 3n; other	Clementi et al.[114]
Cleft palate	30.8	+13; +18; del; +21; 3n; other	Clementi et al.[114]
Club foot, isolated	3.4	Various	Shipp and Benacerraf,[115] Malone et al.[116]
Cardiac anomalies			
Structural anomalies	40	+21; +18; +13; 45,X; other; del(22)(q11.2q11.2)	Stoll et al.[117]
Echogenic focus, isolated	1.5	+21, others	Huggon et al.,[118] Sotiriadis et al.[118a]
Echogenic focus, complex	5–10	+21; +13; others	Sotiriadis et al.,[118a] Bromley et al.[119] Vibhakar et al.[120]
Cystic hygroma	63	45,X; +21; +18; +13; other	Gallagher et al.[121]
Dandy–Walker malformation	60	3n; +18; +13; translocations	Ecker et al.,[122] Kölble et al.[123]
Diaphragmatic hernia, complex	9.5	+18; +13; +i(12p); 4n/2n	Witters et al.[124]
Duodenal atresia	33	+21	Nicolaides et al.,[125] Halliday et al.,[126] Hanna et al.,[127] Rizzo et al.[128]
Echogenic bowel	3–25	+21; 3n; +18; 45,X; +13; others	Penna and Bower,[129] Simon-Boug et al.[129a]
Femur, humerus, short	20[d]	+21; +18;	Nyberg et al.[130]
Holoprosencephaly	55	+13; +18; del(13q); del(18p); del(7q); other	Peebles[131]
Hydrocephaly/ventriculomegaly	16	+21; +18; 3n; other	Nicolaides et al.,[125] Halliday et al.,[126] Hanna et al.[127]
IUGR	20	+18, 3n; +13; other; +21	Nicolaides et al.,[125] Halliday et al.,[126] Hanna et al.[127]

Finding	%	Chromosomal abnormality	Reference
Microcephaly	23	+13; del(7q34); +8 mos	Den Hollander et al.[132]
Neural tube defect, isolated	2.4	Various	Kennedy et al.[133]
Neural tube defect, complex	6.5	+18; other	Kennedy et al.[133]
Nuchal translucency (first trimester)	35[d]	+21; +18; 45,X; +13; 3n; other	Snijders et al.[108]
Nuchal fold (second trimester)	40[d]	+21; +18; 3n	Benacerraf[134]
Oligohydramnios	14	3n; +13; other	Halliday et al.,[126] Hanna et al.[127]
Polyhydramnios	12	+18; +21; +13; other	Halliday et al.,[126] Hanna et al.[127]
Teratoma	nk	dup(1q)	Wax et al.[135]
Tetraphocomelia	nk	PCS	Van den Berg and Francke[136]
Tracheoesophageal fistula/esophageal atresia	63	+18; +21; other	Nicolaides et al.,[125] Hanna et al.,[127] Rizzo et al.[128]
Two vessel cord, complex	5.5	+13; +18; other	Saller et al.,[137] Hanna et al.[126]
Urogenital anomalies			
Renal structural defect	nk	+18; +13; 45,X; 3n; +9 mos; del(10q); del(18q); del(22)(q11.2q11.2)	Wellesley and Howe[138]
Hydronephrosis/multicystic kidneys	12	+21; +18; +13; del; 45,X, del(22q11.2q11.2) other	Nicolaides et al.,[139] Wellesley and Howe[135]
Pyelectasis, isolated	0–2	+21; other	Corteville et al.,[140] Wickstrom et al.[141]

[a]Complex and isolated anomalies are defined as with, or without, other abnormal ultrasound findings.
[b]Percentage of cases with a chromosomal abnormality.
[c]Listed in the approximate order in which the abnormalities might be encountered.
[d]Risks presented are based on fixed cutoffs to define the presence or absence of the marker. Patient-specific risks are also available.
3n = triploidy; 4n/2n = tetraploid mosaicism; nk = not known; PCS = premature chromatid separation (diagnostic for Roberts syndrome, SC phocomelia syndrome).

Table 6.14. Ultrasound abnormalities and frequency of fetal aneuploidy

Defect	Nicolaides et al.[125] Isolated # Aneupl/Total	Nicolaides et al.[125] Multiple # Aneupl/Total (%)	Halliday et al.[126] Isolated # Aneupl/Total (%)	Hanna et al.[127] Primary U/S Abn. # Aneupl/Total (%)	Rizzo et al.[128] Primary U/S Abn. # Aneupl/Total (%)	Overall Frequency[a] # Aneupl/Total (%)
Abdominal wall defect	1/30	41/86 (48)	3/45 (7)	38/196 (19)	7/161 (44)	90/373 (24)
Agenesis of corpus callosum	—	—	—	0/2 (0)	8/19 (42)	8/21 (38)
Choroid plexus cyst	1/49	33/72 (46)	0/21 (—)	21/514 (4)	—	55/656 (8)
Congenital heart disease						166/339 (49)
Unspecified	0/4	101/152 (66)	8/42 (19)	10/60 (17)	20/34 (59)	
Ventricular septal defect	—	—	—	8/21 (38)	9/13 (69)	
Atrioventricular canal	—	—	—	2/2 (100)	8/11 (82)	
Cystic hygroma	0/4	35/45 (73)	11/21 (52)	65/108 (60)	22/33 (67)	133/211 (63)
Diaphragmatic hernia	0/38	17/41 (41)	2/17 (12)	8/72 (11)	2/5 (40)	29/173 (17)
Duodenal atresia	1/6	9/17 (53)	3/10 (30)	10/45 (22)	8/15 (53)	31/93 (33)
Echogenic bowel	—	—	—	5/34 (15)	—	5/34 (15)
Facial cleft	0/8	31/56 (55)	1/7 (14)	—	3/11 (28)	35/82 (43)
Holoprosencephaly	0/7	15/51 (29)	3/9 (33)	9/19 (47)	6/12 (50)	33/98 (34)
Hydrocephaly	2/42	40/144 (28)	7/30 (23)	25/256 (9)	—	74/472 (16)
Hydronephrosis	—	—	—	8/110 (7)	—	8/110 (7)
Hydrops (nonimmune)	7/104	18/106 (17)	23/57 (40)	37/116 (32)	6/17 (35)	91/400 (22)
Intrauterine growth retardation	4/251	133/424 (31)	8/37 (22)	71/389 (18)	—	216/1101 (20)
Limb anomalies	0/18	195/457 (43)	4/29 (14)	3/39 (8)	3/6 (50)[b]	205/549 (37)
Microcephaly	0/1	8/51 (16)	0/1 (0)	5/28 (18)	—	13/81 (16)
NTD (various types)	—	—	1/33 (3)	4/57 (7)	2/6 (33)	7/96 (7)
Nuchal fold/thickness/edema	0/12	53/132 (40)	5/21 (24)	15/75 (20)	—	73/240 (30)
Oligohydramnios	—	—	1/14 (7)	14/97 (14)	—	15/111 (14)
Polyhydramnios	—	—	2/9 (22)	23/194 (12)	—	25/203 (12)
Renal anomalies	9/482	87/360 (24)	3/29 (10)	7/107 (7)	3/6 (50)	106/978 (11)
Tracheoesophageal fistula/esophageal atresia	0/1	18/23 (78)	—	4/10 (40)	3/6 (50)	25/40 (63)
Two-vessel cord	—	—	—	5/72 (6)	—	5/72 (7)

[a]Combined isolated and/or multiple ultrasound abnormalities.

[b]Club feet.

Abn. = abnormality; # Aneupl/Total = number of aneuploidy cases divided by total cases with the abnormality; U/S = ultrasound.

be detected prenatally through routine ultrasound screening,[147] and a chromosomal abnormality is the cause in approximately 40 percent of the prenatally identified cases.[117] The specific types of heart defects that are present in the common aneuploidies has been reviewed by Yates,[148] and a list of the risks associated with specific cardiac defects has been developed by Allan et al.[149] The association between tetralogy of Fallot, double-outlet right ventricle (DORV), and other conotruncal abnormalities with the deletion of 22q11 (DiGeorge/velocardial facial syndrome) is noteworthy. The types of cardiac defects found with 22q11 deletion may not be limited to conotruncal defects, and Manjii et al.[150] proposed that FISH testing using a 22q11 probe be carried out for all cases with prenatally detected heart defects (except hypoplastic left heart and echogenic focus).

Other abnormalities identifiable on ultrasound associated with very high risk for aneuploidy are tracheoesophageal fistula/esophageal atresia, Dandy–Walker malformation, and holoprosencephaly.

High Risk for Fetal Aneuploidy (20–35 percent)

A common purpose for amniocentesis is to identify the cause and full significance of intrauterine growth retardation (IUGR) identified by ultrasound. IUGR, in the absence of any other biochemical or screening tests, will occasionally signal the presence of pregnancies affected by trisomies 13 and 18, but the finding is not a strong indicator for trisomy 21. More severe IUGR is associated with an even greater chance for aneuploidy.[151] Combined data from three large series[125–127] suggest an overall risk of 20 percent for a cytogenetic abnormality in cases with IUGR. A broad range of abnormal karyotypes is possible.

Comparable levels of risk are associated with an ultrasound finding of microcephaly. Other anomalies that can be considered to be associated with a high risk for fetal aneuploidy include facial clefts, duodenal atresia ("double bubble" anomaly), some limb anomalies, and omphalocele (but not gastroschisis).

There is also a high risk for aneuploidy when femur length, humerus length, or both, are shorter than that expected for the gestational age.[130] These biometric measurements can be combined with serum screening tests and nuchal fold measurement to modify individual patient's risk for aneuploidy.[144]

Moderate Risk for Fetal Aneuploidy (10–19 percent)

Hyperechogenic bowel is often a nonspecific finding seen in some fetuses with intestinal obstruction and meconium ileus secondary to cystic fibrosis.[129] However, it may also be an indicator for fetal Down syndrome or other chromosomal abnormality. Estimates for the risk for fetal aneuploidy when "echogenic bowel" is observed have been somewhat variable, probably reflecting the variable criteria used to define hyperechogenicity and ascertainment bias.

Moderate risks for fetal aneuploidy can also be assigned when there is ultrasound detection of renal anomalies (including hydronephrosis), oligohydramnios or polyhydramnios, hydrocephaly/ventriculomegaly, and diaphragmatic hernia (in association with other anomalies).

Low Risk for Fetal Aneuploidy (<10 percent)

At the low end of the risk spectrum, isolated clubfoot and neural tube defects are rarely attributable to aneuploidy. Isolated choroid plexus cysts, single umbilical artery, pyelectasis, and echogenic intracardiac focus are relatively common findings that suggest only a modest increase in risk. However, each of these findings has much greater significance when they are observed in the presence of additional ultrasound anomalies.

The finding of any ultrasound anomaly, including these common low-risk factors, should prompt a thorough examination to determine whether additional anomalies are present.

History of Repeated Fetal Losses: Parents' Karyotype Unknown

In studies of couples experiencing multiple spontaneous abortions, a mean of 5.1 percent (range, 2.2–7.4 percent) were found to have a chromosomal abnormality in one of the partners.[152] There appears to be a positive correlation between the number of spontaneous abortions and the frequency of parental chromosome aberrations. Also, couples with a history of a stillborn or a malformed infant reportedly have a greater frequency of chromosomal abnormalities (16.7 percent) than couples with no such history (5.4 percent).[153]

These observations are consistent with that presented in a review by De Braekeleer and Dao.[154] Data were gathered on 22,199 couples (44,398 individuals). Of the couples with a history of two or more spontaneous abortions, 4.7 percent were found to have a chromosome rearrangement. Translocations (reciprocal and Robertsonian) and inversions were associated with a high risk of fetal loss. The frequencies of reciprocal translocations, Robertsonian translocations, and inversions were 15 times, 6 times, and 26 times higher, respectively, than the general population frequency (which was based on those reported in consecutive newborn series).

It is therefore appropriate to perform cytogenetic analyses on blood specimens from individuals who have a history of either two or more losses, a stillbirth, or a malformed infant. Ideally, these studies would be completed before the time of amniocentesis. However, this risk factor is often recognized only in a genetic counseling session immediately before amniocentesis. In this situation, there is an increased risk for a fetus with an unbalanced karyotype in the current pregnancy, and therefore amniocentesis should be considered.

History of Repeated Fetal Losses: Parents' Karyotype Normal

Warburton et al.[155] identified 273 women who had more than one spontaneous abortion karyotyped. They analyzed their data to determine whether a chromosomally abnormal loss constituted a risk factor for future pregnancies. They concluded that a chromosomally abnormal loss did not increase the subsequent risk for trisomy. This finding was unexpected, given the fact that a previous liveborn child with a chromosomal abnormality is considered to increase the risk (see above). The spectrum of chromosomal abnormalities present in spontaneous abortions differs markedly from that seen at birth, and the data of Warburton et al. do not exclude an increased risk for the specific chromosomal abnormalities that are compatible with a full-term livebirth. Amniocentesis is therefore often considered by women who have a history of a spontaneous abortion, if it was established that the prior abortus carried a chromosomal abnormality that was compatible with a livebirth.

Male or Female Subfertility

Cytogenetic Causes

Male or female infertility or subfertility may be associated with chromosomal abnormalities. The overall frequencies of chromosomal abnormalities in infertile or subfertile men with a sperm count below 10 million/mL were reported to be 7.1 percent in a study of 496 infertile men[156] and 10.3 percent in another study of 952 males.[157] Both studies showed higher frequencies of chromosomal abnormalities in men with azoospermia than in those with oligospermia (14–15 percent versus 5–7 percent). The azoospermia group showed mostly sex chromosomal abnormalities, such as XXY, XX male, XYY, and mosaics.

The importance of two complete X chromosomes for fertility in human females is evident from studies of Turner syndrome. Reduced fertility or infertility has also been associated with 45,X mosaics and X-chromosome structural abnormalities. In fact, 45,X or XXX mosaics and structural abnormalities in one X chromosome, such as partial deletion of the short arm of one X, have often been reported in females with a history of repeated spontaneous abortions.[152]

Therefore, it appears that couples with a history of infertility or subfertility carry an increased risk of having a chromosomal abnormality themselves, and consequently, an increased risk of bearing a fetus with abnormal chromosomes. Again, if parental chromosome studies cannot be performed first, couples with such a history should be offered prenatal diagnosis.

Reduced Ovarian Complement

Surgical removal of part, or all, of an ovary or congenital absence of an ovary is associated with early menopause. In mice, unilateral oophorectomy is also associated with an early rise in the proportion of conceptions that are aneuploid[158] and there are some human data to suggest that the prevalence of Down syndrome is increased in the pregnancies of women with a reduced ovarian complement.[159–161] Risk for aneuploidy may therefore be dependent on the time from menopause (i.e., biologic age rather than chronologic age),[158] perhaps the consequence of reduced selection within diminished oocyte pools.[100] Freeman et al.[161] concluded that women with reduced ovarian complement should be offered prenatal cytogenetic diagnosis.

Abnormal Parental Karyotype (Other Than a Balanced Structural Rearrangement)

If one of the parents has a trisomic mosaicism, or a sex-chromosome aneuploidy that does not abrogate reproductive ability (e.g., 47,XYY or 47,XXX), the risk of having offspring with an abnormal karyotype is increased.

Trisomy 21 mosaicism has been found in both mothers and fathers of patients with Down syndrome.[96,99,100,152,162] Several of these mosaic parents had two affected children with trisomy 21. Prenatal cytogenetic diagnosis should therefore be offered when an individual has been established as being mosaic.

Because the vast majority of XYY males and XXX females remain unidentified (because of the absence of diagnostic signs), prenatal diagnosis for this indication is rather infrequent. The frequencies of 47,XXX, 47,XXY, and 47,XYY in couples ascertained through fetal wastage are not significantly different from those reported in consecutive liveborns.[154] Although 47,XXX women may be at a higher risk for meiotic nondisjunction, there is no strong indication that 47,XYY men have the same increased risk.[154]

Prenatal diagnosis may also be considered when a parent has a microdeletion syndrome or other abnormal karyotype that is compatible with reproduction.

Prenatal Sex Determination for X-linked Disorders

When a mother is an obligate or a proven carrier of an X-linked disease or is at high risk for being a carrier, prenatal sex determination is justified. Fetal sexing becomes obsolete for X-linked disorders when a definitive prenatal diagnosis becomes available. However, prenatal sex determination might be sufficient when the cost of a direct test for the disorder is very high or when information about the carrier status of female offspring is not sought.

The sex of the fetus should always be based on karyotype analysis and not solely on interphase FISH or sex chromatin/Y-chromatin body determination of noncultivated amniotic fluid cells. One study reported a 20 percent maternal cell contamination rate in noncultivated amniotic fluid cells using dual-color X and Y probes for FISH, compared with 0.2 percent for maternal cell contamination in cultured amniocytes.[163] Examination of X and Y chromatin in noncultivated amniotic fluid cells is also not reliable.[152]

Fetal sex determination solely for social reasons should not be an acceptable indication for prenatal diagnosis.

Prenatal Diagnosis for a Nonchromosomal Disorder

Increasing numbers of amniocenteses are being performed for the purpose of diagnosing a genetic disorder other than those identifiable through karyotyping. Included in this category are some disorders (such as fragile X, Fanconi anemia, and ataxia telangiectasia) that have, in the past, been diagnosed using special cytogenetic protocols. For a discussion of the cytogenetic diagnoses of these disorders, see earlier editions of this chapter. Current biochemical and molecular genetic tests are discussed elsewhere in this edition and the Web site for Gene Tests provides an excellent resource for currently available tests.[164]

When a midtrimester amniocentesis is performed for such a noncytogenetic indication, karyotype analysis of amniocytes is routinely offered by most geneticists.

Miscellaneous

It remains to be determined whether maternal exposure to radiation before conception increases the frequency of aneuploid progeny. Several investigations have suggested some association, but none have showed statistical significance.[152] Histories of cancer chemotherapy and other environmental exposures to mutagens are often a source of concern to patients. These patients should be counseled carefully about the limitations of prenatal cytogenetic diagnosis in order to avoid creating a false sense of security.

Advanced paternal age is now generally not considered to be a valid indication for prenatal cytogenetic diagnosis, as several studies have found no evidence for a positive effect of paternal age.[152]

Finally, anxiety is often used as an indication for prenatal diagnosis when there is no other medical indication for testing. As with concerns about mutagens, couples with this request must be fully informed about the limitations of prenatal diagnosis.

INTERPRETATION ISSUES: CHROMOSOME MOSAICISM AND PSEUDOMOSAICISM

General Considerations

Cultured amniotic fluid cells (AFC) (amniocytes) are believed to be derived from fetal skin, urinary and respiratory tract, placenta and membranes.[165] The presence of one, or more, karyotypically abnormal cells in otherwise normal AFC chromosome preparations may reflect "true mosaicism," which is defined as the presence of multiple fetal cell lines. Alternatively, the abnormal cells could indicate "pseudomosaicism" (i.e., abnormality either arising in culture or presumed to be derived from extrafetal tissue and not representative of the fetus.)

Mosaicism involving trisomy can arise by one of two mechanisms.[166] First, the trisomy may have a meiotic origin, with loss of one copy in a postzygotic cell. This mechanism can sometimes result in a situation in which the normal cell line is represented by two copies of a chromosome that were both derived from the same parent (uniparental disomy or UPD). The second mechanism involves a normal postzygotic (somatic) cell experiencing a nondisjunction event resulting in an extra copy of a chromosome in one daughter cell and a monosomy in the other. UPD can again arise if there is a reduplication of the chromosome in the monosomic cell or loss of the appropriate chromosome in the trisomic line. Monosomy involving an autosome is generally associated with cell nonviability; therefore, only two cell lines are usually observed; the original euploid population plus the trisomic line. The timing of nondisjunctional events is important. Events occurring after the commitment of the cells into fetal and extrafetal compartments can result in a dichotomy between the chromosome constitution of the placental tissue and the fetus (confined placental mosaicism, CPM, or confined fetal mosaicism CFM). Within the placenta and within the fetus, further nonrandom distributions of normal and abnormal cells may occur. In addition, there may be cell selection pressures that favor the proliferation of normal diploid cells, relative to the proliferation of the trisomic line (or visa versa).

The phenotype associated with any particular type of mosaicism can be expected to he highly variable, reflecting the differences in the proportions of normal and abnormal cells. In general, the fetal abnormalities that might be present in mosaic cases can be expected to be consistent with that seen in nonmosaic trisomy or partial trisomy. However, a number of unique aspects to the mosaic situation also need to be considered:

1. CPM may cause placental insufficiency and therefore may be associated with intrauterine growth retardation (IUGR) or fetal death.[167]
2. The presence or extent of a normal cell line in the placenta may be important in determining whether an otherwise abnormal pregnancy might survive in utero.[168–171]
3. UPD may cause specific abnormalities when involving chromosomes carrying imprinted genes (chromosomes 6, 7, 11, 14, 15, 20, and perhaps others).[168]
4. UPD may allow the expression of a recessive disorder when two identical recessive alleles (associated with isodisomy) are present.[168]
5. Impaired cell proliferation of the trisomic cells could be associated with tissue-specific developmental abnormalities.[172]
6. There may be additional clinical features that are apparent only when multiple cell lines are present. Examples are asymmetrical growth and pigmentary anomalies ("hypomelanosis of Ito").[173,174]

Diagnosing Mosaicism

A diagnosis of true mosaicism should be made only when two cell populations with different karyotypes are found in multiple (at least two) independent culture vessels. For in situ harvesting, the finding of an identical aneuploidy in cells from one, or more, colonies from a minimum of two different culture vessels should be the major criterion for the diagnosis of true chromosome mosaicism. Two aneuploid colonies in the same culture do not establish a diagnosis of mosaicism because cell migration can occur within a culture vessel.

With in situ harvesting, there can be three different types of chromosome pseudomosaicism: (1) one cell or one region in a colony with an abnormal karyotype; (2) all the cells of an entire single colony with an identical aberrant karyotype; and (3) multiple colonies within the same culture vessel showing an identical abnormal karyotype.[175] In the flask method, one cannot distinguish whether multiple cells are derived from one initial colony or multiple colonies. Thus, with trypsinized AFC and the flask method, there are only two types of pseudomosaicism (i.e., multiple cells showing an identical abnormality and a single cell showing an aberrant karyotype).

Chromosome mosaicism can never be excluded entirely. For example, examination of 14 colonies or 14 fetal cells can detect only 20 percent of chromosome mosaicism at the 95 percent confidence level. Table 6.15 presents the 90, 95, and 99 percent confidence levels to detect different percentages of chromosome mosaicism.[176] This table was not specifically designed for studying chromosome mosaicism in AFC. However, it is applicable for the in situ method, where N refers to the number of colonies rather than to the number of cells to be examined. Twenty AFCs in the flask method usually represent fewer than twenty colonies, because multiple cells derived from the same colony may well be analyzed. Claussen et al.[177] developed tables for a 95 percent (Table 6.15) and a 99 percent probability for detection of chromosome mosaicism with the flask method, but this requires that the number of the colonies in the flask be recorded before harvesting. A table also exists for the situation in which part of the analysis is based on colonies and part on the flask method.[178]

Guidelines for the diagnosis of mosaicism are presented later in this chapter.

Pseudomosaicism

Frequency of Pseudomosaicism

Pseudomosaicism is much more common than true mosaicism. In three large surveys,[179–181] the frequency of true chromosome mosaicism in cultured AFC ranged from 0.1 to 0.3 percent (Table 6.16). The frequency of pseudomosaicism with multiple cells showing an identical abnormality but restricted to one culture vessel ranged from 0.64 to 1.1 percent. The occurrence of a single cell or a single colony with an aberrant karyotype is not at all rare, ranging from 2.47 to 7.10 percent. In a series of 12,000 cases studied at the Prenatal Diagnosis Laboratory of New York City (PDL), there were 24 cases of chromosome mosaicism (0.2 percent), 126 cases of multiple-cell pseudomosaicism (1.05 percent), and 801 cases of single-cell pseudomosaicism (6.68 percent).[182] When these frequencies are compared with three previous surveys, they are similar to those reported in the Canadian survey[181] (Table 6.17).

Of the 126 cases diagnosed as multiple-cell pseudomosaicism (MCPM) (Table 6.18), there were 77 structural abnormalities versus 49 numerical abnormalities (a ratio of 3:2). In the structural category, there were more balanced reciprocal translocations than deletions. Monosomy X was seen more frequently than additional sex chromosomes.

Of the 801 cases diagnosed as having single-cell pseudomosaicism (SCPM) (Table 6.19), 79 cases had two or more different types of SCPM; this resulted in 888 cells with

Table 6.15. The percentage of mosaicism excluded with 90, 95, and 99 percent confidence if a specified number of cells are evaluated and found to have identical karyotypes

No. of Cells Counted	Mosaicism Excluded at Confidence Level (%)			No. of Cells Counted	Mosaicism Excluded at Confidence Level(%)		
	90 (%)	95 (%)	99 (%)		90 (%)	95 (%)	99 (%)
<4	—	—	—	36	7	8	13
5	38	—	—	37	7	8	12
6	32	41	—	38	6	8	12
7	29	35	—	39	6	8	12
8	26	32	46	40	6	8	11
9	23	29	41	41	6	8	11
10	21	26	37	42	6	7	11
11	19	24	35	43	6	7	11
12	18	23	32	44	6	7	10
13	17	21	30	45	5	7	10
14	16	20	29	46	5	7	10
15	15	19	27	47	5	7	10
16	14	18	26	48	5	7	10
17	13	17	24	49	5	6	9
18	13	16	23	50–55	5	6	9
19	12	15	22	56	5	6	8
20	11	14	21	57–58	4	6	8
21	11	14	20	59–63	4	5	8
22	10	13	19	64–73	4	5	7
23	10	13	19	74	4	4	7
24	10	12	18	75	4	4	6
25	9	12	17	76–89	3	4	6
26	9	11	17	90–98	3	4	5
27	9	11	16	99–112	3	3	5
28	8	11	16	113	3	3	4
29	8	10	15	114–148	2	3	4
30	8	10	15	149–151	2	2	4
31	8	10	14	152–227	2	2	3
32	7	9	14	228–229	2	2	2
33	7	9	14	230–298	1	2	2
34	7	9	13	299–458	1	1	2
35	7	9	13	>459	1	1	1

Source: Hook, Table 1, 1977.[176] Reproduced by permission from the University of Chicago Press.

Note: The table provides the level of mosaicism (or greater) that is excluded with the given confidence level when N cells are counted. The population of cells is assumed to be a random sample. To determine the number of cells to count to exclude a specific level of mosaicism ($\times$ % or greater), choose the lowest value N for which $\times$ % appears in the appropriate column. For example, to exclude 10% mosaicism, with 90% confidence, 22 cells must be counted; for 95% confidence, 29 cells are needed; and for 99% confidence, 44 cells.

SCPM. Among the 888 cells with SCPM, there were 590 with a structural abnormality and 298 with a numerical abnormality (trisomy or monosomy X), showing a ratio of almost 2:1 between a structural and a numerical abnormality. Deletions (all terminal, including 49 broken at the centromere) were the most common abnormalities of SCPM. Among numerical SCPMs, monosomy X was a rather frequent finding. However, this could reflect ascertainment bias because the loss of an X in an XY specimen, or the loss of an autosome, tends to be disregarded.

Table 6.16. The percentage of mosaicism that will be detected with 95% probability for cells analyzed from a mixture of clones (flask method)

Number of Cells	Number of Clones (k)																			
	1	2	3	4	5	**6**	7	8	9	10	11	12	13	14	15	16	17	18	19	20
1	95	95	95	95	95	95	95	95	95	95	95	95	95	95	95	95	95	95	95	95
2	95	91	88	86	85	84	83	83	82	82	82	81	81	81	81	80	80	80	80	80
3	95	86	81	77	75	73	72	71	70	70	69	69	68	68	68	67	67	67	67	67
4	95	83	75	71	68	65	64	63	62	61	60	60	59	59	58	58	58	58	57	57
5	95	80	71	66	62	60	58	56	55	54	54	53	52	52	51	51	51	50	50	50
6	95	79	69	63	58	56	53	52	50	49	49	48	47	47	46	46	46	45	45	45
7	95	79	67	60	56	52	50	48	47	46	45	44	43	43	42	42	41	41	41	41
8	95	78	66	58	53	**50**	47	45	44	43	42	41	40	40	39	39	38	38	38	37
9	95	78	65	57	52	48	45	43	42	40	39	38	38	37	37	36	36	35	35	35
10	95	78	65	56	50	47	44	42	40	38	37	36	36	35	34	34	33	33	33	32
11	95	78	64	55	49	45	42	40	38	37	36	35	34	33	33	32	32	31	31	30
12	95	78	64	55	49	44	41	39	37	36	34	33	32	32	31	31	30	30	29	29
14	95	78	64	54	48	43	40	37	35	33	32	31	30	29	29	28	28	27	27	26
15	95	78	64	54	47	42	39	36	34	33	31	30	29	28	28	27	27	26	26	25
16	95	78	64	54	47	42	38	36	34	32	30	29	28	28	27	26	26	25	25	24
17	95	78	64	54	47	42	38	35	33	31	30	29	28	27	26	25	25	24	24	24
18	95	78	64	54	46	41	38	35	32	31	29	28	27	26	25	25	24	24	23	23
19	95	78	64	53	46	41	37	34	32	30	29	28	26	26	25	24	24	23	23	22
20	95	78	64	53	46	41	37	34	32	30	28	17	26	25	24	24	23	23	22	22
30	95	78	64	53	46	40	36	32	30	28	26	24	23	22	21	20	20	19	19	18
40	95	78	64	53	46	40	35	32	29	27	25	23	22	21	20	19	18	18	17	16
50	95	78	64	53	46	40	35	32	29	27	25	23	21	20	19	18	17	17	16	16
60	95	78	64	53	46	40	35	32	29	26	24	23	21	20	19	18	17	16	16	15
70	95	78	64	53	46	40	35	32	29	26	24	23	21	20	19	18	17	16	15	15
80	95	78	64	53	46	40	35	32	29	26	24	23	21	20	19	18	17	16	15	15
90	95	78	64	53	46	40	35	32	29	26	24	23	21	20	19	18	17	16	15	15
100	95	78	64	53	46	40	35	32	29	26	24	23	21	20	19	18	17	16	15	14

Source: Claussen et al., Table 2, 1984.[177] Reproduced by permission from Springer-Verlag.

Note: This table is used to determine the number of cells that should be analyzed from a single flask. k = total number of clones in the flask before harvesting. For example, if there are 6 clones in the flask ($k = 6$), to detect 50% mosaicism at 95% confidence level, eight cells must be analyzed. This number is obtained by looking down the column corresponding to $k = 6$ and reaching the first percentage not greater than 50 (shown in bold).

Table 6.17. The frequency of mosaicism and pseudomosaicism

Origin of Data	Mosaicism		Pseudomosaicism Multiple Cells		Pseudomosaicism Single Cell	
	N	(%)	N	(%)	N	(%)
U.S. survey[179]	62,279	0.25	48,442	0.70	30,754	2.47
European survey[180]	44,170	0.1	44,170	0.64	44,170	2.83
Canadian survey[181]	12,386	0.3	12,386	1.10	12,386	7.1
PDL data[182]	12,000	0.2	12,000	1.05	12,000	6.68

N = number of cases studied.

Table 6.18. The frequency of multiple-cell pseudomosaicism (MCPM)

Type of Abnormality	No. of Cells
Structural	77
Balanced	46
Reciprocal translocation	43
Robertsonian translocation	1
Inversion	2
Unbalanced	30
Deletion	15
Additional chromosomal material	12
Isochromosome	1
Fragment or marker	2
Mixed balanced and unbalanced	1
Numerical	49
Autosomal trisomy	32
Extra sex chromosome	6
XXX	4
XXY	2
Involving 45,X	11
Missing an X	4
Missing a Y	7
Total cases of MCPM	126/12,000 (1.05%)

Source: Data from Hsu et al., 1992.[182]

Table 6.19. Single-cell pseudomosaicism (SCPM)

Type of Abnormality	No. of Cells
Structural	590
Balanced	100
Reciprocal translocation	81
Robertsonian translocation	12
Inversion	7
Unbalanced	490
Deletion	339
Additional chromosomal material	79
Isochromosome	16
Fragment or marker	56
Numerical	298
Autosomal trisomy	221
Extra sex chromosome	17
XXX	13
XXY	3
XYY	1
Involving 45,X	60
Missing an X	29
Missing a Y	31
Total number of cells with SCPM	888
Total number of cases with SCPM	801[a]
Frequency of SCPM	6.68% (801/12,000)

Source: Data from Hsu et al., 1992.[182]
[a]79 cases had two or more different types of SCPM.

Significance of Pseudomosaicism

Given that true mosaicism can never be entirely excluded, there is a concern that clinically significant abnormalities might be inappropriately dismissed as pseudomosaicism. How concerned should we be?

SCPM and MCPM involving nonspecific structural abnormalities are unlikely to be important. A low level of random chromosome breakage is expected. Furthermore, true mosaicism involving a structural abnormality is relatively rare (see below). In the case of balanced rearrangements, the risk associated with a true mosaicism would be minimal.

A greater concern exists for autosomal trisomy pseudomosaicism. There is a nonrandom involvement of specific chromosomes in these cases. The U.S. survey combined with PDL data[179–182] shows that trisomy 2 and trisomy 7 are each involved in more than 10 percent of the MCPM cases (Table 6.20). These two trisomies are also the most commonly encountered in SCPM (Table 6.21). Trisomy 2 and trisomy 7 are also among the most frequently seen trisomies in first-trimester CVS cultures (villus mesenchyme).[109] It is extremely unlikely that the preferential involvement of chromosomes 2 and 7 in both amniocytes and CVS cultures is coincidental. When encountered in CVS cultures, the origin of the extra chromosome is generally a somatic cell error,[183,184] but the presence of these trisomic cells is considered to be an accurate indication of chromosomal mosaicism in the placenta (but not necessarily the fetus). It is therefore reasonable to think that the

Table 6.20. The frequency of trisomy chromosome in pseudomosaicism (multiple cell)

Chromosome	Number	(%)
1	0	0.0
2	34	23.0
3	2	1.3
4	1	0.7
5	4	2.7
6	1	0.7
7	16	10.8
8	5	3.4
9	8	5.4
10	5	3.4
11	4	2.7
12	2	1.4
13	6	4.0
14	3	2.0
15	4	2.7
16	2	1.3
17	9	6.1
18	3	2.0
19	2	1.3
20	9	6.1
21	7	4.7
22	4	2.7
X	13	8.8
Y	14	2.7
Total	148	

Source: Data from Hsu and Perlis, 1984[179] and Hsu et al., 1992.[182]

Table 6.21.   The frequency of trisomy chromosome in
pseudomosaicism (single cell)

Chromosome	Number	(%)
1	16	2.3
2	102	14.6
3	23	3.3
4	17	2.4
5	27	3.9
6	20	2.9
7	44	6.3
8	27	3.9
9	36	5.2
10	23	3.3
11	25	3.6
12	27	3.9
13	23	3.3
14	22	3.2
15	21	3.0
16	22	3.2
17	30	4.3
18	24	3.4
19	20	2.9
20	42	6.0
21	35	5.0
22	19	2.7
X	36	5.2
Y	15	2.2
Total	696	

Source: Data from Hsu and Perlis, 1984,[179] and Hsu et al., 1992.[182]

occasional finding of trisomy 2 and trisomy 7 cells in amniotic fluid cells also often represents cell lines that are derived from extrafetal tissues. It seems likely that some of the other abnormalities characterized as pseudomosaicism are similarly derived from extrafetal tissues. We therefore emphasize that the abnormalities that are classified as pseudomosaicism should not be viewed solely as artifacts arising during cell culture.

The clinical significance of these cells remains unclear. Studies have linked placental mosaicism to IUGR and poor pregnancy outcomes,[185,186] but there is no direct evidence that trisomy 2 or trisomy 7 pseudomosaicism in amniocytes is associated with an adverse outcome. However, as discussed below in the section on true autosomal mosaicism, there is a special concern for low-level trisomy 16 mosaicism or pseudomosaicism that may well be clinically significant.

In theory, SCPM and MCPM involving gain of a sex chromosome could also potentially reflect true mosaicism. Based on the phenotypes associated with nonmosaic gain of a sex chromosome, the clinical consequences of this type of true mosaicism would be minimal. Loss of a sex chromosome may well reflect random somatic cell loss and is quite common. Although theoretically possible, there is currently no direct evidence that pseudomosaicism involving loss of a sex chromosome is associated with an increased risk for Turner syndrome characteristics, infertility, or other clinical conditions that can be found in true mosaic cases.

Concerns about pseudomosaicism need to be considered in the context of the patient anxiety that the information will cause. In the absence of direct evidence that a particular pseudomosaicism is clinically significant, it is justifiable and appropriate to interpret the results as part of a range of cytogenetic diversity that is expected to be present in a normal population.

Summary Conclusions and Recommendations for Pseudomosaicism

1. Most nonspecific structural chromosomal abnormalities that are classified as pseudomosaicism will be clinically insignificant.
2. Some autosomal trisomies may reflect cell lines present in extra-fetal tissues.
3. With the exception of those involving chromosome 16, there is little direct evidence that autosomal trisomy pseudomosaicism is likely to be clinically significant.
4. Similarly, there is no direct evidence that the SCPM and MCPM involving gain or loss of a sex chromosome is associated with increased risk for abnormality.

True Mosaicism Involving Gain or Loss of Autosomes

In evaluating the risk associated with the prenatally detected rare autosomal trisomies, it is necessary to rely heavily on published case reports. Most cases included in this compilation did not appear to be subject to the ascertainment bias that is associated with referral through ultrasound detection of fetal anomalies. However, the data are subject to publication bias; only the cases with the most unusual findings or comprehensive follow-up tend to be published. For our assessment of risk for the common autosomal mosaicisms (chromosomes 13, 18, and 21) our summary of risk is based on a survey in which cases ascertained because of abnormal ultrasound findings were excluded.[187] These estimates of risk can therefore be viewed as being the most objective.

Chromosome 1

Nonmosaic trisomy 1 appears to be incompatible with even rudimentary fetal development,[188] but rare cases of trisomy 1 mosaicism have been described.[189,190] These presumably arise through chromosome 1 nondisjunction in somatic cells. We are unaware of any reports of trisomy 1 mosaicism in amniocytes.

Chromosome 2

Trisomy 2 is a relatively common finding in the analysis of CVS, and the additional chromosome 2 may be attributed to either meiotic or mitotic error.[183] In CVS specimens, this trisomy is often present in the villus mesenchyme (longer-term cultures) but absent in cytotrophoblasts (direct preparations).[109] A high proportion of trisomy 2 cells in placental tissue appear to be associated with IUGR and fetal and neonatal death.[183,191] Although a specific phenotype has been proposed for upd(2)mat,[192] there are also examples of normal individuals with upd(2)mat.[193,194] This strongly suggests that any abnormalities noted in individuals with upd(2)mat are more likely to be attributable to the effect of a coexisting trisomic cell line rather than to the UPD.

A total of 12 cases of trisomy 2 mosaicism have been reported in AFC cultures.[195,196] In four of the eight cases, the indication for amniocentesis was elevated MSAFP. In eleven of the twelve cases there was an abnormal pregnancy outcome. The phenotype may include minor craniofacial anomalies, digital anomalies, wide-spaced nipples, ventriculomegaly, and developmental delay.[196]

Chromosome 3

Trisomy 3 is occasionally seen in CVS specimens but appears to be confined largely to direct preparations (cytotrophoblasts). Only three cases of trisomy 3 mosaicism in amniocytes have been described.[195,196a] In one, multiple congenital anomalies were present in the liveborn infant and in another case IUGR was noted.

Chromosome 4

Prenatal diagnosis of trisomy 4 mosaicism seems to be extremely rare. This mosaicism has been diagnosed twice in CVS[197] and four times in amniocytes.[195,198–200] In the second trimester, the diagnosis has been associated with both abnormal[198,199] and normal[195,200] pregnancy outcomes.

Chromosome 5

Trisomy 5 mosaicism is sometimes observed in CVS specimens.[109] Of five cases with second-trimester trisomy 5 mosaicism, two cases (40 percent), both liveborns, were abnormal, with IUGR and congenital heart disease.[195] Facial dysmorphism was also present in one and an ear pit in the other. Trisomy 5 mosaicism was confirmed in both cases.

Chromosome 6

Upd(6)pat is associated with transient neonatal diabetes,[192] and UPD should be considered in rare cases that show this particular mosaicism. There are only seven reported cases of trisomy 6 mosaicism, of which three were identified through CVS.[201–203] Among the four cases identified through cytogenetic analysis of amniocytes,[195,204] one showed an abnormal phenotype.[204]

Chromosome 7

Mosaic trisomy 7 is the most commonly encountered mosaicism in CVS specimens, in which it may be confined to cytotrophoblasts or mesenchyme tissue and is only rarely found in both.[109] In most cases, the additional chromosome 7 is mitotic in origin.[184] However, there are some cases in which the abnormality is attributable to meiotic error; in some of these cases (theoretically, one-third), upd(7) is present. Some individuals with Silver–Russell syndrome have upd(7)mat but the precise genetic basis for this disorder remains to be established.[205] Imprinted genes at 7p11.2–p13 and perhaps also at 7q32 may account for some cases.[205,206,206a] Occult trisomy 7 may also be causal.[207] Skewed X-inactivation is sometimes present in females with Silver–Russell syndrome, which may reflect impaired growth or selection against trisomic cells.[208,208a]

In seven cases of trisomy 7 diagnosed in amniotic fluid cells, only two cases were associated with an abnormal phenotype.[195,209] Data from both prenatal and postnatal diagnosed cases indicate that trisomy 7 mosaicism is associated with a variably expressed phenotype that can include hypotonia, abnormal face, renal anomalies, sparse hair, and pigmentary anomalies ("hypomelanosis of Ito").[209]

Chromosome 8

In contrast to the situation seen in spontaneous abortion tissues, the additional chromosome 8 present in viable mosaic and nonmosaic trisomy 8 pregnancies is usually mitotic in origin.[210,211] There appears to be considerable potential for tissue-specific variation in the proportion of abnormal cells,[212] which can lead to false-negative results in the analysis of both CVS and AFC.[201,213–215]

Of 14 cases with trisomy 8 mosaicism in AFC,[195] only one case with 77 percent trisomy 8 cells was reported to be phenotypically abnormal, the remaining thirteen cases all resulted in either grossly normal abortuses (eight cases) or grossly normal liveborns (five cases). It is known that a clinical diagnosis of trisomy 8 syndrome is difficult because of the subtle abnormalities associated with this disorder (i.e., thick lips, prominent ears, absent or dysplastic patellae, and deep plantar skin furrows). What appears to be the low risk of an abnormal outcome or the high probability of finding a grossly normal appearing offspring following a prenatal diagnosis of 46/47,+8 in amniocytes may be explained by the difficulty in recognizing these subtle clinical features. In cases with fibroblasts and/or placental studies, trisomy 8 mosaicism was confirmed in the majority of cases (72.7 percent).

Chromosome 9

Trisomy 9, nonmosaic or mosaic, is a distinct clinical entity. Of twenty-seven cases of trisomy 9 mosaicism diagnosed through amniotic fluid specimens,[195,216,216a] sixteen (59 percent) resulted in grossly abnormal offspring (fifteen abortuses and one liveborn). In these sixteen abnormal cases, eight had multiple congenital anomalies, eight had facial dysmorphism, four had congenital heart defects, three had urogenital abnormalities, three had skeletal abnormalities, and three had IUGR. Comparison of the major phenotypic abnormalities noted in the prenatal versus the postnatal cases show rather comparable features. Of twenty cases with successful cytogenetic follow-up studies, trisomy 9 mosaicism was confirmed in the majority of cases (75 percent).

Chromosome 10

Chromosome 10 mosaicism is sometimes encountered in CVS cell cultures, rarely in direct preparations.[109] In only one instance has a prenatal diagnosis of trisomy 10 mosaicism, through CVS, been confirmed in fetal tissues,[217] and we are unaware of any such cases diagnosed through amniocentesis.

Chromosome 11

Chromosome 11 is known to carry imprinted genes, and upd(11)pat is associated with Beckwith–Weidemann syndrome.[192] A concern therefore exists that trisomy 11 mosaicism could be associated with UPD in the normal cell line. This particular mosaicism appears to be very rare. Only two second-trimester cases are known,[195] both of which were associated with a low frequency of trisomic cells; both had normal pregnancy outcomes.

Chromosome 12

Chromosome 12 mosaicism is rare in CVS specimens,[109] but there are five reports of postnatally diagnosed trisomy 12 mosaicism.[218] The phenotype appears to be highly variable. Among twenty-four cases with trisomy 12 mosaicism in AFC,[195,219] seven (26 percent) had abnormal outcome. This included five offspring (three liveborns, one premature infant, and 1 abortus) with congenital heart disease, facial dysmorphism in two, skeletal abnormalities in two, renal abnormality in one, tracheoesophageal fistula in one, and fetal demise with IUGR in one. Of seven grossly normal liveborns, three had follow-up from five months to five years; all were reported to be developmentally normal. The overall cytogenetic confirmation rate was 64 percent from fibroblasts and/or placental tissues.

Chromosome 13

The survey of common trisomy mosaicism[187] identified twenty-five cases of trisomy 13 mosaicism in amniocytes. This survey excluded cases with prior abnormal ultrasound findings and other factors that would constitute ascertainment bias. Abnormal outcomes were noted in ten (40 percent), with a higher probability of abnormality when the proportion of abnormal cells was high. The overall rate of positive confirmatory studies was six of thirteen cases (46 percent). There were four cases in which trisomy 13 mosaicism was diagnosed at amniocentesis (mean proportion of abnormal cells 9 percent) and the pregnancy was continued. In all four cases there were no abnormalities noted at birth and, in the three cases with follow-up cytogenetic analyses, no abnormal cells were detected.

Chromosome 14

Upd(14)mat and upd(14)pat are associated with different abnormal phenotypes,[77,78] and it is likely that additional anomalies would be present in cases in which there is a residual trisomy 14 cell line. Of five cases with a trisomy 14 mosaicism in amniotic fluid cells,[195] two (both abortuses) resulted in abnormal offspring; one had multiple congenital anomalies and facial dysmorphism and the other had hydrocephaly.

Chromosome 15

Trisomy 15 is usually attributable to meiotic error,[211] and mosaic cases can be expected to show UPD in a proportion of the cases. Upd(15)mat is a cause of Prader–Willi syndrome and upd(15)pat is associated with Angelman syndrome.[192] These diagnoses therefore also need to be considered when a trisomy 15 cell line is identified in CVS or amniocytes. Among thirteen second-trimester cases with trisomy 15 mosaicism,[195,220] seven (54 percent) resulted in abnormal offspring (six abortuses, one liveborn). There were heart defects (four), IUGR (three) (one of them had arrhinencephaly, hand contractures, low-set ears), and malrotation of the intestine and a two-vessel cord (one). Two abortuses showed upd(15)mat, which would be consistent with Prader–Willi syndrome had these pregnancies been continued.

Chromosome 16

Although there are now a substantial number of documented prenatal diagnoses of trisomy 16 mosaicism, this diagnosis is associated with a highly variable set of pregnancy outcomes and counseling is therefore complex.[107,220a] Most cases have been identified through CVS and outcomes in these cases frequently included fetal death, IUGR and/or a diverse spectrum of birth defects (some of which involved only a single organ). Sometimes there was an entirely normal liveborn infant.

   The extra chromosome present in trisomy 16 and trisomy 16 mosaicism is nearly always the result of a maternal meiotic error[221] and the possible effect of UPD needs to be considered. Although it has been predicted that imprinted genes exist on chromosome 16, none has yet been identified.[192] Yong et al.[222] reported that cases of trisomy 16 mosaicism in which upd(16)mat was present were more likely to show IUGR and major fetal malformations compared with cases with a biparental diploid cell line. However, after excluding case reports that may show ascertainment bias, this association lacked statistical significance. The proportions of trisomic cells in the fetus and in the placenta are probably important factors in determining pregnancy outcome. Peñaherrera et al.[223] noted extremely skewed X-inactivation patterns in many female fetuses and newborns with trisomy 16 mosaicism. These data would be consistent with the hypothesis that there is substantial selection against trisomic cells, reducing the size of the early embryonic cell pool. Extreme skewing appeared to be more common in cases with abnormal outcomes. Malformations and IUGR could therefore reflect the poor viability and depletion of cells in developing tissues rather than a direct consequence of the gene imbalance.

Excluding multiple reports that relate to the same patients, we are aware of forty-one cases of trisomy 16 mosaicism in AFC cultures.[107,223–225] Elevated MSAFP is a common reason for referral.[107] Maternal serum hCG is often grossly elevated, and inhibin-A seems to follow a similar pattern.[226] Of the forty-one pregnancies, abnormality was noted in thirty-four (83 percent). IUGR was noted in eighteen (44 percent). Among the twenty-five pregnancies that were not electively terminated, there were five (25 percent) neonatal deaths. Preterm delivery was common with at least sixteen (64 percent) of the births before 37 weeks of gestational age. Fetal abnormalities or malformations in newborns were noted in twenty-eight of the forty-one cases (68 percent). These were generally consistent with that expected in 16p or 16q duplications.[107]

The forty-one cases included three that, technically, should be classed as pseudomosaicism because the abnormal cell line was not detected in multiple independent cultures.[107,225] All three of these cases had grossly elevated maternal serum hCG, abnormal pregnancy outcomes consistent with this diagnosis, and follow-up studies that confirmed trisomy 16 mosaicism. In addition, eight of the forty-one cases had 10 percent, or less, abnormal cells in the AFC cultures. Therefore, low levels of trisomy 16 should not be dismissed as clinically insignificant.

Confirmatory rates for trisomy 16 mosaicism are high when follow-up studies are carried out on placental tissue (eighteen of nineteen studies positive), amnion (four of four) and cord (four of five). In contrast, the presence of trisomic cells is inconsistently found in fibroblasts (nine of twenty-two) and is rarely present in blood (two of twenty-two).

Chromosome 17

Chromosome 17 mosaicism appears to be uncommon in CVS preparations.[109] There have been sixteen reported instances of trisomy 17 mosaicism in AFC cultures.[195,227–231,232] In two cases,[230,231] mild dysmorphic features were noted. Confirmatory cytogenetic studies established the presence of trisomy 17 cells in the skin fibroblasts in these two cases.

Chromosome 18

The survey of common trisomies in AFC[187] identified thirty-one cases of trisomy 18 mosaicism with abnormal outcomes in seventeen (54 percent). These amniocenteses were performed because of advanced maternal age (thirty women) or choroid plexus cysts (one). Abnormal outcomes were more common in the cases with high proportions of abnormal cells. Eight of twelve cases had positive confirmatory studies. In the three cases with trisomy 18 mosaicism (mean proportion of abnormal cells in AFC, 9 percent) and a liveborn infant, no abnormalities were seen at birth. In two of these three cases, follow-up cytogenetic analyses were performed and no abnormal cells were detected.

Chromosome 19

We are aware of only one case of trisomy 19 mosaicism in AFC cultures, and no follow-up information was available in that case.[195]

Chromosome 20

Trisomy 20 mosaicism is sometimes encountered in CVS. The abnormal cell line is most often limited to direct preparations, with only a few cases showing the presence in both cytotrophoblasts and villus mesenchyme.[109] The proportion of cases in which the additional chromosome is meiotic is not known. Both upd(20)mat and upd(20)pat have been observed.[232–235] Thus far, only one imprinted gene, *GNAS1,* has been assigned to chromosome 20. Mutation of this gene and UPD has been implicated in several human endocrine disorders.[233] Although the upd(20)mat cases share the common characteristic of prenatal and/or postnatal growth failure, this could be attributable to the presence of a trisomic cell line rather than to the UPD.[235]

The most common autosomal trisomy mosaicism encountered in AFC cultures involves a cell line with an additional copy of chromosome 20. Despite the large number of reports, prenatal counseling in these cases remains problematic. Table 6.22 summarizes data from 318 published cases.[187,236–238] Of the 294 cases with outcome information, abnormality was noted in 22 (7.5 percent). No specific pattern of abnormality emerged, although hypotonia, cardiac anomalies, and urinary tract anomalies were each documented in several cases. Facial dysmorphism was noted in 7 of the 22 cases with abnormalities. Serial high-resolution ultrasound examinations with special emphasis on the renal and cardiovascular systems may be helpful in the management of these cases.

Recent case reports have focused on the longer-term follow-up of prenatally diagnosed trisomy 20 mosaicism.[239,240] Hypomelanosis of Ito was noted in these children. There are also reports documenting developmental delay,[237,241,242] but, again, this is an inconsistent finding and the risk is poorly defined.[239]

Further confounding this diagnosis is the inability to routinely confirm the presence of a trisomic line through follow-up cytogenetic testing. The overall confirmatory rate for the 214 cases receiving these studies was only 15.4 percent (Table 6.23). Cases with an abnormal phenotype may be more likely to show the presence of the trisomy 20 cell line in these follow-up studies.[187] The suspicion of urinary tract involvement, together with the data in Table 6.23, indicates that cytogenetic confirmation in abortuses should involve studies on kidney, skin, and placental tissues (including membranes). For confirmation in liveborns, placental tissues, including membranes, skin (foreskin in male), cord fibroblasts, blood cells, and urine sediment should all be studied. The urinary sediment may contain cells that were shed from the kidneys.

Chromosome 21

Ninety-seven cases of trisomy 21 mosaicism are included in the common mosaicism in amniocytes survey.[187] Indications for amniocentesis were advanced maternal age (sixty-nine pregnancies), serum screen-positive for Down syndrome (nineteen pregnancies), parental anxiety (two pregnancies), elevated MSAFP (three pregnancies) and a prior child with a chromosomal abnormality (two pregnancies). Cases with ultrasound-identified cardiac defects or other visible anomalies were excluded from the study. Forty-nine (51 percent) had abnormal outcomes, with a spectrum of anomalies consistent with Down

Table 6.22.   A summary of prenatally diagnosed cases with 46/47,+20: pregnancy outcome

Total number of cases: 318 (from 317 pregnancies including one pair of twins)
Pregnancy outcome:
    Pregnancy continued: 251
    Pregnancy terminated: 55
    Spontaneously aborted: 4
    Unknown: 7

Phenotype	No. of Cases
Grossly normal	272 (237 liveborns; 37 abortuses)
Grossly abnormal	22 (10 liveborns; 12 abortuses)
Other	2
Turner phenotype	1 abortus with 45,X/46,X+20
Hydrops	1 abortus with Rh incompatibility
Abnormality rate	22/294 (7.5%)

Abnormal liveborns
    4 IUGR (one with hypotonia)
    1 unilateral cleft lip
    1 Williams syndrome
    1 facial asymmetry, microcephaly, low-set abnormal ears, other anomalies
    1 structural CNS abnormalities and seizures
    1 facial dysmorphism, hypotonia, failure to thrive, developmental delay at 16 months
    1 hypotonia, micrognathia
Abnormal abortuses
    3 fetal demise (spontaneous abortion)
    1 IUGR
    1 facial dysmorphism and microcephaly
    1 renal anomaly (megapelvis and kinky ureters)
    1 slight facial dysmorphism and microretrognathia
    1 facial dysmorphism
    1 facial dysmorphism, congenital heart disease (transposition of great arteries, pulmonary stenosis,
        hypoplasia of right ventricle, and hypoplasia of tricuspid and bicuspid valves), anal fistula,
        camptodactyly
    1 micrognathia, abnormal ears, renal anomalies (pelvic horseshoe kidneys), and congenital heart disease
        (stenosis of ductus Botalli, hypoplasia of right ventricle, and hypertrophy of ventricle walls)
    1 slight facial dysmorphism, epicanthal folds, microretrognathia, abnormal ears, and meandering of left ureter
    1 occipital and cervical meningocele

Source: Data from Hsu et al., 1987,[236] Hsu et al., 1991,[237] Hsu, 1998,[238] and Wallerstein et al., 2000. [187]

syndrome. The presence of a trisomic cell line was confirmed in twenty-four of fifty-four (44 percent) cases receiving these studies. In the thirteen cases with trisomy 21 mosaicism (mean proportion of abnormal cells in amniocytes 17 percent) and a liveborn infant, abnormalities were present at birth in six. Among the thirteen liveborns, confirmatory studies were performed in five (all with abnormalities) and the trisomic cell line was confirmed in four.

Chromosome 22

The additional copy of chromosome 22 appears to be generally attributable to a meiotic error.[211] Both upd(22)mat and upd(22)pat have been observed, but there are no known imprinted genes on chromosome 22. Trisomy 22 mosaicism is a relatively well-defined en-

Table 6.23. Summary of prenatally diagnosed cases with 46/47,+20 cytogenetic confirmation studies

Overall confirmation rate	33/214 (15.4%)
Tissues studied with recovery of trisomy 20 cells (33 cases)	
Blood	1
Skin	9
Placenta/membrane/amnion/cord	13
Urine sediment	6
Second amniotic fluid	1
Kidney	6
Other fetal tissue	4
Tissues studied with normal cells only (181 cases)	
Blood	102
Skin	46
Placenta/membrane/amnion/cord	47
Urine sediment	4
Second amniotic fluid	7
Other fetal tissue	4
No study or unsuccessful study (49 cases)	

Source: Data from Hsu et al., 1987, 1991,[236,237] Hsu, 1998,[238] and Wallerstein et al., 2000.[187]

tity.[243,243a] Of twelve cases with trisomy 22 mosaicism in AFC,[195,244] eight (67 percent) had an abnormal outcome. This included two liveborns with congenital heart defects and dysmorphic features, one neonatal death with IUGR and hydrocephaly, one premature infant with IUGR, three abortuses with dysmorphic features and/or skeletal anomalies, and one fetal demise. Four cases (two liveborns and two abortuses) had two or more features of trisomy 22 syndrome (such as abnormal ears or ear tags, heart defects, and long fingers).

Autosomal Monosomy Mosaicism

Thirteen cases of autosomal monosomy mosaicism have been diagnosed prenatally.[152,238] This included five cases involving chromosome 21, three for chromosome 22, two cases for chromosome 17, and one case each involving chromosomes 9, 19, and 20. Of seven cases with phenotypic information and four cases with successful cytogenetic follow-up studies, one case with monosomy 22 mosaicism was reported to have multiple congenital anomalies (including congenital heart disease), and the mosaicism was confirmed by blood culture. One case involving chromosome 21 was also confirmed cytogenetically but was reported to be phenotypically normal.

Autosomal monosomy in amniocytes has generally been considered to be an in vitro artifact. However, as noted, it appears that it can represent true mosaicism and may be associated with congenital anomalies. If cells with autosomal monosomy are detected in two or more culture vessels, and if the missing chromosome is a 21 or a 22, further workup is indicated. This includes FISH studies of a large number of interphase nuclei, percutaneous umbilical blood sampling (PUBS), and/or ultrasound examination.

Complex and Variegated Aneuploidy

There is an isolated report of AFC 46,XX/47,XY+3/48,XXY+18 mosaicism.[245] At birth, the karyotype was confirmed and the phenotype was consistent with trisomy 18. The highly unusual combination of 46,XY/47,XY+4/47,XY+6 confirmed mosaicism has been reported.[246] In addition, double trisomy[247] and even triple trisomy[248] have been noted in pregnancies with normal outcomes. Mitotic instability has also been described in which the cells develop many different aneuploid lines apparently as a result of premature chromatid separation.[249,249a]

Summary Conclusions and Recommendations for Mosaicism Involving Gain or Loss of Autosomes

1. The risks for abnormal outcome appear to be very high (>60 percent) for mosaic trisomies 2, 16, and 22; high (40–59 percent) for trisomies 4, 5, 9, 13, 14, 15, 18, and 21; and moderately high (20–29 percent) for trisomies 6, 7, and 12 (Table 6.24). In categories with a small number of cases (three or fewer), the risk was not well defined.
2. Comparison of the phenotype of prenatally diagnosed abnormal cases and postnatally diagnosed cases with the same diagnosis shows considerable concordance.
3. When the percentages of trisomic cells were recorded for the category of "normal outcome" versus "abnormal outcome," it appears that cases with a relatively high proportion of trisomic cells are more likely to be associated with an abnormal outcome than those with a low proportion of trisomic cells.
4. Because many anomalies are prenatally detectable with ultrasound, a high-resolution ultrasound examination of the fetus should be performed in all prenatally diagnosed cases.
5. For cytogenetic confirmation, both fibroblasts (from skin, other fetal tissues, and/or cord) and placental tissues should be studied. When both fetal and extrafetal tissues are studied, a cytogenetic confirmation can usually be achieved.
6. Except for trisomy 8, 9, 13, 18, and 21 mosaicism, PUBS is of limited value in further workup of the diagnosis.
7. DNA studies for uniparental disomy are recommended when mosaicism involves a chromosome with established imprinting effects (chromosomes 6, 7, 11, 14, and 15). There are insufficient data to know whether this is necessary in cases of chromosome 20 mosaicism.
8. Mosaicism involving monosomy 21 or 22, and aneuploidy involving more than one chromosome are very rare but may be clinically significant.

Mosaicism Involving an Autosomal Structural Abnormality

Frequency

Among 179,663 prenatal diagnosis cases collected from ten institutions and two publications, 555 (0.3 percent) were diagnosed as having true chromosome mosaicism.[250] Of these, fifty-seven (10.3 percent of all mosaic cases) were mosaic for an autosomal structural abnormality (excluding mosaicism involving a marker chromosome). In a multicenter study,[250] pregnancy outcomes were reviewed for ninety-five cases with mosaicism involving an autosomal structural abnormality and a normal cell line (Table 6.25).

Balanced Structural Rearrangement

Of twenty-one cases mosaic for a balanced structural rearrangement,[250] including thirteen cases of a reciprocal translocation, four cases of a Robertsonian translocation, and four

Table 6.24. Summary of pregnancy outcomes and confirmation rate for trisomy mosaicism diagnosed in amniocytes

Trisomy	No. of Cases	Pregnancy Outcome			Phenotypic Outcome			Positive Cytogenetic Confirmation Studies (%)
		Continued	Term.	Normal	Abn.	FD/Sb	Abn./Total (%)	
1	0	—	—	—	—	—	— —	— —
2	12	8	4	1	8*	3	11/12 (92)	8/9 (89)
3	3	3	0	1	2ᵃ	0	2/3 (66)	1/3 (33)
4	4	3	1	2	2ᵇ	0	2/4 (50)	1/4 (25)
5	5	5	0	3	2ᶜ	0	2/5 (40)	2/4 (50)
6	4	3	1	3	1ᵈ	0	1/4 (25)	1/2 (50)
7	9	9	0	7	2ᵉ	0	2/9 (22)	4/7 (57)
8	14	5	9	13	1*	0	1/14 (7)	8/11 (73)
9	27	4	23	11	16*	0	16/27 (59)	15/20 (75)
10	0	—	—	—	—	—	—	—
11	2	1	1	2	0	0	0/2 (0)	0/2 (0)
12	24	13	11	17	5*	2	7/24 (29)	10/15 (67)
13	25	4	21	15	10	2	10/25 (40)	6/13 (46)
14	5	3	2	3	2ᶠ	0	2/5 (40)	0/3 (0)
15	13	5	8	5	7*	0	7/13 (54)	9/11 (82)
16	41	25	16	7	34*	0	34/41 (83)	18/19 (95)
17	16	14	2	14	2ᵍ	0	2/16 (13)	2/15 (13)
18	31	3	28	14	17	3	17/31 (54)	8/12 (66)
19	1	1	0	1	0	0	0/1 (0)	—
20	318	251	55	272	22	3	22/318 (7)	33/214 (15)
21	97	13	84	48	49	5	49/97 (50)	24/54 (44)
22	12	7	5	4	7*	1	8/12 (67)	6/9 (67)

*See text for details.

ᵃOne liveborn had bilateral cleft lip and palate, tetralogy of Fallot, pulmonary stenosis, microphthalmia, abnormal left ear, and vertebral abnormalities and died at 18 months from heart defects; one liveborn with IUGR.

ᵇOne liveborn had facial dysmorphism, short neck, ventricular septal defect, and pectus excavatum; one abortus with cyclopia, alobar holoprosencephaly, skeletal anomalies and other defects.

ᶜOne liveborn had IUGR, heart murmur, and ear pit; the other liveborn had IUGR, facial dysmorphism, and ventricular septal defect.

ᵈOne abortus with short femurs, micrognathia, posterior malrotation of the ears, and bilateral camptomelia.

ᵉOne liveborn had mild developmental delay at 7 years of age and was noted to have facial asymmetry and hypomelanosis of Ito; one liveborn with sparse hair, short left palpebral fissure, ptosis, strabismus, enamel dysplasia, low-set posteriorly rotated ears, undescended testes, and pigmentary anomalies at age 3 years.

ᶠOne abortus had hydrocephaly; one abortus had low-set ears, simian lines, clinodactyly, equinovarus, abnormal hip, and rocker-bottom feet.

ᵍOne liveborn with prominent forehead, temporal narrowing, retrognathism, hypoplastic columella, short hands and feet, simian crease, abnormal ears; one abortus with micrognathia, large mouth, and long philtrum.

FD = fetal demise; Sb = stillbirth.

cases of an inversion (three cases with a pericentric inversion and one with a paracentric inversion), all resulted in phenotypically normal liveborns.

Unbalanced Structural Rearrangement

Unbalanced structural rearrangements include supernumerary structurally abnormal chromosomes. We discuss supernumerary chromosomes in more detail below (see "Interpretation Issues: Chromosome Rearrangements" and "De novo Supernumerary Chromosomes (Including Mosaic Cases)."

Table 6.25. Mosaicism with an autosomal structural abnormality

Type of Abnormal Cell Line in Mosaicism	No. Cases	Pregnancy Outcome		Phenotype		Abn./Total (%)	Cytogenetic Confirmation (%)
		Cont.	Term.	Normal	Abnormal		
Balanced rearrangement							
Reciprocal translocation	13	11	2	13	0	0/13 (0.0)	3/8 (37.5)
Robertsonian translocation	4	4	0	4	0	0/4 (0.0)	2/2 (100)
Inversion	4	4	0	4	0	0/4 (0.0)	1/4 (25.0)
Unbalanced rearrangement							
Reciprocal translocation	1	1	—		1-LB (MCA, MR)	1/1 (0.0)	1/1 (100.0)
Robertsonian translocation[a]	4	2	2	3 (2-LB; 1-AB)	1-LB (micrognathia; hyperlobation of lung)	1/4 (25.0)	3/4 (75.0)
Terminal deletion *not* involving a fragile site	10	6	4	8 (5-LB; 3-AB)	2 (1-LB, del(11)(q24) MCA) (1-AB, 18p− microcephaly)	2/10 (20.0)	5/8 (62.5) (both phenotypically abnormal cases confirmed)
Terminal deletion involving a fragile site	5	4	1	4 (all LB)	1(AB, del(16)(q23) cystic hygroma)	1/5 (20.0)	1/3 (33.3) (phenotypically abnormal case confirmed)
Interstitial deletion							
del(18)(q12.2q21.1)	1	0	1		1 (AB-MCA)	1/1 (100.0)	1/1 (100.0)
del(18)(q21q23)	1	1	0	1 (LB)		0/1 (0.0)	0/1 (100.0)
Ring chromosome							
46,r(12)	1	1	0	1 (LB)		0/1 (0.0)	1/1 (100.0)
46,r(22)	2	0	2	1 (AB)	1 (AB, single umbilical artery, clinodactyly)	1/2 (50.0)	1/2 (50.0) (phenotypically abnormal AB case confirmed)

Isochromosome							
46,i(20q)	19	19	0	19 (all LB)		0/19 (0.0)	0/15 (0.0)
46,i(17p)	1	0	1		1 (AB-MCA)	1/1 (100.0)	1/1 (100.0)
47,+i(12p)	7	0	7	2 (2 AB)	5 (AB, Pallister–Killian syndrome)	5/7 (71.4)	4/6 (66.7)
47,+i(18p)	4	2	2	3 (2-AB; 1-LB)	1 (AB-MCA)	1/4 (25.0)	3/3 (100.0) (phenotypically abnormal AB case confirmed)
47,+i(9p)	1	0	1		1 (AB-MCA)	1/1 (100.0)	1/1 (100.0)
Other							
46,dir dup(3)(q23q27)	1	1	0		1 (LB, deLange syndrome)	1/1 (100.0)	1/1 (100.0)
46,dup(12q)	1	1	0		1 (LB-MCA)	1/1 (100.0)	1/1 (100.0)
46,add(p or q)	8	5	3	4[b] (3-LB; 1-AB)	4[c] (1-LB; 2-AB, 1-hydrops fetalis)	4/8 (50.0)	3/5[d] (60.0)
47,+mar	7	1	6	3[e] (all AB)	4[f] (3-AB; 1-LB)	4/7 (57.1)	4/4[g] (100)

Source: Data from Hsu et al., 1996.[250]

aIncluding two rob(14q14q) and one rob(21q21q).

bOne each of 6q+; 13p+; 14p+, and 22p+.

c12p+ (AB) with facial dysmorphism; 15p+ (LB) with MCA, 16p+ (AB) with webbed neck and long philtrum; 22p+ (intra-uterine fetal demise at 28 weeks) with hydrops fetalis.

dThe three confirmed cases included two phenotypically abnormal and one phenotypically normal case.

eOne each of 47,+del(17)(p12); 47, inv dup(15); and 47,+r(19).

fOne each of 47,+17p+ (AB) with MCA and Dandy–Walker malformation; 47,+del(17)(p12) (AB) with microcephaly and low set ears; 47,+dup(20)(pter → q11) (AB) with microcephaly, micrognathia, IUGR; 47,+22q− (LB) with cat eye syndrome.

gThe four confirmed cases included three phenotypically abnormal cases and one phenotypically normal case.

AB = abortus; Abn. = abnormal; Cont. = continued; LB = liveborn; MCA = multiple congenital abnormalities; MR = mental retardation; Term. = terminated.

A relatively commonly encountered structural abnormality involves a mosaicism in which one copy of chromosome 20 is replaced by an isochromsome 20q. Chen[251] reviewed twenty-three such cases and noted that several have shown abnormal phenotypes, but no consistent pattern emerges. This chromosomal abnormality has never been confirmed in postnatal blood studies. However, there is one report of confirmation in umbilical cord tissue, buccal smear, and urinary sediment cells.[252]

The 1996 survey of structural chromosome mosaicism[250] documented five cases mosaic for an unbalanced translocation (one unbalanced reciprocal and four unbalanced Robertsonian, three of which involved a homologous chromosome). Two cases resulted in phenotypically abnormal offspring.

When mosaicism involves a cell line with a terminal deletion, the chromosome breakpoint often appears to be at, or close to, a fragile site. Of fifteen terminal deletions, five appeared to involve a fragile site (one case each for 2q11, 2q31, and 16q23 and two for 10q23).[250] One case (an abortus) mosaic for del(16)(q23) had a cystic hygroma. The other four cases were all phenotypically normal at birth. Four additional cases of 10q23 deletions have been described, each with normal pregnancy outcomes.[253,254] In their review of the significance of fragile sites, Sutherland and Baker[253] concluded that there are insufficient data to be entirely reassuring about these deletion mosaicisms even when the fragile site is known to be segregating in the family. Of special concern is the 11q23.2 (FRA11B) site. A deletion at this fragile site is associated with Jacobsen syndrome.[255]

Of the 10 cases mosaic for a terminal deletion *not* involving a fragile site (one case each for 1q22, 4p12, 4q33, 9q11, 11q24, 12p12, 18p11, both 18q11 and 18p11, and two cases for 18p-),[250] two had abnormal outcomes; one was a liveborn with a 46/46,del(11)(q24) karyotype and multiple congenital anomalies and the other an abortus with a 46/46,18p− karyotype and microcephaly. There were two cases with a mosaic interstitial deletion.[231] A del(18)(q12.2q21.1) karyotype was associated with multiple congenital anomalies identified in an abortus. The second case involved a del(18)(q21.q23) abnormality and a normal-appearing liveborn.

The overall risk for an abnormal outcome in a case with an unbalanced structural abnormality, excluding 46/46,i(20q) and supernumerary chromosomes was approximately 32 percent (12 of 38).[250] The data from this study showed a suggestive correlation between the percentage of abnormal cells and an abnormal phenotype (median of 15.4 percent for the normal outcome group versus a median of 64.0 percent for the abnormal outcome group).

For cytogenetic confirmation for most of the subcategories of autosomal mosaicism discussed, fibroblast culture appeared to be a better than blood culture.

Summary Conclusions and Recommendations for Mosaicism Involving an Autosomal Structural Abnormality

1. The risks for an abnormality associated with mosaicism involving balanced rearrangement is low.
2. Risks associated with some mosaic unbalanced rearrangements (i(20q), i(12q), and others) are relatively well defined, whereas for others there remains considerable uncertainty.
3. When mosaicism involving a terminal deletion is diagnosed in AFC, the chromosome breakpoint should be evaluated to determine whether it is in the region of a known fragile site. If the breakpoint is at a fragile site, parental chromosome stud-

ies should be undertaken with cell culture conditions appropriate for fragile site induction.

4. Confirmatory studies should generally include tissue fibroblast cultures.

Sex Chromosome Mosaicism

Frequency

Mosaicism involving a sex chromosome is more common than autosomal mosaicism.[250] The three most commonly seen sex chromosome mosaics are 45,X/46,XX, 45,X/46,XY, and 46,XY/47,XXY. The relative prevalence of the most common sex chromosome mosaicisms is summarized in Table 6.26.

45,X/46,XY Mosaicism

One hundred percent of 151 *postnatally* diagnosed cases with 45,X/46,XY mosaicism were phenotypically abnormal. Among these patients, 42 percent of patients had mixed gonadal dysgenesis, 42 percent had a female phenotype but with some features of Turner syndrome, and 15 percent of patients had a male phenotype but with incomplete masculinization.[258] However, this represents biased ascertainment because phenotypically normal individuals with 45,X/46,XY are not likely to seek medical attention. In contrast, among eighty-five *prenatally* diagnosed cases of 45,X/46,XY mosaicism with outcome information[238,258,259] (Table 6.27), only six cases (7.1 percent) resulted in phenotypically abnormal fetuses. This included mixed gonadal dysgenesis in three, phenotypic female with the possibility of Turner syndrome developing in two, and one phenotypic male with hypoplastic scrotum and penile chordee. The vast majority (seventy-four cases, or 92.9 percent) resulted in grossly normal male offspring. The drastic difference in the phenotypic outcome between postnatal and prenatal diagnosis is clearly due to the differences in ascertainment.

When a prenatal diagnosis of 45,X/46,XY mosaicism is established in AFC, a high-resolution ultrasound examination of the fetus with special emphasis on the external genitalia should be recommended. The identification of male external genitalia is reassuring. When a liveborn with 45,X/46,XY is found to be a phenotypic female, a careful follow-up should be performed, including a workup to rule out an intra-abdominal gonad, which may contain testicular tissues and which may have malignant potential. In addition, a phenotypic female child with 45,X/46,XY may develop features of Turner syndrome.

Table 6.26.   Major sex chromosome mosaicism diagnosed in amniocytes

Karyotype	No. of Cases	Abnormal Phenotype/ Total Cases with Information (%)	Number with Cytogenetic Confirmation/ Total Successful Studies (%)
45,X/46,XX	250	25/165 (15.2)	89/105 (84.8)
45,X/46,XY	104	6/85 (7.1)	45/60 (75.0)
46,XY/47,XXY	61	2/37 (5.4)	35/35 (100.0)
45,X/47,XXX	31	5/13 (38.5)	13/13 (100.0)
46,XY/47,XYY	28	2/17 (11.8)	11/14 (78.6)
46,XX/47,XXX	26	0/22 (0)	10/10 (100.0)
45,X/47,XYY	10	1/8 (12.5)	6/6 (100.0)
45,X/46,XY/47,XYY	9	0/7 (0)	5/6 (83.3)
45,X/46,XX/47,XXX	7	0/3 (0)	4/4 (100.0)

Source: Data from Hsu, 1992, 1998,[152,238] Robinson et al., 1992,[256] Koeberl et al., 1995,[257] and Huang et al., 2002.[259a]

45,X/46,XX Mosaicism

More than 250 cases have been diagnosed through amniocentesis. Of 165 prenatal cases with available outcome information,[152,238,256,257,259a] 25 (15.2 percent) had an abnormal outcome. This included 3 stillbirths and 22 cases with an abnormal phenotype, of which 14 showed some features of Turner syndrome and 8 had anomalies possibly not related to Turner syndrome (Table 6.26). The majority of cases (more than 84 percent) with a 45,X/46,XX prenatal diagnosis appeared to result in phenotypically normal females, either at birth or at termination. However, even in patients with a nonmosaic 45,X complement, the major features of Turner syndrome (such as short stature and sexual infantilism) are not apparent until later in childhood or adolescence. According to Robinson et al.,[256] girls with 45,X mosaicism identified at newborn screening, by and large, have normal pubertal development. As with 45,X/46,XY mosaicism, cases of 45,X/46,XX mosaicism diagnosed prenatally represent an unbiased sample of patients who probably have a much more favorable prognosis than that seen in cases studied postnatally (and ascertained, most likely, on the basis of a clinical finding). A cohort of these cases will need long-term follow-up before it can be established whether or not a prenatal diagnosis of 45,X/46,XX mosaicism is associated with reduced fertility.[260]

46,XY/47,XXY Mosaicism

Of sixty-one cases, thirty-seven had outcome information (Table 6.26). Thirty-five were associated with a normal male phenotype; only two had abnormal outcomes. One liveborn had IUGR and one showed clubfeet, which was not likely to have been related to the XXY mosaicism. Again, as with 45,X Turner syndrome, the typical features for 47,XXY Klinefelter syndrome, such as hypogonadism and infertility, cannot be recognized perinatally.

Other Sex Chromosome Mosaicism Involving a 45,X Cell Line (Excluding 45,X/46,XX or 45,X/46,XY)

There were thirty-one cases with 45,X/47,XXX, ten with 45,X/47,XYY, nine with 45,X/46,XY/47,XYY, and seven with 45,X/46,XX/47,XXX (Table 6.26). Of thirteen cases

Table 6.27. 45,X/46,XY mosaicism diagnosed in amniocytes

Phenotypic Male (81 Cases)	Intersex (1 Case, Abortus)	Phenotypic Female (3 Cases)
Normal male genitalia (79) (61 liveborns; 16 abortuses; 1 stillborn; 1 fetal demise)	Mixed gonadal dysgenesis Ambiguous genitalia	Normal female genitalia (2) (1 liveborn; 1 abortus)
Phenotypic male with hypospadias and mixed gonadal dysgenesis (1) (abortus)		Phenotypic female with mixed gonadal dysgenesis (abortus) (1)
Phenotypic male with hypoplastic scrotum and penile chordee (1) (abortus)		

Source: Data from Hsu, 1992, 1998, 1989, 1994,[152,238,259,258] and Huang et al., 2002.[259a]

of 45,X/47,XXX and with some information on phenotypic outcome, five cases were reported to be abnormal. This included two liveborns with Turner features, one liveborn small for gestational age, an abortus with minor abnormalities, and an abortus reported to be abnormal, but with no details given. All eight informative cases of 45,X/47,XYY and seven of 45,X/46,XY/47,XYY were reported to have normal male external genitalia. These observations were quite comparable to what has been observed in cases with 45,X/46,XY mosaicism. One abortus with 45,X/47,XYY had clubbed feet, an anomaly that was probably not related to the chromosomal abnormalities.

The overall cytogenetic confirmation rates for these cases of mosaicism were excellent (75–100 percent) (Table 6.26).

Mosaicism Involving an Additional Sex Chromosome Other than XXY

There were twenty-eight cases with 46,XY/47,XYY and twenty-six with 46,XX/47,XXX (Table 6.26). Among seventeen informative cases of XY/XYY, two were reported to be abnormal, including one liveborn with a short neck, right hydronephrosis, and undescended testes and one abnormal abortus (no details given) associated with oligohydramnios. Of twenty-two cases of XX/XXX with information, none were reported to be phenotypically abnormal. Cytogenetic confirmation of mosaicism was achieved in 78–100 percent of cases with follow-up studies.

Mosaicism Involving a Structurally Abnormal X

Mosaicism involving a cell line with a structurally abnormal X and a normal 46,XX cell line appears to carry a low risk for recognizable malformation at birth. This conclusion is based on:

- Four cases with a normal 46,XX cell line and a second cell line with a structurally abnormal X (two with i(Xq), and one each with r(X) and Xp−). All four cases resulted in liveborns with a normal female phenotype.[152]
- Two cases with a normal 46,XX cell line, a second cell line of 45,X, and a third cell line with a structurally abnormal X (i(Xq) and der(X)). Both cases also resulted in normal female liveborns.[152]

When no normal 46,XX cell line is present, risks for an abnormal outcome appear to be rather high. Data are available for fifteen cases with outcome information, of which five were abnormal (33 percent). Specifics of the cases with no normal cell line are as follows:[152, 259a]

- Six cases of 45,X/46,X,i(Xq). Two of three abortuses appeared to be normal females; one had no information. One liveborn was lost to follow-up. Cytogenetic confirmation of mosaicism was achieved in three abortuses.
- Two cases of 45,X/46,X,i(Xq)/47,X,i(Xq),i(Xq). One abortus was associated with a Turner phenotype and one had no noticeable abnormalities. Both abortuses were phenotypically female, and both were cytogenetically confirmed.
- Seven cases with 45,X/46,Xr(X). All seven pregnancies were terminated. Two abnormal female abortuses were reported to have Turner features (one had cystic hygroma), and five had no information. In two cases in which cytogenetic studies were performed, the prenatal diagnosis was confirmed.
- Six cases with mosaicism involving a structurally altered X and 45,X line. One case with 45,X/46,XXq− was associated with an abnormal female abortus with edema;

the mosaicism was confirmed. Two cases were terminated, and no postmortem information was available. There were three cases of 45,X/46,X,+der(X) (including one pair of twins). The twins were both reported as normal females, with mosaicism confirmed. The third pregnancy was terminated and the female abortus showed multiple congenital abnormalities.

A special concern exists when a small r(X) or other small structurally abnormal X chromosome is present (mosaic or nonmosaic). In a proportion of these cases, a severe phenotype can be present, which can include mental retardation and other anomalies not normally seen in Turner syndrome.[261–264] Disomic expression of X-chromosome genes (functional disomy of X) due to absence of the X-inactivation-specific transcript (XIST) or failure to express XIST can account for this severe phenotype.[265–267]

Mosaicism Involving a Structurally Abnormal Y Chromosome

There were seven such cases, including three of 46,XY/46,X,del(Y)(q11 or q12), one of 45,X/46,r(Y), one of 46,XY/46,X,i(Yq) and two 45,X/46,X,idic(Y).[152,259a] All three cases with del(Y)(q11 or q12) and the two with idic(Y) mosaicism resulted in normal male liveborns and four of the five cases were cytogenetically confirmed. The other two cases had no information (one liveborn and one abortus).

Summary Conclusions and Recommendations for Mosaicism Involving a Sex Chromosome

1. These aneuploidies are common and, as expected, most cases show a normal phenotype at birth.
2. Follow-up of 45,X/46,XY mosaicism should include ultrasound evaluation of fetal gender and comprehensive evaluation at birth, which may include ruling out an intra-abdominal gonad.
3. Long-term clinical significance of most prenatally diagnosed sex chromosome aneuploidy remains uncertain.
4. The risk associated with mosaicism involving a structurally abnormal X is probably higher when no normal cell line is present. Because of functional disomy, there is a special concern when a small r(X) or other small X-derived chromosome is present.
5. Most sex chromosomal abnormalities identified in AFC are confirmed in follow-up studies.

Other Types of Mosaicism

Diploid/Triploid Mosaicism

Diploid/triploid mosaicism may arise as the result of an inclusion of the second polar body into a diploid embryo cell at an early stage of development, chimerism of diploid and triploid zygotes, or incorporation of a second sperm into an embryonic blastomere.[268,268a] Clinical features include mental and growth retardation, truncal obesity, asymmetry, and digit and facial anomalies.[269] At least three cases with diploid/triploid mosaicism have been diagnosed in AFC.[152] One was spontaneously aborted, with multiple congenital anomalies; one resulted in an abnormal stillborn; and the third appeared to be normal. Cytogenetic confirmation of diploid/triploid mosaicism was achieved in the first two cases but failed in the third. Failure to detect diploid/triploid mosaicism through the analysis of AFC has also been described.[269a]

Diploid/Tetraploid Mosaicism

Diploid/tetraploid mosaicism is a very rare disorder that is associated with mental retardation, reduced peripheral limb muscle bulk, asymmetry, seizures and skin pigmentary anomalies, and various other anomalies.[270–275] Three cases of nonmosaic tetraploidy were diagnosed prenatally; one was confirmed with flow cytometry of several fetal tissues,[276] another was initially diagnosed by FISH in noncultivated AFC,[277] and the third was confirmed in fetal lymphocytes.[278]

Tetraploidy is a frequent observation among the AFC; two-thirds of all cases show more than 10 percent of the cultured cells to be tetraploid.[279] Occasionally, the frequency of tetraploid cells is more than 80 percent and it is not possible to distinguish between in vitro and in vivo origin. Therefore, most cytogeneticists now regard tetraploidy in amniotic fluid cultures as clinically insignificant. It is probably both justified and practical for cytogeneticists not to be overly concerned about tetraploidy. However, if the frequency of tetraploidy in multiple primary cultures is very high, a high-resolution ultrasound scan is recommended.

Marker Chromosome Mosaicism

The risk for an abnormal pregnancy outcome when a de novo supernumerary marker chromosome is identified is probably not related to whether the marker is mosaic or nonmosaic because all cases probably start as nonmosaic 47,+mar. A subsequent loss of the marker chromosome would result in 46/47,+mar mosaicism (for further discussion, see "De Novo Supernumerary Chromosomes (Including Mosaic Cases)" on p. 267).

Guidelines for the Diagnosis of Mosaicism

Suggested approaches for the management of cases with suspected amniocyte mosaicism have been published and updated.[182,280] These guidelines are designed to balance maximum detection of clinically significant mosaicism with realistic and practical levels of analysis. The approach is based on three levels of evaluation: standard, moderate, and extensive. Extensive workup is indicated when there is a suspicion of mosaicism involving an abnormality in which there have been two, or more, well-documented reports of confirmed amniocyte mosaicism with abnormal pregnancy outcome.

Table 6.28 provides a further update to these guidelines. Trisomy involving chromosomes 7 and 17 have now been added to the category of cases requiring extensive workup. As noted above, the existence and significance of true mosaicism involving these two chromosomes has now been established.

Genetic Counseling and Chromosome Mosaicism

In genetic counseling for prenatal diagnosis of chromosome mosaicism, certain points must be kept in mind:

1. The frequency of noticeable abnormalities in prenatally diagnosed mosaic cases (Table 6.29) is likely to be underestimated, because it is difficult to recognize minor dysmorphic features in midtrimester fetuses and among liveborns. A physical evaluation at birth would not reveal mental retardation, subtle abnormalities, or yet-undeveloped characteristics.

Table 6.28. Guidelines for the management of cases with suspected amniocyte mosaicism

Flask Method	In Situ Method
A. Indications for extensive workup	A. Indications for extensive workup
1. Autosomal trisomy involving a chromosome 2, 5, 7, 8, 9, 12, 13, 14, 15, 16, 17, 20, 21, or 22 (SC, MC)	1. Autosomal trisomy involving a chromosome 2, 5, 7, 8, 9, 12, 13, 14, 15, 16, 17, 20, 21, or 22 (SC$_o$, MC$_o$)
2. Unbalanced structural rearrangement (MC)	2. Unbalanced structural rearrangement (MC$_o$)
3. Marker chromosome (MC)	3. Marker chromosome (MC$_0$)
B. Indications for moderate workup	B. Indications for moderate workup
4. Extra sex chromosome (SC, MC)	4. Extra sex chromosome (SC$_o$, MC$_o$)
5. Autosomal trisomy involving a chromosome 1, 3, 4, 6, 10, 11, or 19 (SC, MC)	5. Autosomal trisomy involving a chromosome 1, 3, 4, 6, 10, 11, or 19 (SC$_o$, MC$_o$)
6. 45,X (MC)	6. 45,X (SC$_o$, MC$_o$)
7. Monosomy (other than 45,X) (MC)	7. Monosomy (other than 45,X) (SCo, MC$_o$)
8. Marker chromosome (SC)	8. Marker chromosome (SC$_o$)
9. Balanced structural rearrangement (MC)	9. Balanced structural rearrangement (MC$_o$)
	10. Unbalanced structural rearrangement (SC$_o$)
C. Standard, no additional work-up	C. Standard, no additional workup
10. 45,X (SC)	11. Balanced structural rearrangement (SC$_o$)
11. Unbalanced structural rearrangement (SC)	12. Break at centromere with loss of one arm (SC$_o$)
12. Balanced structural rearrangement (SC)	13. All single-cell abnormalities
13. Break at centromere with loss of one arm (SC)	

Source: Modified from Hsu and Benn, 1999.[280]

Note: A = 40 cells (20 cells from each of two flasks, excluding cells analyzed from the culture with the initial observation of abnormality) or 24 colonies (excluding colonies analyzed from the vessel with the initial observation). B = 20 cells (from the flask without the initial observation) or 12 colonies (from vessels without the initial observation). C = 20 cells (10 from each of two independent cultures) or 15 colonies (from at least two independent vessels).

SC = Single cell (single flask); MC = multiple cells (single flask); SC$_o$ = single colony (single dish); MC$_o$ = multiple colonies (single dish).

2. The proportion of each cell line in the amniotic fluid culture does not accurately reflect the proportion in the different somatic tissues of the fetus.

3. In some cases, the abnormal cell line may be derived from extra-embryonic tissues and may not be found in any fetal tissue. It may therefore be impossible to predict the phenotypic spectrum of the fetus, a limitation that must be communicated.

4. Because major congenital abnormalities are prenatally detectable with high-resolution ultrasound, this procedure should be performed in all mosaic cases diagnosed in amniocytes.

5. Except for mosaicism of trisomy 8, 9, 13, 18, or 21 or sex chromosome mosaicism, fetal blood sampling (PUBS) is of limited value in the evaluation of chromosome mosaicism.

6. The counseling should be nondirective (see also Chapter 1).

7. UPD may need to be excluded when the mosaicism involved a cell line with trisomy 6, 7, 11, 14, 15, or 20.

8. For cytogenetic confirmation of the mosaicism, fibroblast cultures are generally better than blood cultures.

It is important that cytogeneticists and clinical geneticists recognize the value of confirmatory studies on placental tissues as well as studies of fetal or liveborn tissues. These studies are often reassuring for patients, may inform about future risks, and also further our understanding of mosaicism.

Table 6.29. A summary of chromosome mosaicism and the percentage of abnormal outcome in cases diagnosed in amniocytes

Type of Mosaicism	No. with Abnormal Outcome/ Total Cases with Information (%)
Autosome	
Trisomy 20 mosaicism (only)	22/294 (7.5)
Trisomy mosaicism (excluding 46/47,+20)	173/345 (50.1)
Monosomy mosaicism	1/7 (14.3)
Mosaicism with a balanced structural abnormality	0/21 (0)
Mosaicism with an unbalanced structural abnormality	
(excluding 46/46,i(20q))	24/55 (43.6)
46/46,i(20q)	4/2 (17.4)
Sex chromosome	
45,X/46,XX	25/165 (15.2)
45,X/46,XY	6/85 (7.1)
46,XY/47,XXY	2/37 (5.4)
45,X mosaic without Y (exclusive 45,X/46,XX)	5/15 (33.3)
45,X mosaic with Y (exclusive 45,X/46,XY)	1/15 (6.7)
46,XY/47,XYY	2/17 (11.8)
46,XX/47,XXX	0/22 (0)
46,XX/46,X, Abnormal X	0/6 (0)
45,X,/Abnormal X mosaic	5/15 (33.3)
46,XY/46,X, Abnormal Y	0/5 (0)
Triploid/diploid	2/3 (66.7)
Total number of cases excluding marker chromosome	
mosaicism with outcome information: 1,130 cases	

Long-term follow-up of all mosaic liveborns remains as an important responsibility for all geneticists and the physicians who care for these children.

INTERPRETATION ISSUES: CHROMOSOME REARRANGEMENTS

When a structural rearrangement (exclusive of inv(9), which is a common polymorphism) is diagnosed in AFC, every effort should be made to study both parents' chromosomes. The karyotypes from the parents and the AFC should be compared, a determination made whether the rearrangement is balanced or unbalanced, and chromosome breakpoints assigned. The studies on the parents should be carried out regardless of whether or not the fetal karyotype appears, on initial impression, to be balanced or unbalanced.

Supernumerary marker chromosomes detected in AFC are often familial in origin, and in some instances a parent is a low-level mosaic for the marker. It is therefore sometimes necessary to search for an identical marker with 50–100 cells from each parent analyzed. In the cases with balanced Robertsonian translocations involving chromosomes 14 and 15, and also for small supernumerary marker chromosomes involving chromosome 15, molecular genetic studies to rule out UPD may also be appropriate (see below).

Familial Structural Rearrangements

The observation that an autosomal chromosome rearrangement is familial in origin is usually highly reassuring. Unequal crossover during meiosis may lead to minute duplication(s) and/or deletion(s), which could lead to an abnormal phenotype.[281] This would be of concern for the alternate segregation of both balanced and normal chromosome complements. Indeed, Horsthemke et al.[282] described two families in which fathers with

15q11–q13 balanced translocations produced offspring with 15q11–q13 microdeletions and a Prader–Willi syndrome phenotype. The deletions were postulated to have arisen through unequal crossover and were not identified at the time of amniocentesis (at which time normal karyotypes were reported). There is also the highly unusual situation in which there is transmission of a translocation and a sex-dependent expression of a disorder attributable to disrupted imprinting.[283,284]

These mechanisms are exceptional, and there are no direct data to show that, overall, the commonly encountered autosomal familial, seemingly balanced, structural rearrangements in AFC are associated with a measurably increased risk for abnormality. In counseling the prospective parents after finding a seemingly similar "balanced" reciprocal translocation like the one detected in the phenotypically normal parent, some caution is suggested. It should be indicated that there is a very remote possibility that this seemingly balanced reciprocal translocation could in fact be unbalanced at the submicroscopic or gene functional level.

Familial X/autosomal translocations are of greater concern. There is a possibility that a phenotypically normal carrier mother could have a carrier daughter with anomalies because of differences in X-chromosome inactivation patterns.[285] X-autosome translocations in males are associated with infertility,[286] and there are reports of a variably expressed premature ovarian failure in the females with familial X/autosome translocations.[287,288]

De Novo Structural Rearrangements

De novo structural chromosome rearrangements will be considered in three major categories: (1) apparently balanced rearrangements, including reciprocal translocations, Robertsonian translocations, and inversions; (2) apparently unbalanced rearrangements; and (3) small supernumerary chromosomes. Frequencies of de novo rearrangements diagnosed in newborns and prenatally are shown in Table 6.30. For every 10,000 amniocenteses, six to nine cases with a de novo balanced rearrangement and four to nine cases with a de novo unbalanced rearrangement can be expected.

Apparently Balanced De Novo Rearrangements

The finding of an apparently balanced de novo chromosome rearrangement in amniocytes poses a counseling dilemma. A significant excess of balanced de novo rearrangements (about eight times the newborn incidence) was observed among mentally retarded individuals.[289] Apparently balanced de novo rearrangements do appear to be associated with mental and/or physical abnormality.[294,295] This association between an increased risk for mental retardation and/or congenital anomalies may be due to one, or more, of the following factors: (1) a position effect of rearranged genetic material (disturbance of gene expression or imprinting); (2) mutation at the translocation or rearranged site; and (3) minute chromosome deletion or duplication not detectable by conventional cytogenetic methods.

Warburton[47] conducted a North American survey to evaluate risk following a prenatally detected de novo rearrangement. Thirteen of 195 (6.7 percent) informative cases with a de novo balanced non-Robertsonian translocations and inversions had an abnormal phenotype (Table 6.31). Two of fifty-one (3.9 percent) de novo balanced Robertsonian translocations had abnormal pregnancy outcomes. These rates can be compared to an overall background estimate of 2–3 percent for congenital anomalies. Less than 40 percent of the infants reported to be normal in Warburton's study[47] had follow-up information beyond 1 year of age. Those who were reported to be normal at birth remained normal at 1 year of age.

Table 6.30. The frequency (%) of de novo rearrangements diagnosed in newborns and at amniocentesis

Source of Data	No. Studied	Balanced de novo				Unbalanced de novo			Reference
		Reciprocal Translocation	Robertsonian Translocation	Inversion		Robertsonian Translocation	Others	+ Markers	
Newborns	59,452	0.026	0.009	0.002		0.005	0.007	0.005	Jacobs[289]
	76,952	—	—	—		0.005	0.018	0.019	Warburton[290,291]
	54,806	0.053	0.027	0.013		0.005	0.035	0.038	Hook and Cross[292]
Amniocenteses	23,495	0.055	0.026	—		—	—	—	Wassman et al.[293]
	337,357	0.047	0.011	0.009		—	—	—	Warburton[47]
	44,000	0.052	0.013	0.009		0.007	0.009	0.038	Hsu[238]

265

Table 6.31. The phenotypic outcome of de novo balanced rearrangement diagnosed at amniocentesis

	No. of Cases	Total with Known Outcome		Livebirths		Elective Abortions		Fetal Death	
		Normal	Abn (%)	Normal	Abn.	Normal	Abn.	Normal	Abn.
Reciprocal translocation	163	153	10 (6.1)	134	8	16	2	3	0
Inversion	32	29	3 (9.4)	28	1	1	1	0	1
Subtotal	195	182	13 (6.7)	162	9	17	3	3	1
Robertsonian translocation	51	49	2 (3.9)	48	2	1	0	0	0
Total	246	231	15 (6.1)	210	11	18	3	3	1

Source: Warburton, Table 2, 1991.[47] Reproduced by permission from the University of Chicago Press.
Note: Data are limited to cases with known pregnancy outcomes and excludes cases ascertained through abnormal ultrasound findings.
Abn. = abnormal

MacGregor et al.[296] presented outcome data on eight cases of de novo balanced reciprocal translocations. Except for one, which was terminated at 18 weeks of gestation with a diagnosis of anencephaly, all these cases proceeded to term. All seven children were reported to be normal at follow-up examination; their ages ranged from 16 months to 10 years. Three school-aged children were reported to be performing satisfactorily in a class appropriate to their age.

Wassman et al.[293] had follow-up data for thirteen cases with a de novo balanced translocations (ten reciprocal and three Robertsonian). Four were evaluated at ages up to 6–8 months, and four others were examined at 3 to 3.5 years of age. All thirteen cases were reported to be normal at birth, and the eight with additional follow-up information remained normal (six had a reciprocal translocation and two had a Robertsonian translocation).

There were two conflicting earlier reports on the mental development of children with a de novo balanced translocation ascertained at birth. One report[297] indicated normal physical and mental development in five children with de novo balanced translocations (three reciprocal and two Robertsonian). The other reported a significantly lower IQ in ten children with a de novo balanced translocation (seven reciprocal and three Robertsonian), compared with twenty children with familial translocations ($p < 0.01$).[298] All children in the study attended regular school.

For de novo balanced rearrangements other than Robertsonian translocations, the positions of the chromosome breakpoints may play a role in determining the risks for an abnormal offspring. One example is the finding of blepharophimosis sequence (BPES) in two cases with a reciprocal translocation involving 3q23 as a breakpoint.[299] The BPES gene is located at 3q23 band, and a deletion of 3q23 band has been detected in many cases of BPES syndrome.

The risk figures developed by Warburton[47] for de novo chromosome rearrangements included a number of cases with X-autosome translocations in females. These translocations can be associated with abnormal gonadal development, notably when the X-chromosome breakpoint is within q13–q22 or q22–q26 critical regions.[300,301] Atypical X-inactivation patterns could also lead to functional gene imbalances and an abnormal phenotype.[285] Unfortunately, there are insufficient data on cases ascertained through amniocentesis to provide a separate estimate of the risk associated with de novo X/autosome translocations.

Unbalanced de novo Rearrangements (Excluding Supernumerary Marker Chromosomes)

When a de novo unbalanced chromosome rearrangement is diagnosed, FISH can usually help to identify the exact duplication and/or deficiency present. The finding of an unbalanced rearrangement is generally associated with a high probability of an abnormal phenotype (60 percent or more).[291] Schinzel's *Catalogue of Unbalanced Chromosome Aberrations*[302] is an invaluable resource for data on the phenotypes associated with specific imbalances. A high-resolution ultrasound examination of the fetus may help to identify major congenital abnormalities and therefore may assist parents in making an informed decision regarding termination or maintaining the pregnancy. Some unbalanced karyotypes appear to be associated with a normal phenotype and the registry maintained by the National Genetics Reference Laboratory, Wessex, provides a catalogue of such cases.[302a]

De Novo Supernumerary Chromosomes (Including Mosaic Cases)

The presence of an additional supernumerary marker chromosome is a relatively common finding in AFC. The term *supernumerary marker chromosome* has been used to refer to any unidentifiable small chromosome present in addition to the normal chromosome complement. This definition encompasses a diverse range of cytogenetic abnormalities.

Based on conventional cytogenetic techniques for chromosome identification, the overall incidence of supernumerary marker chromosomes in AFC ranges from 0.6 to 1.5 per 1,000 (Table 6.32).[27,47,238,290–292,303–305] Two newborn studies showed rather different frequencies of supernumerary marker chromosomes.[22,306] A report in 1981 showed an overall incidence of 0.18/1,000,[306] whereas a 1991 study reported an overall frequency of 0.72/1,000.[22] This difference may be partly related to the chromosome banding improvements in the 1991 study, as well as counting more cells (five cells per case in the 1991 study versus three cells per case in the 1981 study). There appear to be more de novo marker chromosomes than inherited markers in AFC (Table 6.32). There is also an association of supernumerary markers with increased maternal age.[292] In AFC, the ratio of satellited to nonsatellited de novo markers is almost 1:1.[47]

Table 6.32.   The incidence of supernumerary marker chromosomes

Source of Data	No. Studied	Overall	De Novo	Inherited	Reference
		Incidence (per 1,000)			
Amniocentesis	52,965	0.60	—	—	Ferguson-Smith and Yates[27]
	76,952	0.65	0.4	0.25	Warburton[290,291]
	75,000	0.64	0.32–0.40	0.23–0.32	Hook and Cross[292]
	10,000	1.5	0.9	0.6	Sachs et al.[303]
	377,357	—	0.4	—	Warburton[47]
	44,000	0.82	0.52	0.25	Hsu[238]
Amniocentesis and CVS (combined)	Amnio 34,908 + CVS 4,197	0.8	0.4	0.3	Blennow et al.[304]
	Amnio 11,055 + CVS 1,644	1.1	0.7	0.39	Brondum–Nielson and Mikkelsen[305]
Newborns	59,452	0.18	0.05	0.1	Jacobs[306]
	34,919	0.72	—	—	Nielsen and Wohlert[22]

Before the use of molecular cytogenetic techniques for the identification of marker chromosomes, risks used in counseling were largely based on the gross morphologic characteristics of the markers. A satellited de novo marker appeared to carry a better prognosis than a nonsatellited de novo marker chromosome (10.9 versus 14.7 percent).[47] A minute or a fragment-like dot marker primarily made of C-banding positive chromatin material was associated with a lower risk for fetal abnormalities[47,152] presumably because of the absence of euchromatic material.[307–309]

Today, using molecular cytogenetic techniques (FISH, multicolor FISH, spectral karyotyping) in combination with banding studies (Giemsa (G), Constitutive heterochromatin (C), Reverse (R), Quinacrine (Q), Distamyacine/DAPI (DA/DAPI), and nucleolar organizer region (NOR) staining), the origins of all marker chromosomes are potentially identifiable.[309a] Marker chromosomes can be derived from any chromosome. However, there is a nonrandom involvement of specific chromosomes, and knowing the most likely candidate chromosomes can greatly facilitate characterization.

In a study based on 39,105 consecutive prenatal diagnoses in Sweden, Blennow et al.[304] found thirty-one supernumerary chromosomes, of which twelve were inherited, fourteen were de novo, and five were of unknown origin. Among the fourteen de novo cases, five were derived from chromosome 15, five were derived from other identified chromosomes, and four were not characterized. Therefore, it would appear that about half of all de novo markers are derived from chromosome 15. The frequent involvement of chromosome 15 in supernumerary chromosomes had been noted previously by Buckton et al.[310] in studies before the widespread use of FISH. Supernumerary chromosomes derived from chromosome 15 are commonly, but technically incorrectly, referred to as inv dup(15) chromosomes. More accurately, they can be described as dic(15;15) or psu dic(15;15). They contain variable amounts of chromosome-15-derived material and can be classified into two major subtypes. First, a large form that contains the Prader–Willi syndrome (PWS)/Angelman syndrome (AS) critical region, is de novo in origin, is usually comprised of maternally derived chromosome 15, and is associated with mental retardation, seizures, growth retardation and dysmorphic features.[311–313] The second subtype is smaller, may be inherited or de novo in origin, and lacks the PWS/AS critical region. The de novo cases also usually contain maternally derived chromosome 15 material.[314] Generally, although not invariably, small dic(15;15) supernumerary chromosomes are associated with a normal phenotype (see also "Uniparental Disomy in Familial and De Novo Rearrangements" below). Therefore, cytogenetic characterization of dic(15;15) chromosomes requires FISH analysis with chromosome 15 PWS/AS gene region and pericentromeric probes.

Supernumerary chromosomes derived from chromosome 22 are also common. These appear to be a heterogeneous group that can include variable amounts of 22q euchromatin.[315] Cases with no detectable euchromatin appear to be associated with a normal phenotype.[315] Cases with larger amounts of euchromatin are associated with cat eye syndrome[316–318] but severity of the phenotype does not appear to correlate directly with the extent of the additional chromosome-22-derived material.[315]

Other common supernumerary markers are isochromosomes, i(12p), i(18p) and i(9p).[250,302] A prenatal diagnosis of +i(12p) is indicative of Pallister–Killian syndrome.[319] Most, but not all, of these cases will show fetal abnormalities on ultrasound (polyhydramnios, diaphragmatic hernia, micromelia, overgrowth, and other anomalies).[320] In cases in which the diagnosis is suspected on the basis of the ultrasound findings, detection of the i(12p) cell line is often difficult due to mosaicism.

At least ten prenatally diagnosed cases of de novo +i(18p) have been reported.[250] Six were nonmosaic and four were mosaic, with a normal cell line. Five of the six non-mosaic +i(18p) and three of the four mosaic 46/47,+i(18p) were reported to be grossly normal either at birth or at termination. However, this does not rule out the possibility of 47,+i(18p) syndrome because the major features are mental retardation and other neuro-logic abnormalities that become evident only later in life.[321] A high risk for an abnormal outcome has been quoted for prenatal cases with +i(18p).[250,304,321]

The +i(9p) abnormality is also a relatively well defined disorder, and some of the as-sociated features may be identified through ultrasonography.[302,322]

Many other uncommon supernumerary chromosomes have been described.[323–326] Crolla[324] reviewed the findings in 168 cases of autosomal supernumerary marker chro-mosomes (excluding those derived from chromosome 15, common chromosome-22-derived markers associated with cat eye syndrome, and i(12p), i(18p) and i(9p)). He con-cluded that the risk for an abnormal phenotype is approximately 7 percent when the marker is derived from an acrocentric chromosome and approximately 28 percent when derived from a non-acrocentric chromosome. These risk figures may be useful when the most com-monly recognized origins for a marker have been excluded and complete characterization is not possible.

Uniparental Disomy in Familial and De Novo Rearrangements

Imprinted genes are known to be present on chromosomes 6, 7, 11, 14, 15, and 20, and may be present on others. In addition to the previously discussed potential for UPD in mosaic cases, the issue also needs to be considered when a prenatal diagnosis of a re-arrangement involving these chromosomes is encountered.

Balanced Robertsonian Translocations

Kotzot[327] reviewed the data from 12 studies[327–338] that looked for UPD in prenatal diag-nosis specimens with Robertsonian translocations. In addition, data are available from one other study.[339] The combined data from these thirteen reports yielded 500 cases includ-ing seven that involved homologous chromosomes (isochromosomes) (Table 6.33). UPD was observed in eight cases (1.6 percent), five of which involved homologs. The very high risk for UPD when the translocation involves homologs is consistent with case reports and systematic surveys of individuals with an abnormal phenotype.[327] The three cases of UPD in nonhomologous Robertsonian translocations were all observed in rob(13q14q) ex-changes. However, it cannot be concluded that the risk is confined to rob(13q14q) translo-cations; cases ascertained through testing of individuals with an abnormal phenotype have also involved various other nonhomologous Robertsonian translocations involving chro-mosome 14 and/or chromosome 15.[340] Assuming that the unspecified cases in Table 6.33 involved homologous and nonhomologous chromosome rearrangements in the same pro-portions as that reported in the fully characterized cases, the overall risk for UPD in a pa-tient with a homologous Robertsonian translocation was 56 percent and for a nonhomologous Robertsonian translocation 0.6 percent.

Balanced Non-Robertsonian Translocations and Supernumerary Chromosomes

There have been isolated case reports of UPD in individuals with balanced non-Robert-sonian translocations,[340] but the limited systematic searches that have been carried out to

Table 6.33. Incidence of UPD in carriers of Robertsonian translocations ascertained at prenatal diagnosis

Type of Translocation	No. of Diagnoses	Normal	UPD
rob(13q14q)	252	249	3
rob(13q15q)	18	18	
rob(13q21q)	3	3	
rob(13q22q)	1	1	
rob(14q15q)	36	36	
rob(14q21q)	40	40	
rob(14q22q)	11	11	
rob(15q21q)	2	2	
rob(15q22q)	7	7	
rob(13q13q)	2	0	2
rob(14q14q)	3	0	3
rob(15q15q)	1	1	
rob(22q22q)	1	1	
Unspecified	123	123	
Nonhomologous[a]	491	488	3 (0.6%)
Homologous[a]	9	4	5 (56%)
Grand total	500	492	8 (1.6%)

Source: Data from Han et al., 1994,[328] Corviello et al., 1995,[329] Page and Shaffer, 1997,[330] Harrison et al., 1998,[331] Papenhausen et al., 1991,[332] Exeler et al., 1991,[333] Eggermann et al., 1999,[334] Trabanelli et al., 2000,[335] Pereira et al., 2000,[336] Berend et al., 2000,[337] Jay et al., 2001,[338] Kotzot, 2002,[327] and Silverstein et al., 2002.[339]

[a]The unspecified cases are assumed to have the same proportions of homologous (2%) and nonhomologous (98%) Robertsonian translocations as that found in the characterized cases.

identify such cases have failed to identify any additional cases.[327] Therefore, the risk for UPD when a balanced translocation is prenatally identified is probably low.

A special concern exists when a supernumerary chromosome derived from chromosome 15 is identified. As discussed above, this finding is generally associated with a normal pregnancy outcome when the marker is small. However, there have been reports of both upd(15)mat (associated with Prader–Willi syndrome) and upd(15)pat (associated with Angelman syndrome) in individuals with supernumerary dic(15;15) chromosomes.[341] Cotter et al.[342] reviewed all reported cases of Prader–Willi and Angelman syndrome with supernumerary chromosomes. They identified twenty-three cases in which the supernumerary chromosome was derived from chromosome 15 and these diagnoses were present (or could be inferred). The origin of the supernumerary chromosome had been established in nineteen cases and in each instance it was de novo. At amniocentesis, upd(15)mat was observed in two of seventeen cases with de novo supernumerary dic(15;15).[343] The risk for upd(15) therefore appears to be high (provisionally, 12 percent) when a de novo dic(15;15) is found. There was no evidence for UPD in nine cases with familial supernumerary dic(15;15) chromosomes.[343] However, as Cotter et al.[342] point out, it would be prudent to offer UPD15 studies when a familial dic(15;15) is encountered, at least until a larger number of cases has been studied.

A risk for UPD may also exist when other supernumerary chromosomes are present.[327] However, from a practical standpoint, the presence or absence of UPD may be moot if the karyotype is also associated with a significant chromosome imbalance and is expected to result in an abnormal phenotype because of the imbalance.

Summary Conclusions and Recommendations for Chromosome Rearrangements

1. Familial balanced chromosome rearrangements are generally not associated with a measurably increased risk for abnormality, although some notable exceptions have been documented. The risk associated with a familial balanced X/autosomal translocation is uncertain.
2. Risk associated with a de novo unbalanced rearrangement will depend on the specific imbalance, and molecular cytogenetic techniques should be used to fully characterize the karyotype.
3. De novo balanced reciprocal translocations and inversions appear to carry a risk of approximately 7 percent for phenotypically abnormal offspring. This figure is based on limited long-term follow-up of prenatally identified cases. The risk associated with a de novo balanced X/autosomal translocation is uncertain and will depend on the X-chromosome breakpoint and X-inactivation patterns.
4. De novo supernumerary marker chromosomes can be characterized using FISH and additional chromosome banding techniques.
5. Prenatally diagnosed rob(14q14q) and rob(15q15q) are at high risk for clinically significant UPD, and molecular studies are indicated in these rare cases. The risk for UPD for other Robertsonian translocations involving chromosomes 14 or 15 is approximately 0.6 percent, and UPD studies should therefore also be considered.
6. UPD studies should also be offered when a small supernumerary dic(15;15) chromosome is identified.

INTERPRETATION ISSUES: CHROMOSOME POLYMORPHISMS

Chromosome polymorphisms or heteromorphisms are structural chromosome variants that are widespread in human populations and have no effect on the phenotype. These variants are most often found at the centromeric regions of chromosomes 1, 9, and 16, the distal part of the long arm of the Y chromosome, and the short arms (satellite regions) of the acrocentric chromosomes. A rare chromosome polymorphism could be misdiagnosed as a structural aberration. For the most part, examination of parental karyotypes and further study of the variant chromosome by use of a combination of different banding techniques and FISH can distinguish chromosome polymorphism from structural abnormality.

Because there are an average of five Q- and C-banding variants per individual,[344] chromosome polymorphisms can be very useful for diagnosing maternal cell contamination (see below) or in situations in which a possible mix-up or cross-contamination of cases is suspected.

Polymorphisms of Chromosomes 1, 9, 16, and Y

The polymorphisms of chromosomes 1, 9, 16, and Y involve primarily the constitutive heterochromatic regions (i.e., the secondary constriction region of chromosomes 1, 9, and 16), and the distal two-thirds of the long arm of the Y chromosome. Major polymorphisms, such as a complete pericentric inversion of the constitutive heterochromatic region, a greatly enlarged heterochromatic region (qh+, twice or more the size of 16p), a large Y (larger than chromosome 18), a small Y (smaller than a G-group chromosome), and a pericentric inversion of Y, can be recognized with the common banding techniques (G-, Q- and C-banding).

Table 6.34. The incidence of inv(1), inv(9), 1qh1, 9qh1, and 16qh1 in four racial/ethnic groups

Racial/Ethnic Group	No. of Cases	Inversion		qh+[a]		
		inv(1)	inv(9)	1qh+	9qh+	16qh+
European origin	2,334	0.04%	0.73%	0.09%	0.26%	0.04%
African origin	1,795	0.06%	3.57%	0.06%	0.28%	0.11%
Hispanic origin	1,737	[b]	2.41%	0.17%	0.35%	0.29%
Asian origin	384	[b]	0.26%	[b]	[b]	[b]
Total	6,250	0.32%	1.98%	0.10%	0.27%	0.13%

Source: Data from Hsu et al., 1987.[345]

[a]qh+ = twice or more the size of 16p.

[b]No cases with such polymorphism were detected in this small series.

The incidence of the common chromosome polymorphisms varies among different racial/ethnic groups (Table 6.34).[345] Although the overall incidence of a complete pericentric inversion of 9qh is approximately 1.98 percent, the incidence is highest in the African American population (3.59 percent), moderate in those of Hispanic origin (2.4 percent), and relatively low in persons of European (0.73 percent) or Asian (0.26 percent) origin. Among other heterochromatic polymorphisms, 9qh+ is seen more frequently than 1qh+ or 16qh+. An inv(1), 1qh−, 9qh−, 16qh−, and inv(16) are rare.[345]

An extra euchromatic band in the qh region of chromosome 9 was first reported by Madan.[346] This variant chromosome 9 has been associated with a relatively large qh block.[346–348] An extra euchromatic band in the 9qh region is frequently visible when a 9qh+ is large (more than twice the size of 16p), and the G-banded metaphase cell shows >400 bands. It seems to have no phenotypic effect.[238] Several other reports described an extra G-positive band on the long arm of chromosome 9 within the 9qh regions (sandwiched between two blocks of heterochromatin); all had no apparent phenotypic effect.[349–353] Homologous sequences at 9p12 and 9q13–21.1 appear to be involved in a diverse set of chromosome 9 pericentromeric rearrangements[353a] but there is no convincing evidence that these are causal in reproductive failure or are associated with specific abnormal phenotypes.

The Y chromosome is more polymorphic in Asian Americans (3.36 percent) and Hispanic Americans (1.85 percent) than among European Americans or African Americans (Table 6.35). The incidence of pericentric inversions of Y was found to be 1 per 1,000 males. A pericentric inv(Y) appears to be more prevalent in Asian American and Hispanic American populations.[345,354]

Table 6.35. The incidence of large Y, small Y, and inv(Y) in four racial/ethnic groups

Racial/Ethnic Group	No. of Cases	Yq+[a]	Yq−[b]	inv(Y)
European origin	1,139	0.53%	0.53%	[c]
African origin	909	0.66%	0.11%	[c]
Hispanic origin	877	0.57%	1.00%	0.23%
Asian origin	208	1.92%	0.96%	0.48%
Total	3,133	0.67%	0.57%	0.10%

Source: Data from Hsu et al., 1987.[345]

[a]Yq+ = A Y larger than chromosome 18.

[b]Yq− = A Y smaller than a G-group chromosome.

[c]No cases with such polymorphism were detected.

Satellited Y chromosomes have been reported occasionally.[355] Eight cases of Yqs were observed among 22,136 males in one prenatal series (i.e., 1 in 2,767 males).[238] A Yqs does not appear to cause any phenotypic abnormalities.[355]

Polymorphisms of Acrocentric Chromosomes

The size of satellites, stalks, and short arms of the acrocentric chromosomes varies a great deal. Occasionally, the entire short arm can be absent, with no visible satellites remaining. In 33,000 genetic amniocenteses, 21ps− and 13ps− were the most frequently seen variants in the ps− category, with frequencies of 0.73 and 0.33 per 1,000, respectively.[238] 22ps−, 14ps−, and 15ps− occurred less often, with frequencies of 0.27, 0.14, and 0.12 per 1,000. The absence of the short arm of an acrocentric chromosome appears to have no deleterious effect.

Among the acrocentric chromosomes, polymorphisms in satellites, stalks, and short arms have been described most frequently in chromosome 15. The short arm of chromosome 15 possesses a large amount of 5-methylcytosine and stains positively with DA/DAPI. Using a variety of staining techniques (Q-, C-, NOR-, and DA/DAPI), Wachtler and Musil[356] reported up to six highly polymorphic regions of the short arm of chromosome 15. Chen et al.[357] found eight polymorphic variants in human chromosome 15, and Babu et al.[358] noted at least five classes of different intensities with DA/DAPI staining of 15p. Proximal 15q (bands q12–3) can also show considerable variation in appearance by G-banding and FISH.[359]

A large short arm (not a large satellite) of an acrocentric chromosome can be of diagnostic concern. Y/autosomal translocations have been described in which the heterochromatic region (fluorescent region) of the Y chromosome (Yq12) is translocated to the short arm of a D or G group chromosome.[258] Most of these translocations are familial in origin. 46,XY individuals with these translocations show a normal male phenotype, and 46,XX individuals with these translocations show a normal female phenotype. The most commonly encountered examples are t(Y;15)(q12;p11–12)[258,360] and t(Y;22)(q12;p11–12).[258] More than 60 cases of these types of translocation have been reported in multiple families. Segregation of the translocation in both males and females and/or, FISH analyses using probes for SRY, Yq12 sequences, and nucleolar organizer region (NOR) DNA sequences can be used to help determine whether any particular Y/autosomal translocation encountered prenatally is likely to be clinically significant.

Using different chromosome banding techniques, a short arm, stalk, or satellite polymorphism can usually be distinguished from a structural abnormality. A practical first step in the evaluation of a polymorphic acrocentric chromosome would be to search for satellite associations involving the short arm of the chromosome in question. Cytogenetic studies of the parents' chromosomes should determine the origin and assist in the characterization of an unusual polymorphism.

Polymorphism of Other Chromosomes, "Common" Inversions, and Translocations

Polymorphisms of constitutive heterochromatin have been found at the centromeric region of many autosomes other than 1, 9, and 16. A large heterochromatic region has been reported for chromosome 3,[361] chromosome 4,[362,363] chromosome 5,[364,365] and chromosome 6.[366] An additional G-band-positive and C-band-negative segment has been found in the proximal region of the short arm of chromosome 16 (resulting in 16p+) in eleven instances; nine were familial, and two were of unknown origin.[367–371] The extra euchromatic material on 16p was shown to be late in replicating.[372] Chromosome variants have also been reported for 17p, 18p, and 20p, which resulted in 17ph+,[373] 18ph+,[374–377] and 20ph+,[378,379] respectively. Centromeric heteromorphisms in chromosome 19 are also known.[380–382]

In addition to pericentric inversion of chromosomes 1, 9, and Y, pericentric inversion of chromosome 2, involving p11 and q13, has been seen many times.[74,80,383] MacDonald and Cox[383] reported an incidence of 1 in 600 in AFC analyses and 1 in 1,800 in blood cultures. In 44,000 prenatal diagnoses, inv(2)(p11q13) was observed in 119 cases, giving an incidence of 0.043 percent (4 in 10,000).[238] Other inversions that may be occasionally encountered are inv(10)(p11.2q21.2),[74,83] inv(8)(p23q22),[74,84] and inv(5)(p13q13)[74,384,385] (see also, "Indications for Prenatal Cytogenetic Diagnosis: Chromosome Inversion" above).

Other than Robertsonian translocations, t(11;22)(q23.3;q11.2) is the only specific translocation expected to be commonly encountered. The risks for unbalanced segregation have been established (Table 6.8). Rare translocations that involve acrocentric satellite regions and various nonacrocentrics are also sometimes seen (in addition to the satellited Y chromosomes previously discussed). Exchanges have been reported with terminal bands of 1p,[386] 2p,[387] 2q,[388] 4p,[389] 4q,[390–393] 5p,[394] 10p,[395] 10q,[396] 12p,[397] 17p,[398] Xp,[399] and Xq.[400] Most, but not all, individuals with satellited nonacrocentrics are phenotypically normal. The possibility that the satellited nonacrocentric represents the unbalanced segregation product of a balanced reciprocal exchange in a parent must be considered. It may therefore be necessary to perform FISH analyses with subtelomeric probes on the carrier parent's chromosomes and the amniotic fluid cells to fully evaluate these cases. Interstitial insertions of satellite regions can also occur.[401–406]

Summary Conclusions and Recommendations for Polymorphisms

1. Common polymorphisms show different frequencies in different populations and are useful for the identification of individual cell lines.
2. Rare polymorphisms can generally be distinguished from structural chromosomal abnormalities by using various chromosome staining techniques, FISH, and, if necessary, performing chromosome analyses on the parents.
3. There are specific inversions, Y/acrocentric short arm, acrocentric short arm/telomere, and t(11;22)(q23.3;q11.2) translocations that are seen recurrently in human populations.

FACTORS AFFECTING DIAGNOSTIC SUCCESS RATE AND ACCURACY

Maternal Cell Contamination

Maternal cell contamination (MCC) of AFC cultures is a potentially serious source of error in prenatal diagnosis. According to the data collected from three large surveys,[180,181,407] and PDL's data[238] (Table 6.36), in a combined sample of 189,323 genetic amniocenteses, the overall frequency of MCC was 0.24 percent. Because MCC would generally not be recognized when the fetal sex is female, the true incidence of MCC is therefore approximately twice the observed figure.

In the 1983 U.S. survey of MCC,[407] there were 112 cases detected through an admixture of XY and XX cells, and 22 cases were ascertained as the result of an unexpected pregnancy outcome (i.e., a 46,XX diagnosis had been reported, but the liveborn had a dif-

Table 6.36.   The frequency of maternal cell contamination (MCC) in amniocytes

Reference	No. of Cases with MCC	No. of Samples	(%)
U.S. Survey[407]	134	91,131	0.15
European Study[180]	79	45,806	0.17
Canadian Study[181]	22	12,386	0.18
PDL Data[238]	210	40,000	0.53
Total	445	189,323	0.24

ferent chromosome constitution). Although most of the unexpected pregnancy outcomes were cases in which XX had been diagnosed prenatally and XY males were born, at least four cases of trisomy 21 were missed, apparently because of MCC.[152,407]

The data from the 1983 U.S. survey of MCC[407] showed that the incidence of MCC was reduced by 2.5 times when the first few milliliters of amniotic fluid were not used for cell culture. This indicates that fragments of maternal tissue picked up by the needle could be the main source of MCC. This suggestion is supported by the repeated finding of MCC in AFC from consecutive pregnancies of a patient with fibroids, in which the shedding of cells or fibroid fragments into the amniocentesis needle was thought to cause the MCC.[408]

The 1983 U.S. survey of MCC[407] also made the following observations:

1. MCC is more frequent when wider-gauge needles are used for the amniocentesis. The incidence of MCC in the group using a wider needle (20 gauge or less) was 0.15 percent, whereas the incidence was 0.11 percent in the group using a smaller needle (21 gauge or greater). The difference, however, was not statistically significant. In both groups, a needle stylet was said to be in place at the time of the insertion.

2. The incidence of MCC was more common in cultures established from bloody fluids. Approximately 35 percent of all cases with MCC were associated with bloody samples.

3. Cultures with MCC showed no unusual growth patterns. The harvesting time did not differ from cultures without MCC.

4. MCC was detected in more than one culture in 41 percent of the MCC cases.

5. In the majority of cases in which MCC caused misdiagnosis, only one culture and/or fewer than 20 cells had been examined.

6. A comparison of chromosome polymorphisms of the AFC and of parental cells, especially the mother's, can be helpful in confirming MCC.

Considerable variability in terms of the observed frequency of MCC exists among laboratories.[181,407] Among 40,000 cases analyzed at PDL over 16 years, the MCC rate remained unchanged at 0.5 percent (a total of 210 cases with XY and XX admixture were detected). Approximately half of the cases showed multiple XX cells in one flask, and one-quarter of the cases showed either one single XX cell or multiple XX cells in two or more culture vessels.[238] All cases with follow-up information were reported to be normal males.[238]

Regarding the sensitivity in detection of MCC and mosaicism using the flask method versus the in situ method for cell culture, the data from the U.S. survey on MCC[407] and from the U.S. survey on mosaicism[179] indicated that the overall detection rates were not noticeably different. The rate for MCC detection was slightly higher for the in situ method, but it was slightly lower for detecting chromosome mosaicism with the same method.[152]

It should be emphasized that whereas nearly all cases with an admixture of XY and XX cells turn out to be MCC in XY fetuses, the remote possibility of XX/XY chimerism or mosaicism still exists. In fact, four such cases have been identified through prenatal diagnosis.[152,409,410]

Using FISH and simultaneous dual-color X- and Y-specific chromosome probes, the overall rate of MCC in noncultivated AFC was 21.4 percent,[158] compared with 0.2 percent in cultured amniotic fluid cells. A major difference in MCC percentage is observed in moderately bloody versus slightly bloody amniotic fluid. Fifty-five percent of moderately bloody amniotic fluid specimens, compared with 16 percent of slightly bloody amniotic fluid specimens, exhibited XX nuclei in ≥20 percent of cells. Fortunately, for prenatal cytogenetic diagnosis using cultured AFC, the frequency of MCC is drastically reduced.

Several reports have described different DNA methods to detect MCC in noncultivated and cultured AFC.[411–413] Although these methods may not be practical in routine cytogenetic diagnosis, they may be useful in prenatal diagnosis of genetic disorders using noncultivated AFC, where MCC can be the potential source of a major diagnostic error.

Summary Conclusions and Recommendations for MCC

1. The frequency of MCC can be reduced using a smaller-gauge needle for amniocentesis (preferably 21 gauge or greater), initially having the stylet in place, and discarding (or separating) the first 1 or 2 mL of amniotic fluid.
2. Cytogenetic analysis should include cells from at least two independent primary cultures, with chromosome analysis of a minimum of twenty metaphases in the flask method or ten to fifteen colonies in the in situ method.
3. When an admixture of XY and XX cells is found, a comparison of the Q-banding chromosome polymorphisms of the 46,XX amniotic fluid cells with the mother's cells can be informative.
4. An ultrasound examination to confirm the presence of male genitalia should be performed in cases in which MCC is suspected.

Twin Pregnancy

The overall twin pregnancy rate in the United States has been steadily increasing, and for the year 2000 the prevalence was 29.3 per 1,000 pregnancies.[414,415] More than 70 percent of these cases are expected to be dizygotic.[152,416] The incidence of dizygotic twinning increases with maternal age, with a peak between the ages of 35 and 39 years.[416] Because many of the women seeking prenatal diagnosis are of advanced maternal age, a twin pregnancy can be expected in more than 3 percent of the referrals for amniocentesis.

With routine ultrasound examination before amniocentesis, twin pregnancies are nearly always identified before the procedure. Under ultrasound guidance, separate aspiration of amniotic fluid samples from each of two sacs has been very successful. In diamniotic cases, addition of indigo carmine during the amniocentesis procedure can help establish that fluid from the two independent sacs has been sampled. A management and counseling dilemma occurs when one twin is found to be normal and the other abnormal. Many instances of selective termination of an abnormal fetus have been reported[417–419,419a] (see also discussions in chapters 26 and 32).

Mycoplasma Contamination of Cell Cultures

Mycoplasma infection has been a rather frequent problem in cell culture, especially in continuous cell lines; the incidence of such infection in continuous cell lines may be as high as 15 percent.[420] Mycoplasma contamination was a major problem in cultured AFC in the 1970s. In a study by Schneider and Stanbridge,[421] mycoplasma RNA was detected in more than half of the AFC cultures.

The seriousness of mycoplasma contamination is largely due to its insidious damaging effect on the cells. The contaminated cells may at first show no noticeable difference in terms of cell growth or cell morphology, but they exhibit a significant increase in chromosome gaps, breaks, rearrangements, and other types of aneuploidy.[420,421]

A cost-effective method for the detection of mycoplasma is in situ fluorescent DNA staining with Hoechst 33258 or 4,6-diamidino-2-phenylindole (DAPI).[321] Using this procedure, mycoplasma-contaminated cultures will show small, brightly fluorescent particles that are primarily associated with the cytoplasm.

For practical purposes, once mycoplasma contamination is diagnosed, immediate disposal of the contaminated culture is probably the method of choice. When all cultures from a given case are infected, it is better to request a repeat amniocentesis immediately than to attempt to salvage the cultures with antibiotics. Meanwhile, all likely sources of the infection should be removed, and incubators should be emptied and cleaned.

It appears that mycoplasma infection in amniocytes has not been a major concern for most cytogenetic laboratories during the past 20 years. It is not known whether this reflects a true reduction of such infections, improved quality of tissue culture reagents, or is related to an overall shortened cell culture time, which in turn does not allow mycoplasma infection to become evident.

Toxic Syringes or Tubes

AFC culture failure has been associated with syringe or tube toxicity and was reported as early as 1976.[422,423] Although many of the known toxic vessels may have been reformulated, this issue remains a problem. When there is repeated culture failure, the possibility of a toxic syringe or tube must be considered. Anecdotal reports have also implicated agents used to sterilize the skin at the needle insertion site as an additional factor in cell culture failure.

Other Causes of Culture Failure

AFC culture failure is not always attributable to laboratory conditions, syringes, and tubes. Cell culture failure rates may be higher for chromosomally abnormal pregnancies.[424,425] Cell culture failure is not uncommon when fetal death has occurred, when there is very heavy blood contamination of the specimen, or when the sample volume is inadequate. Failure rates are also higher for early- (<14 weeks) and late- (>24 weeks) gestational-age specimens.[426,427]

Technical Standards for Prenatal Cytogenetics Laboratories

Basic guidelines on the technical aspects of prenatal cytogenetic diagnosis were proposed by the International Workshop on Prenatal Diagnosis in 1979.[428] Today, many of the earlier recommendations are considered minimal requirements. The proposal that prenatal cytogenetic diagnosis should be an integral part of a collaborative antenatal genetic program using expertise in obstetrics, ultrasonography, genetic counseling, cytogenetics, and clinical genetics is now well recognized and practiced in the majority of medical centers.

The American College of Medical Genetics has adopted specific standards and guidelines for clinical cytogenetics laboratories performing AFC analyses, and these are periodically revised.[429] The basic elements of good cytogenetic laboratory practice include the following:

1. The laboratory should demonstrate its competency in all aspects of testing before formally offering a diagnostic service. This is achieved by coprocessing a series of specimens in the new laboratory in parallel with an established laboratory.
2. The training, qualifications, and experience of the staff should be consistent with this complex testing.
3. A minimum of three containers should be set up as primary cultures for both flask and in situ methods.
4. The cultures should be grown and maintained in two different incubators.
5. To avoid contamination of all the cultures of a specimen, two different batches or types of tissue culture media (including fetal calf serum) should be used.
6. The status of each cell culture should be determined within 10 days to assess the need for a repeat amniocentesis.
7. The final cytogenetic diagnosis should be derived through the analysis of cells from at least two primary-culture containers in both flask and in situ methods.
8. In the flask method, generally twenty metaphases (with a minimum of fifteen) should be examined (preferably ten from each culture). In the in situ method, fifteen metaphases from ten to fifteen colonies (preferably one from each colony) should be examined.
9. All cells to be analyzed should be banded with G, Q, or R banding. A minimum of 400 bands per haploid set is required. Ideally, one karyotype should show 550 bands per haploid set.
10. A minimum of two banded metaphases should be karyotyped by photography or with an automated system. Three other cells should be mapped directly under the microscope.
11. The karyotypes should show at least one pair of each chromosome without overlapping and should be clearly identifiable by its banding pattern. Otherwise, additional karyotypes or partial karyotypes should be appended.
12. Ninety to ninety-five percent of the cases should be completed within 14 days (preferably within 10).
13. There should be a minimum success rate of 95 percent in cell culture and chromosome analysis, based on a moving average of consecutive cases over a 3-month period.
14. Documentation should include the numbers of cells reviewed, information about any numerical and structural abnormalities observed, and microscope slide coordinates.
15. Backup cultures should be maintained, pending the need for additional studies.
16. The laboratory should provide peripheral blood chromosome analyses on parents when structural chromosomal abnormalities or unusual heteromorphisms are detected.
17. The laboratory should be able to provide a variety of different staining techniques and FISH analyses.

18. Reports should provide karyotype descriptions using the International System for Human Cytogenetic Nomenclature (ISCN) and be written such that they are also fully interpretable by noncytogeneticists.
19. Records should be maintained in a manner that will maximize their usefulness for patients and their families.
20. Whenever possible, information on pregnancy outcome should be obtained for each case. Abnormal results should be confirmed either after termination or at birth.

There are no specific recommendations regarding the number of cases that an individual technologist should handle. The number should not compromise accuracy or the ability to provide additional counts, FISH, or other studies when potentially abnormal cases are encountered. There should also be provision for training and continuing education of both laboratory staff and those who are involved with referral of tests to the laboratory.

The occasional need to perform additional cell counts, FISH, or other supplemental staining techniques used to reach a cytogenetic diagnosis are an integral part of the prenatal cytogenetic testing procedure. As such, these procedures should not be viewed as adjunctive or reflexive in nature (i.e., requiring further physician authorization and patient contact before they are performed).

Error Rates in Prenatal Cytogenetic Diagnosis through Amniocentesis

Because the error rates for prenatal cytogenetic diagnosis through amniocentesis differ in different laboratories and all laboratories tend to keep their error unreported, an accurate current overall error rate is not known. Nevertheless, it is likely that the overall error rates have been reduced possibly 10–30 times in the past 30 years. Because the overall error rates were reported to be 0.1–0.6 percent in the 1970s and early 1980s,[152] at least a few reports of error rates of 0.01–0.02 percent were reported in the 1990s.[430,431] The vast majority of errors were incorrect sex assignment due either to maternal cell contamination, laboratory error, or typographic mistakes.[152] At least four cases of trisomy 21 were misdiagnosed as 46,XX because of maternal cell contamination.[152] Not all inconsistencies between the sex established through karyotyping and phenotype are attributable to laboratory problems. Follow-up cytogenetic confirmation and FISH analyses using an SRY probe will identify some cases of translocation or deletion of this Y-chromosome critical region.[432,433]

A routine prenatal cytogenetic diagnosis is designed primarily to detect numerical abnormalities and major structural aberrations. Low-level chromosome mosaicism can be missed.[434] UPD will not be detected. A subtle structural abnormality or microdeletion syndrome may easily go undetected, and an accurate diagnosis requires FISH studies. In one report, three cases, each with a subtle structural abnormality, were diagnosed as having a normal diploid karyotype in studies performed on 10,500 amniotic fluid samples.[435] Furthermore, a misdiagnosis could be attributed to a vanishing twin that is sampled at amniocentesis.[431,436]

CONCLUSION

Nearly all women who choose to receive prenatal cytogenetic diagnosis through amniocentesis receive a normal test result. These women can be reassured that their fetus is unaffected with Down syndrome or other serious aneuploidy. Women who do have an affected pregnancy can choose elective termination. Alternatively, they can benefit from predelivery guidance in the care of their child, receive modified delivery plans that integrate neonatal specialty services, and can be prepared through family support and other coping resources. The past 35 years of providing these services have clearly demonstrated these benefits and shown the widespread acceptability of prenatal testing.

Important changes have been made in redefining the population of women who would most benefit from amniocentesis. Maternal serum screening and ultrasound examinations have substantially assisted in identifying women at greatest risk for fetal aneuploidy while simultaneously reducing the need for amniocentesis for others. Steady progress has also been made in understanding the clinical significance of many of the rare cytogenetic diagnoses. However, those who provide these services still regularly encounter novel findings, and it is important that this information continue to be shared through publication. Molecular cytogenetic testing has augmented traditional karyotyping and expanded the range of chromosomal abnormalities that are prenatally diagnosable. We envisage an important role for microarray technology, which has the potential to lead to rapid diagnoses of aneuploidy, identification of microdeletion syndromes, and the detection of subtelomeric abnormalities that are currently not routinely diagnosed.[437]

The results of amniocentesis testing are currently delivered to patients through a counseling session that is sensitive to their individual ethical values and respects their decision making. It is essential that this aspect of the service, together with the quality of the testing, never be compromised.

ACKNOWLEDGMENTS

We thank Michael Benn for assistance in compiling the references.

REFERENCES

1. Serr DM, Sachs L, Danon M. Diagnosis of sex before birth using cells from the amniotic fluid. Bull Res Council Isr 1955;58:137.
2. Fuchs F, Riis R. Antenatal sex determination. Nature 1956;177:330.
3. Steele MW, Breg WR. Chromosome analysis of human amniotic fluid cells. Lancet 1966;1:383.
4. Niazi M, Coleman DV, Loeffler FE. Trophoblast sampling in early pregnancy culture of rapidly dividing cells from immature placental villi. Br J Obstet Gynaecol 1981;88:1081.
5. Simoni G, Brambati B, Danesino C, et al. Efficient direct chromosome analyses and enzyme determinations from chorionic villi samples in the first trimester of pregnancy. Hum Genet 1983;63:349.
6. Egan JFX, Benn PA, Borgida A, et al. Efficacy of screening for fetal Down syndrome in the US from 1974 to 1997. Obstet Gynecol 2000;96:979.
7. Wald NJ, Kennard A, Hackshaw A, et al. Antenatal screening for Down's syndrome. J Med Screen 1997;4:181. www.ncchta.org/fullmono/mon201.pdf.
8. Benn PA. Advances in prenatal screening for Down syndrome. I. General principles and second trimester testing. Clin Chim Acta.2002;323:1.
9. Benn PA. Advances in prenatal screening for Down syndrome. II. First trimester testing, integrated testing and future directions. Clin Chim Acta.2002;324:1.
10. Shipp TD, Benacerraf BR. Second trimester screening for chromosomal abnormalities. Prenat Diagn 2002;22:296.
11. Sergovich F, Valentine GH, Chen AL, et al. Chromosome aberrations in 2159 consecutive newborn babies. N Engl J Med 1969;280:851.
12. Lubs HA, Ruddle FH. Chromosomal abnormalities in the human population: estimation of rates based on New Haven newborn study. Science 1970;169:495.
13. Gerald PS, Walzer S. Chromosome studies of normal newborn infants. In: Jacobs PA, Price WH, Law P, eds. Human population cytogenetics. Edinburgh: Edinburgh University Press, 1970:143.
14. Friedrich U, Nielsen J. Chromosome studies in 5,049 consecutive newborn children. Clin Genet 1973;4:333.

15. Jacobs PA, Melville M, Ratcliff S, et al. A cytogenetic survey of 11,680 newborn infants. Ann Hum Genet 1974;37:359.

16. Nielsen J, Silesen I. Incidence of chromosome aberrations among 11,148 newborn children. Hum Genet 1975;30:1.

17. Hamerton JL, Canning N, Ray M, et al. A cytogenetic survey of 14,069 newborn infants. Clin Genet 1975;8:223.

18. Lin CC, Gedeon MM, Griffith P, et al. Chromosome analysis on 930 consecutive newborn children using quinacrine fluorescent banding technique. Hum Genet 1976;31:313.

19. Maeda T, Ohno M, Takada M, et al. A cytogenetic survey of consecutive liveborn infants: incidence and type of chromosome abnormalities. Jpn J Hum Genet 1978;23:217.

20. Buckton KE, O'Riordan ML, Ratcliffe S, et al. A G-band study of chromosomes in liveborn infants. Ann Hum Genet 1980;43:223.

21. Nielsen J, Wohlert M, Faaborg-Andersen J, et al. Incidence of chromosome abnormalities in newborn children: comparison between incidence in 1969–1974 and 1980–1982 in the same area. Hum Genet 1982;61:98.

22. Nielsen J, Wohlert M. Chromosome abnormalities found among 34,910 newborn children: results from a 13-year incidence study in Arhus, Denmark. Hum Genet 1991;87:81.

23. Jacobs PA, Browne C, Gregson N, et al. Estimates of the frequency of chromosome abnormalities detectable in unselected newborns using moderate levels of banding. J Med Genet 1992;29:103.

24. Hook EB, Hamerton JL. The frequency of chromosome abnormalities detected in consecutive newborn studies: differences between studies: results by sex and severity of phenotypic involvement. In: Hook EB, Porter I eds. Population cytogenetics, studies in humans. New York: Academic Press, 1985:63.

25. Bray I, Wright DE, Davies CJ, et al. Joint estimation of Down syndrome risk and ascertainment rates: a meta-analysis of nine published data sets. Prenat Diagn 1998;18:9.

26. Hook EB. Rates of chromosome abnormalities at different maternal ages. Obstet Gynecol 1981;58:282.

27. Ferguson-Smith MA, Yates JRW. Maternal age specific rates for chromosome aberrations and factors influencing them: report of a collaborative European study on 52,965 amniocenteses. Prenat Diagn (special issue) 1984;4:5.

28. Shreinemachers DM, Cross PK, Hook EB. Rates of trisomies 21, 18, 13 and other chromosome abnormalities in about 20,000 prenatal studies compared with estimated rates in livebirths. Hum Genet 1982;61:318.

29. Hook EB, Warburton D. The distribution of chromosomal genotypes associated with Turner's syndrome: livebirth prevalence rates and evidence for diminished fetal mortality and severity in genotypes associated with structural X abnormalities or mosaicism. Hum Genet 1983;64:24.

30. Hook EB, Cross PK, Regal RR. The frequency of 47,+21, 47, +18 and 47, +13 at the upper-most extremes of maternal ages: results on 56,094 fetuses studied prenatally and comparisons with data on live births. Hum Genet 1984;68:211.

31. Hook EB, Cross PK, Jackson L, et al. Maternal age-specific rates of 47, +21 and other cytogenetic abnormalities diagnosed in the first trimester of pregnancy in chorionic villus biopsy specimens: comparison with rates expected from observations at amniocentesis. Am J Hum Genet 1988;42:797.

32. Leschot NJ, Wolf H, Van Prooijen-Knegt AC, et al. Cytogenetic findings in 1250 chorionic villus samples follow-up of the first 1000 pregnancies. Br J Obstet Gynaecol 1989;96:663.

33. Kratzer PG, Golbus MS, Schonberg SA, et al. Cytogenetic evidence for enhanced selective miscarriage of trisomy 21 pregnancies with advancing maternal age. Am J Med Genet 1992;44:657.

34. Snijders RJM, Holzgreve W, Cuckle H, et al. Maternal age-specific risks for trisomies at 9–14 weeks' gestation. Prenat Diagn 1995;14:543.

35. Macintosh MCM, Wald NJ, Chard T, et al. Selective miscarriage of Down's syndrome fetuses in women 35 years and older. Br J Obstet Gynaecol 1995;102:798.

36. Cuckle HS, Wald NJ. Thompson SG. Estimating a woman's risk of having a pregnancy associated with Down's syndrome using her age and serum alpha-fetoprotein level. Br J Obstet Gynaecol 1987;94:387.

37. Hecht CA, Hook EB. The imprecision in the rates of Down syndrome by 1-year maternal age intervals: a critical analysis of rates used in biochemical screening. Prenat Diagn 1994;14:729.

38. *Idem.* Rates of Down syndrome at livebirth by one-year maternal age intervals in studies with apparent close to complete ascertainment in populations of European origin: a proposed revised rate schedule for use in genetic and prenatal screening. Am J Med Genet 1996;62:376.

39. Huether CA, Ivanovich J, Goodwin BS, et al. Maternal age specific risk rate estimates for Down syndrome among live births in whites and other races from Ohio and metropolitan Atlanta. J Med Genet 1998;35:482.

40. Morris JK, Mutton DE, Alberman E. Revised estimates of the maternal age specific live birth prevalence of Down's syndrome. J Med Screen 2002;9:2.
41. Hook EB, Topol BB, Cross PK. The natural history of cytogenetically abnormal fetuses detected at mid trimester amniocentesis which are not terminated electively: new data and estimates of the excess and relative risk of late fetal death associated with 47,+21 and some other abnormal karyotypes. Am J Hum Genet 1989;45:855.
42. Hook EB, Mutton DE, Ide R, et al. The natural history of Down syndrome conceptuses diagnosed parentally that are not electively terminated. Am J Hum Genet 1995;57:875.
43. Morris JK, Wald NJ, Watt HC. Fetal loss in Down syndrome pregnancies. Prenat Diagn 1999;19:142.
44. Cuckle HS. Wald NJ. Screening for Down's syndrome. In: Lilford R, ed. Prenatal diagnosis and prognosis. London: Butterworth, 1990;67.
45. Cuckle H. Down syndrome fetal loss rate in early pregnancy. Prenat Diagn 1999;19:1175.
46. Benn PA, Egan JFX. Survival of Down syndrome in utero. Prenat Diagn 2000;20:432.
47. Warburton D. De novo balanced chromosome rearrangements and extra marker chromosomes identified at prenatal diagnosis: clinical significance and distribution of breakpoints. Am J Hum Genet 1991;49:995.
48. Hsu LYF, Hirschhorn K. Numerical and structural chromosome abnormalities. In: Wilson JG, Clark-Fraser F, eds. Handbook of teratology, vol. 2. New York: Plenum Press, 1977;41.
49. Boué J, Boué A, Lazar P. Retrospective and prospective epidemiological studies of 1500 karyotyped spontaneous human abortions. Teratology 1975;12:11.
50. Creasy MR, Crolla JA, Alberman ED. A cytogenetic study of human spontaneous abortions using banding techniques. Hum Genet 1976;3:177.
51. Takahara H, Ohama K, Fujiwara A. Cytogenetic study in early spontaneous abortions. Hiroshima J Med Sci 1977;26:291.
52. Carr DH, Gedeon MM. Q-banding of chromosomes in human spontaneous abortions. Can J Genet Cytol 1978;20:415.
53. Geisler M, Kleinebrecht J. Cytogenetic and histologic analyses of spontaneous abortions. Hum Genet 1978;45:239.
54. Kajii T, Ferrier A, Niikaula N, et al. Anatomic and chromosomal anomalies in 639 spontaneous abortuses. Hum Genet 1980;55:87.
55. Hassold T, Chen N, Funkhouser J, et al. A cytogenetic study of 1000 spontaneous abortions. Ann Hum Genet 1980;44:151.
56. Andrews T, Dunlop W, Roberts DF. Cytogenetic studies in spontaneous abortuses. Hum Genet 1984;66:77.
57. Warburton D, Kline J, Stein Z, et al. Cytogenetic abnormalities in spontaneous abortions of recognized conception. In: Porter IH, Willey A, eds. Perinatal genetics diagnosis and treatment. New York: Academic Press, 1986:133.
58. Warburton D, Kline J, Stein Z. Monosomy X: a chromosomal anomaly associated with young maternal age. Lancet 1980;1:17.
59. Kajii T, Ohama K, Mikama K. Anatomic and chromosomal anomalies in 944 induced abortuses. Hum Genet 1978;43:247.
60. Mueller RF, Sybert VP, Johnson J, et al. Evaluation of a protocol for post-mortem examination of stillbirths. N Engl J Med 1983;309:586.
61. Ellis PM, Bain AG. Cytogenetics in the evaluation of perinatal death. Lancet 1984;1:630.
62. Machin GA, Crolla JA. Chromosome constitution of 500 infants dying during the perinatal period. Hum Genet 1974;23:183.
63. Bauld R, Sutherland GR, Bain AD. Chromosome studies in investigation of stillbirths and neonatal deaths. Arch Dis Child 1974;49:782.
64. Kuleshov NP. Chromosome anomalies of infants dying during the perinatal period and premature newborn. Hum Genet 1976;31:151.
65. Alberman ED, Creasy MR. Frequency of chromosomal abnormalities in miscarriages and perinatal deaths. J Med Genet 1977;14:313.
66. President's Commission for the Study of Ethical Problems in Medicine and Biomedical and Behavioral Sciences. Screening and counseling for genetic conditions. Washington, DC: Government Printing Office, 1983.
67. Wald NJ, Cuckle HS, Densem JW, et al. Maternal serum screening for Down's syndrome in early pregnancy. BMJ 1988;297:883.
68. Haddow JE, Palomaki GE, Knight GJ, et al. Reducing the need for amniocentesis in women 35 years of age or older with serum markers for screening. N Engl J Med 1994;330:1114.

69. Cuckle H. Time for a total shift to first-trimester screening for Down's syndrome. Lancet 2001;358:1658.

70. Benn P. Improved antenatal screening for Down's syndrome. Lancet 2003;361:794.

71. American College of Medical Genetics. ACMG Position Statement on Multiple Marker Screening in Women 35 and Older. www.acmg.net/Pages/ACMG_Activities/policy_statements_pages/current/Multiple_Marker_Screening_in_Women_35_and_Older_Position_Statement_on.asp.

72. American College of Obstetrics and Gynecology. Committee opinion no 141. Down syndrome screening. Washington, DC: American College of Obstetrics and Gynecology, 1994.

73. Boué A, Gallano P. A collaborative study of the segregation of inherited chromosome structural rearrangements in 1356 prenatal diagnoses. Prenat Diagn (special issue) 1984;4:45.

74. Daniel A, Hook EB, Wulf G. Risks of unbalanced progeny at amniocentesis to carriers of chromosome rearrangements: data from United States and Canadian laboratories. Am J Med Genet 1989;33:14.

75. Daniel A, Boué A, Gallano P. Prospective risk in reciprocal translocation in heterozygotes at amniocentesis as determined by potential chromosome imbalance sizes: data of the European collaborative prenatal diagnosis centers. Prenat Diagn 1986;6:315.

76. Ledbetter DH, Engel E. Uniparental disomy in humans: development of an imprinting map and its implications for prenatal diagnosis. Hum Mol Genet 1995;4:1757.

77. Ralph A, Scott F, Tiernan C, et al. Maternal uniparental isodisomy for chromosome 14 detected prenatally. Prenat Diagn 1999;19:681.

78. Kurosawa K, Sasaki H, Sato Y, et al. Paternal UPD14 is responsible for a distinctive malformation complex. Am J Med Genet 2002;110:268.

79. Kaiser P. Pericentric inversions: problems and significance for clinical genetics. Hum Genet 1984;68:1.

80. Djalali M, Steinbach P, Bellerdiek J, et al. The significance of pericentric inversions of chromosome 2. Hum Genet 1986;72:32.

81. Magee AC, Humphreys MW, McKee S, et al. De novo direct duplication 2 (p12–p21) with paternally inherited pericentric inversion 2p11.2 2q12.2. Clin Genet 1998;54:65–69.

82. Lacbawan FL, White BJ, Anguiano A, et al. Rare interstitial deletion (2)(p11.2p13) in a child with pericentric inversion (2)(p11.2q13) of paternal origin. Am J Med Genet 1999;87:139.

83. Collinson MN, Fisher AM, Walker J, et al. Inv(10) (p11.2q21.2), a variant chromosome. Hum Genet 1997;101:175.

84. Smith AC, Spuhler K, Williams TM, et al. Genetic risk for recombinant 8 syndrome and the transmission rate of balanced inversion 8 in the Hispanic population of the southwest United States. Am J Hum Genet 1987;41:1083.

85. Madan K, Seabright M, Lindenbaum RH, et al. Paracentric inversions in man. J Med Genet 1984;21:407.

86. Mules EH, Stamberg J. Reproductive outcomes of paracentric inversion carriers: report of a liveborn dicentric recombinant and literature review. Hum Genet 1984;67:126.

87. Callen DF, Woollatt E, Sutherland GR. Paracentric inversions in man. Clin Genet 1985;27:87.

88. Fryns JP, Kleczkowska A, Van den Berghe H. Paracentric inversions in man. Hum Genet 1986;73:205.

89. Madan K Nieuwint AWM. Reproductive risks for paracentric inversion heterozygotes: Inversion or insertion? That is the question. Am J Med Gent 2002;107:340.

90. Pettinati MJ, Rao PN, Phalen MC et al. Paracentric inversions in humans: a review of 446 paracentric inversions with presentation of 120 new cases. Am J Med Genet 1995;55:171.

91. Madan K, Menko FH. Intrachromosomal insertions: a case report and a review. Hum Genet 1992;89:1.

92. Van Hemel JO, Eussen HJ. Interchromosomal insertions: identification of five cases and a review. Hum Genet 2000;107:415.

93. Arbuzova S, Cuckle H, Mueller R, et al. Familial Down syndrome: evidence supporting cytoplasmic inheritance. Clin Genet 2001;60:456.

94. Medical Research Council of Canada. Diagnosis of genetic disease by amniocentesis during the second trimester of pregnancy: a Canadian study. Report no. 5. Ottawa: Supply Services, 1977.

95. Mikkelsen M, Stene J. Previous child with Down syndrome and other chromosome aberrations. In: Murken J, Stengel-Rutkowski S, Schwinger EW eds. Prenatal diagnosis: proceedings of the Third European Conference on Prenatal Diagnosis of Genetic disorders. Stuttgart: Enke, 1979:22.

96. Stene J, Stene E, Mikkelsen M. Risk for chromosome abnormality at amniocentesis following a child with a non-inherited chromosome aberration. Prenat Diagn (special issue) 1984;4:81.

97. Uehara S, Yaegashi N, Maeda T et al. Risk of recurrence of fetal chromosome aberrations: analysis of trisomy 21, trisomy 18, trisomy 13, and 45,X in 1,076 Japanese mothers. J Obstet Gynaecol Res 1999;25:373.

98. Jewell AF, Keene WE, Ferre MM, et al. Analysis of the recurrence risks for trisomies 13 and 18. Am J Hum Genet 1996;59(Suppl):A121.

99. Uchida IA, Freeman VCP. Trisomy 21 Down syndrome: Parental mosaicism. Hum Genet 1985;70:246.

100. Warburton D. In: Hassold T, Epstein CJ eds. Molecular and cytogenetic studies of non-disjunction. New York: Alan Liss, 1989;165.

101. Pangalos CG, Talbot CC Jr, Lewis JG, et al. DNA polymorphism analysis in families with recurrence of free trisomy 21. Am J Hum Genet 1992;51:1015.

102. Steinberg C, Zackai EH, Eunpu DL, et al. Recurrence risk for de novo 21q21q translocation Down syndrome: a study of 112 families. Am J Med Genet1984;17:523.

103. Barkai G, Arbuzova S, Berkenstadt M, et al. Frequency of Down's syndrome and neural tube defects in the same family. Lancet 2003;361:1331.

103a. Olsen JH, Winther JF. Down's syndrome and neural tube defects in the same families. Lancet 2003;361:1316.

104. Feuchtbaum LB, Cunningham G, Waller K, et al. Fetal karyotyping for chromosome abnormalities after an unexplained elevated maternal serum alpha-fetoprotein screening. Obstet Gynecol 1995;86:248.

105. Saller DN, Canick JA, Schwartz S, et al. Multiple-marker screening in pregnancies with hydropic and non-hydropic Turner syndrome. Am J Obstet Gynecol 1992:1021.

106. Benn PA, Gainey A, Ingardia CJ, et al. Second trimester maternal serum analytes in triploid pregnancies: correlation with phenotype and sex chromosome complement. Prenat Diagn 2001;21:680.

107. Benn PA. Trisomy 16 and trisomy 16 mosaicism: a review. Am J Med Genet 1998;79:121.

108. Snijders RJM, Noble P, Sebire N, et al. UK multicenter project on assessment of risk for trisomy 21 by maternal age and fetal nuchal-translucency thickness at 10–14 weeks of gestation. Lancet 1998;351:343.

109. Hahnemann JM, Vejerslev LO. European collaborative research on mosaicism in CVS (EUCROMIC): fetal and extrafetal cell lineages in 192 gestations with CVS mosaicism involving single autosomal trisomy. Am J Med Genet 1997;70:179.

110. Hunter A, Soothill P. Gastroschisis: an overview. Prenat Diagn 2002;22:869–873.

111. Kilby MD, Lander A, Usher-Somers M. Exomphalos (omphalocele). Prenat Diagn 1998;18:1283.

112. Gupta JK, Lilford RJ. Assessment and management of fetal agenesis of the corpus callosum. Prenat Diagn 1995;15:301.

113. Gupta JK, Cave M, Lilford RJ, et al. Clinical significance of fetal choroid plexus cysts. Lancet 1995; 346:724.

114. Clementi M, Tenconi R, Bianchi F, et al. Evaluation of prenatal diagnosis of cleft lip with or without cleft palate and cleft palate by ultrasound: experience from 20 European registries. Prenat Diagn 2000;20:870.

115. Shipp TD, Benacerraf BR. The significance of prenatally identified isolated clubfoot: Is amniocentesis indicated? Am J Obstet Gynecol 1998;178:600.

116. Malone FD, Marino T, Bianchi DW, et al. Isolated clubfoot diagnosed prenatally: is karyotyping indicated? Obstet Gynecol 2000;95:437.

117. Stoll C, Garne E, Clementi M, et al. Evaluation of prenatal diagnosis of associated congenital heart diseases by fetal ultrasonographic examination in Europe. Prenat Diagn 2001;21:243.

118. Huggon IC, Cook AC, Simpson JM, et al. Isolated echogenic foci in the fetal heart as marker of chromosomal abnormality. Ultrasound Obstet Gynecol 2001;17:11.

118a. Sotiriadis A, Makrydimas G, Ioannidis JPA. Diagnostic performance of intracardiac echogenic foci for Down syndrome: a meta-analysis. Obstet Gynecol 2003;101:1009.

119. Bromley B, Lieberman E, Shipp TD, et al. Significance of an echogenic intracardiac focus in fetuses at high and low risk for aneuploidy. J Ultrasound Med 1998;17:127.

120. Vibhakar NI, Budorick NE, Scioscia AL, et al. Prevalence of aneuploidy with cardiac intraventricular echogenic focus in an at-risk population. J Ultrasound Med 1999;18:265.

121. Gallagher PG, Mahoney MJ, Gosche JR. Cystic hygroma in the fetus and newborn. Semin Perinatol 1999;23:341.

122. Ecker JL, Shipp TD, Bromley B, et al. The sonographic diagnosis of Dandy–Walker and Dandy–Walker variant: associated findings and outcomes. Prenat Diagn 2000;20:328.

123. Kölble N, Wisser J, Kurmanavicius J, et al. Dandy–Walker malformation: prenatal diagnosis and outcome. Prenat Diagn 2000;20:318.

124. Witters I, Legius E, Moerman PH, et al. Associated malformations and chromosomal anomalies in 42 cases of prenatally diagnosed diaphragmatic hernia. Am J Med Genet 2001;103:278.

125. Nicolaides KH, Snijders RJM, Gosden CM, et al. Ultrasonographically detectable markers of fetal chromosomal abnormalities. Lancet 1992;340:704.

126. Halliday J, Lumley J, Bankier A. Karyotype abnormalities in fetuses diagnosed as abnormal on ultrasound before 20 weeks' gestational age. Prenat Diagn 1994;14:689.

127. Hanna JS, Neu RL, Lockwood DH. Prenatal cytogenetics results from cases referred for 44 different types of abnormal ultrasound findings. Prenat Diagn 1996;16:109.

128. Rizzo N, Pittalis MC, Pilu G, et al. Distribution of abnormal karyotypes among malformed fetuses detected by ultrasound throughout gestation. Prenat Diagn 1996;16:159.

129. Penna L, Bower S. Hyperechogenic bowel in the second trimester fetus: a review. Prenat Diagn 2000;20:909.

129a. Simon-Bouy B, Satre V, Ferec C, et al. Hyperechogenic fetal bowel: a large French collaborative study of 682 cases. Am J Genet 2003;209:213.

130. Nyberg DA, Resta RG, Luthy DA, et al. Humerus and femur length shortening in the detection of Down's syndrome. Am J Obstet Gynecol. 1993;168:534.

131. Peebles DM. Holoprosencephaly. Prenat Diagn 1998;18:477.

132. Den Hollander NS, Wessels MW, Los FJ, et al. Congenital microcephaly detected by prenatal ultrasound: genetic aspects and clinical significance. Ultrasound Obstet Gynecol 2000;15:282.

133. Kennedy D, Chitayat D, Winsor EJT, et al. Prenatally diagnosed neural tube defects: ultrasound, chromosome, and autopsy or postnatal findings in 212 cases. Am J Med Genet 1998;77:317.

134. Benacerraf B. The significance of the nuchal fold in the second trimester fetus. Prenat Diagn 2002;22:798.

135. Wax JR, Benn PA, Steinfeld JD, et al. Prenatally diagnosed sacrococcygeal teratoma: a unique expression of trisomy 1q. Cancer Genet Cytogenet 2000;117:84.

136. Van Den Berg DJ, Francke U. Roberts syndrome: a review of 100 cases and a new rating system for severity. Am J Med Genet 1993;47:1104.

137. Saller DN, Keene CL, Sun CJ, et al. The association between single umbilical artery with cytogenetically abnormal pregnancies. Am J Obstet Gynecol 1990;163:922.

138. Wellesley D, Howe DT. Fetal renal anomalies and genetic syndromes. Prenat Diagn 2001;21:992.

139. Nicolaides KH, Cheng HH, Abbas A, et al. Fetal renal defects: associated malformations and chromosome defects. Fetal Diagn Ther 1992;7:1.

140. Corteville JE, Dicke JM, Crane JP. Fetal pyelectasis and Down syndrome: is genetic amniocentesis warranted? Obstet Gynecol 1992;79:770.

141. Wickstrom EA, Thangavelu MA, Parilla BV, et al. A prospective study of the association between isolated fetal pyelectasis and chromosomal abnormality. Obstet Gynecol 1996;88:397.

142. Nicolaides KH, Azar G, Byrne D, et al. Fetal nuchal translucency: ultrasound screening for chromosomal defects in first trimester of pregnancy. BMJ 1992;304:867.

143. Nicolaides KH, Heath V, Cicero S. Increased fetal nuchal translucency at 11–14 weeks. Prenat Diagn 2002;22:308.

144. Benn PA, Kaminsky LM, Ying J, et al. Combining second-trimester biochemical and ultrasound screening for Down syndrome. Obstet Gynecol 2002;100:1168.

145. Edmonds LD, Levy MJ. Temporal trends in the prevalence of congenital malformations at birth based on the Birth Defects Monitoring Program, United States, 1979–87. MMWR 1990;39:19.

146. Hoffman JI, Kaplan S. The incidence of congenital heart disease. J Am Coll Cardiol 2002;39:1890.

147. Garne E, Stoll C, Clementi M, et al. Evaluation of prenatal diagnosis of congenital heart diseases by ultrasound: experience from 20 European registries. Ultrasound Obstet Gynecol 2001;17:386.

148. Yates R. Fetal cardiac abnormalities and their association with aneuploidy. Prenat Diagn 1999;19:563.

149. Allan LD, Sharland GK, Milburn A, et al. Prospective diagnosis of 1006 consecutive cases of congenital heart disease in the fetus. J Am Coll Cardiol 1994;23:1452.

150. Manji S, Robertson JR, Wiktor A, et al. Prenatal diagnosis of 22q11.2 deletion when ultrasound examination reveals a heart defect. Genet Med 2001;3:65.

151. Moran CJ, Tay JB, Morrison JJ. Ultrasound detection and perinatal outcome of fetal trisomies 21, 18, and 14 in the absence of a routine fetal anomaly scan or biochemical screening. Ultrasound Obstet Gynecol 2002;20:482.

152. Hsu LYF. Prenatal diagnosis of chromosomal abnormalities through amniocentesis. In: Milunsky A, ed. Genetic disorders and the fetus: diagnosis, prevention, and treatment. 3rd ed. Baltimore: Johns Hopkins University Press, 1992:155.

153. Schwartz S, Palmer C. Chromosomal findings in 164 couples with repeated spontaneous abortions: with special consideration to prior reproductive history. Hum Genet 1983;62:28.

154. De Braekeleer M, Dao T-N. Cytogenetic studies in couples experiencing repeated pregnancy losses. Hum Reprod 1990;5:519.

155. Warburton D, Kline J, Stein Z, et al. Does the karyotype of a spontaneous abortion predict the karyotype of a subsequent abortion?: Evidence from 273 women with two karyotyped spontaneous abortions. Am J Hum Genet 1987;41:465.

156. Retief AE, VanZyl JA, Menkveld R, et al. Chromosome studies in 496 infertile males with a sperm count below 10 million/ml. Hum Genet 1984;66:162.
157. Bourrouillou G, Dastugue N, Columbies P. Chromosome studies in 952 infertile males with a sperm count below 10 million/ml. Hum Genet 1985;71:366.
158. Brook JD, Gosden RG, Chandley AC. Maternal ageing and aneuploid embryos: evidence from the mouse that biological and not chronological age is the important influence. Hum Genet 1984;66:41.
159. Reyes FI, Koh KS, Faiman C. Fertility in women with gonadal dysgenesis. Am J Obstet Gynecol 1976; 126:668.
160. King CR, Magenis E, Bennett S. Pregnancy and the Turner syndrome. Obstet Gynecol 1978;52:617.
161. Freeman SB, Yang Q, Allran K et al. Women with reduced ovarian complement may have an increased risk for a child with Down syndrome. Am J Hum Genet 2000;66:1680.
162. James RS, Ellis K, Pettay et al. Cytogenetic and molecular study of four couples with multiple trisomy 21 pregnancies. Eur J Hum Genet 1998;3:207.
163. Winsor EJT, Silver MP, Theve R, et al. Maternal cell contamination in uncultured amniotic fluid. Prenat Diagn 1996;16:49.
164. Gene Tests. http://www.genetests.org.
165. Gosden CM. Cell culture. In: Brock DJH, Rodeck CH, Ferguson-Smith MA (eds). Prenatal diagnosis and screening. London: Churchill Livingstone, 1992:85.
166. Kalousek DK. Pathogenesis of chromosomal mosaicism and its effect of early human development. Am J Med Genet 2000;91:39.
167. Kalousek DK, Dill FJ. Chromosomal mosaicism confined to the placenta in human conceptions. Science 1983;221:665.
168. Engel E. A new genetic concept: uniparental disomy and its potential effect, isodisomy. Am J Med Genet1980;6:137.
169. Kalousek DK, Barrett IJ, McGillvray BC. Placental mosaicism and intrauterine survival of trisomies 13 and 18. Am J Hum Genet 1989;44:338.
170. Moore GE, Ruangvutilert P, Chatzimmeletiou K, et al. Examination of trisomy 13, 18 and 21 foetal tissues at different gestational ages using FISH. Eur J Hum Genet 2000;8:223.
171. Schuring-Blom GH, Boer K, Leschot NJ. A placental diploid cell line is not essential for ongoing trisomy 13 or 18 pregnancies. Eur J Hum Genet 2001;9:286.
172. Lau AW, Brown CJ, Peñaherrera M, et al. Skewed X-chromosome inactivation is common in fetuses or newborns associated with confined placental mosaicism. Am J Hum Genet 1997;61:1353.
173. Jones, KL. Smith's recognizable patterns of human malformation, 5th edition. Philadelphia: Saunders, 1997.
174. Küster W, König A. Hypomelanosis of Ito: no entity but a cutaneous sign of mosaicism. Am J Med Genet 1999;85:346.
175. Boué J, Nicholas H, Barichard F, et al. Le clonage des cellules du liquide amniotique, aide dans l'interpretation des mosaiques chromosomiques en diagnostic prenatal. Ann Genet 1979;22:3.
176. Hook EB. Exclusion of chromosome mosaicism: tables of 90%, 95% and 99% confidence limits and comments on use. Am J Hum Genet 1977;29:94.
177. Claussen U, Schäfer H, Trampisch HJ. Exclusion of chromosomal mosaicism in prenatal diagnosis. Hum Genet 1984;67:23.
178. Sikkema-Raddatz B, Castedo S, Te Meerman GJ. Probability tables for exclusion of mosaicism in prenatal diagnosis. Prenat Diagn 1997;17:115–18.
179. Hsu LYF, Perlis T. United States survey on chromosome mosaicism and pseudomosaicism in prenatal diagnosis. Prenat Diagn (special issue) 1984;4:97.
180. Bui TH, Iselius L, Lindsten J. European collaborative study on prenatal diagnosis: mosaicism, pseudomosaicism and single abnormal cells in amniotic fluid cell cultures. Prenat Diagn (special issue) 1984;4:145.
181. Worton RG, Stern R. A Canadian collaborative study of mosaicism in amniotic fluid cell cultures. Prenat Diagn (special issue) 1984;4:131.
182. Hsu LYF, Kaffe S, Jenkins EC, et al. Proposed guidelines for diagnosis of chromosome mosaicism in amniocytes based on data derived from chromosome mosaicism and pseudomosaicism. Prenat Diagn 1992;12:555.
183. Wolstenholme J. Confined placental mosaicism for trisomies 2,3,7,8,16 and 22: their incidence, likely origins and mechanisms for cell lineage compartmentalisation. Prenat Diagn 1966;16:511.
184. Kalousek DK, Langlois S, Robinson WP, et al. Trisomy 7 CVS mosaicism: pregnancy outcome, placental and DNA analysis in 14 cases. Am J Med Genet 1996;65:348.

185. Kalousek DK Vekemens M. Confined placental mosaicism. J Med Genet 1996;33:529.

186. Stipoljev F, Latin V, Kos M, et al. Correlation of confined placental mosaicism with fetal intrauterine growth retardation. Fetal Diagn Ther 2001;16:4.

187. Wallerstein R, Yu M-T, Neu RL, et al. Common trisomy mosaicism diagnosed in amniocytes involving chromosomes 13,16,20 and 21: karyotype-phenotype correlations. Prenat Diagn 2000;20:103.

188. Hanna JS, Shires P, Matile G. Trisomy 1 in a clinically recognized pregnancy. Am J Med Genet 1997;68:98.

189. Neu RL, Kousseff BG, Madan S, et al. Monosomy, trisomy fragile sites and rearrangements of chromosome no. 1 in a mentally retarded male with multiple congenital anomalies. Clin Genet 1988;33:73.

190. Howard PJ, Cramp CE, Fryer AE. Trisomy 1 mosaicism only detected on a direct chromosome preparation in a neonate. Clin Genet 1995;48:313.

191. Wolstenholme J, White I, Strgiss S, et al. Maternal uniparental heterodisomy for chromosome 2: detection through "atypical" maternal AFP/hCG levels, with an update on a previous case. Prenat Diagn 2001;21:813.

192. Engel E, Antonarakis SE. Genomic imprinting and uniparental disomy in medicine: clinical and molecular aspects. New York: Wiley-Liss, 2002.

193. Bernasconi F, Karaguzel A, Celep F, et al. Normal phenotype with maternal isodisomy in a female with two isochromosomes: i(2p) and i(2q). Am J Hum Genet 1996;59:1114.

194. Heide E, Heide KG, Rodewald A. Maternal uniparental disomy (UPD) for chromosome 2 discovered by exclusion of paternity. Am J Med Genet 2000;92:260.

195. Hsu LYF, Yu M-T, Neu RL, et al. Rare trisomy mosaicism diagnosed in amniocytes, involving an autosome other than chromosomes 13, 18, 20, and 21: karyotype/phenotype correlations. Prenat Diagn 1997;17:210.

196. Sago H, Chen E, Conte WJ, et al. True trisomy 2 mosaicism in amniocytes and newborn liver associated with multiple system abnormalities. Am J Med Genet 1997;72:343.

196a. Zaslav A, Pierno G, Fougner A, et al. Prenatal diagnosis of trisomy 3 mosaicism. Am J Hum Genet 2003;73(Suppl):594.

197. Kuchinka BD, Barrett IJ, Moya G, et al. Two cases of confined placental mosaicism for chromosome 4, including one with maternal uniparental disomy. Prenat Diagn 2001;21:36.

198. Van Allen MI, Ritchie S, Toi A, et al. Trisomy 4 in a fetus with cyclopia and other anomalies. Am J Med Genet 1993;46:193.

199. Marion JP, Fernhoff PM, Jeffrey K, et al. Pre- and postnatal diagnosis of trisomy 4 mosaicism. Am J Med Genet 1990;37:362.

200. Zaslav A-L, Blumenthal D, Wilner JP, et al. Prenatal diagnosis of trisomy 4 mosaicism. Am J Med Genet 2000;95:318.

201. Ledbetter DH, Zachary JM, Simpson JL, et al. Cytogenetic results from the U.S. collaborative study on CVS. Prenat Diagn 1992;12:317.

202. Vejerslev LO, Mikkelsen M. The European collaborative study on mosaicism in chorionic villus sampling: data from 1986 to 1987. Prenat Diagn 1989;9:575.

203. Miller KR, Mühlhaus K, Herbst RA, et al. Patient with trisomy 6 mosaicism. Am J Med Genet 2001;100:103.

204. Wallerstein R, Oh T, Durcan J, et al. Outcome of prenatally diagnosed trisomy 6 mosaicism. Prenat Diagn 2002;22:722.

205. Monk D, Bentley L, Hitchins M, et al. Chromosome 7p disruption in Silver–Russell syndrome: delineating an imprinted candidate gene region. Hum Genet 2002;111:376.

206. Hannula K, Lipsanen-Nyman M, Kontiokari T, et al. A narrow segment of maternal uniparental disomy of chromosome 7q31-qter in Silver-Russell syndrome delimits a candidate gene region. Am J Hum Genet 2001;68:247.

206a. Riegel M, Baumer A, Schnizel A. No evidence of submicroscopic deletion or segmental uniparental disomy within the candidate regions of non-uniparental disomy Silver-Russell syndrome cases. Clin Genet 2003; 252:254.

207. Joyce CA, Sharp A, Walker JM, et al. Duplication of 7p12.1–p13 including GRB10 and IGFBP1, in a mother and daughter with features of Silver–Russell syndrome. Hum Genet 1999;105:273.

208. Sharp A, Moore G, Eggermann T. Evidence from skewed X inactivation for trisomy mosaicism in Silver–Russell syndrome. Eur J Hum Genet 2001;9:887.

208a. Beever CL, Peñaherrera MS, Langlois S, Robinson WR. X Chromosome inactivation patterns in Russell-Silver syndrome patients and their mothers. Am J Med Genet 2003;231:235.

209. Kivirikko S, Salonen R, Salo A, et al. Prenatally detected trisomy 7 mosaicism in a dysmorphic child. Prenat Diagn 2002;22:541.

210. Karadima G, Bugge M, Nicolaides P et al. Origin of nondisjunction in trisomy 8 and trisomy 8 mosaicism. Eur J Hum Genet 1988;6:432.

211. Robinson WP, Bernasconi F, Lau A, et al. Frequency of meiotic trisomy depends on involved chromosome and mode of ascertainment. Am J Med Genet 1999;84:34.

212. Van Haelst MM, van Oppstal D, Lindhout D, et al. Management of prenatal detected trisomy 8 mosaicism. Prenat Diagn 2001;21:1075.

213. Schneider M, Klein-Vogler U, Tomiuk J, et al. Pitfall: amniocentesis fails to detect mosaic trisomy 8 in male newborn. Prenat Diagn 1994;60:651.

214. Hanna JS, Neu RL, Barton JR. Difficulties in prenatal detection of mosaic trisomy 8. Prenat Diagn 1995;15:1196.

215. Southgate WM, Wagner CL, Heilds SM, et al. Mosaic trisomy 8: a cautionary note regarding missed antenatal diagnosis. J Perinatol 1998;18:78.

216. Van Den Berg C, Ramlakhan SK, van Opstal D, et al. Prenatal diagnosis of trisomy 9: cytogenetic, FISH and DNA studies. Prenat Diagn 1997;17:933.

216a. Chen C-P, Chern S-R, Town D-D, et al. Fetoplacental and fetoamniotic chromosomal discrepancies in prenatally detected mosaic trisomy 9. Prenat Diagn 2003;23:1019.

217. Knoblaunch H, Sommer D, Zimmer C, et al. Fetal trisomy 10 mosaicism: ultrasound, cytogenetic and morphologic findings in early pregnancy. Prenat Diagn 1999;19:379.

218. DeLozoier-Blanchet CD, Roeder E, Denis-Arrue R, et al. Trisomy 12 mosaicism confirmed in multiple organs from a liveborn child. Am J Med Genet 2000;95:444.

219. Brosens JJ, Overton C, Lavery SA, et al. Trisomy 12 mosaicism diagnosed by amniocentesis. Acta Obstet Gynecol Scand 1996;75:79.

220. Zaslav AL, Fallet S, Brown S, et al. Prenatal diagnosis of low level trisomy 15 mosaicism: review of literature. Clin Genet 1998;53:286.

220a. Yong PJ, Barrett IJ, Kalousek DK, et al. Clinical aspects, prenatal diagnosis, and pathogenesis of trisomy 16 mosiacism. J Med Genet 2003;175:182.

221. Hassold T, Merrill M, Adkins K, et al. Recombination and maternal age-dependent nondisjunction: molecular studies of trisomy 16. Am J Hum Genet 1995;57:867.

222. Yong PJ, Marion SA, Barrett IJ, et al. Evidence for imprinting on chromosome 16: the effect of uniparental disomy on the outcome of mosaic trisomy 16 pregnancies. Am J Med Genet 2002;112:123.

223. Peñaherrera MS, Barrett IJ, Brown CJ, et al. An association between skewed X-chromosome inactivation and abnormal outcome in mosaic trisomy 16 confined predominantly to the placenta. Clin Genet 2000;58:436.

224. Hsu W-T, Shchepin, Mao R, et al. Mosaic trisomy 16 ascertained through amniocentesis: evaluation of 11 new cases. Am J Med Genet 1998;80:473.

225. Hohler PM, Neiswanger K, Thomas L, et al. Variable outcomes in 5 cases of mosaic trisomy 16. Am J Hum Genet 2000;67:A148.

226. Benn PA, Collins R. Abnormal maternal serum inhibin-A levels in trisomy 16 mosaic pregnancies. Am J Hum Genet 1999;65:A172.

227. Djalali M, Barbi, G, Mueller-Navia J, et al. Further observations of true mosaic trisomy 17 ascertained in amniotic fluid cell cultures. Prenat Diagn 1998;18:1191–94.

228. Butler MG, Neu RL, Mitchell K. Trisomy 17 detected in amniotic fluid cells but not in newborn infant. Am J Med Genet 1996;65:247.

229. Butler MG. Trisomy 17 mosaicism in a four-year seven-month old white girl: follow up report. Prenat Diagn 1999;19:689.

230. Genuardi M, Tozzi C, Pomponi MG, et al. Mosaic trisomy 17 in amniocytes: phenotypic outcome, tissue distribution, and uniparental disomy studies. Eur J Hum Genet 1999;7:421.

231. Lesca G, Boggio D, Bellec V, et al. Trisomy 17 mosaicism in amniotic fluid cells not found at birth in blood but present in skin fibroblasts. Prenat Diagn 1999;19:263.

231a. Collado FK, Fisher AJ, Bombard AT. Counselling patients with trisomy 17 mosaicism found at genetic amniocentesis. Prenat Diagn 2003; 944–951.

232. Spinner NB, Rand E, Bucan M, et al. Paternal uniparental isodisomy for human chromosome 20 and absence of external ears. Am J Hum Genet 1994;55:A118.

233. Bastepe M, Lane AH, Juppner H. Paternal uniparental isodisomy of chromosome 20q—and the resulting changes in GNAS1 methylation—as a plausible cause of pseudohypoparathyroidism. Am J Hum Genet 2001;68:1283.

234. Salafsky IS, MacGregor SN, Claussen U, et al. Maternal UPD 20 in an infant from pregnancy with mosaic trisomy 20. Prenat Diagn 2001;21:860.

235. Velissariou V, Antoniadi T, Gyftodimou J, et al. Maternal uniparental isodisomy 20 in a foetus with trisomy 20 mosaicism: clinical, cytogenetic and molecular analysis. Eur J Hum Genet 2002;20:694.

236. Hsu LYF, Kaffe S, Perlis TE. Trisomy 20 mosaicism in prenatal diagnosis: a review and update. Prenat Diagn 1987;7:581.

237. Hsu LYF, Kaffe S, Perlis TE. A revisit of trisomy 20 mosaicism in prenatal diagnosis: an overview of 103 cases. Prenat Diagn 1991;11:7.

238. Hsu LYF. Prenatal diagnosis of chromosomal abnormalities through amniocentesis. In: Milunsky A, ed. Genetic disorders and the fetus: diagnosis, prevention, and treatment, 4th ed. Baltimore: Johns Hopkins University Press, 1998:179.

239. Baty BJ, Olson SB, Magenis RE, et al. Trisomy 20 mosaicism in two unrelated girls with skin hypopigmentation and normal intellectual development. Am J Med Genet 2001;99:210.

240. Warren NS, Soukup S, King JL, et al. Prenatal diagnosis of trisomy 20 by chorionic villus sampling (CVS): a case report with long term outcome. Prenat Diagn 2001;21:1111.

241. Miny P, Karabacak Z, Hammer P, et al. Chromosome analyses from urinary sediment: postnatal confirmation of a prenatally diagnosed trisomy 20 mosaicism. N Engl J Med 1989;320:809.

242. Reish O, Wolach B, Ameil A, et al. Dilemma of trisomy 20 mosaicism detected prenatally: is it an innocent finding? Am J Med Genet 1998;77:71.

243. Crowe CA, Schwartz S, Black CJ, et al. Mosaic trisomy 22: a case presentation and literature review of trisomy 22 phenotypes. Am J Med Genet 1997;71:406.

243a. Tinkle BT, Walker ME, Blough-Pfau RI, et al. Unexpected survival in a case of prenatally diagnosed nonmosaic trisomy22: clinical report and review of the natural history. Am J Med Genet 2003;90:95.

244. Berghella V, Wapner RJ, Yang-Feng T, Mahoney MJ. Prenatal confirmation of true fetal trisomy 22 mosaicism by fetal skin biopsy following normal fetal blood sampling. Prenat Diagn 1998;18:384.

245. Van Ravenswaaij-Arts CMA, Tuerlings JHAM, Van Heyst AFJ, et al. Misinterpretation of trisomy 18 as a pseudomosaicism at third-trimester amniocentesis of a child with a mosaic 46,XY/47,XY+3/ 48,XXY,+18 karyotype. Prenat Diagn 1997;17:375.

246. Wieczorek D, Prott EC, Robinson WP, et al. Prenatally detected trisomy 2 and 6 mosaicism: cytogenetic results and clinical phenotype. Prenat Diagn 2003;23:128.

247. Bartels I, Franke U, Braukle I, et al. Normal outcome of a pregnancy with mosaicism for double trisomy in amniotic fluid cells. Prenat Diagn 1997;17:877.

248. Mascarello JT, Jones MC, Catanzarite VA et al. Mosaic triple trisomy in amniocytes from a phenotypically normal fetus. Prenat Diagn 1994;14:163.

249. Kajii T, Kawai T, Takumi T, et al. Mosaic variegated aneuploidy with multiple congenital abnormalities: homozygosity for total premature chromatid separation trait. Am J Med Genet 1998;78:245.

249a. Plaja A, Mediano C, Cano L, et al. Prenatal diagnosis of a rare chromosomal instability syndrome: variegated aneuploidy related to premature centromere division (PCD). Am J Med Genet 2003;85:86.

250. Hsu LYF, Yu MT, Richkind KE, et al. Incidence and significance of chromosome mosaicism involving an autosomal structural abnormality diagnosed prenatally through amniocentesis: a collaborative study. Prenat Diagn 1996;16:1.

251. Chen C-P. Detection of mosaic isochromosome 20q in amniotic fluid in a pregnancy with fetal arthrogryposis multiplex congenita and normal karyotype in fetal blood and postnatal samples of placenta, skin, and liver. Prenat Diagn 2003;23:80.

252. Pfeiffer RA, Ulmer R, Rauch A, et al. True fetal mosaicism of an isochromosome of the long arm of a chromosome 20: the dilemma persists. Prenat Diagn 1997;17:1171.

253. Sutherland GR, Baker E. The clinical significance of fragile sites on human chromosomes. Clin Genet 2000;58:157.

254. Zaslav AL, Fox JE, Jacob et al. Significance of a prenatally diagnosed del(10)(q23). Am J Med Genet 2002;107:174.

255. Jones C, Penny L, Mattina T, et al. Association of a chromosome deletion syndrome with a fragile site within the proto-oncogene CBL2. Nature 1995;7:553–56.

256. Robinson A, Bender BG, Linden MG. Prenatal diagnosis of sex chromosome abnormalities. In: Milunsky A, ed. Genetic disorders and the fetus, 3rd ed. Baltimore: Johns Hopkins University Press, 1992:211.

257. Koeberl DD, McGillivray B, Sybert VP. Prenatal diagnosis of 45,X/46,XX mosaicism and 45,X: implications for postnatal outcome. Am J Hum Genet 1995;57:661.

258. Hsu LYF. Phenotype/karyotype correlations of Y chromosome aneuploidy with emphasis on structural aberrations in postnatally diagnosed cases. Am J Med Genet 1994;53:108.

259. Hsu LYF. Prenatal Diagnosis of 45,X/46,XY mosaicism: A review and update. Prenat Diagn 1989;9:31.

259a. Huang B, Thangavelu M, Bhatt S, et al. Prenatal diagnosis of 45,X and 45.X mosaicism: the need for thorough cytogenetic and clinical evaluations. Prenat Diagn 2002;22:105.

260. Devi AS, Metzger DA, Luciano AA, Benn PA. 45,X/46,XX mosaicism in patients with idiopathic premature ovarian failure. Fertil Steril 1998;70:89.

261. Kushnick T, Irons TG, Wiley JE, et al. 45X/46X,r(X) with syndactyly and severe mental retardation. Am Med Genet 1987;28:567.

262. Grompe M, Rao N, Elder FF, et al. 45,X/46,X,+r(X) can have a distinct phenotype different from Ullrich–Turner syndrome. Am J Hum Genet 1992;42:39.

263. Van Dyke DL, Wiktor A, Palmer CG, et al. Ullrich–Turner syndrome with a small ring X chromosome and presence of mental retardation. Am J Hum Genet 1992;43:996.

264. Le Caignec C, Boceno M, Joubert M, et al. Prenatal diagnosis of a small supernumerary, XIST-negative mosaic ring X chromosome identified by fluorescence in situ hybridization in an abnormal male fetus. Prenat Diagn 2003;23:143.

265. Migeon BR, Luo S, Jani M, Jeppsen P. The severe phenotype of females with tiny ring X chromosomes is associated with inability of these chromosomes to undergo X inactivation. Am J Hum Genet 1994;55:497.

266. Wolff DJ, Brown CJ, Schwartz S, et al. Small marker X chromosomes lack the X inactivation center: implications for karyotype/phenotype correlations. Am J Hum Genet 1994;55:87.

267. Yorifuji T, Muroi J, Kawai M, et al. Uniparental and functional X disomy in Turner syndrome patients with unexplained mental retardation and X derived marker chromosomes. J Med Genet 1998;35:539.

268. Muller U, Weber JL, Berry P, Kupke KG. Second polar body incorporation in to a blastomere results in 46,XX/69,XXX diploid-triploid mixoploidy. J Med Genet 1993;30:597.

268a. Daniel A, Wu Z, Darmanian A, Collins F, et al. Three different origins for apparent triploid and diploid mosaics. Prenat Diagn 2003;529:534.

269. Van de Laar I, Rabelink G, Hochstenbach R, et al. Diploid/ triploid mosaicism in dysmorphic patients. Clin Genet 2002;62:376.

269a. Flori E, Doray B, Rudolf G, et al. Failure of prenatal diagnosis of diploid triploid mosaicism after amniocentesis. Clin Genet 2003;328:331.

270. Wullich B, Henn W, Groterath E, et al. Mosaic tetraploidy in a liveborn infant with features of the DiGeorge anomaly. Clin Genet 1991;40:353.

271. Veenema H, Tasseron EWK, Geraedts JPM. Mosaic tetraploidy in a male neonate. Clin Genet 1982;22:295.

272. Quiroz E, Orozco A, Salamanca F. Diploid-tetraploid mosaicism in a malformed boy. Clin Genet 1985;27:183.

273. Aughton DJ, Saal HM, Delach JA, et al. Diploid/tetraploid mosaicism in a liveborn infant demonstrable only in the bone marrow: case report and literature review. Clin Genet 1988;33:299.

274. López Pajares I, Delicado A, Diaz de Bustamante A, et al. Tetraploidy in a liveborn infant. J Med Genet 1990;27:782.

275. Edwards MJ, Park JP, Wurster-Hill DH, et al. Mixoploidy in humans: two surviving cases of diploid-tetraploid mixoploidy and comparison with diploid-triploid mixoploidy. Am J Med Genet 1994;52:324.

276. Coe SJ, Kapur R, Luthardt F, et al. Prenatal diagnosis of tetraploidy: a case report. Am J Med Genet 1993;45:378.

277. Goyert GL, Charfoos DA, Ward BE, et al. Prenatal identification of a tetraploid fetus using FISH. Am J Hum Genet 1993;53(Suppl):abstract 1414.

278. Teyssier M, Gaucherand P, Buenerd A. Prenatal diagnosis of a tetraploid fetus. Prenat Diagn 1997;17:474.

279. Milunsky A. The prenatal diagnosis of chromosomal disorders. In: Milunsky A, ed. Genetic disorders and the fetus. New York: Plenum Press, 1979:93.

280. Hsu LYF, Benn PA. Revised guidelines for the diagnosis of mosaicism in amniocytes. Prenat Diagn 1999;19:1081.

281. Wenger SL, Steele MW, Boone LY, et al. "Balanced" karyotypes in six abnormal offspring of balanced reciprocal translocation normal carrier parents. Am J Med Genet 1995;55:47.

282. Horsthemke B, Maat-Kievit A, Leegers E, et al. Familial translocations involving 15q11–q13 can give rise to interstitial deletions causing Prader–Willi or Angelman syndrome. J Med Genet 1996;33:848.

283. Tommerup N, Brandt CA, Pedersen S, et al. Sex dependent transmission of Beckwith–Wiedemann syndrome associated with a reciprocal translocation t(9;11)(p11.2;p15.5). J Med Genet 1993;30:958.

284. Tommerup N. Mendelian cytogenetics. Chromosome rearrangements associated with Mendelian disorders. J Med Genet 1993;30:713.

285. Schmidt M, Du Sart D. Functional disomies of the X chromosome influence the cell selection and hence the X inactivation pattern in females with balanced X-autosome translocations: a review of 122 cases. Am J Med Genet 1992;42:161.

286. Elejalde BR, de Elejalde MM. Phenotypic manifestation of X-autosome translocations. In: Sandberg AA, ed. Cytogenetics of the mammalian X chromosome, part B. New York: Alan R. Liss, 1983:225.

287. Madan K, Hompes PGA, Schoemaker J, et al. X-autosome translocation with a breakpoint in Xq22 in a fertile woman and her 47,XXX infertile daughter. Hum Genet 1981;59:290.

288. Devi A, Benn PA. X-chromosome abnormalities in women with premature ovarian failure. J Reprod Med 1999;44:321.

289. Jacobs PA. Correlation between euploid structural chromosome rearrangements and mental subnormality in humans. Nature 1974;249:164.

290. Warburton D. De novo structural rearrangements: implications for prenatal diagnosis. In: Willey AM, Carter TP, Kelly S, et al., eds. Clinical genetics: problems in diagnosis and counseling. New York: Academic Press, 1982:63.

291. Warburton D. Outcome of cases of de novo structural rearrangements diagnosed at amniocentesis. Prenat Diagn (special issue) 1984;4:69.

292. Hook EB, Cross PK. Extra structurally abnormal chromosomes (ESAC) detected at amniocentesis: frequency in approximately 75,000 prenatal cytogenetic diagnoses and association with maternal and paternal age. Am J Hum Genet 1987;40:83.

293. Wassman ER, Cheyovich DL, Nakahara Y. "Possibly" de novo translocations: prenatal risk counseling. Am J Obstet Gynecol 1989;161:698.

294. Funderburk SJ, Spence MA, Sparkes RS. Mental retardation associated with "balanced" chromosome rearrangements. Am J Hum Genet 1977;29:136.

295. Tharapel AV, Summit RL, Wilroy RS, et al. Apparently balanced de novo translocations in patients with abnormal phenotypes: report of 6 cases. Clin Genet 1977;11:255.

296. MacGregor DJ, Imrie S, Tolmie JL. Outcome of de novo balanced translocations ascertained prenatally. J Med Genet 1989;26:590.

297. Nielsen J, Krag-Olsen B. Follow-up of 32 children with autosomal translocations found among 11,148 consecutively newborn children from 1964–1974. Clin Genet 1981;20:48.

298. Tierney I, Axworthy D, Smith L, et al. Balanced rearrangements of the autosomes: results of a longitudinal study of a newborn survey population. J Med Genet 1984;21:45.

299. Ishikiriyama S, Goto M. Blepharophimosis sequence (BPES) and microcephaly in a girl with del(3)(q22.2q23): a putative gene responsible for microcephaly close to the BPES gene? Am J Med Genet 1993;47:487.

300. Therman E, Laxova R, Susman B. The critical region on the human Xq. Hum Genet 1990;85:455.

301. Waters JJ, Campbell PL, Crocker AJM, et al. Phenotypic effects of balanced X-autosome translocations in females: a retrospective survey of 104 cases reported from UK laboratories. Hum Genet 2001;108:318.

302. Schinzel A. Catalogue of unbalanced chromosome aberrations in man, 2nd ed. Berlin: Walter de Gruyter, 2001.

302a. National Genetics Laboratory, Wessex. Chromosome anomaly register. www.ngrl.co.uk/wessex/register.htm

303. Sachs ES, Van Hemel JO, Den Hollander JC, et al. Marker chromosomes in a series of 10,000 prenatal diagnoses, cytogenetic and follow-up studies. Prenat Diagn 1987;7:81.

304. Blennow E, The-Hung B, Kristoffersson U, et al. Swedish survey on extra structurally abnormal chromosomes in 39105 consecutive prenatal diagnoses: prevalence and characterization by fluorescence in situ hybridization. Prenat Diagn 1994;14:1019.

305. Brondum-Nielsen K, Mikkelsen M. A 10-year survey, 1980–1990, of prenatally diagnosed small supernumerary marker chromosomes, identified by FISH analysis: outcome and follow-up of 14 cases diagnosed in a series of 12699 prenatal samples. Prenat Diagn 1995;15:615.

306. Jacobs PA. Mutation rates of structural chromosome rearrangements in man. Am J Hum Genet 1981;33:44.

307. Steinbach P, Djalali M, Hansmann I, et al. The genetic significance of accessory bisatellited marker chromosomes. Hum Genet 1983;65:155.

308. Kaffe S, Hsu LYF. Supernumerary marker chromosomes in a series of 19000 prenatal diagnoses: pregnancy outcome of satellited vs. non-satellited de novo markers. Am J Hum Genet 1988;43:A237.

309. Djalali M. The significance of accessory bisatellited marker chromosomes in amniotic fluid cell cultures. Ann Genet 1990;33:141.

309a. Heng HHQ, Ye CJ, Fang F, et al. Analysis of marker or complex chromosomal rearrangements present in pre- and post-natal karyotypes utilizing a combination of G-banding, spectral karyotyping and flourescence in situ hybridization. Clin Genet 2003;358:367.

310. Buckton KE, Spowart G, Newton MS, et al. Forty four probands with an additional "marker" G chromosome. Hum Genet 1985;69:353.

311. Robinson WP, Binkert F, Gine R, et al. Clinical and molecular analysis of five inv dup(15) patients. Eur J Hum Genet 1993;1:37.

312. Leana-Cox J, Jenkins L, Palmer CG, et al. Molecular cytogenetic analysis of inv dup(15) chromosomes, using probes specific for the Prader–Willi/Angelman syndrome region: clinical implications. Am J Hum Genet 1994;54:748.

313. Crolla JA, Harvey JF, Sitch FL, et al. Supernumerary marker 15 chromosomes: a clinical, molecular and FISH approach to diagnosis and prognosis. Hum Genet 1995;95:161.

314. Huang B, Crolla JA, Christian SL, et al. Refined molecular characterization of the breakpoints in small inv dup(15) chromosomes. Hum Genet 1997;99:11.

315. Crolla JA, Howard P, Mitchell C, et al. A molecular and FISH approach to determining karyotype and phenotype correlations in six patients with supernumerary marker (22) chromosomes. Am J Med Genet 1997;72:440.

316. McDermid HE, Duncan AMV, Brasch KR, et al. Characterization of the supernumerary chromosome in cat eye syndrome. Science 1986;232:646.

317. Mears AJ, Duncan AMV, Budarf ML, et al. Molecular characterization of the marker chromosome associated with cat eye syndrome. Am J Hum Genet 1994;55:134.

318. Mears AJ, El Shanti H, Murray JC, et al. Minute supernumerary ring chromosome 22 associated with cat eye syndrome: further delineation of the critical region. Am J Hum Genet 1995;57:667.

319. Schinzel A. Tetrasomy 12p (Pallister–Killian syndrome). J Med Genet 1991;28:122.

320. Doray B, Girard-Lemaire F, Gasser B, et al. Pallister–Killian syndrome: difficulties of prenatal diagnosis. Prenat Diagn 2002;22:470.

321. Callen DF, Freemantle CJ, Ringenbergs ML, et al. The isochromosome 18p syndrome: confirmation of cytogenetic diagnosis in nine cases by in situ hybridization. Am J Hum Genet 1990;47:493.

322. Schaefer GB, Domek DB, Morgan MA, et al. Tetrasomy of the short arm of chromosome 9: prenatal diagnosis and delineation of the phenotype. Am J Med Genet 1991;38:612.

323. Crolla JA, Long F, Rivera H, et al. FISH and molecular study of autosomal supernumerary marker chromosomes excluding those derived from chromosomes 15 and 22. I. Results of 26 new cases. Am J Med Genet 1998;75:355.

324. Crolla JA. FISH and molecular studies of autosomal supernumerary marker chromosomes excluding those derived from chromosome 15. II. Review of the literature. Am J Med Genet 1998;75:367.

325. Hastings RJ, Nisbet DL, Waters K, et al. Prenatal detection of extra structurally abnormal chromosomes (ESACs): new cases and a review of the literature. Prenat Diagn 1999;19:436.

326. Stankiewicz P, Bocian E, Jakubow-Durska K, et al. Identification of supernumerary marker chromosomes derived from chromosomes 5, 6, 19, and 20 using FISH. J Med Genet 2000;37:114.

327. Kotzot D. Review and meta-analysis of systematic searches for uniparental disomy (UPD) other than UPD 15. Am J Med Genet 2002;111:366.

328. Han J-Y, Choo KHA, Shaffer LG. Molecular cytogenetic characterization of 17 rob(13q14q) Robertsonian translocations by FISH, narrowing the region containing the breakpoints. Am J Hum Genet 1994;55:960.

329. Corviello DA, Panucci E, Mantero MM, et al. Maternal uniparental disomy for chromosome 14. Am J Hum Genet 1995;57:A111.

330. Page SL, Shaffer LG. Nonhomologous Robertsonian translocations form predominantly during female meiosis. Nat Genet 1997;15:231.

331. Harrison KJ, Allingham-Hawkins DJ, Hummel J, et al. Risk of uniparental disomy in Robersonian translocations carriers: identification of UPD14 in a small cohort. Am J Hum Genet 1998;63:A11.

332. Papenhausen PR, Tepperberg JH, Mowrey PN, et al. UPD risk assessment: three cytogenetic subgroups. Am J Hum Genet 1999;65:A353.

333. Exeler JR, Meschede D, Lemmens M, et al. Low prevalence of uniparental disomy in association with prenatally diagnosed balanced Robertsonian translocations. Cytogenet Cell Genet 1999;85:148.

334. Eggermann T, Wolf M, Spaich C, et al. Search for uniparental disomy 14 in balanced Robertsonian translocation carriers. Clin Genet 1999;56:464.

335. Trabanelli C, Gualandi F, Ravani A, et al. UPD risk in prenatally identified Robertsonian translocations: a collaborative study. Eur J Hum Genet 2000;8(suppl):297.

336. Pereira CR, Kennedy DL, Mak-Tam E, et al. Uniparental disomy testing in a clinical setting. Am J Hum Genet 2000;67:1927.

337. Berend SA, Horwitz J, McCaskill C, et al. Identification of uniparental disomy following prenatal detection of Robertsonian translocations and isochromosomes. Am J Hum Genet 2000;66:1787.

338. Jay AM, Roberts E, Davies T, et al. Prenatal testing for uniparental disomy. Prenat Diagn 2001;21:512.

339. Silverstein S, Lerer I, Sagi M, et al. Uniparental disomy in fetuses diagnosed with balanced Robertsonian translocations: risk estimate. Prenat Diagn 2002;22:649.

340. Kotzot D. Complex and segmental uniparental disomy (UPD): review and lessons from rare chromosome complements. J Med Genet 2001;38:497.

341. Robinson WP, Wagstaff J, Bernasconi F, et al. Uniparental disomy explains the occurrence of the Angelman or Prader–Willi syndrome in patients with an additional small inv dup(15) chromosome. J Med Genet 1993;30:756.

342. Cotter PD, Ledesma CT, Dietz LG, et al. Prenatal diagnosis of supernumerary marker 15 chromosomes and exclusion of uniparental disomy for chromosome 15. Prenat Diagn 1999;19:726.

343. Christian SL, Mills P, Das S, et al. High risk uniparental disomy 15 associated with amniotic fluid containing de novo small supernumerary marker 15 chromosomes. Am J Hum Genet 1998;63:A11.

344. McKenzie WH, Lubs HA. Human Q&C chromosomal variations: distribution and incidence. Cytogenet Cell Genet 1975;14:97.

345. Hsu LYF, Benn PA, Tannenbaum HL, et al. Chromosome polymorphisms of 1, 9, 16, and Y in four major ethnic groups: a large prenatal study. Am J Med Genet 1987;26:95.

346. Madan K. An extra band in human 9qh+ chromosomes. Hum Genet 1978;43:259.

347. Docherty Z, Hultén MA. Extra euchromatic band in the qh region of chromosome 9. J Med Genet 1985;22:156.

348. Reddy KS. Variants of chromosome 9 with additional euchromatic bands: two case reports. Am J Med Genet 1996;64:536.

349. Roland B, Chernos JE, Cox DM. 9qh+ variant band in two families. Am J Med Genet 1992;42:137.

350. Hoo JJ. A new chromosome 9 variant: an extra band within the 9qh region. Clin Genet 1992;41:157.

351. Docherty Z, Hultén MA. Rare variant of chromosome 9. Am J Med Genet 1993;45:105.

352. Knight LA, Soon GM, Tan M. Extra G positive band on the long arm of chromosome 9. J Med Genet 1993;30:613.

353. Verma RS, Luke S, Brennan JP, et al. Molecular topography of the secondary constriction region (qh) of human chromosome 9 with an unusual euchromatic band. Am J Hum Genet 1993;52:981.

353a. Starke H, Siedel J, Henn W, et al. Homologous sequences at human chromosome 9 bands p12 and q13–21.1 are involved in different patterns of pericentric rearrangements. Eur J Hum Genet 2002;790:800.

354. Shapiro LR, Petterson RO, Wilmot PL, et al. Pericentric inversion of the Y chromosome and prenatal diagnosis. Prenat Diagn 1984;4:463.

355. Schmid M, Haaf T, Solleder E, et al. Satellited Y chromosomes: structure, origin, and clinical significance. Hum Genet 1984;67:72.

356. Wachtler F, Musil R. On the structure and polymorphism of the human chromosome no. 15. Hum Genet 1980;56:115.

357. Chen TR, Kao ML, Marks J, et al. Polymorphic variants in human chromosome 15. Am J Med Genet 1981;9:61.

358. Babu A, Macera MJ, Verma RS. Intensity heteromorphisms of human chromosome 15p by DA/DAPI technique. Hum Genet 1986;73:298.

359. Delach JA, Rosengren SS, Kaplan L, et al. Comparison of high resolution chromosome banding and fluorescence in situ hybridization (FISH) for the laboratory evaluation of Prader–Willi syndrome and Angelman syndrome. Am J Med Genet 1994;52:85.

360. Schmid M, Schmidtke J, Kruse K, et al. Characterization of a Y/15 translocation by banding methods, distamycin A, treatment of lymphocytes and DNA restriction endonuclease analysis. Clin Genet 1983;24:234.

361. Petrovic V. A new variant of chromosome 3 with unusual staining properties. J Med Genet 1988;25:781.

362. Bardhan S, Singh DN, Davis K. Polymorphism in chromosome 4. Clin Genet 1981;20:44.

363. Docherty Z, Bowser-Riley SM. A rare heterochromatic variant of chromosome 4. J Med Genet 1984;21:470.

364. Seabright M, Gregson NM, Johnson M. A familiar polymorphic variant of chromosome 5. J Med Genet 1980;17:444.

365. Fineman RM, Issa B, Weinblatt V. Prenatal diagnosis of a large heteromorphic region in a chromosome 5: implications for genetic counseling. Am J Med Genet 1989;32:498.

366. Madan K, Bruinsma AH. C-band polymorphism in human chromosome no. 6. Clin Genet 1979;15:193.

367. Thompson PW, Roberts SH. A new variant of chromosome 16. Hum Genet 1987;76:100.

368. Pinel I, Diaz de Bustammante A, Urioste M, et al. An unusual variant of chromosome 16. Hum Genet 1988;80:194.

369. Bryke CR, Breg WR, Potluri VR, et al. Duplication of euchromatin without phenotypic effects: a variant of chromosome 16. Am J Med Genet 1990;36:43.

370. Jahal SM, Schneider NR, Kukolich MK, et al. Euchromatic 16p+ heteromorphism: first report in North America. Am J Med 1990;37:548.

371. Croci G, Camurri L, Franchi F. A familial case of chromosome 16p variant. J Med Genet 1991;28:60.
372. Thompson PW, Roberts SH, Rees SM. Replication studies in the 16p+ variant. Hum Genet 1990;84:371.
373. Kubien E, Kieczkowska A. Familial occurrence of chromosome variant 17ph+. Clin Genet 1977;12:39.
374. Hoo JJ, Robertson A. 18ph+ is a normal chromosomal variant. Clin Genet 1987;32:79.
375. Verma RS, Agarwal AK, Madahar CJ, et al. Tandemly repeated DNA sequences of centromere resulting in 18p+. Prenat Diagn 1989;9:863.
376. Pittalis MC, Santarini L, Bovicelli L. Prenatal diagnosis of a heterochromatic 18p+ heteromorphism. Prenat Diagn 1994;14:72.
377. Zelante L, Notarangelo A, Dallapiccola B. The 18ph+ chromosome heteromorphism. Prenat Diagn 1994;14:1096.
378. Fryns JP, Kleczkowska A, Smeets E, et al. A new centromeric heteromorphism in the short arm of chromosome 20. J Med Genet 1988;25:636.
379. Park JP, Rawnsley BE. Prenatal detection of chromosome 20 variants (20ph+,20ps). Prenat Diagn 1996;16:771.
380. Crossen PE. Variation in the centromeric banding of chromosome 19. Clin Genet 1975;8:218.
381. Friedrich U. Centromere heteromorphism in chromosome 19. Clin Genet 1985;28:358.
382. Alessandro ED, DeMatteis Vaccarella C, LoRe ML, et al. Pericentric inversion of chromosome 19 in three families. Hum Genet 1988;80:203.
383. MacDonald IM, Cox DM. Inversion of chromosome 2 (p11q13): Frequency and implications for genetic counseling. Hum Genet 1985;69:281.
384. Kleczkowska A, Fryns JP, Van den Berghe H. Pericentric inversions in man: personal experience and review of the literature. Hum Genet 1987;75:333.
385. Vargas-Moyeda E, Rivera H, Garcia-Cruz D, et al. Inv(5)(p13q13) in a four generation pedigree. J Genet Hum 1987;35:305.
386. Habibian R, Hajianpour MJ, Shaffer LG, et al. Genotype-phenotype correlation in satellited 1p chromosome: importance of fluorescence in situ hybridization (FISH) applications. Am J Hum Genet 1994;55:A106.
387. Elliott J, Barnes ICS. A satellited chromosome 2 detected at prenatal diagnosis. J Med Genet 1992;29:213.
388. Lamb AN, Pettenati M, Hanna J, et al. Six cases of satellited long arm of chromosome 2 detected during prenatal chromosome diagnosis. Am J Hum Genet 1995;57:A282.
389. Arn PH, Younie L, Russo L, et al. Reproductive outcome in 3 families with a satellited chromosome 4 with review of literature. Am J Med Genet 1995;57:420.
390. Babu VR, Roberson JR, Van Dyke DL, et al. Interstitial deletion of 4q35 in a familial satellited 4q in a child with developmental delay. Am J Hum Genet 1987;41:A113.
391. Mihelick K, Jackson-Cook C, Hays P, et al. Craniorachischisis in a fetus with familial satellited 4q. Am J Hum Genet 1984;36:105A.
392. Miller I, Songster G, Fontana S, et al. Satellited 4q identified in amniotic fluid cells. Am J Hum Genet 1995;55:237.
393. Shah HO, Verma RS, Conte RA, et al. Fishing for origin of satellite on the long arm of chromosome 4. Am J Hum Genet 1997;61:A375.
394. Dev VG, Byrne J, Bunch G. Partial translocation of NOR and its activity in a balanced carrier and in her cri-du-chat fetus. Hum Genet 1979;51:277.
395. Faivre L, Morichon-Delvallez N, Viot G, et al. Prenatal diagnosis of a satellited non-acrocentric chromosome derived from a maternal translocation (10;13)(p13;p12) and review of the literature. Prenat Diagn 1999;19:282.
396. O'Malley DP, Diehn T, Bullard B, et al. Satellited chromosome 10 detected prenatally in fetus and mosaic in a parent. Am J Hum Genet 1997;65:A159.
397. Willatt L, Green AJ, Trump D. Satellites on the terminal short arm of chromosome 12 (12ps), inherited through several generations in three families: a new variant without phenotypic effect. J Med Genet 2001;38:723.
398. Killos LD, Lese CM, Mills PL, et al. A satellited 17p with telomere deleted and no apparent clinical consequence. Am J Hum Genet 1997;61:A130.
399. Stetten G, Sroka B, Schmidt M, et al. Translocation of the nucleolus organizer region to the human X-chromosome. Am J Hum Genet 1986;39:245.
400. Chen C-P, Devriendt K, Chern S-R, et al. Prenatal diagnosis of inherited satellited non-acrocentric chromosomes. Prenat Diagn 2000;20:384.
401. Gutternbach M, Haaf T, Steinlein C, et al. Ectopic NORs on human chromosomes 5qter and 8q11: rare chromosomal variants detected in two families. J Med Genet 1999;36:339.

402. Watt JL, Couzin DA, Lloyd DJ, et al. A familial insertion involving an active nucleolar organizer within chromosome 12. J Med Genet 1984;21:379.

403. Prieto F, Badia L, Beneyto M, et al. Nucleolus organizer regions (NORs) inserted in 6q15. Hum Genet 1989;81:289.

404. Park VM, Gustashaw KM, Wather TM. The presence of interstitial telomeric sequences in constitutional chromosome abnormalities. Am J Hum Genet 1992;50:914.

405. Norris FM, Mercer B, Pertile MD. Interstitial insertion of NORs into Yq and 22q: two case studies. Bull Hum Genet Soc Australas 1995;8:48.

406. Gutternbach M, Nassar N, Feichtinger W, et al. An interstitial nucleolus organizer region in the long arm of chromosome 7: cytogenetic characterization and familial segregation. Cytogenet Cell Genet 1998;80:104.

407. Benn PA, Hsu LYF. Maternal cell contamination of amniotic fluid cell cultures: results of a U.S. nation-wide survey. Am J Med Genet 1983;15:297.

408. Benn PA, Gilbert F, Hsu LYF. Maternal cell contamination of amniotic fluid cultures from two consecutive pregnancies complicated by fibroids. Prenat Diagn 1984;4:151.

409. Freiberg AS, Blumberg B, Lawce H, et al. XX/XY chimerism encountered during prenatal diagnosis. Prenat Diagn 1988;8:423.

410. Yaron Y, Feldman B, Kramer RL, et al. Prenatal diagnosis of 46,XY/46,XX mosaicism: a case report. Am J Med Genet 1999;84:12.

411. Craig I, Ross M, Edwards JH, et al. Detecting maternal cell contamination in prenatal diagnosis. Lancet 1989;1:1074.

412. Rebello MT, Abas A, Nicolaides K, et al. Maternal contamination of amniotic fluid demonstrated by DNA analysis. Prenat Diagn 1994;14:109.

413. Smith GW, Graham CA, Nevin J, et al. Detection of maternal cell contamination in amniotic fluid cell cultures using fluorescent labelled microsatellites. J Med Genet 1995;32:61.

414. Martin JA, Park MM. Trends in twin and triplet births, 1980–97. National Vital Statistics Reports 1999;47:1.

415. Egan JFX. Personal communication, 2003.

416. MacGillivray I, Nylander POS, Corney G, et al. Human multiple reproduction. London: WB Saunders, 1975.

417. Golbus MS, Cunningham N, Goldberg JD, et al. Selective termination of multiple gestations. Am J Med Genet 1988;31:339.

418. Appelman Z, Caspi B. Chorionic villus sampling and selective termination of a chromosomally abnormal fetus in a triplet pregnancy. Prenat Diagn 1992;12:215.

419. Berkowitz R. Selective termination of an abnormal fetus in multiple gestations. Prenat Diagn 1995; 15:1085.

419a. Evans MI, Goldberg JD, Horenstein J, et al. Selective termination for structural, chromosomal, and Mendelian anomalies: international experience. Am J Obstet Gynecol 1999;181:893.

420. McGarrity GJ. Mycoplasmal infection of cell cultures. Passing (Bulletin of Coriell Institute for Medical Research), 1987;1:5.

421. Schneider EL, Stanbridge EJ. Mycoplasma contamination of cultured amniotic fluid cells: potential hazard to prenatal chromosome diagnosis. Science 1975;184:477.

422. Garver KL, Marchese SL, Boas EG. Amniotic fluid culture failure: possible role of syringe. N Engl J Med 1976;295:286.

423. BD Medical Systems. Current information regarding BDTM syringes and amniocentesis. 2003. http: www.bd.com/injections/amnio.

424. Persutte WH, Lenke RP. Failure of amniotic-fluid-cell growth: is it related to fetal aneuploidy? Lancet 1995;345:96.

425. Reid R, Sepulveda W, Kyle PM, et al. Amniotic fluid culture failure: clinical significance and association with aneuploidy. Obstet Gynecol 2996;87:588–592.

426. Sundberg K, Jorgensen FS, Tabor A, et al. Experience with early amniocentesis. J Perinat Med 1995; 23:149.

427. Lam YH, Tang MHY, Sin SY, et al. Clinical significance of amniotic-fluid-cell culture failure. Prenat Diagn 1998;18:343.

428. Hamerton JL, Boué A, Cohen MM, et al. Chromosome disease. In: Hamerton JL, Simpson NE, eds. Prenatal diagnosis: past, present and future (report of an international workshop). Prenat Diagn (special issue) 1980:11.

429. American College of Medical Genetics. www.acmg.net/Pages/ACMG_Activities/stds-2002/stdsmenu.htm

430. Association of Clinical Cytogeneticists. National external quality assessment scheme in clinical cytogenetics 1988/89. United Kingdom: Association of Clinical Cytogeneticists, 1990:9.

431. Griffiths MJ, Miller PR, Stibbe HM. A false-positive diagnosis of Turner syndrome by amniocentesis. Prenat Diagn 1996;16:463.
432. McElreavey K, Cortes LS. X-Y Translocations and sex differentiation. Semin Reprod Med 2001;19:133.
433. Margarit E, Soler A, Carrio A, et al. Molecular, cytogenetic, and clinical characterization of six XX males including one prenatal diagnosis. J Med Genet 1998;35:727.
434. Beverstock GC, Hansson K, Helderman van den Enden ATJM, et al. A near false-negative finding of mosaic trisomy 21—a cautionary tale. Prenat Diagn 1998;18:742.
435. Berry AC, Docherty Z, Bobrow M. Abnormal chromosome complement after normal amniocentesis result. Lancet 1992;340:1361.
436. Landy HJ, Weiner S, Corson SL, et al. The "vanishing twin": ultrasonographic assessment of fetal disappearance in the first trimester. Am J Obstet Gynecol 1986;155:14.
437. Abbott M-A, Benn P. Prenatal genetic diagnosis of Down's syndrome. Expert Rev Mol Diagn 2002;2:605.

Jeff M. Milunsky, M.D., F.A.C.M.G.

7

Prenatal Diagnosis of Sex Chromosome Abnormalities

Sex chromosome abnormalities (SCAs) are the most common chromosome abnormalities present at birth. It is estimated that annually over 10,000 babies with SCAs are born in the United States. Historically, many affected individuals remained undiagnosed throughout their lifetime, but prenatal diagnosis has greatly increased the awareness and identification of SCAs. Genetic counseling after the prenatal diagnosis of SCAs often presents a challenge even for the experienced genetics professional. Knowledge of the phenotypic variability within each karyotype group and the range of associated developmental and behavioral problems is essential to provide the most complete counseling. As in any genetic counseling, sensitivity, empathy, nondirectiveness, and an understanding of the cultural and family dynamic is important. For several of the SCAs presented in this chapter, appearance and lifespan may be normal, with no associated anatomic abnormalities. Although many different SCAs exist, the most frequent karyotypes include 45,X; 47,XXY; 47,XXX; 47,XYY; and sex chromosome mosaicism.

INCIDENCE

SCAs occur in one in every 300–400 births, making them about twice as frequent in newborns as trisomy 21. The incidence from amniocentesis studies of mothers 35 years of age is even greater and is estimated to be 1 in 250.[1,2] Twenty-five percent of all chromosome abnormalities detected at amniocentesis involve variations of the sex chromosomes. Results of studies from chorionic villus sampling (CVS) and early amniocentesis procedures in older women are similar.[3,4] The few studies in women younger than 35 have shown SCAs to comprise about one-third of chromosome abnormalities.[5]

ASCERTAINMENT BIAS

It is imperative that the counseling of parents faced with fetal SCA be based on current knowledge as opposed to older, biased information. Much of the literature published before 1980 is replete with studies of institutionalized individuals with SCAs that reported increased incidences of mental retardation and instability. As a result, a series of stereotypes about sex chromosome aneuploid individuals evolved. In most of these studies the possibility of normal adaptation was not generally considered.

Another bias was derived from published case reports in which individuals with medical or psychologic abnormalities were karyotyped and found to have an abnormality of the X or Y chromosome. In many cases, it was concluded that the resultant phenotype was due to the sex chromosome complement, despite the absence of causal evidence. An additional confounder was that the psychologic abnormalities described in these studies were not specific to SCAs and were common in the general population with normal karyotypes. Because only those with physical or behavioral phenotypic abnormalities were identifiable, the remaining vast majority with SCAs without abnormalities were not generally studied.

Such biased portraits of sex chromosome aneuploidy are being displaced by information from long-term prospective studies on individuals with X and Y chromosomal abnormalities. Between 1964 and 1975, researchers from seven centers around the world screened almost 200,000 consecutive newborn livebirths for the presence of these chromosomal abnormalities. As a result, 307 individuals were identified representing various cultures, ethnic groups, and socioeconomic levels. The individuals were followed from birth into young adulthood, and these represent the only unbiased studies performed on such a group.[6–9] From these studies has come an appreciation for the variability of these conditions, as well as the knowledge that most individuals with sex chromosome aneuploidy fall within the normal range of development.

PATTERNS OF INHERITANCE

In most cases, the birth of a child with an SCA to parents with normal karyotypes is considered to be a sporadic event. The recurrence risk is generally low, although it is possible that a familial tendency toward nondisjunction may exist, which could increase the risk slightly. Advanced maternal age risks exist for XXY, XXX, and their variants. In all cases, prenatal diagnosis is recommended for any subsequent pregnancies.

The advent of artificial reproductive technologies, specifically epididymal sperm aspiration with intracytoplasmic sperm injection (ICSI), has allowed some males with SCAs to have children. Mosaicism often makes reproductive counseling difficult in these circumstances. Couples with infertility using these technologies may be faced with the prenatal diagnosis of SCA. Hence, prenatal diagnosis is recommended for any ICSI pregnancy.

A few conditions involving the X and Y chromosomes may have a mendelian pattern of inheritance and are discussed below.

PRENATAL DIAGNOSIS

Because SCAs yield the most common abnormal karyotypes in newborns, it is important that parents be counseled about the possibility of such an incidental finding before prenatal diagnosis is performed. When they do receive such a diagnosis, this preparation enables them to better understand and use the information provided more effectively.[10]

For all prenatal conditions involving the X or Y chromosome, an ultrasound study should be performed to ensure that the karyotype and phenotype of the fetus are in accordance. If they are not, additional studies should be performed.

There are occasional structural modifications of the X or Y chromosome that may be familial. Whenever such a condition is diagnosed, parental chromosome analysis is recommended.

TURNER SYNDROME

Turner syndrome is defined as the loss or partial loss of an X chromosome in a female that produces short stature, gonadal dysgenesis, and various somatic abnormalities. About 99 percent of conceptions with Turner syndrome miscarry; the overall frequency among female livebirths is 1 in 1,500 to 1 in 2,500.[11] Various sex chromosome complements have been associated with the Turner phenotype (Table 7.1).

The Turner phenotype is thought to be due to the presence of one active copy of a "Turner gene" or "Turner genes" on the X chromosome. It is probable that these genes normally escape X inactivation and have functional Y chromosome homologs.[12]

Turner syndrome may be suspected prenatally through ultrasound. Usual findings can include nuchal cystic hygroma, increased nuchal translucency, nonimmune hydrops, and cardiac or renal abnormalities (see chapter 23). A low or elevated maternal serum α-fetoprotein may be found in fetal Turner syndrome. Many fetuses with Turner syndrome have normal sonographic features and are detected inadvertently through karyotyping as a routine part of CVS or amniocentesis, most commonly performed for advanced maternal age. Genetic counseling following a prenatal diagnosis of this disorder requires communication of the key clinical features and anticipated management issues.

Diagnosis and Management

Diagnosis and management of Turner syndrome requires an initial comprehensive evaluation followed by annual evaluations for life.[13–15] Recent advances in management have greatly improved the prognosis and quality of life for these individuals.

The diagnosis of Turner syndrome is made through chromosome analysis. For any individual with a 45,X cell line plus a marker or fragment, molecular SRY (sex-determining region Y) probe analysis should also be performed to rule out the presence of Y chromosomal material. This study should also be performed if there is any evidence of virilization. When Y chromosomal material is found with a 45,X cell line, there is a 15–25 percent risk of gonadal neoplasia developing, and a gonadectomy is recommended (see "45,X/46,XY" below). There is no need to routinely perform Y chromosome molecular analysis on females with 45,X karyotypes and typical features of Turner syndrome.[16]

A hallmark of Turner syndrome is *short stature*. Typically there is mild intrauterine growth restriction, decreased growth rate in childhood, and no adolescent growth spurt. Final adult height averages about 143 cm. Growth hormone therapy is routinely offered for this condition. Growth hormone is usually initiated between 2 and 5 years of age, when

Table 7.1. The incidence of various karyotypes among females with Turner syndrome

Karyotype	Incidence
45,X	50%
46,X,i(Xq)	17%
45,X/46,XX	15%
45,X/46,X,r(X)	7%
45,X/46,XY	4%
46,XXq−, 46,XXp−, 46,X,i(Xp)	7%

Source: Data from Saenger, 1993.[11]

height falls below the fifth percentile on standard growth curves. The injections are continued until appropriate bone age or satisfactory height has been reached, which is usually in midadolescence. Growth hormone therapy may add approximately 8–10 cm to the individual's height.[17]

Gonadal dysgenesis is usually present at birth. During the first 12 weeks of gestation, the ovaries appear normal. This is followed by a decline in the number of follicles with very few, if any, remaining at birth. The ovaries present as streaked tissue and do not produce estrogen. Most females with Turner syndrome will need hormone replacement therapy. Supplemental estrogen is usually initiated at approximately 14–15 years of age and is timed to minimize compromising growth while coordinating puberty with that of peers. Estrogen supplementation promotes the development of secondary sex characteristics and, combined with progesterone, establishes and maintains menses throughout adulthood. Pregnancy is possible for many adult women with Turner syndrome through the use of donor eggs, and their pregnancy rate is equal to that of women with other causes of premature ovarian failure.[18] Fertility among women with the 45,X karyotype and without recognized mosaicism is not common.[19] Spontaneous puberty occurs in 5–10 percent of women with Turner syndrome.[20,21] There is a high incidence of miscarriage and an increased likelihood of chromosomal errors and anatomic defects in the offspring of fertile 45,X women; thus, prenatal diagnosis is recommended.[22]

An increased risk of *cardiovascular malformations* is associated with Turner syndrome.[23] Coarctation of the aorta occurs in about 20 percent of patients and is usually surgically corrected in infancy. Bicuspid aortic valves are found in almost 50 percent of cases.[11] This condition requires prophylactic antibiotics before surgery and dental procedures to prevent subacute bacterial endocarditis. Adults are at increased risk for aortic dissection, particularly if there is a history of aortic root enlargement, cardiac lesions, or hypertension. All individuals with Turner syndrome should have a baseline echocardiogram at diagnosis and cardiac follow-up throughout their lifetime. Individuals with and without evidence of structural cardiac malformations should be monitored for hypertension on a lifelong basis.[23] Lifespan is typically not significantly reduced in Turner syndrome except in cases of serious cardiac malformation.

Renal malformations can contribute to hypertension, hydronephrosis, and urinary tract infection. Horseshoe kidney is the most common renal malformation seen with the nonmosaic 45,X karyotype. Renal collecting system abnormalities are most frequently seen in mosaic Turners or those with an X chromosome structural anomaly.[24] A renal ultrasound in infancy or at diagnosis should be performed on all patients, and follow-up should be instituted where applicable.

Lymphedema of the hands/feet and *webbing of the neck* are frequent features of Turner syndrome. The presence of lymphedema in a female newborn is an indication for karyotyping. It is estimated that one-third of postnatally diagnosed cases of Turner syndrome is ascertained in this way. The lymphedema typically resolves by 1 year of age, but may persist beyond childhood.

Hypothyroidism develops in 10–30 percent of patients. It is most often associated with autoimmune antibodies and is most common in females with the 46,X,i(Xq) karyotype.[25] All patients should have thyroid function tests at diagnosis and every 1–2 years thereafter.

During infancy and childhood, recurrent *otitis media* occurs in over 50 percent of girls. Since it may progress to complications and subsequent hearing loss, aggressive treatment with tubes and/or antibiotics is recommended. Sensorineural hearing loss (especially high frequency) is prevalent among adults.[26] Periodic hearing evaluations are recommended for all individuals with Turner syndrome. Various *disorders of the eye* have been reported. An ophthalmologic evaluation in childhood is important to rule out strabismus, amblyopia, and ptosis. Vision should be routinely evaluated.

Autoimmune diseases are more common in Turner syndrome. These include gastrointestinal disorders such as ulcerative colitis, Crohn disease, and celiac disease.[27] Glucose intolerance with insulin resistance is a common finding, and there is a significantly elevated risk of clinical diabetes.[28] The risk of cancer, except cancer of the large bowel, is not increased in women with Turner syndrome.[28]

Some *other medical issues* that should be addressed at an annual physical examination include evaluation for hypertension, weight control through diet and exercise, and monitoring for skeletal abnormalities such as scoliosis, kyphosis, and lordosis, as well as osteoporosis. Cholesterol and a lipid panel should be monitored, since there is an increased risk for dyslipidemia. If physical features are dysmorphic, plastic surgery may be considered for the neck, face, or ears; however, since keloids tend to form in many individuals with Turner syndrome, this issue needs to be addressed and patients should be cautioned before any surgical procedures are undertaken.

Cognitive/Psychologic Development

The intellectual and psychosocial characteristics of Turner syndrome can be quite variable, but patterns of development and adaptation have been identified. The early childhood of some 45,X girls may be marked by delays in walking and the acquisition of other motor skills. This decreased coordination can persist into childhood and may interfere with success in sports and athletics.[29] Early language development is generally unaffected,[30] and most girls with Turner syndrome do not show evidence of language impairment.

Although early reports associated Turner syndrome with mental retardation, it is now understood that for the vast majority of females with Turner karyotypes, this is not the case. A large review of studies of IQ in girls with Turner syndrome revealed that the mean verbal IQ was not significantly different from that of controls, whereas the mean performance IQ was reduced by 12 points.[31] The impairment of perceptual and spatial thinking suggested by these results was described as "space–form blindness" in 1966 and has been associated with a number of related cognitive impairments, including difficulty mentally rotating geometric shapes, orienting to left–right directions, drawing human figures, and solving arithmetic problems.[32,33] Not all subjects with Turner syndrome demonstrate this impairment of spatial thinking. Brain MRI studies have demonstrated decreases in parietal gray and occipital white matter accompanied by increased cerebellar gray matter in females with Turner syndrome.[34] Neuropsychologic profiles have identified strengths in verbal processing, with the aforementioned weaknesses in visuospatial processing, consistent with the Non-Verbal Learning Disabilities syndrome.[35]

Approximately 50 percent of girls with Turner syndrome require some degree of special education in the course of their public schooling.[31] Mathematics and handwriting skills are commonly identified problem areas.[36] However, learning difficulties in girls with Turner syndrome are not limited to any single academic area. No educational intervention specifically designed for these girls is available, and such therapy should be no different from that provided to chromosomally normal girls. When any learning difficulties are identified, early and intensive intervention is recommended. These identified cognitive deficits have been shown to persist into adulthood in women with Turner syndrome, with or without estrogen replacement therapy.[37]

Difficulties of psychologic adaptation and the existence of distinct personality styles in females with Turner syndrome have been described, including the tendency to be unassertive and overcompliant.[38,39] The spatial thinking deficits experienced by some girls with Turner syndrome may contribute to their social immaturity because of difficulties interpreting the subtle nuances of facial expressions and gestures.[38,40] In one study of 6,483 females with schizophrenia, Turner syndrome was found with a threefold greater frequency than in the general female population.[40a] These authors noted that almost all the women with Turner syndrome and schizophrenia had a mosaic karyotype. We reported two unrelated female patients with both these disorders, each of whom had an Xp22.3 deletion.[40b] Whether or not a gene involved in the pathogenesis of paranoid schizophrenia resides at this location remains to be determined.

Behavioral characteristics of Turner syndrome appear to vary with the developmental level. Preadolescent girls with Turner syndrome have been reported to have increased activity level and difficulty concentrating.[41] Adolescents with Turner syndrome have been observed to be more anxious, depressed, and more socially withdrawn and to have fewer friends than short-stature controls.[42,43] The psychosocial adaptation of adults with Turner syndrome has been characterized by strong female gender identification but also shyness and insecurity, a tendency to date less often and later than peers, and decreased likelihood of developing a satisfying sexual relationship or marrying. Although psychosocial tendencies have been identified, individual variability is significant. As with all individuals with an SCA, girls with Turner syndrome benefit greatly from a stable and supportive environment. Even though social difficulties appear to be an area of vulnerability, many girls and women with Turner syndrome have demonstrated strong psychosocial adaptation throughout their lifetime. In a volunteer sample of adults with Turner syndrome in Seattle, 75 percent had attended college, although many obtained jobs that appeared to be below their level of education.[44]

As with any child, girls with Turner syndrome will develop a stronger sense of self-esteem if they experience success and are encouraged to develop their own special abilities. Such success is seldom found in competitive sports, but it may be found in a variety of other avenues. Social activities, particularly those available through well-supervised programs such as Girl Scouts, church or synagogue youth organizations, can facilitate the successful development of a variety of social relationships. When psychologic distress, such as anxiety or depression, becomes apparent, immediate intervention increases the probability of a successful outcome. Turner syndrome support groups can help counter the sense of isolation sometimes experienced by these girls and their families. Open discussion and sharing of information and experiences promote understanding and acceptance.

Karyotype Variations

Half of all individuals with Turner syndrome have a 45,X karyotype. Many chromosomal variants can also produce a Turner syndrome phenotype. The most prevalent forms are listed in Table 7.1 and discussed below.

45,X

It is estimated that about 1.5 percent of known conceptuses are 45,X, and of these, less than 1 percent survive to birth with the clinical manifestations of Turner syndrome. Monosomy X accounts for approximately 15 percent of all spontaneous miscarriages. The mechanism of chromosome loss is unknown. Among 45,X karyotypes, approximately 80 percent retain the maternal X and 20 percent retain the paternal X.[45] Imprinting does not appear to play a role in the phenotype. Advanced maternal age is not associated with an increased incidence of Turner syndrome.

The 45,X karyotype is usually found in individuals with Turner syndrome who are the most severely affected, but the clinical features can be quite varied. Mental retardation is not typically associated with this karyotype.

46,X,i(Xq)

Isochromosome Xq is the most common structural rearrangement of the X chromosome and is present in approximately 15–20 percent of individuals with Turner syndrome. It can exist as 46,X,i(Xq) or as 45,X/46,X,i(Xq) mosaicism. The isochromosome usually consists of two q arms joined at the centromere, with no short arm material present. In some cases, however, the isochromosome can be dicentric, although only one centromere is active and small amounts of short arm material may then be present in duplicate.[46,47] In all cases, females have a Turner phenotype with short stature, but their remaining somatic features may be less pronounced than in instances of a pure 45,X cell line. Not all individuals with 46,X,i(Xq) will have ovarian dysgenesis, and some may be fertile. Individuals with i(Xq) have a higher incidence of autoimmune disorders, including Hashimoto thyroiditis,[25] inflammatory bowel disease, and diabetes mellitus.

Isochromosome Xq is rarely found in spontaneous abortions but is frequent in postnatal diagnoses of Turner syndrome. This is known as the fetoprotective effect and its etiology is unknown. The i(Xq) is equally likely to be derived from either parent.[48]

46,X,del(Xq) or 46,X,Xq−

The critical region for gonadal development is Xq13–26,[49,50] and thus a deletion in this area of the long arm of the X chromosome usually results in gonadal dysgenesis and primary amenorrhea in females. Short stature may also be present, but height is often normal; it has been proposed that height is correlated to the closeness of the breakpoint to Xq13.[51] The somatic features of Turner syndrome may or may not be present.[52]

46,X,r(X)

Ring X chromosomes result from the loss of both ends of the chromosome, with a subsequent union of the shortened arms. The resultant ring X is unstable. It is usually associated with a 45,X cell line, and the prognosis is that for monosomy X.[53] Identification of r(X) is through the use of X chromosome probes.[54]

In patients with a small r(X), mental retardation has been reported, an otherwise infrequent occurrence in Turner syndrome. In these cases, it is thought that the X inactivation center (XIST) at Xq21 is lost resulting in both X chromosomes being active.[55–60] Additional features include facial dysmorphism, syndactyly, cardiac and skeletal anomalies.

45,X/46,XY

The 45,X/46,XY karyotype can produce phenotypes from females with Turner syndrome with or without mental retardation, to males with ambiguous genitalia and/or gonadal dysgenesis, to almost normal males (see "45,X Mosaicism" below). Prenatal counseling should address all of the points listed below for Turner syndrome fetuses and should also include discussion of gonadal surveillance.

Other Variants

Karyotypes that are rare and can produce Turner syndrome include 46,X,del(Xp); 46,X,i(Xp); and 46,XX,+ marker (see "Structural Abnormalities of the X Chromosome" on page 320).

Prenatal Counseling for Turner Syndrome

Genetic counseling of parents with an intrauterine diagnosis of Turner syndrome includes the following points:

1. Short stature will probably be present. The use of human growth hormone therapy should be discussed.
2. Gonadal dysgenesis resulting in infertility will probably be present. Hormonal therapy can enable these girls to experience normal pubertal development. Pregnancy using egg donation may be an option.
3. Other physical abnormalities may be present, including cardiac malformations, webbed neck, and renal anomalies. A careful ultrasound at about 18–20 weeks can help in differentiating those who are seriously affected from those with milder manifestations. The ultrasound should also include visualization of the genitals to identify any individuals in whom there is a discrepancy between karyotype and phenotype. Medical management of the various other complications of Turner syndrome should be discussed.
4. Mental retardation is not characteristic of Turner syndrome, but may be encountered with specific karyotypes (e.g., r(X)).
5. There is a risk for difficulty in motor or learning skills. Anticipatory guidance and early intervention may be helpful. Management is no different from that given to chromosomally normal children with similar developmental problems.
6. Variability among girls with Turner syndrome is considerable. A precise prediction about any child's prognosis is not possible.

45,X Mosaicism

Mosaicism arises from mitotic nondisjunction or anaphase lag occurring after fertilization and is more frequent in Turner syndrome than in most other chromosomal disorders. The incidence of 45,X mosaicism is greater in liveborns than in abortuses, which suggests that the presence of a second cell line can increase the chances of survival. 45,X mosaicism occurs in approximately 15 percent of individuals presenting with some stigmata of Turner syndrome. Prenatally, 45,X mosaicism is the most common sex chromosomal mosaicism diagnosed, with many of these girls being minimally affected. There are many different 45,X mosaic karyotypes possible and the phenotype within each type of mosaicism is variable. The following are discussed: 45,X/46,XX; 45,X/47,XXX; 45,X/46,XX/47,XXX; and 45,X/46,XY.

45,X/46,XX

45,X/46,XX mosaicism presents with variable phenotypes. It generally has a better prognosis than when all cells are 45,X. There is a tremendous ascertainment bias in the medical literature in descriptions of the phenotypes of a selected group of postnatally diagnosed females with this karyotype, the vast majority having been identified because of a clinical abnormality. In contrast, of those 45,X/46,XX mosaics detected prenatally, most have a normal phenotype at birth. The prevalence of 45,X/46,XX mosaicism is tenfold higher among amniocenteses diagnoses than in postnatal diagnoses, suggesting that most individuals with mosaicism escape detection.[61]

At birth, the degree of mosaicism should be confirmed in peripheral blood. The initial management stages of Turner syndrome, include an echocardiogram and a renal ultrasound. Later management will depend on the type of Turner stigmata present in the mosaic individual. The most common finding is short stature, but most are predicted to attain an adult height greater than the fifth percentile.[61] Many 45,X/46,XX mosaics undergo spontaneous pubertal development and are fertile. Some of these females are likely to experience an early menopause and may have an increased number of miscarriages.[62]

Prenatal counseling for the parents of a 45,X/46,XX fetus includes the following:

1. Variability of the phenotype is considerable, ranging from that of classic Turner syndrome to an intermediate phenotype to normal. The degree of mosaicism as determined by CVS or amniocentesis bears little relationship to clinical severity. The prognosis is generally better than that for the fetus with the pure 45,X karyotype.
2. There is an increased likelihood of short stature.
3. Pubertal development may be normal, but reproductive capability may be decreased. Early menopause is possible. Prenatal diagnosis is desirable if the mosaic woman becomes pregnant, as there is probably an increased risk for numerical chromosome abnormalities in her offspring.
4. IQ is often similar to that of siblings. Mental retardation is not expected.

45,X/47,XXX

45,X/47,XXX mosaics have a combination of a Turner syndrome cell line and a triple X cell line. Phenotype can reflect some features of each syndrome with some Turner stigmata, but stature may be unaffected. Many are phenotypically normal. Females with 45,X/47,XXX karyotype can complete spontaneous puberty with menarche and hence are typically fertile.[63]

45,X/46,XX/47,XXX

There are few data on unselected individuals with 45,X/46,XX/ 47,XXX mosaicism. Normal phenotypes have been reported, as well as cases with manifestations of Turner syndrome.

45,X/46,XY and Variants

When diagnosed in utero, the 45,X/46,XY karyotype or its variants (45,X/46,XY/47,XYY or 45,X/46,X,idic(Y) or 45,X/47,XYY or 45,X/48,XYYY) present a serious genetic counseling challenge because possible abnormalities of sexual differentiation. Postnatally identified individuals have displayed phenotypes ranging from females with Turner syndrome phenotypes to individuals with ambiguous genitalia with or without mental retardation, to almost normal phenotypic males. As in other forms of sex chromosome mosaicism, the phenotype of postnatally diagnosed cases represents marked ascertainment bias.[64]

Several larger reviews of prenatally diagnosed 45,X/46,XY fetuses give less biased information.[65–67] The phenotype in these individuals was normal male at birth in over 90 percent of cases. Because these patients have not been followed into adulthood, their fertility status as well as the incidence of gonadoblastoma is not yet known. There was no relation between the degree of mosaicism and the presence or severity of abnormalities.

The most likely product of a 45,X/46,XY fetus with normal male genitals on ultrasound is a phenotypically normal male.[68] However, the determination of male fetal sex does not rule out the presence of ambiguous genitalia or the existence of ovotestes or other gonadal disorders. Dysgenetic gonads in any individual who possesses Y chromosomal material are at an estimated 20–25 percent risk for malignant transformation. These abnormal cells develop initially as gonadoblastomas that subsequently have about a 50 percent risk of becoming malignant germinomas. There is a gene on the Y chromosome involved in the development of these tumors. It is referred to as GBY (gonadoblastoma locus on the Y chromosome) and has been localized to a region near the centromere on Yp.[69]

It is recommended that all 45,X/46,XY individuals with genital abnormalities undergo a gonadectomy at the time of diagnosis to remove all abnormal gonadal tissue (this includes phenotypic females with streak gonads, those with ambiguous genitalia, and phenotypic males with undescended testicles). When normal gonadal tissue is present in such males, the risk of neoplasia is unknown. An approach to the management of males with the 45,X/46,XY karyotype and one or more malformations of the external genitalia has been proposed.[70] Repeated palpation of the testis is recommended during childhood. Routine testicular biopsy before puberty is not recommended. Testicular biopsy is not sensitive enough to detect carcinoma in situ before puberty. Ultrasonography of the testis should be performed yearly from age 10 years, and bilateral testicular biopsy should be performed when puberty is completed. Annual follow-up with testicular ultrasonography until the age of 20 is recommended when no evidence of carcinoma in situ is found. A follow up testicular biopsy at age 20 should also be performed. If carcinoma in situ is found in the first biopsy, more intensive surveillance is recommended and treatment with orchidectomy or local irradiation should be considered. Adult men have an increased risk of neoplasia and should have regular examinations.

When a diagnosis of 45,X/46,XY mosaicism or variant is made prenatally, the following counseling is recommended:

1. If normal male genitals are visualized, the expectation is for a phenotypically normal male. If normal male genitalia are not visualized after adequate ultrasonography, there is a significant risk for ambiguous genitalia, a need for surgical reconstruction, and probable infertility. There is a risk of gonadoblastoma.
2. A pelvic and testicular ultrasound in infancy is indicated for all individuals, including those with a normal male phenotype. A follow-up MRI may be necessary to further define the anatomy.
3. Surveillance with ultrasound usually commences at 10 years, and testicular biopsy is recommended after puberty to seek for evidence of carcinoma in situ.
4. Short stature may occur.
5. Mental retardation may be part of the male phenotype.
6. There is no direct correlation between the proportion of 45,X cells and the phenotype.

47,XXY AND VARIANTS

The addition of an extra X chromosome to a normal male chromosome constitution produces the 47,XXY karyotype. This is commonly referred to as Klinefelter syndrome, although the full constellation of the clinical features first described by Dr. Klinefelter in 1942, including testicular dysgenesis, elevated urinary gonadotropins, and gynecomastia, are often not present.

Klinefelter syndrome is the most common cause of hypogonadism in males and is the most common SCA. The fetal survival rate is approximately 97 percent, making the newborn incidence about 1 per 600 male births. In the United States, this incidence amounts to about eight to nine births per day, or at least 3,000 males per year with 47,XXY. Affected males who are diagnosed come to attention in one of three ways: (1) a karyotype is performed as part of an infertility evaluation or the presence of gynecomastia (2) a karyotype is performed as part of an evaluation for learning and behavioral disorders in childhood, or (3) it is inadvertently diagnosed prenatally. The majority are never identified.

It has been suggested that the dup Xq11–Xq22 may be sufficient for the expression of Klinefelter syndrome.[71] The presence of the extra X chromosome can be attributed to either maternal or paternal nondisjunction in a gamete. Approximately 50 percent of the additional X chromosomes come from the father, and 50 percent of cases are maternally derived. There is no imprinting effect. Advanced maternal age is associated with 47,XXY, but to a lesser degree than in autosomal aneuploidy.[72] It now appears that the frequency of XY sperm increases with age in fathers of boys with Klinefelter syndrome, implicating an advanced paternal age effect.[73]

Clinical Features and Management

The main features of the 47,XXY syndrome include tall stature, small testes, infertility, and a risk for developmental and behavioral disorders. There is considerable variability in clinical findings.

The newborn with 47,XXY typically has no significant dysmorphism. There is no increased incidence of birth defects. Genitalia are usually normal. Boys with this karyotype tend to be tall, with increased length of the lower extremities. Height velocity is increased by 5 years of age, and by adolescence, most are at or above the 75th percentile.

Sexual development is normal in the prepubertal years, and the initiation of pubertal changes with normal pituitary gonadal function is similar to that of peers. By 14 years of age, both follicle-stimulating hormone (FSH) and luteinizing hormone (LH) are elevated. There is an adolescent elevation in testosterone, which begins to plateau at about this same age, with serum testosterone levels then remaining in the low or low-normal adult range. By midpuberty, the boys are hypergonadotropic, with FSH and LH levels five to ten times above the normal range.[74] The testes initially begin to enlarge during early pubertal development, but by midpuberty, testicular growth ceases and the mean testicular volume is about 3 mL. Testicular prostheses are available for occasional cases in which the presence of small testes can contribute to psychologic problems, such as poor body image or lowered self-esteem.

Azoospermia or oligospermia and infertility are almost always present in adults. Testicular histology reveals hyalinization and fibrosis of the seminiferous tubules. The penis is usually normal in size. Sexual function is normal, although decreased testosterone levels may also decrease libido.

Gynecomastia may be present in 50 percent of patients, but it is usually only slightly above the physiologic norm. Occasionally, a simple mastectomy may be required if the gynecomastia persists.

Testosterone supplementation is recommended, usually beginning at early to midadolescence. Although this intervention does not reduce gynecomastia, it does promote and sustain development of secondary sex characteristics, especially facial and body hair and often assists in increasing muscle mass, energy, and drive. Importantly, testosterone supplementation helps prevent osteoporosis in men, a condition to which they are subject throughout adulthood because of insufficient testosterone levels. It can also promote a general sense of well-being and decreases emotional lability. Therapy can be provided through intramuscular injections given twice or three times per month, depending on age and dose, or through the use of transdermal patches.

There is an increased risk of various health problems for men with Klinefelter syndrome. Osteoporosis may occur, caused by decreased bone mineral content as a result of androgen insufficiency; this can be prevented with supplemental testosterone therapy. If osteoporosis occurs in an untreated man, testosterone can halt its progress but cannot reverse the decrease in bone mass. Adults with Klinefelter syndrome are thought to be more susceptible to autoimmune diseases. An increased incidence of systemic lupus erythematosus, thyroid disorders, and diabetes mellitus has been reported.[75] Some studies have not found an increased risk for breast cancer,[76] while others have noted an increased incidence of breast cancer comparable to that of normal females.[77,78] There is an elevated risk for extragonadal germ-cell tumors in the mediastinum from early adolescence until young adulthood.[79] In 47,XXY young men with respiratory symptoms or precocious pubertal development, the possibility of a such a tumor should be considered.[80] The mortality rate due to cerebrovascular disease may be increased.[77]

All 47,XXY men should have a thorough annual physical examination that addresses ongoing medical concerns, if any, as well as associated risk factors.

Notwithstanding their azoospermia or oligospermia, men with Klinefelter syndrome may be able to sire children through epididymal sperm aspiration and retrieval of viable sperm, intracytoplasmic sperm injection (ICSI), and IVF. However, their offspring, conceived through ICSI, have an increased risk of being born with an SCA. Multiple studies on the offspring of pregnancies through ICSI have largely concluded that there is no increased risk of congenital malformations in the subsequent offspring.[81–83] Some authors, although not observing a significantly increased risk of congenital malformations among offspring of ICSI pregnancies, consider that the results be "treated with caution," given their low numbers in some of their groups understudy.[83a] The authors of a Belgium study initially reported their 7-year experience with ICSI in 1,987 children, among whom they found no increased incidence of congenital malformations.[81] Subsequently they also found no indication that children sired by ICSI had a lower psychomotor developmental quotient than children born after IVF.[84] The same group had earlier noted a significantly higher rate of de novo chromosomal abnormalities among ICSI offspring detected prenatally, more especially reflecting an increased number of SCA.[84a] Two different studies noted an increased frequency of hypospadias (e.g., relative risk 3.0) in ICSI offspring.[84b,84c] Of particular note is the small increase in overall congenital malformations observed in children born after IVF only.[85] However, of potentially most concern are studies of children born after IVF in which early reports reflect a significant increased frequency of imprinting disorders, including Angelman syndrome,[85a,85b] Beckwith–Wiedemann syndrome,[85c,85d] and retinoblastoma.[85e,85f] Much more study is necessary before final conclusions can be reached about the frequency of disorders resulting from imprinting defects and IVF/ICSI. However, there is already a need for heightened awareness.[85g]

In a prospective epidemiologic prenatal study of 7,332 women who had an amniocentesis in our center, 231 had gestational diabetes.[85h] Women with gestational diabetes had a 7.7 times greater likelihood of having an infant with a numerical sex chromosome defect than those without gestational diabetes.

Cognitive/Psychological Development

The 47,XXY karyotype carries a risk for cognitive problems that include slightly reduced IQ, language skills, and reading ability. Although most 47,XXY boys have IQ scores in the average range, IQs typically are about 10 points lower than those of siblings.[86] Verbal IQs are frequently lower than performance IQs, reflecting difficulty with language processing. Language impairment associated with the 47,XXY karyotype is well documented and frequently appears first as delayed early language milestones, such as the emergence of single words or short sentences.[87,88] Impairments of verbal memory, fluency, and speed of verbal information processing have been documented in school-age 47,XXY boys.[87–92] In young adulthood, there appears to be increases in verbal IQ relative to performance IQ in some Klinefelter patients.[93]

Because reading skills are closely associated with language skills, it is not surprising that reading disability is found with increased frequency in this group of males. Three studies of unselected propositi reported that thirty-two of forty-three 47,XXY boys (74 percent) experienced reading disability requiring educational intervention.[88,89,94] Most 47,XXY boys remain in regular education classrooms with some supportive tutoring in reading or other areas of academic deficiency. Some 47,XXY boys require more time than their peers on tasks such as handwriting and timed activities. No specific educational intervention has been designed for 47,XXY boys; when reading difficulties are encountered, intervention proceeds as it would with chromosomally normal boys.

Motor skills among 47,XXY males tend to be lower than those of their peers.[95] Slight delays in age of onset of independent walking may be followed by a tendency toward reduced speed and coordination during childhood. Consequently, few have found success in competitive sports. Individual sports such as swimming, hiking, and cycling are often more satisfying than team sports. Fine motor abilities are generally stronger than gross motor skills.[95]

The language difficulties of 47,XXY males may partially underlie the psychologic tendency toward shyness, unassertiveness, and immaturity.[91,96,97] As is the case with all individuals with SCAs, 47,XXY boys and adolescents tend to be more vulnerable to a stressful environment than their siblings. For 47,XXY adolescents, limited academic, athletic, and social success can result in many frustrations, although most move toward full independence from families and enter adulthood without evidence of serious psychiatric difficulty. One study of unselected 47,XXY adolescents reported that, despite fewer friendships than peers, many developed important friendships, and more than half dated girls in high school, although steady romantic relationships were few.[97] However, it has been found that adults with Klinefelter syndrome appear to do as well as a control group in terms of socioeconomic status and degree of education.[98] Heterosexual orientation is predominant, although sexual drive is diminished.[99]

The early identification of a 47,XXY boy allows parents to understand his developmental risks and to provide early intervention as needed. This may include the provision of speech and language therapy even before school age for patients in which delays have been noted. During the grade school years, early intervention for language and reading problems may forestall greater difficulties later in a boy's academic career. Low self-esteem, sometimes leading to depression, has been noted in some 47,XXY boys and adolescents; in these cases, early counseling or psychotherapy can again help ameliorate difficulties before they become more serious. Participation in noncompetitive sports and clubs and organizations that facilitate the comfortable development of social relationships can also be invaluable to 47,XXY boys and adolescents.

Prenatal Counseling for 47,XXY

Prenatal counseling for parents of a 47,XXY fetus includes the following points:

1. Phenotype is generally normal. Height will be increased.
2. 47,XXY men will be infertile, but can avail themselves of the latest reproductive technologies (currently including epididymal sperm aspiration and ICSI) in order to potentially sire children. Pubertal development is normal, but testes will be small. There is a risk for gynecomastia. Testosterone supplementation is desirable, starting in midadolescence and continuing throughout the lifetime.
3. Mental retardation is not characteristic of 47,XXY.
4. There is a risk for developmental problems, the severity of which cannot be predicted, including delays in speech, motor, and learning skills. Reading is a likely area of difficulty. These problems are not unique to 47,XXY boys, and treatment and management are the same as for karyotypically normal children. Anticipatory guidance and early intervention can be helpful.
5. 47,XXY males tend to be shy, and social integration may be difficult. They are usually heterosexually oriented.
6. There is considerable variability, and precise predictions of physical or psychological development are not possible.

47,X,i(Xq),Y

The 47,X,i(Xq),Y karyotype consists of monosomy for Xp and trisomy for Xq. In general, the typical clinical manifestations of 47,XXY are present except that stature is not increased. Intelligence is generally normal.[100]

47,XXY Mosaicism

46,XY/47,XXY

46,XY/47,XXY mosaicism is the most common form of Klinefelter mosaicism. Developmental risks are generally lessened, and fertility may be normal.

Prenatal counseling for 46,XY/47,XXY mosaicism includes the following points:

1. The prognosis is better than that for the nonmosaic 47,XXY karyotype. The degree of mosaicism in CVS tissue or amniotic fluid cells does not necessarily reflect the degree to which a boy may be affected.
2. Phenotype will probably be normal.
3. Fertility is possible. A semen analysis in late adolescence can clarify reproductive competency. Testosterone supplementation is probably not needed.
4. Developmental risks are lessened, compared with the 47,XXY karyotype. Anticipatory guidance and early intervention are appropriate, if needed.
5. No precise predictions about any individual can be made.

Other 47,XXY Mosaicism

Other types of mosaicism can include 46,XX/47,XXY; 46,XX/46,XY/47,XXY; 46,XY/48,XXXY; 45,X/46,XY/47,XXY; and 47,XXY/48,XXXY. Prenatal counseling is difficult because of variability. The phenotype may reflect features of more than one cell line.

48,XXYY

This is the most common variant of Klinefelter syndrome. The males are taller than 47,XXY males and have disproportionately longer lower extremities. Facial characteristics are variable, and skeletal abnormalities are usually minor. Some reports have indicated an increased association with this karyotype and leg ulcers or varicose veins. They have hypergonadotropic hypogonadism similar to 47,XXY males, with increased levels of FSH and LH and decreased testosterone. Their genitalia may be small, and they are infertile. Body hair is often sparse and there is a risk for gynecomastia. Testosterone therapy is similar to that for 47,XXY males. Central precocious puberty has been reported.[101]

IQ is diminished, typically ranging from 60 to 80; however, at least 10 percent of these males have IQs from 80 to 111. They often have delayed speech and motor skills.

Behavior is often shy and reserved, but there are numerous reports of impulsive and aggressive tendencies. Because of ascertainment bias of screenings among confined populations, the assumptions of aberrant behavior may be overstated.

48,XXXY

This relatively rare finding includes the addition of another extra X chromosome to the Klinefelter karyotype. The features are more severe than 47,XXY. Stature is usually tall. Facial anomalies have included hypertelorism, epicanthal folds, simplified ears, and mild prognathism. Skeletal abnormalities previously reported have included clinodactyly, elbow abnormalities, and radioulnar synostosis. Hypogonadism is similar to 47,XXY, and these males can benefit from testosterone therapy. Genitalia are small, and gynecomastia is frequent.

Moderate mental retardation is usually reported, in the 40- to 60-point range, but a boy with an IQ as high as 79 has been described.[102] Language development is consistently delayed. Motor delays are common, and these boys often have poor coordination.

Behavior is usually consistent with the level of intelligence and may be immature for chronological age. Most reports describe them as passive, pleasant, and cooperative.

49,XXXXY

Pentasomy 49,XXXXY is the most severe variant of Klinefelter syndrome; it includes distinctive features of coarse facies, marked hypogenitalism, skeletal abnormalities, and moderate to severe mental retardation.[103] This rare disorder, with an estimated incidence of 1 of 85,000 male births has been reported in association with cystic hygroma on prenatal ultrasound.[104,105]

Facial appearance often includes hypertelorism, epicanthal folds, broad nasal bridge, low-set and malformed ears, and prognathism. Cleft palate or bifid uvula has been reported to be a common finding.[103] Progressive, severe myopia is described. The neck is short and broad, while the thorax is narrow. Cardiac defects usually consist of patent ductus arteriosus or ventricular septal defect in about 15–20 percent of these males. Short stature is a frequent finding. Other skeletal involvement includes radioulnar synostosis, genu valgus, pes cavus, and hyperextensible joints with hypotonia. The genitalia are hypoplastic, and cryptorchidism is frequent.

Mental retardation is characteristic, with IQs ranging from 20 to 70; but there are a few reports of boys with IQs in the 67–78 range.[106–109] Speech is often severely impaired, and motor skills are usually poor.

Behavior is generally placid with pleasant disposition, but aggressiveness has also been reported.[102,110]

As with other poly X karyotypes, the prognosis may be better than reports have indicated. There is a need for case reports of boys who have been prenatally diagnosed or identified shortly after birth.

49,XXXYY

This unusual polysomy X and Y karyotype has been reported only five times.[102] Affected males had normal to tall stature, facial dysmorphism, gynecomastia, small testes, and moderate to severe mental retardation. Behavior was described as generally passive with occasional aggressive outbursts.

47,XXX

The addition of an X chromosome to a normal female 46,XX karyotype produces 47,XXX, also called triple X syndrome. About 70 percent of conceptions survive, yielding an incidence of 1 in every 1,000 female births. In the United States, an estimated five to six girls are born daily with 47,XXX (almost 2,000 girls per year). Because the features of this syndrome are not medically significant, very few individuals are ever identified with 47,XXX except for those diagnosed prenatally.

The presence of the extra X chromosome is maternally derived in over 90 percent of cases. Advanced maternal age is a factor in meiosis I but not in meiosis II. There does not appear to be a paternal age effect.

Because so few 47,XXX females have been identified and followed prospectively, only a small amount of information about their growth and development is available:

Clinical Features and Medical Management

Females with the 47,XXX karyotype show considerable variability in clinical presentation. There are few definitive features or characteristics.

The only significant physical characteristic is tall stature, with many reaching the 80th percentile by adolescence. Head circumference is usually in the 25th to 35th percentile. Pubertal development is normal, and they are usually fertile. Premature ovarian failure has also been reported in 47,XXX females.[111] Because they have a chromosome abnormality, they are at a slightly increased risk to have a child with a chromosome aberration; therefore, prenatal diagnosis is advisable.

Cognitive/Psychological Development

Although physically indistinguishable from other infants early in life, 47,XXX girls frequently experience slight delays in language and neurodevelopment. Deficits in motor skills persist into childhood, in which 47,XXX girls have been found to have lower levels of muscle tone, balance, strength, and coordination than their unaffected siblings[29] and seldom find satisfaction in competitive athletic activities. Language delays similarly persist and sometimes require speech and language intervention by school age.

IQ scores fall on average about 15–20 points below those of siblings and controls,[86,90,112] although considerable variability has been noted, with some 47,XXX girls possessing IQ scores in the high average range. In addition, 47,XXX girls frequently demonstrate learning disabilities requiring special education intervention. One summary from several studies of unselected 47,XXX girls noted that 71 percent required educational intervention.[113] The nature of educational problems experienced by 47,XXX girls is quite variable; not infrequently, educational assistance is required in several different subjects.

The impeded motor and language development of 47,XXX girls, combined with school failure, frequently results in a lack of self-confidence and lowered self-esteem.[114] Behavioral and psychiatric problems have been found to be increased in this group.[97,115] Adolescence is a particularly difficult period, because the successful achievement of independence from family can be quite difficult, and psychologic problems can be common.[97,115,116] Considerable variability has been found in the 47,XXX population. Those from stable and supportive environments tend to have stronger psychological development. Although difficulty forming interpersonal relationships is not unusual, many form meaningful personal attachments, marry, have children, and are economically self-sufficient.

No specific educational or psychologic intervention has been designed for 47,XXX girls or women. As noted, their difficulties are quite varied, and therefore, educational and psychologic interventions must be provided as needed and designed specific to the problems demonstrated. This is particularly important during their early developmental years, when the rapid response to identified language and motor delays may help ameliorate some difficulties later.

Prenatal Counseling for 47,XXX

Prenatal counseling for parents of a 47,XXX fetus includes the following points:

1. The phenotype is normal. Tall stature is likely.
2. Pubertal development and reproductive competency will probably be normal.
3. Mental retardation is not characteristic of 47,XXX.
4. There is a risk for developmental problems in speech, motor skills, and learning abilities. These problems are not unique to 47,XXX girls, and treatment and management should be no different than that given chromosomally normal children with similar problems. Anticipatory guidance and early intervention can be helpful.
5. There is considerable variability, and precise predictions about any individual's prognosis is not possible.

47,XXX Mosaicism

46,XX/47,XXX

Mosaicism for 47,XXX with a normal 46,XX cell line lessens the phenotypic implications as compared with those with a 47,XXX chromosome complement. Prenatal counseling should include the above points, but the likelihood of developmental risks is reduced. There is an increased risk among mosaics for offspring with abnormal karyotypes, a risk that may be greater than for nonmosaic 47,XXX females.[117] Prenatal diagnosis is recommended.

See "45,X Mosaicism," above, for 45,X/47,XXX and 45,X/46,XX/47,XXX.

Other 47,XXX Mosaicism

Mosaicism involving other cell lines such as tetrasomy X or pentasomy X can occur, with a relatively more severe prognosis than 46,XX/47,XXX.

48,XXXX

The addition of two extra X chromosomes results in a 48,XXXX chromosome constitution, also called tetrasomy X, and has been described in more than 40 cases. There are no specific abnormal or consistent clinical features.[102,118,119]

Stature is variable; above-average height is common. Microcephaly has been described. Facial abnormalities are usually minor and may include hypertelorism, epicanthal folds, depressed nasal bridge, and strabismus. Skeletal abnormalities often consist of clinodactyly and radioulnar synostosis, but they can also be more severe. Genitalia are normal, but there may be incomplete development of secondary sex characteristics. Menarche, menstrual dysfunction, and fertility are variable; three 48,XXXX women are known to have reproduced.

Mental retardation of 48,XXXX females is characteristic; the reported IQ range is 35–75. One instance of low average intelligence in an adult woman has been documented.[120]

Behavioral characteristics are varied; some females are reported to be pleasant and cooperative, while others are said to be aggressive and socially inappropriate. There is a risk for unstable behavior in adult women.

The range of features of this condition may be milder than previously described as a result of ascertainment bias. There are no reports of long follow-up of a prenatally diagnosed 48,XXXX patient.

49,XXXXX

Pentasomy X is rare, and of the approximately 25 cases described, all have involved girls <16 years of age. The characteristic phenotype of 49,XXXXX includes mental retardation, short stature, coarse facial features, and skeletal abnormalities.[102,121]

Intrauterine and postnatal growth deficiency are common features. Craniofacial abnormalities include microcephaly, hypertelorism, low-set ears, upslanting palpebral fissures, epicanthal folds, and depressed nasal bridge. Congenital heart defects have consisted of patent ductus arteriosus or ventricular septal defect. The skeleton is usually severely affected with radioulnar synostosis, joint laxity and dislocations, and talipes equinovarus. External genitalia are normal, but in several cases, the uterus has been small and hypoplasia or malformations of kidneys have been described. Pubertal development is delayed, and fertility is assumed to be reduced. There are no reports of 49,XXXXX females who have become pregnant.

Mental retardation has ranged from IQs of 20 to 75; the average IQ is 50. There are severe speech and language deficits. There is no distinct behavioral phenotype. Several of the girls have been described as shy and cooperative.

Features of those diagnosed in utero may be milder than postnatal reports; however, no 49,XXXXX prenatally diagnosed pregnancies have been continued to term and documented in the literature. Thus, no unbiased reports are available.

47,XYY

The addition of a Y chromosome to a normal male 46,XY chromosome constitution does not produce a discernible phenotype. Males with 47,XYY cannot be characterized by discriminating physical or behavioral features. The first diagnosis of this condition, therefore, was a karyotypic and not a phenotypic discovery.

The incidence of 47,XYY is about 1 in every 1,000 male births. In the United States, an estimated five to six boys are born daily with 47,XYY (almost 2,000 boys per year). Because the features of this syndrome are not medically significant, few individuals are ever identified with 47,XYY, except for those inadvertently diagnosed prenatally, or karyotyped because of significant learning and/or behavioral disorders during childhood.

The presence of the extra Y chromosome is paternally derived in all cases, and the extra Y originates at meiosis II.[122] There is no paternal age effect.

Because so few 47,XYY males have been identified and followed prospectively, there is a paucity of reliable information about their growth and development.

Historical Perspective

For years, great interest and concern was directed at the association between 47,XYY males and aggressive, antisocial behavior. This interest began when early chromosome screening studies in the 1960s identified a fourfold to five-fold increase of 47,XYY men in mental and penal institutions.[123] Unfortunately, this sample represented less than 1 percent of all men with the extra Y chromosome and reflected a strong bias of ascertainment (see "Conclusions"). The stereotype image that resulted from these studies was highly biased and incorrect. Results from unselected newborn studies over the past 20 years have provided a more balanced picture of the behavioral adaptation of 47,XYY males. It is now known that the majority of 47,XYY men do not demonstrate marked psychopathology.

Clinical Features and Medical Management

Males with the 47,XYY karyotype show considerable variability in clinical presentation. There are few definitive features or characteristics. The only significant physical characteristic is tall stature, which may manifest in childhood. Final height is greater than that of parents or siblings. Pubertal development is normal, and these men are usually fertile. Severe facial acne has occasionally been reported. Because they have a chromosome abnormality, they are at a slightly increased risk to have a child with a chromosome aberration; therefore, prenatal diagnosis for their partners is advisable.

Cognitive/Psychological Development

Motor and language impairment and increased learning difficulties characterize 47,XYY males much as they do 47,XXY males.[95] Mild delays in achievement of early motor milestones have been reported.[124] 47,XYY boys tend to have impaired motor development characterized by reduced gross motor speed and coordination. Consequently, most are not accomplished athletes.[95] Language delays are common and sometimes predictive of later school learning problems. Approximately half of 47,XYY boys require special education intervention, the majority involving persistent reading and spelling difficulties.[86] IQ scores on average fall 10–15 points below controls and, while variability is large, most are within the average range.[86] There may be an increase in the pervasive developmental disorder spectrum in 47,XYY males,[125] but large unbiased studies are not available.

Behavioral and psychological development of 47,XYY boys is variable. Distractibility, hyperactivity, and a low tolerance for frustration characterize some during childhood and early adolescence.[9] Attention deficits and impulsive tendencies include difficulty organizing school work, talking out loud, or acting before thinking. Despite these difficulties of impulse control, marked psychiatric disturbance or aggression has not characterized most 47,XYY propositi.[86] There is an increased frequency of antisocial behavior reported in adolescents and adults with 47,XYY.[126] Property offenses constitute the majority of criminal convictions of 47,XYY males.[126]

No specific educational or psychologic intervention has been designed for 47,XYY boys or men. As noted, their difficulties are quite varied, and therefore, educational and psychologic interventions must be provided as needed and designed specifically for the problems encountered. This is particularly important during their early developmental years, when the rapid response to identified language and motor delays may help ameliorate some difficulties later.

Prenatal Counseling for 47,XYY

Prenatal counseling for parents of a 47,XYY fetus includes the following points:

1. The phenotype is normal. Tall stature is likely.
2. Pubertal development and reproductive competency will almost certainly be normal.
3. Mental retardation is not characteristic of 47,XYY.
4. There is a significant risk for developmental problems in speech, neuromotor skills, and learning abilities. Behavioral problems are common. These problems are not unique to 47,XYY boys, and treatment and management should be no different than that given chromosomally normal children with similar problems. Anticipatory guidance and early intervention can be helpful.
5. There is considerable variability, and precise predictions about any individual's prognosis is not possible.

46,XY/47,XYY Mosaicism

Mosaicism for 47,XYY with a normal cell line lessens the phenotypic implications as compared to the 47,XYY male. Prenatal counseling should include the above points, but the likelihood of developmental risks is reduced. There is an increased risk among mosaics for offspring with abnormal karyotypes and prenatal diagnosis for the partner of the mosaic man is recommended.

Polysomy Y Karyotypes

Karyotypes with more than one extra Y chromosome are rare conditions characterized by hypogonadism, developmental delay or mental retardation, and aberrant behavior. As is the case with other infrequently occurring SCAs involving multiple X and Y chromosomes, prenatally diagnosed pregnancies with these karyotypes have not been continued and reported. It is possible that the phenotype may be milder than that described in the few case reports currently available.

48,XYYY

Eight cases of 48,XYYY have been reported in the literature.[102] The common characteristics include tall stature, frequent respiratory infections, abnormal dentition, radioulnar synostosis and hypogonadism with azoospermia. They have borderline to low normal IQs (range, 65–86). Behavior has been characterized by impulsiveness and poor emotional stability. 48,XYYY detected through amniocentesis and chromosome analysis from products of conception has been reported following ICSI treatment in a chromosomally normal couple.[127]

49,XYYYY

Eleven cases of 49,XYYYY and mosaic variants in children have been reported.[102,128,129] Physical features include facial anomalies, speech delay, radioulnar synostosis, and scoliosis. Craniofacial dysmorphism includes trigonocephaly, hypertelorism, epicanthal folds, upslanting palpebral fissures, and low-set ears. External genitalia appear normal. These children have hypotonia and speech and motor delay, and appear to have a more severe degree of mental retardation then those with other polysomy Y karyotypes. Behavior is described as impulsive and aggressive.

49,XXYYY

A single case report of this karyotype described a 7-year-old boy with microcephaly, facial dysmorphism, radioulnar synostosis, and mental retardation with an IQ of 46.[130]

STRUCTURAL ABNORMALITIES OF THE X CHROMOSOME

To identify and define the extent of a structural rearrangement, several techniques use chromosome-specific or unique DNA sequence probes.

Xp Deletions: del(Xp) or Xp−

Deletions of the short arm of the X chromosome are rare in females. Such deletions can be terminal or interstitial. In cases in which the entire short arm is missing, Turner syndrome is the result. A telomeric deletion of Xp produces secondary amenorrhea and infertility. When the deleted segment is a terminal deletion between Xp21 and Xpter, it is possible to have normal ovarian function and none of the somatic features of Turner syndrome except for short stature.[131] When the deletion is closer to the centromere (proximal Xp21), gonadal function is lost and the Turner phenotype is present.

Only a few cases of interstitial deletions of Xp in females have been reported and have included minor dysmorphism, and in two of our cases, paranoid schizophrenia.[40b]

In males with deletion of Xp, the phenotype is dependent on the genes that have been deleted. Reports have cited males with a deletion at Xp22 who had steroid sulfatase deficiency, Kallmann syndrome, chondrodysplasia punctata, and mental retardation.[132–134]

Xq Deletions—del (Xq) or Xq−

A deletion of Xq in the Xq13–26 region in a female can result in a Turner syndrome phenotype with or without short stature (see "45,X" above). A telomeric deletion at Xq28 usually results in premature ovarian failure and infertility.[135,136]

In males, most deletions of the long arm of X have involved band Xq21. All have had mental retardation, usually associated with choroideremia or other abnormalities.[137,138] Deletions involving Xq22.3 result in a contiguous gene syndrome whose main features include mental retardation, mid-face hypoplasia, Alport syndrome, and elliptocytosis.[139] A deletion of Xq25 was described in a male with mental retardation and X-linked lymphoproliferative disease.[140] Several males with an Xq26 deletion have been described with familial situs ambiguus.[141] Myotubular myopathy and male hypogenitalism have been described with a deletion in Xq28.[142]

Xp Duplications—dup(Xp)

Duplications of part of the short arm of the X chromosome have been reported in both females and males, and the effects are varied. When associated with a Y chromosome, these genetic males are disomic for part of the short arm of the X chromosome. External genitalia may be male or female.[143] All of these individuals have been reported to have mental retardation, multiple congenital anomalies, and short stature. Several of the 46,dup(X),Y males had sex reversal in cases in which the duplication was associated with Xp21.1–21.2.[144,145]

When the duplicated Xp is associated with the presence of another X chromosome, anomalies are usually less severe. Several 46,X,dup(Xp) carrier women have reproduced and are phenotypically normal, but their offspring usually have mental retardation, multiple congenital anomalies, and gonadal dysgenesis.[146]

Xq Duplications—dup(Xq)

Duplication of part of the long arm of the X chromosome affects males more severely than females. They usually have mental retardation and short stature, and may have minor congenital anomalies.[147,148]

Females with a duplication of part of the long arm of the X chromosome may have short stature and gonadal dysgenesis with primary or secondary amenorrhea. Microcephaly, mental retardation, and hypotonia may also be present. Some females may be protected from genetic imbalance through preferential inactivation of the duplicated X. Many are normal relatives of phenotypically abnormal males, but a few females with abnormal phenotypes have been reported.[149] De novo dup (X)(q22.3q26) has been described in a female with microcephaly, hypotonia, developmental delay, and multiple dysmorphic features.[150]

Isochromosome Xp—i(Xp)

Isochromosome Xp is a rare condition that results from a duplication of the short arm of X and an absence of any Xq material. The p arms are joined at the centromere. Females have three copies of Xp and one copy of Xq. Affected individuals are infertile with Turner syndrome stigmata but have normal stature. This can also occur as 45,X/46,X,i(Xp) or 45,X/46,X,idic(Xp) mosaicism; in the latter case, part of the Xq arm has also been duplicated.[151,152] A 16-year-old female with short stature, normal development, Turner syndrome stigmata, diabetes, and Hashimoto thyroiditis has been described with an isochromosome consisting of the terminal short and proximal long arm of the X chromosome.[153]

Isochromosome Xq—i(Xq)

Isochromosome Xq in a female may be present as 46,X,i(Xq) or 45,X/46,X,i(Xq), and both types produce Turner syndrome (see "Turner Syndrome" above). In males, isoXq has been reported in concurrence with an additional X chromosome (see "47,XXY" above).

Marker X

Marker X or fragment X chromosomes are identified using molecular probes. In a female fetus with a marker X, the prognosis is for Turner syndrome. In some cases, the presence of a marker X in conjunction with a 45,X cell line (45,X/46,X,+mar) can result in Turner syndrome with mental retardation, similar to 45,X/46,XX,r(X) noted above.[154] In a male fetus with a small r(X) chromosome, congenital anomalies may also be present.[155]

Inversion X—inv(X)

Inversion X, in which the order of the genes on the X chromosome is changed, is the rarest of the X structural abnormalities. The phenotype can be normal, especially if the inversion is familial rather than de novo. Inversion X carriers are often ascertained through prenatal diagnosis when the inv(X) in the fetus is detected and parental chromosomes are checked.[156] Carriers of inv (X) are at risk for duplications and deletions of the X chromosome in their offspring.[157]

Carriers of paracentric inversions are at risk for spontaneous abortions. Their risk for abnormal offspring is not high, but prenatal diagnosis is recommended.[158] Most pericentric inversions of the X chromosome are familial and usually have normal phenotypes. Carriers are advised to have prenatal diagnosis to detect duplications and deletions in offspring. If the inversion is at the critical region (Xq13–Xq26), the female carrier may be infertile. Male carriers usually have a normal phenotype and fertility. However, a male with a pericentric inversion of the X chromosome (46,Y,inv(X)(p11.2q21.3)) inherited from his normal mother, has been described with short stature, mild mental retardation, prepubescent macro-orchidism and submucous cleft palate.[159] It is unclear if his additional anomalies are related to his karyotype. De novo pericentric inversions may result in more severe consequences.

X;autosome Translocations

X;autosome translocations are rare, probably because of the lethality of disrupted genes and loss of dosage compensation.[160] They can exist in two forms, balanced and unbalanced, and are associated with a variety of clinical findings ranging from normal phenotypes to multiple congenital anomalies and mental retardation. All twenty-two autosomes have been reported to be involved at least once, but those most commonly involved include chromosomes 1, 2, 9, 11, 15, 21, and 22. Breakpoints on the X chromosome have occurred in the proximal, medial, and distal regions of the p and q arms.

Balanced X;autosome Translocations

Female carriers of balanced X;autosome chromosomal rearrangements have varied clinical manifestations ranging from a normal phenotype to multiple congenital malformations and mental retardation. The major determinant of clinical phenotype is dependent on the X-inactivation pattern.[161] In a majority of cases, the translocated X is early replicating and thus active in all cells, while the normal X is inactivated.. A normal phenotype usually results; such individuals are often identified through abnormal offspring.[162] In other cases in which the translocated X is late replicating in a proportion of cells, the inactivation spreads to the autosome. These cases are frequently associated with mental retardation and other abnormalities.[163] Primary or secondary amenorrhea is found in a significant proportion of females with balanced X;autosome translocations,[164–166] especially if the breakpoint occurs in the Xq13–q26 segment, defined as the critical region.[49,167]

In many balanced X;autosome translocations, females have been reported to exhibit X-linked recessive conditions because the normal X is inactivated, and thus all genes on the translocated X are expressed. Some of these conditions include Hunter syndrome, Duchenne or Becker muscular dystrophy, and Menkes syndrome.[163,168–170]

Fertile females with balanced X;autosome translocations have a risk for offspring with unbalanced translocations, which can result in multiple congenital anomalies and mental retardation. Genetic counseling and prenatal diagnosis should be provided to these women.

Male carriers of balanced X;autosome translocations are usually phenotypically normal but severely subfertile or infertile.[171,172] They may be sons of carrier mothers, or the translocation may be de novo.

When a balanced X;autosome translocation is found during prenatal diagnosis, the chromosomes of the parents should be checked. If it is found in a normal parent, the prognosis is optimistic, although the possibility of an undetected duplication or deletion in the fetus cannot be ruled out. If neither parent carries the translocation, then nonpaternity should be considered. The translocation might also be de novo. In this case, there is cause for concern, as an apparently balanced translocation can actually be unbalanced and undetected. Unbalanced translocations often present with congenital malformations and mental retardation.

Unbalanced X;autosome Translocations

In unbalanced X;autosome translocations, a variety of phenotypes is observed. Clinical manifestations are dependent on the autosome involved, the breakpoints on the X and on the autosome, and on the spread of inactivation to the autosome on the derivative X.[173] The inactivation can spread partially or wholly over the attached autosomal fragment, resulting in monosomy and/or trisomy. The individual with the unbalanced X;autosome translocation usually has multiple congenital anomalies and mental retardation, reflecting the aneuploidy of the autosomal segment attached to the X chromosome.[160,174] A smaller proportion of cases may have only gonadal dysgenesis or mild abnormalities.[175]

When an unbalanced X;autosome translocation is detected during prenatal diagnosis, parents need to be counseled about the risk for congenital malformations and/or mental retardation. The chromosomes of the parents should be checked. If a parent carries a balanced form of the translocation, the family should be advised of risks for genetic imbalance in future pregnancies. If neither parent carries a translocation, future pregnancy risks for imbalance are reduced. Nonpaternity should also be considered.

X;X Translocations

Translocations between two X chromosomes are rare occurrences. They exist as either 46,X,t(X;X) or 45,X/46,X,dic(X). Most frequently, a duplication of almost the entire X chromosome occurs with a deletion of part of the arm at the breakpoint. Such duplication/deficiency of X chromosome material leads to abnormal positioning of genes, monosomy for one part of X, and trisomy for another. The phenotypes range from Turner syndrome to only ovarian dysgenesis without other Turner syndrome stigmata.[176,177]

STRUCTURAL ABNORMALITIES OF THE Y CHROMOSOME

Yp Deletions—del(Yp)

Individuals with Yp deletions usually show no evidence of masculinization when the deletion includes the loss of the testis determining factor (SRY gene). The phenotype is usually female and includes features of Turner syndrome but with normal stature.[178] There is a risk for gonadoblastoma.[179]

Yq Deletions—del(Yq)

Individuals with deletions of Yq are phenotypic males. Deletions that occur in the heterochromatic region of the long arm of the Y chromosome (Yqh) are usually familial and are not associated with phenotypic abnormalities. However, when a Yq deletion occurs de novo, this may result in various dysmorphic features, testicular maldevelopment, infertility, and short stature.[179,180] It is postulated that the Y chromosome gene that contributes to height is located at the most proximal portion of Yq.[181,182] The azoospermic factor (AZF) is located at Yq11.23 at the interface of the euchromatin and heterochromatin; a loss of this gene results in sterility.[183] There is no apparent risk for gonadoblastoma. When Yq− is detected in utero, the father's chromosomes should be checked. If the deletion is de novo, concern for malformations is justified.

Y chromosome microdeletions are a well known cause of oligospermia or azoospermia.[184–186] Epididymal sperm aspiration and ICSI are now allowing some of these men to sire children with vertical transmission of their Y microdeletions.[187] However, transmission of Y chromosome microdeletions in this manner has been shown to have potential additional features, including sexual ambiguities and Turner stigmata caused by concomitant 45,X/46,XY mosaicism.[188] Hence, prenatal diagnosis is recommended for all ICSI pregnancies.

Isochromosome Yp—i(Yp)

Isochromosome Yp results in a duplication of the short arm of Y and an absence of any Yq material. Only a few cases of 46 X,i(Yp) have been reported, and all were either phenotypically infertile males or males with ambiguous genitalia.

Some cases of 45,X/46,X,i(Yp) have been described with the phenotype varying from an incompletely masculinized male to a Turner phenotype female[189] (see "45,X/46,XY" above). Because it is difficult to distinguish i(Yp) from Yq− cytogenetically, molecular probe analysis is necessary to diagnose this condition.

Isochromosome Yq—i(Yq)

Isochromosome Yq is a very rare occurrence in which the p arm of the Y chromosome is deleted and Yq is present in duplicate. Such individuals have lost the SRY gene on Yp and are phenotypic females usually with Turner syndrome features.[179]

The isochromosome may be associated with a 45,X cell line, and affected individuals are phenotypic females with Turner syndrome features.

Isodicentric Yp—idic(Yp)

When isodicentric Yp occurs, two complete short arms of the Y chromosome are present. Most cases have breakpoints in Yq11, proximal to the heterochromatic fluorescent region at Yq12, and identical portions of the q arm are also present in duplicate. In such cases, the heterochromatin is lost, and the chromosome is nonfluorescent; these chromosomes are often called Ynf. One centromere is inactive. The chromosome is unstable and usually associated with a 45,X cell line (see 45,X/46,XY Mosaicism section), with similar phenotypes and the attendant risk for gonadoblastoma.[190–194] Very rarely, microcephaly and mental retardation have been reported.[195]

Occasionally, there is a breakpoint in the terminal heterochromatin on Yq, resulting in a large isodicentric Yp with a central fluorescent region between the centromeres. Because of the presence of two centromeres, these chromosomes are unstable. All reported cases have been mosaic for a 45,X cell line (see above).

Isodicentric Yq—idic(Yq)

An isodicentric Yq chromosome has two complete long arms and two identical partial short arms. The breakpoint is in the short arm of Y, so there is a partial but variable loss of Yp. Two centromeres are present, with one usually inactivated. These chromosomes are unstable and are associated with a 45,X cell line.[190,194] Depending on the amount of Yp deleted, some cases are reported as male with incomplete masculinization, some are reported as female with streak gonads, and others have ambiguous genitalia. Most individuals have short stature. There is an increased risk for gonadoblastoma (see "45,X/46,XY" above).

Ring Y—r(Y)

Ring Y chromosomes have deletions of both arms and are usually diagnosed using Y probe molecular technology.[196] Spectral karyotyping has also been used to identify a ring (Y) in the prenatal diagnosis of an unidentified extra-structurally abnormal chromosome.[197] They are usually, but not always, associated with a 45,X cell line, and the phenotypic variations are those of 45,X/46,XY mosaicism (see "45,X/46,XY" above). Familial transmission of a ring Y chromosome by ICSI was revealed by prenatal diagnosis of a 45,X/46,X,r(Y) karyotype in the son of an oligospermic male with the same karyotype.[198] When no mosaicism is detected and the karyotype is 46,X,r(Y), most individuals are phenotypic males with short stature and are at risk for abnormalities of the gonads or genitalia.

Marker Y—mar(Y)

Marker Y or fragment Y chromosomes are identified using molecular probes. In a female fetus with a marker Y, there is a risk for gonadal malignancy. In a male fetus, short stature may be present.[199] A marker Y chromosome was investigated by FISH in a 20-month-old infant with psychomotor retardation, dysmorphism, and ambiguous genitalia, who was found to have an extra Xp21-pter segment replacing most of Yq (46,X,der(Y)t(X;Y)(p21;q11)). The patient's phenotype was consistent with the spectrum seen with similar Xp duplications in whom sex reversal with female or ambiguous genitalia has occurred in spite of an intact Yp or SRY gene.[200] Marker Y chromosomes are often associated with a 45,X/46,XY cell lines, and the phenotype may vary from a Turner female to an almost normal male (see "45,X/46,XY" above).

Inversion Y—inv(Y)

Inversion Y cases occur with a frequency of about 1 in 1,000 in the general population and typically have no phenotypic effects.[201] When diagnosed prenatally, the father's chromosomes should be checked. The pericentric inversion of the Y chromosome has also rarely been described in subfertile males with Y microdeletions or disruptions in the DAZ gene critical region.[202,203]

Satellited Yq—Yqs

A satellited Yq condition stems from a translocation between Yqter and the p arm of an acrocentric autosome that is not missing satellite material. Hence, the translocation is unbalanced, but there is no apparent deleterious effect, so the phenotype is normal. This is a rare condition and is often familial.[204,205] When diagnosed prenatally, the father's chromosomes should be checked.

Y;autosome Translocations

The frequency of Y;autosome translocations in the general population is about 1 in 2,000.[206] Chromosome 15 is more often the recipient of a Y translocation than other chromosomes. In such cases, the heterochromatic fluorescent region on the Yq arm is translocated onto the short arm of chromosome 15. These translocations between Yqh and 15p in 46,XY males are often familial and generally have no phenotypic effects.[207] When such a translocation is found in 46,XX females, a normal phenotype is usual; however, there is a possibility that Yp material may be present that could affect phenotype. Any time a Y;15 translocation is prenatally detected, parental chromosomes should be checked and a careful ultrasound should be performed looking for the presence of normal male genitalia. In the case of females, molecular probes can identify the presence or absence of Yp material.[179]

Balanced Y;autosome reciprocal translocations are generally associated with a male phenotype and either infertility or azoospermia, although fertility has been reported in about 20 percent of cases.[179,208]

Unbalanced Y;autosome translocations may be de novo[209] or may be present in offspring of balanced Y;autosome translocation carriers. There is a risk for congenital malformations, dysmorphic features, azoospermia, and infertility. Genital phenotypes range from male to ambiguous genitalia to female (see "45,X Males" below).[210,211]

X;Y Translocations

In most X;Y translocations, a portion of the Yq arm has been translocated to the normal Xp arm. The most common translocation in females is Xp22;Yq11, in which the patients are most often phenotypic females with small stature and at risk for spontaneous abortions.[212] These women can give birth to 46,XY sons with this translocation on the X chromosome who also have a normal Y chromosome. Such males are short, usually mentally retarded, infertile, and may have ichthyosis and minor facial abnormalities that correlate with the partial deletion of Xp.[213]

Other types of X;Y translocations that result in abnormal X chromosomes produce phenotypes ranging from males with short stature and hypogonadism to females with streak gonads. A paternal Y-to-X translocation of the region involving the SRY gene has been present in over 90 percent of 46,XX males[214] (see "46,XX Males" below).

A few rare cases of X;Y translocations resulting in a derivative Y chromosome have been reported.[215] These are males with genital abnormalities, mental retardation, and facial anomalies.

In all cases of X;Y translocations, it is important to use cytogenetic and molecular technology to determine breakpoints on the X and Y chromosomes and the resultant addition/loss of genes.

Y;Y Translocations

Translocations between two Y chromosomes are rare. Most cases have been mosaic for a 45,X cell line. Phenotype has been male or ambiguous genitalia with azoospermia or infertility.

46,XX MALES

Males with the clinical features of Klinefelter syndrome who have an apparently normal cytogenetic female karyotype are commonly referred to as 46,XX males. Their population frequency is 1 in 20,000 male births.[216] About one-third have gynecomastia, and facial hair may be sparse.[217]

These patients are shorter than 47,XXY males and do not have disproportionately long extremities. Their genitalia are generally normal male, but there is an increased risk for hypospadias or ambiguous genitalia. The testes are uniformly small, and azoospermia and infertility have been present in all cases.[218] Testicular histology resembles that of the 47,XXY condition, and management of testosterone deficiency is the same.[219]

Their IQ is generally higher than that of a 47,XXY male, and they have fewer learning disabilities. Behavior problems have not been noted.

There are two forms of the 46,XX male syndrome: Y-positive and Y-negative. About 90 percent of these males have part of the short arm of the Y chromosome containing the *SRY* gene translocated to the paternal X chromosome. This Y chromosome material undergoing the X–Y interchange is not always cytogenetically visible, but can be detected with the use of FISH using Yp DNA probes. In a few cases of Y-positive 46,XX males, cryptic mosaicism (46,XX/47,XXY) may occur in which the Y has been lost in most cells but is present at least in the Sertoli cells.[220]

At least 10 percent of 46,XX males do not have the *SRY* gene translocated, and hence they are Y-negative.[221] These males are more likely to have genital abnormalities along with infertility. Their sex reversal is thought to be due to an autosomal or X-chromosomal gene mutation. Others with 46,XX who are negative for Y sequences are true hermaphrodites with ambiguous genitalia, dysgenetic gonads or ovotestes, and occasional müllerian duct remnants (see "46,XX True Hermaphrodites" below). It has been postulated that Y-negative males and XX true hermaphrodites have a common origin.[222–225] A 46,XX male with velocardiofacial syndrome (22q11.2 microdeletion) has been reported with no Y DNA detected by PCR testing of twenty-four distinct loci spanning the Y chromosome.[226] No previous cases of velocardiofacial syndrome and sex reversal have been described.[226]

It is important that all fetuses diagnosed prenatally have an ultrasound performed between the 18th and 20th week to determine whether the image of the genitals is appropriate for the fetal karyotype. If a discrepancy between fetal chromosomal sex and the ultrasound image of male genitals exists, the parents need to be informed of the above possibilities. A further consideration in the differential diagnosis would be the adrenogenital syndrome, in which 46,XX females may have masculinized external genitalia.

Genetic counseling for parents of a 46,XX male fetus is dependent on the presence or absence of Y chromosomal material.

For 46,XX males who are Y-positive:

1. The prognosis is that given for Klinefelter syndrome.
2. Recurrence risk is unlikely since a Y-to-X translocation or XX/XXY mosaicism is considered a sporadic occurrence.

For 46,XX males who are Y negative:

1. The possibility of genital abnormalities, need for surgical repair, and probable infertility should be discussed.
2. A pelvic ultrasound should be performed in the first 2 years to rule out gonadal

abnormalities. If intra-abdominal ovotestes are found, a gonadectomy should be considered. If no gonadal dysgenesis is found, the testes should be examined and surveillance continued through puberty, monitoring for signs of malignancy.

3. There is an increased risk for gynecomastia.
4. Recurrence risk is significant. It can be as high as 25–50 percent for familial cases.

45,X MALES

In the relatively few cases seen, 45,X males have been Y-positive through the translocation of SRY to an autosome, a mechanism different from the usual X–Y interchange in 46,XX males.[227] These males have small testes and are sterile. They may have other congenital anomalies, depending on the loss of autosomal material at the site of the translocation.

47,XXX MALES

47,XXX males are very rare and probably arise from an abnormal X–Y interchange occurring either during or before paternal meiosis with the addition of maternal X–X nondisjunction.[228] In the two cases reported, the phenotype is that of a normal male.[228] Infertility is expected because gonadal biopsies revealed testicular dysgenesis. In one case, DNA from Yp containing the testis determining factor was present, but Yq location of the gene for spermatogenesis was missing. The older of the two males with a 47,XXX karyotype showed a phenotype similar to that of Klinefelter syndrome. A 53-year-old male with complex mosaicism for 45,X/46,XX/47,XXX/48,XXXX with between zero and two copies of SRY in each cell line has been reported.[229] His clinical features included hypoplastic scrotal testes, normally formed small penis, scant pubic hair, gynecomastia, age-appropriate male height, and mental retardation (verbal IQ of 56).

46,XY FEMALES

The absence of male genitalia on ultrasound examination of a 46,XY fetus suggests the existence of a 46,XY female. There are at least five differential diagnoses possible, most of which include dysgenetic gonads, infertility, and an increased risk for the development of gonadoblastoma.

Androgen Insensitivity Syndrome or Testicular Feminizing Syndrome

The molecular basis of androgen insensitivity in the majority of cases has been elucidated.[230,231] The most common explanation for a 46,XY female is the androgen insensitivity syndrome, formerly called the testicular feminizing syndrome. This is an X-linked recessive inborn error of metabolism caused by a mutation in the androgen receptor gene located at Xq11–12.[232] It is a form of male pseudohermaphroditism in which female external genitalia are present with a normal male karyotype. It exists in two forms, complete and incomplete (partial and mild).

In the complete form, the phenotype is feminine with female external genitalia, a vagina that is short and ends blindly,[233] and breast development at puberty. Typically, there is no uterus or cervix. Axillary and pubic hair are scanty or absent. The internal genitalia consist of testes that are inguinal, intra-abdominal, or labial. MRI can be used to locate the undescended testes and confirm uterine agenesis in these cases.[234] These individuals are at an increased risk for malignant transformation of the gonads, but the risk for neoplasia is low before 25 years of age.[235] The current recommendation is to the leave the testes in place to allow for spontaneous puberty and then to remove them after breast development is complete. Estrogen supplementation is necessary after the gonadectomy. There is feminine psychosocial orientation, and intelligence is normal. Affected 46,XY fetuses can be diagnosed by androgen-receptor studies of cells from amniotic fluid or through molecular analysis of the gene. Variable expressivity in this condition has been documented because of the somatic mosaicism of androgen receptor mutations.[236]

In the incomplete form of androgen insensitivity syndrome, there is partial impairment of the androgen-receptor function. The phenotype is predominantly female with clitoromegaly and a short, blind-ending vagina. At puberty, there is less breast development than in the complete form and there may be partial virilization. In these cases, the testes in the abdomen or inguinal canal are removed before puberty and estrogen supplementation is begun at the age of normal puberty.[237]

Other forms of incomplete androgen insensitivity produce a more masculine phenotype. These include Reifenstein syndrome and several other forms of underdeveloped males.

Swyer Syndrome or Complete Gonadal Dysgenesis

Male pseudohermaphroditism can also be a result of 46,XY gonadal dysgenesis, commonly known as Swyer syndrome. The complete form is termed 46,XY pure gonadal dysgenesis. These patients have a female phenotype with degeneration of the ovaries and poorly developed secondary sexual characteristics. The gonads are fibrous streaks containing no follicles or normal germ cells. There is a high risk for gonadoblastoma developing, and thus, a gonadectomy is warranted at the time of diagnosis. The internal organs consist of bilateral fallopian tubes, a uterus, and a vagina. Females with Swyer syndrome are of normal to tall stature without somatic Turner syndrome anomalies. These females are a result of submicroscopic mutations or deletions in the *SRY* gene on Yp.[238–240] Recurrence risk is low as familial mutations are rarely described.[241] Successful pregnancies in 46,XY women with gonadal dysgenesis using ovum or embryo donations have been described.[242,243]

Another form of Swyer syndrome is gonadal dysgenesis in which the Y chromosome is intact. It is speculated that these 46,XY females are the result of mutations in autosomal or X-linked genes involved in sex determination.[238,244] Autosomal dominant inheritance has been described in a large family with 46,XY gonadal dysgenesis.[245] The recurrence risk for this form of gonadal dysgenesis is up to 50 percent because it segregates in a pattern consistent with male limited autosomal dominant conditions.

Mixed Gonadal Dysgenesis or 46,XY Partial Gonadal Dysgenesis

A 46,XY female can also be a result of mixed gonadal dysgenesis, also called 46,XY partial gonadal dysgenesis.[246] These individuals are characterized by a female Turner phenotype and ambiguous external genitalia with hypertrophy of the clitoris. There is virilization at puberty. The gonads are intra-abdominal and asymmetric, with a streak gonad on one side and a dysgenetic testicle on the other side.[247] As with all forms of gonadal dysgenesis and the presence of Y chromosomal material, the risk for gonadal neoplasia is high. The gonads should be removed as soon after diagnosis as possible.

5α-Reductase Deficiency

5α-Reductase deficiency, formerly called pseudovaginal perineoscrotal hypospadias, is an autosomal recessive disorder that produces female external genitalia at birth in the presence of a 46,XY normal male karyotype. It is a result of a deficiency of the enzyme that converts testosterone to an active form during fetal development. The gonads are normal male, and virilization occurs at puberty. No gynecomastia is present and no testicular neoplasia has been reported. Phenotypic variation has been reported and correlated with different mutations in the 5α-reductase gene that result in partially functional enzymes.[248] Most of these males have been raised as females, and there is a gender identity change at puberty from female to male. Phenotypes with ambiguous genitalia or undermasculinization have also been reported.[249]

True Hermaphroditism

About 20 percent of true hermaphrodites have a 46,XY karyotype, and in one-third of these cases, the genitals present as female. The gonads contain both male and female structures. Development of secondary sex characteristics may be incomplete and hypertrophy of the clitoris may occur. A gonadectomy is advised (see True Hermaphroditism section).

Other Sex Reversal Syndromes

Several other genetic syndromes are associated with a female phenotype in the presence of a 46,XY karyotype. When Xp21 is duplicated, sex reversal occurs in conjunction with multiple congenital abnormalities and mental retardation (see "Xp Duplication" above). This is thought to be due to an additional copy of the DSS (dosage-sensitive sex reversal) gene. The *Dax1* gene has been implicated as being responsible for the dosage-sensitive sex reversal.[250,251] Campomelic dwarfism is a lethal bone and cartilage malformation present at birth that often presents with sex reversal. This disorder is caused by a mutation in an SRY-related gene known as SOX9 located on chromosome 17q.[252,253] An individual with Denys–Drash syndrome presents as a phenotypically normal 46,XY female in whom progressive neuropathy and Wilms tumor develop.[254] Smith–Lemli–Opitz syndrome,[255] chromosome 9p deletions,[256] 10q deletions,[257] and some rare autosomal recessive disorders[258] have been associated with sex reversal in some cases.

TRUE HERMAPHRODITISM

True hermaphroditism is a rare condition in which both male and female tissues are present in the gonads of an individual. The presence of undifferentiated tissue or gonadal stroma is insufficient to diagnose this condition. Follicles, as well as seminiferous tubules, must be clearly identifiable. Patients are subclassified into categories according to the type and location of the gonads: unilateral (an ovotestis on one side and a testis or ovary on the other); lateral (a testis on one side and an ovary on the other); or bilateral (ovotestis on both sides). The positions of the gonads are pelvic or abdominal, inguinal, or labioscrotal.

True hermaphroditism is genetically heterogeneous.[259] The karyotype may be 46,XX (70 percent); 46,XX/46,XY (20 percent); or 46,XY (10 percent).[260,261] The 46,XX cases have no detectable Y chromosomal material, making this condition distinct from the more common 46,XX males. However, low level cryptic mosaicism for Y-derived sequences including SRY has been documented.[262] Because there have been several instances of 46,XX true hermaphrodites and 46,XX males existing in the same pedigree, it has been hypothesized that these disorders may have a common genetic basis.[221–224]

The 46,XX/46,XY karyotype, known as chimerism, is the occurrence of two or more genotypes from different zygotes existing in the same individual. It is either dispermic or tetragametic. When both 46,XX and 46,XY cells are diagnosed prenatally, it is essential to rule out maternal cell contamination in the amniotic fluid of a male fetus. A careful ultrasound can confirm the presence of male genitalia. Further examination by fetal blood sampling may be considered (see chapter 2).

The external genitalia of true hermaphrodites are most often ambiguous but can vary from almost normal female to almost normal male. Internally, müllerian and wolffian derivatives usually coexist. Breast development occurs at puberty, and virilization may also occur. There may be incomplete development of the secondary sex characteristics. Menarche occurs in over half of true hermaphrodites. The ovarian tissue is usually composed of normal follicles and can be functional, whereas the testes are histologically abnormal, containing only Sertoli cells without evidence of spermatogenesis. Pregnancies have been reported in some females (most of whom were 46,XX),[263,264] but male fertility is reduced. Stature is normal (female), and intelligence is normal.

Gender assignment is usually made shortly after birth, when cytogenetic, hormonal, and histologic evaluations have been completed. It is recommended that reconstructive surgery occur by 2 years of age. A gonadectomy should be performed to remove all gonadal tissue that is inappropriate for the assigned sex.[265] If the remaining gonadal tissue is dysgenetic, there is an increased risk for malignancy and it too should be removed. Hormonal supplementation usually begins in both sexes at the time of puberty.

In prenatal counseling of true hermaphrodites, the issue of intersexuality must be discussed to include the possibility of surgical repair of the genitalia, potential for gonadal malignancy, and probable infertility. It is possible that this condition may be milder when diagnosed in utero than when ascertained after birth. There has been at least one report of a phenotypically normal prenatally diagnosed XX/XY chimera[266] and one prenatal report of a 46,XX/47,XXY male with hypospadias and testicular tissue with no evidence of ovarian components.[267]

The recurrence risk of true hermaphroditism varies. Chimerism is rare and the recurrence risk is small. In the case of 46,XX or 46,XY karyotypes, the mechanism responsible for abnormal development is not known. Because it is possible that this may be caused by autosomal recessive inheritance, the recurrence risk could be as high as 25 percent.

CONCLUSION

With the cytogenetic breakthrough in 1956, when Tjio and Levan first demonstrated that the diploid number of human chromosomes was 46 and not 48, as previously believed, a series of studies ensued with the discovery of individuals with chromosomal abnormalities. The suspicion that abnormalities of the sex chromosomes were associated with behavioral abnormality led to a series of chromosome screening studies in mental and penal institutions during the early 1960s in which captive populations were required to participate in a relatively simple chromosome analysis involving a quick scraping of buccal mucosa, with anomalies confirmed by subsequent chromosome analysis. Over 100 such studies of adult groups were conducted, most in the United States, the United Kingdom, and Europe. The incidence of 47,XXY men and 47,XXX women was found to be fourfold to fivefold greater in mentally retarded, imprisoned felons or psychotic groups, than the background incidence in the newborn population.[268] Among prison populations, an increased representation of men with SCAs, particularly 47,XYY, was reported.[23] Although these studies of institutionalized populations marked an important first step toward understanding the influence of sex chromosomes on behavior, their results were frequently misinterpreted. The several hundred subjects represented in these studies actually comprised less than 1 percent of all living individuals with SCAs and provided no information or consideration of the other 99 percent, many of whom were undoubtedly more "normal." Nonetheless, the information from these skewed studies led to a series of stereotypes in which 47,XXX women were viewed as psychotic, 47,XXY men were considered mentally retarded and prone to homosexuality, and 47,XYY men were described as overly aggressive "super males."[269]

Results from unselected newborn studies over the past 25 years have provided a more balanced picture of the behavioral adaptation of individuals with sex chromosome abnormalities. These prospective studies of individuals identified at birth with sex chromosome abnormalities have replaced the biased literature.[6–9] In this chapter, emphasis has been given to these studies over individual case reports, although our understanding of individuals with more than one additional chromosome or rare structural abnormalities is primarily limited to the latter.

Genetic counseling of couples carrying a fetus with an SCA must take into consideration the possibility that the couple have acquired some of the early, distorted literature or have received advice from a professional who is unfamiliar with more recent studies. While the frequency of prenatal diagnosis of SCAs (1 in 250) warrants discussion in preamniocentesis or pre-CVS counseling, too often parents have received no information about this possibility and have never heard of these conditions. In many cases, both the expectant parents and genetic counselors are unprepared for their occurrence, and a flurry of activity follows the diagnosis, during which both parents and counselors search for information about these conditions. These are the circumstances, unfortunately, under which distorted information is first encountered and subsequently provided to the parents. In general, it is best that parents be counseled by geneticists and genetic counselors who are responsible for understanding the complex literature about individuals with SCAs. A significant correlation has been found between the decision to continue a pregnancy and the type of SCA and the presence of fetal abnormalities on ultrasound.[270] In addition, more recently, a significant trend has been observed with a higher rate of pregnancy continuation.[270]

When the decision to continue the pregnancy is made, parents often request more information concerning anticipatory guidance, as well as about disclosure to the child and to others.[271] References that are appropriate for parents include several publications and booklets about the most common types of SCAs.[10,271,272] The question of whether to join a support group is often raised. In general, support groups are often helpful when a specific problem is encountered or when additional information is needed. Families with a fetal diagnosis of an SCA generally do not need such support because their child is at risk for developmental problems that may or may not occur.

Individual characteristics and risks are associated with each primary SCA. Nonetheless, general conclusions about these conditions can be drawn and are offered here as a final summary:

1. Given the great phenotypic variability of individuals with SCA, it is difficult to offer an accurate prognosis—prenatal or postnatal—for this group of disorders.
2. Mental retardation is not characteristic of the common SCA, although IQ in general is slightly diminished. Mental retardation is associated with only some SCAs, but cognitive problems are common.

3. Parents who elect to continue a pregnancy should realize that their child will be at an increased risk for some developmental problems of unpredictable severity.

4. The neurocognitive and behavioral problems of this group are not unique to them, and their management is the same as for a euploid individual with the same problems.

5. The environment in which these children grow is of great importance, because children with SCAs appear more vulnerable to a stressful and unsupportive family environment.

ACKNOWLEDGMENT

My thanks are due to the late Arthur Robinson, M.D., who pioneered so much of this work, and to Mary G. Linden, M.S., and Bruce G. Bender, Ph.D., who joined him in contributions to the chapter in the previous edition, on which this updated chapter is largely based.

REFERENCES

1. Ferguson-Smith MA, Yates JRW. Maternal age specific rates for chromosome aberrations and factors influencing them: report of a collaborative European study on 52,965 amniocenteses. Prenat Diagn 1984;4 (special issue):5.
2. Hsu LYF. Prenatal diagnosis of chromosome abnormalities through amniocentesis. In: Milunsky A, ed. Genetic disorders and the fetus, 4th ed. Baltimore: Johns Hopkins University Press, 1998:179.
3. Lockwood DH, Neu RL. Cytogenetic analysis of 1375 amniotic fluid specimens from pregnancies with gestational age less than 14 weeks. Prenat Diagn 1993;13:801.
4. Hook EB, Cross PK, Jackson L, et al. Maternal age-specific rates of 47,121 and other cytogenetic abnormalities diagnosed in the first trimester of pregnancy in chorionic villus biopsy specimens: Comparison with rates expected from observations at amniocentesis. Am J Hum Genet 1988;42:797.
5. Tabor A, Philip J. Incidence of fetal chromosome abnormalities in 2264 low-risk women. Prenat Diagn 1987;7:355.
6. Robinson A, Lubs HA, Bergsma D. Sex chromosome aneuploidy: prospective studies on children. Birth Defects 1979;15(1).
7. Stewart DA. Children with sex chromosome aneuploidy: follow-up studies. Birth Defects 1982;18(4).
8. Ratcliffe SG, Paul N. Prospective studies on children with sex chromosome aneuploidy. Birth Defects 1986;22(3).
9. Evans JA, Hamerton JL, Robinson A. Children and young adults with sex chromosome aneuploidy. Birth Defects 1990;26(4).
10. Linden MG, Bender BG, Robinson A. Intrauterine diagnosis of sex chromosome aneuploidy. Obstet Gynecol 1996;87:468.
11. Saenger P. The current status of diagnosis and therapeutic intervention in Turner's syndrome. J Clin Endocrinol Metab 1993;77:297.
12. Zinn AR, Page DC, Fisher EMC. Turner syndrome: the case of the missing sex chromosome. Trends Genet 1993;9:90.
13. Rosenfeld RG, Tesch L-G, Rodriguez-Rigau LJ, et al. Recommendations for diagnosis, treatment, and management of individuals with Turner syndrome. Endocrinologist 1994;4:351.
14. Committee on Genetics. Health supervision for children with Turner syndrome. Pediatrics 1995;96:1166.
15. Saenger P, Wikland KA, Conway GS, et al. Recommendations for the diagnosis and management of Turner syndrome. J Clin Endocrinol Metab 2001;86:3061.
16. Page DC. Y chromosome sequences in Turner's syndrome and risk of gonadoblastoma or virilisation. Lancet 1994;343:240.
17. Rosenfeld RG, Frane J, Attie KM, et al. Six-year results of a randomized prospective trial of human growth hormone and oxandrolone in Turner syndrome. J Pediatr 1992;21:49.

18. Press F, Shapiro H, Cowell CA, et al. Outcome of ovum donation in Turner's syndrome patients. Fertil Steril 1995;64:995.

19. Birkebaek NH, Cruger D, Hansen J, et al. Fertility and pregnancy outcome in Danish women with Turner syndrome. Clin Genet 2002;61:35.

20. Swapp GH, Johnston AW, Watt JL, et al. A fertile women with non-mosaic Turner's syndrome: case report and review of the literature. Br J Obstet Gynecol 1989;96:876.

21. Hovatta O. Pregnancies in women with Turner's syndrome. Ann Med 1999;31:106.

22. Tarani L, Lampariello S, Raguso G, et al. Pregnancy in patients with Turner's syndrome: six new cases and review of literature. Gynecol Endocrinol 1998;12:83.

23. Sybert VP. Cardiovascular malformations and complications in Turner syndrome. Pediatrics 1998;101:E11.

24. Bilge I, Kayserili H, Emre S, et al. Frequency of renal malformations in Turner syndrome: analysis of 82 Turkish children. Pediatr Nephrol 2000;14:1111.

25. Elsheikh M, Wass JA, Conway GS. Autoimmune thyroid syndrome in women with Turner's syndrome: the association with karyotype. Clin Endocrinol 2001;55:223.

26. Gungor N, Boke B, Belgin E, et al. High frequency hearing loss in Ullrich–Turner syndrome. Eur J Pediatr 2000;159:740.

27. Bonamico M, Pasquino AM, Mariani P, et al. Prevalence and clinical picture of celiac disease in Turner syndrome. J Clin Endocrinol Metab 2002;87:5495.

28. Gravholt CH, Juul S, Naeraa RW, et al. Morbidity in Turner syndrome. J Clin Epidemiol 1998;51:147.

29. Salbenblatt JA, Meyers DC, Bender BG, et al. Gross and fine motor development in 45,X and 47,XXX females. Pediatrics 1989;84:678.

30. Bender B, Puck M, Salbenblatt J, et al. Cognitive development of unselected girls with complete and partial X monosomy. Pediatrics 1984;73:175.

31. Rovet JF. Psychological characteristics of children with Turner syndrome. Contemp Pediatr 1992;March/April:13.

32. Money J, Alexander D. Turner's syndrome: further demonstration of the presence of specific cognitional deficiencies. J Med Genet 1966;3:47.

33. Ross JL, Stefanatos G, Roeltgen D, et al. Ullrich–Turner syndrome: neurodevelopmental changes from childhood through adolescence. Am J Med Genet 1995;58:74.

34. Brown WE, Kesler SR, Eliez S, et al. Brain development in Turner syndrome: a magnetic resonance imaging study. Psychiatry Res 2002;116:187.

35. Hepworth SL, Rovet JF. Visual integration difficulties in a 9-year-old girl with Turner syndrome: parallel verbal disabilities? Neuropsychol Dev Cogn Sect C Child Neuropsychol 2000;6:262.

36. Berch D, Bender B. Turner's and other chromosomal syndromes. In: Yates KO, Ris MD, Taylor HG, eds. Pediatric neuropsychology: research, theory, and practice. New York: Guilford Press, 1999.

37. Ross JL, Stefanatos GA, Kushner H, et al. Persistent cognitive deficits in adult women with Turner syndrome. Neurology 2002;58:218.

38. McCauley E, Kay T, Eto J, et al. The Turner syndrome: cognitive deficits, affective discrimination and behavior problems. Child Dev 1987;58:464.

39. McCauley E, Ross JL, Kushner H, et al. Self-esteem and behavior in girls with Turner syndrome. Dev Behav Pediatr 1995;16:82.

40. Mazzocco MM, Baumgardner T, Freund LS, et al. Social functioning among girls with fragile X or Turner syndrome and their sisters. J Autism Dev Disord 1998,28:509.

40a. Prior TI, Chue PS, Tibbo P. Investigation of Turner syndrome in schizophrenia. Am J Med Genet 2000;96:373.

40b. Milunsky J, Huang XL, Wyandt HE, et al. Schizophrenia susceptibility gene locus at Xp22.3. Clin Genet 1999;55:455.

41. Rovet J, Ireland L. Behavioral phenotype in children with Turner syndrome. J Pediatr Psychol 1994;19:779.

42. McCauley E, Ito J, Kay T. Psychological functioning in girls with Turner syndrome and short stature. J Am Acad Child Psychiatry 1986;25:105.

43. McCauley E, Feuillan P, Kushner H, et al. Psychosocial development in adolescents with Turner syndrome. J Dev Behav Pediatr 2001;22:360.

44. Sybert VP. The adult patient with Turner syndrome. In: Albertsson-Wikland K, Ranke MB, eds. Turner syndrome in a life span perspective: research and clinical aspects. In: Proceedings of the 4th International Symposium on Turner Syndrome, Gothenburg, Sweden, May 18–21, 1995. Amsterdam: Elsevier, 1995:205.

45. Uematsu A, Yorifuji T, Muroi J, et al. Parental origin of normal X chromosomes in Turner syndrome pa-

tients with various karyotypes: implications for the mechanism leading to generation of a 45,X karyotype. Am J Med Genet 2002;111:134.

46. Melaragno MI, Fakih LMA, Cernach MCSP, et al. Isodicentric X chromosome and mosaicism: report on two cases of 45,X/46,X,idic(Xq)/47,X,idic(Xq),idic (Xq) and review of the literature. Am J Med Genet 1993;47:357.

47. Wolff DJ, Miller AP, Van Dyke DL, et al. Molecular definition of breakpoints associated with human Xq chromosomes: implications for mechanisms of formation. Am J Hum Genet 1996;58:154.

48. Jacobs PA, Betts PR, Cockwell AE, et al. A cytogenetic and molecular reappraisal of a series of patients with Turner syndrome. Ann Hum Genet 1990;54:209.

49. Sarto GE, Thurman E, Patau K. X-inactivation in man: a woman with t(Xq-;12q1). Am J Hum Genet 1973;25:262.

50. Therman E, Laxova R, Susman B. The critical region on the human Xq. Hum Genet 1990;85:455.

51. Geerkens C, Just W, Vogerl W. Deletions of Xq and growth deficit: a review. Am J Med Genet 1994;50:105.

52. Therman E, Susman B. The similarity of phenotypic effects caused by Xp and Xq deletions in the human female: a hypothesis. Hum Genet 1990;85:175.

53. Collins A, Cockwell AE, Jacobs PA, et al. A comparison of the clinical and cytogenetic findings in nine patients with a ring (X) cell line and 16 45,X patients. J Med Genet 1994;31:528.

54. Dennis N, Coppin B, Turner C, et al. A clinical, cytogenetic and molecular study of 47 females with r(X) chromosomes. Ann Hum Genet 2000;64:277.

55. Grompe M, Rao N, Elder FFB, et al. 45,X/46,X1r(X) can have a distinct phenotype different from Ullrich–Turner syndrome. Am J. Med Genet 1992;42:39.

56. Van Dyke DL, Wiktor A, Palmer CG, et al. Ullrich–Turner syndrome with a small ring X chromosome and presence of mental retardation. Am J Med Genet 1992;43:996.

57. Migeon BR, Luo S, Jani M, et al. The severe phenotype of females with tiny ring X chromosomes is associated with inability of these chromosomes to undergo X inactivation. Am J Hum Genet 1994;55:497.

58. Wolff DJ, Brown CJ, Schwartz S, et al. Small marker X chromosomes lack the X inactivation center: implications for karyotype/phenotype correlations. Am J Hum Genet 1994;55:87.

59. Matsuo M, Muroya K, Adachi M, et al. Clinical and molecular studies in 15 females with ring X chromosomes: implications for r(X) formation and mental development. Hum Genet 2000;107:433.

60. Leppig KA, Disteche CM. Ring X and other structural X chromosome abnormalities: X inactivation and phenotype. Semin Reprod Med 2001;19:147.

61. Koeberl DD, McGillivray B, Sybert VP. Prenatal diagnosis of 45,X/46,XX mosaicism and 45,X: implications for postnatal outcome. Am J Hum Genet 1995;57:661.

62. Devi AS, Metzger DA, Luciano AA, et al. 45,X/46,XX mosaicism in patients with idiopathic premature ovarian failure. Fertil Steril 1998;70:89.

63. Blair J, Tolmie J, Hollman AS, et al. Phenotype, ovarian function, and growth in patients with 45,X/47,XXX Turner mosaicism: implications for prenatal counseling and estrogen therapy at puberty. J Pediatr 2001;139:724.

64. Pettenati MJ, Wheeler M, Bartlett DJ, et al. 45,X/47,XYY mosaicism: clinical discrepancy between prenatally and postnatally diagnosed cases. Am J Med Genet 1991;39:42.

65. Chang HJ, Clark RD, Bachman H. The phenotype of 45,X/46,XY mosaicism: an analysis of 92 prenatally diagnosed cases. Am J Hum Genet 1990;46:156.

66. Hsu LYF. Prenatal diagnosis of 45,X/46,XY mosaicism: a review and update. Prenat Diagn 1989;9:31.

67. Wheeler M, Peakman D, Robinson A, et al. 45,X/46,XY mosaicism: Contrast of prenatal and postnatal diagnosis. Am J Med Genet 1988;29:565.

68. Telvi L, Lebbar A, Del Pino O, et al. 45,X/46,XY mosaicism: report of 27 cases. Pediatrics 1999;104:304.

69. Lau Y, Chou P, Iezzoni J, et al. Expression of a candidate gene for the gonadoblastoma locus in gonadoblastoma and testicular seminoma. Cytogenet Cell Genet 2000;91:160.

70. Muller J, Ritzen EM, Ivarsson SA, et al. Management of males with 45,X/46,XY gonadal dysgenesis. Horm Res 1999;52:11.

71. Kleczkowska A, Fryns JP, Van den Berghe H. X-chromosome polysomy in the male. Hum Genet 1988;80:16.

72. Jacobs PA, Hassold TJ. The origin of numerical chromosome abnormalities. Adv Genet 1995;33:101.

73. Lowe X, Eskenazi B, Nelson DO, et al. Frequency of XY sperm increases with age in fathers of boys with Klinefelter syndrome. Am J Hum Genet 2001;69:1046.

74. Salbenblatt JA, Bender BG, Puck MH, et al. Pituitary-gonadal function in Klinefelter syndrome before and during puberty. Pediatr Res 1985;19:82.

75. Schwartz JD, Root AW. The Klinefelter syndrome of testicular dysgenesis. Endocrinol Metab Clin North Am 1991;20:153.

76. Hasle H, Mellemgaard, Nielsen J, et al. Cancer incidence in men with Klinefelter syndrome. Br J Cancer 1995;71:416.

77. Price WH, Clayton JF, Wilson J, et al. Causes of death in X chromatin positive males (Klinefelter's syndrome). J Epidemiol Commun Health 1985;39:330.

78. Swerdlow AJ, Hermon C, Jacobs PA, et al. Mortality and cancer incidence in persons with numerical sex chromosome abnormalities: a cohort study. Ann Hum Genet 2001;65:177.

79. Hasle H, Jacobsen BB, Asschenfeldt P, et al. Mediastinal germ cell tumour associated with Klinefelter syndrome: a report of a case and review of the literature. Eur J Pediatr 1992;151:735.

80. Kurzrock EA, Tunuguntla HS, Busby JE, et al. Klinefelter's syndrome and precocious puberty: a harbinger for tumor. Urology 2002;60:514.

81. Bonduelle M, Camus M, DeVos A, et al. Seven years of intracytoplasmic sperm injection and follow-up of 1987 subsequent children. Hum Reprod 1999; Suppl 1:243.

81a. Bonduelle M, Liebaers I, Deketelaere V, et al. Neonatal data on a cohort of 2889 infants born after ICSI (1991–1999) and of 2995 infants born after IVF (1983–1999). Hum Reprod 2002;17:671.

81b. Hansen M, Kurinczuk JJ, Bower C, et al. The risk of major birth defects after intracytoplasmic sperm injection and in vitro fertilization. N Engl J Med 2002;346:725.

82. Sutcliffe AG, Taylor B, Saunders K, et al. Outcome in the second year of life after in-vitro fertilisation by intracytoplasmic sperm injection: a UK case-control study. Lancet 2001;357:2080.

83. Pinborg A, Loft A, Schmidt L, et al. Morbidity in a Danish National cohort of 472 IVF/ICSI twins, 1132 non-IVF/ICSI twins and 634 IVF/ICSI singletons: health-related and social implications for the children of their families. Hum Reprod 2003;18:1234.

83a. Ludwig M, Katalinic A. Pregnancy course and health of children born after ICSI depending on parameters of male factor infertility. Hum Reprod 2003;18:351.

84. Bonduelle M, Ponjaert I, Steirteghem Av, et al. Developmental outcome at 2 years of age for children born after ICSI compared with children born after IVF. Hum Reprod 2003;18:342.

84a. Bonduelle M, Van Assche E, Joris H, et al. Prenatal testing in ICSI pregnancies: incidence of chromosomal anomalies in 1586 karyotypes and relation to sperm parameters. Hum Reprod 2002;17:2600.

84b. Wennerholm UB, Bergh C, Hamberger L, et al. Incidence of congenital malformations in children born after ICSI. Hum Reprod 2000:15:944.

84c. Ericson A, Kallen B. Congenital malformations in infants born after IVF: a population-based study. Hum Reprod 2001;16:504.

85. Anthony S, Buitendijk SE, Dorrepaal CA, et al. Congenital malformations in 4224 children conceived after IVF. Hum Reprod 2002;17:2089.

85a. Cox GF, Burger J, Lip V, et al.. Intracytoplasmic sperm injection may increase the risk of imprinting defects. Am J Hum Genet 2002:71;162.

85b. Orstavik KH, Eiklid K, Van Der Hagen CB, et al. Another case of imprinting defect in a girl with Angelman syndrome who was conceived by intracytoplasmic sperm injection. Am J Hum Genet 2003;72;218.

85c. Gicquel C, Gaston V, Mandelbaum J, et al. In vitro fertilization may increase the risk of Beckwith–Wiedemann syndrome related to the abnormal imprinting of the KCNQ1OT gene. Am J Hum Genet 2003;72:1338.

85d. Maher ER, Brueton LA, Bowdin SC, et al. Beckwith–Wiedemann syndrome and assisted reproduction technology (ART). J Med Genet 2003; 40:62.

85e. Moll AC, Imhof SM, Cruysberg JR, et al. Incidence of retinoblastoma in children born after in-vitro fertilisation. Lancet 2003;361:309.

85f. Gosden R, Trasler J, Lucifero D, et al. Rare congenital disorders, imprinted genes, and assisted reproductive technology. Lancet 2003;361:1975.

85g. BenEzra D. In-vitro fertilisation and retinoblastoma. Lancet 2003;361:273.

85h. Moore LL, Bradlee ML, Singer MR, et al. Chromosomal anomalies among the offspring of women with gestational diabetes. Am J Epidemiol 2002;155:719.

86. Robinson A, Bender BG, Linden MG. Summary of clinical findings in children and young adults with sex chromosome anomalies. In: Evans JA, Hamerton JL, Robinson A, eds. Children and young adults with sex chromosome aneuploidy: follow-up, clinical, and molecular studies. Birth Defects 1990;26:225.

87. Bender B, Fry E, Pennington B, et al. Speech and language development of 41 children with sex chromosome anomalies. Pediatrics 1983;71:262.

88. Graham JM, Bashir AS, Stark RE, et al. Oral and written language abilities of XYY boys: implications for anticipatory guidance. Pediatrics 1988;81:795.

89. Bender BG, Linden M, Robinson A. Cognitive and academic skills in children with sex chromosome abnormalities. Read Writ 1991;3:127.

90. Bender BG, Linden MG, Robinson A. Neuropsychological impairment in 42 adolescents with sex chromosome abnormalities. Am J Med Genet 1993;48:169.

91. Mandoki MW, Sumner GS, Hoffman RP, et al. A review of Klinefelter's syndrome in children and adolescents. J Am Acad Child Adolesc Psychiatry 1991;30:167.

92. Geschwind DH, Boone KB, Miller BL, et al. Neurobehavioral phenotype of Klinefelter syndrome. Ment Retard Dev Disabil Res Rev 2000;6:107.

93. Boone KB, Swerdloff RS, Miller BL, et al. Neuropsychological profiles of adults with Klinefelter syndrome. J Int Neuropsychol Soc 2001;7:446.

94. Ratcliffe SG, Murray L, Teague P. Edinburgh study of growth and development of children with sex chromosome abnormalities III. Birth Defects Orig Artic Ser 1986;22:73.

95. Salbenblatt JA, Meyers DC, Bender BG, et al. Gross and fine motor development in 47,XXY and 47,XYY males. Pediatrics 1987;80:240.

96. Nielsen J, Sillesen I, Sorensen AM, et al. Follow-up until age 4 to 8 of 25 unselected children sex chromosome abnormalities, compared with sibs and controls. Birth Defects Orig Artic Ser 1979;15:15.

97. Bender BG, Harmon RJ, Linden MG, et al. Psychosocial adaptation of 39 adolescents with sex chromosome abnormalities. Pediatrics 1995;96:302.

98. Porter ME, Gardner HA, DeFeudis P, et al. Verbal deficits in Klinefelter (XXY) adults living in the community. Clin Genet 1998;33:246.

99. Sorensen K. Physical and mental development of adolescent males with Klinefelter syndrome. Horm Res 1992;37 (suppl 3):55.

100. Arps S, Koske-Westphal R, Meinecke P, et al. Isochromosome Xq in Klinefelter syndrome: report of 7 new cases. Am J Med Genet 1996;64:580.

101. Bertelloni S, Battini R, Baroncelli GI, et al. Central precocious puberty in 48,XXYY Klinefelter syndrome variant. J Pediatr Endocrinol Metab 1999;12:459.

102. Linden MG, Bender BG, Robinson A. Sex chromosome tetrasomy and pentasomy. Pediatrics 1995;96:672.

103. Peet J, Weaver DD, Vance GH. 49,XXXXY: a distinct phenotype: three new cases and review. J Med Genet 1998;35:420.

104. Sepulveda W, Ivankovic M, Be C, et al. Sex chromosome pentasomy (49,XXXXY) presenting as cystic hygroma at 16 weeks' gestation. Prenat Diagn 1999;19:257.

105. Schluth C, Doray B, Girard-Lemaire F, et al. Prenatal sonographic diagnosis of the 49,XXXXY syndrome. Prenat Diagn 2002;22:1177.

106. Sheridan MK, Radlinski SS. Brief report: a case study of an adolescent male with XXXXY Klinefelter's syndrome. J Autism Dev Disord 1988;18:449.

107. Sheridan MK, Radlinski SS, Kennedy MD. Developmental outcome in 49,XXXXY Klinefelter syndrome. Dev Med Child Neurol 1990;32:532.

108. Hersh JH, Bloom AS, Yen F, et al. Mild intellectual deficits in a child with 49,XXXXY. Res Dev Disabil 1988;9:171.

109. Lomelino CA, Reiss AL. 49,XXXXY syndrome: behavioural and developmental profiles. J Med Genet 1991;28:609.

110. Borghraef M, Fryns JP, Smeets J, et al. The 49,XXXXY syndrome: clinical and psychological follow-up data. Clin Genet 1988;33:429.

111. Holland CM. 47,XXX in an adolescent with premature ovarian failure and autoimmune disease. J Pediatr Adolesc Gynecol 2001;14:77.

112. Rovet J, Netley C. The triple X syndrome in childhood. Recent empirical findings. Child Dev 1983;54:831.

113. Netley C. Summary overview of behavioral development in individuals with neonatally identified X and Y aneuploidy. In: Ratcliffe SG, Paul N, eds. Prospective studies on children with sex chromosome aneuploidy. Birth Defects 1986;22:293.

114. Linden MG, Bender BG, Harmon RJ, et al. 47,XXX: What is the prognosis? Pediatrics 1988;82:619.

115. Bender BG, Linden MG, Harmon RJ. Neuropsychological and functional cognitive skills of 35 unselected adults with sex chromosome abnormalities. Am J Med Genet 2001;102:309.

116. Harmon RJ, Bender BG, Linden MG, et al. Transition from adolescence to early adulthood: adaptation and psychiatric status of women with 47,XXX. J Am Acad Child Adolesc Psychiatry 1998;37:286.

117. Neri G. A possible explanation for the low incidence of gonosomal aneuploidy among the offspring of triplo-X individuals. Am J Med Genet 1987;18:357.

118. Cammarata M, Di Simone P, Graziano L, et al. Rare sex chromosome aneuploidies in humans: report of six patients with 48,XXYY, 49,XXXXY, and 48,XXXX karyotypes. Am J Med Genet 1999;85:86.

119. Rooman RP, Van Driessche K, Du Caju MV. Growth and ovarian function in girls with 48,XXXX karyotype: patient report and review of the literature. J Pediatr Endocrinol Metab 2002;15:1051.

120. Blackston RD, Grinzaid KS, Saxe DF. Reproduction in 48,XXXX women. Am J Med Genet 1994;52:379.

121. Kassai R, Hamada I, Furuta H, et al. Penta X syndrome: a case report with review of the literature. Am J Med Genet 1991;40:51.

122. Robinson DO, Jacobs PA. The origin of the extra Y chromosome in males with a 47,XYY karyotype. Hum Mol Genet 1999;8:2205.

123. Hook EB. Extra sex chromosomes and human behavior: the nature of the evidence regarding XYY, XXY, XXYY, and XXX genotypes. In: Vallet HL, Porter IY, eds. Genetic aspects of sexual differentiation. New York: Academic Press, 1979:437.

124. Bender B, Puck M, Salbenblatt J, et al. The development of four unselected 47,XYY boys. Clin Genet 1984;25:435.

125. Nicolson R, Bhalerao S, Sloman L. 47,XYY karyotypes and pervasive developmental disorders. Can J Psychiatry 1998;43:619.

126. Gotz MJ, Johnstone EC, Ratcliffe SG. Criminality and antisocial behaviour in unselected men with sex chromosome abnormalities. Psychol Med 1999;29:953.

127. Venkataraman G, Craft I. Triple-Y syndrome following ICSI treatment in a couple with normal chromosomes: case report. Hum Reprod 2002;17:2560.

128. Shanske A, Sachmechi I, Patel DK, et al. An adult with 49,XYYY karyotype: case report and endocrine studies. Am J Med Genet 1998;80:103.

129. DesGroseilliers M, Lemyre E, Dallaire L, et al. Tetrasomy Y by structural rearrangement: clinical report. Am J Med Genet 2002;111:401.

130. Das GP, Shukla A, Verma IC. Phenotype of 49,XXYY. Clin Genet 1993;43:196.

131. Schwinger E, Kirchstein M, Greiwe M, et al. Short stature in a mother and daughter with terminal deletion of Xp22.3. Am J Med Genet 1996;63:239.

132. Bick DP, Schorderet DF, Price PA, et al. Prenatal diagnosis and investigation of a fetus with chondrodysplasia punctata, ichthyosis, and Kallmann syndrome due to an Xp deletion. Prenat Diagn 1992;12:19.

133. Meindl A, Hosenfeld D, Bruckl W, et al. Analysis of a terminal Xp22.3 deletion in a patient with six monogenic disorders: Implications for the mapping of X linked ocular albinism. J Med Genet 1993;30:838.

134. Weissortel R, Strom TM, Dorr HG, et al. Analysis of an interstitial deletion in a patient with Kallmann syndrome, X-linked ichthyosis and mental retardation. Clin Genet 1998;54:45.

135. Bates A, Howard PJ. Distal long arm deletions of the X chromosome and ovarian failure. J Med Genet 1990;27:722.

136. Marozzi A, Manfredini E, Tibiletti MG, et al. Molecular definition of Xq common-deleted region in patients affected by premature ovarian failure. Hum Genet 2000;107:304.

137. Wells S, Mould S, Robins D, et al. Molecular and cytogenetic analysis of a familial microdeletion of Xq. J Med Genet 1991;28:163.

138. May M, Colleaux L, Murgia A, et al. Molecular analysis of four males with mental retardation and deletions of Xq21 places the putative MR region in Xq21.1 between DXS233 and CHM. Hum Mol Genet 1995;4:1465.

139. Jonsson J, Renieri A, Gallagher P, et al. Alport syndrome, mental retardation, midface hypoplasia, and elliptocytosis: a new X-linked contiguous gene deletion syndrome? J Med Genet 1998;35:273.

140. Wyandt HE, Grierson HL, Sanger WG, et al. Chromosome deletion of Xq25 in an individual with X-linked lymphoproliferative disease. Am J Med Genet 1989;33:426.

141. Ferrero GB, Gebbia M, Pilia G, et al. A submicroscopic deletion in Xq26 associated with familial situs ambiguus. Am J Hum Genet 1997;61:395.

142. Bartsch O, Kress W, Wagner A, et al. The novel contiguous gene syndrome of myotubular myopathy (MTM1), male hypogenitalism and deletion in Xq28: report of the first familial case. Cytogenet Cell Genet 1999;85:310.

143. Baumstark A, Barbi G, Djalali M, et al. Xp-duplications with and without sex reversal. Hum Genet 1996;97:79.

144. Zhang A, Weaver DD, Palmer CG. Molecular cytogenetic identification of four X chromosome duplications. Am J Med Genet 1997;68:29.

145. Vasquez AI, Rivera H, Mayorquin A, et al. Sex reversal due to Xp disomy by t(X;Y)(p21;q11). Genet Couns 1999;10:301.

146. Tuck-Miller CM, Martinez JE, Batista DAS, et al. Duplication of the short arm of the X chromosome in mother and daughter. Hum Genet 1993;91:395.

147. Thode A, Parrington MW, Yip M-Y, et al. A new syndrome of mental retardation, short stature and an Xq duplication. Am J Med Genet 1988;30:239.

148. Rao PN, Klinepeter K, Stewart W, et al. Molecular cytogenetic analysis of a duplication Xp in a male: further delineation of a possible sex influencing region on the X chromosome. Hum Genet 1994;94:149.

149. Aughton DJ, AlSaadi AA, Johnson JA, et al. Dir dup(X)(q13-qter) in a girl with growth retardation, microcephaly, developmental delay, seizures, and minor anomalies. Am J Med Genet 1993;46:159.

150. Armstrong L, McGowan-Jordan J, Brierley K, et al. De novo dup(X)(q22.3q26) in a girl with evidence that functional disomy of X material is the cause of her abnormal phenotype. Am J Med Genet 2003;116A:71.

151. Jalal SM, Dahl R, Erickson L, et al. Cytogenetic and clinical characteristics of a case involving complete duplication of XpterRXq13. J Med Genet 1996;33:237.

152. Dalton P, Coppin B, James R, et al. Three patients with a 45,X/46,X,psu dic (Xp) karyotype. J Med Genet 1998;35:519.

153. Uehara S, Hanew K, Harada N, et al. Isochromosome consisting of terminal short arm and proximal long arm X in a girl with short stature. Am J Med Genet 2001;99:196.

154. Cole H, Huang B, Salbert BA, et al. Mental retardation and Ullrich-Turner syndrome in cases with 45,X/46,X,+mar: additional support for the loss of the X-inactivation center hypothesis. Am J Med Genet 1994;52:136.

155. Callen DF, Eyre HJ, Dolman G, et al. Molecular cytogenetic characterization of a small ring X chromosome in a Turner patient and in a male patient with congenital abnormalities: role of X inactivation. J Med Genet 1995;32:113.

156. Brothman AR, Newlin A, Phillips SE, et al. Prenatal detection of an inverted X chromosome in a male. Clin Genet 1993;44:139.

157. Abeliovich D, Dagan J, Kimchi-Sarfaty C, et al. Paracentric inversion X(q21.2q24) associated with mental retardation in males and normal ovarian function in females. Am J Med Genet 1995;55:359.

158. Pettenati MJ, Rao PN, Phelan MC, et al. Paracentric inversions in humans: a review of 446 paracentric inversions with presentation of 120 new cases. Am J Med Genet 1995;55:171.

159. Sloan-Bena F, Philippe C, LeHeup B, et al. Characterization of an inverted X chromosome (p11.2q21.3) associated with mental retardation using FISH. J Med Genet 1998;35:146.

160. Sivak LE, Esbenshade J, Brothman AR, et al. Multiple congenital anomalies in a man with (X;6) translocation. Am J Med Genet 1994;51:9.

161. Schmidt M, Du Sart D. Functional disomies of the X chromosome influence the cell selection and hence the X inactivation pattern in females with balanced X-autosome translocations: a review of 122 cases. Am J Med Genet 1992;42:161.

162. Preis W, Barbi G, Liptay S, et al. X/autosome translocation in three generations ascertained through an infant with trisomy 16p due to failure of spreading of X-inactivation. Am J Med Genet 1996;61:117.

163. Waters JJ, Campbell PL, Crocker AJ, et al. Phenotypic effects of balanced X-autosome translocations in females: a retrospective survey of 104 cases reported from UK laboratories. Hum Genet 2001;108:318.

164. Mattei MG, Mattei JF, Ayme S, et al. X-autosome translocation: cytogenetic characteristics and their consequences. Hum Genet 1982;61:295.

165. Liu J. Balanced X;3 translocation associated with gonadal dysgenesis: clinical report and a review. Am J Med Genet 1991;40:121.

166. Prueitt RL, Chen H, Barnes RI, et al. Most X;autosome translocations associated with premature ovarian failure do not interrupt X-linked genes. Cytogenet Genome Res 2002;97:32.

167. Summitt RL, Tipton RE, Wilroy RS, et al. X-autosome translocations: a review. Birth Defects Orig Artic Ser 1978;14:219.

168. Mossman J, Blunt S, Stephens R, et al. Hunter's disease in a girl: association with X:5 chromosomal translocation disrupting the Hunter gene. Arch Dis Child 1983;58:911.

169. Boyd Y, Buckle V, Holt S, et al. Muscular dystrophy in girls with X;autosome translocations. J Med Genet 1986;23:484.

170. Verga V, Hall BK, Wang S, et al. Localization of the translocation breakpoint in a female with Menkes syndrome to Xq13.2–q13.3 proximal to PGK-1. Am J Hum Genet 1991;48:1133.

171. Madan K. Balanced structural changes involving the human X: effect on sexual phenotype. Hum Genet 1983;63:216.

172. Kalz-Fuller B, Sleegers E, Schwanitz G, et al. Characterization, phenotypic manifestations and X-inactivation pattern in 14 patients with X-autosome translocations. Clin Genet 1999;55:362.

173. Sharp AJ, Spotswood HT, Robinson RO, et al. Molecular and cytogenetic analysis of the spreading of X inactivation in X;autosome translocations. Hum Mol Genet 2002;11:3145.

174. Nothwang HG, Schroer A, van der Maarel S, et al. Molecular cloning of Xp11 breakpoints in two unrelated mentally retarded females with X;autosome translocations. Cytogenet Cell 2000;90:126.

175. Kulharya AS, Roop H, Kukolich MK, et al. Mild phenotypic effects of a de novo deletion Xpter-Xp22.3 and duplication 3pter-33p23. Am J Med Genet 1995;45:16.

176. Letterie GS. Unique unbalanced X;X translocation (Xp22;p11.2) in a woman with primary amenorrhea but without Ullrich-Turner syndrome. Am J Med Genet 1995;59:414.

177. Marozzi A, Manfredini E, Tibiletti MG, et al. Molecular definition of Xq common-deleted region in patients affected by premature ovarian failure. Hum Genet 2000;107:304.

178. Epstein CJ. Mechanisms leading to the phenotype of Turner syndrome. In: Rosenfeld RG, Grumbach MM, eds. Turner syndrome. New York: Marcel Dekker, 1990:13.

179. Hsu LYF. Phenotype/karyotype correlations of Y chromosome aneuploidy with emphasis on structural aberrations in postnatally diagnosed cases. Am J Med Genet 1994;53:108.

180. Podruch PE, Yen F-S, Dinno ND, et al. Yq− in a child with livedo reticularis, snub nose, microcephaly, and profound mental retardation. J Med Genet 1982;19:377.

181. Salo P, Kaarianinen H, Page DC, et al. Deletion mapping of stature determinants on the long arm of the Y chromosome. Hum Genet 1995;95:283.

182. Kirsch S, Weiss B, Schon K, et al. The definition of the Y chromosome growth-control gene (GCY) critical region: relevance of terminal and interstitial deletions. J Pediatr Endocrinol Metab 2002;5:1295.

183. Reijo R, Alagappan RK, Patrizio P, et al. Severe oligozoospermia resulting from deletions of azoospermia factor gene on Y chromosome. Lancet 1996;347:1290.

184. Pryor JL, Kent-First M, Muallem A, et al. Microdeletions in the Y chromosome of infertile men. N Engl J Med 1997;336:534.

185. Simoni M. Molecular diagnosis of Y chromosome microdeletions in Europe: state-of-the-art and quality control. Hum Reprod 2001;16:402.

186. Pieri Pde C, Pereira DH, Glina S, et al. A cost-effective screening test for detecting AZF microdeletions on the human Y chromosome. Genet Test 2002;6:185.

187. Cram DS, Ma K, Bhasin S, et al. Y chromosome analysis of infertile men and their sons conceived through intracytoplasmic sperm injection: vertical transmission of deletions and rarity of de novo deletions. Fertil Steril 2000;74:909.

188. Patsalis PC, Sismani C, Quintana-Murci L, et al. Effects of transmission of Y chromosome AZFc deletions. Lancet 2002;360:1222.

189. Robinson DO, Dalton P, Jacobs PA, et al. A molecular and FISH analysis of structurally abnormal Y chromosomes in patients with Turner syndrome. J Med Genet 1999;36:279.

190. Tuck-Miller CM, Chen H, Martinez JE, et al. Isodicentric Y chromosome: cytogenetic, molecular, and clinical studies and review of the literature. Hum Genet 1995;96:119.

191. Giltay JC, Ausems MG, van Seumeren I, et al. Short stature as the only presenting feature in a patient with an isodicentric (Y)(q11.23) and gonadoblastoma: a clinical and molecular cytogenetic study. Eur J Pediatr 2001;160:154.

192. Stankiewicz P, Helias-Rodzewicz Z, Jakubow-Durska K, et al. Cytogenetic and molecular characterization of two isodicentric Y chromosomes. Am J Med Genet 2001;101:20.

193. Hernando C, Carrera M, Ribas I, et al. Prenatal and postnatal characterization of Y chromosome structural anomalies by molecular cytogenetic analysis. Prenat Diagn 2002;22:802.

194. Morava E, Hermann R, Czako M, et al. Isodicentric Y chromosome in an Ullrich–Turner patient without virilization. Am J Med Genet 2000;91:99.

195. Allanson JE, Graham GE. Sex chromosome abnormalities. In: Emery and Rimoin's principles and practice of medical genetics, vol. 1, 4th ed. New York: Churchill Livingstone, 2002:1184.

196. Pohlschmidt M, Rappold G, Krause M, et al. Ring Y chromosome: molecular characterization by DNA probes. Cytogenet Cell Genet 1991;56:65.

197. Yaron Y, Carmon E, Goldstein M, et al. The clinical application of spectral karyotyping (SKY trade mark) in the analysis of prenatally diagnosed extra structurally abnormal chromosomes. Prenat Diagn 2003;23:74.

198. Bofinger MK, Needham DF, Saldana LR, et al. 45,X/46,X,r(Y) karyotype transmitted by father to son after intracytoplasmic sperm injection for oligospermia: a case report. J Reprod Med 1999;44:645.

199. Johnson VP, McDonough PG, Cheung SW, et al. Sex chromosome marker: clinical significance and DNA characterization. Am J Med Genet 1991;39:97.

200. Vasquez AI, Rivera H, Mayorquin A, et al. Sex reversal due to Xp disomy by t(X;Y)(p21;q11). Genet Couns 1999;10:301.

201. Shapiro LR, Pettersen RO, Wilmot PL, et al. Pericentric inversion of the Y chromosome and prenatal diagnosis. Prenat Diagn 1984;4:463.

202. Tomomasa H, Adachi Y, Iwabuchi M, et al. Pericentric inversion of the Y chromosome of infertile male. Arch Androl 2000;45:181.

203. Causio F, Canale D, Schonauer LM, et al. Breakpoint of a Y chromosome pericentric inversion in the DAZ gene area: a case report. J Reprod Med 2000;45:591.
204. Wilkinson TA, Crolla JA. Molecular cytogenetic characterization of three familial cases of satellited Y chromosomes. Hum Genet 1993;91:389.
205. Kuhl H, Rottger S, Heilbronner H, et al. Loss of the Y chromosomal PAR2-region in four familial cases of satellited Y chromosomes (Yqs). Chromosome Res 2001;9:215.
206. Nielsen J, Rasmussen K. Y/autosomal translocations. Clin Genet 1976;9:609.
207. Alitolo T, Tiihonen J, Hakola P, et al. Molecular characterization of a Y;15 translocation segregating in a family. Hum Genet 1988;79:29.
208. Pabst B, Glaubitz R, Schalk T, et al. Reciprocal translocation between Y chromosome long arm euchromatin and the short arm of chromosome 1. Ann Genet 2002;45:5.
209. Alves C, Carvalho F, Cremades N, et al. Unique (Y;13) translocation in a male with oligozoospermia: cytogenetic and molecular studies. Eur J Hum Genet 2002;10:467.
210. Farah SB, Ramos CF, DeMello MP, et al. Two cases of Y; autosome translocations: a 45,X male and a clinically trisomy 18 patient. Am J Med Genet 1994;49:388.
211. Gimelli G, Cinti R, Varone P, et al. The phenotype of a 45,X male with Y/18 translocation. Clin Genet 1996;49:37.
212. Yen PH, Tsai SP, Wenger SL, et al. X/Y translocations resulting from recombination between homologous sequences on Xp and Yp. Proc Natl Acad Sci USA 1991;88:8944.
213. Shankman S, Spurdle AB, Morris D, et al. Presence of Y chromosome sequences and their effect on the phenotype of six patients with Y chromosome anomalies. Am J Med Genet 1995;55:269.
214. McElreavey K, Cortes LS. X-Y translocations and sex differentiation. Semin Reprod Med 2001;19:133.
215. Bardoni B, Floridia G, Guioli S, et al. Functional disomy of Xp22-pter in three males carrying a portion of Xp translocated to Yq. Hum Genet 1993;91:333.
216. de la Chapelle A. The etiology of maleness in XX men. Hum Genet 1981;58:105.
217. Wachtel SS, Bard J. The XX testis. Pediatr Adolesc Endocrinol 1981;8:116.
218. Margarit E, Soler A, Carrio A, et al. Molecular, cytogenetic, and clinical characterisation of six XX males including one prenatal diagnosis. J Med Genet 1998;35:727.
219. Van Dyke DC, Hanson JW, Moore JW, et al. Clinical management issues in males with sex chromosomal mosaicism and discordant phenotype/sex chromosomal patterns. Clin Pediatr 1991;30:15.
220. Ferguson-Smith MA, Cooke A, Affara NA, et al. Genotype-phenotype correlation in XX males and their bearing on current theories of sex determination. Hum Genet 1990;84:198.
221. Abusheikha N, Lass A, Brinsden P. XX males without SRY gene and with infertility. Hum Reprod 2001;16:717.
222. Abbas NE, Toublanc JE, Boucekkine C, et al. A possible common origin of "Y-negative" human XX males and XX true hermaphrodites. Hum Genet 1990;84:356.
223. Toublanc JE, Boucekkine C, Abbas N, et al. Hormonal and molecular genetic findings in 46,XX subjects with sexual ambiguity and testicular differentiation. Eur J Pediatr (Suppl) 1993;2:S70.
224. Turner F, Fechner PPY, Fuqua JS, et al. Combined Leydig cell and Sertoli cell dysfunction in 46,XX males lacking the sex determining region Y gene. Am J Med Genet 1995;57:440.
225. Ramos ES, Moreira-Filho CA, Vicente YA, et al. SRY-negative true hermaphrodites and an XX male in two generations of the same family. Hum Genet 1996;97:596.
226. Phelan MC, Rogers RC, Crawford EC, et al. Velocardiofacial syndrome in an unexplained XX male. Am J Med Genet 2002;116A:77.
227. Andersson M, Page DC, Pettay D, et al. Y;autosome translocations and mosaicism in the etiology of 45,X maleness: assignment of fertility factor to distal Yq11. Hum Genet 1988;79:2.
228. Scherer G, Schempp W, Fraccaro M, et al. Analysis of two 47,XXX males reveals X–Y interchange and maternal or paternal nondisjunction. Hum Genet 1989;81:247.
229. Ogata T, Matsuo M, Muroya K, et al. 47,XXX male: a clinical and molecular study. Am J Med Genet 2001;98:353.
230. Nitsche EM, Hiort O. The molecular basis of androgen insensitivity. Horm Res 2000;54:327.
231. Brinkmann AO. Molecular basis of androgen insensitivity. Mol Cell Endocrinol 2001;179:105.
232. Loy CJ, Yong EL. Sex, infertility and the molecular biology of the androgen receptor. Curr Opin Obstet Gynecol 2001;13:315.
233. Damiani D, Mascolli MA, Almeida MJ, et al. Persistence of Mullerian remnants in complete androgen insensitivity syndrome. J Pediatr Endocrinol Metab 2002;15:1553.
234. Tanaka YO, Mesaki N, Kurosaki Y, et al. Testicular feminization: role of MRI in diagnosing this rare male pseudohermaphroditism. J Comput Assist Tomogr 1998;22:884.

235. Sakai N, Yamada T, Asao T, et al. Bilateral testicular tumors in androgen insensitivity syndrome. Int J Urol 2000;7:390.

236. Holterhus PM, Wiebel J, Sinnecker GH, et al. Clinical and molecular spectrum of somatic mosaicism in androgen insensitivity syndrome. Pediatr Res 1999;46:684.

237. Griffin JE. Androgen resistance: the clinical and molecular spectrum. N Engl J Med 1992;326:611.

238. Schafer AJ. Sex determination and its pathology in man. Adv Genet 1995;33:275.

239. Hawkins JR, Taylor A, Goodfellow PN, et al. Evidence for increased prevalence of SRY mutations in XY females with complete rather than partial gonadal dysgenesis. Am J Hum Genet 1992;51:979.

240. Uehara S, Hashiyada M, Sato K, et al. Complete XY gonadal dysgenesis and aspects of the SRY genotype and gonadal tumor formation. J Hum Genet 2002;46:279.

241. Jordan BK, Jain M, Natarajan S, et al. Familial mutation in the testis-determining gene SRY shared by an XY female and her normal father. J Clin Endocrinol Metab 2002;87:3428.

242. Frydman R, Parneix I, Fries N, et al. Pregnancy in a 46,XY patient. Fertil Steril 1988;50:813.

243. Sauer MV, Lobo RA, Paulson RJ. Successful twin pregnancy after embryo donation to a patient with XY gonadal dysgenesis. Am J Obstet Gynecol 1989;161:380.

244. Kempe A, Engels H, Schubert R, et al. Familial ovarian dysgerminomas (Swyer syndrome) in females associated with 46 XY-karyotype. Gynecol Endocrinol 2002;16:107.

245. Le Caignec C, Baron S, McElreavey K, et al. 46,XY gonadal dysgenesis: evidence for autosomal dominant transmission in a large kindred. Am J Med Genet 2003;116A:37.

246. Berkovitz GD, Fechner PY, Zacur HW, et al. Clinical and pathologic spectrum of 46,XY gonadal dysgenesis: its relevance to the understanding of sex differentiation. Medicine (Baltimore) 1991;70:375.

247. Kim KR, Kwon Y, Joung JY, et al. True hermaphroditism and mixed gonadal dysgenesis in young children: a clinicopathologic study of 10 cases. Mod Pathol 2002;15:1013.

248. Nordenskjold A, Ivarsson SA. Molecular characterization of 5α-reductase type 2 deficiency and fertility in a Swedish family. J Clin Endocrinol Metab 1998;82:3236.

249. Sinnecker GHG, Hiort O, Dibbelt L, et al. Phenotypic classification of male pseudohermaphroditism due to steroid 5α-reductase 2 deficiency. Am J Med Genet 1996;63:223.

250. Swain A, Narvaez V, Burgoyne P, et al. Dax1 antagonizes Sry action in mammalian sex determination. Nature 1998;391:761.

251. Goodfellow PN, Camerino G. DAX-1 an "antitestis" gene. EXS 2001;97:57.

252. Moog U, Jansen NJ, Scherer G, et al. Acampomelic campomelic syndrome. Am J Med Genet 2001;104:239.

253. Giordano J, Prior HM, Bamforth JS, et al. Genetic study of SOX9 in a case of campomelic dysplasia. Am J Med Genet 2001;98:176.

254. Koziell A, Charmandari E, Hindmarsh PC, et al. Frasier syndrome, part of the Denys–Drash continuum or simply a WT1 gene associated disorder of intersex and nephrology? Clin Endocrinol 2000;52:801.

255. Bick DP, McCorkle D, Stanley WS, et al. Prenatal diagnosis of Smith–Lemli–Opitz syndrome in a pregnancy with low maternal serum oestriol and a sex-reversal fetus. Prenat Diagn 1999;19:68.

256. Raymond CS, Parker ED, Kettlewell JR, et al. A region of human chromosome 9p required for testis development contains two genes related to known sexual regulators. Hum Mol Genet 1999;8:989.

257. Wulfsberg EA, Weaver RP, Cunniff CM, et al. Chromosome 10qter deletion syndrome: a review and report of three new cases. Am J Med Genet 1989;32:364.

258. Teebi AS, Miller S, Ostrer H, et al. Spastic paraplegia, optic atrophy, microcephaly with normal intelligence, and XY sex reversal: a new autosomal recessive syndrome. J Med Genet 1998;35:759.

259. Modan-Moses D, Litmanovitch T, Rienstein S, et al. True hermaphroditism with ambiguous genitalia due to a complicated mosaic karyotype: clinical features, cytogenetic findings, and literature review. Am J Med Genet 2003;116A:300.

260. Krob G, Braum A, Kuhnle U. True hermaphroditism: geographical distribution, clinical findings, chromosomes and gonadal histology. Eur J Pediatr 1994;153:2.

261. Torres L, López M, Méndez JP, et al. Molecular analysis in true hermaphrodites with different karyotypes and similar phenotypes. Am J Med Genet 1996;63:348

262. Queipo G, Zenteno JC, Pena R, et al. Molecular analysis in true hermaphroditism: demonstration of low-level hidden mosaicism for Y-derived sequences in 46,XX cases. Hum Genet 2002;111:278.

263. Williamson HO, Phansey SA, Mathur RS. True hermaphroditism with term vaginal delivery and a review. Am J Obstet Gynecol 1981;141:262.

264. Starceski PJ, Sieber WK, Lee PA. Fertility in true hermaphroditism. Adolesc Pediatr Gynecol 1988;1:55.

265. Hadjiathanasiou CG, Brauner R, Lortat-Jacob S, et al. True hermaphroditism: genetic variants and clinical management. J Pediatr 1994;125:738.

266. Freiberg AS, Blumberg B, Lawce H, et al. XX/XY chimerism encountered during prenatal diagnosis. Prenat Diagn 1988;8:423.

267. Cheng W-F, Huang S-C, Ko T-M. Prenatal diagnosis of 46,XX/47,XXY mosaicism: a case report. Prenat Diagn 1995;15:64.

268. Polani PE. Abnormal sex chromosomes, behaviour and mental disorder. In: Tanner JM, ed. Developments in psychiatric research. London: Hodder and Stoughton, 1977:89.

269. Bender BG, Berch DB. Overview: Psychological phenotypes and sex chromosome abnormalities. In: Berch DB, Bender BG, eds. Sex chromosome abnormalities and human behavior. Boulder, CO: Westview Press, 1990:1.

270. Christian SM, Koehn D, Pillay R, et al. Parental decisions following prenatal diagnosis of sex chromosome aneuploidy: a trend over time. Prenat Diagn 2000;20:37.

271. Linden MG, Bender BG, Robinson A. Clinical manifestations of sex chromosome anomalies. Compr Ther 1990;16:3.

272. Milunsky A. Your genetic destiny: know your genes, secure your health, save your life., Cambridge: Perseus Books, 2001.

Stuart Schwartz, Ph.D. 　　　　　　　　　　　　　　　　　 8

Molecular Cytogenetics and Prenatal Diagnosis

DNA–DNA hybridization on metaphase chromosomes had its origin in 1969, when Pardue and Gall used a radioactive DNA probe to detect repetitive sequences.[1] The widespread use of nonradioactive hybridization techniques can be traced to the pioneering work of Pinkel et al. in 1986 and Landegent et al. in 1987.[2,3] Briefly stated, the objective of nonradioactive in situ hybridization is the hybridization of a labeled, denatured, single-stranded DNA probe to a single-stranded target DNA that has been denatured in place on a microscope slide. Probes are labeled with biotin or digoxigenin and detected by fluorochrome-labeled antibodies; more typically, the probes are labeled directly with a fluorochrome. Less commonly, hybridization is detected using nonfluorescent enzymatic methods. Fluorescent labels are combined with fluorescent microscopy (fluorescence in situ hybridization [FISH]). The use of fluorescent microscopy allows the detection of more than one probe, each labeled with a different color. The technology has now advanced so that combinatorial fluorescence with twenty-four different colors can be visualized on the same metaphase spread, thereby highlighting each chromosome pair.[4,5] The target DNA may include either metaphase or interphase cells. Interphase cells can be derived from cultured or direct (noncultivated) cells; preparations from tissue specimens may be examined either as dispersed cells or still in the original tissue architecture (e.g., paraffin sections).

A vast variety of types of DNA can be used as probes for FISH analysis, including: (1) repetitive DNA segments such as alpha-satellite DNA from the centromeric regions of chromosomes[2]; (2) whole chromosome libraries, constructed either by the flow sorting of individual chromosomes or by the use of somatic cell hybrids with a single human chromosome, in which DNA from the entire chromosome is used as a probe[6–8]; and (3) single-copy probes, in which a unique segment of genomic DNA is used.[9] Single-copy probes, which can be <1 kb or >1 Mb, as in some yeast artificial chromosomes (YACs), have been used most extensively to study microdeletion syndromes. Owing to the sequencing of the Human Genome, single copy probes as bacterial artificial chromosomes (BACs) can be used to study almost any chromosomal segment.

The advent of molecular cytogenetics over the past fifteen years has revolutionized both the research and clinical studies of chromosomes. Its influence has been seen in the evaluation of somatic abnormalities in neoplasia and constitutional abnormalities detected

341

in peripheral blood samples obtained postnatally and amniotic fluid (AF) and chorionic villus samples (CVS) obtained prenatally. This chapter will focus on the use of FISH in prenatal diagnosis. The applications of FISH in prenatal diagnosis include studies of both metaphase chromosomes and interphase cells. FISH analysis of metaphase chromosomes has been used to: (1) detect or confirm the presence of cytologically suspected microdeletion syndromes; (2) characterize structurally abnormal chromosomes; and (3) define the origin of marker chromosomes. The primary prenatal application of FISH to interphase cells has been the detection of aneuploidy. These prenatal studies have involved: (1) amniotic fluid cells (AFC); (2) chorionic villi; (3) fetal cells obtained transcervically or from maternal blood; and (4) preimplantation embryos. This chapter will discuss each of these applications in turn.

MICRODELETIONS

One of the most common uses of FISH over the past several years has been in the detection of microdeletions associated with contiguous gene syndromes. The term *contiguous gene syndromes* was first coined by Schmickel in 1986, to define a deletion of a contiguous stretch of DNA that contains multiple genes.[10] These deletions produce syndromes that are usually clinically recognizable and can be detected by either high-resolution chromosome analysis or FISH. The prototypic example of a contiguous gene syndrome was described by Francke et al.[11] Males with a Xp21 deletion may have one, several, or all of the following syndromes and abnormalities, depending on the size of the deletion: Duchenne muscular dystrophy, chronic granulomatous disease, McLeod phenotype, retinitis pigmentosa, mental retardation, glycerol kinase deficiency, adrenal hypoplasia, and Åland eye disease.

Many contiguous gene deletions have been described clinically and identified cytogenetically: Prader–Willi syndrome, DiGeorge syndrome, velocardiofacial syndrome, Williams syndrome, Miller–Dieker syndrome, Smith–Magenis syndrome, Langer–Gideon syndrome, and Aniridia–Wilms tumor association.[12–23] A summary of the phenotypic features and cytogenetic observations is provided in Table 8.1. The utility of FISH in studying these disorders varies, depending on the specific disorders.

Table 8.1. Microdeletion syndromes (contiguous gene syndromes) detectable by FISH

Syndrome	Principal Features	Cytogenetic Location	Detectable by Cytogenetics
Alagille[23]	Dysmorphic facial features, cholestasis, arteriohepatic dysplasia	20p11.23–20p12.2	+/−
Alpha-thalassemia and mental retardation[21]	α-Thalassemia, mental retardation	16p13.3	+/−
Angelman[13]	Hypotonia, feeding difficulties, ataxia, seizures, microcephaly, mental retardation	15q11.2–q13	+/−
Aniridia–Wilms tumor[19]	Aniridia, Wilms tumor, genitourinary abnormalities, mental retardation	11p13	+
Diamond–Blackfan anemia with neurologic signs[19a,19b]	Psychomotor retardation, microcephaly and hypotonia with anemia due to congenital pure red-blood-cell aplasia and skeletal malformations	19q13.2	+/−

Table 8.1. Microdeletion syndromes (contiguous gene syndromes) detectable by FISH (continued)

Syndrome	Principal Features	Cytogenetic Location	Detectable by Cytogenetics
DiGeorge/velocardiofacial[14]	Abnormalities in third and fourth branchial arches, thymic hypoplasia, parathyroid hypoplasia, conotruncal defects	22q11.2	+/−
Greig cephalopolysyndactyly[20]	Craniosynostosis, polysyndactyly, mental retardation	16p13.3	+/−
Kallmann[20a]	Hypogonadotropic hypogonadism and anosmia	Xp22.3	−
Langer-Gideon[18]	Trichorhinophalangeal syndrome, multiple cartilaginous exostosis, mental retardation	8q24.1	+/−
Learning disability and attention deficit/hyperkinetic disorder (ADHD)[18a]	Severe learning disability/ADHD/mild mental retardation, short stature, skeletal abnormalities	Xp22.3	+/−
Mental retardation, nonspecific[18b]	Mental retardation	Xp21.3-p22.1	−
Microdeletion 22q13[18c,18d]	Mental retardation, delayed speech, hypotonia and dyamorphic features	22q13.3	+/−
Microphthalmia with linear skin defects[18e]	Microphthalmia, linear skin defects	Xp22.3	+/−
Miller–Dieker[17]	Lissencephaly, dysmorphic facial features, mental retardation	17p13.3	+/−
Monosomy 1p36[18f]	Severe psychomotor retardation, microcephaly, seizures and visual impairment	1p36	+/−
Potocki–Shaffer[15b,15c]	Parietal foramina, multiple exostoses, mental retardation, craniofacial abnormalities	11p13.11	+/−
Prader–Willi[12]	Hypertonia, feeding difficulties, obesity, hypogonadism, mental retardation	15q11.2-q13	+/−
Rubenstein-Taybi[22]	Dysmorphic facial features, broad thumbs and first toes, mental retardation	16p13	+/−
Saethre–Chotzen[18g,18h]	Craniosynostosis	7p21.1	+/−
Smith–Magenis[16]	Dysmorphic facial features, short broad hands, delayed speech, bizarre behavioral abnormalities, peripheral neuropathy, mental retardation	17p11.2	+/−
Steroid sulfatase deficiency[16a,16b]	Ichthyosis, corneal opacity, cryptorchidism	Xp22.3	+/−
Williams[15]	Gregarious personality, dysmorphic facial features, transient infantile hypercalcemia, congenital heart disease, premature aging of the skin, mental retardation	7q11.23	−
Wolf–Hirschhorn[15a]	Dysmorphic, multiple congenital anomalies, mental retardation and failure to thrive	4p16.3	+/−

+ = detectable by classical cytogenetics; +/− = detectable by classical cytogenetics in some cases; − = not detectable by classical cytogenetics.

Both Prader–Willi syndrome (PWS) and Angelman syndrome (AS) can involve deletions in 15q11.2–15q13; when deletions are identified in either PWS or AS, they are indistinguishable cytogenetically.[12,13] However, these syndromes are clearly distinct entities. The basis for the phenotypic differences between PWS and AS is the parental origin of the deletion. The origin of the deletion is paternal in PWS and is maternal in AS. Although the vast majority of deletions can be detected cytogenetically, some deletions can be detected only by FISH. The SNRPN probe is the most useful in detecting a deletion.

Several syndromes are associated with a characteristic deletion of chromosome 22 (22q11.2–22q11.22), including DiGeorge syndrome, velocardiofacial syndrome, and conotruncal heart defects.[14] Only a small proportion of these deletions can be detected with high-resolution cytogenetics. However, use of a D22S75 or TUPLE I probe can detect the deletion.

Williams syndrome is a developmental disorder involving the central nervous system and vascular connective tissue. The pathogenetic deletion in 7q11.23 cannot be detected with cytogenetic analysis but can be detected with FISH using an elastin gene probe.[15]

Smith–Magenis syndrome is a developmental disorder involving dysmorphic facial features, short broad hands, delayed speech, bizarre behavioral abnormalities, peripheral neuropathy, and mental retardation. Deletions in 17p11.2 can generally be detected cytogenetically but should always be confirmed by FISH using a probe containing D17S379, which is localized to this region.[16] Miller–Dieker syndrome presents with type I lissencephaly and dysmorphic facial features.[17] The deletion in 17p13.3 can be detected in some patients, but not all, with cytogenetic analysis. FISH with probe D17S258, localized to 17p13.3, has been shown to be an excellent DNA probe to detect the deletion associated with this syndrome. The deletions in all of the aforementioned syndromes can be detected by FISH, using commercially available probes that are both easy to use and very effective for diagnosis (Table 8.1). Other contiguous gene deletions are also well defined, but no commercial FISH probes are available for diagnostic studies. In most cases, however, DNA probes have been localized to the deleted areas by several different investigators and have been used successfully for FISH. Langer–Gideon syndrome is a combination of trichorhinophalangeal (TRP) syndrome (sparse scalp hair, bulbous/pear-shaped nose, and cone-shaped phalangeal epiphyses) with multiple cartilaginous exostoses and mental retardation. In some patients, a deletion in 8q24.1 can be detected cytogenetically.[18] A deletion in 11p13 can be seen in the Aniridia–Wilms tumor association.[19] These are almost all invariably detectable by standard cytogenetic analysis. Several rare deletions include Grieg cephalopolysyndactyly, α-thalassemia, and mental retardation, Rubenstein–Taybi syndrome, and Alagille syndrome. In some cases, the deletions can be detected by cytogenetics, but with the appropriate probes, the deletions can be detected with FISH.[20–23]

Descriptions of the most common microdeletions and their detection by FISH have been described above, and FISH is most effective in detecting these syndromes in postnatal populations. In these populations the clinical phenotype dictates which probes should be tested, and if patients should be referred to rule out a syndrome because of specific features (e.g., hypotonia, congenital heart disease) the appropriate FISH probes can be used. For prenatal diagnostic studies, FISH probes have always been effectively used if there is a question posed by the G-banding patter, especially involving the microdeletions. Figure 8.1 illustrates the confirmation of a deletion of 17p11.2 using FISH in an AF specimen. Initial G-banding suggested the presence of this deletion, which is found in the Smith–Magenis syndrome. In addition, a number of fetuses identified prenatally because of either abnormal ultrasound or because of family history have been studied with ap-

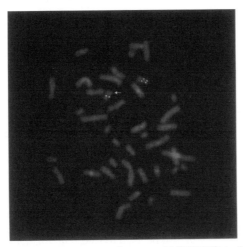

Fig. 8.1. Example of FISH to a single-copy target, using a cosmid (D17S379) to the Smith-Magenis "critical region" localized to 17p11.2 on a metaphase spread from an amniotic fluid sample. One chromosome 17 shows two hybridization signals, one with the probe to the critical region and one with a control probe; therefore, this chromosome is normal. However, the other chromosome 17, denoted by an arrow, hybridizes only the control probe. Thus, this chromosome is deleted for the critical region.

propriate microdeletion/microduplication FISH probes. All of the same probes used postnatally can be used prenatally; however, lack of prenatal ascertainment of these syndromes precludes their use in most prenatal cases. One microdeletion that has been most frequently and successfully prenatally detected is the deletion of chromosome 22. This deletion is most often detected prenatally because of the presence of a conotruncal heart defect (tetralogy of Fallot, interrupted aortic arch); it has also been seen in association with uropathy, and polyhydramnios, as well as studied due to the presence of a familial deletion. In 1997 Davidson et al. used FISH with probe D22S75 to detect a 22q11 deletion in a fetus detected prenatally to have an interrupted aortic arch type B.[24] Subsequent to this report a number of cases, detected prenatally, have been reported. In a larger study in 2001, Manji et al. examined forty-six cases with a heart defect but without a visible chromosome anomaly and found that 5 had del(22q).[25] They emphasized the need for FISH analysis on all fetuses with cardiac defects (except hypoplastic left heart and echogenic focus). In 2002 Boudjemline et al. screened 151 consecutive fetuses with tetralogy of Fallot (with or without pulmonary atresia) for a 22q11 deletion.[26] They noted that 25 (16.6 percent) of those studied had a deletion detected by FISH. However, they also looked for a number of additional features in these fetuses (e.g., increased nuchal translucency [NT], intrauterine growth retardation [IUGR], polyhydramnios, extracardiac malformations, and abnormalities of the pulmonary arteries). They determined that increased NT, polyhydramnios, and IUGR were more frequently in fetuses with 22q deletions and by using these findings the efficiency of screening for the 22q deletions prenatally could be improved. Devriendt et al. also noted that in several patients with 22q deletions detected prenatally, polyhydramnios was present and could be used for the ascertainment of patients for study by FISH.[27]

Other microdeletions/duplications have also been studied and detected prenatally. Kashork et al.[28] studied nine cases with a probe for the steroid sulfatase gene (STS) to determine if a microdeletion involving that gene was present. All nine cases were ascertained because of a low or absent maternal unconjugated estriol (uE$_3$), which has been associated with placental sulfatase deficiency. They detected six deletions and one partial deletion in the nine cases. The previous two microdeletions have been studied because of the specific ascertainment of these patients; however, abnormalities are also studied because of the familial nature of the disorders. For example, approximately 5–10 percent of patients with DiGeorge and velocardiofacial syndromes (22q deletions) show familial transmissions.[29] Therefore, FISH studies can be used prenatally for an affected parent who has a 50 percent chance of producing an affected offspring. Both Driscoll et al.[29] and Van Hemel et al.[30] successfully used FISH to monitor at-risk pregnancies for 22q deletions. Kashork et al.[32] tested seventeen prenatal CVS specimens with interphase FISH to detect the submicroscopic duplication in 17p12 associated with Charcot–Marie–Tooth type 1A. Seven duplications were detected using this interphase analysis. Previously this group also showed the effectiveness of this analysis in AFC.[32] Inoue et al. reported on three families with Pelizaeus–Merzbacher disease (PMD).[33] They used interphase FISH with a probe for the proteolipid protein 1 gene (*PLP1*) revealing a *PLP1* duplication in two cases studied prenatally. FISH analysis can also be used to study microdeletion syndromes that have resulted from cryptic rearrangements. These cryptic rearrangements have been identified in both Prader–Willi/Angelman syndromes and in Miller–Dieker syndromes.[31] The increased frequency of diagnosis of microdeletion syndromes, both postnatally and prenatally, have provided a greater understanding of these syndromes. This, in turn, has shown an increased need for the application of FISH probes in prenatal diagnosis. As more microdeletions and microduplications are delineated and their prenatal detection understood, this method will be used more frequently.

SUBTLE/CRYPTIC REARRANGEMENTS

The detection of subtle chromosomal rearrangements with standard banding analysis can often be difficult. This is especially true for prenatal diagnostic studies in which the specimens cannot be analyzed easily with high-resolution procedures. However, even high-resolution analysis is not always sufficient for the interpretation of small structural rearrangements or complex karyotypes. Several studies have demonstrated the effectiveness of FISH with chromosomal libraries or single-copy probes for confirming or clarifying the G-banded interpretation of subtle or cryptic constitutional translocations.[34–37]

Subtle rearrangements can involve alteration of euchromatin and genes interstitially or can involve the terminal regions. A variety of studies over the past few years have shown the importance of cryptic subtelomeric rearrangements in postnatal studies. The telomeric regions on every chromosome are similar and consist of simple tandem repeats (TTAGGG)n that vary between 500 and 3000 copies at each chromosome arm and have been shown to be conserved among vertebrates. The telomere-associated repeat (TAR) is located immediately internal to the terminal telomeric repeated DNA segment, and homologous recombination may occur within both the telomeric regions. The unique DNA sequence for each chromosome arm (subtelomeric sequences) is attached to the telomeric associated repeats and is estimated to be anywhere from 100 to 300 kb from the end of the chromosome. These subtelomeric sequences vary among all of the chromosome arms and can be used as FISH probes for the analysis of telomeric cryptic rearrangements and deletions. These telomeric regions are thought to be gene-rich, and the loss of these regions is correlated with dysmorphic features and mental retardation.

In 1996 two groups generated a complete set of unique sequence telomeric probes for the submicroscopic detection of subtelomeric chromosomal abnormalities.[38] These probes consist of unique sequences of DNA from the subtelomeric region approximately 100–300 kb from the end of the chromosome. A probe for each chromosome arm has been developed, with a few exceptions; there are no probes for the individual acrocentric short arms and no unique probes for Xp and Yp since they share similar sequences, as do Xq and Yq. In 2000, Knight et al. reported on newer probes for some of the regions that have been developed and that are closer to the end of the chromosome.[39] Overall, in several postnatal studies more than 1,000 individuals have been examined with telomeric probes, showing an overall frequency of approximately 5 percent with a range of 0–13.3 percent in these studies.[40–45] However, subtelomeric studies are very costly and extremely time-consuming. Although there is more than one technology, the most common is to use probes provided by Vysis, Inc., which uses a total of fifteen probe hybridizations per study. Though the postnatal studies are time-consuming, this would create considerably more work on prenatal studies. However, recently Souter et al. published two prenatal cases involving cryptic rearrangement (one studied at 24 weeks and the other at 36 weeks) that were resolved using a panel of telomere-specific probes.[46] In this report, the authors state the technical feasibility of multiple simultaneous screening of subtelomeric regions.

Although the majority of subtle/cryptic rearrangements do involve the telomeric regions, there have also been a number of cryptic abnormalities involving interstitial regions. At present there is no adequate FISH technology to routinely detect random subtle deletions or duplications prenatally (specific and recurrent microdeletions/duplications that can be detected have been mentioned above). However, cryptic deletions associated with specific chromosomal rearrangements can possibly be delineated prenatally. Warburton demonstrated that 6.7 percent of prenatally detected de novo *balanced* reciprocal translocations and inversions had phenotypic abnormalities.[47] Kumar et al. showed that in two of three postnatal de novo "balanced rearrangements," a subtle deletion could be delineated.[48] Building on this study Astbury et al. delineated deletions in 9 of 15 ascertained "balanced rearrangements."[49] One of two prenatally detected cases had a deletion. These studies indicated that, by using data from the Human Genome Project (http://genome. ucsc.edu) along with FISH using BACs, deletions in seemingly balanced rearrangements could be detected. However, caution must be used in the prenatal setting because of the time constraints of these studies.

Before the development of FISH, precise characterization of subtle rearrangements was tedious. Additional work, involving multiple cell harvests, and additional chromosome banding techniques, together with a high degree of analytical skill at the microscope, was necessary for interpretation of these subtle rearrangements. This work is time-consuming and laborious. These obstacles were especially formidable in the area of prenatal diagnosis, in which time is of the essence. Thus, the advent of FISH was especially advantageous in the analysis of subtle rearrangements detected prenatally. Several studies have shown the value of this application.[34–36,50,51] When a carrier of a subtle translocation decides to have prenatal testing, application of FISH provides a definitive advantage for determining whether the fetus has an unbalanced karyotype. As the technology continues to improve and more probes become available, the delineation of cryptic aberrations will continue to expand.

An example of the utility of FISH is shown in Figure 8.2, which shows a subtle translocation between chromosomes 15 and 16 in a carrier father [46,XY,t(15;16) (q26.3;q24.1)]. Although this translocation could be detected with standard banding, its elucidation in a prenatal specimen would have been problematic. Prenatal cytogenetic analysis of a subsequent pregnancy revealed what appeared to be a der(16) and an un-

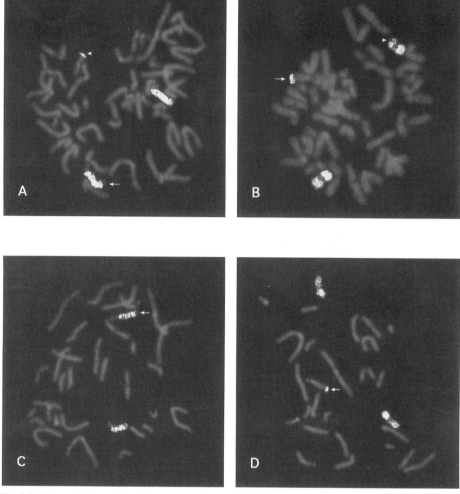

Fig. 8.2. Characterization of a subtle translocation between chromosomes 15 and 16 [t(15;16)(q26.3;q24.1)] by FISH in a carrier and unbalanced offspring. *A*, Hybridization with a chromosome 15 library in the balanced translocation. *B*, Hybridization with a chromosome 16 library in the balanced translocation. *C*, Hybridization with a chromosome 15 library in the unbalanced karyotype [der(16)t(15;16)(q26.3;q24.1)]. *D*, Hybridization with a chromosome 16 library in the unbalanced karyotype.

balanced karyotype. This impression was easily confirmed using chromosomes 15 and 16 specific painting probes. FISH analysis allowed for much more expeditious handling of this prenatal diagnostic case and in most cases similar rearrangements could even be more easily delineated using subtelomeric probes.

IDENTIFICATION OF MARKER CHROMOSOMES

Determining the origin of chromosomal material that cannot be identified by conventional banding (i.e., "marker chromosome") has been greatly facilitated by molecular cytogenetic studies, and FISH in particular. Classification of such marker chromosomes is important for phenotype/karyotype correlations, which is imperative for proper counseling (see also chapter 6). Although many techniques may be used to determine the origin of marker chromosomes, FISH using repetitive alpha-satellite DNA probes is the least complicated and most effective technique. Additional samples are not needed, because unstained slides or fixed pellets are usually available and amenable to analysis. If necessary, previously banded slides can be used immediately, saving time in prenatal cases.

Although marker chromosomes have been identified prenatally, the majority of this work has been done in postnatal studies. The frequency of marker chromosomes identified at birth is 0.14–0.72 in 1,000 births, whereas their frequency in prenatal diagnostic studies is slightly elevated to 0.65–1.5 in 1,000.[47,52–54] The elevated frequency seen in prenatal studies is most likely associated with the advanced maternal age seen in the prenatal population. Approximately 40 percent of prenatally detected markers are inherited and thought to be heterochromatic; approximately 60 percent are de novo.[47] Marker chromosomes may be autosomal or sex chromosomal in origin. The autosomal markers can be further subdivided into satellited or nonsatellited markers. Our approach for analyzing these markers and determining their significance is illustrated and detailed in Figure 8.3.

Sex chromosome markers are routinely identified by FISH, and numerous cases have now been reported.[55] The majority of these markers have been identified postnatally in patients with 45,X,+mar karyotype and a presumptive diagnosis of Ullrich–Turner syndrome. In these cases, the determination of the markers is important not only for establishing phenotype–karyotype correlations, but also for clinical care. Females with a 45,X/46,XY karyotype have a 10–20 percent chance of having a gonadal dysgerminoma or gonadoblastoma develop.[56,57] Therefore, it is presumed that female patients with a marker derived from a Y chromosome have an increased risk for developing gonadoblastoma. Alternatively, patients, with Ullrich–Turner syndrome who have a marker chromosome derived from an X chromosome are at an increased risk for mental retardation.[58–60] Studies have shown that patients with a small ring X chromosome who lack the XIST gene fail to have normal inactivation of their X-chromosome genes and are at increased risk for mental retardation,

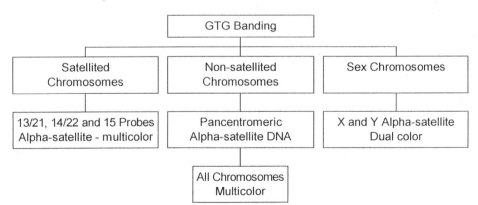

Fig. 8.3. Flow chart illustrating our approach for analyzing a marker of unknown etiology. The metaphase spread is initially analyzed with G-banding to determine whether the marker is a satellited or nonsatellited derivative of an autosomal chromosome or if it is derived from a sex chromosome (i.e., only one normal sex chromosome is seen). Satellited markers are studied with 13/21, 14/22, and chromosome 15 alpha-satellite probes; sex chromosome markers are studied with both X and Y chromosome alpha-satellite probe; and nonsatellited markers are studied with a pericentromeric probe to first determine whether alpha-satellite DNA is present and then, if needed, with chromosome-specific alpha-satellite DNA probes. When possible, a multiple-color approach for this analysis is taken, using two or three colors. This approach allows for the conservation of slides and material and, more importantly, permits a more immediate answer.

although if limited euchromatin is present they will display a mild phenotype.[61–63] To date, twenty-seven cases of sex chromosome markers ascertained through prenatal diagnosis and studied with FISH have been reported. Eleven (41 percent) were derived from an X chromosome and 16 (59 percent) were derived from a Y chromosome (Table 8.2).[55,64–77] Unfortunately, phenotypic follow-up of these pregnancies has been too limited to make substantial conclusions, although there are interesting trends in the Y-derived chromosomes. Fourteen of the sixteen pregnancies with Y-derived chromosome markers proceeded to term, with thirteen resulting in the birth of a male infant. Twelve of these males appeared normal at birth; one had hypospadias and seminiferous tubules without germinal cells. One of the fourteen pregnancies resulted in a child with Turner syndrome. Less follow-up was available for the X-derived markers; however, one of these pregnancies ended as a stillbirth and several appeared normal at birth or showed phenotypic features associated with Turner syndrome. Two marker X chromosomes were found as supernumerary chromosomes in males [47,XY,+der(X)], both were lacking Xist on the der(X).

Numerous autosomal markers ascertained either prenatally or postnatally have also now been routinely examined with FISH.[73,78–90] These studies have shown that markers can be derived from all of the chromosomes, but little is known about the mechanism of formation of these markers or their phenotypic consequences in many cases. Before the

Table 8.2. Patients with sex chromosome markers ascertained through prenatal testing by FISH

Clinical Findings	Karyotype	Reference
Livebirth—normal male	45,X/46,X,mar(Y)	Cole et al.[64]
TOP—no follow-up	45,X/46,X,r(X)	Bajalica et al.[65]
Livebirth—male with hypospadius, seminiferous tubules	45,X/46,X,i(Yp)	Slim et al.[66]
Livebirth—normal male (1 year)	45,X/46,X,der(Y)	Qu et al.[67]
TOP—no follow-up	45,X/46,X,idic(Y)	Bernstein et al.[68]
TOP—normal infant	45,X/46,X,der(X)	Amiel et al.[69]
Livebirth—normal male	46,X,mar(X)	Ameil et al.[69]
Stillbirth	45,X/46,X,mar(X)	Schwartz et al.[55]
Livebirth—normal male	45,X/46,X,i(Yp)	Schwartz et al.[55]
TOP—normal male	45,X/46,X,i(Y)	Schwartz et al.[55]
Livebirth—normal male	45,X/46,X,psudic(Y)	Schwartz et al.[55]
Livebirth—normal male	45,X/46,X,i(Yp)	Schwartz et al.[55]
TOP—male with slight facial dysmorphism	46,X,i(Yp)	Wang et al.[70]
Livebirth—normal male (3 years)	46,X,r(Y)	Yaron et al.[71]
Livebirth—normal male	46,X,del(Y)	Hernando et al.[72]
Livebirth—normal male	45,X/46,X,i(Yp)	Hernando et al.[72]
Livebirth—Turner syndrome	45,X/46,X,r(X)	Li et al.[73]
Livebirth—Turner syndrome	45,X/46,X,r(X)	Li et al.[73]
Livebirth—Down syndrome	46,X,+21/47,X,der(X),+21	Li et al.[73]
Livebirth—Turner syndrome	45,X/46,X,der(Y)	Li et al.[73]
Livebirth—normal male	45,X/46,X,der(Y)	Li et al.[73]
Livebirth—normal male	45,X/46,X,r(Y)	Li et al.[73]
Ultrasound—normal male	46,X,der(Y)	Velagaleti et al.[74]
Livebirth—normal female	47,XX,+der(X)	Viersbach et al.[75]
Livebirth—abnormal female	47,XX,+der(X)	Viersbach et al.[75]
Livebirth—normal male	45,X/46,X,der(Y)	Hoshi et al.[76]
Livebirth—abnormal male	47,XY,+der(X)	Le Caignec et al.[77]

TOP = termination of pregnancy

use of FISH, Warburton reported the overall risk of an abnormal phenotype for a prenatally detected marker chromosome to be 13 percent.[47] Subdivided by type, the risk is 10.9 percent for a satellited marker, 14.7 percent for a nonsatellited marker, and 4.5 percent for a minute nonsatellited marker. Demonstrated below, however, the use of FISH has aided the characterization of markers and helped to provide an understanding of the phenotypic consequences of some of these markers. Crolla et al. have indicated that de novo supernumerary marker chromosomes derived from the acrocentric chromosomes (excluding 15) has an associated 7 percent risk compared with 20 percent for small marker chromosomes from nonacrocentric chromosomes.[89,90]

In our prenatal and postnatal collaborative studies, we have examined 400 autosomal markers, of which the chromosome of origin was determined in approximately 75 percent of the cases. Approximately 70 percent were satellited and 30 percent were nonsatellited. Characterization and determination of the significance of satellited markers can be done in the manner shown in Figure 8.4. Approximately 17 percent of satellited markers are derived from chromosome 13 or 21, 24 percent from chromosome 14 or 22, and 59 percent from chromosome 15. Approximately 90 percent of these markers are bisatellited. The presumption is that a monocentromeric, bisatellited marker consists of only repetitive sequences and has no phenotypic effects. However, dicentric markers with euchromatic material between the two centromeres may have a deleterious phenotypic effect. For example, studies by Leana-Cox et al. indicated that patients with markers derived from chromosome 15 that do not contain the Prader–Willi/Angelman syndrome critical region are phenotypically normal, whereas patients with a chromosome 15 marker that contains this region have an abnormal phenotype.[91] Therefore, chromosome 15 markers should be studied with the FISH probes localized to this region (D15S11, SNRPN, D15S10, and GABRB3) to determine their phenotypic significance. We recommend that all such satellited markers should also be similarly studied (see Figure 8.5).

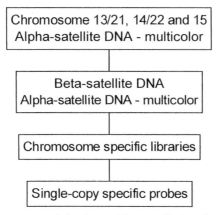

Fig. 8.4. Flow chart illustrating our approach for characterizing a satellited marker. The first step is multiple-color FISH with alpha-satellite DNA probes for chromosomes 13/21, 14/22, and 15. The currently available alpha-satellite DNA probes cannot differentiate between alpha-satellite DNA from chromosomes 13 and 21 or between chromosomes 14 and 22. The next step is hybridization with beta-satellite DNA probes to confirm by FISH whether the markers are monosatellited or bisatellited. The markers can be characterized best by using simultaneous two-color alpha- and beta-satellite DNA probes. If a marker is dicentric, or monocentric and monosatellited, we then evaluate it with chromosome-specific libraries and single-copy specific probes. For example, a dicentric chromosome 15 [inv dup(15)] identified by alpha-satellite DNA probes should be studied with chromosome 15q11–15q13 specific probes (e.g., SNRPN) to characterize the euchromatin between the centromeres.

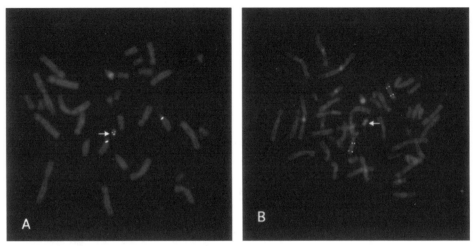

Fig. 8.5. A dicentric chromosome 15. *A*, Hybridized with a chromosome 15 alpha-satellite DNA probe demonstrating two signals, confirming that it is dicentric. *B*, Hybridized with a single-copy SNRPN probe, indicating that it is present on the normal chromosome 15 but not on the marker chromosome. The arrow indicates the marker chromosome.

Nonsatellited chromosome markers are more problematic, both in their identification and their phenotypic implications. Multiple studies have shown that marker chromosomes have been derived from all of the autosomal chromosomes. Our suggested approach for analyzing and subgrouping these markers is shown on the flow diagram in Figure 8.6. A rare subset of this group of markers appears to lack alpha-satellite DNA.[92] Nonetheless, recognition of these unusual markers is important because they are invariably associated

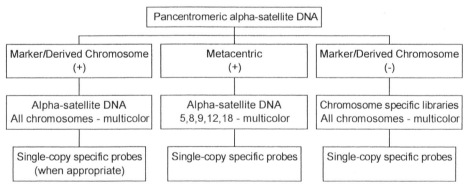

Fig. 8.6. Flow chart illustrating our approach for analyzing a nonsatellited marker. The first step in studying a nonsatellited chromosome marker is to perform FISH with pericentromeric alpha-satellite DNA. This FISH analysis, which indicates the presence of alpha-satellite DNA, together with concurrent G-banding studies, will help subdivide these markers into the following groups: markers without alpha-satellite DNA; metacentric marker chromosome (isochromosome); and ring chromosome or derived chromosomes with alpha-satellite DNA. Identification and characterization of isochromosomes can be done successfully with a combination of alpha-satellite DNA, chromosomal libraries, and single-copy probes. The ring (or derived) chromosomes can be identified with chromosome-specific alpha-satellite DNA probes. However, follow-up studies to define the size of the ring are limited in many cases. Appropriate probes are not available for follow-up studies for most chromosomes. However, in some cases (for example, where a ring is derived from chromosome 15), probes within the PWS/AS region can be used for further characterization and phenotypic correlations.

with an abnormal phenotype. Several different metacentric marker chromosomes, another subgroup, have been identified and found to be associated with an abnormal phenotype. These markers include iso(5p), iso(8p), iso(9p), iso(12p), and iso(18p).

An example of the use of FISH is seen in Figure 8.7, which shows the hybridization of a nonsatellited marker chromosome with a chromosome 7 specific alpha-satellite DNA probe, confirming its origin from that chromosome. The elastin gene probe, which is localized distally to the chromosome 7 alpha-satellite probe, was not present on the marker, thereby reducing the possibility that this marker will be associated with an abnormal phenotype. However, additional studies would need to be done to conclude this.

Marker chromosomes may be formed in different ways. For example, two ring chromosomes derived from chromosome 4 were found to have been formed by very different mechanisms.[93] One marker contained only centromeric and pericentromeric sequences, while the other contained centromeric sequences and other noncontiguous DNA sequences from both the long and short arms of the chromosome. Without single-copy probes to precisely delineate these markers, phenotypic-karyotype correlations would be of limited value.

The majority of the markers reported in the literature have been ascertained postnatally in individuals with phenotypic abnormalities, creating considerable ascertainment bias. However, enough work has been done to show specific phenotypes with some specific marker chromosomes. FISH with a combination of repetitive, single-copy and chromosomal libraries have been used to identify conclusively a number of markers that are associated with specific phenotypic syndromes, including iso(18p), iso(12p) seen in Pallister–Killian syndrome, der(11)t(11;22), and inv dup(15).

Several individual case reports have been published illustrating the use of FISH for the elucidation of prenatally detected markers. For example, markers identified by FISH as an i(12p) associated with Pallister–Killian syndrome and a marker identified as a dic(22) associated with cat-eye syndrome have been reported.[94,95] Both Thangavelu et al. and Müller-Navia et al. used microdissection to elucidate the origin of prenatally detected marker chromosomes.[96,97] In our collaborative studies, more than 155 markers detected

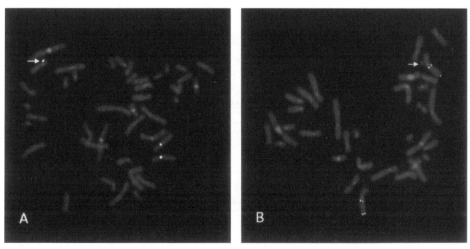

Fig. 8.7. A nonsatellited marker chromosome *A*, Hybridized with a chromosome 7 alpha-satellite DNA probe, demonstrating its origin from this chromosome. *B*, Lack of hybridization of the elastin gene, indicating that this gene is not present on the marker.

prenatally have been identified, and this number is certainly increased when adding the cases from the literature. Unfortunately, all of these markers have not been identified or fully characterized by FISH. In addition, many do not have appropriate clinical follow-up. However, many of these markers were delineated by FISH, and data overall show that 80 percent of these markers were derived from an acrocentric chromosome. Approximately 29 percent of the prenatally detected markers were familial; all of these were derived from an acrocentric chromosome, and more than two-thirds of the de novo markers were derived from an acrocentric chromosome. Postnatal outcome information was available for almost all of the familial cases, and the majority had a normal phenotype. As many as 28 percent of the de novo prenatal markers could be abnormal; however, this number is inflated because of ascertainment difficulties. However, both our data and those from the Crolla study suggest that the nonsatellited markers are more likely to be associated with an abnormal phenotype.[89,90] A large number of cases must be followed systematically before an adequate phenotype–karyotype correlation can be established for prenatally ascertained marker chromosomes.

STRUCTURAL REARRANGEMENTS: DUPLICATIONS

Although unbalanced chromosomal duplications are generally observed in studies of phenotypically abnormal individuals, they have also been observed in a few phenotypically normal individuals. Unbalanced duplications can occur as a consequence of various structural rearrangements. They most commonly result from the meiotic malsegregation of a rearrangement in a phenotypically normal balanced carrier. When these are detected prenatally, the identity of the chromosomes involved will allow for appropriate counseling. However, the duplications may also result from either de novo interchromosomal or intrachromosomal rearrangements. It has been difficult to determine the chromosomal origin of the extra material and the exact breakpoints of the duplicated segments using routine banding techniques. Both classical and molecular cytogenetic methodologies should be used to characterize the duplicated chromosomal material in these de novo rearrangements and allow for the appropriate counseling when they are ascertained prenatally.

As is the case for most of the structural rearrangements studied with FISH, relatively little work has been done using prenatally ascertained cases. However, even the postnatal study of these rearrangements has been limited; the majority of these rearrangements have been reported as single cases. Our recent survey of 136 patients with interchromosomal or intrachromosomal duplications is the largest systematic study of these rearrangements.[98] We found that the majority of duplications (96 of 136; 71 percent) were intrachromosomal. These intrachromosomal duplications could be subgrouped into four types of intrachromosomal rearrangements: (1) The most common rearrangements were direct tandem duplications identified in 57 percent of the cases. (2) Inverted tandem duplications were detected in nine percent of the cases. (3) A small number of patients (5 percent) had a duplication and insertion from one portion of the chromosome to another. (4) A simultaneous duplication and deletion of chromosomal material (e.g., isochromosome) was seen in 28 percent of the cases. The identity of the vast majority of these duplications could be inferred from the initial banding pattern; the origin of all but one of these could be confirmed with the use of only a single chromosomal library.

Although we were able to determine the origin of thirty-one of the forty interchromosomal duplications using high-resolution analysis and FISH with a single chromosome library, identification of the other five cases required use of multiple chromosome libraries.

In one case, we used twenty different libraries to determine the origin of the extra material. These studies were done before the availability of m-FISH/SKY and this latter case could be easily resolved with a multicolor analysis. In our current study, m-FISH is used to determine the chromosome origin of duplicated material for any case that cannot be resolved with four individual chromosome libraries.

No matter how unequivocal the banding pattern may be or how routine and expected a specific abnormality may be, the impression from routine cytogenetic studies should always be confirmed with FISH. When necessary, FISH with single-copy probes should be done to clarify the identity of an abnormal observation. The use of single-copy probes is exemplified by the studies of Jalal et al., who showed that patients with proximal duplications of 15q that do not contain the PWS/AS critical region are likely not to have an abnormal phenotype.[99] This is also true for other pericentromeric chromosomal regions such as 9p, 9q, and 16p.

Twenty-eight of the 136 duplications ascertained in these studies were prenatally detected.[98,100,101] A variety of chromosomes was involved, all of which were delineated or confirmed with the appropriate FISH studies. A useful example demonstrating the use of FISH for the determination of these structural abnormalities involves the case given below. Cytogenetic analysis of AFC, obtained during the course of evaluating a fetus for hydrocephalus, revealed an abnormal chromosome 8. G-banding studies suggested that it was an inverted duplication of the short arm of chromosome 8. FISH analysis with a whole chromosome 8 painting probe confirmed that all of the duplicated material originated from chromosome 8 (see Figure 8.8). Additional FISH studies with an 8p subtelomeric probe revealed that 8p subtelomeric DNA sequences were deleted in the abnormal chromosome. Based on the G-banding and FISH studies, it was determined that this patient had an inverted duplication of the short arm of one chromosome 8, and breakpoints were assigned to 8p11.2 and 8p23.1. Multiple patients with duplications of 8p with concurrent deletions of 8p23 have been reported in the literature, and therefore, appropriate counseling could be given.[102–104] We strongly recommend that FISH be used to study all chromosomal abnormalities detected during the course of prenatal diagnostic studies.[105,106]

PRENATAL DIAGNOSIS: INTERPHASE ANALYSIS

FISH has been used for cases in which metaphase chromosomes are not available for study, either by design or due to poor growth. The analysis of interphase cells from cultured specimens has been used successfully over the past several years, especially in the analysis of bone marrow transplantations and from noncultivated specimens, such as amniocytes.

The obvious advantage of interphase analysis of noncultivated AFC ("direct analysis") is that it provides a result more quickly because it obviates the need to wait for the growth of cells. When applied to prenatal diagnosis, this can reduce the necessary time from 7 to 10 days for metaphase analysis to just 24–48 hours for interphase analysis. The technology for analysis of noncultivated amniocytes was first introduced by Klinger et al. in 1992.[107] A list of several studies that examined the uses of these cells, along with the probes used and the success of the studies, is provided in Table 8.3.[107–124] These studies examined not only the feasibility of interphase FISH analysis but also many of the factors affecting the hybridization and detection of the signals.[107–125] Cells derived from prenatal studies performed late in gestation ($>$25 weeks) do not hybridize as well and provide an increased number of dead cells and cellular debris on the slide. These factors all in-

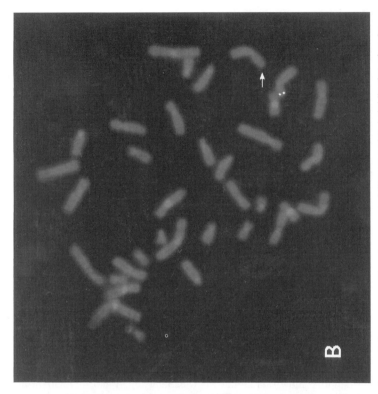

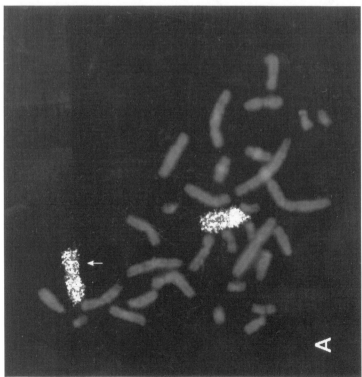

Fig. 8.8. An inverted duplicated chromosome 8 showing: *A*, Hybridization of the entire abnormal chromosome with a chromosome 8 library; and *B*, hybridization of an 8p subtelomeric probe to the normal chromosome 8, but not to the inv dup(8) chromosome.

Table 8.3. Interphase prenatal diagnosis by FISH: noncultivated amniocytes

Reference	Number Studied	Number Abnormal	Probes Used	Comments
Klinger et al.[107]	526	21	13,18,21,X and Y Single-copy probes	Five probes used on 117/526 samples
Ward et al.[110]	4,500	107	13,18,21,X and Y Single-copy probe	73.3% (107/146) detection rate
Carelli et al.[117]	13,883	464	13,18,21,X and Y	83.9% (464/553) detection rate for the study
			Single-copy probe	92.8% (161/181) detection in 1994
Bryndorf et al.[118]	2,000	40	13,18,21,X and Y Single-copy probes	Unable to reproduce results of Ward et al.[110] and Carelli et al.[117]
Weremowicz et al.[121]	911	80	13, 21—single copy 18, X, Y—alpha sat	84% (80/89) detection rate
Tepperberg et al.[122]	5,348	574	13, 21—single copy 18,X,Y—alpha sat	Literature of 29,039 cases; 6,576 new cases; 5,348 with AneuVysion probes
				Overall 1 false positive; 9 false negative
Sawa et al.[123]	2,319		13, 21—single copy 18,X,Y—alpha sat	87.6% detection rate
				Successful for use in third trimester
Witters et al.[124]	5,049	—	Only 21 used initially 13,18,X and Y later	Strategy to only use 21 probe initially followed by other probes in findings of ultrasound abnormalities proved successful

crease the difficulties with FISH analysis. Similarly, too few cells are often available from pregnancies at less than 15 weeks of gestation to be useful with this protocol. Bloody specimens will lower the hybridization efficiency because of cell crowding, and may be problematic because of the possibility of maternal cell contamination, although the studies examining the effect of maternal cell contamination have indicated that the low frequency of maternal cells detected should not hinder the evaluation.[126,127]

Prenatal interphase FISH analysis is generally effective and provides rapid and reliable results. In most cases, only a limited amount of material is needed. Interphase FISH studies appear to be especially useful for high-risk populations (e.g., fetal ultrasound abnormalities, advanced maternal age, increased risk conferred by triple marker screening, women ascertained after 20 weeks, and families with increased anxiety). Since the publication by Ward et al.[110] of the first large-scale application of interphase FISH for prenatal diagnosis, this technique has been used increasingly by most clinical laboratories. This method has become part of protocols of most laboratories.[122] In their initial study, Ward et al.[110] reported the detection of 107 of the 146 aneuploidies (73.3 percent) in their population. They reported that thirty-two abnormal cases were uninformative, seven cases yielded false-negative results for autosomal aneuploidies, and one case yielded a false-positive result for a sex chromosome aneuploidy.[110,128] In 1995, they updated this information by presenting data on more than 13,883 clinical specimens.[117] They found that interphase FISH studies were informative for 12,387 cases (89.2 percent), with a false-positive rate of 0.008 percent and a false-negative rate of 1.5 percent (7 of 471). Technologic refinements and increased technologist experience has increased both the accuracy and detection rates of FISH studies. For example, their accuracy increased from 99.8 percent (9,466 of 9,481) in 1991–1993 to 100 percent (2,906 of 2,906) in 1994 and their detection rate of abnormalities has improved from 79.6 percent (464 of 553) to 92.8 percent (168 of 181). Bryndorf et al.,[118] using the same probe set as Ward et al.[110], compared the results of FISH and conventional cytogenetics on 2,000 AF specimens. They were not able to reproduce the results of Ward et al.[110] and Carelli et al.[117] in their study. They found that the clinical utility of interphase FISH was affected by high rates of (1) unsuccessful hybridizations, (2) hybridization with less than fifty scorable nuclei, and (3) visibly contaminated samples.

Philip et al. suggested that if interphase FISH were considered a screening test, classical cytogenetic analysis should follow all abnormal or indeterminate results as in any screening test.[129] Using this scenario, they predicted that the accuracy of interphase FISH is potentially higher than that of other screening methods used for prenatal detection of trisomy 21. The limitations to their suggestion are the inability of interphase FISH to detect most structural rearrangements and the need to perform two amniocenteses. With respect to the first limitation, FISH will not detect all chromosomal abnormalities. Evans et al. surveyed the results of 72,994 prenatal cases from seven centers in four countries during 1990–1993.[130] There were 2,613 abnormalities detected during this period, of which only 1,745 (66.8 percent; range from centers, 52.6–84.5 percent) would have been detected by FISH with the 13, 18, 21, X, and Y single-copy probe set. Thus, one-third of the karyotype abnormalities would be missed. They recommend against replacement of complete karyotyping by interphase FISH because it would result in an unacceptably high false-negative rate for chromosomal abnormalities as a whole. A similar study by one of the groups in the above international collaboration published similar findings and conclusions in a study of 12,454 prenatal cytogenetic cases (7,529 amniocenteses and 4,925 CVS).[131] It should be noted that the numbers presented here may be somewhat misleading because not all undetectable abnormalities missed by FISH would have an impact on fetal development and well-being.

A number of studies validating the technology (Table 8.3) have been undertaken since the publication of these initial studies.[122] A number of technologic advances has led to improvements of these studies including: (1) a direct labeled probe set consisting of three repetitive DNA probes (18, X, and Y) and two single copy DNA probes localized to the long arms of chromosome 13 and 21; and (2) significantly improved methods for preparing noncultivated cells for analysis. As indicated above, although this technology can provide answers within 24 hours of obtaining a sample, it is limited in that it can only detect aneuploidies for a limited number of chromosomes (13, 18, 21, X, and Y). In a collaborative study of eight centers for 5 years a total of 146,128 amniocentesis were performed, revealing a total of 4,163 abnormalities; however, only 69.4 percent of these would have been detected using interphase analysis of noncultivated AFC.[132] A similar number (65–70 percent) has been proposed in a position statement by the American College of Medical Genetics (ACMG) and the American Society of Human Genetics (ASHG) (see below). However, they indicate that the detection rate will increase to 80 percent with increasing age because of the association of increased age and nondisjunction.[133] In 2001 Tepperberg reported on a 2–year multicenter retrospective analysis and review of literature of the AneuVysion assay (Vysis, Inc.). Using the data from the 29,039 studies, they were able to document that these probes revealed only one false-positive (0.003 percent) and seven false-negative (0.024 percent) results.[122] They conclude, similarly to most other investigators that this technology is an effective test for aneuploidy of the testable chromosomes in cases of advanced maternal age, or pregnancies indicated to be at increased risk due to maternal screening results or ultrasound findings.

At present, most laboratories use interphase FISH analysis routinely for prenatal diagnosis, but base this use on the preferences of their patients. Still in most cases it is used: (1) to reassure patients who have an unusually high degree of anxiety, or (2) to test for fetuses with an increased risk due to late gestational age, advanced maternal age, abnormal screening assays, or ultrasound findings. This latter group has always appeared to be an excellent population to study and is still a mainstay for the use of this technology.[134] Isada et al. studied fifty cases ascertained for abnormal ultrasound findings and detected eight abnormal fetuses (16 percent) by interphase FISH studies, a considerably higher frequency than in most study populations.[112]

As with any clinical test, specific guidelines must be met before using interphase FISH in the clinical laboratory. The laboratory must test the available probe sets and optimize one for use in its own studies. There are now a variety of commercial probes available for this testing, including the most commonly used, a three-color system available commercially through Vysis, Inc. Standards for evaluating samples need to be instituted and followed. Ward et al. suggested that at least fifty cells should be evaluated and that 80 percent of cells should demonstrate two signals to be considered disomic and 70 percent of cells should show three signals to be considered trisomic.[110] This pattern of analysis has become fairly standard in most laboratories. The conditions for hybridization can be difficult and must be well established on controls before proceeding with clinical testing, although in the past several years this technology has become much more routine. The evaluation of signals is a learned skill, as technologists become better evaluators with time.

Figure 8.9 shows four cells with varying signal patterns. The cell in the upper left corner clearly has only two signals, whereas the cell in the lower right has three areas of hybridization. The other two cells must be interpreted as having only two signals because the double signals are too close together to be considered separate signals. This part of the evaluation can be difficult for laboratories, and criteria for this evaluation must be

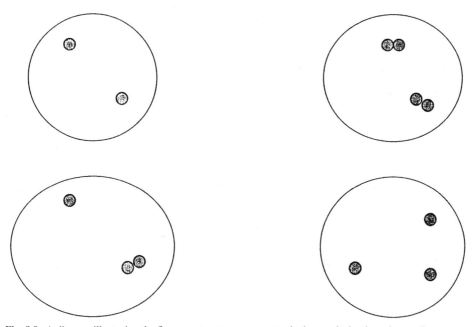

Fig. 8.9. A diagram illustrating the fluorescent patterns encountered when analyzing interphase cells.

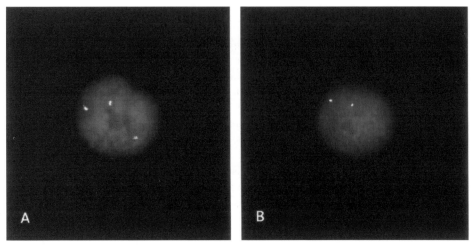

Fig. 8.10. Examples of interphase FISH using a repetitive probe to the centromere of chromosome 18. *A*, The results are consistent with trisomy 18. *B*, The results are disomic for chromosome 18.

carefully established and maintained. Figure 8.10 shows examples of interphase FISH showing results that are consistent with trisomy 18 (Figure 8.10*A*) and that are disomic for chromosome 18 (Figure 8.10*B*).

Although studies show both low false-positive and false-negative rates from recent studies, interphase FISH for prenatal diagnosis continues to be mainly an adjunct protocol for classic cytogenetic studies because of the inability to detect most structural abnormalities.[110,130,132,133] The recommendations regarding prenatal interphase fluorescence in situ hybridization articulated initially by the ACMG[135] included the following:

1. The investigational nature of FISH testing should be described clearly to all patients and health care providers.
2. Proper informed consent should be obtained following explanations of the purpose, accuracy, potential risks, and limitations of FISH testing.
3. Until accepted as a standard laboratory technique, FISH should be used in prenatal interphase cytogenetics only in conjunction with standard cytogenetic analysis.
4. Irreversible therapeutic action should not be initiated on the basis of FISH analysis alone.
5. Well-designed, multicenter, prospective trials should be undertaken to assess the reproducibility, sensitivity, specificity, and positive and negative predictive values, as well as the general applicability of FISH analysis in prenatal diagnosis.
6. Appropriate quality assurance/quality control for reagents and techniques in the development of standardized protocols must be established for FISH analysis.

In a published position paper in 2000, the ASHG/ACMG updated this statement and noted that prenatal screening for common autosomal trisomies and sex chromosome anomalies is becoming more routine as an initial study.[133] They indicated that among patients presenting with advanced maternal age (AMA >35) the clinical sensitivity of this test approaches 80 percent, but is reduced for all prenatal patients to approximately 65–70 percent. Increased use of FISH as an initial evaluation would need either the cost of this test to be significantly lower or technical enhancements to the available probe sets. They also indicated that decisions based on prenatal testing should be accompanied by two of the following three pieces of information: (1) FISH results, (2) routine chromosome analysis, and (3) clinical information.

CHORIONIC VILLUS SAMPLES (CVS)

Interphase FISH studies of noncultivated CVS have been reported less frequently than those with AF samples, possibly because it is relatively easy to obtain a complete karyotype analysis on direct CVS preparations within 24 hours of obtaining a specimen. Most of the interphase studies done on CVS have been small in both scope and number of patients analyzed (see Table 8.4).[136–143] Through 1995, approximately sixty or fewer patients had been examined in each study. Although these studies demonstrated the feasibility of interphase FISH on direct CVS cells for rapid analysis, the numbers are too small to make substantial conclusions. In 1996 Bryndorf et al. reported a study of 2,709 noncultivated CVS with interphase FISH.[140] Their novel approach was to examine, with interphase FISH, noncultivated mesenchymal chorionic villus cells within 24 hours rather than using conventional chromosome analysis on cytotrophoblasts during the same time interval. This approach was taken because studies have shown that, although direct studies of cytotrophoblasts can be done in 24 hours, there is a 1–2 percent false-positive rate and a 0.04 percent false-negative rate associated with this approach.[144] Bryndorf et al. also found that the technician time required by the two protocols was similar, taking about 1 hour of technician time. This study revealed that, on average, 99 percent of the nuclei had a hybridization pattern consistent with the sex of the fetus and that >94 percent of the nuclei demonstrated the appropriate pattern for fetuses with sex chromosome abnormalities. Cases needed to have >45 nuclei scored, with an abnormal number of hybridization signals seen in >60 percent of the cells to permit an abnormal diagnosis to be made. An informative disomic sample was defined as having three signals in <20 percent of the nuclei examined. Overall, 93 percent of the 2,709 samples were informative. The detection rate for the numerical abnormalities was 82 percent (80 of 97); there were two false-positive sex chromosome aberrations and four false-negative results (all mosaics). These results indicate the efficacy of CVS-interphase FISH studies.

Although there is less interest in performing interphase FISH on CVS samples than for AFC, several other laboratories have reported these findings. Cai et al. reported the

Table 8.4. Selected interphase prenatal diagnosis by FISH: CVS studies

Reference	Number Studied	Number Abnormal[a]	Comments
Evans et al.[136]	49	1	10% failure rate
Bryndorf et al.[140]	2,709[b]	80	94% technically successful
Cai et al.[141]	239	3	Successful in high-risk pregnancies 100% positive and negative predictive value
Quilter et al.[142]	100	12	FISH an accurate and less labor-intensive alternative to direct chromosome analysis of CVS
Fiddler et al.[143]	—		Useful and rapid assessment of fetal assessment before decisions about fetal reduction

[a]Detected by FISH.
[b]Includes 39 abnormal placental specimens.

successful use of probes for chromosomes 13, 18, 21, X, and Y in 239 CVS samples and indicated its importance in high-risk pregnancies.[141] In a smaller study of 100 CVS samples, Quilter et al. concluded that FISH with commercial probes was an accurate and less labor-intensive alternative to direct chromosome analysis of CVS.[142] In a study of multiple-gestation pregnancies using interphase FISH, Fiddler et al. concluded that FISH may provide rapid and useful assessment of fetal status in decision making regarding fetal reduction.[143] However, they did caution that there was an associated risk of obstetrical difficulty of ensuring a sample representative of each fetus following CVS. In addition to delineating chromosomal anomalies, some laboratories do use FISH in direct CVS preparations to assess fetal sex, but this approach is not used as frequently as it is for AFC studies. As is the case for AFC interphase FISH, each clinical laboratory must find the optimal probe set, develop standards for both disomic and aneuploid cases, and analyze the appropriate number of controls before using this approach as an adjunct procedure.

The guidelines espoused by the ACMG for AFC are also applicable to these CVS samples.[133] In their article, Bryndorf et al. suggested that based on earlier ACMG guidelines, the most effective way to use interphase FISH in the United States, as an adjunctive tool to conventional cytogenetics, is to offer the assay to pregnant women with an elevated risk of fetal aneuploidy.[140] However, in 2000, Bryndorf et al, indicated that 72 percent of the terminations of chromosomally abnormal pregnancies were based on FISH and ultrasound results rather than on conventional cytogenetic results, indicating how the attitude concerning this technology has changed in the past several years.[145]

Because of the potential of an inconclusive (or questionable) finding in CVS analysis, a number of groups have devised confirmatory tests involving FISH in the past several years. Mavrou et al. successfully used FISH analysis to study fetal nucleated erythrocytes isolated from CVS in 41 cases.[146] They indicated that this technique could be used as a quick and accurate method for the immediate verification of CVS results of mosaicism, thus avoiding amniocentesis. In a similar study Schuring-Blom et al. used FISH to study nucleated red blood cells from CVS washings to study six nonmosaic 45,X cases and seven trisomy 18 cases.[147] Their results also confirmed that the application of this technology could confirm a CVS diagnosis, minimize the risk of a false-positive result, and prevent a further invasive technique.

INTERPHASE STUDIES: FETAL CELLS IN MATERNAL BLOOD

It has always been a desire not only to provide prenatal diagnostic studies as early as possible but also to do this in the least invasive way possible. Attempts to analyze fetal cells obtained from the maternal circulation have been ongoing since the 1950s.[148] The intention here is to highlight the use of interphase FISH for analyzing these circulating fetal cells, more fully discussed in chapter 28.

FISH is currently the method of choice for analyzing the limited number of fetal nucleated red blood cells generally isolated from the maternal circulation. Using the common probe sets, FISH was shown to be effective for the diagnosis of trisomy 18, trisomy 21, and 47,XYY in fetal red blood cells.[149–151] In a summary of their initial work, Simpson and Elias detected seven of eight trisomic pregnancies in a group of sixty-nine pregnancies studied (see chapter 2).[152] FISH has been used as a tool for evaluating different methods of cell separation as well as different laboratory conditions for FISH analysis. For example, using FISH, Ganshirt-Ahlert et al. successfully identified five cases of trisomy 18 and ten cases of trisomy 21 in fetal cells sorted using a combination of triple-density gradient and magnetic sorting of antitransferring receptor antibody-labeled cells together with FISH analysis.[153] Zheng et al. combined simultaneous immunophenotyping of cells with mouse antifetal hemoglobin antibody with FISH (with X- and Y-specific DNA probes) to determine fetal sex.[154] This enabled the selective FISH analysis of fetal cells, even in the presence of excess maternal cells. In an effort to establish fetal nucleated red-blood-cell detection in maternal blood, Oosterwijk et al. demonstrated the successful detection of noninvasive prenatal diagnosis of trisomy 13, before CVS in the first trimester.[155] A number of different studies have now presented a variety of techniques to enrich for fetal cells in these samples. Bischoff et al. effectively demonstrated the use of five-color interphase FISH to analyze rare fetal aneuploidy in enriched flow-sorted cells isolated from maternal blood.[156] The common thread among these studies is the successful use of interphase FISH to detect either chromosomal trisomies or to identify fetal sex.[157–162] An analysis of these research studies suggests that interphase FISH is the method of choice for diagnosing aneuploidy in the fetal blood cells.

The majority of the recent data for this work come from the National Institute of Child Health Development Fetal Cell Isolation Study (NIFTY), which is a prospective multicenter project studying fetal cells recovered from maternal cells (see chapter 28).[163] Studies from 2,744 blood samples revealed a false-positive rate of gender identification in 11.1 percent; 74.4 percent of the cases of aneuploidy were detected by FISH and the false-positive rate of aneuploidy was estimated to be approximately 0.6–4.1 percent. Although controversy exists about whether fetal cells in the maternal blood can be reliably used for prenatal diagnosis with enrichment of fetal cells, the studies still emphasize that FISH offers the greatest promise for studying the limited number of cells likely to be available.[163–165]

INTERPHASE ANALYSIS: TRANSCERVICAL AND UTERINE CAVITY SAMPLES

FISH technology not only allows for more rapid prenatal diagnosis of certain types of abnormalities than current standard methods, but also may allow diagnosis to be at earlier stages of pregnancy. More than 20 years ago, Rhine et al. showed the potential of obtaining fetal cells from the uterine cavity early in pregnancy.[166] Obtaining fetal cells either from the uterine cavity or transcervically allows for early diagnosis of genetic disorders using minimally invasive procedures that are simple and easy to master.

In 1993, Adinolfi et al. initially demonstrated the efficacy of using FISH to study these fetal cells.[167] Subsequent studies focused on the usefulness of these samples for prenatal evaluation of fetal sex and determination of the frequency of fetal cells in these samples. Ville et al. used FISH on cells recovered by endocervical lavage to correctly predict the fetal sex in eight of ten cases.[168] A study of eleven samples obtained by lavage and eleven obtained by a cytobrush showed reliable determination of fetal sex by FISH (ten of eleven and nine of eleven, respectively).[169] However, in some cases, as few as 2 percent of the cells showed the fetal karyotype. In addition, two chromosomal abnormalities were detected in their study: a trisomy 21 fetus and a triploid fetus. Other work by this group used FISH to aid in confirming the isolation of fetal cells from transcervical samples by micromanipulation.[170] FISH analysis confirmed the isolation of fetal cells, making these samples more appropriate for prenatal diagnosis. Ishai et al. used two-color FISH with X and Y probes to successfully confirm fetal sex and assess maternal cell contamination in two groups of women studied by uterine cavity lavage.[171] In both groups, fetal sex could be determined in all cases studied and maternal contamination was assessed to be 5–10 percent. Massari et al. recovered fetal DNA from seventeen of thirty-nine (55 percent) transcervical cell samples obtained by endocervical canal flushing.[172] Examination of possible chromosome 21 aneuploidy was done on all seventeen samples using two-color FISH. Sixty to 100 nuclei were examined in each case and one fetus with trisomy 21 was detected and subsequently confirmed by direct cytogenetic analysis of a CVS sample. Chang et al. compared FISH results on transcervical cells collected by uterine lavage with cytogenetic results from CVS samples from thirty-six women.[173] They confirmed one abnormality, but could identify male fetuses in only thirteen of the fifteen cases and concluded that a specific fetal cell marker is necessary to avoid false-negative results. Fejgin et al. used a Pap smear fetal brush to obtain fetal cells and confirmed the findings by FISH on these samples by full chromosomal analysis in twenty-nine of thirty cases (one male was not identified).[174] In a study of twenty-five women by ErgIn et al., FISH was successfully used to detect the status of aneuploidy and fetal sex from transcervical cell samples (overall fetal sex was identified in eleven of twelve fetuses from uterine lavage and eight of ten from endocervical lavage).[175]

Cioni et al. detected Y FISH signals in 80 percent of known male pregnancies and none of the female pregnancies of the eighty-one pregnancies studied after obtaining transcervical samples by intrauterine lavage.[176] Most recently Bussani et al. revealed correct fetal sexing by FISH in forty-one of the forty-five male fetuses of the eighty-nine transcervical samples obtained (although PCR analysis detected forty-three of forty-five).[177] They concluded that both FISH and PCR techniques allowed the detection of common aneuplodies, confirming the power of this minimally invasive technique for obtaining transcervical cells. Overall, these studies have been limited in scope, but in general these studies confirm the use and potential use of FISH in these samples with some limitation.

INTERPHASE ANALYSIS: PREIMPLANTATION GENETIC DIAGNOSIS (PGD)

As efforts to perform prenatal testing are moved to earlier and earlier stages of pregnancy, fewer and fewer fetal cells will be available for analysis, and the more valuable FISH will become as an analytical tool. Grifo et al. presented work in 1992 showing the feasibility of using FISH for analyzing an in vitro fertilized (IVF) embryo before transfer.[178] Using both human and mouse Y-chromosome-specific probes, they studied human polyploid embryos that failed to divide and single-cell mouse blastomeres. In both cases, FISH successfully determined the sex of the embryo. In concurrent studies, Griffin et al. introduced FISH as a way of studying single human blastomeres.[179] Subsequently, dual-color fluorescence was established as the method of choice for embryo sexing by some laboratories.[180,181] The current status of preimplantation genetics is discussed in chapter 27; however, the application of FISH will be discussed briefly below.

Improvements in FISH technology have allowed it to become more advantageous than PCR alone for embryo sexing.[182] Technical advances have reduced the signal overlap and increased the efficiency of FISH. In addition, the introduction of directly labeled probes has allowed the determination of the sex of human preimplantation embryos in just 2 hours.[183,184] However, investigators have also introduced methods to allow sequential PCR and FISH analysis of single cells.[185,186]

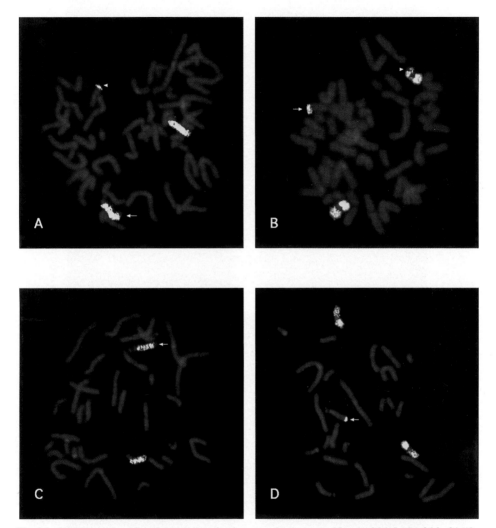

Fig. 8.2. Characterization of a subtle translocation between chromosomes 15 and 16 [t(15;16)(q26.3;q24.1)] by FISH in a carrier and unbalanced offspring: (*A*) hybridization with a chromosome 15 library in the balanced translocation; (*B*) hybridization with a chromosome 16 library in the balanced translocation; (*C*) hybridization with a chromosome 15 library in the unbalanced karyotype [der(16)t(15;16)(q26.3;q24.1)]; and (*D*) hybridization with a chromosome 16 library in the unbalanced karyotype.

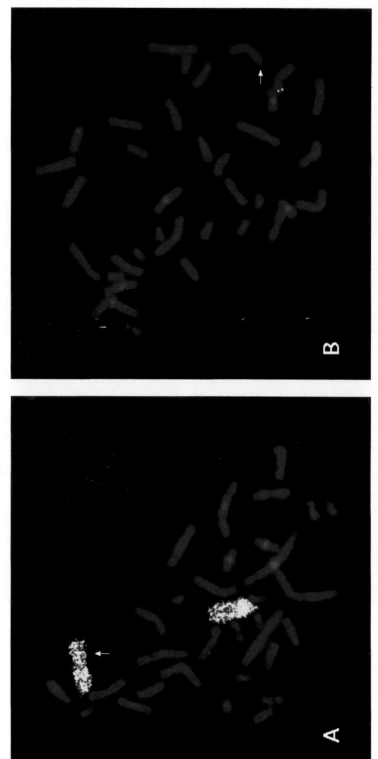

Fig. 8.8. An inverted duplicated chromosome 8 showing: (*A*) hybridization of the entire abnormal chromosome with a chromosome 8 library; and (*B*) hybridization of an 8p subtelomeric probe to the normal chromosome 8, but not to the inv dup (8) chromosome.

The vast majority of preimplantation FISH studies have been used for determination of sex in preimplantation embryos at risk for an X-linked disorders.[187] Through 1995, FISH was used in fourteen centers for determining embryonic sex; it was used to study cleavage-stage embryo biopsies and involved seventy cycles, resulting in fifteen pregnancies, eight deliveries, and eleven newborns.[188] The FISH studies of single blastomeres and whole embryos revealed four different chromosomal patterns: (1) normal chromosomes, all of the nuclei uniformly diploid; (2) diploid mosaics, in which the majority of the nuclei were aneuploid, but some normal diploid cells are present; (3) chromosomally abnormal, in which each of the nuclei demonstrate a chromosomal abnormality; and (4) chaotic, in which all of the nuclei showed a different chromosomal complement.[189] Because these studies demonstrated the frequent occurrence of chromosomal mosaicism, the authors recommended that for a chromosomal diagnosis at least two cells should be analyzed to reduce the chance of misdiagnosis.[189–191]

The aneuploidy technology and probes used are extremely useful, have been continually improved, and have been used successfully for the PGD of aneuploidy. Munne and Weier demonstrated that FISH with probes from chromosomes 13, 18, 21, X, and Y could be used for interphase PGD analysis.[192] They demonstrated no false-positive and 14 percent false-negative findings, which indicated that transferring an abnormal embryo could be minimized. Subsequent to this report, a number of other studies validating this work have also been done. Verlinsky et al. used FISH with DNA probes for chromosomes 13, 18, and 21 to study first and second polar bodies to lessen the chance of implanting an aneuploid fetus.[193] Of 3,651 oocytes obtained, FISH provided successful results in 80.9 percent of the cases of which 43.1 percent were aneuploid. Only oocytes without aneuploidy were implanted, and no children with aneuploidy for chromosomes 13, 18, and 21 resulted. The goal of aneuploid analysis in PGD is not only to not implant trisomy 13, 18, and 21 embryos, but also to maximize the number of viable embryos that are implanted. As such, some of the FISH analysis is done not only using the standard five DNA probes listed, but to also use probes for chromosomes 16 and 22. Trisomy 16 is the frequent aneuploidy detected in spontaneously lost pregnancies and by eliminating aneuploidy for 13, 16, 18, 21, 22, X, and Y, the rate of successful implantation has increased.

CONCLUSION

FISH has become an essential part of the cytogenetics laboratory for both prenatal and postnatal diagnosis. A variety of DNA probes are available for studies, ranging from a chromosome-specific library to single-copy probes ≤ 1 kb. Different tissues can be studied involving the analysis of metaphase chromosomes or undivided interphase cells.

For constitutional studies, FISH is extensively used with metaphase chromosomes to define structurally abnormal chromosomes. This can involve subtle deletions, duplications, or cryptic rearrangement of chromosomal material. FISH is frequently used for the detection of microdeletions associated with the contiguous gene syndromes. It has also been used extensively to define and characterize extrachromosomal material, whether present as interchromosomal or intrachromosomal duplications or supernumerary marker chromosomes. The appropriate probes for these studies include alpha-satellite DNA chromosome libraries and /or single-copy probes.

In prenatal studies, FISH is also commonly used to study interphase cells in which metaphase chromosomes are not available for study, especially by design. The most fre-

quent use has been in the "direct analysis" of noncultivated AF interphase cell for the
rapid prenatal diagnosis of aneuploidy.

REFERENCES

1. Pardue ML, Gall JG. Molecular hybridization of radioactive DNA to the DNA of cytological preparations. Proc Natl Acad Sci USA 1969;64:600.
2. Pinkel D, Straume T, Gray JW. Cytogenetic analysis using quantitative high sensitivity fluorescence hybridization. Proc Natl Acad Sci USA 1986;83:2934.
3. Landegent JE, Jansen IDW, Dirks RW, et al. Use of whole cosmid cloned genomic sequences for chromosomal localization by nonradioactive in-situ hybridization. Hum Genet 1987;77:366.
4. Schrock E, du Manoir S, Veldman T, et al. Multi-color spectral karyotyping of human chromosomes. Science 1996;273:494.
5. Speicher MR, Ballard SG, Ward DC. Karyotyping human chromosomes by combinatorial multi-fluor FISH. Nat Genet 1996;12:368.
6. Cremer T, Lichter P, Borden J, et al. Detection of chromosome aberrations in metaphase and interphase tumor cells by in-situ hybridization using chromosome specific library probes. Hum Genet 1988;80:235.
7. Pinkel D, Landegent J, Collins C, et al. Fluorescence in-situ hybridization with human chromosome-specific libraries: detection of trisomy 21 and translocations of chromosome 4. Proc Natl Acad Sci USA 1988;85:9138.
8. Lichter P, Cremer T, Borden J, et al. Delineation of individual human chromosomes in metaphase and interphase cells by in-situ suppression hybridization using recombinant DNA libraries. Hum Genet 1988;80:224.
9. Lichter P, Tang CJC, Call K, et al. High-resolution mapping of human chromosome 11 by in-situ hybridization with cosmid clones. Science 1990;247:64.
10. Schmickel RD. Contiguous gene syndromes. a component of recognizable syndromes. J Pediatr 1986;109:231.
11. Francke U, Ochs HD, de Martinville B, et al. Minor Xp21 chromosome deletion in a male associated with expression of Duchenne muscular dystrophy, chronic granulomatous disease, retinitis pigmentosa, and McLeod syndrome. Am J Hum Genet 1985;37:250.
12. Butler MG. Prader-Willi syndrome: current understanding of cause and diagnosis. Am J Med Genet 1990;35:319.
13. Williams CA, Frias JL. The Angelman ("happy puppet") syndrome. Am J Med Genet 1982;11:453.
14. Lindsay EA, Greenberg F, Shaffer LG, et al. Submicroscopic deletion at 22q11.2: variability of the clinical picture and delineation of a commonly deleted region. Am J Med Genet 1995;56:191.
15. Ewart AK, Morris CA, Atkinson D, et al. Hemizygosity at the elastic locus in a developmental disorder, Williams syndrome. Nat Genet 1993;5:11.
15a. Zollino M, Lecce R, Fischetto R, et al. Mapping the Wolf–Hirschhorn syndrome phenotype outside the currently accepted WHS critical region and defining a new critical region, WHSCR-2. Am J Hum Genet 2003;72:590.
15b. Bartsch O, Wuyts W, Van Hul W, et al. Delineation of a contiguous gene syndrome with multiple exostoses, enlarged parietal foramina, craniofacial dysostosis, and mental retardation, caused by deletions on the short arm of chromosome 11. Am J Hum Genet 1996;58:734.
15c. Hall CR, Wu Y, Sahffer LG, et al. Familial case of Potocki–Shaffer syndrome associated with microdeletion of EXT2 and ALX4. Clin Genet 2001;60:356.
16. Greenberg F, Guzetta V, Montes de Oca-Luna R, et al. Molecular analysis of the Smith–Magenis syndrome: a possible contiguous gene syndrome associated with del(17)(p11.2). Am J Med Genet 1991;49:1207.
16a. Aviram-Goldring A, Goldman B, Netanelov-Shapira I, et al. Deletion patterns of the STS gene and flanking sequences in Israeli X-linked ichthyosis patients and carriers: analysis by polymerase chain reaction and fluorescence in situ hybridization techniques. Int J Dermatol 2000;39:182.
16b. Valdes-Flores M, Kofman-Alfaro SH, Jimenez-Vaca AL, et al. Carrier identification by FISH analysis in isolated cases of X-linked ichthyosis. Am J Med Genet 2001;102:146.
17. Kuwano A, Ledbetter SA, Dobyns WB, et al. Detection of deletions and cryptic translocations in Miller–Dieker syndrome by in-situ hybridization. Am J Hum Genet 1991;49:707.
18. Yamamoto Y, Oguro N, Miyao M, et al. Tricho-rhino-phalangeal syndrome type I with severe mental retardation due to interstitial deletion of 8p23.3–24.13. Am J Med Genet 1989;32:133.

18a. Boycott KM, Parslow MI, Ross JL, et al. A familial contiguous gene deletion syndrome at Xp22.3 characterized by severe learning disabilities and ADHD. Am J Med Genet 2003;122A:139.

18b. des Portes V, Carrie A, Billuart P, et al. Inherited Microdeletion in Xp21.3–22.1 involved in non-specific mental retardation. Clin Genet 1998;53:136.

18c. Wong AC, Ning Y, Flint J, et al. Molecular characterization of a 130–kb terminal microdeletion at 22q in a child with mild mental retardation. Am J Hum Genet 1997;60:113.

18d. Wilson HL, Wong AC, Shaw SR, et al. Molecular characterization of the 22q13 deletion syndrome supports the role of haploinsufficiency of SHANK3/PROSAP2 in the major neurological symptoms. J Med Genet 2003;40:575.

18e. Enright F, Campbell P, Stallings RL, et al. Xp22.3 Microdeletion in a 19-year old girl with clinical features of MLS syndrome. Pediatr Dermatol 2003;20:153.

18f. Zenker M, Rittinger O, Grosse KP, et al. Monosomy 1p36: a recently delineated, clinically recognizable syndrome. Clin Dysmorphol 2002;11:43.

18g. Johnson D, Horsley SW, Moloney DM, et al. A comprehensive screen for TWIST mutations in patients with craniosynostosis identifies a new microdeletion syndrome of chromosome band 7p21.1. Am J Hum Genet 1998;63:1282.

18h. Kosan C, Kunz J. Identification and characterization of the gene TWIST NEIGHBOR (TWISTNB) located in the microdeletion syndrome 7p21 region. Cytogenet Genome Res 2002;97:167.

19. Francke U, Holmes LB, Atkins L, et al. Aniridia-Wilms' tumor association: evidence for specific deletion of 11p13. Cytogenet Cell Genet 1979;24:185.

19a. Cario H, Bode H, Gustavsson P, et al. A microdeletion syndrome due to a 3–Mb deletion on 19q13.2: Diamond–Blackfan anemia associated with microcephaly, hypotonia, and psychomotor retardation. Clin Genet 1999;55:487.

19b. Tentler D, Gustavsson P, Elinder G, et al. A Microdeletion in 19q13.2 associated with mental retardation, skeletal malformations, and Diamond–Blackfan anaemia suggest a novel contiguous gene syndrome. J Med Genet 2000;37:128.

20. Pettigrew AL, Greenberg F, Caskey CT, et al. Grieg syndrome associated with an interstitial deletion of 7p: confirmation of the localization of Grieg syndrome to 7p13. Hum Genet 1991;87:452.

20a. Massin N, Pecheux C, Eloit C, et al. X chromosome-linked Kallmann syndrome: clinical heterogeneity in three siblings carrying an intragenic deletion of the KAL-1 gene. J Clin Endocrinol Metab 2003;88:2003.

21. Wilke AOM, Buckle VJ, Harris PC, et al. Clinical features and molecular analysis of the α-thalassemia/mental retardation syndromes. I. Cases due to deletions involving chromosome band 16p13.3. Am J Hum Genet 1990;46:1112.

22. Breuning MH, Dauwerse HG, Fugazza G, et al. Rubinstein–Taybi syndrome caused by submicroscopic deletions within 16p13.13. Am J Hum Genet 1993;52:249.

23. Anad F, Burn J, Matthews D, et al. Alagille syndrome and deletion of 20p. J Med Genet 1990;227:729.

24. Davidson A, Khandelwal M, Punnett HH. Prenatal diagnosis of the 22q11 deletion syndrome. Prenat Diagn 1997;17:380.

25. Manji S, Roberson JR, Wiktor A, et al. Prenatal diagnosis of 22q11.2 deletion when ultrasound examination reveals a heart defect. Genet Med 2001;3:65.

26. Boudjemline Y, Fermont L, Le Bidois J, et al. Can we predict 22q11 status of fetuses with tetralogy of Fallot? Prenat Diagn 2002;22:231.

27. Devriendt K, Van Schoubroeck D, Eyskens B, et al. Polyhydramnios as a prenatal symptom of the DiGeorge/velo-cardio-facial syndrome. Prenat Diagn 1998;18:68.

28. Kashork CD, Sutton VR, Fonda Allen JS, et al. Low or absent unconjugated estriol in pregnancy: an indicator for steroid sulfatase deficiency detectable by fluorescence in situ hybridization and biochemical analysis. Prenat Diagn 2002;22:1028.

29. Driscoll DA, Salvin J, Sellinger B, et al. Prevalence of 22q11 microdeletions in DiGeorge and velocardiofacial syndromes: implications for genetic counseling and prenatal diagnosis. J Med Genet 1993;30:813.

30. Van Hemel JO, Schaap C, Van Opstal D, et al. Recurrence of DiGeorge syndrome: prenatal detection by FISH of a molecular 22q11 deletion. J Med Genet 1995;32:657.

31. Kuwano A, Ledbetter SA, Dobyns WB, et al. Detection of deletions and cryptic translocations in Miller–Dieker syndrome by in-situ hybridization. Am J Hum Genet 1991;49:707.

32. Kashork CD, Chen KS, Lupski JR, et al. Prenatal diagnosis of Charcot–Marie–Tooth disease type 1A. Ann NY Acad Sci 1999;883:457.

33. Inoue K, Osaka H, Thurston VC, et al. Genomic rearrangements resulting in PLP1 deletion occur by non-

homologous end joining and cause different dysmyelinating phenotypes in males and females. Am J Hum Genet 2002;71:838.

34. Speleman F, Van Roy N, Wiegant J, et al. Detection of subtle reciprocal translocations by fluorescence in-situ hybridization. Clin Genet 1992;41:169.

35. Sullivan BA, Leana-Cox J, Schwartz S. Clarification of subtle reciprocal rearrangements using fluorescence in-situ hybridization. Am J Med Genet 1993;47:223.

36. Bernstein R, Bocian ME, Cain MJ, et al. Identification of a cryptic t(5;7) reciprocal translocation by fluorescent in-situ hybridization. Am J Med Genet 1993;46:77.

37. Shaffer LG, Spikes AS, Macha M, et al. Identification of a subtle chromosomal translocation in a family with recurrent miscarriages and a child with multiple congenital anomalies. J Reprod Med 1996;41:367.

38. Knight SJ, Horsley SW, Regan R, et al. Development and clinical application of an innovative fluorescence in situ hybridization technique which detects submicroscopic rearrangements involving telomeres. Eur J Hum Genet 1997;5:1.

39. Knight SJ, Lese CM, Precht KS, et al. An optimized set of human telomere clones for studying telomere integrity and architecture. Am J Hum Genet 2000;67:320.

40. Knight SJ, Regan R, Nicod A, et al. Subtle chromosomal rearrangements in children with unexplained mental retardation. Lancet 1999;354:1676.

41. Rossi E, Piccini F, Zollino M, et al. Cryptic telomeric rearrangements in subjects with mental retardation associated with dysmorphism and congenital malformations. J Med Genet 2001;38:417.

42. Joyce CA, Dennis NR, Cooper S, et al. Subtelomeric rearrangements: results from a study of selected and unselected probands with idiopathic mental retardation and control individuals by using high-resolution G-banding and FISH. Hum Genet 2001;109:440.

43. Anderlid BM, Schoumans J, Anneren G, et al. Subtelomeric rearrangements detected in patients with idiopathic mental retardation. Am J Med Genet 2002;107:275.

44. Jalal SM, Harwood AR, Sekhon GS, et al. Utility of subtelomeric fluorescent DNA probes for detection of chromosome anomalies in 425 patients. Genet Med 2003;5:28.

45. Popp S, Schulze B, Granzow M, et al. Study of 30 patients with unexplained developmental delay and dysmorphic features or congenital abnormalities using conventional cytogenetics and multiplex FISH telomere (M-TEL) integrity assay. Hum Genet 2002;111:31.

46. Souter VL, Glass IA, Chapman DB, et al. Multiple fetal anomalies associated with subtle subtelomeric chromosomal rearrangements. Ultrasound Obstet Gynecol 2003;21:609.

47. Warburton D. De novo balanced chromosome rearrangements and extra marker chromosomes identified at prenatal diagnosis: clinical significance and distribution of breakpoints. Am J Hum Genet 1991;49:995.

48. Kumar A, Becker LA, Depinet TW, et al. Molecular characterization and delineation of subtle deletions in de novo "balanced" F chromosomal rearrangements. Hum Genet 1998;103:173.

49. Astbury C, Christ L, Aughton D, et al. Detection of cryptic deletions in *de novo* 'balanced' chromosome rearrangements: further evidence for their role in phenotypic abnormalities. Genetics in Medicine 2004, in press.

50. Jauch A, Daumer C, Lichter P, et al. Chromosomal in-situ suppression hybridization of human gonosomes and autosomes and its use in clinical cytogenetics. Hum Genet 1990;85:145.

51. Senger G, Chudoba I, Friedrich U, et al. Prenatal diagnosis of a half-cryptic translocation using chromosome microdissection. Prenat Diagn 1997;17:369.

52. Ferguson-Smith MA, Yates YRW. Maternal age specific rates for chromosome aberrations and factors influencing them: a report of a collaborative European study on 52,965 amniocenteses. Prenat Diagn 1994;4:5.

53. Hook EB, Cross PK. Extra structurally abnormal chromosomes (ESAC) detected at amniocentesis: frequency in approximately 75,000 prenatal cytogenetic diagnoses and association with maternal and paternal age. Am J Hum Genet 1987;40:83.

54. Sachs ES, van Hemel JO, den Hollander JC, et al. Marker chromosomes in a series of 10,000 prenatal diagnoses. Prenat Diagn 1987;7:81.

55. Schwartz S, Depinet TW, Leana-Cox J, et al. Sex chromosome markers: characterization using fluorescence in-situ hybridization and review of the literature. Am J Med Genet 1997;93:366.

56. Scully RE. Gonadoblastoma: a review of 74 cases. Cancer 1970;25:1340.

57. Nagel T, Carnage M, Tagatz G, et al. Gonadal tumors in patients with gonadal dysgenesis and sex chromosome rings and fragments. Am J Obstet Gynecol 1984;150:76.

58. Kushnick T, Irons TG, Wiley JE, et al. 45X/46X,r(X) with syndactyly and severe mental retardation. Am J Med Genet 1987;28:567.

59. Grompe M, Rao N, Elder FFB, et al. 45,X/46,X+r(X) can have a distinct phenotype different from Ullrich–Turner syndrome. Am J Med Genet 1992;42:39.

60. Van Dyke DL, Witkor A, Palmer G, et al. Ullrich–Turner syndrome with a small ring X chromosome and presence of mental retardation. Am J Med Genet 1992;43:996.

61. Migeon B, Luo S, Stasiowski BA, et al. Deficient transcription of XIST from tiny ring X chromosomes in females with severe phenotypes. Proc Natl Acad Sci USA 1993;90:12025.

62. Wolff DJ, Brown H, Schwartz S, et al. Small marker X chromosomes lack the X inactivation center: implications for karyotype/phenotype correlations. Am J Hum Genet 1994;55:87.

63. Jani MM, Torchia BS, Pai GS, et al. Molecular characterization of tiny ring X chromosomes from females with functional X chromosomes disomy and lack of cis X inactivation. Genomics 1995;27:182.

64. Cole H, Stevens C, Brown J, et al. The identification of marker chromosomes using cytogenetic and molecular techniques. Am J Hum Genet 1990;47:A28.

65. Bajalica S, Bui TH, Koch J, et al. Prenatal investigation of 46,X/46,X,r(?) karyotype in amniocytes using fluorescence in-situ hybridization with an X-centromere probe. Prenat Diagn 1992;12:61.

66. Slim R, Soulie J, Hotmar J, et al. Prenatal identification of an isochromosomes for the short arm of the Y i(Yp), by cytogenetic and molecular analyses. Prenat Diagn 1994;14:23.

67. Qu J, Dallaire L, Fetni R, et al. Prenatal identification of a 45,X/46,Xder(Y) mosaicism and confirmation by high resolution cytogenetics and fluorescence in-situ hybridization. Prenat Diagn 1992;12:909.

68. Bernstein R, Steinghaus KA, Cain MJ. Prenatal application of fluorescent in-situ hybridization (FISH) for identification of a mosaic Y chromosome marker, idic(Yp). Prenat Diagn 1992;12:709.

69. Amiel A, Fejgin M, Appelman Z, et al. Fluorescent in-situ hybridization (FISH) as an aid to marker chromosome identification in prenatal diagnosis. Eur J Obstet Gynecol Reprod Biol 1995;59:103.

70. Wang BBT, Loh-Chung Y, Willow P, et al. Prenatal identification of i(Yp) by molecular cytogenetic analysis. Prenat Diagn 1995;15:1115.

71. Yaron Y, Carmon E, Goldstein M, et al. The clinical application of spectral karyotyping (SKY) in the analysis of prenatally diagnosed extra structurally abnormal chromosomes (ESACs). Prenat Diagn 2003;23:74.

72. Hernando C, Carrera M, Ribas I, et al. Prenatal and postnatal characterization of Y chromosome structural anomalies by molecular cytogenetic analysis. Prenat Diagn 2002;22:802.

73. Li MM, Howard-Peebles PN, Killos LD, et al. Characterization and clinical implications of marker chromosomes identified at prenatal diagnosis. Prenat Diagn 2000;20:138.

74. Velagaleti GV, Tharapel SA, Martens PR, et al. Rapid identification of marker chromosomes using primed in situ labeling (PRINS). Am J Med Genet 1997;71:130.

75. Viersbach R, Engels H, Gamerdinger U, et al. Delineation of supernumerary marker chromosomes in 38 patients. Am J Med Genet 1998;76:351.

76. Hoshi N, Tonoki H, Handa Y, et al. Prenatal identification of mos 45,X/46,X,+mar in a normal male baby by cytogenetic and molecular analysis. Prenat Diagn 1998;18:1316.

77. Le Caignec C, Boceno M, Joubert M, et al. Prenatal diagnosis of a small supernumerary, XIST-negative, mosaic ring X chromosome identified by fluorescence in situ hybridization in an abnormal male fetus. Prenat Diagn 2003;23:143.

78. Callen DF, Ringenbergs ML, Fowler JCS, et al. Small marker chromosomes in man: origin from pericentric heterochromatin of chromosomes 1, 9, and 16. J Med Genet 1990;27:155.

79. Schad CR, Kraker WJ, Jalal SM, et al. Use of fluorescent in-situ hybridization for marker chromosome identification in congenital and neoplastic disorders. Am J Clin Pathol 1991;96:203.

80. Callen DF, Eyre HJ, Ringenbergs ML, et al. Chromosomal origin of small ring marker chromosomes in man: characterization by molecular genetics. Am J Hum Genet 1991;48:769.

81. Callen DF, Eyre H, Yip MY, et al. Molecular cytogenetic and clinical studies of 42 patients with marker chromosomes. Am J Med Genet 1992;43:709.

82. Rauch A, Pfeiffer RA, Trautmann U, et al. A study of ten small supernumerary (marker) chromosomes identified by fluorescence in-situ hybridization (FISH). Clin Genet 1992;42:84.

83. Crolla JA, Dennis NR, Jacobs PA. A non-isotopic in-situ hybridization of the chromosomal origin of 15 supernumerary marker chromosomes in man. J Med Genet 1992;29:699.

84. Plattner R, Heerema NA, Howard-Peebles PN, et al. Clinical findings in patients with marker chromosomes identified by fluorescence in-situ hybridization. Hum Genet 1993;91:589.

85. Plattner R, Heerema NA, Yurov YB, et al. Efficient identification of marker chromosomes in 27 patients by stepwise hybridization with alpha-satellite DNA probes. Hum Genet 1993;91:131.

86. Blennow E, Bui TH, Kristoffersson U, et al. Swedish survey on extra structurally abnormal chromosomes

in 39,105 consecutive prenatal diagnoses: prevalence and characterization by fluorescence in-situ hybridization. Prenat Diagn 1994;14:1019.

87. Brondum-Nielson K, Mikkelsen M. A 10–year old survey, 1980–1990, of prenatally diagnosed small supernumerary marker chromosomes, identified by FISH analysis: outcome and follow-up of 14 cases diagnosed in a series of 12,699 prenatal samples. Prenat Diagn 1995;15:615.

88. Blennow E, Brondum-Nielson K, Telenius H, et al. Fifty probands with extra structurally abnormal chromosomes characterized by fluorescence in-situ hybridization. Am J Med Genet 1995;55:85.

89. Crolla JA, Long F, Rivera H, et al. FISH and molecular study of autosomal supernumerary marker chromosomes excluding those derived from chromosomes 15 and 22. I. Results of 26 new cases. Am J Med Genet 1998;75:355.

90. Crolla JA. FISH and molecular studies of autosomal supernumerary marker chromosomes excluding those derived from chromosome 15. II. Review of the literature. Am J Med Genet 1998;75:367.

91. Leana-Cox J, Jenkins L, Palmer CG, et al. Molecular cytogenetic analysis of inv dup(15) chromosomes, using probes specific for the Prader–Willi/Angelman syndrome region: clinical implications. Am J Hum Genet 1994;54:748.

92. Depinet TW, Zackowski JL, Earnshaw WC, et al. Characterization of neo-centromeres in marker chromosomes lacking detectable alpha-satellite DNA. Hum Mol Genet 1997;6:1195.

93. Fang YY, Eyre HJ, Bohlander SK, et al. Mechanisms of small ring formation suggested by the molecular characterization of two small accessory ring chromosomes derived from chromosome 4. Am J Hum Genet 1995;57:1137.

94. Reeser SL, Donnenfeld AE, Miller RC, et al. Prenatal diagnosis of the derivative chromosome 22 associated with cat eye syndrome by fluorescence in-situ hybridization. Prenat Diagn 1994;14:1029.

95. McLean S, Stanley W, Stern H, et al. Prenatal diagnosis of Pallister-Killian syndrome: Resolution of cytogenetic ambiguity by use of fluorescent in-situ hybridization. Prenat Diagn 1992;12:985.

96. Thangavelu M, Pergament E, Espinosa III R, et al. Characterization of marker chromosomes by microdissection and fluorescence in-situ hybridization. Prenat Diagn 1994:14:583.

97. Müller-Navia J, Nebel A, Schleiermacher E. Complete and precise characterization of marker chromosomes by application of microdissection in prenatal diagnosis. Hum Genet 1995;96:661.

98. Tarvin R, Christ L, Curtis C, et al. Delineation of the origin and structure of chromosomal duplications: analysis of 136 cases. Am J Hum Genet 2003;71:A315.

99. Jalal SM, Persons DL, Dewald GW, et al. Form of 15q proximal duplication appears to be a normal euchromatic variant. Am J Med Genet 1994;52:495.

100. Leana-Cox J, Levin S, Surana R, et al. Characterization of de novo duplications in eight patients by using fluorescence in-situ hybridization with chromosome-specific DNA libraries. Am J Hum Genet 1993;52:1067.

101. Wolff DJ, Raffel LJ, Ferre MM, et al. Prenatal ascertainment of an inherited dup(18p) associated with an apparently normal phenotype. Am J Med Genet 1991;41:319.

102. Henderson KG, Dill FJ, Wood S. Characterization of an inversion duplication of the short arm of chromosome 8 by fluorescent in-situ hybridization. Am J Med Genet 1992;44:615.

103. Minelli A, Floridia G, Rossi E, et al. D8S7 is consistently deleted in inverted duplications of the short arm of chromosome 8 (inv dup 8p). Hum Genet 1993;92:391.

104. Dill FJ, Schertzer M, Sandercock J, et al. Inverted tandem duplication generates a duplication deficiency of chromosome 8p. Clin Genet 1987;32:109.

105. Neumann AA, Robson LG, Smith A. A 15p+ variant shown to be a t(Y;15) with fluorescence in-situ hybridization. Ann Genet 1992;4:227.

106. Siffroi JP, Molina-Gomez F, Viguie F, et al. Prenatal diagnosis of partial 2p trisomy by 'de novo' duplication 2p (13.1→21): confirmation by FISH. Prenat Diagn 1994;14:1097.

107. Klinger K, Landes G, Shook D, et al. Rapid detection of chromosome aneuploidies in uncultured amniocytes by using fluorescence in-situ hybridization (FISH). Am J Hum Genet 1992;51:55.

108. Christensen B, Bryndorf T, Philip J, et al. Rapid prenatal diagnosis of trisomy 18 and triploidy in interphase nuclei of uncultured amniocytes by non-radioactive in-situ hybridization. Prenat Diagn 1992;12:241.

109. Zheng YL, Ferguson-Smith A, Warner JP, et al. Analysis of chromosome 21 copy number in uncultured amniocytes by fluorescence in-situ hybridization using a cosmid contig. Prenat Diagn 1992;12:931.

110. Ward BE, Gersen SL, Carelli MP, et al. Rapid prenatal diagnosis of chromosomal aneuploidies by fluorescence in-situ hybridization: clinical experience with 4500 specimens. Am J Hum Genet 1993;52:854.

111. Davies AF, Barber L, Murer-Orlando M, et al. FISH detection of trisomy 21 in interphase by the simultaneous use of two differentially labelled cosmid contigs. J Med Genet 1994;31:679.

112. Isada NB, Hume Jr, RF, Reichler A, et al. Fluorescent in-situ hybridization and second-trimester sonographic anomalies: uses and limitations. Fetal Diagn Ther 1994;9:367.

113. Cacheux V, Tachdjian G, Druart L, et al. Evaluation of X, Y, 18, and 13/21 alpha satellite DNA probes for interphase cytogenetic analysis of uncultured amniocytes by fluorescence in-situ hybridization. Prenat Diagn 1994;14:79.

114. Spathas DH, Divane A, Maniatis GM, et al. Prenatal detection of trisomy 21 in uncultured amniocytes by fluorescence in-situ hybridization: a proactive study. Prenat Diagn 1994;14:1049.

115. Gersen SL, Carelli MP, Klinger KW, et al. Rapid prenatal diagnosis of 14 cases of triploidy using FISH with multiple probes. Prenat Diagn 1995;15:1.

116. Verlinsky Y, Ginsberg N, Chmura M, et al. Cross-hybridization of the chromosome 13/21 alpha-satellite DNA probe to chromosome 22 in the prenatal screening of common chromosomal aneuploidies by FISH. Prenat Diagn 1995;15:831.

117. Carelli MP, Lamb AN, Estabrooks LL, et al. Prenatal interphase FISH analysis of amniocytes: longitudinal study of accuracy and detection rates. Am J Hum Genet 1995;56:A50.

118. Bryndorf T, Christensen B, Vad M, et al. Prenatal detection of chromosome aneuploidies by fluorescence in situ hybridization: experience with 2000 uncultured amniotic fluid samples in a prospective preclinical trial. Prenat Diagn 1997;17:333.

119. Jalal SM, Law ME, Carlson RO, et al.: Prenatal detection of aneuploidy by directly labeled multicolored probes and interphase fluorescence in situ hybridization. Mayo Clin Proc 1998;73:132.

120. Eiben B, Trawicki W, Hammans W, et al. Rapid prenatal diagnosis of aneuploidies in uncultured amniocytes by fluorescence in situ hybridization: evaluation of >3,000 cases. Fetal Diagn Ther 1999;14:193.

121. Weremowicz S, Sandstrom DJ, Morton CC, et al. Fluorescence in situ hybridization (FISH) for rapid detection of aneuploidy: experience in 911 prenatal cases. Prenat Diagn 2001;21:262.

122. Tepperberg J, Pettenati MJ, Rao PN, et al. Prenatal diagnosis using interphase fluorescence in situ hybridization (FISH): 2–year multi-center retrospective study and review of the literature. Prenat Diagn 2001;21:293.

123. Sawa R, Hayashi Z, Tanaka T, et al. Rapid detection of chromosome aneuploidies by prenatal interphase FISH (fluorescence in situ hybridization) and its clinical utility in Japan. J Obstet Gynaecol Res 2001;27:41.

124. Witters I, Devriendt K, Legius E, et al. Rapid prenatal diagnosis of trisomy 21 in 5049 consecutive uncultured amniotic fluid samples by fluorescence in situ hybridisation (FISH). Prenat Diagn 2002;22:29.

125. Schwartz S, Micale MM. Preparation of amniocytes for interphase fluorescence in-situ hybridization (FISH). In: Boyle AL, ed. Current protocols in human genetics. New York: Wiley, 1995:8.9.1.

126. Nub S, Brebaum D, Grond-Ginsbach C. Maternal cell contamination in amniotic fluid samples as a consequence of the sampling technique. Hum Genet 1994;93:121.

127. Rebello MT, Abas A, Nicolaides K, et al. Maternal contamination of amniotic fluid demonstrated by DNA analysis. Prenat Diagn 1994;14:109.

128. Benn P, Ciarleglio L, Lettieri L, et al. A rapid (but wrong) prenatal diagnosis. N Engl J Med 1992;326:1638.

129. Philip J, Bryndorf T, Christensen B. Prenatal aneuploidy detection in interphase cells by fluorescence in-situ hybridization (FISH). Prenat Diagn 1994;14:1203.

130. Evans MI, Henry GP, Miller WA, et al. International, collaborative assessment of limitations of chromosome-specific probes (CSP) and fluorescent in-situ hybridization (FISH): analysis of expected detections in 73,000 prenatal cases. Am J Hum Genet 1994;55:A45.

131. Hume RF Jr, Kilmer-Ernst P, Wolfe HM, et al. Prenatal cytogenetic abnormalities: correlations of structural rearrangements and ultrasonographically detected fetal anomalies. Am J Obstet Gynecol 1995;173:1334.

132. Feldman B, Ebrahim SA, Hazan SL, et al. Routine prenatal diagnosis of aneuploidy by FISH studies in high-risk pregnancies. Am J Med Genet 2000;9:233.

133. Test and Technology Transfer Committee, American College of Medical Genetics. Technical and clinical assessment of fluorescence in situ hybridization: an ACMG/ASHG position statement. I. Technical considerations. Genet Med 2000;2:356.

134. Schwartz S. Efficacy and applicability of interphase fluorescence in-situ hybridization for prenatal diagnosis. Am J Hum Genet 1993;52:851.

135. American College of Medical Genetics. Prenatal interphase fluorescence in-situ hybridization (FISH) policy statement. Am J Hum Genet 1993;53:526.

136. Evans MI, Klinger KW, Isada NB, et al. Rapid prenatal diagnosis by fluorescent in-situ hybridization of chorionic villi: an adjunct to long-term culture and karyotype. Am J Obstet Gynecol 1992;167:1522.

137. Lebo RV, Flandermeyer RR, Diukman R, et al. Prenatal diagnosis with repetitive in-situ hybridization probes. Am J Med Genet 1992;43:848.

138. Rao PN, Hayworth R, Cox K, et al. Rapid detection of aneuploidy in uncultured chorionic villus cells using fluorescence in-situ hybridization. Prenat Diagn 1993;13:233.

139. Bryndorf T, Christensen B, Xiang Y, et al. Fluorescence in-situ hybridization with a chromosome 21–specific cosmid contig: 1–day detection of trisomy 21 in uncultured mesenchymal chorionic villus cells. Prenat Diagn 1994;14:87.

140. Bryndorf T, Christensen B, Vad M, et al. Prenatal detection of chromosome aneuploidies in uncultured chorionic villus samples by FISH. Am J Hum Genet 1996;59:918.

141. Cai LS, Lim AS, Tan A. Rapid one-day fluorescence in situ hybridisation in prenatal diagnosis using uncultured amniocytes and chorionic villi. Ann Acad Med Singapore 1999;28:502.

142. Quilter CR, Holman S, AL-Hammadi RM, et al. Aneuploidy screening in direct chorionic villus samples by fluorescence in situ hybridisation: the use of commercial probes in a clinical setting. BJOG 2001;108:215.

143. Fiddler M, Frederickson MC, Chen PX, et al. Assessment of fetal status in multiple gestation pregnancies using interphase FISH. Prenat Diagn 2001;21:196.

144. Simoni G, Sirchia SM. Confined placental mosaicism. Prenat Diagn 1994;14:1185.

145. Bryndorf T, Lundsteen C, Lamb A, et al. Rapid prenatal diagnosis of chromosome aneuploidies by interphase fluorescence in situ hybridization: a one-year clinical experience with high-risk and urgent fetal and postnatal samples. Acta Obstet Gynecol Scand 2000;79:8.

146. Mavrou A, Zheng YL, Kolialexi A, et al. Fetal nucleated erythrocytes (NRBCs) in chorionic villus sample supernatant fluids: an additional source of fetal material for karyotype confirmation. Prenat Diagn 1997;17:643.

147. Schuring-Blom GH, Hoovers JM, van Lith JM, et al. FISH analysis of fetal nucleated red blood cells from CVS washings in cases of aneuploidy. Prenat Diagn 2001;21:864.

148. Holzgreve W, Garritsen HS, Ganshirt-Ahlert D. Fetal cells in the maternal circulation. J Reprod Med 1992;37:410.

149. Price J, Elias S, Wachtel SS, et al. Prenatal diagnosis using fetal cells isolated from maternal blood by multi-parameter flow cytometry. JAMA 1993;270:2357.

150. Elias S, Price J, Dockter M, et al. First trimester prenatal diagnosis of trisomy 21 in fetal cells from maternal blood. Lancet 1992;340:1033.

151. Cacheux V, Milesi-Fluet C, Tachdjian G, et al. Detection of 47,XYY trophoblast fetal cells in maternal blood by fluorescence in-situ hybridization after using immunomagnetic lymphocyte depletion and flow cytometry sorting. Fetal Diagn Ther 1992;7:190.

152. Simpson JL, Elias S. Isolating fetal cells from maternal blood: advances in prenatal diagnosis through molecular technology. JAMA 1993;270:2357.

153. Ganshirt-Ahlert D, Borjesson-Stoll R, Burschyk M, et al. Detection of fetal trisomies 21 and 18 from maternal blood using triple gradient and magnetic cell sorting. Am J Reprod Immunol 1993;30:194.

154. Zheng YL, Carter NP, Price CM, et al. Prenatal diagnosis from maternal blood: simultaneous immunophenotyping and FISH of fetal nucleated erythrocytes isolated by negative magnetic cell sorting. J Med Genet 1993;30:1051.

155. Oosterwijk JC, Mesker WE, Ouwerkerk-Van Velzen MC, et al. Prenatal diagnosis of trisomy 13 on fetal cells obtained from maternal blood after minor enrichment. Prenat Diagn 1998;18:1082.

156. Bischoff FZ, Lewis DE, Nguyen DD, et al. Prenatal diagnosis with use of fetal cells isolated from maternal blood: five-color fluorescent in situ hybridization analysis on flow-sorted cells for chromosomes X, Y, 13, 18, and 21. Am J Obstet Gynecol 1998;179:203.

157. Bianchi DW, Mahr A, Zickwolf GK, et al. Detection of fetal cells with 47,XY,+21 karyotype in maternal and peripheral blood. Hum Genet 1992;90:368.

158. Yagel S, Shpan P, Dushnik M, et al. Trophoblasts circulating in maternal blood as candidates for prenatal genetic evaluation. Hum Reprod 1994;9:1184.

159. Reading JP, Huffman JL, Wu JC, et al. Nucleated erythrocytes in maternal blood: quantity and quality of fetal cells in enriched populations. Hum Reprod 1995;10:2510.

160. Simpson JL, Lewis DE, Bischoff F, et al. Detection of fetal cells in maternal blood: towards a non-invasive prenatal diagnosis. Contracep Fertil Sex 1995;23:445.

161. Zheng YL, Craigo SD, Price CM, et al. Demonstration of spontaneously dividing male fetal cells in maternal blood by negative magnetic cell sorting and FISH. Prenat Diagn 1995;15:573.

162. Simpson JL, Lewis DE, Bischoff FZ, et al. Isolating fetal nucleated red blood cells from maternal blood: The Baylor experience–1995. Prenat Diagn 1995;15:907.

163. Bianchi DW, Simpson JL, Jackson LG, et al. Fetal gender and aneuploidy detection using fetal cells in maternal blood: analysis of NIFTY I data. National Institute of Child Health and Development Fetal Cell Isolation Study. Prenat Diagn 2002;22:609.

164. Hamada H, Arinami T, Sohda S, et al. Mid-trimester fetal sex determination from maternal periph-eral blood by fluorescence in-situ hybridization without enrichment of fetal cells. Prenat Diagn 1995; 15:78.

165. Björkqvist AM, Slunga-Tallberg A, Wessman M, et al. Prenatal sex determination by in-situ hybridiza-tion on fetal nucleated cells in maternal whole venous blood. Clin Genet 1994;46:352.

166. Rhine SA, Cain JL, Cleary RF, et al. Prenatal sex detection with endocervical smear: successful result utilizing Y-body fluorescence. Am J Obstet Gynecol 1975;122:155.

167. Adinolfi M, Davies A, Sharif S, et al. Detection of trisomy 18 and Y-derived sequences in fetal nucleated cells obtained by transcervical flushing. Lancet 1993;342:403.

168. Ville Y, Lochu P, Rhali H, et al. Are desquamated trophoblastic cells retrieved from the cervix suitable for a prenatal diagnosis? Contracept Fertil Sex 1994;22:475.

169. Adinolfi M, Sherlock J, Tutschek B, et al. Detection of fetal cells in transcervical samples and prenatal diagnosis of chromosomal abnormalities. Prenat Diagn 1995:15;943.

170. Tutschek B, Sherlock J, Halder A, et al. Isolation of fetal cells from transcervical samples by microma-nipulation: molecular confirmation of their fetal origin and diagnosis of fetal aneuploidy. Prenat Diagn 1995;15:951.

171. Ishai D, Amiel A, Diukman R, et al. Uterine cavity lavage: Adding FISH to conventional cytogenetics for embryonic sexing and diagnosing common chromosomal aberrations. Prenat Diagn 1995;15:961.

172. Massari A, Novelli G, Colosimo A, et al. Non-invasive early prenatal molecular diagnosis using retrieved transcervical trophoblast cells. Hum Genet 1996;97:150.

173. Chang SD, Lin SL, Chu KK, et al. Minimally-invasive early prenatal diagnosis using fluorescence in situ hybridization on samples from uterine lavage. Prenat Diagn 1997;17:1019.

174. Fejgin MD, Diukman R, Cotton Y, et al. Fetal cells in the uterine cervix: a source for early non-invasive prenatal diagnosis. Prenat Diagn 2001;21:619.

175. ErgIn T, Baltaci V, Zeyneloglu HB, et al. Non-invasive early prenatal diagnosis using fluorescent in situ hybridization on transcervical cells: comparison of two different methods for retrieval. Eur J Obstet Gy-necol Reprod Biol 2001;95:37.

176. Cioni R, Bussani C, Scarselli B, et al. Detection of fetal cells in intrauterine lavage samples collected in the first trimester of pregnancy. Prenat Diagn 2002;22:52.

177. Bussani C, Cioni R, Scarselli B, et al. Strategies for the isolation and detection of fetal cells in transcer-vical samples. Prenat Diagn 2002;22:1098.

178. Grifo JA, Boyle A, Tang YX, et al. Preimplantation genetic diagnosis. Arch Pathol Lab Med 1992;116:393.

179. Griffin DK, Handyside AH, Penketh RJA, et al. Fluorescent in-situ hybridization to interphase nu-clei of human preimplantation embryos with X and Y chromosome-specific probes. Hum Reprod 1991;6:101.

180. Griffin DK, Wilton LJ, Handyside AH, et al. Dual fluorescent in-situ hybridization for the simultaneous detection of X and Y chromosome-specific probes for the sexing of human preimplantation embryonic nuclei. Hum Genet 1992;89:18.

181. Delhanty JDA. Preimplantation diagnosis. Prenat Diagn 1994;14:1217.

182. Grifo JA, Tang YX, Munne S, et al. Healthy deliveries from biopsied human embryos. Hum Reprod 1994;9:912.

183. Munne S, Weier HUG, Grifo J, et al. Chromosome mosaicism in human embryos. Biol Reprod 1994; 51:373.

184. Harper JC, Coonen E, Ramaekers FC, et al. Identification of the sex of human preimplantation embryos in two hours using an improved spreading method and fluorescent in-situ hybridization (FISH) using di-rectly labelled probes. Hum Reprod 1994;9:721.

185. Muggleton-Harris AL, Glazier AM, Pickering S, et al. Genetic diagnosis using polymerase chain reac-tion and fluorescent in-situ hybridization analysis of biopsy cells from both the cleavage and blastocyst stages of individual cultured human preimplantation embryos. Hum Reprod 1995;10:183.

186. Rechitsky S, Freidine M, Verlinsky Y, et al. Allele dropout in sequential PCR and FISH analysis of single-cells (cell recycling). J Assist Reprod Genet 1996;13:115.

187. Coonen E, Domoulin JC, Dreesen JC, et al. Clinical application of FISH for sex determination of em-bryos in preimplantation diagnosis of X-linked diseases. J Assist Reprod Genet 1996;13:133.

188. Harper JC. Preimplantation diagnosis of inherited disease by embryo biopsy: an update of the world fig-ures. J Assist Reprod Genet 1996;13:90.

189. Harper JC, Delhanty JD. Detection of chromosomal abnormalities in human preimplantation embryos using FISH. J Assist Reprod Genet 1996;13:137.

190. Harper JC, Coonen E, Handyside AH, et al. Mosaicism of autosomes and sex chromosomes in morphologically normal, monosomic preimplantation human embryos. Prenat Diagn 1995;15:41.
191. Munne S, Dailey T, Finkelstein M, et al. Reduction in signal overlap results in increased FISH efficiency: implications for preimplantation genetic diagnosis. J Assist Reprod Genet 1996;13:149.
192. Munne S, Weier HU. Simultaneous enumeration of chromosomes 13, 18, 21, X, and Y in interphase cells for preimplantation genetic diagnosis of aneuploidy. Cytogenet Cell Genet 1996;75:263.
193. Verlinsky Y, Cieslak J, Ivakhnenko V, et al. Preimplantation diagnosis of common aneuploidies by the first- and second-polar body FISH analysis. J Assist Reprod Genet 1998;15:285.

Edmund C. Jenkins, Ph.D., F.A.C.M.G., and
W. Ted Brown, M.D., Ph.D., F.A.C.M.G.

9

Prenatal Diagnosis of the Fragile X Syndrome

The excess of males affected with nonspecific mental retardation has been known for some time. In 1938 Penrose first noted an excess of mentally retarded males among persons institutionalized for mental retardation, and found that there were approximately 25 percent more males with mental retardation than females.[1] The explanation for the excess of males with mental retardation was thought to be X-linked disorders,[2] more than seventy-six of which are now known (nonspecific mental retardation).[2a] Most of these disorders are relatively rare, and approximately half of the cases of X-linked mental retardation seem to be due to FXS.[3] Although Martin and Bell[4] and Renpenning et al.[5] described families with characteristic X-linked pedigrees, and Davison[6] suggested that nonspecific mental retardation may have an X-linked etiology, it was Lehrke[7] and Turner and Turner,[2] who underlined the significance of X linkage by concluding that various mutations of the X chromosome may be the reason for nonspecific mental retardation in more than 20 percent of affected males.

Since the fragile X mental retardation-1 (FMR1) gene was cloned in 1991,[8–11] much new information has come to light about fragile X syndrome (FXS). Fragile X is considered to be the most common inherited cause of mental retardation and is thought to be responsible for 2–8 percent, and most likely about 5 percent of mental retardation.[12] It was the first example of a class of "dynamic mutations" that exhibit "anticipation" or increased severity and earlier onset from one generation to the next because of the amplification of a triplet repeat region.[13] For fragile X, the gene becomes hypermethylated and inactivated when triplet expansion exceeds 200 repeats. This chapter summarizes some of this information in general and reviews the recent advances made in the prenatal detection of FXS in particular.

THE FIRST REPORTS OF THE MARKER OR FRAGILE X CHROMOSOME

The first observation of a marker or fragile X chromosome in a family with X-linked mental retardation was made by Lubs in 1969.[14] Although Escalante and Frota-Pessoa[15] described a marker C chromosome in a family with three retarded brothers in 1973, the importance of Lubs's observation was not realized until 1976–1977, when Giraud et al.[16]

and Harvey et al.[17] demonstrated the marker in twenty-five affected males, one affected female, and thirteen normal females from ten families.

The fragile X site (fra(X)) is located at band Xq27.3,[18,19] and it may appear as a gap or break.[20] Fra(X) has also been observed rarely as a triradial,[21,22] which resembles a "bisatellite" configuration.[23]

CHARACTERIZATION OF THE XQ27.3 FRAGILE SITE INDUCTION SYSTEM

Sutherland and Hecht[24] discovered that a folate-deficient culture medium was necessary to induce fra(X)(q27.3). Sutherland[20] suggested that the formation of the fragile X site may be due to (1) interference with DNA spiralization, (2) viral DNA modification, or (3) the relationship of thymidine monophosphate (TMP) production to DNA synthesis. Support for the third hypothesis came independently from Glover[25] and Tommerup et al.,[26,27] who demonstrated fragile site induction using 5-fluorodeoxyuridine. This antimetabolite interferes with thymidylate synthase activity by limiting or blocking the formation of TMP from uridine monophosphate. The disruption of folic acid metabolism, whether through the action of an antimetabolite such as trimethoprim[28] or through folate depletion,[29] achieves the same results. Krumdieck and Howard-Peebles[30] hypothesized that the induction of fragility is caused by specific structural collapses along the linear axis of the chromosome, due to the misincorporation of uracil into DNA, whereas Taylor and Hagerman[31] suggested that depleted levels of TMP lead to uracil misincorporation, which may halt DNA replication or may cause faulty repair and thus result in extensively nicked or gapped DNA. They also suggested that the formation of fra(X) may be due to the prevention of normal chromosome condensation because of abnormal protein–DNA interactions.

Sutherland et al.[32,33] showed that excess thymidine and guanosine in vitro induce fra(X) and other folate-sensitive fragile sites. He and his associates hypothesized that Z-DNA may be related to the occurrence of common fragile sites, which are strongly induced by aphidicolin,[34] the DNA polymerase α-inhibitor, and only weakly induced by folate-deficient systems. They further hypothesized that the amount of amplification of a naturally occurring polypurine/polypyrimidine sequence could be related to the different frequencies of fragile sites. Such differences can be familial, particularly with regard to fra(X).[35,36] More recently, Dobkin et al.[37] hypothesized that fragile site development may be related to the tendency for long triplet repeats to form hairpins, which are more likely to form in long CGG repeats because of a lower nucleosome-binding affinity as compared with long CTG repeats (which do not show fragile sites) having a higher nucleosome-binding capacity.

One of the most widely used induction systems for demonstrating the fragile site at Xq27.3 involves the addition of excess thymidine to the cell culture, reported initially by Sutherland et al.[32] in 1985, with specific application to the prenatal detection of fra(X) communicated in 1987.[38] At the end of the cytogenetics "era" of fragile X detection in the early 1990s, most laboratories used multiple fragile site induction systems to demonstrate fra(X)(q27.3) because at times the fragile site had been demonstrated by one system and not the other (e.g., Jenkins et al.[39]). The use of multiple induction systems for whole blood was recommended by an ad hoc committee at the Fourth International Workshop on Fragile X and X-Linked Mental Retardation.[40] A summary of a variety of induction systems, along with some information on their mechanisms of action, can be found in reports by Wilmot[41] and by Jacky et al.[40]

THE ESTIMATED INCIDENCE/PREVALENCE OF FRAGILE X SYNDROME

An analysis of two epidemiologic studies, by Blomquist et al.[42,43] and by Webb et al.,[44] led Brown and Jenkins[3] to estimate that the prevalence of affected males with the fragile X mutation (FRAXA) was approximately 1 per 1,000. In light of the discovery of a common fragile site at Xq27.2 (FRAXD),[45] Webb and Bundey[46] reanalyzed their data[44] and concluded that the prevalence of FXS in schoolchildren from 11 to 16 years of age when examined was 1 in 1,039 for both sexes.

After FMR1 was cloned in 1991,[8–11] new epidemiologic studies were conducted based on molecular rather than cytogenetic analyses. Estimates of the prevalence of FXS were revised in 1996 by Turner et al.[47] to significantly lower levels of 1:4,000 for males and 1:6,000 for females. The true prevalence is a matter of some debate and is likely to be higher (see Brown[48] and Rousseau et al.[49] for further discussion).

THE FRAGILE X PHENOTYPE

The physical and mental characteristics of affected fragile X males have been well described in many previous reports, including the proceedings of nine international workshops on fragile X and X-linked mental retardation.[50–57,57a] Most affected adult males are moderately to severely mentally impaired, with mean IQs that typically range from 20 to 50 (reviewed by Bennetto and Pennington[58]). Selected characteristics of FXS have been developed into screening instruments or checklists for the identification and genetic counseling, when appropriate, of fragile X males and their families. These instruments have helped reduce some of the costs of screening/testing.[59–61]

Some individuals with autism have the fragile X mutation. We conducted a multicenter survey of autistic individuals, in which we found that 24 of 183 autistic males (13 percent) had FXS.[62] A subsequent survey showed that approximately 8 percent of both male and female autistic individuals have the fragile X mutation.[63] A summary of 17 surveys of 1,243 autistic male subjects overall found that 4 percent (range, 0–16 percent) had FXS.[64] A variety of conceptual and methodologic issues may explain the wide range of findings,[65] including sample size, ascertainment bias, the type of method used to detect the fragile site, and changing definitions of autism. Females with autism are less common than males, but one study of forty autistic females found 5 percent were positive for FXS.[66] Fragile X males are commonly diagnosed with autism. In our original study, we found that five of twenty-two subjects (23 percent) found to have FXS, had a previous diagnosis of autism.[67] A summary of fourteen studies of 479 FXS male subjects found that a mean of 24 percent had autism (range, 7–60 percent).[65] A longitudinal study of fifty-five young boys with FXS found that 25 percent had autism and that over time those with autism had a lower trajectory of developmental age progression than nonautistic FXS subjects.[68] These studies have found that approximately one-fourth of male FXS subjects meet the full criteria for autism and indicate a strong association of autism and FXS.

Cohen et al.[69] showed increased development rates of adaptive skills in males with mosaicism versus full-mutation fragile X. They also observed a trend for an increased presence of autism in the full-mutation group of fragile X males. Finally, Dobkin et al.[70] reported that adaptive behavior correlated more closely with mosaicism found in skin fibroblast cultures. This is not surprising, because skin is closer embryologically to brain than lymphocytes.

Several groups have reported abnormal brainstem auditory evoked responses in people with fragile X syndrome.[71–73] When compared with a control group, Arinami et al.[72]

found that individuals with fragile X had longer wave V latencies and prolonged III–V interpeak intervals. Among seventy-five male individuals (forty-four with no disability, eighteen with mental retardation, and thirteen with the fragile X mutation), Miezejeski et al.[74] found no differences between individuals with fragile X and those without mental retardation. Increased latencies were observed, however, in persons who were sedated. Therefore, sedation effects may explain increased latencies for fragile X individuals in previous reports.

MALE AND FEMALE CARRIERS

Sherman et al.[75,76] first observed that fragile X female carriers had 20 percent more normal sons than expected. Also, a family has been reported that was cytogenetically positive but unaffected,[77] whereas an affected male has been described who was cytogenetically negative but DNA-linkage positive for fragile X.[78] Now that the fragile X mutation has been not only located (FRAXA) but also cloned and designated "fragile X mental retardation-1" or "FMR1" mutation, nonpenetrant males as well as unaffected females with FRAXA will be more easily and rapidly identified.

Our understanding of the genetic mechanism of the fragile X mutation has increased substantially in recent years. We now know, for example, that nonpenetrant transmitting grandfathers have premutations with less than 200 CGG repeats that are not hypermethylated. There are examples of cases in which male individuals carried 200 or more repeats but were not methylated and thus were unaffected.[79–81] Unaffected female carriers, on the other hand, may have either premutations or full mutations, both premutations and full mutations, or a combination. Of those with the full mutation, approximately one-half are mentally retarded, although usually less severely than males. This is because of random X inactivation as well as a combination of X inactivation and the occurrence of mosaicism.

Hagerman et al.[82,83] observed that, of forty-two women who were cytogenetically positive for FRAXA (presumably full mutations by DNA) and who were sisters of fra(X)-positive males, approximately one-fourth had IQs lower than 70, one-fourth had IQs ranging from 70 to 85, one-fourth had learning disabilities, and one-fourth were not affected. Therefore, it seems that female penetrance may be as high as 75 percent in cytogenetically positive (full mutation) sisters of fragile X males.[82–84] A clinical follow-up of cytogenetically positive fragile X fetuses subsequently showed that three of four were mentally retarded.[85] Because of this high degree of expression, this disorder is now considered X-linked dominant but with reduced penetrance.

Approximately 90 percent of all affected female carriers will exhibit the fragile X chromosome.[76] There is a loose association between the presence of mental impairment and the inactivation of the normal X chromosome.[86,87] This does not, however, account for all cases lacking mental impairment among carrier females. This is because females who inherit the mutation from a premutation carrier father are nearly always only premutation carriers as well and are thus unaffected. These females would be cytogenetically negative but linkage-positive in older studies. The molecular technology that has become available now allows one to test for FMR1 status in potential carrier females.

Affected female carriers may exhibit a characteristic profile of cognitive deficits. A number of groups have reported increased verbal and decreased performance scores on the Wechsler IQ test. Relatively low subtest scores were observed on arithmetic digit, block design, and object assembly.[88–90] Wolff et al.[91] reported reduced arithmetic abilities in a group of fifteen nonretarded female carriers. Reiss et al.[92] found that 40 percent of a group of thirty-five carriers had chronic recurrent depression, and approximately 30 percent exhibited schizoid features, including inappropriate affect, odd communication, and social isolation. Using magnetic resonance imaging, Reiss et al.[93] reported neuroanatomic differences between monozygotic twin girls who had full FMR1 mutations and were discordant for mental retardation. Again, with the application of FMR1 probes, it is expected that all carriers will be more easily and rapidly identified, and it is not unlikely that the degree of mental impairment in female carriers will be predictable because of X-inactivation.

PREMUTATION CARRIERS

The prevalence of fragile X premutation carriers has been reported to be as high as 1:259 for females and 1:755 for males.[95a] Usually premutation carriers have normal intelligence, although depression has been observed among some females and about 20 percent exhibit premature ovarian failure (early menopause). Recently, Hagerman et al.[96] described five transmitting males (premutation carriers) over the age of 50 with development of progressive intention tremor and cerebellar ataxia. Progressive cognitive and behavioral problems occurred, including memory loss and dementia. This newly emergent syndrome has been termed "fragile X-associated tremor/ataxia syndrome" (FXTAS). Molecular studies have found elevated mRNA and reductions of fragile X mental retardation 1 protein (FMRP) levels.[95]

EXPERIENCE IN PRENATAL TESTING FOR FRAGILE X

Cytogenetics

Since the initial retrospective prenatal diagnosis in amniotic fluid (AF) cultures by Jenkins et al.[97] and prospective prenatal diagnoses in fetal whole blood and AF cell cultures by Webb et al.[98] and Shapiro et al.,[99] respectively, it is estimated that thousands of prenatal fragile X tests have now been conducted worldwide, using cultures of chorionic villus samples (CVS), AF, and percutaneous umbilical blood samples (PUBS). The frequency of requests for prenatal (as well as postnatal) diagnosis of fragile X in families with possible X-linked mental retardation, regardless of whether fragile X syndrome was previously documented in the family, has been increasing steadily.[100–102] As indicated in Table 9.1, twenty different laboratories or groups of investigators have reported the detection of the fragile X chromosome in 148 fetuses at risk (149 specimens; 2 specimens from one case).

Among 149 specimens, 57 percent were AF, 28 percent were CVS, and 15 percent were PUBS. The reliability or sensitivity of cytogenetic prenatal detection has been calculated[101–113] as $r = P/(P + FN)100$, where P is the total number of fra(X) specimens detected prenatally and FN is the number of false-negative specimens detected postnatally. Therefore, r for PUBS is $r = 24/(24 + 1)100 = 96$ percent. The r values for AF, CVS, and PUBS are listed in Table 9.1 and summarize the experience of all twenty-one laboratories. Although it seems that the most reliable tissue type is PUBS, these samples accounted for the smallest number of specimens tested. Although the r value for PUBS was 96 percent overall, there were variations between laboratories. For example, r values for our laboratory are much higher than the overall values for AF and CV, as seen in the bottom line of Table 9.1. In fact, the r values for AF and CVS in our laboratory were 95.0

Table 9.1. Cytogenetic identification of fragile X chromosome in 149 AF, CVS, and PUBS reported by twenty-one laboratories or groups of investigators

Lab/Group	Initial Report	AF	CVS	PUBS	Total	False Negative	False Positive
Jenkins et al.[97a]	1981	19	15	0	34	1 AFf 1 CVSm	0
Webb et al.[98a]	1981	0	0	11	11	1 CVSm 1 PUBSm	0
Shapiro et al.[99a]	1982	29	4	2	35	2 AFm 1 AFf 1 AFm or f[b] 3 CVSm	0
Schmidt et al.[a]	1982	6	0	0	6	0	0
Tejada et al.[a]	1983	1	0	0	1	0	0
Wilson et al.[a]	1984	1	0	0	1	0	0
Hogge et al.[a]	1984	1	0	0	1	0	0
Tommerup et al.[a]	1985	1	1	0	2	0	1 AFm
Von Koskull et al.[104,105]	1985	5	5	0	10	1 CVSm 1 CVSf lnk 1	1(2)[c] AFm lnk 2
Rocchi et al.[a]	1985	1	0	2	3	1 AFm	0
Webb G, et al.[a]	1986	4	0	0	4	0	0
Howard-Peebles[106]	1986	7	5	0	12	1 AFm	0
Sutherland et al.[a]	1987	2	2	0.00	4	1 CVSm (inconclusive)	0.00
Purvis-Smith et al.[a]	1988	4	6	0.00	10	1 AFf	0.00
McKinley et al.[a]	1988	0.00	0.00	3	3	0.00	0.00
Kennerknecht et al.[a]	1991	0.00	3	0.00	3	1 CVSf	0.00
Devillard et al.[a]	1992	3	0.00	0.00	3	0.00	0.00
Tarleton et al.[107]	1992	0.00	0.00	0.00	0.00	1 CVSf[d]	0.00
Liou et al.[108]	1993	0.00	0.00	4	4 AF neg. but PUBS pos.	3 AFm 1AFf	0.00
Baranov et al.[109]	1993	0	0	1	1	0	0
Grasso et al.[110]	1996	0.0	0.0	1	1	0.0	
Total number	—	84	41	24	149	12 AF 10 CVS 1 PUBS	2 AF
Percentage		56.4	27.5	16.1	100		
r value[e]		84/96	41/51	24/25	86.6		98.7
		87.5	80.4	96.0	—		
		(95.0)[f]	(93.8)		(94.4)		(100.0)

[a]Initial citations are listed chronologically; updates are referred to in Jenkins et al., 1991[101,103]; others are given in this chapter.
[b]As reported in Jenkins et al., 1995.[111]
[c]One cytogenetically unconfirmed; one no material.
[d]Referred to as inconclusive (thus not positive), resolved by Southern analysis.
[e]r explained in text.
[f]r values for Jenkins et al.
f = female; m = male; lnk = linkage.

and 93.8 percent, which are nearly the same as the overall r value for PUBS. Early in prenatal testing, AF was the most referred specimen, but currently, most specimens are CVS.

The preceding calculations were based on the retrospective ascertainment of risks, whereas other calculations of the accuracy of a prenatal diagnosis of fragile X were made based on prospective estimates of risk. For prenatal cytogenetic diagnosis from amniocentesis specimens, the overall analysis revealed a predictive value[114] of 100 percent for fragile X-positive results because there were no false positives in 23 cases. For a fragile X-negative result, the value was 97 percent (143/147).

Regarding the potential causes of false-negative findings, a variety of factors have been identified, including the type of fragile site induction system, the number of cells analyzed, the type of culture medium, interlaboratory variability, and the possibility that fragile sites unrelated to FMR1 were being observed, such as FRAXD, FRAXE, and FRAXF. FRAXA corresponds to fra(X)(q27.3), whereas FRAXD is referred to as a common fragile site and is located at Xq27.2.[115] We observed it only once in 760 cases (or 1 cell in nearly 80,000[116]) in cultures that were exposed to conditions for fra(X)(q27.3) induction. FRAXE has been found to be related to individuals with mild mental impairment and can be distinguished from FRAXA molecularly, but not cytogenetically, whereas FRAXF has not been correlated with any known syndrome and is also indistinguishable cytogenetically from FRAXA.

Cytogenetic Testing No Longer Recommended for Fragile X Diagnosis

Although the reliability of the prenatal cytogenetic test was approximately 95 percent for detection of the fragile X mutation in peripheral umbilical blood samples and amniotic fluid specimens, reliance on cytogenetic testing is no longer recommended for the detection of the fragile X mutation because of the possibility of overlap with FRAXD–F. Furthermore, cytogenetic testing is both more labor-intensive and more time-consuming. Although cytogenetic testing was good for detecting males with full mutations both prenatally and postnatally, it was not reliable in detecting full mutations in females. Finally, it could neither detect nor size premutations in either sex.

Currently, it is recommended that cytogenetic studies should no longer be used for the detection of the fragile X mutation[111,115,117] either prenatally or postnatally. However, standard cytogenetic analysis of individuals with mental retardation of unknown etiology is still appropriate, along with constitutional chromosomal analysis in AF and CVS cultures from women at increased risk for a chromosome abnormality (e.g., advanced maternal age and Down syndrome). Note that the full mutation identified by Wilkin et al.[118] in Table 9.2 was also mosaic for Turner syndrome.

In addition, laboratory technologists should remain alert to the possibility that spontaneous (noninduced) fragile X chromosomes may occur during standard cytogenetic analysis. To date, we are aware of five such instances, which were subsequently proven to be from full-mutation fetuses.[112,125,126] When spontaneously occurring fragile X chromosomes are observed, immediate characterization of the pregnant woman's carrier status is now possible and recommended.

Prenatal detection from 1981 through 1991 was primarily cytogenetic with some complementation by DNA linkage studies. Although accuracy was improved with the use of linkage studies, many times, it was not possible to obtain sufficient information in a timely fashion. Linkage studies were best done preconceptionally, not at the time of CVS or amniocentesis.

TRANSMISSION ELECTRON MICROSCOPY (TEM) OF THE FRAGILE SITE

It became possible in the late 1990s to study the ultrastructure of longitudinal serial sections of complete metaphases using transmission electron microscopy (TEM).[128,129] Increased detail was revealed of chromosomes that exhibited the fragile site at Xq27.3, as well as those that did not, using bright-field or fluorescence analysis. Some of these chro-

Table 9.2. Genomic (Southern blot analysis) and PCR prenatal detection of the FMR1 full mutation in AF, CVS, and PUBS reported by sixteen laboratories or groups of investigators

Lab/Report	Initial Report	AF	CVS	PUBS	Total	False Negative	False Positive
Hirst et al.[a]	1991	0	1	0	1	0	0
Dobkin et al.[b]	1991	13	31	0	44	0	0
Rousseau et al.[a]	1991	1	10	1	12	0	0
Sutherland et al.[a]	1991	0	1	0	1	0	0
Murphy et al.a (in Howard-Peebles[c])	1992	1	1	0	2	0	0
Howard-Peebles	1992	5	5	0	10	0	0
Maddalena et al.[a] (in Jenkins et al.[112])							
Tarleton et al.[107]	1992	1	0	0	1	0	0
Sutcliffe et al.[a]	1992	0	1	0	1	0	0
Baranov et al.[a]	1993	0	0	1	1	0	0
Suzumori et al.[a]	1993	0	1	0	1	0	0
Yamauchi et al.[a]	1993	0	1	0	1	0	0
Ryynanen et al.[a]	1994	?	?	?	14	0	0
von Koskull[a]	1994	0	5	0	5	0	0
Puissant et al.[119]	1994	?	?	?	2	0	0
Castellvi-Bel et al.[120]	1995	0	2	0	2	0	0
Grasso et al.[110]	1996	0	9[d]	3	12	0	0
Appelman et al.[121]	1999	0	1	0	1	0	0
Drasinover et al.[122]	2000	?	?	0	5	0	0
Kallinen et al.[123]	2000	?	?	0	18	0	0
Pesso et al.[124]	2000	?	?	0	9	0	0
Wilkin et al.[118]	2000	0	1	0	1	0	0
Toledano-Alhadef et al.[94]	2001	?	?	0	5	0	0
Total		21	70	5	149	0	0

[a]Citations given in Jenkins et al., 1992[112] or in references of this chapter.

[b]Updated for Institute for Basic Research in Developmental Disabilities, Staten Island, NY, through January 1, 2003, in Table 9.3.

[c]Information on the laboratory of Shapiro et al., 1991.[102]

[d]Three confirmed with PUBS.

[e]This case also exhibited mosaicism for Turner syndrome: 45,X[19]/46,XX[31].

mosomes that did not exhibit the fragile site during bright-field or fluorescence analysis did exhibit differences in density in the locus of the fragile site using TEM. The frequency of the fragile site using Q- and G-banding analysis, from the same sample prepared for TEM studies, was 20 percent. It is possible that such density differences visualized with TEM, without a constriction or gap, would increase the total number of X chromosomes that revealed fragility.

Molecular Genetic Testing

Southern blot methods for direct genomic analysis of DNA became the standard prenatal diagnostic fragile X test after its validation in the early 1990s. Using probes such as StB12.3,[130] information on both the size and methylation status of the repeat region was provided. PCR technology was developed to provide more accurate sizing of the triplet repeat region and to provide information more quickly with much less sample. Early attempts to amplify the triplet repeat by PCR were not successful[131] because the region was high in GC content. A PCR method that amplified normal-sized and most premutation alleles was developed by Fu et al.,[132] but this method could not amplify full mutations. A nonradioactive protocol that allowed sizing of normal, premutation, and most full-mutation alleles was developed by Brown et al.[133,134] The method called for replacing deoxyguanidine triphosphate (dGTP) with 7-deaza-2-dGTP and used chemiluminescence. It provided rapid, cost-effective analysis of carrier status and prenatal samples.

CURRENT MOLECULAR PRENATAL FRAGILE X DETECTION PROTOCOLS

PCR and Southern Analyses of Amniotic Fluid and Chorionic Villus Samples

After validating the procedure, we recommend using PCR alone when it can be demonstrated that the mother's normal allele was transmitted to the fetus, which is the case when the fetus is male, or when the father's allele is different in size from the mother's normal allele, which is the case when the fetus is female. This information can be provided within a short time after the specimen arrives in the laboratory. In practice, this generally takes 3–5 working days. Similarly, when the normal alleles of both parents can be identified clearly, PCR alone may be used. For all other combinations, follow-up/confirmation with direct genomic Southern analysis is recommended, which at this time requires 2–5 weeks in our laboratory, depending on the sample size and the time taken to culture cells when necessary.[133,134]

Dobkin et al.[135,136] developed a hybrid Southern–PCR procedure that can reduce turnaround time by 2–4 weeks. Diagnostic *Eco*RI–Eag I restriction fragments from less than 50,000 cells, or 200 ng of DNA, can be fractionated by agarose gel electrophoresis and detected by PCR amplification of the array of fragments in serial sections of the gel matrix.

When using CVS, it has been recommended that samples be obtained close to 12 weeks to ensure that methylation has occurred[137] and that the FMR1 gene product can be distinguished immunocytochemically in control cells compared with full-mutation cells.[138] On the other hand, using specimens obtained between 10 and 12 weeks, we have thus far been able to characterize the mutation, either premutation or full mutation, with the combination of PCR and Southern analysis. CVS analysis was effective in identifying potentially affected fetuses, even though methylation was incomplete or absent in most samples. When the affected chromosome was transmitted, it was difficult to distinguish between full-mutation and mosaic cases using Southern analysis of CVS. This was not critical because both individuals with full mutations and those with mosaicism are usually affected. Also, because of incomplete methylation, it may be difficult to distinguish between a premutation carrier and mosaicism because of the problem of identifying a full-mutation allele.

Southern analysis is preferred for the identification of individuals with mosaicism. For both CVS and AF samples, we have not experienced significant problems. We have found that approximately 40 percent of our samples that exhibited a full-sized mutation were also mosaic. Most of our CVS samples with the full mutation have exhibited incomplete or absent methylation patterns. This is in agreement with the concept that the FMR1 mutation usually is methylated sometime after 10 weeks of gestation.

The remote possibility exists that a case may arise in which it will be difficult to distinguish between a large premutation and a full mutation. When CVS analysis is ambiguous, follow-up amniocentesis would be recommended for clarification. Thus far, we have not encountered such a situation. Increased amplification is still measurable using the PCR and Southern analysis combination, whether or not methylation has commenced.

If insufficient quantities of CVS material are obtained, the likely success of direct analysis by PCR is reduced. If we obtain less than 10 mg of dissected material, or receive only cultured material, this requires culturing the cells for both PCR and providing sufficient DNA for Southern analysis measurements and increases the turnaround time. Furthermore, careful dissection of CVS is necessary to reduce the chance of maternal cell contamination.

As can be seen in Table 9.2, twenty-two laboratories or groups of investigators have reported nearly 150 full mutations genomically identified using either Southern analysis or a combination of PCR and Southern analyses to characterize the FMR1 mutation in AF, CVS, or PUBS samples. Excluding problems of maternal cell contamination, there have been no false negatives or false positives to date. This is in contrast to cytogenetic testing, in which there were twenty-three false negatives and two false positives. It is clear that molecular genetic testing for full mutations alone is superior to cytogenetic testing.

Our experience in prospective prenatal FMR1 mutation through January 1, 2003, is listed in Tables 9.2 and 9.3. Excluding maternal cell contamination,[112] the absence of false negatives or false positives indicates that the protocol is highly reliable. There is still room for improvement relative to reducing Southern analysis turnaround time.

A Protocol for Prenatal Testing Using Monoclonal Antibodies to Show Whether the FMR1 Gene Product, FMRP, Is Present or Absent

FXS results from the lack of the fragile X mental retardation protein (FMRP). It is generally cytoplasmic[139] and is thought to act as a regulator of translation and it associates with mRNAs and ribosomes. As reviewed by Todd and Malter[140] FMRP may have a role in the central nervous system in the transport, localization, and activity-dependent translocation of bound mRNAs.

Willemsen et al.[141] reported use of an immunocytochemical procedure for detection of the full mutation in whole blood lymphocytes from fragile X males. This procedure employs mouse monoclonal antibodies against FMRP and was adapted for the immunocytochemical detection of FMRP in prenatal samples. They have used this protocol to detect full mutations in CVS material that is at 12.5 weeks of gestation and in amniotic fluid cells.[142,143] Using a modification of this method, we have confirmed that FMRP can be detected in cultured CVS samples. Clear differences between immunostaining intensities

Table 9.3. Results of 314 prospective prenatal studies of FMR1 by a combination of PCR and Southern blot analyses at the Institute for Basic Research in Developmental Disabilities (Staten Island, NY)

Sample	Total	CVS	AF	Full Mutation	Intermediate	Premutation	Revertant	Normal
2002	44	38	6	14	3	3	0	24
Cumulative	314	234	80	119	16	18	5	156
2002 (male)	23	20	3	7	3	0	0	13
Cumulative (male)	147	116	31	53	8	11	1	74
2002 (female)	21	18	3	7	0	3	0	11
Cumulative (female)	166	117	49	66	8	7	4	81
TOP[a] (male)	16	—	—	14	0	2	0	0
TOP (female)	13	—	—	13	0	0	0	0

[a]TOP = termination of pregnancy

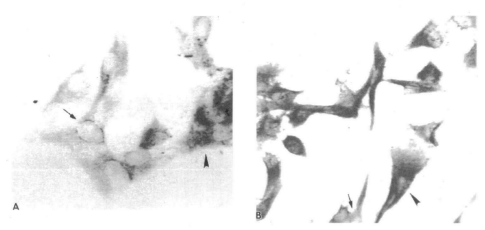

Fig. 9.1. *A,* Cultured cells from products of conception of a full-mutation male fetus stained with mouse monoclonal antibodies, mAb1A1 (provided by Dr. Mandel, INSERM), specific for FMRP, FMR1 gene protein product. The methodology was a modification of a three-step immunocytochemical procedure by Jenkins et al.[145] using alkaline phosphatase/fuchsin. Most of the cells were more lightly stained (arrow), whereas others were more heavily stained, similar to control cells from CVS cultures (B), which had more heavily stained cells, indicating the presence of FMRP (arrowhead). *B,* Cultured cells from CVS samples from a normal fetus. Most cells were more heavily stained (arrowhead), indicating the presence of FMRP, as compared with the more lightly stained cells (arrow) in this figure and in (*A*).

in cells from a full-mutation male fetus compared with controls were demonstrable, as indicated in Figure 9.1. Variations in staining intensity were present, but cells with the full mutation could be clearly identified.

The results in Table 9.4 showed that most cells from control female CVS samples were heavily stained (primarily cytoplasmic), whereas most cells from a full-mutation male fetus were stained much less intensely.[144] The gradation from heavy to light in the full-mutation male cells may reflect histiotypic mosaicism for the full mutation/methylation, as well as technical variations in the developing time. These confirmatory results suggest that the use of this method may allow fragile X results to be available on the same day the specimen is received. Additional information showing that full mutation male fetuses may be identified immunocytochemically as early as 10 weeks of gestation via chorionic villus samples, or later using amniotic fluid samples, can be found in reports by Jenkins et al.[145] and Willemsen et al.[146] Finally, Lambiris et al.[147] have also demonstrated the feasibility of FMRP detection in fetal blood lymphocytes that can be distinguished from fetal erythrocytes.

Table 9.4. Monoclonal antibody detection of FMRP in prenatal material shows variation in intensity of staining but identifies full-mutation specimen

Case	Intensity of Staining			Total Cell Number
	Heavy	Moderate	Light	
1 CVS normal (female)	340 (68%)	155 (31%)	5 (1%)	500
2 CVS normal (female)	308 (62)	182 (36)	10 (2)	500
3 POC full mutation (female)	177 (35)	210 (42)	113 (23)	500

Source: Jenkins et al., 1999.[145]

Polar Body Analysis Feasibility

The feasibility of polar body-based preimplantation genetic diagnosis (PGD) of the fragile X mutation was reported by Verlinsky et al.[148] (see also chapter 27). They removed the first and second polar bodies from embryos following maturation and fertilization of oocytes and analyzed the polar bodies using a multiplex nested PCR approach that involved simultaneous testing for mutations with X-linked markers. For two pregnancies that were predicted to be FMR1 mutation-free regarding the maternal contribution, one was a misdiagnosis as a result of allele dropout. Another type of PGD was also reported by Black et al.[149] to be unreliable because PCR failed to amplify the FMR-1 allele in 30–50 percent of single embryonic cells in contrast to amplifying DYZ1 and amelogenin. Thus, this approach has not yet been demonstrated to be a reliable alternative to CVS and amniocentesis for prenatal diagnosis.

THE NATURE OF THE FRAGILE X MUTATION: AN UPDATE ON PROGRESS IN MOLECULAR STUDIES

In the past, several hypotheses have been proposed to explain the nature of the fragile X mutation.[150–159] Brown et al.[150,151] suggested that heterogeneity was part of the nature of the fragile X mutation and presented evidence for heterogeneity of DNA linkage. Nussbaum et al.[156] hypothesized that the fragile X mutation includes a long pyrimidine-rich DNA sequence that undergoes unequal crossing over, resulting in rearrangement, duplication (or amplification), or deletion. Laird et al.[158] hypothesized that a mutation occurred at the fragile X locus, but to be expressed, it had to be "imprinted" by going through a female meiosis. This would allow for inactivation of the fragile X chromosome and subsequent incomplete reactivation. Incomplete reactivation would result in a lack of production of the FMR1 protein.[11] Laird et al. suggested that the mutation could be an epigenetic phenomenon, the result of abnormal methylation, and as such, there was no absolute need for a variation in the DNA sequence.

Initial molecular evidence in 1991 regarding the nature of the fragile X locus provided some support for the hypotheses just summarized. Vincent et al.[160] and Bell et al.[161] identified a CpG island (an indication of a promotor region near a gene) that was hypermethylated in affected fra(X) males as compared with being unmethylated in controls and nonpenetrant, transmitting male carriers; these results are consistent with Laird's hypothesis. Soon afterward, Heitz et al.[8] isolated a yeast artificial chromosome clone that bracketed the fragile X locus. Then, Oberlé et al.[9] and Yu et al.[10] reported the isolation of probes near the CpG island. Both found significant size increases within the regions detected by these probes in fragile X males. Normal, non-fra(X) males did not exhibit this size amplification, whereas nonpenetrant, transmitting carrier males had a 100–500 base pair (bp) increase in base size, and their affected grandsons exhibited a large size increase of 1,000–4,000. These results offered support for Nussbaum's hypothesis. The size of the amplification or insertion varied in affected individuals, indicating molecular heterogeneity. The possible relationship between this heterogeneity and the heterogeneity observed for DNA-linkage studies[151,152] has yet to be resolved.

Finally, Verkerk et al.[11] used a cosmid clone that they isolated from the fragile X region, to identify a complementary DNA (cDNA) clone from a fetal brain cDNA library, which included the region of size increase. They reported that the total message was 4.8 kb, and they named the gene FMR1. They found that the gene was expressed in lymphocytes and brain but not in liver, lung, or kidney. In fragile X males, it either was unexpressed or was expressed at reduced levels. A large number of CGG repeats was identified near the 5' end of the sequenced cDNA. If translated, they would encode long stretches of arginine. Because, in this regard, the protein would be basic, similar to histones and other nucleic acid binding proteins, it was hypothesized that the gene may be regulatory and affect the expression of other genes. However, subsequent analysis showed the CGG repeat region was transcribed but not translated.[162]

A PCR-based method was developed by Pieretti et al.[163] to detect the expression of the FMR1 gene by analysis of cDNA made from messenger RNA (mRNA) using a set of downstream primers that did not include the CGG repeat region. They found that sixteen of twenty males affected with fragile X lacked expression. The 20 percent that had some expression reflected mosaicism. Therefore, most affected males seemed to lack FMR1 expression. We now know that 20–40 percent of males exhibit mosaicism for the full mutation, including both size mosaicism (the presence of premutation and normal-sized alleles along with full mutations) and methylation mosaicism (the presence of both methylated and unmethylated forms of some larger alleles).

Using probes for regions downstream of the gene, Hirst et al.,[164] Dobkin et al.,[165] Rousseau et al.,[130] and Sutherland et al.[166] showed that prenatal diagnosis for both affected males and females was possible by direct probe analysis of genomic Southern blots. These demonstrations opened a new molecular era in prenatal fragile X diagnosis.

Partial success in PCR analysis of the FMR1 CGG repeat region with size increases up to approximately 500 bp was obtained by Fu et al.[132] A method for PCR analysis of fragile X full mutations with size increases up to 6,000 bp was developed, and its feasibility was demonstrated[167] in a retrospective prenatal diagnosis of a fragile X-positive male fetus. These PCR methods opened the way for rapid, efficient, and inexpensive prenatal diagnosis and carrier screening tests for fragile X mutations.

The FMR1 gene contains a highly polymorphic triplet CGG repeat that ranges from 6 to 45 in unaffected people, from 46 to 55 in an intermediate range, from 56 to 200 in premutation carriers, and from 200 to 2,000+ in full-mutation affected individuals.[168] Sizes in the range of 46 to 55 are an intermediate zone of alleles that can be stably or unstably inherited. The smallest premutation known to expand to a full mutation had 59 repeat alleles. More than 70 percent of intermediate alleles are stable when ascertained from women with no family history of fragile X. Increased instability was observed for larger intermediate repeats: 19 percent at a repeat number of 49–54; 30.9 percent at 55–59, and 80 percent at 60–65.[168,169] This triplet repeat is present in the first exon of seventeen in the gene that collectively spans 38 kb. When the repeat exceeds 200, hypermethylation of the upstream CpG island promoter occurs and blocks production of the gene product, FMRP.[163]

Both males and females may carry premutations, but those expanding to full mutations are found to occur only after female transmission. The likelihood of expansion to the full mutation is correlated with the size of the female premutation,[126,127] and it also has been shown to be related to the stability of the premutation as indicated by its AGG interspersion pattern.[170] Although most affected male individuals seem to be nonmosaic full mutations, as many as 40 percent[168] may be mosaic for exhibiting full mutation, premutation, and alleles within the normal range. Finally, reduction in the size of the expansion from a premutation size to a normal size has been observed with an estimated frequency of approximately 1 percent.[171–173] All these factors add to the challenge and complexity of prenatal fragile X diagnosis.

CONCLUSIONS

Although the cytogenetic era for fragile X detection has effectively ended, traditional chromosomal analysis should be performed when individuals who are suspected of having the fragile X mutation are found to be negative. In addition, laboratory personnel should remain alert to the possibility of spontaneous fragile X chromosome observations, which may indicate the unexpected presence of the FMR1 full mutation. When this occurs, the pregnant woman's status can be assessed immediately via molecular testing.

Although the current protocol for FMR1 evaluation, involving a combination of PCR and Southern analysis, has been shown to be 100 percent reliable, reductions in turnaround time are still being made with regard to Southern analysis. It is possible that a combination of Southern analysis and monoclonal antibody studies (currently applicable to male samples only) will result in significantly reduced turnaround times and even same-day analysis for many samples.

Additional research is needed to improve predictions of subsequent cognitive defects for both males and females with mosaicism as well as with full mutations. This includes additional genotype/phenotype correlations and the determination of the best tissue types amenable to providing such correlations prenatally.

Finally, additional research is needed to determine the function of the gene product so that therapeutic gene replacement strategies may be provided in the future, at which time large-scale screening programs would also become more feasible.[174] However, it is also thought that carrier screening for a number of single gene disorders is cost effective at this time and should be made available to all pregnant women.[94,175,176] The need for larger-scale screening was pointed out by Bailey et al.,[177,178] who conducted a small survey of 140 parents whose first child with fragile X syndrome was diagnosed between 1990 and 1999. The survey showed that about half the families did not have their first child diagnosed with fragile X until more than a year had elapsed from the time of their first concerns about their child's development and behavior. This resulted in half the families having additional pregnancies before they knew of their increased risk. Therefore, there is not only a need to develop gene therapy for individuals with fragile X but there is currently a need to provide increased screening for the fragile X mutation and premutation.

ACKNOWLEDGMENTS

We thank Ms. Anne Glicksman for help in tabulating our experience at IBR, Mr. Lawrence Black for his assistance in obtaining interlibrary loan requests, and Dr. Milen Velinov and Ms. Charlotte J. Ducan for their constructive comments during the preparation of the manuscript. This work was funded in part by the New York State Office of Mental Retardation and Developmental Disabilities and, in part, by grant MCJ360587 from the Maternal and Child Health Program (Title V, Social Security Act), Health Resources and Services Administration, Department of Health and Human Services.

REFERENCES

1. Penrose LS. A clinical and genetic study of 1,280 cases of mental defect. Special Report Series No. 299. London: Medical Research Council, 1938.
2. Turner G, Turner B. X-linked mental retardation. J Med Genet 1974;11:109.
2a. Hamel BCJ, Chiurazzi P, Lubs HA. Syndromic XLMR Genes (MRXS): update 2000. Am J Med Genet 2000;94:361.
3. Brown WT. Jenkins EC (1999): Fragile X Syndrome. In: Adelman G, Smith BH, Birkhäuser XX, eds. Elsevier's encyclopedia of neuroscience, 2nd ed., Boston (available in 1998 as CD-ROM).

4. Martin JP, Bell J. A pedigree of mental defect showing sex-linkage. J Neurol Psychiatry 1943;6:154.

5. Renpenning H, Gerrard JW, Zalewski WA, et al. Familial sex-linked mental retardation. Can Med Assoc J 1962;87:954.

6. Davison BC. Familial idiopathic severe subnormality: The question of a contribution by X-linked genes: genetic studies in mental subnormality. Br J Psychiatry 1973;8:1.

7. Lehrke R. A theory of X-linkage of major intellectual traits. Am J Ment Defic 1972;76:626.

8. Heitz D, Rousseau F, Devys D, et al. Isolation of sequences that span the fragile X and identification of a fragile-X related CpG island. Science 1991;251:1236.

9. Oberlé I, Rousseau F, Heitz D, et al. Instability of a 550-base pair DNA segment and abnormal methylation in fragile X syndrome. Science 1991;252:1097.

10. Yu S, Pritchard M, Kremer E, et al. Fragile X genotype characterized by an unstable region of DNA. Science 1991;252:1179.

11. Verkerk AJMH, Pieretti M, Sutcliffe JS, et al. Identification of a gene (FMR-1) containing a CGG repeat coincident with a breakpoint cluster region exhibiting length variation in fragile X syndrome. Cell 1991;65:905.

12. Sherman S. Epidemiology. In: Hagerman RJ, Hagerman PJ, eds. Fragile X syndrome: diagnosis, treatment and research, 3rd ed. Baltimore: Johns Hopkins University Press, 2002:136.

13. Yaron Y, Orr-Urtreger A. New genetic principles. Clin Obstet Gynecol 2002;45:593.

14. Lubs HA. A marker X chromosome. Am J Hum Genet 1969;21:231.

15. Escalante JA, Frota-Pessoa O. Retaramento mental. In: Becak W, Frota-Pessoa O, eds. Genetica medica. Sao Paulo: Sarvier, 1973:300.

16. Giraud F, Ayme S, Mattei JF, et al. Constitutional chromosomal breakage. Hum Genet 1976;34:125.

17. Harvey J, Judge C, Wiener W. Familial X-linked mental retardation with an X chromosome abnormality. J Med Genet 1977;14:46.

18. Brookwell R, Turner G. High resolution banding and the locus of the Xq fragile site. Hum Genet 1983; 63:77.

19. Krawczun MS, Jenkins EC, Brown WT. High resolution preparations of fragile X chromosomes using acridine orange: localization and expression of the fragile site. Hum Genet 1985;69:209.

20. Sutherland GR. Heritable fragile sites on human chromosomes. I. Factors affecting expression in lymphocyte culture. Am J Hum Genet 1979;31:125.

21. Jenkins EC, Duncan CJ, Krawczun MS, et al. Frequency of tri- or multiradial configurations in fragile X identification. Am J Med Genet 1986;23:531.

22. Subrt I, Stirská K. Frequency of tri- and multiradial configurations in fragile X chromosomes. Hum Genet 1988;78:196.

23. Sutherland GR, Hecht F. Cytogenetics of the fragile X. In: Motulsky AG, Harper PS, Bobrow M, eds. Fragile sites on human chromosomes. New York: Oxford University Press, 1985:53.

24. Sutherland GR. Fragile sites on human chromosomes: demonstration of their dependence in the type of tissue culture medium. Science 1977;197:265.

25. Glover TW. FUdR induction of the X chromosome fragile site: Evidence for the mechanism of folic acid and thymidine inhibition. Am J Hum Genet 1981;33:234.

26. Tommerup N, Nielsen KB, Mikkelsen M. Marker X chromosome induction in fibroblasts by FUdR. Am J Med Genet 1981;9:263.

27. Tommerup N, Poulsen H, Brondum-Nielsen K. 5-Fluoro-29-deoxyuridine induction of the fragile site on Xq28 associated with X linked mental retardation. J Med Genet 1981;18:374.

28. Lejeune J, Legrand N, Lafourcade J, et al. The fragile X effect of trimethoprim treatment (in French). Ann Genet 1982;25:149.

29. Glover TW. The fragile X chromosome: factors influencing its expression in vitro. In: Sandberg AA, ed. Progress and topics in cytogenetics, vol. 3B. New York: Alan R. Liss, 1983:415.

30. Krumdieck CL, Howard-Peebles PN. On the nature of folic acid-sensitive fragile sites in human chromosomes: an hypothesis. Am J Med Genet 1983;16:23.

31. Taylor WH, Hagerman PJ. Biochemistry of fragile X. In: Hagerman R, McBogg P, eds. The fragile X syndrome: diagnosis, biochemistry, and treatment. Denver: Spectra Press, 1983:151.

32. Sutherland GR, Baker E, Fratini A. Excess thymidine induces folate sensitive fragile sites. Am J Med Genet 1985;22:433.

33. Sutherland GR, Baker E. Induction of fragile sites in fibroblasts. Am J Hum Genet 1986;38:573.

34. Glover TW, Berger C, Coyle J, et al. DNA polymerase inhibition by aphidicolin induces gaps and breaks at common fragile sites in human chromosomes. Hum Genet 1984;67:136.

35. Soudek D, Partington MW, Lawson JS. The fragile X syndrome. I. Familial variation in the proportion of lymphocytes with the fragile site in males. Am J Med Genet 1984;17:241.

36. Jenkins EC, Kastin BR, Krawczun MS, et al. Fragile X chromosome frequency is consistent temporally and within replicate cultures. Am J Med Genet 1986;23:475.
37. Dobkin C, Zhong N, Brown WT. The molecular basis of fragile sites. Am J Hum Genet 1996;59:478.
38. Sutherland GR, Baker E, Purvis-Smith W, et al. Prenatal diagnosis of the fragile X using thymidine induction. Prenat Diagn 1987;7:197.
39. Jenkins EC, Duncan CJ, Sanz MM, et al. Progress toward an internal control system for fra(X) induction by FUdR in whole blood cultures. Pathobiology 1990;58:236.
40. Jacky PB, Ahuja YR, Anyane-Yeboa K, et al. Guidelines for the preparation and analysis of the fragile X chromosome in lymphocytes. Am J Med Genet 1991;38:400.
41. Wilmot PL. Review of cytogenetic data for fragile X detection: lymphocytes and other tissues. In: Wiley AM, Murphy PD, eds. Fragile X/cancer cytogenetics. New York: Wiley-Liss, 1991:15.
42. Blomquist HK, Gustavson KH, Nordenson L, et al. Fragile site X chromosomes and X-linked mental retardation in severely retarded boys in a Northern Swedish county: a prevalence study. Clin Genet 1982;60:278.
43. Blomquist HK, Gustavson KH, Holmgren G, et al. Fragile X syndrome in mildly mentally retarded children in a Northern Swedish county: a prevalence study. Clin Genet 1983;24:393.
44. Webb T, Bundey S, Thake A, et al. The frequency of the fragile X chromosome among school children in Coventry. J Med Genet 1986;23:396.
45. Sutherland GR, Baker E. The common fragile site in band q27 of the human chromosome is not coincident with the fragile X. Clin Genet 1990;37:167.
46. Webb T, Bundey S. Prevalence of fragile X syndrome. J Med Genet 1991; 28;358.
47. Turner G, Webb T, Wake S, et al. Prevalence of fragile X syndrome. Am J Med Genet 1996;64:196.
48. Brown WT. Invited editorial on the FRAXE syndrome: is it time for routine screening? Am J Hum Genet 1996;58:903.
49. Rousseau F, Rouillard P, Morel ML, et al. Prevalence of carriers of premutation-sized alleles of the FMR1 gene and implication for the population genetics of the fragile X syndrome. Am J Hum Genet 1995;57: 1006.
50. Opitz JM, Sutherland GR. Conference report: International Workshop of the Fragile X and X-Linked Mental Retardation. Am J Med Genet 1984;17:5.
51. Turner G, Opitz JM, Brown WT, et al. Conference report: Second International Workshop on the Fragile X and on X-Linked Mental Retardation. Am J Med Genet 1986;23:11.
52. Neri G, Opitz, JM, Mikkelsen M, et al. Conference report: Third International Workshop of the Fragile X and X-Linked Mental Retardation. Am J Med Genet 1988;30:1.
53. Brown WT, Jenkins E, Neri G, et al. Conference report: Fourth International Workshop on the Fragile X and X-Linked Mental Retardation. Am J Med Genet 1991;38:158.
54. Mandel J-L, Hagerman R, Froster U, et al. Conference Report: Fifth International Workshop on the Fragile X and X-Linked Mental Retardation. Am J Med Genet 1992;43:5.
55. Sutherland GR, Brown WT, Hagerman R, et al. Conference Report: Sixth International Workshop on the Fragile X and X-Linked Mental Retardation. Am J Med Genet 1994;51:281.
56. Tranebjaerg L, Lubs HA, Borghgraef M, et al. Conference Report: Seventh International Workshop on the Fragile X and X-Linked Mental Retardation. Am J Med Genet 1996;64:1.
57. Holden JJA, Percy M, Allingham-Hawkins D, et al. Conference Report: Eighth International Workshop on the Fragile X Syndrome and X-Linked Mental Retardation. Am J Med Genet 1999;83:221.
57a. Fryns JP, Borghgraef M, Brown WT, et al. Conference Report: Ninth International Workshop on Fragile X Syndrome and X-linked Mental Retardation. Am J Med Genet 2000;94:345.
58. Bennetto L, Pennington BF. Neuropsychology. In Fragile X syndrome: diagnosis, treatment and research, 3rd ed. Hagerman R, Hagerman P, eds. Baltimore: Johns Hopkins University Press, 2002.
59. Turner G, Robinson H, Laing S, et al. Preventive screening for the fragile X syndrome. N Engl J Med 1986;315:607.
60. Hagerman RJ, Amiri K, Cronister A. The fragile X checklist. Am J Med Genet 1991;38:283.
61. Nolin SL, Snider DA, Jenkins EC, et al. Fragile X screening program in New York State. Am J Med Genet 1991;38:251.
62. Brown WT, Jenkins EC, Cohen IL, et al. Fragile X and autism: a multicenter survey. Am J Med Genet 1986;23:334.
63. Cohen IL, Brown WT, Jenkins EC, et al. Fragile X syndrome in females with autism. Am J Med Genet 1989;34:302.
64. Dykens EM, Volkmar FR. Medical conditions associated with autism. In: Cohen DJ, Volkmar FR, eds. Handbook of autism and pervasive developmental disorder, 2nd ed. New York. Wiley, 1997:388.

65. Cohen IL, Sudhalter V, Pfadt A, et al. Why are autism and the fragile-X syndrome associated? Conceptual and methodological issues. Am J Hum Genet 1991;48:195.

66. Bailey A, Bolton P, Butler L, et al. Prevalence of the fragile X anomaly amoungst autistic twins and singletons. J Child Psychol Psychiatr 1993:34: 673.

67. Brown WT, Jenkins EC, Friedman E et al. Autism is associated with the fragile X syndrome. J Autism Dev Dis 1982;12:303.

68. Bailey DB, Hatton DD, Skinner M, Mesibov G. Autistic behavior, FMR1 protein and developmental trajectories in young males with fragile X syndrome. J Autism Dev Dis 2001:31:165.

69. Cohen IL, Nolin SL, Sudhalter V, et al. Mosaicism for the FMR1 gene influences adaptive skills development in fragile X-affected males. Am J Med Genet 1996;64:365.

70. Dobkin C, Nolin SL, Cohen I, et al. Tissue differences in fragile X mosaics: mosaicism in blood cells may differ greatly from skin. Am J Med Genet 1996;64:296.

71. Gillberg C, Pearsson E, Wahlstrom J. The autism-fragile-X syndrome (AFRAX): a population-based study of ten boys. J Ment Defic Res 1986;30:27.

72. Arinami T, Sato M, Nakajima S, et al. Auditory brain-stem responses in the fragile X syndrome. Am J Hum Genet 1988;43:46.

73. Wisniewski KM, Segan SM, Miezejeski CM. The fra(X) syndrome: neurological, electrophysiological, and neuropathological abnormalities. Am J Med Genet 1991;38:476.

74. Miezejeski CM, Heany G, Belser R, et al. Longer brainstem auditory evoked response latencies of individuals with fragile X syndrome related to sedation. Am J Med Genet 1997,74:167.

75. Sherman SL, Morton NE, Jacobs PA, et al. The marker (X) syndrome: a cytogenetic and genetic analysis. Ann Hum Genet 1984;48:21.

76. Sherman SL, Jacobs PA, Morton NE, et al. Further segregation analysis of the fragile X syndrome with special reference to transmitting males. Hum Genet 1985;69:289.

77. Voelckel MA, Philip N, Piquet C, et al. Study of a family with fragile site of the X chromosome at Xq27–28 without mental retardation. Hum Genet 1989;81:353.

78. Sklower Brooks S, Cohen I, Ferrando C, et al. Cytogenetically negative, linkage positive "fragile X" syndrome. Am J Med Genet 1991;38:370.

79. Hagerman RJ, Hull CE, Safanda JF, et al. High functioning fragile X males: demonstration of an unmethylated fully expanded FMR-1 mutation associated with protein expression. Am J Med Genet 1994;51:298.

80. Jenkins E, Dobkin C, Ding X, et al. Fragile X frequency levels correlate with size of the repeat expansion in lymphocyte, lymphoblastoid and clonal lymphoblastoid cultures from an unmethylated mosaic full mutation male individual (abstract P35). In: Proceedings of the 7th International Workshop on the Fragile X and X-Linked Mental Retardation, 1995.

81. Wang Z, Taylor AK, Bridge J. FMR1 fully expanded mutation with minimal methylation in a high functioning fragile X male. J Med Genet 1996;33:376.

82. Hagerman RJ, Jackson C, Amiri K, et al. Fragile X girls: Physical and neurocognitive status and outcome. Pediatrics 1992;89:395.

83. Hagerman RJ. Physical and behavioral phenotype. In: Hagerman R, Hagerman P, eds. Fragile X syndrome: diagnosis, treatment and research, 3rd ed. Baltimore: Johns Hopkins University Press, 2002:3.

84. Cronister A, Hagerman RJ, Wittenberger M, et al. Mental impairment in cytogenetically positive fragile X females. Am J Med Genet 1991;38:503.

85. Brown WT, Jenkins EC, Goonewardena P, et al. Prenatally detected fragile X females: long-term follow-up studies show high risk of mental impairment. Am J Med Genet 1992;43(1/2):96.

86. Tuckerman E, Webb T, Bundey SE. Frequency and replication status of the fragile X, fra(X)(q27/28), in a pair of monozygotic twins of markedly differing intelligence. J Med Genet 1985;22:85.

87. Tuckerman E, Webb T. The inactivation of the fragile X chromosome in female carriers of the Martin Bell syndrome as studied by two different methods. Clin Genet 1989;36:25.

88. Kemper MB, Hagerman RJ, Ahmad RS, et al. Cognitive profiles and the spectrum of clinical manifestations in heterozygous fra(X) females. Am J Med Genet 1986;23:139.

89. Miezejeski CM, Jenkins EC, Hill AL, et al. Verbal vs. nonverbal ability, fragile X syndrome, and heterozygous carriers. Am J Hum Genet 1984;36:227.

90. Idem. A profile of cognitive deficit in females from fragile X families. Neuropsychologia 1986;24:405.

91. Wolff PH, Gardiner J, Lappen J, et al. Variable expression of the fragile X syndrome in heterozygous females of normal intelligence. Am J Med Genet 1988;30:213.

92. Reiss A, Hagerman RJ, Vinogradov W, et al. Psychiatric disability in female carriers of the fragile X chromosome. Arch Gen Psychiatry 1988;45:25.

93. Reiss AL, Abrams MT, Greenlaw R, et al. Neurodevelopmental effects of the FMR-1 full mutation in human. Nature Med 1995;1:159.
94. Toledano-Alhadef H, Basel-Vanagaite L, Magal N, et al. Fragile-X carrier screening and the prevalence of premutation and full-mutation carriers in Israel. Am J Hum Genet 2001;69:351.
95. Jacquemont S, Hagerman RJ, Leehey M, et al. Fragile X premutation tremor/ataxia syndrome: molecular, clinical, and neuroimaging correlates. Am J Hum Genet 2003;72:869.
95a. Sherman S. Epidemiology. In: Fragile X Syndrome: Diagnosis, Treatment and Research. Eds: RJ Hagerman, PJ Hagerman, Baltimore, The Johns Hopkins University Press, p. 145.
96. Hagerman RJ, Leehey M, Heinrichs W, et al. Intention tremor, Parkinsonism and generalized brain atrophy in older male carriers of fragile X. Neurology 2001;57:127.
97. Jenkins EC, Brown WT, Duncan C, et al. Feasibility of fragile X chromosome prenatal diagnosis demonstrated. Lancet 1981;2:1292.
98. Webb T, Butler D, Insley J, et al. Prenatal diagnosis of Martin–Bell syndrome associated with fragile site at Xq27–28. Lancet 1981;2:1423.
99. Shapiro LR, Wilmot PL, Brenholz P, et al. Prenatal diagnosis of the fragile X chromosome. Lancet 1982;1:99.
100. Wilmot PL, Shapiro LR. Family history of mental retardation for which fragile X cannot be documented: is prenatal diagnosis for fragile X indicated? Am J Hum Genet 1990;47(3):A126.
101. Jenkins EC, Krawczun MS, Brooks SE, et al. Laboratory aspects of prenatal fra(X) detection. In: Willey AM, Murphy PD, eds. Fragile X/cancer cytogenetics. New York: Wiley-Liss, 1991:27.
102. Shapiro LR, Wilmot PL, Shapiro DA, et al. Cytogenetic diagnosis of the fragile X syndrome: efficiency utilization, and trends. Am J Med Genet 1991;38:408.
103. Jenkins EC, Houck GE Jr, Jeziorowska A, et al. Prenatal detection of fragile X: experience of 10 years including introduction of molecular testing. In: Hagerman RJ, McKenzie P, eds. Proceedings of the International Fragile X Conference, 1992:349.
104. Von Koskull H, Nordstrom A-M, Salonen R, et al. Prenatal diagnosis and carrier detection in fragile X. Am J Med Genet 1992;43:174.
105. Von Koskull H, Gahmberg N, Salonen R, et al. FRAXA locus in fragile X diagnosis: family studies, prenatal diagnosis, and diagnosis of sporadic cases of mental retardation. Am J Med Genet 1994;51:486.
106. Howard-Peebles PN. Prenatal diagnosis of fragile X: Experience in three laboratories. In: Hagerman RJ, McKenzie P, eds. Proceedings of the International Fragile X Conference Proceedings, 1992:348.
107. Tarleton J, Wong S, Heitz D, et al. Difficult diagnosis of the fragile X syndrome made possible by direct detection of DNA mutations. J Med Genet 1992;29:726.
108. Liou J-D, Chen C-P, Breg WR, et al. Fetal blood sampling an cytogenetic abnormalities. Prenat Diagn 1993;13:1.
109. Baranov VS, Aseev MV, Rakisheva ZB, et al. Molecular diagnosis of the fragile X-chromosome syndrome (Martin-Bell syndrome) in patients of native populations of the former USSR. Genetika 1993;29(6):102.
110. Grasso M, Perrnoi L, Colella S, et al. Prenatal diagnosis of 30 fetuses at risk for fragile X syndrome. Am J Med Genet 1996;64:187.
111. Jenkins EC, Houck GE Jr, Ding X-H, et al. An update on fragile X prenatal diagnosis: End of the cytogenetic testing era. Dev Brain Dysfunct 1995;8:293.
112. Jenkins EC, Shapiro LR, Brown WT. Prenatal diagnosis of the fragile X syndrome. In: Milunsky A, ed. Genetics disorders and the fetus, 3rd ed. Baltimore: Johns Hopkins University Press, 1992:241.
113. Jenkins EC, Krawczun MS, Stark-Houck SL, et al. Improved prenatal detection of fra(X)(q27.3): Methods for prevention of false negatives in chorionic villus and amniotic fluid cell cultures. Am J Med Genet 1991;38:447.
114. Shapiro LR, Wilmot PL, Fisch GS. Prenatal cytogenetic diagnosis of the fragile X syndrome in amniotic fluid: calculation of accuracy. Am J Med Genet 1992;43:170.
115. Sutherland GR, Richards RI. Fragile X syndrome: the most common cause of familial mental retardation. Acta Paediatr Sin 1994;35:94.
116. Jenkins EC, Genovese M, Duncan CJ, et al. Fra(X)(q27.2), the common fragile site, observed in only one of 760 cases studied for the fragile X syndrome. Am J Med Genet 1992;43:136.
117. Neville L, Cochrane J, Fitzgerald P, et al. Fragile X mental retardation syndrome: DNA diagnosis and carrier detection in New Zealand families. NZ Med J 1995;108:404.
118. Wilkin H, Tuohy J, Theewis W. Prenatal diagnosis of fragile X and Turner mosaicism in a 12-week fetus. Prenat Diagn 2000;20:854,55.

119. Puissant H, Malinge MC, Larget-Piet A, et al. Molecular analysis of 53 fragile X families with the probe StB12.3. Am J Med Genet 1994;53:370.

120. Castellvi-Bel S, Mila M, Soler A, et al. Prenatal diagnosis of fragile X syndrome: (CGG)n expansion and methylation of chorionic villus samples. Prenat Diagn 1995;15:801.

121. Appelman Z, Vinkler C, Caspi B. Chorionic villus sampling in multiple pregnancies. Eur J Obstet Gynecol. 1999;85:97.

122. Drasinover V, Ehrlich S, Magal N, et al. Increased transmission of intermediate alleles of the *FMR1* gene compared with normal alleles among female heterozygotes. Am J Med Genet 2000;93:155.

123. Kallinen J, Heinonen S, Mannermaa A, et al. Prenatal diagnosis of fragile X syndrome and the risk of expansion of a premutation. Clin Genet 2000;58:111.

124. Peso R, Berkenstadt M, Cuckle H, et al. Screening for fragile X syndrome in women of reproductive age. Prenat Diagn 2000;20:611.

125. Jenkins EC, Brown WT, Krawczun MS, et al. Recent experience in prenatal fra(X) detection. Am J Med Genet 1988;30:329.

126. Tommerup N, Reintoft I, Reske-Nielsen E, et al. Unsuspected prenatal diagnosis of the fragile X. Am J Med Genet 1988;30:25A.

127. Brown WT, Nolin S, Houck Jr G, et al. Prenatal diagnosis and carrier screening for fragile X by PCR. Am J Med Genet 1996;64:191.

128. Wen GY, Jenkins EC, Yao X-L, et al. Transmission electron microcopy of chromosomes by longitudinal section preparation: application to fragile X chromosome analysis. Am J Med Genet 1997;68:445–449.

129. Wen GY, Jenkins EC, Goldberg EM, et al. Ultrastructure of the fragile X chromosome: new observations on the fragile site. Am J Med Genet 1999;83(4):331.

130. Rousseau F, Heitz D, Biancalana V, et al. Direct diagnosis by DNA analysis of the fragile X syndrome of mental retardation. N Engl J Med 1991;325:1673.

131. Kremer EJ, Pritchard M, Lynch M, et al. Mapping of DNA instability at the fragile X to a trinucleotide repeat sequence p(CCG)n. Science 1991;252:1711.

132. Fu YH, Kuhl DPA, Pizzuti A, et al. Variation of the CGG repeat at the fragile X site results in genetic instability: resolution of the Sherman paradox. Cell 1991;57:1047.

133. Brown WT, Houck G Jr, Jeziorowska A, et al. Rapid fragile X carrier screening and prenatal diagnosis by a nonradioactive PCR test. JAMA 1993;270:1569.

134. Nolin S, Dobkin C, Brown WT. Molecular analysis of fragile X syndrome. In: Cracopoli NC, Haines JL, Korf BR, eds. Current protocols in human genetics. New York: Wiley, 2003;9:5.

135. Dobkin CS, Ding X, Li SY, et al. Fragile X prenatal diagnosis by a novel Southern-PCR hybrid procedure. Am J Hum Genet 1996;59:A320.

136. Dobkin C, Ding X, Li S-Y, et al. Accelerated fragile X prenatal diagnosis by PCR restriction fragment detection. Am J Med Genet 1999; 83:338.

137. Suzumori K, Yamauchi M, Seki N, et al. Prenatal diagnosis of a hypermethylated @REF:full fragile X mutation in chorionic villi of a male fetus. J Med Genet 1993;30:785.

138. Willemsen R, Oosterwijk JC, Los FJ, et al. Prenatal diagnosis of fragile X syndrome. Lancet 1996;348:967.

139. Devys D, Lutz Y, Rouyer N, et al. The FMR-1 protein is cytoplasmic, most abundant in neurons and appears normal in carriers of a fragile premutation. Nat Genet 1993;4:335.

140. Todd PK, Malter JS. Fragile X mental retardation protein in plasticity and disease. J Neurosci Res 2002;70:633.

141. Willemsen R, Smits A, Mohkamsing S, et al. Rapid antibody test for diagnosing fragile X syndrome: a validation of the technique. Hum Genet 1997;99:308.

142. Willemsen R, Oosterwijk JC, Los FJ, et al. Prenatal diagnosis of fragile X syndrome. Lancet 1996;348:967.

143. Willemsen R, Los F, Mohkamsing S, et al. Rapid antibody test for prenatal diagnosis of fragile X syndrome on amniotic fluid cells: a new appraisal. J Med Genet 1997;34:250.

144. Jenkins EC, Wen GY, Li S-Y, et al. Studies of fragile X protein (FMRP) detection in cells form prenatal samples indicate variation in immunocytochemical staining intensities. In: Proceedings of the 4th Joint Clinical Genetics Meeting, 28th Annual March of Dimes Clinical Genetics Conference/American College of Medical Genetics 4th Annual Meeting, 1997:A7.

145. Jenkins EC, Wen GY, Kim KW, et al. Prenatal fragile X detection using cytoplasmic and nuclear-specific monoclonal antibodies. Am J Med Genet 1999;83:342.

146. Willemsen R, Bontekoe CJM, Severijnen L-A, et al. Timing of the absence of *FMR1* expression in full mutation chorionic villi. Hum Genet 2002;110:601.

147. Lambiris N, Peters H, Bollmann R, et al. Rapid FMR1-protein analysis of fetal blood: an enhancement of prenatal diagnosis. Hum Genet 2002;110:601.

148. Verlinsky Y, Rechitsky S, Verlinsky O, et al. Polar body-based preimplantation diagnosis for X-linked disorders. Reproductive BioMedicine Online 2002; 4(1):38. www.rbmonline.com.

149. Black SH, Levinson G, Harton GL, et al. Preimplantation genetic testing (PGT) for fragile X (fraX). Am J Hum Genet 1995;57:A153.

150. Brown WT, Gross AG, Chan CB, et al. Genetic heterogeneity in the fragile X syndrome. Hum Genet 1985;71:11.

151. Brown WT, Gross AG, Chan CB. DNA linkage studies in the fragile X syndrome suggests heterogeneity. Am J Med Genet 1986;23:643.

152. Pembrey ME, Winter RM, Davies KE. A premutation that generates a defect at crossing over explains the inheritance of fragile X mental retardation. Am J Med Genet 1985;21:709.

153. Hoegerman SF, Rary JM. Speculation on the role of transposable elements in human genetic disease with particular attention to achondroplasia and the fragile X syndrome. Am J Med Genet 1986;23:685.

154. Winter RM, Pembrey ME. Analysis of linkage relationships between genetic markers around the fragile X markers around the fragile X locus with special reference to the daughters of normal transmitting males. Hum Genet 1986;74:93.

155. Brown WT, Sherman SL, Dobkin CS. Hypothesis regarding the nature of the fragile X mutation: a reply to Winter and Pembrey. Hum Genet 1987;75:294.

156. Nussbaum RL, Airhart SD, Ledbetter DH. Recombination and amplification of pyrimidine-rich sequences may be responsible for initiation and progression of the Xq27 fragile site: an hypothesis. Am J Med Genet 1986;23:715.

157. Laird CD. Proposed mechanism of inheritance and expression of the human fragile-X syndrome of mental retardation. Genetics 1987;117:587.

158. Laird C, Jaffe E, Karpen G, et al. Fragile sites in human chromosomes as regions of late-replicating DNA. Trends Genet 1987;3:274.

159. Israel MH. Autosomal suppressor gene for fragile-X: An hypothesis. Am J Med Genet 1987;26:19.

160. Vincent A, Heitz D, Petit C, et al. Abnormal pattern detected in fragile-X patients by pulsed-field gel electrophoresis. Nature 1991;349:624.

161. Bell MV, Hirst MC, Nakahon Y, et al. Physical mapping across the fragile X: hypermethylation and clinical expression of the fragile X syndrome. Cell 1991;64:861.

162. Eichler EE, Richards S, Gibbs R, et al. Fine structure of the human FMR1 gene. Hum Mol Genet 1993;2:1147.

163. Pieretti M, Zhang F, Fu YH, et al. Absence of expression of the FMR-1 gene in fragile X syndrome. Cell 1991;66:1.

164. Hirst M, Knight S, Davies K, et al. Prenatal diagnosis of fragile X syndrome. Lancet 1991;338:956.

165. Dobkin CS, Ding X-H, Jenkins EC, et al. Prenatal diagnosis of fragile X syndrome. Lancet 1991;338:957.

166. Sutherland GR, Gedeon A, Kornman L, et al. Prenatal diagnosis of fragile X syndrome by direct detection of the unstable DNA sequence. N Engl J Med 1991;325:1720.

167. Pergolizzi RG, Erster SH, Goonewardena P, et al. Detection of full fragile X mutation. Lancet 1992; 339:271.

168. Nolin SL, Lewis FA, Ye LL, et al. Familial transmission of the FMR1 CGG repeat. Am J Hum Genet 1996;59:1252.

169. Nolin S, Brown WT, Glicksman A, et al. Expansion of the fragile X CGG repeat in females with premutation or intermediate alleles. Am J Hum Genet 2003;72:454.

170. Zhong N, Ju W, Pietrofesa J, et al. Fragile X "Gray Zone" alleles: AGG patterns, expansion risks, and associated haplotypes. Am J Med Genet 1996;64:261.

171. Brown WT, Houck GE Jr, Ding X, et al. Reverse mutations in the fragile X syndrome. Am J Med Genet 1996;64:287.

172. Malzac P, Biancalana V, Voelckel MA, et al. Unexpected inheritance of the (CGG)n trinucleotide expansion in a fragile X syndrome family. Eur J Hum Genet 1996;4:8.

173. Vaisanen M-L, Haataja R, Leisti J. Decrease in the CGGn trinucleotide repeat mutation of the fragile X syndrome to normal size range during paternal transmission. Am J Hum Genet 1996;59:540.

174. Evans MI, Wapner RJ. Future Directions. Clin Obstet Gynecol 2002;45:730.

175. Ryynänen M, Heinonen S, Makkonen M, et al. Feasibility and acceptance of screening for fragile X mutations in low-risk pregnancies. Eur J Hum Genet 1999;7:212.

176. Kallinen J, Maria K, Heinonen S, et al. Wide scope prenatal diagnosis at Kuopio Universtiy Hospital 19976–1998: integration of gene tests and fetal karyotyping. Br J Obstet Gynaecol 2001;108:505.

177. Bailey DB, Skinner D, Sparkman K, et al. Delayed diagnosis of fragile X syndrome—United States, 1990–1999. Morb Mortal 2002;51:740.

178. Bailey DB, Skinner D, Sparkman KL. Discovering fragile X syndrome: family experiences and perceptions. Pediatrics 2003;111(2):407.

Thomas W. Prior, Ph.D., Aubrey Milunsky,
MB.B.Ch., D.Sc., F.R.C.P., F.A.C.M.G., D.C.H.,
Cindy L. Vnencak-Jones, Ph.D., and
John A. Phillips III, M.D.

10

Molecular Genetics and Prenatal Diagnosis

Molecular genetic techniques, including restriction endonucleases, DNA hybridization, Southern blots, polymerase chain reaction (PCR) amplification, and DNA sequence analysis, have been used to characterize the DNA alterations that cause a variety of genetic disorders. Use of these techniques facilitates prenatal detection of a rapidly increasing number of Mendelian and mitochondrial disorders (see Table 10.1). Future applications will be pertinent to almost every medical subspecialty. Consideration of some basic molecular aspects will facilitate comprehension of the ensuing discussion on prenatal DNA diagnostics.

BACKGROUND: DNA AND GENE STRUCTURE

DNA Structure

Human chromosomes contain DNA and histone and nonhistone proteins. DNA is made up of three components: (1) bases, which are the purines adenine (A) and guanine (G) and the pyrimidines thymine (T) and cytosine (C); (2) a five-carbon deoxyribose sugar; and (3) a phosphate backbone. The sugar phosphate backbone consists of a phosphate molecule attached to the 5′ carbon of the deoxyribose sugar with the 3′ carbon of the sugar attached to the phosphate of the next molecule. Phosphate bonding to the 3′ carbons gives direction to the DNA strand as bases are added 5′ to 3′. Hydrogen bonding between AT and GC bases on complementary DNA strands stabilizes the conformation of the double helix. The pairing of A=Ts is formed by two hydrogen bonds, whereas the pairing of G/C forms three hydrogen bonds. Notice that hydrogen bonds occur between the bases of complementary strands that run in antiparallel directions (i.e., 5′ → 3′ on one strand and 3′ → 5′ on the complementary strand). For example, 5′TCGA3′on one strand corresponds to 3′AGCT5′on the other, forming the double-stranded molecule. Units of three bases, called triplets, constitute a codon, which by convention, is read from the "coding" DNA strand that has the same sequence as the mRNA. These codons are units of the genetic code that direct the cellular machinery to add specific amino acids during translation of the mRNA encoded by the gene. Codons are arranged in a linear sequence within the exons of genes.[1,2] A final important point regarding DNA structure is that as the temperature increases, denaturation of the two DNA strands occurs, first between A=T pairs then between G/C pairs. The G/C base pairs melt at higher temperatures because their three hydrogen bonds make them more stable than A=T base pairs, which have two hydrogen bonds. Advantage is taken of these differences in melting temperature by a variety of methods used to detect DNA mutations.

Gene Structure

Genes are divided into segments called exons and introns (Figure 10.1). Exons are portions of genes that are contained in the mature mRNA. Because exons are sequences that are contained in mature RNA, they include: (1) 5′ untranslated sequences, (2) internal exons whose codons encode for amino acids in the translated protein product, and (3) 3′ untranslated sequences. In contrast, introns or intervening sequences (IVS) contain only noncoding DNA sequences, which are transcribed but then removed from the mRNA by splicing before translation.[3] Thus, mutations that are differences between the sequences of copies of a gene, called alleles, can occur within exons or introns of a gene. Missense mutations are single base changes in exons which result in a change in the amino acid normally found in the protein. A change in the amino acid may affect the overall three-dimensional structure of the protein or the stability of the protein or it may alter the function of the protein product. Mutations can also affect untranslated portions of exons or introns or other sequences of DNA that flank the gene but are not contained in the exons. Although these mutations in noncoding sequences can affect different steps in gene expression, or mRNA processing because they do not reside in the translated exons, they may not be detectable by analysis of the gene's protein product.

Many human genes occur in groups of related genes called gene families or clusters. Examples of gene clusters are the α- and β-globin and growth hormone gene clusters. The

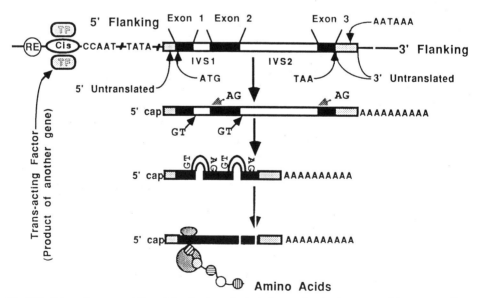

Fig. 10.1. Schematic representation of the structure of a typical gene showing its exons and introns as well as selected sequences that are important in various steps of its expression.

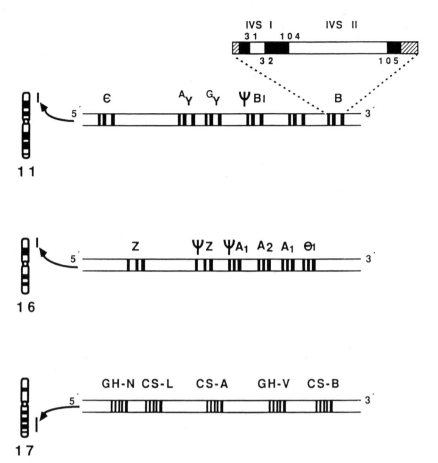

Fig. 10.2. α-Globin (AG), β-globin (NAG), and growth hormone (GH) gene clusters. For every gene shown, the black boxes represent coding regions (exons), small white boxes represent introns, and hatched boxes are the 5′ and 3′ untranslated regions. The large white boxes represent pseudogenes, which are not expressed because of DNA sequence alterations. The numbers below the areas of the coding sequences represent the corresponding amino acid encoded by that sequence.

human α-globin gene cluster on chromosome 16 contains the paired α-globin loci and the ζ locus. The human β-globin gene cluster on chromosome 11 contains the β, δ, γ^G, γ^A, and ϵ loci.[3–5] The growth hormone gene cluster on chromosome 17 contains five loci that are evolutionarily related (Figure 10.2).[6,7] Frequently, pseudogenes that are inactive but stable sequences derived by mutation of an ancestral active gene are also found in gene clusters (see $\psi\alpha$ and $\psi\beta$ in Figure 10.2). These pseudogenes have homology to and resemble related, active genes but have acquired DNA sequence alterations that prevent their expression.

THE NATURE AND MECHANISMS OF HUMAN GENE MUTATION

CpG Dinucleotides Are Hot Spots for Nucleotide Substitutions

In the genomes of eukaryotes (higher organisms that have a well-defined nucleus), 5-methylcytosine (^{5m}C) occurs predominantly in CpG dinucleotides, the majority of which appear to be methylated.[8,9] Methylation of such cytosines results in a high level of muta-

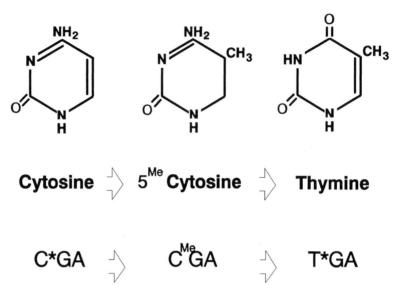

Fig. 10.3. The structure of cytosine, 5me cytosine, and thymine. Note the tendency for C → T substitutions.

tion because of the propensity of ^{5m}C to undergo deamination to form thymine (Figure 10.3). Deamination of ^{5m}C probably occurs with the same frequency as either cytosine or uracil. However, whereas uracil DNA glycosylase activity in eukaryotic cells is able to recognize and excise uracil, thymine is a "normal" DNA base that is thought to be less readily detectable as a substitution for C and hence escapes removal by cellular DNA repair mechanisms. One consequence of the hypermutability of ^{5m}C is the paucity of CpG in the genomes of many eukaryotes, and heavily methylated vertebrate genomes exhibit "CpG suppression."[9] For example, in vertebrate genomes, the frequency of CpG dinucleotides is 20–25 percent of the frequency predicted from observed mononucleotide frequencies.[10] The distribution of CpG in the genome is also nonrandom; about 1 percent of the vertebrate genome consists of a fraction that is CpG-rich and that accounts for ~15 percent of all CpG dinucleotides.[11] In contrast to most of the scattered CpG dinucleotides, these "CpG islands" represent unmethylated domains that, in many cases, coincide with transcribed regions. The evolution of the heavily vertebrate genome has been accompanied by the progressive loss of CpG dinucleotides or "CpG suppression" as a direct consequence of their methylation in the germ line.[9]

The CpG hypermutability observed in inherited disease implies that these sites are methylated in the germ line, resulting in ^{5m}Cs that are prone to deamination. Evidence that ^{5m}C deamination is directly responsible for these mutational events is that several cytosine residues known to have undergone a germ-line mutation in the LDL receptor gene (hypercholesterolemia) and the tumor protein 53 (TP53) gene (various types of tumor) are indeed methylated in the germ line.[12] Last, the most mutable single nucleotide, which occurs within a CpG dinucleotide, is found in achondroplasia.[12a] Achondroplasia is transmitted as an autosomal dominant trait and is the most common form of short-limbed dwarfism. Essentially, almost all cases of achondroplasia are due to a single base change at nucleotide 1138 in the fibroblast growth factor receptor 3 gene (*FGFR3*). The mutation rate at nucleotide 1138 is at least two to three orders of magnitude higher than other known

CpG spots in the human genome. The mutation results in the substitution of glycine at codon 380 by an arginine. The net effect of the amino acid substitution is to reduce the rate of endochondrial bone growth.

Non-CpG Point Mutation Hot Spots

Because a variety of DNA sequence motifs are known to play an important role in the breakage and rejoining of DNA and could be potential determinants of single base-pair changes, the DNA sequence environment of mutations has been analyzed. Some trinucleotide and tetranucleotide motifs are significantly overrepresented within 10 bp on either side of the mutation hot spots. These motifs include TTT, CTT, TGA, TTG, CTTT, TCTT, and TTTG. In addition, Cooper and Krawczak[13] screened a region of ±10 bp around 219 non-CpG base substitution sites with known sequence environment for triplets and quadruplets that occurred at significantly increased frequencies. Only one trinucleotide (CTT) was found to occur at a frequency significantly higher than expected. Interestingly, CTT is the topoisomerase I cleavage site consensus sequence described by Bullock et al.,[14] and it was observed thirty-six times in the vicinity of a point mutation, whereas the expected frequency was twenty.

Strand difference in base substitution rates reveals some asymmetry, suggesting a strand difference for single base-pair substitutions. For example, the relative dinucleotide mutability of CT to CC and AG to GG differ by almost fivefold. This finding suggests that, at least within gene coding regions, the two strands are differentially methylated and/or differentially repaired. Holmes et al.[15] demonstrated in vitro the existence of a strand-specific correction process in human and *Drosophila* cells whose efficiency depends on the nature of the mispair.

Single nucleotide substitutions that affect mRNA splicing are nonrandomly distributed, and this nonrandomness can be related to the resulting phenotype.[15] Naturally occurring point mutations that affect mRNA splicing fall into different categories (Figure 10.4). First, mutations can occur in 5' or 3' consensus splice sites. These mutations usually reduce the amount of correctly spliced mature mRNA and/or lead to the use of alternative splice sites in the vicinity. The use of alternative splice sites can cause production of mRNAs that either lack a portion of the coding sequence ("exon skipping") or contain additional sequences of intronic origin ("cryptic splice site utilization"). Second, mutations within an intron or exon that may serve to activate cryptic splice sites can lead to the production of abnormal mRNAs. Third, mutations within a branch-point sequence can reduce normal splicing. Fourth, changes in other intronic sequences that are binding sites for proteins regulating splicing can cause alternative splicing.[16] Last, base changes occurring in exon sequences called exon splicing enhancers (ESEs) may also disrupt normal splicing.[17,18] ESEs are 6–8 nucleotide sequences found within exons, and in concert with the SR proteins enhance the use of adjacent splice sites. ESEs can be disrupted by single nonsense, missense, or silent point mutations. Disruption of ESEs has been identified in a number of genes and may be a very common mechanism for the alteration of normal gene splicing.

Transcription of an mRNA is initiated at the cap site (+1), so named because of the posttranscriptional addition of 7-methylgluanine at this position to protect the transcript from exonucleolytic degradation. Mutations at the cap site can either reduce transcription or cause initiation of transcription at a different but incorrect site. In the latter case, the transcript can be incomplete and/or unstable.

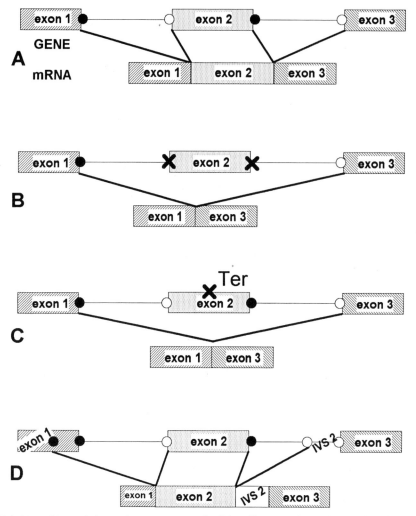

Fig. 10.4. Normal (*A*) and abnormal (*B–D*) patterns of splicing. Genes are shown above and resulting mRNA products below. *A*, Normal splicing. *B*, Exon skipping due to defects in either 3′ splice site of IVS1 or 5′ splice site IVS2. *C*, Exon skipping due to terminator mutation in exon 2. *D*, Alternative splicing that deletes a portion of exon 1 due to the use of a cryptic 5′ splice site (left) and includes a portion of IVS2 due to the use of a cryptic 3′ splice site (right). Rectangles = exons; horizontal lines = introns; solid and open circles = 5′ and 3′ splice sites, respectively.

A number of mutations in Met (ATG) translational initiation codons have been reported, with a preponderance of Met-to-Val substitutions. Whether the mutant mRNA is translated depends on a complex interplay of the different structural features of an mRNA that serves to modulate its translation.[19] Until fairly recently, it was thought that an AUG codon was an absolute requirement for translational initiation in mammals. However, some exceptions are now known—for example, ACG, CUG. The scanning model of translational initiation predicts that the 40S ribosomal subunit initiates at the first AUG codon to be encountered within an acceptable Kozak consensus sequence context (GCC A/G CCAUGG).[19] Another type of mutation that interferes with correct initiation is the creation of a cryptic ATG codon (in the context of a favorable Kozak consensus sequence shown above).

The first reported example of a mutation in a termination codon was that in the α_2-globin gene causing Hemoglobin Constant Spring, an abnormal hemoglobin that occurs frequently in Southeast Asia.[20] The associated α-globin chain is 172 amino acids in length, rather than the normal 141 amino acids, as a result of a TAA-to-CAA transition in the translation termination codon that causes a readthrough mutation.

All polyadenylated mRNA in higher eukaryotes possess the sequence AAUAAA, or a close homologue, 10–30 nucleotides upstream of the polyadenylation site. This motif is thought to play a role in 3′ end formation through endonucleolytic cleavage and polyadenylation of the mRNA transcript. Several single bp-substitutions are now known in the cleavage/polyadenylation signal sequences of the α_2- and β-globin genes, and all of these cause a relatively mild form of thalassemia.

Single base changes that result in new stop codons are known as nonsense mutations and are often associated with severe phenotypic consequences. An mRNA carrying a premature stop codon is usually rapidly degraded by a form of RNA surveillance known as nonsense-mediated mRNA decay.[21] However exon skipping in exons that contain nonsense mutations has also been reported by Deitz et al.[22] For example, exon B was deleted or skipped from fibrillin transcripts of a patient with Marfan syndrome whose exon B of the fibrillin gene contained a TAT-to-TAG nonsense mutation.

Regulatory Mutations

Most mutations causing human genetic disease lie within the coding regions of exons. A different class of mutation is represented by those affecting regulatory regions of genes. These mutations disrupt the normal processes of gene activation and transcriptional initiation and serve either to increase or decrease the level of mRNA/gene product synthesized rather than altering its nature.

Single nucleotide substitutions in the promoter region 5′ to the β-globin gene produce β-thalassemia by causing a moderate reduction in globin synthesis. The known naturally occurring mutations are clustered around two regions that are implicated in regulation of expression of the human β-globin gene. One is a CACCC motif located -91 to -86 and the other is the TATA box found at about -30 bp upstream to the transcriptional initiation site.

In addition to mutations in the remote promoter element known as the "locus control region" (LCR), Gastier et al.[23] reported a mutation at -530 that causes reduced β-globin synthesis. This mutation causes a ninefold increase in the binding capacity of BP1, a protein that may function as a repressor of expression of the β-globin gene.

Gene Deletions

Gene deletions cause many different inherited conditions in humans, and these may be broadly categorized on the basis of the length of DNA deleted. Some deletions consist of only one or a few base pairs, while others may span several hundred kilobases.[13]

The term *homologous recombination* describes recombination occurring at meiosis or mitosis between identical or similar DNA sequences. It can involve recombination of homologous but nonallelic DNA sequences. This type of recombination is one cause of deletions of the α-globin genes that underlie α-thalassemia. Repetitive DNA sequences can also produce this type of deletion by promoting unequal crossovers through homologous unequal recombination. For example, the *Alu* repeat is the most abundant repetitive element in the human genome and *Alu* repeats are involved in recombinations that cause deletions of the LDLR and complement component 1 inhibitor genes (CINH).

Hemoglobin (Hb) Lepore is the classic example of a gene fusion. Hb Lepore is an abnormal molecule, which has the first 50–80 amino acid residues of δ-globin at its N terminal and the last 60–90 amino acid residues of β-globin at its C terminal.

Nonhomologous or illegitimate recombination occurs between two sequences that show minimal sequence homology. This kind of recombination underlies some gross DNA rearrangements, in which the breakpoints share only a few nucleotides of homology.

The endpoints of some deletions are found to be marked by short repeated sequences. These short tandem repeats have been shown to be prone to slipped strand mispairing during DNA replication. This occurs when the normal pairing between the two complementary strands of a double helix is altered by the staggering of the repeats on the two strands, leading to incorrect pairing of repeats and a deletion of the intervening sequence on the newly synthesized strand. This slipped strand mispairing mechanism has been shown to generate deletions in the Kearns–Sayre syndrome (KSS), a mitochondrial encephalomyopathy characterized by external ophthalmoplegia, ptosis, ataxia, and cataracts.[24] About one-third of the cases of KSS are due to a common 4,977-bp deletion that is associated with two perfect 13-bp direct repeats. The deletion result is the elimination of the intervening sequence between two perfect 13-bp repeats. Because the mitochondrial genome is recombination-deficient, it has been postulated that the common deletion occurs by the replication slippage mechanism.

Gene Conversion

Gene conversion is the alteration of one allele so that it acquires one or more changes from the other allele.[25] The result is similar to that of a double crossover event. The difference between the two processes is that the modification of one allele (the target) after gene conversion is nonreciprocal because the other allele (the source) is left unchanged. Pseudogenes have been shown to be sources of deleterious mutations by gene conversion. The majority of the point mutations occurring in steroid 21-hydroxylase deficiency arise by gene conversion between the functional 21-hydroxylase gene, CYP21B, and the closely related pseudogene, CYP21A. The two genes occur on tandem DNA sequences, and the point mutations are copied from the pseudogene into the functional gene. Approximately 75 percent of the mutations in the functional gene have been transferred from the pseudogene by gene conversions. About 20 percent of the mutations are the result of an unequal crossover during meiosis, which deletes a 30-kb gene segment that encompasses the 3′ end of the pseudogene and the 5′ end of the functional gene, producing a nonfunctional chimeric pseudogene.[25a]

Expansion of Unstable Repeat Sequences

Trinucleotide repeat expansions are the molecular basis for increasing recognition of a growing number of human genetic diseases, including fragile X syndrome, myotonic dystrophy, Huntington disease, spinal bulbar muscular atrophy, Friedreich ataxia, and of other inherited ataxias. Trinucleotide repeats undergo a unique process of dynamic mutation, whereby the polymorphic repeat sequences are unstable and expand beyond the normal size range. The effects of the expansion are varied and may result in a loss of gene expression, a gain of function, or abnormal RNA processing. Genetic anticipation, mosaicism, and phenotypic heterogeneity are common features of these disorders.

Summary

There are various kinds of mutations in the human genome and many potential mechanisms for their production. Single-base-pair substitutions account for the majority of gene defects. Among them, the hypermutability of CpG dinucleotides represents an important and frequent cause of mutation in humans. Point mutations can affect protein function and stability, transcription, translation, mRNA stability, and mRNA splicing and processing. Mutations in regulatory elements are of particular significance because they often reveal DNA domains that are bound by regulatory proteins. Mutations that affect mRNA splicing likewise contribute to our understanding of sequences important in transcript splicing. Additional splicing mutations whose phenotype results primarily or exclusively from ESE disruption may be even more prevalent. There is a growing list of disorders caused by abnormal copy number of trinucleotide repeats within the 5′ or 3′ untranslated regions or coding sequences of genes. However, the mechanisms by which the numbers of these trinucleotide repeats expand or contract during meiosis and mitosis are not completely understood. The study of mutations in human genes is vital in understanding the pathophysiology of hereditary disorders, providing improved diagnostic tests, and designing appropriate therapeutic approaches.

MOLECULAR GENETIC TECHNIQUES USED IN PRENATAL DIAGNOSIS

To determine if a fetus has inherited a mutation that will cause a genetic disease, one must overcome several problems related to DNA and gene structure and the variety of different possible mutations. First, the amount of DNA that is present in each cell by itself poses a problem. Because the haploid DNA complement of each cell is 3×10^9 base pairs, the average gene compromises only 1/100,000 of the total nuclear DNA. Second, the presence of related DNA sequences such as those found in gene clusters can make the process of detecting a mutation in one member of the gene cluster difficult. Third, the variety of mutations at the locus and allelic heterogeneity that occurs in different diseases must be considered in all DNA diagnostic tests. Although these and other factors pose problems for prenatal diagnosis, a variety of molecular genetic techniques enable detection of a growing list of mutations that cause heritable disorders.

The basic tools of gene diagnosis are restriction endonucleases, gene segments, oligonucleotides, and DNA polymerase. Restriction endonucleases are used to produce genomic DNA fragments that are suitable for size analysis and can be separated by size using gel electrophoresis. The fragments resulting from endonuclease cleavage are denatured and transferred to a membrane to form a Southern blot. Gene segments and oligonucleotides can be labeled and used as probes that anneal to and detect specific genomic fragments. Oligonucleotides and DNA polymerase can be used to amplify selected genomic segments using PCR amplification. These amplified segments or amplicons can be analyzed to detect mutations. Applications of these tools to directly or indirectly detect gene alterations are illustrated by the following examples and the genetic diseases are listed in Table 10.1.

Table 10.1. Selected monogenic disorders detectable by DNA analysis (see Appendix)

Disease	Mode	OMIM No.	Reference
Aarskog–Scott syndrome	XL	305400	26
Abdominal aortic aneurysm	AD, AR	100070	27
Achondrogenesis, type II	AR	200610	28
Achondroplasia	AD	100800	29
Adenine monophosphate deaminase 1	AD	102770	31
Adenine phosphoribosyltransferase deficiency	AR	102600	30
Adrenoleukodystrophy, autosomal neonatal form	AR	202370	34
Adrenoleukodystrophy, X-linked	XL	300100	35
Adenomatous polyposis of the colon	AD	175100	32
Adenosine deaminase deficiency	AR	102700	33
Agammaglobulinemia, Bruton	XL	300300	36
Agammaglobulinemia, Swiss	XL	300400	37
Albinism, ocular, type 1	XL	300500	38
Albinism, oculocutaneous, type 1	AR	203100	39
Albinism, oculocutaneous, type 2	AR	203200	40,41
Albinism, oculocutaneous, type 3	AR	203290	42
Albright hereditary osteodystrophy-3	AD	600430	43
Aldolase deficiency	AR	103850	44
α_1-Antitrypsin deficiency	AR	107400	45–50
Alport syndrome, autosomal	AR	203780	51
Alport syndrome, X-linked	XL	301050	52–54
Alzheimer disease, type 3	AD	104311	55
Alzheimer disease, type 4	AD	600759	56
Amyloidosis, type 1	AD	176300	58–60
Amyotrophic lateral sclerosis	AD	105400	61
Androgen insensitivity	XL	313700	62
Angelman syndrome	AD, de novo	105830	63
Angioneurotic edema, hereditary	AD	106100	64,65
Aniridia	AD	106200	66
Anophthalmos	XL	301590	67
Antithrombin III deficiency	AD	107300	57
Apert syndrome	AD	101200	68
Apolipoprotein E	AD	107741	69
Arachnodactyly, contractural	AD	121050	70
Argininosuccinic aciduria	AR	207900	71
Arthrogryposis, multiplex congenita, distal, type 1	AD	108120	72
Arthrogryposis, multiplex congenita, distal, type 2	XL	301830	73
Ataxia telangiectasia	AR	208900	74
Azoospermia	AD	415000	75
Bardet–Biedl syndrome, type 2	AR	209900	76
Barth syndrome	XL	302060	77
Basal-cell nevus syndrome	AD	109400	78
Beare–Stevenson syndrome	AD	123790	79
Beckwith–Wiedemann syndrome	AD	130650	80
Blepharophimosis, ptosis	AD	110100	81
Bloom syndrome	AR	210900	82
Branchio-otorenal dysplasia	AD	113650	83
Breast cancer (*BRAC1*)	AD	113705	84
Breast cancer (*BRAC2*)	AD	600185	85
Campomelic dysplasia	AR	211970	86
Canavan disease	AR	271900	85,87
Carbamylphosphate synthetase 1 deficiency	AR	237300	88–90
Carnitine palmitoyltransferase deficiency	AR	255110	92

Table 10.1. Selected monogenic disorders detectable by DNA analysis (see Appendix) (continued)

Disease	Mode	OMIM No.	Reference
Cartilage-hair hypoplasia	AR	250250	91
Cat eye syndrome	AD, de novo	115470	93
Cerebrotendinous xanthomatosis	AR	213700	94
Charcot–Marie–Tooth disease	XL	302800	98
Charcot–Marie–Tooth disease, type 1A	AD	118200	95,96
Charcot–Marie–Tooth disease, type 4A	AR	214400	97
Chediak–Higashi syndrome	AR	214500	99
Chondrodysplasia punctata	XL	302950	100
Choroideremia	XL	303100	101
Chronic granulomatous disease	XL	306400	102–104
Citrullinemia	AR	215700	105
Clasped thumb and mental retardation	XL	303350	106
Coffin–Lowry syndrome	XL	303600	107
Coloboma-renal syndrome	AD	120330	108
Congenital adrenal hyperplasia	AR	201910	24a,110
Congenital adrenal hypoplasia	XL	300200	111
Congenital nephrosis	AR	256300	111a
Conotruncal heart malformations	AR	217095	112
Coproporphyria, hereditary	AD	121300	113
Corneal dystrophy, granular type	AD	121900	114
Cowden syndrome	AD	158350	115
Craniosynostosis, Shprintzen–Goldberg	AD	182212	116
Craniosynostosis, type II	AD	123101	117
Creutzfeldt–Jakob disease	AD	123400	118
Cri du chat syndrome	AD	123450	119
Crouzon disease	AD	123500	120
Cystic fibrosis	AR	219700	109,121–123
Deafness, nonsyndromic	XL	304700	124
Dentatorubral-pallidoluysian atrophy	AD	125370	125,126
Denys–Drash syndrome	AD	194080	127,128
Diabetes mellitus, maturity-onset diabetes of youth (MODY), type I	AD	125850	129
Diabetes mellitus, MODY, type II	AD	125851	130
Diabetes mellitus, non-insulin-dependent	AD	138190	131
Dyskeratosis congenita	XL	305000	132
Dystonia, type I	AD	128100	133
Ectrodactyly	AD	183600	137
Ectodermal dysplasia, anhidrotic	XL	305100	134–136
EEC syndrome	AD	129900	138
Ehlers–Danlos syndrome, type I	AD	130000	139
Ehlers–Danlos syndrome, type II	AD	130010	140
Ehlers–Danlos syndrome, type III	AD	130020	141
Ehlers–Danlos syndrome, type IV	AD	130050	142
Ehlers–Danlos syndrome, type VI	AR	225400	143
Ehlers–Danlos syndrome, type VII	AD	130060	144,145
Epidermolysis bullosa simplex, Dowling–Meara	AD	131760	146
Epidermolysis bullosa simplex, Koebner	AD	131900	147,148
Epidermolysis bullosa simplex, Weber–Cochayne	AD	131800	149,150
Exudative vitreoretinopathy, familial	AD	133780	151
Fabry disease	XL	301500	152
Factor V Leiden mutation	AD	227400	153
Factor XI deficiency	AR	264900	154
Familial adenomatous polyposis	AD	175100	155

Table 10.1. Selected monogenic disorders detectable by DNA analysis (see Appendix) (continued)

Disease	Mode	OMIM No.	Reference
Familial dysautonomia	AR	256800	156
Familial isolated growth hormone deficiency	AD	173100	23,320,321
Fanconi anemia	AR	227650	157
Fragile X syndrome	XL	309550	23,158,159
Friedreich ataxia	AR	229300	160
Fucosidosis	AR	230000	161,162
Fumarate hydratase deficiency	AD	136850	12,162
Galactosemia	AR	230400	163
Gaucher disease	AR	230800	164–167
Gerstmann–Straussler disease	AD	137440	168
Glaucoma, open-angle, type 1A	AD	137750	169
Glaucoma, primary open-angle	AD	137760	170
Glucocorticoid receptor deficiency	AD	138040	171
Glutaric aciduria, type IIA	AR	231680	12,172
Glycerol kinase deficiency	XL	307030	173,174
Glycogen storage disease, type I/Ia	AR	232200	175
Glycogen storage disease, type II	AR	232300	176
Glycogen storage disease, type III	AR	232400	177
Glycogen storage disease, type IV	AR	232500	178
Glycogen storage disease, type V	AD	153460	179
Glycogen storage disease, type VI	AR	232700	180
Glycogen storage disease, type VII	AR	232800	181
Gonadal dysgenesis, 46,XY	XL	306100	182
Greig syndrome	AD	175700	183
Hallervorden–Spatz syndrome	AR	234200	184
Hemangioma, familial cavernous	AD	116860	185
Hemochromatosis	AR	235200	186
Hemophilia A	XL	306700	193,194
Hemophilia B	XL	306900	195,196
Hemoglobin C	AR	141900	187
Hemoglobin E	AR	141900	188
Hemoglobin O	AR	141900	189
Hemoglobin S	AR	141900	190–192
Hereditary hemorrhagic telangiectasia	AD	187300	197
Hereditary neuropathy with liability to pressure palsies	AD	162500	198
Hermansky–Pudlak syndrome	AR	203300	199
Hirschsprung disease	AD	142623	200,201
Holoprosencephaly, type III	AD	142945	202
Holt–Oram syndrome	AD	142900	203
Homocystinuria	AR	236200	204
Hunter syndrome	XL	309900	205
Huntington disease	AD	143100	206–209
Hurler syndrome	AR	252800	210
Hydrocephalus	XL	307000	211
Hypercholesterolemia	AD	143890	212
Hyperhomocysteinemia (MTHFR deficiency)	AR	236250	213
Hyperkalemic periodic paralysis	AD	170500	214
Hyperlipoproteinemia, type I	AR	238600	215
Hyperoxaluria, type I	AR	259900	216
Hypochondroplasia	AD	146000	217
Hypoglycemia, persistent hyperinsulinemic, of infancy	AD	601820	218,219
Hypoparathyroidism	XL	307700	220
Hypophosphatasia, infantile	AR	241500	221

Table 10.1. Selected monogenic disorders detectable by DNA analysis (see Appendix) (continued)

Disease	Mode	OMIM No.	Reference
Hypophosphatemic rickets	XL	307800	222
Ichthyosis	XL	308100	223,224
Incontinentia pigmenti, type I	XL	308300	225
Incontinentia pigmenti, type II	XL	308310	226
Isovaleric acidemia	AR	243500	227
Jackson–Weiss syndrome	AD	123150	228
Kallmann syndrome	XL	308700	229
Kell antigen	AD	110900	230
Kennedy disease	XL	313200	231
Kniest dysplasia	AD	156500	232
Krabbe disease	AR	245200	233
Lamellar ichthyosis	AR	242300	234
Langer–Giedion	AD	150230	235
Leber congenital amaurosis	AR	204000	236
Leber hereditary optic neuropathy	XL	308900	237,238
Leprechaunism	AR	246200	239
Lesch–Nyhan syndrome	XL	308000	240,241
Leydig cell hypoplasia	AD	152790	242
Li–Fraumeni syndrome	AD	151623	243
Long-chain 3-hydroxyl-CoA dehydrogenase deficiency	AD	143450	244
Long-QT syndrome	AD	192500	245
Long-QT syndrome	AR	220400	246
Lowe syndrome	XL	309000	247
Macular dystrophy, retinal, type I	AD	136550	248
Malignant hyperthermia	AD	145600	249
Maple syrup urine disease	AR	248600	250
Marfan syndrome	AD	154700	251,252
Maroteaux–Lamy syndrome	AR	253200	253
McCune–Albright syndrome	AD	174800	254
Meckel–Gruber syndrome	AR	249000	255
Medium chain acyl-CoA dehydrogenase deficiency	AR	201450	256
Medullary thyroid carcinoma	AD	155240	200
Menkes disease	XL	309400	257
Metachromatic leukodystrophy	AR	250100	258
Metaphyseal chondrodysplasia, Schmid type	AD	156500	259
Methylmalonic acidemia	AR	251000	260
Migraine hemiplegic, familial	AD	141500	261
Miller–Dieker syndrome	AR	247200	262
Morquio syndrome, type B	AR	253010	263
Multiple endocrine neoplasia, type 1	AD	131100	264
Multiple endocrine neoplasia, type 2A	AD	171400	263
Multiple endocrine neoplasia, type 2B/3	AD	162300	265
Multiple epiphyseal dysplasia	AD	132400	266
Multiple exostoses	AD	133700	267
Muscular dystrophy, Duchenne and Becker	XL	310200	268–272
Muscular dystrophy, Emery–Dreifuss	XL	310300	273
Muscular dystrophy, facioscapulohumeral	AD	158900	274
Muscular dystrophy, Fukuyama	AR	253800	275
Muscular dystrophy, limb-girdle	AR	253600	276
Muscular dystrophy, oculopharyngeal	AD	164300	277
Myotonia congenita	AD	160800	278
Myotonia congenita	AR	255700	279
Myotonic dystrophy	AD	160900	280–284

Table 10.1. Selected monogenic disorders detectable by DNA analysis (see Appendix) (continued)

Disease	Mode	OMIM No.	Reference
Myotubular myopathy	XL	310400	285
Nail-patella syndrome	AD	161200	286
Nemaline myopathy	AD	161800	287
Nephrogenic diabetes insipidus	XL	304800	288
Nephrosis, congenital (Finnish)	AR	256300	289
Nesidioblastosis	AR	256450	218,219
Neurofibromatosis, type I	AD	162200	290,291
Neurofibromatosis, type II	AD	101000	292
Neuronal ceroid lipofuscinosis, juvenile	AR	204200	293
Niemann–Pick disease	AR	257200	294
Nonketotic hyperglycinemia	AR	238300	295
Norrie disease	XL	310600	296–299
Optic atrophy, type 1	AD	165500	300
Ornithine transcarbamylase deficiency	XL	311250	301,302
Osteoarthrosis, precocious	AD	165720	303
Osteogenesis imperfecta, type I	AD	166200	304–306
Osteogenesis imperfecta, type II	AD	166210	307
Osteogenesis imperfecta, type III	AR	259420	308
Osteogenesis imperfecta, type IV	AD	166220	306,309
Ovarian cancer	AD	167000	310
Ovarian failure, premature	AD	176440	311
Pallister–Hall syndrome	AD, de novo	260350	312
Pancreatitis, hereditary	AD	167800	313
Pearson syndrome	Mit	557000	314
Pelizaeus–Merzbacher disease	XL	312080	315
Pfeiffer syndrome	AD	101600	230,316
Pituitary dwarfism, type I	AR	262400	320,321
Pituitary dwarfism, type II	AR	262500	22
Pituitary specific transcription factor defects (Pit-1)	AD, AR	173110	322
Phenylketonuria	AR	261600	317–319
Polycystic kidney disease	AD	173900	323–324,327–328
Polycystic liver disease	AD	174050	329
Porphyria, acute intermittent	AD	176000	331
Porphyria, congenital erythropoietic	AR	263700	332
Porphyria, cutanea tarda	AD	176100	330
Prader–Willi syndrome	AD	176270	333
Precocious puberty, male-limited	AD	176410	334
Progeria	AD	176670	12b
Propionicacidemia, type I	AR	232000	335
Propionicacidemia, type II	AR	232050	336
Protein C deficiency	AD	176860	337
Protein C deficiency	AD	176880	338
Pseudoachondroplasia	AD	177170	339
Pycnodysostosis	AR	265800	340
Pyruvate kinase deficiency	AR	266200	341
Retinitis pigmentosa	AR	268000	344
Retinitis pigmentosa	XL	312600	345
Retinitis pigmentosa 1	AD	180100	342
Retinitis pigmentosa 4	AD	180380	343
Retinoblastoma	AD	180200	346,347
Retinoschisis, juvenile	XL	312700	348
Rh C genotyping	AD	111700	349
Rh D genotyping	AD	111680	350

Table 10.1. Selected monogenic disorders detectable by DNA analysis (see Appendix) (continued)

Disease	Mode	OMIM No.	Reference
Rh E genotyping	AD	111690	351
Rieger syndrome	AD	180500	351,352
Rubinstein–Taybi syndrome	AD	180849	353
Saethre–Chotzen syndrome	AD	101400	354
Salla disease	AR	269920	355
Sandhoff disease	AR	268800	356
Sanfilippo syndrome, type B	AR	252920	357
Severe combined immune deficiency	AR	601457	358
Sex-determining region Y	Y-linked	480000	360,361
Sex reversal, dosage sensitive	XL	300018	359
Short chain acyl-CoA dehydrogenase deficiency	AR	201470	362
Sickle cell anemia	AR	141900	190–192
Sideroblastic anemia	XL	301300	363
Simpson–Golabi–Behmel syndrome	XL	312870	364
Sly syndrome	AR	253220	365
Spastic paraplegia	AR	270800	367
Spastic paraplegia	XL	312900	368
Spastic paraplegia-3	AD	182600	366
Spinal and bulbar muscular atrophy	XL	313200	369
Spinal muscular atrophy, types I/II/III	AR	253300	370,371
Spinocerebellar ataxia, type I	AD	164400	372
Spinocerebellar ataxia, type II	AD	183090	373
Spinocerebellar ataxia, type III	AD	109150	374
Spondyloepiphyseal dysplasia	AD	183900	375
Spondylometaepiphyseal dysplasia congenita, Strudwick type	AD	184250	376
Stickler syndrome	AD	108300	377,378
Supravalvular aortic stenosis	AD	185500	379
Tay–Sachs disease	AR	272800	380–383
Thalassemia, alpha	AR	141800	190,384
Thalassemia, beta	AR	141900	191,385
Thanatophoric dysplasia	AD	187600	386
Thyroid hormone β-receptor deficiency	AD	190160	387
Treacher Collins syndrome	AD	154500	388,389
Trichorhinophalangeal syndrome, type I	AD	190350	390
Triosephosphate isomerase deficiency	AD	190450	391
Tuberous sclerosis	AD	191100	392,393
Tyrosinemia, type I	AR	276700	394
Usher syndrome, type I	AR	276900	395
Usher syndrome, type II	AR	276901	396
Usher syndrome, type III	AR	276902	397
Van der Woude syndrome	AD	119300	398
Vas deferens, congenital bilateral aplasia	AR	277180	399
Velocardiofacial syndrome	AD	192430	400
Very-long-chain acyl-CoA dehydrogenase deficiency	AR	201475	401
von Hippel–Lindau disease	AD	193300	401,402
von Willebrand disease	AD	193400	403
Waardenburg syndrome, type I	AD	193500	404
Waardenburg syndrome, type II	AD	193510	405
Werner syndrome	AR	277700	406
Williams syndrome	AD	194050	379
Wilms tumor	AD	194070	127,128
Wilson disease	AR	277900	407

Table 10.1. Selected monogenic disorders detectable by DNA analysis (see Appendix) (continued)

Disease	Mode	OMIM No.	Reference
Wiskott–Aldrich syndrome	XL	301000	408
Wolf–Hirschhorn syndrome	AD	194190	409,410
Wolman disease	AR	278000	411
Xeroderma pigmentosum	AR	278700	412

Note: This list is by necessity incomplete because of the rapid progress being made in genetics. To obtain current information on disorders that can be detected by molecular techniques, the reader should consult electronic databases that are regularly updated. Among these databases, there are two, GeneTests and OMIM, that are dedicated to genetic disorders. GeneTests (http://www.genetests.org) maintains a voluntary listing of laboratories that offer molecular tests on a service or research basis and includes contact information for regional genetic services. Online Mendelian Inheritance in Man, or OMIM (http://www3.ncbi.nlm.nih.gov/omim/), contains more comprehensive information on genetic disorders, including clinical synopses, references, and database links to MEDLINE and the Genome Database.

Specimens for Prenatal Diagnosis

Specimens submitted for prenatal testing of the fetal DNA most often include chorionic villi or cultured chorionic villi or amniotic fluid cells.

Direct Detection of Mutations

Many mutations can be directly detected because they alter a restriction endonuclease site, change the size of a fragment, or alter a PCR product size and/or sequence. The use of a variety of methods detecting these specific changes is discussed and illustrated below.

Restriction Endonuclease Analysis and Southern Blots

The basic tools of molecular genetics for the past two decades have been restriction endonucleases, Southern blots, and probes.[413–415] Restriction endonucleases are bacterial enzymes that protect bacteria from invasion by foreign DNA (Table 10.2). They prevent viral infection by recognizing specific nucleotide sequences of four or more bases and cleave the double-stranded viral DNA at that site. Molecular geneticists take advantage of the thousands of restriction endonuclease sites in human DNA and use restriction enzymes to cleave long strands of DNA into fragments of reproducible size.[416] Despite the morphologic differences between cells from different organs within the human body, DNA contained within each cell (amniotic fluid cells, chorionic villi, leukocytes, fibroblasts, solid tissue, etc.) is identical. After purification from cells or tissue, the DNA is quantitated and microgram quantities are digested with a restriction endonuclease specific for the analysis and for which fragments of reproducible size have been well characterized. The digested DNA is subjected to agarose-gel electrophoresis to separate the DNA fragments by size[417] (Figure 10.5). After electrophoresis, the DNA fragments can be visualized by a variety of techniques, including gel staining with ethidium bromide and exposure to ultraviolet light.

Because thousands of DNA fragments of varying size are generated from the digestion, a smear spanning the length of the gel, as opposed to discrete bands, is seen. DNA hybridization is then done to identify the specific DNA fragment of interest. Originally described by Southern in 1975,[417] this method involves treatment of the gel with alkali to render the patient's DNA single-stranded (denatured). Next, the DNA is transferred from

Table 10.2. Selected restriction endonucleases and their specificities

Endonuclease	Sequence Cleaved
*Bam*HI	↓ GGATCC CCTAGG
*Bgl*II	↓ ↑ AGATCT TCTAGA
*Eco*RI	↓ ↑ GAATTC CTTAAG
*Hinc*II	↓↑ GTPyPuAC CAPuPyTG
*Hind*III	↓ ↑ AAGCTT TTCGAA
*Hinf*I	↓ ↑ GANTC CTNAG
*Hpa*I	↓↑ GTTAAC CAATTG
*Mbo*II	↑ ↓ TCTTCNNNNNNNN AGAAGNNNNNNNNN
*Mst*II	↓ ↑ CCTNAGG GGANTCC
*Pst*I	↑ CTGCAG GACGTC
*Sst*I	↑ ↓ GAGCTC CTCGAG
*Taq*I	↑ TCGA AGCT
*Xba*I	↓ ↑ TCTAGA AGATCT ↑

Note: The sequence recognized and cleaved by a restriction endonuclease is usually palindromic (i.e., it reads the same in opposite directions on the two DNA strands). Arrows represent sites of cleavage.

the gel to a filter membrane either by diffusion, using a salt solution passed through the gel and the filter into blotting paper, or by vacuum or electrophoretic transfer. Once transferred, the DNA fragments are firmly attached to the membrane either by baking or chemical treatment. The filter-bound DNA is then placed in a hybridization solution containing a single-stranded radiolabeled or otherwise tagged DNA, cDNA, or RNA probe. During incubation, the single-stranded probe anneals to single-stranded DNA fragments with com-

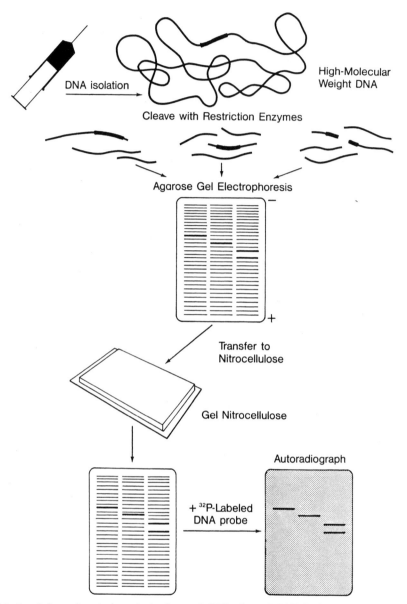

Fig. 10.5. Restriction endonuclease analysis of genomic DNA. Genomic DNA is digested with one or more restriction endonucleases and the resulting DNA fragments are separated by size through agarose-gel electrophoresis and blotted to nitrocellulose. The nitrocellulose-bound DNA fragments are then hybridized to a radiolabeled gene probe, and the resulting radioactive double-stranded DNA molecules are visualized by autoradiography.

plementary DNA sequences to form hybrid molecules. After hybridization, the excess probe is removed from the membrane and the membrane is exposed to film by autoradiography, and genomic DNA fragments containing sequences that are complementary to the probe appear as bands on the autoradiograph. The sizes and number of bands seen are determined by the number and locations of restriction endonuclease sites in the segment under study. Applications of Southern blotting to detect chromosome fragments, deletions, rearrangements, and point mutations will be illustrated by the following examples.

Detection of Gene Deletions. Familial isolated growth hormone (GH) deficiency type 1A (IGHD 1A) is an endocrine disorder that is caused by deletion of the GH genes. This disorder has an autosomal recessive mode of inheritance, and affected individuals have severe growth retardation due to complete deficiency of GH. Most cases respond only briefly to GH replacement therapy due to their tendency to develop high titers of anti-GH antibodies.[7]

Restriction analysis of the GH gene (GH1) is complicated by the fact that it is one of the five GH-related genes (5'-GH1:CSHP1:CSH1:GH2:CSH2-3') contained in the GH gene cluster (see Fig. 10.2). Although these other genes share extensive sequence homology, only the GH1 locus encodes GH. The GH1 gene is flanked by consistent *BamHI* sites that are 3.8 kb apart. Although the CSHP1, CSH1, GH2, and CSH2 genes are sufficiently homologous to hybridize to the GH1 probe, they all are contained in *Bam*HI-derived fragments that differ in size from that of GH1. Autoradiograms of DNAs from IGHD 1A subjects lack the 3.8-kb fragments that normally contain the GH1 genes (Figure 10.6). In addition, the intensity of the 3.8-kb bands in DNA from the heterozygous parents is intermediate between that of controls and their affected children. These results show that IGHD 1A subjects are homozygous and their parents are heterozygous for GH1 gene deletions. Because these deletions preclude production of any GH, affected individuals tend to be immunologically intolerant to exogenous GH.

Hereditary neuropathy with liability to pressure palsies (HNPP) is an autosomal dominant disorder characterized by recurrent focal neuropathy. Patients with HNPP typically have a deletion of the PMP gene on chromosome 17p11.2-12 due, in all likelihood, to unequal crossing over during germ-cell meiosis.[418] Diagnosis can be accomplished using fluorescent in situ hybridization[418a] or by quantitative PCR multiplex assay.[418b,418c]

Detection of Gene Expansions. The molecular defect in patients with fragile X syndrome can be detected by Southern blot analysis. In contrast to IGHD-1A, in which there is a deletion of genetic information resulting in the disease state, in fragile X syndrome, there is an expansion of a repetitive trinucleotide (CGG) DNA segment in the FMR-1 gene.[158,159,419,420] Fragile X syndrome is the most common cause of inherited mental retardation (see chapter 9) and the fragile site at band Xq27.3 can be determined in lymphocytes of affected males when cultured in folate deficient media.[421] The FMR-1 gene mapped to this location encodes an mRNA-binding protein with domains that function to mediate nucleocytoplasmic shuttling of RNA[422] and is prominently expressed in brain and testis.[423]

In the majority of patients with fragile X syndrome, the disease results from a massive postzygotic expansion of the CGG repeat located in the 5' untranslated region of the FMR-1 gene (Figure 10.7).[424] When the repeat number exceeds about 230, the DNA becomes abnormally methylated and the gene becomes nonfunctional. Thus, the repeat expansion and methylation result in the full mutation observed in affected patients. Varying degrees of methylation can lead to a "mosaic" male. Although some FMR-1 protein may be produced from the unmethylated alleles, phenotypically, the majority of these males have moderate to severe mental retardation.[425] In the normal population, the CGG repeat number is polymorphic and varies from 6 to 50, with the most common alleles having 29–30 repeats. Carriers have premutations that are unmethylated, transcriptionally active, and 50–200 repeats. However, the fragile site analysis[426] has been replaced by the more

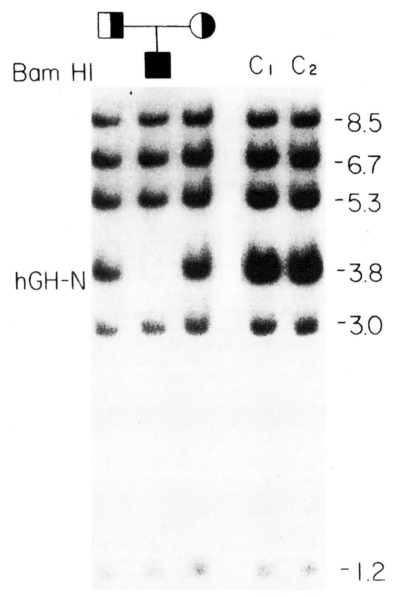

Fig. 10.6. Autoradiogram patterns of DNA from a child (solid symbol) with isolated growth hormone deficiency, his parents (half solid symbols), and two controls (C₁ and C₂) after digestion with *Bam*HI and hybridization to the GH cDNA probe. Note that the GH gene (hGH-N) is deleted in the child.

sensitive molecular analysis, which facilitates identification of the majority of carriers. Premutations are unstable and at risk for expansion into a full mutations when maternally transmitted. The risk for expansion increases as the repeat number increases.[427,428] It appears very low (<5 percent) for alleles less than 60 repeats. However, alleles greater than 100 repeats almost always expand to full mutations. Interestingly, female carriers of premutations have been shown to be at risk for premature ovarian failure,[429–431] which is present

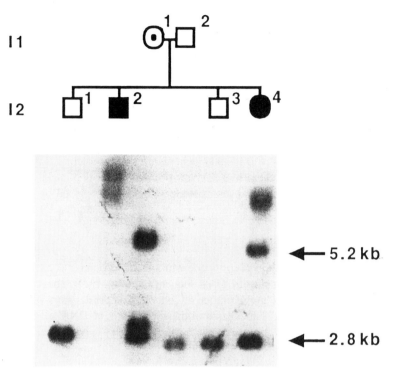

Fig. 10.7. Autoradiogram patterns obtained from a fragile X syndrome family after digestion of DNA with restriction endonucleases *Eco*RI and *Eag*I. Normal females demonstrate bands corresponding DNA fragments 5.2 and 2.8 in length and represent the inactive and active X chromosomes, respectively. Normal males have a single band corresponding to DNA fragments 2.8 kb in length. Additional bands in carrier females represent "premutation" alleles. Full-mutation alleles observed in affected males and females are characterized by smears as opposed to discrete bands.

in ~20 percent of women who carry premutation expansions. Although premutation carrier males, referred to as normal transmitting males, will always transmit the premutation allele to each of their daughters, they are not at risk for having affected daughters. However, male carriers of premutations (>50 years of age) may develop a neurodegenerative disorder, characterized by cerebellar ataxia and/ or intention tremor, cognitive decline, and other features.[432]

Detection of Gene Rearrangements. Hemophilia A is an example of a disease that can result from a gene rearrangement. Hemophilia A is an X-linked recessive bleeding disorder caused by a deficiency of coagulation factor VIII; it affects approximately 1 in 10,000 males. The disease results from mutations in the factor VIII gene that are heterogeneous in both type and position within the gene. However, intragenic inversion mutations have been found to be common to 45 percent of patients with severe disease (factor VIII activity levels <1 percent).[433] The inversion results from an intrachromosomal recombination involving DNA sequences in intron 22 of the factor VIII gene and homologous sequences upstream to the factor VIII gene. As a result of this recombination, the orientation of exons 1–22 is reversed, while exons 23–26 remain unaltered but now separated from the rest of the gene. Accurate diagnosis is achieved by rapid PCR, long-distance PCR, and Southern blot when necessary.[434,434a,434b]

Detection of Point Mutations. Sickle cell anemia is an autosomal recessive disorder characterized by episodic sickle crises caused by irreversible sickling and destruction of red blood cells, resulting in abdominal and musculoskeletal pain. The disease occurs predominantly in blacks, who have a carrier frequency of about 1 in 15 and a disease frequency between 1 in 396 and 1 in 600 births.[434c,434d] The point mutation responsible for sickle cell anemia is a substitution of thymidine for adenine in the sixth codon of the β-globin gene changing G<u>A</u>G (glutamine) to G<u>T</u>G (valine). This substitution alters an *Mst*II recognition site (CCTG<u>A</u>GG) and which encodes codons 5–7 of the β-globin molecule. Digestion of genomic DNA containing this mutation would yield restriction fragments of 1.35 kb rather than the 1.15-kb fragments generated from the normal β-globin sequence (Figure 10.8). However, Southern blot analysis for the diagnosis of sickle cell anemia[435] and other disorders due to a base-pair substitution has been replaced by PCR amplified products or other methods to detect the A → T or other transversions.[436]

Polymerase Chain Reaction

The PCR, as described by Saiki et al.[436] and Mullis and Faloona,[437] is a primer-directed enzymatic amplification of a specific DNA sequence (Figure 10.9). The specificity of the PCR reaction results from the use of unique oligonucleotide primer pairs whose sequences are complementary to DNA sequences on opposite strands of DNA yet flank the DNA segment to be amplified.[438] The reaction is carried out in a DNA thermal cycler that can rapidly increase or decrease the reaction temperature. Each reaction tube contains deoxyribonucleotide triphosphates (dNTPs), a pair of oligonucleotide primers, Tris buffer supplemented with $MgCl_2$, template DNA, and DNA polymerase. The DNA polymerase first used in PCR was isolated from the bacteria *Thermus aquaticus*. However, currently available are DNA polymerases derived from a variety of organisms, including *Pyrococcus furiosus* and *Thermococcus litoralis*. The advantage of all of these is their ability to sustain viability at temperatures >95°C. However, they can differ in their half-life and

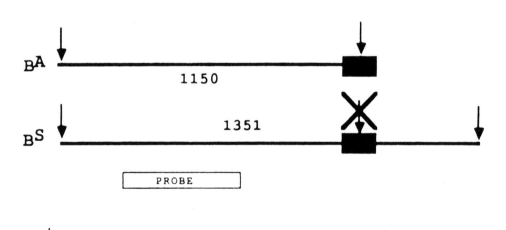

Fig. 10.8. The size of genomic DNA fragments obtained after *Mst*II digestion of the β-globin gene. The locations of the $β^S$ mutation (center arrow), which eliminates an *Mst*II site that normally occurs at codons 5–7 of the $β^A$-globin gene and probe sequences used in Southern blot analysis are indicated.

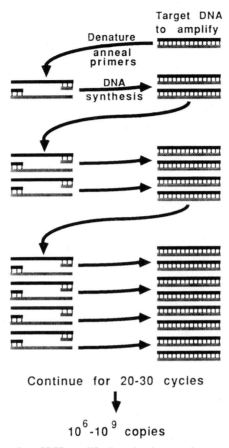

Fig. 10.9. Schematic representation of PCR amplification, showing complementary genomic strands to be amplified and their corresponding primers after annealing. Different temperatures are used to denature (94 percent), anneal (45 percent), and elongate (72 percent), enabling rapid accumulation of multiple copies with succeeding cycles of amplification.

their efficiency of base incorporation, making one polymerase more suitable than another depending on the type of assay that is to be performed.

The PCR reaction begins with an initial denaturation phase at 94°C to render the template DNA single-stranded by breaking the hydrogen bonds between the complementary purine and pyrimidine bases of the two strands of the double helix (Figure 10.10). The initial denaturation phase is followed by 20–30 repetitive cycles of short denaturing, annealing, and extension periods. After the denaturing period at 94°C, the primers are allowed to anneal to opposite strands of the DNA template by lowering of the temperature from 94 to 65°C. The annealing temperature used is a function of the GC content of the oligonucleotide primers. The greater the number of complementary G/C base pairs in the sequence, the higher the annealing temperature. During the extension period at 72°C, DNA polymerase directs DNA synthesis. After this primer-directed synthesis, the strands of DNA are again denatured at 94°C to begin yet another round of amplification. With each amplification cycle, the number of copies synthesized of that specific region of DNA doubles. Potentially, after 30 cycles, 10^6 to 10^9 copies are achieved. The amplification yields enough DNA for subsequent analysis using simple gel electrophoresis or gel elec-

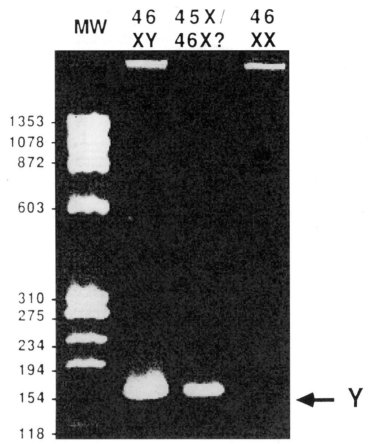

Fig. 10.10. Polyacrylamide-gel analysis of PCR product of DNA from a family similar to that shown in Figure 10.6 after amplification using Y-chromosome-specific primers.

trophoresis coupled with restriction endonuclease digestion, allele-specific hybridization, or DNA sequencing.

Direct Detection of Chromosome Fragments. An example of the utility of PCR amplification is detection of Y-chromosome fragments in Turner syndrome. We used the PCR and Y-specific oligonucleotide primers to determine whether a chromosomal fragment was derived from an X or Y (see Figure 10.10).[194] Note that the affected subject, who was mosaic and had a 45,X/46X +frag karyotype, has easily detectable Y chromosomal material in DNA derived from peripheral blood. Such studies can be done in hours; require small amounts of blood, amniotic fluid, or chorionic villi; and avoid the use of Southern blots or probes. This technique has been applied to determine the sex of fetuses at risk for X-linked disorders.

Direct Detection of Gene Deletions. Cystic fibrosis (CF) is an autosomal recessive disorder characterized by chronic lung disease and pancreatic insufficiency (see chapter 15). The genetic abnormality underlying CF was discovered in 1989 by characterization of the cystic fibrosis transmembrane conductance regulator (*CFTR*) gene.[122,439,440] About 70 percent of abnormal *CFTR* genes have a 3-bp deletion in exon 10, causing the loss of pheny-

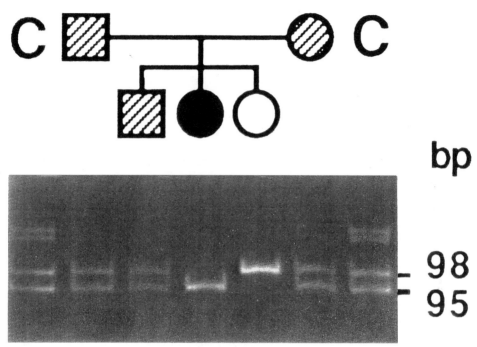

bp

98
95

Fig. 10.11. Polyacrylamide-gel analysis of PCR products obtained from blood spots collected on newborn screening forms from a family with CF. Upper symbols indicate heterozygous control subjects (C) and parents; lower symbols represent (left to right) carrier son, affected daughter, and unaffected daughter. Fragment sizes are shown on right. Additional upper fragments seen in heterozygotes are due to heterodimer formation, which occurs when different strands of 95- and 98-bp PCR products anneal.

lalanine at codon 508 (ΔF508). Detection of the ΔF508 mutation by PCR amplification of exon 10 followed by polyacrylamide-gel electrophoresis of the amplified products and staining with ethidium bromide is shown in Figure 10.11. Using this procedure, the altered mobility from the 3-bp deletion in exon 10 resulting in the loss of phenylalanine at codon 508 (ΔF508) in the CFTR gene can be seen easily.[441] This and other tests for specific *CFTR* gene mutations are usually done to confirm that a patient has CF or for carrier studies of individuals with a family history of CF. The heteroduplexes seen in heterozygotes in Figure 10.11 are sensitive indicators that the allelic PCR products of the CFTR alleles differ in size. Such differences in the size of the forward and reverse strands from two different alleles cause "bubbles" to form in the heteroduplex that affect its migration.

PCR can also be used to detect large deletions associated with the allelic disorders Duchenne muscular dystrophy (DMD) and Becker muscular dystrophy (BMD). The combined incidence of these X-linked disorders is 1 in 3,500 boys. Both disorders are characterized by progressive muscle wasting, with DMD being more severe and associated with early death.[442] The gene that is defective in DMD and BMD is dystrophin, which has been mapped to Xp21, spans >2,000 kb, contains 79 exons, and has an mRNA product of 14,000 nucleotides in length.[269,443–445] About 65 percent of dystrophin gene mutations are intragenic deletions clustered in two hot spots containing the 5′ terminal and exons 44–53.[446,447] With the ability to identify deletions in 65 percent of the affected patients, accurate direct DNA testing can be used for these cases. By using full-length dystrophin cDNA clones to probe Southern blots it is possible to directly detect deletions and duplications. The cDNA probes detect the site of the mutation itself, so meiotic recombination events are irrelevant. Therefore, the chance of diagnostic error is greatly reduced. The deletions are simply detected by examination of Southern blots for the presence or absence of each exon containing genomic restriction fragments that hybridize to the cDNA probe. However, the Southern blotting technique requires isotope and is tedious and time consuming. A deletion screen can be quickly administered using a multiplex PCR.[448,449] The technique facilitates amplification of specific deletion prone exons within the DMD gene up to a millionfold from nanogram amounts of genomic DNA. When any one of the coding sequences is deleted from a patient's sample, no ethidium-bromide-stained amplification product, corresponding to the specific exon, is present on the gel (Figure 10.12). Multiplex PCR, using primer sets for about twenty different exons, now detects approximately 98 percent of the deletions in the dystrophin gene. In contrast to Southern blotting, which may require several cDNA hybridizations and take several weeks to obtain results, the PCR can be completed in 1 day. This makes the technique ideal for prenatal diagnosis, when time is critical.

The identification of a deletion in a patient with DMD not only confirms the diagnosis but also allows one to perform accurate carrier detection in the affected family. Carrier status is determined by gene dosage, which shows whether a female at risk exhibits no reduction or 50 percent reduction in hybridization intensity in the bands that are deleted for the affected male. A 50 percent reduction (single-copy intensity) for the deleted band or bands on the autoradiograph indicates a deletion on one of her X chromosomes and she would therefore be a carrier. Dosage determinations can be made from Southern blots or using a quantitative PCR.[450]

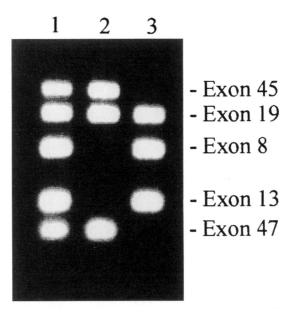

Fig. 10.12. Multiplex DNA amplification of Duchenne muscular dystrophy exons 8, 13, 19, 45, and 47. Lane 1: normal control; lane 2: DMD patient deleted for exons 8 and 13; lane 3: DMD patient deleted for exons 45 and 47.

Detection of Gene Expansions. Similar to fragile X syndrome, the cause of Huntington disease (HD) is an expansion of a trinucleotide repeat.[451] HD is a late-onset autosomal dominant neurodegenerative disorder characterized by involuntary choreic movements, psychiatric disorders, and dementia; it has an incidence of 1 in 10,000. In HD, the polymorphic repetitive segment is a CAG repeat located in exon 1 that encodes a polyglutamine tract near the N terminal of the huntingtin protein. Huntingtin contains 3,144 amino acids, is widely expressed throughout the brain and non-neural tissues,[452] and is located primarily in the cytoplasm, but a nuclear function has also been observed.[453] Structural analysis of the HD gene promoter region is consistent with the gene being a housekeeping gene. Although on a cellular level mutant huntingtin is widely expressed in both neural and non-neural tissue, there is regional specific neuronal loss in the neurons in the caudate and putamen.

HD is caused by a toxic gain-of-function mechanism. The gain of function could be due either to an overactivity of the normal function or perhaps to the introduction of a novel function of the protein. The pathogenic process relation to the expansion may involve a novel interaction with other proteins or multimerization of the protein, leading to large insoluble aggregates. In HD brains, intranuclear inclusions of the truncated mutant protein aggregates have been identified. These alterations are ultimately associated with, but not necessarily causative of, cell death. Unlike fragile X, however, the HD allele is transcribed at equal amounts as the normal allele.[454] Normal alleles are defined as alleles with #36 CAG repeats. These alleles are not pathologic and segregate as a stable polymorphic repeat in >99 percent of meiosis. The most common normal allele lengths contain 17 and 19 CAG repeats.

Mutable normal alleles are defined as alleles with 27–35 CAG repeats, and this repeat range is often referred to as the meiotic instability range.[455,456] These alleles have yet to be convincingly associated with an HD phenotype; however, they can be meiotically unstable in sperm, and pathologic expansion of paternally derived alleles in this size range have been described. Approximately 1.5–2 percent of the general population carries alleles in this size range. The likelihood that transmission of an allele in this range will expand into an HD allele depends on several factors, which include sex of the transmitting individual, the size of the allele, and the molecular configuration of the region surrounding the CAG repeat and its haplotype. This risk may be as high as 10 percent for paternal alleles carrying a CAG repeat of 35. HD alleles with reduced penetrance are defined as alleles with 36–39 CAG repeats. Repeat sizes in this range are often referred to as being in the reduced penetrance range.[457] Alleles in this size range are meiotically unstable and are associated with the HD phenotype in both clinically and neuropathologically documented cases. However in rare cases, these alleles may also manifest reduced penetrance and have been found in elderly asymptomatic individuals.

HD alleles with full penetrance are defined as alleles with ≥40 CAG repeats (Fig. 10.13). Although a large repeat number contributes significantly to the age of onset in juvenile-onset patients, the repeat number is less correlated with the age of onset in the elderly and thus implies that other genetic or environmental factors may contribute to the age of onset in that group.[456] Interestingly, the expansion of HD alleles demonstrates a sex-of-parent effect, with 69 percent of paternal transmission demonstrating expansion compared with 32 percent of maternal transmission. In addition, 21 percent of paternal transmitted expansions increase by >5 repeats as compared to <2 percent of those inherited via maternal transmission.[457]

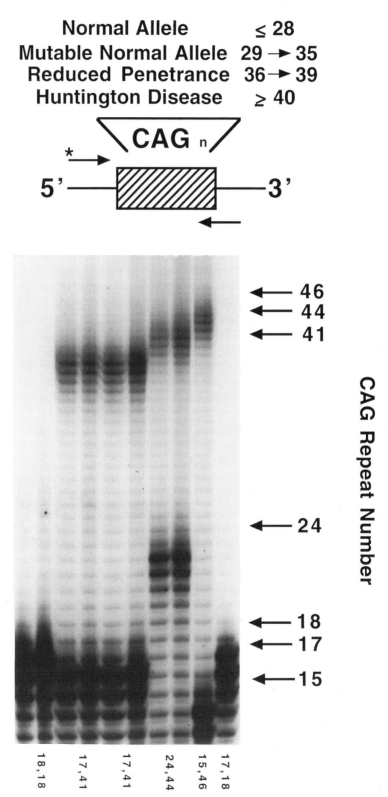

Fig. 10.13. Autoradiogram patterns obtained after PCR amplification of the CAG repeat in the Huntington gene using a ^{32}P-radiolabeled oligonucleotide PCR primer. Lanes 1 and 2: symptomatic patient with no expanded CAG repeat; lanes 3–6: presymptomatic patient with expanded HD alleles; lanes 7 and 8: symptomatic patient with expanded HD alleles; lane 9: HD positive control; lane 10: normal control.

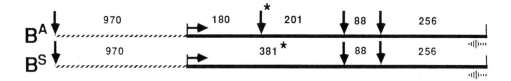

PCR   Primers

5'- ATCACTTAGACCTCACCCTGTGGAGCCA - 3'➡

➡ 3'-CAAATCTTACCCTTTGTCTGCTTACT - 5'

↓= Mst II Restriction Sites

Fig. 10.14. Size of PCR amplification products containing portions of β-globin genes after digestion with *Mst*II. The *Mst*II sites are indicated by arrows (asterisk indicates site of β^S mutation, which eliminates an *Mst*II site), and the primer sequences are shown below.

Prenatal testing for this late-onset disease is possible, yet it is complicated by profound ethical questions (see also chapters 1 and 32).

Detection of Point Mutation. In prenatal testing for the hemoglobin S allele, PCR requires much less material and offers a rapid 1- to 2-day turnaround time. As is illustrated in Figure 10.14, a 725-bp fragment containing the potential A → G substitution is amplified, an aliquot of the amplified product is digested with restriction endonuclease *Mst*II, and the digested products are subjected to gel electrophoresis. The presence of the mutation results in the loss of hemoglobin A associated fragments at 180 and 201 and the observance of hemoglobin S specific 301-bp fragment (Figure 10.15).

A second example using PCR and restriction endonuclease analysis for the detection of a base-pair substitution is in the case of medium-chain acyl-CoA dehydrogenase (MCAD) deficiency. MCAD is a rare autosomal recessive disorder of fatty acid oxidation, with an estimated incidence of 1 in 12,000–15,000 births. Onset of symptoms usually occurs in infancy or early childhood, when intermittent hypoglycemia, metabolic acidosis, lethargy, and coma are precipitated by fasting. Although this enzyme plays a central role in fat metabolism, some symptoms are due in part to secondary carnitine deficiency. Treatment is effective and consists of prevention of fasting and supplementation with oral L-carnitine. Although several mutations have been identified in the MCAD gene, an A → G substitution of codon 329 (K329E) represents >90 percent of those reported.[458] The K329E mutation does not create or remove a restriction endonuclease site but can be detected by *Nco*I digestion of PCR amplification products containing a segment of the MCAD gene and a modified oligonucleotide primer[459] (Figure 10.16). Note that the modified forward primer with a mismatch 5 bases upstream from its 3' end contains a portion (CCATG) of the *Nco*I recognition site (CCATG<u>G</u>). When normal MCAD alleles are amplified by the CCATG<u>A</u>, amplified products are not cut by *Nco*I, thus producing the uncut 63-bp fragments. However, amplified products derived from alleles containing the K329E mu-

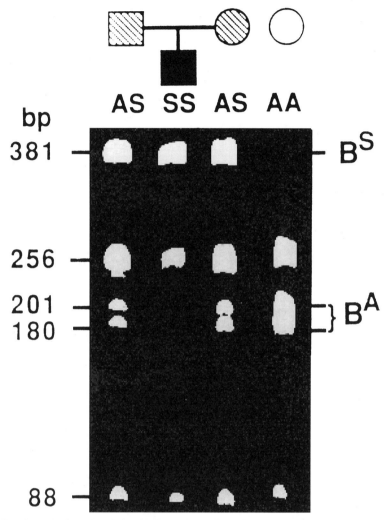

Fig. 10.15. Polyacrylamide-gel analysis of PCR products of DNA from a subject with sickle cell anemia (solid), his parents (hatched), and a control (open symbol) after *Mst*II digestion.

tation yield CCAT<u>G</u>G products that are cleaved by *Nco*I to produce 43- and 20-bp fragments (Figure 10.17).

A third example using PCR and restriction endonuclease analysis is for the detection of the spinal muscular atrophy deletion. The autosomal recessive disorder proximal spinal muscular atrophy (SMA) is a severe neuromuscular disease characterized by degeneration of alpha motor neurons in the spinal cord, which results in progressive proximal muscle weakness and paralysis. SMA is the second most common fatal autosomal recessive disorder (after cystic fibrosis), with an estimated prevalence of 1 in 10,000 livebirths.[460] Childhood SMA is subdivided into three clinical groups on the basis of age of onset and clinical course; type I SMA (Werdnig–Hoffmann) is characterized by severe, generalized muscle weakness and hypotonia at birth or within the first 3 months. Death from respiratory failure usually occurs within the first 2 years. Type II children are able to sit, although

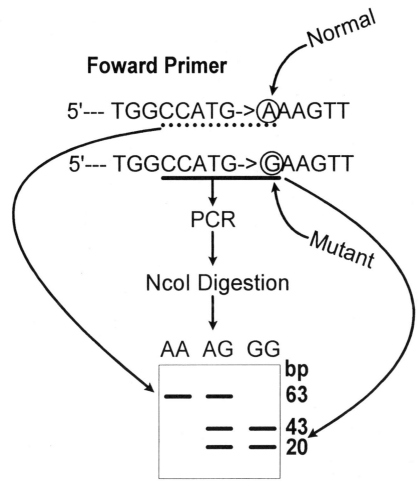

Fig. 10.16. Detection of the K329E MCAD mutation. Normal MCAD alleles yield CCATG<u>A</u> PCR products that are not cut by *Nco*I and are 63 bp, while K329E alleles yield CCATG<u>G</u> products that are cleaved into 43- and 20-bp fragments.

they cannot stand or walk unaided, and they survive beyond 4 years. Type III SMA (Kugel-berg–Welander) is a milder form, with onset during infancy or youth: patients learn to walk unaided.

The survival motor neuron (SMN) gene comprises 9 exons and has been shown to be the primary SMA-determining gene.[461] Two almost identical SMN genes are present on 5q13: the telomeric or *SMN1* gene, which is the SMA-determining gene, and centromeric or *SMN2* gene. The *SMN1* gene exon 7 is absent in about 95 percent of affected patients, while small more subtle mutations have been identified in the remaining affected patients. Although mutations of the *SMN1* gene are observed in the majority of patients, no phenotype–genotype correlation was observed because *SMN1* exon 7 is absent in the majority of patients independent of the type of SMA. This is due to the fact that routine diagnostic methods do not distinguish between a deletion of *SMN1* and a conversion event whereby *SMN1* is replaced by a copy of *SMN2*. There have been several studies that have shown that the *SMN2* copy number influences the severity of the disease.[462–464] The copy

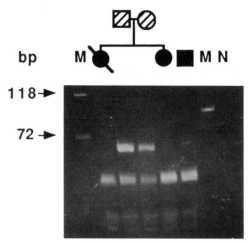

Fig. 10.17. DNA fragments generated after PCR amplification, digestion with *Nco*I, and electrophoresis in a polyacrylamide gel. Both parents' (denoted by hatches) DNAs are heterozygous and yield fragments of 63 and 43 bp. Both of their affected children's samples yield patterns containing only 43-bp fragments that are identical to the positive control.

number varies from 0 to 3 copies in the normal population, with approximately 10 percent of normals having no *SMN2*. However, patients with milder type II or III have been shown to have more copies of *SMN2* than do patients with type I. It has been proposed that the extra *SMN2* in the more mildly affected patients arise through gene conversions, whereby the *SMN2* gene is copied either partially or totally into the telomeric locus.

Five base-pair changes exist between *SMN1* and *SMN2* transcripts, and none of these differences change amino acids. Because virtually all individuals with SMA have at least one *SMN2* gene copy, the obvious question that arises is why do individuals with *SMN1* mutations have an SMA phenotype? It has now been shown that the *SMN1* gene produces predominantly full-length transcript, whereas the *SMN2* copy produces predominantly an alternatively transcribed (exon 7 deleted) product. The inclusion of exon 7 in *SMN1* transcripts and exclusion of this exon in *SMN2* transcripts is caused by a single nucleotide difference at +6 in SMN exon 7. Although the C-to-T change in *SMN2* exon 7 does not change an amino acid, it does disrupt an ESE, which results in the majority of transcripts lacking exon 7.[17,18] Therefore, SMA arises because the *SMN2* gene cannot compensate for the lack of *SMN1* expression when SMN1 is mutated. However, the small amount of full-length transcripts generated by *SMN2* are able to produce a milder type II or III phenotype when the copy number of *SMN2* is increased.

Recent evidence supports a role for SMN in snRNP (small nuclear ribonuclear protein) biogenesis and function.[465] Based on recent reports, SMN has been shown to be required for pre-mRNA splicing. Immunofluorescence studies using a monoclonal antibody to the SMN protein have revealed that the SMN protein is localized to novel nuclear structures called "gems," which display similarity to and possibly interact with coiled bodies, which are thought to play a role in the processing and metabolism of small nuclear RNAs. snRNPs and possibly other splicing components require regeneration from inactivated to activated functional forms. The function of SMN is in the reassembly and regeneration of these splicing components. Mutant SMNs, such as those found in patients with SMA, lack the splicing-regeneration activity of wild-type SMN. SMA may actually be the result of

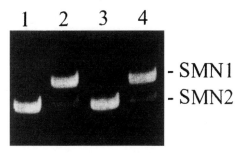

Fig. 10.18. Restriction enzyme digestion of PCR product distinguishes *SMN1* from *SMN2*. Lanes 1 and 3: SMA patients deleted for *SMN1*; lanes 2 and 4: normal controls with *SMN1* present.

a genetic defect in spliceosomal snRNP biogenesis in motor neurons. Consequently, the motor neurons of patients with SMA have an impaired capacity to produce specific mRNAs; as a result they become deficient in proteins that are necessary for the growth and function of these cells.

The molecular diagnosis of the SMA consists of the detection of the absence of exons 7 of the *SMN1* gene (Figure 10.18). Although this is a highly repetitive region and there is the almost identical centromeric *SMN2* copy of the *SMN1* gene, there is an exonic base pair difference and one can distinguish *SMN1* from the *SMN2* by restriction enzyme digestion. The absence of detectable *SMN1* in patients with SMA is being used as a powerful diagnostic and prenatal test for SMA.

Direct Detection Using Allele-Specific Oligonucleotides. Tay–Sachs disease is an autosomal recessive disease characterized by the accumulation of GM_2 ganglioside primarily in the lysosomes of neurons (see chapter 11). A deficiency in hexosaminidase A is the underlying cause of the disease. Three mutations in the hexosaminidase A (Hex A) gene— $G \rightarrow C$ substitution in exon 12, a $G \rightarrow A$ substitution in exon 7, and a 4-bp insertion in exon 11—represent approximately 95–99 percent of abnormal Hex A genes in Ashkenazi Jews.[380,466,467] Because both the $G \rightarrow C$ and the $G \rightarrow A$ substitutions alter a restriction endonuclease site, they can be easily detected by restriction endonuclease digestion of amplified products after gel electrophoresis.[378]

The 4-bp insertion in exon 11 of the Hex A gene can be easily detected by PCR amplification coupled with dot-blot hybridization using allele-specific oligonucleotides (ASOs) to distinguish the normal and mutant alleles (Figure 10.19). This method is similar to Southern blot analysis. The PCR amplification products of both alleles are denatured and applied to the filter membrane and blotted by vacuum. ASOs corresponding to the normal (5′GAACCGTATATCCTATGGC3′) and mutant (5′GAACCGTATAT<u>CTATC</u>-CTA3′) alleles are radiolabeled with ^{32}P and hybridized to small circular areas or dots on the membrane. After the removal of excess unbound probe by washing, the radiolabeled probe that has annealed to complementary sequences in the PCR-amplified products will appear as blackened circles, and three patterns can be observed on the autoradiogram. First, PCR-amplified products from homozygous normal individuals will yield a positive signal only after hybridization with the ASO complementary to the normal allele. Second, PCR products from affected individuals homozygous for the mutation will yield a positive signal only after hybridization with the ASO complementary to the mutant allele. Third, samples from heterozygotes for the mutation yield a positive signal after hybridization with both of these probes. PCR amplification coupled with ASO hybridization

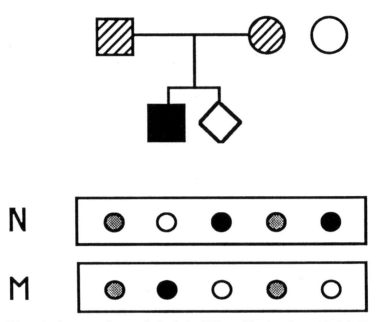

Fig. 10.19. Schematic of an autoradiogram obtained after PCR amplification of exon 11 of the Hex A gene coupled with hybridization to detect a 4-bp insertion. The presence or absence of a signal after hybridization with normal and mutant allele ASOs is used to determine the genotype of each individual (see text).

is a highly sensitive technique and is capable of detecting as small as a single base difference. This technique is most useful in instances in which the mutation does not either create or destroy a restriction endonuclease recognition site, no modified primer is easily generated, and direct DNA sequencing of PCR products is too labor-intensive. This method is adaptable for high volume throughout[468] and is used for the detection of many genetic diseases, including α_1-antitrypsin deficiency, β-thalassemia, cystic fibrosis, Lesch–Nyhan syndrome, and phenylketonuria.[48,122,123,469–471]

DNA Sequence Analysis of Amplified DNA

One of the most widespread uses of PCR is to generate amplified products for direct DNA sequence analysis. DNA sequence analysis of amplified products enables the base-by-base sequence determination of the amplified fragment, which is then a reflection of the sequence in the patient's genomic DNA. All types of mutation can be detected using this method, including missense, nonsense, insertion, and deletion mutations. Sanger or dideoxy DNA sequencing uses randomly incorporated 2', 3' dideoxynucleotides of A, C, G, or T containing no 3' OH group, thereby inhibiting 3' extension of the growing chain.[472] When one of the dideoxynucleotides is incorporated, the 3' end of the reaction is no longer a substrate for chain elongation, the growing DNA chain is terminated and DNA fragments of varying length are produced. Original cycle sequencing used ^{32}P end-labeled primer and a separate reaction mix was required for each terminating dideoxynucleotide. Current methods of cycle sequencing of double-stranded DNA, which rely on the principle of PCR to produce products by chain elongation, use fluorescence-labeled dideoxynucleotides, each A, C, G, and T labeled with a unique dye. The reaction mix can now be performed in a single tube, and the reaction products are detected fluorescently as they

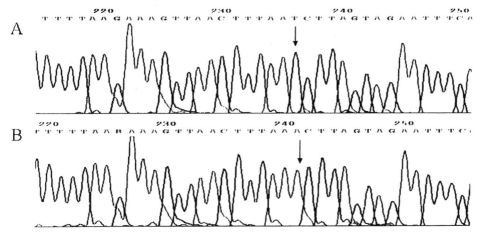

Fig. 10.20. Automated DNA sequencing using fluorescence-labeled dideoxynucleotides. This shows a typical output of sequence data from an ABI377 automated DNA sequencer. Note the individual in *A* has a T, whereas the individual in *B* has an A substitution.

pass an exciting source and an emission detector after electrophoretic separation, either by vertical polyacrylamide- or capillary-gel electrophoresis. Instrument computer software now is capable of separating the fluorescent dye colors and assigning a base (A, C, G, or T) to each terminating dye peak in the chromatogram (Figure 10.20). The sequence of the PCR product can then be read from the chromatogram and compared with a known or wild-type sequence.

Indirect Detection of Mutations

In some inherited disorders, the gene responsible for the disease has not yet been elucidated. However, the chromosomal locations of many of these genes have been mapped. As a result, the transmission of a defective gene can be tracked in a family through the use of DNA polymorphisms. The DNA polymorphisms identified in each family act to flag the abnormal gene so that, in the case of prenatal testing, the normal, carrier, or affected status of the fetus can be determined. This process is referred to as DNA linkage analysis. This technique is most useful for diseases in which the gene has not yet been isolated but is quite helpful for diseases in which the gene has already been identified but for which a multitude of different mutations have been identified, thus preventing the feasibility of direct mutation analysis for each family.

DNA Polymorphisms

The majority of variation occurring between individuals at the DNA level is the normal variation associated with DNA polymorphisms, which occur about every 250–500 nucleotides in noncoding regions of the genome. By definition, DNA polymorphisms are changes within the DNA present in the population at frequencies of greater than 1 percent.[473,474] DNA polymorphisms, in some cases, can lead to differences in the number and location of restriction enzyme recognition sites (Figure 10.21). The resulting differences in DNA fragment sizes are referred to as restriction-fragment-length polymorphisms (RFLPs) and are easily detected by PCR.

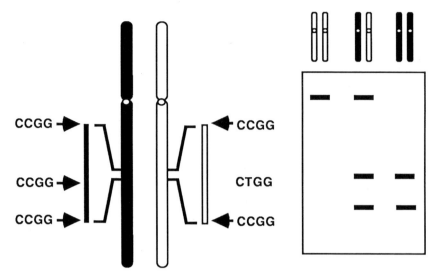

Fig. 10.21. Schematic representation of a restriction-fragment-length polymorphism. Note that the substitution of a T for a C on the white chromosome eliminates its middle CG *Msp*I recognition site and yields a single, larger fragment, which can be used as a chromosome-specific marker after Southern blotting, as shown on the right.

An example of how a DNA polymorphism produces an RFLP is shown in Figure 10.21, in which the black chromosome has three *Msp*I recognition sites (CCGG). Cleavage of DNA from this chromosome segment results in two DNA fragments of different sizes. The electrophoretic pattern of DNA from an individual homozygous for this RFLP pattern is shown on the extreme right as it would appear on a Southern blot after hybridization with a probe contained within this region. In contrast, the homologous (white) chromosome has a polymorphic C-to-T substitution so that the middle *Msp*I site (CCGG) is replaced by CTGG and now is no longer recognized by the enzyme. Thus, after digestion with *Msp*I, a single DNA fragment is obtained and the pattern of an individual homozygous for the lack of this site is shown under the two white chromosomes in the right panel. In the middle of the panel, the pattern of a heterozygote (i.e., an individual having both a black and a white chromosome) is shown. In contrast to homozygous individuals, with two black or two white chromosomes, it is only in the heterozygous individual that the two chromosomes can be distinguished and their transmission followed to the offspring.

A second type of common DNA polymorphism are dinucleotide, trinucleotide, and tetranucleotide repeats, also called microsatellites. Microsatellites are small simple repeats of 1–6 bases (i.e., AGAG, CAGCAG, CGGGCGGG) and are found throughout the genome. As such, they provide a source of highly polymorphic markers and their high frequency in the genome has facilitated the identification of many genes, the positioning of genes on the chromosomes in relation to each other, and traditional linkage studies for diagnostic analysis. In addition, because of their highly polymorphic nature, they can also be used for identity testing associated with paternity and forensic studies.

A third type of common DNA polymorphisms are single-nucleotide polymorphisms (SNPs). SNPs occur about every 1,300 nucleotides and extensive data on the location and characterization of SNPs throughout the genome is available at www.ncbi.nlm.nih.gov/

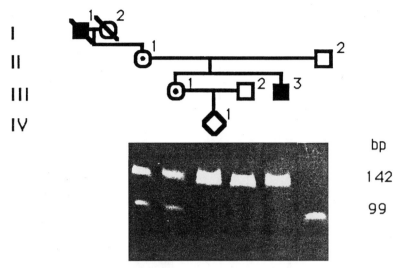

Fig. 10.22. DNA fragments generated after PCR amplification of intron 18 of the factor VIII gene and restriction endonuclease digestion with *Bcl*I. Digested PCR-amplified products are subjected to polyacrylamide-
gel electrophoresis and stained with ethidium bromide for visualization. Those that do not contain the polymorphic *Bcl*I recognition sequence are referred to as the 1 allele and remain 142 bp in length. PCR products
of alleles containing the *Bcl*I recognition sequence will generate a 99- and 43-bp (not shown) fragment. In
this family, the abnormal factor VIII gene is linked to the 1 allele (see text).

SNP. The SNPs have been most useful in mapping complex genetic disorders. The SNPs,
which do not alter restriction enzyme sites, are detected by DNA sequencing.

Linkage Analysis Using RFLPS. The transmission of mutant genes can be indirectly detected by genetic linkage analysis using DNA polymorphisms as markers. When a gene
and a DNA polymorphism are close to each other on a chromosome, they are said to be
linked. The closer genes are physically, the more likely they will cosegregate. Rough estimates indicate that an RFLP and gene that are 10^6 bp apart have 99 percent probability
of segregating together without being separated by genetic recombination. When the disease gene and a specific polymorphism are on the same chromosome, the polymorphism
and disease are in coupling. When the disease gene and the polymorphism are on opposite chromosomes, the disease and the polymorphism are said to be in repulsion.

For linkage analysis to be informative for a family, various family members must be
heterozygous for the polymorphic markers linked to the disease gene so that the linkage
phase can be determined and the polymorphism in coupling with the abnormal gene and
the polymorphism in repulsion with the abnormal gene can be determined. Once the linkage phase has been determined, the transmission or lack of transmission of disease genes
to the fetus can be inferred.

Indirect Analysis for an X-Linked Disease. Although common inversion mutations in the
factor VIII gene have been described, most patients with hemophilia A have "private" or
family-specific mutations. This heterogeneity makes direct detection of all mutations for
each family impractical. Linkage analysis using RFLPs that lie either within the factor
VIII gene or outside the factor VIII gene but closely linked provides an alternative method
to determine the carrier status of at-risk females and ultimately at-risk fetuses.

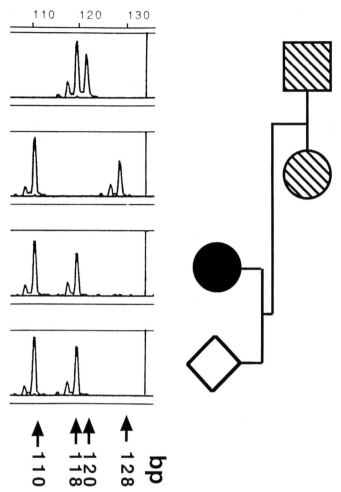

Fig. 10.23. A chromatogram of fluorescently labeled PCR products for marker D2S143, illustrating prenatal testing for carbamyl phosphate synthetase I deficiency. The pattern generated from the fetal DNA is the same as the one generated from the affected child.

For example, a polymorphic *Bcl*I recognition site lies within intron 18 (IVS18) of the factor VIII gene.[194] Because half of females are heterozygous for this *Bcl*I IVS18 RFLP, its analysis often enables inference of the factor VIII status of their offspring. For example, the PCR reaction is used to amplify a 143-bp fragment containing the polymorphic *Bcl*I site within IVS18. The amplified products are digested with *Bcl*I and the products are subjected to gel electrophoresis (Figure 10.22).

Individual II-1 is the daughter of an affected male and is therefore an obligate carrier of hemophilia A. Digestion of the PCR products generated from her DNA with *Bcl*I shows that she is heterozygous for this PCR RFLP because 99- and 143-bp fragments are seen in which the *Bcl*I recognition site is (1 allele) and is not (2 allele) present, respectively. Because she donated her 1 allele to her affected son her abnormal factor VIII gene is coupled with the 1 allele. Because this is an intragenic PCR RFLP, the likelihood of genetic recombination between the mutation in the gene and this site in II-1 is negligible.

Thus, the diagnostic accuracy is >99 percent. Examination of the PCR products from II-I's DNA after *Bcl*I digestion also shows a 1,2 (heterozygous) pattern. These results suggest that III-1 is a carrier, because she inherited the 2 allele from her father and her mother's 1 allele, which is contained in her abnormal factor VIII gene. DNA extracted directly from chorionic villi or cultured chorionic villi or amniocytes can be used to determine the carrier status of the fetus (IV-1). In this case, the pattern of the fetal DNA indicates a 1 allele. Because the 1 allele is contained in the abnormal factor VIII gene, if the fetus is male, it would be predicted to be affected. However, if the fetus is female, it would have received a 1 allele from both parents and would be a carrier of hemophilia A. Thus, the fetal sex must be known to interpret the results.

DNA Linkage Analysis for an Autosomal Recessive Disease. Carbamyl phosphate synthetase I deficiency (CPSID) is an autosomal recessive disease of ureagenesis[475] (see chapter 13). Common mutations in the CPSI gene have been described,[476] but most are thought to be family-specific. For this reason, linkage analysis is used for the prenatal diagnosis of CPSID. In this case, PCR is used to amplify several polymorphic dinucleotide repeat markers linked to the CPSI gene.[89] To separate the fragments that differ by as few as two bases, one of the two oligonucleotide primers used in a PCR can be fluorescently labeled, and amplified fragments can be separated on a 4.25 percent polyacrylamide denaturing gel on an ABI 377 instrument. Figure 10.23 illustrates the results of a prenatal analysis in a CPSID family. In this case, both the father (120/122) and the mother (110/128) are heterozygous and informative for marker D2S143, which lies 3×10^6 bp 3' to the CPSI gene. The genotype of the affected child is 110/120, indicating that the abnormal paternal CPSI gene is coupled with the 120-bp allele while the abnormal maternal CPSI gene is coupled to the 110-bp allele. The fetal DNA yields a 110/120 pattern, which is identical to the DNA from the previously affected child. The fetus is predicted to be affected with CPSID with an accuracy of 94 percent.

Diagnostic Pitfalls Associated with Linkage Analysis. One can use such RFLPs to detect the transmission of any mutation within a family through linkage analysis without actually knowing the nature of the mutation. However, to do this, DNA samples are needed from multiple family members, often including an affected patient, a normal sibling, or, alternatively, spouses or grandparents. These samples are needed to establish the linkage

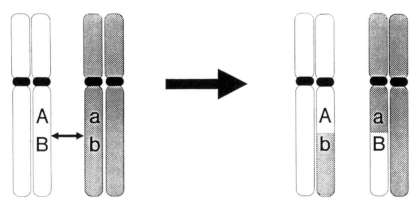

Fig. 10.24. Recombination event during meiosis in which sister chromatids exchange homologous segments. Note that the recombinant chromatids have reversed the coupling phase of the AB (ab) and ab (aB) alleles.

phase between the mutation and the RFLP being used as a marker. In addition, for the studies to be informative, certain members of the family will have to be heterozygous for the markers used to enable inference of the coupling phase. Occasionally, specimens must be obtained from deceased family members. In these cases, not only is it difficult to acquire archived material, but also the quality of the DNA recovered may not be suitable for analysis.

The distance between the RFLP being used as a marker and the mutant gene is critical. The greater the distance between the two, the greater the chance that an erroneous diagnosis will be made. This is because the probability of recombination increases with increasing genetic distance between the RFLP and the gene being analyzed. A single recombination between the gene and RFLP during meiosis will cause a reversal of the linkage phase and cause an error in the inferred genotype of the fetus (Figure 10.24). The map distance between two loci that corresponds to a 1 percent chance of recombination is called a centimorgan (cM). An estimate of the relationship between the map distance and physical distance is that two loci separated by a distance of $\sim 10^6$ bp have about a ~ 1 percent chance of recombination[477] (Figure 10.25). In the case of a second CPSI family depicted in Figure 10.26, marker D2S355 was used. This marker lies 4×10^6 bp or 4 cM 5′ to the CPSI gene. In this case, one of the PCR primers was radiolabeled with ^{32}P, resulting in the radiolabeling of all PCR products. Both the mother and father are informative for this analysis, 1/3 and 2/4, respectively. Both affected siblings had inherited the same maternal 1 allele but they had received alternate paternal alleles of 2 or 4. These results suggest that a recombinational event between the *CPSI* gene and marker D2S355 had occurred in one of the paternal gametes.

Correct identification of the biologic father is essential for linkage studies to be accurate. False assignment of biologic paternity can cause erroneous assignments of linkage phase between mutant alleles and DNA polymorphisms and can result in errors in prenatal diagnoses. This problem is serious for autosomal dominant and recessive disorders involving families with a single affected individual. Although in X-linked recessive

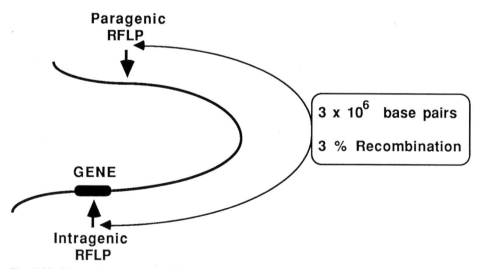

Fig. 10.25. Schematic representation of intragenic and paragenic RFLPs, showing the correlation between physical distance and recombination.

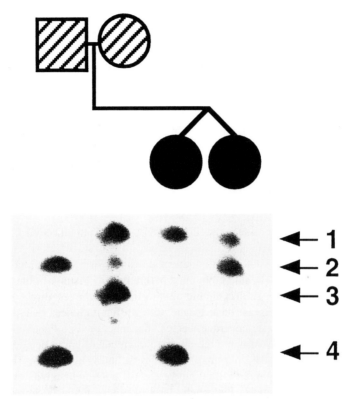

Fig. 10.26. Autoradiogram generated from PCR products for marker D2S355 from a family with carbamyl phosphate synthetase I deficiency. Although both daughters are thought to have this disease, they have inherited different paternal alleles, indicating that a recombination event has occurred.

disorders, false paternity of males does not affect the accuracy of prenatal diagnosis of females who are carriers, false paternity can result in errors in determining the carrier status of females.

Genetic heterogeneity (occurrence of the same phenotype from different genetic mechanisms) presents a possible source of error in all linkage studies, especially those involving small kindreds. The major assumption made, when performing the indirect linkage analysis, is that the disease is linked to the polymorphic loci. Because many mendelian disorders are caused by heterogeneous mutations at the same as well as different loci, phenotypes that appear clinically identical can be caused by mutations at nonlinked loci. For example, referring to the family in Figure 10.26, while it is possible that a recombination event has occurred in one paternal gamete, it is also possible that the mutation causing the disease in these children is not found at the CPSI locus and could also explain the lack of genotypic concordance observed at the CPSI locus between the two affected sibs.

General Laboratory Issues

Sampling Problems

Fetal DNA necessary for prenatal diagnostic studies can be isolated from cultured amniotic fluid cells or chorionic villus biopsies (CVS) or directly from CVS tissue. Amounts of DNA needed for different studies varies and could be the limiting factor in an analysis. For Southern blot analysis, 3–4 culture flasks are requested as opposed to PCR analysis, in which only one small cultured flask is needed. Alternatively, the CVS sampling procedure provides an advantage regarding DNA yield. Cultures are usually not needed because 10–60 μg of fetal DNA are usually obtained from each CVS tissue sample.[478,479]

Although CVS material may be useful, because it offers prenatal testing earlier in gestation and can provide an adequate amount of material without culturing, maternal contamination can be a problem and can lead to erroneous results. If detected, the final results are delayed because the backup flasks representing the cultured tissue must be analyzed. Only through culturing of CVS tissue can maternal cells not teased away at the time of collection be outgrown by the rapidly dividing fetal cells.

Informed Consent

Legal, ethical, and policy issues concerning DNA analysis are discussed in detail in chapters 31 and 32.

Because of the implications of genetic test results, for both individuals and their families, informed consent should be obtained before genetic testing. In the case of most genetic tests, the patient or subject should be informed that the test might yield information regarding a carrier or disease state that requires difficult choices regarding their current or future health, insurance coverage, career, marriage, or reproductive options. The objective of informed consent is to preserve the individual's right to decide whether to have a genetic test. This includes the right of refusal if the individual decides the potential harm (stigmatization or undesired choices) outweighs the potential benefits of the test.[480]

When obtaining samples for genetic tests, it is recommended that the following be clarified: (1) description of current test including its purpose, limitations (e.g., possibility of false-positive and false-negative results and predictive value); (2) possible outcomes of the test; (3) how the results will be communicated; and (4) anticipated use of samples, including whether samples will be used only for the purpose for which they were collected and then be destroyed. If samples will be retained after testing, the scope of permission needs to include using samples or results in counseling and testing relatives, the possibility of future test refinements, and subjects' expectations that their samples will be analyzed using these new tests, and that the results will be communicated to them. The duration of storage of samples should also be clarified.[480]

Privacy and Confidentiality (see also chapter 32)

Consent forms related to genetic molecular diagnosis should respect the patient's right for privacy.[480] In some cases, the need to obtain a detailed family history of medical and genetic information can pose problems, especially when information needed on certain relatives is not offered voluntarily. Usually, requests for medical information from relatives are made by the interested family member. Because samples from relatives often need to be analyzed to infer the genotype, the inclusion of results of these relatives in the laboratory reports is both necessary and problematic. Logical inferences that can be made regarding the disease status or nonpaternity of patients or their relatives pose serious problems regarding confidentiality. Careful attempts to address these issues should be covered in the consent process before sampling. If samples will be retained after testing, the scope of permission to use samples or results in counseling and testing relatives should be made clear.

Time Required for Sample Analysis

In studies in which PCR analysis coupled with restriction endonuclease and/or gel electrophoresis is performed, results can be obtained within 48 hours of receipt of the sample. In PCR studies requiring more extensive analysis such as allele-specific oligonucleotide hybridization or DNA sequencing, results are usually obtained within 1 week. Other studies requiring Southern blot analysis may take as long as 2 weeks. If direct CVS tissue is not used in the analysis, an additional 2–3 weeks may be required to culture enough cells before sending for DNA analysis.

Quality Control

In the clinical molecular diagnostics laboratory, quality control measures must be established to ensure the accuracy of the results. Of vital importance is an in-depth procedure manual listing each assay. Each procedure should contain specimen requirements, specimen processing, controls, recipes and storage conditions for all materials and reagents, and a step-by-step procedure with interpretation of the data. In addition, documentation of scheduled calibration as well as routine and preventive maintenance checks on all equipment and instrumentation is required. Further, documentation of personnel competency and laboratory proficiency in all assays is essential. In laboratories in which PCR analysis is used, quality control is especially challenging in preventing the contamination of highly abundant PCR products in the "pre-PCR" area of the laboratory. Several preventive measures can be taken, the most important of which is physical separation of pre- and post-PCR areas of the laboratory with designated equipment for each. Lastly, it is imperative that laboratories participate in proficiency testing. Proficiency testing for DMD, cystic fibrosis, factor V Leiden, prothrombin, fragile X, hemochromatosis, Huntington disease, myotonic dystrophy, multiple endocrine neoplasia type 2 (MEN2), spinal muscular atrophy, spinocerebellar ataxia, *MTHFR*, *BRCA1* and *BRCA2*, hemoglobin S/C, and Prader–Willi/Angelman is offered through the College of American Pathologists (CAP). These proficiency specimens are sent to participants twice per year. For rarer disorders not offered through the CAP, blinded samples distributed to the technologists is an alternative means.

NEW DIRECTIONS

Preimplantation genetic diagnosis (PGD) refers to genotype analysis of an oocyte before fertilization by study of the polar body[481] or embryonic blastomere[482,483] (see full discussion in chapter 27). The list of disorders successfully detected or excluded has grown rapidly (chapter 27). Although PGD offers great hope for couples at risk for a child with a genetic disease, erroneous results from amplification inefficiency, cell preparation or cross-contamination, and differential amplification of alleles in the heterozygous state continue to pose great challenges for investigators using these procedures.[484–493]

SUMMARY

It has been more than 25 years since the first prenatal diagnosis using DNA analysis was done for sickle cell anemia.[494] Since that time, accurate tests using different methods of DNA analysis have been developed for many inherited diseases (see Table 10.1). Because of the Human Genome Project, the number of applications has increased dramatically. This initiative in gene mapping and sequencing will identify all DNA markers and genes contained in the human genome. These maps are providing countless DNA segments, oligonucleotides, and PCR primers that can be used to detect mutations underlying many inherited disorders, both single and polygenic, as well as acquired gene rearrangements associated with neoplasia and aging.

There is no question that the gene discoveries have had their largest impact on improved genetic testing. The application of DNA-based assays, for several of the genetic diseases described in this chapter, has significantly improved the accuracy of diagnosis and has provided families with more accurate risk estimates. Today, through genetic counseling, at-risk family members are able to make family-planning decisions with information that was not available a short time ago. It is to be hoped that in the near future, we will observe a direct effect of the testing on therapy. The type of therapy will often be determined by the specific gene mutation. Molecular therapies (such as antisense oligonucleotides, antibiotics, chimeric RNA/DNA, etc.) will be applied according to and require knowledge of the exact mutation. At least four ideas are important in understanding diagnostic applications that use DNA analysis:

1. When DNA changes in a gene are detected, one must determine if these represent DNA variations not associated with disease or mutations that affect expression of the gene. This is particularly important for missense mutations that have not previously been reported in the literature.
2. Different mutations found in the same gene from different patients are examples of allelic heterogeneity. In a growing number of disorders, including retinitis pigmentosa, defects at many different genes or locus heterogeneity can cause the disease in different families. Allelic and locus heterogeneity can often explain clinical variation at a molecular level, and both must be considered in molecular studies done for prenatal diagnosis to maximize its accuracy.
3. Gene diagnosis is applicable to many clinical disorders, both genetic and acquired. Requisites are a portion of the gene involved or a segment of DNA that lies close to the gene.
4. It is imperative that the results of the genetic tests be accurately conveyed to the affected individual or family members at-risk. This type of communication often requires the expertise of a clinical geneticist or genetic counselor.

REFERENCES

1. Watson JD, Crick FHC. Molecular structure of nucleic acids. Nature 1953;171:737.
2. Lewin B. Genes VI. New York: Oxford University Press, 1997.
3. Maniatis T, Fritsch EF, Laver J, et al. The molecular genetics of human hemoglobins. Annu Rev Genet 1980;14:145.
4. Deisseroth A, Nienhuis A, Turner P, et al. Localization of the human α-globin structural gene to chromosome 16 in somatic cell hybrids by molecular hybridization assay. Cell 1977;12:205.
5. Deisseroth A, Nienhuis A, Lawrence J, et al. Chromosomal localization of human β-globin gene on human chromosome 11 in somatic cell hybrids. Proc Natl Acad Sci USA 1978;75:1456.
6. Chen EY, Liao Y-C, Smith DH, et al. The human growth hormone locus: nucleotide sequence, biology, and evolution. Genomics 1989;4:479.
7. Phillips JA III. Inherited defects in growth hormone synthesis and action. In: Scriver CR, Beaudet AL, Sly WS, et al., eds. The metabolic basis of inherited disease, 7th ed. New York: McGraw-Hill, 1995:3023.
8. Grippo P, Iaccarino M, Parisi E, et al. Methylation of DNA in developing sea urchin embryos. J Mol Biol 1968;36:195.
9. Cooper DN. Eukaryotic DNA methylation. Hum Genet 1983;64:315.

10. Nussinov R. Eukaryotic dinucleotide preference rules and their implications for degenerate codon usage. J Mol Biol 1981;149:125.

11. Bird AP. CpG-rich islands and the function of DNA methylation. Nature 1986;321:209.

12. Rideout WM, Coetzee GA, Olumi AF, et al. 5-Methylcytosine as an endogenous mutagen in the human LDL receptor and p53 genes. Science 1990;249:1288.

12a. Bellus GA, Hefferon TW, Ortiz RI, et al. Achondroplasia is defined by recurrent G380R mutations of FGFR3. Am J Hum Genet 1995;56:369.

13. Cooper DN, Krawczak M. Human gene mutations. Oxford: BIOS Scientific, 1993.

14. Bullock P, Champoux JJ, Botchan M. Association of crossover points with topoisomerase I cleavage sites: a model for non-homologous recombination. Science 1985;230:954.

15. Holmes J, Clark S, Modrich P. Strand-specific mismatch correction in nuclear extracts of human and Drosophila melanogaster cell lines. Proc Natl Acad Sci USA 1990;87:5837.

16. Cogan JD, Prince MA, Lekhakula S, et al. A novel mechanism of aberrant pre-mRNA splicing in humans. Hum Mol Genet 1997;6:909.

17. Coulter LR, Lancree MA, Cooper TA. Identification of a new class of exonic splicing enhancers by in vivo selection. Mol Cell Biol 1997;17:2143.

18. Cooper TA, Mattox W. The regulation of splice site selection, and its role in human disease. Am J Hum Genet 1997;61:259.

19. Kozak M. Structural features in eukaryotic mRNAs that modulate the initiation of translation. J Biol Chem 1991;266:19867.

20. Clegg JB, Weatherall DJ, Milner PG. Haemoglobin constant spring: a chain termination mutant? Nature 1971;234:337.

21. Hentze MW, Kulozik AE. A perfect message: RNA surveillance and nonsense-mediated decay Cell 1999;96:307.

22. Dietz HC, Valle D, Francomano CA, et al. The skipping of consecutive exons in vivo induced by nonsense mutations. Science 1993;259:680.

23. Gastier JM, Berg MA, Vesterhus P, et al. Diverse deletions in the growth hormone receptor gene cause growth hormone insensitivity syndrome. Hum Mutat 2000;16:323.

24. Schmiedel J, Jackson S, Schafer J, et al. Mitochondrial cytopathies. J Neurol 2003;250:267.

25. Vogel F, Motulsky AG. Human genetics: problems and approaches, 3rd ed. Berlin: Springer Verlag, 1997.

25a. Speiser PW, White PC. Congenital adrenal hyperplasia. N Engl J Med 2003;349:776.

26. Orrico A, Galli L, Falciani M, et al. A mutation in the pleckstrin homology (PH) domain of the FGD1 gene in an Italian family with faciogenital dysplasia (Aarskog–Scott syndrome). FEBS Lett 2000; 478:216.

27. Tromp G, Wu Y, Prockop DJ, et al. Sequencing of cDNA from 50 unrelated patients reveals that mutations in the triple-helical domain of type III procollagen are an infrequent cause of aortic aneurysms. J Clin Invest 1993;91:2539.

28. Vissing H, D'Alessio M, Lee B, et al. Glycine to serine substitution in the triple helical domain of proalpha-1(II) collagen results in a lethal perinatal form of short-limbed dwarfism. J Biol Chem 1989; 264:18265.

29. Horton WA, Lunstrum GP. Fibroblast growth factor receptor 3 mutations in achondroplasia and related forms of dwarfism. Rev Endocr Metab Disord 2002;3:381.

30. Hidaka Y, Palella TD, O'Toole TE, et al. Human adenine phosphoribosyltransferase: identification of allelic mutations at the nucleotide level as a cause of complete deficiency of the enzyme. J Clin Invest 1987;80:1409.

31. Morisaki T, Gross M, Morisaki H, et al. Molecular basis of AMP deaminase deficiency in skeletal muscle. Proc Natl Acad Sci USA 1992;89:6457.

32. Bertario L, Russo A, Sala P, et al. Multiple approach to the exploration of genotype–phenotype correlations in familial adenomatous polyposis. J Clin Oncol 2003;21:1698.

33. Berkvens TM, Gerritsen EJA, Oldenburg M, et al. Severe combined immune deficiency due to a homozygous 3.2-kb deletion spanning the promoter and first exon of the adenosine deaminase gene. Nucleic Acids Res 1987;15:9365.

34. Dodt G, Braverman N, Wong C, et al. Mutations in the PTS1 receptor gene, PXR1, define complementation group 2 of the peroxisome biogenesis disorders. Nat Genet 1995;9:115.

35. Depreter M, Espeel M, Roels F. Human peroxisomal disorders. Microsc Res Tech 2003;61:203.

36. Okoh MP, Kainulainen L, Heiskanen K, et al. Novel insertions of Bruton tyrosine kinase in patients with X-linked agammaglobulinemia. Hum Mutat 2002;20:480.

37. Leonard WJ. X-linked severe combined immunodeficiency: from molecular cause to gene therapy within seven years. Mol Med Today 2000;6:403.

38. Camand O, Boutboul S, Arbogast L, et al. Mutational analysis of the OA1 gene in ocular albinism. Ophthalmic Genet 2003;24:167.

39. Oetting WS, King RA. Molecular basis of albinism: mutations and polymorphisms of pigmentation genes associated with albinism. Hum Mutat 1999;13:99.

40. Camand O, Marchant D, Boutboul S, et al. Mutation analysis of the tyrosinase gene in oculocutaneous albinism. Hum Mutat 2001;17:352.

41. Rinchik EM, Bultman SJ, Horsthemke B, et al. A gene for the mouse pink-eyed dilution locus and for human type II oculocutaneous albinism. Nature 1993;361:72.

42. Boissy RE, Zhao H, Oetting WS, et al. Mutation in and lack of expression of tyrosinase-elated protein-1 (TRP-1) in melanocytes from an individual with brown oculocutaneous albinism: A new subtype of albinism classified as "OCA3." Am J Hum Genet 1996;58:1145.

43. Phelan MC, Rogers RC, Clarkson KB, et al. Albright hereditary osteodystrophy and del(2)(q37.3) in four unrelated individuals. Am J Med Genet 1995;58:1.

44. Kishi H, Mukai T, Hirono A, et al. Human aldolase A deficiency associated with a hemolytic anemia: thermolabile aldolase due to a single base mutation. Proc Natl Acad Sci USA 1987;84:8623.

45. Verlinsky Y, Kuliev A. Preimplantation polar body diagnosis. Biochem Mol Med 1996;58:13.

46. Braun A, Meyer P, Cleve H, et al. Rapid and simple diagnosis of the two common alpha 1-proteinase inhibitor deficiency alleles Pi*Z and Pi*S by DNA analysis. Eur J Clin Chem Clin Biochem 1996;34:761.

47. Kidd VJ, Woo SLC. Recombinant DNA probes used to detect genetic disorders of the liver. Hepatology 1984;4:731.

48. Norman MR, Mowat AP, Hutchison DC. Molecular basis, clinical consequences and diagnosis of alpha-1 antitrypsin deficiency. Ann Clin Biochem 1997;34:230.

49. Abbott CM, Lovegrove JU, Whitehouse DB, et al. Prenatal diagnosis of alpha-1-antitrypsin deficiency by PCR of linked polymorphisms: a study of 17 cases. Prenat Diagn 1992;12:235.

50. Hejtmancik JF, Holcomb JD, Howard J, et al. In vitro amplification of the α_1-antitrypsin gene: application to prenatal diagnosis. New York: John Wiley, 1989:177.

51. Buzza M, Dagher H, Wang YY, et al. Mutations in the COL4A4 gene in thin basement membrane disease. Kidney Int 2003;63:447.

52. Dagher H, Yan Wang Y, Fassett R, et al. Three novel COL4A4 mutations resulting in stop codons and their clinical effects in autosomal recessive Alport syndrome. Hum Mutat 2002;20:321.

53. Szpiro-Rapia S, Bobrie G, Guilloud-Bataille M, et al. Linkage studies in X-linked Alport's syndrome. Hum Genet 1988;81:85.

54. Zhou J, Barker DF, Hostikka SL, et al. Single base mutation in $\alpha5(IV)$ collagen chain gene converting a conserved cysteine to serine in Alport syndrome. Genomics 1991;9:10.

55. Howell WM, Brookes AJ. Evaluation of multiple presenilin 2 SNPs for association with early-onset sporadic Alzheimer disease. Am J Med Genet 2002;111:157.

56. Levy-Lahad E, Wijsman EM, Nemens E, et al. A familial Alzheimer's disease locus on chromosome 1. Science 1995;269:970.

57. Vinazzer H. Hereditary and acquired antithrombin deficiency. Semin Thromb Hemost 1999;25:257.

58. Lobato L. Portuguese-type amyloidosis (transthyretin amyloidosis, ATTR V30M). J Nephrol 2003;16:438.

59. Carvalho F, Sousa M, Fernandes S, et al. Preimplantation genetic diagnosis for familial amyloidotic polyneuropathy (FAP). Prenat Diagn 2001;21:1093.

60. Hiltunen T, Kiuru S, Hongell V, et al. Finnish type of familial amyloidosis: cosegregation of $Asp_{187} \rightarrow$ Asn mutation of gelsolin with the disease in three large families. Am J Hum Genet 1991;49:522.

61. Majoor-Krakauer D, Willems PJ, Hofman A. Genetic epidemiology of amyotrophic lateral sclerosis. Clin Genet 2003;63:83.

62. McPhaul MJ. Molecular defects of the androgen receptor. Recent Prog Horm Res 2002;57:181.

63. Matsuura T, Sutcliffe JS, Fang P, et al. De novo truncating mutations in E6-AP ubiquitin-protein ligase gene (UBE3A) in Angelman syndrome. Nat Genet 1997;15:74.

64. Freiberger T, Kolarova L, Mejstrik P, et al. Five novel mutations in the C1 inhibitor gene (C1NH) leading to a premature stop codon in patients with type I hereditary angioedema. Hum Mutat 2002;19:461.

65. Cicardi M, Igarashi T, Kim MS, et al. Restriction fragment length polymorphism of the C1 inhibitor gene in hereditary angioneurotic edema. J Clin Invest 1987;80:1640.

66. Azuma N, Yamaguchi Y, Handa H, et al. Mutations of the PAX6 gene detected in patients with a variety of optic-nerve malformations. Am J Hum Genet 2003;72:1565.

67. Ng D, Hadley DW, Tifft CJ, et al. Genetic heterogeneity of syndromic X-linked recessive microphthalmia-anophthalmia: is Lenz microphthalmia a single disorder? Am J Med Genet 2002;110:308.

68. Chun K, Teebi AS, Azimi C, et al. Screening of patients with craniosynostosis: molecular strategy. Am J Med Genet 2003;120A:470.

69. Emi M, Wu LL, Robertson MA, et al. Genotyping and sequence analysis of apolipoprotein E isoforms. Genomics 1988;3:373.

70. Gupta PA, Putnam EA, Carmical SG, et al. Ten novel FBN2 mutations in congenital contractural arachnodactyly: delineation of the molecular pathogenesis and clinical phenotype. Hum Mutat 2002;19:39.

71. Linnebank M, Tschiedel E, Haberle J, et al. Argininosuccinate lyase (ASL) deficiency: mutation analysis in 27 patients and a completed structure of the human ASL gene. Hum Genet 2002;111:350.

72. Sung SS, Brassington AM, Grannatt K, et al. Mutations in genes encoding fast-twitch contractile proteins cause distal arthrogryposis syndromes. Am J Hum Genet 2003;72:681.

73. Zori RT, Gardner JL, Zhang J, et al. Newly described form of X-linked arthrogryposis maps to the long arm of the human X chromosome. Am J Med Genet 1998;78:450.

74. Mitui M, Campbell C, Coutinho G, et al. Independent mutational events are rare in the ATM gene: haplotype prescreening enhances mutation detection rate. Hum Mutat 2003;22:43.

75. Raicu F, Popa L, Apostol P, et al. Screening for microdeletions in human Y chromosome: AZF candidate genes and male infertility. J Cell Mol Med 2003;7:43.

76. Carmi R, Elbedour K, Stone EM, et al. Phenotypic differences among patients with Bardet–Biedl syndrome linked to three different chromosome loci. Am J Med Genet 1995;59:199.

77. Bione S, D'Adamo P, Maestrini E, et al. A novel X-linked gene, G4.5. [sic] is responsible for Barth syndrome. Nat Genet 1996;12:385.

78. Lam CW, Leung CY, Lee KC, et al. Novel mutations in the PATCHED gene in basal cell nevus syndrome. Mol Genet Metab 2002;76:57.

79. Vargas RA, Maegawa GH, Taucher SC, et al. Beare–Stevenson syndrome: two South American patients with FGFR2 analysis. Am J Med Genet 2003;121A:41.

80. Hatada I, Ohashi H, Fukushima Y, et al. An imprinted gene p57(KIP2) is mutated in Beckwith–Wiedemann syndrome. Nat Genet 1996;14:171.

81. Dollfus H, Stoetzel C, Riehm S, et al. Sporadic and familial blepharophimosis–ptosis–epicanthus inversus syndrome: FOXL2 mutation screen and MRI study of the superior levator eyelid muscle. Clin Genet 2003;63:117.

82. Ellis NA, Groden J, Ye TZ, et al. The Bloom's syndrome gene product is homologous to RecQ helicases. Cell 1995;83:655.

83. Abdelhak S, Kalatzis V, Heilig R, et al. A human homologue of the Drosophila eyes absent gene underlies branchio-oto-renal (BOR) syndrome and identifies a novel gene family. Nat Genet 1997;15:157.

84. Dite GS, Jenkins MA, Southey MC, et al. Familial risks, early-onset breast cancer, and BRCA1 and BRCA2 germline mutations. J Natl Cancer Inst 2003;95:448.

85. Gorski B, Debniak T, Jakubowska A, et al. Usefulness of polymorphic markers in exclusion of BRCA1/BRCA2 mutations in families with aggregation of breast/ovarian cancers. J Appl Genet 2003;44:419.

86. Preiss S, Argentaro A, Clayton A, et al. Compound effects of point mutations causing campomelic dysplasia/autosomal sex reversal upon SOX9 structure, nuclear transport, DNA binding, and transcriptional activation. J Biol Chem 2001; 276:27864.

87. Zeng BJ, Wang ZH, Ribeiro LA, et al. Identification and characterization of novel mutations of the aspartoacylase gene in non-Jewish patients with Canavan disease. J Inherit Metab Dis 2002;25:557.

88. Summar ML, Hall LD, Eeds AM, et al. Characterization of genomic structure and polymorphisms in the human carbamylphosphate synthetase I gene. Gene 2003;311:51.

89. Caldovic L, Morizono H, Panglao MG, et al. Null mutations in the N-acetylglutamate synthase gene associated with acute neonatal disease and hyperammonemia. Hum Genet 2003;112:364.

90. Vella S, Steiner F, Schlumbom V, et al. Mutation of ornithine transcarbamylase (H136R) in a girl with severe intermittent orotic aciduria but normal enzyme activity. J Inherit Metab Dis 1997;20:517.

91. Ridanpaa M, Jain P, McKusick VA, et al. The major mutation in the RMRP gene causing CHH among the Amish is the same as that found in most Finnish cases. Am J Med Genet 2003;121:81.

92. Thuillier L, Rostane H, Droin V, et al. Correlation between genotype, metabolic data, and clinical presentation in carnitine palmitoyltransferase 2 (CPT2) deficiency. Hum Mutat 2003;21:493.

93. McDermid HE, Duncan AMV, Brasch KR, et al. Characterization of the supernumerary chromosome in cat eye syndrome. Science 1986;232:646.

94. Lamon-Fava S, Schaefer EJ, Garuti R, et al. Two novel mutations in the sterol 27-hydroxylase gene causing cerebrotendinous xanthomatosis. Clin Genet 2002;61:185.

95. Middleton-Price HR, Harding AE, Monteiro C, et al. Linkage of hereditary motor and sensory neuropathy type I to the pericentromeric region of chromosome 17. Am J Hum Genet 1990;46:92.

96. Zhou L, Griffin JW. Demyelinating neuropathies. Curr Opin Neurol 2003;16:307.

97. Nelis E, Erdem S, Van Den Bergh PY, et al. Mutations in GDAP1: autosomal recessive CMT with demyelination and axonopathy. Neurology 2002;59:1865.

98. Takashima H, Nakagawa M, Umehara F, et al. Gap junction protein beta 1 (GJB1) mutations and central nervous system symptoms in X-linked Charcot–Marie–Tooth disease. Acta Neurol Scand 2003;107:31.

99. Ward DM, Shiflett SL, Kaplan J. Chediak–Higashi syndrome: a clinical and molecular view of a rare lysosomal storage disorder. Curr Mol Med 2002;2:469.

100. Shimozawa N, Nagase T, Takemoto Y, et al. Genetic heterogeneity of peroxisome biogenesis disorders among Japanese patients: Evidence for a founder haplotype for the most common PEX10 gene mutation. Am J Med Genet 2003;120:40.

101. McTaggart KE, Tran M, Mah DY, et al. Mutational analysis of patients with the diagnosis of choroideremia. Hum Mutat 2002;20:189.

102. Heyworth PG, Noack D, Cross AR. Identification of a novel NCF-1 (p47-phox) pseudogene not containing the signature GT deletion: significance for A47 degrees chronic granulomatous disease carrier detection. Blood 2003;101:3337.

103. Kaneda M, Sakuraba H, Ohtake A, et al. Missense mutations in the gp91-phox gene encoding cytochrome b558 in patients with cytochrome b positive and negative X-linked chronic granulomatous disease. Blood 1999;93:2098.

104. Jirapongsananuruk O, Niemela JE, Malech HL, et al. CYBB mutation analysis in X-linked chronic granulomatous disease. Clin Immunol 2002;104:73.

105. Gao HZ, Kobayashi K, Tabata A, et al. Identification of 16 novel mutations in the argininosuccinate synthetase gene and genotype-phenotype correlation in 38 classical citrullinemia patients. Hum Mutat 2003;22:24.

106. Weller S, Gartner J. Genetic and clinical aspects of X-linked hydrocephalus (L1 disease): mutations in the L1CAM gene. Hum Mutat 2001;18:1.

107. Abidi F, Jacquot S, Lassiter C, et al. Novel mutations in Rsk-2, the gene for Coffin–Lowry syndrome (CLS). Eur J Hum Genet 1999;7:20.

108. Sanyanusin P, Schimmenti LA, McNoe LA, et al. Mutation of the PAX2 gene in a family with optic nerve colobomas, renal anomalies and vesicoureteral reflux. Nat Genet 1995;9:358.

109. Richards CS, Bradley LA, Amos J, et al. Standards and guidelines for CFTR mutation testing. Genet Med 2002;4:379.

110. Mao R, Nelson L, Kates R, et al. Prenatal diagnosis of 21-hydroxylase deficiency caused by gene conversion and rearrangements: pitfalls and molecular diagnostic solutions. Prenat Diagn 2002;22:1171.

111. Yates JRW, Gillard EF, Cooke A, et al. A deletion of Xp21 maps congenital adrenal hypoplasia distal to glycerol kinase deficiency. Cytogenet Cell Genet 1987;46:723.

111a. Kestila M, Jarvela I. Prenatal diagnosis of congenital nephrotic syndrome (CNF, NPHS1). Prenat Diagn 2003;23:323.

112. Devriendt K, Eyskens B, Swillen A, et al. The incidence of a deletion in chromosome 22q11 in sporadic and familial conotruncal heart disease. Eur J Pediatr 1996;155:721.

113. Lamoril J, Puy H, Whatley SD, et al. Characterization of mutations in the CPO gene in British patients demonstrates absence of genotype–phenotype correlation and identifies relationship between hereditary coproporphyria and harderoporphyria. Am J Hum Genet 2001;68:1130.

114. Munier FL, Korvatska E, Djemai A, et al. Kerato-epithelin mutations in four 5q31-linked corneal dystrophies. Nat Genet 1997;15:247.

115. McGarrity TJ, Wagner Baker MJ, Ruggiero FM, et al. GI polyposis and glycogenic acanthosis of the esophagus associated with PTEN mutation positive Cowden syndrome in the absence of cutaneous manifestations. Am J Gastroenterol 2003;98:1429.

116. Robinson PN, Booms P, Katzke S, et al. Mutations of FBN1 and genotype-phenotype correlations in Marfan syndrome and related fibrillinopathies. Hum Mutat 2002;2053.

117. Cohen MM Jr. Craniofacial disorders caused by mutations in Homeobox genes MSX1 and MSX2. J Craniofac Genet Dev Biol 2000;20:19.

118. Brandel JP, Preece M, Brown P, et al. Distribution of codon 129 genotype in human growth hormone-treated CJD patients in France and the UK. Lancet 2003;362:128.

119. Overhauser J, Huang X, Gersh M, et al. Molecular and phenotypic mapping of the short arm of chromosome 5: sublocalization of the critical region for the cri-du-chat syndrome. Hum Mol Genet 1994;3:247.

120. Glaser RL, Jiang W, Boyadjiev SA, et al. Paternal origin of FGFR2 mutations in sporadic cases of Crouzon syndrome and Pfeiffer syndrome. Am J Hum Genet 2000;66:768.

121. Beaudet AL, Feldman GL, Fernbach SD, et al. Linkage disequilibrium, cystic fibrosis, and genetic counseling. Am J Hum Genet 1989;44:319.

122. Scotet V, Barton DE, Watson JB, et al. Comparison of the CFTR mutation spectrum in three cohorts of patients of Celtic origin from Brittany (France) and Ireland. Hum Mutat 2003;22:105.

123. Vrettou C, Tzetis M, Traeger-Synodinos J, et al. Multiplex sequence variation detection throughout the CFTR gene appropriate for preimplantation genetic diagnosis in populations with heterogeneity of cystic fibrosis mutations. Mol Hum Reprod 2002;8:880.

124. Ng ISL, Pace R, Richard MV, et al. Methods for analysis of multiple cystic fibrosis mutations. Hum Genet 1991;87:613.

125. Jin H, May M, Tranebjaerg L, et al. A novel X-linked gene, DDP, shows mutations in families with deafness (DFN-1), dystonia, mental deficiency and blindness. Nat Genet 1996;14:177.

126. Oyangi S. Hereditary dentatorubral-pallidoluysian atrophy. Neuropathology 2000;20:S42.

127. Heathcott RW, Morison IM, Gubler MC, et al. A review of the phenotypic variation due to the Denys–Drash syndrome–associated germline WT1 mutation R362X. Hum Mutat 2002;19:462.

128. Schumacher V, Schuhen S, Sonner S, et al. Two molecular subgroups of Wilms' tumors with or without WT1 mutations. Clin Cancer Res 2003;9:2005.

129. Yamagata K, Furuta H, Oda N, et al. Mutations in the hepatocyte nuclear factor-4-alpha gene in maturity-onset diabetes of the young (MODY1). Nature 1996;384:458.

130. Frayling TM, Lindgren CM, Chevre JC, et al. A genome-wide scan in families with maturity-onset diabetes of the young: evidence for further genetic heterogeneity. Diabetes 2003;52:872.

131. Kusari J, Verma US, Buse JB, et al. Analysis of the gene sequences of the insulin receptor and the insulin-sensitive glucose transporter (GLUT-4) in patients with common-type non-insulin-dependent diabetes mellitus. J Clin Invest 1991;88:1323.

132. Marrone A, Mason PJ. Dyskeratosis congenita. Cell Mol Life Sci 2003;60:507.

133. Risch N, Tang H, Katzenstein H, et al. Geographic distribution of disease mutations in the Ashkenazi Jewish population supports genetic drift over selection. Am J Hum Genet 2003;72:812.

134. Nishibu A, Hashiguchi T, Yotsumoto S, et al. A frameshift mutation of the ED1 gene in sibling cases with X-linked hypohidrotic ectodermal dysplasia. Dermatology 2003;207:178.

135. Vincent MC, Biancalana V, Ginisty D, et al. Mutational spectrum of the ED1 gene in X-linked hypohidrotic ectodermal dysplasia. Eur J Hum Genet 2001;9:355.

136. Zonana J. Hypohidrotic (anhidrotic) ectodermal dysplasia: molecular genetic research and its clinical applications. Semin Dermatol 1993;12:241.

137. Brunner HG, Hamel BC, Van Bokhoven H. The p63 gene in EEC and other syndromes. J Med Genet 2002;39:377.

138. Brunner HG, Hamel BC, Bokhoven Hv H. P63 gene mutations and human developmental syndromes. Am J Med Genet 2002;112:284.

139. Wenstrup RJ, Langland GT, Willing MC, et al. A splice-junction mutation in the region of COL5A1 that codes for the carboxyl propeptide of pro-alpha-1(V) chains results in the gravis form of the Ehlers–Danlos syndrome (type I). Hum Mol Genet 1996;5:1733.

140. De Paepe A, Nuytinck L, Hausser I, et al. Mutations in the COL5A1 gene are causal in the Ehlers–Danlos syndromes I and II. Am J Hum Genet 1997;60:547.

141. Narcisi P, Richards AJ, Ferguson SD, et al. A family with Ehlers–Danlos syndrome type III/articular hypermobility syndrome has a glycine 637-to-serine substitution in type III collagen. Hum Mol Genet 1994;3:1617.

142. Kroes HY, Pals G, van Essen AJ. Ehlers–Danlos syndrome type IV: unusual congenital anomalies in a mother and son with a COL3A1 mutation and a normal collagen III protein profile. Clin Genet 2003;63:224.

143. Yeowell HN, Walker LC. Mutations in the lysyl hydroxylase 1 gene that result in enzyme deficiency and the clinical phenotype of Ehlers–Danlos syndrome type VI. Mol Genet Metab 2000;71:212.

144. Raff ML, Craigen WJ, Smith LT, et al. Partial COL1A2 gene duplication produces features of osteogenesis imperfecta and Ehlers–Danlos syndrome type VII. Hum Genet 2000;106:19.

145. Giunta C, Superti-Furga A, Spranger S, et al. Ehlers–Danlos syndrome type VII: clinical features and molecular defects. J Bone Joint Surg Am 1999;81:225.

146. Schuilenga-Hut PH, Vlies P, Jonkman MF, et al. Mutation analysis of the entire keratin 5 and 14 genes in patients with epidermolysis bullosa simplex and identification of novel mutations. Hum Mutat 2003;21:447.

147. Smith F. The molecular genetics of keratin disorders. Am J Clin Dermatol 2003;4:347.

148. Lanschuetzer CM, Flausegger A, Pohla-Gubo G, et al. A novel homozygous nonsense deletion/insertion mutation in the keratin 14 gene (Y248X; 744delC/insAG) causes recessive epidermolysis bullosa simplex type Kobner. Clin Exp Dermatol 2003;28:77.

149. Ciubotaru D, Bergman R, Baty D, et al. Epidermolysis bullosa simplex in Israel: clinical and genetic features. Arch Dermatol 2003;139:498.

150. Chao SC, Yang MH, Lee SF. Novel KRT14 mutation in a Taiwanese patient with epidermolysis bullosa simplex (Kobner type). J Formos Med Assoc 2002;101:287.

151. Robitaille J, MacDonald ML, Kaykas A, et al. Mutant frizzled-4 disrupts retinal angiogenesis in familial exudative vitreoretinopathy. Nat Genet 2002;32:326.

152. Yasuda M, Shabbeer J, Osawa M, et al. Fabry disease: novel alpha-galactosidase A 3-terminal mutations result in multiple transcripts due to aberrant 3'-end formation. Am J Hum Genet 2003;73:162.

153. Welbourn JT, Maiti S, Paley J. Factor V Leiden detection by polymerase chain reaction-restriction fragment length polymorphism with mutagenic primers in a multiplex reaction with Pro G20210A: a novel technique. Hematology 2003;8:73.

154. Mitchell M, Harrington P, Cutler J, et al. Eighteen unrelated patients with factor XI deficiency, four novel mutations and a 100% detection rate by denaturing high-performance liquid chromatography. Br J Haematol 2003;121:500.

155. Solomon CH, Pho LN, Burt RW. Current status of genetic testing for colorectal cancer susceptibility. Oncology (Huntingt) 2002;16:161.

156. Indo Y. Genetics of congenital insensitivity to pain with anhidrosis (CIPA) or hereditary sensory and autonomic neuropathy type IV: clinical, biological and molecular aspects of mutations in TRKA (NTRK1) gene encoding the receptor tyrosine kinase for nerve growth factor. Clin Auton Res 2002;12:I20.

157. Rischewski J, Schneppenheim R. Screening strategies for a highly polymorphic gene: DHPLC analysis of the Fanconi anemia group A gene. J Biochem Biophys Methods 2001;47:53.

158. Kremer EJ, Pritchard M, Lynch M, et al. Mapping of DNA instability at the fragile X to a trinucleotide repeat sequence p(CCG)n. Science 1991;252:1711.

159. O'Donnell WT, Warren ST. A decade of molecular studies of fragile X syndrome. Annu Rev Neurosci 2002;25:315.

160. Sharma R, Bhatti S, Gomez M, et al. The GAA triplet-repeat sequence in Friedreich ataxia shows a high level of somatic instability in vivo, with a significant predilection for large contractions. Hum Mol Genet 2002;11:2175.

161. Willems PJ, Seo HC, Coucke P, et al. Spectrum of mutations in fucosidosis. Eur J Hum Genet 1999;7:60.

162. Bourgeron T, Chretien D, Poggi-Bach J, et al. Mutation of the fumarase gene in two siblings with progressive encephalopathy and fumarase deficiency. J Clin Invest 1994;93:2514.

163. Dobrowolski SF, Banas RA, Suzow JG, et al. Analysis of common mutations in the galactose-1-phosphate uridyl transferase gene: new assays to increase the sensitivity and specificity of newborn screening for galactosemia. J Mol Diagn 2003;5:42.

164. Tayebi N, Stubblefield BK, Park JK, et al. Reciprocal and nonreciprocal recombination at the glucocerebrosidase gene region: implications for complexity in Gaucher disease. Am J Hum Genet 2003;72:519.

165. Orvisky E, Park JK, Parker A, et al. The identification of eight novel glucocerebrosidase (GBA) mutations in patients with Gaucher disease. Hum Mutat 2002;19:458.

166. Diaz GA, Gelb BD, Risch N, et al. Gaucher disease: the origins of the Ashkenazi Jewish N370S and 84GG acid beta-glucosidase mutations. Am J Hum Genet 2000;66:1821.

167. Hatton CE, Cooper A, Whitehouse C, et al. Mutation analysis in 46 British and Irish patients with Gaucher's disease. Arch Dis Child 1997;77:17.

168. Mishra RS, Gu Y, Bose S, et al. Cell surface accumulation of a truncated transmembrane prion protein in Gerstmann–Straussler–Scheinker disease P102L. J Biol Chem 2002;277:24554.

169. Michels-Rautenstrauss K, Mardin C, et al. Novel mutations in the MYOC/GLC1A gene in a large group of glaucoma patients. Hum Mutat 2002;20:479.

170. WuDunn D. Genetic basis of glaucoma. Curr Opin Ophthalmol 2002;13:55.

171. Bray PJ, Cotton RG. Variations of the human glucocorticoid receptor gene (NR3C1): pathological and in vitro mutations and polymorphisms. Hum Mutat 2003;21:557.

172. Goodman SI, Binard RJ, Woontner MR, et al. Glutaric academia type II: gene structure and mutations of the electron transfer flavoprotein:ubiquinone oxidoreductase (ETF:QO) gene. Mol Genet Metab 2002;77:86.

173. Hellerud C, Adamowicz M, Jurkiewicz D, et al. Clinical heterogeneity and molecular findings in five Polish patients with glycerol kinase deficiency: investigation of two splice site mutations with computerized splice junction analysis and Xp21 gene-specific mRNA analysis. Mol Genet Metab 2003;79:149.

174. Dipple KM, Zhang YH, Huang BL, et al. Glycerol kinase deficiency: evidence for complexity in a single gene disorder. Hum Genet 2001;109:55.

175. Lei KJ, Shelly LL, Pan CJ, et al. Mutations in the glucose-6-phosphatase gene that cause glycogen storage disease type 1a. Science 1993;262:580.

176. Shieh JJ, Terzioglu M, Hiraiwa H, et al. The molecular basis of glycogen storage disease type 1a: structure and function analysis of mutations in glucose-6-phosphatase. J Biol Chem 2002;277:5047.

177. Shen J, Bao Y, Chen YT. A nonsense mutation due to a single base insertion in the 3-prime-coding region of glycogen debranching enzyme gene associated with a severe phenotype in a patient with glycogen storage disease type IIIa. Hum Mutat 1997;9:37.

178. Bao Y, Kishnani P, Wu JY, et al. Hepatic and neuromuscular forms of glycogen storage disease type IV caused by mutations in the same glycogen-branching enzyme gene. J Clin Invest 1996;97:941.

179. Dimaur S, Andreu AL, Bruno C, et al. Myophosphorylase deficiency (glycogenosis type V; McArdle disease). Curr Mol Med 2002;2:189.

180. Burwinkel B, Bakker HD, Herschkovitz E, et al. Mutations in the liver glycogen phosphorylase gene (PYGL) underlying glycogenosis type VI. Am J Hum Genet 1998;62:785.

181. Nakajima H, Raben N, Hamaguchi T, et al. Phosphofructokinase deficiency; past, present and future. Curr Mol Med 2002;2:197.

182. Harley VR, Layfield S, Mitchell CL, et al. Defective importin beta recognition and nuclear import of the sex-determining factor SRY are associated with XY sex-reversing mutations. Proc Natl Acad Sci USA 2003;100:7045.

183. Kroisel PM, Petek E, Wagner K. Phenotype of five patients with Greig syndrome and microdeletion of 7p13. Am J Med Genet 2001;102:243.

184. Hayflick SJ, Westaway SK, Levinson B, et al. Genetic, clinical, and radiographic delineation of Hallervorden–Spatz syndrome. N Engl J Med 2003;348:33.

185. Laurans MS, DiLuna ML, Shin D, et al. Mutational analysis of 206 families with cavernous malformations. J Neurosurg 2003;99:38.

186. Neff LM. Current directions in hemochromatosis research: towards an understanding of the role of iron overload and the HFE gene mutations in the development of clinical disease. Nutr Rev 2003;61:38.

187. Fischel-Ghodsian N, Hirsch PC, Bohlman MC. Rapid detection of the hemoglobin C mutation by allele-specific polymerase chain reaction (letter). Am J Hum Genet 1990;47:1023.

188. Thein SL, Lynch JR, Old JM, et al. Direct detection of haemoglobin E with MnlI. J Med Genet 1987;24:110.

189. Little PFR, Whitelaw E, Annison G, et al. The detection and use of hemoglobin mutants in the direct analysis of human globin genes. Blood 1980;55:1060.

190. Boehm CD, Antonarakis SE, Phillips JA III, et al. Prenatal diagnosis using DNA polymorphisms: report on 95 pregnancies at risk for sickle-cell disease or β-thalassemia. N Engl J Med 1983;308:1054.

191. Boehm CD. Use of polymerase chain reaction for diagnosis of inherited disorders. Clin Chem 1989;35:1843.

192. Wilson JT, Milner PF, Summer ME, et al. Use of restriction endonucleases for mapping the allele for beta-S-globin. Proc Natl Acad Sci USA 1982;79:3628.

193. Gitschier J, Drayna D, Tuddenham EGD, et al. Genetic mapping and diagnosis of haemophilia A achieved through a BclI polymorphism in the factor VIII gene. Nature 1985;314:738.

194. Kogan SM, Doherty M, Gitschier J. An improved method for prenatal diagnosis of genetic diseases by analysis of amplified DNA sequences: application to hemophilia A. N Engl J Med 1987;317:985.

195. Connor JM, Pettigrew AF, Shiach C, et al. Application of three intragenic DNA polymorphisms for carrier detection in haemophilia B. J Med Genet 1986;23:300.

196. Bottema CDK, Koeberl DD, Sommer SS. Direct carrier testing in 14 families with haemophilia B. Lancet 1989;II:526.

197. McAllister KA, Grogg KM, Johnson DW, et al. Endoglin, a TGF-beta binding protein of endothelial cells, is the gene for hereditary haemorrhagic telangiectasia type 1. Nat Genet 1994;8:345.

198. Lupski JR, Montes de Oca-Luna R, Slaugenhaupt S, et al. DNA duplication associated with Charcot–Marie–Tooth disease type 1A. Cell 1991;66:219.

199. Oh J, Bailin T, Fukai K, et al. Positional cloning of a gene for Hermansky–Pudlak syndrome, a disorder of cytoplasmic organelles. Nat Genet 1996;14:300.

200. Mulligan LM, Kwok JBJ, Healey CS, et al. Germ-line mutations of the RET proto-oncogene in multiple endocrine neoplasia type 2A. Nature 1993;363:458.

201. Puffenberger EG, Hosoda K, Washington SS, et al. A missense mutation of the endothelin-B receptor gene in multigenic Hirschsprung's disease. Cell 1994;79:1257.

202. Roessler E, Belloni E, Gaudenz K, et al. Mutations in the human Sonic Hedgehog gene cause holopros-encephaly. Nat Genet 1996;14:357.

203. Li QY, Newbury-Ecob RA, Terrett JA, et al. Holt–Oram syndrome is caused by mutations in TBX5, a member of the Brachyury (T) gene family. Nat Genet 1997;15:21.

204. Hu FL, Gu Z, Kozich V, et al. Molecular basis of cystathionine beta-synthase deficiency in pyridoxine responsive and nonresponsive homocystinuria. Hum Mol Genet 1993;2:1857.

205. Chase DS, Morris AH, Ballabio A, et al. Genetics of Hunter syndrome: carrier detection, new mutations, segregation and linkage analysis. Ann Hum Genet 1986;50:349.

206. Hayden MR, Kastelein JJP, Wilson RD, et al. First-trimester prenatal diagnosis for Huntington's disease with DNA probes. Lancet 1987;1:1284.

207. Quarrell OWJ, Tyler A, Upadhyaya M, et al. Exclusion testing for Huntington's disease in pregnancy with a closely linked DNA marker. Lancet 1987;I:1281.

208. Fahy M, Robbins C, Bloch M, et al. Different options for prenatal testing for Huntington's disease using DNA probes. J Med Genet 1989;26:353.

209. McIntosh I, Curtis A, Millan FA, et al. Prenatal exclusion testing for Huntington disease using the poly-merase chain reaction. Am J Med Genet 1989;32:274.

210. Scott HS, Guo XH, Hopwood JJ, et al. Structure and sequence of the human alpha-L-iduronidase gene. Genomics 1992;13:1311.

211. Fryns JP, Spaepen A, Cassiman JJ, et al. X linked complicated spastic paraplegia, MASA syndrome, and X linked hydrocephalus owing to congenital stenosis of the aqueduct of Sylvius: Variable expression of the same mutation at Xq28. J Med Genet 1991;28:429.

212. Hobbs HH, Leitersdorf E, Goldstein JL, et al. Multiple CRM-mutations in familial hypercholesterolemia: evidence for 13 alleles, including four deletions. J Clin Invest 1988;81:909.

213. Goyette P, Sumner JS, Milos R, et al. Human methylenetetrahydrofolate reductase: isolation of cDNA, mapping and mutation identification. Nat Genet 1994;7:195.

214. Ptacek LJ, Tyler F, Trimmer JS, et al. Analysis in a large hyperkalemic periodic paralysis pedigree supports tight linkage to a sodium channel locus. Am J Hum Genet 1991;49:378.

215. Beg OU, Meng MS, Skarlatos SI, et al. Lipoprotein lipase (Bethesda): a single amino acid substitution (ala176-to-thr) leads to abnormal heparin binding and loss of enzymic activity. Proc Natl Acad Sci USA 1990;87:3474.

216. Danpure CJ, Rumsby G. Strategies for the prenatal diagnosis of primary hyperoxaluria type I. Prenat Diagn 1996;16:587.

217. Bellus GA, McIntosh I, Smith EA, et al. A recurrent mutation in the tyrosine kinase domain of fibrob-last growth factor receptor 3 causes hypochondroplasia. Nat Genet 1995;10:357.

218. Thomas PM, Cote GJ, Hallman DM, et al. Homozygosity mapping, to chromosome 11p, of the gene for familial persistent hyperinsulinemic hypoglycemia of infancy. Am J Hum Genet 1995;56:416.

219. Thomas P, Ye Y, Lightner E. Mutation of the pancreatic islet inward rectifier Kir6.2 also leads to famil-ial persistent hyperinsulinemic hypoglycemia of infancy. Hum Mol Genet 1996;5:1809.

220. Thakker RV, Davies KE, Whyte MP, et al. Mapping of the X-linked idiopathic hypoparathyroid gene to Xq26-Xq27 by linkage studies (abstract). Cytogenet Cell Genet 1989;51:1089.

221. Orimo H, Nakajima E, Hayashi Z, et al. First trimester prenatal molecular diagnosis of infantile hy-pophosphatasia in a Japanese family. Prenat Diagn 1996;16(6):559.

222. Thakker RV, Davies KE, Read AP. Linkage analysis of two cloned DNA sequences, DXS197 and DXS207, in hypophosphatemic rickets families. Genomics 1990;8:189.

223. Conary JT, Lorkowski G, Schmidt B. Genetic heterogeneity of steroid sulfatase deficiency revealed with cDNA for human steroid sulfatase. Biochem Biophys Res Commun 1987;144:1010.

224. Gillard EF, Affara NA, Yates JR, et al. Deletion of a DNA sequence in eight of nine families with X-linked ichthyosis (steroid sulphatase deficiency). Nucleic Acids Res 1987;15:3977.

225. Sefiani A, Abel L, Heuertz S, et al. The gene for incontinentia pigmenti is assigned to Xq28. Genomics 1989;4:427.

226. Smahi A, Hyden-Granskog C, Peterlin B, et al. The gene for the familial form of incontinentia pigmenti (IP2) maps to the distal part of Xq28. Hum Mol Genet 1994;3:273.

227. Vockley J, Parimoo B, Tanaka K. Molecular characterization of four different classes of mutations in the isovaleryl-CoA dehydrogenase gene responsible for isovaleric acidemia. Am J Hum Genet 1991;49:147.

228. Rutland P, Pulleyn LJ, Reardon W, et al. Identical mutations in the FGFR2 gene cause both Pfeiffer and Crouzon syndrome phenotypes. Nat Genet 1995;9:173.

229. Bick D, Franco B, Sherins RJ, et al. Brief report: Intragenic deletion of the KALIG-1 gene in Kallmann's syndrome. N Engl J Med 1992;326:1752.

230. Lee S, Wu X, Reid ME, et al. Molecular basis of the Kell (K1) phenotype. Blood 1995;85:912.

231. La Spada AR, Wilson EM, Lubahn DB, et al. Androgen receptor gene mutations in X-linked spinal and bulbar muscular atrophy. Nature 1991;352:77.

232. Winterpacht A, Hilbert M, Schwarze U, et al. Kniest and Stickler dysplasia phenotypes caused by collagen type II gene (COL2A1) defect. Nat Genet 1993;3:323.

233. Sakai N, Inui K, Fujii N, et al. Krabbe disease: isolation and characterization of a full-length cDNA for human galactocerebrosidase. Biochem Biophys Res Commun 1994;198:485.

234. Huber M, Rettler I, Bernasconi K, et al. Mutations of keratinocyte transglutaminase in lamellar ichthyosis. Science 1995;267:525.

235. Ludecke HJ, Wagner MJ, Nardmann J, et al. Molecular dissection of a contiguous gene syndrome: localization of the genes involved in the Langer–Giedion syndrome. Hum Mol Genet 1995;4:31.

236. Perrault I, Rozet JM, Calvas P, et al. Retinal-specific guanylate cyclase gene mutations in Leber's congenital amaurosis. Nat Genet 1996;14:461.

237. Singh G, Lott MT, Wallace DC. A mitochondrial DNA mutation as a cause of Leber's hereditary optic neuropathy. N Engl J Med 1989;320:1300.

238. Huoponen K, Vilkki J, Aula P, et al. A new mtDNA mutation associated with Leber hereditary optic neuroretinopathy. Am J Hum Genet 1991;48:1147.

239. Longo N, Langley SD, Still MJ, et al. Prenatal analysis of the insulin receptor gene in a family with leprechaunism. Prenat Diagn 1995;15(11):1070.

240. Gibbs DA, Crawfurd MD, Headhouse-Benson CM, et al. First-trimester diagnosis of Lesch Gibbs DA, Crawfurd Nyhan syndrome. Lancet 1984;2:1180.

241. Sinnett D, Lavergne L, Melancon SB, et al. Lesch Gibbs DA, Crawfurd Nyhan syndrome: molecular investigation of three French Canadian families using a hypoxanthine-guanine phosphoribosyltransferase cDNA probe. Hum Genet 1988;81:4.

242. Kremer H, Kraaij R, Toledo SPA, et al. Male pseudohermaphroditism due to a homozygous missense mutation of the luteinizing hormone receptor gene. Nat Genet 1995;9:160.

243. Malkin D, Li FP, Strong LC, et al. Germ line p53 mutations in a familial syndrome of breast cancer, sarcomas, and other neoplasms. Science 1990;250:1233.

244. Ushikubo S, Aoyama T, Kamijo T, et al. Molecular characterization of mitochondrial trifunctional protein deficiency: formation of the enzyme complex is important for stabilization of both alpha- and beta-subunits. Am J Hum Genet 1996;58:979.

245. Wang Q, Curren ME, Splawski I, et al. Positional cloning of a novel potassium channel gene: KVLQT1 mutations cause cardiac arrhythmias. Nat Genet 196;12:17.

246. Neyroud N, Tesson F, Denjoy I, et al. A novel mutation in the potassium channel gene KVLQT1 causes the Jervell and Lange–Nielsen cardioauditory syndrome. Nat Genet 1997;15:186.

247. Wadelius C, Fagerholm P, Pettersson U, et al. Lowe oculocerebrorenal syndrome: DNA-based linkage of the gene to Xq24-q26, using tightly linked flanking markers and the correlation to lens examination in carrier diagnosis. Am J Hum Genet 1989;44:241.

248. Small KW, Hermsen V, Gurney N, et al. North Carolina macular dystrophy and central areolar pigment epithelial dystrophy: one family, one disease. Arch Ophthalmol 1992;110:515.

249. Gillard EF, Otsu K, Fujii J, et al. Polymorphisms and deduced amino acid substitutions in the coding sequence of the ryanodine receptor (RYR1) gene in individuals with malignant hyperthermia. Genomics 1992;13:1247.

250. Fisher CR, Fisher CW, Chuang DT, et al. Occurrence of a Tyr393 → Asn (Y393N) mutation in the EIα

gene of the branched-chain α-keto acid dehydrogenase complex in maple syrup urine disease patients from a Mennonite population. Am J Hum Genet 1991;49:429.

251. Kainulainen K, Pulkkinen L, Savolainen A, et al. Location on chromosome 15 of the gene defect causing Marfan syndrome. N Engl J Med 1990;323:935.

252. Dietz HC, Pyeritz RE, Hall BD, et al. The Marfan syndrome locus: confirmation of assignment to chromosome 15 and identification of tightly linked markers at 15q15-q21.3. Genomics 1991;9:355.

253. Wicker G, Prill V, Brooks D, et al. Mucopolysaccharidosis VI (Maroteaux–Lamy syndrome): an intermediate clinical phenotype caused by substitution of valine for glycine at position 137 of arylsulfatase B. J Biol Chem 1991;266:21386.

254. Patten JL, Johns DR, Valle D, et al. Mutation in the gene encoding the stimulatory G protein of adenylate cyclase in Albright's hereditary osteodystrophy. N Engl J Med 1990;322:1412.

255. Paavola P, Salonen R, Weissenbach J, et al. The locus for Meckel syndrome with multiple congenital anomalies maps to chromosome 17q21-q24. Nat Genet 1995;11:213.

256. Ding J-H, Roe CR, Lafolla AK, et al. Medium-chain acyl-coenzyme a dehydrogenase deficiency and sudden infant death. N Engl J Med 1991;325:61.

257. Kaler SG, Gallo LK, Proud VK, et al. Occipital horn syndrome and a mild Menkes phenotype associated with splice site mutations at the MNK locus. Nat Genet 1994;8:195.

258. Gieselmann V, Zlotogora J, Harris A, et al. Molecular genetics of metachromatic leukodystrophy. Hum Mutat 1994;4:233.

259. Warman ML, Abbott M, Apte SS, et al. A type X collagen mutation causes Schmid metaphyseal chondrodysplasia. Nat Genet 1993;5:79.

260. Jansen R, Ledley FD. Heterozygous mutations at the mut locus in fibroblasts with mut^0 methylmalonic acidemia identified by polymerase-chain-reaction cDNA cloning. Am J Hum Genet 1990;47:808.

261. Ophoff RA, Terwindt GM, Vergouwe MN, et al. Familial hemiplegic migraine and episodic ataxia type-2 are caused by mutations in the Ca(2+) channel gene CACNL1A4. Cell 1996;87:543.

262. Batanian JR, Ledbetter SA, Wolff RK, et al. Rapid diagnosis of Miller-Dieker syndrome and isolated lissencephaly sequence by the polymerase chain reaction. Hum Genet 1990;85:555.

263. Oshima A, Yoshida K, Shimmoto M, et al. Human β-galactosidase gene mutations in Morquio B disease. Am J Hum Genet 1991;49:1091.

264. Nakamura Y, Larsson C, Julier C, et al. Localization of the genetic defect in multiple endocrine neoplasia type I with a small region of chromosome II. Am J Hum Genet 1989;44:751.

265. Norum RA, Lafreniere RG, O'Neal LW, et al. Linkage of the multiple endocrine neoplasia type 2B gene (MEN2B) to chromosome 10 markers linked to MEN2A. Genomics 1990;8:313.

266. Briggs MD, Hoffman SMG, King LM, et al. Pseudoachondroplasia and multiple epiphyseal dysplasia due to mutations in the cartilage oligomeric matrix protein gene. Nat Genet 1995;10:330.

267. Ahn J, Lucecke HJ, Lindow S, et al. Cloning of the putative tumour suppressor gene for hereditary multiple exostoses (EXT1). Nat Genet 1995;11:137.

268. den Dunnen JT, Bakker E, Klein Breteler EG, et al. Direct detection of more than 50% of the Duchenne muscular dystrophy mutations by field inversion gels. Nature 1987;329:640.

269. Koenig M, Hoffman EP, Bertelson CJ, et al. Complete cloning of the Duchenne muscular dystrophy (DMD) cDNA and preliminary genomic organization of the DMD gene in normal and affected individuals. Cell 1987;50:509.

270. Hentemann M, Reiss J, Wagner M, et al. Rapid detection of deletions in the Duchenne muscular dystrophy gene by PCR amplification of deletion-prone exon sequences. Hum Genet 1990;84:228.

271. Bieber FR, Hoffman EP. Duchenne and Becker muscular dystrophies: genetics, prenatal diagnosis, and future prospects. Clin Perinatol 1990;17:845.

272. Beggs AH, Koenig M, Boyce FM, et al. Detection of 98% of DMD/BMD gene deletions by polymerase chain reaction. Hum Genet 1990;86:45.

273. Yates JRW, Affara NA, Jamieson DM, et al. Emery–Dreifuss muscular dystrophy: Localisation to Xq27.3 → qter confirmed by linkage to the factor VIII gene. J Med Genet 1986;23:587.

274. Wijmenga C, Padberg GW, Moerer P, et al. Mapping of facioscapulohumeral muscular dystrophy gene to chromosome 4q35-qter by multipoint linkage analysis and in situ hybridization. Genomics 1991;9:570.

275. Toda T, Miyake M, Kobayashi K, et al. Linkage-disequilibrium mapping narrows the Fukuyama-type congenital muscular dystrophy (FCMD) candidate region to less than 100 kb. Am J Hum Genet 1996;59:1313.

276. Richard I, Broux O, Allamand V, et al. Mutations in the proteolytic enzyme calpain 3 cause limb-girdle muscular dystrophy type 2A. Cell 1995;81:27.

277. Brais B, Xie YG, Sanson M, et al. The oculopharyngeal muscular dystrophy locus maps to the region of

the cardiac alpha and beta myosin heavy chain genes on chromosome 14q11.2-q13. Hum Mol Genet 1995;4:429.

278. George AL Jr, Crackower MA, Abdalla JA, et al. Molecular basis of Thomsen's disease (autosomal dominant myotonia congenita). Nat Genet 1993;3:305.

279. Koch MC, Steinmeyer K, Lorenz C, et al. The skeletal muscle chloride channel in dominant and recessive human myotonia. Science 1992;257:797.

280. Shaw DJ, Harper PS. Myotonic dystrophy: Developments in molecular genetics. Br Med Bull 1989;45:745.

281. Norman AM, Floyd JL, Meredith AL, et al. Presymptomatic detection and prenatal diagnosis for myotonic dystrophy by means of linked DNA markers. J Med Genet 1989;26:750.

282. Milunsky JM, Skare JC, Milunsky A. Presymptomatic and prenatal diagnosis of myotonic muscular dystrophy with linked DNA probes. Am J Med Sci 1991;301:231.

283. Aslanidis C, Jansen G, Amemiya C, et al. Cloning of the essential myotonic dystrophy region and mapping of the putative defect. Nature 1992;355:548.

284. Brook JD, McCurrach ME, Harley HG, et al. Molecular basis of myotonic dystrophy: expansion of a trinucleotide (CTG) repeat at the 3′ end of a transcript encoding a protein kinase family member. Cell 1992;68:799.

285. Laporte J, Hu LJ, Kretz C, et al. A gene mutated in X-linked myotubular myopathy defines a new putative tyrosine phosphatase family conserved in yeast. Nat Genet 1996;13:175.

286. Campeau E, Watkins D, Rouleau GA, et al. Linkage analysis of the nail-patella syndrome. Am J Hum Genet 1995;56:243.

287. Laing NG, Wilton SD, Akkari PA, et al. A mutation in the alpha tropomyosin gene TPM3 associated with autosomal dominant nemaline myopathy. Nat Genet 1995;9:75.

288. Rosenthal W, Seibold A, Antaramian A, et al. Molecular identification of the gene responsible for congenital nephrogenic diabetes insipidus. Nature 1992;359:233.

289. Olsen AS, Georgescu A, Johnson S, et al. Assembly of a 1-Mb restriction-mapped cosmid contig spanning the candidate region for Finnish congenital nephrosis (NPHS1) in 19q13.1. Genomics 1996;34:223.

290. Pulst SM. Prenatal diagnosis of the neurofibromatoses. Clin Perinatol 1990;17:829.

291. Ward K, O'Connell P, Carey JC, et al. Diagnosis of neurofibromatosis I by using tightly linked, flanking DNA markers. Am J Hum Genet 1990;46:943.

292. Rouleau GA, Seizinger BR, Wertelecki W, et al. Flanking markers bracket the neurofibromatosis type 2 (NF2) gene on chromosome 22. Am J Hum Genet 1990;46:323.

293. International Batten Disease Consortium. Isolation of a novel gene underlying Batten disease, CLN3. Cell 1995;82:949.

294. Levran O, Desnick RJ, Schuchman EH. Niemann-Pick disease: a frequent missense mutation in the acid sphingomyelinase gene of Ashkenazi Jewish type A and B patients. Proc Natl Acad Sci 1991;88:3748.

295. Koyata H, Hiraga K. The glycine cleavage system: Structure of a cDNA encoding human H-protein, and partial characterization of its gene in patients with hyperglycinemias. Am J Hum Genet 1991;48:351.

296. Gal A, Uhlhaas S, Glaser D, et al. Prenatal exclusion of Norrie disease with flanking DNA markers. Am J Med Genet 1988;31:448.

297. Curtis D, Blank CE, Parsons MA, et al. Carrier detection and prenatal diagnosis in Norrie disease. Prenat Diagn 1989;9:735.

298. de La Chapelle A, Sandal E-M, Lindlof M, et al. Norrie disease caused by a gene deletion allowing carrier detection and prenatal diagnosis. Clin Genet 1985;28:317.

299. Zhu D, Antonarakis SE, Schmeckpeper BJ, et al. Microdeletion in the X-chromosome and prenatal diagnosis in a family with Norrie disease. Am J Med Genet 1989;33:485.

300. Lunkes A, Hartung U, Magarino C, et al. Refinement of the OPA1 gene locus on chromosome 3q28-q29 to a region of 2–8 cM, in one Cuban pedigree with autosomal dominant optic atrophy type Kjer. Am J Hum Genet 1995;57:968.

301. Fox J, Hack AM, Fenton WA, et al. Prenatal diagnosis of ornithine transcarbamylase deficiency with use of DNA polymorphisms. N Engl J Med 1986;315:1205.

302. Grompe M, Caskey CT, Fenwick RG. Improved molecular diagnostics for ornithine transcarbamylase deficiency. Am J Hum Genet 1991;48:212.

303. Palotie A, Vaisanen P, Ott J, et al. Predisposition to familial osteoarthrosis is linked to type II collagen gene. Cytogenet Cell Genet 1989;51:1058.

304. Pope FM, Cheah KS, Nicholls AC, et al. Lethal osteogenesis imperfecta congenita and a 300 base pair gene deletion for an alpha 1 (I)-like collagen. BMJ 1984;288:431.

305. Tsipouras P, Myers JC, Ramirez F, et al. Restriction fragment length polymorphism associated with pro

$\alpha 2$(I) gene of human type I procollagen: application to a family with an autosomal dominant form of osteogenesis imperfecta. J Clin Invest 1983;72:1262.

306. Tsipouras P, Schwartz R, Goldberg JD, et al. Prenatal prediction of osteogenesis imperfecta (OI type IV): Exclusion of inheritance using a collagen gene probe. J Med Genet 1987;24:406.

307. Byers PH, Tsipouras P, Bonadio JF, et al. Perinatal lethal osteogenesis imperfecta (OI type II): A biochemically heterogeneous disorder usually due to new mutations in the genes for type I collagen. Am J Hum Genet 1988; 42:237.

308. Starman BJ, Eyre D, Charbonneau H, et al. Osteogenesis imperfecta: The position of substitution for glycine by cysteine in the triple helical domain of the pro-alpha-1(I) chains of type I collagen determines the clinical phenotype. J Clin Invest 1989;84:1206.

309. Pope FM, Daw SCM, Narcisa P, et al. Prenatal diagnosis and prevention of inherited abnormalities of collagen. Inherit Metab Dis 1989;12:135.

310. Simard J, Tonin P, Durocher F, et al. Common origins of BRCA1 mutations in Canadian breast and ovarian cancer families. Nat Genet 1994;8:392.

311. Amati P, Gasparini P, Zlotogora J, et al. A gene for premature ovarian failure associated with eyelid malformation maps to chromosome 3q22-q23. Am J Hum Genet 1996;58:1089.

312. Kang S, Graham JM Jr, Olney AH, et al. GLI3 frameshift mutations cause autosomal dominant Pallister–Hall syndrome. Nat Genet 1997;15:266.

313. Whitcomb DC, Gorry MC, Preston RA, et al. Hereditary pancreatitis is caused by a mutation in the cationic trypsinogen gene. Nat Genet 1996;14:141.

314. McShane MA, Hammans SR, Sweeney M, et al. Pearson syndrome and mitochondrial encephalomyopathy in a patient with a deletion of mtDNA. Am J Hum Genet 1991;48:39.

315. Maenpaa J, Lindahl E, Aula P, et al. Prenatal diagnosis in Pelizaeus–Merzbacher disease using RFLP analysis. Clin Genet 1990;37:141.

316. Muenke M, Schell U, Hehr A, et al. A common mutation in the fibroblast growth factor receptor 1 gene in Pfeiffer syndrome. Nat Genet 1994;8:269.

317. Lidsky AS, Guttler F, Woo SLC. Prenatal diagnosis of classic phenylketonuria by DNA analysis. Lancet 1985;1:549.

318. Sommer SS, Cassady JD, Sobell JL, et al. A novel method for detecting point mutations or polymorphisms and its application to population screening for carriers of phenylketonuria. Mayo Clin Proc 1989;64:1361.

319. Labrune P, Melle D, Rey F, et al. Single-strand conformation polymorphism for detection of mutations and base substitutions in phenylketonuria. Am J Hum Genet 1991;48:1115.

320. Phillips JA III, Hjelle BL, Seeburg PH, et al. A molecular basis for familial isolated growth hormone deficiency. Proc Natl Acad Sci USA 1981;78:6372.

321. Vnencak-Jones CL, Phillips JA III, De-fen W. Use of polymerase chain reaction in detection of growth hormone gene deletions. J Clin Endocrinol Metab 1990;70:1550.

322. Tatsumi K, Miyai K, Notomi T, et al. Cretinism with combined hormone deficiency caused by a mutation in the PIT1 gene. Nat Genet 1992;1:56.

323. Reeders ST, Gal A, Propping P, et al. Prenatal diagnosis of autosomal dominant polycystic kidney disease with a DNA probe. Lancet 1986;II:6.

324. Ceccherini I, Lituania M, Cordone MS, et al. Autosomal dominant polycystic kidney disease: prenatal diagnosis by DNA analysis and sonography at 14 weeks. Prenat Diagn 1989;9:751.

325. Breuning MH, Snijdewint FGM, Brunner H, et al. Map of 16 polymorphic loci on the short arm of chromosome 16 close to the polycystic kidney disease gene (PKD1). J Med Genet 1990;27:603.

326. Breuning MH, Snijdewint FGM, Dauwerse JG, et al. Two step procedure for early diagnosis of polycystic kidney disease with polymorphic DNA markers on both sides of the gene. J Med Genet 1990;27:614.

327. Germino GG, Barton NJ, Lamb J, et al. Identification of a locus which shows no genetic recombination with the autosomal dominant polycystic kidney disease gene on chromosome 16. Am J Hum Genet 1990;46:925.

328. Harris PC, Thomas S, Ratcliffe PJ, et al. Rapid genetic analysis of families with polycystic kidney disease 1 by means of a microsatellite marker. Lancet 1991;338:1484.

329. Pirson Y, Lannoy N, Peters D, et al. Isolated polycystic liver disease as a distinct genetic disease, unlinked to polycystic kidney disease 1 and polycystic kidney disease 2. Hepatology 1996;23:249.

330. Garey JR, Harrison LM, Franklin KF, et al. Uroporphyrinogen decarboxylase: a splice site mutation causes the deletion of exon 6 in multiple families with porphyria cutanea tarda. J Clin Invest 1990;86:1416.

331. Grandchamp B, Picat C, de Rooij F, et al. A point mutation G-to-A in exon 12 of the porphobilinogen

deaminase gene results in exon skipping and is responsible for acute intermittent porphyria. Nucleic Acids Res 1989;17:6637.

332. Deybach JC, de Verneuil H, Boulechfar S, et al. Point mutations in the uroporphyrinogen III synthase gene in congenital erythropoietic porphyria (Gunther's disease). Blood 1990;75:1763.

333. Donlon TA, Lalande M, Wyman A, et al. Isolation of molecular probes associated with the chromosome 15 instability in the Prader–Willi syndrome. Proc Natl Acad Sci USA 1986;83:4408.

334. Shenker A, Laue L, Kosugi S, et al. A constitutively activating mutation of the luteinizing hormone receptor in familial male precocious puberty. Nature 1993;365:652.

335. Ohura T, Miyabayashi S, Narisawa K, et al. Genetic heterogeneity of propionic acidemia: analysis of 15 Japanese patients. Hum Genet 1991;87:41.

336. Lamhonwah A-M, Troxel CE, Schuster S, et al. Two distinct mutations at the same site in the PCCB gene in propionic acidemia. Genomics 1990;8:249.

337. Romeo G, Hassan HJ, Staempfli S, et al. Hereditary thrombophilia: identification of nonsense and missense mutations in the protein C gene. Proc Natl Acad Sci USA 1987;84:2829.

338. Ploos van Amstel HK, Huisman MV, Reitsma PH, et al. Partial protein S gene deletion in a family with hereditary thrombophilia. Blood 1989;73:479.

339. Hecht JT, Nelson LD, Crowder E, et al. Mutations in exon 17B of cartilage oligomeric matrix protein (COMP) cause pseudoachondroplasia. Nat Genet 1995;10:325.

340. Gelb BD, Shi GP, Chapman HA, et al. Pyknodysostosis, a lysosomal disease caused by cathepsin K deficiency. Science 1996;273:1236.

341. Neubauer B, Lakomek M, Winkler H, et al. Point mutations in the L-type pyruvate kinase gene of two children with hemolytic anemia caused by pyruvate kinase deficiency. Blood 191;77:1871.

342. Olsson JE, Samanns C, Jimenez J, et al. Gene of type II autosomal dominant retinitis pigmentosa maps on the long arm of chromosome 3. Am J Med Genet 1990;35:595.

343. Dryja TP, McGee TL, Hahn LB, et al. Mutations within the rhodopsin gene in patients with autosomal dominant retinitis pigmentosa. N Engl J Med 1990;323:1302.

344. McLaughlin ME, Sandberg MA, Berson EL, et al. Recessive mutations in the gene encoding the beta-subunit of rod phosphodiesterase in patients with retinitis pigmentosa. Nat Genet 1993;4:130.

345. Teague PW, Aldred MA, Jay M, et al. Heterogeneity analysis in 40 X-linked retinitis pigmentosa families. Am J Hum Genet 1994;55:105.

346. Scheffer H, te Meerman GJ, Kruize YCM, et al. Linkage analysis of families with hereditary retinoblastoma: nonpenetrance of mutation, revealed by combined use of markers within and flanking the RB1 gene. Am J Hum Genet 1989;45:252.

347. Yandell DW, Campbell TA, Dayton SH, et al. Oncogenic point mutations in the human retinoblastoma gene: their application to genetic counseling. N Engl J Med 1989;321:1689.

348. Sieving PA, Bingham EL, Roth MS, et al. Linkage relationship of X-linked juvenile retinoschisis with Xp22.1-p22.3 probes. Am J Hum Genet 1990;47:616.

349. Mouro I, Colin Y, Cherif-Zahar B, et al. Molecular genetic basis of the human Rhesus blood group system. Nat Genet 1993;5:62.

350. Colin Y, Cherif-Zahar B, Le Van Kim C, et al. Genetic basis of the RhD-positive and RhD-negative blood group polymorphism as determined by Southern analysis. Blood 1991;78:2747.

351. Semina EV, Reiter R, Leysens NJ, et al. Cloning and characterization of a novel bicoid-related homeobox transcription factor gene, RIEG, involved in Rieger syndrome. Nat Genet 1996;14:392.

352. Phillips JC, Del Bono EA, Haines JL, et al. A second locus for Rieger syndrome maps to chromosome 13q14. Am J Hum Genet 1996;59:613.

353. Petrij F, Giles RH, Dauwerse HG, et al. Rubinstein–Taybi syndrome caused by mutations in the transcriptional co-activator CBP. Nature 1995;376:348.

354. Howard TD, Paznekas WA, Green ED, et al. Mutations in TWIST, a basic helix-loop-helix transcription factor, in Saethre–Chotzen syndrome. Nat Genet 1997;15:36.

355. Schleutker J, Sistonen P, Aula P. Haplotype analysis in prenatal diagnosis and carrier identification of Salla disease. J Med Genet 1996;33(1):36.

356. Neote K, McInnes B, Mahuran DJ, et al. Structure and distribution of an Alu-type deletion mutation in Sandhoff disease. J Clin Invest 1990;86:1524.

357. Zhao HG, Li HH, Bach G, et al. The molecular basis of Sanfilippo syndrome type B. Proc Natl Acad Sci USA 1996;93:6101.

358. Schwartz K, Gauss GH, Ludwig L, et al. RAG mutations in human B cell-negative SCID. Science 1996;274:97.

359. Bardoni B, Zanaria E, Guioli S, et al. A dosage sensitive locus at chromosome Xp21 is involved in male to female sex reversal. Nat Genet 1994;7:497.

360. Gosden JR, Gosden CM, Christie S, et al. The use of cloned Y chromosome-specific DNA probes for fetal sex determination in first trimester prenatal diagnosis. Hum Genet 1984;66:347.

361. Pinckert TL, Lebo RV, Golbus MS. Rapid determination of fetal sex by deoxyribonucleic acid amplification of Y chromosome-specific sequences. Am J Obstet Gynecol 1989;161:693.

362. Naito E, Indo Y, Tanaka K. Identification of two variant short chain acyl-coenzyme A dehydrogenase alleles, each containing a different point mutation in a patient with short chain acyl-coenzyme A dehydrogenase deficiency. J Clin Invest 1990;85:1575.

363. Cotter PD, Baumann M, Bishop DF. Enzymatic defect in "X-linked" sideroblastic anemia: molecular evidence for erythroid delta-aminolevulinate synthase deficiency. Proc Natl Acad Sci USA 1992;89: 4028.

364. Pilia G, Hughes-Benzie RM, MacKenzie A, et al. Mutations in GPC3, a glypican gene, cause the Simpson–Golabi–Behmel overgrowth syndrome. Nat Genet 1996;12:241.

365. Tomatsu S, Fukuda S, Sukegawa K, et al. Mucopolysaccharidosis type VII: characterization of mutations and molecular heterogeneity. Am J Hum Genet 1991;48:89.

366. Dube MP, Mlodzienski MA, Kibar Z, et al. Hereditary spastic paraplegia: LOD-score considerations for confirmation of linkage in a heterogeneous trait. Am J Hum Genet 1997;60:625.

367. Hentati A, Pericak-Vance MA, Hung WY, et al. Linkage of "pure" autosomal recessive familial spastic paraplegia to chromosome 8 markers and evidence of genetic locus heterogeneity. Hum Mol Genet 1994;3:1263.

368. Jouet M, Rosenthal A, Armstrong G, et al. X-linked spastic paraplegia (SPG1), MASA syndrome and X-linked hydrocephalus result from mutations in the L1 gene. Nat Genet 1994;7:402.

369. Yapijakis C, Kapaki E, Boussiou M, et al. Prenatal diagnosis of X-linked spinal and bulbar muscular dystrophy in a Greek family. Prenat Diagn 1996;16:262.

370. Gilliam TC, Brzustowicz LM, Castilla LH, et al. Genetic homogeneity between acute and chronic forms of spinal muscular atrophy. Nature 1990;345:823.

371. Melki J, Sheth P, Abdelhak S, et al. Mapping of acute (type I) spinal muscular atrophy to chromosome 5q12-q14. Lancet 1990;336:271.

372. Banfi S, Servadio A, Chung M, et al. Identification and characterization of the gene causing type 1 spinocerebellar ataxia. Nat Genet 1994;7:513.

373. Pulst SM, Nechiporuk A, Nechiporuk T, et al. Moderate expansion of a normally biallelic trinucleotide repeat in spinocerebellar ataxia type 2. Nat Genet 1996;14:269.

374. Giunti P, Sweeney MG, Harding AE. Detection of the Machado–Joseph disease/spinocerebellar ataxia three trinucleotide repeat expansion in families with autosomal dominant motor disorders, including the Drew family of Walworth. Brain 1995;118:1077.

375. Lee B, Vissing H, Ramirez F, et al. Identification of the molecular defect in a family with spondyloepiphyseal dysplasia. Science 1989;244:978.

376. Tiller GE, Weis MA, Lachman RS, et al. A dominant mutation in the type II collagen gene (COL2A1) produces spondyloepimetaphyseal dysplasia (SEMD), Strudwick type. Am J Hum Genet 1993;53(Suppl.): A209.

377. Brunner HG, van Beersum SEC, Warman ML, et al. A Stickler syndrome gene is linked to chromosome 6 near the COL11A2 gene. Hum Mol Genet 1994;3:1561.

378. Richards AJ, Yates JRW, Williams R, et al. A family with Stickler syndrome type 2 has a mutation in the COL11A1 gene resulting in the substitution of glycine 97 by valine in alpha-1(XI) collagen. Hum Mol Genet 1996;5:1339.

379. Ewart AK, Jin W, Atkinson D, et al. Supravalvular aortic stenosis associated with a deletion disrupting the elastin gene. J Clin Invest 1994;93:1071.

380. Arpaia E, Dumbrille-Ross A, Maler T, et al. Identification of an altered splice site in Ashkenazic Tay–Sachs disease. Nature 1988;333:85.

381. Mahuran DJ, Triggs-Raine BL, Feigenbaum AJ, et al. The molecular basis of Tay–Sachs disease: Mutation identification and diagnosis. Clin Biochem 1990;23:409.

382. Paw BH, Wood LC, Neufeld EF. A third mutation at the CpG dinucleotide of codon 504 and a silent mutation at codon 506 of the HEX A gene. Am J Hum Genet 1991;48:1139.

383. Triggs-Raine BL, Archibald A, Gravel RA, et al. Prenatal exclusion of Tay–Sachs disease by DNA analysis. Lancet 1990;I:1164.

384. Higgs DR, Weatherall DJ. Alpha-thalassemia. Curr Top Hematol 1985;4:37.

385. Cai SP, Kan YW. Identification of the multiple beta-thalassemia mutations by denaturing gradient gel electrophoresis. J Clin Invest 1990;85:550.

386. Tavormina PL, Shiang R, Thompson LM, et al. Thanatophoric dysplasia (types I and II) caused by distinct mutations in fibroblast growth factor receptor 3. Nat Genet 1995;9:321.

387. Sakurai A, Takeda K, Ain K, et al. Generalized resistance to thyroid hormone associated with a mutation in the ligand-binding domain of the human thyroid hormone receptor beta. Proc Natl Acad Sci USA 1989;86:8977.

388. Dixon MJ, Read AP, Donnai D, et al. The gene for Treacher Collins syndrome maps to the long arm of chromosome 5. Am J Hum Genet 1991;49:17.

389. Jabs EW, Li X, Coss CA, et al. Mapping the Treacher Collins syndrome locus to 5q31.3 → 5q33.3. Genomics 1991;11:193.

390. Hou J, Parrish J, Ludecke HJ, et al. A 4-megabase YAC contig that spans the Langer–Giedion syndrome region on human chromosome 8q24.1: use in refining the location of the trichorhinophalangeal syndrome and multiple exostoses genes (TRPS1 and EXT1). Genomics 1995;29:87.

391. Daar IO, Artymiuk PJ, Phillips DC, et al. Human triose-phosphate isomerase deficiency: a single amino acid substitution results in a thermolabile enzyme. Proc Natl Acad Sci USA 1986;83:7903.

392. Connor JM, Pirrit LA, Yates JRW, et al. Linkage of the tuberous sclerosis locus to a DNA polymorphism detected by v-abl. J Med Genet 1987;24:544.

393. Kumar A, Wolpert C, Kandt RS, et al. A de novo frame-shift mutation in the tuberin gene. Hum Mol Genet 1995;4:1471.

394. Phaneuf D, Lambert M, Laframboise R, et al. Type 1 hereditary tyrosinemia: evidence for molecular heterogeneity and identification of a causal mutation in a French Canadian patient. J Clin Invest 1992;90:1185.

395. Kaplan J, Gerber S, Bonneau D, et al. A gene for Usher syndrome type I (USH1A) maps to chromosome 14q. Genomics 1992;14:979.

396. Kimberling WJ, Weston MD, Moller C, et al. Localization of Usher syndrome type II to chromosome 1q. Genomics 1990;7:245.

397. Sankila EM, Pakarinen L, Kaariainen H, et al. Assignment of an Usher syndrome type III (USH3) gene to chromosome 3q. Hum Mol Genet 1995;4:93.

398. Schutte BC, Sander A, Malik M, et al. Refinement of the Van der Woude gene location and construction of a 3.5-Mb YAC contig and STS map spanning the critical region in 1q32-q41. Genomics 1996;36:507.

399. Anguiano A, Oates RD, Amos JA, et al. Congenital bilateral absence of the vas deferens: a primarily genital form of cystic fibrosis. JAMA 1992;267:1794.

400. Demczuk S, Levy A, Aubry M, et al. Excess of deletions of maternal origin in the DiGeorge/velocardiofacial syndromes: a study of 22 new patients and review of the literature. Hum Genet 1995;96:9.

401. Aoyama T, Souri M, Ueno I, et al. Cloning of human very-long-chain acyl-coenzyme A dehydrogenase and molecular characterization of its deficiency in two patients. Am J Hum Genet 1995;57:273.

402. Maher ER, Bentley E, Yates JRW, et al. Mapping of the von Hippel–Lindau disease locus to a small region of chromosome 3p by genetic linkage analysis. Genomics 1991;10:957.

403. Bernardi F, Marchetti G, Patracchini P, et al. RFLPs studies in coagulation FVIII and von Willebrand factors. Cytogenet Cell Genet 1987;46:580.

404. Tassabehji M, Read AP, Newton VE, et al. Waardenburg's syndrome patients have mutations in the human homologue of the Pax-3 paired box gene. Nature 1992;355:635.

405. Tassabehji M, Newton VE, Read AP. Waardenburg syndrome type 2 caused by mutations in the human microphthalmia (MITF) gene. Nat Genet 1994;8:251.

406. Yu CE, Oshima J, Fu YH, et al. Positional cloning of the Werner's syndrome gene. Science 1996;272:258.

407. Bowcock AM, Farrer LA, Herbert JM, et al. DNA markers at 13q14-q22 linked to Wilson's disease. In: Albertini A, Paoletti R, Reisfeld RA, eds. Molecular probes. New York: Raven, 1989:51.

408. Schwartz M, Mibashan RS, Nicolaides KH, et al. First-trimester diagnosis of Wiskott–Aldrich syndrome by DNA markers. Lancet 1989;II:1405.

409. Gusella JF, Tanzi RE, Bader PI, et al. Deletion of Huntington's disease-linked G8 (D4S10) locus in Wolf–Hirschhorn syndrome. Nature 1985;318:75.

410. Quarrell OWJ, Snell RG, Curtis MA, et al. Paternal origin of the chromosomal deletion resulting in Wolf–Hirschhorn syndrome. J Med Genet 1991;28:256.

411. Fujiyama J, Sakuraba H, Kuriyama M, et al. A new mutation (LIPA Tyr22X) of lysosomal acid lipase gene in a Japanese patient with Wolman disease. Hum Mutat 1996;8:377.

412. Alapetite C, Benoit A, Moustacchi E, et al. The comet assay as a repair test for prenatal diagnosis of Xeroderma pigmentosum and trichothiodystrophy. J Invest Derm 1997;108(2):154.

413. Antonarakis SE, Phillips JA III, Kazazian HH Jr. Genetic diseases: diagnosis by restriction endonuclease analysis. J Pediatr 1982;100:845.

414. Phillips JA III. Clinical applications of gene mapping and diagnosis. In: Childs B, Holtzman NA, Kazazian HH, et al., eds. Progress in medical genetics. Philadelphia: WB Saunders, 1987:68.

415. Phillips JA III. Diagnosis at the bedside by gene analysis. South Med J 1990;83:868.

416. Malcolm ADB. The use of restriction enzymes in genetic engineering. Genet Eng 1981;2:129.

417. Southern E. Detection of specific sequences among DNA fragments separated by gel electrophoresis. J Mol Biol 1975;98:503.

418. Chance PF, Pleasure D. Charcot–Marie–Tooth syndrome. Arch Neurol 1993;50:1180.

418a. Mohammed MS, Shaffer LG. Fluorescence in situ hybridization (FISH) for identifying the genomic rearrangements associated with three myelinopathies: Charcot–Marie–Tooth disease, hereditary neuropathy with liability to pressure palsies, and Pelizaeus–Merzbacher disease. Methods Mol Biol 2003;217:219.

418b. Thiel CT, Kraus C, Rauch A, et al. A new quantitative PCR multiplex assay for rapid analysis of chromosome 17p11.2-12 duplications and deletions leading to HMSN/HNPP. Eur J Hum Genet 2003;11:170.

418c. Lorentzos P, Kaiser T, Kennerson ML, et al. A rapid and definitive test for Charcot–Marie–Tooth 1A and hereditary neuropathy with liability to pressure palsies using multiplexed real-time PCR. Genet Test 2003;7:135.

419. Rousseau F, Heitz D, Biancalana V, et al. Direct diagnosis by DNA analysis of the fragile X syndrome of mental retardation. N Engl J Med 1991;325:1673.

420. Verkerk AJMH, Pieretti M, Sutcliffe JS, et al. Identification of a gene (FMR-1) containing a CGG repeat coincident with a breakpoint cluster region exhibiting length variation in fragile X syndrome. Cell 1991;65:905.

421. Sutherland GR. Fragile sites on human chromosomes: demonstration of their dependence on the type of tissue culture medium. Science 1977;197:265.

422. Eberhart DE, Malter HE, Feng Y, et al. The fragile X mental retardation protein is a ribonucleoprotein containing both nuclear localization and nuclear export signals. Hum Mol Genet 1996;5:1083.

423. Hinds HL, Ashley CT, Sutcliffe JS, et al. Tissue specific expression of FMR-1 provides evidence for a functional role in fragile X syndrome. Nat Genet 1993;3:36.

424. Reyniers E, Vits L, DeBoulle K, et al. The full mutation in the FMR-1 gene of male fragile X patients is absent in their sperm. Nat Genet 1993;4:143.

425. Rousseau F, Heitz D, Tarleton J, et al. A multicenter study on genotype–phenotype correlations in the fragile X syndrome, using direct diagnosis with probe StB 12.3: the first 2,253 cases. Am J Hum Genet 1994;55:225.

426. Sherman SL, Morton NE, Jacobs PA, et al. The marker (X) chromosome: a cytogenetic and genetic analysis. Ann Hum Genet 1984;48:21.

427. Eichler EE, Holden JJA, Popovich BW, et al. Length of uninterrupted CGG repeats determines instability in the FMR1 gene. Nat Genet 1994;8:88.

428. Murray A, Macpherson JN, Pound MC, et al. The role of size, sequence and haplotype in the stability of FRAXA and FRAXE alleles during transmission. Hum Mol Genet 1997;6:173.

429. Turner G, Robinson H, Wake S, et al. Dizygous twinning and premature ovarian failure in fragile X syndrome. Lancet 1994;344:1500.

430. Schwartz CE, Deon J, Howard-Peebles PN, et al. Obstetrical and gynecological complication in fragile X carriers: a multicenter study. Am J Med Genet 1994;51:400.

431. Conway GS, HeHiarachchi S, Murray A, et al. Fragile X premutation in familial premature ovarian failure. Lancet 1995;346:309.

432. Jacquemont S, Hagerman RJ, Leehey M, et al. Fragile X permutation tremor/ataxia syndrome: molecular, clinical and neuroimaging correlates. Am J Hum Genet 2003;72:869.

433. Lakich D, Kazazian HH, Antonarakis SE, et al. Inversions disrupting the factor VIII gene are a common cause of severe hemophilia A. Nat Genet 1993;5:236.

434. Bagnall RD, Waseem N, Green PM, et al. Recurrent inversion breaking intron 1 of the factor VIII gene is a frequent cause of severe hemophilia A. Blood 2002;99:168.

434a. Andrikovics H, Klein I, Bors A, et al. Analysis of large structural changes of the factor VIII gene, involving intron 1 and 22, in severe hemophilia A. Haematologica 2003;88:778.

434b. Ahmed R, Kannan M, Choudhry VP, et al. Mutation reports: Intron 1 and 22 inversions in Indian haemophilics. Ann Hematol 2003;82:546.

434c. Lorey FW, Arnopp J, Cunningham GC. Distribution of hemoglobinopathy variants by ethnicity in a multiethnic state. Genet Epidemiol 1996;13:501.

435. Chang JC, Kan YW. A sensitive new prenatal test for sickle cell anemia. N Engl J Med 1982;307:30.

436. Saiki RK, Scharf S, Faloona F, et al. Enzymatic amplification of β-globin genomic sequences and restriction site analysis for diagnosis of sickle cell anemia. Science 1985;230:1350.

437. Mullis KB, Faloona FA. Specific synthesis of DNA in vitro via a polymerase-catalyzed chain reaction. Methods Enzymol 1987;155:335.

438. Saiki RK, Chang CA, Levenson CH, et al. Diagnosis of sickle cell anemia and β-thalassemia with enzymatically amplified DNA and nonradioactive allele-specific oligonucleotide probes. N Engl J Med 1988;319:537.

439. Riordan JR, Rommens JM, Kerem B-S, et al. Identification of the cystic fibrosis gene: cloning and characterization of complementary DNA. Science 1989;245:1066.

440. Rommens JM, Iannuzzi MC, Kerem B-S, et al. Identification of the cystic fibrosis gene: chromosome walking and jumping. Science 1989;245:1059.

441. Campbell PW III, Phillips JA III, Krishnamani MRS, et al. Cystic fibrosis: relationship between clinical status and F508. J Pediatr 1991;118:239.

442. Emery AEH. The muscular dystrophies. In: Emery AEH, Rimoin DL, eds. Principles and practice of medical genetics. Edinburgh: Churchill Livingstone, 1997:2337.

443. Love DR, Davies KE. Duchenne muscular dystrophy: the gene and the protein. Mol Biol Med 1989;6:7.

444. Francke U, Ochs HD, de Martinville B, et al. Minor Xp21 chromosome deletion in a male associated with expression of Duchenne muscular dystrophy, chronic granulomatous disease, retinitis pigmentosa and Macleod syndrome. Am J Hum Genet 1985;37:250.

445. Hoffman EP, Brown RH Jr, Kunkel LM. Dystrophin: The protein product of the Duchenne muscular dystrophy locus. Cell 1987;51:919.

446. Darras BT, Blattner P, Harper JF, et al. Intragenic deletions in 21 Duchenne muscular dystrophy (DMD)/Becker muscular dystrophy (BMD) families studied with the dystrophin cDNA: location of breakpoints on HindIII and BglII exon-containing fragment maps, meiotic and mitotic origin of mutations. Am J Hum Genet 1988;43:620.

447. Forrest SM, Cross GS, Flint T, et al. Further studies of gene deletions that cause Duchenne and Becker muscular dystrophies. Genomics 1988;2:109.

448. Chamberlain JS, Gibbs RA, Ranier JE, et al. Deletion screening of the Duchenne muscular dystrophy locus via multiplex DNA amplification. Nucleic Acids Res 1988;16:11141.

449. Chamberlain JS, Gibbs RA, Ranier JE, et al. Multiplex amplification for diagnosis of Duchenne's muscular dystrophy. In: Current communications in molecular biology: polymerase chain reaction. Cold Spring Harbor, NY: Cold Spring Harbor Laboratory Press, 1989:75.

450. Prior TW, Friedman KJ, Highsmith WE, et al. Molecular probe protocol for determining carrier status in Duchenne and Becker muscular dystrophies. Clin Chem 1990;36:441.

451. Huntington's Disease Collaborative Research Group. A novel gene containing a trinucleotide repeat that is expanded and unstable on Huntington's disease chromosomes. Cell 1993;72:971.

452. Strong TV, Tagle DA, Valdes JM, et al. Widespread expression of the human and rat Huntington's disease gene in brain and nonneural tissues. Nat Genetics 1993;5:259.

453. DeRooij KE, Dorsman JC, Smoor MA, et al. Subcellular localization of the Huntington's disease gene product in cell lines by immunofluorescence and biochemical subcellular fractionation. Hum Mol Genet 1996;5:1093.

454. Schilling G, Sharp AH, Loev SJ, et al. Expression of the Huntington's disease (1T15) protein product in HD patients. Hum Mol Genet 1995;4:1365.

455. Kremer B, Goldberg P, Andrew SE, et al. A worldwide study of the Huntington's disease mutation: the sensitivity and specificity of measuring CAG repeats. N Engl J Med 1994;330:1401.

456. Duyao M, Ambrose C, Myers R, et al. Trinucleotide repeat length instability and age of onset in Huntington's disease. Nat Genet 1993;4:387.

457. Nance M. Huntington disease: another chapter rewritten. Am J Hum Genet 1996;59:1.

458. Yokota I, Coates PM, Hale DE, et al. Molecular survey of a prevalent mutation, A to G transition and identification of five infrequent mutations in the medium chain acyl-CoA dehydrogenase (MCAD) gene in 55 patients with MCAD deficiency. Am J Hum Genet 1991;49:1280.

459. Matsubara Y, Narisawa K, Miyabayashi S, et al. Identification of a common mutation in patients with medium-chain acyl-CoA dehydrogenase deficiency. Biochem Biophys Res Commun 1990;171:498.

460. Pearn J. Incidence, prevalence, and gene frequency studies of chronic childhood spinal muscular atrophy. J Med Genet 1978;15:409.

461. Lefebvre S, Burglen L, Reboullet S, et al. Identification and characterization of a spinal muscular atrophy-determining gene. Cell 1995;80:155.

462. McAndrew PE, Parsons DW, Simard LR, et al. Identification of proximal spinal muscular atrophy carriers and patients by analysis of SMNT and SMNC gene copy number. Am J Hum Genet 1997;60:1411.

463. Mailman MD, Heinz JW, Papp AC, et al. Molecular analysis of spinal muscular atrophy and modification of the phenotype by SMN2. Genet Med 2002;4:20.

464. Velasco E, Valero C, Valero A, Moreno F, Hernandez-Chico C. Molecular analysis of the SMN and NAIP genes in Spanish spinal muscular atrophy (SMA) families and correlation between number of copies of cBCD 541 and SMA phenotype. Hum Mol Genet 1996;5:257.

465. Liu Q, Dreyruss G. A novel nuclear structure containing the survival of motor neurons protein. EMBO J 1996;15:3355.

466. Paw BH, Kaback MM, Neufeld EF. Molecular basis of adult-onset G_{M2} gangliosidoses in patients of Ashkenazi Jewish origin: Substitution of serine for glycine at position 269 of the α-subunit of β-hexosaminidase. Proc Natl Acad Sci USA 1989;86:2413.

467. Myerowitz R, Costigan FC. The major defect in Ashkenazi Jews with Tay Sachs disease is an insertion in the gene for the α-chain of β-hexosaminidase. J Biol Chem 1988;263:18587.

468. Shuber AP, Michalowky LA, Nass GS, et al. High throughput parallel analysis of hundreds of patient samples for more than 100 mutations in multiple disease gene. Hum Mol Genet 1997;6:337.

469. Kazazian HH Jr, Boehm CD. Molecular basis and prenatal diagnosis of β-thalassemia. Blood 1988;72:1107.

470. Gibbs RA, Nguyen PN, McBride LJ, et al. Identification of mutations leading to the Lesch-Nyhan syndrome by automated direct DNA sequencing of in vitro amplified cDNA. Proc Natl Acad Sci USA 1989;86:1919.

471. DiLella AG, Huang WM, Woo SLC. Screening for phenylketonuria mutations by DNA amplification with the polymerase chain reaction. Lancet 1988;I:497.

472. Gyllensten UB, Erlich HA. Generation of single-stranded DNA by the polymerase chain reaction and its application to direct sequencing of the HLA-DQA locus. Proc Natl Acad Sci USA 1988;85:7652.

473. Jeffreys AJ. DNA sequence variants in the $^G\gamma$-, $^A\gamma$, δ- and β-globin genes of man. Cell 1979;18:1.

474. Ewens WJ, Spielman RS, Harris H. Estimation of genetic variation at the DNA level from restriction endonuclease data. Proc Natl Acad Sci USA 1981;78:3748.

475. Brusilow SW, Horwich AL. Urea cycle enzymes. In: Scriver CS, Beaudet AL, Sly WS, et al., eds. The metabolic basis of inherited disease, 6th ed. New York: McGraw-Hill, 1989.

476. Hoshide R, Matsuura T, Haraguchi Y, et al. Carbamyl phosphate synthetase I deficiency: one base substitution in an exon of the CPS I gene causes a 9 base pair deletion due to aberrant splicing. J Clin Invest 1993;91:1884.

477. Summar et al. Personal communication, 1997.

478. Rodeck CH, Morsman JM. First-trimester chorion biopsy. Br Med Bull 1983;39:338.

479. Humphries SE, Williamson R. Application of recombinant DNA technology to prenatal detection of inherited defects. Br Med Bull 1983;39:343.

480. American College of Medical Genetics. Statement on storage and use of genetic materials. Am J Hum Genet 1995;57:1499.

481. Coutelle C, Williams C, Handyside A, et al. Genetic analysis from DNA from single human oocytes: a model for preimplantation diagnosis of cystic fibrosis. Br Med J 1989;299:22.

482. Navidi W, Arnheim N. Using PCR in preimplantation genetic disease diagnosis. Hum Reprod 1991;6:836.

483. Handyside AH, Lesko JG, Tarin JJ et al. Birth of a normal girl after in vitro fertilization and preimplantation diagnostic testing for cystic fibrosis. N Engl J Med 1992;327:905.

484. Kristjansson K, Chong SS, van den Veyver IB, et al. Preimplantation single cell analysis of dystrophin gene deletions using whole genome amplification. Nat Genet 1994;6:19.

485. Liu J, Lissens W, Selber SJ, et al. Birth after preimplantation diagnosis of the cystic fibrosis ΔF508 mutation by polymerase chain reaction in human embryos resulting from intracytoplasmic sperm injection with epididymal sperm. JAMA 1994;272:1858.

486. Snabes MC, Chong SS, Subramanian SB et al. Preimplantation single cell analysis of multiple genetic loci by whole-genome amplification. Proc Natl Acad Sci USA 1994;91:6181.

487. Ao A, Ray P, Harper J, et al. Clinical experience with preimplantation genetic diagnosis of cystic fibrosis. Prenat Diagn 1996;16:137.

488. Soussis I, Harper JC, Handyside AH, et al. Obstetric outcome of pregnancies resulting from embryos biopsied for preimplantation diagnosis of inherited disease. Br J Obstet Gynecol 1996;103:784.

489. Eldadah ZA, Grifs JA, Dietz HC. Marfan syndrome as a paradigm for transcript-targeted preimplantation diagnosis of heterozygous mutations. Nat Med 1995;8:798.

490. Gibbons WE, Gitlin SA, Lanzendorf SE. Strategies to respond to polymerase chain reaction deoxyribonucleic acid amplification failure in a preimplantation genetic diagnosis program. Am J Obstet Gynecol 1995;175:1088.

491. Dreesen JCFM, Bras M, Coonen E, et al. Allelic dropout caused by allele specific amplification failure in single-cell PCR of the cystic fibrosis ΔF508 deletion. J Assist Reprod Genet 1996;13:112.

492. Gitlin SA, Lanzendorf SE, Gibbons WE. Polymerase chain reaction amplification specificity: Incidence of allele dropout using different DNA preparation methods for heterozygous single cells. J Assist Reprod Genet 1996;13:107.

493. Ray PF, Winston RML, Handyside AH. Reduced allele dropout in single-cell analysis for preimplantation genetic diagnosis of cystic fibrosis. J Assist Reprod Genet 1996;13:104.

494. Kan YW, Dozy AM. Antenatal diagnosis of sickle cell anemia by DNA analysis of amniotic fluid cells. Lancet 1978;2:910.

Bryan G. Winchester, M.A., Ph.D., and
Elisabeth P. Young, B.Sc.

11

Prenatal Diagnosis of
Disorders of Lipid Metabolism

Most disorders of lipid metabolism are the result of defects in enzymes or nonenzymatic proteins located in lysosomes or peroxisomes[1–7] (Tables 11.1 through 11.4). In addition, mutations in plasma lipoproteins or lipoprotein receptors result in changes in the concentration of certain lipids in the blood and tissues, which can contribute to diseases, such as coronary heart disease[8] (see Table 11.5). Although defects in the metabolism of the different classes of lipids may appear initially to give rise to distinct clinical presentations and biochemical abnormalities, the metabolic pathways for these compounds are interconnected. Therefore, a defect in one pathway can have an impact on another to produce secondary effects and atypical symptoms. Lipids play important roles in many cellular processes, including development, differentiation and intracellular signaling.[9,10] Consequently, defects in their metabolism will affect many systems and give rise to a wide range of symptoms, including developmental delay and other neuropathies.

There has been a continual increase in the number of requests for diagnostic investigation of infants or children with developmental delay or unexplained regression. Defects in the lysosomal and peroxisomal metabolism of lipids remain largely untreatable. A few disorders in which there is little or no involvement of the central nervous system (CNS) can be treated by enzyme replacement therapy, by direct administration of recombinant human enzyme, or by bone marrow transplantation. The levels of cholesterol and other lipids in the lipoprotein-associated disorders can sometimes be controlled by drugs. In the absence of treatment for most of the lipid disorders, genetic counseling with the option of prenatal diagnosis is very important for families affected by one of these disorders. Reliable prenatal diagnosis depends on accurate diagnosis in the index case and a robust test for assaying the fetal material from the pregnancy at risk. A reliable method for the detection of carriers among family members will often be necessary. It is essential that the laboratory carrying out the prenatal diagnosis is experienced in handling fetal biopsies and carrying out and interpreting the assay procedure.

This chapter briefly describes the molecular basis and any genotype/phenotype correlation of each disorder and how this information is used for accurate diagnosis of patients, carrier detection and prenatal diagnosis. Detailed information regarding each disorder can be found in Scriver et al.,[11] Blau et al.,[12] and Applegarth et al.[13]

Table 11.1. Lysosomal disorders of lipid metabolism

Disorder	Major Storage Products	Measured Defect	Prenatal Diagnosis
GM_1 gangliosidosis	GM_1 ganglioside, glycoproteins, oligosaccharides	Acid β-galactosidase	CVS/CAC
Galactosialidosis	Glycoproteins oligosaccharides	Acid β-galactosidase and sialidase	CVS/CAC
GM_2 gangliosidosis			
B variant (Tay-Sachs/B1 variant)	GM_2 ganglioside	Hexosaminidase A	CVS/CAC
O variant (Sandhoff)	GM_2 ganglioside, GA_2, globoside	Hexosaminidase A and B	CVS/CAC
AB variant	GM_2 ganglioside, GA_2	GM_2 activator protein Lipid loading/Ab mutations	Cultured CVS Mutations
Fabry disease	Trihexosylceramide	α-galactosidase	CVS/CAC
Gaucher disease SAP-C deficiency	Glucosylceramide	β-glucosidase mutations/Ab	CVS/CAC Mutations
Metachromatic leukodystrophy	Sulfatide	Arylsulfatase A or SAP-B (SAP-1)	CVS/CAC Cultured CVS Mutations
Multiple sulfatase deficiency	Sulfatide, mucopolysaccharides	Most sulfatases	CVS/CAC
Krabbe disease	Galactosylceramide, psychosine	Galactocerebrosidase	CVS/CAC
Niemann–Pick disease			
Types A and B	Sphingomyelin, cholesterol	Sphingomyelinase	CVS/CAC
Type C (NPC1 and NPC2)	Cholesterol, sphingomyelin, glycolipids	Cholesterol esterification	Cultured CVS Mutations
Farber disease	Ceramide	Acid ceramidase	CVS/CAC Lipid loading
Wolman disease and cholesteryl ester storage disease	Cholesteryl esters and triglycerides	Acid lipase	CVS/CAC
Prosaposin deficiency	Glycosphingolipids	Lipid loading in fibroblasts	Cultured CVS Mutations

CAC = cultured amniotic fluid cells; CVS = chorionic villi samples; SAP = sphingolipid activator protein; Ab = antibody detection.

Table 11.2. Neuronal ceroid lipofuscinoses

Gene	Clinical Type	Storage	Prenatal Diagnosis
CLN 1	Infantile, late infantile and juvenile	GROD	Enzyme assay, DNA (histology)
CLN2	Late infantile	CL	Enzyme assay, DNA (histology)
CLN3	Juvenile	FP	DNA, histology
CLN4	Adult	CL/FP/GROD	—
CLN5	Finnish variant late infantile	FP/CL	DNA, histology
CLN6	Early juvenile/variant late infantile	FP/CL	DNA, histology
CLN7	Early juvenile / variant late infantile	FP/CL	DNA, histology
CLN8	Northern epilepsy	CL	DNA, histology

GROD = granular osmiophilic deposits; CL = curvilinear profiles; FP = fingerprint profiles.

Table 11.3.   Biochemical abnormalities in patients with peroxisome biogenesis disorders

Abnormal Metabolite or Function	Analysis Material	Zellweger Spectrum		
		Severe Form	Milder Forms	
		Zellweger Syndrome	Pseudo-Zellweger-Infantile Refsum Neonatal ALD	Rhizomelic Chrondrodysplasia Punctata
Very-long-chain fatty acids	Plasma, fibroblasts, chorion cells, amniocytes	↑ ↑	↑	—
Phytanic acid	Plasma, fibroblasts, chorion cells, amniocytes	↑	↑	↑ ↑
Pipecolic acid	Plasma, fibroblasts, chorion cells, amniocytes	↑ ↑	↑	—
Bile acid intermediates	Plasma, urine	↑ ↑	↑	—
Plasmalogen	Erythrocytes	↓	↓	↓ ↓
Plasmalogen biosynthesis	Fibroblasts, chorion cells, amniocytes	↓	↓	↓ ↓
Catalase import (PTS1 enzyme)	Fibroblasts, chorion cells, amniocytes	↓ ↓	↓ , ↓	—
Thiolase processing	Fibroblasts, chorion cells, amniocytes	↓	↓ or —	↓
Thiolase import (PTS2 enzyme)	Fibroblasts, chorion cells, amniocytes	↓ or —	↓ or —	↓

Source: After Brosius and Gartner, 2002.[7] Reprinted with permission.
    ↓ = decreased; ↓ ↓ = strongly decreased; ↑ = increased; ↑ = strongly increased; — = not affected;
PTS = peroxisomal targeting signal.

LYSOSOMAL STORAGE DISEASES: LIPIDOSES

The defects in lysosomal storage diseases were initially delineated in the 1960s, but our understanding of the molecular and cellular bases of these diseases continues to grow (Figure 11.1). Reliable methods for diagnosing patients and prenatal diagnosis in pregnancies at risk are available for all the lipidoses. The genes encoding most disease-associated lysosomal proteins have been cloned and disease-causing mutations, often family-specific, have been identified. This has permitted accurate early diagnosis and more reliable carrier detection, particularly for the X-linked disorders (e.g., Fabry disease and Hunter disease [MPS II]). It also raises the possibility of preimplantation diagnosis of affected embryos (see chapter 27). For most lysosomal disorders, mutation analysis has provided some insight into the causes of the clinical variability, although other genetic and environmental factors can clearly affect the severity and age of onset. Molecular genetics has also revealed that the so-called pseudodeficiencies of lysosomal enzymes are due to mutations or polymorphisms (pseudodeficiency alleles) that drastically decrease the activity of an enzyme without actually causing disease.[14] The decrease in enzymatic activity due to a pseudodeficiency allele or a disease-causing mutation cannot be distinguished by enzymatic assay, but a simple DNA test for the presence of the pseudodeficiency allele can usually resolve the problem.

The lysosomal catabolism of membrane-bound glycosphingolipids is brought about by soluble hydrolases in the lumen of lysosomes. Nature has developed two strategies for coping with this heterologous system, association of the enzymes with the lysosomal mem-

Table 11.4. Single peroxisomal enzyme protein deficiencies

Peroxisomal Function	Disorder/Clinical Phenotype	Enzyme/Protein Deficiency (*GENE*)[Reference]	Prenatal Diagnostic Tests
Fatty acid β-oxidation	X-Adrenoleukodystrophy	ALDP (*ABCD1*)	↑ VLCFA, DNA
	NALD-like	Straight chain acyl-CoA oxidase (*AOX*) (362)	↑ VLCFA, enzyme, DNA
	ZS/NALD-like	ᴅ-Bifunctional protein (*DBP*) (363–365)	↑ VLCFA, enzyme, DNA
	Late-onset neuropathy	α-methyl-acyl-CoA racemase (*AMACR*) (365)	‡ ↑ pristanic acid and C27 bile acid intermediates, enzyme, DNA*
Ether phospholipid synthesis	Rhizomelic chondrodysplasia punctata type 2	Dihydroxyacetone phosphate acyltransferase-DHAPAT (*DHAPAT*) (310)	↓ Plasmalogen analysis DHAPAT activity DNA
	Rhizomelic chondrodysplasia punctata type 3	Alkyl-DHAP synthase deficiency (315)	↓ Plasmalogen analysis Alkyl-DHAP activity DNA
Fatty acid α-oxidation	Refsum disease	Phytanoyl-CoA hydroxylase deficiency	↑ Phytanic acid Phytanoyl-CoA hydroxylase assay DNA
Isoprenoid biosynthesis	Classical MK-deficiency Hyper IgD/periodic fever syndrome	Mevalonate kinase deficiency (*MVK*) (366–368)	Mevalonate kinase assay DNA
Pipecolic acid degradation	Isolated hyperpipecolic acidemia	Isolated hyperpipecolic acidemias (310)	‡
Glutaryl-CoA metabolism	Glutaric aciduria type 3	Glutaryl-CoA oxidase deficiency (369)	‡
Hydrogen peroxide metabolism	Acatalasemia	Catalase deficiency (370)	Yes
Glyoxylate detoxification	Hyperoxaluria type 1	Alanine:glyoxylate aminotransferase deficiency (*AXGT*) (371,372)	Alanine:glyoxylate aminotransferase assay in liver DNA

‡Prenatal diagnosis not reported.
Key reference if not mentioned in text.

461

Table 11.5. Monogenic lipoprotein-associated disorders

Disorder (Inheritance)	Main Features	Observed Plasma Lipoprotein Pattern	Gene Responsible	Key Reference
Apolipoprotein disorders				
Apo-A deficiencies				
Type I (AR)	CHD, corneal clouding	↓HDL	Apo-A-I and C-III	381
Type II (AR)	CHD, corneal clouding	↓HDL	Apo-A-I, C-III, A-IV[a]	382
Type III (AR)		↓HDL	Apo-A-I	383
Hypobetalipoproteinemia (AD)	Fat malabsorption, retinal degeneration, anemia, neuromuscular weakness, Mild	↓apo-B lipoproteins (chylomicrons, VLDL LDL)	Apo-B	373
Familial ligand-defective apo-B, FLBD (AD)	Mild increased risk for CHD	↑LDL	Apo-B	373
Apolipoprotein C-II deficiency (AR)	Acute pancreatitis, anemia, eruptive xanthomas	↑Chylomicrons, VLDL	Apo-C-II	384
Type III Hyperlipoproteinemia (dysbetalipoproteinemia) (AR and AD)	Cutaneous xanthomas, atherosclerosis	↑Chylomicron remnants, VLDL	Apo-E	385
Enzyme disorders				
Familial lipoprotein lipase deficiency (AR)	Abdominal pain, HSM, pancreatitis, cutaneous xanthomas	↑Chylomicrons	Lipoprotein lipase	384
Hepatic triglyceride lipase (AR)	Increased risk for CHD	Altered HDL	HTGL	384
Familial LCAT deficiency and fish-eye disease (AR)	Corneal clouding, anemia, proteinuria, uremia	↓HDL	LCAT	386
Receptor/transport disorders				
Familial hypercholesterolemia (AD)	CHD, tendon xanthomas	↑LDL	LDL receptor[b]	374
Cholesteryl ester transfer protein deficiency (NK)	Normal	Altered HDL	CETP	383
Abetalipoproteinemia (AR)	Fat malabsorption, retinal degeneration, anemia, neuromuscular weakness	↓Apo-B lipoproteins (chylomicrons, VLDL, LDL)	Large subunit of microsomal triglyceride transfer protein	387 / 373
Other				
Tangier disease (AR) ATP-binding cassette transporter 1 ABC1	Corneal clouding, orange Tonsils, neuropathy	↓HDL	ABC1	388

ABC1 = ATP-binding cassette transporter; 1; AD = autosomal dominant; apo = apolipoprotein; AR = autosomal recessive; CETP = cholesterol ester transfer protein; CHD = coronary heart disease; HDL = high-density lipoproteins; HSM = hepatosplenomegaly; HTGL = hepatic triglyceride lipase; LCAT = lecithin cholesterol acyltransferase; LDL = low-density lipoproteins; VLDL = very-low-density lipoproteins.

[a] A-I, C-III, and A-IV are adjacent genes

[b] Homozygotes are more affected.

462

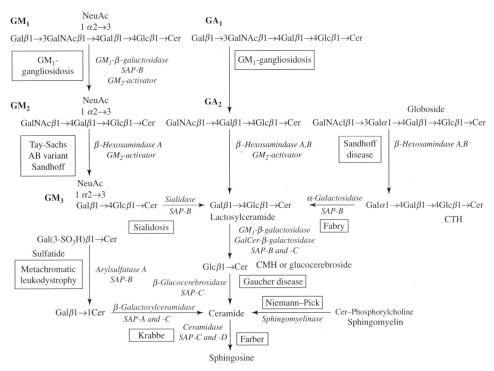

Fig. 11.1. Lysosomal catabolism of some glycosphingolipids. Cer = ceramide; CTH = ceramide trihexoside; Gal = galactose; Glc = glucose; NAc = N-acetyl; NeuAc = N-acetyl neuraminic acid; SAP = sphingolipid activator protein.

brane and the use of nonenzymic protein detergents and cofactors. β-Glucocerebrosidase, which cleaves the β-glucosylceramide core linkage found in most extraneural glycosphingolipids, associates with the membrane, enabling it to interact directly with its predominantly hydrophobic substrate. If the glycan of a glycosphingolipid is longer than a tetrasaccharide, it can be hydrolyzed by the glycosidases alone, but the degradation of shorter glycans requires the assistance of a nonenzymic protein cofactor or sphingolipid activator protein (saposin, or SAP).[15,16] To date, two genes are known to encode sphingolipid activator proteins. One encodes the GM_2 activator protein, which facilitates the action of hexosaminidase A on ganglioside GM_2[17] and is deficient in the AB-variant of GM_2-gangliosidosis. The other gene encodes prosaposin (or sap-precursor),[18] which is proteolytically processed sequentially from the N-terminal end to four homologous saposins, A–D, with specificities for different sphingolipids. A deficiency of prosaposin leads to the accumulation of a range of glycosphingolipids.[19] The activities of SAP-B, the GM_2 activator protein and β-glucocerebrosidase, are also stimulated by acidic lipids, such as phosphatidylserine or phosphatidylinositol and bis(monoacyl)glycerophosphate. In the laboratory most lipid hydrolases are assayed using water-soluble synthetic substrates, obviating the need for detergents, or, by using natural substrates in the presence of added detergent. Consequently, a deficiency of a sphingolipid activator protein can be missed using such assays. If there is strong clinical indication of a lipidosis but the enzyme activity appears to be normal, a deficiency of a sphingolipid activator protein should be considered. In contrast multiple deficiencies of lysosomal hydrolases can arise because of defects in the posttranslational modification of lysosomal enzyme precursors. In mucolipidosis II (I-cell disease) and III, the soluble lysosomal hydrolases fail to acquire the lysosomal recognition marker, mannose-6-phosphate, and are diverted from the lysosomes to the extracellular compartment in many cell types, including fibroblasts, white blood cells, cultured amniotic fluid cells (CAC) and chorionic villi (CV). The assay of two or more relevant enzymes can distinguish between mucolipidosis II/III and a genuine single enzyme deficiency. Similarly, in multiple sulfatase deficiency (mucosulfatidosis), the activities of all lysosomal sulfatases, including arylsulfatase A, which is deficient in metachromatic leukodystrophy, are defective. This is due to a defect in the enzyme that catalyses the modification of a common active site cysteine, which is essential for sulfatase activity.[20]

The availability of enzyme replacement therapy for the non-neuronal form of Gaucher disease, type 1[21] and Fabry disease[22,23] will continue to lead to a decrease in requests for prenatal diagnosis of these disorders. Enzyme replacement therapy for Niemann–Pick B using recombinant human sphingomyelinase is imminent. Treatment by substrate deprivation[24,25] is under trial for Gaucher disease type 1,[26] Fabry disease, and Niemann–Pick C disease, and is being used on a named patient basis for GM$_2$-gangliosidosis. Bone marrow transplantation is considered an option for metachromatic leukodystrophy, globoid cell leukodystrophy, Gaucher disease type 3, and Hurler disease (MPS I).[27] Because early commencement of treatment is beneficial, considerable effort is going into developing methods for newborn screening of lysosomal storage diseases.[28] Early diagnosis and therapy will make a significant impact on genetic counseling and prenatal diagnosis of the lipidoses.

There are several reviews of the diagnosis of lysosomal storage diseases[12,29–33] and two comprehensive reviews of the prenatal diagnosis of lysosomal storage diseases.[34,35]

GM$_1$-Gangliosidosis/MPS IVB

A deficiency of acidic β-galactosidase (EC 3.2.1.23) is the underlying defect in two autosomal recessive, lysosomal storage diseases, GM$_1$-gangliosidosis and Morquio disease type B (mucopolysaccharidosis IVB).[36,37] These disorders represent the two extremes in a spectrum of clinical phenotype resulting from mutations in the β-galactosidase gene. β-Galactosidase has a relatively wide specificity and acts on $\beta1 \rightarrow 4$ galactosidic linkages in N-glycans and keratan sulfate and $\beta1 \rightarrow 3$ and $\beta1 \rightarrow 4$ galactosidic linkages in glycolipids. Therefore, a deficiency of the enzyme leads to a mixture of storage products, the composition of which depends on the underlying mutations. A secondary deficiency of β-galactosidase can arise from defects in the protective protein-cathepsin A (galactosialidosis).[38] The hydrolysis of GM$_1$-ganglioside and lactosylceramide are stimulated in vitro by saposin B and saposins B and C, respectively,[39] but mutations in saposin B do not give rise to the GM$_1$-gangliosidosis or Morquio disease phenotype. A second, genetically distinct lysosomal β-galactosidase, galactocerebrosidase, which acts on galactosylceramide and galactosylsphingosine, is deficient in globoid cell leukodystrophy.

Historically, GM$_1$-gangliosidosis has been classified into three forms, infantile type 1, late infantile/juvenile type 2, and adult/chronic type 3, with the majority of patients having type 1. GM$_1$-ganglioside and its asialo derivative GA$_1$ accumulate in the brain in all three types, and galactose-terminated oligosaccharides are excreted in the urine of types 1 and 2. Some glycosaminoglycan derived from keratan sulfate is excreted in the urine of patients with type 1, who have severe skeletal dysplasia, but it is not believed to contribute to the pathology. The amount of residual enzymic activity and the level of storage material correlate with the severity and rate of neurologic deterioration. In contrast, keratan sulfate is the major storage product in patients with Morquio B, but it is different from that excreted by patients with GM_1-gangliosidosis type 1. Patients with Morquio B have extensive skeletal dysplasia but normal intelligence. There is no CNS involvement consistent with lack of storage of GM_1-ganglioside. However, the biochemical and clinical distinction between the GM_1-gangliosidosis and Morquio B disease is disappearing, as more cases are investigated in depth. More than 40 different mutations have been found in the *BGAL* gene,[40] including nonsense, frameshift and splice-site mutations, duplications, insertions and a predominance of missense mutations. GM_1-gangliosidosis is extremely heterogeneous, and there is no obvious relationship between the type and position of the mutation and the phenotype. Most mutations give rise to no activity in expression studies, and combinations of such mutations give rise to the severe infantile form of the disease. Mutations with measurable residual activity are associated with the juvenile, adult and Morquio B variants[41] in either homozygotes or compound heterozygotes. The second allele can modify the rate of progression of the disease in adult GM_1-gangliosidosis, and individuals homozygous for the mild mutations may be asymptomatic.[42] A common mutation and mutations in a specific domain of β-galactosidase are associated with the Morquio B phenotype.[40,41] Currently, there is no effective treatment for GM_1-gangliosidosis, but substrate depletion using drugs that can cross the blood–brain barrier may be applicable. In contrast, Morquio B disease in which there is no neurologic involvement should be amenable to enzyme replacement therapy.

Definitive diagnosis of GM_1-gangliosidosis and Morquio B disease is based on demonstrating a deficiency of acidic β-galactosidase activity in leukocytes, or cultured skin fibroblasts, typically using the synthetic substrate, 4-methylumbelliferyl-β-D-galactopyranoside.[37] Carriers can be identified by testing for the mutations in the index case. Prenatal diagnosis of GM_1-gangliosidosis and Morquio B disease can be achieved by assaying the β-galactosidase activity directly in chorionic villi samples (CVS), cultured chorionic villi cells (CCV) and in CAC.[34,35,37]

GM_2-Gangliosidoses

The GM_2-gangliosidoses are characterized by massive accumulation of GM_2-gangliosides and related lipids in lysosomes, predominantly in neurons, due to a deficiency of β-N-acetyl-D-hexosaminidase (EC 3.2.1.52) activity.[43] Three gene products are involved in the lysosomal catabolism of GM_2-gangliosides, the α- and β-subunits of β-N-acetyl-D-hexosaminidase (*HEXA* and *HEXB*) on chromosomes 15 and 5, respectively, and the GM_2-activator protein (*GM2A*) also on chromosome 5.[43,44] The monomeric subunits of β-N-acetyl-D-hexosaminidase have inactive catalytic sites but combine to form active dimers, known as hexosaminidase A ($\alpha\beta$), hexosaminidase B ($\beta\beta$), and hexosaminidase S ($\alpha\alpha$). All these forms of hexosaminidase are specific for the hydrolysis of terminal, nonreducing β-glycosidically linked N-acetylglucosamine or N-acetylgalactosamine. However, they have different substrate specificities because of differences in the specificities of the catalytic sites on the α- and β-subunits. The α-subunit catalytic site can act on neutral or negatively charged glycolipids, oligosaccharides, glycosaminoglycans, and synthetic substrates. In contrast, the β-subunit acts preferentially on neutral, water-soluble, natural, and synthetic substrates. To be degraded in vivo, lipophilic GM_2-gangliosides must combine with the GM_2-activator protein, which lifts the gangliosides out of membranes and presents the hydrophilic oligosaccharide moiety to the water-soluble enzyme.[39,45] Only hexosaminidase A ($\alpha\beta$) can act on the GM_2-ganglioside/GM_2-activator protein complex. In addition to GM_2-ganglioside, a range of other glycolipids and oligosaccharides accumulate in the GM_2-gangliosidoses, depending on which gene is mutated. GM_2-gangliosidosis can arise from a defect in any of the three genes, *HEXA, HEXB* or *GM2A*.[44] The resultant forms or variants of GM_2-gangliosidosis are very similar clinically, but all present with a wide range of severity and age of onset. No effective therapy is available for treating these disorders. All three genes have been cloned, and the identification of a wide range of different mutations in each gene has provided a basis for much of the clinical variation in GM_2-gangliosidosis. The crystal structures of human hexosaminidase B[46,47] and the GM_2-activator protein[48] have been elucidated recently, allowing the subsequent molecular modeling of hexosaminidase A. These structures show how the active dimers are formed, the molecular basis of their substrate specificities, and how point mutations in the genes cause the different forms of GM_2-gangliosidosis.

Mutations in the *HEXA* gene lead to a deficiency of hexosaminidase A ($\alpha\beta$) and hexosaminidase S ($\alpha\alpha$) but the hexosaminidase B ($\beta\beta$) activity is normal. Patients with a deficiency of hexosaminidase A are called B variants because hexosaminidase B is present. More than 100 different mutations have been reported in the *HEXA* gene,[43,46] database at http://www.medgen.mcgill.ca. Combinations of null alleles, such as all the nonsense mutations and the deletions and insertions that produce frameshifts and most of the splice-site mutations, give rise to the severe infantile form of GM_2-gangliosidosis, or classic infantile Tay–Sachs disease. The incidence of infantile Tay–Sachs disease is high in certain ethnic groups because of founder effects; it has been estimated to be 1 in 2,500 live births in Ashkenazi Jews[43] with three mutations accounting for more than 98 percent of mutant alleles.[48a] Many other combinations of null alleles cause infantile Tay–Sachs disease in individual non-Jewish families. If the family is consanguineous, the patients are generally homozygous for a rare mutation, if not they are usually compound heterozygotes for a recurrent mutation and a rare mutation. Typical patients with Tay–Sachs disease present between 3 and 6 months of age with loss of interest in surroundings, hypotonia, poor head control, apathy, and an abnormal startle response to sharp sounds.[43] Deafness, blindness, seizures, and generalized spasticity are usually evident by 18 months of age. Bilateral cherry-red spots in the macula caused by perimacular lipid deposition and macrocephaly are almost always present. Death from respiratory infection usually occurs between 3 and 5 years. The number of Jewish cases has dropped because of screening programs, and most patients diagnosed now are non-Jewish.

Juvenile patients and adult patients with deficiency of hexosaminidase A have been described.[43,49] Juvenile patients usually present between 2 and 8 years of age with ataxia and progressive psychomotor retardation. Loss of speech, progressive spasticity, athetoid posturing of hands and extremities, and minor motor seizures become evident. Neuronal storage of GM_2-ganglioside similar to classic Tay–Sachs disease can be found. A number of adult patients with spinocerebellar degeneration (ataxia, muscle atrophy, pes cavus, foot drop, spasticity, and dysarthria) with or without psychoses have been demonstrated to have a defect in hexosaminidase A.[50,51] Some of these patients were originally considered to be healthy people with low hexosaminidase A activity.[52] Any infant, child, or adult with psychomotor retardation and regression with no known cause should be a candidate for enzymatic testing for hexosaminidase A levels. The tests are simple and reliable and will result in a diagnosis of a small, but significant, number of people.

Most patients are readily diagnosed using the fluorogenic substrate 4-methylumbelliferyl-2-acetamido-2-deoxy-β-D-glucopyranoside (MU-β-GlcNAc),[53,54] but others can be diagnosed only using the natural substrate or a sulfated fluorogenic substrate, 4-methy-lumbelliferyl-6-sulfo-2-acetamido-2-deoxy-β-D-glucopyranoside (MU-β-GlcNAcS).[55] For prenatal diagnosis, it has become the substrate of choice. The diagnosis of patients with a defect in the α-chain of hexosaminidase A requires accurate determination of hexosaminidase A in the presence of hexosaminidase B. Methods for differentiating the two isozymes have been developed because both hexosaminidase A and B hydrolyze MU-β-GlcNAc. They include heat denaturation (hexosaminidase A is unstable),[53] pH-inactivation of hexosaminidase A,[56] and separation of hexosaminidases A and B on small ion-exchange columns.[57] Many laboratories use the heat denaturation method, which has proved to be useful for diagnosis in most cases. Most patients of all age groups have a severe deficiency of hexosaminidase A, usually 0–10 percent of the total hexosaminidase activity, compared with 58–70 percent of the total hexosaminidase activity in controls. Some juvenile patients have been reported to have up to 25 percent hexosaminidase A activity,[58,59] but with hindsight these may have been B1 variants.

B1 Variant

Some patients have near normal levels of hexosaminidase A activity when measured with the neutral, synthetic substrate, MU-β-GlcNAc but a marked deficiency of hexosaminidase A activity with either the natural substrate or MU-β-GlcNAcS.[60] These patients, who were probably undiagnosed in the past, are called B1 variants to differentiate them from classic Tay–Sachs patients, the B variant. This change in specificity of the enzyme was shown to be due to a mutation, R178H (DN allele), which inactivates the α-subunit[61] but does not affect the association of the α- and β-subunits or the activity of the β-subunit. As a result, the mutant dimeric hexosaminidase A behaves like hexosaminidase B and hydrolyzes uncharged substrates predominantly. Homozygotes for this B1 mutation have the juvenile disease, but compound heterozygotes for the B1 mutation and a null allele have a more severe phenotype with late infantile onset.[62,63] Two other mutations, which occur in the same codon, R178C and R178L, produce a more severe, acute B1-like phenotype. Arginine 178 is in the active site cleft of the α-subunit and another mutation in the α-subunit active site, D258H, also results in the B1 variant phenotype.[64]

Pseudodeficiency

Two benign mutations in the *HEXA* gene[65] lead to a pseudodeficiency of hexosaminidase A,[66] in which the α-subunit loses activity toward synthetic substrates but retains activity toward GM_2-ganglioside and does not, therefore, cause disease. The loss of activity toward the synthetic substrates is due to a decrease in stability rather than to a change in substrate recognition which is suprising because the mutations are in the active site of the enzyme. These two mutations are responsible for most false-positive results in the enzyme-based screening for Tay–Sachs carriers. Fortunately, their frequency in the Ashkenazi Jewish population is very low.

Hexosaminidase S

Hexosaminidase S ($\alpha\alpha$), which is also deficient in the B variant, is more active than hexosaminidase A toward sulfated glycolipids such as SM_2 in the presence of the GM_2-activator protein and sulfated oligosaccharides.[67] Mice with the double knockout of *Hexa* and *Hexb* show signs of mucopolysaccharidosis as well as GM_2-gangliosidosis. This suggests that β-hexosaminidase has a role in the degradation of glycosaminoglycans.[68] Human patients with deficiencies of both the α- and β-subunits of hexosaminidase have not been reported.

Carrier Detection

Reliable Tay–Sachs disease carrier identification in serum samples has led to the mass screening of Ashkenazi Jewish communities around the world. Currently, more than 1,000,000 people have been screened to determine whether they are carriers of this autosomal recessive disease.[69] Because of the success of the Tay–Sachs carrier-testing program in the Ashkenazi Jewish population, most patients diagnosed with Tay–Sachs disease today are not Jewish. The carrier frequency is about 1 in 25 in Ashkenazi Jews and about 1 in 150 in the general population. Accurate heterozygote detection is possible by demonstrating intermediate levels of hexosaminidase A activity in serum and leukocytes. Carrier identification in the Jewish population can also be performed by mutation analysis because three mutations account for 98 percent of the mutant alleles.[43,44,48a] Mutation analysis has some important advantages. It can identify mutations causing infantile and adult forms, and the so-called pseudodeficiency mutations.[70,71] After a mutation has been identified in a family, other family members can be tested by rapid, accurate DNA analysis.

Serum and plasma are not suitable for carrier detection in pregnant women. However, carriers can be identified accurately by studies of hexosaminidase A in mixed leukocytes.[69] Also some noncarrier women taking oral contraceptives have been found to have reduced hexosaminidase A so leukocyte studies are again recommended.

Tay–Sachs disease was among the first lysosomal storage diseases to be diagnosed prenatally using CVS.[72] In noncultivated CV, measurement of hexosaminidase A directly using MU-β-GlcNAcS is the most accurate method to diagnose a fetus affected with Tay–Sachs disease. Most studies can be completed within hours of sampling.[73] Cultured CV cells can be used to confirm the preliminary studies on direct CVS. The assay is also reliable in CAC. Prenatal diagnosis of Tay–Sachs disease is available for couples with previously affected children and couples identified at risk in carrier testing programs,[43] with the latter group in the majority. The proportion of fetuses identified with Tay–Sachs disease is considerably less than the expected 25 percent because tests are carried out in pregnancies in which it is not known definitely that both parents are carriers (e.g., when there are inconclusive heterozygote screening results and to reassure an obligate carrier with a new partner). When both mutations are known, DNA-based diagnosis is very reliable, highly specific, and preferred.[48a] It is also particularly important for exclusion of the pseudodeficiency alleles.

Mutations in β-subunit

Mutations in the β-subunit lead to a combined deficiency of β-hexosaminidase A and B or Sandhoff disease (GM$_2$-gangliosidosis 0 variant). More than 25 mutations have been reported.[44,46] Most are associated with the severe infantile form of the disease, which is clinically identical to classic infantile Tay–Sachs disease, with the possible exception of the presence of hepatomegaly in some cases.[43] There is no ethnic predilection for this autosomal recessive disease. Juvenile and adult cases also have been described.[43,74] GM$_2$-ganglioside and its asialo derivative (GA$_2$) accumulate in the brain, and globoside, a major red blood cell glycosphingolipid, accumulates in the visceral organs.[43] There is less than 10 percent of the total, normal, hexosaminidase activity, measured with MU-β-GlcNAc substrate in serum, plasma, leukocytes, fibroblasts, or tissues[43,44,75] of affected children. A significant amount of residual activity is found if MU-β-GlcNAcS is used for the diagnosis of Sandhoff disease because of the presence of excess α-chains that combine to form hexosaminidase S ($\alpha\alpha$), which is able to hydrolyze the MU-β-GlcNAcS. Carriers have a lower total hexosaminidase activity but a higher percentage of hexosaminidase A than controls. Leukocytes and plasma can be used for carrier identification[76,77] but, as in Tay–Sachs disease, plasma is not suitable for carrier detection in pregnant women or women taking the oral contraceptive pill. Reliable carrier detection is achieved by DNA analysis. Prenatal diagnosis is possible by measuring the total hexosaminidase activity with MU-β-GlcNAc in CV directly, CCV cells, and CAC. A mutation in the β-subunit causing a pseudodeficiency of hexosaminidase A and B can cause problems with enzymic diagnosis, especially when it occurs in the same family as a Sandhoff mutation.[78] The problem can be resolved by DNA analysis.

Variant AB

A deficiency of the GM$_2$-activator protein due to mutations in *GM2A* gene (variant AB) prevents the formation of the GM$_2$-ganglioside/GM$_2$-activator protein complex and a loss of hexosaminidase A activity toward GM$_2$-ganglioside.[17] Five mutations in the *GM2A* gene leading to a deficiency of the GM$_2$-activator protein have been discovered to date.[39,44,46] They all occur in the homozygous state and lead to a severe infantile form of GM$_2$-gangliosidosis. The activities of hexosaminidases A and B toward the synthetic soluble substrates are unaffected, making diagnosis of this variant difficult both prenatally and postnatally. GM$_2$-activator activity can be measured in vitro by its ability to stimulate hydrolysis of GM$_2$-ganglioside by purified hexosaminidase A[60] or by the hydrolysis of radiolabeled GM$_2$-ganglioside in cells in culture.[79] A deficiency of the GM$_2$-activator protein can also be demonstrated by an ELISA method.[80] Identification of the mutation in the index case is essential for reliable carrier detection and can be helpful for prenatal diagnosis.

Fabry Disease

Fabry disease is an X-linked lipidosis resulting from a deficiency of α-galactosidase A (EC 3.2.1.22).[81] It is characterized biochemically by the progressive accumulation within lysosomes of glycosphingolipids with terminal α-galactosyl residues: globotriaosylceramide and to a lesser extent galabiosylceramide and blood group AB- and B-related glycolipids. Storage occurs predominantly in the endothelial, perithelial, and smooth muscle cells of blood vessels, but there is deposition in many other cell types. Fine sudanophilic, periodic acid–Schiff (PAS)-positive granules and foamy storage cells are found in tissues of patients, and bone marrow samples show granular material in the histiocytes. The levels of storage products in the urine and plasma are elevated in most but not all patients with Fabry disease. The elevation reflects the clinical severity and progression of the disease and may be used to monitor the progress of the disease and conversely treatment.[82]

Male hemizygotes with Fabry disease usually present with pain in the extremities, lack of sweating, unexplained proteinuria, attacks of fever, corneal atrophy, and the presence of purple skin lesions.[81] Similar purple skin lesions have been found in patients with fucosidosis, GM$_1$-gangliosidosis, sialidosis, galactosialidosis, and Schindler disease (α-galactosaminidase deficiency). Although most patients present in the second decade of life, some present before 5 years of age and others in the fourth decade of life. As the disease progresses, there are symptoms and signs related to easy fatigability (due to storage in skeletal muscle), poor vision (corneal opacities, tortuosity of retinal and conjunctival vessels, and cataracts), and high blood pressure (due to continued vascular storage). The storage can lead to cardiac or renal failure in the third or fourth decade. There is negligible residual α-galactosidase activity and mostly no detectable α-galactosidase protein in male hemizygotes with typical clinical presentation. A group of atypical patients, who lack the typical early symptoms, present with a late-onset cardiomyopathy or cardiomegaly. These patients and other patients, who may be asymptomatic or mildly affected, do generally have residual activity. Paradoxically, several male patients with classic clinical symptoms have been reported with normal activity in vitro. The α-galactosidase activity in female heterozygotes for all variants ranges from near zero to normal due to random inactivation of the X-chromosome. Heterozygotes can reliably be detected only by molecular genetic techniques.[83] Only a few female heterozygotes are asymptomatic, and some are as severely affected as typical hemizygotes. Their symptoms may be confined to a single organ because of the pattern of the X-inactivation (e.g., in some female patients the characteristic corneal and retinal changes may be the only indication). The extreme of this mosaicism is seen in two identical female twin carriers who showed very different phenotypes because of uneven X-inactivation.[84] There is no correlation between activity measured in plasma or white blood cells, genotype, and severity in heterozygotes.

The *GLA* gene has been fully characterized[85,86] and over 200 different mutations have been reported. Most mutations are private and all except a few missense mutations give rise to null alleles and the classic phenotype in hemizygotes. The "cardiac variants" have missense mutations that give rise to residual α-galactosidase A activity.[87,88] Other atypical patients with a slower course of the disease or limited range of symptoms have missense mutations,[89] suggesting that there is a spectrum of phenotypes depending on the amount and distribution of the residual α-galactosidase A activity. Some of the mutations found in these variants are also found in patients with the classic phenotype,[90] and intrafamilial variation is found with some null alleles,[91] suggesting that other factors affect the phenotype. Manifesting females with decreased α-galactosidase A activity but no proven mutations in the *GLA* gene are also known,[92] and 0.5 percent of normal individuals have a mutation that gives rise to elevated plasma α-galactosidase A.[93] It is important to be aware of these genetic variations when making an enzymatic diagnosis of Fabry disease.

The X-ray structure of the closely related enzyme, α-*N*-acetylgalactosaminidase (α-NAGAL), has been elucidated[94] and a model of α-galactosidase A constructed based on this structure.[95] Location of known mutations in the α-galactosidase A protein on the model has shown that they fall into two classes, active site mutations decreasing the enzymic activity and ones that destabilize the folding of the protein. This model will be useful in predicting the effect of novel mutations and in formulating rational approaches for therapy in individual patients.

The definitive diagnosis of Fabry disease is based on demonstrating a deficiency of α-galactosidase A activity in leukocytes,[96] serum or plasma,[97] or cultured skin fibroblasts.[98] The fluorogenic substrate, 4-methylumbelliferyl-α-D-galactopyranoside (MU-α-Gal) is widely used as the substrate. α-*N*-acetylgalactosaminidase (also called α-galactosidase B) also acts on this synthetic substrate and a specific inhibitor, *N*-acetylgalactosamine,[99] is added to the assay to eliminate this activity, which could mask a deficiency of α-galactosidase A. Heterozygote detection in family members is now carried out by DNA analysis.

Prenatal diagnosis of Fabry disease can be made by measuring α-galactosidase A activity in CV directly, CCV and CAC.[81,100] Fetal sex determination is performed to support the diagnosis of an affected male and to exclude females from further testing, although there is no way to predict which females will have significant health problems related to their carrier status for Fabry disease. If the family mutation in the α-galactosidase A gene is known, then detection of the mutation in the fetal sample provides confirmation and is essential for the genetic variants mentioned above.

The major cause of death in patients with typical Fabry disease is renal failure, and hemodialysis and renal transplantation have become life-saving procedures.[101–103] Although transplantation improves renal clearance, no improvement of other symptoms is observed consistently.[104] Fabry disease is amenable to enzyme replacement therapy because of the lack of major CNS involvement, and two forms of recombinant human α-galactosidase are in use for enzyme replacement therapy.[22,23] Although the results of two trials and extended treatment of patients are encouraging,[105] the consequences of long-term treatment of adults and early treatment of children are not yet available. Undoubtedly, the availability of enzyme replacement therapy and possibly substrate deprivation[106] or enzyme stabilization by substrate and substrate analogues[107] will affect the demand and necessity for prenatal diagnosis of Fabry disease.

Gaucher Disease

Gaucher disease is the most prevalent lysosomal storage disease, with a frequency of about 1 in 50,000 in the Caucasian population[108] but a carrier frequency of about 1 in 15 in the Ashkenazi Jewish population. It results from a deficiency of acidic β-glucosidase (EC 3.2.1.45), which catalyzes the hydrolysis of the β-glucosidic linkage in glucosylceramide and its deacylated derivative, glucosylsphingosine in the presence of saposin C.[109,110] The deficiency of β-glucosidase leads to the accumulation of these glycolipids in cells of the monocyte/macrophage system, and large lipid-laden histiocytes (Gaucher cells) are found in tissues from most patients. There is marked elevation in the liver, spleen, and brain of the major storage product, glucosylceramide, which is widely distributed normally at low levels as an intermediate in the biosynthesis and catabolism of glycosphingolipids. This results in enlargement of the liver and spleen and storage in bone marrow in most patients. Plasma and erythrocyte glucosylceramide is increased.[111] High concentrations of glucosylsphingosine, which is not normally present in detectable amounts, are found in the liver and spleen of all patients with Gaucher disease but in the brain only of patients with the neuronopathic forms of the disease.[109,112] It is the effect of the brain-specific storage products on neuronal loss rather than the accumulation of glucosylceramide that cause the neuronopathic forms.[113] The structures of the storage products reflect their tissue of origin, with only the brain storage products in the neuronopathic forms of the disease being of neural origin.

The gene for acidic β-glucosidase, *GBA*, has been fully characterized,[114,115] and more than 200 mutations, mostly missense, have been described.[116–118] The existence of a pseudogene with a high degree of homology close to the functional gene causes problems in the detection of pathogenic mutations in the functional gene.[119,120] Recombinant alleles are found in ~20 percent of patients.[116] Genotyping is providing some insight into the molecular basis of the different phenotypes.[109,116,118]

Three main clinical phenotypes of Gaucher disease are recognized on the basis of the absence (type 1) or presence and rate of progression of neurologic involvement (acute type 2 and chronic type 3).[109,118] Type 1 is the most common subtype and is particularly prevalent in Ashkenazi Jews, in whom the predicted prevalence is ~1 in 850.[118] Patients usually present with splenomegaly and thrombocytopenia, resulting in easy bruising and possibly bone pain, but without neurologic disease.[109,110] The age of enzymatic diagnosis ranges from less than 2 to 84 years of age. Most of the health problems of these patients result from continued spleen enlargement and moderate to severe bone deterioration caused by the replacement of healthy bone marrow with marrow filled with Gaucher cells. Some patients have a more severe type of Gaucher disease resulting in liver disease and lung infiltration. Although many patients with type 1 Gaucher disease live a full life, some have a rapid rate of glucosylceramide accumulation resulting in death in the second or third decade of life. Pathologic changes have been observed in brain samples from the few adult patients who came to autopsy.[121] There is wide variation in the age of onset and severity, even within families, making prediction of the clinical course very difficult even with genotyping. Four common mutations (N370S, c.84–85insG, IVS2+1G → A, and L444P) account for more than 93 percent of the mutations in type 1 Jewish patients but only 49 percent in non-Jewish type 1 patients.[116] The most common mutation, N370S, produces sufficient enzyme with residual activity to protect against neurologic disease, and individuals homozygous for N370S may even be asymptomatic.[122] The null alleles, c.84–85insG and IVS2+1G → A, are never found homoallelically and are found only rarely in non-Jewish type 1 patients. Other mutations found in combination with null alleles in patients with type 1 disease are deduced or have been shown to produce residual activity. Homozygosity for the L444P mutation is generally but not exclusively associated with the neuronopathic forms of the disease.

The acute neuronopathic, form of Gaucher disease, type 2, is very rare (<1 in 500,000 livebirths),[123] with rapidly progressing visceral and CNS disease. Patients usually present in the first few months of life with hepatosplenomegaly, slow development, strabismus, swallowing difficulties, laryngeal spasm, opisthotonos, and a picture of "pseudobulbar palsy."[109] Some patients die at birth from fetal hydrops.[124] Most cases have continual problems with respiration and chronic bronchopneumonia, which result in death by 18 months of age (mean age, 9 months).

The subacute neuronopathic form of Gaucher disease, type 3, is characterized by a later age of onset of neurologic symptoms and a more chronic course than type 2.[125] Although rare, with an incidence of approximately 1 in 100,000 live births,[123] a large number of cases has been reported in the Norrbotten region of Sweden.[126] These patients are homozygous for the L444P mutation, which is polymorphic in this population. Children generally present in early childhood with hepatosplenomegaly similar to type 1 Gaucher disease. However, by early adolescence, dementia, seizures, and extrapyramidal and cerebellar signs become evident. They all have a horizontal gaze palsy.[127] The age of onset of the neurologic signs can vary greatly, with some apparent only at an older age or after splenectomy.[126] In some cases, the degree of splenomegaly is very minimal. In one family one second cousin had type 2 Gaucher disease and the other had type 3, with no evidence of spleen enlargement or glucosylceramide storage.[128]

Recently, a rare type 4, with the genotype D409H/D409H, has been described with hydrocephalus and calcification of heart valves with only mild to moderate involvement of liver, spleen, and bones.[129]

Diagnosis of all the types of Gaucher disease is based on demonstrating a deficiency of acidic β-glucosidase activity in leukocytes, platelets or cultured skin fibroblasts.[130–132] A great variety of substrates and conditions for assay have been described, but the fluorogenic substrate 4-methylumbelliferyl-β-glucopyranoside (MU-β-Glc), is widely used with bile salt detergents such as sodium taurocholate plus oleic acid or Triton X-100 included in the assay. The presence of isoenzymes of β-glucosidase necessitates careful control of the assay conditions, particularly pH. Fluorescent derivatives of glucosylceramide and the radiolabeled natural substrate can also be used. Patients usually have less than 15 percent of normal activity, with no significant difference between clinical subtypes.[133] The residual β-glucosidase activity in patients with type 1 Gaucher disease is stimulated by the sphingolipid activator protein SAP-C and phosphatidylserine, whereas samples from patients with type 2 disease are not.[134]

Prenatal diagnosis of Gaucher disease can be achieved by measuring the acidic β-glucosidase activity directly in CV, in CCV cells and CAC using natural or synthetic substrates in the presence of bile salts.[123,135,136] If the mutations in the parents are known, DNA analysis can be used to confirm the diagnosis, but it must be remembered that a precise genotype/phenotype correlation does not exist, especially for type 1. Prediction of phenotype is complicated if one parent is affected with type 1 and the other is a carrier.[123] Prenatal testing may be undertaken for families who have had an affected child or for couples identified to be at risk by population screening for carriers of Gaucher disease.

Identification of carriers by enzymic assay is unreliable, and when the mutations in the family are known, heterozygotes should be identified by DNA testing. On account of the high incidence of type 1 Gaucher disease and the prevalence of a small number of mutations in Ashkenazi Jews, carrier screening by mutation analysis has been incorporated into many Jewish genetic disease screening programs. Five mutations account for approximately 97 percent of the carriers in this population.[109] Only about 75 percent of the mutations in the non-Jewish population can be detected by this approach because of the large number of private mutations. Therefore, assessment of the risk of Gaucher disease by mutation analysis for reproductive decision-making is accurate if both parents are Ashkenazi Jews but less informative if one parent is non-Jewish.[137]

A further complication for counseling and reproduction decision making is the availability of treatment for some forms of Gaucher disease. The principal cause of visceral storage in Gaucher disease is the accumulation of β-glucosylceramide in macrophages. It is possible to deliver replacement enzyme to these cells and to disperse the storage either by bone marrow transplantation (BMT)[138,139] or by direct intravenous administration of recombinant human β-glucosidase that has been modified for targeting to macrophages.[21,140] Although BMT is potentially a one-off permanent treatment, it has been superseded by enzyme replacement therapy (ERT) for type 1 because of the considerable risk associated with the BMT procedure and the difficulty of finding matched donors. It may have some value in the treatment of type 3.[141] ERT for type 1 is safe and effective in decreasing or preventing the visceral aspects of type 1 Gaucher disease, but many patients on treatment still have appreciable symptoms.[142] ERT will also clear the visceral disease in type 3, but there is no clear evidence that it can reverse the CNS disease. However, inhibitors of glucosyltransferase can cross the blood–brain barrier, and on the basis of favorable results in a cell model of Gaucher disease[143] and animal models of other sphingolipidoses,[144] a clinical trial of substrate deprivation using N-butyldexynojirimycin has been carried out with encouraging results.[26,145,146]

Metachromatic Leukodystrophy

Metachromatic leukodystrophy (MLD) is an autosomal recessive disorder resulting from a defect in the release of the sulfate moiety from sulfatide (3-sulfo-galactosylceramide) (see Figure 11.1).[147] The hydrolytic release of the sulfate moiety is catalyzed by the lysosomal enzyme sulfatide sulfatase or arylsulfatase A (ASA, EC 3.1.6.1).[148,149] in the presence of saposin B.[150] Therefore, MLD can arise from a defect in either arylsulfatase A or, more rarely, in saposin B.[151] Sulfatide occurs mainly in the myelin sheath of the central and peripheral nervous systems and to a lesser extent in gallbladder, kidney, and liver. The defect in MLD leads to the accumulation of sulfatide in the lysosomes of cells of these tissues and the deposition of storage granules, which appear metachromatic and stain strongly positive with PAS and Alcian blue. The disruption of the turnover of myelin ultimately leads to demyelination in the central and peripheral nervous systems, which is responsible for the predominantly neurologic symptoms of MLD.

There is great variation in the severity and age of onset of MLD, but most patients have the late infantile form. These children present between 1 and 2 years of age with genu recurvatum and impairment of motor function.[147,152,153] Examination reveals reduced or absent tendon reflexes. Within a span of months or years, nystagmus, signs of cerebellar dysfunction, dementia, tonic seizures, optic atrophy, and quadriparesis will develop in such a child. Death usually comes before 10 years of age. Patients with the juvenile form usually present between 5 and 12 years of age with ataxia and intellectual deterioration. These patients continue to have psychomotor deterioration and usually die 4 to 6 years after diagnosis. Adult patients present with psychoses, ataxia, weakness, and dementia after 18 years of age.[154] Some patients are noted to have emotional lability, apathy, or change in character. The neurologic deterioration continues until death occurs in the fourth or fifth decade of life. Some are initially misdiagnosed as having multiple sclerosis. Decreased nerve-conduction velocities and detection of demyelination by MRI or CT scan are useful diagnostically. Although saposin-B stimulates the hydrolysis of many glycolipids, the clinical symptoms of patients with a deficiency of saposin-B are predominantly those associated with MLD, with a few exceptions.[155]

The genes for arylsulfatase A[156] and SAP-B[157] have been cloned. More than sixty mutations have been identified in the *ASA* gene, many of which are private mutations, indicating a genetic basis for the clinical heterogeneity of MLD. Three recurrent mutations occur in European patients with a high frequency, and other mutations are associated with ethnic groups.[147] The functional significance of many mutations has been assessed by in vitro expression studies. Patients with infantile MLD have two null alleles, whereas juvenile or adult patients have at least one allele with residual enzymic activity.[158] There is a good inverse correlation between residual enzymic activity and severity of disease. At least six different mutations have been identified in the saposin-B portion of the prosaposin gene, which encodes a common precursor for the four specific saposins.[155]

Confirmation of a clinical diagnosis of MLD is made by demonstrating a deficiency of ASA in leukocytes or cultured cells,[159–161] using a synthetic, colorimetric substrate, nitrocatechol sulfate (NCS). Serum[162] and other tissues have also been used. Support for the diagnosis can be obtained by the detection of metachromatic granules in urine by staining with toluidine blue and by quantitative measurement of excreted sulfatide.[163,164] However, the enzymic diagnosis of MLD is complicated by two factors.[33,147,165] First, a defect in saposin-B cannot be detected using nitrocatechol sulfate because its hydrolysis is not dependent on the presence of a saposin. These patients have normal ASA activity using this substrate and with the natural radiolabeled substrate if a detergent is included in the assay. The detection of metachromatic granules or increased secretion of sulfatide in the urine provides support. The profile of excreted glycolipids can also give a clue because glycolipids, such as globotriaosylceramide and digalactosylceramide, should be present in addition to sulfatide because of the broad specificity of saposin-B.[166] Diagnosis can be confirmed by an ELISA for saposin B[167] or a sulfatide loading test in cultured cells.[168–170]

If the test is being carried out on a patient from a family with a known mutation in saposin-B, diagnosis can be confirmed by DNA analysis.

The second serious complication with the enzymic diagnosis of MLD is that a significant number of healthy people have ASA levels near those found in affected patients. This is due to homozygosity for a benign pseudodeficiency allele (Pd allele), which gives residual enzymic activity of 5–15 percent of the normal activity. These individuals do not excrete excessive sulfatide or show any clinical symptoms of MLD.[171] About 1–2 percent of the European population are homozygous for the Pd allele, with a carrier frequency of about 1 in 7 in most ethnic groups. The Pd allele can lead to the incorrect identification of patients and carriers in some families. The molecular basis of the Pd allele has been shown to be a mutation in the polyadenylation signal that results in the production of only about 10 percent messenger RNA.[172] It is usually, but not always, found *cis* with another polymorphism that abolishes a glycosylation site on the protein but is believed not to affect the catalytic properties of the enzyme. A simple DNA test is available for the detection of the Pd allele, and it is essential to carry out this test if a low level of ASA activity is found. Compound heterozygotes for the Pd allele and an MLD allele will have ASA activity lower than Pd homozygotes but they do not have the neurologic problems associated with MLD or excrete excessive sulfatide. However, detection of homozygosity for the Pd allele in a symptomatic patient by DNA analysis does not preclude diagnosis of MLD, because disease-causing mutations in the *ASA* gene occur on chromosomes carrying the Pd allele.[33,173–176] It has been estimated that one-fifth of MLD mutations occur on a Pd background.[14] Identification of carriers in families with MLD must include DNA tests for the Pd allele and the mutations in the index case. It is important to genotype the parents of an affected child to establish whether the disease-causing mutations are on a Pd background. With this knowledge it is possible to make an accurate prenatal diagnosis of MLD in a subsequent pregnancy by demonstrating a deficiency of ASA in CV or CCV cells or CAC together with DNA analysis for the Pd allele and the MLD mutations. When both parents are heterozygous for an allele containing both the Pd allele and the MLD mutation, as occurs in consanguineous couples, it is essential to analyze the fetal DNA for both mutations. The sulfatide loading test carried out with CCV or CAC is also very helpful in resolving difficult situations.

Bone marrow transplantation is considered an option for presymptomatic patients and those with mild neurologic manifestations.[27,177] It is assumed that sufficient bone marrow–derived monocytes can cross the blood–brain barrier to form perivascular microglia, which can secrete replacement enzyme for the deficient glial cells.

Multiple Sulfatase Deficiency

The lysosomal sulfatases, including arylsulfatase A, undergo a specific posttranslational modification to generate the active site, the conversion of an active site cysteine to C_α-formylglycine (FGly).[20] The enzyme catalyzing this reaction (FGly$_\alpha$-generating enzyme, FGE) has been purified and its gene (*SUMF1*) identified.[178,179] Mutations in this gene lead to a multiple deficiency of lysosomal and other sulfatases, called multiple sulfatase deficiency or multiple sulfatidosis (MSD).[180–185] This results in the disruption of the lysosomal catabolism of sulfated glycolipids and glycosaminoglycans and cholesterol sulfate. Children with MSD present with clinical features similar to those of late infantile metachromatic leukodystrophy, but features such as coarse facies, low-level dysostosis multiplex and stiff joints reminiscent of a mucopolysaccharidosis contribute to the phenotype. There is increased urinary excretion of dermatan sulfate (a substrate for arylsulfatase B and iduronate sulfatase) and heparan sulfate (a substrate for heparan sulfamidase and iduronate sulfatase) and glycopeptides. Confusion with patients with a mucopolysaccharidosis is possible, especially in young patients.[186] Within the first 2 years of life, patients demonstrate slow development, skeletal changes, coarse facial features, hepatosplenomegaly, and ichthyosis (due to the deficiency of arylsulfatase C). Vacuolated lymphocytes and Alder–Reilly bodies are found. Death usually occurs within a few years of onset of symptoms after rapid neurodegeneration.

Diagnosis is made by demonstrating deficiencies of several sulfatases in plasma, leukocytes or fibroblasts.[182,183] The pattern of sulfatase deficiencies varies, reflecting the clinical and biochemical heterogeneity of MSD. In general, the greater the decrease in the activities, the more severe is the phenotype. Parents of affected children do not have intermediate levels of sulfatases because the primary defect is not being measured. This has also prevented carrier detection in other members of an affected family. Now that the gene has been cloned and mutations identified in individual patients,[178,179] carrier detection will be feasible. Prenatal diagnosis has been made by assaying sulfatases in CAC and CV and fetal blood (author personal experience). The availability of DNA analysis will greatly improve the reliability of prenatal diagnosis for families in which the mutations are known. No therapy is currently available for these children.

Krabbe Disease (Globoid-Cell Leukodystrophy)

Krabbe disease results from a deficiency of galactocerebrosidase (EC 3.2.1.46) (GALC), which catalyzes the hydrolysis of the β-galactosidic linkages in various galactolipids, such as galactosylceramide, galactosylsphingosine, monogalactosyldiglyceride, and possibly lactosylceramide (see Figure 11.1). Galactosylceramide and its sulfated derivative, sulfatide, are found almost exclusively in myelin. Therefore, a deficiency of galactocerebrosidase leads to a progressive, cerebral degenerative disease affecting the white matter of the central and peripheral nervous systems.[187,188] Pathologic examination of the brain[189,190] shows that most but not all patients have characteristic, multinucleated globoid cells, containing undigested galactosylceramide. There is extensive depletion of glycolipids in the white matter, but the total concentration of galactosylceramide in the brain does not increase. The toxic metabolite galactosylsphingosine (psychosine) is also a substrate for galactocerebrosidase and it has been postulated that its accumulation is responsible for the early destruction of the oligodendroglia.[191,192]

The majority of patients have a severe infantile disease, but patients with a later onset, even in adulthood, have been described.[188,193–195] The onset in infancy usually occurs before 6 months of age, with irritability, hypertonicity, bouts of hypothermia, mental regression, and possibly optic atrophy and seizures.[196] This can be followed by increased hypertonicity, opisthotonos, hyperpyrexia, and blindness. Most patients die before 2 years of age.[188,193–195] Cerebrospinal fluid protein is highly elevated (values of 100–500 mg/dL are not unusual) and nerve-conduction velocities are decreased. The age of onset and progress of the disease are highly variable even in patients with the same genotype.

The *GALC* gene has been cloned,[197] and more than sixty mutations have been found.[187,188] The majority of patients are compound heterozygotes, but several missense mutations have been found in homozygous form, permitting their designation as null or mild alleles, with the caveat of marked variability of phenotype. A 30-kb deletion accounts for 40–50 percent of the alleles in infantile patients of European ancestry and 35 percent in infantile Mexican patients.[198] Some mutations, which presumably produce enzyme with residual activity, are homoallelic in juvenile/adult or adult patients. Patients, who are compound heterozygotes for one of these mutations and the large deletion have a juvenile or adult phenotype, but with tremendous variation in severity. The *GALC* gene is highly polymorphic, and about 80 percent of disease-causing mutations occur on alleles with at least one polymorphism. These polymorphisms affect the activity in normal and mutant alleles. The most common polymorphism has a frequency of 40–50 percent in the general population and decreases activity by up to 70 percent. The common deletion is always found in association with another polymorphism. These polymorphisms are responsible for the wide reference ranges of activities in carriers and normal individuals and for some but certainly not all, of the variation within a disease genotype.

Diagnosis is based on demonstrating a marked deficiency of galactocerebrosidase (GALC) activity in leukocytes or cultured fibroblasts[29,199–201] using the radiolabeled, natural substrate, galactosylceramide. A number of nonradioactive substrates have also been developed for the diagnosis of Krabbe disease.[202–205] Carrier detection is by DNA testing because of the wide range of galactocerebrosidase activity in normal individuals due to polymorphisms in the gene. Healthy people with enzyme values almost as low as those measured in affected children[201,206] occur, as well as obligate carriers with values clearly in the normal range.

Prenatal diagnosis for Krabbe disease has been performed for more than 1,000 pregnancies at risk worldwide.[188] Galactocerebrosidase can be assayed in CV directly, and in CCV and CAC.[203,205] Knowledge of the levels of activity in the index case and in the obligate heterozygote parents is essential for interpretation of the results. A method based on the uptake and use of [^{14}C]fatty-acid-labeled sulfatide in CAC has also been used to accurately identify fetuses affected with Krabbe disease.[207] However, in families in whom the genotype is known, the enzyme assay can now be combined with detection of specific mutations.

A number of patients with Krabbe disease have had BMT.[177] Although some juvenile patients have shown a clear positive effect of the transplantation, others have died from complications of the procedure. Typical infantile patients are not considered good candidates for transplantation because of the rapid course of their disease.

Niemann–Pick Disease

Niemann–Pick disease (NPD) consists of a group of autosomal recessive, lysosomal, lipid storage diseases, which have in common the storage of sphingomyelin, cholesterol, and possibly other lipids in many tissues of the body.[208–214] In Niemann–Pick disease types A and B, a primary deficiency of acidic sphingomyelinase (E.C. 3.1.4.12) due to mutations in the *ASM* gene leads to the lysosomal accumulation of sphingomyelin (see Figure 11.1).[213] In contrast, in Niemann–Pick disease type C, mutations in two genes, *NPC1* and *NPC2/HEI*, lead to altered trafficking of endocytosed cholesterol.[214]

There is massive accumulation of sphingomyelin in the liver and spleen of all patients with a deficiency of sphingomyelinase, but types A and B differ in their severity and neurologic involvement. NPD A is a severe neurovisceral disease, whereas there is only visceral involvement in NPD B with a chronic course. Patients with NPD type A usually present before 6 months of age with hepatomegaly and a slowing of motor and mental progress. This is followed by a general deterioration of neurologic function and health. About half of the children have a macular cherry-red spot, similar to that seen in

Tay–Sachs disease. Death from respiratory infections usually occurs by 4 years of age. A higher incidence of NPD type A is found in children of Ashkenazi Jewish ancestry, in which the carrier frequency is about 1 in 80. Patients with NPD type B can present with hepatomegaly within the first few years of life, but adults can also be diagnosed because of their hepatomegaly. Continued storage of sphingomyelin and other lipids, especially cholesterol, in liver, spleen, and lungs causes many health problems. There is no obvious mental deterioration or retardation, although some have been found to have a cherry-red spot in the macular region.[215,216] Complementation and molecular genetic studies have shown that NPD type A and NPD type B are allelic variants within the *ASM* gene. More than fifty different mutations have been identified in the *ASM* gene.[213] Patients with NPD A have two null alleles, three of which account for 92 percent of the mutations in Ashkenazi Jewish patients with NPD type A. A common mild mutation found in patients with type B has sufficient residual activity to prevent neurologic symptoms. Combinations of a milder allele and a null allele or two mild mutations are found in patients with NPD B. Patients with a more protracted neuropathic form of the disease than NPD A have a combination of mutations that produce less sphingomyelinase activity than typical NPD B mutations. This suggests that there is a continuous spectrum of clinical phenotypes, but this particular genotype does not always give an identical clinical course.[217]

Diagnosis of NPD A and B can be made by assaying acid sphingomyelinase in leukocytes or cultured cells using sphingomyelin radiolabeled in the choline moiety as the substrate. Several synthetic substrates have also been developed for the diagnosis of NPD,[212,218,219] but [^{3}H]choline-labeled sphingomyelin is still widely used because of its sensitivity, ease of assay, and specificity[29,220] NPD types A and B cannot be distinguished by measuring the amount of residual acid sphingomyelinase in a conventional assay in vitro, but more residual activity is found in NPD type B than in type A cells when the activity is measured by loading cells with labeled sphingomyelin and measuring the rate of hydrolysis.[221] This is consistent with the less severe phenotype of NPD type B. Heterozygote detection is unreliable by enzyme assay and should be based on DNA analysis.

Prenatal diagnosis of NPD types A and B can be made by assaying acid sphingomyelinase in CV samples directly.[220] Higher specific activities are obtained in CCV and CAC, but this delays the result. If the mutations are known in the index case and/or in the parents, mutation analysis on the CV sample is effective.

The genetic and metabolic basis of NPD type C is quite distinct from that of NPD types A and B. The lysosomal accumulation of unesterified cholesterol results from a defect in the processing and intracellular transport of endocytosed LDL-derived cholesterol and not from a primary defect in acid sphingomyelinase.[214] NPD type C is more common than NPD types A and B combined and is panethnic. NPD type C is extremely heterogeneous clinically. Most patients have progressive neurologic disease with mild but variable visceral enlargement. The classic phenotype presents in childhood with ataxia, vertical supranuclear palsy, variable hepatosplenomegaly, dysarthria, dystonia and psychomotor regression.[209,214] Death occurs in the second or third decade. Variants include an acute form with hydrops, an early form with fatal neonatal liver disease, an early-onset form with hypotonia and delayed motor development and adult variants. A small group of patients with severe pulmonary involvement and early death[222] were shown by complementation studies to be genetically distinct.[223] The two groups have been called NPC1 and NPC2, with about 95 percent of cases belonging to the NPC1 group.[208] Recently, the two genes affected in these groups have been identified, *NPC1*[224] and *NPC2/HE1*.[225] More than 100 disease-causing mutations have been identified in the *NPC1* gene.[220,226–228] There are some common mutations, and there is some correlation between genotype and residual NPC1 protein and clinical phenotype.[220,229,230] However, the genotype of many patients is incomplete, despite complete sequencing of the gene.[220] Several mutations have also been identified in the much smaller gene, *NPC2/HEI*.[231] A group of patients concentrated in Nova Scotia have a homogeneous subacute phenotype and were originally designated as NPD type D.[232] However, complementation studies[233] and subsequently the discovery of a point mutation in the *NPC1* gene[234] showed that they are an allelic variant of NPC1, and the term NPD type D has been discontinued. The proteins encoded by *NPC1* and *NPC2* are presumed to act closely to one another in the intracellular pathway for endocytosed cholesterol but their precise functions are not known, although it is an area of very active research.[235,236]

The diagnosis of NPC is complicated because there are two genetic defects, neither of which is a simple enzyme deficiency.[220] If the genetic defect (i.e., NPC1 or NPC2) has been established in the index case and the mutations are known, diagnosis of other patients within the family and detection of carriers can be made by mutation analysis. Otherwise, a defect in the trafficking of cholesterol has to be demonstrated using cultured fibroblasts. The "filipin" test detects the accumulation of unesterified cholesterol in perinuclear vesicles in fixed cells stained with filipin by fluorescence microscopy. Alternatively, the kinetics of LDL-induced cholesterol ester formation can be measured using labeled oleate.[226] Although these tests can detect both NPC1 and NPC2 with marked clinical defects, they may have to be modified to detect the less typical clinical variants, which account for ~20 percent of the NPC1 cases.[237]

These cell-based assays can be applied successfully to the prenatal diagnosis of NPC1 and NPC2 in CCV for families with the classic, marked phenotype but not to the variant cases. Cultured amniocytes can also be used, but the result will be obtained much later in the pregnancy and there is a risk of a false-negative result with epithelial-like amniotic cells.[220,238] Because heterozygotes can show abnormal filipin staining comparable to that seen in the variants, it is advisable to examine the parents' cells at the same time. If the genetic defect has been established in the index case and the mutations are known, then prenatal diagnosis by mutation analysis on CV samples is fast and reliable for both NPC1 and NPC2.[214,220,231,239] Unfortunately, determining the full genotype of many patients with NPC1 has proved difficult because of the size and complexity of the gene. The problem with NPC2 is knowing that it is NPC2, because very few laboratories can carry out the complementation test. For these reasons, the prenatal diagnosis of NPC2 remains a complex procedure that should be undertaken only in very experienced laboratories.

Several therapeutic strategies have been considered for the various types of NPD but none has been really effective. Liver transplantation was tried in one 4-month-old patient with NPD A, but the results did not demonstrate a clear benefit from this drastic procedure.[240] Another patient with NPD C underwent orthotopic liver transplantation with no evidence of improvement.[241] Because of the serious nature, without neurologic complications, of NPD B, this disease might be a good candidate for effective therapy by bone marrow transplantation if a suitable donor is available. Some patients with NPD B were given amniotic membrane implants, and a significant improvement in some clinical parameters was obtained.[242] This has not been confirmed by others. Some patients with NPD C have been placed on low-cholesterol diets and cholesterol-lowering drugs, but the results have not been encouraging. Enzyme replacement therapy (ERT) is a possibility for NPD B, and a trial of substrate deprivation is taking place for NPD C.

Farber Disease

Farber disease is a rare, autosomal recessive, lysosomal sphingolipid storage disorder caused by a deficiency of acid ceramidase, also called N-acylsphingosine amidohydrolase (EC 3.5.1.23).[243,244] The alkaline ceramidase present in most cells is not affected in this disorder. Ceramide is formed during the catabolism of all sphingolipids within the lyso-somes[245] (see Figure 11.1) and the deficiency of acid ceramidase leads to the intralyso-somal accumulation of ceramide in most tissues, including heart, liver, lung, and spleen. Extremely high levels of ceramide have been observed in the urine,[246] but it is not increased in the plasma of patients.[244]

Farber disease is also called Farber lipogranulomatosis because of the formation of the subcutaneous nodules near joints and other pressure points.[244] The characteristic features include progressive hoarseness due to laryngeal involvement, painful swollen joints, subcutaneous nodules, and pulmonary infiltrations. Initial signs appear between 2 and 4 months of age, and death usually occurs before 2 years of age, but survival to the age of 16 years is known. Psychomotor development in the few patients described so far has been mostly normal, although deterioration has been observed in the later phases of this disorder.[244,247] Conversely, very severe forms, with corneal clouding, hepatosplenomegaly, marked histiocytosis, and death before 6 months of age have been reported.[244,248,249] A rare subtype has been attributed to a deficiency of the sphingolipid activator protein precursor prosaposin.[244] Variable severity probably signals the existence of juvenile and perhaps even adult forms of this disorder, but too few patients have been described to define the clinical spectrum of this disease. The acid ceramidase gene has been cloned[250] and mutations identified in patients.[251–254] It is not yet possible to make any deductions about a genotype–phenotype correlation because of the small number of patients analyzed.[253] The clinical severity does not correlate with the residual activity measured under non-physiologic conditions,[255] but there is a good correlation with the level of lysosomal storage of ceramide.[256]

Patients can be diagnosed by measuring the accumulation of ceramide in cultured fibroblasts either by including [^{14}C]stearic acid-labeled sulfatide in the medium for 1–3 days[169] or by the enzymic determination of extracted, unlabeled ceramide.[257] The residual acid ceramidase can also be measured using synthetic substrates in the presence of added detergent.[258,259] A novel mass spectrometric method for measuring glycosphingolipids in extracts of cultured fibroblasts may also be applicable to the diagnosis of Farber disease.[260] Reliable carrier detection should be based on mutation analysis. Prenatal diagnosis has been carried out by measuring the ceramidase activity in CV[261] and CAC[262] or by lipid-loading tests in CAC.[263] No effective therapy is available. Two patients have undergone bone marrow transplantation, but the overall outcome was unfavorable.[244]

Wolman Disease and Cholesteryl Ester Storage Disease

Wolman disease, or primary familial xanthomatosis with involvement and calcification of the adrenals, is an autosomal recessive disease marked by severe failure to thrive, diarrhea, vomiting, and hepatosplenomegaly evident in the first few weeks of life.[264–268] Death usually occurs within 6 months from cachexia complicated by peripheral edema. Although most patients have calcification of the adrenals, some severely affected patients do not.[269] Foam cells are found in the bone marrow and other organs. The organs contain cells loaded with neutral lipids, especially cholesterol esters and triglycerides.

Cholesteryl ester storage disease (CESD) can be a relatively mild disorder, characterized by liver enlargement, short stature, chronic gastrointestinal bleeding, chronic anemia, headaches, and abdominal pain.[268,270–273] Patients usually have no calcification of the adrenals, but they may have sea-blue histiocytosis.[274] Some die in their juvenile years, but others live to adulthood with few health problems. Levels of cholesterol esters are markedly elevated in the liver; levels of triglycerides are only moderately elevated.

Patients with both Wolman disease and CESD have a marked deficiency of acid lipase (EC 3.1.1.13) activity in all tissues examined, including liver, spleen, leukocytes, lymphocytes, and cultured skin fibroblasts.[271,275–277] A variety of substrates has been used in the in vitro assays. These include radiolabeled triglycerides and cholesterol esters as well as fatty acid esters of 4-methylumbelliferone and p-nitrophenol.

Prenatal diagnosis is possible by direct enzyme assay of CV and CCV and CAC using synthetic substrates[278–280] and radiolabeled cholesterol oleate[281]

The gene for acid lipase has been cloned,[282] and a number of mutations have been identified.[268,282,283] The relationship between genotype and phenotype in Wolman disease and CESD is still a matter of debate.[282,284,285]

In common with many of the other lysosomal storage disorders, mutation analysis is the preferred approach to accurate carrier detection in family members even though some heterozygotes can be identified by enzyme analysis. There is a report of successful bone marrow transplantation in a case of Wolman disease.[286]

The Neuronal Ceroid Lipofuscinoses

The neuronal ceroid lipofuscinoses (NCL), also collectively known as Batten disease, encompass a group of severe, progressive degenerative disorders characterized by the accumulation of an autofluorescent material composed of ceroid and lipofuscin.[287] Clinically, the patients show progressive visual failure, neurodegeneration, epilepsy, and premature death. The inheritance is autosomal recessive. Until recently, a diagnosis of NCL was made on the basis of the age at onset of symptoms, clinical features, and ultrastructural morphology, but in the past few years rapid advances have been made in identifying the genes involved in the different subtypes (see Table 11.2). The gene, *CLN1*, encoding for the lysosomal enzyme palmitoyl protein thioesterase is mutated in patients with infantile NCL (INCL, NCL1),[288] and in cases of classic late infantile NCL (LINCL, NCL2), mutations are found in the gene, *CLN2*,[289] encoding tripeptidyl peptidase I.[290] Mutations in the *CLN3* gene are associated with juvenile NCL (JNCL, NCL3),[291] and approximately 90 percent of the affected alleles show a 1-kb deletion.[292,293] Mutations in the *CLN5* gene are found in a late infantile onset variant, (vLINCL, NCL5) particularly prevalent in Finnish patients,[294] while in a third group of patients also presenting in the late infancy, mutations have been found in the *CLN6* gene, (vLINCL, NCL6).[295] Another type of NCL (NCL8), in which the patients have progressive epilepsy with mental retardation, is again predominantly a Finnish disease with mutations in the *CLN8* gene.[296] The genes *CLN3*, *CLN5*, and *CLN8* encode putative membrane proteins whose function is still unknown. They do not appear to have homology to known membrane transporters, channels, receptors or ligands. The protein product of *CLN6* is unknown but work on the murine model of NCL6 indicates this too is a transmembrane protein.[295] There is another group of patients, from Turkey, with a late infantile presentation (vLINCL, NCL7), and these families were thought to represent a distinct genetic locus which was designated *CLN7*.

However a recently reported Turkish patient with a late infantile presentation was excluded from all the known NCL loci but was subsequently shown to be linked to the *CLN8* locus, which suggests that *CLN7* and *CLN8* may be allelic.[297]

Historically, a diagnosis of Batten disease was made on the ultrastructural morphology and composition of the storage material, a skin biopsy, or the white-cell buffy coat being readily available sources of material. Usually this enabled the subtype to be defined. In patients classified as having INCL, with onset of symptoms in the first or second year of life, granular osmiophilic deposits (GROD) were observed by electron microscopy (EM). Curvilinear bodies (CL) were found in biopsies from patients with LINCL and in patients with JNCL vacuolated lymphocytes were seen under light microscopy and fingerprint profiles (FP) under EM. In other patients with a late infantile presentation, the storage material was shown to be a mixture of FP and CL, and in the northern Finnish patients with epilepsy who had mutations in the *CLN8* gene, rectilinear profiles (RL) were evident. Adult patients have also been found in whom the storage material is usually a mixture of FP and CL, but in some patients only GROD is evident. Very little progress has been made in identifying the gene, *CLN4*, underlying this subtype (called Kuf disease), but it is now clear that patients with GROD have mutations in the *CLN1* gene and a palmitoyl protein thioesterase deficiency.

To offer reliable prenatal diagnosis for the NCLs it is essential to have studied the index case and to define the subtype of NCL as accurately as possible. Postnatal diagnosis should include histology, enzymology, and mutation analysis. All these approaches can be used, as appropriate, either singly or in combination in prenatal diagnosis.

As stated previously, EM of the leukocyte buffy coat will reveal characteristic ultrastructural morphology, allowing a diagnosis of NCL to be made. The presence of GROD indicates a palmitoyl protein thioesterase deficiency, which can be confirmed in leukocytes and/or fibroblasts using a synthetic substrate.[298] Once the enzyme deficiency is proven, mutation analysis of the *NCL1* gene will define the mutation, which allows accurate carrier detection in family members. Carrier detection is not possible on histology and is not always possible by enzyme analysis. Classic LINCL can be diagnosed in the same way. The presence of only CL would indicate a tripeptidyl peptidase I deficiency that, once proven, should lead to mutation analysis of the *CLN2* gene. Vacuolated lymphocytes and only FP in the buffy coat would be consistent with JNCL; this can be confirmed by mutation analysis of the *CLN3* gene. The presence of a mixed FP/CL profile would indicate NCL5, NCL6, or NCL7 and mutation analysis of these genes should be made. There are no biochemical tests available for these last four subtypes.

Prenatal diagnosis for Batten disease was first made for NCL2 on noncultivated amniotic cells.[299,300] EM of these cells showed the characteristic CL profile in both pregnancies. The first pregnancy reported was not terminated, and the diagnosis was confirmed postnatally by EM of a skin biopsy and lymphocytes.[301] In the second pregnancy the prenatal diagnosis was confirmed by EM studies in the aborted fetus.[300] Skin, amnion, umbilical vessels, blood, liver, and brain showed the classical CL profile. Subsequently, inclusions have been found in CV from two fetuses affected with NCL1.[302,303]

Currently, prenatal diagnosis is available by analysis of CV directly, CCV, CAC and, as reported in the cases of LINCL, noncultivated amniotic cells. For NCL1 and NCL2, assay of the palmitoyl protein thioesterase[304] or the tripeptidyl peptidase[305] in CV directly is very fast and reliable. However, it is reassuring to confirm this result either by histologic analysis and/or mutation analysis if the mutation is known and sufficient material is available. Abnormal histology has been found in CV, in a pregnancy at risk for NCL6;

the pregnancy was terminated. The diagnosis was confirmed histologically on the termination products (Anderson G, Histopathology, Great Ormond Street Hospital, personal communication). This pregnancy was monitored before mutation analysis of the *CLN6* gene was available. At present, histologic and mutation analysis (if the mutation is known) of CV is the preferred approach to prenatal diagnosis of NCL3, NCL5, NCL6, NCL7, and NCL8. This allows a diagnosis to be made in the first trimester.

There is no effective treatment for these disorders. BMT has been performed in two patients, one with LINCL and one with JNCL.[306] Although the patient with LINCL was less severely affected than his older sister was at 5 years of age the BMT did not prolong his life, and he died before his older sister, who had not been treated (Lake B, personal communication). There have been no follow-up reports on the patient with JNCL. There has been a suggestion that phosphocysteamine may be helpful in patients with NCL1,[307] but so far there have been no follow-up reports of this in the literature.

Peroxisomal Disorders

Peroxisomes are present in nearly all eukaryotic cells. They are bound by a single membrane, which contains at least ten peroxisome-specific integral membrane proteins. The peroxisomal matrix contains more than fifty different proteins, which are largely responsible for the metabolic functions of the peroxisome. These include the biosynthesis of plasmalogens (ether phospholipids), bile acids, cholesterol and polyunsaturated fatty acids and catabolic functions such as β-oxidation of very-long-chain fatty acids (VLCFAs), glyoxylate metabolism, and oxidation of pipecolic, glutaric, and phytanic acids. Peroxisomal disorders fall into two classes: those in which the biogenesis of the peroxisome is defective, leading to multiple defects in peroxisomal function, and those in which a single protein is defective and a single metabolic function is disrupted (see Tables 11.3 and 11.4). There are several excellent reviews of the structure, function, and disorders of peroxisomes.[6,7,308–312] Disorders in peroxisome biogenesis or in a peroxisomal metabolic pathway result in severe diseases with a wide range of clinical features and an estimated overall incidence of 1 in 20,000–100,000.[309] Symptoms can include dysmorphic facies, hepatomegaly, cataracts, retinopathy, psychomotor delay, hypotonia, seizures, and hearing problems.

Disorders of Peroxisome Biogenesis

The biogenesis of peroxisomes is a complex process[7,309] in which the matrix proteins are synthesized on ribosomes in the cytosol and transported to the peroxisome by transporters that recognize a specific peroxisomal targeting signal (PTS) at the carboxy terminal (PTS1) or occasionally the amino terminal (PTS2) on the matrix proteins. The peroxisomal membrane proteins are transported by a different and less well understood mechanism. Peroxins are the proteins involved in these processes; they are encoded by the *PEX* genes.[313] At least fifteen human *PEX* genes have been identified. The peroxisome biogenesis disorders fall into twelve complementation groups and the *PEX* genes defective in eleven of these groups are known. Eight of them encode proteins involved in the import of matrix proteins. Although the precise pathophysiology of these disorders is not known, there is a correlation between severity of the disease and the degree of loss of function of peroxins. Two clinical spectra are recognized. The Zellweger spectrum is a continuum from the Zellweger syndrome, which is the most severe phenotype, to the milder forms, neonatal adrenoleukodystrophy and infantile Refsum disease. They are characterized by defects in

PTS1 protein import alone or both the PTS1 and PTS2 protein import and occur in eleven of the complementation groups. The largest complementation group for Zellweger syndrome results from mutations in the *PEX1* gene. The other phenotypic pattern is represented by classical rhizomelic chondrodysplasia punctata and its milder forms,[7,309] which result from mutations in the *PEX7* gene, which encodes the PTS2 receptor.

The biochemical phenotypes of the peroxisome biogenesis disorders reflect the disruption of peroxisome function, and diagnosis is based on measuring abnormal concentrations of typical peroxisomal metabolites in plasma or red blood cells[314] (see Table 11.3). The most common metabolites measured areVLCFAs, which are elevated in the Zellweger spectrum (and all β-oxidation defects due to single enzyme deficiencies except α-methylacyl-CoA racemase deficiency) but not in the rhizomelic chondrodysplasia punctata group.[309] Rhizomelic chondrodysplasia punctata may also arise as a result of an isolated enzyme deficiency.[315] The measurement of several metabolites is often necessary to be sure of a diagnosis of a particular phenotype together with complementary tests[309,314] (see Table 11.3). Microscopic examination of cells for the absence or presence of peroxisomes can be very useful.[312] Immunologic methods have been developed for detecting deficiencies of specific proteins,[316] but the absence of one protein may have secondary effects on the transport of other proteins, giving rise to overlap of clinical symptoms. Further, it is becoming clear that different mutations in the same *PEX* gene can give rise to a wide range of clinical phenotypes. Therefore, a precise diagnosis for these overlapping disorders will come from DNA analysis once the defective *PEX* gene and mutations in the index case have been established.[317] Prenatal diagnosis of peroxisome biogenesis disorders can be made by using combinations of the same metabolic assays, immunodetection of peroxisomal proteins, and DNA analysis in CAC and CCV samples.[309,312,318–322] Diagnosis of rhizomelic chondrodysplasia punctata cannot be made by measuring VLCFAs and requires measurement of plasmalogen synthesis and phytanic acid oxidation studies.

Isolated Enzyme Deficiencies

Several single peroxisomal enzyme deficiencies involved in different aspects of peroxisomal metabolism have been identified.[310] They can be diagnosed by a combination of metabolite measurement and enzymic assay or DNA analysis (see Table 11.4). Prenatal diagnosis has been carried out for all of the disorders except the very rare defects in pipecolic acid metabolism, α-methylacyl-CoA racemase deficiency and glutaric aciduria. Two disorders are more common, X-linked adrenoleukodystrophy and Refsum disease, and are discussed in more detail.

Two genetically distinct forms of adrenoleukodystrophy exist: X-linked adrenoleukodystrophy (X-ALD)[323–327] and the autosomal recessive adrenoleukodystrophy that occurs in neonatal ALD (NALD) and can complicate infantile Refsum disease.[309] There are defects in nervous system myelination and the adrenal cortex and high levels of VCLFAs in both forms. However, peroxisome biogenesis is defective in the recessive forms, and there are multiple deficiencies of peroxisomal proteins. Clinically they fall within the Zellweger spectrum and should be considered as a peroxisome biogenesis disorder (see above). Peroxisomes are normal in X-linked adrenoleukodystrophy; the only biochemical abnormality appears to be in VLCFA metabolism.

X-linked adrenoleukodystrophy is the most common peroxisomal disorder, with an incidence of 1 in 20,000–50,000 males; it is clinically heterogeneous. About 35 percent of the cases have a childhood cerebral form, with the first symptoms, including behavioral changes, loss of vision, gait disturbances, dysarthria, and dysphagia, appearing between 4 and 10 years of age. Symptoms of Addison disease, including melanoderma, hypotension, and a failure of adrenocorticotrophic hormone (ACTH) to induce a rise in plasma cortisol, are noted after the initial diagnosis. Mental and motor regression is soon noted. Another 35–49 percent of male patients present in the second or third decade of life with symptoms of peripheral neuropathy, disturbances in bladder and bowel function, and progressive spastic paraparesis. They also can have adrenal insufficiency and hypogonadism. The commonest adult-onset form of ALD is called adrenomyeloneuropathy (AMN),[327–329] which is characterized by gait disturbance due to involvement of the spinal cord and peripheral nerves. The clinical phenotype of X-ALD is highly variable even within families. About half of heterozygotes have mild neurologic symptoms, with a smaller group having more severe symptoms. Adrenal sufficiency is almost unknown in females.

In patients with ALD, the cerebral white matter, peripheral nerves, and adrenal cortex have characteristic inclusions consisting of electron-dense leaflets enclosing an electron-lucent space. Lipids extracted from adrenal cortex and brain white-matter macrophages contain a high proportion of VLCFAs (C24–C30).[330] This led to diagnostic tests for patients and carriers using easily obtainable samples such as plasma and cultured skin fibroblasts.[331–333] Most commonly, the ratio of hexacosanoate (C26:0) to behenic acid (C22:0) in the total lipids from plasma and cultured skin fibroblasts has been used. Patients with ALD, AMN, and neonatal ALD show an average sevenfold to tenfold increase in this ratio in cultured skin fibroblasts. The biochemical defect in ALD and AMN is a decreased capacity to oxidize VLCFAs,[334,335] and the initial diagnosis of X-ALD is based on measuring VLCFAs in plasma. This will identify males accurately, but some female carriers have normal levels, and DNA analysis is necessary for carrier identification and useful for confirmation of diagnosis. The gene defective in X-ALD has been cloned.[336] It encodes a peroxisomal membrane protein (ALDP) with homology to the ATP-binding cassette transporter superfamily (ABC) and has been called *ABCD1*. ALDP is one of four peroxisomal proteins in the D subclass of these transporters.[327] It is not known how defects in ALDP lead to accumulation of VLCFAs. More than 500 mutations have been identified in the *ABCD1* gene in families (see www.xald.nl). Although the identification of mutations has greatly improved diagnosis and carrier detection, there is no clear correlation between genotype and phenotype. A novel neonatal phenotype similar to a peroxisomal biogenesis disorder has been shown to be due to a novel contiguous gene deletion *ABCD1:DXS1357E*.[337]

The prenatal diagnosis of X-linked ALD and neonatal ALD can be made by measuring VLCFAs in CV and CAC[338,339] by biochemical and immunologic methods[340] or DNA analysis if the mutation is known.[341,342] Currently, it is not possible to predict whether a male fetus diagnosed with X-linked ALD will have the milder AMN or boyhood form.

It is possible to lower the plasma VLCFAs in patients with X-linked ALD and AMN by dietary restriction of VLCFAs along with an increase in monounsaturated fatty acids (oleic and erucic acids).[327,343,344] Clinical trials suggest that the onset of neurologic disease can be delayed if treatment is started in the presymptomatic phase. Clinical improvement in patients with milder disease and in heterozygous females is sometimes noted, but dietary therapy seems to have little effect on patients with significant peripheral and CNS degeneration. BMT has been tried in patients with X-linked ALD,[327,345,346] and this may prove useful for some patients with a perfectly matched donor and moderate nervous system involvement.

Refsum disease (heredopathia atactica polyneuritiformis) is an autosomal recessive disease characterized by cerebellar ataxia, peripheral neuropathy, retinitis pigmentosa, and skin and skeletal changes.[347,348] Most patients present before 20 years of age with nerve deafness, anosmia, ichthyosis, night blindness, and weakness in the extremities. Phytanic acid (a 20-carbon branched-chain acid) accumulates in the liver and kidney of the patients.[349] Plasma contains a large amount of phytanic acid, and this may constitute 5–30 percent of the total fatty acids. This increase in phytanic acid is due to a defect in phytanoyl-CoA hydroxylase, which oxidizes (α-oxidation) phytanic acid to pristanic acid, which is further degraded by β-oxidation.[350–353] The gene encoding phytanoyl-CoA hydroxylase (*PHYH*) has been isolated,[354] and mutations have been identified in many patients.[355,356] However, some patients, who have been diagnosed clinically and biochemically with Refsum disease, do not have mutations in the *PHYH* gene.[357] A subset of these patients was found to have mutations in the *PEX7* gene, which is normally associated with the severe rhizomelic chondrodysplasia punctata.[358] These patients were shown to have deficiencies of plasmalogen biosynthesis and the peroxisomal thiolase, indicators of a peroxisome biogenesis disorder. Thus, mutations in *PEX7* can give rise to a relatively mild Refsum phenotype or the severe rhizomelic chondrodysplasia punctata phenotype. This diversity in clinical phenotype for allelic variants emphasizes the need to use more than one test for the diagnosis of a peroxisomal disorder. Patients described as having infantile Refsum disease should be classified with the peroxisomal biogenesis disorders, because they have a decreased number of peroxisomes.

Patients with classic Refsum disease can be diagnosed by finding increased cerebrospinal fluid protein (average, 275 mg/dL) and elevated phytanic acid (up to 25 μg/mL) in plasma. Confirmation of the diagnosis can be made by finding severely decreased levels of [^{14}C]phytanic acid oxidation in cultured skin fibroblasts[351] or by direct enzyme assay.[353] Patients usually oxidize less than 5 percent of normal levels, and carriers may have less than normal activity.[351] However, normal activity has been found in fibroblasts from two obligate heterozygotes.[359] Phytanoyl-CoA hydroxylase is also deficient in peroxisome biogenesis disorders, including infantile Refsum disease. Prenatal diagnosis for classic Refsum disease is possible by measuring phytanic acid oxidation in CAC and CCV cells, by enzyme assay, and by DNA analysis. However, because there is effective treatment, this is rarely done.

Refsum disease is one of the few lipid storage diseases for which there is effective therapy. Phytanic acid cannot be synthesized by humans and is completely dietary in origin. Because phytanic acid and phytol, which is not absorbed very well, are components of chlorophyll, reduction of dairy products, ruminant fats, and other products containing chlorophyll will lower plasma phytanic acid and decrease clinical problems.[347,360] Because dietary treatment should be started as soon as possible, a combination of plasmapheresis and dietary control may be used to bring the plasma level of phytanic acid down more quickly. Most patients show a marked clinical improvement but there is usually only partial restoration of peripheral nerve functions.[347]

In peroxisomal disorders, the biochemical and clinical consequences of a defect in a particular protein can arise from an isolated defect in that protein or secondarily from a multiprotein deficiency in peroxisome biogenesis disorders. This leads to overlap of clinical phenotypes, making a definitive diagnosis more demanding. It has been recommended by the European Concerted Action on Peroxisomes[361] that a combined approach of one microscopic and one biochemical and/or genetic method should always be used for the prenatal diagnosis of peroxisomal disorders.

Lipoprotein-Associated Disorders

This group of genetic disorders is exemplified by changes in plasma lipids due to defects in the protein lipid-carriers (lipoproteins), lipoprotein receptors, or enzymes responsible for the hydrolysis and clearance of lipoprotein-lipid complexes (see Table 11.5).[8] The proteins responsible for the maintenance of normal plasma and tissue lipids, which are primarily triglycerides and free and esterified cholesterol, include the apolipoproteins A-I, A-II, A-IV, B, C-I, C-II, C-III, D, E, and LP(a) as well as lipoprotein lipase, hepatic triglyceride lipase, lecithin cholesterol acyltransferase, cholesterol ester transfer protein, low-density lipoprotein receptor, chylomicron remnant receptor, and scavenger receptor (see Table 11.5). The normal structure and metabolism of plasma lipoproteins have been reviewed recently.[373] With the exception of familial hypercholesterolemia,[374] defects in these proteins tend to be rare. Most of the disorders can be managed by a combination of dietary control, cholesterol-lowering drugs and, in some cases, vitamin supplementation. Homozygotes for familial hypercholesterolemia, who frequently die by the age of 20 from myocardial infarction after coronary heart disease from childhood, are an exception.[374] Many of the disorders do not affect children, although early diagnosis through screening programs and family histories could result in dietary management to prevent the onset of serious, life-threatening coronary heart disease later in life. Most of the genes encoding these proteins have been cloned, and mutations and informative polymorphisms[375,376] have been identified. This information can be used to identify carriers of autosomal recessive disorders or asymptomatic or mildly affected members of families with autosomal dominant disorders. It could also be used to improve screening for people at risk in the general population. Prenatal diagnosis by DNA analysis of fetal samples from pregnancies at risk is possible if a reliable DNA test is available. Although this would offer the advantage of dietary intervention soon after birth,[376] not many prenatal tests are carried out for these disorders because of the possibility of testing and treating babies at risk soon after birth. Again the exception is prenatal diagnosis for homozygosity for familial hypercholesterolemia, which has been performed by a functional assay in CAC[377] or by measurement of the cholesterol in fetal blood.[378] If the mutation(s) in the LDL receptor or the haplotype of the mutated chromosome is known, prenatal diagnosis can be carried out reliably by DNA analysis.[379,380] The investigation of these disorders is yielding a better understanding of the delicate balance between diet and de novo lipid synthesis and of the functions of the many proteins responsible for transporting and processing cholesterol and triglycerides.

ACKNOWLEDGMENTS

We acknowledge the dedication, experience, and friendship of our colleagues in the Enzyme Diagnostic Laboratory at Great Ormond Street Hospital, London, with whom we have worked for many years and without whom this chapter could not have been written. We would also like to thank Professors Peter Clayton and David Muller, both of the Institute of Child Health, for reading and making helpful comments on the sections on peroxisomal disorders and lipoprotein-associated disorders, respectively.

REFERENCES

1. Winchester B. Lysosomal metabolism of glycoconjugates. In: Lloyd JB, Mason RW, eds. Subcellular biochemistry: biology of the lysosome, vol. 27. New York: Plenum Press, 1996:191.

2. Kolter T, Sandhoff K. Sphingolipids: their metabolic pathways and the pathobiochemistry of neurodegenerative diseases. Angew Chem Int Ed Engl 1999;38:1532.

3. Scriver CR, Beaudet AL, Sly WS, et al., eds. Part 16 Lysosomal Disorders. In: The metabolic and molecular bases of inherited disease, 8th ed. New York: McGraw-Hill, 2001:3371.

4. Powers JM, Moser HW. Peroxisomal disorders: genotype, phenotype, major neuropathologic lesions and pathogenesis. Brain Pathol 1998;8:101.

5. Scriver CR, Beaudet AL, Sly WS, et al., eds. Part 15 peroxisomes. In: The metabolic and molecular bases of inherited disease, 8th edition. New York: McGraw-Hill, 2001:3181.

6. Baumgartner MR, Saudubray JM. Peroxisomal disorders. Semin Neonatol 2002;7:85.

7. Brosius U, Gartner J. Cellular and molecular aspects of Zellweger syndrome and other peroxisomal biogenesis disorders. Cell Mol Life Sci 2002;59:1058.

8. Scriver CR, Beaudet AL, Sly WS, et al., eds. Part 12 Lipids. In: The metabolic and molecular bases of inherited disease, 8th ed. New York: McGraw-Hill, 2001:2705.

9. Hakomori S. The glycosynapse. Proc Natl Acad Sci USA 2002;99:225.

10. Simons K, Toomre, D. Lipid rafts and signal transduction. Nat Rev Mol Cell Biol 2000;1:31.

11. Scriver CR, Beaudet AL, Sly WS, et al. eds. The metabolic and molecular bases of inherited disease, 8th ed. New York: McGraw-Hill, 2001.

12. Blau N, Duran M, Blaskovics ME, et al. Physician's guide to the laboratory diagnosis of metabolic diseases, 2nd ed. New York: Springer, 2002.

13. Applegarth DA, Dimmick JF, Hall JG, eds. Organelle diseases. London: Chapman Hall, 1997.

14. Thomas GH. "Pseudodeficiencies" of lysosomal hydrolases. Am J Hum Genet 1994;54:934.

15. Kishimoto Y, Hiraiwa M, O'Brien JS. Saposins: structure, function, distribution and molecular genetics. J Lipid Res 1992;33:1255.

16. Schuette CG, Pierstorff B, Huettler S, et al. Sphingolipid activator proteins: proteins with complex functions in lipid degradation and skin biogenesis. Glycobiology 2001;11:81R.

17. Conzelmann E, Sandhoff K. AB variant of infantile GM_2 gangliosidosis: deficiency of a factor necessary for stimulation of hexosaminidase A-catalyzed degradation of ganglioside GM_2 and glycolipid A2. Proc Natl Acad Sci USA 1978;75:3979.

18. O'Brien JS, Kretz KA, Dewji N. Coding of two sphingolipid activator proteins (SAP-1 and SAP-2) by same genetic locus. Science 1988;241:1098.

19. Harzer K, Paton BC, Poulos A, et al. Sphingolipid activator protein deficiency in a 16-week-old atypical Gaucher disease patient and his fetal sibling: biochemical signs of combined sphingolipidoses. Eur J Pediatr 1989;149:31.

20. Schmidt B, Selmer T, Ingendoh A, et al. A novel amino acid modification in sulfatases that is defective in multiple sulfatase deficiency. Cell 1995;82:271.

21. Barton NW, Brady RO, Dambrosia, JM, et al. Replacement therapy for inherited enzyme deficiency: macrophage-targeted glucocerebrosidase for Gaucher's disease. N Engl J Med 1991;324:1464.

22. Schiffman R, Kopp JB, Austin HA, et al. Enzyme replacement in Fabry disease: a randomised controlled trial. JAMA 2001;285:2743.

23. Eng CM, Guffon N, Wilcox WR, et al. Safety and efficacy of recombinant human alpha-galactosidase A replacement therapy in Fabry's disease. N Engl J Med 2001;345:9.

24. Butters TD, Mellor HR, Narita K, et al. Small-molecule therapeutics for the treatment of glycolipid lysosomal storage disorders. Phil Trans R Soc Lond B Biol Sci 2003;358:927.

25. Abe A, Wild SR, Lee WL et al. Agents for the treatment of glycosphingolipid storage disorders. Curr Drug Metab 2001;2:331.

26. Cox T, Lachmann R, Hollak C, et al. Novel oral treatment of Gaucher's disease with N-butyldeoxynojirimycin (OGT 918) to decrease substrate biosynthesis. Lancet 2000;355:1481.

27. Krivit W. Stem cell bone marrow transplantation in patients with metabolic storage diseases. Adv Pediatr 2002;49:359.

28. Chang MH, Bindloss CA, Grabowski GA, et al. Saposins A, B, C, and D in plasma of patients with lysosomal storage disorders. Clin Chem 2000;46:167.

29. Wenger DA, Williams C. Screening for lysosomal disorders. In: Hommes FA, ed. Techniques in diagnostic human biochemical genetics. New York: Wiley-Liss, 1991:587.

30. Clarke LA. Clinical diagnosis of lysosomal storage diseases. In: Applegarth DA, Dimmick JF, Hall JG, eds. Organelle diseases. London: Chapman Hall, 1997:43.

31. Weibel TD, Brady RO. Systematic approach to the diagnosis of lysosomal storage disorders. Ment Retard Dev Disabil Res Rev 2001;7:190.

32. Wraith JE. Lysosomal disorders. Semin Neonatol 2002;7:75.

33. Wenger DA, Coppola S, Liu SL. Insights into the diagnosis and treatment of lysosomal storage diseases. Arch Neurol 2003;60:322.

34. Lake BD, Young, EP, Winchester BG. Prenatal diagnosis of lysosomal storage diseases. Brain Pathol 1998;8:133.

35. Kleijer WJ. Inborn errors of metabolism. In: Rodeck CH, Whittle MJ, eds. Fetal medicine: basic science and clinical practice. London: Churchill Livingstone 1999:525.

36. Callahan JW. Molecular basis of GM1 gangliosidosis and Morquio disease, type B: structure–function studies of lysosomal beta-galactosidase and the non-lysosomal beta-galactosidase-like protein. Biochim Biophys Acta 1999;455:85.

37. Suzuki Y, Oshima A, Nanba E. β-Galactosidase deficiency (β-galactosidosis): GM$_1$-gangliosidosis and Morquio B disease. In: Scriver CR, Beaudet AL, Sly WS, et al., eds. The metabolic and molecular bases of inherited disease, 8th ed. New York: McGraw-Hill, 2001:3775.

38. D'Azzo A, Andria G, Strisciuglio P, et al. Galactosialidosis. In: Scriver CR, Beaudet AL, Sly WS, et al., eds. The metabolic and molecular bases of inherited disease, 8th ed. New York: McGraw-Hill, 2001:3811.

39. Kolter T, Sandhoff K. Recent advances in the biochemistry of sphingolipidoses. Brain Pathol 1998;8:79.

40. Bagshaw RD, Zhang S, Hinek A, et al. Novel mutations (Asn484Lys, Thr500Ala, Gly438Glu) in Morquio B disease. Biochim Biophys Acta 2002;1588:247.

41. Paschke E, Milos I, Kreimer-Erlacher H, et al. Mutation analyses in 17 patients with deficiency in acid β-galactosidase: three novel point mutations and high correlation of mutation W273L with Morquio disease type B. Hum Genet 2001;109:159.

42. Chakraborty S, Rafi MA, Wenger DA. Mutations in the lysosomal β-galactosidase gene that cause the adult form of GM1 gangliosidosis. Am J Hum Genet 1994;54:1004.

43. Gravel RA, Kaback MM, Proia RL, et al. The GM$_2$ gangliosidoses. In: Scriver CR, Beaudet AL, Sly WS, et al., eds. The metabolic and molecular bases of inherited disease, 8th ed. New York: McGraw-Hill, 2001:3827.

44. Mahuran DJ. Biochemical consequences of mutations causing the GM$_2$ gangliosidoses. Biochim Biophys Acta 1999;1455:105.

45. Sandhoff K, Kolter T. Biosynthesis and degradation of mammalian glycosphingolipids. Phil Trans R Soc Lond B Biol Sci 2003;358:847.

46. Mark BL, Mahuran DJ, Cherney MM, et al. Crystal structure of human β-hexosaminidase B: understanding the molecular basis of Sandhoff and Tay-Sachs disease. J Mol Biol 2003;327:1093.

47. Maier T, Strater N, Schuette CG, et al. The X-ray crystal structure of human β-hexosaminidase B provides new insights into Sandhoff disease. J Mol Biol 2003;328:669.

48. Wright CS, Li SC, Rastinejad F. Crystal structure of human-GM$_2$-activator protein with a novel beta-cup topology. J Mol Biol 2000;304:411.

48a. Bach G, Tomczak J, Risch N, et al. Tay-Sachs Screening in the Jewish Ashkenazi population: DNA testing is the preferred procedure. Am J Med Genet 2001;99:70.

49. Johnson WG. The clinical spectrum of hexosaminidase deficiency diseases. Neurology 1981;31:1453.

50. Willner JP, Grabowski GA, Gordon RE, et al. Chronic GM$_2$ gangliosidosis masquerading as atypical Friedreich ataxia: clinical, morphologic and biochemical studies of nine cases. Neurology 1981;31:787.

51. Harding AE, Young EP, Schon F. Adult onset supranuclear ophthalmoplegia, cerebellar ataxia, and neurogenic proximal muscle weakness in a brother and sister: another hexosaminidase A deficiency syndrome. J Neurol Neurosurg Psychiatry 1987;50:687.

52. Navon R, Padeh B, Adam A. Apparent deficiency of hexosaminidase A in healthy members of a family with Tay–Sachs disease. Am J Hum Genet 1973;25:287.

53. Okada S, O'Brien JS. Tay–Sachs disease: generalized absence of a beta-D-N-acetylhexosaminidase component. Science 1969;165:698.

54. O'Brien JS, Okada S, Chen A, et al. Tay–Sachs disease: detection of heterozygotes and homozygotes by serum hexosaminidase assay. N Engl J Med 1970;283:15.

55. Fuchs W, Navon R, Kaback MM, et al. Tay–Sachs disease: one-step assay of β-N-acetylhexosaminidase in serum with a sulphatedchromogenic substrate. Clin Chim Acta 1983;133:253.

56. Saifer A, Rosenthal AL. Rapid test for the detection of Tay–Sachs disease heterozygotes and homozygotes by serum hexosaminidase assay. Clin Chim Acta 1973;43:417.

57. Robinson D, Stirling JL. N-Acetyl-β-glucosaminidases in human spleen. Biochem J 1968;107:321.

58. Okada S, Veath ML, O'Brien JS. Juvenile GM$_2$ gangliosidosis: partial deficiency of hexosaminidase A. J Pediatr 1970;77:1063.

59. Suzuki Y, Suzuki K. Partial deficiency of hexosaminidase component A in juvenile GM_2 gangliosidosis. Neurology 1970;20:848.

60. Kytzia HJ, Hinrichs U, Maire I, et al. Variant of GM_2-gangliosidosis with hexosaminidase A having a severely changed substrate specificity. EMBO J 1983;2:1201.

61. Ohno K, Suzuki K. Mutation in the GM_2-gangliosidosis B1 variant. J Neurochem 1988;50:316.

62. Eiris J, Chabas A, Coll MJ, et al. Late infantile and juvenile form of GM_2-gangliosidosis variant B1. Rev Neurol 1999;29:435.

63. Grosso S, Farnetani MA, Berardi R, et al. GM_2 gangliosidosis variant B1neuroradiological findings. J Neurol 2003;250:17.

64. Bayleran J, Hechtman P, Kolodny E, et al. Tay-Sachs disease with hexosaminidase A: characterization of the defective enzyme in two patients. Am J Hum Genet 1987;41:532.

65. Cao Z, Petroulakis E, Salo T, et al. Benign *HEXA* mutations, C739T (R247W) and C745T (R249W), cause β-hexosaminidase A pseudodeficiency by reducing the α-sub-unit protein levels. J Biol Chem 1997;272:14975.

66. Vidgoff J, Buist NR, O'Brien JS. Absence of β-N-acetyl-D-hexosaminidase A activity in a healthy woman. Am J Hum Genet 1973;25:372.

67. Hepbildikler ST, Sandhoff R, Kolzer M, et al. Physiological substrates for human lysosomal hexosaminidase S. J Biol Chem 2002;277:2562.

68. Sango K, McDonald MP, Crawley JN, et al. Mice lacking both sub-units of lysosomal β-hexosaminidase display gangliosidosis and mucopolysaccharidosis. Nat Genet 1996;14:348.

69. Kaback MM, Zeiger RS. Heterozygote detection in Tay-Sachs disease: a prototype community screening program for the prevention of genetic disorder. In: Volk BW, Aronson SM, eds. Sphingolipids, sphingolipidoses and allied disorders. New York: Plenum Press, 1972:613.

70. Triggs-Raine BL, Mules EH, Kaback MM, et al. A pseudodeficiency allele common in non-Jewish Tay-Sachs carriers: implications for carrier screening. Am J Hum Genet 1992;51:793.

71. Cao Z, Natowicz MR, Kaback MM, et al. A second mutation associated with apparent β-hexosaminidase A pseudodeficiency: identification and frequency estimation. Am J Hum Genet 1993;53:1198.

72. Pergament E, Ginsberg N, Verlinsky Y, et al. Prenatal Tay–Sachs diagnosis by chorionic villi sampling. Lancet 1983;2:286.

73. Grebner EE, Wenger DA. Use of 4-methylumbelliferyl-6-sulpho-2-acetamido-2-deoxy-β-D-glucopyranoside for prenatal diagnosis of Tay-Sachs disease using chorionic villi. Prenat Diagn 1987;7:419.

74. Thomas PK, Young EP, King RHM. Sandhoff disease mimicking adult-onset bulbospinal neuropathy. J Neurol Neurosurg Psychiatry 1989;52:1103.

75. Sandhoff K, Andreae U, Jatzkewitz H. Deficient hexosaminidase activity in an exceptional case of Tay–Sachs disease with additional storage of kidney globoside in visceral organs. Life Sci 1968;7:283.

76. Suzuki Y, Koizumi Y, Togari H, et al. Sandhoff disease: diagnosis of heterozygous carriers by serum hexosaminidase assay. Clin Chim Acta 1973;48:153.

77. Lowden JA, Ives EJ, Keene DL, et al. Carrier detection in Sandhoff disease. Am J Hum Genet 1978;30:38.

78. Dreyfus JC, Poenaru L, Vibert M, et al. Characterization of a variant β-hexosaminidase: "hexosaminidase Paris". Am J Hum Genet 1977;29:287.

79. Raghavan S, Krusell A, Lyerla TA, et al. GM_2-ganglioside metabolism in cultured human skin fibroblasts: unambiguous diagnosis of GM_2-gangliosidosis. Biochim Biophys Acta 1985;834:238.

80. Banerjee A, Burg J, Conzelmann E, et al. Enzyme-linked immunosorbent assay for the ganglioside GM2-activator protein: screening of normal human tissues and body fluids, of tissues of GM_2-gangliosidosis, and for its subcellular localization. Hoppe Seylers Z Physiol Chem 1984;365:347.

81. Desnick RJ, Ioannou YA, Eng CM. α-Galactosidase A deficiency: Fabry disease. In: Scriver CR, Beaudet AL, Sly WS, et al., eds. The metabolic and molecular bases of inherited disease, 8th ed. New York: McGraw-Hill, 2001:3733.

82. Mills K, Johnson A, Winchester B. Synthesis of novel internal standards for the quantitative determination of plasma ceramide trihexoside in Fabry disease by tandem mass spectrometry. FEBS Lett 2002; 515:171.

83. Whybra C, Kampmann C, Willers I, et al. Anderson-Fabry disease: clinical manifestations of disease in female heterozygotes. J Inherit Metab Dis 2001;24:715.

84. Redonnet-Vernhet I, Ploos van Amstel JK, Jansen RP et al. Uneven X-inactivation in a female monozygotic twin pair with Fabry disease and discordant expression of a novel mutation in the alpha-galactosidase A gene. J Med Genet 1996;33:682.

85. Bishop DF, Calhoun DH, Bernstein HS, et al. Human alpha-galactosidase A: nucleotide sequence of a cDNA clone encoding the mature enzyme. Proc Natl Acad Sci USA 1986;83:4859.

86. Kornreich R, Bishop DF, Desnick RJ. The gene encoding alpha-galactosidase A and gene rearrangements causing Fabry disease. Trans Assoc Am Phys 1989;102:30.

87. Ishii S, Sakuraba H, Suzuki Y. Point mutations in the upstream region of the alpha-galactosidase A gene exon 6 in an atypical variant of Fabry disease. Hum Genet 1992;89:29.

88. Sakuraba H, Oshima A, Fukuhara Y, et al. Identification of point mutations in the alpha-galactosidase A gene in classical and atypical hemizygotes with Fabry disease. Am J Hum Genet 1990;47:784.

89. Okumiya T, Kawamura O, Itoh R, et al. Novel missense mutation (M72V) of α-galactosidase gene and its expression product in an atypical Fabry hemizygote. Hum Mutat 1998;S1:S213.

90. Ashton-Prolla P, Tong B, Shabbeer J, et al. Fabry disease: twenty two novel mutations in the α-galactosidase A gene and genotype/phenotype correlations in severely and mildly affected hemizygotes and heterozygotes. J Invest Med 2000;48:227.

91. Knol IE, Ausems MG, Lindhout D, et al. Different phenotypic expression in relatives with Fabry disease caused by a W226X mutation. Am J Med Genet 1999;82:436.

92. Handa Y, Yotsumoto S, Isobe E, et al. A case of symptomatic heterozygous female Fabry's disease without detectable mutation in the alpha-galactosidase gene. Dermatology 2000;200:262.

93. Fitzmaurice TF, Desnick RJ, Bishop DF. Human α-galactosidase A: high plasma activity expressed by the $-30G \rightarrow A$ allele. J Inherit Metab Dis 1997;20:643.

94. Garman SC, Hannick L, Zhu A, et al. The 1.9 A° structure of α-N-acetylgalactosaminidase: molecular basis of glycosidase deficiency diseases. Structure 2002;10:425.

95. Garman SC, Garboczi DN. Structural basis of Fabry disease. Mol Genet Metab 2002;77:3.

96. Kint JA. Fabry's disease, alpha-galactosidase deficiency. Science 1970;167:1268.

97. Mapes CA, Anderson RL, Sweeley CC. Galactosylgalactosylglucosylceramide: galactosyl hydrolase in normal human plasma and its absence in patients with Fabry's disease. FEBS Lett 1970;7:180.

98. Romeo G, Migeon BR. Genetic inactivation of the α-galactosidase locus in carriers of Fabry's disease. Science 1970;170:180.

99. Mayes JS, Scheerer JB, Sifers RN, et al. Differential assay for lysosomal α-galactosidases in human tissues and its application to Fabry's disease. Clin Chim Acta 1981;112:247.

100. Brady RO, Uhlendorf BW, Jacobson CB. Fabry's disease: antenatal detection. Science 1971;172:174.

101. Clarke JT, Guttmann RD, Wolfe LS, et al. Enzyme replacement therapy by renal allotransplantation in Fabry's disease. N Engl J Med 1972;287:1215.

102. Desnick RJ, , Simmons RL, Allen KY, et al. Correction of enzymatic deficiencies by renal transplantation: Fabry's disease. Surgery 1972;72:203.

103. Philippart M, Franklin SS, Gordon A. Reversal of an inborn sphingolipidosis (Fabry's disease) by kidney transplantation. Ann Intern Med 1972;77:195.

104. Spence MW, MacKinnon KE, Burgess JK, et al. Failure to correct the metabolic defect by renal allotransplantation in Fabry's disease. Ann Intern Med 1976;84:13.

105. Pastores GM, Thadhani R. Advances in the management of Anderson–Fabry disease: enzyme replacement therapy. Expert Opin Biol Ther 2002;2:325.

106. Abe A, Gregory S, Lee L, et al. Reduction of globotriaosylceramide in Fabry mice by substrate deprivation. J Clin Invest 2000;105:1563.

107. Frustacia A, Chimenti C, Ricci R, et al. Improvement in cardiac function in the cardiac variant of Fabry's disease with galactose-infusion therapy. N Engl J Med 2001;345:25.

108. Meikle PJ, Hopwood JJ, Clague AE, et al. Prevalence of lysosomal storage disorders.JAMA 1999;281:249.

109. Beutler E, Grabowski GA. Gaucher disease: In: Scriver CR, Beaudet AL, Sly WS, et al., eds. The metabolic and molecular bases of inherited disease, 8th ed. New York: McGraw-Hill, 2001:3635.

110. Zimran A. Gaucher's disease. Baillieres Clin Haematol 1997;10:whole book.

111. Nilsson O, Hakansson G, Dreborg S, et al. Increased cerebroside concentration in plasma and erythrocytes in Gaucher disease: significant differences between Type I and Type III. Clin Genet 1982;22:274.

112. Orvisky E, Sidransky E, McKinney CE, et al. Glucosylsphingosine accumulation in mice and patients with type 2 Gaucher disease begins early in gestation. Pediatr Res 2000;48:233.

113. Conradi N, Kyllerman M, Mansson J-E, et al. Late-infantile Gaucher disease in a child with myoclonus and bulbar signs: neuropathological and neurochemical findings. Acta Neuropathol (Berlin) 1991;82:152.

114. Sorge J, West C, Westwood B, et al. Molecular cloning and nucleotide sequence of human glucocerebrosidase cDNA. Proc Natl Acad Sci USA 1985;82:7289.

115. Tsuji S, Choudary PV, Martin BM, et al. Nucleotide sequence of cDNA containing the complete coding sequence for human lysosomal glucocerebrosidase. J Biol Chem 1986;261:50.

116. Koprivica V, Stone DL, Park JK, et al. Analysis and classification of 304 mutant alleles in patients with type 1 and type 3 Gaucher disease. Am J Hum Genet 2000;66:1777.

117. Qi X, Grabowski GA. Molecular and cell biology of acid β-glucosidase and prosaposin. Prog Nucleic Acid Res Mol Biol 2001;66:203.

118. Elstein D, Abrahamov A, Hadas-Halpern I, et al. Gaucher's disease. Lancet 2001;358:324.

119. Grabowski GA, Horowitz M. Gaucher's disease: molecular, genetic and enzymological aspects. Baillieres Clin Haematol 1997;10:635.

120. Cormand B, Diaz A, Grinberg D, et al. A new gene-pseudogene fusion allele due to a recombination in intron 2 of the glucocerebrosidase gene causes Gaucher disease. Blood Cells Mol Dis 2000;26:409.

121. Soffer D, Yamanaka T, Wenger DA, et al. Central nervous system involvement in adult-onset Gaucher's disease. Acta Neuropathol 1980;49:1.

122. Cox TM, Schofield JP. Gaucher's disease: clinical features and natural history. Baillieres Clin Haematol 1997;10:657.

123. Grabowski GA. Gaucher disease; considerations in prenatal diagnosis. Prenat Diagn 2000;20:60.

124. Sun CC, Panny S, Combs J, et al. Hydrops fetalis associated with Gaucher disease. Pathol Res Pract 1984;179:101.

125. Vellodi A, Bembi B, de Villemeur TB, et al. Management of neuronopathic Gaucher disease: a European consensus. J Inherit Metab Dis 2001;24:319.

126. Svennerholm L, Dreborg S, Erikson A. Gaucher disease of the Norrbottnian type (type III): phenotypic manifestations. In: Desnick RJ, Gatt S, Grabowski GA, eds. Gaucher disease: a century of delineation and research. New York: Alan R. Liss, 1982:67.

127. Harris CM, Taylor DS, Vellodi A. Ocular motor abnormalities in Gaucher disease. Neuropediatrics 1999;30:289.

128. Wenger DA, Roth S, Kudoh T, et al. Biochemical studies in a patient with subacute neuropathic Gaucher disease without visceral glucosylceramide storage. Pediatr Res 1983;17:344.

129. Abrahamov A, Elstein D, Gross-Tsur V, et al. Gaucher's disease variant characterised by progressive calcification of heart valves and unique genotype. Lancet 1995;346:1000.

130. Kampine JP, Brady RO, Kanfer JN et al. Diagnosis of Gaucher's disease and Niemann–Pick disease with small samples of venous blood. Science 1967;155:86.

131. Beutler E, Kuhl W, Matsumoto F, et al. Acid hydrolases in leukocytes and platelets of normal subjects and in patients with Gaucher's and Fabry's disease. J Exp Med 1976;143:975.

132. Beutler E, Kuhl W, Trinidad F, et al. β-Glucosidase activity in fibroblasts from homozygotes and heterozygotes for Gaucher's disease. Am J Hum Genet 1971;23:62.

133. Wenger DA, Olson GC. Heterogeneity in Gaucher disease. In: Callahan JW, Lowden JA, eds. Lysosomes and lysosomal storage diseases. New York: Raven Press, 1981:157.

134. Wenger DA, Roth S. Homozygote and heterozygote identification. In: Desnick RJ, Gatt S, Grabowski JA, eds. Gaucher disease: a century of delineation and research. New York: Alan R. Liss, 1982:551.

135. Schneider EL, Ellis WG, Brady RO, et al. Infantile (type II) Gaucher's disease: in utero diagnosis and fetal pathology. J Pediatr 1972;81:1134.

136. Besley GTN, Ferguson-Smith ME, Frew C, et al. First trimester diagnosis of Gaucher disease in a fetus with trisomy 21. Prenat Diagn 1988;8:471.

137. Wallerstein R, Starkman A, Jansen V. Carrier screening for Gaucher disease in couples of mixed ethnicity. Genet Test 2001;5:61.

138. Rappeport JM, Ginns EI. Bone-marrow transplantation in severe Gaucher's disease. N Engl J Med 1984;311:84.

139. Erikson A, Groth CG, Mansson J-E, et al. Clinical and biochemical outcome of marrow transplantation for Gaucher disease of the Norrbottnian type. Acta Paediatr Scand 1990;79:680.

140. Grabowski GA, Pastores G, Brady RO, et al. Safety and efficacy of macrophage targeted recombinant glucocerebrosidase therapy. Pediatr Res 1993;33:139A.

141. Ringden O, Groth CG, Erikson A, et al. Ten years' experience of bone marrow transplantation for Gaucher disease. Transplantation 1995;59:864.

142. Grabowski GA, Leslie N, Wenstrup RJ. Enzyme therapy for Gaucher disease: the first 5 years. Blood Rev 1998;12:115.

143. Platt FM, Neises GR, Dwek RA, et al. N-Butyldeoxynojirimycin is a novel inhibitor of glycolipid biosynthesis. J Biol Chem 1994;269:8362.

144. Platt FM, Jeyakumar M, Andersson U, et al. Substrate reduction therapy in mouse models of the gly-cosphingolipidoses. Phil Trans R Soc Lond B Biol Sci 2003;358:947.

145. Moyses C. Substrate reduction therapy, clinical evaluation in type1 Gaucher disease. Phil Trans R Soc Lond B Biol Sci 2003;358:955.

146. Zimran A, Elstein D. Gaucher disease and the clinical experience with substrate reduction therapy. Phil Trans R Soc Lond B Biol Sci 2003;358:961.

147. Von Figura K, Gieselmann V, Jaeken J. Metachromatic leukodystrophy. In: Scriver CR , Beaudet AL, Sly WS, et al., eds. The metabolic and molecular bases of inherited disease, 8th ed. New York: McGraw-Hill, 2001:3695.

148. Austin J, Armstrong D, Shearer L. Metachromatic form of diffuse cerebral sclerosis. V. The nature and significance of low sulfatase activity: a controlled study of brain, liver and kidney in four patients with metachromatic leukodystrophy (MLD). Arch Neurol 1965;13:593.

149. Jatzkewitz H, Mehl E. Cerebroside-sulphatase and arylsulphatase A deficiency in metachromatic leukody-strophy (ML). J Neurochem 1969;16:19.

150. Mehl E, Jatzkewitz H. Ein cerebrosidsulfatase aus schweineniere. Hoppe Seylers Z Physiol Chem 1964;339:260.

151. Shapiro LJ, Aleck KA, Kaback MM, et al. Metachromatic leukodystrophy without arylsulfatase A defi-ciency. Pediatr Res 1979;13:1179.

152. Hagberg B. Clinical symptoms, signs and tests in metachromatic leukodystrophy. In: Folch-Pi J, Bauer H, eds. Brain lipids and lipoproteins and the leukodystrophies. Amsterdam: Elsevier, 1963:134.

153. Percy AK, Kaback MM, Herndon RM. Metachromatic leukodystrophy: comparison of early- and late-onset forms. Neurology 1977;27:933.

154. Muller D, Pilz H, Muelen VT. Studies on adult metachromatic leukodystrophy. Part I. Clinical, morpho-logical and histochemical observations in two cases. J Neurol Sci 1969;9:567.

155. Sandhoff K, Kolter T, Harzer K. Sphingolipid activator proteins. In: Scriver CR, Beaudet AL, Sly WS, et al., eds. The metabolic and molecular bases of inherited disease, 8th ed. New York: McGraw-Hill, 2001:3371.

156. Stein C, Gieselmann V, Kreysing J, et al. Cloning and expression of human arylsulfatase A. J Biol Chem 1989;264:1252.

157. Dewji NN, Wenger DA, O'Brien JS. Nucleotide sequence of cloned cDNA for human sphingolipid acti-vator protein-1 precursor. Proc Natl Acad Sci USA 1987;84:8652.

158. Polten A, Fluharty AL, Fluharty CB, et al. Molecular basis of different forms of metachromatic leukody-strophy. N Engl J Med 1991;324:18.

159. Percy AK, Brady RO. Metachromatic leukodystrophy: diagnosis with samples of venous blood. Science 1968;161:594.

160. Porter MT, Fluharty AL, Kihara H. Metachromatic leukodystrophy: arylsulfatase-A deficiency in skin fi-broblast cultures. Proc Natl Acad Sci USA 1969;62:887.

161. Lee-Vaupel M, Conzelmann E. A simple chromogenic assay for arylsulfatase A. Clin Chim Acta 1987;164:171.

162. Beratis NG, Aron AM, Hirschhorn K. Metachromatic leukodystrophy: detection in serum. J Pediatr 1973;83:824.

163. Molzer B, Sundt-Heller R, Kainz-Korschinsky M, et al. Elevated sulfatide excretion in heterozygotes of metachromtic leukodystrophy: dependence on reduction of arylsulphatase A activity. Am J Med Genet 1992;44:523.

164. Whitfield PD, Sharp PC, Johnson DW, et al. Characterization of urinary sulfatides in metachromatic leukodystrophy using electrospray ionization-tandem mass spectrometry. Mol Genet Metab 2001;73:30.

165. Wenger DA, Coppola S, Liu SL. Lysosomal storage disorders: diagnostic dilemmas and prospects for therapy. Genet Med 2002;4:412.

166. Li SC, Kihara H, Serizawa S, et al Activator protein required for the enzymatic hydrolysis of cerebroside sulfate: deficiency in urine of patients affected with cerebroside sulfatase activator deficiency and iden-tity with activators for the enzymatic hydrolysis of GM_1 ganglioside and globotriaosylceramide. J Biol Chem 1985;260:1867.

167. Wenger DA, DeGala G, Williams C, et al. Clinical, pathological and biochemical studies on an infantile case of sulfatide/GM1 activator protein deficiency. Am J Med Genet 1989;33:255.

168. Kudoh T, Sattler M, Malmstrom J, et al. Metabolism of fatty acid-labeled cerebroside sulfate in cultured cells from controls and metachromatic leukodystrophy patients: use in the prenatal identification of a false positive fetus. J Lab Clin Med 1981;98:704.

169. Kudoh T, Wenger DA. Diagnosis of metachromatic leukodystrophy, Krabbe disease and Farber disease after uptake of fatty acid-labeled cerebroside sulfate into cultured skin fibroblasts. J Clin Invest 1982;70:89.

170. Schlote W, Harzer K, Christomanou H, et al. Sphingolipid activator protein 1 deficiency in metachromatic leucodystrophy with normal arylsulphatase A activity: a clinical, morphological, biochemical, and immunological study. Eur J Pediatr 1991;150:584.

171. Penzien JM, Kappler J, Herschkowitz N, et al. Compound heterozygosity for metachromatic leukodystrophy and arylsulfatase A pseudodeficiency alleles is not associated with progressive neurological disease. Am J Hum Genet 1993;52:557.

172. Gieselmann V, Polten A, Kreysing J, et al. Arylsulfatase A pseudodeficiency: loss of a polyadenylation signal and N-glycosylation site. Proc Natl Acad Sci USA 1989;86:9436.

173. Gieselmann V. An assay for the rapid detection of the arylsulfatase A pseudodeficiency allele facilitates diagnosis and genetic counseling for metachromatic leukodystrophy. Hum Genet 1991;86:251.

174. Barth ML, Ward C, Harris A, et al. Frequency of arylsulphatase A pseudodeficiency-associated mutations in a healthy population. J Med Genet 1994;31:667.

175. Leistner S, Young E, Meaney C, et al. Pseudodeficiency of arylsulphatase A: strategy for clarification of genotype in families of subjects with low ASA activity and neurological symptoms. J Inherit Metab Dis 1995;18:710.

176. Regis S, Filocamo M, Stroppiano M, et al. A 9-bp deletion (2320del9) on the background of the arylsulfatase A pseudodeficiency allele in a metachromatic leucodystrophy patient and in a patient with nonprogressive neurological symptoms. Hum Genet 1998;102:50.

177. Krivit W, Peters C, Shapiro EG. Bone marrow transplantation as effective treatment of central nervous system disease in globoid cell leukodystrophy, metachromatic leukodystrophy, adrenoleukodystrophy, mannosidosis, fucosidosis, aspartyglucosaminuria, Hurler, Maroteaux–Lamy and Sly syndromes and Gaucher disease type III. Curr Opin Neurol 1999;12:167.

178. Dierks T, Schmidt B, Borissenko LV, et al. Multiple sulfatase deficiency is caused by mutations in the gene encoding the human C (alpha)-formylglycine generating enzyme. Cell 2003;113:435.

179. Cosma MP, Pepe S, Annunziata I, et al. The multiple sulfatase deficiency gene encodes an essential and limiting factor for the activity of sulfatases. Cell 2003;113:445.

180. Austin J. Studies in metachromatic leukodystrophy. XII. Multiple sulphatase deficiency. Arch Neurol 1973;28:258.

181. Couchot J, Pluot M, Schmauch MA et al. La mucosulfatidose: étude de trois cas familiaux. Arch Fr Pediatr 1974;31:775.

182. Eto Y, Rampini S, Wiesmann U, et al. Enzymic studies of sulphatases in tissues of the normal human and in metachromatic leukodystrophy with multiple sulphatase deficiencies: arylsulphatases A, B, and C, cerebroside sulphatase, psychosine sulphatase and steroid sulphatases. J Neurochem 1974;23:1161.

183. Minami R, Fujibayashi S, Tachi N, et al. Activities of sulfatases for the degradation of acidic glycosaminoglycans in cultured skin fibroblasts from two siblings with multiple sulfatase deficiency. Clin Chim Acta 1983;129:175.

184. Eto Y, Tokoro T, Liebaers I, et al. Biochemical characterization of neonatal multiple sulfatase deficient (MSD) disorder cultured skin fibroblasts. Biochem Biophys Res Commun 1982;106:429.

185. Hopwood JJ, Ballabio A. Multiple sulfatase deficiency and the nature of the sulfatase family. In: Scriver CR, Beaudet AL, Sly WS, et al., eds. The metabolic and molecular bases of inherited disease, 8th ed. New York: McGraw-Hill, 2001:3725.

186. Burk RD, Valle D, Thomas GH et al. Early manifestations of multiple sulfatase deficiency. J Pediatr 1984;104:574.

187. Wenger DA, Rafi MA, Luzi P, et al. Krabbe disease: genetic aspects and progress towards therapy. Mol Genet Metab 2000;70:1.

188. Wenger DA, Suzuki K, Suzuki Y, et al. Galactosylceramide lipidosis: globoid cell leukodystrophy (Krabbe disease). In: Scriver CR, Beaudet AL, Sly WS, et al., eds. The metabolic and molecular bases of inherited disease, 8th ed. New York: McGraw-Hill, 2001:3669.

189. Collier J, Greenfield J. The encephalitis periaxialis of Schilder: a clinical and pathological study, with an account of two cases, one of which was diagnosed during life. Brain 1924;47:489.

190. Dunn HG, Dolman CL, Farrell DF, et al. Krabbe's leukodystrophy without globoid cells. Neurology 1976;26:1035.

191. Suzuki K. Twenty five years of the "psychosine hypothesis": a personal perspective of its history and present status. Neurochem Res 1998;23:251.

192. Im D-S, Heise CE, Nguyen T, et al. Identification of a molecular target of psychosine and its role in globoid cell formation. J Cell Biol 2001;153:429.

193. Young E, Wilson J, Patrick AD, et al. Galactocerebrosidase deficiency in globoid cell leukodystrophy of late onset. Arch Dis Child 1972;47:449.

194. Crome L, Hanefeld F, Patrick D, et al. Late onset globoid cell leukodystrophy. Brain 1973;96:841.

195. Kolodny EH, Raghavan S, Krivit W. Late-onset Krabbe disease (globoid cell leukodystrophy): clinical and biochemical features of 15 cases. Dev Neurosci 1991;13:232.

196. Hagberg B. The clinical diagnosis of Krabbe's infantile leukodystrophy. Acta Paediatr Scand 1963;52:213.

197. Chen YQ, Rafi MA, de Gala G, et al. Cloning and expression of cDNA encoding human galactocerebrosidase, the enzyme deficient in globoid cell leukodystrophy. Hum Mol Genet 1993;2:1841.

198. Rafi MA, Luzi P, Chen YQ, et al. A large deletion together with a point mutation in the GALC gene is a common mutant allele in patients with infantile Krabbe disease. Hum Mol Genet 1995;4:1285.

199. Suzuki K, Suzuki Y. Globoid cell leukodystrophy (Krabbe's disease): deficiency of galactocerebroside β-galactosidase. Proc Natl Acad Sci USA 1970;66:302.

200. Suzuki Y, Suzuki K. Krabbe's globoid cell leukodystrophy: deficiency of galactocerebrosidase in serum, leukocytes and fibroblasts. Science 1971;171:73.

201. Malone MJ, Szoke MC, Looney GL. Globoid leukodystrophy. I. Clinical and enzymatic studies. Arch Neurol 1975;32:606.

202. Besley GTN, Bain AD. Krabbe's globoid cell leukodystrophy: studies on galactosylceramide beta-galactosidase and non-specific beta galactosidase of leucocytes, cultured skin fibroblasts, and amniotic fluid cells. J Med Genet 1976;13:195.

203. Besley GTN, Bain AD. Use of a chromogenic substrate for the diagnosis of Krabbe's disease, with special reference to its application in prenatal diagnosis. Clin Chim Acta 1978;88:229.

204. Besley GTN, Gatt S. Spectrophotometric and fluorimetric assays of galactocerebrosidase activity, their use in the diagnosis of Krabbe's disease. Clin Chim Acta 1981;110:19.

205. Zeigler M, Zlotogora J, Regev R, et al. Prenatal diagnosis of Krabbe disease using a fluorescent derivative of galactosylceramide. Clin Chim Acta 1984;142:313.

206. Wenger DA, Riccardi VM. Possible misdiagnosis of Krabbe disease. J Pediatr 1976;88:76.

207. Kudoh T, Wenger DA. Prenatal diagnosis of Krabbe disease: galactosylceramide metabolism in cultured amniotic fluid cells. J Pediatr 1982;101:754.

208. Vanier MT, Suzuki K. Recent advances in elucidating Niemann–Pick C disease. Brain Pathol 1998; 8:163.

209. Kolodny EH. Niemann–Pick disease. Curr Opin Hematol 2000;7:48.

210. Crocker AC, Farber S. Niemann–Pick disease: a review of 18 patients. Medicine (Baltimore) 1958;37:1.

211. Crocker AC. The cerebral defect in Tay–Sachs disease and Niemann–Pick disease. J Neurochem 1961;7:69.

212. Wenger DA. Niemann-Pick disease. In: Glew RH, Peters SP, eds. Practical enzymology of the sphingolipidoses. New York: Alan R. Liss, 1977:39.

213. Schuchman EH, Desnick RJ. Niemann–Pick disease types A and B: acid sphingomyelinase deficiencies. In: Scriver CR, Beaudet AL, Sly WS, et al., eds. The metabolic and molecular bases of inherited disease, 8th ed. New York: McGraw-Hill, 2001:3589.

214. Patterson MC, Vanier MT, Suzuki K, et al. Niemann-Pick disease type C: a lipid trafficking disorder. In: Scriver CR, Beaudet AL, Sly WS, et al., eds. The metabolic and molecular bases of inherited disease, 8th ed. New York: McGraw-Hill, 2001:3611.

215. Hammersen G, Oppermann H,Harms E, et al. Oculo-neural involvement in an enzymatically proven case of Niemann–Pick disease type B. Eur J Pediatr 1979;132:77.

216. Lipson MH, O'Donnell J, Callahan JW, et al. Ocular involvement in Niemann–Pick disease type B. J Pediatr 1986;108:582.

217. Pavlu H, Elleder M. Two novel mutations in patients with atypical phenotypes of acid sphingomyelinase deficiency. J Inherit Metab Dis 1997;20:615.

218. Gatt S, Dinur T, Barenholz Y. A fluorometric determination of sphingomyelinase by use of fluorescent derivatives of sphingomyelin, and its application to diagnosis of Niemann–Pick disease. Clin Chem 1980;26:93.

219. He X, Chen F, Dagan A, et al. A fluorescence-based, high-performance liquid chromatographic assay to determine acid sphingomyelinase activity and diagnose types A and B Niemann–Pick disease. Anal Biochem 2003;314:116.

220. Vanier MT. Prenatal diagnosis of Niemann–Pick diseases types A, B and C. Prenat Diagn 2002;22:630.

221. Rodriguez-Lafrasse C, Vanier MT. Sphingosylphosphorylcholine in Niemann–Pick disease brain: accumulation in type A but not type B. Neurochem Res 1999;24:199.

222. Schofer O, Mischo B, Puschel W, et al. Early-lethal pulmonary form of Niemann–Pick type C disease belonging to a second rare genetic complementation group. Eur J Pediatr 1998;157:45.

223. Steinberg SJ, Mondal D, Fensom AH. Co-cultivation of Niemann–Pick disease type C fibroblasts be-

longing to complementation groups alpha and beta stimulates LDL-derived cholesterol esterification. J Inherit Metab Dis 1996;19:769.

224. Carstea ED, Morris JA, Coleman KG, et al. Niemann–Pick C1 disease gene: homology to mediators of cholesterol homeostasis. Science 1997;277:228.

225. Naureckiene S, Sleat DE, Lackland H, et al. Identification of HE1 as the second gene of Niemann–Pick C disease. Science 2000;290:2298.

226. Sun X, Marks DL, Park WD, et al. Niemann-Pick C variant detection by altered sphingolipid trafficking and correlation with mutations within a specific domain of NPC1. Am J Hum Genet 2001;68:1361.

227. Millat G, Marcais C, Tomasetto C, et al. Niemann–Pick C1 disease: correlations between NPC1 mutations, levels of NPC1 protein and phenotypes emphasize the functional significance of the putative sterol-sensing domain and of the cysteine-rich luminal loop. Am J Hum Genet 2001;68:1373.

228. Tarugi P, Ballarini G, Bembi B, et al. Niemann–Pick type C disease: mutations of NPC1 gene and evidence of abnormal expression of some mutant alleles in fibroblasts. J Lipid Res 2002;43:1908.

229. Millat G, Marcais C, Rafi MA, et al. Niemann–Pick C1 disease: the I1061T substitution is a frequent mutant allele in patients of Western European descent and correlates with a classic juvenile phenotype. Am J Hum Genet 1999;65:1321.

230. Yamamoto T, Ninomiya H, Matsumoto M, et al. Genotype–phenotype relationship of Niemann–Pick disease type C: a possible correlation between clinical onset and levels of NPC1 protein in isolated skin fibroblasts. J Med Genet 2000;37:707.

231. Millat G, Chikh K, Naureckiene S, et al. Niemann–Pick disease type C: spectrum of HE1 mutations and genotype/phenotype correlations in the NPC2 group. Am J Hum Genet 2001;69:1013.

232. Jan MM, Camfield PR. Nova Scotia Niemann–Pick disease (type D): clinical study of 20 cases. J Child Neurol 1998;13:75.

233. Greer WL, Riddell DC, Byers DM, et al. Linkage of Niemann–Pick disease type D to the same region of human chromosome 18 as Niemann–Pick disease type C. Am J Hum Genet 1997;61:139.

234. Greer WL, Riddell DC, Gillan TL, et al. The Nova Scotia (type D) form of Niemann–Pick disease is caused by a G30976T transversion in NPC1. Am J Hum Genet 1998;63:52.

235. Ioannou YA. Multidrug permeases and subcellular cholesterol transport. Nat Rev Mol Cell Biol 2001;2:657.

236. Garver WS, Heidenreich RA. The Niemann–Pick C proteins and trafficking of cholesterol through the late endosomal/lysosomal system. Curr Mol Med 2002;2:485.

237. Vanier MT, Rodriguez-Lafrasse C, Rousson R, et al. Type C Niemann–Pick disease: spectrum of phenotypic variation in disruption of intracellular LDL-derived cholesterol processing. Biochim Biophys Acta 1991;1096:328.

238. Vanier MT, Rodriguez-Lafrasse C, Rousson R, et al. Prenatal diagnosis of Niemann–Pick type C disease: current strategy from an experience of 37 pregnancies at risk. Am J Hum Genet 1992;51:111.

239. Tsukamoto H, Yamamoto T, Nishigaki T, et al. SSCP analysis by RT-PCR for the prenatal diagnosis of Niemann–Pick disease type C. Prenat Diagn 2001;21:55.

240. Daloze P, Delvin EE, Glorieux FH, et al. Replacement therapy for inherited enzyme deficiency: liver orthotopic transplantation in Niemann–Pick disease type A. Am J Med Genet 1977;1:229.

241. Gartner JC Jr, Bergman I, Malatack JJ, et al. Progression of neurovisceral storage disease with supranuclear ophthalmoplegia following orthotopic liver transplantation. Pediatrics 1986;77:104.

242. Scaggiante B, Pineschi A, Sustersich M, et al. Successful therapy of Niemann–Pick disease by implantation of human amniotic membrane. Transplantation 1987;44:59.

243. Sugita M, Dulaney JT, Moser HW. Ceramidase deficiency in Farber's disease (lipogranulomatosis). Science 1972;178:1100.

244. Moser HW, Linke T, Fensom AH, et al. Acid ceramidase deficiency: Farber lipogranulomatosis. In: Scriver CR, Beaudet AL, Sly WS, et al., eds. The metabolic and molecular bases of inherited disease, 8th ed. New York: McGraw-Hill, 2001:3573.

245. Chen WW, Moser AB, Moser HW. Role of lysosomal acid ceramidase in the metabolism of ceramide in human skin fibroblasts. Arch Biochem Biophys 1981;208:444.

246. Iwamori M, Moser HW. Above-normal urinary excretion of urinary ceramides in Farber's disease, and characterization of their components by high-performance liquid chromatography. Clin Chem 1975;21:725.

247. Toppet M, Vamos-Hurwitz E, Jonniaux G, et al. Farber's disease as a ceramidosis: clinical, radiological and biochemical aspects. Acta Paediatr Scand 1978;67:113.

248. Pierpont MEM, Wenger DA, Moser HW. Heterogeneity of clinical expression of Farber's lipogranulomatosis. Am J Hum Genet 1983;35 (suppl):111A.

249. Antonarakis SE, Valle D, Moser HW, et al. Phenotypic variability in siblings with Farber disease. J Pediatr 1984;104:406.

250. Koch J, Gartner S, Li CM, et al. Molecular cloning and characterization of a full-length complementary DNA encoding human acid ceramidase: identification of the first molecular lesion causing Farber disease. J Biol Chem 1996;271:33110.

251. Li C-M, Park J-H, He X, et al. The human acid ceramidase gene (ASAH): structure, chromosomal location, mutation analysis and expression. Genomics 1999;62:223.

252. Zhang Z, Mandal AK, Mital A, et al. Human acid ceramidase gene: novel mutations in Farber disease. Mol Genet Metab 2000;70:301.

253. Bär J, Linke T, Ferlinz K, et al. Molecular analysis of acid ceramidase deficiency in patients with Farber disease. Hum Mutat 2001;17:199.

254. Muramatsu T, Sakai N, Yanagihara L, et al. Mutation analysis of the acid ceramidase gene in Japanese patients with Farber disease. J Inherit Metab Dis 2002;25:585.

255. Van Echten-Deckert G, Klein A, Linke T, et al. Turnover of endogenous ceramide in cultured normal and Farber fibroblasts. J Lipid Res 1997;38:2569.

256. Levade T, Moser HW, Fensom AH, et al. Neurodegenerative course in ceramidase deficiency (Farber disease) correlates with the residual lysosomal ceramide turnover in cultured living patient cells. J Neurol Sci 1995;134:108.

257. Chatelut M, Feunteun J, Harzer K, et al. A simple method for screening for Farber disease on cultured skin fibroblasts. Clin Chim Acta 1996;245:61.

258. Bernardo K, Hurwitz R, Zenk T, et al. Purification, characterization and biosynthesis of human acid ceramidase. J Biol Chem 1995;270:11098.

259. He X, Li CM, Park JH, et al. A fluorescence-based high-performance liquid chromatographic assay to determine acid ceramidase activity. Anal Biochem 1999;274:264.

260. Fujiwaki T, Yamaguchi S, Sukegawa K, et al. Application of delayed extraction matrix-assisted laser desorption ionization time-of-flight mass spectrometry for analysis of sphingolipids in cultured skin fibroblasts from sphingolipidosis patients. Brain Dev 2002;24:170.

261. Akhunov VS, Gargaun SS, Krasnopolskaya XD. First-trimester enzyme exclusion of Farber disease using a micromethod with [3H]ceramide. J Inherit Metab Dis 1995;18:616.

262. Fensom AH, Benson PF, Neville BRG, et al. Prenatal diagnosis of Farber's disease. Lancet 1979;2:990.

263. Levade T, Enders H, Schliephacke M, et al., A family with a combined Farber and Sandhoff, isolated Sandhoff and isolated fetal Farber disease: postnatal exclusion and prenatal diagnosis of Farber disease using lipid loading tests on intact cultured cells. Eur J Pediatr 1995;154:643.

264. Abramov A, Schorr S, Wolman M. Generalized xanthomatosis with calcified adrenals. Am J Dis Child 1956;91:282.

265. Wolman M, Sterk VV, Gatt S, et al. Primary familial xanthomatosis with involvement and calcification of the adrenals: report of two more cases in siblings of a previously described infant. Pediatrics 1961;28:742.

266. Crocker AC, Vawter GF, Neuhauser EBD, et al. Wolman's disease: three new patients with a recently described lipidosis. Pediatrics 1965;35:627.

267. Kyriakides EC, Filippone N, Paul B, et al. Lipid studies in Wolman's disease. Pediatrics 1970;46:431.

268. Assmann G, Seedorf U. Acid lipase deficiency: Wolman disease and cholesteryl ester storage disease. In: Scriver CR, Beaudet AL, Sly WS, et al., eds. The metabolic and molecular bases of inherited disease, 8th ed. New York: McGraw-Hill, 2001:3551.

269. Schaub J, Janka GE, Christomanou H, et al. Wolman's disease: clinical, biochemical and ultrastructural studies in an unusual case without striking adrenal calcification. Eur J Pediatr 1980;135:45.

270. Schiff L, Schubert WK, McAdams AJ, et al. Hepatic cholesterol ester storage disease, a familial disorder. I. Clinical aspects. Am J Med 1968;44:538.

271. Burke JA, Schubert WK. Deficient activity of hepatic acid lipase in cholesterol ester storage disease. Science 1972;176:309.

272. Partin JC, Schubert WK. The ultrastructure and lipid composition of cultured skin fibroblasts in cholesterol ester storage disease. Pediatr Res 1972;6:393.

273. Beaudet AL, Ferry GD, Nichols BL Jr, et al. Cholesterol ester storage disease: clinical, biochemical, and pathological studies. J Pediatr 1977;90:910.

274. Besley GTN, Broadhead DM, Lawlor E, et al. Cholesterol ester storage disease in an adult presenting with sea-blue histiocytosis. Clin Genet 1984;26:195.

275. Patrick AD, Lake BD. Deficiency of an acid lipase in Wolman's disease. Nature 1969;222:1067.

276. Kyriakides EC, Paul B, Balint JA. Lipid accumulation and acid lipase deficiency in fibroblasts from a family with Wolman's disease, and their apparent correction in vitro. J Lab Clin Med 1972;80:810.

277. Beaudet AL, Lipson AH, Ferry GD, et al. Acid lipase in cultured fibroblasts: cholesterol ester storage disease. J Lab Clin Med 1974;84:54.

278. Patrick AD, Willcox P, Stephens R, et al. Prenatal diagnosis of Wolman's disease. J Med Genet 1976;13:49.

279. Coates PM, Cortner JA, Mennuti MT, et al. Prenatal diagnosis of Wolman disease. Am J Med Genet 1978;2:397.

280. Van Diggelen OP, von Koskull H, Ammala P, et al. First trimester diagnosis of Wolman's disease. Prenat Diagn 1988;8:661.

281. Wenger D. Prenatal diagnosis of disorders of lipid metabolism. In Milunsky A ed. Genetic disorders and the fetus, 4th ed. Baltimore: Johns Hopkins University Press, 1998:394.

282. Anderson RA, Sando GN. Cloning and expression of cDNA encoding human lysosomal acid lipase/cholesteryl ester hydrolase. Similarities to gastric and lingual lipases. J Biol Chem 1991;266:22479.

283. Zschenker O, Jung N, Rethmeier J, et al. Characterization of lysosomal acid lipase mutations in the signal peptide and mature polypeptide region causing Wolman disease. J Lipid Res 2001;42:1033.

284. Lohse P, Maas S, Sewell AC et al. Molecular defects underlying Wolman disease appear to be more heterogeneous than those resulting in cholesteryl ester storage disease. J Lipid Res 1999;40:221.

285. Lohse P, Maas S, Lohse P, et al. Compound heterozygosity for a Wolman mutation is frequent among patients with cholesteryl ester storage disease. J Lipid Res 2000;41:23.

286. Krivit W, Peters C, Dusenbery K, et al. Wolman disease successfully treated by bone marrow transplantation. Bone Marrow Transplant 2000;26:567.

287. Santavuori P. Neuronal ceroid-lipofuscinoses in childhood. Brain Dev 1988;10:80.

288. Vesa J, Hellsten E, Verkruyse LA, et al. Mutations in the palmitoyl protein thioesterase gene causing infantile neuronal ceroid lipofuscinosis. Nature 1995;376:584.

289. Sleat D, Donnelly R, Lackland H, et. al. Association of mutations in a lysosomal protein with classical late-infantile neuronal ceroid lipofuscinosis. Science 1997;277:1802.

290. Vines D, Warburton M. Classical late infantile neuronal ceroid lipofuscinosis fibroblasts are deficient in lysosomal tripeptidyl peptidase I. FEBS Lett 1999;443:131.

291. The International Batten Disease Consortium. Isolation of a novel gene underlying Batten disease, *CLN3*. Cell 1995;82:949.

292. Mitchison HM, O'Rawe AM, Taschner PEM, et al. Batten disease gene CLN3 linkage disequilibrium mapping in the Finnish population and analysis of European haplotypes. Am J Hum Genet 1995;56:654.

293. Munroe PB, Mitchison HM, O'Rawe AM, et al. Spectrum of mutations in the Batten disease gene, CLN3. Am J Hum Genet 1997;61:310.

294. Savukoski M, Klockars T, Holmberg V, et al. CLN5, a novel gene encoding a putative transmembrane protein mutated in Finnish variant late infantile neuronal ceroid lipofuscinosis. Nat Genet 1998;19:286.

295. Wheeler RB, Sharp JD, Schultz RA, et al. The gene mutated in variant late-infantile neuronal ceroid lipofuscinosis (CLN6) and in *nclf* mutant mice encodes a novel predicted transmembrane protein. Am J Hum Genet 2002;70:537.

296. Ranta S, Zhang Y, Ross B, et al. The neuronal ceroid lipofuscinosis in human EPMR and *mnd* mutant mice are associated with mutations in *CLN8*. Nat Genet 1999;23:233.

297. Mitchell WA, Wheeler RB, Sharp DE, et al. Turkish variant late infantile neuronal ceroid lipofuscinosis (*CLN7*) may be allelic to *CLN8*. Eur J Paediatr Neurol 2001;5 (suppl A):21.

298. Voznyi YV, Keulemans JLM, Mancini GMS, et al. A new simple enzyme assay for pre- and postnatal diagnosis of infantile neuronal ceroid lipofuscinosis (INCL) and its variants. J Med Genet 1999;36:471.

299. Macleod PM, Dolman CL, Nickel RE, et al. Prenatal diagnosis of neuronal ceroid lipofuscinosis. N Engl J Med 1984;310:595.

300. Chow CW, Borg J, Billson VR, et al. Fetal tissue involvement in the late infantile type of neuronal ceroid lipofuscinosis. Prenat Diagn 1993;13:833.

301. Macleod PM, Dolman CL, Nickel RE, et al. Prenatal diagnosis of neuronal ceroidlipofuscinoses. Am J Hum Genet 1985;22:781.

302. Rapola J, Salonen R, Ammala P, et al. Prenatal diagnosis of infantile neuronal ceroid-lipofuscinosis, INCL: morphological aspects. J Inherit Metab Dis 1993;16:349.

303. Munroe PB, Rapola J, Mitchison HM, et al. Prenatal diagnosis of Batten's disease. Lancet 1996;347:1014.

304. Van Diggelen OP, Keulemans JLM, Winchester B, et al. A rapid fluorogenic palmitoyl-protein thioesterase assay: pre- and postnatal diagnosis in INCL. Mol Genet Metab 1999;66:240.

305. Young EP, Winchester BG, Logan WP, et al. Exclusion of late infantile neuronal ceroid lipofuscinosis (LINCL) in a fetus by assay of tripeptidyl peptidase I in chorionic villi. Prenat Diagn 2000;20:337.
306. Lake BD, Steward CG, Oakhill A, et al. Bone marrow transplantation in late infantile Batten disease and juvenile Batten disease. Neuropaediatrics 1997;28:80.
307. Zhang Z, Butler JDeB, Levin S, et al. Lysosomal ceroid depletion by drugs: therapeutic implications for a hereditary neurodegenerative disease of childhood. Nat Med 2001;7:478.
308. Powers JM, Moser HW. Peroxisomal disorders: genotype, phenotype, major neuropathologic lesions and pathogenesis. Brain Pathol 1998;8:101.
309. Gould SJ, Raymond GV, Valle D. The peroxisome biogenesis disorders. In: Scriver CR, Beaudet AL, Sly WS, et al., eds. The metabolic and molecular bases of inherited disease, 8th ed. New York: McGraw-Hill, 2001:3181.
310. Wanders RJ, Barth PG, Heymans HAS. Single peroxisomal enzyme deficiencies. In: Scriver CR, Beaudet AL, Sly WS, et al., eds. The metabolic and molecular bases of inherited disease, 8th ed. New York: McGraw-Hill, 2001:3219.
311. Moser, HW. Molecular genetics of peroxisomal disorders. Front Biosci 2000;5:D298.
312. Depreter M, Espeel M, Roels F. Human peroxisomal disorders. Microsc Res Tech 2003;61:203.
313. Distel B, Erdmann R, Gould SJ, et al. A unified nomenclature for peroxisome biogenesis factors. J Cell Biol 1996;135:1.
314. Schutgens RB, Schrakamp G, Wanders RJ, et al. Prenatal and perinatal diagnosis of peroxisomal disorders. J Inherit Metab Dis 1989;12 S1:118.
315. Brookhyser KM, Lipson MH, Moser AB, et al. Prenatal diagnosis of rhizomelic chondrodysplasia punctata due to an isolated alkyldihydroacetonephosphate acyltransferase synthase deficiency. Prenat Diagn 1999;19:383.
316. Wanders RJ, Dekker C, Ofman R, et al. Immunoblot analysis of peroxisomal proteins in liver and fibroblasts from patients. J Inherit Metab Dis 1995;18 S1:101.
317. Maxwell MA, Nelson PV, Chin SJ, et al. A common PEX1 frameshift mutation in patients with disorders of peroxisome biogenesis correlates with the severe Zellweger syndrome phenotype. Hum Genet 1999;105:38.
318. Roels F, Verdonck V, Pauwels M, et al. Light microscopic visualization of peroxisomes and plasmalogens in first trimester chorionic villi. Prenat Diagn 1987;7:525.
319. Wanders RJ, van Wijland MJ, van Roermund CW, et al. Prenatal diagnosis of Zellweger syndrome by measurement of very long chain fatty acid (C26:0) β-oxidation in cultured chorionic villous fibroblasts: implications for early diagnosis of other peroxisomal disorders. Clin Chim Acta 1987;165:303.
320. Wanders RJ, Schutgens RB, van den Bosch H, et al. Prenatal diagnosis of inborn errors in peroxisomal β-oxidation. Prenat Diagn 1991;11:253.
321. Suzuki Y, Shimozawa N, Kawabata I, et al. Prenatal diagnosis of peroxisomal disorders biochemical and immunocytochemical studies on peroxisomes in human amniocytes. Brain Dev 1994;16:27.
322. Zhang Z, Suzuki Y, Shimozawa N, et al. Prenatal diagnosis of peroxisome biogenesis disorders by means of immunofluorescence staining of cultured chorionic villous cells. Clin Genet 1999;56:467.
323. Schaumburg HH, Powers JM, Raine CS, et al. Adrenoleukodystrophy: a clinical and pathological study of 17 cases. Arch Neurol 1975;32:577.
324. Moser HW, Moser AB, Kawamura N, et al. Adrenoleukodystrophy: studies of the phenotype, genetics and biochemistry. Johns Hopkins Med J 1980;147:217.
325. Moser HW, Moser AE, Singh I, et al. Adrenoleukodystrophy: survey of 303 cases: biochemistry, diagnosis, and therapy. Ann Neurol 1984;16:628.
326. Fournier B, Smeitink JAM, Dorland L, et al. Peroxisomal disorders: a review. J Inherit Metab Dis 1994;17:470.
327. Moser HW, Smith KD, Watkins PA, et al. X-linked adrenoleukodystrophy. In: Scriver CR, Beaudet AL, Sly WS, et al., eds. The metabolic and molecular bases of inherited disease, 8th ed. New York: McGraw-Hill, 2001:3257.
328. Griffin JW, Goren E, Schaumburg H et al. Adrenomyeloneuropathy: a probable variant of adrenoleukodystrophy. I. Clinical and endocrinological aspects. Neurology 1977;27:1107.
329. Schaumburg HH, Powers JM, Raine CS, et al. Adrenomyeloneuropathy: a probable variant of adrenoleukodystrophy. II. General pathologic, neuropathologic, and biochemical aspects. Neurology 1977;27:1114.
330. Igarashi M, Schaumburg HH, Powers JM, et al. Fatty acid abnormality in adrenoleukodystrophy. J Neurochem 1976;26:851.

331. Tonshoff B, Lehnert W, Ropers H-H. Adrenoleukodystrophy: diagnosis and carrier detection by determination of long-chain fatty acids in cultured fibroblasts. Clin Genet 1982;22:25.

332. Moser HW, Moser AB, Trojak JE, et al. Identification of female carriers of adrenoleukodystrophy. J Pediatr 1983;103:54.

333. O'Neill BP, Moser HW, Saxena KM, et al. Adrenoleukodystrophy: clinical and biochemical manifestations in carriers. Neurology 1984;34:798.

334. Singh I, Moser AE, Moser HW, et al. Adrenoleukodystrophy: Impaired oxidation of very long chain fatty acids in white blood cells, cultured skin fibroblasts, and amniocytes. Pediatr Res 1984;18:286.

335. Lazo O, Contreras M, Bhushan A, et al. Adrenoleukodystrophy: impaired oxidation of fatty acids due to peroxisomal lignoceroyl-CoA ligase deficiency. Arch Biochem Biophys 1989;270:722.

336. Mosser J, Douar AM, Sarde CO, et al. Putative X-linked adrenoleukodystrophy gene shares unexpected homology with ABC transporters. Nature 1993;361:726.

337. Corzo D, Gibson W, Johnson K, et al. Contiguous deletion of the X-linked adrenoleukodystrophy gene (ABCD1) and DXS1357E: a novel neonatal phenotype similar to peroxisomal biogenesis disorders. Am J Hum Genet 2002;70:1520.

338. Boue J, Oberle I, Heilig R, et al. First trimester prenatal diagnosis of adrenoleukodystrophy by determination of very long chain fatty acid levels and by linkage analysis to a DNA probe. Hum Genet 1985;69:272.

339. Moser AB, Moser HW. The prenatal diagnosis of X-linked adrenoleukodystrophy. Prenat Diagn 1999;19:46.

340. Wanders RJ, Mooyer PW, Dekker C, et al. X-linked adrenoleukodystrophy: improved prenatal diagnosis using both biochemical and immunological methods. J Inherit Metab Dis 1998;21:285.

341. Imamura A, Suzuki Y, Song XQ, et al. Prenatal diagnosis of adrenoleukodystrophy by means of mutation analysis. Prenat Diagn 1996;16:259.

342. Matsumoto T, Tsuru A, Amamoto N, et al. Mutation analysis of the ALD gene in seven Japanese families with X-linked adrenoleukodystrophy. J Hum Genet 2003;48:125.

343. Moser AB, Borel J, Odone A, et al. A new dietary therapy for adrenoleukodystrophy: biochemical and preliminary clinical results in 36 patients. Ann Neurol 1987;21:240.

344. Aubourg P, Adamsbaum C, Lavallard-Rousseau MC, et al. A two-year trial of oleic and erucic acids ("Lorenzo's oil") as treatment for adrenomyeloneuropathy. N Engl J Med 1993;329:745.

345. Moser HW, Tutschka PJ, Brown FR III, et al. Bone marrow transplant in adrenoleukodystrophy. Neurology 1984;34:1410.

346. Aubourg P, Blanche S, Jambaque I, et al. Reversal of early neurologic and neuroradiologic manifestations of X-linked adrenoleukodystrophy by bone marrow transplantation. N Engl J Med 1990;322:1860.

347. Wanders RJA, Jakobs C, Skjeldal OH. Refsum disease. In: Scriver CR, Beaudet AL, Sly WS, et al., eds. The metabolic and molecular bases of inherited disease, 8th ed. New York: McGraw-Hill, 2001:3303.

348. Wierzbicki AS, Lloyd MD, Schofield CJ, et al. Refsum's disease: a peroxisomal disorder affecting phytanic acid α-oxidation. J Neurochem 2002;80:727.

349. Steinberg D, Herndon JH Jr, Uhlendorf BW, et al. Refsum's disease: nature of the enzyme defect. Science 1967;156:1740.

350. Herndon JH Jr, Steinberg D, Uhlendorf BW, et al. Refsum's disease: characterization of the enzyme defect in cell culture. J Clin Invest 1969;48:1017.

351. Herndon JH, Steinberg D, Uhlendorf BW. Refsum's disease: defective oxidation of phytanic acid in tissue cultures derived from homozygotes and heterozygotes. N Engl J Med 1969;281:1034.

352. Hutton D, Steinberg D. Localization of the enzymatic defect in phytanic acid storage disease (Refsum's disease). Neurology 1973;23:1333.

353. Jansen GA, Wanders RJ, Watkins PA, et al. Phytanoyl-coenzyme A hydroxylase deficiency: the enzyme defect in Refsum disease. N Engl J Med 1997;337:133.

354. Jansen GA, Ofman R, Ferdinandusse S, et al. Refsum disease is caused by mutations in the phytanoyl-CoA hydroxylase gene. Nat Genet 1997;17:190.

355. Mihalik SJ, Morrell JC, Kim D, et al. Identification of PAHX, a Refsum disease gene. Nat Genet 1997;17:185.

356. Mukherji M, Chien W, Kershaw NJ, et al. Structure-function analysis of phytanoyl-CoA 2-hydroxylase mutations causing Refsum's disease. Hum Mol Genet 2001;10:1971.

357. Wierzbicki AS, Mitchell J, Lambert-Hammill M, et al. Identification of genetic heterogeneity in Refsum's disease. Eur J Hum Genet 2000;8:649.

358. van den Brink DM, Brites P, Haasjes J, et al. Identification of *PEX7* as the second gene involved in Refsum disease. Am J Hum Genet 2003;72:471.

359. Poulos A. Diagnosis of Refsum's disease using (1-^{14}C)phytanic acid as substrate. Clin Genet 1981;20:247.

360. Refsum S. Heredopathia atactica polyneuritiformis. Phytanic-acid storage disease, Refsum's disease: a biochemically well-defined disease with a specific dietary treatment. Arch Neurol 1981;38:605.

361. Roels F. Screening, prevention, treatment, and pathogenesis of congenital peroxisomal disorders. Eur Concert Act Final Rep 2003;1.

362. Suzuki Y, Iai M, Kamei A, et al. Peroxisomal acyl CoA oxidase deficiency. J Pediatr 2002;140:128.

363. Suzuki Y, Zhang Z, Shimozawa N, et al. Prenatal diagnosis of peroxisomal D-3-hydroxyacyl-CoA dehydratase/D-3-hydroxyacyl-CoA-dehydrogenase bifunctional protein deficiency. J Hum Genet 1999;44:143.

364. Van Grunsven EG, van Berkel E, Moojier PA, et al. Peroxisomal bifunctional protein deficiency revisited: resolution of its true enzymatic and molecular basis. Am J Hum Genet 1999;64:99.

365. Ferdinandusse S, Denis S, Clayton PT, et al. Mutations in the gene encoding peroxisomal α-methylacyl-CoA racemase cause adult-onset sensory motor neuropathy. Nat Genet 2000;24:188.

366. Hoffmann GF, Brendel SU, Scharfschwerdt SR, et al. Mevalonate kinase assay using DEAE-cellulose column chromatography for first-trimester prenatal diagnosis and complementation analysis in mevalonic aciduria. J Inherit Metab Dis 1992;15:738.

367. Houten SM, van Woerden CS, Wijburg FA, et al. Carrier frequency of the V377I (1129G $\rightarrow$ A) MVK mutation, associated with hyper-IgD and periodic fever syndrome in the Netherlands. Eur J Hum Genet 2003;11:196.

368. Simon A, Cuisset L. Vincent MF, et al. Molecular analysis of the mevalonate kinase gene in a cohort of patients with the hyper-igd and periodic fever syndrome: its application as a diagnostic tool. Ann Intern Med 2001;135:338.

369. Knerr I, Zschocke J, Trautmann U, et al. Glutaric aciduria type III: a distinctive non-disease? J Inherit Metab Dis 2002;25:483.

370. Eaton JW, Mouchou M. Acatalasemia. In Scriver CR, Beaudet AL, Sly WS, et al, eds. The metabolic and molecular bases of inherited disease, 7th ed. New York: McGraw-Hill, 1995:2371.

371. Rumsby G. Biochemical and genetic diagnosis of the primary hyperoxalurias: a review. Mol Urol 2000;4:349.

372. Danpure C. Primary hyperoxaluria. In: Scriver CR, Beaudet AL, Sly WS, et al., eds. The metabolic and molecular bases of inherited disease, 8th ed. New York: McGraw-Hill, 2001:3323.

373. Havel RJ, Kane JP. Introduction: structure and metabolism of plasma lipoproteins. In: Scriver CR, Beaudet AL, Sly WS, et al., eds. The metabolic and molecular bases of inherited disease, 8th ed. New York: McGraw-Hill, 2001:2705.

374. Goldstein JL, Hobbs HL, Brown MS. Familial hypercholesterolemia. In: Scriver CR, Beaudet AL, Sly WS, et al., eds. The metabolic and molecular bases of inherited disease, 8th ed. New York: McGraw-Hill, 2001:2863.

375. Humphries S, King-Underwood L, Gudnason V, et al. Six DNA polymorphisms in the low-density lipoprotein-receptor gene: their genetic relationship and an example of their use for identifying affected relatives of patients with familial hypercholesterolaemia. J Med Genet 1993;30:273.

376. Heath KE, Luong L-A, Leonard JV, et al. The use of a highly informative CA repeat polymorphism within the abetalipoproteinaemia locus (4q22–24). Prenat Diagn 1997;17:1181.

377. Brown MS, Kovanen PT, Goldstein JL, et al. Prenatal diagnosis of homozygous familial hypercholesterolaemia: expression of a genetic disease in utero. Lancet 1978;i:526.

378. De Gennes JL, Daffos F, Dairou F, et al. Direct fetal blood examination for prenatal diagnosis of homozygous familial hypercholesterolaemia. Arteriosclerosis 1985;5:440.

379. Reshef A, Meiner V, Dann EJ, et al. Prenatal diagnosis of familial hypercholesterolaemia caused by the "Lebanese" mutation at the low density lipoprotein receptor locus. Hum Genet 1992;89:237.

380. De Oliveira e Silva ER, Haddad L, Kwiterovich PO Jr, et al. Applicability of LDLR flanking microsatellite polymorphisms for prenatal diagnosis of homozygous state for familial hypercholesterolaemia. Clin Genet 1998;53:375.

381. Norum RA, Lakier JB, Goldstein S, et al. Familial deficiency of apolipoproteins A-I and C-III and precocious coronary-artery disease. N Engl J Med 1982;306:1513.

382. Ordovas JM, Cassidy DK, Civeira F, et al. Familial apolipoprotein A-I, C-III and A-IV deficiency and premature atherosclerosis due to deletion of a gene complex on chromosome 11. J Biol Chem 1989;264:16339.

383. Tall AR, Breslow JL, Rubin EM. Genetic disorders affecting high plasma high-density lipoproteins. In: Scriver CR, Beaudet AL, Sly WS, et al., eds. The metabolic and molecular bases of inherited disease, 8th ed. New York: McGraw-Hill, 2001:2915.

384. Brunzell JD, Deeb SS. Familial lipoprotein lipase deficiency, apoC-II deficiency, and hepatic lipase deficiency. In: Scriver CR, Beaudet AL, Sly WS, et al., eds. The metabolic and molecular bases of inherited disease, 8th ed. New York: McGraw-Hill, 2001:2789.

385. Mahley RW, Rall SC Jr. Type III hyperlipoproteinaemia (dysbetalipoproteinaemia). The role of apolipoprotein E in normal and abnormal lipoprotein metabolism. In: Scriver CR, Beaudet AL, Sly WS, et al., eds. The metabolic and molecular bases of inherited disease, 8th ed. New York: McGraw-Hill, 2001:2835.

386. Santamarina-Fojo S, Hoeg JM, Assmann G, et al. Lecithin cholesterol acyltransferase deficiency and fish-eye disease In: Scriver CR, Beaudet AL, Sly WS, et al., eds. The metabolic and molecular bases of inherited disease, 8th ed. New York: McGraw-Hill, 2001:2817.

387. Wetterau JR, Aggerbeck LP, Bouma ME, et al. Absence of microsomal triglyceride transfer protein in individuals with abetalipoproteinemia. Science 1992;258:999.

388. Assmann G, von Eckardstein A, Brewer BH. Familial analphalipoproteinemia disease. In: Scriver CR, Beaudet AL, Sly WS, et al., eds. The metabolic and molecular bases of inherited disease, 8th ed. New York: McGraw-Hill, 2001:2937.

Gideon Bach, Ph.D.

12

Prenatal Diagnosis of Disorders of Mucopolysaccharide Metabolism

The mucopolysaccharidoses (MPSs) are a group of eleven genetically distinct disorders in which mucopolysaccharides accumulate because of defective lysosomal hydrolases participating in the degradation of these substrates. They are all progressive disorders involving multiple organ systems as a result of the storage and excretion of excess mucopolysaccharides. The mode of inheritance is autosomal recessive for all except Hunter syndrome (MPS II), which is X-linked recessive. Considerable heterogeneity is recognized in the clinical manifestations in each of these disorders, from severe to mild forms, that are sometimes also delineated as infantile (severe), juvenile (intermediate), and adult (mild) forms. These variations stem mostly from allelic mutations in genes of the relevant lysosomal hydrolases, leading to either complete deficiency of the relevant protein or its activity, resulting in a severe phenotype or structural mutations leaving some residual activity in less affected patients. In the past 15 years almost all of the relevant genes involved in the various MPSs have been cloned and characterized. Subsequently, disease-causing mutations have been discovered for each of these disorders, facilitating diagnosis (including prenatal diagnosis) and unambiguous heterozygote identification in high-risk families.

The cloning of the MPS genes enabled the design of animal models ("knockout mice") for investigating the basis for the physiologic and biochemical abnormalities occurring in these diseases and for the development of therapeutic procedures for these patients. Therapy experiments were extensively studied in recent years, which enhanced the need for early diagnosis of these patients as a crucial step for successful treatment. Indeed, newborn screening for babies affected with MPS has been established in a few centers in the world.[1,2] For older patients the detection of a patient affected with MPS is achieved by urine analysis for excess mucopolysaccharides excretion.[3]

The characteristics of the eleven types, the most common allelic variants, and the chromosomal localization of each of these genes are summarized in Table 12.1.

HURLER SYNDROME (α-L-IDURONIDASE DEFICIENCY; MUCOPOLYSACCHARIDOSIS IH)

The various features characterizing Hurler syndrome include early corneal clouding and apparently normal development for most of the first year of life. Thereafter, psychomotor

Table 12.1. The classification of the mucopolysaccharidoses

Number	Eponym	Clinical Manifestations	Enzyme Deficiency	Gene Locus
IH	Hurler	Corneal clouding, dysostosis multiplex, organomegaly, heart disease, mental retardation, death in childhood	α-L-iduronidase	4p16.3
IS	Scheie	Corneal clouding, stiff joints, normal intelligence, normal lifespan	α-L-iduronidase	
IH/S	Hurler–Scheie	Phenotype intermediate between IH and IS	α-L-iduronidase	
II (severe)	Hunter (severe)	Dysostosis multiplex, organomegaly, no corneal clouding, mental retardation, death before 15 years of age	Iduronate sulfatase	Xq28
II (mild)	Hunter (mild)	Normal intelligence, short stature, survival mostly 20–30 years	Iduronate sulfatase	
III A	Sanfilippo A	Profound mental deterioration, hyperactivity, relatively mild somatic manifestations	Heparan N-sulfatase (heparan sulfamidase)	17q25.3
III B	Sanfilippo B	Phenotype similar to III A	α-N-acetylglucosaminidase	17q21
III C	Sanfilippo C	Phenotype similar to III A	acetyl-CoA- α-Glucosaminide-acetyltransferase	14
IIID	Sanfilippo D	Phenotype similar to IIIA	N-acetylglucosamine-6-sulfatase	12q14
IVA	Morquio A	Distinctive skeletal abnormalities, corneal clouding, odontoid hypoplasia, milder forms known to exist	Galactose-6-sulfatase	16q24.3
IVB	Morquio B	Spectrum of severity as in IVA	β-galactosidase	3p21.33
VI	Maroteaux–Lamy	Dysostosis multiplex, corneal clouding, normal intelligence, survival to teens in severe form, milder forms known to exist	N-acetylgalactosamine-4-sulfatase (arylsulfatase B)	5q11–13
VII	Sly	Dysostosis multiplex, hepatosplenomegaly, wide spectrum of severity	β-glucuronidase	7q21.11
IX		Short stature, soft tissues masses, particularly in the limbs, mild dysmorphic craniofacial features.	Hyaluronidase (HYAL1)	3p21.2–21.3

deterioration becomes evident, causing profound retardation, associated with skeletal and connective-tissue abnormalities leading to spinal deformity, stiff joints, chest deformity, deafness, dwarfism, and coarse facies. Other features include hepatosplenomegaly, recurrent infections of the upper respiratory tract, and cardiomyopathy, all of which are progressive and almost invariably lead to death by 10 years of age.[4,5] An estimate of the incidence of Hurler syndrome is 1 per 100,000 births.[6]

Mucopolysaccharides accumulate in various tissues and cells in Hurler syndrome, primarily dermatan sulfate and heparan sulfate.[7] The basic defect in this disorder is a specific deficiency of α-L-iduronidase.[8,9] Earlier studies identifying a Hurler corrective factor[10] showed this to be α-L-iduronidase.[8] In various patients with Hurler syndrome, no cross-reactive material of α-L-iduronidase was detected.

The iduronidase gene was cloned[11–13] after the purification of the enzyme. Numerous mutations have been characterized in patients with Hurler syndrome, some of which occur commonly.[4,14,15] Generally this type is characterized with either the absence of the enzyme protein or an active enzyme. Multiple mutations have been found in Arab patients with Hurler syndrome in a small geographic region in Israel.[16] The cause of this phenomenon is not well understood. The diagnosis of Hurler syndrome is made by direct assay for α-L-iduronidase activity in various tissues, including leukocytes, lymphocytes, cultured fibroblasts, amniocytes, and serum.[4] Appropriate oligosaccharides derived from dermatan or heparan sulfate are also used.[17] The characterization of mutations causing this disorder is a useful tool for its diagnosis, including heterozygote identification in high-risk families. Heterozygote detection is also feasible by measuring α-L-iduronidase activity in leukocytes or cultivated skin fibroblasts in which intermediate activity has been found.[12,13,18–22]

The prenatal diagnosis of Hurler syndrome was accomplished first by Fratantoni et al.[23] and subsequently by others.[24,25] However, the enzyme activity of heterozygote fetuses might overlap with those of affected fetuses. It was therefore suggested in such cases that a [^{35}S]sulfate accumulation test be performed for final confirmation.[26] This latter procedure is of particular importance also in cases in which one of the parents possesses the pseudodeficiency mutation (very low iduronidase activity in apparently healthy individuals) in addition to the Hurler-causing mutation in this gene.[25] An important breakthrough in prenatal diagnosis has been achieved through the use of chorionic villus sampling (CVS), which is performed at 10–11 weeks of pregnancy.[27,28] This technique has been used for early detection of fetuses affected with Hurler syndrome as well as other MPSs.[28] Prenatal diagnosis by CVS (see chapter 5) requires complete removal of any maternal tissue, because even traces of maternal contamination might result in misdiagnosis. Preimplantation diagnosis (see chapter 27) is another important advance in very early prenatal diagnosis of inherited diseases.[29]

At present, prenatal diagnosis is performed either by routine enzyme assays using the sensitive fluorescent substrates or by mutation analysis, which also can be used as an important tool for the confirmation of the enzyme diagnosis.

In the past decade considerable progress has been achieved in the therapy of this disease as well as the other MPSs. Experimental therapy has been performed on animal model as well as on human patients. Significant improvement of some features in patients with Hurler syndrome, as well as other MPSs, was achieved by bone marrow transplantation,[30–34] but the great risk of this procedure, mainly due to graft-versus-host disease, should be noted. Thus, ethical considerations of this procedure have been raised.[34] Recent advances in gene therapy, in which the normal gene is injected into cells of patients or attempts are made to correct the mutation in situ were also extensively studied, and are believed to yield the most hopeful approach for the successful treatment of these inherited disorders.[35,36] Enzyme replacement therapy for the various α-L-iduronidase deficiency types has been recently used successfully,[37–39] although the blood–brain barrier poses the major difficulty in successful treatment of the mental deficiency of these patients. Moreover, immune tolerance appears to develop in some MPS1 patients after long-term enzyme replacement therapy.[39a] Finally, antibiotic drugs, especially gentamicin, which are capable of suppressing stop codon mutations, has been shown in vitro to restore some activity of the mutated iduronidase and reduce substrate accumulation.[40]

SCHEIE SYNDROME (α-L-IDURONIDASE DEFICIENCY; MUCOPOLYSACCHARIDOSIS IS)

Scheie syndrome is the mild subtype. The essential clinical features include severe corneal clouding, deformity of the hands, and involvement of the aortic valve, with normal intelligence. Other somatic features of Hurler syndrome may also be found, but life expectancy usually is normal. Scheie syndrome is extremely rare (the estimated incidence being about 1 per 500,000 births),[4] but undiagnosed patients undoubtedly exist.

Mucopolysaccharide accumulates in cells and tissues, and a basic deficiency of α-L-iduronidase occurs, as it does in Hurler syndrome.[8] Hopwood et al. reported kinetic differences in the residual activity of α-L-iduronidase of patients with Hurler syndrome, as compared with patients with Scheie syndrome.[17] The Scheie and Hurler mutations are allelic, and the failure of complementation after cell-fusion studies involving Hurler and Scheie cells is consistent with this view. The statements made for heterozygote detection and prenatal diagnosis in Hurler syndrome apply equally to Scheie syndrome. The question, of course, is whether prenatal diagnosis is an appropriate approach. This decision is clearly a parental one. In most patients with Scheie syndrome, mutation analysis demonstrated compound heterozygosity of a "severe mutation" and a second mutation allowing the presence of trace enzyme activities.[41,42]

Patients with Scheie syndrome have normal intelligence and a reasonable lifespan; therefore, surgery to correct aortic valvular disease, carpal tunnel syndrome, glaucoma, and corneal disease is important.

HURLER–SCHEIE COMPOUND DISEASE (α-L-IDURONIDASE DEFICIENCY MUCOPOLYSACCHARIDOSIS IH/S)

The allelic subgroup Hurler–Scheie compound disease is not well defined and is essentially an intermediate clinical form. The clinical phenotype has features in common with both the Hurler and the Scheie syndromes but sometimes is intermediate in severity.[4,43] The incidence of this compound disorder has been calculated to be about 1 per 115,000 births.[44]

Mucopolysaccharide storage in cells and tissues is again characteristic of this type, and the basic enzymatic deficiency of α-L-iduronidase is found in cultivated skin fibroblasts, as in other tissues of these patients.[8] This disorder therefore represents a genetic compound for two different alleles at the locus for α-L-iduronidase, although homozygosity for one mutation is equally plausible. Indeed, most patients with the MPS I/H type were characterized to be compound heterozygotes for two different mutations, but homozygosity for one mutation was also identified.[42]

HUNTER SYNDROME (IDURONATE SULFATASE DEFICIENCY; MUCOPOLYSACCHARIDOSIS II)

There are severe and mild forms of Hunter syndrome, a sex-linked mucopolysaccharide disorder.[4,5] The most prominent difference between these forms is that patients with the mild form have normal intelligence and mostly longer life expectancy than the severe form. In addition to mental retardation, the essential features of the severe form include coarse facies, dwarfism, stiff joints, retinal degeneration, hepatosplenomegaly, and recurrent infections of the ear and upper respiratory tract. Clinically, the patients are similar to Hurler patients, but corneal clouding is observed only rarely.[45] Heart disease due to valvular, myocardial, and ischemic factors is the most common cause of death, often occurring in the first or second decade of life.[46,47] The typical signs are not always prominent in patients with the mild form of Hunter syndrome,[48,49] and these patients usually have normal intelligence; survival is known to have reached 87 years of age in one case. Nevertheless, most patients with the mild form have visceral symptoms similar to those of patients with the severe form. Both mild and severe forms have been described in one sibship.[50] Life expectancy is longer with the mild disorder than with the severe form, but for most patients, it is not beyond the second decade of life. The incidence of Hunter syndrome is about 0.66 per 100,000 births,[4] but Schaap and Bach reported a relatively high frequency among Ashkenazi and Moroccan Jews in Israel.[51] Genetic analysis of families of patients with Hunter syndrome in these ethnic groups indicated an excess of individuals bearing the mutant allele (heterozygotes or affected hemizygotes). This phenomenon was attributed to a possible selection in favor of the Hunter allele in these populations.[52]

Sex-linked inheritance in Hunter syndrome is well established and demonstrable by the cloning of single cells from cultivated skin fibroblasts.[53–55] Cases of female patients with Hunter syndrome have been reported;[56,57] however, at least one was later reevaluated and found to be affected by multisulfatase-deficient syndrome, and a second was not fully evaluated (Bach G, unpublished data). Other female patients with Hunter syndrome had chromosomal aberrations involving the long arm of one X chromosome; they included a 3-year-old girl with the severe form bearing a balanced translocation 46XX,t (X:5) with the X breakpoint between q26 and q27[58] and a girl aged 2.5 years with a mild form bearing a partial deletion of the long arm of one X chromosome.[59] Girls affected with Hunter syndrome and normal karyotype were also reported.[60,61]

The mucopolysaccharide storage in this disorder (dermatan and heparan sulfate) is due to the deficient activity of the hydrolase—iduronate 2 sulfate sulfatase (IDS).[62,63] Both the mild and severe forms of Hunter syndrome manifest the same enzymatic deficiency[62,64] because of allelic mutations at the IDS locus on the X chromosome. In heterozygotes, there is no mucopolysaccharide accumulation in cultured fibroblasts, where, on average, 50 percent of the cells should contain the X chromosome with the Hunter mutation as the active X. This is obviously due to cross-correction,[65] so that cells with the normal X secrete the enzyme into the medium, which is later recaptured by the "Hunter cells," thus preventing storage.

IDS has been purified from human liver and characterized in various human tissues.[66] This allowed the isolation of the IDS complementary DNA (cDNA) clone[67] and the characterization of mutations causing IDS deficiency. Numerous mutations were characterized in patients with Hunter syndrome in both the severe and mild subtypes. It should be noted that approximately 20 percent of these patients show full or partial deletions of the IDS gene or other rearrangements.[68] These patients are all affected by the severe form of the disease, whereas other patients had point mutations (missense or nonsense) resulting in either mild or severe manifestations.[69] There are mutation "hot spots" in this gene that are CpG sites, resulting in more frequent mutations in these sites.[70] The molecular analysis may be complicated because of the presence of a second IDS-related locus in Xq28.[71] Metabolic correction had been achieved by retrovirus-mediated gene transfer.[72,73]

The disorder is diagnosed by the assay of IDS in serum, leukocytes, and cultivated skin fibroblasts.[64,74–76] Heterozygote detection is of utmost importance in this disorder and is possible by cloning cultivated skin fibroblasts and assaying IDS[53,54] or by the analysis of hair roots.[77–79] However, these techniques are laborious and complicated. Tonnesen introduced a technique of heterozygote detection in cultured skin fibroblasts by incubating the cells with radioactive sulfate in the presence of fructose-l-phosphate and thus blocking the uptake of the secreted enzyme from the cells with the normal X into the affected cells.[80] Therefore, the "affected" cells will accumulate radioactively labeled mucopolysaccharides. This yielded a 90 percent detection rate. Lymphocytes and serum have been used for enzyme assays for heterozygote detection[64] but have yielded a detection rate of only 50 percent. Zlotogora and Bach used a substrate of highly specific radioactivity and, incubating under linear conditions, succeeded in detecting more than 90 percent of obligate heterozygotes by enzyme assay in serum.[81] After the identification of mutations causing Hunter disease, DNA analysis is the most efficient tool for heterozygote identification, but similar to other disorders in this group, many mutations causing Hunter disease are expected (see above), although some are relatively more common. The characterization of numerous mutations hitherto should simplify this search.

The prenatal diagnosis of Hunter syndrome was first achieved by demonstrating increased [^{35}S]mucopolysaccharide accumulation and correction of the defect by the Hunter "corrective factor."[23] At present the diagnosis is performed by the enzyme assay, which can be performed directly in cell-free amniotic fluid for a rapid prenatal diagnosis,[82] using in recent years a fluorescent substrate that increases the sensitivity of the enzyme determination.[83] However, because in a female heterozygote fetus the enzyme level in the fluid might be low enough, it is advisable to do a karyotype. Zlotogora and Bach reported the possibility of obtaining accurate prenatal diagnosis through the assay of IDS in the maternal serum.[84] When the fetus is not affected with Hunter syndrome, the level of this enzyme rises constantly in the maternal serum from as early as the sixth week of pregnancy, whereas in pregnancies in which the fetus is affected, the enzyme remains unchanged. Chorionic villus biopsies are also used for early prenatal diagnosis of this disorder.[85,86] Mutation analysis is an important tool for prenatal diagnosis because it is accurate, rapid, and sensitive. Mutation analysis is also preferred for the delineation of affected male fetuses to females with low enzyme activity due to skewed X chromosome inactivation.

Experimental treatment of this disease has been tried using various approaches; in the past, plasma and lymphocyte infusions, as well as the use of skin grafts from a histocompatible sibling have been evaluated.[30,31,87–91] Because the mild form does not involve the central nervous system, bone marrow transplantation in these cases might be very beneficial, although there are serious risks for this procedure, as mentioned above. Enzyme replacement therapy showed encouraging results[92] and probably will be used broadly in the future, particularly for the mild form. Gene therapy for this condition is also under experimental trials.[72]

SANFILIPPO SYNDROME (MUCOPOLYSACCHARIDOSIS III)

There are four clinically indistinguishable, phenotypically variable, but enzymatically distinct forms of Sanfilippo syndrome: types A, B, C, and D.[4,5] The main feature of this disorder is psychomotor retardation, which manifests in infancy or early childhood and is progressive, leading to severe retardation and usually the loss of speech.[93] Hepatosplenomegaly, joint stiffness, dwarfism, and skeletal changes occur but are not as striking as in Hurler syndrome.[94] Corneal clouding may be evident only on slit-lamp examination. Typical features of these types are severe behavior problems, hyperactivity, and aggression, accompanied by sleep disturbances.[95] As in other disorders in this group, heterogeneity in the clinical picture is noted, although the C and D types are relatively rare. Generally, type A is more severe and more rapidly progressive than the other types. During the first 6 years of life a clinician may have difficulty distinguishing a male with Sanfilippo syndrome from one with Hunter syndrome. The frequency of these disorders is not as clear as with the other MPSs. Sanfilippo is believed to be underdiagnosed because, unlike the other MPSs, the major clinical manifestation in this condition is mental retardation without prominent skeletal abnormalities or other physical features found in all the other MPSs. A relatively high frequency of all four types of Sanfilippo syndrome was reported in the Netherlands, with an estimated frequency of 1:24,000 livebirths.[96] Of these, approximately 50 percent were type A, 30 percent type B, 25 percent type C, and the remaining type D. This differentiation between the subtypes represents the general distribution of this disease.

Mucopolysaccharide storage results from the failure of degradation of heparan sulfate. The four missing enzymes in the various types of Sanfilippo syndrome participate specifically in the degradation of heparan sulfate. In type A, the basic defect is a deficiency of heparan sulfatase (heparin sulfamidase).[97–99] Type B is characterized by a deficiency of the hydrolase N-acetyl-α-glucosaminidase.[99,100] In type C, the lysosomal enzyme acetyl-CoA:α-glucosaminide-N-acetyltransferase (CoA is coenzyme A) is deficient.[101,102] This enzyme transfers acetyl residues onto the exposed amine group of the glucosamine residues resulting from the removal of N-sulfate by the heparin sulfamidase. The N-acetyl-α-glucosaminidase residues can then be cleaved by the N-acetyl-α-glucosaminidase. In type D, N-acetyl-α-D-glucosaminide-6-sulfatase is the deficient hydrolase,[103] which is a distinct enzyme from the N-acetylgalactosamine-6-sulfatase (see "Morquio Syndrome").

The genes for Sanfilippo A, B, and D have been cloned.[104–107] The gene for Sanfilippo C has not yet been cloned, but cytogenetic analysis of a patient with this type bearing a translocation of 14;21 indicates its localization on chromosome 14.[108] The cloning of these genes led to the identification of mutations in the three subtypes of Sanfilippo.

The preliminary diagnosis of the various types of Sanfilippo syndrome is accomplished by the identification of the excretion of excess heparan sulfate in urine. The accumulation of [^{35}S]mucopolysaccharide is demonstrable in cultured fibroblasts, and the correction of this storage by the high-uptake forms of the deficient enzymes,[65] but compared with MPS I and II the [^{35}S] accumulation in cultured cells of these patients is less profound and might be difficult to demonstrate. The precise diagnosis is achieved by the appropriate enzyme analysis in peripheral blood leukocytes, or lymphocytes as well as cultivated fibroblasts,[4,5,109–121] and/or by mutation analysis. A fluorescent substrate was synthesized for the diagnosis of type A, replacing the radioactive substance previously used. This substrate enables a more sensitive and faster diagnosis, including prenatal diagnosis.[122,123] Prenatal diagnosis of all four types of Sanfilippo syndrome is possible by the determination of enzyme activity in cultured amniotic fluid cells or chorionic villi, or by mutation analysis, which can be performed also in noncultivated cells because of the high sensitivity of this procedure.

Regarding therapy, leukocyte transfusion has been tried without success.[124] Partial success was reported with bone marrow transplantation, but no effective improvement of mental deficiency was achieved. Recently, experimental enzyme replacement therapy has been performed in an animal model of type B and D.[125,126] Gene therapy is also experimental.[127]

MORQUIO SYNDROME (MUCOPOLYSACCHARIDOSIS IV)

There are two clinically similar types of Morquio syndrome: types A and B. Physical signs of abnormality are not manifested at birth. Development of skeletal changes in the rib cage or limbs usually signals the presence of this disorder between 1 and 2 years of age. Coarse facies, knock-knees, dwarfism with a short trunk, pectus carinatum, short neck, kyphosis, corneal clouding, deafness, joint laxity, and severe skeletal involvement constitute the main clinical features.[4,5] Involvement of the spinal cord with compression occurs invariably and may even lead to quadriplegia in infancy.[128] Intellectual development usually is normal. Similar to other MPSs, heterogeneity in the clinical spectrum was reported for both Morquio type A and type B.[4,5,129,130] Those with the severe form of this disease rarely survive beyond 50 years of age. The major complications include paralysis from compression of the spinal cord, cardiorespiratory insufficiency, paralysis of respiratory muscles, and involvement of the heart valves.

The disorder is the result of defective degradation of keratan sulfate, a mucopolysaccharide found mainly in cartilage, nucleus pulposus, and cornea, causing these tissues to be specifically affected.[4,5] The type A syndrome is caused by a deficiency of N-acetylgalactosamine-6-sulfatase.[131–134] It should be noted that keratan sulfate does not contain N-acetylgalactosamine-6-sulfated residues, but it has been shown that the same enzyme also can desulfate galactose-6-sulfate found in keratan sulfate.[135] As mentioned previously, N-acetyl-glucosamine-6-sulfatase, which is deficient in Sanfilippo D syndrome was shown to be a different enzyme.[133,135] Kinetic differences in the residual activity of the enzyme in patients with mild versus severe forms were noted.[136] The *GALANS* gene has been cloned and characterized.[137–139] This was the basis for the identification of various mutations in patients with Morquio syndrome type A, mild and severe. In Morquio syndrome type B, β-galactosidase is the deficient hydrolase.[140–142] This enzyme also is deficient in GM_1 gangliosidosis, resulting in the accumulation and excretion of GM_1 ganglioside, together with keratan sulfate and oligosaccharides with terminal β-galactoside residues. In contrast, in Morquio syndrome type B, no impairment in the breakdown of the ganglioside is observed. This probably stems from two different allelic mutations of β-galactosidase. Paschke and Kresse[143] reported that the residual β-galactosidase in Morquio syndrome type B is capable of degrading GM_1 ganglioside and might in fact be grossly stimulated by a GM_1 activator protein. This activator, on the other hand, did not stimulate the breakdown of keratan sulfate. In GM_1 gangliosidosis, the mutation obviously leads to an inability to break down both keratan sulfate and GM_1 ganglioside. Hoogeveen et al.[144] showed that the immunoprecipitable protein corresponding to β-galactosidase undergoes different processing in Morquio syndrome type B and GM_1 gangliosidosis. Mutations in the β-galactosidase gene resulting in Morquio type B manifestations were identified. Most of these patients are compound heterozygotes with a null allele and a second allele coding for an enzyme with some residual activity.

The two types of Morquio syndrome can be diagnosed by appropriate enzyme determinations in leukocytes, lymphocytes, or cultured fibroblasts as well as by mutation analysis, if a mutation is identified. In type B, intermediate β-galactosidase activities in leukocytes and fibroblasts were reported.[139] No particular difficulties are encountered in prenatal diagnosis of either type. Mutation analysis is an important aid for the diagnosis of both types.

In the absence of any effective therapy, only orthopedic surgery and neurosurgery are helpful in relieving the spinal and skeletal problems. Correction of the storage in cultured cells by a retroviral construct of the appropriate cDNA was reported recently,[145,146] this is the first essential step for trials of gene therapy in Morquio type A and B.

MAROTEAUX–LAMY SYNDROME (GALACTOSAMINE-4-SULFATASE DEFICIENCY: MUCOPOLYSACCHARIDOSIS VI)

Maroteaux–Lamy syndrome is characterized by the somatic signs of Hurler syndrome with prominent growth retardation, but is associated with the retention of normal intelligence.[4,5,147,148] Both severe and mild forms of the disease have been described.[149–156] Initial clinical manifestations arise most often between 2 and 3 years of age because of poor growth. Skeletal changes, including knock-knees, lumbar kyphosis, and pectus carinatum, are most striking and are associated with coarse facies, stiff joints, corneal clouding, cardiac involvement, hepatomegaly, and often splenomegaly. Death usually is caused by heart failure in the second or third decade of life. Severe involvement of the femoral heads is typical. In the milder forms of this disorder, some manifestations may be absent and others may be only minimally evident.

The primary enzymatic deficiency in this disorder is of arylsulfatase B.[157–160] This enzyme was identified as galactosamine-4-sulfatase.[161,162] The N-acetylgalactosamine-4-sulfate residues occur in dermatan sulfate and in chondroitin-4-sulfate; therefore, these two mucopolysaccharides accumulate in this syndrome. Arylsulfatase B has been purified and the cDNA has been cloned.[163,164] As a consequence, mutations in mild and severe patients were identified.

The enzymatic defect is evident in leukocytes, lymphocytes and cultured fibroblasts,[158] making heterozygote detection potentially possible.[165] Mutation analysis is essential for the accurate identification of heterozygotes. Prenatal diagnosis has been accomplished,[166,167] but the presence of relatively high activity of arylsulfatase C in the chorion villi complicates the prenatal diagnosis by CVS of MPS VI by enzyme determination.[168]

Regarding therapy, Krivit et al. performed bone marrow transplantation on a severely affected 13-year-old girl, using tissue donated from her compatible sibling.[169] Evidence of biochemical improvement was associated with a decrease in hepatomegaly, return to normal cardiac function after the cessation of digoxin therapy, and improvement in visual acuity and joint mobility. Encouraging results of bone marrow transplantation were also reported in several other patients.[170,171]

Enzyme replacement therapy in a cat model of the disease showed encouraging results, especially if the treatment started from birth compared with cats treated at a later age.[172]

β-GLUCURONIDASE DEFICIENCY (MUCOPOLYSACCHARIDOSIS VII)

Sly et al. described the first patient with β-glucuronidase deficiency.[173] At 7 weeks of age, this African-American child showed coarse facies, hepatosplenomegaly, thoracolumbar gibbus, puffy hands and feet, and other features. Psychomotor development was normal for the first 2–3 years after birth but deteriorated thereafter. A number of other patients with β-glucuronidase deficiency have also been described, with marked variation in the clinical phenotype.[4,5,174–183] Variable and mixed features of the MPSs in general have been noted in these cases, including coarse facies, hepatosplenomegaly, hernias, kyphosis, recurrent respiratory infections, short stature, and developmental delay. Corneal clouding has been a variable finding.

The essential defect is the deficiency of β-glucuronidase, which results in the impairment of the degradation of dermatan sulfate, chondroitin sulfate, and heparan sulfate.[183] The cDNA and the gene for human β-glucuronidase were isolated and characterized.[184,185] This permitted the characterization of mutations in patients with β-glucuronidase deficiency.

Heterozygote detection using leukocytes, lymphocytes, serum, or cultivated skin fibroblasts is possible,[186] as is prenatal diagnosis.[187] The molecular techniques are also efficient tools for the purpose. In severe manifestations of this disorder increased nuchal translucency was found in the fetus, adding an interesting approach for prenatal diagnosis in these cases.[174]

Many experimental efforts have been made in this MPS, with the aim of developing effective therapy. Most of these studies were performed on a mouse model. These experiments included bone marrow transplantations, gene therapy (as well as neonatal hepatic gene therapy), the transfection of a viral construct into brain tissues, and transplantation of hepatic cells.[188–200] Indeed, encouraging results were reported, indicating that this syndrome, as well as others in this group should be candidates for therapy.

HYALURONIDASE DEFICIENCY (MUCOPOLYSACCHARIDOSIS IX)

This MPS is the most recently described[201] and is caused by a deficiency of hyaluronidase, a lysosomal endoglycosidase catalyzing the degradation of hyaluronic acid, a nonsulfated, high-molecular-weight mucopolysaccharide.[4] One patient, a 14-year-old girl, has been described. At 7.5 years of age, she presented with soft-tissue masses, particularly in her limbs, that exacerbated with age. She had mild growth retardation, but generally her health was good. She had mild dysmorphic craniofacial features with a flattened nasal bridge and no neurologic involvement. The patient had complete deficiency of plasma hyaluronidase and a parallel increase of hyaluronic acid in the plasma. Her parents showed 50 percent reduction, on the average, of the hyaluronidase activity.

Six hyaluronidase-like genes were recently described in humans and mice.[202] HYALl is the one that was demonstrated to be mutated in the patient mentioned above.[203]

REFERENCES

1. Meikele PJ, Ranierri E, Ravenscroft EM, et al. Newborn screening for lysosomal storage disorders. Southeast Asian J Trop Med Public Health 1999;2:104.
2. Ranierri E, Gerace RL, Ravenscroft EM, et al. Pilot neonatal screening program for lysosomal storage disorders, using lamp-1. Southeast Asian J Trop Med Public Health 1999;2:111.
3. Gallegos-Arreola MP, Machorro-Lazo MV, Flores-Martinez SE, et al. Urinary glycosaminoglycan excretion in healthy subjects and in patients with mucopolysaccharidoses. Arch Med Res 2000;31:505.
4. Neufeld EF, Muenzer J. The mucopolysaccharidoses. In: Scriver CR, Beaudet AL, Sly WS, et al., eds. The metabolic and molecular bases of inherited disease, 8th ed. New York: McGraw-Hill, 2001:3421.
5. Neufeld EF, Muenzer J. The mucopolysaccharidoses. In: Scriver CR, Beaudet AL, Sly WS, et al., eds. The metabolic and molecular bases of inherited disease, 7th ed. New York: McGraw-Hill, 1995:2465.
6. Lowry RB, Renwick DHG. The relative frequency of the Hurler and Hunter syndromes. N Engl J Med 1971;284:221.
7. Dorfman A, Matalon R. The mucopolysaccharidoses. In: Stanbury JB, Wyngaarden JB, Fredrickson DS, eds. The metabolic basis of inherited disease, 3rd ed. New York: McGraw-Hill, 1972:1218.
8. Bach G, Friedman R, Weissman B, et al. The defect in the Hurler and Scheie syndromes: deficiency of α-L-iduronidase. Proc Natl Acad Sci USA 1972;69:2048.
9. Matalon R, Dorfman A. Hurler's syndrome: an α-L-iduronidase deficiency. Biochem Biophys Res Commun 1972;47:959.
10. Barton RW, Neufeld EF. The Hurler corrective factor. J Biol Chem 1971;246:7773.

11. Scott HS, Anson DS, Osborn AM, et al. Human α-L-iduronidase: DNA isolation and expression. Proc Natl Acad Sci USA 1991;88:9665.

12. Scott HS, Guo XH, Hopwood JJ, et al. Structure and sequence of the human α-L-iduronidase gene. Genomics 1992;13:1311.

13. Stoltzfus LJ, Sosa-Pineda B, Moskowitz SM, et al. Cloning and characterization of DNA encoding canine α-L-iduronidase. J Biol Chem 1992;267:6570.

14. Scott HS, Litjens T, Hopwood JJ, et al. A common mutation for mucopolysaccharidosis type I associated with a severe Hurler syndrome phenotype. Hum Mutat 1992;1:103.

15. Scott HS, Bunge S, Gal A, et al. Molecular genetics of mucopolysaccharidosis type I: diagnostic, clinical and biological implications. Hum Mutat 1995;6:288.

16. Bach G, Moskowitz SM, Tieu PT, et al. Molecular analysis of Hurler syndrome in Druze and Muslim Arab patients in Israel: multiple allelic mutations of the IDUA gene in a small geographic area. Am J Hum Genet 1993;53:330.

17. Hopwood JJ, Muller V, Pollard AC. Post and prenatal assessment of α-L-iduronidase deficiency with a radiolabeled natural substrate. Clin Sci 1979;56:591.

18. Liem KO, Hooghwinkel GJ. The use of α-L-iduronidase activity in leukocytes for the detection of Hurler and Scheie syndromes. Clin Chim Acta 1975;60:259.

19. Wapner RS, Brandt IK. Hurler syndrome: α-L-iduronidase activity in leukocytes as a method for heterozygote detection. Pediatr Res 1976;10:629.

20. Omura K, Higami S, Tada K. α-L-iduronidase activity in leukocytes: diagnosis of homozygotes and heterozygotes of the Hurler syndrome. Eur J Pediatr 1976;122:103.

21. Dulaney JT, Milunsky A, Moser HW. Detection of the carrier state of Hurler's syndrome by assay of α-L-iduronidase in leukocytes. Clin Chim Acta 1976;69:305.

22. Mandelli J, Wajner A, Pires R, et al. detection of mucopolysaccharidosis type I heterozygotes on the basis of the biochemical properties of plasma α-L-iduronidase. Clin Chim Acta 2001;12:81.

23. Fratantoni JC, Neufeld EF, Uhlendorf BW, et al. Intrauterine diagnosis of the Hurler and Hunter syndromes. N Engl J Med 1969;280:686.

24. Crawford M, Dean MF, Hunt DM, et al. Early prenatal diagnosis of Hurler's syndrome with termination of pregnancy and confirmatory findings on the fetus. J Med Genet 1973;10:144.

25. Gatti R, Borrone C, Filocamo M, et al. Prenatal diagnosis of mucopolysaccharidosis I: a special difficulty arising from an unusually low enzyme activity in mother's cells. Prenat Diagn 1985;5:149.

26. Hall CW, Liebars I, Di Natale P, et al. Enzymic diagnosis of the genetic mucopolysaccharide storage disorders. Methods Enzymol 1978;30:443.

27. Simoni G, Brambati B, Danesino C, et al. Efficient direct chromosome analyses from chorionic villi samples in the first trimester of pregnancy. Hum Genet 1983;63:349.

28. Mikkelson M, Somergaard FT, Tonnesen T, et al. First trimester biopsies of chorionic villi for prenatal diagnosis: experience of two laboratories. Clin Genet 1984;26:263.

29. Lissens W, Sermon K, Staessen C, et al. Preimplantation diagnosis of inherited disease. J Inherit Metab Dis 1996;19:709.

30. Hobbs JR, Hugh-Jones K, Barrett AJ, et al. Reversal of clinical features of Hurler's disease and biochemical improvement after treatment by bone marrow transplantation. Lancet 1981;2:709.

31. Hopwood JJ, Vellodi A, Scott HS, et al. Long term clinical progress in bone marrow transplant mucopolysaccharidosis type I patients with defined genotype. J Inherit Metab Dis 1993;16:1024.

32. Grewal SS, Krivit W, Defor TE, et al. Outcome of second hematopoietic cell transplantation in Hurler syndrome. Bone Marrow Transplant 2002;29:491.

33. Braunlin EA, Rose AG, Hopwood JJ, et al. Coronary artery patency following long term successful engraftment 14 years after bone marrow transplantation in the Hurler syndrome. Am J Cardiol 2001;88:1075.

34. Braunlin EA, Stauffer NR, Peters CH, et al. Usefulness of bone marrow transplantation in the Hurler syndrome. Am J Cardiol 2003;92:882.

35. Di Natali P, Di Domenico C, Villani GR, et al. In vitro gene therapy of mucopolysaccharidosis type I by lentiviral vectors. Eur J Biochem 2002;269:2764.

36. Pan D, Aronovich E, McIvor ES, et al. Retroviral vector design toward hematopoietic stem cell gene therapy for mucopolysaccharidosis type I. Gene Ther 2000;7:1875.

37. Kakkis ED, Muenzer J, Tiller GE, et al. Enzyme replacement therapy in mucopolysaccharidosis I. N Eng J Med 2001;344:182.

38. Wraith JE. Enzyme replacement therapy in mucopolysaccharidosis type I: progress and emerging difficulties. J Inherit Metab Dis 2001;24:245.

39. Kakkis ED, Schuchman E, He X, et al. Enzyme replacement therapy in feline mucopolysaccharidosis I. Mol Genet Metab 2001;72:199.

39a. Kakavanos R, Turner CT, Hopwood JJ, et al. Immune tolerance after long-term enzyme-replacement therapy among patients who have mucopolysaccharidosis I. Lancet 2003;361:1608.

40. Keeling KM, Brooks DA, Hopwood JJ, et al. Gentamicin-mediated suppression of Hurler syndrome stop mutations restores a low level of α-L-iduronidase activity and reduces lysosomal glycosaminoglycan accumulation. Hum Mol Genet 2001;10:291.

41. Scott HS, Litjens T, Nelson PV, et al. Identification of mutations in the α-L-iduronidase gene that cause Hurler and Scheie syndrome. Am J Hum Genet 1993;53:973.

42. Tieu PT, Bach G, Matynia A, et al. Four novel mutations underlying mild or intermediate forms of α-L-iduronidase deficiency (MPS IS and MPS IH/S). Hum Mutat 1995;6:55.

43. Kajii T, Matsuda K, Osawa T, et al. Hurler/Scheie genetic compound (mucopolysaccharidosis IH/IS) in Japanese brothers. Clin Genet 1974;6:394.

44. McKusick VA, Neufeld EF, Kelly TE. The mucopolysaccharide storage diseases. In: Stanbury JB, Wyngaarden JB, Fredrickson DS, eds. The metabolic basis of inherited disease, 4th ed. New York: McGraw-Hill, 1978:1282.

45. Spranger J, Cantz M, Gehler J, et al. Mucopolysaccharidosis II (Hunter disease) with corneal opacities: report of two patients at the extremes of a wide clinical spectrum. Eur J Pediatr 1978;129:11.

46. Spranger J. The systemic mucopolysaccharidoses. Ergeb Inn Med Kinderheilkd 1972;32:165.

47. Lichenstein JR, Bilbrey GL, McKusick VA. Clinical and probable genetic heterogeneity within mucopolysaccharidosis II: report of a family with a mild form. Johns Hopkins Med J 1972;131:425.

48. Karpati G, Carpenter S, Eitan AA, et al. Multiple peripheral nerve entrapment: an unusual phenotypic variant of the Hunter syndrome (mucopolysaccharidosis II) in a family. Arch Neurol 1974;31:418

49. McKusick VA. Genetic nosology: three approaches. Am J Hum Genet 1978;30:105.

50. Yatziv S, Erickson RP, Epstein CJ. Mild and severe Hunter syndrome (MPS II) within the same sibship. Clin Genet 1977;11:319.

51. Schaap T, Bach G. The incidence of mucopolysaccharidosis in Israel: Is Hunter's disease a "Jewish disease"? Hum Genet 1981;56:221.

52. Zlotogora J, Schaap T, Zeigler M, et al. Hunter syndrome among Ashkenazi Jews in Israel: evidence for prenatal selection favoring the Hunter allele. Hum Genet 1985;71:329.

53. Capobianchi MR, Romeo G. Mosaicism for sulfoiduronate sulfatase deficiency in carriers of Hunter's syndrome. Experientia 1976;32:459.

54. Migeon BR, Sprenkle JA, Liebaers I, et al. X-linked Hunter syndrome: the heterozygous phenotype in cell culture. Am J Hum Genet 1977;29:448.

55. Frederik PM, Fortuin JJH, Klepper D, et al. Autoradiographic detection of mucopolysaccharide accumulation in single fibroblasts. Histochem J 1977;9:89.

56. Milunsky A, Neufeld EF. The Hunter syndrome in a 46XX girl. N Engl J Med 1973;288:106.

57. Neufeld EF, Liebaers I, Epstein CJ, et al. The Hunter syndrome in females: is there an autosomal recessive form of iduronate sulfate deficiency? Am J Hum Genet 1977;29:455.

58. Mossman J, Blunt S, Stephens R, et al. Hunter's disease in a girl: association with X:5 chromosome translocation disrupting the Hunter gene. Arch Dis Child 1983;58:911.

59. Broadhead DM, Krik JM, Burt AJ, et al. Full expression of Hunter disease in a female with an X-chromosome deletion leading to non-random inactivation. Clin Genet 1986;30:392.

60. Clarke JTR, Willard HF, Teshima I, et al. Hunter disease (mucopolysaccharidosis type I) in a karyotypically normal girl. Clin Genet 1990;37:355.

61. Winchester B, Young E, Geddes S, et al. Female twin with Hunter disease due to nonrandom inactivation in the X-chromosome: a consequence of twinning. Am J Med Genet 1992;44:834.

62. Bach G, Eisenberg R Jr, Cantz M, et al. The defect in the Hunter syndrome: deficiency of sulfoiduronate sulfatase. Proc Natl Acad Sci USA 1973;70:2134.

63. Sjoberg I, Fransson LA, Matalon R, et al. Hunter's syndrome: a deficiency of L-iduronate-sulfate sulfatase. Biochem Biophys Res Commun 1973;54:1125.

64. Liebaers I, Neufeld EF. Iduronate sulfatase activity in serum, lymphocytes, and fibroblasts: simplified diagnosis in the Hunter syndrome. Pediatr Res 1976;10:733.

65. Cantz M, Kresse H, Barton RW, et al. Corrective factors for inborn errors of mucopolysaccharide metabolism. Methods Enzymol 1972;28:884.

66. Bielicki J, Freeman C, Clements PR, et al. Human liver iduronate-2-sulfatase: purification, characterization and catalytic properties. Biochem J 1990;271:75.

67. Wilson PJ, Morris CP, Anson DS, et al. Hunter syndrome: isolation of an iduronate-2-sulfatase cDNA clone and analysis of patient DNA. Proc Natl Acad Sci USA 1990;87:8531.
68. Hopwood JJ, Bunge S, Morris CP, et al. Molecular basis of mucopolysaccharidosis type II: mutations in the iduronate-2-sulfatase gene. Hum Mutat 1993;2:435.
69. Bonuccelli G, Di Natali P, Carsolini F, et al. The effect of 4 mutations on the expression of iduronate-2-sulfatase in mucopolysaccharidosis type II. Biochim Biophys Acta 2001;1537:233.
70. Rothman M, Bunge S, Beck M, et al. Mucopolysaccharidosis type II (Hunter syndrome): mutation "hot spots" in the iduronate-2-sulfatase gene. Am J Hum Genet 1996;59:1202.
71. Bondeson ML, Malmgnen H, Dahle N, et al. Presence of an IDS-related locus (IDS2) in Xq28 complicates the mutational analysis of Hunter syndrome. Eur J Hum Genet 1995;3:219.
72. Braun SE, Aronovich EL, Anderson RA, et al. Metabolic correction and cross-correction of mucopolysaccharidosis type II (Hunter syndrome) by retroviral-mediated gene transfer and expression of human iduronate-2-sulfatase. Proc Natl Acad Sci USA 1993;90:11830.
73. Braun SE, Pan D, Aronovich EL, et al. Preclinical studies of lymphocyte gene therapy for mild Hunter syndrome (mucopolysaccharidosis type II). Hum Gene Ther 1996;7:283.
74. Neufeld EF, Liebaers I, Lim TW. Iduronate sulfatase determination for the diagnosis of the Hunter syndrome and the detection of the carrier state. In: Volk BW, Schneck L, eds. Current trends in sphingolipidoses and allied disorders, vol. 68. New York: Plenum Press, 1976:253.
75. Archer IM, Harper PS, Wustman FS. An improved assay for iduronate-2-sulfatase in serum and its use in the detection of Hunter syndrome. Clin Chim Acta 1981;112:107.
76. Dean MF. The iduronate sulfatase activities of cells and tissue fluids from patients with Hunter syndrome and normal controls. J Inherit Metab Dis 1983;6:108.
77. Yataka T, Fluharty AL, Stevens RL, et al. Iduronate sulfatase analysis of hair roots for identification of Hunter syndrome heterozygotes. Am J Hum Genet 1978;30:575.
78. Nwokoro N, Neufeld EF. Detection of Hunter heterozygotes by enzymatic analysis of hair roots. Am J Hum Genet 1979;31:42.
79. Archer IM, Rees DW, Oladimeji A, et al. Detection of female carriers of Hunter syndrome: comparison of serum and hair-root analysis. J Inherit Metab Dis 1982;2:15.
80. Tonnesen T, Lykkelund C, Guttler F. Diagnosis of Hunter syndrome carriers: radioactive sulfate incorporation into fibroblasts in the presence of fructose-1-phosphate. Hum Genet 1982;60:167.
81. Zlotogora J, Bach G. Heterozygote detection in Hunter syndrome. Am J Med Genet 1984;17:661.
82. Liebaers I, Di Natale P, Neufled EF. Iduronate sulfatase in amniotic fluid: an aid in the prenatal diagnosis of the Hunter syndrome. J Pediatr 1977;90:423.
83. Voznyi YV, Keulemans JL, van Diggelen OP. A fluorimetric enzyme assay for the diagnosis of MPS II (Hunter disease). J Inherit Metab Dis 2001;24:675.
84. Zlotogora J, Bach G. Hunter syndrome: activity of iduronate sulfate sulfatase in the serum of pregnant heterozygotes: prospects for prenatal diagnosis. N Engl J Med 1984;311:331.
85. Lykkelund C, Sondergaard F, Therkelsen AJ, et al. Feasibility of first trimester prenatal diagnosis of Hunter syndrome. Lancet 1983;2:1147.
86. Harper PS, Bamforth S, Rees D, et al. Chorion biopsy for prenatal testing in Hunter syndrome. Lancet 1984;2:812.
87. Erickon RP, Sandman R, Van B, et al. Inefficacy of fresh frozen plasma therapy of mucopolysaccharidosis II. Pediatrics 1972;50:693.
88. Dekaban AS, Holden KP, Constantopoulos G. Effects of fresh plasma or whole blood transfusions on patients with various types of mucopolysaccharidosis. Pediatrics 1972;50:688.
89. Dean MF, Muir H, Benson PF, et al. Increased breakdown of glycosaminoglycans and appearance of corrective enzyme after skin transplants in Hunter syndrome. Nature 1975;257:609.
90. Yatziv S, Statter M, Abewliuk P, et al. A therapeutic trial of fresh plasma infusions over a period of 22 months in two siblings with Hunter's syndrome. Isr J Med Sci 1975;11:802.
91. Brown FR, Hall CW, Neufeld EF, et al. Administration of iduronate sulfatase by plasma exchange to patients with Hunter syndrome: a clinical study. Am J Med Genet 1982;13:309.
92. Muenzer J, Lamsa JC, Garcia A, et al. Enzyme replacement therapy in mucopolysaccharidosis type II (Hunter syndrome): preliminary report. Acta Paediatr 2002;91:98.
93. Sanfilippo SJ, Posodin R, Langer LO Jr, et al. Mental retardation associated with acid mucopolysacchariduria (heparitin sulfate type). J Pediatr 1963;63:837.
94. Van De Kamp JJP. The Sanfilippo syndrome: a clinical and genetical study of 75 patients in the Netherlands. Doctoral thesis. S'Gravenhage, JH Pasmanas, 1979.

95. Fraser J, Wraith JE, Delatycki MB. Sleep disturbance in mucopolysaccharidosis type III (Sanfilippo syndrome): a survey of managing clinicians. Clin Genet 2002;62:418.

96. Kresse H. Mucopolysaccharidosis III A (Sanfilippo disease): deficiency of heparin sulfamidase in skin fibroblasts and leukocytes. Biochem Biophys Res Commun 1973;54:1111.

97. Matalon R, Dorfman A. Sanfilippo A syndrome: sulfamidase deficiency in cultured skin fibroblasts and liver. J Clin Invest 1974;54:905.

98. Gordon BA, Feleki V, Budreau CH, et al. Defective heparin sulfate metabolism in the Sanfilippo syndrome and assay of this defect in the assessment of the mucopolysaccharidosis patient. Clin Biochem 1975;8:184.

99. Von Figura K, Kresse H. The Sanfilippo B corrective factor: a *N*-acetyl-α-D-glucosaminidase. Biochem Biophys Res Commun 1972;48:262.

100. O'Brien JS. Sanfilippo syndrome: profound deficiency of alpha-glucosaminidase activity in organs and skin fibroblasts from type B patients. Proc Natl Acad Sci USA 1972;69:1720.

101. Kresse H, Von Figura K, Klein U. New biochemical subtype of the Sanfilippo syndrome: Characterization of the storage material in cultured fibroblasts of Sanfilippo C patients. Eur J Biochem 1978;92:333.

102. Klein U, Kresse H, Von Figura K. Sanfilippo syndrome type C: Deficiency of acetyl-CoA:α-glucosaminide-*N*-acetyltransferase in skin fibroblasts. Proc Natl Acad Sci USA 1978;75:5178.

103. Kresse H, Paschke E, Von Figura K, et al. Sanfilippo disease type D: Deficiency of N-acetylglucosamine-6-sulfate sulfatase required for heparan sulfate degradation. Proc Natl Acad Sci USA 1980;77:6622.

104. Scott HS, Blanch L, Guo XH, et al. Cloning of the sulphamidase gene and identification of mutations in Sanfilippo A syndrome. Nat Genet 1995;11:465.

105. Zhao HG, Li HH, Bach G, et al. The molecular basis of Sanfilippo syndrome type B. Proc Natl Acad Sci USA 1996;93:6101.

106. Weber B, Blanch L, Clements PR, et al. Cloning and expression of the gene involved in Sanfilippo B syndrome. Hum Mol Genet 1996;5:771.

107. Robertson DA, Freeman C, Nelson PV, et al. Human glucosamine-6-sulfatase cDNA reveals homology with steroid sulfatase. Biochem Biophys Res Commun 1988;157:218.

108. Zaremba J, Kleijer WJ, Huijmans JG, et al. Chromosomes 14 and 21 as possible candidates for mapping the gene for Sanfilippo disease Type IIIC. J Med Genet 1992;29:514.

109. Kresse H, von Figura K, Klein H, et al. Enzymatic diagnosis of the genetic mucopolysaccharide storage disorders. Methods Enzymol 1982;83:559.

110. Hopwood JJ, Elliot H. Radiolabeled oligosaccharides as substrates for the estimation of sulfaminidase and the detection of Sanfilippo type A syndrome. Clin Chim Acta 1981;112:55.

111. Thompson JN, Roden L, Reynertson R. Oligosaccharide substrates for heparin sulfamidase. Anal Biochem 1986;152:412.

112. Marsh J, Fenson AH. 4-Methylumbelliferyl-α-*N*-acetylglucosaminidase activity for diagnosis of Sanfilippo B disease. Clin Genet 1985;27:258.

113. Pallini R, Leder IG, di Natale P. Sanfilippo type C diagnosis: assay of acetyl-CoA: α-glucosaminide *N*-acetyltransferase using [^{14}C]glucosamine as substrate and leukocytes as enzyme source. Pediatr Res 1984;18:543.

114. Freeman C, Hopwood JJ. Sanfilippo D syndrome: Estimation of *N*-acetyl-glucosamine-6-sulfatase activity with a radiolabeled monosulfated disaccharide substrate. Anal Biochem 1989;176:244.

115. Elliot E, Hopwood JJ. Detection of Sanfilippo D syndrome by the use of radio-labeled monosaccharide sulfate as the substrate for the estimation of *N*-acetyl-glucosamine-6-sulfate sulfatase. Anal Biochem 1984;138:205.

116. Von Figura K, Logering M, Mersmann G, et al. Sanfilippo B disease: serum assay for detection of homozygous and heterozygous individuals in three families. J Pediatr 1973;83:607.

117. Liem KO, Giesberts AH, van de Kamp JJP, et al. Sanfilippo B disease in two related sibships: biochemical studies in patients, parents and sibs. Clin Genet 1976;10:273.

118. Matalon R, Deanching M, Marback R, et al. Carrier detection for Sanfilippo A syndrome. J Inherit Metab Dis 1988;11:158.

119. Toone JR, Applegarth DA. Carrier detection in Sanfilippo A syndrome. Clin Genet 1988;33:401.

120. Stone J, Brimble A, Pennock CA. Carrier detection for Sanfilippo A syndrome. J Inherit Metab Dis 1990;13:184.

121. Hopwood JJ, Elliot H. The diagnosis of the Sanfilippo C syndrome using monosaccharide and oligosaccharide substrates to assay acetyl-CoA: 2-amino-2-deoxy-α-glucoside *N*-acetyltransferase activity. Clin Chim Acta 1981;112:67.

122. Kaprova EA, Vozni YV, Keulemans JLM, et al. A fluorometric enzyme assay for the diagnosis of Sanfilippo type A (MPS IIIA). J Inherit Metab Dis 1996;19:278.

123. Kleijer WJ, Karpova EA, Geilen GC, et al. Prenatal diagnosis of Sanfilippo A syndrome: Experience in 35 pregnancies at risk and the use of a new fluorogenic substrate for the heparin sulphamidase assay. Prenat Diagn 1996;16:829.

124. Moser HW, O'Brien JS, Atkins L, et al. Infusion of normal HL-A identical leukocytes in Sanfilippo disease type B: estimate of infused cell survival by assays of α-N-acetylglucosaminidase activity and cytogenetic techniques: effect of glycosaminoglycan excretion in the urine. Arch Neurol 1974;31:329.

125. Yu WH, Zhao KW, Ryazantsev S, et al. Short term enzyme replacement in the murine model of Sanfilippo syndrome type B. Mol Genet Metab 2000;71:573.

126. Downs-Kelly E, Jones MZ, Alroy J, et al. Caprine mucopolysaccharidosis IIID: a preliminary trial of enzyme replacement therapy. J Mol Neurosci 2000;15:251.

127. Fu H, Samulski RJ, McCown TJ, et al. Neurological correction of lysosomal storage in mucopolysaccharidosis IIIB mouse model by adeno-associated virus-mediated gene delivery. Mol Ther 2002;5:42.

128. Gilles FH, Deuel RK. Neuronal cytoplasmic globules in the brain in Morquio's syndrome. Arch Neurol 1971;25:393.

129. Dale F. Unusual forms of familial osteochondrodystrophy. Acta Radiol 1931;12:337.

130. Nelson J, Broadhead D, Mossman J. Clinical findings in 12 patients with MPS IVA (Morquio disease). Clin Genet 1988;33:111.

131. Matalon R, Arbogast B, Justice P, et al. Morquio's syndrome: deficiency of a chondroitin sulfate N-acetyl hexosamine sulfate sulfatase. Biochem Biophys Res Commun 1974;61:759.

132. Singh J, DiFerrante N, Niebes P, et al. N-Acetyl-galactosamine-6-sulfate sulfatase in man: absence of the enzyme in Morquio disease. J Clin Invest 1976;57:1036.

133. Horwitz AL, Dorfman A. The enzymatic defect in Morquio's disease: the specificity of N-acetylhexosamine sulfatases. Biochem Biophys Res Commun 1978;80:819.

134. Yukata T, Okada S, Kato T, et al. Galactose-6-sulfate sulfatase activity in Morquio syndrome. Clin Chim Acta 1982;122:169.

135. DiFerrante N, Ginsberg LC, Donnelly PV, et al. Deficiencies of glucosamine-6-sulfatase or galactosamine-6-sulfatase are responsible for different mucopolysaccharidoses. Science 1978;199:79.

136. Glossl J, Maroteaux P, DiNatale P, et al. Different properties of residual N-acetylgalactosamine-6-sulfate sulfatase in fibroblasts (patients with mild and severe forms of Morquio disease, type A). Pediatr Res 1981;15:976.

137. Tomtsu S, Fukuda S, Masue M, et al. Morquio disease: isolation, characterization and expression of full length cDNA for human N-acetylgalactosamine-6-sulfate sulfatase. Biochem Biophys Res Commun 1991;181:677.

138. Nakashima Y, Tomatsu S, Hori T, et al. Mucopolysaccharidosis IV A: molecular cloning of the human N-acetylgalactosamine-6-sulfatase gene and analysis of the 5' flanking region. Genomics 1994;29:99.

139. Morris CP, Guo XH, Apostolou S, et al. Morquio A syndrome: cloning, sequence and structure of the human N-acetylgalactosamine-6-sulfatase gene. Genomics 1994;22:652.

140. Arbisser AL, Donnelly KA, Scott CI, et al. Morquio-like syndrome with β-galactosidase deficiency and normal hexosamine sulfatase activity: mucopolysaccharidosis IV B. Am J Med Genet 1977;32:258.

141. Groebe H, Krins M, Schmidberger H, et al. Morquio syndrome (mucopolysaccharidosis IV B) associated with β-galactosidase deficiency: report of two cases. Am J Hum Genet 1980;32:258.

142. Van der Horst GTJ, Kleijer WJ, Hoogeveen AT, et al. Morquio type B syndrome: a primary defect in β-galactosidase. Am J Hum Genet 1983;16:261.

143. Paschke E, Kresse H. Morquio disease type B: activation of GM_1 activator protein. Biochem Biophys Res Commun 1982;109:569.

144. Hoogeveen AT, Graham-Kawashima H, d'Azzo A, et al. Processing of human β-galactosidase in GM_1 gangliosidosis and Morquio B syndrome. J Biol Chem 1984;259:1974.

145. Toietta G, Severini GM, Traversari C, et al. Various cells retrovirally transduced with N-acetylgalactosamine-6-sulfate sulfatase correct Morquio skin fibroblasts in vitro. Hum Gene Ther 2001;12:2007.

146. Sena-Estivis M, Camp SM, Alroy J, et al. Correction of acid-galactosidase deficiency in GM_1 gangliosidosis human fibroblasts by retroviral vector mediated gene transfer: high efficiency of release and cross correction by murine enzyme. Hum Gene Ther 2000;11:715.

147. Maroteaux P, Leveque B, Marie J, et al. Une nouvelle dysotose avec elimination urinarie de chondroitine-sulfate B. Presse Med 1963;71:1849.

148. Spranger J, Koch F, McKusick VA. Mucopolysaccharidosis VI (Maroteaux–Lamy's disease). Helv Paediatr Acta 1970;25:337.

149. Glover GA, Tanaka KR, Turner JA, et al. Mucopolysaccharidosis, an unusual cause of cardiac valvular disease. Am J Cardiol 1968;22:133.

150. DiFerrante N, Hyman BH, Klish W, et al. Mucopolysaccharidosis VI (Maroteaux–Lamy disease): clinical and biochemical study of a mild variant case. Johns Hopkins Med J 1975;135:42.

151. Quigley HA, Kenyon KR. Ultrastructural and histochemical studies of a newly recognized form of systemic mucopolysaccharidosis (Maroteaux–Lamy syndrome, mild phenotype). Am J Ophthalmol 1974;77:809.

152. Peterson DI, Bacchus A, Seaich L, et al. Myelopathy associated with Maroteaux–Lamy syndrome. Arch Neurol 1975;32:127.

153. Pilz H, Von Figura K, Goebel HH. Deficiency of arylsulfatase B in two brothers aged 40 and 38 years (Maroteaux–Lamy syndrome, type B). Ann Neurol 1978;6:315.

154. Vestermark S, Tonnesen T, Andersen MS, et al. Mental retardation in a patient with Maroteaux–Lamy. Clin Genet 1987;31:114.

155. Taylor HR, Hollows FC, Hopwood JJ, et al. Report of a mucopolysaccharidosis occurring in Australian aborigines. J Med Genet 1978;15:455.

156. Whiley CB. The mucopolysaccharidoses. In Beighton P ed. Heritable disorders of connective tissue, 5th ed. St Louis: CV Mosby, 1993:367.

157. Stumpf DA, Austin JH, Crocker AC, et al. Mucopolysaccharidosis type VI (Maroteaux–Lamy syndrome): arylsulfatase B deficiency in tissues. Am J Dis Child 1973;126:747.

158. Fluharty AL, Steven RL, Sanders DL, et al. Arylsulfatase B deficiency in Maroteaux–Lamy syndrome cultured fibroblasts. Biochem Biophys Res Commun 1974;59:455.

159. O'Brien JF, Cantz M, Spranger J. Maroteaux-Lamy disease (mucopolysaccharidosis VI) subtype A: deficiency of N-acetyl-galactosamine-4-sulfatase. Biochem Biophys Res Commun 1974;60:1170.

160. Shapira E, De Gregorio RP, Matalon R, et al. Reduced arylsulfatase B activity of the mutant enzyme protein in Maroteaux–Lamy syndrome. Biochem Biophys Res Commun 1975;62:448.

161. Gibson GJ, Saccone GTP, Brooks DA, et al. Human N-acetylgalactosamine-4-sulfate sulfatase: purification, monoclonal antibody production and native and subunit Mr values. Biochem J 1987;248:755.

162. Tsuji M, Nakanishi Y Habachi H, et al. the common identity of UDP-N-acety-galactosamine-4-sulfatase, nitrocatechol sulfatase (arylsulfatase) and chondroitin-4-sulfatase. Biochim Biophys Acta 1980;612:373.

163. Peters C, Schmidt B, Rommerskirch W, et al. Phylogenetic conservation of arylsulfatases: cDNA cloning and expression of human arylsulfatase B. J Biol Chem 1990;265:3374.

164. Schuchman EH, Jackson CE, Desnick RJ. Human arylsulfatase B: MOPAC cloning, nucleotide sequence of a full length cDNA and regions of amino acid identity with arylsulfatase A and C. Genomics 1990;6:149.

165. Beratis NG, Turnes BM, Weiss R, et al. Arylsulfatase B deficiency in Maroteaux–Lamy syndrome: cellular studies and carrier identification. Pediatr Res 1975;9:475.

166. Kleijer WJ, Wolffers GM, Hoogeveen A, et al. Prenatal diagnosis of Maroteaux–Lamy syndrome. Lancet 1977;2:50.

167. Van Dyke DL, Fluharty AL, Schafer IA, et al. Prenatal diagnosis of Maroteaux–Lamy syndrome. Am J Med Genet 1981;8:235.

168. Sanguinetti N, Marsh J, Jackson M, et al. The arylsulfatases of chorionic villi: potential problems in the first trimester diagnosis of metachromatic leukodystrophy and Maroteaux–Lamy diseases. Clin Genet 1986;30:302.

169. Krivit W, Pierpont ME, Ayazk K, et al. Bone marrow transplantation in the Maroteaux–Lamy syndrome (mucopolysaccharidosis VI). N Engl J Med 1984; 311:1606.

170. McGovern MM, Lundman MD, Short MP, et al. Status of bone marrow transplantation in Maroteaux–Lamy syndrome: status 40 months after BMT. Birth Defects 1986;22:42.

171. Ucakhan OO, Brodie SE, Desnick R, et al. Long-term follow-up of corneal graft survival following bone marrow transplantation in the Maroteaux–Lamy syndrome. CLAO J 2001;27:234.

172. Auclair D, Hopwood JJ, Brooks DA, et al. Replacement therapy in mucopolysaccharidosis type VI: advantages of early onset of therapy. Mol Genet Metab 2003;78:163.

173. Sly WS, Quinton BA, McAlister WH, et al. β-Glucuronidase deficiency: report of clinical, radiologic and biochemical features of a new mucopolysaccharidosis. J Pediatr 1973;82:249.

174. Geipel A, Berg C, Germer U, et al. Mucopolysaccharidosis VII (Sly disease) as a cause of increased nuchal translucency and non immune fetal hydrops: study of a family and technical approach to prenatal diagnosis in early and late pregnancy. Prenat Diagn 2002;22:493.

175. Gehler J, Cantz M, Tolksdorf M, et al. Mucopolysaccharidosis VII (β-glucuronidase deficiency). Hum Genet 1974;23:149.

176. Danes BS, Degnan M. Different clinical and biochemical phenotypes associated with β-glucuronidase deficiency. Birth Defects 1974;10:251.

177. Beaudet AL, DiFerrante N, Ferry GD, et al. Variation in the phenotype expression of β-glucuronidase deficiency. J Pediatr 1978;86:388.

178. Gitzelman R, Wiesmann UN, Spycher MA, et al. Unusually mild course of β-glucuronidase deficiency in two brothers (mucopolysaccharidosis VII). Helv Paediatr Acta 1978;33:413.

179. Sewell AC, Gehler J, Mittermaier G, et al. Mucopolysaccharidosis type VII (β-glucuronidase deficiency): a report of a new case and survey of those in the literature. Clin Genet 1982;21:366.

180. Sheets JE, Falk RE, Ng WG, et al. β-Glucuronidase deficiency. Am J Dis Child 1985;139:57.

181. de Kremer RD, Givogri I, Argarana CE, et al. Mucopolysaccharidosis type VII (β-glucuronidase deficiency): a chronic variant with an oligosymptomatic severe skeletal dysplasia. Am J Med Genet 1992;44:145.

182. Kagie M, Kleijer WJ, Huijmans JGM, et al. β-Glucuronidase deficiency as a cause of fetal hydrops. Am J Med Genet 1992;42:693.

183. Hall CW, Cantz M, Neufeld EF. A β-glucuronidase deficiency mucopolysaccharidosis: studies in cultured fibroblasts. Arch Biochem Biophys 1973;155:32.

184. Oshima A, Kyle JW, Miller RD, et al. Cloning, sequencing and expression of cDNA for human β-glucuronidase. Proc Natl Acad Sci USA 1987;84:685.

185. Miller RD, Hoffman JW, Powell PP, et al. Cloning and characterization of human β-glucuronidase gene. Genomics 1990;7:280.

186. Glaser JH, Sly WS. β-Glucuronidase deficiency mucopolysaccharidosis: methods for enzymatic diagnosis. J Lab Clin Med 1973;82:969.

187. Poenaru L, Castelnau L, Mossman J, et al. Prenatal diagnosis of a heterozygote for mucopolysaccharidosis type VII (β-glucuronidase deficiency). Prenat Diagn 1982;2:251.

188. Kyle JW, Birkenmeir EH, Gwynn B, et al. Correction of murine mucopolysaccharidosis VII by human β-glucuronidase transgene. Proc Natl Acad Sci USA 1990;87:3914.

189. Vogler C, Sands MS, Levy B, et al. Enzyme replacement with recombinant β-glucuronidase in murine mucopolysaccharidosis type VII: impact of therapy during the first six weeks of life on subsequent lysosomal storage, growth and survival. Pediatr Res 1996;39:1050.

190. Sly WS. Gene therapy on the sly. Nat Genet 1993;4:105.

191. Wolfe JH, Schuchman EH, Stramm LE, et al. Restoration of normal lysosomal function in mucopolysaccharidosis type VII cells by retroviral vector-mediated gene transfer. Proc Natl Acad Sci USA 1990;87:2877.

192. Wolfe JH, Sands MS, Barker JE, et al. Reversal of pathology in murine mucopolysaccharidosis type VII by somatic cell gene transfer. Nature 1992;360:749.

193. Ponder KP, Melnczek JR, Xu L, et al. Therapeutic neonatal hepatic gene therapy in mucopolysaccharidosis VII dogs. Proc Natl Acad Sci USA 2002;99:13102.

194. Elliger SS, Elliger CA, Lang C, et al. Enhanced secretion and uptake of β-glucuronidase improves adeno-associated viral-mediated gene therapy of mucopolysaccharidosis type VII mice. Mol Ther 2002;5:617.

195. Brooks AI, stein CS, Hughes SM, et al. Functional correction of established central nervous system deficits in an animal model of lysosomal storage disease with feline immunodeficiency virus based vectors. Proc Nat Acad Sci USA 2002;99:6216.

196. Vogler C, Barker J, Sands MS, et al. Murine mucopolysaccharidosis VII: impact of therapies on the phenotype, clinical course, and pathology in a model of a lysosomal storage disease. Pediatr Dev Pathol 2001;4:421.

197. Daly TM, Ohlemiller KK, Roberts MS, et al. Prevention of systemic clinical disease in MPS VII mice following AAV-mediated neonatal gene transfer. Gene Ther 2001;8:1291.

198. Wolfe JH, Sands MS, Harel N, et al. Gene transfer of low levels of β-glucuronidase corrects hepatic lysosomal storage in a large animal model of mucopolysaccharidosis VII. Mol Ther 2000;2:552.

199. Casal ML, Wolfe JH. In utero transplantation of fetal liver cells in the mucopolysaccharidosis type VII mouse results in low level chimerism, but overexpression of β-glucuronidase, can delay onset of clinical signs. Blood 2001;97:1625.

200. Ross CJ, Bastedo L, Maier SA, et al. Treatment of a lysosomal storage disease, mucopolysaccharidosis VII, with microencapsulated recombinant cells. Hum Gene Ther 2000;11:2117.

201. Natowicz MR, Short MP, Wang Y, et al. Clinical and biochemical manifestations of hyaluronidase deficiency. N Engl J Med 1996;335:1029.

202. Csoka AB, Frost GI, Stern R. The six hyaluronidase-like genes in human and mouse genomes. Matrix Biol 2001;20:499.

203. Triggs-Raine B, Salo TJ, Zhang H, et al. Mutations in HYAL1, a member of a tandemly distributed multigene family encoding disparate hyaluronidase activity, cause a newly described lysosomal disorder, mucopolysaccharidosis IX. Proc Nat Acad Sci USA 1999;96:6296.

Vivian E. Shih, M.D., and Roseann Mandell, B.A.

13

Disorders of the Metabolism of Amino Acids and Related Compounds

The clinical manifestations of amino acid and organic acid metabolic disorders vary from few or no symptoms to serious and fatal diseases. Many of these disorders affect the nervous system, and mental retardation is a major finding. Acute metabolic crisis and dysmorphism have been described with increasing frequency. Newborn screening, simple diagnostic tests, and effective treatment are available for many of these disorders, and early intervention can improve the clinical outlook for these patients. Several books offer extensive reviews.[1–3] The opportunities for prenatal diagnosis continue to increase in parallel with technologic refinements (see Table 13.1).

Prenatal diagnosis of amino acid metabolic disorders has been achieved mainly by using one or a combination of the following tests: (1) measurement of enzyme activity in amniotic fluid cells (AFCs), chorionic villi (CV), fetal liver, or fetal blood; (2) detection of abnormal metabolites, including amino acids, organic acids, and acylcarnitines in amniotic fluid (AF); and (3) DNA analysis. Free amino acids have generally been measured in AF obtained by transabdominal amniocentesis early in the second trimester. Prenatal quantitation of amino acids in AF has been useful in the early detection of only a few hereditary disorders of amino acid metabolism. It should be noted that abnormal patterns of amino acids or organic acids in AF often reflect a maternal metabolic disorder. For instance, the greatly increased phenylalanine concentration in AF from women with untreated phenylketonuria[4] is of maternal origin (maternal PKU syndrome) and is well known to be the cause of fetal damage. So far other metabolic disorders have not been found to have similar deleterious fetal effects.

Organic acid profiles of normal AF measured by gas chromatography–mass spectrometry are generally characterized by over thirty major intermediary metabolites.[5] Abnormal metabolites often accumulate in AF from affected fetuses. Accurate prenatal diagnosis of many of these disorders can be made by employing a sensitive stable isotope dilution technique developed for the specific metabolites.[6,7] The introduction of electrospray tandem mass spectrometry (MS-MS) to clinical medicine and newborn screening has greatly improved the diagnosis of a variety of inherited metabolic disorders. The technique uses a small amount of sample, and results can be available in a few days. In a retrospective study of acylcarnitine profiling by MS-MS using stored AF collected from a group of high-risk pregnancies, Shigematsu et al were able to correctly identify affected

Table 13.1. Prenatal diagnosis of disorders of the metabolism of amino acids and related compounds

Disorder	Prenatal Diagnosis[a]	Tissue with Enzyme Defect	Body Fluid with Abnormal/Excess Metabolites[b]	DNA Analysis
Disorders of the urea cycle				
N-Acetylglutamate synthetase deficiency	Possible	Fetal liver	—	Gene
Carbamylphosphate synthetase deficiency	Made	Fetal liver	—	Gene/haplotype
Ornithine carbamyltransferase deficiency	Made	Fetal liver	—	Gene/RFLP
Argininosuccinate synthetase deficiency (citrullinemia type I)	Made	AF cells/CV	AF	Gene
Citrin deficiency (citrullinemia type II)	Possible	—	—	Gene
Argininosuccinate lyase deficiency (argininosuccinic aciduria)	Made	AF cells/CV	AF	—
Arginase deficiency (hyperargininemia)	Made	Fetal blood	Fetal blood	Gene
Disorders of ornithine metabolism				
Hyperornithinemia, hyperammonemia, and homocitrullinuria (HHH syndrome)	Made	AF cells/CV	—	Gene
Ornithine aminotransferase deficiency (gyrate atrophy)	Possible	AF cells/CV	—	Gene
Disorders of lysine metabolism				
Familial hyperlysinemia	Not indicated	—	—	Gene
Saccharopinuria	Possible	AF cells	—	—
Disorders of sulfur amino acid metabolism				
Methionine adenosyltransferase deficiency (hypermethioninemia)	Not indicated	—	—	Gene
Cystathionine β-synthase deficiency (homocystinuria)	Made	AF cells/CV	—	Gene
γ-Cystathionase deficiency	Not indicated	—	—	Gene
Molybdenum cofactor defect	Made	AF cells/CV	AF	Gene/linkage
Sulfite oxidase deficiency	Possible	AF cells	AF	Gene
Disorders of phenylalanine metabolism				
Phenylketonuria (PKU)	Made	Fetal liver	—	Gene/haplotype
Tetrahydrobiopterin (BH$_4$) deficiency				
Guanosine triphosphate cyclohydrolase (GTPCH) deficiency	Made	Fetal liver	AF	—
6-Pyruvolyltetrahydrobiopterin synthase (PTPS) deficiency	Made	Fetal blood	AF	—
Dihydropteridine reductase (DHPR) deficiency	Made	AF cells/CV	AF	Gene/RFLP

Table 13.1. Prenatal diagnosis of disorders of the metabolism of amino acids and related compounds (continued)

Disorder	Prenatal Diagnosis[a]	Tissue with Enzyme Defect	Body Fluid with Abnormal/Excess Metabolites[b]	DNA Analysis
Disorders of tyrosine metabolism				
Hereditary tyrosinemia type I (hepatorenal)	Made	AF cells/CV	AF	Gene
Hereditary tyrosinemia type II (Richner–Hanhart syndrome)	Possible	Fetal liver	—	Gene/RFLP
4-Hydroxyphenylpyruvate oxidase deficiency	Possible	Fetal liver	—	Gene
Nonketotic hyperglycinemia	Made	Placenta	AF[b]	Gene
Disorders of branched-chain amino acid metabolism				
Maple syrup urine disease (branched-chain ketoaciduria)	Made	AF cells/CV	—	Gene
Hypervalinemia	Possible	—	—	—
Disorders of organic acid metabolism				
Propionic acidemia	Made	AF cells	AF/maternal urine	Gene
Methylmalonic acidemia (B_{12}-nonresponsive)	Made	AF cells/CV	AF/maternal urine	Gene
Isovaleric acidemia	Made	AF cells	AF	—
Isolated 2-methylbutryl coenzyme A dehydrogenase deficiency	Made	—	AF	—
β-Ketothiolase deficiencies (Ketolytic disorders)				
Acetoacetyl-CoA thiolase (T2) deficiency	Made	—	—	Gene
Succinyl-CoA 3-ketoacid CoA transferase (SCOT) deficiency	Made	AF cells/CV	—	—
Biotin-resistant 3-methylcrotonylglycinuria	Possible	—	—	—
3-Methylglutaconyl-CoA hydratase deficiency (3-methylglutaconic aciduria)	Possible	—	—	—
3-Hydroxy-3-methylglutaryl-CoA lyase deficiency	Made	AF cells/CV	AF	Gene
3-Hydroxyisobutyric aciduria	Possible	AF cells	AF	—
Glutaric aciduria type I	Made	AF cells/CV	AF	Gene
Acyl-CoA dehydrogenase deficiencies				
Short-chain acyl-CoA dehydrogenase (SCAD) deficiency	Possible	—	—	—
Medium-chain acyl-CoA dehydrogenase (MCAD) deficiency	Made	AF cells	AF	Gene
Very-long-chain acyl-CoA dehydrogenase (VLCAD) deficiency	Made	AF cells/CV	AF	—
Long chain hydroxy acyl-CoA dehyrogenase (LCHAD) deficiency	Made	AF cells/CV	AF	Gene

Glutaric aciduria type II (ethylmalonic–adipic aciduria)	Made	AF cells	AF	Gene
4-Hydroxybutyric aciduria	Made	AF cells/CV	AF	—
Mevalonic aciduria	Made	CV	AF/maternal urine	Gene
Fumarase deficiency	Made	AF cells/CV	AF	Gene
L-2-hydroxyglutaric aciduria	Made	—	AF	—
D-2-hydroxyglutaric aciduria	Made	—	AF	—
Canavan disease (N-acetylaspartic aciduria)	Made	AF cells/CV[b]	AF	Gene
Prolidase deficiency	Made	AF cells	—	Gene
Disorders of proline metabolism				
Hyperprolinemia type I	Not indicated	—	—	—
Hyperprolinemia type II	Possible	AF cells	—	—
Histidinemia	Not indicated	—	—	Gene
Renal transport disorders				
Hartnup	Not indicated	—	—	—
Iminoglycinuria	Not indicated	—	—	—
Cystinuria	Possible	—	—	Gene

[a]Possible: enzyme activity is present in normal fetal tissue or normal skin fibroblasts.
[b]Both false positive and false negative results.
AF = amniotic fluid; CV = chorionic villi

fetuses with propionic acidemia, methylmalonic aciduria, isovaleric acidemia, and glutaric aciduria.[8] It is anticipated that tandem mass spectrometry will be a reliable and efficient technology applicable to prenatal diagnosis of the organic acidopathies, fatty acid oxidation defects, and amino acid disorders.

Mutation analysis is the definitive diagnostic test if the DNA mutation in the family is known. Linkage analysis using haplotype markers can be useful when the mutation is unknown, but may be less accurate because of the possibility of recombination.

DISORDERS OF THE UREA CYCLE

The urea cycle converts ammonia to urea and is an important pathway in nitrogen metabolism. Disorders of the urea cycle, as a group, are relatively common hereditary metabolic disorders. The clinical features in these disorders are similar. Three clinical phenotypes have been described: the neonatal, infantile and late-onset types. The most severely affected patients become ill shortly after birth, with feeding problems, rapid respiration, seizures, and lethargy progressing to coma and death. In patients presenting later in infancy the history is typically characterized by a gradual onset of vomiting, feeding problems, hepatomegaly, and psychomotor retardation. A third type is characterized by the late onset of symptoms from childhood to adulthood.

Hyperammonemia has been observed in all of the urea cycle disorders and is believed to cause many of the clinical manifestations seen in these patients. Acute hyperammonemic crisis is a life-threatening situation, and aggressive treatment to remove ammonia is imperative. Long-term management involves dietary protein restriction and medications to promote waste nitrogen disposal. Early initiation of therapy has greatly prolonged survival and improved the intellectual achievement of children with urea cycle defects. Enzyme therapy in the form of liver transplantation has given promising results in selected patients.[9–12]

N-Acetylglutamate Synthetase Deficiency

Deficiency of N-acetylglutamate synthetase is a rare disorder presenting with hyperammonemia and variable other features.[13–17] The human N-acetylglutamate synthase gene has been identified on chromosome 17q21.31, and a number of mutations in the gene have been described.[18–21]

N-acetylglutamate is a cofactor for carbamylphosphate synthetase and has a regulatory function in urea synthesis. Confirmation of N-acetylglutamate synthetase deficiency requires enzyme assay in a liver biopsy specimen. This enzyme is not expressed in cultured cells. DNA testing is now possible. No cases of attempted prenatal diagnosis have been reported.

Carbamylphosphate Synthetase Deficiency

The majority of patients with carbamylphosphate synthetase (CPS) deficiency have symptoms develop in the neonatal period. Known outcomes have included death in infancy and survival with retardation and/or neurologic deficits.[22,23] Patients with later onset often have less severe symptoms and have survived into adulthood.[24–27]

The basic defect is a deficiency of hepatic CPS activity.[28] Inheritance is autosomal recessive. The gene structure of human CPS has been described and a number of mutations detected.[29] Prenatal diagnosis is often performed by linkage analysis or direct mutational analysis of the CPS gene.[30–32]

Ornithine Carbamoyltransferase Deficiency

Ornithine carbamoyltransferase (OCT) deficiency is the most common disorder of the urea cycle and is transmitted as an X-linked trait.[33,34] Unusual male-to-female transmission has been reported.[35,36] The hemizygous affected male in general has a clinically severe disease and rarely survives the neonatal hyperammonemia without treatment. A small percentage of affected males became symptomatic with hyperammonemic coma during childhood or as late as the fourth decade.[35,37,38] Heterozygous females have clinical manifestations varying from the severe involvement seen in the male to recurrent episodes of hyperammonemia with possible death in later childhood, to a mere dislike of high-protein foods.

Ornithine carbamoyltransferase activity is markedly deficient in the liver of severely affected males.[22,39,40] Heterozygous females, because of random inactivation of the X chromosome (lyonization), may have varying degrees of OCT deficiency. Increased orotic acid and orotidine in blood or urine following a protein or allopurinol load has been used as one of the diagnostic criteria for partial OCT deficiency.[41,42] Over 240 mutations and polymorphisms have now been identified in the OCT gene.[43] Normal cultured AFCs do not contain OCT activity, and orotic acid, which is markedly increased in the urine of patients with OTC deficiency, has not been found to be elevated in the AF from affected fetuses.[44] Molecular diagnostic advances have made the prenatal diagnosis of OCT deficiency more readily available.[33,45–51] Preimplantation genetic diagnosis has been performed.[52,53]

Argininosuccinate Synthetase Deficiency (Citrullinemia, type 1)

Citrullinemia is an autosomal recessive disorder, and three clinical phenotypes (neonatal, infantile, and late onset) have been recognized.[23,33] The enzyme defect in citrullinemia is a deficiency of argininosuccinate synthetase activity which is evident in liver,[54] cultured skin fibroblasts,[55] and cultured long-term lymphoid cells.[56] Altered enzyme kinetics have been demonstrated in some cases.[55,57,58] The gene for argininosuccinate synthetase has been identified in chromosome 9q34, and over 20 mutations and deletions identified.[59–63]

Prenatal diagnosis has been made by measurement of argininosuccinate synthetase activity in cultured AFCs and in CV biopsy.[64–69] By both direct assay and [^{14}C]citrulline incorporation assay, the enzyme activity is quite variable in the different types of cells grown from normal AF,[70,71] and distinction between an affected and an unaffected fetus may not be easy. Direct enzyme assay on at least 10 mg of CV can be performed at 11–12 weeks of gestation.[72] Elevation of the citrulline concentration in AF is an adjunctive finding.[69,73] and the use of the citrulline/ornithine + arginine ratio seems more discriminatory than the citrulline level alone.[72] Prenatal diagnosis by molecular (DNA) techniques is clearly the best choice in families with known mutations.[74,75]

Citrin Deficiency (Citrullinemia, Type 2)

Citrullinemia type 2 was originally reported as an adult-onset citrullinemia, mainly in Japanese patients, with a liver-specific argininosuccinate synthetase deficiency.[76,77] Clinical features included a sudden disturbance of consciousness, restlessness, drowsiness, and coma. Most patients died within a few years of onset, mainly from cerebral edema.[78] Recent studies have identified a deficiency of the citrin protein as the underlying cause. The SLC25A13 gene located on chromosome 7q21.3 encodes citrin, a mitochondrial transporter of aspartate/glutamate.[77,78] Citrin deficiency has also been identified in patients with citrullinemia who come from different ethnic background, with neonatal intrahepatic cholestasis and other forms of severe hepatic dysfunction.[79–82] For prenatal diagnosis, mutation analysis of the SLC25A13 gene would be the technique of choice. No cases of attempted prenatal diagnosis have been reported.

Argininosuccinate Lyase Deficiency (Argininosuccinic Aciduria)

The clinical presentation of argininosuccinate lyase deficiency is similar to the other urea cycle disorders, ranging from neonatal hyperammonemic encephalopathy to late onset with seizures, episodic hyperammonemia, and developmental delay.[33,34] There are two unique features in this disorder: (1) abnormal, friable, short hair (trichorexis nodosa), which has been described in a number of patients,[83,84] and (2) hepatomegaly with progressive liver fibrosis.[34,85,86] Patients discovered by newborn screening or late onset seem to have mild variants with good outcome.[87–89] This aminoaciduria was an incidental finding in two asymptomatic adult siblings (Shih VE, unpublished data).

The enzyme defect is evident in erythrocytes,[90] cultured skin fibroblasts,[91] and liver.[85] Obligate heterozygotes often have intermediate activity of argininosuccinate lyase.[91,92]

Prenatal diagnosis has been accomplished by measuring argininosuccinate lyase activity in cultured AFCs[93,94] and in cultured and noncultivated chorionic villous tissue.[95] However, there have been both false-negative and false-positive results.[73,95–97] Detection of argininosuccinate in the AF as early as 12 weeks gestation has proven to be a simple, fast and reliable way of identifying an affected fetus for both severe and mild argininosuccinate lyase deficiency.[73,89,93,94,97–99] It should be noted that AF argininosuccinate can be of maternal origin.[73,100] Moreover, increased excretion of argininosuccinate in maternal urine has been observed with an affected fetus and is potentially useful for prenatal diagnosis[93,101] (Shih VE, unpublished data).

Arginase Deficiency (Hyperargininemia)

Arginase deficiency is clinically characterized by progressive loss of psychomotor skills and spastic diplegia.[102,103] Rarely, it presents as neonatal encephalopathy and cerebral edema.[104] The enzyme defect, arginase A1 deficiency, is evident in erythrocytes, leukocytes, and liver.[102,105–107] Studies of the molecular pathology of arginase deficiency have shown extensive heterogeneity.[108,109]

In this autosomal recessive disorder, obligate heterozygotes have been found with intermediate levels of arginase activity in erythrocytes.[103,110] The A1 arginase is not expressed in cultured skin fibroblasts[111,112] or AFCs.[105]

For the purpose of prenatal diagnosis of arginase deficiency, fetal blood sampling permits the direct assay of arginase activity in erythrocytes.[113] Prenatal diagnosis has been accomplished by finding a marked elevation of the fetal plasma arginine level and deficient fetal RBC arginase activity; a heterozygous fetus and an unaffected fetus was also identified using these techniques.[114,115] Prenatal diagnosis by DNA analysis is applicable to families with informative restriction fragment length polymorphism (RFLP) or known mutations. A heterozygous fetus has been identified by molecular prenatal diagnosis.[116]

DISORDERS OF ORNITHINE METABOLISM

Hyperornithinemia, Hyperammonemia, and Homocitrullinuria (HHH Syndrome)

The clinical features of the HHH syndrome are similar to those of other hyperammonemic syndromes, namely, protein intolerance, psychomotor retardation, and episodic lethargy and ataxia.[117] The same approach to treatment used for urea cycle disorders applies to this disorder.

This autosomal recessive syndrome is a disorder of compartmentation. The basic defect is an impaired transport of ornithine into the mitochondrion.[118,119] Failure of ornithine to reach the mitochondrial ornithine carbamyltransferase and ornithine aminotransferase would cause functional deficiency of both enzymes, resulting in hyperammonemia and hyperornithinemia. A gene encoding a mitochondrial ornithine transporter has been mapped to 13q14, and a number of mutations described, including a common F188 deletion mutation in French-Canadian HHH patients.[120–124] Defective use of ornithine in cultured amniocytes[119] has been used to identify one affected fetus[125] and to correctly predict several unaffected fetuses.[125–127] Molecular (DNA) diagnosis is available for families with known mutations.

Ornithine Aminotransferase Deficiency Associated with Gyrate Atrophy of the Choroid and Retina

Gyrate atrophy of the choroid and retina is a rare type of retinitis pigmentosa, clinically characterized by progressive night blindness and loss of peripheral vision, leading to blindness between 40 and 60 years of age.[128,129] These patients have normal intelligence. Affected patients have hyperornithinemia as a result of ornithine aminotransferase (OAT) deficiency.[130,131] The goal of treatment is to lower the plasma ornithine level by a low-arginine (precursor of ornithine) diet. OAT requires pyridoxal phosphate as a cofactor. In some patients, high doses of pyridoxine can result in the reduction of plasma ornithine. Only long-term treatment may slow progression of the retinal degeneration.[128,132] The OAT deficiency is demonstrable in liver,[133] cultured fibroblasts,[131,134,135] and cultured lymphoblasts.[136] Heterozygotes have intermediate activity of OAT in cultured fibroblasts.[135,137,138] The molecular defect is quite heterogeneous.[139,140] Prenatal diagnosis is possible by measurement of OAT activity in cultured AFCs,[141] CV tissue and cultured CV,[142] or by mutation analysis. There have been no reported cases of prenatal diagnosis.

DISORDERS OF LYSINE METABOLISM

Familial Hyperlysinemia

Initial reports of patients with persistent hyperlysinemia described clinical features varying from normal to severe psychomotor retardation and seizures.[143] However, a study of ten patients identified through newborn screening programs or family surveys showed that no adverse mental or physical effects could be attributed to the metabolic abnormality.[144] The hyperlysinemia is caused by deficient activity of a bifunctional protein, referred to as α-aminoadipic semialdehyde synthase, which catalyzes the first two steps of the lysine-degradation pathway. A mutation in the gene encoding this enzyme has been identified in the genomic DNA from a patient with hyperlysinemia.[145] Enzyme activity is present in normal cultured skin fibroblasts.[146,147] Although heterozygote detection and prenatal diagnosis are potentially possible, there appears to be no indication for such testing.

Saccharopinuria

Several patients have been described with saccharopinuria and hyperlysinemia; two were mentally retarded, one had spastic diplegia, one had speech delay, hyperactive behavior, and minor neurologic abnormalities.[148–150] The activity of saccharopine dehydrogenase was reduced in cultured fibroblasts from these patients.[151,152] Lysine-oxoglutarate reductase activity was also partially impaired in one case and not detectable in another.[150] The causal relationship between the biochemical and clinical abnormalities remains to be established. Nonetheless, prenatal diagnosis is possible by measurement of the enzyme activities in cultured AFCs.[153]

DISORDERS OF SULFUR AMINO ACID METABOLISM

There are a number of disorders in the metabolic pathway from methionine to inorganic sulfate. Disorders involving defects of vitamin B_{12} and folate metabolism are discussed in chapter 17.

Hypermethioninemia Due to Methionine Adenosyltransferase (MAT) Deficiency

Hypermethioninemia is a rare metabolic disorder. The majority of patients have been discovered as a result of routine newborn screening for the hypermethioninemia associated with cystathionine β-synthase deficiency.[154] There appear to be no clinical consequences resulting from the hypermethioninemia in the thirty patients reported[155] except for two patients,[155,156] who had demyelination by MRI. The enzyme defect is a partial deficiency of hepatic methionine adenosyltransferase activity. This enzyme activity is normal, however, in erythrocytes, cultured skin fibroblasts, and lymphoblasts derived from these patients.[157,158] Over fifteen mutations have been identified in the *MAT1* gene.[159–162] Prenatal diagnosis has not been attempted for this seemingly benign metabolic disorder.

Homocystinuria Due to Cystathionine β-Synthase Deficiency

Homocystinuria due to cystathionine β-synthase (CBS) deficiency is a relatively common metabolic disorder. Information on more than 600 cases has been compiled and extensively reviewed.[163–165]

CBS deficiency is a multisystem disease and includes phenotypic features of gradual appearance of Marfan-like habitus with arachnodactyly and dislocated lenses, mental retardation, psychotic behavior, episodes of arterial and venous thromboses, osteoporosis, skeletal abnormalities, and fair brittle hair. In mildly affected patients, dislocation of the ocular lenses may be the only finding. Vascular complications resulting in heart attack or stroke are often the cause of death. Lowering the plasma homocysteine levels in CBS-deficient patients significantly reduced the risk of cardiovascular complications even when levels remained several times higher than the normal population mean.[166] Early treatment of patients detected by newborn screening has greatly reduced these complications.[167]

Patients have been divided into two clinical types, pyridoxine-responsive and pyridoxine-nonresponsive, based on changes in methionine and homocystine levels following pyridoxine administration. Pyridoxine-responsive patients in general have milder clinical manifestations than pyridoxine-nonresponsive patients. Women with homocystinuria, in contrast to women with phenylketonuria, have borne normal children. A total of 108 pregnancies among 47 women has been recorded, most occurring in women with the pyridoxine-responsive type.[164,168]

The deficiency of CBS activity has been demonstrated in multiple tissues, including liver,[169] cultured skin fibroblasts[170] and short-term cultivated lymphocytes,[171,172] but not in noncultivated leukocytes. The CBS activity in cultured skin fibroblasts of a number of obligate heterozygotes overlapped the control range,[173,174] making the distinction between heterozygotes and normal individuals difficult by this measurement alone. More than 120 mutations of the CBS gene have been identified.[165,175,176] The G307S mutation is prevalent in pyridoxine-nonresponsive patients of Celtic ethnic origin,[177] whereas the I278T mutation is prevalent among pyridoxine-responsive patients.[178] These two mutations account for approximately 50 percent of affected alleles in patients with CBS deficiency.

The activity of CBS is readily demonstrable in cultured AFCs[170,179] but is too low to be measured in noncultivated CV.[154] Prenatal diagnosis has been made using cultured AFCs[179,180] and cultured CV (Kraus J, personal communication, 1997). An unaffected child has been correctly predicted in several other monitored pregnancies.[180–183] DNA diagnosis is possible in families with known mutation.

γ-Cystathionase Deficiency

γ-Cystathionase deficiency was first observed in a mentally retarded patient.[184] However, subsequent studies[165] indicate no characteristic clinical phenotype and no defined relationship to mental retardation. The enzyme defect is evident only in liver tissue[185] and cultured lymphocytes.[186,187] The expression of this enzyme in cultured skin fibroblasts has not been confirmed.[186,188–190] Maternal γ-cystathionase deficiency does not seem to be deleterious to the pregnant woman or the fetus.[191] Four mutations have been described.[192] This autosomal recessive biochemical disorder is without clinical manifestations and thus at present does not raise questions about prenatal diagnosis.

Combined Sulfite Oxidase Deficiency and Xanthine Oxidase Deficiency (A Defect in Molybdenum Cofactor Synthesis)

The combined deficiency of sulfite oxidase and xanthine oxidase is a rare metabolic disorder associated with severe neurologic impairment. Most patients manifested intractable neonatal seizures and developmental delay. Facial dysmorphism and dislocated lenses were observed in most patients in the first few months of life. One-half of the reported patients died in early childhood.[193] There is no effective treatment.

The basic defect is in the synthesis of the molybdenum cofactor, which in humans is shared by the two molybdoenzymes, sulfite oxidase and xanthine oxidase. In addition to the abnormal sulfur-containing metabolites (sulfite, thiosulfate, and sulfocysteine), these patients also excrete an increased amount of xanthine and have hypouricemia. Molybdenum cofactor deficiency is inherited in an autosomal recessive manner and can be diagnosed by the combination of the characteristic metabolite pattern and sulfite oxidase deficiency in cultured skin fibroblasts. Xanthine oxidase is not expressed in cultured fibroblasts.

Prenatal diagnosis of this disorder has been made by finding increased sulfocysteine in AF and sulfite oxidase deficiency in cultured AFCs.[193,194] An unaffected fetus was correctly predicted in two other monitored pregnancies.[195,196] Sulfite oxidase activity is low in cultured amniocytes, and large numbers of cells are needed for prenatal diagnosis. On the other hand, abundance of sulfite oxidase activity in chorionic villous tissue makes first-trimester diagnosis possible.[197,198] Cofactor synthesis is a complex pathway that involves four different genes. Mutations causing disease have been identified in the *MOCS1*, *MOCS2*, and *GEPH* genes. Over thirty mutations in the genes responsible for molybdenum cofactor biosynthesis have been identified in affected patients.[199] In families with known mutations, prenatal diagnosis can best be done by mutation analysis or linkage studies.[200,201]

Sulfite Oxidase Deficiency

Isolated sulfite oxidase deficiency is clinically indistinguishable from molybdenum cofactor deficiency.[202–206] A deficiency of sulfite oxidase activity is evident in liver, kidney, and brain.[204,207] The enzyme protein was absent in liver tissue of the first patient, indicating that the deficiency of sulfite oxidase activity is secondary to the lack of a structural enzyme protein.[208] The human sulfite oxidase gene has been cloned[209] and three single base substitutions have been identified.[210] Because xanthine oxidase is not affected, uric acid production is normal.

Sulfite oxidase deficiency can be confirmed in cultured skin fibroblasts.[203] Prenatal diagnosis is possible by enzyme assay or by detection of the abnormal metabolite S-sulfocysteine in AF.[194] Over twenty mutations have been described in the gene encoding sulfite oxidase.[211] DNA diagnosis has been performed, with identification of both an affected and unaffected fetus,[212] and will be possible in families with known mutations.

DISORDERS OF PHENYLALANINE METABOLISM

Phenylketonuria (PKU)˙

PKU is among the most common of the amino acid disorders, with a frequency varying from a high of 1 per 4,500 newborns in Belfast, Northern Ireland, to a low of 1 per 64,000 in Denmark. In the United States the incidence is approximately 1 per 14,000 newborns.[213] With early detection by newborn screening and early institution of a low-phenylalanine diet, mental retardation can be prevented. It has become apparent, however, that some degree of cognitive deficit may be seen, even in successfully treated patients.[214] Behavioral changes or loss of IQ points[215,216] have been observed in a number of patients after the termination of diet therapy.

Maternal PKU is a serious clinical problem. Offspring of untreated pregnant women with PKU suffer from brain damage in utero and most often have microcephaly and mental retardation, and sometimes congenital heart disease as well.[217] It appears that in order to prevent the teratogenic effects of high levels of phenylalanine, it is necessary to start the dietary treatment before conception or during early pregnancy.[218–221]

The enzyme defect in PKU is a deficiency of hepatic phenylalanine hydroxylase activity.[222] Activity of this enzyme is not expressed in cultured normal skin fibroblasts.[223,224] Heterozygote detection has been attempted by several methods, including measuring the fasting plasma phenylalanine/tyrosine ratio,[225] oral or intravenous phenylalanine loading,[226] and calculating the in vivo conversion of deuterium-labeled phenylalanine to labeled tyrosine.[227] The reliability of these tests is limited. DNA analysis would be a definitive way to determine the genotype of an individual. Analysis of the phenylalanine hydroxylase gene has identified over 80 polymorphic patterns (haplotypes) and over 400 mutations.[228–230]

Prenatal diagnosis of PKU has been made by haplotype and mutation analysis.[231–234] In Caucasians, 86 percent of PKU families are heterozygous for one or more RFLPs. Haplotype analysis in Asians is of limited value because only 32 percent of families are heterozygous for one or more RFLP sites.[235,236] Preimplantation genetic diagnosis of phenylketonuria has been reported.[237]

Hyperphenylalaninemia Due to Tetrahydrobiopterin Deficiency

Tetrahydrobiopterin (BH$_4$) deficiency is a rare cause of hyperphenylalaninemia, occurring in about 2 percent of newborns with increased blood phenylalanine levels.[230] Clinically,

BH$_4$ deficiency is characterized by progressive encephalopathy and disabling dystonia despite treatment with a low-phenylalanine diet. Mental retardation, myoclonic seizures, hypertonicity of the extremities, drooling, and swallowing difficulties are frequently observed. BH$_4$ is a cofactor for three aromatic amino acid hydroxylases mediating the conversion of phenylalanine to tyrosine, tyrosine to L-DOPA, and tryptophan to 5-hydroxytryptophan. BH$_4$ deficiency leads to phenylalanine accumulation and, more importantly, deficiency of the neurotransmitters dopamine and serotonin. Therapy includes the combined use of neurotransmitter precursors with BH$_4$, folic acid, or folinic acid. Results were encouraging in a small number of patients.[238–240]

BH$_4$ deficiency can be a result of either reduced biosynthesis or impaired recycling of this cofactor. Deficiencies of four enzymes have been identified: guanosine triphosphate cyclohydrolase I (GTPCH)[241]; 6-pyruvoyl tetrahydrobiopterin synthase (PTPS)[242]; dihydropteridine reductase (DHPR)[243]; and pterin-4α-carbinolamide dehydratase (PCD or primpterinuria).[244] PTPS and DHPR deficiencies are associated with mild hyperphenylalaninemia and are often detected by newborn screening. GTPCH deficiency is rare. Diagnosis of the variants of BH$_4$ deficiency can best be made by the pattern of urine pterins[245–247] and can be confirmed by enzyme assays. Deficiency of DHPR activity can be demonstrated in cultured fibroblasts.[243,248] GTPCH deficiency is evident in cultured lymphocytes.[241,249] PTPS deficiency can be confirmed by enzyme analysis in erythrocytes.

Prenatal diagnosis is possible for the BH$_4$ deficiency disorders and can be achieved by analysis of AF pterins (neopterin and biopterin), often in combination with enzyme assay.[250] PTPS activity is not expressed in cultured amniocytes; however, Niederwieser et al.[251] made the first prenatal diagnosis by finding high neopterin and low biopterin in the AF and confirmed it by measurement of PTPS in fetal erythrocytes. GTPCH is not expressed in amniocytes, and prenatal diagnosis has been made by finding reduced neopterin and biopterin in AF.[252] DHPR deficiency on the other hand, is detectable in AFCs and CV, and increased biopterin in AF has been demonstrated in an at-risk fetus.[253] The cDNA for DHPR has been cloned and sequenced,[254,255] and prenatal diagnosis by RFLP analysis[256] and by direct mutation analysis of CV has been reported.[257] The gene encoding the PCD protein has been characterized and seven mutations described,[258] but no attempts at prenatal diagnosis have been reported. There is an international register of BH$_4$ deficient patients and a mutation database.[259,260]

DISORDERS OF TYROSINE METABOLISM

Hereditary Tyrosinemia Type I (Hepatorenal type)

Hereditary tyrosinemia type I is characterized clinically by hepatomegaly and liver dysfunction in early infancy. Other complications include coagulation defect, renal tubular dysfunction and the consequent rickets, and a high risk of liver cancer. Acute episodes of peripheral neuropathy are more common in Canadian patients than in Norwegian patients. Most patients die from liver failure in early childhood. Therapy with a phenylalanine and tyrosine-restricted diet has limited effects. A new drug—2-(2-nitro-4-trifluoromethylbenzoyl)-1,3-cyclohexanedione (NTBC)—was recently approved by the FDA and has been effective in reducing the harmful metabolites and has greatly improved the outlook for these patients. It is now the treatment of choice rather than liver transplantation.

Hereditary tyrosinemia is an autosomal recessive disease. It has been described in various ethnic groups, but is so highly prevalent among French-Canadians from the Lac St. John-Chicoutimi district of Quebec[261] that newborns in Quebec are routinely screened for this disorder. The enzyme defect is a deficiency of fumarylacetoacetate hydrolase (FAH) activity, which is evident in liver tissue,[262,263] kidney,[264] erythrocytes,[265] lymphocytes, and fibroblasts.[265,266] The FAH gene is located at 15q23–25,[267,268] and over thirty mutations have been identified.[269,270] A guanine-to-adenine change in the splice-donor sequence in intron 12 of the gene was detected in 86 percent of French-Canadian patients from Quebec.[271]

Prenatal diagnosis of hereditary tyrosinemia has been made by finding increased succinylacetone in AF as early as twelve weeks of gestation.[272–276] However, it is important that the sensitive stable isotope technique be used to avoid false-negative results.[274,277,278] In Quebec, thirty-six pregnancies were monitored by succinylacetone in AF and eight affected fetuses were correctly diagnosed, with no false-negative cases.[270] In one additional case the succinylacetone level in AF was within the normal range, but the outcome was an affected offspring.[279] This patient was later determined to be a compound heterozygote for two known mutations; the normal AF succinylacetone level remains unexplained.[280] The diagnosis can also be made by measuring fumarylacetoacetase activity in cultured AFCs[277,278,281] or in chorionic villous biopsy.[265,276,282] Prenatal diagnosis of both an affected and unaffected fetus by mutation analysis has been reported.[283]

Other Types of Tyrosinemia

Tyrosinemia type II (Richner–Hanhart syndrome) has clinical manifestations entirely different from those of hereditary tyrosinemia type I. The salient features in type II are oculocutaneous manifestations of corneal erosions and plaques and keratotic lesions of the palms and soles. Mild to severe mental retardation is seen in some patients. Plasma tyrosine levels are usually much higher than in tyrosinemia type I. There is no hepatorenal involvement. Therapy with a low-tyrosine, low-phenylalanine diet has resulted in rapid resolution of the oculocutaneous lesions, but no change in intellectual performance or behavior has been observed.[270] The enzyme defect is a deficiency of hepatic cytosol tyrosine aminotransferase activity. The cDNA for the human tyrosine aminotransferase has been cloned, and characteristic RFLPs[284] and several point mutations have been described.[285] Untreated maternal tyrosinemia II with plasma tyrosine level over 1100 μmol/L may have an adverse effect on the developing fetus[286]; one woman treated during pregnancy with a protein-restricted diet had a normal infant.[287]

A rare third type of tyrosinemia caused by hepatic 4-hydroxphenylpyruvate dioxidase (HPD) deficiency has been described. Most patients presented with neurologic symptoms. A number of patients were detected by newborn screening, and those treated from infancy with a low-tyrosine, low-phenylalanine diet have had normal development.[288] DNA analysis has revealed at least four mutations in patients with HPD deficiency.[289]

Prenatal diagnosis of tyrosinemia types II and III would require fetal liver biopsy or DNA analysis when applicable. Analysis of tyrosyl metabolites in AF may or may not be helpful.

NONKETOTIC HYPERGLYCINEMIA

Nonketotic hyperglycinemia (NKH) is a relatively common and devastating hereditary metabolic disease with autosomal recessive inheritance. The incidence of NKH is 1 in 55,000 newborns in Finland and 1 in 63,000 in British Columbia, Canada, with a calculated carrier frequency of approximately 1 in 125.[290] Symptoms usually appear within hours after birth and include marked hypotonia, apnea, seizures, and coma. Early death in the first few months of life is common, and those who survive are severely retarded. In rare cases, neurologic symptoms appear later in childhood. There is no effective treatment.

The metabolic defect in NKH is in the glycine cleavage system (GCS), a mitochondrial enzyme complex consisting of four individual protein components encoded on four different chromosomes. The gene for the P-protein has been mapped to 9p13 and the T-protein to 3q21.1–21.2. H-protein deficiency and L-protein deficiency are rare. The molecular defect in NKH is heterogeneous. A number of mutations have been identified in the glycine cleavage enzyme subunits.[291–298] Over 80 percent of NKH patients have a defect in the P-protein with approximately 15 percent having a defect in the T-protein. The P-protein mutation S564I is frequent in Finnish patients with NKH,[292] and the T-protein mutation H42R has been described in the Israeli-Arab population.[299]

The GCS enzyme is not expressed in normal cultured cells, including cultured chorionic villi. Prenatal diagnosis has been attempted by measuring the glycine level or the molar ratio of glycine and serine in AF, however, this test has proven to be unreliable in predicting the phenotype of the fetus.[300,301] Measurements of placental GCS activity and enzyme protein subunits have provided prenatal diagnosis of NKH.[302–304] Activity of the glycine cleavage system can be assayed directly in CVS tissue,[301,302] however, both false-negative and false-positive prenatal diagnosis have been reported.[305,306] Prenatal diagnosis using molecular analysis is the approach of choice in families with known mutations.[307]

Transient neonatal nonketotic hyperglycinemia and leukodystrophy with vanishing white matter are two other diseases in which glycine is increased in CSF and/or plasma, however, GCS deficiency has not been proven in these disorders. It is important that the diagnosis of "classic" NKH be confirmed before prenatal diagnosis is attempted.

DISORDERS OF BRANCHED-CHAIN AMINO ACID METABOLISM

Many disorders have been described in the metabolic pathways of the branched-chain amino acids, which include leucine, isoleucine, and valine. Except for the disorders described in this section, the others have no specific amino acid abnormalities and will be discussed in the section on organic acid disorders.

Maple Syrup Urine Disease (Branched-Chain Ketoaciduria, Leucinosis)

Classic maple syrup urine disease (MSUD) represents the most severe form of MSUD, with neonatal onset of symptoms. These patients usually behave normally in the first 2–3 days of life; however, poor feeding, lethargy, seizures, and ketoacidosis become apparent within 1 week. An odor resembling maple syrup in the wet diaper is characteristic.[308] Recurrent metabolic crises and severe neurologic damage is inevitable in the absence of treatment. In the intermittent milder form of MSUD and the thiamine-responsive form, the onset of symptoms may be later in life.[309–311] In these variant forms, symptoms and biochemical change may appear only intermittently, often preceded by infection or diet indiscretion; death can result from these acute episodes. In a rare form of MSUD, patients are retarded, but do not have the acute symptoms.[312] Early diagnosis by newborn screening and long-term therapy with a diet restricted in the branched-chain amino acids, thiamine administration, and aggressive intervention during acute metabolic decompensation have greatly improved the outcome of these patients. Several early treated women with MSUD have given birth to normal infants.[313,314]

The enzyme defect in this autosomal recessive disorder is a deficiency of branched-chain α-ketoacid dehydrogenase activity. The diagnosis can be confirmed by measuring leucine oxidation or by direct assay of enzyme activity in leukocytes, established lymphoid cells, and cultured fibroblasts.[315] In classic MSUD, the enzyme activity is less than 2 percent; in the milder forms, the residual enzyme is 2–15 percent.

The branched-chain α-ketoacid dehydrogenase is a multienzyme complex, consisting of six individual enzymes. Four molecular phenotypes can be defined based on the affected subunits of the BCKD complex. More than sixty mutations have been identified in patients with MSUD.[315] MSUD is prevalent among Pennsylvania Mennonites, with a frequency of 1 in 176 newborns[316] compared with 1 in 200,000 in the general population. All Mennonite patients studied have the same missense mutation (Tyr 393 to Asn) in the E_1 α-subunit.[317] There is a strong correlation between mutations in the E_2-subunit and thiamine-responsive MSUD.[315]

Heterozygote detection by assaying both intact leukocytes and cultured skin fibroblasts for leucine or branched-chain α-ketoacid decarboxylation has been achieved with varying degrees of success.[318–321]

Attempts at prenatal diagnosis by measuring AF metabolites have not been successful.[322] Prenatal diagnosis has been made by measuring [1-^{14}C]leucine oxidation in cultured AFCs[315, 323–327] (Shih VE, Mandell R, unpublished data) and in intact CV.[328] Poorly growing cells, normally low in leucine oxidation, may give erroneous results when used for prenatal diagnosis.[326] Prenatal diagnosis of E3 deficiency by mutation analysis has been reported.[329] When applicable, DNA analysis is the method of choice for both identification of carrier status and prenatal diagnosis. If the pregnancy is continued, measurement of plasma branched-chain amino acids and allo-isoleucine in the first 24 to 48 hours of life allows early diagnosis and early treatment.

Hypervalinemia

Only four children with hypervalinemia have been described; the major clinical finding is psychomotor retardation.[330–332] The enzyme defect in this disorder is a deficiency of valine transaminase activity. This defect is evident in peripheral blood leukocytes and cultured skin fibroblasts.[333–335] Prenatal diagnosis remains only a potential possibility.

DISORDERS OF ORGANIC ACIDS

The organic acid disorders included in this section are defects in the intermediary metabolism of amino acid and fatty acid oxidation. Many are in the metabolic pathway of the branched-chain amino acids. Clinically, hypoglycemia and recurrent metabolic acidosis with or without ketosis are the most common symptoms. Diagnosis can be made by gas or liquid chromatographic profiling of urinary organic acids[336–338] or plasma acylcarnitines.[8,339]

Propionic Acidemia (Propionyl CoA Carboxylase Deficiency)

Isolated propionic acidemia is a relatively common organic acid disorder. It often presents in the neonatal period with symptoms of hyperammonemia (see "Urea Cycle Disorders" on page 524) and metabolic ketoacidosis. Infants surviving the initial illness have recurrent acute metabolic decompensation, cardiomyopathy, and mental retardation. Pancytopenia, neutropenia, and failure to thrive are frequent findings in chronically ill patients. Therapy includes fluid and electrolyte management, during the acute phase and long-term dietary protein restriction and carnitine supplementation.[340,341]

Propionic acidemia is an autosomal recessive disease caused by propionyl-CoA carboxylase deficiency. This enzyme is a tetrapeptide, composed of α- and β-subunits.

Genetic heterogeneity has been demonstrated by complementation analysis in fibroblasts.[342,343] Heterozygote detection is possible in certain cases by assaying the enzyme activity in cultured skin fibroblasts.[344,345] Propionyl-CoA carboxylase requires biotin as a cofactor and is among the multiple carboxylases affected in the biotin metabolic disorders (see chapter 17).

Prenatal diagnosis has been made by measurement of propionyl-CoA carboxylase activity in cultured AFCs[346–351] and by detection of abnormal metabolites in AF.[69,350,352–356] Experience with prenatal diagnosis of propionic acidemia in over 100 at-risk pregnancies has established that stable isotope dilution analysis of abnormal metabolites in AF is rapid and accurate. Diagnosis of an affected fetus in the eleventh week of gestation was accomplished using metabolite analysis after the results of the enzyme assay in CV suggested a heterozygous phenotype.[69] Propionylcarnitine was also increased in AFs from affected pregnancies.[8,357] Increased methylcitrate has been detected in the urine of women carrying an affected fetus[358] but has not been proven to be a reliable test for prenatal diagnosis. The gene for the α-subunit of propionyl-CoA carboxylase is located on 13q32, and the gene for the β-subunit is on 3q13.3–q22. Over eighty mutations have been reported among patients in Europe and North America.[359] When applicable, DNA analysis can be used for prenatal diagnosis.[360]

Methylmalonic Acidemia (Methylmalonyl CoA Mutase Deficiency)

Methylmalonic acidemia (MMA) is a relatively common organic acid disorder, with an incidence of approximately 1 in 20,000 newborns.[361,362] Depending on the response to B_{12} administration, MMA can be divided into two types. The B12 responsive type is due to defects in the synthesis of the cobalamin cofactor is discussed in chapter 17. The clinical and biochemical features of B_{12}-nonresponsive methylmalonic acidemia caused by methylmalonyl-CoA mutase deficiency include failure to thrive, vomiting with recurrent ketosis, neutropenia, hyperglycinemia, and severe hypotonia, and are similar to those seen in propionic acidemia (see "Propionic Acidemia" above).

Methylmalonyl-CoA mutase deficiency is an autosomal recessive disorder, and the enzyme defect is evident in leukocytes and cultured skin fibroblasts. There are two types of the apoenzyme defect. Patients with the more severe mut^0 type have either much reduced or no enzyme protein; patients with the mut^- type produce a structurally abnormal enzyme protein. The gene for this enzyme has been mapped to chromosome 6[363] and over twenty mutations have been described.[364]

Prenatal diagnosis of methylmalonic acidemia has been made by enzyme assay in cultured AFCs[346,348,349,353] and noncultured AFCs[349] and CV.[365,366] False-negative results from CV [^{14}C]propionate incorporation assay have been reported.[69] Metabolite measurement in AF using the sensitive stable isotope dilution assay for methylcitrate and methylmalonate provides a fast and accurate means of diagnosis.[69,354,355,367–369] Acylcarnitine profiling in AF can also be useful for prenatal diagnosis.[8] Increased midtrimester urine methylmalonic acid has been found in women pregnant with an affected child but may not be suitable for prenatal diagnosis.[346,367,368,370,371] DNA diagnosis is a possibility in families with known mutation.

Isovaleric Acidemia

Isovaleric acidemia is an autosomal recessive disorder characterized by the early onset of poor feeding, recurrent vomiting, and ketoacidosis. An offensive odor resembling "sweaty feet" is noticeable during these episodes.[372,373] Mild mental retardation may also occur.

A low-protein diet minimizes the recurrence of symptoms; in more severe cases glycine and carnitine supplements may also be helpful.[374–377] One case of maternal isovaleric acidemia with three pregnancies has been described without harmful effects on the fetus[378] (Shih VE, unpublished data).

The enzyme defect in isovaleric acidemia is a deficiency of isovaleryl-CoA dehydrogenase activity, which is demonstrable in cultured fibroblasts.[379,380] Heterozygotes have intermediate levels of enzyme activity.[381]

At least twenty-five at-risk pregnancies have been monitored. Four prenatal diagnoses of affected fetuses have been made by finding an increased amount of isovalerylglycine in AF using a sensitive isotope dilution technique[275,382,383] or by measurement of $^{14}CO_2$ liberation from [2–^{14}C]leucine in cultured AFCs or chorionic villous tissue.[379,383–385] Increased maternal urine isovalerylglycine has been shown during pregnancy with both affected and unaffected fetuses and thus may not be a reliable index for prenatal diagnosis of isovaleric acidemia.[382] AF levels of acylcarnitines using the ratio of isovalerylcarnitine to propionylcarnitine have been used for prenatal diagnosis of five affected and five unaffected cases.[8]

Isolated 2-Methylbutryl Coenzyme A Dehydrogenase Deficiency

This disorder of L-isoleucine degradation was first described by Gibson et al. in a 4-month-old infant who presented with mild hypoglycemia, lethargy, and apnea.[386] Lab findings included increased plasma short-chain acylcarnitine and increased urine 2-methylbutyrylglycine (2-MBG) and 2-methylbutyrylcamitine (2-MBC). Prenatal diagnosis in a subsequent pregnancy showed an increased concentration of 2-MBG in AF obtained at 15 weeks of gestation, suggesting an affected fetus. Increased plasma C5-acylcarnitine and increased urine 2-MBG were confirmed in the newborn.[386]

The β-Ketothiolase Deficiencies (Ketolytic Disorders)

Ketones are generated from fatty acids and ketogenic amino acids (branched-chain amino acids) and have an important role in energy metabolism. Ketolysis is mediated by the β-ketothiolases. Mitochondrial acetoacetyl-CoA thiolase (T2) and succinyl-CoA 3-ketoacid CoA transferase (SCOT) are two major enzymes in this group.

T2 deficiency[387,388] or SCOT deficiency[389] results in recurrent ketoacidosis often starting in the first 2 years of life. Patients are asymptomatic between episodes but may have persistent ketonuria. Mental retardation and dystonia have been observed in T2 deficiency, and cardiomyopathy has been reported in SCOT deficiency.[390] The diagnosis of β-ketothiolase deficiencies is confirmed by demonstrating a reduction of enzyme activity in leukocytes or cultured skin fibroblasts. These are autosomal recessive traits.

Prenatal diagnosis has been made in SCOT deficiency by enzyme assay in cultured AFCs[391] and in CV.[392] Molecular techniques were used for prenatal diagnosis of T2 deficiency.[393] Prenatal diagnosis by molecular analysis is possible for families with known mutation.

Biotin-Resistant 3-Methylcrotonylglycinuria

The clinical features in biotin-resistant 3-methylcrotonylglycinuria are quite variable and range from hypoglycemia, recurrent metabolic acidosis, and dietary protein intolerance to a lack of clinical manifestations.[394,395] A number of asymptomatic women were discovered postpartum because of a false-positive screening test in their newborn infants (maternal 3-methylcrotonylglycinuria)[396] (Shih VE, unpublished data). Both mother and child were normal.

The diagnosis of biotin-resistant 3-methylcrotonylglycinuria is made by the detection of large amounts of urinary 3-hydroxyisovalerate and 3-methylcrotonylglycine, without other metabolites seen in propionic acidemia. The deficiency of 3-methylcrotonyl-CoA carboxylase activity is evident in liver, cultured fibroblasts, and leukocytes.[397,398] Prenatal diagnosis is thus potentially possible if indicated.

3-Methylglutaconic Aciduria

3-Methylglutaconic aciduria has been associated with a variety of clinical phenotypes, and at least four types have been delineated. Type 1 is associated with 3-methylglutaconyl-CoA hydratase deficiency. Patients had developmental delay, hypoglycemia, and metabolic acidosis. A number of mutations in the gene encoding methylglutaconyl-CoA hydratase have been described.[399]

Patients with other types of 3-methylglutaconic aciduria often have multisystem diseases, including Barth syndrome (X-linked cardiomyopathy, growth retardation, and neutropenia)[400, 401]; severe deficiency of respiratory chain complexes[402,403]; Costeff syndrome (optic atrophy and other severe neurologic impairment) in Iraqi Jews[404]; and a syndrome of neuropsychiatric disorder, seizures, deafness and blindness in Saudi Arabian patients.[405] The enzyme defect and underlying cause of 3-methylglutaconic aciduria in these patients is unknown.

Prenatal diagnosis of 3-methylglutaconyl-CoA hydratase deficiency is potentially possible by enzyme assay or mutation analysis. Chitayat et al.[406] monitored a pregnancy at risk for 3-methylglutaconic aciduria type 4 (Barth syndrome) and found normal AF 3-methylglutaconic acid in an unaffected fetus. For Barth syndrome, prenatal diagnosis strategy should be based on DNA analysis for the responsible gene.[407] There have been no reports of prenatal diagnosis for the other types of 3-methylglutaconic aciduria.

3-Hydroxy-3-Methylglutaryl-CoA Lyase Deficiency

The clinical manifestations of 3-hydroxy-3-methylglutaryl-CoA (HMG-CoA) lyase deficiency include hepatomegaly, vomiting, episodic hypoketotic hypoglycemia, metabolic acidosis, and often hyperammonemia.[408–410] Neonatal death has resulted from these symptoms. Fatal cardiomyopathy was reported in one case.[411] The majority of patients who survived the neonatal episode or had a later onset of the disease have had normal psychomotor development.

The urine organic acid pattern in HMG-CoA lyase deficiency includes marked increases of urinary 3-hydroxy-3-methlglutaric acid, 3-methylglutaconic acid, 3-methylglutaric acid, and 3-hydroxyisovaleric acid. 3-Methylglutarylcarnitine is also increased in urine. However, unexplained elevations of these organic acids have been observed in a few patients with carbamylphosphate synthetase deficiency but with normal HMG-CoA lyase activity.[412,413]

A deficiency of HMG-CoA lyase activity is demonstrable in leukocytes[414] cultured skin fibroblasts,[415–417] and liver.[418,419] Obligate heterozygotes have been found to have reduced levels of HMG-CoA lyase activity.[414,417]

Prenatal diagnosis has been made by finding the abnormal organic acid pattern in AF at 16 weeks of gestation[415] and by enzyme determination in cultured AFCs and in chorionic villous tissue.[420,421] Prenatal molecular diagnosis has also been made.[422]

3-Hydroxyisobutyric Aciduria

Less than a dozen patients with 3-hydroxyisobutyric aciduria have been reported. The patients presented with facial dysmorphisms, vomiting, recurrent acidosis, and hypotonia. One patient had acute encephalopathy at 4 months and severe brain damage.[423] One patient had a mild clinical course.[424] The metabolic defect in this disorder is in the oxidation of valine and based on the complex urine organic acid patterns, a defect in the further metabolism of methylmalonyl semialdehyde is likely.[424,425] For prenatal diagnosis, measurement of AF 3-hydroxyisobutyrate is potentially possible. A mild increase of this organic acid was found in the AF of affected twins.[426]

Glutaric Acidemia Type I

The major clinical manifestations in glutaric acidemia type I are perinatal macrocephaly, progressive movement disorder consisting of choreoathetosis and dystonia, and recurrent metabolic encephalopathy.[427–432] Neuroimaging findings include prominent Sylvian fissure, frontotemporal atrophy, and subdural effusion.[433–435] Glutaric aciduria has also been found in asymptomatic family members.[429] A case of adult onset glutaric aciduria type I presented with a leukoencephalopathy.[436]

The enzyme defect is a deficiency of glutaryl-CoA dehydrogenase activity, causing the accumulation of glutaric acid and 3-hydroxyglutaric acid in body fluids. Assay of glutaryl-CoA dehydrogenase activity in leukocytes,[437–439] cultured fibroblasts,[437,440] or liver[441] confirms the diagnosis. This is an autosomal recessive disorder, and heterozygotes have intermediate levels of glutaryl-CoA dehydrogenase activity. The gene encoding this enzyme is on chromosome 19p12.2, and over eighty mutations have been identified.[442–446] The R402W mutation is common in European patients.[447] Glutaric acidemia type I in the Old Order Amish of Lancaster County, Pennsylvania, is due to a single mutation, A421V.[448] A G-to-T transversion at the donor splice site of intron 1 is associated with the Island Lake variant of glutaric acidemia type I.[449] The carrier frequency of glutaric aciduria type I in this population based on 3 years of newborn screening results is very high at 1 in 17.[450]

Prenatal diagnosis has been made by finding increased glutaric acid in AF and deficient glutaryl-CoA dehydrogenase activity in cultured AFCs.[451] This disorder was excluded in six at-risk pregnancies by measurement of glutaryl-CoA dehydrogenase activity in CV.[452,453] Prenatal diagnosis can be accomplished by AF acylcarnitine profiling[8] and DNA analysis.[454,455] Abnormal prenatal sonographic findings have also been described.[455]

Acyl-CoA Dehydrogenase Deficiencies

The process of fatty acid transport and mitochondrial oxidation involves multiple enzymes and is an important source of energy during fasting or insufficient gluconeogenesis.

Four types of mitochondrial acyl-CoA dehydrogenase deficiencies have been described: short-chain (SCAD), medium-chain (MCAD), very-long-chain (VLCAD), and long-chain hydroxy (LCHAD) acyl CoA dehydrogenase deficiencies. Hypoglycemia with inappropriately mild ketosis is the hallmark of this group of disorders. Patients have been misdiagnosed as having Reye syndrome and are at risk for sudden death. The accumulated metabolites may be toxic. Clinical manifestations of the long-chain fatty acid oxidation defects often include cardiomyopathy, liver dysfunction, myopathy, and in some cases, retinopathy. HELLP syndrome often develops during pregnancy in women carrying an affected fetus.[456] MCAD deficiency is one of the most common inborn errors of metabolism with a frequency of 1 in 6,500–20,000. It is known to be an important cause of "sudden infant death." The principle of treatment is a low-fat diet and avoidance of long fasting, with symptomatic treatment during metabolic crisis.

The diagnosis of fatty acid oxidation defects can be suspected by their characteristic plasma acylcarnitine profile and confirmed by enzyme measurement or by molecular analysis. Prenatal diagnosis of MCAD deficiency has been made by enzyme assay in cultured amniocytes[457–459] and by mutation analysis.[460] In MCAD deficiency, a missense mutation, 985A → G is highly prevalent in patients of Northwestern European background.[461] Molecular analysis in these families is recommended for both carrier identification and prenatal diagnosis. Preimplantation genetic diagnosis for MCAD deficiency has been reported.[462]

Prenatal diagnosis of LCHAD has been made by enzyme assay in cultured CVS cells[463] and cultured AFCs.[464] Prenatal diagnosis of VLCAD has been performed in seven pregnancies in six families by measuring enzyme activity in either cultured trophoblasts and amniocytes or in noncultured trophoblasts with correct identification of four affected fetuses.[465] Successful prenatal diagnosis of eight pregnancies at risk for LCHAD deficiency using molecular techniques has been reported.[466] Incubation of amniocytes with stable isotopically labeled palmitate and quantification of labeled acylcarnitine using tandem mass spectrometry has been used successfully for prenatal diagnosis of MCAD and VLCAD.[467] AF acylcarnitines were not diagnostic in one case of VLCAD deficiency.[467]

Nearly twenty disorders in fatty acid oxidation have been described. Prenatal diagnosis of most of these disorders, including those discussed above, can be performed by the analysis of metabolites (acylcarnitine, acylglycine) in AF, measurement of enzyme activity or enzyme protein, and DNA analysis in CV or cultured AFCs.[468]

Glutaric Aciduria Type II (Multiple Acyl-CoA Dehydrogenase Disorder, Ethylmalonic–Adipic Aciduria)

The clinical and biochemical findings in glutaric aciduria type II clearly indicate heterogeneity in these patients. Clinical disease can present as early as the first day of life,[469,470] and severe hypoglycemia and metabolic acidosis often lead to death within the first week. A number of these infants were born with facial dysmorphism, macrocephaly, polycystic kidneys, and congenital heart disease.[471] Some patients with milder forms of the disease have had an onset of symptoms later in infancy,[472,473] in childhood,[474–476] or in adulthood.[477–480]

Glutaric aciduria type II is an autosomal recessive disorder of the respiratory chain affecting the functions of multiple enzymes in fatty acid β-oxidation (acyl-CoA dehydrogenases), and in the metabolism of branched-chain amino acids, lysine and tryptophan, and sometimes sarcosine. The underlying defect in the majority of cases is either a deficiency of the α- or β-subunits of electron transfer flavoprotein (ETF) or a deficiency of ETF:ubiquinone oxidoreductase (ETF-QO). In rare patients the defect is suspected to be in the metabolism of the riboflavin cofactor of these flavin-containing enzymes.[481]

Prenatal diagnosis has been made by the detection of increased glutarate in AF and/or enzyme assay in cultured AFCs.[482–487] Measurement of AF glutaric acid alone may not be reliable.[488] Immunoblot analysis has been used to identify a fetus with a deficiency of the ETF β-subunit.[489] Prenatal diagnosis by acylcarnitine profile in AF using glutarylcarnitine, isovalerylcarnitine, hexanoylcarnitine, and propionylcarnitine may be useful.[8,488] The abnormal acylcarnitines may be present in maternal urine, but this is not reliable for prenatal diagnosis.[488,490] The structure of the ETF:QO gene on chromosome 4q33 has recently been described and twenty-one different disease-causing mutations identified.[491] Detection of known mutations in certain families is applicable to prenatal diagnosis. Ultrasonographic studies to detect fetal renal anomalies in association with glutaric aciduria type II can support the diagnosis of an affected fetus.[492,493]

4-Hydroxybutyric Aciduria

4-Hydroxybutyric aciduria is a rare disorder of γ-aminobutyric acid (GABA) metabolism with severe neurologic impairment, including mild psychomotor retardation, mild to marked hypotonia, and movement disorder.[494–500]

The enzyme defect is a deficiency of succinic semialdehyde dehydrogenase activity, which can be shown in lymphocytes and cultured lymphoblasts.[501,502] Prenatal diagnosis can best be done by analysis of the abnormal metabolite in AF and measurement of succinic semialdehyde dehydrogenase activity in cultured AFCs or CVS cells.[503,504]

Mevalonic Aciduria

Mevalonic aciduria caused by mevalonate kinase deficiency is a rare disorder of cholesterol biosynthesis.[505] Its clinical features range from mild to severe failure to thrive, recurrent diarrhea, anemia, hepatosplenomegaly, cataracts, dysmorphic features, and developmental delay.[506] A more moderate mevalonic aciduria has also been described in patients with hyperimmunoglobulinemia D and periodic fever syndrome (HIDS) that is apparent during acute crisis. These patients have no neurologic abnormalities and a partial mevalonate kinase deficiency.[507,508] The gene encoding mevalonate kinase is located on chromosome 12 q24. Ten mutations have been identified in patients with severe mevalonic aciduria, and additional mutations have been described in HIDS patients.[509]

Prenatal diagnosis of severe mevalonic aciduria has been accomplished by finding markedly increased levels of mevalonic acid in maternal urine and in AF in the seventeenth week of gestation.[505,510–512] A normal mevalonic acid level by stable isotope dilution assay in the AF at the tenth week of gestation and adequate enzyme activity in CV correctly predicted an unaffected fetus.[512] Molecular prenatal diagnosis is possible with known mutations.

Fumarase Deficiency

Fumarase deficiency is a rare autosomal recessive metabolic disorder of the citric acid cycle. Clinical features include congenital brain malformation, cerebral atrophy, psychomotor retardation, and hypotonia.[513–524]

The enzyme defect is expressed in skin fibroblasts, lymphoblasts, liver, muscle, and brain. Parents have intermediate levels of activity. Because fumaric acid is present in urine in normal neonates and is increased in association with other pathophysiologic conditions, enzyme confirmation of fumarase deficiency is essential. Recent DNA analysis has revealed a number of mutations in fumarase deficiency.[522,525–527]

Prenatal DNA testing performed in two at-risk pregnancies in one family with known mutation correctly identified both affected and unaffected fetuses.[528] Using stable-isotope dilution GC-MS, increased fumaric acid has also been detected in the AF of two affected pregnancies.[529] Measurement of fumarase activity in cultured AFCs or CV has excluded fumarase deficiency in several families.[528,530] Because some patients have considerable residual fumarase activity, molecular and/or metabolite analysis is preferred for prenatal diagnosis.

L-2-hydroxyglutaric Aciduria

Since first reported by Duran et al. in 1980,[531] more than twenty cases of L-2-hydroxyglutaric aciduria have been described. All patients had similar neurologic findings.[532–538] Patients were normal in the first year and gradually showed developmental delay. Seizures and cerebellar dysfunctions such as abnormal gait and dysarthria were common findings. Neuroimaging studies showed loss of subcortical white matter and cerebellar atrophy. Large amounts of L-2-hydroxyglutaric acid in cerebrospinal fluid (CSF), plasma, and urine, and a mild increase of lysine in CSF and plasma were found in all patients. This disorder appears to be transmitted as an autosomal recessive trait and has been observed in different ethnic groups. The enzyme defect has not been identified. Prenatal diagnosis is possible by finding the abnormal metabolite in AF, and a positive prenatal diagnosis has been reported.[539,540]

D-2-Hydroxyglutaric Aciduria

D-2-Hydroxyglutaric aciduria is a rare organic acid disorder.[541] The clinical features in these patients ranged from mild symptoms to severe illness, with infantile onset of encephalopathy, seizures, and hypotonia.[542] The level of D-2-hydroxyglutaric acid was increased in CSF, blood, and urine. The underlying defect remains elusive, but prenatal testing by metabolite measurement has successfully identified an affected fetus and two unaffected fetuses[543] (Shih VE, Jakobs C, unpublished data).

Combined D-2- and L-2-Hydroxyglutaric Aciduria

A recent report described three patients with combined D-2- and L-2-hydroxyglutaric aciduria with neonatal onset of metabolic encephalopathy. Prenatal diagnosis was not successful.[544]

N-Acetylaspartic Aciduria (Canavan Disease)

Canavan disease is a neurodegenerative disease clinically characterized by developmental delay, hypotonia, and progressive macrocephaly.[545] This autosomal recessive metabolic disease is due to aspartoacylase deficiency, which results in excessive amounts of *N*-acetylaspartate in the blood, CSF, and urine of patients.[546–549] The enzyme defect can be demonstrated in the brain and in skin fibroblasts.[547,550] The cDNA for human aspartoacylase has been cloned.[551] This disorder is prevalent among Ashkenazi Jews, and two missense mutations (854A → C, 693C → A) account for the molecular defect in approximately 98 percent of such patients.[552–555]

For prenatal diagnosis, DNA analysis, where applicable[556,557] (Shih VE, unpublished data), is the test of choice. *N*-acetylaspartate can be measured in AF by stable isotope dilution technique.[558–560] Normal AF *N*-acetylaspartate values increase with gestational age[559]; thus, comparison with age-matched control ranges is important. One false-negative result by metabolite analysis has been reported.[560] Mildly increased *N*-acetylaspartate in AF was found at 16 and 20 weeks of gestation in a heterozygous fetus.[561] There has been a report of increased *N*-acetylaspartate in maternal urine in a woman carrying an affected fetus after 4 months of gestation.[562] Testing by enzyme assay in cultured cells has been unreliable and given erratic results.[563–565]

MISCELLANEOUS DISORDERS

Prolidase Deficiency

Prolidase deficiency is an autosomal recessive disorder with variable clinical features. The major clinical manifestations are facial dysmorphism, hepatomegaly, failure to thrive, skin lesions) including multiple progressive ulcers of the lower extremities), telangiectasis, and erythematous rashes.[566–568] Mental retardation was present in about half of the reported cases.[566] About one-fourth of patients were asymptomatic.[567] A deficiency of prolidase activity is evident in blood cells, cultured skin fibroblasts, and skin.[566, 569–571] The gene for human prolidase has been cloned and characterized, and several molecular defects have been demonstrated in prolidase deficiency.[572–577] Prenatal diagnosis of an affected fetus has been reported in one family by finding low prolidase activity in AFCs.[568]

Disorders of Proline Metabolism

There are two types of hyperprolinemia. Type I, characterized by a moderate degree of hyperprolinemia, is now considered a benign biochemical disorder.[578] The hyperprolinemia in type II is of a more marked degree, and in addition there is an accumulation of Δ-pyrroline-5-carboxylate. The clinical consequences of this disorder are variable. Approximately one-half of the reported patients with type II were normal. The rest had mental retardation and seizures or abnormal electroencephalograms.[579]

A block in either of the first two steps of the proline metabolic pathways causes hyperprolinemia. The enzyme defect in type I is proline oxidase deficiency, which has been demonstrated only in liver.[580] In type II, deficient Δ-pyrroline-5-carboxylate dehydrogenase activity has been shown in cultured skin fibroblasts.[581] Therefore, prenatal diagnosis of type II is potentially possible.

Histidinemia

Histidinemia caused by histidase deficiency is one of the more common amino acid metabolic disorders, with a frequency of approximately 1 per 20,000 newborns.[582] Information derived from following children with histidinemia detected by routine newborn screening has shown that this biochemical disorder is not associated with clinical manifestations.[582,583] Histidase activity is not expressed in cultured skin fibroblasts.[584] The gene for histidase has been identified, and several gene mutations have been described in histidinemic patients.[585,586] There appears to be no indication for prenatal diagnosis of this benign metabolic disorder.

Disorders of Renal Amino Acid Transport

There are four known renal amino acid transport disorders: cystinuria, affecting the transport of cystine and dibasic amino acids; Hartnup disorder, affecting the transport of neutral amino acids; familial iminoglycinuria, affecting the transport of glycine, proline, and hydroxyproline; and dicarboxylic aminoaciduria, affecting the transport of glutamic acid and aspartic acid. These patients excrete large amounts of the amino acid(s) involved.

Cystinuria is the only renal amino acid transport disorder that is associated with a clinical disease, namely urinary stones. The renal and intestinal transport of cystine and the dibasic amino acids (lysine, ornithine, and arginine) are affected. Molecular studies have identified a transporter gene (SLC3A1) of cystine and the dibasic amino acids, and a number of mutations and polymorphisms have been described in patients with cystinuria.[587–589] Recently, mutations in an additional gene, SLC7A9, have been identified in cystinuria.[590–592] Mutations in SLC3A1 and SLC7A9 have been found in all patients with cystinuria studied so far.[591,592] The new classification of cystinuria based on the genotypes is type A, two SLC3A1 mutations; type B, two SLC7A9 mutations; and type AB, a rare occurrence of one mutation in each of these two genes. No attempts at prenatal diagnosis for cystinuria have been reported.

ACKNOWLEDGMENTS

Supported in part by The Mary L. Efron Fund.

REFERENCES

1. Blau N, Duran M, Blaskovics NE, et al., eds. Physician's guide to the laboratory diagnosis of metabolic diseases, 2nd ed. Berlin: Springer, 2003.
2. Fernandes J, Saudubray J-M, van den Berghe G, eds. Inborn metabolic diseases, 3rd ed. Berlin Heidelberg New York: Springer-Verlag, 2000.
3. Scriver CR, Beaudet AL, Sly WS, et al., eds. The metabolic and molecular bases of inherited disease, 8th ed. New York: McGraw-Hill, 2001.
4. Thomas GH, Parmley TH, Stevenson RE, et al. Developmental changes in amino acid concentrations in human amniotic fluid: abnormal findings in maternal phenylketonuria. Am J Obstet Gynecol 1971;111:38.
5. Ng KJ, Andersen BD, Bianchine JR. Capillary gas chromatographic-mass spectrometric profiles of trimethylsilyl derivatives of organic acids from amniotic fluids of different gestational age. J Chromatogr 1982;228:43.
6. Sweetman L. Prenatal diagnosis of the organic acidurias. J Inherit Metab Dis 1984;7 (suppl 1):18.
7. Millington DS, Norwood DL, Kodo N, et al. Application of fast atom bombardment with tandem mass spectrometry and liquid chromatography/mass spectrometry to the analysis of acylcarnitines in human urine, blood, and tissue. Anal Biochem 1989;180:331.
8. Shigematsu Y, Hata I, Nakai A, et al. Prenatal diagnosis of organic acidemias based on amniotic fluid levels of acylcarnitines. Pediatr Res 1996;39:680.
9. Largillere C, Houssin D, Gottrand F, et al. Liver transplantation for ornithine transcarbamylase deficiency in a girl. J Pediatr 1989;115:415.
10. Todo S, Starzl T, Tzakis A, et al. Orthotopic liver transplantation for urea cycle enzyme deficiency. Hepatology 1992;15:419.
11. Whitington PF, Alonso EM, Boyle JT, et al. Liver transplantation for the treatment of urea cycle disorders. J Inherit Metab Dis 1998;21 Suppl 1:112.
12. Saudubray JM, Touati G, Delonlay P, et al. Liver transplantation in urea cycle disorders. Eur J Pediatr 1999;158 (suppl 2):S55.
13. Bachmann C, Krahenbuhl S, Colombo JP, et al. N-acetylglutamate synthetase deficiency: a disorder of ammonia detoxification. N Engl J Med 1981;304:543.
14. Bachmann C, Columbo JP, Jaggi K. N-acetylglutamate synthetase (NAGS) deficiency: diagnosis, clinical observations and treatment. In: Lowenthal A, Mori A, Marescau B, eds. Urea cycle diseases. New York: Plenum Press, 1982:39.
15. Bachmann C, Brandis M, Weissenbarth-Riedel E, et al. N-acetylglutamate synthetase deficiency, a second case. J Inherit Metab Dis 1988;11:191.
16. Vockley J, Vockley CM, Lin SP, et al. Normal N-acetylglutamate concentration measured in liver from a new patient with N-acetylglutamate synthetase deficiency: physiologic and biochemical implications. Biochem Med Metab Biol 1992;47:38.
17. Guffon N, Vianey-Saban C, Bourgeois J, et al. A new neonatal case of N-acetylglutamate synthase deficiency treated by carbamylglutamate. J Inherit Metab Dis 1995;18:61.
18. Elpeleg O, Shaag A, Ben-Shalom E, et al. N-acetylglutamate synthase deficiency and the treatment of hyperammonemic encephalopathy. Ann Neurol 2002;52:845.
19. Caldovic L, Morizono H, Gracia Panglao M, et al. Cloning and expression of the human N-acetylglutamate synthase gene. Biochem Biophys Res Commun 2002;299:581.

20. Caldovic L, Morizono H, Panglao MG, et al. Null mutations in the *N*-acetylglutamate synthase gene associated with acute neonatal disease and hyperammonemia. Hum Genet 2003;112:364.

21. Haberle J, Schmidt E, Pauli S, et al. Mutation analysis in patients with *N*-acetylglutamate synthase deficiency. Hum Mutat 2003;21:593.

22. Brusilow SW, Horwich AL. Urea Cycle Enzymes. In: Scriver CR, Beaudet AL, Sly WS, Valle D, eds. The metabolic and molecular bases of inherited disease, 7th ed. New York: McGraw-Hill, 1995:1187.

23. Leonard JV. Urea cycle disorders. In: Fernandes J, Saudubray JM, van den Berghe G, eds. Inborn metabolic diseases, 2nd ed. Berlin: Springer-Verlag, 1995:167.

24. Batshaw M, Brusilow S, Walser M. Treatment of carbamyl phosphate synthetase deficiency with keto analogues of essential amino acids. N Engl J Med 1975;292:1085.

25. Call G, Seay AR, Sherry R, et al. Clinical features of carbamyl phosphate synthetase I deficiency in an adult. Ann Neurol 1984;16:90.

26. Horiuchi M, Imamura Y, Nakamura N, et al. Carbamoylphosphate synthetase deficiency in an adult: deterioration due to administration of valproic acid. J Inherit Metab Dis 1993;16:39.

27. Lo WD, Sloan HR, Stots JF, et al. Late clinical presentation of partial carbamyl phosphate synthetase I deficiency. Am J Dis Child 1993;147:267.

28. Jones ME. Regulation of pyrimidine and arginine biosynthesis in mammals. Adv Enzyme Regul 1971;9:19.

29. Haberle J, Schmidt E, Pauli S, et al. Gene structure of human carbamylphosphate synthetase 1 and novel mutations in patients with neonatal onset. Hum Mutat 2003;21:444.

30. Summar ML. Molecular genetic research into carbamoyl-phosphate synthase I: molecular defects and linkage markers. J Inherit Metab Dis 1998;21 (suppl 1):30.

31. Finckh U, Kohlschutter A, Schafer H, et al. Prenatal diagnosis of carbamoyl phosphate synthetase I deficiency by identification of a missense mutation in CPS1. Hum Mutat 1998;12:206.

32. Aoshima T, Kajita M, Sekido Y, et al. Carbamoyl phosphate synthetase I deficiency: molecular genetic findings and prenatal diagnosis. Prenat Diagn 2001;21:634.

33. Brusilow SW, Horwich AL. Urea cycle enzymes. In: Scriver CR, Beaudet AL, Sly WS, Valle D, eds. The metabolic and molecular bases of inherited disease, 8th ed. New York: McGraw-Hill, 2001:1909.

34. Leonard JV. Disorders of the urea cycle. In: Fernandes J, Saudubray JM, van den Berghe G, eds. Inborn metabolic diseases, 3rd ed. Berlin: Springer-Verlag, 2000:213.

35. Finkelstein JE, Hauser ER, Leonard CO, et al. Late onset transcarbamylase deficiency in male patients. J Pediatr 1990;117:897.

36. Komaki S, Matsuura T, Oyanagi K, et al. Familial lethal inheritance of a mutated paternal gene in females causing X-linked ornithine transcarbamylase (OTC) deficiency. Am J Med Genet 1997;69:177.

37. Dimagno EP, Lowe JE, Snodgrass PJ, et al. Ornithine transcarbamylase deficiency: a cause of bizarre behavior in a man. N Engl J Med 1986;315:744.

38. Shih VE, Safran AP, Ropper AH, et al. Ornithine carbamoyltransferase deficiency: unusual clinical findings and novel mutation. J Inherit Metab Dis 1999;22:672.

39. Campbell AGM, Rosenberg LE, Snodgrass PJ, et al. Ornithine transcarbamylase deficiency: a cause of lethal neonatal hyperammonemia in males. N Engl J Med 1973;228:1.

40. Short EM, Conn HO, Snodgrass PJ, et al. Evidence for X-linked dominant inheritance of ornithine transcarbamylase deficiency. N Engl J Med 1973;288:7.

41. Hauser ER, Finkelstein JE, Valle D, et al. Allopurinol-induced orotidinuria: a test for mutations at the ornithine carbamoyltransferase locus in women. N Engl J Med 1990;322:1641.

42. Pelet A, Rotig A, Bonaiti-Pellie C, et al. Carrier detection in a partially dominant X-linked disease: ornithine transcarbamylase deficiency. Hum Genet 1990;84:167.

43. Tuchman M, Jaleel N, Morizono H, et al. Mutations and polymorphisms in the human ornithine transcarbamylase gene. Hum Mutat 2002;19:93.

44. Jakobs C, Sweetman L, Nyhan WL, et al. Stable isotope dilution analysis of orotic acid and uracil in amniotic fluid. Clin Chim Acta 1984;143:123.

45. Matsuura T, Hoshide R, Fukushima M, et al. Prenatal monitoring of ornithine transcarbamoylase deficiency in two families by DNA analysis. Inherit Metab Dis 1993;16:31.

46. Hoshide R, Matsuura T, Sagara Y, et al. Prenatal monitoring in a family at high risk for ornithine transcarbamylase (OTC) deficiency: a new mutation of an A-to-C transversion in position +4 of intron 1 of the OTC gene that is likely to abolish enzyme activity. Am J Med Genet 1996;64:459.

47. Plante RJ, Tuchman M. Polymorphisms in the human ornithine transcarbamylase gene useful for allele tracking. Mutations in brief no. 193. Online. Hum Mutat 1998;12:289.

48. Watanabe A, Sekizawa A, Taguchi A, et al. Prenatal diagnosis of ornithine transcarbamylase deficiency by using a single nucleated erythrocyte from maternal blood. Hum Genet 1998;102:611.

49. Yoo HW, Kim GH. Prenatal molecular evaluation of six fetuses in four unrelated Korean families with or-nithine transcarbamylase deficiency. J Korean Med Sci 1998;13:179.

50. Topaloglu AK, Sansaricq C, Fox JE, et al. Prenatal molecular diagnosis of severe ornithine carbamoyl-transferase deficiency due to a novel mutation, E181G. J Inherit Metab Dis 1999;22:82.

51. Climent C, Rubio V. H intragenic polymorphisms and haplotype analysis in the ornithine transcarbamy-lase (OTC) gene and their relevance for tracking the inheritance of OTC deficiency. Hum Mutat 2002;20:407.

52. Ray PF, Gigarel N, Bonnefont JP, et al. First specific preimplantation genetic diagnosis for ornithine tran-scarbamylase deficiency. Prenat Diagn 2000;20:1048.

53. Verlinsky Y, Rechitsky S, Verlinsky O, et al. Preimplantation diagnosis for ornithine transcarbamylase de-ficiency. Reprod Biomed Online 2000;1:45.

54. McMurray WC, Mohyruddin F, Bayer SM, et al. Citrullinuria: a disorder of amino acid metabolism asso-ciated with mental retardation. International Copenhagen Congress on the Scientific Study of Mental Re-tardation 1964. Denmark, August 7–14.

55. Tedesco TA, Mellman WJ. Argininosuccinate synthetase activity and citrulline metabolism in cells cul-tured from a citrullinemic subject. Proc Natl Acad Sci USA 1967;57:169.

56. Spector EB, Bloom AD. Citrullinemic lymphocytes in long term culture. Pediatr Res 1973;7:700.

57. Kennaway NG, Harwood PJ, Ramberg DA, et al. Citrullinemia: enzymatic evidence for genetic hetero-geneity. Pediatr Res 1975;9:554.

58. Saheki T, Ueda A, Hosoya M, et al. Qualitative and quantitative abnormalities of argininosuccinate syn-thetase in citrullinemia. Clin Chim Acta 1981;109:325.

59. Su T-S, Beaudet AL, O'Brien WE. Abnormal mRNA for argininosuccinate synthetase in citrullinaemia. Nature 1983;301:533.

60. Sase M, Kobayashi K, Imamura Y, et al. Level of translatable messenger RNA coding for argininosucci-nate synthetase in the liver of the patients with quantitative-type citrullinemia. Hum Genet 1985;69:130.

61. Kobayashi K, Rosenbloom C, Beaudet AL, et al. Additional mutations in argininosuccinate synthetase caus-ing citrullinemia. Mol Biol Med 1991;8:95.

62. Kobayashi K, Kakinoki H, Fukushige T, et al. Nature and frequency of mutations in the argininosuccinate synthetase gene that cause classical citrullinemia. Hum Genet 1995;96:454.

63. Haberle J, Pauli S, Linnebank M, et al. Structure of the human argininosuccinate synthetase gene and an improved system for molecular diagnostics in patients with classical and mild citrullinemia. Hum Genet 2002;110:327.

64. Fleisher LD, Harris CJ, Mitchell DA, et al. Citrullinemia: prenatal diagnosis of an affected fetus. Am J Hum Genet 1983;35:85.

65. Kamoun P, Parvy P, Dinh DP, et al. Citrulline in amniotic fluid and the prenatal diagnosis of citrullinemia. Prenat Diagn 1983;3:53.

66. Kleijer WJ, Blom W, Huijmans JG, et al. Prenatal diagnosis of citrullinemia: elevated levels of citrulline in the amniotic fluid in the three affected pregnancies. Prenat Diagn 1984;4:113.

67. Christensen E, Brandt NJ, Philip J, et al. Exclusion of citrullinaemia in the first trimester of pregnancy by direct assay of argininosuccinate synthetase in chorionic villi. Prenat Diagn 1985;5:299.

68. Northrup H, Beaudet AL, O'Brien WE. Prenatal diagnosis of citrullinaemia: review of a 10-year experi-ence including recent use of DNA analysis. Prenat Diagn 1990;10:771.

69. Kamoun P, Chadefaux B. Eleventh week amniocentesis for prenatal diagnosis of some metabolic diseases. Prenatal Diagn 1991;11:691.

70. Jacoby LB, Shih VE, Struckmeyer C, et al. Variation in argininosuccinate synthetase activity in amniotic fluid cell cultures: implications for prenatal diagnosis of citrullinemia. Clin Chim Acta 1981;116:1.

71. Cathelineau L, Pham Dinh D, Boue J, et al. Improved method for the antenatal diagnosis of citrullinemia. Clin Chim Acta 1981;116:111.

72. Chadefaux-Vekemans B, Rabier D, Chabli A, et al. Improving the prenatal diagnosis of citrullinemia using citrulline/ornithine+arginine ratio in amniotic fluid. Prenat Diagn 2002;22:456.

73. Mandell R, Packman S, Laframboise R, et al. Use of amniotic fluid amino acids in prenatal testing for argininosuccinic aciduria and citrullinemia. Prenatal Diagnosis 1996;16:419.

74. Kakinoki H, Kobayashi K, Terazono H, et al. Mutations and DNA diagnoses of classical citrullinemia. Hum Mutat 1997;9:250.

75. Hong KM, Paik MK, Yoo OJ, et al. The first successful prenatal diagnosis on a Korean family with cit-rullinemia. Mol Cells 2000;10:692.

76. Kobayashi K, Shaheen N, Kumashiro R, et al. A search for the primary abnormality in adult-onset type II citrullinemia. Am J Hum Genet 1993;53:1024.

77. Kobayashi K, Sinasac DS, Iijima M, et al. The gene mutated in adult-onset type II citrullinaemia encodes a putative mitochondrial carrier protein. Nature Genet 1999;22:159.

78. Yasuda T, Yamaguchi N, Kobayashi K, et al. Identification of two novel mutations in the SLC25A13 gene and detection of seven mutations in 102 patients with adult-onset type II citrullinemia. Hum Genet 2000;107:537.

79. Ohura T, Tazawa Y, Kobayashi K, et al. Neonatal intrahepatic cholestasis caused by citrin deficiency: clinical features of 14 patients. Am J Hum Genet 2001;69:217.

80. Ohura T, Kobayashi K, Tazawa Y, et al. Neonatal presentation of adult-onset type II citrullinemia. Hum Genet 2001;108:87.

81. Tomomasa T, Kobayashi K, Kaneko H, et al. Possible clinical and histologic manifestations of adult-onset type II citrullinemia in early infancy. J Pediatr 2001;138:741.

82. Tazawa Y, Kobayashi K, Ohura T, et al. Infantile cholestatic jaundice associated with adult-onset type II citrullinemia. J Pediatr 2001;138:735.

83. Farrell G, Rauschkolb EW, Moure J, et al. Argininosuccinic aciduria. Tex Med 1969;65:90.

84. Kvedar JC, Baden HP, Baden LA, et al. Dietary management reverses grooving and abnormal polarization of hair shafts in argininosuccinase deficiency. Am J Med Genet 1991;40:211.

85. Solitaire GB, Shih VE, Nelligan DJ, et al. Argininosuccinic aciduria: clinical, biochemical, anatomical and neuropathological observations. J Ment Defic Res 1969;13:153.

86. Mori T, Nagai K, Mori M, et al. Progressive liver fibrosis in late-onset argininosuccinate lyase deficiency. Pediatr Dev Pathol 2002;5:597.

87. Widhalm K, Koch S, Scheibenreiter S, et al. Long-term follow-up of 12 patients with the late-onset variant of argininosuccinic acid lyase deficiency: no impairment of intellectual and psychomotor development during therapy. Pediatrics 1992;89:1182.

88. Ficicioglu CH, Mandell R, Shih VE. Argininosuccinate lyase deficiency: long-term outcome of 12 patients detected by newborn screening. Pediatr Res 2000;47 (suppl):240A.

89. Kleijer WJ, Garritsen VH, Linnebank M, et al. Clinical, enzymatic, and molecular genetic characterization of a biochemical variant type of argininosuccinic aciduria: prenatal and postnatal diagnosis in five unrelated families. J Inherit Metab Dis 2002;25:399.

90. Tomlinson S, Westall RG. Argininosuccinic aciduria, argininosuccinase and arginase in human blood cells. Clin Sci 1964;26:261.

91. Shih VE, Littlefield JW, Moser HW. Argininosuccinase deficiency in fibroblasts cultured from patients with argininosuccinic aciduria. Biochem Genet 1969;3:81.

92. Coryell ME, Hall WK, Theraos TG, et al. A familial study of a human enzyme defect, argininosuccinic aciduria. Biochem Biophys Res Commun 1964;14:307.

93. Goodman SI, Mace JW, Turner B, et al. Antenatal diagnosis of argininosuccinic aciduria. Clin Genet 1973;4:236.

94. Fleisher LD, Rassin DK, Desnick RJ, et al. Argininosuccinic aciduria: prenatal studies in a family at risk. Am J Hum Genet 1979;31:439.

95. Vimal CM, Fensom AH, Heaton D, et al. Prenatal diagnosis of argininosuccinic aciduria by analysis of cultured chorionic villi. Lancet 1984;1:521.

96. Fensom AH, Benson PF, Baker JE, et al. Prenatal diagnosis of argininosuccinic aciduria: effect of mycoplasma contamination on the indirect assay for argininosuccinate lyase. Am J Hum Genet 1980;32:761.

97. Chadefaux B, Rabier D, Kamoun P. Pitfalls in the prenatal diagnosis of argininosuccinuria. Am J Med Genet 1988;30:999.

98. Donn SM, Thoene JG. Prospective prevention of neonatal hyperammonaemia in argininosuccinic aciduria by arginine therapy. J Inherit Metab Dis 1985;8:18.

99. Chadefaux B, Ceballos I, Rabier D, et al. Prenatal diagnosis of argininosuccinic aciduria by assay of argininosuccinate in amniotic fluid at the 12th week of gestation. Am J Med Genet 1990;35:594.

100. Ward JC, Meyers CM, Shih VE, et al. Successful pregnancy in a woman with argininosuccinic aciduria (ASU): biochemical investigations and outcome. Am J Hum Genet 1990;47:A82.

101. Hartlage PL, Coryell ME, Hall WK, et al. Argininosuccinic aciduria: perinatal diagnosis and early dietary management. J Pediatr 1974;85:86.

102. Terheggen HG, Schwenk A, Lowenthal A, et al. Argininaemia with arginase deficiency. Lancet 1969;2:748.

103. Cederbaum SD, Shaw KNF, Spector EB, et al. Hyperargininemia with arginase deficiency. Pediatr Res 1979;13:827.

104. Picker JD, Puga AC, Levy HL, et al. Arginase deficiency with lethal neonatal expression: evidence for the glutamine hypothesis of cerebral edema. J Pediatr 2003;142:349.

105. Cederbaum SD, Shaw KNF, Valente M. Hyperargininemia. J Pediatr 1977;90:569.
106. Snyderman SE, Sansaricq C, Chen WJ, et al. Argininemia. J Pediatr 1977;90:563.
107. Naylor EW, Orfanos AP, Guthrie R. A simple screening test for arginase deficiency (hyperargininemia). J Lab Clin Med 1977;89:876.
108. Grody WW, Klein D, Dodson AE, et al. Molecular genetic study of human arginase deficiency. Am J Hum Genet 1992;50:1281.
109. Iyer R, Jenkinson CP, Vockley JG, et al. The human arginases and arginase deficiency. J Inherit Metab Dis 1998;21 (suppl 1):86.
110. Colombo JP, Terheggen HG, Lowenthal A, et al. Argininaemia. In: Hommes FA, Van den Bergh CJ, eds. Inborn errors of metabolism. London: Academic Press, 1973:239.
111. Van Elsen AF, Leroy JG. Arginase isozymes in human diploid fibroblasts. Biochem Biophys Res Comm 1975;62:191.
112. Van Elsen AF, Leroy JG. Human hyperargininemia: a mutation not expressed in skin fibroblasts? Am J Hum Genet 1977;29:250.
113. Spector EB, Kiernan M, Bernard B, et al. Properties of fetal and adult red blood cell arginase: a possible prenatal diagnostic test for arginase deficiency. Am J Hum Genet 1980;32:79.
114. Caruso U, Cerone R, Schiaffino M, et al. Prenatal Diagnosis of Argininemia: experience on Two Pregnancies in the Same Family. International Pediatrics 1994;9:77.
115. Hewson S, Clarke JTR, Cederbaum S. Prenatal diagnosis for arginase deficiency: A case study. J Inherit Metab Dis, 2003;26:607.
116. Cardoso ML, Silva E, Fortuna A, et al. Argininemia: molecular prenatal diagnosis. J Inherit Metab Dis 2001;24 (suppl 1):43.
117. Shih VE. Hyperornithinemias. In: Fernandes J, Saudubray JM, van den Berghe G, eds. Inborn metabolic diseases, 2nd ed. Berlin Heidelberg New York: Springer-Verlag, 1995:183.
118. Hommes FA, Ho CK, Roesel RA, et al. Decreased transport of ornithine across the inner mitochondrial membrane as a cause of hyperornithinaemia. J Inherit Metab Dis 1982;5:41.
119. Shih VE, Mandell R, Herzfeld A. Defective ornithine metabolism in cultured skin fibroblasts from patients with the syndrome of hyperornithinemia, hyperammonemia and homocitrullinuria. Clin Chim Acta 1982;118:149.
120. Camacho J, Obie C, Biery B, et al. Hyperornithinaemia–hyperammonaemia–homocitrullinuria syndrome is caused by mutations in a gene encoding a mitochondrial ornithine transporter. Nat Genet 1999;22:151.
121. Shih VE, Ficicioglu CH. Genotype and phenotype findings in the hyperornithinemia–hyperammonemia–homocitullinuria (HHH) syndrome. J Inherit Metab Dis 2000;23 (suppl 1):72.
122. Tsujino S, Kanazawa N, Ohashi T, et al. Three novel mutations (G27E, insAAC, R179X) in the ORNT1 gene of Japanese patients with hyperornithinemia, hyperammonemia, and homocitrullinuria syndrome. Ann Neurol 2000;2000:625.
123. Salvi S, Dionisi-Vici C, Bertini E, et al. Seven novel mutations in the ORNT1 gene (SLC25A15) in patients with hyperornithinemia, hyperammonemia, and homocitrullinuria syndrome. Hum Mutat 2001; 18:460.
124. Miyamoto T, Kanazawa N, Hayakawa C, et al. A novel mutation, P126R, in a Japanese patient with HHH syndrome. Pediatr Neurol 2002;26:65.
125. Shih VE, Laframboise R, Mandell R, et al. Neonatal form of the hyperornithinemia, hyperammonemia and homocitrullinuria (HHH) syndrome and prenatal diagnosis. Prenat Diagn 1992;12:717.
126. Chadefaux B, Bonnefont JP, Shih VE, et al. Potential for the prenatal diagnosis of hyperornithinemia, hyperammonemia, and homocitrullinuria syndrome. Am J Med Genet 1989;32:264.
127. Gray RGF, Green A, Hall S, et al. Prenatal exclusion of the HHH Syndrome. Prenat Diagn 1995;15:474.
128. Valle D, Simell O. The hyperornithinemias. In: Scriver CR, Beaudet AL, Sly WS, Valle D, eds. The metabolic and molecular basis of inherited disease, 8th ed. New York: McGraw-Hill, 2001:1857.
129. Shih VE, Stockler-Ipsiroglu S. Disorders of ornithine and creatine metabolism. In: Fernandes J, Saudubray JM, van den Berghe G, eds. Inborn metabolic diseases, 3rd ed. New York: Springer-Verlag, 2000:233.
130. Simell O, Takki K. Raised plasma ornithine and gyrate atrophy of the choroid and retina. Lancet 1973;1:1030.
131. Trijbels JMF, Sengers RCA, Bakkaren JAJM, et al. L-Ornithine-ketoacidtransaminase deficiency in cultured fibroblasts of a patient with hyperornithineaemia and gyrate atrophy of the choroid and retina. Clin Chim Acta 1977;79:371.
132. Kaiser-Kupfer M, Caruso R, Valle D. Gyrate atrophy of the choroid and retina: further experience with long-term reduction of ornithine levels in children. Arch Ophthalmol 2002;120:146.

133. Sipila I, Simell O, O'Donnell JJ. Gyrate atrophy of the choroid and retina with hyperornithinemia: characterization of mutant liver-L-ornithine: 2-oxoacid aminotransferase kinetics. J Clin Invest 1981;67:1805.

134. Kennaway NG, Weleber RG, Buist NRM. Gyrate atrophy of choroid and retina: deficient activity of ornithine ketoacid aminotransferase in cultured skin fibroblasts. N Engl J Med 1977;297:1180.

135. Shih VE, Berson EL, Mandell R, et al. Ornithine ketoacid transaminase deficiency in gyrate atrophy of the choroid and retina. Am J Hum Genet 1978;30:174.

136. Valle D, Kaiser-Kupfer MK, Del Valle LA. Gyrate atrophy of the choroid and retina: deficiency of ornithine aminotransferase in transformed lymphocytes. Proc Natl Acad Sci USA 1977;74:5159.

137. Sengers RCA, Trijbels JMF, Brussart JH, et al. Gyrate atrophy of the choroid and retina and ornithine-ketoacid amino transferase deficiency. Pediatr Res 1976;10:894.

138. Shih VE, Mandell R, Berson EL. Pyridoxine effects on ornithine ketoacid transaminase activity in fibroblasts from carriers of two forms of gyrate atrophy of the choroid and retina. Am J Hum Genet 1988;43:929.

139. Ramesh V, Gusella JF, Shih VE. Molecular pathology of gyrate atrophy of the choroid and retina due to ornithine aminotransferase deficiency. Mol Biol Med 1991;8:81.

140. Mashima Y, Shiono T, Tamai M, et al. Heterogeneity and uniqueness of ornithine aminotransferase mutations found in Japanese gyrate atrophy patients. Curr Eye Res 1996;18:792.

141. Shih VE, Schulman JD. Ornithine-ketoacid transaminase activity in human skin and amniotic fluid cell culture. Clin Chim Acta 1970;27:73.

142. Roschinger W, Endres W, Shin YS. Characteristics of L-ornithine: 2-oxoacid aminotransferase and potential prenatal diagnosis of gyrate atrophy of the choroid and retina by first trimester chorionic villus sampling. Clin Chim Acta 2000;296:91.

143. Ghadimi H. The hyperlysinemias. In: Stanbury JB, Wyngaarden JB, Frederickson DS, eds. The metabolic basis of inherited disease. New York: McGraw-Hill, 1978:387.

144. Dancis J, Hutzler J, Ampola MG, et al. The prognosis of hyperlysinemia: an interim report. Am J Hum Genet 1983;35:438.

145. Sacksteder KA, Biery BJ, Morrell JC, et al. Identification of the alpha-aminoadipic semialdehyde synthase gene, which is defective in familial hyperlysinemia. Am J Hum Genet 2000;66:1736.

146. Dancis J, Hutzler J, Woody NC, et al. Multiple enzyme defects in familial hyperlysinemia. Pediatr Res 1976;10:686.

147. Dancis J, Hutzler J, Cox RP. Familial hyperlysinemia: enzyme studies, diagnostic methods, comments on terminology. Am J Hum Genet 1979;31:290.

148. Carson NAJ, Scally BG, Neill DW. Saccharopinuria: a new inborn error of lysine metabolism. Nature 1968;218:678.

149. Simell O, Visakorpi JK, Donner M. Saccharopinuria. Arch Dis Child 1972;47:52.

150. Cederbaum SD, Shaw KNF, Dancis J, et al. Hyperlysinemia with saccharopinuria due to combined lysine-ketoglutarate reductase and saccharopine dehydrogenase deficiencies presenting as cystinuria. J Pediatr 1979;95:234.

151. Fellows FCK, Carson NAJ. Enzyme studies in a patient with saccharopinuria: a defect of lysine metabolism. Pediatr Res 1974;8:42.

152. Simell O, Johansson T, Aula P. Enzyme defect in saccharopinuria. J Pediatr 1973;82:54.

153. Gray RGF, Bennett MJ, Green A, et al. Studies on a case of persistent hyperlysinaemia with a possible method for prenatal diagnosis. J Inherit Metab Dis 1983;6:115.

154. Mudd SH, Levy HL, and Kraus JP. Disorders of transsulfuration. In: Scriver CR, Beaudet AL, Sly WS, Valle D, eds. The metabolic and molecular bases of inherited disease, 8th ed. New York: McGraw-Hill, 2001:2007.

155. Mudd SH, Levy HL, Tangerman A, et al. Isolated persistent hypermethioninemia. Am J Hum Genet 1995;57.

156. Surtees R, Leonard J, Austin S. Association of demyelination with deficiency of cerebrospinal-fluid S-adenosylmethionine in inborn errors of methyl-transfer pathway. Lancet 1991;338:1550.

157. Gaull GE, Bender AN, Vulovic D, et al. Methioninemia and myopathy: a new disorder. Ann Neurol 1981;9:423.

158. Gahl WA, Bernardini I, Finkelstein JD, et al. Transsulfuration in an adult with hepatic methionine adenosyltransferase deficiency. J Clin Invest 1988;81:90.

159. Ubagai T, Lei K-J, Huang S, et al. Molecular mechanisms of an inborn error of methionine pathway: methionine adenosyltransferase deficiency. J Clin Invest 1995;96:1943.

160. Chamberlin ME, Ubagai T, Mudd SH, et al. Demyelination of the brain is associated with methionine adenosyltransferase I/III deficiency. J Clin Invest 1996.

161. Chamberlin ME, Ubagai T, Mudd SH, et al. Methionine adenosyltransferase I/III deficiency: novel mutations and clinical variations. Am J Hum Genet 2000;66:347.

162. Kim SZ, Santamaria E, Jeong TE, et al. Methionine adenosyltransferase I/III deficiency: two Korean compound heterozygous siblings with a novel mutation. J Inherit Metab Dis 2002;25:661.

163. McKusick VA. Heritable disorders of connective tissue. St. Louis: Mosby, 1972.

164. Mudd SH, Skovby F, Levy HL, et al. The natural history of homocystinuria due to cystathionine β-synthase deficiency. Am J Hum Genet 1985;37:1.

165. Mudd SH, Levy HL, Kraus JP. Disorders of transsulfuration. In: Scriver CR, Beaudet AL, Sly WS, Valle D, eds. The metabolic and molecular bases of inherited disease, 8th ed. New York: McGraw-Hill, 2001:2007.

166. Yap S, Naughten ER, Wilcken B, et al. Vascular complications of severe hyperhomocysteinemia in patients with homocystinuria due to cystathionine β-synthase deficiency: effects of homocysteine-lowering therapy. Semin Thromb Hemost 2000;26:335.

167. Yap S, Naughten E. Homocystinuria due to cystathionine beta-synthase deficiency in Ireland: 25 years' experience of a newborn screened and treated population with reference to clinical outcome and biochemical control. J Inherit Metab Dis 1998;21:738.

168. Lamon JM, Lenke RR, Levy HL, et al. Selected metabolic diseases. In: Schulman JD, Simpson JL, eds. Genetic diseases in pregnancy. New York: Academic Press, 1981:1.

169. Finkelstein JD, Mudd SH, Irreverre F, et al. Homocystinuria due to cystathionine synthetase deficiency: the mode of inheritance. Science 1964;146:785.

170. Uhlendorf BW, Mudd SH. Cystathionine synthase in tissue culture derived from human skin: enzyme defect in homocystinuria. Science 1968;160:1007.

171. Goldstein JL, Campbell BK, Gartler SM. Cystathionine synthase activity in human lymphocytes: induction by phytohemagglutinin. J Clin Invest 1972;51:1034.

172. Goldstein JL, Campbell BK, Gartler SM. Homocystinuria: heterozygote detection using phytohemagglutinin-stimulated lymphocytes. J Clin Invest 1973;52:218.

173. Uhlendorf BW, Conerly EB, Mudd SH. Homocystinuria: studies in tissue culture. Pediatr Res 1973;7:645.

174. Bittles AH, Carson NAJ. Homocystinuria: studies on cystathionine β-synthase, S-adenosylmethionine synthase, and cystathionase activities in skin fibroblasts. J Inherit Metab Dis 1981;4:3.

175. Kraus JP, Janosik M, Kozich V, et al. Cystathionine beta-synthase mutations in homocystinuria. Hum Mutat 1999;13:362.

176. Kraus JP, Kozich V, Janosik M. www.uchsc.edu/sm/cbs/cbsdata/mutations.htm.

177. Hu F, Gu Z, Kozich V, et al. Molecular basis of cystathionine β-synthase deficiency in B_6 responsive and nonresponsive homocystinuria. Hum Mol Genet 1993;2:1857.

178. Shih VE, Fringer JM, Mandell R, et al. A missense mutation (I278T) in the cystathionine β-synthase gene prevalent in pyridoxine responsive homocystinuria and associated with mild clinical phenotype. Am J Hum Genet 1995;57:34.

179. Fowler B, Borresen AL, Boman N. Prenatal diagnosis of homocystinuria. Lancet 1982;2:875.

180. Fowler B, Jakobs C. Post- and prenatal diagnostic methods for the homocystinurias. Eur J Pediatr 1998;157 (suppl 2):S88.

181. Bittles AH, Carson NAJ. Tissue culture techniques as an aid to prenatal diagnosis and genetic counselling in homocystinuria. J Med Genet 1973;10:120.

182. Fleisher LD, Longhi RC, Tallan HH, et al. Homocystinuria: investigations of cystathionine synthase in cultured fetal cells and the prenatal determination of genetic status. J Pediatr 1974;85:677.

183. Fensom AH, Benson PF, Crees MJ, et al. Prenatal exclusion of homocystinuria (cystathionine β-synthase deficiency) by assay of phytohaemagglutinin-stimulated fetal lymphocytes. Prenat Diagn 1983;3:127.

184. Harris H, Penrose LS, Thomas DHH. Cystathioninuria. Ann Hum Genet 1959;23:442.

185. Frimpter GW. Cystathioninuria: nature of the defect. Science 1965;149:1095.

186. Pascal TA, Gaull G, Beratis NG, et al. Cystathionase in long term lymphoid cell lines: evidence for altered enzyme protein in cystathioninuria. Pediatr Res 1975;9:315.

187. Pascal TA, Gaull GE, Beratis NG, et al. Cystathionase deficiency: evidence for genetic heterogeneity in primary cystathioninuria. Pediatr Res 1978;12:125.

188. Bittles AH, Carson NAJ. Cystathionase deficiency in fibroblast cultures in a patient with primary cystathioninuria. J Med Genet 1974;11:121.

189. Mudd SH. Discussion. In: Carson NAJ, Raine DN, eds. Inherited disorders of sulphur metabolism. Edinburgh: Churchill Livingstone, 1971:311.

190. Pascal TA, Gaull GE, Beratis NG, et al. Vitamin B_6-responsive and unresponsive cystathioninuria: two variant molecular forms. Science 1975;190:1209.

191. Vargas JE, Mudd SH, Waisbren SE, et al. Maternal gamma-cystathionase deficiency: absence of both teratogenic effects and pregnancy complications. Am J Obstet Gynecol 1999;181:753.

192. Wang J, Hegele RA. Genomic basis of cystathioninuria (MIM 219500) revealed by multiple mutations in cystathionine gamma-lyase (CTH). Hum Genet 2003;112:404.

193. Johnson JL, Duran M. Molybdenum cofactor deficiency and isolated sulfite oxidase deficiency. In: Scriver CR, Beaudet AL, Sly WS, Valle D, eds. The metabolic and molecular bases of inherited disease, 8th ed. New York: McGraw-Hill, 2001:3163.

194. Ogier H, Wadman SK, Johnson JL, et al. Antenatal diagnosis of combined xanthine and sulphite oxidase deficiencies. Lancet 1983;1:1363.

195. Desjacques P, Mousson B, Vianey-Liaud C, et al. Combined deficiency of xanthine oxidase and sulphite oxidase: diagnosis of a new case followed by an antenatal diagnosis. J Inherit Metab Dis 1985;8:117.

196. Bamforth FJ, Johnson JL, Davidson AGF, et al. Biochemical investigation of a child with molybdenum cofactor deficiency. Clin Biochem 1990;23:537.

197. Gray RF, Green A, Basu SN, et al. Antenatal diagnosis of molybdenum cofactor deficiency. Am J Obstet Gynecol 1990;163:1203.

198. Johnson JL, Rajagopalan KV, Lanman JT, et al. Prenatal diagnosis of molybdenum cofactor deficiency by assay of sulphite oxidase activity in chorionic villus samples. J Inherit Metab Dis 1991;14:932.

199. Reiss J, Johnson JL. Mutations in the molybdenum cofactor biosynthetic genes MOCS1, MOCS2, and GEPH. Hum Mutat 2003;21:569.

200. Reiss J, Christensen E, Dorche C. Molybdenum cofactor deficiency: first prenatal genetic analysis. Prenat Diagn 1999;19:386.

201. Shalata A, Mandel H, Dorche C, et al. Prenatal diagnosis and carrier detection for molybdenum cofactor deficiency type A in northern Israel using polymorphic DNA markers. Prenat Diagn 2000;20:7.

202. Irreverre F, Mudd SH, Heizer WE, et al. Sulfite oxidase deficiency: studies of a patient with mental retardation, dislocated lenses and abnormal urinary excretion of S-sulfo-L-cysteine, sulfite and thiosulfate. Biochem Med 1967;1:187.

203. Shih VE, Abroms IF, Johnson JL, et al. Sulfite oxidase deficiency: biochemical and clinical investigations of a hereditary metabolic disorder in sulfur metabolism. N Engl J Med 1977;297:1022.

204. Vianey-Liaud C, Desjacques P, Gaulme J, et al. A new case of isolated sulphite oxidase deficiency with rapid fatal outcome. J Inherit Metab Dis 1988;11:425.

205. Vilarinho L, Ramos Alves J, Dorche C, et al. Citrullinaemia and isolated sulphite oxidase deficiency in two siblings. J Inherit Metab Dis 1994;17:638.

206. Barbot C, Martins E, Vilarinho L, et al. A mild form of infantile isolated sulphite oxidase deficiency. Neuropediatrics 1995;26:322.

207. Mudd SH, Irreverre F, Laster L. Sulfite oxidase deficiency in man: demonstration of the enzymatic defect. Science 1967;156:1599.

208. Johnson JL, Rajagopalan KV. Human sulfite oxidase deficiency: characterization of the molecular defect in a multicomponent system. J Clin Invest 1976;58:551.

209. Garrett RM, Bellissimo DB, Rajagopalan KV. Molecular cloning of human liver sulfite oxidase. Biochim Biophys Acta 1995;1262:147.

210. Johnson JL, Garrett RM, Rajagopalan KV. The biochemistry of molybdenum cofactor deficiency and isolated sulfite oxidase deficiency. Int Pediatr 1997;12:23.

211. Johnson JL, Coyne KE, Garrett RM, et al. Isolated sulfite oxidase deficiency: identification of 12 novel SUOX mutations in 10 patients. Hum Mutat 2002;20:74.

212. Johnson JL, Rajagopalan KV, Renier WO, et al. Isolated sulfite oxidase deficiency: mutation analysis and DNA-based prenatal diagnosis. Prenat Diagn 2002;22:433.

213. Veale AMO. Screening for phenylketonuria. In: Bickel H, Guthrie R, Hammersen G, eds. Neonatal screening for inborn errors of metabolism. Berlin: Springer, 1980:7.

214. Dobson JC, Kushida E, Williamson M, et al. Intellectual performance of 36 phenylketonuria patients and their nonaffected siblings. Pediatrics 1976;58:53.

215. Waisbren SE, Schnell RR, Levy HL. Diet termination in children with phenylketonuria: a review of psychological assessments used to determine outcome. J Inherit Metab Dis 1980;3:149.

216. Seashore MR, Friedman E, Novelly RA, et al. Loss of intellectual function in children with phenylketonuria after relaxation of dietary phenylalanine restriction. Pediatrics 1985;75:226.

217. Lenke RR, Levy HL. Maternal phenylketonuria and hyperphenylalaninemia: an international survey of the outcome of untreated and treated pregnancies. N Engl J Med 1980;303:1202.

218. Bickel H. Maternal phenylketonuria, problems-experiences-recommendations. Eppingen: Pentadruck, 1980.

219. Lenke RR, Levy HL. Maternal phenylketonuria: results of dietary therapy. Am J Obstet Gynecol 1982;142:548.

220. Rohr FJ, Doherty LB, Waisbren SE, et al. New England Maternal PKU Project: prospective study of untreated and treated pregnancies and their outcomes. J Pediatr 1987;110:391.

221. Rouse B, Matalon R, Koch R, et al. Maternal phenylketonuria syndrome: congenital heart defects, microcephaly, and developmental outcomes. J Pediatr 2000;136:57.

222. Kaufman S. Phenylketonuria: biochemical mechanisms. In: Agranoff BW, Aprison MH, eds. Advances in neurochemistry. New York: Plenum Press, 1976:1.

223. Bartholome K, Ertel E. Immunological detection of phenylalanine hydroxylase in phenylketonuria. Lancet 1976;2:862.

224. Bartholome K, Ertel E. Immunological detection of phenylalanine hydroxylase in phenylketonuria. Lancet 1978;1:454.

225. Saraiva JM, Seakins JWT, Smith I. Plasma phenylalanine and tyrosine levels revisited in heterozygotes for hyperphenylalaninaemia. J Inherit Metab Dis 1993;16:105.

226. Guldberg P, Henriksen KF, Lou HC, et al. Aberrant phenylalanine metabolism in phenylketonuria heterozygotes. J Inherit Metab Dis 1998;21:365.

227. Lehmann WD, Theobald N, Heinrich HC, et al. Detection of heterozygous carriers for phenylketonuria by a L-[^{2}H$_5$]phenylalanine stable isotope loading test. Clin Chim Acta 1984;138:59.

228. Woo SLC. Collection of RFLP haplotypes at the human phenylalanine hydroxylase (PAH) locus. Am J Hum Genet 1988;43:781.

229. Cotton RGH, Scriver CR, McKusick VA. Locus-specific mutation databases: a resource. Genome Digest 1996;3:6.

230. Scriver CR, Kaufman S. Hyperphenylalaninemia: Phenylalanine hydroxylase deficiency. In: Scriver CR, Beaudet AL, Sly WS, Valle D, eds. The metabolic and molecular bases of inherited disease, 8th ed. New York: McGraw-Hill, 2001:1667.

231. Lidsky AS, Guttler F, Woo SL. Prenatal diagnosis of classic phenylketonuria by DNA analysis. Lancet 1985;1:549.

232. Ledley FD, Koch R, Jew K, et al. Phenylalanine hydroxylase expression in liver of a fetus with phenylketonuria. Pediatrics 1988;113:463.

233. Wang T, Okano Y, Eisensmith RC, et al. Missense mutations prevalent in Orientals with phenylketonuria: molecular characterization and clinical implications. Genomics 1991;10:449.

234. Goltsov AA, Eisensmith RC, Naughton ER, et al. A single polymorphic STR system in the human phenylalanine hydroxylase gene permits rapid prenatal diagnosis. Hum Mol Genet 1993;2:577.

235. Daiger SP, Reed L, Huang S-Z, et al. Polymorphic DNA haplotypes at the phenylalanine hydroxylase (PAH) locus in Asian families with phenylketonuria (PKU). Am J Med Genet 1989;45:319.

236. Chen SH, Hsiao KJ, Lin LH, et al. Study of restriction fragment length polymorphisms at the human phenylalanine hydroxylase locus and evaluation of its potential application in prenatal diagnosis of phenylketonuria. Hum Genet 1989;81:226.

237. Verlinsky Y, Rechitsky S, Verlinsky O, et al. Preimplantation testing for phenylketonuria. Fertil Steril 2001;76:346.

238. Dhondt J-L. Tetrahydrobiopterin deficiencies: preliminary analysis from an international survey. J Pediatr 1984;104:501.

239. Irons M, Levy HL, O'Flynn M, et al. Folinic acid therapy in dihydropteridine reductase deficiency. J Pediatr 1987;110:61.

240. Fukuda K, Tanaka T, Hyodo S, et al. Hyperphenylalaninaemia due to impaired dihydrobiopterin biosynthesis: leukocyte function and effect of tetrahydrobiopterin therapy. J Inherit Metab Dis 1985;8:49.

241. Niederwieser A, Blau N, Wang M, et al. GTP cyclohydrolase I deficiency, a new enzyme defect causing hyperphenylalaninemia with neopterin, biopterin, dopamine, and serotonin deficiencies and muscular hypotonia. Eur J Pediatr 1984;141:208.

242. Niederwieser A, Leimbacher W, Curtius HC, et al. Atypical phenylketonuria with "dihydrobiopterin synthetase" deficiency: absence of phosphate eliminating enzyme activity demonstrated in liver. Eur J Pediatr 1985;144:13.

243. Kaufman S, Holtzman NA, Milstien S, et al. Phenylketonuria due to a deficiency of dihydropteridine reductase. N Engl J Med 1975;293:785.

244. Dhondt JL, Guibaud P, Rolland MO, et al. Neonatal hyperphenylalaninaemia presumably caused by a new variant of biopterin synthetase deficiency. Eur J Pediatr 1988;147:153.

245. Dhondt J-L, Largilliere C, Ardouin P, et al. Diagnosis of variants of hyperphenylalaninemia by determination of pterins in urine. Clin Chim Acta 1981;110:205.

246. Niederwieser A, Curtius HC. Tetrahydrobiopterin biosynthetic pathway and deficiency. Enzyme 1987;38:302.

247. Blau N. Inborn errors of pterin metabolism. Annu Rev Nutr 1988;8:185.

248. Leeming RJ, Barford PA, Blair JA, et al. Blood spots on Guthrie cards can be used for inherited tetrahydrobiopterin deficiency screening in hyperphenylalaninaemic infants. Arch Dis Child 1984;59:58.

249. Blau N, Joller P, Atares M, et al. Increase of GTP cyclohydrolase I activity in mononuclear blood cells by stimulation: detection of heterozygotes of GTP cyclohydrolase I deficiency. Clin Chim Acta 1985;148:47.

250. Blau N, Kierat L, Matasovic A, et al. Antenatal diagnosis of tetrahydrobiopterin deficiency by quantification of pterins in amniotic fluid and enzyme activity in fetal and extrafetal tissue. Clin Chim Acta 1994;226:159.

251. Niederwieser A, Shintaku H, Hasler T, et al. Prenatal diagnosis of "dihydrobiopterin synthase" deficiency, a variant form of phenylketonuria. Eur J Pediatr 1986;145:176.

252. Dhondt JL, Tilmont P, Ringel J, et al. Pterins analysis in amniotic fluid for the prenatal diagnosis of GTP cyclohydrolase deficiency. J Inherit Metab Dis 1990;13:879.

253. Blau N, Niederwieser A, Curtius HC, et al. Prenatal diagnosis of atypical phenylketonuria. J Inherit Metab Dis 1989;12:295.

254. Dahl HHM, Hutchison W, McAdam W, et al. Human dihydropteridine reductase: characterisation of a cDNA clone and its use in analysis of patients with dihydropteridine reductase deficiency. Nucleic Acids Res 1987;15:1921.

255. Lockyer J, Cook RG, Milstien S, et al. Structure and expression of human dihydropteridine reductase. Proc Natl Acad Sci USA 1987;84:3329.

256. Dahl HHM, Wake S, Cotton RGH, et al. The use of restriction fragment length polymorphisms in prenatal diagnosis of dihydropteridine reductase deficiency. J Med Genet 1988;25:25.

257. Smooker PM, Cotton RG, Lipson A. Prenatal diagnosis of DHPR deficiency by direct detection of mutation. Prenat Diagn 1993;13:881.

258. Blau N, Thony B, Cotton RGH, et al. Disorders of tetrahydrobiopterin and related biogenic amines. In: Scriver CR, Beaudet AL, Sly WS, Valle D, eds. The metabolic and molecular bases of inherited disease. New York: McGraw-Hill, 2001:1725.

259. Blau N, Barnes I, Dhondt JL. International database of tetrahydrobiopterin deficiencies. J Inherit Metab Dis 1996;19:8.

260. Blau N, Thöny B, Dianzani I. www.bh4.org/biomdb1.html.

261. Partington M, Scriver CR, Sasskortsak A. Conference on hereditary tyrosinemia. Can Med Assoc J 1967;97:1045.

262. Lindblad B, Lindstedt S, Steen G. On the enzymic defects in hereditary tyrosinemia. Proc Natl Acad Sci USA 1977;74:4641.

263. Kvittingen EA, Jellum E, Stokke O. Assay of fumarylacetoacetate fumarylhydrolase in human liver-deficiency activity in a case of hereditary tyrosinemia. Clin Chim Acta 1981;114:311.

264. Berger R, Van Faasen H, Taanman JW, et al. Type I tyrosinemia: lack of immunologically detectable fumarylacetoacetase enzyme protein in tissues and cell extracts. Pediatr Res 1987;22:394.

265. Holme E, Lindblad B, Lindstedt S. Possibilities for treatment and for early prenatal diagnosis of hereditary tyrosinaemia. Lancet 1985;1:527.

266. Kvittingen EA, Halvorsen S, Jellum E. Deficient fumarylacetoacetate fumarylhydrolase activity in lymphocytes and fibroblasts from patients with hereditary tyrosinemia. Pediatr Res 1983;14:541.

267. Phaneuf D, Labelle Y, Berube Bérubé D, et al. Cloning and expression of the cDNA encoding human fumarylacetoacetate hydrolase, the enzyme deficient in hereditary tyrosinemia: assignment of the gene to chromosome 15. Am J Hum Genet 1991;48:525.

268. Agsteribbe E, van Faassen H, Hartog MV, et al. Nucleotide sequence of cDNA encoding human fumarylacetoacetase. Nucleic Acids Res 1990;18:1887.

269. Ploos van Amstel JK, Bergman AJ, van Beurden EA, et al. Hereditary tyrosinemia type 1: novel missense, nonsense and splice consensus mutations in the human fumarylacetoacetate hydrolase gene; variability of the genotype–phenotype relationship. Hum Genet 1996;97:51.

270. Mitchell GA, Grompe M, Lambert M, et al. Hypertyrosinemia. In: Scriver CR, Beaudet AL, Sly WS, Valle D, eds. the metabolic and molecular bases of inherited disease, 8th ed. New York: McGraw-Hill, 2001:1777.

271. Grompe M, St-Louis M, Demers SI, et al. A single mutation of the fumarylacetoacetate hydrolase gene in French Canadians with hereditary tyrosinemia type I. N Engl J Med 1994;331:353.

272. Gagne R, Lescault A, Grenier A, et al. Prenatal diagnosis of hereditary tyrosinaemia: measurement of succinylacetone in amniotic fluid. Prenat Diagn 1982;2:185.

273. Pettit BR, Mackenzie F, King GS, et al. The antenatal diagnosis and aid to the management of hereditary tyrosinaemia by use of a specific and sensitive GC-MS assay for succinylacetone. J Inherit Metab Dis 1984;7:135.

274. Jakobs C, Dorland L, Wikkerink B, et al. Stable isotope dilution analysis of succinylacetone using electron capture negative ion mass fragmentography: an accurate approach to the pre- and neonatal diagnosis of hereditary tyrosinemia type I. Clin Chim Acta 1988;171:223.

275. Jakobs C. Prenatal diagnosis of inherited metabolic disorders by staple isotope dilution GC-MS analysis of metabolites in amniotic fluid: review of four years' experience. J Inherit Metab Dis 1989;12:267.

276. Jakobs C, Stellaard F, Kvittingen EA, et al. First-trimester prenatal diagnosis of tyrosinemia type I by amniotic fluid succinylacetone determination. Prenat Diagn 1990;10:133.

277. Steinmann B, Gitzelmann R, Kvittingen EA, et al. Prenatal diagnosis of hereditary tyrosinemia. N Engl J Med 1984;310:855.

278. Kvittingen EA, Steinmann B, Gitzelmann R, et al. Prenatal diagnosis of hereditary tyrosinemia by determination of fumarylacetoacetase in cultured amniotic fluid cells. Pediatr Res 1985;19:334.

279. Grenier A, Cederbaum S, Laberge C, et al. A case of tyrosinaemia type I with normal level of succinylacetone in the amniotic fluid. Prenat Diagn 1996;16:239.

280. Poudrier J, Lettre F, St-Louis M, et al. Genotyping of a case of tyrosinaemia type I with normal level of succinylacetone in amniotic fluid. Prenat Diagn 1999;19:61.

281. Pettit BR, Kvittingen EA, Leonard JV. Early prenatal diagnosis of hereditary tyrosinaemia I. Lancet 1985;1:1038.

282. Kvittingen EA, Guibaud PP, Divry P, et al. Prenatal diagnosis of hereditary tyrosinaemia type I by determination of fumarylacetoacetase in chorionic villus material. Eur J Pediatr 1986;144:597.

283. Mustonen A, Ploos van Amstel HK, Berger R, et al. Mutation analysis for prenatal diagnosis of hereditary tyrosinaemia type 1. Prenat Diagn 1997;17:964.

284. Westphal EM, Natt E, Grimm T, et al. The human tyrosine aminotransferase gene: characterization of restriction fragment length polymorphisms and haplotype analysis in a family with tyrosinemia type II. Hum Genet 1988;79:260.

285. Natt E, Kida K, Odievre M, et al. Point mutations in the tyrosine aminotransferase gene in tyrosinemia type II. Proc Natl Acad Sci USA 1992;89:9297.

286. Cerone R, Fantasia AR, Castellano E, et al. Pregnancy and tyrosinaemia type II. J Inherit Metab Dis 2002;25:317.

287. Francis DE, Kirby DM, Thompson GN. Maternal tyrosinaemia II: management and successful outcome. Eur J Pediatr 1992;151:196.

288. Ellaway CJ, Holme E, Standing S, et al. Outcome of tyrosinaemia type III. J Inherit Metab Dis 2001;24:824.

289. Ruetschi U, Cerone R, Perez-Cerda C, et al. Mutations in the 4-hydroxyphenylpyruvate dioxygenase gene (HPD) in patients with tyrosinemia type III. Hum Genet 2000;106:654.

290. Applegarth DA, Toone JR. Non-ketotic hyperglycinemia (glycine encephalopathy): laboratory diagnosis. Mol Genet Metab 2001;74:139.

291. Kure S, Narisawa K, Tada K. Structural and expression analyses of normal and mutant mRNA encoding glycine decarboxylase: three-base deletion in mRNA causes nonketotic hyperglycinemia. Biochem Biophys Res Commun 1991;174:1176.

292. Kure S, Takayanagi M, Narisawa K, et al. Identification of a common mutation in Finnish patients with nonketotic hyperglycinemia. J Clin Invest 1992;90:160.

293. Tada K, Kure S. Nonketotic hyperglycinemia: molecular lesion and pathophysiology. Int Pediatr 1993;8:52.

294. Nanao K, Okamura-Ikeda K, Motokawa Y, et al. Identification of the mutations in the T protein gene causing typical and atypical nonketotic hyperglycinemia. Hum Genet 1994;93:655.

295. Kure S, Shinka T, Sakata Y, et al. A one-base deletion (183delC) and a missense mutation (D276H) in the T-protein gene from a Japanese family with nonketotic hyperglycinemia. J Hum Genet 1998:135.

296. Toone JR, Applegarth DA, Coulter-Mackie MB, et al. Identification of the first reported splice site mutation (IVS7-1G → A) in the aminomethyltransferase (T-protein) gene (AMT) of the glycine cleavage complex in 3 unrelated families with nonketotic hyperglycinemia. Hum Mutat 2001;17:76.

297. Toone JR, Applegarth DA, Coulter-Mackie MB, et al. Recurrent mutations in P- and T-proteins of the glycine cleavage complex and a novel T-protein mutation (N145I): a strategy for the molecular investigation of patients with nonketotic hyperglycinemia (NKH). Mol Genet Metab 2001;72:322.

298. Toone JR, Applegarth DA, Kure S, et al. Novel mutations in the P-protein (glycine decarboxylase) gene in patients with glycine encephalopathy (non-ketotic hyperglycinemia). Mol Genet Metab 2002;76:243.

299. Kure S, Mandel H, Rolland MO, et al. A missense mutation (His42Arg) in the T-protein gene from a large Israeli-Arab kindred with nonketotic hyperglycinemia. Hum Genet 1998;102:430.

300. Mesavage C, Nance CS, Flannery DB, et al. Glycine/serine ratios in amniotic fluid: an unreliable indicator for the prenatal diagnosis of nonketotic hyperglycinemia. Clin Genet 1983;23:354.

301. Toone JR, Applegarth DA, Levy HL. Prenatal diagnosis of non-ketotic hyperglycinaemia: experience in 50 at-risk pregnancies. J Inherit Metab Dis 1994;17:342.

302. Hayasaka K, Tada K, Fueki N, et al. Prenatal diagnosis of nonketotic hyperglycinemia: enzymatic analysis of the glycine cleavage system in chorionic villi. J Pediatr 1990;116:444.

303. Toone JR, Applegarth DA, Levy HL. Prenatal diagnosis of non-ketotic hyperglycinemia by assay of CVS glycine cleavage enzyme and amniotic fluid glycine. 8th International Congress of Human Genetics, 1991.

304. Toone JR, Applegarth DA, Levy HL. Prenatal diagnosis of non-ketotic hyperglycinemia. J Inherit Metab Dis 1992;15:713.

305. Applegarth DA, Toone JR, Rolland MO, et al. Non-concordance of CVS and liver glycine cleavage enzyme in three families with non-ketotic hyperglycinaemia (NKH) leading to false negative prenatal diagnoses. Prenat Diagn 2000;20:367.

306. Kure S, Rolland MO, Leisti J, et al. Prenatal diagnosis of non-ketotic hyperglycinaemia: enzymatic diagnosis in 28 families and DNA diagnosis detecting prevalent Finnish and Israeli-Arab mutations. Prenat Diagn 1999;19:717.

307. Applegarth DA, Rolland MO, Toone JR, et al. Molecular prenatal diagnosis of non-ketotic hyperglycinemia (glycine encephalopathy). Prenat Diagn 2002;22:266.

308. Menkes JH, Hurst PL, Craig JM. A new syndrome: progressive familial cerebral dysfunction with an unusual urinary substance. Pediatrics 1954;14:462.

309. Scriver CR, Mackenzie S, Clow CL, et al. Thiamine responsive maple syrup urine disease. Lancet 1971;1:310.

310. Chuang DT, Ku LS, Cox RP. Thiamin-responsive maple-syrup-urine disease: decreased affinity of the mutant branched-chain alpha-keto acid dehydrogenase for alpha-ketoisovalerate and thiamin pyrophosphate. Proc Natl Acad Sci USA 1982;79:3300.

311. Scriver CR, Clow CL, George H. So-called thiamin-responsive maple syrup urine disease: 15-year followup of the original patient. J Pediatr 1985;107:763.

312. Schulman JD, Lustberg TJ, Kennedy JL, et al. A new variant of maple syrup urine disease (branched chain ketoaciduria): clinical and biochemical evaluation. Am J Med 1970;49:118.

313. McKnight L, McKnight SA. Maple syrup urine disease: M.S.U.D. Parents Newsletter 1990,7:1.

314. Grunewald S, Hinrichs F, Wendel U. Successful outcome of a pregnancy in a woman with maple syrup urine disease (maternal MSUD). 7th International Congress of Inborn Errors of Metabolism. Vienna, Austria, 1997:P193.

315. Chuang DT, Shih VE. Maple syrup urine disease (branched-chain ketoaciduria). In: Scriver CR, Beaudet AL, Sly WS, Valle D, eds. The metabolic and molecular bases of inherited disease, 8th ed. New York: McGraw-Hill, 2001:1971.

316. Marshall L, DiGeorge A. Maple syrup urine disease in the old order Mennonites. Am J Hum Genet 1981;33:139A.

317. Matsuda I, Nobukuni Y, Mitsubuchi H, et al. A T-to-A substitution in the E1 α subunit gene of the branched-chain α-ketoacid dehydrogenase complex in two cell lines derived from Mennonite maple syrup urine disease patients. Biochem Biophys Res Commun 1990;172:646.

318. Dancis J, Hutzler J, Levitz M. Detection of the heterozygote in maple syrup urine disease. J Pediatr 1965;66:595.

319. Langenbeck U, Rudiger HW, Schulze-Schencking M, et al. Evaluation of a heterozygote test for maple syrup urine disease in leucocytes and cultured fibroblasts. Humangenetik 1971;11:304.

320. Langenbeck U, Grimm T, Rudiger HW, et al. Heterozygote tests and genetic counseling in maple syrup urine disease. Humangenetik 1975;27:315.

321. Shih VE, Mandell R, Scholl ML. Historical observation in maple syrup urine disease. J Pediatr 1974;85:868.

322. Jakobs C, Sweetman L, Nyhan WL. Hydroxy acid metabolites of branched-chain amino acids in amniotic fluid. Clin Chim Acta 1984;140:157.

323. Dancis J, Hutzler J, Snyderman SE, et al. Enzyme activity in classical and variant forms of maple syrup urine disease. J Pediatr 1972;81:312.

324. Wendel U, Wohler W, Goedde HW, et al. Rapid diagnosis of maple syrup urine disease (branched chain ketoaciduria) by micro-enzyme assay in leukocytes and fibroblasts. Clin Chim Acta 1973;45:433.

325. Fensom AH, Benson PF, Baker JE. A rapid method for assay of branched-chain keto acid decarboxylation in cultured cells and its application to prenatal diagnosis of maple syrup urine disease. Clin Chim Acta 1978;87:169.

326. Cox RP, Hutzler J, Dancis J. Antenatal diagnosis of maple-syrup-urine disease. Lancet 1978;1:212.

327. Wendel U, Claussen U. Antenatal diagnosis of maple-syrup-urine disease. Lancet 1979;1:161.

328. Kleijer WJ, Horsman D, Mancini GMS, et al. First-trimester diagnosis of maple syrup urine disease on intact chorionic villi. N Engl J Med 1985;313:1608.

329. Hong YS, Kerr DS, Liu TC, et al. Deficiency of dihydrolipoamide dehydrogenase due to two mutant alleles (E340K and G101del): analysis of a family and prenatal testing. Biochim Biophys Acta 1997;1362:160.

330. Wada Y, Taka K, Minagawa A, et al. Idiopathic hypervalinemia: probably a new entity of inborn error of valine metabolism. Tohoku J Exp Med 1963;81:46.

331. Reddi OS, Reddy SV, Reddy KR. A sibship with hypervalinemia. Hum Genet 1977;39:139.

332. Sweetman L. Disorders of the Branched Chain Amino Acids. In: Kelley VC, ed. Practice of Pediatrics, Volume 6. Philadelphia: Harper & Row, 1984:1.

333. Tada K, Wada Y, Arakawa T. Hypervalinemia. Its metabolic lesion and therapeutic approach. Am J Dis Child 1967;113:64.

334. Dancis J, Hutzler J, Tada K, et al. Hypervalinemia. A defect in valine transamination. Pediatrics 1967;39:813.

335. Dancis J. The antepartum diagnosis of genetic disease. J Pediatr 1968;72:301.

336. Goodman SI, Markey SP. Diagnosis of organic acidemias by gas chromatography-mass spectrometry. New York: Liss, 1981.

337. Chalmers RA, Lawson AM. Organic acids in man. Analytical chemistry, biochemistry and diagnosis of the organic acidurias. London: Chapman and Hall, 1982.

338. Hoffmann G, Aramaki S, Blum-Hoffmann E, et al. Quantitative analysis for organic acids in biological samples: Batch isolation followed by gas chromatographic-mass spectrometric analysis. Clin Chem 1989; 35:587.

339. Millington DS. Tandem Mass Spectrometry in Clinical Diagnosis. In: Blau N, Duran M, Blaskovics NE, Gibson KM, eds. Physician's Guide to the Laboratory Diagnosis of Metabolic Diseases. 3rd ed. Berlin: Springer, 2003:57.

340. Roe CR, Bohun TP. L-Carnitine therapy in propionic acidemia. Lancet 1982;1:1411.

341. Fenton WA, Rosenberg LE. Disorders of propionate and methylmalonate metabolism. In: Scriver CR, Beaudet AL, Sly WS, Valle D, eds. The metabolic and molecular bases of inherited disease, 7th ed. New York: McGraw-Hill, 1995:1423.

342. Gravel RA, Lam KF, Scully KJ, et al. Genetic complementation of propionyl-CoA carboxylase deficiency in cultured human fibroblasts. Am J Hum Genet 1977;29:378.

343. Wolf B. Biochemical characterization of mutant propionyl CoA carboxylases from two minor genetic complementation groups. Biochem Genet 1979;17:703.

344. Hsia YE, Scully KJ, Rosenberg LE. Inherited propionyl-CoA carboxylase deficiency in "ketotic hyperglycinemia." J Clin Invest 1971;50:127.

345. Wolf B, Rosenberg LE. Heterozygote expression in propionyl coenzyme A carboxylase deficiency. J Clin Invest 1978;62:931.

346. Morrow G, Schwartz RH, Hallock JA, et al. Prenatal detection of methylmalonic acidemia. J Pediatr 1970;77:120.

347. Gompertz D, Goodey PA, Thom H, et al. Prenatal diagnosis and family studies in a case of propionicacidaemia. Clin Genet 1975;8:244.

348. Willard HF, Ambani LM, Hart AC, et al. Rapid prenatal and postnatal detection of inborn errors of propionate, methylmalonate, and cobalamin metabolism: a sensitive assay using cultured cells. Hum Genet 1976;34:277.

349. Morrow G, Revsin B, Lebowitz J, et al. Detection of errors in methylmalonyl-CoA metabolism by using amniotic fluid. Clin Chem 1977;23:791.

350. Naylor G, Weetman L, Nyhan WL, et al. Isotope dilution analysis of methylcitric acid in amniotic fluid for the prenatal diagnosis of propionic and methylmalonic acidemia. Clin Chim Acta 1980;107:175.

351. Mandon G, Mathieu M. Fifteen years of prenatal diagnosis of inherited metabolic diseases: the Lyon experience. J Inherit Metab Dis 1989;12:257.

352. Sweetman L, Weyler W, Shafai T, et al. Prenatal diagnosis of propionic acidemia. JAMA 1979;242:1048.

353. Fensom AH, Benson PF, Chalmers RA, et al. Experience with prenatal diagnosis of propionic acidaemia and methylmalonic aciduria. J Inherit Metab Dis 1984;7:127.

354. Holm J, Ponders L, Sweetman L. Prenatal diagnosis of propionic and methylmalonic acidaemia by stable isotope dilution analysis of amniotic fluid. J Inherit Metab Dis 1989;12:271.

355. Jakobs C, Ten Brink HJ, Stellaard F. Prenatal diagnosis of inherited metabolic disorders by quantitation of characteristic metabolites in amniotic fluid: facts and future. Prenat Diagn 1990;10:265.

356. Coker M, Duran M, De Klerk JB, et al. Amniotic fluid odd-chain fatty acids are increased in propionic acidaemia. Prenat Diagn 1996;16:941.

357. Van Hove JL, Chace DH, Kahler SG, et al. Acylcarnitines in amniotic fluid: application to the prenatal diagnosis of propionic acidaemia. J Inherit Metab Dis 1993;16:361.
358. Aramaki S, Lehotay D, Nyhan WL, et al. Methylcitrate in maternal urine during a pregnancy with a fetus affected with propionic acidaemia. J Inherit Metab Dis 1989;12:86.
359. Perez B, Desviat LR, Rodriguez-Pombo P, et al. Propionic acidemia: identification of twenty-four novel mutations in Europe and North America. Mol Genet Metab 2003;78:59.
360. Muro S, Perez-Cerda C, Roddriguez-Pombo P, et al. Feasibility of DNA based methods for prenatal diagnosis and carrier detection of propionic acidaemia. J Med Genet 1999;36:412.
361. Coulombe JT, Shih VE, Levy HL. Massachusetts metabolic disorders screening program. II. methylmalonic aciduria. Pediatrics 1981;67:26.
362. Scriver CR, Beaudet AL, Sly WS, et al., eds. The metabolic and molecular bases of inherited disease, 7th ed. New York: McGraw-Hill, 1995.
363. Ledley FD, Lumetta MR, Zoghbi HY, et al. Mapping of human methylmalonyl CoA mutase (MUT) locus on chromosome 6. Am J Hum Genet 1988;42:839.
364. Ledley FD, Rosenblatt DS. Mutations in mut methylmalonic acidemia: clinical and enzymatic correlations. Hum Mutat 1997;9:1.
365. Kleijer WJ, Thoomes R, Galjaard H, et al. First-trimester (chorion biopsy) diagnosis of citrullinaemia and methylmalonicaciduria. Lancet 1984;1:1340.
366. Fowler B, Giles L, Sardharwalla IB, et al. First trimester diagnosis of methylmalonic aciduria. Prenat Diagn 1988;8:207.
367. Trefz FK, Schmidt H, Tauscher B, et al. Improved prenatal diagnosis of methylmalonic acidemia: mass fragmentography of methylmalonic acid in amniotic fluid and maternal urine. Eur J Pediatr 1981;137:261.
368. Zinn AB, Hine DG, Mahoney MJ, et al. The stable isotope dilution method for measurement of methylmalonic acid: a highly accurate approach to the prenatal diagnosis of methylmalonic acidemia. Pediatr Res 1982;16:740.
369. Tada K, Aikawa J, Igarashi Y, et al. A survey on prenatal diagnosis of inherited metabolic diseases in Japan. J Inherit Metab Dis 1989;12:260.
370. Ampola MG, Mahoney MJ, Nakamura E, et al. Prenatal therapy of a patient with vitamin-B_{12}-responsive methylmalonic acidemia. N Engl J Med 1975;293:313.
371. Bakker HD, Van Gennip AH, Duran M, et al. Methylmalonate excretion in a pregnancy at risk for methylmalonic acidemia. Clin Chim Acta 1978;86:349.
372. Tanaka K, Budd MA, Efron ML, et al. Isovaleric acidemia: a new genetic defect of leucine metabolism. Proc Natl Acad Sci USA 1966;56:236.
373. Budd MA, Tanaka K, Holmes LB, et al. Isovaleric acidemia: clinical features of a new genetic defect of leucine metabolism. N Engl J Med 1967;277:321.
374. Kreiger I, Tanaka K. Therapeutic effects of glycine in isovaleric acidemia. Pediatr Res 1976;10:25.
375. Roe CR, Millington DS, Maltby DA, et al. L-Carnitine therapy in isovaleric acidemia. J Clin Invest 1984;74:2290.
376. Naglak M, Salvo R, Madsen K, et al. The treatment of isovaleric acidemia with glycine supplement. Pediatr Res 1988;24:9.
377. Berry GT, Yudkoff M, Segal S. Isovaleric acidemia: medical and neurodevelopmental effects of long-term therapy. J Pediatr 1988;113:58.
378. Shih VE, Aubry RH, DeGrande G, et al. Maternal isovaleric acidemia. J Pediatr 1984;105:77.
379. Shih VE, Mandell R, Tanaka K. Diagnosis of isovaleric acidemia in cultured fibroblasts. Clin Chim Acta 1973;48:437.
380. Rhead WJ, Tanaka K. Demonstration of a specific mitochondrial isovaleryl-CoA dehydrogenase deficiency in fibroblasts from patients with isovaleric acidemia. Proc Natl Acad Sci USA 1980;77:580.
381. Tanaka K, Mandell R, Shih VE. Metabolism of [1-^{14}C] and [2-^{14}C] leucine in cultured skin fibroblasts from patients with isovaleric acidemia: characterization of metabolic defects. J Clin Invest 1976;58:164.
382. Hine DG, Hack AM, Goodman SI, et al. Stable isotope dilution analysis of isovalerylglycine in amniotic fluid and urine and its application for the prenatal diagnosis of isovaleric acidemia. Pediatr Res 1986;20:222.
383. Dumoulin R, Divry P, Mandon G, et al. A new case of prenatal diagnosis of isovaleric acidaemia. Prenat Diagn 1991;11:921.
384. Blaskovics ME, Ng WG, Donnell GD. Prenatal diagnosis and a case report of isovaleric acidemia. J Inherit Metab Dis 1978;1:9.
385. Kleijer WJ, VanDerKraan M, Huijmans JGM, et al. Prenatal diagnosis of isovaleric acidaemia by enzyme and metabolite assay in the first and second trimesters. Prenat Diagn 1995;15:527.

386. Gibson KM, Burlingame TG, Hogema B, et al. 2-Methylbutyryl-coenzyme A dehydrogenase deficiency: a new inborn error of L-isoleucine metabolism. Pediatr Res 2000;47:830.
387. Robinson BH, Sherwood WG, Taylor J, et al. Acetoacetyl CoA thiolase deficiency: a cause of severe ketoacidosis in infancy simulating salicylism. J Pediatr 1979;95:228.
388. Schutgens RBH, Middleton B, vd Blij JF, et al. Beta-ketothiolase deficiency in a family confirmed by in vitro enzymatic assays in fibroblasts. Eur J Pediatr 1982;139:39.
389. Tildon JT, Cornblath M. Succinyl-CoA: 3-ketoacid CoA-transferase deficiency: a cause for ketoacidosis in infancy. J Clin Invest 1972;51:493.
390. Mitchell FA, Fukao T. Inborn errors of ketone body metabolism. In: Scriver CR, Beaudet AL, Sly WS, Valle D, eds. The metabolic and molecular bases of inherited disease, 8th ed. New York: McGraw-Hill, 2001:2327.
391. Fukao T, Song X-Q, Watanabe H, et al. Prenatal diagnosis of succinyl-coenzyme A: 3-ketoacid coenzyme A transferase deficiency. Prenat Diagn 1996;16:471.
392. Rolland MO, Guffon N, Mandon G, et al. Succinyl-CoA:acetoacetate transferase deficiency. identification of a new case; prenatal exclusion in three further pregnancies. J Inherit Metab Dis 1998;21:687.
393. Fukao T, Wakazono A, Song XQ, et al. Prenatal diagnosis in a family with mitochondrial acetoacetyl-coenzyme A thiolase deficiency with the use of the polymerase chain reaction followed by the heteroduplex detection method. Prenat Diagn 1995;15:363.
394. Pearson MA, Aleck KA, Heidenreich RA. Benign clinical presentation of 3-methylcrotonylglycinuria. J Inherit Metab Dis 1995;18:640.
395. Mourmans J, Bakkeren J, de Jong J, et al. Isolated (biotin-resistant) 3-methylcrotonyl-CoA carboxylase deficiency: four sibs devoid of pathology. J Inherit Metab Dis 1995;18:643.
396. Gibson KM, Bennett MJ, Naylor EW, et al. 3-Methylcrotonyl-coenzyme A carboxylase deficiency in Amish/Mennonite adults identified by detection of increased acylcarnitines in blood spots of their children. J Pediatr 1998;132:519.
397. Stokke O, Eldjarn L, Jellum E, et al. β-methylcrotonyl-CoA carboxylase deficiency: a new metabolic error in leucine degradation. Pediatrics 1972;49:726.
398. Bartlett K, Bennett MJ, Hill RP, et al. Isolated biotin-resistant 3-methylcrotonyl CoA carboxylase deficiency presenting with life-threatening hypoglycaemia. J Inherit Metab Dis 1984;7:182.
399. Ly TB, Peters V, Gibson KM, et al. Mutations in the AUH gene cause 3-methylglutaconic aciduria type I. Hum Mutat 2003;21:401.
400. Kelley RI, Cheatham J, P., Clark BJ, et al. X-linked dilated cardiomyopathy with neutropenia, growth retardation, and 3-methylglutaconic aciduria. J Pediatr 1991;119:738.
401. Christodoulou J, McInnes RR, Jay V, et al. Barth syndrome: clinical observations and genetic linkage studies. Am J Med Genet 1994;50:255.
402. Besley GTN, Lendon M, Broadhead DM, et al. Mitochondrial complex deficiencies in a male with cardiomyopathy and 3-methylglutaconic aciduria. J Inherit Metab Dis 1995;18:221.
403. Ibel H, Endres W, Hadorn HB, et al. Multiple respiratory chain abnormalities associated with hypertrophic cardiomyopathy and 3-methylglutaconic aciduria. Eur J Pediatr 1993;152:665.
404. Elpeleg ON, Costeff H, Joseph A, et al. 3-Methylglutaconic aciduria in the Iraqi-Jewish "optic atrophy plus" (Costeff) syndrome. Dev Med Child Neurol 1994;36:167.
405. al Aqeel A, Rashed M, Ozand PT, et al. 3-Methylglutaconic aciduria: ten new cases with a possible new phenotype. Brain Dev 1994;16:23.
406. Chitayat D, Chemke J, Gibson KM, et al. 3-Methylglutaconic aciduria: a marker for as yet unspecified disorders and the relevance of prenatal diagnosis in a "new" type ("type 4"). J Inherit Metab Dis 1992;15:204.
407. Cardonick EH, Kuhlman K, Ganz E, et al. Prenatal clinical expression of 3-methylglutaconic aciduria: Barth syndrome. Prenat Diagn 1997;17:983.
408. Faull K, Bolton P, Halpern B, et al. Patient with defect in leucine metabolism. N Engl J Med 1976;294:1013.
409. Gibson KM, Breuer J, Nyhan WL. 3-Hydroxy-3-methylglutaryl-coenzyme A lyase deficiency: review of 18 reported patients. Eur J Pediatr 1988;148:180.
410. Ozand PT, Al Aqeel A, Gascon G, et al. 3-Hydroxy-3-methylglutaryl-coenzyme A (HMG-CoA) lyase deficiency in Saudi Arabia. J Inherit Metab Dis 1991;14:174.
411. Gibson KM, Cassidy SB, Seaver LH, et al. Fatal cardiomyopathy associated with 3-hydroxy-3-methylglutaryl-CoA lyase deficiency. J Inherit Metab Dis 1994;17:291.
412. Hammond J, Wilcken B. 3-Hydroxy-3-methylglutaric, 3-methylglutaconic and 3-methylglutaric acids can be non-specific indicators of metabolic disease. J Inherit Metab Dis 1984;7:117.

413. Sweetman L, Williams JC. Branched chain organic acidurias. In: Scriver CR, Beaudet AL, Sly WS, Valle D, eds. The metabolic and molecular bases of inherited disease. 7th ed. New York: McGraw-Hill, 1995:1387.

414. Wysocki SJ, Hahnel R. 3-Hydroxy-3-methylglutaric aciduria: 3-hydroxy-3-methylglutaryl-coenzyme A lyase levels in leucocytes. Clin Chim Acta 1976;73:373.

415. Duran M, Schutgens RB, Ketel A, et al. 3-Hydroxy-3-methylglutaryl coenzyme A lyase deficiency: postnatal management following prenatal diagnosis by analysis of maternal urine. J Pediatr 1979;95:1004.

416. Sovik O, Sweetman L, Gibson KM, et al. Genetic complementation analysis of 3-hydroxy-3-methylglutaryl–coenzyme A lyase deficiency in cultured fibroblasts. Am J Hum Genet 1984;36:791.

417. Gibson KM, Lee CF, Kamali V, et al. 3-Hydroxy-3-methylglutaryl-CoA lyase deficiency as detected by radiochemical assay in cell extracts by thin-layer chromatography, and identification of three new cases. Clin Chem 1990;36:297.

418. Robinson BH, Oei J, Sherwood WG, et al. Hydroxymethylglutaryl CoA lyase deficiency: features resembling Reye syndrome. Neurology 1980;30:714.

419. Norman EJ, Denton MD, Berry HK. Gas-chromatographic/mass spectrometric detection of 3-hydroxy-3-methylglutaryl-CoA lyase deficiency in double first cousins. Clin Chem 1982;28:137.

420. Chalmers RA, Tracey BM, Mistry J, et al. Prenatal diagnosis of 3-hydroxy-3-methylglutaric aciduria by GC-MS and enzymology on cultured amniocytes and chorionic villi. J Inherit Metab Dis 1989;12:286.

421. Chalmers R, Mistry J, Penketh R, et al. First trimester prenatal diagnosis of 3-hydroxy-3-methylglutaric aciduria. J Inherit Metab Dis 1989;12:283.

422. Mitchell GA, Jakobs C, Gibson KM, et al. Molecular prenatal diagnosis of 3-hydroxy-3-methylglutaryl CoA lyase deficiency. Prenat Diagn 1995;15:725.

423. Sasaki M, Iwata H, Sugai K, et al. A severely brain-damaged case of 3-hydroxyisobutyric aciduria. Brain Dev 2001;23:243.

424. Boulat O, Benador N, Girardin E, et al. 3-Hydroxyisobutyric aciduria with a mild clinical course. J Inherit Metab Dis 1995;18:204.

425. Ko FJ, Nyhan WL, Wolff J, et al. 3-Hydroxyisobutyric aciduria: an inborn error of valine metabolism. Pediatr Res 1991;30, No.4:322.

426. Chitayat D, Meagher-Villemure K, Mamer OA, et al. Brain dysgenesis and congenital intracerebral calcification associated with 3-hydroxyisobutyric aciduria. J Pediatr 1992;121:86.

427. Goodman SI, Markey SP, Moe PG, et al. Glutaric aciduria: a "new" disorder of amino acid metabolism. Biochem Med 1975;12:12.

428. Goodman SI, Frerman FE. Organic acidemias due to defects in lysine oxidation: 2-ketoadipic acidemia and glutaric acidemia. In: Scriver CR, Beaudet AL, Sly WS, Valle D, eds. The metabolic and molecular bases of inherited disease, 7th ed. New York: McGraw-Hill, 1995:1451.

429. Amir N, Elpeleg ON, Shalev RS, et al. Glutaric aciduria type I: Enzymatic and neuroradiologic investigations of two kindreds. J Pediatr 1989;114:983.

430. Bergman I, Finegold D, Gartner JC, Jr., et al. Acute profound dystonia in infants with glutaric acidemia. Pediatrics 1989;83:228.

431. Hoffman GF, Trefz FK, Barth PG, et al. Glutaryl-CoA dehydrogenase deficiency: a distinct encephalopathy. Pediatrics 1991;88:1194.

432. Hauser SE, Peters H. Glutaric aciduria type 1: an underdiagnosed cause of encephalopathy and dystonia-dyskinesia syndrome in children. J Paediatr Child Health 1998;34:302.

433. Haworth JC, Booth FA, Chudley AE, et al. Phenotypic variability in glutaric aciduria type I: Report of fourteen cases in five Canadian Indian kindreds. J Pediatr 1991;118:52.

434. Morton DH, Bennett MJ, Seargeant LE, et al. Glutaric aciduria type I: a common cause of episodic encephalopathy and spastic paralysis in the Amish of Lancaster County, Pennsylvania. Am J Med Genet 1991;41:89.

435. Kyllerman M, Skjeldal OH, Lundberg M, et al. Dystonia and dyskinesia in glutaric aciduria type I: clinical heterogeneity and therapeutic considerations. Mov Disord 1994;9:22.

436. Bahr O, Mader I, Zschocke J, et al. Adult onset glutaric aciduria type I presenting with a leukoencephalopathy. Neurology 2002;59:1802.

437. Goodman SI, Kohlhoof JG. Glutaric aciduria: inherited deficiency of glutaryl-CoA dehydrogenase activity. Biochem Med 1975;13:138.

438. Gregersen N, Brandt NJ, Christensen E, et al. Glutaric aciduria: biochemical and morphologic consideration. J Pediatr 1977;90:746.

439. Whelan DT, Hill R, Ryan ED, et al. L-Glutaric acidemia: investigation of a patient and his family. Pediatrics 1979;63:88.

440. Dunger DB, Snodgrass GJ. Glutaric aciduria type I presenting with hypoglycaemia. J Inherit Metab Dis 1984;7:122.

441. Christensen E. Improved assay of glutaryl-CoA dehydrogenase in cultured cells and liver: application to glutaric aciduria type I. Clin Chim Acta 1983;129:91.

442. Goodman SI, Kratz LE, DiGiulio KA, et al. Cloning of glutaryl-CoA dehydrogenase cDNA, and expression of wild type and mutant enzymes in Escherichia coli. Hum Mol Genet 1995;4:1493.

443. Goodman SI, Stein DE, Schlesinger S, et al. Glutaryl-CoA dehydrogenase mutations in glutaric acidemia (type I): review and report of thirty novel mutations. Hum Mutat 1998;12:141.

444. Schwartz M, Christensen E, Superti-Furga A, et al. The human glutaryl-CoA dehydrogenase gene: report of intronic sequences and of 13 novel mutations causing glutaric aciduria type I. Hum Genet 1998;102:452.

445. Tang NL, Hui J, Law LK, et al. Recurrent and novel mutations of GCDH gene in Chinese glutaric acidemia type I families. Hum Mutat 2000;16:446.

446. Zschocke J, Quak E, Guldberg P, et al. Mutation analysis in glutaric aciduria type I. J Med Genet 2000;37:177.

447. Busquets C, Soriano M, de Almeida IT, et al. Mutation analysis of the GCDH gene in Italian and Portuguese patients with glutaric aciduria type I. Mol Genet Metab 2000;71:535.

448. Biery BJ, Stein DE, Morton HD, et al. Gene structure and mutations of glutaryl-coenzyme A dehydrogenase: impaired association of enzyme subunits that is due to an A421V substitution causes glutaric acidemia type 1 in the Amish. Am J Hum Genet 1996;59:1006.

449. Greenberg CR, Reimer D, Singal R, et al. A G-to-T transversion at the +5 position of intron 1 in the glutaryl CoA dehydrogenase gene is associated with the Island Lake variant of glutaric acidemia type I. Hum Mol Genet 1995;4:493.

450. Greenberg CR, Prasad AN, Dilling LA, et al. Outcome of the first 3-years of a DNA-based neonatal screening program for glutaric acidemia type 1 in Manitoba and northwestern Ontario, Canada. Mol Genet Metab 2002;75:70.

451. Goodman SI, Gallegos DA, Pullin CJ, et al. Antenatal diagnosis of glutaric acidemia. Am J Hum Genet 1980;32:695.

452. Christensen E. First trimester prenatal exclusion of glutaryl-CoA dehydrogenase deficiency (glutaric aciduria type 1). J Inherit Metab Dis 1989;12:277.

453. Holme E, Kyllerman M, Lindstedt S. Early prenatal diagnosis in two pregnancies at risk for glutaryl-CoA dehydrogenase deficiency. J Inherit Metab Dis 1989;12:280.

454. Busquets C, Coll MJ, Merinero B, et al. Prenatal molecular diagnosis of glutaric aciduria type I by direct mutation analysis. Prenat Diagn 2000;20:761.

455. Lin SK, Hsu SG, Ho ES, et al. Novel mutation and prenatal sonographic findings of glutaric aciduria (type I) in two Taiwanese families. Prenat Diagn 2002;22:725.

456. Wilcken B, Leung KC, Hammond J, et al. Pregnancy and fetal long-chain 3-hydroxyacyl coenzyme A dehydrogenase deficiency. Lancet 1993;341:407.

457. Bennett MJ, Allison F, Lowther GW, et al. Prenatal diagnosis of medium-chain acyl-coenzyme A dehydrogenase deficiency. Prenat Diagn 1987;7:135.

458. Bennett MJ, Allison F, Pollitt RJ, et al. Prenatal diagnosis of medium-chain acyl-CoA dehydrogenase deficiency in family with sudden infant death. Lancet 1987;1:440.

459. Hale DE, Stanley CA, Coates PM. Genetic defects of acyl-CoA dehydrogenases: studies using an electron transfer flavoprotein reduction assay. In: Tanaka K, Coates PM, eds. Fatty acid oxidation: clinical, biochemical, and molecular aspects. New York: Alan R. Liss, 1990:333.

460. Gregersen N, Winter V, Jensen PK, et al. Prenatal diagnosis of medium-chain acyl-CoA dehydrogenase (MCAD) deficiency in a family with a previous fatal case of sudden unexpected death in childhood. Prenat Diagn 1995;16:82.

461. Tanaka K, Gregersen N, Ribes A, et al. A survey of the newborn populations in Belgium, Germany, Poland, Czech Republic, Hungary, Bulgaria, Spain, Turkey, and Japan for the G985 variant allele with haplotype analysis at the medium chain Acyl-CoA dehydrogenase gene locus: clinical and evolutionary consideration. Pediatr Res 1997;41:201.

462. Sermon K, Henderix P, Lissens W, et al. Preimplantation genetic diagnosis for medium-chain acyl-CoA dehydrogenase (MCAD) deficiency. Mol Hum Reprod 2000;6:1165.

463. Perez-Cerda C, Merinero B, Jimenez A, et al. First report of prenatal diagnosis of long-chain 3-hydroxy-acyl-CoA dehydrogenase deficiency in a pregnancy at risk. Prenat Diagn 1993;13:529.

464. Sluysmans T, Tuerlinckx D, Hubinont C, et al. Very long chain acyl-coenzyme A dehydrogenase deficiency in two siblings: evolution after prenatal diagnosis and prompt management. J Pediatr 1997;131:444.

465. Vianey-Saban C, Divry P, Brivet M, et al. Mitochondrial very-long-chain acyl-coenzyme A dehydrogenase deficiency: clinical characteristics and diagnostic considerations in 30 patients. Clin Chim Acta 1998;269:43.

466. Ibdah JA, Zhao Y, Viola J, et al. Molecular prenatal diagnosis in families with fetal mitochondrial tri-functional protein mutations. J Pediatr 2001;138:396.

467. Nada MA, Vianey-Saban C, Roe CR, et al. Prenatal diagnosis of mitochondrial fatty acid oxidation defects. Prenat Diagn 1996;16:117.

468. Rinaldo P, Studinski AL, Matern D. Prenatal diagnosis of disorders of fatty acid transport and mitochondrial oxidation. Prenat Diagn 2001;21:52.

469. Przyrembel H, Wendel U, Becker K, et al. Glutaric aciduria type II: report on a previously undescribed metabolic disorder. Clin Chim Acta 1976;66:227.

470. Coude FX, Charpentier G, Thomassin G, et al. Neonatal glutaric aciduria Type II: an X-linked recessive inherited disorder. Hum Genet 1981;59:263.

471. Frerman FE, Goodman SI. Defects of electron transfer flavoprotein and electron transfer flavoprotein-ubiquinone oxidoreductase: glutaric acidemia type II. In: Scriver CR, Beaudet AL, Sly WS, Valle D, eds. The metabolic and molecular bases of inherited disease, 8th ed. New York: McGraw-Hill, 2001:2357.

472. Mantagos S, Genel M, Tanaka K. Ethylmalonic-adipic aciduria. J Clin Invest 1979;64:1580.

473. Mooy PD, Geisberts MAH, van Gelderen HH, et al. Glutaric aciduria type II: multiple defects in isolated muscle mitochondria and deficient β-oxidation in fibroblasts. J Inherit Metab Dis 1984;2:101.

474. Gregersen N, Solvaa S, Rasmussen R, et al. General (medium-chain) acyl-CoA dehydrogenase deficiency (non-ketotic dicarboxylic aciduria): quantitative urinary excretion pattern of 23 biologically significant organic acids in three cases. Clin Chim Acta 1983;132:181.

475. Bougneres PF, Rocchiccioli F, Kolvraa S, et al. Medium-chain acyl-CoA dehydrogenase deficiency in two siblings with a Reye-like syndrome. J Pediatr 1985;106:918.

476. Curcoy A, Olsen RK, Ribes A, et al. Late-onset form of beta-electron transfer flavoprotein deficiency. Mol Genet Metab 2003;78:247.

477. Dusheiko G, Kew MC, Joffe BI, et al. Recurrent hypoglycemia associated with glutaric aciduria type II in an adult. N Engl J Med 1979;301:1405.

478. Harpey JP, Charpentier C, Goodman SI, et al. Multiple acyl-CoA dehydrogenase deficiency occurring in pregnancy and caused by a defect in riboflavin metabolism in the mother. J Pediatr 1983;103:394.

479. Turnbull DM, Bartlett K, Stevens DL, et al. Short-chain acyl-CoA dehydrogenase deficiency associated with a lipid-storage myopathy and secondary carnitine deficiency. N Engl J Med 1984;311:1232.

480. Bell RB, Brownell AKW, Roe CR, et al. Electron transfer flavoprotein: ubiquinone oxidoreductase (ETF:QO) deficiency in an adult. Neurology 1990;40:1779.

481. Gregersen N, Rhead W, Christensen E. Riboflavin responsive glutaric aciduria type II. In: Tanaka K, Coates PM, eds. Fatty acid oxidation: clinical, biochemical, and molecular aspects. New York: Alan R. Liss, 1990:477.

482. Niederwieser A, Steinmann B, Exner U, et al. Multiple acyl-CoA dehydrogenation deficiency (MADD) in a boy with nonketotic hypoglycemia, hepatomegaly, muscle hypotonia and cardiomyopathy. Helv Paediatr Acta 1983;38:9.

483. Mitchell G, Saudubray JM, Benoit Y, et al. Antenatal diagnosis of glutaric aciduria type II. Lancet 1983;1:1099.

484. Jakobs C, Sweetman L, Wadman SK, et al. Prenatal diagnosis of glutaric aciduria type II by direct chemical analysis of dicarboxylic acids in amniotic fluid. Eur J Pediatr 1984;141:153.

485. Bennett MJ, Curnock DA, Engel PC, et al. Glutaric aciduria type II: biochemical investigation and treatment of a child diagnosed prenatally. J Inherit Metab Dis 1984;7:57.

486. Boue J, Chalmers RA, Tracey BM, et al. Prenatal diagnosis of dysmorphic neonatal-lethal type II glutaricaciduria. Lancet 1984;1:846.

487. Chalmers RA, Tracey BM, King GS. The prenatal diagnosis of glutaric aciduria type II using quantitative GC-MS. J Inherit Metab Dis 1985;8:145.

488. Sakuma T, Sugiyama N, Ichiki T, et al. Analysis of acylcarnitines in maternal urine for prenatal diagnosis of glutaric aciduria type 2. Prenat Diagn 1991;11:77.

489. Yamaguchi S, Shimizu N, Orii T, et al. Prenatal diagnosis and neonatal monitoring of a fetus with glutaric aciduria type II due to electron transfer flavoprotein (β-subunit) deficiency. Pediatr Res 1991;30, No.5:439.

490. Manning NJ, Bonham JR, Downing M, et al. Normal acylcarnitines in maternal urine during a pregnancy affected by glutaric aciduria type II. J Inherit Metab Dis 1999;22:88.

491. Goodman SI, Binard RJ, Woontner MR, et al. Glutaric acidemia type II: gene structure and mutations of the electron transfer flavoprotein:ubiquinone oxidoreductase (ETF:QO) gene. Mol Genet Metab 2002;77:86.

492. Kjaergaard S, Graem N, Larsen T, et al. Recurrent fetal polycystic kidneys associated with glutaric aciduria type II. APMIS 1998;106:1188.

493. Chisholm CA, Vavelidis F, Lovell MA, et al. Prenatal diagnosis of multiple acyl-CoA dehydrogenase deficiency: association with elevated alpha-fetoprotein and cystic renal changes. Prenat Diagn 2001;21:856.

494. Jakobs C, Bojasch M, Monch E, et al. Urinary excretion of γ-hydroxybutyric acid in a patient with neurological abnormalities: the probability of a new inborn error of metabolism. Clin Chim Acta 1981;111:169.

495. Jakobs C, Kneer J, Rating D, et al. 4-Hydroxybutyric aciduria: a new inborn error of metabolism. II. Biochemical findings. J Inherit Metab Dis 1984;7:92.

496. Rating D, Hanefeld F, Siemes H, et al. 4-Hydroxybutyric aciduria: a new inborn error of metabolism. I. Clinical review. J Inherit Metab Dis 1984;7:90.

497. Pattarelli PP, Nyhan WL, Gibson KM. Oxidation of [U-^{14}C]succinic semialdehyde in cultured human lymphoblasts: measurement of residual succinic semialdehyde dehydrogenase activity in 11 patients with 4-hydroxybutyric aciduria. Pediatr Res 1988;24, No.4:455.

498. Rahbeeni Z, Ozand PT, Rashed M, et al. 4-Hydroxybutyric aciduria. Brain Dev 1994;16 (suppl):64.

499. Gibson KM, Christensen E, Jakobs C, et al. The clinical phenotype of succinic semialdehyde dehydrogenase deficiency (4-hydroxybutyric aciduria): case reports of 23 new patients. Pediatrics 1997; 99:567.

500. Pearl PL, Gibson KM, Acosta MT, et al. Clinical spectrum of succinic semialdehyde dehydrogenase deficiency. Neurology 2003;60:1413.

501. Gibson KM, Jansen I, Sweetman L, et al. 4-Hydroxybutyric aciduria: a new inborn error of metabolism. III. Enzymology and inheritance. J Inherit Metab Dis 1984;7:95.

502. Gibson KM, Sweetman L, Nyhan WL, et al. Defective succinic semialdehyde dehydrogenase activity in 4-hydroxybutyric aciduria. Eur J Pediatr 1984;142:257.

503. Gibson KM, Baumann C, Ogier H, et al. Pre- and postnatal diagnosis of succinic semialdehyde dehydrogenase deficiency using enzyme and metabolite assays. J Inherit Metab Dis 1994;17:732.

504. Jakobs C, Ogier H, Rabier D, et al. Prenatal detection of succinic semialdehyde dehydrogenase deficiency (4-hydroxybutyric aciduria). Prenat Diagn 1993;13:150.

505. Sweetman L, Hoffmann G, Gibson KM, et al. Mevalonic aciduria: A newly recognized inborn error of cholesterol biosynthesis. Pediatr Res 1985;19:322A.

506. Hoffmann GF, Charpentier C, Mayatepek E, et al. Clinical and biochemical phenotype in 11 patients with mevalonic aciduria. Pediatrics 1993;91:915.

507. Houten SM, Kuis W, Duran M, et al. Mutations in MVK, encoding mevalonate kinase, cause hyperimmunoglobulinaemia D and periodic fever syndrome. Nat Genet 1999;22:175.

508. Prietsch V, Mayatepek E, Krastel H, et al. Mevalonate kinase deficiency: enlarging the clinical and biochemical spectrum. Pediatrics 2003;111:258.

509. Houten SM, Wanders RJ, Waterham HR. Biochemical and genetic aspects of mevalonate kinase and its deficiency. Biochim Biophys Acta 2000;1529:19.

510. Hoffmann G, Gibson KM, Brandt IK, et al. Mevalonic aciduria: an inborn error of cholesterol and nonsterol isoprene biosynthesis. N Engl J Med 1986;314:1610.

511. Kozich V, Gibson KM, Zeman J, et al. Mevalonic aciduria. J Inherit Metab Dis 1991;14:265.

512. Hoffmann GF, Sweetman L, Bremer HJ, et al. Facts and artifacts in mevalonic aciduria: development of a stable isotope dilution GCMS assay for mevalonic acid and its application to physiological fluids, tissue samples, prenatal diagnosis and carrier detection. Clin Chim Acta 1991;198:209.

513. Christensen E, Brandt NJ, Skovby F, et al. Fumaric aciduria due to fumarase deficiency. Society for the Study Inborn Errors of Metabolism 24th Annual Symposium. Amersfoort, The Netherlands, 1986:72.

514. Zinn AB, Kerr DS, Hoppel CL. Fumarase deficiency: a new cause of mitochondrial encephalomyopathy. N Engl J Med 1986;315:469.

515. Petrova-Benedict R, Robinson BH, Stacey TE, et al. Deficient fumarase activity in an infant with fumaricacidemia and its distribution between the different forms of the enzyme seen on isoelectric focusing. Am J Hum Genet 1987;40:257.

516. Chaves-Carballo E. Fumaric aciduria (FA): An organic aciduria associated with mitochondrial encephalomyopathy in infancy. Pediatr Res 1987;21:489A.

517. Walker V, Mills GA, Hall MA, et al. A fourth case of fumarase deficiency. J Inherit Metab Dis 1989;12:331.

518. Gellera C, Uziel G, Rimoldi M, et al. Fumarase deficiency is an autosomal recessive encephalopathy affecting both the mitochondrial and the cytosolic enzymes. Neurology 1990;40:495.

519. Shih VE, Mandell R, Krishnamoorthy KS. Trial of dietotherapy in fumarase deficiency. 8th International Congress of Human Genetics. Washington, DC, 1991.

520. Elpeleg ON, Amir N, Christensen E. Variability of clinical presentation in fumarate hydratase deficiency. J Pediatr 1992;121:752.

521. Remes AM, Rantala H, Hiltunen JK, et al. Fumarase deficiency: two siblings with enlarged cerebral ventricles and polyhydramnios *in utero*. Pediatrics 1992; 89:730.

522. Bourgeron T, Chretien D, Poggi-Bach J, et al. Mutation of the fumarase gene in two siblings with progressive encephalopathy and fumarase deficiency. J Clin Invest 1994;93:2514.

523. Narayanan V, Diven W, Ahdab-Barmada M. Congenital fumarase deficiency presenting with hypotonia and areflexia. J Child Neurol 1996;11:252.

524. Bonioli E, Di Stefano A, Peri V, et al. Fumarate hydratase deficiency. J Inherit Metab Dis 1998;21:435.

525. Coughlin EM, Chalmers RA, Slaugenhaupt SA, et al. Identification of a molecular defect in a fumarase deficient patient and mapping of the fumarase gene. Am J Hum Genet 1993;53:896A.

526. Gellera C, Cavadini S, Dethlefs S, et al. Fatal mitochondrial encephalopathy caused by fumarase deficiency: molecular-genetic study. VI International Inborn Errors of Metabolism Congress. Milan, Italy, 1994.

527. Shih VE, Coughlin EM, Chalmers RA, et al. Genotype and phenotype findings in fumarate hydratase deficiency. Society for the Study of Inborn Errors of Metabolism 33rd Annual Symposium. Toledo, Spain, 1995.

528. Coughlin EM, Christensen E, Kunz PL, et al. Molecular analysis and prenatal diagnosis of human fumarase deficiency. Mol Genet Metab 1998;63:254.

529. Manning NJ, Olpin SE, Pollitt RJ, et al. Fumarate hydratase deficiency: increased fumaric acid in amniotic fluid of two affected pregnancies. J Inherit Metab Dis 2000;23:757.

530. Stacey TE, Robinson BH, Petrova-Benedict R, et al. Fumaric aciduria: microcephaly and severe developmental retardation caused by deficiency of mitochondrial and cytosolic fumarase activities. Annual Symposium of the SSIEM 1986:71.

531. Duran M, Kamerling JP, Bakker HD, et al. L-2-Hydroxyglutaric aciduria: an inborn error of metabolism? J Inherit Metab Dis 1980;3:109.

532. Barth PG, Hoffmann GF, Jaeken J, et al. L-2-Hydroxyglutaric acidemia: a novel inherited neurometabolic disease. Ann Neurol 1992;32:66.

533. Barth PG, Hoffmann GF, Jaeken J, et al. L-2-Hydroxyglutaric acidaemia: clinical and biochemical finding in 12 patients and preliminary report on L-2-hydroxyacid dehydrogenase. J Inherit Metab Dis 1993;16:753.

534. Larnaout A, Hentati F, Belal S, et al. Clinical and pathological study of three Tunisian siblings with L-2-hydroxyglutaric aciduria. Acta Neuropathol 1994;88:367.

535. Wilcken B, Pitt J, Heath D, et al. L-2-Hydroxyglutaric aciduria: three Australian cases. J Inherit Metab Dis 1993;16:501.

536. Divry P, Jakobs C, Vianey-Saban C, et al. L-2-Hydroxyglutaric aciduria: two further cases. J Inherit Metab Dis 1993;16:505.

537. Kaabachi N, Larnaout A, Rabier D, et al. Familial encephalopathy and L-2-hydroxyglutaric aciduria. J Inherit Metab Dis 1993;16:893.

538. Hoffmann CF, Jakobs C, Holmes B, et al. Organic acids in cerebrospinal fluid and plasma of patients with L-2-hydroxyglutaric aciduria. J Inherit Metab Dis 1995;18:189.

539. Gibson KM, ten Brink HJ, Schor DS, et al. Stable-isotope dilution analysis of D- and L-2-hydroxyglutaric acid: application to the detection and prenatal diagnosis of D- and L-2-hydroxyglutaric acidemias. Pediatr Res 1993;34:277.

540. Moroni I, D'Incerti L, Farina L, et al. Clinical, biochemical and neuroradiological findings in L-2-hydroxyglutaric aciduria. Neurol Sci 2000;21:103.

541. Jakobs C, Verhoeven NM, van der Knaap MS. Various organic acidurias. In: Blau N, Duran M, Blaskovics M, eds. Physician's guide to the laboratory diagnosis of metabolic diseases. London: Chapman and Hall, 1996:163.

542. van der Knaap MS, Jacobs C, Hoffmann GF, et al. D-2-hydroxyglutaric aciduria: further clinical delineation. J Inherit Metab Dis 1999;22:404.

543. Craigen WJ, Sekul EA, Levy ML, et al. D-2-Hydroxyglutaric aciduria in a neonate with seizures and central nervous system dysfunction. Pediatr Neurol 1994;10:49.

544. Muntau AC, Roschinger W, Merkenschlager A, et al. Combined D-2- and L-2-hydroxyglutaric aciduria with neonatal onset encephalopathy: a third biochemical variant of 2-hydroxyglutaric aciduria? Neuropediatrics 2000;31.

545. Matalon R, Michals K, Kaul R. Canavan disease: from spongy degeneration to molecular analysis. J Pediatr 1995;127:511.

546. Kvittingen EA, Guldal G, Borsting S, et al. *N*-acetylaspartic aciduria in a child with a progressive cerebral atrophy. Clin Chim Acta 1986;158:217.

547. Hagenfeldt L, Bollgren I, Venizelos N. *N*-acetylaspartic aciduria due to aspartoacylase deficiency: a new etiology of childhood leukodystrophy. J Inherit Metab Dis 1987;10:135.

548. Matalon R, Michals K, Sebesta D, et al. Aspartoacylase deficiency and *N*-acetylaspartic aciduria in patients with Canavan disease. Am J Med Genet 1988;29:463.

549. Divry P, Vianey-Liaud C, Gay C, et al. *N*-Acetylaspartic aciduria: report of three cases in children with a neurological syndrome associating macrocephaly and leucodystrophy. J Inherit Metab Dis 1988;11:307.

550. Matalon R, Kaul R, Casanova J, et al. Aspartoacylase deficiency: the enzyme defect in Canavan disease. J Inherit Metab Dis 1989;12:329.

551. Kaul R, Gao GP, Balamurugan K, et al. Cloning of the human aspartoacylase cDNA and a common missense mutation in Canavan disease. Nat Genet 1993;118.

552. Elpeleg ON, Anikster Y, Barash V, et al. The frequency of the C854 mutation in the aspartoacylase gene in Ashkenazi Jews in Israel. Am J Hum Genet 1994;55:287.

553. Kaul R, Gao GP, Balamurugan K, et al. Canavan disease: molecular basis of aspartoacylase deficiency. J Inherit Metab Dis 1994;17:295.

554. Kaul R, Gao GP, Aloya M, et al. Canavan disease: mutations among Jewish and non-Jewish patients. Am J Hum Genet 1994;55:34.

555. Matalon R, Matalon KM. Canavan disease prenatal diagnosis and genetic counseling. Obstet Gynecol Clin North Am 2002;29:297.

556. Elpeleg ON, Shaag A, Anikster Y, et al. Prenatal detection of Canavan disease (aspartoacylase deficiency) by DNA analysis. J Inherit Metab Dis 1994;17:664.

557. Matalon R, Kaul R, Gao GP, et al. Prenatal diagnosis for Canavan disease: the use of DNA markers. J Inherit Metab Dis 1995;18:215.

558. Jakobs C, ten Brink HJ, Divry P, et al. Prenatal diagnosis of Canavan disease. Eur J Pediatr 1992;151:620.

559. Kelley RI. Prenatal detection of Canavan disease by measurement of *N*-acetyl-L-aspartate in amniotic fluid. J Inherit Metab Dis 1993;16:918.

560. Bennett MJ, Gibson KM, Sherwood WG, et al. Reliable prenatal diagnosis of Canavan disease (aspartoacylase deficiency): comparison of enzymatic and metabolite analysis. J Inherit Metab Dis 1993;16:831.

561. Besley GT, Elpeleg ON, Shaag A, et al. Prenatal diagnosis of Canavan disease: problems and dilemmas. J Inherit Metab Dis 1999;22:263.

562. Ozand PT, Gascon GG, Al Aqeel A, et al. Prenatal detection of Canavan disease. Lancet 1991;337:735.

563. Matalon R, Kaul R, Michals K. Canavan disease: Biochemical and molecular studies. J Inherit Metab Dis 1993;16:744.

564. Rolland MO, Mandon G, Bernard A, et al. Unreliable verification of prenatal diagnosis of Canavan disease: aspartoacylase activity in deficient and normal fetal skin fibroblasts. J Inherit Metab Dis 1994;17:748.

565. Matalon R, Michals-Matalon K. Prenatal diagnosis of Canavan disease. Prenat Diagn 1999;19:669.

566. Freij BJ, Levy HL, Dudin G. Clinical and biochemical characteristics of prolidase deficiency in siblings. Am J Med Genet 1984;19:561.

567. Milligan A, Graham-Brown RAC, Burns DA, et al. Prolidase deficiency: a case report and literature review. Br J Dermatol 1989;121:405.

568. Mandel H, Abeling N, Gutman A, et al. Prolidase deficiency among an Israeli population: prenatal diagnosis in a genetic disorder with uncertain prognosis. Prenat Diagn 2000;20:927.

569. Naughten ER, Proctor SP, Levy HL. Congenital expression of prolidase defect in prolidase deficiency. Pediatr Res 1984;18:259.

570. Kodama H, Umemura S, Shimomura M, et al. Studies on a patient with iminopeptiduria. I. Identification of urinary iminopeptides. Physiol Chem Phys 1976;8:463.

571. Endo F, Tanoue A, Kitano A, et al. Biochemical basis of prolidase deficiency: polypeptide and RNA phenotypes and the relation to clinical phenotypes. J Clin Invest 1990;85:162.

572. Tanoue A, Endo F, Kitano A, et al. A single nucleotide change in the prolidase gene in fibroblasts from two patients with polypeptide positive prolidase deficiency. J Clin Invest 1990;86:351.

573. Tanoue A, Endo F, Matsuda I. Structural organization of the gene for human prolidase (peptidase D) and demonstration of a partial gene deletion in a patient with prolidase deficiency. J Biol Chem 1990;265:11306.

574. Ledoux P, Scriver C, Hechtman P. Four novel PEPD alleles causing prolidase deficiency. Am J Hum Genet 1994;54:1014.

575. Ledoux P, Scriver CR, Hechtman P. Expression and molecular analysis of mutations in prolidase deficiency. Am J Hum Genet 1996;59:1035.

576. Kikuchi S, Tanoue A, Endo F, et al. A novel nonsense mutation of the PEPD gene in a Japanese patient with prolidase deficiency. J Hum Genet 2000;45:102.

577. Forlino A, Lupi A, Vaghi P, et al. Mutation analysis of five new patients affected by prolidase deficiency: the lack of enzyme activity causes necrosis-like cell death in cultured fibroblasts. Hum Genet 2002;111:314.

578. Phang JM, Yeh GC, Scriver CR. Disorders of proline and hydroxyproline metabolism. In: Scriver CR,

Beaudet AL, Sly WS, Valle D, eds. The metabolic and molecular basis of inherited disease, 7th ed. New York: McGraw-Hill, 1995:1125.

579. Phang JM, Hu CA, Valle D. Disorders of proline and hydroxyproline metabolism. In: Scriver CR, Beaudet AL, Sly WS, Valle D, eds. The metabolic and molecular basis of inherited disease, 8th ed. New York: McGraw-Hill, 2001:1821.

580. Efron ML. Familial hyperprolinemia. Report of a second case, associated with congenital renal malformation, hereditary hematuria and mild mental retardation, with demonstration of an enzyme defect. N Engl J Med 1965;272:1243.

581. Valle D, Goodman SI, Applegarth DA, et al. Type II Hyperprolinemia, Δ1-pyrroline-5-carboxylic acid dehydrogenase deficiency in cultured skin fibroblasts and circulating lymphocytes. J Clin Invest 1976;58:598.

582. Levy HL, Shih VE, Madigan PM. Routine newborn screening for histidinemia. N Engl J Med 1974;291:1214.

583. Tada K, Tateda H, Arashima S, et al. Intellectual development in patients with untreated histidinemia. J Pediatr 1982;101:562.

584. Barnhisel ML, Priest RE, Priest JH. Histidase function in human epithelial cells. J Cell Physiol 1970;76:7.

585. Taylor RC, Levy HL, McInnes RR. Histidase and histidinemia clinical and molecular considerations. Mol Biol Med 1991;8:101.

586. Suchi M, Sano H, Mizuno H, et al. Molecular cloning and structural characterization of the human histidase gene (HAL). Genomics 1995;29:98.

587. Calonge MJ, Gasparini P, Chillaron J, et al. Cystinuria caused by mutations in rBAT, a gene involved in the transport of cystine. Nat Genet 1994;6:420.

588. Gasparini P, Calonge MJ, Biscaglia L, et al. Molecular genetics of cystinuria: identification of four new mutations and seven polymorphisms and evidence for genetic heterogeneity. Am J Hum Genet 1993;57:781.

589. Meyomato K, Katai K, Tatsumis S, et al. Mutations of basic amino acid transporter gene associated with cystinuria. Biochem J 1995;310:951.

590. Goodyer P, Boutros M, Rozen R. The molecular basis of cystinuria: an update. Exp Nephrol 2000;8:123.

591. Schmidt C, Albers A, Tomiuk J, et al. Analysis of the genes SLC7A9 and SLC3A1 in unclassified cystinurics: mutation detection rates and association between variants in SLC7A9 and the disease. Clin Nephrol 2002;57:342.

592. Dello Strologo L, Pras E, Pontesilli C, et al. Comparison between SLC3A1 and SLC7A9 cystinuria patients and carriers: a need for a new classification. J Am Soc Nephrol 2002;13:2547.

Yuan-Tsong Chen

14

Prenatal Diagnosis of Disorders of Carbohydrate Metabolism

Inherited disorders of carbohydrate metabolism result from defects in enzymes or transport proteins in the glycolytic pathway, gluconeogenesis, or glycogen metabolism. The defects in glycogen metabolism typically cause an accumulation of glycogen in the tissues, hence the name *glycogen storage disease*. Defects in gluconeogenesis or glycolytic pathway, including galactose and fructose metabolism, however, do not usually result in an accumulation of glycogen in the tissues. Clinical manifestations of the various disorders of carbohydrate metabolism differ markedly. The symptoms range from harmless to lethal. Unlike disorders of lipid metabolism, mucopolysaccharidosis, or other storage diseases, diet therapy has been effective in many of the carbohydrate disorders. For example, early diagnosis and early diet treatment have changed the outcome of type I glycogen storage disease.

Prenatal diagnosis of disorders of carbohydrate metabolism has been achieved largely by measurement of enzyme activity in cultured or noncultivated chorionic villi or amniocytes. For diseases with limited tissue expression of the defective enzyme, biopsy of fetal tissue has been shown to be useful for diagnosis. All genes responsible for the inherited disorders of carbohydrate metabolism have been cloned. Today, gene-based mutation and linkage analyses provide a reliable and accurate alternative for prenatal diagnosis and obviates the need for more invasive procedures, such as fetal liver biopsy.

This chapter presents information on enzymatic defects, clinical manifestations, laboratory findings, treatment, tissue needed for diagnosis, and methods for carrier detection and prenatal diagnosis. The common forms of the carbohydrate diseases, including enzymatic defect, clinical presentation, carrier detection, and prenatal testing, are summarized in Table 14.1. The reader is referred to the text for rare variants of the disease.

GLYCOGEN STORAGE DISEASE

Glycogen storage diseases (GSDs) are inherited disorders that affect glycogen metabolism.[1,2] The glycogen found in GSDs is abnormal in either quantity or quality. Essentially, all known enzymes and some transport proteins involved in the synthesis or degradation of glycogen and glucose have been discovered to cause some type of GSD. The different forms of GSDs have been categorized by numerical type in accord with the chronologic order in which these enzymatic defects were identified.

565

Table 14.1. Prenatal diagnosis of disorders of carbohydrate metabolism

Disorder	Common Name	Enzyme Defect/Deficiency	Clinical Presentation	Carrier Detection	Prenatal Diagnosis
Glycogen storage diseases					
Type Ia	von Gierke	Glucose-6-phosphatase	Growth retardation hepatomegaly, hypoglycemia, elevated blood lactate, cholesterol, triglycerides, and uric acid	Yes	Yes
Type Ib		Glucose-6-phosphate translocase	Same as type Ia, with additional findings of neutropenia and impaired neutrophil function	Possible	Yes
Type II	Pompe				
	Infantile	Acid maltase (acid α-glucosidase)	Cardiomegaly, hypotonia, hepatomegaly; onset: birth to 6 months	Yes	Yes
	Juvenile	Acid maltase (acid α-glucosidase)	Myopathy, variable cardiomyopathy; onset: childhood	Yes	Yes
	Adult	Acid maltase (acid α-glucosidase)	Myopathy, respiratory insufficiency; onset: adulthood	Yes	Has not been done
Type IIIa	Cori or Forbes	Liver and muscle debrancher deficiency (amylo-1,6-glucosidase)	Childhood: hepatomegaly, growth retardation, muscle weakness, hypoglycemia, hyperlipidemia, elevated transaminases; liver symptoms improve with age	Yes	Yes
Type IIIb		Liver debrancher deficiency; normal muscle enzyme activity	Liver symptoms same as in type IIIa; no muscle symptoms	Yes	Yes
Type IV	Andersen	Branching enzyme	Failure to thrive, hypotonia, hepatomegaly, splenomegaly, progressive cirrhosis (death usually before fifth year), elevated transaminases	Yes	Yes
Type V	McArdle	Myophosphorylase	Exercise intolerance, muscle cramps, increased fatigability	Yes	Has not been done

			Clinical features		
Type VI	Hers	Liver phosphorylase	Hepatomegaly, mild hypoglycemi, hyperlipidemia, and ketosis	Has not been done	Not indicated
Type VII	Tarui	Phosphofructokinase	Exercise intolerance, muscle cramps, hemolytic anemia, myoglobinuria	Yes	Has not been done
Type IX	Phosphorylase kinase deficiency	Phosphorylase kinase	Hepatomegaly, mild hypoglycemia, hyperlipidemia, and ketosis	Yes	Has not been done
Galactose disorders	Galactosemia with transferase deficiency	Galactose-1-phosphate uridyltransferase	Vomiting, hepatomegaly, cataracts, aminoaciduria, failure to thrive	Yes	Yes
	Galactokinase deficiency	Galactokinase	Cataracts	Yes	Not indicated
	Generalized uridine diphosphate galactose-4-epimerase deficiency	Uridine diphosphate galactose-4-epimerase	Similar to transferase deficiency with additional findings of hypotonia and nerve deafness	Yes	Yes
Fructose disorders	Essential fructosuria	Fructokinase	Benign	Has not been done	Not indicated
	Hereditary fructose intolerance	Fructose-1-phosphate aldolase	Acute: vomiting, sweating, lethargy; Chronic: failure to thrive, hepatic failure	Yes	Yes
Disorders of gluconeogenesis	Fructose-1,6-diphosphatase deficiency	Fructose-1,6-diphosphatase	Episodic hypoglycemia; apnea, ketosis, acidosis	Possible	Has not been done
	Phosphoenolpyruvate carboxykinase (PEPCK) deficiency	Phosphoenolpyruvate carboxykinase	Hypoglycemia, hepatomegaly, hypotonia, failure to thrive	Has not been done	Has not been done
Other carbohydrate disorders	Pentosuria	L-xylulose reductase	Benign	Yes	Not indicated

Liver and muscle have abundant quantities of glycogen and are the most common and seriously affected tissues. Because carbohydrate metabolism in the liver is responsible for plasma glucose homeostasis, in the GSDs that mainly affect the liver, the presenting features are usually hepatomegaly and hypoglycemia. The types (and associated enzymatic deficiencies) affecting the liver as the major organ are types I (glucose-6-phosphatase), III (debrancher), IV (brancher), VI (liver phosphorylase), and IX (phosphorylase b kinase), type 0 (glycogen synthase deficiency), as well as glucose type XI (transporter-2 deficiency). Some of the liver GSDs (type III, IV) are also associated with liver cirrhosis.

The GSDs that principally affect the muscle can be divided into two groups. The first involves a lysosomal enzyme deficiency (type II GSD) and has three clinical presentations that differ both in ages of onset, organ involvement, and clinical severity. The second group, of which muscle phosphorylase deficiency (McArdle disease) is the prototype, is characterized by muscle pain, exercise intolerance, and susceptibility to fatigue.

The overall frequency of all forms of the GSDs, based on European data, is approximately 1 in 20,000–25,000 live births.[1] Types I, II (lysosomal acid α-glucosidase deficiency), III, VI, and IX are the most common and account for approximately 90 percent of all GSDs.[1,2] Most GSDs are inherited in an autosomal recessive manner. The exception is a form of phosphorylase kinase deficiency,[3] which is X-linked.

Type I (Glucose-6-Phosphatase Deficiency, von Gierke Disease)

Type I GSD, or von Gierke disease,[4] is caused by a deficiency of glucose-6-phosphatase catalytic activity[5] (type Ia) or a defect in the glucose-6-phosphate translocase,[6,7] (type Ib) with excessive accumulation of glycogen in these organs. The stored materials in the liver include not only glycogen but also fat. The lack of glucose-6-phosphatase catalytic activity or translocase in the liver leads to inadequate conversion of glucose-6-phosphate into glucose through normal glycogenolysis and gluconeogenesis. Patients with this disease may present during the neonatal period with hypoglycemia; however, they more commonly present at 3–4 months of age with hepatomegaly and/or hypoglycemic seizures. These children have doll-like faces, with fat cheeks, protuberant abdomens, relatively thin extremities, and short stature. Abdominal enlargement is caused by massive hepatomegaly. The spleen is of normal size. Xanthoma and diarrhea may be present, and epistaxis can be a frequent problem. Frequent epistaxis with prolonged bleeding time is a result of impaired platelet aggregation and adhesion.[8]

The hallmarks of the disease are hypoglycemia, lactic acidosis, hyperuricemia, and hyperlipidemia. Hypoglycemia and lactic acidosis can develop after a short fast. Hyperuricemia is present in young children, but gout rarely develops before puberty. Hyperlipidemia includes elevation of triglycerides, cholesterol, and phospholipids. Hypertriglyceridemia causes the plasma to appear "milky." The lipid abnormality resembles type IV hyperlipidemia and is characterized by increased levels of very-low-density lipoprotein (VLDL); low-density lipoprotein (LDL); increased levels of apolipoproteins B, C, and E; and normal or reduced levels of apolipoproteins A and D.[9,10]

Puberty is often delayed. Virtually all females have ultrasound findings consistent with polycystic ovaries; however, the other clinical features of polycystic ovary syndrome such as acne and hirsutism are not seen.[11] It remains to be seen whether this ovarian finding actually affects ovulation and fertility. Sporadic cases of pregnancy in women with type I GSD have been reported; hypoglycemia symptoms may be exacerbated by pregnancy.[12,13] Secondary to the lipid abnormalities, there is an increased risk of pancreatitis.[14] The dyslipidemia together with elevated erythrocyte aggregation, predispose these patients for atherosclerosis. However, premature atherosclerosis has not yet been clearly documented except for rare cases.[15,16] Impaired platelet aggregation and increased antioxidative defense may function as a protective mechanism to help reduce the risk of atherosclerosis.[17,18] Frequent fractures and radiographic evidence of osteopenia are not uncommon in adult patients, and radial bone mineral content is significantly reduced in the prepubertal patients.

Hepatic adenomas develop in a significant number of patients, and malignant transformation can occur.[19–21] At puberty, symptoms of gout may seem secondary to long-standing hyperuricemia. Other complications include pulmonary hypertension[22,23] and renal disease.

Renal disease is a serious late complication manifested by proteinuria, hypertension, Fanconi-like syndrome, or altered creatinine clearance.[24–27] Glomerular hyperfiltration is often found during the early stage of renal dysfunction. Microalbuminuria and progressive renal damage may develop. Focal segmental glomerulosclerosis and interstitial fibrosis are typically seen on biopsy. Other renal abnormalities include amyloidosis, Fanconi-like syndrome, hypocitraturia, hypercalciuria, and distal renal tubular acidification defect.[28]

Type Ib has a similar clinical course, with the additional problems of neutropenia and impaired neutrophil function, resulting in recurrent bacterial infections. Oral and mucosal ulcerations are common, and in some cases, regional enteritis occurs.[29,30] The neutrophils in type Ib are apoptotic.[31]

The diagnosis of type I disease can be suspected on the basis of clinical presentation and abnormal plasma lactate and lipid values. In addition, administration of glucagon or epinephrine causes little or no rise in blood glucose but increases lactate levels significantly. Before the glucose-6-phosphatase and glucose-6-phosphate translocase genes were cloned, a definitive diagnosis required a liver biopsy to demonstrate a deficiency. Gene-based mutation analysis now provides a noninvasive way of diagnosis for most patients with types Ia and Ib disease.[32]

The treatment of type I GSD seeks to maintain normoglycemia, which corrects most of the metabolic abnormalities and reduces the morbidity associated with this disease. Normoglycemia can be achieved through a number of different approaches. Nocturnal nasogastric infusion of glucose and orally administered uncooked cornstarch are accepted means of treatment.[33–36] The current treatment is uncooked cornstarch at a dose of 1.6 g/kg of body weight every 4 hours for patients younger than 2 years of age,[37–39] and 1.75–2.5 g/kg every 6 hours for older patients. For patients who do not respond to cornstarch, nocturnal nasogastric infusion of glucose plus frequent daytime feeding is effective. Dietary intake of fructose and galactose should also be restricted. Allopurinol is given to lower the levels of uric acid. The hyperlipidemia can be reduced with lipid-lowering drugs such as HMG-CoA reductase inhibitors, and fibrate. Preliminary studies of treating microalbuminuria, an early indicator of renal dysfunction in patients with GSD-I, have also shown angiotensin-converting-enzyme (ACE) inhibitors, like captopril, to be beneficial. Citrate supplement may be beneficial in preventing or ameliorating nephrocalcinosis and development of urinary calculi. With early diagnosis and treatment, growth and puberty can be normal, and it is hoped that the long-term complications can be minimized.

For patients with type Ib GSD, granulocyte colony-stimulating factors have been used successfully to correct the neutropenia, decrease the severity of bacterial infection, and improve the chronic inflammatory bowel disease.[40,41]

Type I GSD is inherited as an autosomal recessive trait. Reduced levels of glucose-6-phosphatase have been reported in carriers through evaluation of the enzyme activity in the intestinal mucosa.[42] Glucose-6-phosphatase is expressed in liver, kidney, and intestine, but not in amniocytes or chorionic villi. Thus, prenatal enzymatic testing for GSD Ia is possible only through enzymatic examination of a fetal liver biopsy.[43] The translocase has a wider tissue distribution and may be present in amniocytes or villi; however, biochemical assay to demonstrate the translocase activity is technically difficult and requires fresh tissue and microsome isolation. No prenatal enzymatic testing of type Ib has been attempted. The gene for glucose-6-phosphatase is located on chromosome 17q21. Three common mutations (R83C, 130X, and Q347X) are responsible for 70 percent of the known disease alleles.[44,45] The gene for glucose-6-phosphate translocase is located on chromosome 11q23. Two mutations within this gene, G339C and 1211delCT, appear to be prevalent in Caucasian patients, while W118R appears to be most common in Japanese patients.[46,47] Today gene-based mutation and linkage analyses using chorionic villi or amniocytes provide a reliable and accurate alternative to the fetal liver biopsy procedure.[48,49]

Type II (Acid Maltase or Acid α-Glucosidase Deficiency, Pompe Disease)

Type II GSD is caused by a deficiency of lysosomal acid α-glucosidase (acid maltase),[50] an enzyme responsible for the degradation of glycogen engulfed in autophagic vacuoles. Three different forms of the disease, presenting with different age of onset and clinical severity, have been identified.[51] In the most severe form, the infantile form, almost no acid maltase activity exists, whereas the juvenile and adult forms show residual activity. The gene that encodes acid maltase has been cloned and is located on chromosome 17q25.[52,53]

The infantile form presents during the first few months of life, with cardiomegaly, hypotonia, hepatomegaly, and macroglossia, which is followed by a rapid, progressively downhill course. Death usually occurs before the second year of life as a result of cardiorespiratory failure. Characteristic electrocardiographic findings include a high-voltage QRS complex, inversion of the T wave, and a shortened PR interval. Blood creatine kinase and lactic dehydrogenase levels are elevated. Light microscopy of muscle or other tissues demonstrates glycogen accumulation. On electron microscopic examination, the glycogen is usually membrane-bound, but it is also found freely disposed in the cytoplasm. The juvenile form presents in early childhood, with progressive muscle weakness, variable cardiomegaly, and death before puberty from respiratory failure.

In the adult form, the patient may be asymptomatic until the second or third decade of life. The presenting symptom may resemble the muscle weakness of limb-girdle muscular dystrophy or a respiratory insufficiency. The blood creatine kinase level is not always elevated, and the muscle biopsy may not demonstrate the characteristic membrane-bound glycogen. The muscle taken for biopsy should be an involved muscle so that the diagnosis is not overlooked.

Definitive diagnosis requires enzyme analysis of skin fibroblasts, muscle, or liver. Leukocytes can also be used; however, one must be aware of potential interference from neutral α-glucosidase activity. In general, enzyme deficiency is more severe in the infantile form than in the late-onset juvenile and adult forms. Measurement of enzyme activity in the blood spot and oligosaccharides in the urine may be useful in screening patients for type II GSD.[54,55]

Definitive therapy is not currently available; a high-protein diet may be useful for the juvenile and adult forms.[56,57] Nocturnal ventilatory support in late-onset patients improves the quality of life and is beneficial during a period of respiratory decompensation. Clinical trials of enzyme replacement therapy are ongoing. Preliminary data have shown that recombinant acid α-glucosidase is capable of improving cardiac and skeletal muscle functions in these patients.[58,59]

Type II GSD is inherited as an autosomal recessive disorder. Carrier detection is possible, using enzyme analysis of skin fibroblasts, muscle, or leukocytes.[60–62] Leukocytes must be used with caution, because correction for nonspecific α-glucosidase is needed.

Prenatal diagnosis of type II GSD has been achieved by measuring enzyme activity in cultured amniotic fluid cells[63,64] or by direct electron microscopic examination of noncultivated cells.[65] Prenatal diagnosis in the first trimester, using noncultivated chorionic villi, has also been reported.[66–71] Maltose is the recommended substrate for the assay because it reacts preferentially with acid α-glucosidase (see Table 14.2). With maltose as the substrate, only one major form of maltase activity, with a pH optimum at 4.0, is demonstrated.[66] A fluorometric method with an artificial substrate can also be used; however, a specific antibody preparation is recommended.[67] As in other enzymatic methods for prenatal diagnosis, maternal cell contamination of chorionic villus sampling (CVS) is a major concern (see also chapter 5). If residual acid α-glucosidase activity is detected, the diagnosis should be confirmed by enzyme assay in the cultured cells and/or by electron microscopic examination of fetal cells. The latter procedure can be used to rule out maternal-cell contamination because it is conducted on the stromal fibrocytes beneath the basement membrane, which are cells of fetal origin.[71]

Table 14.2. Prenatal diagnosis of type II glycogen storage disease: α-glucosidase activities in noncultivated trophoblasts from normal controls and fetuses at risk for the infantile form of type II GSD

Subject	Gestation (weeks)	Enzyme Activity (nmol of glucose formed/min/mg protein)		
		pH 4	pH 6.7	pH 4/pH 6.7 ratio
Control				
1	9	48.3	6.3	7.7
2	8	55.1	12.3	4.5
3	9	91.5	16.2	5.6
4	11	92.5	10.3	9.0
5	9	108.8	12.2	8.9
6	9	124.2	14.0	8.9
7	10	144.2	18.7	7.7
Mean ± SD		94.9 ± 34.8	12.9 ± 4.0	7.5 ± 1.8
Fetus at risk				
Affected				
1	10	0.0	2.8	0.0
2	10	5.0	6.9	0.7
Unaffected				
3	1	75.6	12.9	5.9
4	10	81.3	11.0	7.4

Numerous mutations causing type II GSD are known, some common mutations exist in specific ethnic groups, including Asians and African-Americans.[72,73] For families with previously known mutations or an informative polymorphism, gene-based carrier detection and prenatal diagnosis are straightforward. However, for routine prenatal diagnosis without prior molecular data, enzyme assay on the noncultivated villi is the option of choice for its simplicity and reliability. Mutation analysis may be helpful for exceptional cases, such as when the fetus is at risk for late-onset GSD-II with residual enzyme activity or one of the parents has low enzyme activity.[73]

Type III (Debrancher Deficiency, Limit Dextrinosis, Cori or Forbes Disease)

Type III GSD is caused by a deficiency of glycogen debrancher enzyme activity.[74] A deficiency of debrancher enzyme impairs the release of glucose from glycogen but does not affect glucose released from gluconeogenesis. The glycogen accumulated has a structure that resembles limit dextrin (glycogen with short outer chains). In addition to glycogen, fat accumulates in the liver. At the protein level, most patients affected with GSD-III have low levels or even absence of debranching enzyme.[75,76] The gene that encodes human debrancher has been cloned, and genetic heterogeneity has been demonstrated at the molecular level.[77–79]

Most patients with type III GSD have disease involving both liver and muscle (type IIIa). However, some patients (<15 percent of all those with type III GSD) have only liver involvement, without apparent muscle disease (type IIIb).[76,80] During infancy and childhood, the disease may be indistinguishable from type I GSD, because hepatomegaly, hypoglycemia, hyperlipidemia, and growth retardation are similar predominant features. The liver symptoms improve with age and usually disappear after puberty. Overt liver cirrhosis rarely occurs. Hepatic adenomas have been reported, its prevalence may be as high as 25 percent in French patients. Malignant transformation of adenomas has not been observed, although hepatocellular carcinoma associated with end-stage liver cirrhosis developed in two patients.

Muscle weakness, although minimal during childhood, may become predominant in adults; these patients may show signs of neuromuscular involvement, with slowly progressive weakness and distal muscle wasting.[81,82]

Hypoglycemia, hyperlipidemia, and elevated liver transaminases occur in childhood. The liver transaminases can reach levels of 1,000–2,000 IU. In contrast to type I GSD, blood lactate and uric acid concentrations are usually normal. Glucagon administered 2 hours after a carbohydrate meal provokes a normal rise of blood glucose; after an overnight fast, glucagon may provoke no change in blood glucose.

The serum creatine kinase is useful for identifying patients with muscle involvement, but normal creatine kinase levels do not rule out muscle enzyme deficiency. Definite diagnosis and subtype require both liver and muscle biopsies. Skin fibroblasts or lymphocytes may also be used for diagnosis, either by measuring enzyme activities with a qualitative assay or by a Western blot analysis showing low levels or absence of the debrancher protein.[76,83] In some patients, excess glycogen and deficient debranching enzyme can be demonstrated in erythrocytes.[84,85]

Treatment is symptomatic. If hypoglycemia is present, frequent meals high in carbohydrates, with cornstarch supplements, constitute effective therapy.[86] In the case of muscle involvement, a diet high in protein during the daytime plus overnight protein enteral infusion may be beneficial.[87] The patient does not need to restrict dietary intake of fructose and galactose, as do patients with type I GSD.

Type III GSD is inherited in an autosomal recessive manner. Carrier detection is possible through Western blot analysis (if the proband has an absence of debrancher protein)[76] or by an assay of enzyme activity in erythrocytes.[85]

Prenatal diagnosis has been performed in cultured amniocytes or in chorionic villi by using (a) immunoblot analysis with a polyclonal antibody against purified porcine-muscle debranching enzyme,[88] (b) a qualitative assay for debranching enzyme activity,[88] or (c) enzyme-activity assays.[70,89] The immunoblot method has a limitation: it cannot be offered to a family in which the proband has cross-reactive material for debranching enzyme. The qualitative assay requires a large number of viable cells. The enzyme activity method is technically difficult because debranching enzyme activity is relatively low in cultured amniocytes or chorionic villi.

The gene for debranching enzyme is located on chromosome 1p21. To date, no true frequent mutations have been found except for an ethnic-specific mutation in the Ashkenazi Jewish population and a subtype-specific mutation associated with GSD-IIIb.[90,91] The gene is large and complex, thus both mutation screen and/or sequencing are impractical for routine prenatal diagnosis. However, three highly polymorphic DNA markers of the gene have been identified. Our experience indicates that 70 percent of GSD-III families are either completely informative or partially informative for one of the three markers. Prenatal diagnosis, therefore, is informative only in families with known mutations or in which linkage has been established.[92]

Type IV (Branching Enzyme Deficiency, Amylopectinosis, or Andersen Disease)

Type IV GSD is caused by a deficiency of branching enzyme activity, which results in the accumulation of glycogen with unbranched, long, outer chains in the tissues.[93,94] This form of GSD most frequently presents during the first few months of life, with hepatosplenomegaly and failure to thrive. Hypoglycemia is rarely seen. Progressive liver cirrhosis, with portal hypertension, ascites, esophageal varices, and death, usually occurs before 5 years of age. There are, however, patients who have survived without apparent progressive liver disease.[95–97] The neuromuscular system may also be involved. The presenting signs are hypotonia and decreased or absent deep tendon reflexes. Severe cardiomyopathy, as the predominant symptom, has been reported.[98]

The glycogen branching enzyme gene is on chromosome 3p21. Mutations responsible for different forms of type IV GSD have been identified and may be used in predicting the clinical outcome.[99]

There is no specific treatment for type IV GSD. Liver transplantation has been performed, and may be an effective treatment.[100] On tissue studied after transplantation, there has been a reduction in the amount of amylopectin found; however, because type IV GSD is a multisystem disorder, the long-term success of liver transplantation is not known.

The diagnosis of type IV is established by demonstration of abnormal glycogen (long outer chains, an amylopectin-like polysaccharide) and a deficiency of branching enzyme in liver, muscle, leukocytes, erythrocytes, or fibroblasts.

Type IV GSD is inherited as an autosomal recessive trait. Carrier detection is possible. Partial enzyme deficiency has been observed in obligate carriers by measurement of enzyme activity in leukocytes, erythrocytes, or skin fibroblasts.[101,102]

Prenatal diagnosis is available for the fatal form of GSD by measuring branching enzyme activity in cultured amniocytes or chorionic villi.[103] Direct villi studies are not suitable for prenatal diagnosis, because they give variable and inconsistent results.

DNA mutation analysis can complement the enzyme activity study for prenatal diagnosis, especially in fetuses with high residual enzyme activity overlapping the heterozygote levels.[104]

Type V (Muscle Phosphorylase Deficiency, McArdle Disease, and Myophosphorylase Deficiency)

Type V GSD is caused by a deficiency of muscle phosphorylase activity. A deficiency of myophosphorylase impairs the cleavage of glucosyl molecules from the straight chain of glycogen. The gene for muscle phosphorylase has been cloned and mapped to chromosome 11q13.[105]

Clinical symptoms usually appear in adulthood and are characterized by exercise intolerance with muscle cramps that can be accompanied by attacks of myoglobinuria. Although most patients present with symptoms in the second or third decade of life, many report having had weakness and lack of endurance since childhood. Myoglobinuria can lead to renal failure. The clinical phenotypic variations may be modulated by the genotypes of the angiotensin-converting-enzyme gene.[106]

Serum creatine kinase is usually elevated and increases after exercise. The transaminases, blood ammonia, inosine, hypoxanthine, and uric acid also increase with exercise. These elevations are attributed to accelerated degradation of muscle purine nucleotides. The diagnosis of type V GSD is strongly suggested by an abnormal ischemic exercise test, during which patients have characteristic forearm "contraction," failure of an increase in blood lactate concentration, and exaggerated blood ammonia elevation.

In general, avoidance of strenuous exercise can prevent major episodes of rhabdomyolysis; however, regular and moderate exercise is recommended to improve exercise capacity. A high-protein diet may increase muscle endurance, and creatine supplementation has been shown to improve muscle function in some patients.[107] In general, longevity does not appear to be affected. There have been several reports of a fatal infantile form of phosphorylase deficiency.[108–110] The presenting features were hypotonia, generalized muscle weakness, and progressive respiratory insufficiency. Death occurred before 4 months of age. Congenital joint contracture was observed in one preterm infant.[110] In addition, phosphorylase deficiency has also been reported in a 4-year-old boy presenting with delayed psychomotor development, proximal weakness, elevated creatine kinase, and myopathic electromyographic changes.[111]

Phosphorous magnetic resonance imaging (^{31}P MRI) allows for the noninvasive evaluation of muscle metabolism. Patients with type V GSD have no decrease in intracellular pH and have excessive reductions in phosphocreatine in response to exercise.[112] The diagnosis should be confirmed by enzymatic evaluation of muscle. Carrier studies have been performed in type V by measurement of enzyme activity in biopsy muscle[113] or use of ^{31}P MRI to study muscle metabolism.[114] The common mutations for Caucasian and Japanese patients are now known, thus allowing DNA-based testing.[115,116] There seems to be no indication for prenatal diagnosis of this relatively benign metabolic disorder. Prenatal diagnosis for the rare and fatal infantile form is clearly indicated and may be possible by fetal muscle biopsy or by ultrasound assessment of fetal movement. However, there are no reports in the literature that these have been done.

Type VI (Liver Phosphorylase, Hers Disease)

The enzyme deficient in type VI GSD is liver phosphorylase. A deficiency of phosphorylase impairs the cleavage of glucosyl molecules from the straight chains of glycogen. Liver and muscle phosphorylase are distinct enzymes and are encoded by separate genes. The gene that encodes liver phosphorylase has been cloned and mapped to chromosome 14q21.[117,118]

Most patients with this disease present with hepatomegaly and growth retardation. Hypoglycemia, hyperlipidemia, and hyperketosis, if present, are usually mild. Lactic and uric acids are normal. The heart and skeletal muscle are not involved. The hepatomegaly improves and disappears around puberty. Diagnosis rests on enzyme analysis of the liver.

The treatment for type VI is symptomatic. A high-carbohydrate diet and frequent feedings are effective in preventing hypoglycemia. Puberty is usually normal, and ultimate growth is not affected.

Liver phosphorylase deficiency is inherited as an autosomal recessive genetic condition. Carrier detection has not been accomplished because the readily accessible tissues (leukocytes, erythrocytes, or skin fibroblasts) do not reflect liver phosphorylase deficiency.

Because this is a benign condition, prenatal diagnosis is not indicated.

Type VII (Phosphofructokinase Deficiency, Tarui Disease)

Type VII is caused by a deficiency of muscle phosphofructokinase. Numerous isoenzymes have been isolated from various types of tissues.[119] The gene for muscle phosphofructokinase has been cloned,[120] and mutations have been identified.[121–124] In Ashkenazi Jews, 95 percent of mutant alleles are either a splicing defect or a nucleotide deletion.[123]

The clinical features are very similar to those in McArdle disease. Patients present in adulthood with exercise-induced muscle cramps and myoglobinuria, but in type VII, the erythrocytes may also be involved and hemolysis occurs. Strenuous exercise should be avoided to prevent the acute renal failure that can occur secondary to rhabdomyolysis.

A fatal infantile form of phosphofructokinase deficiency has been reported.[125,126] These patients present in infancy with limb weakness, seizures, cortical blindness, and corneal clouding. Death occurs before 4 years of age from respiratory failure.

To establish a diagnosis, a biochemical or histochemical demonstration of the enzymatic defect in the muscle is required. The absence of the M isoenzyme of phosphofructokinase can also be demonstrated in blood cells and fibroblasts.[127,128]

Type VII GSD is inherited as an autosomal recessive trait. Partial enzyme deficiency has been reported in obligate carriers.[128] Prenatal diagnosis does not seem to be indicated in this relatively benign disorder, except for the rare fatal form of the disease. There are no reports in the literature that this has been accomplished.

Type IX (Phosphorylase b Kinase Deficiency)

A deficiency of phosphorylase b kinase is responsible for several forms of GSD that differ both in tissues affected and in patterns of inheritance.[129] The enzyme consists of four different subunits, which result in multiple tissue-specific isozymes. The enzyme activates glycogen phosphorylase to enhance the breakdown of glycogen. The genes for α, β, and γ subunits have been cloned.[130–133] The genes for both muscle and liver a subunit have been mapped to X chromosome and for β subunit to chromosome 16q12–q13.[134,135] Mutations for different forms of phosphorylase kinase deficiency have been characterized.[136–139]

The most common form of phosphorylase kinase deficiency is the X-linked form, which mainly affects the liver. In this form, patients present with hepatomegaly, growth retardation, and delayed motor development. Hypoglycemia, hyperlipidemia, and hyperketosis are variable and, if present, are usually mild. Blood lactate and uric acid concentrations are normal. Treatment is symptomatic. A high-carbohydrate diet and frequent feedings are effective in maintaining a normal glucose concentration. The symptoms and signs improve with age, and adult patients have normal stature and minimal hepatomegaly.[140]

Other phosphorylase kinase deficiency variants include an autosomal recessive form that affects both liver and muscle, an autosomal recessive form of liver phosphorylase kinase deficiency, which often develops into liver cirrhosis,[141] a mild myopathic form with muscle cramp and myoglobinuria, a severe myopathic form with onset in early infancy,[142] and an isolated myocardial phosphorylase b kinase deficiency.[143,144] The clinical heterogeneity can be explained by the presence of the four subunits expressed in different tissues.

Definitive diagnosis of phosphorylase b kinase deficiency requires demonstration of the enzymatic defect in affected tissues. Phosphorylase b kinase can be measured in leukocytes and erythrocytes,[145,146] but, because the enzyme has many isozymes, the diagnosis can be missed without studies of liver, muscle, or heart.

Intermediate enzyme levels have been reported in carrier mothers in the X-linked form.[3,147] Carrier detection is possible using DNA-based linkage or mutation analysis for several forms of phosphorylase kinase deficiency.[136–140] There seems to be no indication for prenatal diagnosis for this relatively benign disorder. Prenatal diagnosis for the rare fatal form of the disease has not been reported.

Glycogen Synthase Deficiency

Strictly speaking, glycogen synthase deficiency (Type 0) is not a glycogen storage disease, because deficiency of the enzyme leads to decrease glycogen stores. The patients present in infancy with early-morning drowsiness and fatigue and sometimes convulsions associated with hypoglycemia and hyperketonemia. Blood lactate and alanine levels are low, and there is no hyperlipidemia or hepatomegaly. Prolonged hyperglycemia and elevation of lactate with normal insulin levels after the administration of glucose suggest a possible diagnosis of deficiency of glycogen synthetase.[148,149] Treatment consists of frequent meals, rich protein, and nighttime supplementation with uncooked cornstarch. The disease is due to the mutations in the liver glycogen synthase gene, located on chromosome 12p12.2.[150]

Because glycogen synthase deficiency is not expressed in muscle, erythrocytes, and cultured fibroblasts, a definitive diagnosis requires liver biopsy. The disease is inherited in an autosomal recessive manner. Carrier detection and prenatal diagnosis are possible with a gene-based method; however, this has not yet been performed.

Hepatic Glycogenosis with Renal Fanconi Syndrome (Type IX)

This rare form of glycogen storage disease is caused by defects in the facilitative glucose transporter 2 (GLUT-2), which transports glucose in and out of hepatocytes, pancreatic cells, and the basolateral membranes of intestinal and renal epithelial cells.[151] The disease is characterized by proximal renal tubular dysfunction, impaired glucose and galactose utilization, and accumulation of glycogen in liver and kidney. The gene has been cloned and mutations identified[151]; thus, gene-based diagnosis is possible for families with known mutations.

DISORDERS OF GALACTOSE METABOLISM

Galactosemia with Transferase Deficiency

The enzyme deficient in galactosemia with transferase deficiency is galactose-1-phosphate uridyltransferase. This enzyme catalyzes the second step in the galactose–glucose inter-conversion in which galactose-1-phosphate is converted to uridine diphosphate galactose (UDPgal). Transferase deficiency results in the accumulation of galactose-1-phosphate, galactitol, galactonate, and low levels of UDPgal. The gene encoding galactose-1-phosphate uridyl transferase has been cloned and is mapped to chromosome 9p13.[152,153] Mutations have been extensively characterized.[154,155]

Patients with this disease seem normal at birth. Within a few days of feeding with galactose-containing foods (breast milk or milk-based formula), the vomiting, diarrhea, and dehydration develop in the infant. Jaundice, hepatomegaly, and abnormal liver function are present after the first week of life. Slit-lamp examination of the eye reveals cataracts within a few days to a few weeks. *Escherichia coli* or *Klebsiella* sepsis may complicate the course. Some patients, often of African-American descent, present later in infancy in a more insidious manner, with eventual hepatomegaly, failure to thrive, cataracts, and developmental delay. These children may have residual transferase activity in the liver,[156] and frequently they have a history of reduced galactose intake because milk formula causes them to vomit.

Biochemical findings include abnormal liver function, hyperchloremic acidosis, albuminuria, and generalized aminoaciduria. The identification of a reducing substance in the urine, which does not react with glucose oxidase reagent, suggests the diagnosis, but fructose, lactose, and pentose can give similar results. The urinary galactose disappears within a day of discontinuing milk intake. The diagnosis can be established by measurement of both the erythrocyte galactose-1-phosphate levels and the transferase activity. A galactose challenge should not be done.

Elimination of galactose from the diet by using a lactose-free formula reverses growth failure as well as renal and hepatic dysfunction. Cataracts regress, and most patients have no impairment of eyesight. Early diagnosis and treatment has improved the prognosis for galactosemia; however, complications such as ovarian failure, mild speech and language delay, and neurologic defects still occur, perhaps because of endogenous galactose-1-phosphate production.[156–160] Breast-feeding can be complicated by self-intoxication from endogenous lactose production.[161,162]

The enzyme deficiency can be demonstrated in erythrocytes, white blood cells, skin fibroblasts, intestinal mucosa, and the liver. Because of widespread newborn screening for galactosemia, most patients are being identified early.

Galactosemia is inherited as an autosomal recessive trait; the incidence is about 1 in 62,000 newborns. There are several enzymatic variants of galactosemia.[156,163] The common Duarte variant, a single amino acid substitution (N314D) has diminished red-cell enzyme activity but usually no clinical consequences. Some African-American patients have milder symptoms despite the absence of measurable transferase activity in erythrocytes; these patients retain 10 percent enzyme activity in liver and intestinal mucosa, whereas most white patients have no detectable activity in any of these tissues. In African Americans, 62 percent of alleles are represented by the S135L mutation, a mutation that is responsible for the milder disease. In the white population, 70 percent of alleles are represented by the Q188R and K285N missense mutations and are associated with severe disease.[154,155]

Carrier detection is possible in erythrocytes, skin fibroblasts, or leukocytes.[164] Prenatal diagnosis has been accomplished using cultured amniotic fluid cells, using a direct

CVS for measurement of enzyme activity, or by analyzing amniotic fluid galactitol with a mass spectrometric method.[165–172] Because there are variants of galactosemia, the parental and proband's enzyme levels should be well documented to ensure the accuracy of the prenatal test.[171] Prenatal diagnosis and carrier detection are also possible with the DNA-based test.[172]

Galactokinase Deficiency

In galactokinase deficiency, the enzyme deficiency lies in galactokinase, which normally catalyzes the phosphorylation of galactose. The principal metabolites accumulated in this disorder are galactose and galactitol. The gene coding for galactokinase has been cloned and mapped to chromosome 17q24. Mutations leading to galactokinase deficiency have been identified.[173]

In contrast to the multiple systems that are affected in transferase deficiency galactosemia, cataract and rarely pseudotumor are the only consistent manifestations of galactokinase deficiency.[174] The affected infant is otherwise asymptomatic. These patients have an increased concentration of blood galactose levels, with normal transferase activity and an absence of galactokinase activity in erythrocytes. Treatment is dietary control of galactose intake.

The disease is inherited as an autosomal recessive trait. Carrier detection has been performed using erythrocytes or skin fibroblasts for measurement of the enzyme activity.[175] Prenatal diagnosis is possible by measurement of galactokinase activity in cultured amniotic cells but probably is not indicated for this relatively benign and treatable condition.

Uridine Diphosphate Galactose-4-Epimerase (UDPgal-4-Epimerase) Deficiency

The abnormally accumulated metabolites are very much like those seen in transferase deficiency; however, there is also an increase in cellular UDPgal. There are two distinct forms of epimerase deficiency. A benign form was discovered incidentally through a neonatal screening program.[176] Affected persons in this case are healthy; the enzyme deficiency is limited to leukocytes and erythrocytes without deranged metabolism in other tissues. The second form is severe, with clinical manifestations resembling transferase deficiency, with the additional symptoms of hypotonia and nerve deafness.[177,178] The enzyme deficiency is generalized and clinical symptoms respond to restriction of dietary galactose.

Because patients with epimerase deficiency cannot make galactose and it is an essential component of many nervous system structural proteins, patients are placed on a galactose-restricted diet rather than a galactose-free diet.

The gene for UDPgal 4-epimerase has been cloned and mapped to chromosome 1 at 1p35-1pter.[179,180] Carrier detection is possible by measurement of epimerase activity in the erythrocytes.[178] Prenatal diagnosis for the severe form of epimerase deficiency, using an enzyme assay of cultured amniotic fluid cells, has been achieved.[178]

DISORDERS OF FRUCTOSE METABOLISM

Essential Fructosuria

Essential fructosuria is an asymptomatic metabolic anomaly caused by a deficiency of fructokinase activity in the liver, kidney, and intestine.[181] Affected persons are usually discovered on routine urinalysis to have a reducing substance. The identification of fructose by thin-layer paper or gas–liquid chromatography suggests the diagnosis. Liver biopsies conducted solely to demonstrate the enzyme deficiency are probably not warranted.

The disease is inherited as an autosomal recessive trait. The gene coding for fructokinase has been cloned and mutations have been identified.[182] Prenatal diagnosis is not indicated for this benign condition.

Hereditary Fructose Intolerance (Fructose-1-Phosphate Aldolase B Deficiency)

Hereditary fructose intolerance is caused by deficiency of fructose-1-phosphate aldolase B activity in the liver, kidney, and intestine.[181] The enzyme catalyzes the hydrolysis of fructose-1-phosphate into triose phosphate and glyceraldehyde. Deficiency of this enzyme activity causes a rapid accumulation of fructose-1-phosphate and initiates severe toxic symptoms when exposed to fructose. The gene for aldolase B has been cloned and mapped to chromosome 9q22.3.[183,184]

Patients with fructose intolerance are perfectly healthy and asymptomatic until fructose is ingested (usually from fruit, fruit juice, or sweetened cereal). The infant becomes acutely ill, with vomiting, abdominal pain, sweating, lethargy, and even convulsions and coma. Repeated exposure to fructose leads to hepatomegaly and failure to thrive.

The clinical picture is accompanied by deranged metabolism of liver and kidney, manifested by a prolonged clotting time, hypoalbuminuria, elevation of bilirubin and transaminases, and proximal renal tubular dysfunction. Suspicion of the enzyme deficiency is fostered by the presence of a reducing substance in the urine during an attack. The diagnosis is supported by an intravenous fructose tolerance test, which will cause a rapid fall—first of serum phosphate, then of blood glucose—and a subsequent rise of uric acid and magnesium. Definitive diagnosis is made by assay of fructaldolase B activity in the liver. Treatment of acute illness consists of the complete elimination of all sources of sucrose, fructose, and sorbitol from the diet. Liver and kidney dysfunction is reversible, and catch-up in growth is common. Intellectual development is usually unimpaired. As the patient matures, symptoms become milder even after fructose ingestion, and the long-term prognosis is good.

The incidence of hereditary fructose intolerance is approximately 1 in 20,000. Several mutations causing heredity fructose intolerance have recently been identified. A single missense mutation, a G-to-C transversion in exon 5, which results in the normal alanine at position 149 being replaced by a proline, is the most common mutation identified in northern Europeans. This mutation, plus two other point mutations, account for approximately 80–85 percent of hereditary fructose intolerance in Europe and the United States.[185–189] Diagnosis of hereditary fructose intolerance can thus be made by direct DNA analysis. Prenatal diagnosis should be possible from both amniocentesis and chorionic villi, using DNA mutation or linkage analysis.

DISORDERS OF GLUCONEOGENESIS

Fructose-1,6-Diphosphatase Deficiency

Fructose-1,6-diphosphatase deficiency is not a defect in the fructose pathway; instead, it is a defect involved in gluconeogenesis. The disease is characterized by life-threatening episodes of acidosis, hypoglycemia, hyperventilation, convulsions, and coma.[181] In infants and small children, episodes are triggered when oral food intake decreases. The disease resembles hereditary fructose intolerance because of reduced tolerance to fructose. However, there is no aversion to sweets, and renal tubular and liver functions are usually normal. Treatment consists of avoidance of fasting and elimination of fructose and sucrose from the diet. For long-term prevention of hypoglycemia, a slowly released carbohydrate such as cornstarch is useful. Patients who survive childhood seem to develop normally.

The diagnosis is established by demonstrating an enzyme deficiency in either liver or an intestinal biopsy.[190] The enzyme defect may also be demonstrated in leukocytes or cultured lymphocytes.[191] Urine glycerol-3-phosphate and glycerol can also be used in detection of the fructose-1,6-diphosphatase deficiency.[192] Obligate heterozygotes have an intermediate enzyme activity level in the liver. Because fructose-1,6-diphosphatase activity is not expressed in amniotic fluid cells or chorionic villi, prenatal diagnosis by measurement of enzyme activity in these tissues is not possible. The gene coding for fructose-1,6-diphosphatase has been cloned and mapped to chromosome 9q22.[193,194] Mutations have been characterized, and carrier detection and prenatal diagnosis should be possible using the DNA-based test.

Phosphoenolpyruvate Carboxykinase Deficiency

Phosphoenolpyruvate carboxykinase (PEPCK) is a key enzyme in gluconeogenesis. It catalyzes the conversion of oxaloacetate to phosphoenolpyruvate. PEPCK deficiency has been described both as a mitochondrial enzyme deficiency and as a cytosolic enzyme deficiency.[195,196]

The disease has been reported in only six cases. The clinical features are heterogeneous, with hypoglycemia, hepatomegaly, hypotonia, developmental delay, and failure to thrive as the major manifestations.[195–198] Hepatic and renal dysfunction may be present. The diagnosis is based on the reduced activity of PEPCK in liver, fibroblasts, or lymphocytes. Fibroblasts and lymphocytes are not suitable for diagnosing the cytosolic form of PEPCK deficiency because these tissues possess only mitochondrial PEPCK. Prenatal diagnosis is possible for the mitochondrial form of PEPCK deficiency by cultured amniocytes, but this has not yet been done.

Pentosuria

Pentosuria is a benign condition in which pentose L-xylulose is excreted in the urine.[199] The disorder is caused by a deficiency of activity of nicotinamide adenine dinucleotide phosphate (NADP)–linked xylitol dehydrogenase (L-xylulose reductase), an enzyme involved in the glucuronic acid oxidation pathway. This is an autosomal recessive inherited condition that occurs mainly in the Jewish population. The most common clinical problem is the misdiagnosis of pentosuria as diabetes mellitus. The presence in the urine of a reducing substance that does not react with glucose oxidase reagent suggests the diagnosis, but fructose, galactose, and lactose can give similar results. The heterozygote can be recognized by demonstrating either an intermediate level of erythrocyte enzyme activity or increased urinary or serum L-xylulose, or both, in a glucuronolactone loading test.[200] Prenatal diagnosis is not indicated for this innocuous condition.

ACKNOWLEDGMENTS

I thank Denise Peterson and Dr. Deeksha Bali for their conscientious help in the laboratory with the diagnostic studies for these disorders. Research on these disorders has been sponsored by National Institutes of Health Grants DK39078 and M01-RR30, the National

Center for Research Resources, General Clinical Research Centers Program, a grant from the Muscular Dystrophy Association, and a generous contribution to the Duke GSD fund by E.B. Mandel, and Pompe Children Foundation.

REFERENCES

1. Chen Y-T. Glycogen storage diseases. In Scriver CR, et al., eds. The metabolic and molecular bases of inherited disease, 8th ed. New York: McGraw-Hill, 2001:1521.
2. Chen Y-T. Glycogen storage disease and other inherited disorders of carbohydrate metabolism. In: Harrison's principles of internal medicine, 16th ed. in press 2003.
3. Huijing F, Fernandes J. X-Chromosomal inheritance of liver glycogenosis with phosphorylase kinase deficiency. Am J Hum Genet 1969;21:275.
4. Von Gierke E. Hepato-nephro-megalia glykogenia (Glykogenspeicher-krankheit der Leber und Nieren). Beitr Pathol Anat 1929;82:497.
5. Cori GT, Cori CF. Glucose 6-phosphatase of the liver in glycogen storage disease. J Biol Chem 1952;199:661.
6. Narisawa K, Igarashi Y, Otomo H, et al. A new variant of glycogen storage disease type I probably due to a defect in the glucose 6-phosphate transport system. Biochem Biophys Res Commun 1978;83:1360.
7. Lange AJ, Arion WJ, Beaudet AL. Type Ib glycogen storage disease is caused by a defect in the glucose 6-phosphate translocase of the microsomal glucose 6-phosphatase system. J Biol Chem 1980;255:8381.
8. Kao K-J, Coleman RA, Pizzo SV. The bleeding diathesis in human glycogen storage disease type I: in vitro identification of a naturally occurring inhibitor of ristocetin-induced platelet aggregation. Thromb Res 1980;18:683.
9. Alaupovic P, Fernandes J. The serum apolipoprotein profile of patients with glucose 6-phosphatase deficiency. Pediatr Res 1985;19:380.
10. Levy E, Thiabault LA, Roy CC, et al. Circulating lipids and lipoproteins in glycogen storage disease type I with nocturnal intragastric feeding. J Lipid Res 1988;29:215.
11. Lee P, Patel A, Hindmarsh P, Mowat A, et al. The prevalence of polycystic ovaries in the hepatic glycogen storage disease: its association with hyperinsulinism. Clin Endocrinol 1995;42:601.
12. Farber M, Knuppel RA, Binkiewicz A, et al. Pregnancy and von Gierke's disease. Obstet Gynecol 1976;47:226.
13. Johnson MP, Compton A, Drugan A, et al. Metabolic control of von Gierke disease (glycogen storage disease type Ia) in pregnancy: maintenance of euglycemia with cornstarch. Obstet Gynecol 1990;75:507.
14. Michels VV, Beaudet AL. Hemorrhagic pancreatitis in a patient with glycogen storage disease type I. Clin Genet 1980;17:220.
15. Talente G, Coleman R, Alter C, et al. Glycogen storage disease in adults: a retrospective study of clinical and laboratory findings in types Ia, Ib, and III. Ann Intern Med 1994;120:218.
16. Ubels FL, Rake JP, Slaets JP, et al. Is glycogen storage disease 1a associated with atherosclerosis? Eur J Pediatr 2002;161 (suppl 1):S62.
17. Bandsma RH, Rake J-P, Visser G et al. Increased lipogenesis and resistance of lipoproteins to oxidative modification in two patients with glycogen storage disease type Ia. J Pediatr 2002;140:256.
18. Wittenstein B, Klein M, Finckh B, et al. Radical trapping in glycogen storage disease la. Eur J Pediatr 2002;161 (suppl 1):S70.
19. Howell RR, Stevenson RE, Ben-Menachen Y, et al. Hepatic adenomata with type I glycogen storage disease. JAMA 1976;236:1481.
20. Coire CI, Qizilbash AH, Castelli MF. Hepatic adenomata in type Ia glycogen storage disease. Arch Pathol Lab Med 1987;111:166.
21. Limmer J, Fleig WE, Leupold D, et al. Hepatocellular carcinoma in type I glycogen storage disease. Hepatology 1988;8:531.
22. Kishnani P, Bengur AK, Chen YT. Pulmonary hypertension in glycogen storage disease type I. J Inherit Metab Dis 1996;19:213.
23. Humbert M, Labrune P, Simonneau G. Severe pulmonary arterial hypertension in type 1 glycogen storage disease. Eur J Pediatr 2002;161 (suppl 1):S93.
24. Chen Y-T, Coleman RA, Scheinman JI, et al. Renal disease in type I glycogen storage disease. N Engl J Med 1988;318:7.
25. Baker L, Dahiem S, Goldfarb S, et al. Hyperfiltration and renal disease in glycogen storage disease type I. Kidney Int 1989;35:1345.

26. Chen Y-T. Type I glycogen storage disease, kidney involvement, pathogenesis and its treatment. Pediatr Nephrol 1991;5:71.

27. Chen Y-T, Scheinman JI, Park HK, et al. Amelioration of proximal renal tubular dysfunction in type I glycogen storage disease with dietary therapy. N Engl J Med 1990;323:590.

28. Weinstein DA, Somers MJ, Wolfsdorf JI. Decreased urinary citrate excretion in type Ia glycogen storage disease. J Pediatr 2001;138:378–82.

29. Beaudet AL, Anderson DC, Michels VV, et al. Neutropenia and impaired neutrophil migration in type Ib glycogen storage disease. J Pediatr 1980;97:906.

30. Visser G, Rake JP, Fernandes J, et al. Neutropenia, neutrophil dysfunction, and inflammatory bowel disease in glycogen storage disease type Ib: results of the European study on glycogen storage disease type I. J Pediatr 2000;137:187–90.

31. Kuijpers TW, Maianski NA, Tool AT, et al. Apoptotic neutrophils in the circulation of patients with glycogen storage disease type 1b (GSD1b). Blood 2003 [e-pub ahead of print].

32. Chou JY, Matern D, Mansfield BC, Chen YT. Type I glycogen storage diseases: disorders of the glucose-6-phosphatase complex. Curr Mol Med 2002;2:121.

33. Greene HL, Slonim AE, O'Neil JA, et al. Continuous nocturnal intragastric feeding for management of type I glycogen storage disease. N Engl J Med 1976;294:423.

34. Wolfsdorf JI, Crigler JF Jr. Effect of continuous glucose therapy begun in infancy on the long-term clinical course of patients with type I glycogen storage disease. J Pediatr Gastroenterol Nutr 1999;29:136.

35. Chen Y-T, Cornblath M, Sidbury JB. Cornstarch therapy in type I glycogen storage disease. N Engl J Med 1984;310:171.

36. Smit GPA, Berger R, Potasnick R, et al. The dietary treatment of children with type I glycogen storage disease with slow release carbohydrate. Pediatr Res 1984;18:879.

37. Wolfsdorf JI, Keller FJ, Landy H, et al. Glucose therapy for glycogenosis type I in infants: Comparison of intermittent uncooked cornstarch and continuous overnight glucose feedings. J Pediatr 1990;117:384.

38. Hayde M, Widhalm K. Effects of cornstarch treatment in very young children with type I glycogen storage disease. Eur J Pediatr 1990;149:630.

39. Vici CD, Bartuli A, Mazziotta MRM, et al. Early introduction of uncooked cornstarch for the treatment of glycogen storage disease type I. Acta Paediatr Scand 1990;79:978.

40. Wang W, Crist W, Ihle L, et al. Granulocyte colony-stimulating factor corrects the neutropenia associated with glycogen storage disease type Ib. Leukemia 1991;5:347.

41. Schroten H, Roesler J, Breidenbach T, et al. Granulocyte and granulocyte-macrophage colony-stimulating factors for treatment of neutropenia in glycogen storage disease type Ib. J Pediatr 1991;119:748.

42. Field JB, Epstein S, Egan T. Studies in glycogen storage disease. I. Intestinal glucose 6-phosphatase activity in patients with von Gierke's disease and their parents. J Clin Invest 1965;44:1240.

43. Golbus MS, Simpson TJ, Koresawa M, et al. The prenatal determination of glucose 6-phosphatase activity by fetal liver biopsy. Prenat Diagn 1988;8:401.

44. Lei K-J, Shelly LL, Pan C-J, et al. Mutations in the glucose 6-phosphatase gene that cause glycogen storage disease type Ia. Science 1993;262:580.

45. Lei K-J, Chen Y-T, Chen H, et al. Genetic basis of glycogen storage disease type Ia: prevalent mutations at the glucose 6-phosphatase locus. Am J Hum Genet 1995;57:766.

46. Veiga-da-Cunha M, Gerin I, Chen YT, et al. A Gene on chromosome 11q23 coding for a putative glucose 6-phosphate translocase is mutated in glycogen storage disease type Ib and type Ic. Am J Hum Genet 1998;63:976.

47. Kure S, Suzuki Y, Matsubara Y, et al. Molecular analysis of glycogen storage disease type Ib: identification of a prevalent mutation among Japanese patients and assignment of a putative glucose-6-phosphate translocase gene to chromosome 11. Biochem Biophys Res Commun 1998;248:426.

48. Wong LJ. Prenatal diagnosis of glycogen storage disease type Ia by direct mutation detection. Prenat Diagn 1996;16:105.

49. Lam CW, Sin SY, Lau ET, Lam YY, Poon P, Tong SF. 2000. Prenatal diagnosis of glycogen storage disease type Ib using denaturing high performance liquid chromatography. Prenat Diagn 20:765.

50. Hers HG. α-Glucosidase deficiency in generalized glycogen storage disease (Pompe's disease). Biochem J 1963;86:11.

51. Hirschhorn R, Reuser AJ: Glycogen storage disease type II: Acid β-glucosidase (acid maltase) deficiency. In: The metabolic and molecular bases of inherited disease, 8th ed. Scriver CR, et al., eds. New York, McGraw-Hill, 2001:1389.

52. Martiniuk FM, Mehler M, Pellicer A, et al. Isolation of a cDNA for human acid α-glucosidase and detection of genetic heterogeneity for mRNA in three α-glucosidase deficient patients. Proc Natl Acad Sci USA 1986;83:9641.

53. Hoefsloot LH, Hoogeveen-Westerveld M, Kroos MA. Primary structure and processing of lysosomal α-glucosidase: homology with the intestinal sucrase-isomaltase complex. EMBO J 1988;7:1697.

54. Umapathysivam K, Hopwood JJ, Meikle PJ. Determination of acid alpha-glucosidase activity in blood spots as a diagnostic test for Pompe disease. Clin Chem 2001;47:1378.

55. An Y, Young SP, Hillman SL, Van Hove JLK, Chen Y-T, Millington D. Liquid chromatographic assay for a glucose tetrasaccharide, a putative biomarker for the diagnosis of Pompe disease. Anal Biochem 2002;287:136.

56. Slonim AE, Coleman RA, McElligot MA. Improvement of muscle function in acid maltase deficiency by high-protein therapy. Neurology 1983;33:34.

57. Umpleby AM, Wiles CM, Trend P, et al. Protein turnover in acid maltase deficiency before and after treatment with a high protein diet. J Neurol Neurosurg Psychiatry 1987;50:587.

58. Amalfitano A, Bengur AR, Morse RP, et al. Recombinant human acid-β- glucosidase enzyme therapy for infantile glycogen storage disease type II: results of a phase I/II clinical trial. Genet Med 2001;3:132–38.

59. Van den Hout H, Reuser AJJ, Vulto AG, Loonen MCB, Cromme-Dljkhuis A, Van der Ploeg AT. Recombinant human α-glucosidase from rabbit milk in Pompe patients. Lancet 2000;356:397.

60. Hirschhorn K, Nadler HL, Waithe WI, et al. Pompe's disease: detection of heterozygotes by lymphocyte stimulation. Science 1969;166:1632.

61. Engel AG, Gomez MR. Acid maltase levels in muscle in heterozygous acid maltase deficiency and in nonweak and neuromuscular disease controls. J Neurol Neurosurg Psychiatry 1970;33:801.

62. Loonen MCB, Schram AW, Koster JF, et al. Identification of heterozygotes for glycogenosis 2 (acid maltase deficiency). Clin Genet 1981;19:55.

63. Fujimoto A, Fluharty AL, Stevens RL, et al. Two alpha-glucosidases in cultured amniotic fluid cells and their differentiation in the prenatal diagnosis of Pompe's disease. Clin Chim Acta 1976;68:177.

64. Lin C-Y, Hwang B, Hsiao K-J, et al. Pompe's disease in Chinese and prenatal diagnosis by determination of α-glucosidase activity. J Inherit Metab Dis 1987;10:11.

65. Hug G, Soukup S, Ryan M, et al. Rapid prenatal diagnosis of glycogen-storage disease type II by electron microscopy of uncultured amniotic-fluid cells. N Engl J Med 1984;310:1018.

66. Park HK, Kay HH, McConkie-Rosell A, et al. Prenatal diagnosis of Pompe's disease (type II glycogenosis in chorionic villi biopsy using maltose as a substrate. Prenat Diagn 1992;12:169.

67. Poenaru L, Kaplan L, Dumoz J, et al. Evaluation of possible first trimester prenatal diagnosis in lysosomal diseases by trophoblast biopsy. Pediatr Res 1984;18:1032.

68. Besancon A-M, Castelnau L, Nicolesco H, et al. Prenatal diagnosis of glycogenosis type II (Pompe's disease) using chorionic villi biopsy. Clin Genet 1985;27:479.

69. Grubisic A, Shin YS, Meyer W, et al. First trimester diagnosis of Pompe's disease (glycogenosis type II) with normal outcome: assay of acid α-glucosidase in chorionic villous biopsy using antibodies. Clin Genet 1986;30:298.

70. Shin YS, Rieth M, Tausenfreund J, et al. First trimester diagnosis of glycogen storage disease type II and type III. J Inherit Metab Dis 1989;12:289.

71. Hug G, Chuck G, Chen Y-T, et al. Chorionic villi ultrastructure in type II glycogen storage disease Pompe's disease). N Engl J Med 1991;324:342.

72. Kroos MA, Van der Kraan M, Van Diggelen OP, et al. Glycogen storage disease type II: frequency of three common mutant alleles and their associated clinical phenotypes studied in 121 patients. J Med Genet 1995;32(10):836.

73. Kleijer WJ, Van Der Kraan M, Kroos MA, et al. Prenatal diagnosis of glycogen storage disease type II: Enzyme assay or mutation analysis? Pediatr Res 1995;38:103.

74. Illingworth B, Cori GT, Cori CF. Amylo-1,6-glucosidase in muscle-tissue in generalized glycogen storage disease. J Biol Chem 1956;218:123.

75. Chen Y-T, He J-K, Ding J-H, et al. Glycogen debranching enzyme: purification, antibody characterization and immunoblot analyses of type III glycogen storage disease. Am J Hum Genet 1987;41:1002.

76. Ding J-H, deBarsy T, Brown BI, et al. Immunoblot analysis of glycogen debranching enzyme in different subtypes of type III glycogen storage disease. J Pediatr 1990;116:95.

77. Yang B-Z, Ding J-H, Enghild JJ, et al. Molecular cloning and nucleotide sequence of cDNA encoding human muscle glycogen debranching enzyme. J Biol Chem 1992;267:9294.

78. Shen J, Bao Y, Liu H-M, et al. Mutations in exon 3 of the glycogen debranching enzyme gene are associated with glycogen storage disease type III that is differentially expressed in liver and muscle. J Clin Invest 1996;98:352.

79. Shen J, Bao Y, Chen Y-T. A nonsense mutation due to a single base insertion in the 39 coding region of glycogen debranching enzyme gene associated with a severe phenotype in a patient with glycogen storage disease type IIIa. Hum Mutat 1997;9:37.

80. Brown BI, Brown DH. Glycogen storage disease: Types I, III, IV, V, VII and unclassified glycogenoses. In: Dickens F, Randle PJ, Whelan WJ, eds. Carbohydrate metabolism and its disorders, vol. 2. New York: Academic Press, 1968:123.

81. Cornelio F, Bresolin N, Singer PA, et al. Clinical varieties of neuromuscular disease in debrancher deficiency. Arch Neurol 1984;5:289.

82. Moses SW, Gadoth N, Bashan N, et al. Neuromuscular involvement in glycogen storage disease type III. Acta Paediatr Scand 1986;5:289.

83. Brown BI, Brown DH. Definitive assays for glycogen debranching enzyme in human fibroblasts. In: Schotland DL, ed. Diseases of the motor unit. New York: John Wiley, 1982:667.

84. Sidbury JB Jr, Gitzelmann R, Fischer J. The glycogenoses: further observations on glycogen in erythrocytes of patients with glycogenosis. Helv Paediatr Acta 1961;16:506.

85. Shin YS, Ungar R, Rieth M, et al. A simple assay for amylo-1–6-glucosidase to detect heterozygotes for glycogenosis type III in erythrocytes. Clin Chem 1984;30:1717.

86. Borowitz SM, Greene HL. Cornstarch therapy in a patient with type III glycogen storage disease. Am J Hum Genet 1990;47:735.

87. Slonim AE, Weisberg C, Benke P. Reversal of debrancher deficiency myopathy by the use of high-protein nutrition. Ann Neurol 1982;11:420.

88. Yang B-Z, Ding J-H, Brown BI, et al. Definitive prenatal diagnosis for type III glycogen storage disease type III. J Hum Genet 1990;47:735.

89. van Diggelen OP, Janse HC, Smith GPA. Debranching enzyme in fibroblasts, amniotic fluid cells and chorionic villi: pre- and postnatal diagnosis of glycogenosis type III. Clin Chim Acta 1985;419:129.

90. Shaiu W, Kishnani P, Shen J, Chen YT. Genotype–phenotype correlation in two frequent mutations and mutation update in type III glycogen storage disease. Mol Genet Metab 2000;69:16.

91. Shen JJ, Chen YT. Molecular characterization of glycogen storage disease type III. Curr Mol Med 2002;2:167.

92. Shen J, Liu H-M, McConkie-Rosell A, Chen Y-T. Prenatal diagnosis and carrier detection for glycogen storage disease type III using polymorphic DNA markers. Prenat Diagn 1998;18:61.

93. Illingworth B, Cori GT. Structure of glycogens and amylopectins. III. Normal and abnormal human glycogen. J Biol Chem 1952;199:653.

94. Brown BI, Brown DH. Lack of an α-1, 4-glucan: α-1-4-Glucan 6-glycosyl transferase in a case of type IV glycogenosis. Proc Natl Acad Sci USA 1966;56:725.

95. Guerra AS, van Diggelen OP, Carneiro F, et al. A new variant of type IV glycogenosis IV (Andersen disease). Eur J Pediatr 1986;145:179.

96. Greene HL, Brown BI, McClenathan DT, et al. A new variant of type IV glycogenosis: deficiency of branching enzyme activity without apparent progressive liver disease. Hepatology 1988;8:302.

97. McConkie-Rosell A, Wilson C, Piccoli DA, et al. Clinical and laboratory findings in four patients with the non-progressive hepatic form of type IV glycogen storage disease. J Inherit Metab Dis 1996;19:51.

98. Servidei S, Riepe RE, Langston C, et al. Severe cardiopathy in branching enzyme deficiency. J Pediatr 1987;111:51.

99. Bao Y, Kishnani P, Wu J-Y, et al. Hepatic and neuromuscular forms of glycogen storage disease type IV caused by mutations in the same glycogen-branching enzyme gene. J Clin Invest 1996;97:941.

100. Selby R, Starzi TE, Yunis E, et al. Liver transplantation for type IV glycogen storage disease. N Engl J Med 1991;324:39.

101. Shin YS, Steiguber H, Klemm P, et al. Branching enzyme in erythrocytes: detection of type IV glycogenosis homozygotes and heterozygotes. J Inherit Metab Dis 1988;11 (suppl 2):252.

102. Howell RR, Kaback MM, Brown BI. Type IV glycogen storage disease: branching enzyme deficiency in skin fibroblasts and possible heterozygote detection. J Pediatr 1971;78:638.

103. Brown BI, Brown DH. Branching enzyme activity of cultured amniocytes and chorionic villi: prenatal testing for type IV glycogen storage disease. Am J Hum Genet 1989;44:378.

104. Shen J, Lui H-M, McConkie-Rosell A, Chen Y-T. A prenatal diagnosis of glycogen storage disease type IV using PCR-based DNA mutation analysis. Prenat Diagn 1999;19:837.

105. Lebo RV, Gorin F, Fletterick RJ, et al. High resolution chromosome sorting and DNA spot-blot analysis assign McArdle's syndrome to chromosome 11. Science 1984;225:57.
106. Martinuzzi A, Sartori E, Fanin M, et al. Phenotype modulators in myophosphorylase deficiency. Ann Neurol 2003;53:497.
107. Vorgerd M, Zange J, Kley R et al. Effect of high-dose creatine therapy on symptoms of exercise intolerance in McArdle disease: double-blind, placebo-controlled crossover study. Arch Neurol 2002;59:97.
108. Dimauro S, Hartlage PL. Fatal infantile form of muscle phosphorylase deficiency. Neurology 1978;28:1124.
109. de la Marza M, Patten BM, Williams JC, et al. Myophosphorylase deficiency: a new cause of infantile hypotonia simulating infantile muscular atrophy. Neurology 1980;30:402.
110. Milstein JM, Herron TM, Haas JE. Fatal infantile form muscle phosphorylase deficiency. J Child Neurol 1989;4:186.
111. Cornelio F, Bresolin N, Dimauro S, et al. Congenital myopathy due to phosphorylase deficiency. Neurology 1983;33:1383.
112. Ross BD, Radda GK, Gadian DG. Examination of a case of suspected McArdle's syndrome by ^{31}P nuclear magnetic resonance. N Engl J Med 1981;304:1338.
113. Bank WJ, DiMauro S, Rowland LP, et al. Heterozygotes in muscle phosphorylase deficiency. Trans Am Neurol Assoc 1972;97:179.
114. Bogusky RT, Taylor RG, Anderson LJ, et al. McArdle's disease heterozygotes: metabolic adaptation assessed using ^{31}P-nuclear magnetic resonance. J Clin Invest 1986;77:1881.
115. Tsujino S, Shanske S, Nonaka I, et al. The molecular genetic basis of myophosphorylase deficiency (McArdle's disease). Muscle Nerve 1995;3:S23.
116. el-Schahawi M, Tsujino S, Shanske S, et al. Diagnosis of McArdle's disease by molecular genetic analysis of blood. Neurology 1996;47:579.
117. Newgard CB, Fletterick RJ, Anderson LA, et al. The polymorphic locus for glycogen storage disease VI (liver phosphorylase) maps to chromosome 14. Am J Hum Genet 1987;40:351.
118. Newgard CB, Nakano K, Hwang PK, et al. Sequence analysis of cDNA encoding human liver glycogen phosphorylase reveals tissue-specific codon usage. Proc Natl Acad Sci USA 1986;83:8132.
119. Uyeda K. Phosphofructokinase. Adv Enzymol 1979;48:193.
120. Vora S, Hong F, Olender E. Isolation of a cDNA for human muscle 6-phosphofructokinase. Biochem Biophys Res Commun 1986;135:615.
121. Nakajima H, Kono N, Yamasaki T, et al. Genetic defect in muscle phosphofructokinase deficiency. Biol Chem 1990;265:9392.
122. Tsujino S, Servidei S, Tonin P, et al. Identification of three novel mutations in non-Ashkenazi Italian patients with muscle phosphofructokinase deficiency. Am J Hum Genet 1994;54:812.
123. Sherman JB, Raben N, Nicastri C, et al. Common mutations in the phosphofructokinase-M gene in Ashkenazi Jewish patients with glycogenesis VII—and their population frequency. Am J Hum Genet 1994;55:305.
124. Nakajima H, Hamaguchi T, Yamasaki T, et al. Phosphofructokinase deficiency: recent advances in molecular biology. Muscle Nerve 1995;3:S28.
125. Danon MJ, Carpenter S, Manaligod JR, et al. Fatal infantile glycogen storage disease: deficiency of phosphofructokinase and phosphorylase b kinase. Neurology 1981;31:1303.
126. Servidei S, Bonilla E, Diedrich RG, et al. Fatal infantile form of muscle phosphofructokinase deficiency. Neurology 1986;36:1465.
127. Kahn A, Weil D, Cottreau D, et al. Muscle phosphofructokinase deficiency in man: expression of the defect in blood cells and cultured fibroblasts. Ann Hum Genet 1981;45:5.
128. Layzer RB, Rowland LP, Bank WJ. Physical and kinetic properties of human phosphofructokinase from skeletal muscle and erythrocytes. J Biol Chem 1969;244:3823.
129. Van Den Berg IET, Berger R. Phosphorylase b kinase deficiency in man: a review. J Inherit Metab Dis 1990;13:442.
130. Kilimann MW, Zander NF, Kuhn CC, et al. The α and β subunits of phosphorylase kinase are homologous: cDNA cloning and primary structure of the β subunit. Proc Natl Acad Sci USA 1988;85:9381.
131. Zander NF, Meyer HE, Hoffmann-Posorske E, et al. cDNA cloning and complete primary structure of skeletal muscle phosphorylase kinase (α subunit). Proc Natl Acad Sci USA 1988;85:2929.
132. Da Cruz E, Silva EF, Cohen PTW. Isolation and sequence analysis of a cDNA clone encoding the entire catalytic subunit of phosphorylase kinase. FEBS Lett 1987;220:36.
133. Bender PK, Emerson CP. Skeletal muscle phosphorylase kinase catalytic subunit mRNAs are expressed in heart tissue but not in liver. J Biol Chem 1987;262:8799.

134. Francke U, Darras BT, Zander NF, et al. Assignment of human genes for phosphorylase kinase subunits α (PHKA) to Xq12-q13 and β (PHKB) to 16q12-q13. Am J Hum Genet 1989;45:276.

135. Willems PJ, Hendrickx J, Van der Auwera BJ, et al. Mapping of the gene for X-linked liver glycogenosis due to phosphorylase kinase deficiency to human chromosome region Xp22. Genomics 1991;9:565.

136. Wehner M, Clemens PR, Engel AG, et al. Human muscle glycogenosis due to phosphorylase kinase deficiency associated with a nonsense mutation in the muscle isoform of the α subunit. Hum Mol Genet 1994;3:1983.

137. Hendrickx J, Coucke P, Dams E, et al. Mutations in the phosphorylase kinase gene PHKA2 are responsible for X-linked liver glycogen storage disease. Hum Mol Genet 1995;4:77.

138. Hendricks J, Dams E, Coucke P, et al. X-linked liver glycogenosis type II (XLG II) is caused by mutations in PHKA2, the gene encoding the liver alpha subunit of phosphorylase kinase. Hum Mol Genet 1996;5:649.

139. Maichele AJ, Burwinkel B, Maire I, et al. Mutations in the testis/liver isoform of the phosphorylase kinase g subunit (PHKG2) cause autosomal liver glycogenosis in the gsd rat and in humans. Nature Genet 1996;14:337.

140. Willems PJ, Gerver WJM, Berger R, et al. The natural history of liver glycogenosis due to phosphorylase kinase deficiency: a longitudinal study of 41 patients. Eur J Pediatr 1990;149:268.

141. Burwinkel B, Shiomi S, Al Zaben A, et al. Liver glycogenosis due to phosphorylase kinase deficiency: PHKG2 gene structure and mutations associated with cirrhosis. Hum Mol Genet 1998;7:149.

142. Ohtani Y, Matsuda I, Iwamasa T, et al. Infantile glycogen storage myopathy in a girl with phosphorylase kinase deficiency. Neurology 1982;32:833.

143. Eishi T, Takemura T, Sone R, et al. Glycogen storage disease confined to the heart with deficient activity of cardiac phosphorylase kinase: a new type of glycogen storage disease. Hum Pathol 1985;16:193.

144. Servidel S, Metlay LA, Chodosh J, et al. Fatal infantile cardiopathy caused by phosphorylase b kinase deficiency. J Pediatr 1988;113:82.

145. Huijing F. Phosphorylase kinase in leukocytes of normal subjects and of patients with storage disease. Biochim Biophys Acta 1967;148:601.

146. Lederer B, Van Hoof F, Van den Berghe G, et al. Glycogen phosphorylase and its converter enzymes in haemolysates of normal human subjects and of patients with type VI glycogen storage disease: a study of phosphorylase kinase deficiency. Biochem J 1975;147:23.

147. Wallis PG, Sidbury JB, Harris RC. Hepatic phosphorylase defect: studies on peripheral blood. Am J Dis Child 1966;111:278.

148. Aynsley-Green A, Williamson DH, Gitzelman R. Hepatic glycogen synthetase deficiency. Arch Dis Child 1977;52:573.

149. Gitzelmann R, Spycher MA, Feil G, et al. Liver glycogen synthase deficiency: a rarely diagnosed entity. Eur J Pediatr 1996;155:561.

150. Orho M, Bosshard N, Buisl N, et al. Mutations in the liver glycogen synthase gene in children with hypoglycemia due to glycogen storage disease type 0. J Clin Invest 1998;102:507.

151. Santer R, Schneppenheim R, Dombrowski A, et al. Mutations in GLUT2, the gene for the liver-type glucose transporter, in patients with Fanconi–Bickel syndrome. Nat Genet 1997;17:324.

152. Reichardt JKV, Berg P. Cloning and characterization of a cDNA encoding human galactose 1-phosphate uridyl transferase. Mol Biol Med 1988;5:107.

153. Sparkes RS, Sparkes MC, Funderburk SJ, et al. Expression of GALT in 9p chromosome alterations: assignment of GALT locus to 9 cen-9p22. Am J Hum Genet 1980;43:343.

154. Novelli G, Reichardt JK. Molecular basis of disorders of human galactose metabolism: past, present, and future. Mol Genet Metab 2000;71:62.

155. Elsas LJ 2nd, Lai K. The molecular biology of galactosemia. Genet Med 1998;1:40.

156. Holton JB et al. Galactosemia. In: Scriver CR, et al., eds. The metabolic and molecular bases of inherited disease, 8th ed. New York: McGraw-Hill, 2001:1553.

157. Kaufman FR, Gut KO, Donnell GN, et al. Hypergonadotropic hypogonadism in female patients with galactosemia. N Engl J Med 1981;304:994.

158. Friedman JH, Levy HL, Boustany R-M. Late onset of distinct neurologic syndromes in galactosemic siblings. Neurology 1989;39:741.

159. Lo W, Packman S, Nash S, et al. Curious neurologic sequelae in galactosemia. Pediatrics 1984;73:309.

160. Waggon DD, Buist NRM, Donnell GN. Long-term prognosis in galactosaemia: results of a survey of 350 cases. J Inherit Metab Dis 1990;13:802.

161. Brivet M, Raymond JP, Konopka P, et al. Effect of lactation in a mother with galactosemia. J Pediatr 1989;115:280.

162. Brivet M, Migayron R, Roger J, et al. Lens hexitois and cataract formation during lactation in a woman heterozygous for galactosaemia. J Inherit Metab Dis 1989;12:383.

163. Andersen MW, Williams VP, Sparkes MC, et al. Transferase-deficiency galactosemia: Immunochemical studies of the Duarte and Los Angeles variants. Hum Genet 1984;65:287.

164. Donnell GN, Bergren WR, Bretthauer MS, et al. The enzymatic expression of heterozygosity in families of children with galactosemia. Pediatrics 1960;25:572.

165. Fensom AH, Benson PF, Blunt S. Prenatal diagnosis of galactosemia. BMJ 1974;4:386.

166. Holton JB, Raymont CM. Prenatal diagnosis of classical galactosaemia. In: Burman D, Holton JB, Pennock CA, eds. Inherited disorders of carbohydrate metabolism. Lancaster, England: MTP Press, 1980:141.

167. Shin YS, Rieth WE, Schaub J. Prenatal diagnosis of galactosemia and properties of galactose 1-phosphate uridyltransferase in erythrocytes of galactosemic variants as well as in human fetal and adult organs. Clin Chim Acta 1983;128:271.

168. Jakobs C, Warner TG, Sweetman L, et al. Stable isotope dilution analysis of galactitol in amniotic fluid: an accurate approach to the prenatal diagnosis of galactosemia. Pediatr Res 1984;18:714.

169. Roland MO, Mandon G, Farrior JP, et al. Gallates-1-phosphate uridyl transferase activity in chorionic villi: a first trimester prenatal diagnosis of galactosaemia. J Inherit Metab Dis 1986;9:284.

170. Holton JB, Allen JT, Gillet MG. Prenatal diagnosis of disorders of galactose metabolism. J Inherit Metab Dis 1989;12:202.

171. Benson PF, Brandt NJ, Christensen E, et al. Prenatal diagnosis of galactosaemia in six pregnancies: possible complications with rare alleles of the galactose 1-phosphate uridyl transferase locus. Clin Genet 1979;16:311.

172. Elsas LJ. Prenatal diagnosis of galactose-1-phosphate uridyltransferase (GALT)-deficient galactosemia. Prenat Diagn 2001;21:302–3.

173. Stambolian D, Ai Y, Sidjanin D, et al. Cloning of the galactokinase cDNA and identification of mutations in two families with cataracts. Nat Genet 1995;10:307.

174. Bosch AM, Bakker HD, van Gennip AH, et al. Clinical features of galactokinase deficiency. J Inherit Metab Dis 2002;25:629.

175. Pickering WR, Howell RR. Galactokinase deficiency: clinical and biochemical findings in a new kindred. J Pediatr 1972;81:50.

176. Gitzelmann R. Deficiency of uridine diphosphate galactose 4-epimerase in blood cells of an apparently healthy infant. Helv Paediatr Acta 1972;27:125.

177. Holton JB, Gillet MG, MacFaul R, et al. Galactosaemia: a new severe variant due to uridine diphosphate galactose-4-epimerase deficiency. Arch Dis Child 1981;56:885.

178. Henderson MJ, Holton JB, MacFaul R. Further observations in a case of uridine diphosphate galactose-4-epimerase deficiency with a severe clinical presentation. J Inherit Metab Dis 1983;6:17.

179. Lin MS, Oizumi J, Ng WG, et al. Regional mapping of gene for human UDPgal 4-epimerase on chromosome 1 in mouse-human hybrids. Cytogenet Cell Genet 1979;24:217.

180. Daude N, Gallaher TK, Zeschnigk M, et al. Molecular cloning, characterization, and mapping of a full-length cDNA encoding human UDP-galactose 49-epimerase. Biochem Mol Med 1995;56:1.

181. Steimann B et al. Disorders of fructose metabolism. In: Scriver CR, et al., eds. The metabolic and molecular bases of inherited disease, 8th ed. New York: McGraw-Hill, 2001:1489.

182. Bonthron DT, Brady N, Donaldson IA, et al. Molecular basis of essential fructosuria: molecular cloning and mutational analysis of human ketohexokinase (fructokinase). Hum Mol Genet 194;3:1627.

183. Henry I, Gallano P, Besmond C, et al. The structural gene for aldolase B (ALDB) maps to 9q13-32. Ann Hum Genet 1985;49:172.

184. Tolan DR, Penhoet EE. Characterization of the human aldolase B gene. Mol Biol Med 1986;3:245.

185. Cross NCP, de Franchis R, Sebastio G, et al. Molecular analysis of aldolase B genes in hereditary fructose intolerance. Lancet 1990;335:306.

186. Cross NCP, Tolan DR, Cox TM. Catalytic deficiency of human aldolase B in hereditary fructose intolerance caused by a common missense mutation. Cell 1988;53:881.

187. Cross NCP, Cox TM. Molecular analysis of aldolase B genes in the diagnosis of hereditary fructose intolerance. Lancet 1990;335:306.

188. Tolan DR, Brooks CC. Molecular analysis of common aldolase B alleles for hereditary fructose intolerance in North Americans. Biochem Med Metab Biol 1996;48:19.

189. Tolan DR. Molecular basis of hereditary fructose intolerance: mutations and polymorphisms in the human aldolase B gene. Hum Mutat 1995;6:210.
190. Gitzelmann R. Enzymes of fructose and galactose metabolism: galactose 1-phosphate. In: Curtius HC, Roth M, eds. Clinical biochemistry: principles and method. New York: Walter de Gruyter, 1974:1236.
191. Kikawa Y, Shin YS, Inuzuka M, et al. Diagnosis of fructose-1,6-bisphosphatase deficiency using cultured lymphocyte fraction: a secure and noninvasive alternative to liver biopsy. J Inherit Metab Dis 2002;25:41.
192. Iga M, Kimura M, Ohura T, et al. Rapid, simplified and sensitive method for screening fructose-1,6-diphosphatase deficiency by analyzing urinary metabolites in urease/direct preparations and gas chromatography-mass spectrometry in the selected-ion monitoring mode. J Chromatogr B Biomed Sci Appl 2000;746:75.
193. El-Maghrabi MR, Lange AJ, Jiang W, et al. Human fructose 1,6-bisphosphatase gene (FBP1): exon–intron organization, localization to chromosome bands 9q22.2-q22.3, and mutation screening in subjects with fructose 1,6-bisphosphatase deficiency. Genomics 1995;27:520.
194. Kikawa Y, Inuzuka M, Jin BY, et al. Identification of a genetic mutation in a family with fructose 1,6-bisphosphatase deficiency. Biochem Biophys Res Commun 1995;210:797.
195. Clayton PT, Hyland K, Brand M, et al. Mitochondrial phosphoenolpyruvate carboxykinase deficiency. Eur J Pediatr 1986;145:46.
196. Vidnes J, Sovik O. Gluconeogenesis in infancy and childhood. Acta Paediatr Scand 1976;65:307.
197. Hommes FA, Bendien K, Elema JD, et al. Two cases of phosphoenolpyruvate carboxykinase deficiency. Acta Paediatr Scand 1976;65:233.
198. Matsuo M, Maeda E, Nakamura H, et al. Hepatic phosphoenolpyruvate carboxykinase deficiency: a neonatal case with reduced activity of pyruvate carboxylase. J Inherit Metab Dis 1989;12:336.
199. Hiatt HH. Pentosuria. In: Scriver CR, Beaudet AL, Sly WS, et al., eds. The metabolic and molecular bases of inherited disease, 7th ed. New York: McGraw-Hill, 1995:1001.
200. Lane AB, Jenkins T. Human L-xylulose reductase variation: family and population studies. Am J Hum Genet 1985;49:227.

Gerald L. Feldman, M.D., Ph.D., and
Kristin G. Monaghan, Ph.D.

15

Prenatal Diagnosis of Cystic Fibrosis

Written accounts of cystic fibrosis (CF) date back to the eighteenth century; however, it was not defined as a specific disease until the 1930s, when the term *cystic fibrosis of the pancreas* was introduced.[1] The familial recurrence of CF led to the conclusion that CF was inherited in an autosomal recessive manner.[2] In 1985, Romeo and co-workers[3] examined pedigrees contained in Italian church records. Through segregation analysis and the analysis of consanguineous marriages, they were able to confirm the mode of inheritance as autosomal recessive and lack of genetic heterogeneity. CF is an example of a disorder in which the obstetrician and the geneticist can work together, each bringing a different focus and area of specialty.

GENETICS AND PREVALENCE

CF is one of the most common autosomal recessive genetic disorders among Caucasians of European ancestry, affecting approximately 1 in 2,500 live births.[4] An affected individual must inherit two CF mutations, one from each clinically normal carrier parent. The heterozygote (carrier) frequency in Caucasians is approximately 1 in 25.[4] Data on derivative populations in North America indicate a lower incidence of approximately 1 in 3,500 (carrier frequency of 1 in 29).[5]

CF is less common in other ethnic groups, but significant numbers of affected individuals are found in the Ashkenazi Jewish, African-American, and Hispanic populations. The cystic fibrosis carrier frequency is 1 in 29 for persons of Ashkenazi Jewish descent.[6] The incidence in North American African Americans has been estimated to be 1 in 19,000,[7–9] with a carrier frequency of 1 in 69.[8–10] CF is being recognized with increasing frequency in Hispanics; a recent estimate of the incidence in Mexico is between 1 in 8,000 and 1 in 9,000, giving a carrier frequency of approximately 1 in 46.[9,11] Reports have also described CF in Native Americans[12–14] and Arabs.[15–17] CF has been detected worldwide, and the incidence in various populations has been summarized.[18]

CLINICAL CHARACTERISTICS

CF is a multisystem disorder affecting the pulmonary, gastrointestinal, and reproductive systems. CF encompasses a wide spectrum of disease, from meconium ileus and severe respiratory compromise in infants to the later presentation of mild pulmonary symptoms and no evidence of gastrointestinal problems in adults. Abnormal electrolyte transport across epithelial cells results in viscous mucoid secretions that clog epithelial tubules, leading to organ damage.

Pulmonary Manifestations

Most patients with CF have airway obstruction caused by the accumulation of thick mucus in the airways of the lungs and an increased susceptibility to infections. Bronchial gland hypertrophy, with mucous plugging, leads to small-airway obstructive disease. CF is also characterized by persistent coughing, impaired breathing, chronic bronchitis, and recurrent pneumonia. Nasal polyps are common. Pneumothorax is a pulmonary complication occurring in 5–8 percent of patients with CF.[19] The most life-threatening pulmonary manifestation of CF is respiratory failure, an indication of severe lung disease.

Gastrointestinal Manifestations

In approximately 85 percent of patients with CF, obstructed excretory pancreatic ducts develop, resulting in pancreatic insufficiency (PI). This blockage prevents adequate levels of pancreatic enzymes, water, bicarbonate, and electrolytes from reaching the duodenum, resulting in incompletely digested fats and proteins.[20] Almost all infants with meconium ileus have CF; however, only ~10–20 percent of infants with CF have meconium ileus.[21] Of relevance, however, is that only 59 percent of newborns with CF have pancreatic insufficiency.[22] Thus, it is important not to use the presence or absence of pancreatic disease as the sole diagnostic criterion in newborns. Malabsorption often leads to malnutrition, manifested by poor weight gain, growth retardation, delayed puberty, muscle wasting, and deficiencies of vitamins, minerals, and essential fatty acids.[23,24] Additional complications include distal intestinal obstruction syndrome (DIOS), constipation and acquired megacolon, rectal prolapse, cirrhosis of the liver, cholelithiasis, and diabetic (especially in older patients) pancreatitis.[25]

Involvement of the Reproductive System

Almost all male patients with CF are azoospermic due to congenital bilateral absence of the vas deferens (CBAVD; obstructive azoospermia).[26] However, spermatogenesis is normal. Approximately 2 percent of males with infertility have CBAVD, although the frequency of cystic fibrosis mutations in these otherwise asymptomatic males is significantly higher than expected. Thus, men with CBAVD, once believed to be a distinct genetic disorder, likely represent a range of disorders ranging from isolated CBAVD to atypical forms of CF to classic CF.[27] CF DNA testing is indicated for all patients with CBAVD.

Affected females may have decreased fertility caused by viscous cervical mucus, but there are no reproductive-tract abnormalities in females with CF. In fact, a recent study suggests that it is unlikely for CFTR mutations to cause a birth defect with a similar embryologic origin, Congenital Absence of the Uterus and Vagina (CAUV).[27a] However, a significant number of women with CF are fertile and become pregnant. Patients with CF with minimal pulmonary disease and adequate caloric intake appear able to tolerate pregnancy well, although there can be significant maternal complications (exacerbation of lung disease, poor weight gain) and fetal complications (prematurity, low birth weight) in women with severe disease.[28,29]

Diagnosis

The demonstration of increased sweat chloride and sodium in patients with CF[30] led to the development of the sweat chloride test, which remains the primary method of diagnosis.[31] The improvement in and the availability of CF gene analyses over the past 10 years have expanded the clinical spectrum of CF to include individuals with previously unrecognized features of CF. Diagnostic criteria now exist for CF.[32] In addition to the characteristic phenotypic features of CF, a history of CF in a sibling or a positive newborn screening test result, laboratory evidence of a CF abnormality (elevated sweat test, presence of two disease-causing CF mutations or *in vivo* demonstration of characteristic abnormalities in ion transport across the nasal epithelium) should be present. In laboratories outside established CF centers, both false-positive and false-negative sweat test results occur, so caution must be used in confirming a suspected diagnosis of CF.[33]

TREATMENT

In 1938, most people with CF did not live past 1 year of age.[1] This improved to 14 years of age in 1969 and 33.4 years of age in 2001.[34] Today, regression analysis predicts that median survival may have increased to over 40 years for children born in the 1990s, though these numbers may not be applicable to older infants, given the cumulative long-term effects of the disease.[35] Referral to a regional CF Center is recommended for individuals with CF. Patients with treatments initiated prior to the onset of symptomatic lung disease fare better than those whose treatment is delayed. Although the standard treatments involve clearance of lower-airway secretions, pancreatic enzyme replacement, and antibiotics for pulmonary infections, the increasing survival age of patients with CF can be attributed to improved nutrition, new drug therapies, and organ transplantation.

Chest Physiotherapy

The primary treatment for the clearance of pulmonary secretions is chest physiotherapy[36] because clearance of bronchial secretions is essential in daily management of the disease. Postural drainage, often accompanied by manual percussion, deep breathing, directed cough, forced expiration, and physical exercise are beneficial.

Pancreatic Enzyme Supplementation

Pancreatic enzymes have been used for many years[37] to improve the absorption of fats and proteins, alleviating many of the abdominal symptoms experienced by patients with PI. Pancreatic enzyme supplementation can result in improved intestinal absorption, decreasing the frequency of DIOS, constipation, and rectal prolapse. The increased digestion of fats and proteins improves nutrition, leading to reduced morbidity and mortality, by ultimately improving pulmonary function.[38]

Nutritional Management

In addition to PI, patients are at risk for malnutrition because of the decreased food intake and increased metabolic requirements caused by their lung disease.[25] Good nutrition directly affects survival by improving weight gain, growth, muscle mass, and respiratory strength, which slows the deterioration in lung function.[39] Nutritional therapy may include special formulas for infants to enhance weight gain. Patients are encouraged to follow a normal diet without restrictions, especially with regard to fat intake.[23]

Antibiotic Therapy

Aggressive antibiotic therapy has largely accounted for the increased lifespan of patients with CF. Overall, *Pseudomonas aeruginosa* is the most common isolate, followed by *Staphylococcus aureus*, *Stenotrophomonas maltophilia*, and in some cases *Burkholderia cepacia*.[34] Treatments used with varying degrees of success to prevent pulmonary complications include vaccinations, antibiotics (oral, inhaled, or intravenous), bronchodilators, antiinflammatory agents (steroidal and nonsteroidal), amiloride and chloride secretagogues (ATP and UTP), and mucolytic agents (recombinant human deoxyribonuclease [rhDNase]).[25]

Organ Transplantation

Patients with CF can be considered for lung, heart–lung, pancreas, and liver transplantation. Organ transplantation, along with somatic gene therapy trials, are the two most aggressive therapies available for patients with CF. Bilateral lung transplantation, first introduced in 1988, is now the most widely used technique, though it still available as an option for only a minority of patients with CF. Lung transplantation is primarily indicated for patients with end-stage lung disease. About 125 patients in the CF Patient Registry each year receive a bilateral lung transplant.[34] The outcome for lung transplantation is improving and is comparable to patients without CF, with 1-year survival rates of 70–84 percent and 5-year survival rates of 60–65 percent.[40–42] Simultaneous heart–lung–liver transplantation or liver transplantation is a feasible alternative for patients with hepatic fibrosis or cirrhosis.[43–45]

Somatic Gene-Replacement Therapy

The goal of gene therapy in the treatment of CF is the introduction of a normal CF gene into the respiratory epithelial cells of affected patients. Theoretically, this will result in the production of functional CF protein, preventing lung disease. A number of potential methods for transferring genes into human cells have been studied, including direct transfection, virus-mediated transduction and receptor-mediated transfer.[46–48] Most approaches have focused on gene transfer to airway epithelia. While the principle of gene therapy for CF has been proven, and barriers and limitations have been identified, progress has been slow, with either inefficient transfer of the healthy gene or overwhelming host inflammatory response to the viral vector.[48] Several gene therapy trials are ongoing, and more than 180 patients with CF in the United States have participated in these studies, although it is not currently a treatment option for patients with CF.[44,48]

THE CYSTIC FIBROSIS TRANSMEMBRANE CONDUCTANCE REGULATOR (CFTR)

Localization and Identification of the CF Gene

Through linkage analysis of multiple affected individuals using restriction-fragment-length polymorphisms, the CF gene was initially mapped to the long arm of chromosome 7 (7q31.2)[49] and later narrowed down to a 1.0-Mb region.[50,51] The CF gene was identified in 1989[52–54] and was one of the first genes to be identified by positional cloning. The highest RNA levels were detected in the pancreas and nasal polyps; however, transcripts were also found in lung, colon, sweat glands, placenta, liver, parotid gland, and kidney.[53]

The entire gene locus spans more than 250 kb[53,54] and the cDNA contains 27 exons.[53,55] The identification of a disease-causing mutation verified that this candidate was the gene responsible for CF. A 3-bp deletion (designated by delta or Δ) was identified in exon 10, which resulted in the loss of the amino acid phenylalanine at codon 508. This mutation, named ΔF508, was identified on 68 percent of CF chromosomes and was not present on any normal chromosomes.[52,53]

Protein Structure and Function

The CF protein, named the cystic fibrosis transmembrane conductance regulator (CFTR), consists of 1,480 amino acids with a molecular weight of 168 kD.[53] The CFTR is located within the lipid bilayer, predominantly at the apical membrane of secretory epithelial cells and shares homology with a family of proteins involved in active transport across cell membranes.[53] Acting as an ion channel, the CFTR provides a pathway for chloride anions, water, and small hydrophilic solutes[56] across the epithelia, and also regulates other ion channels and cellular processes (for review, see Sheppard and Welsh[57]).

The CFTR consists of two motifs, each with a membrane-spanning domain composed of six hydrophobic segments, and an ATP-binding domain, referred to as the nucleotide binding domain (NBD). The membrane spanning domains form the pore of the channel, while the NBDs bind and cleave ATP, providing an energy source for ion transport. Separating the two motifs is a unique, highly charged regulatory domain, designated the R domain. Phosphorylation of the R domain by cAMP-dependent protein kinase A controls channel activity. Following phosphorylation, ATP hydrolysis at the NBDs results in conformational changes that open and close the Cl-pore, regulating channel gating (for review, see Sheppard and Welsh[57]). The NBDs have a low degree of sequence homology, indicating that they have very different roles in CFTR control. One model suggests that ATP binding at the first NBD controls channel opening, whereas ATP hydrolysis at NBD2 closes the channel.[58,59] The CFTR is returned to its inactive state following dephosphorylation of the R domain.

CFTR MUTATIONS

Disease-causing CFTR mutations result in abnormal chloride anion transport in secretory epithelial cells and underlie the excessive mucous accumulation characteristic of CF.[60] Allelic heterogeneity has been demonstrated for CF, as more than 1200 mutations have been identified; most are rare, having been detected in only one family.[61] The twenty-five most common panethnic CF mutations, which occur on ≥0.1 percent of CF chromosomes, are listed in Table 15.1. This panel of mutations is recommended for population-based CF carrier screening in the United States.[9] Seventy-two percent of Caucasian patients with CF are homozygotes or compound heterozygotes for eight mutations of the CFTR gene (ΔF508, G542X, R553X, W1282X, N1303K, 621+1G → T, 1717–1G → A, and R117H).[62] Fifty percent of the alterations in the CF gene are missense mutations that result in the substitution of one amino acid for another. Twenty percent are frame-shift mutations caused by small insertions or deletions. Fifteen percent of the sequence changes are nonsense mutations, which result in the substitution of a stop codon for an amino acid, producing a shortened protein. The remaining mutations are in-frame deletions, splice-junction defects, and other variations.[63,64]

Although the identification of so many mutations in the CF gene has increased the accuracy of carrier testing and prenatal diagnosis, failure to find two mutated CF genes

Table 15.1. The 25 common CF mutations, included in the ACMG recommended screening panel[9]

Name	Relative Frequency (%)[65]	Consequence[63]	Associated Phenotype
ΔF508	72.42	Deletion of Phe at codon 508	Severe
G542X	2.28	Gly → Stop at codon 542	Severe
G551D	2.25	Gly → Asp at codon 551	Severe
621+1G → T	1.57	Splice mutation	Severe
W1282X	1.50	Trp → Stop at codon 1282	Severe
N1303K	1.27	Asn → Lys at codon 1303	Severe
R553X	0.88	Arg → Stop at codon 553	Severe
ΔI507	0.87	Deletion of Ile at codon 506 or 507	Severe
R117H	0.70	Arg → His at codon 117	Mild
3849+10kbC → T	0.58	Aberrant splicing	Mild
2789+5G → A	0.48	Splice mutation	Mild
1717−1G → A	0.48	Splice mutation	Severe
R347P	0.45	Arg → Pro at codon 347	Variable
711+1G → T	0.43	Splice mutation	Severe
R560T	0.38	Arg → Thr at codon 560; splice mutation?	Severe
A455E	0.34	Ala → Glu at codon 455	Mild
3659delC	0.34	Frameshift	Severe
G85E	0.29	Gly → Glu at codon 85	Variable
R1162X	0.23	Arg → Stop at codon 1162	Severe
2184delA	0.17	Frameshift	Severe
1898+1G → A	0.16	Splice mutation	Severe
R334W	0.14	Arg → Trp at codon 334	Mild
I148T	0.09	Ile → Thr at codon 148	Dependent on presence of 3199del6
3120+1 G → A	0.08	Splice mutation	Severe
1078delT	0.02	Frameshift	Severe

Reflex tests:
1. I506V, I507V, F508C when ΔF508 is detected. (These variants may result in a false-positive homozygous ΔF508 status.)
2. 5T/7T/9T when R117H is detected. (5T influences the severity of the R117H mutation.)

does not rule out the diagnosis of CF. By screening for the twenty-five most common mutations, approximately 90 percent of all CF mutations can be identified in Caucasians.[5] Using a 90 percent detection rate, fewer than 1 percent of patients with CF have no detectable mutation and 18 percent have only a single identifiable mutation. Screening for additional mutations increases the overall mutation detection rate only slightly, because each of those mutations is exceedingly rare (less than 0.1 percent).

As shown in Figure 15.1, ΔF508, ΔI507, the missense mutations G551D, A455E and nonsense mutations G542X and R553X are located in NBD1. The nonsense mutation, W1282X, is located in NBD2. Mutations within the first membrane-spanning domain are thought to reduce the ability of the CFTR to transport chloride anions. Mutations in this domain include R117H, R334W, R347P, 1078delT, I148T, and G85E. Mutations within the second transmembrane domain are hypothesized to affect chloride channel activity more mildly. Mutations in the regulatory domain are less common.[66]

To further understand how mutations affect CFTR function, mutations were divided into general classes according to the functional properties of the protein product with respect to chloride channel function in epithelial cells.[63,67–69] Class I consists of mutations for which the intact CFTR protein product is not synthesized, usually due to premature

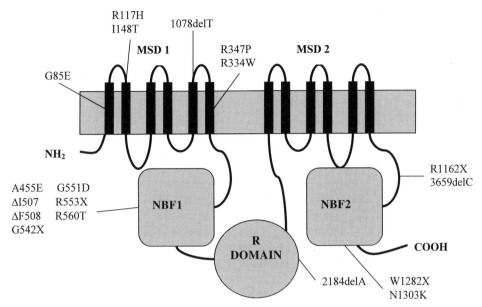

Fig. 15.1. Approximate location of ACOG/ACMG recommended CF mutation panel occurring within the CFTR domain. NBD = nucleotide-binding domain; R = regulatory domain; MSD = membrane-spanning domain

termination signals (e.g., the nonsense mutation G542X, the frameshift mutation 394delTT, and the splice-junction mutation 1717–1G → A). Class II mutations (e.g., ΔF508) result in a protein that is degraded and cannot reach the cell surface. An example of a class III mutation is the missense mutation, G551D. This type of mutation tends to occur in an NBD and affects the binding of ATP. Class IV mutations (e.g., R117H) produce proteins that are oriented correctly in the apical membrane and bind and hydrolyze ATP but do not transport chloride normally. Class V mutations produce decreased amounts of normally functioning CFTR due to aberrant splicing at alternative sites (3849+10kbC → T) or defective processing (A455E). The classification system for CF mutations may assist in improving therapeutic strategies for patients[64] so that it may be possible to design a personalized treatment strategy based on the genotype of each patient with CF.

Ethnic Variation

Not only does the incidence of CF vary markedly among different populations, but the frequency of specific mutations also differs among ethnic groups. The mutation detection rate for the twenty-five mutation core panel in various races/ethnic groups is shown in Table 15.2. Using the American College of Medical Genetics (ACMG) Core Panel of twenty-five mutations permits the detection of approximately 90 percent of CF mutations in non-Hispanic Caucasians.[65]

On average, ΔF508 occurs on 68 percent of all CF chromosomes worldwide[18]; however, the frequency of ΔF508 ranges from ~20 percent in the Ashkenazi Jewish population[70] and Northern Africa[18] to approximately 100 percent in the Faroe Islands of Denmark.[71] The worldwide frequency of most non-ΔF508 mutations is low, although several occur in relatively high frequencies in specific ethnic groups. For example, between

Table 15.2.   CF mutation detection in various ethnic groups based on current mutation screening panel[9,65]

Group	Percentage of Mutations Detected	Carrier Frequency	Disease Frequency
African American	69	1/65	1/15,300
Ashkenazi Jewish	97	1/29	1/3300
Caucasian	90	1/29	1/3300
Hispanic	57	1/46	1/8500
Asian American	Not known*	1/90	1/32,100

*Mutation detection frequency and disease incidence are not known with accuracy for Native Americans or Arab Americans.

48 and 60 percent of CF chromosomes in the Ashkenazi Jewish population carry the non-sense mutation W1282X,[6,70] whereas the worldwide frequency is 2 percent. In people of Ashkenazi Jewish descent, screening for five mutations (ΔF508, G542X, W1282X, N1303K, and 3849+10kb C $\rightarrow$ T) will detect 97 percent of CF alleles.[6] In addition, the mutation, D1152H was reported to be present in high frequency among all Jewish ethnic groups, including the Ashkenazi.[72]

A comprehensive analysis of CF mutations in African-Americans showed that ΔF508 accounted for 48 percent of the CF mutations in this race.[10] The second most common mutation among African Americans was 3120+1G $\rightarrow$ A, which occurred with a frequency of 12 percent. The mutation detection rate among African Americans using the current ACOG/ACMG panel is between 62 and 69 percent, while the mutation detection rate among Hispanic individuals is 57–63 percent.[9] Unfortunately, reports are limited regarding the population-specific mutation frequencies among individuals of Native American, Middle Eastern, and Asian American descent, and the current ACOG/ACMG policy statement does not include disease incidences and/or carrier detection rates for these groups. Based on several small studies, the ACMG core panel will detect 27–63 percent of Arab CF mutations.[15–17] Common mutations reported among this group include 1548delG, I1234V, ΔF508, 3120+1G>A, W1282X, and N1303K. The mutations 1548delG and I1234V, present in high frequency in this population, are not currently included in the recommended mutation screening panel in the United States.

CORRELATION BETWEEN GENOTYPE AND PHENOTYPE

Although CF is a single gene disorder, genotype–phenotype comparisons in this condition are complicated. Analysis of relationships between genotype and phenotype shows a strong correlation between particular mutations and pancreatic function. Between 10 and 15 percent of patients with CF have pancreatic sufficiency (PS), low to normal sweat chloride levels, later age at diagnosis, better nutritional status, and slower decline in pulmonary function.[73,74] Patients with PS CF have a >17 percent chance of developing pancreatitis, which may precede the diagnosis of CF, with an average age of onset of 22 years. No specific mutation is associated with this phenotype.[74] In general, patients with PS have one or two mild mutations, whereas those with two severe mutations have PI and more severe clinical manifestations. Ten percent of CF mutations are mild alleles.[75] The mild allele is presumed to confer a dominant phenotype over the severe allele,[73] although the presence of one mild allele does not ensure pancreatic sufficiency.[76] The pancreatic sufficiency/insufficiency status of each of the twenty-five ACOG/ACMG core panel mutations is included in Table 15.1 and is described as mild and severe, respectively.

Table 15.3. R117H/polyT genotype–phenotype correlations[78,80,82–86]

Genotype	Phenotype Includes
R117H-7T/R117H-7T	Normal, atypical symptoms, CBAVD, PS CF
R117H-5T/R117H-5T	PS CF
R117H-7T/CF mutation	Normal, atypical symptoms, CBAVD, PS CF
R117H-5T/CF mutation	PS CF
5T/5T	Normal, atypical symptoms, CBAVD, PS CF
5T/CF mutation	Atypical symptoms, CBAVD, PS CF

R117H and the Variable Intron 8 PolyT Locus

The CFTR intron 8/exon 9 acceptor-splice site contains a variable number of thymidines known as the polyT allele, with either five, seven, or nine thymidines present at the end of intron 8 (known as 5T, 7T and 9T).[77] The presence of the 5T allele negatively affects RNA splicing, resulting in a CFTR transcript lacking exon 9. The 7T allele is associated with normal splicing and therefore normal levels of functional protein.[78] The 5T allele is present in 5 percent of Caucasians and is associated with a wide range of clinical manifestations including congenital bilateral absence of the vas deferens (see below), mild CF, atypical CF symptoms, as well as in healthy, fertile men.[79–81]

The 5T allele can exist on the same chromosome with the R117H CF mutation, but has not been reported in *cis* with any other CF mutation.[80] R117H has also been reported on a 7T and rarely, a 9T background.[80] A great deal of information regarding genotype–phenotype correlation between the R117H/poly T locus is known (Table 15.3). Homozygosity for R117H and the 7T allele is associated with CBAVD or a normal phenotype.[78,87] It appears that although these individuals may have elevated or borderline sweat chloride levels, clinical CF is rare, but close follow-up may be considered.[87] Homozygosity for R117H *in cis* with the 5T allele or R117H/5T in combination with another CF mutation on the opposite chromosome is associated with PS CF.[78,87] R117H/7T in combination with another CF mutation on the opposite chromosome (such as ΔF508) is associated with a spectrum of phenotypes from normal to CBAVD to PS CF.[82,83] For individuals undergoing routine CF carrier screening, reflex testing to examine the polyT status is recommended when R117H is detected. This will determine which individuals are truly at risk for having CF in combination with a second disease-causing mutation on the opposite chromosome. PolyT testing in the absence of the R117H mutation is not recommended as part of routine screening for CF[9] because this may create confusion in interpreting DNA testing results, especially as it relates to prenatal diagnosis.[88] However, polyT testing may be appropriate for males with CBAVD and patients with other atypical CF symptoms, such as pancreatitis.

Congenital Bilateral Absence of the Vas Deferens

Most males with CF are infertile, because of CBAVD, which is also a cause of infertility in otherwise healthy men. An association between male fertility and the presence of the 3849+10kb C → T mutation has been reported, suggesting that this particular mutation may result in levels of normal CFTR expression necessary to avoid infertility (for review, see Mickle and Cutting[89]). Initial studies reported that of men with CBAVD, approximately one-fourth were compound heterozygotes for two mutant alleles (at least one being a mild mutation), almost half of the men had one identifiable CF mutation, and the remainder had no detectable CF mutation.[90] CFTR mutations are rarely detected in males with CBAVD and renal anomalies[91]; however, recently men with CBAVD, CFTR mutations, and renal agenesis, have been reported.[92] Although some cases of CBAVD may actually represent extremely mild forms of CF, it is recommended that men with CFTR mutations and CBAVD as the only clinical manifestation (even in the presence of positive sweat chloride tests) not be classified with CF.[93,94] However, because the possibility of late-onset CF symptoms cannot be excluded, clinical follow-up of these men may be considered.[94]

Eighty-four percent of males with CBAVD who are heterozygous for a CF mutation and 25 percent with no detectable mutation carry the 5T allele.[77] The 5T allele is present in men with CBAVD at a frequency four times higher than in the general population (20 vs. 5 percent).[79] Of males with CBAVD, 41–48 percent have either two CF mutations or one CF mutation and the 5T allele on the opposite chromosome. Twenty-five to 31 percent have either one mutation or the 5T allele, and approximately 25 percent have neither a CF mutation nor the 5T allele.[84,85] The majority of males with CBAVD have a severe mutation on one chromosome and a mild/variable mutation on the other, with the most common genotype in CBAVD males being ΔF508/R117H (7T) followed by ΔF508/5T.[27]

I148T

The recommended CF mutation screening panel is expected to be modified as new information is learned regarding the phenotype associated with specific mutations and allele frequencies in various populations. One such mutation that is being reexamined is the sequence change I148T. After implementation of CF population-based carrier screening, Rohlfs and co-workers[95] noted more than a one-hundred-fold difference in the frequency of I148T between patients with clinical CF (0.06 percent) and individuals undergoing carrier screening (6.4 percent). This prompted further studies of this allele, resulting in the discovery of another mutation, 3199del6, in *cis* (on the same chromosome) with I148T in patients with clinical CF. Approximately 1 in 55 I148T carriers also have the 3199del6 mutation. The I148T/3199del6 allele appears to be associated with PI CF in individuals with another severe CF mutation on the opposite chromosome. The available data indicates that I148T, in the absence of 3199del6 (even when another mutation is present on the opposite chromosome), is associated with a normal phenotype. However, because the possibility of mild or atypical CF in persons with this genotype cannot be excluded, care must be taken when discussing genotype-phenotype correlations, especially during prenatal diagnosis. When I148T is identified in a CF patient or as part of CF carrier screening, reflex testing for 3199del6 should be performed. New screening panel recommendations will incorporate this information in their updated recommendations.

Modifier Genes

Complications secondary to pulmonary dysfunction are the leading cause of death in patients with CF; however, the degree of respiratory complications in these individuals is highly variable.[96] Twin studies[97] and investigations involving patients with identical mutations do not demonstrate a strong correlation between pulmonary function and CFTR genotype.[62] These results suggest that this aspect of CF is influenced by other factors.[63] Environmental factors, including infection, nutrition, exposures to tobacco smoke, pollutants, age at diagnosis, and compliance and intensity of treatment were originally thought to influence lung function.[98] Recent studies have examined many potential modifier genes for associations between gastrointestinal, liver and pulmonary complications.[96,99] A modifier locus at 19q13 is associated with an increased risk of meconium ileus,[100] and mutations of the mannose-binding lectin and α_1-antitrypsin genes are associated with an increased risk of severe liver disease.[96] Candidate modifiers of pulmonary function include glutathione-S-transferase (functions in the detoxification of aromatic compounds), transforming growth factor β (proinflammatory and antiinflammatory properties), tumor necrosis factor α (contributes to neutrophil-predominant inflammation), β_2-adrenergic receptor (influences airway reactivity), α_1-antitrypsin, β-defensin, and deficiency of mannose-binding lectin (component of the immune defense system).[101–103]

Other Conditions Associated with CFTR Mutations

Although guidelines for making a clinical diagnosis of CF exist,[32] the identification of other conditions associated with CFTR mutations, or "CFTR-opathies" further complicates our understanding of the CFTR genotype as it relates to clinical expression of disease.[86] These conditions include sarcoidosis, asthma, disseminated bronchiectasis, chronic rhinosinusitis, pulmonary emphysema, and idiopathic pancreatitis and have been reported with a wide variety of CF mutations, some of which are unique to the specific conditions.

Summary

The genotype of the patient with CF is useful for predicting pancreatic function. The combination of many different CFTR mutations, absence of clinical CF in patients with two CFTR sequence changes originally thought to be disease-causing mutations, modifier genes, and the lack of a clear association between specific common mutations and symptoms and severity of disease complicates genotype–phenotype correlations. Prenatal counseling after the diagnosis of one or two mild mutations may include the likelihood of long-term pancreatic sufficiency, whereas two severe mutations would indicate early-onset PI. Currently, it is impossible to predict prenatally other manifestations of CF, especially the severity of pulmonary disease, based on genotype information.

METHODS OF DETECTING THE MUTATION

DNA can be extracted from leukocytes isolated from whole blood, dried blood, or fetal cells (amniotic fluid cells or chorionic villus cells, fetal blood cells), but other specimens, such as buccal cells collected on cytology brushes, are also used in some laboratories.[104] It is important to delineate the reason for molecular genetic testing for CF, since the methods may differ significantly. For example, in response to the recommended CF Core mutation panel by the American College of Medical Genetics,[9] commercial companies have developed various detection technologies (Table 15.4). These include PCR-mediated site-directed mutagenesis (PSM), probing with allele-specific oligonucleotides (ASOs), multiplex PCR amplification followed by ASO hybridization, allele-specific priming in PCRs (ASPs), multiplex allele-specific PCR, reverse dot blot detection, automated DNA sequencing, amplification refractory mutation system (ARMS), multiple allele-specific diagnostic assays (MASDA) and electronic microarrays.[105]

For CF mutation analysis, laboratories currently choose between development of home-brew methods or use commercial analyte-specific reagents (ASRs). Laboratories developing genetic tests for clinical use under "home brew" regulations are regulated under

Table 15.4. Methods of mutation detection

Type of Method	Principle	Advantages	Disadvantages
Allele-specific probe hybridization	Individual probes hybridize to each specific mutation	Multiplex possible; can be automated	Design can be complex; not commercially available
Reverse probe hybridization	Probe pairs (wild-type and mutant) are bound to membrane	Multiplex possible; commercially available; high throughput	Difficult to add new mutations
Oligonucleotide ligation assay	Allele-specific PCR followed by ligation with probes to identify mutant and wild-type sequence	Commercially available; high throughput	Detection requires use of automated DNA sequencer
Restriction enzyme digestion and electrophoresis	PCR followed by specific detection of normal or mutant sequence by use of restriction-fragment-length polymorphisms	Not commercially available	Time-consuming; difficult to automate; not commercially available
Allele-specific PCR (amplification refractory mutation system [ARMS])	PCR primers designed to amplify only mutant sequence	Commercially available	Absence of product implies negative result
DNA sequencing	Sequencing of individual exons or complete CFTR	Can theoretically identify all mutations within amplicons	Expensive; cannot identify large deletions (i.e., exons)
Mutation scanning	Scanning to search for sequence alterations	Inexpensive	Cannot identify specific mutations; must have confirmatory test
Electronic microarray	Chip analysis	Relatively easy to add new mutations	Expensive

the provisions of CLIA88.[105] Each method has its own inherent strengths and weaknesses, and an ordering physician should be aware of individual laboratory's methods.

Importantly, however, the ACMG Core Panel of mutations is recommended *only for population-based preconceptual and prenatal CF carrier screening.*[9] For diagnostic CF testing, a few laboratories offer larger mutation panels than the ACMG recommendations, but these extended panels may still fail to identify one or both of the CF mutations in some patients. Extensive sequencing of all exons, intron/exon borders, promoter regions and specific intronic regions with a mutation detection rate as high as 98.7 percent, has been described and is clinically available.[106] Limitations of such technology include the identification of novel sequence changes in which the clinical significance is unknown. Once the mutations in a patient have been identified, specific mutation analyses for that family then becomes available. A reasonable approach for studying patients in whom CF is suspected is to first obtain mutation results for the ACMG Core Panel, because most patients with CF would be expected to have at least one of those mutations. If a mutation is not detected, the likelihood of CF is significantly reduced. However, if the diagnosis of CF remains strong, more extensive CF mutation studies could then be obtained.

In selecting a reference laboratory for population-based preconceptual or CF carrier screening, it is essential to confirm that the laboratory is offering the twenty-five-mutation ACMG recommended mutation panel. Reference laboratories should participate in ACMG/CAP or another comparable proficiency test and should be accredited through the CAP Molecular Pathology Accreditation process or another comparable agency. Laboratories should provide specific proficiency test results and CAP inspection information when requested. Although these processes do not guarantee accuracy, they will provide information that help determine a laboratory's standards.

PRENATAL DIAGNOSIS OF CYSTIC FIBROSIS

Assisted Reproductive Technology (ART) and Preimplantation Genetic Diagnosis (PGD)

ART can be used to achieve pregnancy in couples in whom the male is infertile as a result of CFTR gene mutations. Sperm can be aspirated by microscopic epididymal sperm aspiration (MESA), percutaneous epididymal sperm aspiration (PESA), or open testis biopsy followed by in vitro fertilization (IVF), usually by intracytoplasmic sperm injection (ICSI)[107] The presence of CF mutations in the male with infertility does not negatively affect the rate of pregnancy or healthy livebirths compared with couples undergoing ART for other reasons.[107,108] Because most men with CBAVD have at least one detectable CF mutation, screening for mutations, a detailed family and medical history, and genetic counseling should be offered to all men with CBAVD and couples considering reproduction alternatives.[109] Couples at risk of having an affected child should then be offered prenatal diagnosis either by preimplantation diagnosis, CVS, or amniocentesis.[110]

The first report of preimplantation diagnosis of CF after IVF was in 1992.[111] Three couples in which both parents carried the ΔF508 deletion were treated. One of the two women undergoing embryo transfer became pregnant and gave birth to a normal girl unaffected by CF and free of both parent's ΔF508 alleles. The pregnancy rates for couples undergoing PGD is comparable to couples undergoing regular ICSI.[111,112] During preimplantation diagnosis, the correct genotype of the embryo is essential, and misdiagnosis has been reported because of lack of amplification of a mutant allele (allele drop-out), resulting in a false-negative result. Initially, preimplantation diagnosis for CF was performed only when both parents were ΔF508 carriers because the determination of compound heterozygous embryos is complicated and technically difficult. PGD has been improved with the use of whole genome amplification prior to testing for the mutation of interest,[112] biopsying two blastomeres when only one mutation is identified,[113] analyzing informative, linked microsatellites instead of the disease-causing mutations,[114] and fluorescent-PCR technology (decreases the allele-drop out rate and is 1000× more sensitive than conventional PCR).

Although preimplantation genetic diagnosis of CF has provided couples with an additional option for the prenatal diagnosis of CF, this option currently is limited to couples with financial resources who have access to medical specialists with knowledge of such procedures. Alternative methods of conception available to a known carrier couple to avoid the risk of CF in an offspring include artificial insemination with sperm from a screened male donor, or with an ovum from a screened female donor, and adoption. Many families with a child with CF tend to stop having additional children to avoid the one-in-four risk of having another affected child.[115]

Prenatal Diagnosis

For known carrier couples, prenatal diagnosis with the option of an elective pregnancy termination of an affected fetus remains the main option. Genetic counseling for known CF carrier couples is essential. Studies performed before the actual availability of prenatal diagnosis of CF suggested a potential widespread demand for prenatal diagnosis of CF.[115] However, use has been less than predicted (for review, see Decruyenaere M, Evers-Kiebooms G, Denayer L and Welkenhuysen M[115a]). In one prospective study, 51 percent of parents said they would certainly or probably use prenatal diagnosis in case of pregnancy. Among those rejecting (49 percent), the fear of an unsolvable conflict in case of an affected fetus prevailed. Interestingly, the use of prenatal diagnosis was arranged in 21 percent and actually performed in 17 percent of the cases.[116] However, couples identified through carrier screening programs have drastically different uptakes for prenatal diagnosis and pregnancy termination. Brock,[117] for example, reported that 91 percent of couples identified as carriers through a prenatal screening program opted for prenatal diagnosis, and in 100 percent of cases in which an affected fetus was identified, elective abortion was the parents' choice. The acceptance and uptake of population-based carrier screening now that it is recommended by ACOG and ACMG will depend much on how it is presented to patients.[118] Studies on the uptake of CF carrier screening following the recent guidelines are needed.

Highly accurate prenatal diagnosis is available for families with a previously affected child with known mutations and for couples in which both members are known CF carriers. For couples in which both mutations are known, direct mutation analysis using fetal cells can be performed to determine the fetal genotype. The risk of maternal cell contamination of fetal DNA is a potential cause of erroneous test results, and laboratories should perform additional studies, such as analyzing polymorphic markers, to rule out maternal cell contamination.[105] Because approximately 90 percent of non-Hispanic Caucasian CF mutations are routinely tested in most diagnostic laboratories, the necessity of linkage analysis for this disorder has been markedly reduced. However, linkage analysis with polymorphic markers can be used for families in which one or neither mutation can be identified.[119] Microsatellite polymorphic provide highly accurate linkage analyses with little risk of a crossover.[114] Potential diagnostic pitfalls, such as nonpaternity and uniparental disomy should always be investigated when unusual test results are reported.

The ability to isolate fetal cells from maternal plasma may lead to the future development of noninvasive prenatal genetic testing for CF. The detection of a paternal CF mutation has been reported in fetal cells isolated from maternal plasma at 13 weeks of gestation.[120] Although this technology is promising, because the presence of a maternal mutation present in the mother's genome versus the fetal genome cannot currently be differentiated, this form of noninvasive testing is limited to identifying paternal and de novo fetal mutations.

Uniparental Disomy

Uniparental disomy (UPD), the inheritance of two homologous chromosomes from one parent in a diploid cell, arises from two abnormal cell divisions during meiosis and/or mitosis. Two patients with CF have been described who inherited identical copies of a maternal CF chromosome 7 with no paternal contribution for the genetic material on this chromosome.[121,122] The patient, originally reported by Spence and co-workers,[121] was homozygous for the G542X nonsense mutation.[123] UPD is estimated to account for only 1 in 10,000 CF cases[124]; thus, it is a rare cause of CF. A prenatal procedure generally is not recommended if only one partner is a carrier because the a priori risk of UPD is low.

Echogenic Bowel and CF

Fetal echogenic bowel is detected in 0.2–1.8 percent of all second-trimester pregnancies[125,126] and was initially reported as a normal variant.[127] Although the majority of fetuses with prenatally detected echogenic bowel have a normal outcome, one study reported that nearly one-fourth of pregnancies with this ultrasound finding have an adverse outcome.[128] Echogenic bowel has been found in fetuses with complications including chromosome abnormalities, congenital infections, intrauterine growth retardation, fetal death, intra-amniotic bleeds and CF (for review, see Al-Kouatly et al.[129] and Simon-Bouy B et al.[129a]). One study found that 50–60 percent of fetuses affected with CF (who were at-risk, based on family history) had prenatally detected echogenic bowel.[130] Early studies on the incidence of CF in fetuses with hyperechoic bowel ranged from 0 to 13 percent.[125,131,132] These studies were limited by either small sample size, an undefined or small number of mutations tested for, or lack of information regarding how the diagnosis of CF was made; therefore, the significance of this ultrasound finding as it related to CF was unclear.

More recent studies have reported that the incidence of CF in fetuses with incidentally discovered echogenic bowel ranges from 0.8 percent in the United States[133] to 3–10 percent in France.[129a,134] The French study examined >346,000 pregnancies, of which 142 had echogenic bowel, and identified 14 fetuses affected with CF. DNA testing involved screening for 87 percent of the known mutations in the population followed by an extended analysis with a detection rate of 98.5 percent for all fetuses with one identifiable mutation. The fetal mutations identified were associated with a PI phenotype. Using a bayesian analysis, they report that the remaining carrier risk for a fetus with prenatally detected echogenic bowel is reduced from 1 in 10 to 1 in 500 if no fetal mutation is identified and increased to 24 percent when one mutation is identified. Another study examined 159 cases of prenatally detected echogenic bowel in an ethnically and racially diverse population in the United States.[135] The mutation detection rate in this study was 90 percent for Caucasians of European descent. Two affected fetuses were identified, and both had two severe mutations associated with PI CF. The overall frequency of CF associated with echogenic bowel in this diverse population was 1.3 percent. Using a bayesian calculation, the remaining risk for CF in a Caucasian fetus with echogenic bowel decreased from 1.7 percent to 1 in 5,783 when no fetal mutation was identified and increased to 8 percent when one fetal mutation was identified.

Based on these risks, parental CF mutation studies, along with a fetal karyotype and a search for a congenital infection, should be offered to all pregnant women with this fetal ultrasound finding. Direct fetal studies could be performed if a fetal sample is available; alternatively, both parents could be studied, although mistaken paternity could lead to a false-negative diagnosis if only the parents are studied. Fetal studies would be indicated if one or both of the parents is identified as a CF carrier. If two CF mutations are identified in a fetal sample, the diagnosis of CF is confirmed, whereas identifying only one CF mutation in the fetus creates a dilemma in which a definitive molecular diagnosis cannot be made. In this case DNA testing using an extended mutation panel or DNA sequencing may be useful. To assist with genetic counseling and risk assessment, a bayesian calculation to determine the residual risk in an at-risk fetus may also be performed. This analysis depends on the frequency of CF among fetuses with echogenic bowel, the CF carrier frequency, and the mutation detection rate.

CARRIER DETECTION

Family History of CF

CF carrier detection studies should be offered to relatives of patients with CF who are interested or who are considering a pregnancy. A family history obtained as part of routine primary or obstetrical care should identify individuals with a positive family history of CF. Similarly, if a family history of unilateral or bilateral absence of the vas deferens is obtained, CF carrier testing should also be offered. Ideally, the affected individual is the person in whom testing should first be performed in order to know for certain whether a CF mutation is identifiable within that family. If a mutation is identified, a more accurate risk assessment can be calculated for other family members. Because population screening for CF is now recommended, some individuals may know about other CF carriers in their family even if there is no family history of CF. Individuals with a positive family history of CF and a negative mutation analysis can have a carrier risk calculated that takes into account available information regarding the known family history and the mutation information (see Table 15.2). For most cases in which one partner has a family history positive for CF, the family history in the other partner is usually negative. However, CF screening should still be offered to both individuals, so that a joint risk of having a child with CF can be calculated. For example, a Caucasian couple in which one partner is a known CF carrier and the other partner is not screened has a 1 in 116 chance of having an affected child [(1×0.5) $(1/29 \times 0.5)$]. If that partner is screened and found to be a carrier, their joint risk increases to 1 in 4 [$(1 \times 0.5)(1 \times 0.5)$]. However, if that partner is screened and has a negative mutation analysis, using a Bayesian calculation and assuming a 90 percent CF detection rate, that couple's risk of having an affected child is reduced to 1 in 1124 $(1 \times 0.5)(1/281 \times 0.5)$. For most couples, this is reassuring information, and prenatal diagnosis generally is not indicated under these circumstances. Although initially there was concern regarding pregnancy termination in situations in which a fetus had inherited one CF mutation, this is exceedingly rare in the experience of most laboratories.[136–138]

Population Screening

The identification of the CF gene and its most common mutations introduced the possibility of widespread population screening for CF. Several reservations, however, were raised about the prospect of population-based carrier screening for CF. For some, acting to avoid the birth of children with CF seemed an inappropriate goal, in part because of the improved prognosis of individuals affected with CF and in part because of the belief that a cure for this disease would be developed in the near future.[139] Other concerns were raised about the limitations of the test itself. Even when multiple mutations are screened for, the carrier-detection rate in CF population screening remains, at best, 85–90 percent among those of Caucasian ancestry and is lower in other populations.[18] Thus, some wondered whether this level of sensitivity was sufficient to warrant devoting the resources needed for population-based screening.[140] Others were concerned about the uncertainty that would be faced by couples when only one partner was shown to be a carrier.[141] The projected demand and the perceived difficulties of informing people about CF carrier screening, particularly with regard to the possibility of false-negative results, led some to speculate that geneticists would be overwhelmed by the introduction of CF carrier screening.[142] Additional concerns include the large size of the target population, the relatively high cost of carrier testing, and concerns that misunderstanding test results would lead to unwarranted prenatal procedures and pregnancy terminations. Statements were issued by American professional genetic groups advising a moratorium on widespread carrier testing until pilot studies were completed.[141,143–145] The National Institutes of Health (NIH) and others then funded a series of pilot studies in the United States to determine how to offer voluntary CF carrier screening; other countries instituted similar pilot studies. The results of CF screening trials were reviewed in 1998 and again in 2002.[146,147] An NIH Consensus Development Conference on Genetic Testing for Cystic Fibrosis in April, 1997 recommended that genetic screening for CF in the United States be offered to adults with a family history of CF, to partners of people with CF, to couples currently planning a pregnancy and to couples seeking prenatal care.[148] Recognizing that laboratory testing for CF was not standardized and that educational materials to support such a massive undertaking were not readily available, an NIH-sponsored conference was held shortly thereafter to discuss the implementation of the NIH Consensus Conference recommendations.[149] In the meantime, the ACMG and American College of Obstetrics and Gynecology (ACOG) issued statements that routine prenatal screening for CF was not standard practice and would not be until the above requirements were met.[150,151] Eventually, the ACMG identified and recommended a core panel of mutations for CF population-based CF carrier screening.[9] These recommendations were based on the prevalence of these mutations in more than 20,000 patients with classic CF; any mutation representing 0.1 percent or more of CFTR alleles in this panethnic population was included. This panel included twenty-five mutations and four variants, one of which was known to modify the expression of one of the mutations (Table 15.1). Because the mutation panel is panethnic, the residual remaining carrier risk for an individual is based on their ethnic background and prior carrier risk (Table 15.2). It was anticipated that the composition of the recommended panel would be reviewed and revised appropriately. In a collaborative effort, the ACOG, the ACMG, and the National Human Genome Research Institute's Ethical, Legal and Social Implications program developed the materials and standards needed to ensure the appropriate implementation of these guidelines, which were further refined by these orginizations.[152] Their report recommended CF screening be offered in the United States to:

- Individuals with a family history of CF
- Reproductive partners of individuals who have CF
- Couples in whom one or both partners are Caucasian and are planning a pregnancy or seeking prenatal care. For couples planning pregnancy or seeking prenatal care,

it is recommended that screening should *be offered* to those at higher risk of having children with CF (Caucasians, including Ashkenazi Jews) and in whom the testing is most sensitive in identifying carriers of a CF mutation. It is further recommended that screening should *be made available* to couples in other racial and ethnic groups who are at lower risk and in whom the test may be less sensitive. For couples to whom screening will be offered, it is recommended that this be done when they seek preconception counseling or infertility care, or during the first and early second trimester of pregnancy.

The report noted that the counseling, offer of screening and the couple's decision regarding screening should be discussed and documented in the medical record and that written, informed consent should be obtained only after the woman and her partner have an opportunity to review the educational material and receive pretest counseling. **Documentation of the patient's decision to accept or decline screening should be incorporated into the medical record.** Two different screening strategies were discussed as appropriate: concurrent screening (both partners are tested simultaneously) or sequential screening (one person is tested, then the partner is tested only if the first person is identified as a carrier). The guidelines also stated that patients should receive information that includes a brief description of the following considerations:

- The purpose of screening
- The voluntary nature of the testing
- The range of symptoms and severity of CF, the treatment of the disease, and life expectancy
- The genetics of CF and population estimates of carrier risk in their ethnic or racial group
- The meaning of positive and negative test results
- Factors to consider in deciding to have or not have screening

Finally, the guidelines noted that when both partners are identified as CF carriers during early pregnancy, prenatal diagnosis should be offered. When appropriate or when special expertise is required, referral to a geneticist or a provider with special expertise in CF testing should be made.

Since the implementation of these guidelines, some data are available with regard to uptake and laboratory aspects of testing. For example, CFTR testing has increased significantly and continues to increase.[88] Interpreting and reporting of test results are among the most challenging parts of screening. Accurate interpretation requires that ethnic information and family history be obtained. Risk calculations for an individual with a negative test are not accurate unless that information is available. A predicted, although difficult, situation is the identification of asymptomatic individuals in whom two CF mutations are detected. Many laboratories and physicians have identified such individuals. Referral of the patient to a CF Center is strongly recommended when that occurs.

Of concern is that some laboratories have chosen to include testing for the intron 8 polyT variant (5T/7T/9T) in their initial reporting process,[153] even though the ACMG recommendations clearly indicated that testing for this variant should be performed only as a reflex test when the R117H mutation was identified.[9] The reason that some laboratories have chosen this approach is unclear, although it may be related to the fact that some of the commercially available methods include this variant in an all-or-none single test. Although there are clear indications for studying the status of the polyT variant (see "Correlation between Genotype and Phenotype" above), reporting of the 5T variant in prenatal carrier screening settings has led to many difficult counseling dilemmas, as the goal of the prenatal screening program was to identify individuals at risk for classic CF, not CBAVD.

Another unexpected finding was the discovery that the I148T mutation was appearing about 100 times as often as expected based on its incidence among patients with CF.[95] This suggested that I148T was not a true mutation, but rather a benign polymorphism linked to a causative CF mutation in some patients. Rohlfs et al.[95] identified the likely causative CF mutation in some patients with CF who carried the I148T mutation, called 3199del6. This is one example of how the ACMG Core mutation panel will be revised, because many testing panels do not include 3199del6, it is not one of the twenty-five mutations currently included in the ACMG Core mutation panel and its mutation frequency is so low that it does not meet the inclusion criteria established by the ACMG.

Thus, although there is no clear information about the uptake of CF screening in the United States, it is apparent that many more individuals are choosing to have CF carrier screening performed. Many clinicians may still not be routinely offering this as part of their routine prenatal obstetrical care. Because the ACOG has officially recommended offering CF carrier screening, it will likely the standard of care in the United States, and obstetrical care providers who are not offering CF carrier screening may be at risk for litigation.

Neonatal Screening for CF

Reliable screening of neonates for CF by determination of dried blood-spot immunoreactive trypsin (IRT) levels was first described in 1979.[154] During the subsequent 25 years, there has been much debate regarding whether early diagnosis of CF by newborn screening is beneficial in reducing long-term morbidity and mortality. The underlying premise is that diagnosis of CF in early infancy will allow for aggressive nutritional supplementation and an improvement in long-term pulmonary function. Furthermore, because CF is often difficult to identify, delays mean that children are often not diagnosed until severe malnutrition is already present and the child has been subjected to many invasive evaluations. The identification of the CF gene made possible a different approach to neonatal screening, in which screeners used a combination of IRT determination and direct gene analysis with the same dried blood sample.[155-158] Studies indicate that at least 95 percent of patients with CF can be detected through newborn screening, although false-negative results do occur.[159] Data are accumulating that support the idea that significantly better long-term growth in patients who were diagnosed early through screening does occur.[160-163] Families have benefited from the early diagnosis that newborn screening allows. For the affected child, prompt treatment of symptoms is possible. For the parents of the affected child, additional benefits of newborn screening include the identification of previously undiagnosed siblings with CF, offers the parents the opportunity to obtain genetic counseling in order to make informed decisions about their reproductive future and allows for potential identification of CF carriers in the extended family.[164]

FUTURE

It is clear that CF carrier screening is being carried out in many primary care settings with a high degree of patient satisfaction, an improvement in laboratory methods, and improved reproduction options for individuals with CF or couples at risk for having a child with

CF. There appears to be a high level of interest among couples, although some insurance companies have yet to establish clear policies on whether CF carrier screening is a covered benefit. Studies are currently only beginning to investigate the level of comprehension among patients undergoing CF carrier screening, and, as a result, the manner in which genetic counseling is offered will likely change over time. The ACMG CF Core mutation panel currently being performed will also be modified, as technologies improve and additional information regarding specific CF mutations becomes available. Improved treatments have considerably increased the life expectancy of a child born today with CF. Although gene therapy trials have been less than encouraging so far, it is hoped that continued research will result in successful treatment approaches for CF. Additional studies of modifying loci and genotype–phenotype correlations will be a major factor in determining therapeutic strategies and long-term prognosis for patients with specific CF mutations. In the future one can envision using prenatal diagnosis for CF to predict not only genotype but also therapeutic strategies.[165] As technology advances, noninvasive prenatal diagnosis using fetal DNA extracted from maternal plasma may become a reality.

REFERENCES

1. Andersen DH. Cystic fibrosis of the pancreas and its relation to celiac disease. Am J Dis Child 1938;56:344.
2. Andersen DH, Hodges RG. Celiac syndrome. Am J Dis Child 1946;72:62.
3. Romeo G, Bianco M, Devoto M, et al. Incidence in Italy, genetic heterogeneity, and segregation of cystic fibrosis. Am J Hum Genet 1985;37:338.
4. Kramm ER, Crane MM, Sirkin MG, et al. A cystic fibrosis pilot survey in three New England states. Am J Public Health 1962;52:2041.
5. Korosok MR, Wei W, Farrell PM. The incidence of cystic fibrosis. Stat Med 1996;15:449.
6. Abeliovich D, Lavon IP, Lerer I, et al. Screening for five mutations detects 97% of cystic fibrosis (CF) chromosomes and predicts a carrier frequency of 1:29 in the Jewish Ashkenazi population. Am J Hum Genet 1992;51:951.
7. Kulczycki LL, Schauf V. Cystic fibrosis in blacks in Washington DC. Am J Dis Child 1974;127:64.
8. Phillips OP, Bishop C, Woods D, et al. Cystic fibrosis mutations among African Americans in the southeastern United States. J Natl Med Assoc 1995;87:433.
9. Grody WW, Cutting GR, Klinger KW, et al. Laboratory standards and guidelines for population-based cystic fibrosis carrier screening. Genet Med 2001;149.
10. Macek M, Mackova A, Hamosh A, et al. Identification of common cystic fibrosis mutations in African-Americans with cystic fibrosis increases the detection rate to 75%. Am J Hum Genet 1997;60:1122.
11. Grebe TA, Seltzer WK, DeMarchi J, et al. Genetic analysis of Hispanic individuals with cystic fibrosis. Am J Hum Genet 1994;54:443.
12. Grebe TA, Doane WW, Richter SF, et al. Mutation analysis of the cystic fibrosis transmembrane regulator in Native American populations of the Southwest. Am J Hum Genet 1992;51:736.
13. Mercier B, Raguenes O, Estivill X, et al. Complete detection of mutations in cystic fibrosis patients of Native American origin. Hum Genet 1994;94:629.
14. Yee K, Robinson C, Horlock G, et al. Novel cystic fibrosis mutation L1093P: functional analysis and possible Native American origin. Hum Mutat 2000;15:208.
15. El-Harith EA, Dörk T, Stuhrmann M, et al. Novel and characteristic CFTR mutations in Saudi Arab children with cystic fibrosis. J Med Genet 1997;34:996.
16. Kambouris M, Banjar M, Moggari I, et al. Identification of novel mutations in the CFTR gene causing cystic fibrosis (CF) in Arab populations. Institut Paster del Tunis 1997;74:93.
17. Degeorges M, Megarbane A, Guittard C, et al. Cystic fibrosis in Lebanon: distribution of CFTR mutations among Arab communities. Hum Genet 1997;100:279.
18. Bobadilla J, Macek Jr M, Fine JP and Farrell PM. Cystic fibrosis: a worldwide analysis of CFTR mutations-correlation with incidence data and application to screening. Hum Mutat 2002;19:575.
19. Schidlow DV, Taussig LM, Knowles MR. Cystic fibrosis foundation consensus conference report on pulmonary complications of cystic fibrosis. Pediatr Pulmonol 1993;15:187.

20. Kraisinger M, Hochhaus G, Stecenko A, et al. Clinical pharmacology of pancreatic enzymes in patients with cystic fibrosis and in vitro performance of microencapsulated formulations. J Clin Pharmacol 1994; 34:158.

21. FitzSimmons SC. The changing epidemiology of cystic fibrosis. J Pediatr 1993;122:1.

22. Bronstein M, Sokol R, Abman S, et al. Pancreatic insufficiency, growth and nutrition in infants identified by newborn screening as having cystic fibrosis. J Pediatr 1992;120:533.

23. Ramsey BW, Farrell PM, Pencharz P, et al. Nutritional assessment and management in cystic fibrosis: a consensus report. Am J Clin Nutr 1992;55:108.

24. Johannesson M, Gottlieb C, Hjelte L. Delayed puberty in girls with cystic fibrosis despite good clinical status. Pediatrics 1997;99:29.

25. Ratjen F, Doring G. Cystic fibrosis. Lancet 2003;361:681.

26. Dodge JA. Male fertility in cystic fibrosis. Lancet 1995;346:587.

27. Dörk T, Dworniczak B, Aulehla-Scholz C, et al. Distinct spectrum of CFTR gene mutations in congenital absence of vas deferens. Hum Genet 1997;100:365.

27a. Timmreck LS, Gray MR, Handelin B, et al. Analysis of cystic fibrosis transmembrane conductance regulator in patients with congenital absence of the uterus and vagina. Am J Med Genet 2003;120A:72–76.

28. Gillet D, deBrakeeleer M, Bellis G, et al. Cystic fibrosis and pregnancy: report from French data (1980–1999). BJOG 2002;109:912.

29. Edenborough FP, Wackenzie WE and Stableforth DE. The outcome of 72 pregnancies with cystic fibrosis in the United Kingdom 1977–1996. BJOG 2000;107:254.

30. Di Sant'Agnese PA, Darling RC, Perera GA, et al. Abnormal electrolyte composition of sweat in cystic fibrosis of the pancreas. Pediatrics 1953;12:549.

31. Gibson LE, Cooke RE. A test for concentration of electrolytes in sweat in cystic fibrosis of the pancreas utilizing pilocarpine by iontophoresis. Pediatrics 1959;23:545.

32. Rosenstein BJ and Cutting GR. The diagnosis of cystic fibrosis: a consensus statement. J Pediatr 1998;132:589.

33. LeGrys VA. Sweat testing for the diagnosis of cystic fibrosis: practical considerations. J Pediatr 1996;129:892.

34. Cystic Fibrosis Foundation, Patient Registry 2001 Annual Report, Bethesda, MD: Cystic Fibrosis Foundation, 2002.

35. Elborn JS, Shale DJ, Britton JR. Cystic fibrosis: current survival and population estimates to the year 2000. Thorax 1991;46:881.

36. Ramsey BW. Management of pulmonary disease in patients with cystic fibrosis. N Engl J Med 1996;335:179.

37. Sanchez I, Guiraldes E. Drug management of noninfective complications of cystic fibrosis. Drugs 1995;50:626.

38. Lebenthal E, Rolston DD, Holsclaw DS Jr. Enzyme therapy for pancreatic insufficiency: present status and future needs. Pancreas 1994;9:1–12.

39. Dodge JA. Malnutrition and age-specific nutritional management in cystic fibrosis. Neth J Med 1992; 41:127.

40. Mendeloff EN, Huddleston CB, Mallory GB, et al. Pediatric and adult lung transplantation for cystic fibrosis. J Thorac Cardiovasc Surg 1998;114:404.

41. Vricella LA, Karamichalis JM, Ahmad S, et al. Lung and heart-lung transplantation in patients with end-stage cystic fibrosis: the Stanford experience. Ann Thorac Surg 2002;74:13.

42. Liou TG, Adler FR, Cahill BC, et al. Survival effect of lung transplantation among patients with cystic fibrosis. JAMA 2001;286:2683.

43. Dennis CM, McNeil KD, Dunning J, et al. Heart-lung-liver transplantation. J Heart Lung Transplant 1996;15:536.

44. Cystic Fibrosis Foundation (www.cff.org/about_cf/gene_therapy_and_cf.cfm). Bethesda, MD (accessed May 25, 2003).

45. Milkiewicz P, Skiba G, Kelly D, et al. Transplantation for cystic fibrosis: outcome following early liver transplantation. J Gastroenterol Hepatol 2002;2:208.

46. Knowles MR, Hohneker KW, Zhou Z, et al. A controlled study of adenoviral-vector-mediated gene transfer in the nasal epithelium of patients with cystic fibrosis. N Engl J Med 1995;333:823.

47. Wagner JA, Nepomuceno IB, Messner AH et al. A phase II, double-blind, randomized, placebo-controlled clinical trial of tgAAVCF using maxillary sinus delivery in patients with cystic fibrosis. Hum Gene Ther 2002;11:1349.

48. Griesenbach U, Ferrari S, Geddes DM and Alton EW. Gene therapy progress and prospects: cystic fi-
    brosis. Gene Ther 2002;20:1344.
49. Tsui L-C, Buchwald M, Barker D, et al. Cystic fibrosis locus defined by a genetically linked polymor-
    phic DNA marker. Science 1985;230:1054.
50. Estivill X, Farrall M, Scambler PJ, et al. A candidate for the cystic fibrosis locus isolated by selection for
    methylation-free islands. Nature 1987;326:840.
51. Farrall M, Wainwright BJ, Feldman GL, et al. Recombinations between IRP and cystic fibrosis. Am J
    Hum Genet 1988;43:471.
52. Kerem B, Rommens JM, Buchanan D, et al. Identification of the cystic fibrosis gene: genetic analysis.
    Science 1989;245:1073.
53. Riordan JR, Rommens JM, Kerem B, et al. Identification of the cystic fibrosis gene: cloning and char-
    acterization of complementary DNA. Science 1989;245:1066.
54. Rommens JM, Iannuzzi MC, Kerem B, et al. Identification of the cystic fibrosis gene: chromosome jump-
    ing and walking. Science 1989;245:1059.
55. Zielenski J, Rozmahel R, Bozon D, et al. Genomic sequence of the cystic fibrosis conductance regulator
    (CFTR) gene. Genomics 1991;10:214.
56. Hasegawa HW, Skach W, Baker O, et al. A multifunctional aqueous channel formed by CFTR. Science
    1992;258:1477.
57. Sheppard DN, Welsh MJ. Structure and function of the CFTR chloride channel. Physiol Rev 1999;79:S23.
58. Akabas MH. Cystic fibrosis transmembrane conductance regulator: structure and function of an epithe-
    lial chloride channel. J Biol Chem 2000;275:3729.
59. Zou X, Hwang TC. ATP hydrolysis-coupled gating of CFTR chloride channels: structure and function.
    Biochemistry 2001;40:5579.
60. Tsui L-C. The cystic fibrosis transmembrane conductance regulator gene. Am J Respir Crit Care Med
    1995;151:S47.
61. The Cystic Fibrosis Genetic Analysis Consortium. Cystic Fibrosis Mutation Data Base (www.genet.sick-
    kids.on.ca). Toronto: The Hospital for Sick Children (accessed 15/November, 2003).
62. Cystic Fibrosis Genotype-Phenotype Consortium. Correlation between genotype and phenotype in pa-
    tients with cystic fibrosis. N Engl J Med 1993;329:1308.
63. Tsui L-C. The spectrum of cystic fibrosis mutations. Trends Genet 1992;8:392.
64. Kerem B, Kerem E. The molecular basis for disease variability in cystic fibrosis. Eur J Hum Genet
    1996;4:65.
65. Palomaki GE, Haddow JE, Bradley LA, et al. Updated assessment of cystic fibrosis mutation frequencies
    in non-Hispanic Caucasians. Genet Med 2002;4:90.
66. Schwiebert EM, Benos DJ, Fuller CM. Cystic fibrosis: A multiple exocrinopathy caused by dysfunctions
    in a multifunctional transport protein. Am J Med 1998;104:576.
67. Welsh MJ, Smith AE. Molecular mechanisms of CFTR chloride channel dysfunction in cystic fibrosis.
    Cell 1993;73:1251.
68. Wilschanski M, Zielenski J, Markiewicz D, et al. Correlation of sweat chloride concentration with classes
    of the cystic fibrosis transmembrane conductance regulator gene mutations. J Pediatr 1995;127:705.
69. Tsui LC, Durie P. Genotype and phenotype in cystic fibrosis. Hosp Pract (Off Ed) 1997;32:115.
70. Shoshani T, Augarten A, Gazit E, et al. Association of a nonsense mutation (W1282X), the most com-
    mon mutation in the Ashkenazi Jewish cystic fibrosis patients in Israel, with presentation of severe dis-
    ease. Am J Hum Genet 1992;50:222.
71. Schwartz M, Sørensen N, Brandt NJ. High incidence of cystic fibrosis on the Faroe Islands: a molecular
    and genealogical study. Hum Genet 1995;6:703.
72. Orgad S, Neumann S, Loewenthal R, et al. Prevalence of cystic fibrosis mutations in Israeli Jews. Genet
    Test 2001;5:47.
73. Kerem E, Corey M, Kerem B, et al. The relation between genotype and phenotype in cystic fibrosis:
    analysis of the most common mutation (ΔF508). N Engl J Med 1990;323:1517.
74. Durno C, Corey M, Zielenski J, et al. Genotype and phenotype correlations in patients with cystic fibro-
    sis and pancreatitis. Gastroenterology 2002;123:1857.
75. Kristidis P, Bozon D, Corey M, et al. Genetic determination of exocrine pancreatic function in cystic fi-
    brosis. Am J Hum Genet 1992;50:1178.
76. Walkowiak J, Herzig K-H, Witt M, et al. Analysis of exocrine pancreatic function in cystic fibrosis: one
    mild CFTR mutation does not exclude pancreatic insufficiency. Eur J Clin Invest 2001;31:796.
77. Costes B, Girodon E, Ghanem N, et al. Frequent occurrence of the CFTR intron 8 (TG)n 5T allele in
    men with congenital bilateral absence of the vas deferens. Eur J Hum Genet 1995;3:285.

78. Kiesewetter S, Macek M Jr, Davis C, et al. A mutation in the CFTR produces different phenotypes depending on chromosomal background. Nat Genet 1993;5:274.

79. Chillon M, Casals T, Mercier B, et al. Mutations in the cystic fibrosis gene in patients with congenital absence of the vas deferens. N Engl J Med 1995;332:1475.

80. Friedman KJ, Heim RA, Knowles MR, et al. Rapid characterization of the variable length polythymidine tract in the cystic fibrosis (CFTR) gene: association of the 5T allele with selected CFTR mutations and its incidence in atypical sinopulmonary disease. Hum Mutat 1997;10:108.

81. Noone PG, Pue CA, Zhou Z, et al. Lung disease associated with the IVS8 5T allele of the CFTR gene. Am J Respir Crit Care Med 2000;162:1919.

82. Chmiel JF, Drumm ML, Konstan MW, et al. Pitfall in the use of genotype analysis as the sole diagnostic criterion for cystic fibrosis. Pediatrics 1999;103:823.

83. Taylor CG, Dalton A, Pirzada O. Cystic fibrosis mutations and disease phenotype. Arch Dis Child 2000;83:185.

84. Mak V, Zielenski J, Tsui L-C, et al. Proportion of cystic fibrosis gene mutations not detected by routine testing in men with obstructive azoospermia. JAMA 1999;281:2217.

85. Claustres M, Guittard C, Bozon D, et al. Spectrum of CFTR mutations in cystic fibrosis and in congenital absence of the vas deferens in France. Hum Mutat 2000;16:143.

86. Noone PG, Knowles MR. CFTR-opathies: disease phenotypes associated with cystic fibrosis transmembrane regulator gene mutations. Respir Res 2001;2:328.

87. Massie RJH, Poplawski N, Wilcken B, et al. Intron-8 polythymidine sequence in Australasian individuals with CF mutations R117H and R117C. Eur Respir J 2001;17:1195.

88. Watson MS, Desnick RJ, Grody WW et al. Cystic fibrosis carrier screening: issues in implementation. Genet Med 2002;4:1.

89. Mickle JE, Cutting GR. Genotype-phenotype relationships in cystic fibrosis. Med Clin North Am 2000;84:597.

90. Mercier B, Verlingue C, Lissens W, et al. Is congenital bilateral absence of vas deferens a primary form of cystic fibrosis? Analyses of the CFTR gene in 67 patients. Am J Hum Genet 1995;56:272.

91. Schlegel PN, Shin D, Goldstein M. Urogenital anomalies in men with congenital absence of the vas deferens. J Urol 1996;155:1644.

92. Daudin M, Bieth E, Bujan L, et al. Congenital bilateral absence of the vas deferens: clinical characteristics, biological parameters, cystic fibrosis transmembrane conductance regulator gene mutations, and implications for genetic counseling. Fertil Steril 2000;74:1164.

93. Anguiano A, Oates RD, Amos J, et al. Congenital bilateral absence of the vas deferens: a primarily genital form of cystic fibrosis. JAMA 1992;267:1794.

94. Colin AA, Sawyer SM, Mickle JE, et al. Pulmonary function and clinical observations in men with congenital bilateral absence of the vas deferens. Chest 1996;110:440.

95. Rohlfs EM, Zhou Z, Sugarman EA, et al. The I148T CFTR allele occurs on multiple haplotypes: a complex allele is associated with cystic fibrosis. Genet Med 2002;4:319.

96. Salvatore F, Scudiero O, Castaldo G. Genotype-phenotype correlation in cystic fibrosis: the role of modifier genes. Am J Med Genet 2002;111:88.

97. Santis G, Osborne L, Knight R, et al. Genotype-phenotype relationship in cystic fibrosis: results from the study of monozygotic and dizygotic twins with cystic fibrosis. Pediatr Pulmonol 1992;14 (suppl 8):239.

98. Acton JD and Wilmott RW. Phenotype of CF and the effects of possible modifier genes. Paediatr Respir Rev 2001;2:332.

99. Merlo CA, Boyle MP. Modifier genes in cystic fibrosis lung disease. J Lab Clin Med 2003;141:237.

100. Zielenski J, Corey M, Rozmahel R, et al. Detection of a cystic fibrosis modifier locus for meconium ileus on human chromosome 19q13. Nat Genet 1999;22:128.

101. Garred P, Pressler T, Madsen HO, et al. Association of mannose-binding lectin gene heterogeneity with severity of lung disease and survival in cystic fibrosis. J. Clin Invest 1999;104:431.

102. Arkwright PD, Laurie S, Super M, et al. TGF-β_1 genotype and accelerated decline in lung function of patients with cystic fibrosis. Thorax 2002;55:459–462.

103. Hull J, Thomson AH. Contribution of genetic factors other than CFTR to disease severity in cystic fibrosis. Thorax 1998;53:1018–1021.

104. Richards B, Skoletsky J, Shuber AP, et al. Multiplex PCR amplification from the CFTR gene using DNA prepared from buccal brushes/swabs. Hum Mol Genet 1993;2:159.

105. Richards CS, Bradley LA, Amos J et al. Standards and Guidelines for CFTR mutation testing. Genet Med 2002;4:379.

106. Strom SM, Huang D, Chen C, et al. Extensive sequencing of the cystic fibrosis transmembrane regula-

tor gene: assay validation and unexpected benefits of developing a comprehensive test. Genet Med 2003;5:9.

107. Phillipson GTM, Petrucco OM, Matthews CD. Congenital bilateral absence of the vas deferens, cystic fibrosis analysis and intracytoplasmic sperm injection. Hum Reprod 2000;15:431.

108. McCallum TJ, Milunsky JM, Cunningham DL, et al. Fertility in men with cystic fibrosis: an update on current surgical practices and outcomes. Chest 2000;118:1059.

109. Josserand RN, Bey-Omar F, Rollet J, et al. Cystic fibrosis phenotype evaluation and paternity outcome in 50 males with congenital bilateral absence of vas deferens. Hum Reprod 2003;16:2093.

110. Meschede D, Horst J, Williams C, et al. Genetic testing and counseling for congenital bilateral absence of the vas deferens. Lancet 1994;343:1566.

111. Handyside AH, Lesko JG, Tarin JJ, et al. Birth of a normal girl after in vitro fertilization and preimplantation diagnostic testing for cystic fibrosis. N Engl J Med 1992;327:905.

112. Ao A, Ray P, Harper J, et al. Clinical experience with preimplantation genetic diagnosis of cystic fibrosis (ΔF508). Prenat Diagn 1996;16:137.

113. Goossens V, Sermon K, Lissens W, et al. Clinical application of preimplantation genetic diagnosis for cystic fibrosis. Prenat Diagn 2000;20:571.

114. Eftedal I, Schwartz M. Bendtsen H, et al. Single intragenic microsatellite preimplantation genetic diagnosis for cystic fibrosis provides positive allele identification of all CFTR genotypes for informative couples. Mol Hum Reprod 2001;7:307.

115. Kaback M, Zippin D, Boyd P, et al. Attitudes toward prenatal diagnosis of cystic fibrosis among parents of affected children. In: Lawson D, ed. Cystic fibrosis: horizons. Proceedings of the 9th International Cystic Fibrosis Congress, June 9–15, 1984. Rochester: Wiley, 1984:15.

115a. Decruyenaere M, Evers-Kiebooms G, Denayer L and Welkenhuysen M. Update and impact of carrier testing for cystic fibrosis: a review and theoretical framework about the role of knowledge, health beliefs and coping. Community Genet 1998;1:23–25.

116. Jedlicka-Kohler I, Gotz M, Eichler I. Utilization of prenatal diagnosis for cystic fibrosis over the past seven years. Pediatrics 1994;94:13.

117. Brock DJH. Prenatal screening for cystic fibrosis: 5 years experience reviewed. Lancet 1996;347:148.

118. Farrell PM, Fost N. Prenatal screening for cystic fibrosis: where are we now? J Pediatr 2002;141:758.

119. Feldman GL, Lewiston N, Fernbach SD, et al. Prenatal diagnosis of cystic fibrosis by using linked DNA markers in 138 pregnancies at 1-in-4 risk. Am J Med Genet 1989;32:238.

120. Gonzales-Gonzalez MC, Garcia-Hoyos M, Trujillo MJ, et al. Prenatal detection of a cystic fibrosis mutation in fetal DNA from maternal plasma. Prenat Diagn 2002;22:946.

121. Spence JE, Perciaccante RG, Greig GM, et al. Uniparental disomy as a mechanism for human genetic disease. Am J Hum Genet 1988;42:217.

122. Voss R, Ben-Simon E, Avital A, et al. Isodisomy of chromosome 7 in a patient with cystic fibrosis: could uniparental disomy be common in humans? Am J Hum Genet 1989;45:373.

123. Beaudet AL, Perciaccante RG, Cutting GR. Homozygous nonsense mutation causing cystic fibrosis with uniparental isodisomy. Am J Hum Genet 1991;48:1213.

124. Warburton D. Editorial: Uniparental disomy: a rare consequence of the high rate of aneuploidy in human genes. Am J Hum Genet 1988;42:215.

125. Dicke JM, Crane JP. Sonographically detected hyperechoic fetal bowel: significance and implications for pregnancy management. Obstet Gynecol 1992;80:778.

126. Nyberg DA, Dubinsky T, Resta RG, et al. Echogenic fetal bowel during the second trimester: clinical importance. Radiology 1993;188:527.

127. Fakhry J, Reiser M, Shapiro LR, et al. Increased echogenicity in the lower fetal abdomen: a common normal variant in the second trimester. J Ultrasound Med 1986;5:489.

128. MacGregor SN, Tamura R, Sabbagha R, et al. Isolated hyperechoic fetal bowel: significance and implications for management. Am J Obstet Gynecol 1995;173:1254.

129. Al-Kouatly HB, Chasen ST, Streltzoff J, et al. The clinical significance of fetal echogenic bowel. Am J Obstet Gynecol 2001;185:1035.

129a. Simon-Bouy B, Satre V, Ferec C, Malinge MC, Girodon E, Denamur E, Leporrier N, Lewin P, Forestier F, Muller F and the French Collaborative Group. Hyperchogenic fetal bowel: a large French collaborative study of 682 cases. Am J Med Genet 2003;121A:209–213.

130. Boue A, Muller F, Nezelof C, et al. Prenatal diagnosis in 200 pregnancies with a 1-in-4 risk of cystic fibrosis. Hum Genet 1986;74:288.

131. Sepulveda W, Leung KY, Roberston ME, et al. Prevalence of cystic fibrosis mutations in pregnancies with fetal echogenic bowel. Obstet Gynecol 1996;87:103.

132. Muller F, Dommergues M, Simmon-Buoy B, et al. Cystic fibrosis screening: a fetus with hyperechogenic bowel may be the index case. J Med Genet 1998;35:657.

133. Berlin BM, Norton ME, Sugarman EA, et al. Cystic fibrosis and chromosome abnormalities associated with echogenic fetal bowel. Obstet Gynecol 1999;94:135.

134. Scotet V, De Braekeleer M, Audrezet MP, et al. Prenatal detection of cystic fibrosis by ultrasonography: a retrospective study of more than 346,000 pregnancies. J Med Genet 2002;39:443.

135. Monaghan, K.G., Feldman, G.L. The risk of cystic fibrosis with prenatally detected echogenic bowel in an ethnically and racially diverse North American population. Prenat Diagn 1999;19:604.

136. Brambati B, Tului L, Fattore S. First-trimester fetal screening of cystic fibrosis in low-risk population. Lancet 1993;342:624.

137. Black SH, Bick DP, Maddalena A, et al. Pregnancy screening for cystic fibrosis. Lancet 1993;342:1112.

138. DeMarchi JM, Beaudet AL, Caskey CT, et al. Experience of an academic reference laboratory using automation for analysis of cystic fibrosis mutations. Arch Pathol Lab Med 1994;118:26.

139. Colten HR. Screening for cystic fibrosis: public policy and personal choices. N Engl J Med 1990;322:328.

140. Faden RR, Tambor ES, Chase GA, et al. Attitudes of physicians and genetics professionals toward cystic fibrosis carrier screening. Am J Med Genet 1994;50:1.

141. Workshop on Population Screening for the Cystic Fibrosis Gene. Statement from the National Institutes of Health workshop on population screening for the cystic fibrosis gene. N Engl J Med 1990;323:70.

142. Wilfond BS, Fost N. The cystic fibrosis gene: medical and social implications for heterozygote detection. JAMA 1990;263:2777.

143. Caskey CT, Kaback MM, Beaudet AL. The American Society of Human Genetics statement on cystic fibrosis screening. Am J Hum Genet 1990;46:393.

144. Statement of the American Society of Human Genetics on cystic fibrosis carrier screening. Am J Hum Genet 1992;51:1443.

145. Committee on Obstetrics, Maternal and Fetal Medicine, American College of Obstetricians and Gynecologists. American College of Obstetricians and Gynecologists committee opinion: current status of cystic fibrosis carrier screening. Washington, DC: American College of Obstetricians and Gynecologists, 1992.

146. Haddow JE, Bradley LA, Palomaki GE, et al. Issues in implementing prenatal screening for cystic fibrosis: results of a working conference. Genet Med 1999;1:129.

147. Henneman L, Poppelaars FAM and Kate LP. Evaluation of cystic fibrosis carrier screening programs according to genetic screening criteria. Genet Med 2002;4:241.

148. NIH Consensus Development Conference Statement. Genetic testing for cystic fibrosis. Available at http://consensus.nih.gov/cons/106/106_intro.htm (accessed May 27, 2003).

149. Mennuti MT, Thomson E, Press N. Screening for cystic fibrosis carrier state. Obstet Gynecol 1999;93:456.

150. Holmes LB and Pyeritz RE (for the Clinical Practice Committee of the American College of Medical Genetics). Screening for cystic fibrosis. JAMA 1998;279:1068.

151. American College of Obstetricians and Gynecologists Statement on Cystic Fibrosis Testing. Washington, DC: American College of Obstetricians and Gynecologists, 1998.

152. American College of Obstetricians and Gynecologists and American College of Medical Genetics. Preconception and prenatal carrier screening for cystic fibrosis: clinical and laboratory guidelines. Washington, DC: American College of Obstetricians and Gynecologists, 2001.

153. Strom CM, Huang D, Buller A, et al. Cystic fibrosis screening using the College panel: platform comparison and lessons learned from the first 20,000 samples. Genet Med 2002;4:289.

154. Crossley JR, Elliott RB, Smith PA. Dried blood spot screening for cystic fibrosis in the newborn. Lancet 1979;2:472.

155. Ranieri E, Ryall RG, Morris CP, et al. Neonatal screening strategy for cystic fibrosis using immunoreactive trypsinogen and direct gene analysis. BMJ 1991;302:1237.

156. Gregg RG, Wilfond BS, Farrell PM, et al. Application of DNA analysis in a population screening program for neonatal diagnosis of cystic fibrosis: comparison of screening protocols. Am J Hum Genet 1993;52:616.

157. Larsen J, Campbell S, Faragher EB, et al. Cystic fibrosis screening in neonates: measurement of immunoreactive trypsinogen and direct gene analysis for ΔF508. Eur J Pediatr 1994;153:569.

158. Gregg RG, Simantel A, Farrell PM, et al. Newborn screening for cystic fibrosis in Wisconsin: comparison of biochemical and molecular methods. Pediatrics 1997;99:819.

159. Henry RL, Boulton TJC, Roddick LG. False negative results on newborn screening for cystic fibrosis. J Paediatr Child Health 1990;26:150.

160. Farrell PM. Improving the health of patients with cystic fibrosis through newborn screening. Adv Pediatr 2000;47:79.

161. Farrell PM, Kosorok MR, Rock MJ, et al. Early diagnosis of cystic fibrosis through neonatal screening prevents severe malnutrition and improves long-term growth. Pediatrics 2001;107:1.

162. Wang SS, O'Leary LA, FitzSimmons SC, Khoury MJ. The impact of early cystic fibrosis diagnosis on pulmonary function in children. J Pediatr 2002;141:804.

163. Dankert-Roelse JR, te Meerman GJ. Long term prognosis of patients with cystic fibrosis in relation to early detection by neonatal screening and treatment in a cystic fibrosis centre. Thorax 1995;50:712.

164. Wheeler PG, Smith R, Dorkin H, et al. Genetic counseling after implementation of statewide cystic fibrosis newborn screening: two years' experience in one medical center. Genet Med 2001;3:411.

165. Wilschanski M, Yahav Y, Yaacoy Y, Blau H, Bentur L, Rivlin J, Aviram M, Bdolah-Abrah T, Bebok Z, Shushi L, Karem B, Kerem E. Gentamicin-incuded correction of CFTR function in patients with cystic fibrosis and CFTR stop mutations. N Engl J Med 2003;349:1433–1441.

Phyllis W. Speiser, M.D.

16

Prenatal Diagnosis and Treatment of Congenital Adrenal Hyperplasia

Congenital adrenal hyperplasia (CAH) is a family of autosomal recessive disorders of adrenal steroidogenesis in which there is deficient activity of one of the enzymes necessary for cortisol synthesis. As a result of deficient cortisol synthesis, corticotropin-releasing hormone and adrenocorticotropic hormone (ACTH) secretion are stimulated via negative feedback, with resultant adrenal hyperplasia, overproduction of the adrenal steroids preceding the step that is deficient, and overproduction of the adrenal steroids not requiring the enzymatic step that is deficient. A simplified scheme of adrenal steroidogenesis, showing the series of enzymatic steps required for adrenal steroidogenesis, is depicted in Figure 16.1 Deficiency of each of the enzymatic activities required for cortisol synthesis has been described.[2]

Clinical and genetic heterogeneity of these disorders is well recognized. The signs and symptoms of each deficiency depend on which steroids are deficient and which are produced in excess. Measurement of the serum and urinary steroids help to determine which are overproduced and which are deficient, and the precursor/product ratio helps to localize the site of the disordered enzymatic step. Administration of glucocorticoid results in suppression of the overproduced steroids and restoration of hormonal balance.

Much has been learned in recent years about the enzymes of adrenal steroidogenesis, the genes encoding them, and the genetic mutations resulting in CAH.[2] This chapter focuses on the prenatal diagnosis and treatment of CAH due to 21-hydroxylase (21-OH) deficiency and 11β-hydroxylase (11β-OH) deficiency, which together account for more than 95 percent of cases of CAH, and the prenatal diagnosis of congenital lipoid adrenal hyperplasia, a rare form of the disorder.

21-HYDROXYLASE DEFICIENCY

Deficiency of 21-hydroxylase (21-OH) activity is the most common cause of CAH, accounting for more than 90 percent of cases. Failure to adequately 21-hydroxylate 17-hydroxyprogesterone to 11-deoxycortisol (compound S) results in deficient cortisol, increased ACTH, adrenal hyperplasia, and increased adrenal androgen secretion. Adrenal hyperplasia seems to be mediated by ACTH-stimulated production of several growth factors, including insulinlike growth factors I and II (IGF-I and II).[3] The excessive adrenal androgen production, most markedly androstenedione and by peripheral conversion testos-

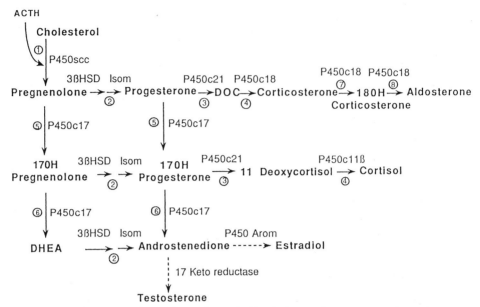

Fig. 16.1. Simplified scheme of adrenal steroidogenesis. Chemical names for enzymes are shown above or to the right of arrow; circled numbers refer to traditional names: $1 = 20, 22$-desmolase; $2 = 3\beta$-hydroxysteroid dehydrogenase/isomerase; $3 = 21$-hydroxylase; $4 = 11\beta$-hydroxylase; $5 = 17\alpha$-hydroxylase; $6 = 17,20$-lyase; $7 = 18$-hydroxylase; $8 = 18$-oxidase. Two unnumbered reactions shown with dotted arrows occur primarily in gonads, not in the adrenal gland. DOC, 11-deoxycorticosterone. *Source*: Adapted from Miller and Levine.[1]

terone, produces the virilization that is the hallmark of this disorder. Beginning in utero, this causes virilization of the affected female fetus, ranging in degree from clitoromegaly, with or without partial fusion of the labioscrotal folds, to complete fusion of the labioscrotal folds, with the appearance of a penile urethra.[4]

In approximately three-fourths of infants with 21-OH deficiency, inadequate 21-hydroxylation of progesterone to 11-deoxycorticosterone (DOC) results in aldosterone deficiency, and salt-wasting crisis may occur, usually during the first few weeks of life.[5] Postnatally, untreated individuals with severe forms of CAH undergo progressive virilization: penile and clitoral enlargement, excessive growth, acne, early onset of pubic hair. Bone-age advancement exceeding the height–age advancement occurs, and ultimately patients with CAH are about 1 to 2 SD below the population mean in stature, regardless of treatment. Disordered puberty and infertility in patients with CAH are well recognized; however, normal puberty and fertility with successful treatment have been achieved.[6–8] Children with bone ages greater than 10 years who are treated may undergo true precocious puberty when adrenal-suppressive treatment is instituted.[9,10]

The diagnosis of 21-OH deficiency is based on elevated baseline and ACTH-stimulated levels of serum 17-hydroxyprogesterone (17-OHP) and adrenal androgens, particularly androstenedione, and their urinary metabolites, pregnanetriol and 17-ketosteroids (17-KS), respectively, and their suppression with glucocorticoid treatment. Elevated plasma renin activity (PRA)/aldosterone ratio is present in subtle or overt salt-wasting.[11]

Genetic Linkage to HLA and Molecular Genetics

21-hydroxylation is mediated by a cytochrome P-450 enzyme, P450c21, which is found in the endoplasmic reticulum and predominantly expressed in adrenal cortical cells. The gene for P450c21 was mapped to chromosome 6 by HLA studies of families of patients with CAH caused by 21-OH deficiency.[12,13] Genetic linkage disequilibrium is observed between HLA and 21-OH deficiency. This phenomenon is the nonrandom association of particular alleles of adjacent genetic loci in an extended haplotype (e.g., increased frequency of Bw47,DR7 associated with deletion of CYP21 and C4B in salt-wasting CAH, frequently observed in Northern European Caucasians, and B14,DR1 in association with duplication of CYP21P and C4A in nonclassic CAH, especially prominent among Ashkenazi Jews).[14] Genetic linkage between CAH caused by 21-OH deficiency and HLA made possible the prenatal prediction of CAH genotype by HLA genotype.[14,15] In addition, HLA testing allowed identification of CAH heterozygotes.[16]

Molecular genetic analysis has demonstrated that there are two human P450c21 genes[17,18]: CYP21P (formerly termed CYP21A, now also CYP21A1) and CYP21 (formerly termed CYP21B, now also CYP21A2). The two genes are highly homologous, but only the CYP21 gene is active; the CYP21P gene has several deleterious mutations that produce an unstable transcript[19] and are inconsistent with normal enzyme function.[20] The two closely homologous 21-OH genes are located in tandem with two highly homologous genes for the fourth component of complement (C4A, C4B)[20] and a gene for an extracellular matrix protein, tenascin-X, which is also duplicated (X, XA).[21] Deficiency of tenascin X and deletion of the corresponding genes is associated with one of the rarer forms of the connective-tissue disease, Ehlers–Danlos syndrome, most of which are caused by mutations in the type V collagen genes.[22] At least one case has been reported of a contiguous gene syndrome including CAH and Ehlers–Danlos syndrome.[22]

CAH due to 21-OH deficiency is caused by mutations in the CYP21 gene; more than seventy such mutations have been identified in patients with 21-OH deficiency summarized in the Human Gene Mutation Databse.[23] Among the various deletions and point mutations reported, approximately 70–75 percent of CAH haplotypes contain sequences identical to those in the CYP21P pseudogene, suggesting that these mutations arose via small-scale gene conversion events.[24]

Rarer mutations that do not seem to have arisen by unequal meiotic recombination between CYP21 and CYP21P have also been reported.[25,26] Approximately 10 percent of alleles have large macroconversions that change a major portion of the active gene sequence into a pseudogene sequence,[27] and approximately 25 percent of affected alleles carry a 30-kb deletion[28] found in association with the haplotype HLA-B47;DR7.[18] Most patients of mixed ethnic background are compound heterozygotes, having inherited different genetic lesions from each parent; those of homogeneous parentage or the product of consanguineous unions are homozygous for either one of the two most common mutations found in classic CAH: the 30-kb deletion or the splice mutation in intron 2, 656G. The severity of disease expression in the compound heterozygote is most often determined by the activity of the less severely affected of the two alleles.[27,29]

The functional effects of mutations in CYP21 gene have been examined. Amino acid substitutions present in patients with late-onset or nonclassic 21-OH deficiency (e.g., P30L, V281L, or P453S) result in an enzyme with 10–50 percent of normal activity[30,31]; the mutation characteristic of simple virilizing 21-OH deficiency (I172N) results in an enzyme with 2 percent of normal activity[32]; and a cluster of mutations in exon 6 found in salt-wasting 21-OH deficiency results in an enzyme with no detectable activity (Figure 16.2).[30]

In general, there is a close correlation between genotype and phenotype. However, patients have been reported who were more or less severely affected than would have been predicted by genotype.[33,34] The mechanism of this is not completely clear but may be due to differing definitions of clinical forms of CAH, variation in splicing with the intron 2

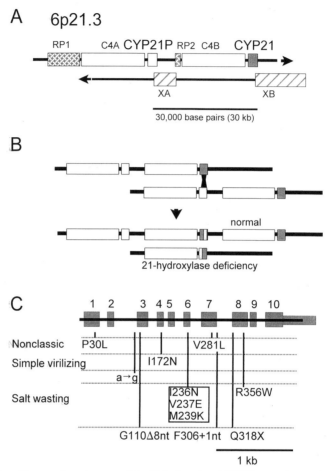

Fig. 16.2. *A,* Map of the genetic region around the 21-hydroxylase (*CYP21*) gene. Arrows denote direction of transcription. *CYP21P,* 21-hydroxylase pseudogene; *C4A* and *C4B,* genes encoding the fourth component of serum complement; *RP1,* gene encoding a putative nuclear protein of unknown function; *RP2,* truncated copy of this gene. *TNXB,* tenascin-X gene and *TNXA,* a truncated copy of this gene, are on the opposite chromosomal strand overlapping the 3′ end of each *CYP21* gene. The 30-kb scale bar is positioned to show the region involved in the tandem duplication location of the *CYP21* genes within the *HLA* major histocompatibility complex on chromosome 6p21.3. *B,* An extended view of the short arm of chromosome 6. Numbers denote distances between genes in kilobase pairs (kb). The *HLA-B* and *HLA-DR* histocompatibility genes flank the *CYP21* gene. The centromere is nearest HLA-DR. *TNF,* tumor necrosis factor (actually two genes, TNF A and B), is situated between the *C4/CYP21* region and HLA-B. There are many other genes in this region with functions as yet unknown. *C,* Diagram showing the location and functional significance of the nine most common mutations (other than deletion) found in patients with CAH due to 21-hydroxylase deficiency. Numbered boxes represent exons. A detailed description of these and other mutations is given in the text. *Source:* Modified from White and Speiser 2000.[2]

mutation, the unrecognized presence of more than one mutation in any single allele, variability in gene copy number and sequence, extra-adrenal 21-OH activity, and the genetic background against which the CYP21 genotype is expressed.

Newborn Screening

Screening for CAH due to 21-OH deficiency became possible with the development of an assay for 17-OHP, using a heel-stick capillary blood specimen impregnated on filter paper.[35] A number of newborn screening programs have been established in the United States, Canada, Europe, Japan, New Zealand, and South America. Results of worldwide screening of several million newborns for CAH due to 21-OH deficiency have been reported. The average incidence of classic CAH in most locales is ~1 in 15,000 livebirths. The world's highest incidence of CAH due to 21-OH deficiency is among the Yupik Eskimos of southwestern Alaska (1 in 282) and the island people of La Reunion, France (1 in 2,141).[36] Salt-wasting is diagnosed in approximately 75 percent of affected newborns. Cost/benefit analysis indicated that newborn screening for classic 21-OH deficiency is variably accurate and cost effective, depending on the timing and type of assays performed, the cutoff designations for affected infants depending on birth weight and gestational age, and whether genotyping is incorporated into the screening procedure.[37–39]

Nonclassic Forms of Congenital Adrenal Hyperplasia

Nonclassic 21-OH deficiency presents in later childhood, at puberty, or in adult life with signs of androgen excess—early appearance of pubic and axillary hair, tall stature, advanced bone age, acne, hirsutism, temporal hairline recession, amenorrhea, or infertility.[40–42] It is relatively rare for females who carry a nonclassic allele to present with clitoromegaly; however, this is more commonly found among those with the P30L mutation.[30] Most cases are diagnosed in female patients. Males may also be affected, although the phenotype is more subtle, and the consequences are usually less severe in men.[43]

Nonclassic 21-OH deficiency results from the combination of a severe CYP21 deficiency gene and a mild CYP21 deficiency gene, or a combination of two mild deficiency genes. Nonclassic 21-OH deficiency may be symptomatic or asymptomatic, and individuals with the same genetic mutations and biochemical abnormalities present with a variable spectrum of disease. Furthermore, androgen excess symptoms may vary in severity over time even in the same individual.[40]

Molecular genetic studies in patients with nonclassic 21-OH deficiency (see Figure 16.2) have revealed that the most common mutation associated with this disorder is a point mutation at codon 281 resulting in a valine-to-leucine shift, found in up to 70 percent of alleles in patients with the HLA-B14,DR1 haplotype.[44] A missense mutation at residue 30 in exon 1, changing proline to leucine, has been identified in 16 percent of haplotypes of patients with nonclassic disease in one population studied.[31] Another point mutation has also been described in nonclassic patients, which may or may not have arisen by gene conversion (codon 453 proline-to-serine).[45] Some mutations have been reported in various phenotypes (especially the intron 2 mutation associated with variable correct splicing, and codon 339 arginine-to-histidine).

The pattern of hormonal abnormality in the nonclassic form of CAH due to 21-OH deficiency demonstrates a less marked elevation in 17-hydroxyprogesterone, androstenendione, and testosterone.[46] There is no clinically significant deficit in cortisol production in response to stress among patients with nonclassic forms of CAH.[47] Nonclassic 21-OH deficiency is among the most frequent autosomal recessive genetic disorders in humans, with a prevalence in Ashkenazi Jews of 3.7 percent (1 in 27) and in a diverse Caucasian population of 0.1 percent (1 in 1,000).[48] Morning salivary 17-OHP was used as a screening test for nonclassic 21-OH deficiency to confirm the frequency of the disorder in one study,[49] and heel-prick blood samples for CYP21 genotyping in another.[38] Studies have indicated a variable incidence of nonclassic 21-OH deficiency in children presenting with early onset of pubic and/or axillary hair, as well as in adolescent and adult females with hirsutism.[50,51] Such variability in the frequency of this disorder may be attributed to ascertainment bias and/or ethnicity of the population studied.

Prenatal Diagnosis and Treatment of Congenital Adrenal Hyperplasia Due to 21-OH Deficiency

Classic CAH due to 21-OH deficiency is the most common cause of ambiguous genitalia in the newborn female. Advances within the past two decades have made possible the prenatal diagnosis and treatment of this disorder, making it among the first genetic disorders amenable to prenatal medical therapy.

The objective of prenatal diagnosis and treatment of 21-OH deficiency is the prevention of ambiguous genitalia in the female fetus affected with the salt-wasting or simple virilizing forms of CAH, thus avoiding the attendant psychologic stress to families and patients caused by the genital ambiguity and the potential complications of surgeries. Moreover, prenatal diagnosis can help avoid possible erroneous male sex assignment in the virilized female, salt-wasting crisis and death in infants with the salt-wasting form, and progressive virilization in undiagnosed infants and children.

Prenatal Diagnosis of 21-OH Deficiency

Prenatal prediction of CAH due to classic 21-OH deficiency has been performed using a number of methods: amniotic fluid (AF) hormone levels, HLA typing of chorionic villus cells and AF cells, and molecular genetic studies of chorionic villus cells and AF cells.

Prenatal diagnosis of CAH was first reported in 1965, based on elevation of amniotic fluid 17-ketosteroids and pregnanetriol.[52] Subsequent reports suggested that elevated 17-OHP concentration in AF was a more accurate test for salt-wasting CAH (reviewed in Pang et al. 1985[53]). Elevated androstenedione (Δ4-A) concentration in AF provides another diagnostic measure. 17-OHP and Δ4-A may be in the normal range in non-salt-wasting classic CAH and in nonclassic CAH due to 21-OH deficiency; therefore, 17-OHP and Δ4-A AF levels are consistently reliable for prenatal prediction only when the fetus is affected with classic salt-wasting CAH. Elevated AF 21-deoxycortisol, may provide a more useful prenatal hormonal measure in non–salt-wasting disease.

The demonstration of the genetic linkage between CAH due to 21-OH deficiency and HLA made possible the prenatal prediction of this disorder by HLA typing of cultured AF cells[15] and cultured chorionic villus cells. Use of chorionic villus cells permits earlier identification of the affected fetus than was possible by amniocentesis (typically at 10 vs. 14 weeks). Recent advances in cell sorting and PCR may allow even earlier detection of fetal sex, and potentially fetal disease status, from maternal blood during the first trimester. In a pregnancy in which the fetus is HLA-identical to the index case with 21-OH deficiency, the fetus will be affected; the fetus that shares one parental haplotype with the index case will be a heterozygous carrier, and the fetus with both haplotypes different from the index case will be homozygous normal.

Molecular genetic analysis using DNA extract from chorionic villus cells or amniocytes for analysis of CYP21 genes for prenatal diagnosis is now the most frequently performed diagnostic procedure, aided by either flanking HLA or microsatellite genotyping. Causative mutations can now be identified on 95 percent of chromosomes using PCR-based CYP21 analysis. Mutations not detected by this approach can be characterized by direct sequencing of CYP21 genes. De novo mutations, found in patients with CAH but not in both parents, are found in 1 percent of disease-causing CYP21B mutations.[54] Pitfalls in the molecular genetic diagnosis include allele "drop out," sample contamination, and inability to detect "phase" (i.e., whether two mutations are situated on the same allele, or on each of two parental alleles).[38]

Prenatal Treatment of Congenital Adrenal Hyperplasia Due to 21-OH Deficiency

Prenatal treatment of CAH to prevent the virilization of an affected female fetus is considered a desirable objective. Because masculinization of the external genitalia begins at about 8 weeks of gestation, treatment to suppress fetal adrenal hormone secretion must begin before that time. Prenatal treatment of CAH was first reported in 1969.[55] Repeated injection of hydrocortisone into a male fetus diagnosed to have CAH on the basis of AF pregnanetriol concentration was associated with a decrease in the AF pregnanetriol level.

Successful prenatal treatment in ameliorating or preventing virilization of a female fetus with classic CAH due to 21-OH deficiency was reported in the mid-1980s.[56,57] In two pregnancies carrying females affected with classic salt-wasting CAH, the mothers were given hydrocortisone or dexamethasone, respectively. Hormonal studies suggested complete suppression of maternal adrenal function in both, and of the fetal adrenal gland in the pregnancy treated with dexamethasone, but incomplete suppression of the fetal adrenal gland in the pregnancy treated with hydrocortisone. At birth, the external genitalia were normal in the infant whose mother was given dexamethasone and minimally virilized in the infant whose mother received hydrocortisone. Postnatally, the diagnosis of 21-OH deficiency was confirmed in both infants.[56] Since the initial report, several hundred at-risk pregnancies have been treated with dexamethasone.[58,59] The protocol used presently consists of early first trimester dosing with 20 μg/kg (prepregnancy weight of the mother)/day divided in three equal doses to the pregnant woman. If the fetus proves to be male by karyotype, or unaffected by CYP21 analysis, dexamethasone is discontinued. Female fetuses are treated to term. Late treatment initiation, stopping dexamethasone in midgestation, and medical noncompliance are all associated with poor treatment outcomes.[58,59]

Fetal Outcome

Treatment has been successful in about 80 percent of the female infants. Among pregnancies treated before 9 weeks of gestation, approximately half had normal genitalia and half were described as being more mildly virilized compared with elder affected sisters who did not receive prenatal dexamethasone. When treatment was initiated after 10 weeks of gestation, only 10 percent of affected females showed any improvement in genital ambiguity. Thus, early treatment is crucial.[58]

To date, there seems to be no serious adverse and clearly attributable complications of prenatal treatment in the infants, either in infants treated throughout the pregnancy or in infants treated prenatally until midgestation. Development seems to be normal, and growth has been consistent with the family pattern and the other affected siblings.[58,59] However, long-term follow-up is limited: the total number of children treated is small and most infants have been followed only for a brief time. Detailed neuropsychologic evaluations have not been reported, although questionnaire surveys indicate that prenatally treated children are somewhat more shy than peers.[60]

Spontaneous abortion, late pregnancy, fetal death, and intrauterine growth retardation (IUGR) occasionally have occurred in short-term treated unaffected pregnancies or longer

Table 16.1. Maternal side effects of prenatal treatment for congenital adrenal hyperplasia with dexamethasone from first trimester until birth

Excess weight gain
Cushingoid facial features
Striae (broad, pigmented with scarring)
Gestational diabetes or abnormal glucose tolerance
Facial hair
Hypertension
Emotional lability, irritability
Abdominal pain
Fatigue
Pedal edema

treated affected pregnancies (Table 16.1); however, the frequency of such events are no different from those observed in untreated pregnancies.[58] An additional possible complication of prenatal treatment is hydrometrocolpos reported in an infant treated prenatally for whom treatment was discontinued for 7 days before amniocentesis.[54] The infant had a small phallus but complete labial fusion and a single opening on the perineum. Hydrometrocolpos developed, and at surgery at 8 weeks the infant was found to have a very small urethral opening and narrow urogenital sinus with retrograde flow of urine into the vagina. Although this has been reported in the absence of prenatal treatment, the authors suggested that the suppression of the androgen-dependent growth of the urethra in the latter part of the pregnancy by the maternal dexamethasone treatment resulted in narrowing of the urogenital sinus.

Hormonal Monitoring

Hormonal measurements have been performed by some investigators to evaluate the adequacy of treatment. Maternal serum or urine cortisol (F), serum or urine estriol, serum 17-OHP, and amniotic fluid levels of 17 OHP, Δ4-A and T have been measured.[59,61] Maternal serum estriol seems to be the most reliable hormonal measurement to evaluate suppression of the fetal adrenal gland. An extremely low maternal level of estriol may indicate overtreatment with dexamethasone.

Maternal Complications of Prenatal Treatment

Maternal side effects may include edema, excessive weight gain, irritability, nervousness, mood swings, hypertension, glucose intolerance, chronic epigastric pain, gastroenteritis, cushingoid facial features, and increased facial hair growth. Overall, adverse side effects of dexamethasone occur in about 10 percent of treated pregnancies, but the incidence of adverse effects increases with dose and duration of treatment (Table 16.2). Marked weight gain is the most common problem in cases of prolonged treatment, while severe striae with permanent scarring is rare.[62] Maternal side effects have prompted decreasing the dose or discontinuing the treatment and may have resulted in noncompliance and unsatisfactory genital outcome.[59] This approach needs to be studied systematically. it has been recommended that a higher dose of dexamethasone be used initially to prevent labioscrotal fusion and formation of a urogenital sinus but that decreasing the dose in the latter part of the second trimester should be considered.

Table 16.2.   Fetal side effects of prenatal treatment for congenital adrenal hyperplasia with dexamethasone

---

Fetal death
Intrauterine growth retardation/failure to thrive
Hydrocephalus
Hydrometrocolpos
Vaginal cyst
Shyness

Note: These side effects may not be directly attributable to dexamethasone.

Current Recommendations for Prenatal Diagnosis and Treatment

The current recommended protocol for prenatal diagnosis and treatment is presented in Figure 16.3. Parents seeking genetic counseling should be fully informed of possible maternal side effects, variable genital outcome, and possible but currently unknown long-term effects in treated children.[63] Mothers with previous medical conditions that may be aggravated by dexamethasone, such as hypertension, overt diabetes, gestational diabetes, or toxemia, probably should not be treated or should be treated only with extreme caution. Ideally, treatment with dexamethasone should be initiated well before the 9th week of gestation, at a dose of approximately 20 μg/kg/day, given in three divided doses. CVS in the 10th week for prenatal diagnosis should be performed with karyotyping, CYP21 genotyping, and analysis of flanking linked markers. If the fetus is a male or an unaffected female, treatment is discontinued. If the fetus is an affected female, or if prenatal diagnosis by CVS is unsuccessful or not performed, treatment is continued. If necessary, amniocentesis is performed at 14–15 weeks with genetic analysis of amniocytes, and a similar decision tree is followed. If only hormonal analysis is available to make the prenatal diagnosis, dexamethasone treatment should be discontinued 5 days before amniocentesis, realizing that this may compromise outcomes.[61]

Maternal monitoring for physical, hormonal, and metabolic changes should begin at the initiation of treatment and should be continued throughout the pregnancy. To evaluate the adequacy of fetal adrenal suppression and fasting blood sugar, serum estriol level should be determined monthly and oral glucose-tolerance tests should be performed during the second and third trimesters. Prompt intervention in the presence of excessive weight gain, increased blood pressure, and glucose intolerance or other side effects should be instituted. Consideration should be given to reducing the dose of dexamethasone during the second and third trimesters, especially if there are adverse effects to the mother.

The safety of the prenatal treatment of CAH remains to be fully defined. It should be offered only to patients who have a clear understanding of the possible risks and benefits and who are able to comply with the need for very close monitoring throughout pregnancy in the setting of an experienced center with institutional review board approval for the trial.[64,65]

11β-HYDROXYLASE DEFICIENCY

Congenital adrenal hyperplasia due to 11β-hydroxylase (11β-OH) deficiency accounts for 5–8 percent of reported cases of CAH. It occurs in approximately 1 in 100,000 births in the general Caucasian population. It is more common among Jews of North African ori-

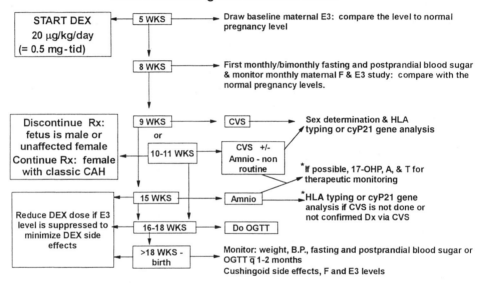

Fig. 16.3. Guidelines for prenatal maternal dexamethasone therapy for fetal virilizing CAH due to 21-hydroxylase deficiency CAH.

gin (1 in 5,000 to 1 in 7,000 births)[66] and also may be more common than recognized previously in other populations.[67]

A deficiency of 11β-OH results in a defect in the conversion of compound S to cortisol and DOC to corticosterone. Similar to 21-OH deficiency, there is virilization secondary to the excessive secretion of the adrenal androgens, resulting in virilization of the female fetus and postnatal virilization of males and females. Hypertension is commonly observed in this disorder, believed to be caused by increased DOC secretion, sodium and water retention, and volume expansion. Hypokalemia also may be present. Glucocorticoid administration suppresses the overproduced adrenal steroids (S, DOC, androgens), preventing continued virilization and resulting in remission of the hypertension in most cases.

The external genitalia of the virilized female may be corrected surgically, as in 21-OH deficiency, and optimal treatment should permit normal growth and pubertal development and fertility.[68]

The 11β-OH deficiency is diagnosed by the presence of elevated baseline and ACTH-stimulated serum levels of S, DOC, and androgens and their urinary metabolites tetra-hydro-11-deoxycortisol (THS), tetrahydro-DOC, and 17-KS, respectively, and their suppression with glucocorticoid therapy. In the untreated state, plasma renin activity and aldosterone often are suppressed because of the sodium- and water-retaining effect of the excessive DOC.

Molecular Genetics

Humans have two mitochondrial 11β-OH isozymes: 11β-hydroxylase and aldosterone synthase encoded by CYP11B1 and CYP11B2, respectively, located on chromosome 8q21-q22. The genes are 95 percent identical in coding sequences and approximately 90 percent identical in introns.[69] The 11β-hydroxylase activity encoded by CYP11B1 and expressed in the zona fasciculata converts 11-deoxycortisol to cortisol and 11-deoxycorticosterone to corticosterone. Aldosterone synthase encoded by CYP11B2 expressed at relatively low levels exclusively in the zona glomerulosa converts corticosterone to aldosterone, and has weak 11β-hydroxylase activity.

CAH caused by 11β-OH deficiency results from mutations in CYP11B1. Numerous mutations have been described in patients with classic CAH caused by 11β-OH deficiency.[70] In Moroccan Jews, almost all affected alleles carry the same mutation, R448H in exon 8, which abolishes enzymatic activity.[71] Genotype–phenotype correlations have been sought in classic 11β-OH deficiency; however, no strict correlation exists between the phenotypic features of hypertension and virilization and the hormonal profile or specific mutations.[72]

Nonclassic 11β-OH Deficiency

Nonclassic 11β-OH deficiency may present in a way similar to that of nonclassic 21-OH deficiency, although precocious pubarche resulting from mild 11β-OH deficiency seems to be quite rare, since these alleles are much rarer in the general population. Hypertension is not a typical feature of mild 11β -OH deficiency. The principles of diagnosis are the same as for the classic form of 11β-OH deficiency, although the hormonal abnormalities are less marked.[67] As expected, the mutations detected in milder forms of the disease are less deleterious than those found in classic 11β-OH deficiency.[73]

Prenatal Diagnosis and Treatment of CAH Due to 11β-OH Deficiency

Prenatal diagnosis of CAH due to 11β-OH deficiency was first reported from Israel.[74] In the affected pregnancies, maternal urinary THS was high during the first trimester and rose further after the first trimester. AF THS and S concentrations and the ratio of AF THS to tetrahydrocortisol (THF) plus tetrahydrocortisone (THE) were also elevated in the pregnancies with affected fetuses. The latter ratio (THS/THF + THE) was the best discriminatory index for an affected fetus. AF androstenedione levels were high in three pregnancies and were borderline elevated in a fourth. Dexamethasone administration to the mother can greatly reduce maternal urinary THS excretion[75] and can allow normal female genital development.[76] Prenatal diagnosis by CYP11B1 DNA analysis of chorionic villus cells or amniocytes has been reported.[76]

CONGENITAL LIPOID ADRENAL HYPERPLASIA

Congenital lipoid adrenal hyperplasia is an even rarer form of CAH that results in a deficiency of all adrenal and gonadal hormones caused by a defect in the earliest stages of steroid hormone synthesis, with an inability to convert cholesterol to pregnenolone. Deficient adrenal steroidogenesis leads to salt-wasting crisis, hyponatremia, hypovolemia, hyperkalemia, and acidosis with death usually in early infancy unless prompt diagnosis and treatment occur. Because there is deficient fetal testicular steroidogenesis in 46,XY patients, males with this disorder have phenotypically normal female genitalia but absent mullerian structures. Some females may undergo female puberty, whereas others will show no evidence of gonadal steroidogenesis. The severity of the phenotype depends on the severity of the underlying mutation.

Molecular Genetics

Mutations in the gene for steroidogenic acute regulatory protein (StAR), a protein that promotes the movement of cholesterol across the mitochondrial membrane, have been reported in patients from various ethnic and genetic backgrounds. The mutations were primarily found in three exons, and two mutations accounted for 70–80 percent of the mutations in Japanese and Palestinian patients.[77] In addition, a heterozygous mutation in CYP11A (also termed CYP11A1) gene encoding the cholesterol side chain cleavage enzyme, accounted for a similar presentation in one reported case.[78]

Prenatal Diagnosis of Congenital Lipoid Hyperplasia

Prenatal diagnosis in pregnancies at risk for lipoid adrenal hyperplasia has been reported using amniotic fluid levels, and also in pregnancies with 46,XY fetuses, by ultrasonographic examination of the external genitalia showing absent phallic structure. Low levels of 17-hydroxyprogesterone, 17-hydroxypregnenolone, cortisol, dehydroepiandrosterone, androstenedione, and estriol in amniotic fluid and female-typical genitalia on ultrasonography in two pregnancies with affected male fetuses suggested the diagnosis that was confirmed after termination of pregnancy or birth.[79]

CONCLUSION

Prenatal diagnosis has been reported in three forms of the disease: CAH due to both 21-hydroxylase and 11β-OH deficiencies, and in lipoid adrenal hypoplasia. Prenatal treatment of pregnancies at risk for affected females with the virilizing disorders must be evaluated carefully to determine the risk/benefit ratio of prenatal treatment.

REFERENCES

1. Miller WL, Levine LS. Molecular and clinical advances in congenital adrenal hyperplasia. J Pediatr 1987;111:1.
2. White PC, Speiser PW. Congenital adrenal hyperplasia due to 21-hydroxylase deficiency. Endocr Rev 2000;21:245.
3. Voutilainen R, Miller WL. Coordinate tropic hormone regulation of mRNAs for insulin-like growth factor II and the cholesterol side-chain-cleavage enzyme, P450scc [corrected], in human steroidogenic tissues. Proc Natl Acad Sci USA 1987;84:1590.
4. Weldon VV, Blizzard RM, Migeon CJ. Newborn girls misdiagnosed as bilaterally cryptorchid males. N Engl J Med 1966;274:829.

5. Fife D, Rappaport EB. Prevalence of salt-losing among congenital adrenal hyperplasia patients. Clin Endocrinol (Oxf) 1983;19:259.

6. Eugster EA, Dimeglio LA, Wright JC, Freidenberg GR, Seshadri R, Pescovitz OH. Height outcome in congenital adrenal hyperplasia caused by 21-hydroxylase deficiency: a meta-analysis. J Pediatr 2001;138:26.

7. Lo J, Grumbach M. Pregnancy outcomes in women with congenital virilizing adrenal hyperplasia. Endocrinol Metab Clin North Am 2001;30:207.

8. Urban MD, Lee PA, Migeon CJ. Adult height and fertility in men with congenital virilizing adrenal hyperplasia. N Engl J Med 1978;299:1392.

9. Pescovitz OH, Comite F, Cassorla F, et al. True precocious puberty complicating congenital adrenal hyperplasia: treatment with a luteinizing hormone-releasing hormone analog. J Clin Endocrinol Metab 1984;58:857.

10. Pescovitz OH, Cassorla F, Comite F, Loriaux DL, Cutler GB Jr. LHRH analog treatment of central precocious puberty complicating congenital adrenal hyperplasia. Ann NY Acad Sci 1985;458:174.

11. Rosler A, Levine LS, Schneider B, Novogroder M, New MI. The interrelationship of sodium balance, plasma renin activity and ACTH in congenital adrenal hyperplasia. J Clin Endocrinol Metab 1977;45:500.

12. Dupont B, Oberfield SE, Smithwick EM, Lee TD, Levine LS. Close genetic linkage between HLA and congenital adrenal hyperplasia. Lancet 1977;2:1309.

13. Levine LS, Zachmann M, New MI, et al. Genetic mapping of the 21-hydroxylase-deficiency gene within the HLA linkage group. N Engl J Med 1978;299:911.

14. Fleischnick E, Awdeh ZL, Raum D, Jr, et al. Extended MHC haplotypes in 21-hydroxylase-deficiency congenital adrenal hyperplasia: shared genotypes in unrelated patients. Lancet 1983;1:152.

15. Pollack MS, Maurer D, Levine LS, et al. HLA typing of amniotic cells: the prenatal diagnosis of congenital adrenal hyperplasia (21-OH-deficiency type). Transplant Proc 1979;11:1726.

16. Lorenzen F, Pang S, New M, et al. Studies of the C-21 and C-19 steroids and HLA genotyping in siblings and parents of patients with congenital adrenal hyperplasia due to 21-hydroxylase deficiency. J Clin Endocrinol Metab 1980;50:572.

17. Higashi Y, Yoshioka H, Yamane M, Gotoh O, Fujii-Kuriyama Y. Complete nucleotide sequence of two steroid 21-hydroxylase genes tandemly arranged in human chromosome: a pseudogene and a genuine gene. Proc Natl Acad Sci USA 1986;83:2841.

18. White PC, New MI, Dupont B. HLA-linked congenital adrenal hyperplasia results from a defective gene encoding a cytochrome P-450 specific for steroid 21-hydroxylation. Proc Natl Acad Sci USA 1984;81:7505.

19. Endoh A, Yang L, Hornsby PJ. CYP21 pseudogene transcripts are much less abundant than those from the active gene in normal human adrenocortical cells under various conditions in culture. Mol Cell Endocrinol 1998;137:13.

20. White PC, New MI, Dupont B. Structure of human steroid 21-hydroxylase genes. Proc Natl Acad Sci USA 1986;83:5111.

21. Bristow J, Tee MK, Gitelman SE, Mellon SH, Miller WL. Tenascin-X: a novel extracellular matrix protein encoded by the human XB gene overlapping P450c21B. J Cell Biol 1993;122:265.

22. Schalkwijk J, Zweers MC, Steijlen PM, et al. A recessive form of the Ehlers–Danlos syndrome caused by tenascin-X deficiency. N Engl J Med 2001;345:1167.

23. The Human Gene Mutation Database. http://archive.uwcm.ac.uk/uwcm/mg/search/120605.html.

24. Donohoue PA, Van Dop C, Jospe N, Migeon CJ. Congenital adrenal hyperplasia: molecular mechanisms resulting in 21- hydroxylase deficiency. Acta Endocrinol Suppl (Copenh) 1986;279:315.

25. Wedell A. Molecular approaches for the diagnosis of 21-hydroxylase deficiency and congenital adrenal hyperplasia. Clin Lab Med 1996;16:125.

26. White PC, Tusie-Luna MT, New MI, Speiser PW. Mutations in steroid 21-hydroxylase (CYP21). Hum Mutat 1994;3:373.

27. Speiser PW, Dupont J, Zhu D, et al. Disease expression and molecular genotype in congenital adrenal hyperplasia due to 21-hydroxylase deficiency. J Clin Invest 1992;90:584.

28. White PC, Vitek A, Dupont B, New MI. Characterization of frequent deletions causing steroid 21-hydroxylase deficiency. Proc Natl Acad Sci USA 1988;85:4436.

29. Wedell A, Thilen A, Ritzen EM, Stengler B, Luthman H. Mutational spectrum of the steroid 21-hydroxylase gene in Sweden: implications for genetic diagnosis and association with disease manifestation. J Clin Endocrinol Metab 1994;78:1145.

30. Tusie-Luna MT, Traktman P, White PC. Determination of functional effects of mutations in the steroid 21-hydroxylase gene (CYP21) using recombinant vaccinia virus. J Biol Chem 1990;265:20916.

31. Tusie-Luna MT, Speiser PW, Dumic M, New MI, White PC. A mutation (Pro-30 to Leu) in CYP21 represents a potential nonclassic steroid 21-hydroxylase deficiency allele. Mol Endocrinol 1991;5:685.

32. Amor M, Parker KL, Globerman H, New MI, White PC. Mutation in the CYP21B gene (Ile-172-Asn) causes steroid 21-hydroxylase deficiency. Proc Natl Acad Sci USA 1988;85:1600.

33. Bormann M, Kochhan L, Knorr D, Bidlingmaier F, Olek K. Clinical heterogeneity of 21-hydroxylase deficiency of sibs with identical 21-hydroxylase genes. Acta Endocrinol (Copenh) 1992;126:7.

34. Wilson RC, Mercado AB, Cheng KC, New MI. Steroid 21-hydroxylase deficiency: genotype may not predict phenotype. J Clin Endocrinol Metab 1995;80:2322.

35. Pang S, Hotchkiss J, Drash AL, Levine LS, New MI. Microfilter paper method for 17 alpha-hydroxyprogesterone radioimmunoassay: its application for rapid screening for congenital adrenal hyperplasia. J Clin Endocrinol Metab 1977;45:1003.

36. Pang S, Shook MK. Current status of neonatal screening for congenital adrenal hyperplasia. Curr Opin Pediatr 1997;9:419.

37. Brosnan CA, Brosnan P, Therrell BL, et al. A comparative cost analysis of newborn screening for classic congenital adrenal hyperplasia in Texas. Public Health Rep 1998;113:170.

38. Fitness J, Dixit N, Webster D, et al. Genotyping of CYP21, linked chromosome 6p markers, and a sex-specific gene in neonatal screening for congenital adrenal hyperplasia. J Clin Endocrinol Metab 1999;84:960.

39. Nordenstrom A, Wedell A, Hagenfeldt L, Marcus C, Larsson A. Neonatal screening for congenital adrenal hyperplasia: 17- hydroxyprogesterone levels and CYP21 genotypes in preterm infants 1. Pediatrics 2001;108:E68.

40. Kohn B, Levine LS, Pollack MS, et al. Late-onset steroid 21-hydroxylase deficiency: a variant of classical congenital adrenal hyperplasia. J Clin Endocrinol Metab 1982;55:817.

41. Migeon CJ, Rosenwaks Z, Lee PA, Urban MD, Bias WB. The attenuated form of congenital adrenal hyperplasia as an allelic form of 21-hydroxylase deficiency. J Clin Endocrinol Metab 1980;51:647.

42. Chrousos GP, Loriaux DL, Mann D, Cutler GB Jr. Late-onset 21-hydroxylase deficiency is an allelic variant of congenital adrenal hyperplasia characterized by attenuated clinical expression and different HLA haplotype associations. Horm Res 1982;16:193.

43. Chrousos GP, Loriaux DL, Sherins RJ, Cutler GB Jr. Unilateral testicular enlargement resulting from inapparent 21- hydroxylase deficiency. J Urol 1981;126:127.

44. Speiser PW, New MI, White PC. Molecular genetic analysis of nonclassic steroid 21-hydroxylase deficiency associated with HLA-B14,DR1. N Engl J Med 1988;319:19.

45. Owerbach D, Sherman L, Ballard AL, Azziz R. Pro-453 to Ser mutation in CYP21 is associated with nonclassic steroid 21-hydroxylase deficiency. Mol Endocrinol 1992;6:1211.

46. New MI, Lorenzen F, Lerner AJ, et al. Genotyping steroid 21-hydroxylase deficiency: hormonal reference data. J Clin Endocrinol Metab 1983;57:320.

47. Feuillan P, Pang S, Schurmeyer T, Avgerinos PC, Chrousos GP. The hypothalamic–pituitary–adrenal axis in partial (late-onset) 21-hydroxylase deficiency. J Clin Endocrinol Metab 1988;67:154.

48. Speiser PW, Dupont B, Rubinstein P, Piazza A, Kastelan A, New MI. High frequency of nonclassical steroid 21-hydroxylase deficiency. Am J Hum Genet 1985;37:650.

49. Zerah M, Pang SY, New MI. Morning salivary 17-hydroxyprogesterone is a useful screening test for nonclassical 21-hydroxylase deficiency. J Clin Endocrinol Metab 1987;65:227.

50. Oberfield SE, Mayes DM, Levine LS. Adrenal steroidogenic function in a black and Hispanic population with precocious pubarche. J Clin Endocrinol Metab 1990;70:76.

51. Temeck JW, Pang SY, Nelson C, New MI. Genetic defects of steroidogenesis in premature pubarche. J Clin Endocrinol Metab 1987;64:609.

52. Jeffcoate TN, Fliegner JR, Russell SH, et al. Diagnosis of the adrenogenital syndrome before birth. Lancet 1965;2:553.

53. Pang S, Pollack MS, Loo M, et al. Pitfalls of prenatal diagnosis of 21-hydroxylase deficiency congenital adrenal hyperplasia. J Clin Endocrinol Metab 1985;61:89.

54. Trautman PD, Meyer-Bahlburg HF, Postelnek J, New MI. Effects of early prenatal dexamethasone on the cognitive and behavioral development of young children: results of a pilot study. Psychoneuroendocrinology 1995;20:439.

55. Nichols J, Gson GG. Antenatal diagnosis of the adrenogenital syndrome. Lancet 1969:2:1068.

56. David M, Forest MG. Prenatal treatment of congenital adrenal hyperplasia resulting from 21-hydroxylase deficiency. J Pediatr 1984;105:799.

57. Evans MI, Chrousos GP, Mann DW, et al. Pharmacologic suppression of the fetal adrenal gland in utero: attempted prevention of abnormal external genital masculinization in suspected congenital adrenal hyperplasia. JAMA 1985;253:1015.

58. New MI, Carlson A, Obeid J, et al. Prenatal diagnosis for congenital adrenal hyperplasia in 532 pregnancies. J Clin Endocrinol Metab 2001;86:5651.

59. Forest MG, David M, Morel Y. Prenatal diagnosis and treatment of 21-hydroxylase deficiency. J Steroid Biochem Mol Biol 1993;45:75.
60. Couper JJ, Hutson JM, Warne GL. Hydrometrocolpos following prenatal dexamethasone treatment for congenital adrenal hyperplasia (21-hydroxylase deficiency). Eur J Pediatr 1993;152:9.
61. Dorr HG, Sippell WG. Prenatal dexamethasone treatment in pregnancies at risk for congenital adrenal hyperplasia due to 21-hydroxylase deficiency: effect on midgestational amniotic fluid steroid levels. J Clin Endocrinol Metab 1993;76:117.
62. Pang S, Clark AT, Freeman LC, et al. Maternal side effects of prenatal dexamethasone therapy for fetal congenital adrenal hyperplasia. J Clin Endocrinol Metab 1992;75:249.
63. Seckl JR, Miller WL. How safe is long-term prenatal glucocorticoid treatment? JAMA 1997;277:1077.
64. Consensus Statement on 21-Hydroxylase Deficiency from The European Society for Paediatric Endocrinology and The Lawson Wilkins Pediatric Endocrine Society. Horm Res 2002;58:188.
65. Clayton PE, Miller WL, Oberfield SE, Ritzen EM, Sippell WG, Speiser PW. Consensus statement on 21-hydroxylase deficiency from the Lawson Wilkins Pediatric Endocrine Society and The European Society for Pediatric Endocrinology. J Clin Endocrinol Metab 2002;87:4048.
66. Rosler A, Leiberman E, Cohen T. High frequency of congenital adrenal hyperplasia (classic 11 beta- hydroxylase deficiency) among Jews from Morocco. Am J Med Genet 1992;42:827.
67. Zachmann M, Tassinari D, Prader A. Clinical and biochemical variability of congenital adrenal hyperplasia due to 11 beta-hydroxylase deficiency: a study of 25 patients. J Clin Endocrinol Metab 1983;56:222.
68. Rosler A, Leiberman E, Sack J, et al. Clinical variability of congenital adrenal hyperplasia due to 11 beta-hydroxylase deficiency. Horm Res 1982;16:133.
69. Mornet E, Dupont J, Vitek A, White PC. Characterization of two genes encoding human steroid 11 beta-hydroxylase (P-450(11) beta). J Biol Chem 1989;264:20961.
70. The Human Gene Mutation Database. http://uwcmml1s.uwcm.ac.uk/uwcm/mg/search/120603.html.
71. White PC, Dupont J, New MI, Leiberman E, Hochberg Z, Rosler A. A mutation in CYP11B1 (Arg-448-His) associated with steroid 11β-hydroxylase deficiency in Jews of Moroccan origin. J Clin Invest 1991;87:1664.
72. White PC. Steroid 11 beta-hydroxylase deficiency and related disorders. Endocrinol Metab Clin North Am 2001;30:61,vi.
73. Joehrer K, Geley S, Strasser-Wozak EM, et al. CYP11B1 mutations causing non-classic adrenal hyperplasia due to 11 beta-hydroxylase deficiency. Hum Mol Genet 1997;6:1829.
74. Rosler A, Leiberman E, Rosenmann A, Ben-Uzilio R, Weidenfeld J. Prenatal diagnosis of 11beta-hydroxylase deficiency congenital adrenal hyperplasia. J Clin Endocrinol Metab 1979;49:546.
75. Rosler A, Weshler N, Leiberman E, et al. 11 Beta-hydroxylase deficiency congenital adrenal hyperplasia: update of prenatal diagnosis. J Clin Endocrinol Metab 1988;66:830.
76. Cerame BI, Newfield RS, Pascoe L, et al. Prenatal diagnosis and treatment of 11beta-hydroxylase deficiency congenital adrenal hyperplasia resulting in normal female genitalia. J Clin Endocrinol Metab 1999;84:3129.
77. Stocco DM. Clinical disorders associated with abnormal cholesterol transport: mutations in the steroidogenic acute regulatory protein. Mol Cell Endocrinol 2002;191:19.
78. Tajima T, Fujieda K, Kouda N, Nakae J, Miller WL. Heterozygous mutation in the cholesterol side chain cleavage enzyme (p450scc) gene in a patient with 46,XY sex reversal and adrenal insufficiency. J Clin Endocrinol Metab 2001;86:3820.
79. Izumi H, Saito N, Ichiki S, Makino Y, Yukitake K, Kaneoka T. Prenatal diagnosis of congenital lipoid adrenal hyperplasia. Obstet Gynecol 1993;81:839.

17

Prenatal Diagnosis of Miscellaneous Biochemical Disorders

INBORN ERRORS OF FOLATE AND COBALAMIN METABOLISM

Disorders of folate metabolism[1–5] and those of vitamin B_{12} (cobalamin, Cbl) metabolism[5–9] are listed in Table 17.1. Advances in the prenatal diagnosis of methylmalonic aciduria, including Cbl-responsive forms, have been summarized.[11–14]

Inborn Errors of Folate Metabolism

Cellular defect of 5-methyltetrahydrofolate uptake[15] is expressed only in stimulated lymphocytes and bone marrow cells. Although dihydrofolate reductase and methenyltetrahydrofolate cyclohydrolase are expressed in cultured fibroblasts, patients with putative defects in these enzymes have not exhibited a deficiency in cultured cells.[2,4] The original patient with putative methionine synthase deficiency had high enzyme levels in cultured fibroblasts. In retrospect, this patient probably did not have a primary defect in methionine synthase. As described below, patients with *cblG* have a defect in the gene for methionine synthase, and prenatal diagnosis has been reported for *cblG*. Prenatal diagnosis has not been reported for dihydrofolate reductase deficiency and methenyltetrahydrofolate cyclohydrolase deficiency, and more case reports are required to validate these diseases as real clinical entities.

Hereditary Malabsorption of Folate

Hereditary malabsorption of folate provides evidence for a specific carrier mechanism for folate, both across the intestine and across the blood–brain barrier. It is unknown whether folate levels are low in this disorder in fetal blood or whether transplacental transfer is sufficient to maintain folate levels in the fetus. Therapy with systemic folinic acid has been only partially successful in this disorder because of the difficulty in getting folate to the brain.[3,16–18] Hereditary malabsorption of folate cannot be diagnosed using cultured cells.

Glutamate Formiminotransferase Deficiency

Glutamate formiminotransferase deficiency has a variable phenotype, ranging from severe neurologic disease[19] to benign excretion of formiminoglutamate (FIGLU). Neither activ-

Table 17.1. Disorders of folate and cobalamin metabolism

Disorders of folate metabolism
  Hereditary folate malabsorption (229050)
  Cellular uptake disorder of 5-methyltetrahydrofolate
  Dihydrofolate reductase (EC 1.5.1.3) deficiency (126060)
  Methenyltetrahydrofolate cyclohydrolase (EC 3.5.4.9) deficiency (251150)
  Methyltetrahydrofolate: homocysteine methyltransferase (methionine synthase) (EC 2.1.1.13) apoenzyme
    deficiency (156570)—not *cblG*
  Methylenetetrahydrofolate reductase (EC 1.5.1.20) deficiency (236250)
  Glutamate formiminotransferase (EC 2.1.2.5.) and formiminotetrahydrofolate cyclodeaminase (EC 4.3.1.4)
    deficiencies (formiminotransferase deficiency syndromes) (229100)
Disorders of cobalamin metabolism
  Intrinsic factor abnormalities (261000)
  Selective intestinal malabsorption of vitamin B_{12} with proteinuria (Imerslund–Gräsbeck syndrome) (defects
    in cubilin and amnionless) (261100)
  Transcobalamin II deficiency (275350)
    cblF: Lysosomal trapping disorder of cobalamin (277380)
  Adenosylcobalamin deficiency: Cbl-responsive methylmalonic aciduria
    cblA: Due to a deficiency in the MMAA gene product (251100)
    cblB: ATP:cob(I)alamin adenosyltransferase deficiency (EC 2.5.1.17), MMAB gene (251110)
    cblH: Similar to *cblA* but complements in somatic cell assay (606169)
  Methylcobalamin deficiency
    cblE: Associated with a defect in methionine synthase reductase (MTRR gene) (236270)
    cblG: Methionine synthase deficiency (MTR gene) (250940)
  Combined adenosylcobalamin and methylcobalamin deficiencies
    cblC (277400); *cblD* (277410): Homocystinuria with methylmalonic aciduria; associated with defects in
      the reduction of cob(III)alamin

Note: The numbers in parentheses after the names of the disorders are the McKusick catalog numbers 1994.[10]

ity of the bifunctional enzyme is expressed in cultured fibroblasts.[4] Mutations in the FTCD gene have recently been described in patients with glutamate formiminotransferase deficiency.[20] This would allow for prenatal diagnosis in families in which the mutations are known. Because of the mild phenotype in most families, prenatal diagnosis is not usually a consideration.

Methylenetetrahydrofolate Reductase Deficiency

Methylenetetrahydrofolate reductase deficiency is the most common and best-characterized inborn error of folate metabolism.[5] There is a wide range of phenotypes, from seizures, apnea, coma, and death in infancy[21] to mild mental retardation and neurologic impairment in adolescence.[22,23] Other phenotypes also have been reported.[24–28] Intermediate hyperhomocysteinemia,[28] associated with a somewhat reduced activity of methylenetetrahydrofolate reductase and a common mutation (677C $\rightarrow$ T) in the gene for this enzyme, has been postulated as a risk factor for vascular disease and neural tube defects.[28–35] Megaloblastic anemia is not a feature of severe reductase deficiency, which is characterized by hyperhomocysteinemia and homocystinuria without hypermethioninemia. The enzyme is expressed in cultured fibroblasts, and the levels of the different folate cofactors can be measured directly.[36,37] There is a direct correlation between the residual proportion of methyltetrahydrofolate in cultured fibroblasts, the residual enzyme activity, and the clinical severity of the disease.[37,38] Lymphocytes have been used for heterozygote detection,[39] in addition to fibroblasts,[40] and the enzyme is expressed in amniocytes and chorionic tissue.[42]

Therapy with folate has been only partially successful.[2,4] One infant showed a good response to multivitamin therapy along with methionine supplements[43] but subsequently deteriorated when the family stopped therapy. Another infant with this disorder had reduced carnitine in serum and muscle.[44] Betaine seems to be the single most beneficial agent, particularly if started early.[41,45–49] The use of very high doses of folic acid has been reported from Japan.[50] The diagnosis of severe methylenetetrahydrofolate reductase deficiency has been excluded by enzyme assay using amniocytes or chorionic villus cells in pregnancies at risk[51,52] and has been reported in an affected fetus, using amniocytes.[42] Treatment of the latter patient with folic acid and betaine resulted in normal development.[46] Using measurement of the specific activity of methylenetetrahydrofolate reductase in confluent cultured amniocytes, our laboratory has excluded the severe disease in nine pregnancies at risk and has made the diagnosis in one. Using cultured CVS cells, we have made the diagnosis in two pregnancies at risk and excluded it in three cases (Three of these five pregnancies tested with cultured CVS cells were also tested in amniocytes and are included in the numbers given above.) Interpretation of prenatal diagnosis of severe methylenetetrahydrofolate reductase deficiency may not be as easy as once thought. In one study, enzyme activity was in the heterozygous range in the prenatal studies, but the activity after birth was very low.[53] In another family, the mother had severely low enzyme function in the range of her affected child, but was herself not clinically affected.[52]

The gene for methylenetetrahydrofolate reductase has been cloned and the first thirty-three mutations causing severe enzyme deficiency have been identified.[5,54–58] This allows prenatal diagnosis using DNA in the families in which both segregating alleles are known. In some families, linkage studies using common polymorphisms in the methylenetetrahydrofolate (*MTHFR*) gene can be used for prenatal diagnosis.

Inborn Errors of Cobalamin Metabolism

The first three disorders of Cbl metabolism listed in Table 17.1 involve the absorption of the vitamin from the gut and its transport to target tissues. Their major clinical manifestation is megaloblastic anemia. The first two disorders present when Cbl stored from transplacental transfer has been exhausted.[6,59–61] The defects cannot be detected using cultured cells. Transcobalamin II (TCII) deficiency presents in the first few weeks of life, and early detection is particularly important.

Transcobalamin II Deficiency

Transcobalamin (TCII) deficiency is associated with megaloblastic anemia and pancytopenia, and with immunologic, gastrointestinal, and mental disorders.[9,62–69] Pharmacologic doses of Cbl allow normal hematologic development. The genetics of TCII has been reviewed extensively.[70] Three different forms of TCII deficiencies have been described: (1) low levels of immunoreactive TCII and absence of unsaturated and endogenous Cbl binding capacity (the most common form); (2) normal immunoreactivity and lack of Cbl binding capacity; and (3) elevated TCII in plasma with unsaturated and endogenous Cbl binding capacity but with nonfunctional TCII.

TCII deficiency presents in the first few weeks of life, an indication that the defect represents a failure to use the Cbl stored in utero. Because Cbl therapy will depress the unsaturated TCII level, a patient's serum must be taken before beginning therapy or after the cessation of therapy for several weeks to obtain relevant data with respect to TCII deficiency. At least one case of TCII deficiency has been misdiagnosed as dihydrofolate reductase deficiency.[4,71]

Patients with TCII deficiency are born healthy and without signs of Cbl deficiency, which suggests that fetal TCII is not physiologically important. The fact that the placenta has receptors for TCII-Cbl[72] suggests that maternal TCII may be important for the transfer of Cbl to the fetus. However, a mother with TCII deficiency gave birth to two normal children,[67] and twins with TCII deficiency had no measurable TCII in cord blood,[73] which suggests that a fetal TCII-like binder might be important. Cord blood contains TCII activity that corresponds to that of the fetus and not that of the mother,[70,74] which leaves unexplained why TCII-deficient infants are healthy at birth. Because cultured fibroblasts have been shown to produce TCII isotypes identical to their genetic serum types[64,75,76] and because TCII is expressed in amniocytes,[77,78] prenatal diagnosis is possible.

With the cloning of the gene for human TCII and the identification of mutations in TCII deficiency, molecular diagnosis is possible for patients in whom mutant alleles are known.[79–84]

Disorders of Cobalamin Utilization

Most of the disorders of Cbl utilization are associated with methylmalonic aciduria (i.e., *cblA*, *cblB*, *cblC*, *cblD*, *cblF*, *cblH*). Both *cblC* and *cblD* have homocystinuria along with methylmalonic aciduria; *cblE* and *cblG* (methylcobalamin deficiencies) have only homocystinuria.[85] Prenatal diagnosis either has been accomplished successfully or is possible for all of these disorders, and prenatal therapy with Cbl has been attempted with some degree of success.[11,86–88]

Lysosomal Trapping of Cobalamin

Lysosomal trapping of cobalamin (*cblF*) has been described in six infants.[7,9,89–92] The first infant had developmental delay and minimal methylmalonic aciduria without homocystinuria and had a good response to therapy with hydroxocobalamin. The second infant had homocystinuria in addition to methylmalonic aciduria, and although she responded well to therapy, she had an unexpected sudden death.[91] Clinical findings in *cblF* have included anemia, failure to thrive, developmental delay, hypotonia, lethargy, hepatomegaly, encephalopathy, recurrent infections, rheumatoid arthritis, and a pigmentary skin abnormality. The disorder is associated with the accumulation of free Cbl in the lysosomal fraction of cells, presumably caused by a defect in the transport of free vitamin out of the lysosome.[89,93] The diagnosis of this disorder can be made on the basis of the accumulation of free Cbl in fibroblasts and on the basis of a low incorporation of both labeled propionate and labeled methyltetrahydrofolate. The diagnosis of *cblF* was excluded prenatally in the first two mothers at risk. In the case of the second mother, *cblF* was excluded in twins.

Defective Synthesis of Adenosylcobalamin

Cbl-responsive methylmalonic aciduria may be caused by defects in the synthesis of adenosylcobalamin. (AdoCbl).[7] At first, the presumed defect in *cblA* was thought to be in a mitochondrial cobalamin reductase, and some evidence has suggested that this might be an nicotinamide adenine dinucleotide phosphate (NADPH)-linked aquacobalamin reductase.[94] Subsequently, a comparative genomic approach was used to clone the responsible gene, *MMAA*, and to find the first mutations from patients in the *cblA* complementation group.[95] The exact function of the MMAA gene product remains unclear, but it may be a component of a transporter, or of an accessory protein involved in the mitochondrial transport of cobalamin. The defect in *cblB* is in cob(I)alamin adenosyltransferase.[96] The responsible gene, *MMAB*, has also been cloned using a comparative genomic approach and the first mutations described in patients from the *cblB* complementation group.[97] We described a single patient whose cultured fibroblasts behaved like those of *cblA* patients but complemented with *cblA* cells.[98] The disorder in this patient was first termed *cblA* and subsequently *cblH*.[9,98,99]

The response to Cbl therapy and the prognosis for the patient depend on the specific defect. Matsui et al.[100] found that more than 90 percent of *cblA* patients and approximately 40 percent of *cblB* patients responded to Cbl supplementation with a decrease in urine or blood methylmalonate, in contrast to patients with Cbl-nonresponsive methylmalonic aciduria. The *cblA* and *cblB* patients also have relatively delayed age of onset, as compared with those with the unresponsive forms. The long-term outcome of patients seemed to be best in the *cblA* group of patients and intermediate in the *cblB* group. Treatment consisted of protein restriction and vitamin supplementation. It was suggested that some patients with *cblA* or *cblB* who are unresponsive to hydroxocobalamin (OHCbl) might respond directly to adenosylcobalamin (AdoCbl). However, treatment with AdoCbl of a 30-month-old girl who was unresponsive to OHCbl failed to give a sustained clinically significant response, which suggests that the cofactor was unavailable to the mutase enzyme.[101]

Prenatal diagnosis has been accomplished in the different types of methylmalonic aciduria through (a) the measurement of elevated methylmalonic acid in amniotic fluid (AF) and in the maternal urine,[102] (b) the measurement of methylmalonic acid in AF and decreased activity of mutase in amniocytes,[103] and (c) a decreased metabolism of propionic and methylmalonic acid in amniocytes.[104] Mutase activity has been assayed in noncultivated amniocytes,[105] and a rapid method in cultured amniocytes was developed to measure the incorporation of [^{14}C]propionic acid into macromolecules.[106] Stable isotope dilution analysis has been used to measure methylcitric acid and methylmalonic acid in amniotic fluid.[10,12,107–109] With the cloning of the genes for these diseases, prenatal diagnosis is possible in families in which the causal mutations are known.

The possibility of prenatal therapy in Cbl-responsive methylmalonic aciduria has been demonstrated.[11,86,88] The elevated concentration of methylmalonic acid in maternal urine was decreased with vitamin therapy, which suggests effective treatment of the fetus. In addition, the levels of odd-chain fatty acids were near the control range in the cord blood and red blood cell lipids of treated fetuses but not in their adipose tissue.[88]

Methylcobalamin Deficiency

An infant with megaloblastic anemia and homocystinuria but no methylmalonic aciduria was described,[110] who had a deficiency of methylcobalamin (MeCbl) in cultured fibroblasts and who responded clinically to therapy with OHCbl. The defect in this patient (*cblE*) was subsequently shown to be in a reducing system required for the synthesis of methionine.[111] The gene, *MTRR*, for the responsible enzyme, methionine synthase reductase was cloned and found to encode an enzyme that is a member of the ferredoxin (flavodoxin) NADP+ reductase family.[112–114] Prenatal diagnosis is possible in this disorder and has been accomplished[87] on the basis of the MeCbl content of cultured amniocytes from the fetus at risk. Prenatal therapy was attempted with OHCbl, and therapy was continued from birth. The patient has continued to develop well. In total, we have attempted prenatal diagnosis in three pregnancies at risk for *cblE* and have made the diagnosis of disease in two of the three. Subsequent studies showed that MeCbl deficiency is heterogeneous, with at least two distinct complementation groups.[9,85] The second group with low in vitro methionine synthase activity has been called *cblG*. The defect in *cblG* has been shown to be in the methionine synthase itself, and with the cloning of the human methionine synthase gene,[115,116] many mutations have been identified, including a common mutation P1173L.[115–117] In our laboratory, using cultured chorionic villus cells, we have excluded *cblG* disease in two pregnancies at risk, and using cultured amniocytes, we have excluded *cblG* disease in three pregnancies at risk. Because of our experience with *cblC* (see below), we always prefer to confirm negative chorionic villus cell results with studies on cultured amniocytes.

Cytosolic Cob(III)alamin Reductase Deficiency Associated with Both Homocystinuria and Methylmalonic Aciduria

An increasing number of patients with combined homocystinuria and methylmalonic aciduria are being described.[9,92,118–127] On the basis of complementation studies,[128] they have been divided into *cblC* and *cblD*. It was originally thought that *cblC* patients presented only during the first year of life, with severe manifestations,[7] but a sibship with *cblC* was described in which the proband presented in adolescence,[129] and there have also been a number of cases first diagnosed in adults.[130,131] Clinical manifestations of these disorders include failure to thrive, feeding difficulties, anemia, and megaloblastic marrow. The *cblD* patients had much milder findings than the original *cblC* patients, with the proband coming to medical attention because of behavioral problems and moderate mental retardation.[132]

Fibroblasts from *cblC* and *cblD* patients are defective in accumulating cobalamin and are presumed to be deficient in one or more cobalamin reductase activity.[94,133–135] Prenatal diagnosis of *cblC* and *cblD* can be accomplished by determining methylmalonic acid levels in amniotic fluid and by the study of the incorporation of labeled propionate, methyltetrahydrofolate, and Cbl by cultured amniocytes. We have established the diagnosis of *cblC* in nine of sixty-three pregnancies at risk, using amniocytes. We have also attempted diagnosis in cultured chorionic villus cells, excluding the diagnosis in sixteen cases (ten of these were subsequently looked at in cultured amniocytes) and making the diagnosis in one. However, in one of the excluded cases, the cultured chorionic villus cells gave a false-negative result and the correct diagnosis was made only in the cultured amniocytes. The diagnosis has also been made using amniotic fluid levels of metabolites in six of thirty pregnancies at risk, some of which were also included in the numbers given above (Rinaldo P, unpublished data). We have also excluded the diagnosis of *cblC* in two pregnancies at risk, using direct chorionic villus sampling.[12] The finding of an unaffected fetus in the published case was verified by the absence of methylmalonic acid in maternal urine or amniotic fluid in the second trimester and by the study of cultured fibroblasts from the baby after birth. The smaller than expected number of *cblC* homozygotes on prenatal diagnosis makes it possible that some affected fetuses are aborted spontaneously early in pregnancy.

There are two reports of pregnancies at risk for methylmalonic aciduria, that were monitored using noncultured chorionic villus tissue.[136,137] The first report excluded methylmalonic aciduria using labeled propionate incorporation as the assay method.[136] The second report demonstrated the variability of propionate incorporation, ranging from 10 to 40 percent of control values in different portions of the same villus tissue from a fetus shown to be affected.[138]

In total, we have attempted the prenatal diagnosis of cobalamin metabolism using cultured chorionic villus cells in twenty-one pregnancies at risk (seventeen *cblC*, one *cblA*, one *cblB*, and two *cblG*), and in all but two *cblC* cases, the tests were negative. However, the cells in one of the samples grew more rapidly than chorionic villus cells and had the appearance of fibroblasts. Maternal contamination was suspected, and studies of cultured amniocytes revealed the diagnosis of *cblC*. (This is the case referred to above.) For these reasons, we prefer to follow normal cultured chorionic villus samples with amniocentesis for the diagnosis of these disorders.

There have been additional reports of prenatal diagnosis in *cblC*.[139,140] These have used the measurement of methylmalonic acid and of total homocysteine in amniotic fluid as well as the incorporation of labeled methyltetrahydrofolate into protein in cultured amniocytes. At present, the most reliable method for the prenatal diagnosis of the inborn errors of cobalamin metabolism involves both the measurement of metabolites in amniotic fluid and the incorporation of precursors in cultured amniocytes.

PRENATAL DIAGNOSIS OF CYSTINOSIS

Cystinosis is an autosomal recessive disorder characterized by the accumulation of free, nonprotein cystine within the lysosomes of most tissues. The cystine accumulates at 10 to 1,000 times the normal levels and forms crystals within the lysosomes. The primary defect in cystinosis is a defective lysosomal transport system for cystine.[141–143] The gene for cystinosis, *CTNS*, codes for the protein cystinosin and is located on the short arm of chromosome 17.[144–148] The major features of cystinosis have been reviewed extensively.[148–153]

Clinical Findings

Children with cystinosis are not symptomatic at birth, but signs of renal Fanconi syndrome develop between 1 and 12 months of life.[148] These signs include failure to grow, dehydration, electrolyte imbalance, vomiting, acidosis, and hypophosphatemic rickets. Affected children have normal intelligence, and their weight is appropriate for their height. They remain short and develop progressive glomerular insufficiency, leading to end-stage renal disease by the end of the first decade. Additional findings in the classic form of cystinosis include photophobia, hypothyroidism, and abnormal sweating. Cystinosis can be diagnosed by examining the cystine content of cultured fibroblasts or leukocytes. After 1 year of age, the diagnosis can also be made by slit-lamp examination for corneal crystals.

There is considerable clinical heterogeneity in cystinosis. Three different forms have been described (infantile nephropathic, late-onset nephropathic, and benign), and the different forms seem to breed true in families. The clinical severity correlates with the extent of the accumulation of cystine.[149,150]

Treatment in cystinosis includes the management of the renal disease and dialysis or transplantation after end-stage renal disease develops. Although storage of cystine does not occur in the transplanted organ, storage in other host tissues may result in retinal blindness, corneal erosions, diabetes mellitus, myopathy, swallowing difficulties, and neurologic disease.[149] It has been shown that cysteamine, a cystine-depleting agent, can retard growth failure and renal deterioration if begun early in life.[148,154–159] However, even if begun before 3 weeks of age, cysteamine does not necessarily prevent the development of the renal Fanconi syndrome.[148,160]

Heterozygote detection has relied on determining the content of free cystine in leukocytes or cultured fibroblasts.

Prenatal Diagnosis

The first prenatal diagnosis of cystinosis was accomplished in 1974 by growing amniocytes for 48 hr in a cystine-free medium containing 10 percent dialyzed fetal bovine serum in the presence of [^{35}S]cystine. The cells were lysed at physiologic pH in the presence of N-ethylmaleimide (NEM), which reacts with free sulfhydryl groups and forms derivatives that are stable at acid pH. Skin fibroblasts and control amniocytes contained most of the label in the form of glutathione-NEM and cysteine-MEM and almost none in cystine. Amniocytes from the cystinotic fetus had much higher levels of nonprotein cystine.[161] A modification of the preceding technique was reported,[162] as was the use of cystine dimethyl ester.[163] There have been other modifications, including the use of high-performance liquid chromatography.[164]

Chorionic villi have been used for direct cystine measurement at 9 weeks of gestational age.[165] The assay used a specific cystine-binding protein.[166] Fresh tissue from the fetus at risk contained 34.7 nmol 2 cystine/mg protein, as compared with 0.09–0.13 nmol 2 cystine/mg protein in control samples. Cultured cells from the fetus at risk contained 9.7 nmol 2 cystine/mg protein, as compared with 0.11–0.18 nmol 2 cystine/mg protein in control cells.[165] A similar technique was used to exclude the diagnosis of cystinosis in another fetus at risk.[167] There are currently more than fifty mutations known in CTNS, with the most common being a large deletion than eliminates the first ten exons of the gene.[148] If both causal mutations are known for a pregnancy at risk, prenatal diagnosis using a molecular approach is theoretically possible.

Because of the therapeutic successes with early cysteamine treatment in cystinosis,[154,155,160] most parents decline prenatal diagnosis, and rapid diagnosis after birth has become important.[148] The measurement of the cystine content of fetal placental tissue[168] and of leukocytes can be used to make the diagnosis.

ACKNOWLEDGMENTS

I thank W.A. Gahl for assistance in the preparation this chapter. The final section, on prenatal diagnosis of cystinosis, is a publication of the Hess B. and Diane Finestone Laboratory in Memory of Jacob and Jenny Finestone.

REFERENCES

1. Rowe PB. Inherited disorders of folate metabolism. In: Stanbury JB, Wyngaarden JB, Frederickson DS, Goldstein JL, Brown MS, eds. The metabolic basis of inherited diseases, 5th ed. New York: McGraw-Hill, 1983:498.
2. Rosenblatt DS. Inherited disorders of folate transport and metabolism. In: Scriver CR, Beaudet AL, Sly WS, Valle D, eds. The metabolic and molecular bases of inherited disease, 7th ed. New York: McGraw-Hill, 1995:3111.

3. Niederweiser A. Inborn errors of pterin metabolism. In: Botez MI, Reynolds EH, eds. Folic acid in neurology, psychiatry and internal medicine. New York: Raven, 1979:349.

4. Erbe RW. Genetic aspects of folate metabolism. Adv Hum Genet 1979;9:293.

5. Rosenblatt D, Fenton WA. Inherited disorders of folate and cobalamin transport and metabolism. In: Scriver CR, Beaudet AL, Sly WS, Valle D, Childs B, Kinzler KW, et al., eds. The metabolic and molecular bases of inherited disease, 8th ed. New York: McGraw-Hill, 2001:3897.

6. Cooper BA. Megaloblastic anaemia and disorders affecting utilisation of vitamin B_{12} and folate in childhood. Clin Haematol 1976;5:631.

7. Fenton WA, Rosenberg LE. Inherited disorders of cobalamin transport and metabolism. In: Scriver CR, Beaudet AL, Sly WS, Valle D, eds. The metabolic and molecular bases of inherited disease, 7th ed. New York: McGraw-Hill, 1995:3129.

8. Rosenblatt DS, Cooper BA. Inherited disorders of vitamin B_{12} metabolism. Blood Rev 1987;1:177–182.

9. Watkins D, Rosenblatt DS. Cobalamin and inborn errors of cobalamin absorption and metabolism. Endocrinologist 2001;11:98.

10. McKusick VA. Mendelian inheritance in man: Catalogs of autosomal dominant, autosomal recessive and X-linked phenotypes, 11th ed. Baltimore: Johns Hopkins University Press, 1994.

11. Sweetman L. Prenatal diagnosis of organic acidurias. J Inherit Metab Dis 1984;7:18.

12. Zammarchi E, Lippi A, Falorni S, et al. cblC disease: case report and monitoring of a pregnancy at risk by chorionic villus sampling. Clin Invest Med 1990;13:139.

13. Van der Meer SB, Spaapen LJM, Fowler B, et al. Prenatal treatment of a patient with vitamin B_{12}-responsive methylmalonic acidemia. J Pediatr 1990;117:923.

14. Jacobs C. Prenatal diagnosis of inherited metabolic disorders by stable isotope dilution GC-MS analysis of metabolites of amniotic fluid: review of four year's experience. J Inherit Metab Dis 1989;12:267.

15. Branda RF, Moldow CF, MacArthur JR, et al. Folate-induced remission in aplastic anemia with familial defect of cellular folate uptake. N Engl J Med 1978;298:469.

16. Poncz M, Colman N, Herbert V, et al. Therapy of congenital folate malabsorption. J Pediatr 1981;98:76.

17. Corbeel L, Van Den Berghe G, Jaeken J, et al. Congenital folate malabsorption. Eur J Pediatr 1985;143:284.

18. Buchanan JA. Fibroblast plasma membrane vesicles to study inborn errors of transport. PhD thesis. Montreal: McGill University, 1984.

19. Arakawa T. Congenital defects in folate utilization. Am J Med 1970;48:594.

20. Hilton JF, Christensen KE, Watkins D, et al. The molecular basis of glutamate formiminotransferase-cyclodeaminase deficiency. Hum Mutat 2003;22:67.

21. Narisawa KY, Wada T, Saito H, et al. Infantile type of homocystinuria with N5,10-methylenetetrahydrofolate reductase defect. Tohoku J Exp Med 1977;121:185.

22. Mudd SH, Uhlendorf BW, Freeman JM, et al. Homocystinuria associated with decreased methylenetetrahydrofolate reductase activity. Biochem Biophys Res Commun 1972;46:905.

23. Freeman JM, Finkelstein JD, Mudd SH. Folate-responsive homocystinuria and "schizophrenia": a defect in methylation due to deficient 5,10-methylenetetrahydrofolate reductase activity. N Engl J Med 1975;292:491.

24. Baumgartner ER, Schweizer K, Wick H. Different congenital forms of defective remethylation in homocystinuria: clinical, biochemical, and morphological studies. Pediatr Res 1977;11:1015.

25. Wong PWK, Justice P, Hruby M, et al. Folic acid non-responsive homocystinuria due to methylenetetrahydrofolate reductase deficiency. Pediatrics 1977;59:749.

26. Kanwar YS, Manaligod JR, Wong PWK. Morphologic studies in a patient with homocystinuria due to 5,10-methylenetetrahydrofolate reductase deficiency. Pediatr Res 1976;10:598.

27. Kang S-S, Wong PWK, Zhou J, et al. Thermolabile methylenetetrahydrofolate reductase in patients with coronary artery disease. Metabolism 1988;37:611.

28. Kang SS, Zhou J, Wong PWK, et al. Intermediate homocysteinemia: a thermolabile variant of methylenetetrahydrofolate reductase. Am J Hum Genet 1988;43:414.

29. Kluijtmans LAJ, van den Heuvel LPWJ, Boers GHJ, et al. Molecular genetic analysis in mild hyperhomocysteinemia: a common mutation in the methylenetetrahydrofolate reductase gene is a genetic risk factor for cardiovascular disease. Am J Hum Genet 1996;58:35.

30. van der Put NMJ, Steegers-Theunissen RPM, Frosst P, et al. Mutated methylenetetrahydrofolate reductase as a risk factor for spina bifida. Lancet 1995;346:1070.

31. Frosst P, Blom HJ, Milos R, et al. A candidate genetic risk factor for vascular disease: a common methylenetetrahydrofolate reductase mutation causes thermoinstability. Nat Genet 1995;10:111.

32. Rosenblatt DS, Lue-Shing H, Arzoumanian A, et al. Methylenetetrahydrofolate reductase (MR) deficiency:

thermolability of residual MR activity, methionine synthase activity, and methylcobalamin levels in cultured fibroblasts. Biochem Med Metab Biol 1992;47:221.

33. Jacques PF, Bostom AG, Williams RR, et al. Relation between folate status, a common mutation in methylenetetrahydrofolate reductase, and plasma homocysteine concentrations. Circulation 1996;93:7.

34. Botto LD, Yang Q. 5,10-methylenetetrahydrofolate reductase gene variants and congenital anomalies: a huge review. Am J Epidemiol 2000;151:862.

35. Rosenblatt DS. Methylenetetrahydrofolate reductase. Clin Invest Med 2001;24:56.

36. Cooper BA, Rosenblatt DS. Folate coenzyme forms in fibroblasts from patients deficient in 5,10-methylenetetrahydrofolate reductase. Biochem Soc Trans 1976;4:921.

37. Rosenblatt D, Cooper BA, Lue-Shing S, et al. Folate distribution in cultured human cells: studies on 5,10-CH_2-H_4PteGlu reductase deficiency. J Clin Invest 1979;63:1019.

38. Baumgartner ER, Stokstad ELR, Wick H, et al. Comparison of folic acid coenzyme distribution patterns in patients with methylenetetrahydrofolate reductase and methionine synthetase deficiencies. Pediatr Res 1985;19:1288.

39. Wong PWK, Justice P, Berlow S. Detection of homozygotes and heterozygotes with methylenetetrahydrofolate reductase deficiency. J Lab Clin Med 1977;90:283.

40. Rosenblatt DS, Erbe RW. Methylenetetrahydrofolate reductase in cultured human cells. II. Studies of methylenetetrahydrofolate reductase deficiency. Pediatr Res 1977;11:1141.

41. Wendel U, Bremer HJ. Betaine in the treatment of homocystinuria due to 5,10-methylenetetrahydrofolate reductase deficiency. Eur J Pediatr 1984;142:147.

42. Christensen E, Brandt NJ. Prenatal diagnosis of 5,10-methylenetetrahydrofolate reductase deficiency. N Engl J Med 1985;313:50.

43. Harpey JP, Rosenblatt DS, Cooper BA, et al. Homocystinuria caused by 5,10-methylenetetrahydrofolate reductase deficiency: a case in an infant responding to methionine, folinic acid, pyridoxine, and vitamin B_{12} therapy. J Pediatr 1981;98:275.

44. Allen RJ, Wong PWK, Rothenberg SP, et al. Progressive neonatal leukoencephalomyopathy due to absent methylenetetrahydrofolate reductase, responsive to treatment. Ann Neurol 1980;8:211.

45. Kang S. Treatment of hyperhomocyst(e)inemia: physiological basis. J Nutr 1996;126 (Suppl 4):1273S.

46. Brandt NJ, Christensen E, Skovby F, et al. Treatment of methylenetetrahydrofolate reductase deficiency from the neonatal period. In: The Society for the Study of Inborn Errors of Metabolism, The Netherlands: Amersfoort, 1986:23 (abstract).

47. Ronge E, Kjellman B. Long term treatment with betaine in methylenetetrahydrofolate reductase deficiency. Arch Dis Child 1996;74:239.

48. Sakura N, Ono H, Nomura H, et al. Betaine dose and treatment intervals in therapy for homocystinuria due to 5,10-methylenetetrahydrofolate reductase deficiency. J Inherit Metab Dis 1998;21:84.

49. Schwahn B, Hafner D, Hohlfeld T, et al. Pharmacokinetics of oral betaine in healthy subjects. J Inherit Metab Dis 2000;23:66.

50. Takenaka T, Shimomura T, Nakayasu H, et al. [Effect of folic acid for treatment of homocystinuria due to 5,10-methylenetetrahydrofolate reductase deficiency] [Japanese]. Rinsho Shinkeigaku 1993;33:1140.

51. Wendel U, Claussen U, Dickmann E. Prenatal diagnosis for methylenetetrahydrofolate reductase deficiency. J Pediatr 1983;102:938.

52. Marquet J, Chadefaux B, Bonnefont JP, et al. Methylenetetrahydrofolate reductase deficiency: prenatal diagnosis and family studies. Prenat Diagn 1994;14:29.

53. Tonetti C, Burtscher A, Bories D, et al. Methylenetetrahydrofolate reductase deficiency in four siblings: a clinical, biochemical, and molecular study of the family. Am J Hum Genet 2000;9:363.

54. Goyette P, Milos R, Ducan AM, et al. Human methylenetetrahydrofolate reductase: isolation of cDNA, mapping and mutation identification. Nat Genet 1994;7:195.

55. Goyette P, Frosst P, Rosenblatt DS, et al. Seven novel mutations in the methylenetetrahydrofolate reductase gene and genotype/phenotype correlations in severe methylenetetrahydrofolate reductase deficiency. Am J Hum Genet 1995;56:1052.

56. Goyette P, Christensen B, Rosenblatt DS, et al. Severe and mild mutations in cis for the methylenetetrahydrofolate (MTHFR) gene, and description of 5 novel mutations in MTHFR. Am J Hum Genet 1996;59:1268.

57. Sibani S, Christensen B, O'Ferrall E, et al. Characterization of six novel mutations in the methylenetetrahydrofolate reductase (MTHFR) gene in patients with homocystinuria. Hum Mutat 2000;15:280.

58. Sibani S, Leclerc D, Weisberg IS, et al. Characterization of mutations in severe methylenetetrahydrofolate reductase deficiency reveals an FAD-responsive mutation. Hum Mutat 2003;21:509.

59. Hall CA. Congenital disorders of vitamin B_{12} transport and their contributions to concepts. II. Yale J Biol Med 1981;54:485.

60. Heidel MA, Siegel SE, Falk RE, et al. Congenital pernicious anemia: report of seven patients with studies of the extended family. J Pediatr 1984;105:564.

61. Cooper BA, Rosenblatt DS. Inherited defects of vitamin B_{12} metabolism. Annu Rev Nutr 1987;7:291.

62. Burman JF, Mollin DL, Sourial NA, et al. Inherited lack of transcobalamin II in serum and megaloblastic anemia: a further patient. Br J Haematol 1979;43:27.

63. Frater-Schroder M, Hitzig WH, Sacher M. Inheritance of transcobalamin (TCII) in two families with TCII deficiency and related immunodeficiency. J Inherit Metab Dis 1981;4:165.

64. Frater-Schroder M, Luthy R, Haurani F, et al. Quantitative messung der neusynthese von transcobalamin II in der fibroblastenkultur-Bedeutung in der diagnose des transcobalamin II-mangels. Schweiz Med Wochenschr 1982;109:1373.

65. Hakami N, Neiman PE, Canellos GP, et al. Neonatal megaloblastic anemia due to inherited transcobalamin II deficiency in two siblings. N Engl J Med 1971;285:1163.

66. Hitzig WH, Dohmann U, Pluss HJ, et al. Hereditary transcobalamin II deficiency: clinical findings in a new family. J Pediatr 1974;85:622.

67. Seligman PA, Steiner LL, Allen RH. Studies of a patient with megaloblastic anemia and an abnormal transcobalamin II. N Engl J Med 1980;303:1209.

68. Thomas PK, Hoffbrand AV, Smith IS. Neurological involvement in hereditary transcobalamin II deficiency. J Neurol Neurosurg Psychiatry 1982;45:74.

69. Hall CA. The neurologic aspects of transcobalamin II deficiency. Br J Haematol 1992;80:117.

70. Frater-Schroder M. Genetic patterns of transcobalamin II and the relationships with congenital defects. Mol Cell Biochem 1983;56:5.

71. Hoffbrand AV, Tripp E, Jackson BFA, et al. Hereditary abnormal transcobalamin II previously diagnosed as congenital dihydrofolate reductase deficiency. N Engl J Med 1984;310:789.

72. Friedman PA, Shia MA, Wallace JK. A saturable high affinity binding site for transcobalamin II–vitamin B_{12} complexes in human placental membrane preparations. J Clin Invest 1977;59:51.

73. Begley JA, Hall CA, Scott CR. Absence of transcobalamin II from cord blood. Blood 1984;63:490.

74. Porck HJ, Frater-Schroder M, Frants KI, et al. Genetic evidence for fetal origin of transcobalamin II in human cord blood. Blood 1983;62:234.

75. Frater-Schroder M, Porck HJ, Erten J, et al. Synthesis and secretion of the human vitamin B_{12}-binding protein, transcobalamin II, by cultured skin fibroblasts and by bone marrow cells. Biochim Biophys Acta 1985;845:421.

76. Frater-Schroder M, Krieg P, Kierat L, et al. Secretion on transcobalamin II, a well characterized vitamin B_{12} binding protein in amniotic fluid cell cultures. Helv Paediatr Acta (Suppl) 1984;50:27.

77. Rosenblatt DS, Hosack A, Matiaszuk N. Expression of transcobalamin II by amniocytes. Prenat Diagn 1987;7:35.

78. Mayes JS, Say B, Marcus DL. Prenatal diagnosis in a family with transcobalamin II deficiency. Am J Hum Genet 1987;41:686.

79. Platica O, Janeczko R, Quadros EV, et al. The cDNA sequence and the deduced amino acid sequence of human transcobalamin II show homology with rat intrinsic factor and human transcobalamin I. J Biol Chem 1991;266:7860.

80. Regec A, Quadros EV, Platica O, et al. The cloning and characterization of the human transcobalamin II gene. Blood 1995;85:2711.

81. Li N, Seetharam S, Seetharam B. Genomic structure of human transcobalamin II: comparison to human intrinsic factor and transcobalamin I. Biochem Biophys Res Commun 1995;208 (2):756.

82. Li N, Seetharam S, Rosenblatt DS, et al. Expression of transcobalamin II mRNA in human tissues and cultured fibroblasts from normal and transcobalamin II-deficient patients. Biochem J 1994;301:585.

83. Li N, Rosenblatt DS, Seetharam B. Nonsense mutations in human transcobalamin II deficiency. Biochem Biophys Res Commun 1994;204:1111.

84. Li N, Rosenblatt DS, Kamen BA, et al. Identification of two mutant alleles of transcobalamin II in an affected family. Hum Mol Genet 1994;3:1835.

85. Watkins D, Rosenblatt DS. Functional methionine synthase deficiency (*cblE* and *cblG*): clinical and biochemical heterogeneity. Am J Med Genet 1989;34:427.

86. Ampola MG, Mahoney MJ, Nakamura E, et al. Prenatal therapy of a patient with vitamin B_{12} responsive methylmalonic acidemia. N Engl J Med 1975;293:313.

87. Rosenblatt DS, Cooper BA, Schmutz SM, et al. Prenatal vitamin B_{12} therapy of a fetus with methylcobalamin deficiency (cobalamin E disease). Lancet 1985;1:1127.

88. Zass R, Leupold MA, Fernandez MA, et al. Evaluation of prenatal treatment in newborns with cobalamin-responsive methylmalonic acidaemia. J Inherit Metab Dis 1995;18:100.

89. Rosenblatt DS, Hosack A, Matiaszuk NV, et al. Defect in vitamin B_{12} release from lysosomes: newly described inborn error of vitamin B_{12} metabolism. Science 1985;228:1319.

90. Rosenblatt DS, Laframboise R, Pichette J, et al. New disorder of vitamin B_{12} metabolism (cobalamin F) presenting as methylmalonic aciduria. Pediatrics 1986;78:51.

91. Shih VE, Axel SM, Tewksbury JC, et al. Defective lysosomal release of vitamin B_{12} (cb1F): a hereditary cobalamin metabolic disorder associated with sudden death. Am J Med Genet 1989;33:555.

92. Rosenblatt DS. Inherited errors of cobalamin metabolism: an overview. In: Bhatt HR, James VHT, Besser GM, Bottazzo GF, Keen H, eds. Advances in Thomas Addison's diseases. Bristol, England: Journal of Endocrinology Ltd., 1994:303.

93. Vassiliadis A, Rosenblatt DS, Cooper BA, et al. Lysosomal cobalamin accumulation in fibroblasts from a patient with an inborn error of cobalamin metabolism (cblF complementation group): visualization by electron microscope radioautography. Exp Cell Res 1991;195:295.

94. Watanabe F, Saido H, Yamaji R, et al. Mitochondrial NADH- or NADP-linked aquacobalamin reductase activity is low in human skin fibroblasts with defects in synthesis of cobalamin coenzymes. J Nutr 1996;126:2947.

95. Dobson CM, Wai T, Leclerc D, et al. Identification of the gene responsible for the *cblA* complementation group of vitamin B_{12}-responsive methylmalonic acidemia based on analysis of prokaryotic gene arrangements. Proc Natl Acad Sci USA 2002;99:15554.

96. Fenton WA, Rosenberg LE. The defect in the *cblB* class of human methylmalonic acidemia: deficiency of cob(I)alamin adenosyltransferase activity in extracts of cultured fibroblasts. Biochem Biophys Res Commun 1981;98:283.

97. Dobson CM, Wai T, Leclerc D, et al. Identification of the gene responsible for the *cblB* complementation group of vitamin B_{12}-dependent methylmalonic aciduria. Hum Mol Genet 2002;11:1.

98. Watkins D, Matiaszuk N, Rosenblatt DS. Complementation studies in the *cblA* class of inborn error of cobalamin metabolism: evidence for interallelic complementation and for a new complementation class (cblH). J Med Genet 2000;37:510.

99. Cooper BA, Rosenblatt DS, Watkins D. Methylmalonic aciduria due to a new defect in adenosylcobalamin accumulation by cells. Am J Hematol 1990;34:115.

100. Matsui SM, Mahoney MJ, Rosenberg LE. The natural history of the inherited methylmalonic acidemias. N Engl J Med 1983;308:857.

101. Batshaw ML, Thomas GH, Cohen SR, et al. Treatment of the cblB form of methylmalonic acidaemia with adenosylcobalamin. J Inherit Metab Dis 1984;7:65.

102. Morrow G, Schwartz RH, Hallock JA, et al. Prenatal detection of methylmalonic acidemia. J Pediatr 1970;77:120.

103. Gompertz D, Goodey PA, Saudubray JM, et al. Prenatal diagnosis of methylmalonic aciduria. Pediatrics 1974;54:511.

104. Mahoney MJ, Rosenberg LE, Linblad B, et al. Prenatal diagnosis of methylmalonic aciduria. Acta Paediatr Scand 1975;64:44.

105. Morrow G, Revsin B, Lebowitz J, et al. Detection of errors in methylmalonyl-CoA metabolism by using amniotic fluid. Clin Chem 1977;23:791.

106. Willard HF, Ambani LM, Hart AC, et al. Rapid prenatal and postnatal detection of inborn errors of propionate, methylmalonate, and cobalamin metabolism: a sensitive assay using cultured cells. Hum Genet 1976;34:277.

107. Sweetman L, Naylor G, Ladner T. Prenatal diagnosis of propionic and methylmalonic acidemia by stable isotope dilution analysis of methylcitric and methylmalonic acid in amniotic fluid. In: Schmidt H, Forstel H, Heizenger K, eds. Stable isotopes. Amsterdam: Elsevier, 1982:287.

108. Trefz FK, Schmidt H, Tauscher B, et al. Improved prenatal diagnosis of methylmalonic acidemia: mass fragmentography of methylmalonic acid in amniotic fluid and maternal urine. Eur J Pediatr 1981;137:261.

109. Zinn AB, Hine DG, Mahoney MJ, Tanaka K. The stable isotope dilution method for measurement of methylmalonic acid: a highly accurate approach to the prenatal diagnosis of methylmalonic acidemia. Pediatr Res 1982;16:740.

110. Schuh S, Rosenblatt DS, Cooper BA, et al. Homocystinuria and megaloblastic anemia responsive to vitamin B_{12} therapy: an inborn error of metabolism due to a defect in cobalamin metabolism. N Engl J Med 1984;310:686.

111. Rosenblatt DS, Cooper BA, Pottier A, et al. Altered vitamin B_{12} metabolism in fibroblasts from a patient with megaloblastic anemia and homocystinuria due to a new defect in methionine biosynthesis. J Clin Invest 1984;74:2149.

112. Leclerc D, Wilson A, Dumas R, et al. Cloning and mapping of a cDNA for methionine synthase reductase, a flavoprotein defective in patients with homocystinuria. Proc Natl Acad Sci USA 1998;95:3059.

113. Wilson A, Leclerc D, Rosenblatt DS, et al. Molecular basis for methionine synthase reductase deficiency in patients belonging to the *cblE* complementation group of disorders in folate/cobalamin metabolism. Hum Mol Genet 1999;8:2009.

114. Zavad'Akova P, Fowler B, Zeman J, et al. CblE type of homocystinuria due to methionine synthase reductase deficiency: clinical and molecular studies and prenatal diagnosis in two families. J Inherit Metab Dis 2002;25:461.

115. Leclerc D, Campeau E, Goyette P, et al. Human methionine synthase: cDNA cloning and identification of mutations in patients of the *cblG* complementation group of folate/cobalamin disorders. Hum Mol Genet 1996;5:1867.

116. Gulati S, Baker P, Li YN, et al. Defects in human methionine synthase in *cblG* patients. Hum Mol Genet 1996;5:1859.

117. Watkins D, Ru M, Hwang H, et al. Hyperhomocysteinemia due to methionine synthase deficiency, *cblG*: structure of the MTR gene, genotype diversity, and recognition of a common mutation, P1173L. Am J Hum Genet 2002;71:143.

118. Ribes A, Vilaseca MA, Briones P, et al. Methylmalonic aciduria with homocystinuria. J Inherit Metab Dis 1984;7:129.

119. Linnell JC, Miranda B, Bhatt HR, et al. Abnormal cobalamin metabolism in a megaloblastic child with homocystinuria, cystathioninuria and methylmalonic aciduria. J Inherit Metab Dis 1983;6 (Suppl 2):137.

120. Carmel R, Goodman SI. Abnormal deoxyuridine suppression test in congenital methylmalonic aciduria-homocystinuria without megaloblastic anemia: divergent biochemical and morphological bone marrow manifestations of disordered cobalamin metabolism in man. Blood 1982;59:306.

121. Carmel R, Bedros AA, Mace JW, et al. Congenital methylmalonic aciduria-homocystinuria with megaloblastic anemia: observations on response to hydroxocobalamin and on the effect of homocysteine and methionine on the deoxyuridine suppression test. Blood 1980;55:570.

122. Dillon MJ, England JM, Gompertz D, et al. Mental retardation, megaloblastic anemia, methylmalonic aciduria and abnormal homocysteine metabolism due to an error in vitamin B_{12} metabolism. Clin Sci Mol Med 1974;47:43.

123. Levy HL, Mudd SH, Schulman JD, et al. A derangement in B_{12} metabolism associated with homocystinemia, cystathioninemia, hypomethioninemia and methylmalonic aciduria. Am J Med 1970;48:390.

124. Anthony M, McLeay AC. A unique case of derangement of vitamin B_{12} metabolism. Proc Aust Assoc Neurol 1976;13:61.

125. Baumgartner ER, Wick H, Maurer R, et al. Congenital defect in intracellular cobalamin metabolism resulting in homocystinuria and methylmalonic aciduria. Helv Paediatr Acta 1979;34:465.

126. Matthews DM, Linnell JC. Cobalamin deficiency and related disorders in infancy and childhood. Eur J Pediatr 1982;138:6.

127. Rosenblatt DS, Aspler AL, Shevell MI, et al. Clinical heterogeneity and prognosis in combined methylmalonic aciduria and homocystinuria (cblC). J Inherit Metab Dis 1997;20:528.

128. Willard HF, Mellman IS, Rosenberg LE. Genetic complementation among inherited deficiencies of methylmalonyl-CoA mutase activity: evidence for a new class of human cobalamin mutant. Am J Hum Genet 1978;30:1.

129. Shinnar S, Singer HS. Cobalamin C mutation (methylmalonic aciduria and homocystinuria) in adolescence: a treatable cause of dementia and myelopathy. N Engl J Med 1984;311:451.

130. Powers JM, Rosenblatt DS, Schmidt RE, et al. Neurological and neuropathologic heterogeneity in two brothers with cobalamin C deficiency. Ann Neurol 2001;49:396.

131. Bodamer OAF, Rosenblatt DS, Appel SH, et al. Adult-onset combined methylmalonic aciduria and homocystinuria (cblC). Neurology 2001;56:1113.

132. Goodman SI, Moe PG, Hammond KB, et al. Homocystinuria with methylmalonic aciduria: two cases in a sibship. Biochem Med 1970;4:500.

133. Mellman I, Willard HF, Youngdahl-Turner P, et al. Cobalamin coenzyme synthesis in normal and mutant fibroblasts: evidence for a processing enzyme activity deficient in cblC cells. J Biol Chem 1979;254:11847.

134. Pezacka EH. Identification and characterization of two enzymes involved in the intracellular metabolism of cobalamin: cyanocobalamin β-ligand transferase and microsomal cob(III)alamin reductase. Biochim Biophys Acta. 1993;1157:167.

135. Pezacka EH, Rosenblatt DS. Intracellular metabolism of cobalamin: altered activities of β-axial-ligand transferase and microsomal cob(III)alamin reductase in *cblC* and *cblD* fibroblasts. In: Bhatt HR, James

VHT, Besser GM, Bottazzo GF, Keen H, eds. Advances in Thomas Addison's diseases. Bristol, London: Journal of Endocrinology Ltd., 1994:315.

136. Fowler B, Giles L, Sardharwalla IB, et al. First trimester diagnosis of methylmalonic aciduria. Prenat Diagn 1988;8:207.

137. Rosenblatt DS. Inborn errors of folate and cobalamin metabolism. In: Milunsky A, ed. Genetic disorders and the fetus, 2nd ed. New York: Plenum, 1986:411.

138. Kleijer WJ, Thoomes R, Galjaard H, et al. First trimester (chorion biopsy) diagnosis of citrullinaemia and methylmalonic aciduria. Lancet 1984;2:1340.

139. Parvy P, Bardet J, Chadefaux-Vekemans B, et al. Free amino acids in amniotic fluid and the prenatal diagnosis of homocystinuria with methylmalonic aciduria. Clin Chem 1995;41:1663.

140. Chadefaux-Vekemans B, Rolland MO, Lyonet S, et al. Prenatal diagnosis of combined methylmalonic aciduria and homocystinuria (cobalamin CblC or CblD mutant). Prenatal Diagn 1994;14:417.

141. Gahl WA, Tietze F, Bashan N, et al. Defective cystine exodus from isolated lysosome-rich fractions of cystinotic leukocytes. J Biol Chem 1982;257:9570.

142. Gahl WA, Bashan N, Tietze F, et al. Cystine transport is defective in isolated leukocyte lysosomes from patients with cystinosis. Science 1982;217:1263–65.

143. Gahl WA, Tietze F, Bashan N, et al. Characteristics of cystine counter-transport in normal and cystinotic lysosome-rich leucocyte granular fractions. Biochem J 1983;216:393.

144. The Cystinosis Collaborative Research Group. Linkage of the gene for cystinosis to markers on the short arm of chromosome 17. Nat Genet 1995;10:246.

145. Jean G, Fuchshuber A, Town MM, et al. High-resolution mapping of the gene for cystinosis, using combined biochemical and linkage analysis. Am J Hum Genet 1996;58:535.

146. Stec I, Peters U, Harms E, et al. Yeast artificial chromosome mapping of the cystinosis locus on chromosome 17p by fluorescence in situ hybridization. Hum Genet 1996;98:321.

147. McDowell G, Isogai T, Tanigami A, et al. Fine mapping of the cystinosis gene using an integrated genetic and physical map of a region within human chromosome band 17p13. Biochem Mol Med 1996; 58:135.

148. Gahl WA, Thoene JG, Schneider JA. Cystinosis. N Engl J Med 2002;347:111.

149. Gahl WA, Schneider JA, Aula PP. Lysosomal transport disorders: cystinosis and sialic acid storage disorders. In: Scriver CR, Beaudet AL, Sly WS, Valle D, eds. The metabolic and molecular bases of inherited disease, 7th ed. New York: McGraw-Hill, 1995:3763.

150. Schneider JA, Seegmiller JE. Cystinosis. In: Stanbury JB, Wyngaarden JB, Frederickson DS, Goldstein JL, Brown MS, eds. The metabolic basis of inherited disease, 5th ed. New York: McGraw-Hill, 1983:1866.

151. Schulman JD. Prenatal diagnosis of cystinosis. In: Milunsky A, ed. Genetic disorders and the fetus. New York: Plenum Press, 1986:427.

152. Thoene JG. Cystinosis. J Inherit Metab Dis 1995;18:380.

153. Gahl WA, Thoene JG, Schneider JA. Cystinosis: a disorder of lysosomal membrane transport. In: Scriver CR, Beaudet AL, Sly WS, Valle D, eds. The metabolic and molecular bases of inherited disease, 8th ed. New York: McGraw-Hill, 2001:5085.

154. da Silva VA, Zurbrugg RP, Lavanchy P, et al. Long-term treatment of infantile nephropathic cystinosis with cysteamine. N Engl J Med 1985;313:1460.

155. Gahl WA, Reed GF, Thoene JG, et al. Cysteamine therapy for children with nephropathic cystinosis. N Engl J Med 1987;316:971.

156. Markello TC, Bernardini IM, Gahl WA. Improved renal function in children with cystinosis treated with cysteamine. N Engl J Med 1993;328:1157.

157. Broyer M, Tete MJ, Guest G, et al. Clinical polymorphism of cystinosis encephalopathy: results of treatment with cysteamine. J Inherit Metab Dis 1996;19:65.

158. Van't Hoff WG, Gretz N. The treatment of cystinosis with cysteamine and phosphocysteamine in the United Kingdom and Eire. Pediatr Nephrol 1995;9:685.

159. Schneider JA, Clark KF, Greene AA, et al. Recent advances in the treatment of cystinosis. J Inherit Metab Dis 1995;18:387.

160. Reznik VM, Adamson M, Adelman RD, et al. Treatment of cystinosis with cysteamine from early infancy. J Pediatr 1991;119:491.

161. Schneider JA, Verroust FM, Kroll WA, et al. Prenatal diagnosis of cystinosis. N Engl J Med 1974;290:878.

162. States B, Blazer B, Harris D, et al. Prenatal diagnosis of cystinosis. J Pediatr 1975;87:558.

163. Steinherz R, Makov N, Narinsky R, et al. Prenatal diagnosis of cystinosis upon exposure of amniotic cells to cystine dimethyl ester. Isr J Med Sci 1985;21:537.

164. Hall NA, Young EP. A high performance liquid chromatography method for the analysis of 35-S-cystine: application to the diagnosis of cystinosis. Clin Chim Acta 1989;184:1.

165. Smith ML, Pellet OL, Cass MM, et al. Prenatal diagnosis of cystinosis utilizing chorionic villus sampling. Prenat Diagn 1987;7:23.

166. Oshima RG, Willis RC, Furlong CE, et al. Binding assays for amino acids. J Biol Chem 1974;249:6033.

167. Gahl WA, Dorfman A, Evans MI, et al. Chorionic biopsy in the prenatal diagnosis of nephropathic cystinosis. In: Fraccaro M, Simmoni G, Brambti B, eds. First trimester fetal diagnosis. Berlin: Springer-Verlag, 1985:260.

168. Smith ML, Clark KF, Davis SE, et al. Diagnosis of cystinosis with use of placenta. N Engl J Med 1989;321:397.

Jennifer M. Puck, M.D.

18

Prenatal Diagnosis of Primary Immunodeficiency Diseases

The immune system is a part of the general defense system that evolved to protect humans from harmful invasion of microorganisms. The phagocytes and lymphocytes and their secreted products constitute a highly specialized and coordinated network responsible for selective recognition and elimination of microorganisms that have passed through the body's outer barriers. The most common causes of immunodeficiency worldwide are acquired. These are most often malnutrition and immunosuppression secondary to infection, not only by human immunodeficiency virus (HIV), but also by measles, tuberculosis, and other agents. Primary disorders of the immune system caused by heritable defects in specific genes are infrequent. Nonetheless, these diseases have been critical in demonstrating the roles played by specific genes and immune pathways in the development of normal immune responses. Moreover, the diagnosis, treatment, and genetic management of families with these diseases have undergone a fundamental shift in the past 10 years, with the identification and molecular cloning of more than 100 newly recognized host defense disease genes. Prenatal diagnosis of specific immunodeficiencies is now beginning to open a broad range of choices for families, only one of which is the termination of an affected pregnancy. Neonatal treatments such as bone marrow transplantation for severe combined immunodeficiency are associated with improved outcome; in utero bone marrow transplantation has been achieved; and gene transfer therapies, such as correcting the defect in an infant's own hematopoietic stem cells, have proven beneficial, although not without the associated risk of leukemia due to insertional mutagenesis.

FAMILY HISTORY

There is a broad range of severity and age at presentation of inherited immunodeficiency disorders. The frequency of these disorders is unknown because they are rare and in some instances not recognized in infants or children who die of infections. Disorders limited to B lymphocytes are more common, but may present later in life than combined T- and B-lymphocyte disorders. Life-threatening immunodeficiencies such as severe combined immunodeficiency are estimated to occur in around 1 in 50,000–100,000 births. Therefore, prenatal evaluation is generally requested in the context of an affected relative. A definitive evaluation of an affected proband in the kindred is a tremendous aid in directing fetal

645

diagnosis. On the other hand, immunodiagnostics have become much more precise in recent years; the significance of a family history of early deaths due to infection must be appreciated and investigated, and review of an affected relative's medical records or an autopsy report can provide important clues.

When encountering a family history of individuals with recurrent infections, it is helpful to know that children with normal immune systems have an average of six to eight respiratory infections per year for the first 10 years of life. Healthy children generally handle these infections well. In contrast, children with impaired host defenses have more severe and even fatal infections, persistent infections, and recurrences despite standard therapy. A very significant indicator of the seriousness of infections is failure to thrive. The timing of infections is also important; infants with immunodeficiency may be protected by transplacentally acquired maternal immunoglobulin G (IgG) for the first 3–6 months of life. Many children with immunodeficiency have chronic skin rashes. A number of primary immunodeficiencies occur in infants with other congenital disorders, such as developmental anomalies of the face, skeleton, heart, or intestine or disorders of pigmentation and hair.

Table 18.1. Infectious agents in different types of immunodeficiency

Pathogen Type	T-Cell Defect	B-Cell Defect	Macrophage Granulocyte Defect	Activation Defect	Complement Defect
Bacteria	Bacterial sepsis	*Streptococcus, Staphylococcus, Haemophilus*	*Staphylococcus, Pseudomonas*		*Neisseria* infections, other pyogenic bacterial infections
Viruses	Cytomegalovirus, Epstein–Barr virus, severe varicella, chronic infections with respiratory and intestinal viruses	Enteroviral encephalitis			
Fungi and parasites	*Candida, Pneumocystis*	Severe intestinal giardiasis	*Candida, Nocardia, Aspergillus*		
Mycobacteria	Disseminated BCGosis			Disseminated and severe typical and atypical mycobacterial disease	
Special features	Aggressive disease with opportunistic pathogens; failure to clear infections	Recurrent sinopulmonary infections; sepsis; chronic meningitis			Autoimmunity

The nature of the pathogens causing infections not only can strongly suggest immunodeficiency, as when an opportunistic pathogen such as *Pneumocystis carinii* is found, but also can point to the specific nature of the immune defect. The infectious agents commonly found in disorders of the various compartments of the immune system are summarized in Table 18.1. Although T cells are essential for controlling viral and fungal diseases, they also provide helper functions to B cells for effective antibody responses and macrophages for activation to kill ingested organisms. Thus, T-cell disorders present as combined T- and B-cell immunodeficiency, with susceptibility to all types of bacterial infections as well as infections with viruses and fungi. Pure B-cell defects produce recurrent sinopulmonary infections, often accompanied by bacterial septicemia. Patients lacking mucosal antibody defenses are also particularly susceptible to invasive disease with enteroviruses, leading to chronic viral meningitis and severe gastroenteritis. Granulocyte disorders predispose to invasive staphylococcal infections because this organism is normally controlled by phagocytosis and superoxide-mediated killing in granulocytes. Finally, complement fixation has recently been recognized as an important mechanism for controlling neisserial species of bacteria, and patients with certain of the complement deficiencies have increased susceptibility to septic arthritis, meningitis, and overwhelming sepsis with these organisms. Immunologic tests to review from probands are listed in Table 18.2.

Autosomal recessive disorders affect both males and females, but low carrier frequencies make it unlikely to find affected relatives other than siblings. Important exceptions occur in cases of consanguineous matings and in population groups that are closely interrelated or are descended from a limited ancestor pool. There are at least nine X-linked immunodeficiencies, including Wiskott–Aldrich syndrome, X-linked chronic granulomatous disease, severe combined immunodeficiency (SCID), agammaglobulinemia, hyper-IgM syndrome, properdin deficiency, and X-linked lymphoproliferative disease. Because the ability to diagnose specific immunodeficiencies has been limited until recently, the family history may be ambiguous. An astute questioner can sometimes elicit a history of maternal male relatives who died at a young age with poor weight gain, diarrhea, or pneumonia. Such patients were not infrequently empirically misdiagnosed as having cystic fibrosis instead of X-linked SCID. Furthermore, the rate of cases caused by new mutations,

Table 18.2. Immunologic tests for patients with suspected immunodeficiency

Type of Defect	Test	Specific Aspects to Note
Any immunodeficiency	Complete blood count; differential count; platelet count	Neutrophil and eosinophil numbers, granule morphology; lymphocyte number; platelet size
Antibody deficiency	Quantitative immunoglobulins; B-cell number	Poor specific antibody responses to vaccinations
T-cell deficiency	Skin tests of delayed type hypersensitivity; T-cell surface marker subsets CD3 or CD11, CD4, CD8; in vitro responses to mitogens	Skin test anergy cannot be diagnosed before 2 years of age; use age-matched normal values for lymphocyte subsets
Phagocyte deficiency	Neutrophil count; neutrophil oxidative function (nitroblue tetrazolium or other test)	
Complement deficiency	CH50 assay	

especially for X-linked disorders, is so significant that the majority of probands with proven X-linked immunodeficiency mutations have no history of affected male relatives.

SPECIFIC IMMUNE DEFECTS

A classification of selected primary immune disorders is presented in Table 18.3. The disease classification[1,2] is partially based on the reports of the International Union if Immunological Societies Committee on Primary Immunodeficiencies.[3] Currently, the availability of molecular diagnostic laboratories performing clinical prenatal testing lags behind the number of diseases for which such tests are possible. The translation of basic discoveries into clinically available services for families depends on availability, cost, evolving diagnostic methods, laboratory regulation and certification, and ability to provide appropriate counseling before and after testing. None of the genetic immunodeficiencies discovered thus far demonstrate a single major or common mutation, such as the Δ508 mutation in cystic fibrosis. Rather, as a rule, a great variety of mutations are observed, primarily changes of one or a few nucleotides, throughout the length of the genes and regulatory and splice sequences. Mutational hot spots at CpG dinucleotides have emerged for many of the genes, but these have not been sufficiently frequent to make single-mutation screening worthwhile. The great variety of mutations, combined with the overall rarity and broad spectrum of genes responsible for immune disorders, has meant that most prenatal diagnosis for these conditions has been conducted in a research setting. For further information about specific diseases, there are Internet resources including mutation databases for an increasing number of the diseases[4–8] and the GeneTests database,[9] which lists molecular diagnostic laboratories performing specialized tests. The Immune Deficiency Foundation[10] and the Modell Foundation[11] also provide information for physicians and families about the diagnosis and treatment of primary immunodeficiencies.

LYMPHOCYTE DEFICIENCIES

T-Cell and Combined Deficiencies

Combined lymphocyte deficiencies include those with primary abnormalities in both T and B cells as well as those in which T-cell defects prevent normal T-cell/B-cell cooperation. Infections in the presence of these disorders do not respond to conventional treatment, and in the most severe forms, designated severe combined immunodeficiency, (SCID), survival beyond the first year of life is rare unless the immune system can be reconstituted, such as by bone marrow transplantation.

The most common form of SCID is the X-linked form, and more than 80 percent of SCID cases in some series are male.[12] In 1993, X-linked SCID was found to be due to defects in *IL2RG*, the gene encoding the γ-chain of the interleukin-2 (IL-2) receptor.[13,14] This transmembrane cytokine receptor protein also participates in the receptor complexes for IL-4, IL-7, IL-9, and IL-15; for this reason it is called the common γ-chain (γc). In X-linked SCID, B cells are usually present, but B-cell function is abnormal, and specific antibody responses do not occur. Healthy carrier females can be identified by nonrandom X chromosome inactivation in their lymphocytes, but not in their granulocytes or non-lymphoid cells.[15,16] This skewed X inactivation is a result of the selective disadvantage of lymphocyte precursors that have inactivated the X chromosome with an intact *IL2RG* gene. However, as expected with X-linked lethal disorders, new mutations are relatively common and can make predictions based on maternal X inactivation testing inaccurate;

Table 18.3. Classification of selected primary immune-deficiency diseases

Category	Designation	Immunologic Abnormality[a]	Gene Defect; Pathogenesis	Genetic Locus	Prenatal Diagnosis Options[b]
Combined lymphocyte defects	X-linked severe combined immune deficiency (XSCID)	Low T cells; abnormal B cells; low Ig	Defect of γ-chain of IL-2 receptor and receptors for other cytokines, IL-4, 7, 9, 15, and 21	IL2RG (SCIDX1), Xq13.1	CVS, amnio: L, G FB: CP
	JAK3 deficiency (JAK3 SCID)	Low T cells; abnormal B cells; low Ig levels	JAK3 intracellular signaling kinase defect	JAK3, 19p13.1	CVS, amnio: L, G FB: CP
	IL-7 receptor deficiency (IL7RA SCID)	Low T cells; abnormal B cells; low Ig; NK cells present	IL-7 α-chain defect	IL7RA, 5p13	CVS, amnio: L, G FB: CP
	Adenosine deaminase (ADA) deficiency	Low T cells and B cells; low Ig	Selective lymphocyte toxicity of purine pathway intermediates	ADA, 20q13.11	CVS, amnio: E, L, G FB: E
	Recombinase activating gene (RAG-1, RAG-2) deficiency	Low T cells; absent B cells; absent Ig	No T- or B-cell receptor rearrangement; blocked lymphocyte development	RAG1, RAG2, 11p13	CVS, amnio: L, G FB: CP
	Artemis recombination protein deficiency (Navajo, Indian SCID)	Absent T, B cells; absent Ig; radiation sensitivity	No B- or T-cell rearrangement; blocked lymphocyte development	DCLRE1C, 10p	CVS, amnio: L, G, FB: CP
	SCID, autosomal recessive, unknown genotype	Low T cells	Unknown; multiple defects	Unknown	FB: CP
	Purine nucleoside phosphorylase (PNP) deficiency	Low T cells, abnormal B cells; low Ig	Lymphocyte toxicity of purine pathway intermediates	PNP, 14q13	CVS, amnio: E FB: E
	MHC class II deficiency	Low CD4 T cells MHC II gene expression	Mutation in factors controlling RFX5, 1q	CIITA, 16p13, FB: CP	CVS, amnio: L, G
	ZAP 70 kinase deficiency	Low CD8 T cells	Thymocyte intracellular kinase defect; blocked maturation of T cells	ZAP70, 2q12	CVS, amnio: L, G FB: CP

Category	Designation	Immunologic Abnormality[a]	Gene Defect; Pathogenesis	Genetic Locus	Prenatal Diagnosis Options[b]
	Reticular dysgenesis	Low T, B cells; low Ig	Unknown bone marrow stem-cell defect	AR	FB: CP
	Omenn syndrome	Low T, B cells; low Ig	RAG-1/RAG-2 defects with residual activity	AR	Unknown
	X-linked hyper-IgM syndrome	Normal to high IgM; low IgA, IgG	Defect of CD40 ligand, expressed on T cells; block in B-cell isotype switch	HIGMX, Xq25-q26	CVS, amnio: L, G
	CD40 deficiency	Normal or high IgM; other antibody isotypes low	No IgG, IgA, IgE B cells	AR CD40 defects, 20q12-q13.2	Potentially CVS, amnio: G
	DiGeorge syndrome	Normal to low T, B cells; normal to low Ig	Embryologic defect of thymic development; variable defects (e.g., heart, parathyroid, face)	22q11.2 and rarely other loci	CVS, amnio: L, FISH
Antibody deficiencies	X-linked agammaglobulinemia	Low B cells; low to absent Ig	Defect of B-cell-specific Bruton tyrosine kinase	XLA, Xq22	CVS, amnio: L, G FB: C
	μ-heavy-chain deficiency	Low B cells; low to absent Ig	Defect of cell surface μ-chain expression	IgHμ, 14q32.3	CVS, amnio: L, G FB: CP
	Other agammaglobulinemias, autosomal recessive	Low to absent B cells and Ig	Defects of μ-heavy-chain gene; λ5 Vpreβ gene; BLNK gene; syk gene	AR	Potentially CVS, amnio: G
	Autosomal deficiency in IgG, IgA, IgE	Selected isotype deficiency	Activation-induced cytidine deaminase deficiency	AICDA, 12p13 AR	Potentially CVS, amnio G
	Immunoglobulin subclass deficiency, most commonly IgA	One or more Ig subtypes low	Unknown defects in B-cell isotype expression; IgG subclass deficiencies associated with Ig heavy- or light-chain gene deletions	Complex	Unknown
	Common variable immunodeficiency	Normal to low B cells; one or more Ig subtypes low	Unknown late-onset variable defects in B- and T-cell function and regulation	Complex; rare families with dominant deletion in ICOS, 2q33	Unknown
	Hyper-IgE syndrome	High IgE, boils, pneumonia with lung cysts	Unknown	Unknown	Unknown

(continued)

Table 18.3. Classification of selected primary immune-deficiency diseases (continued)

Category	Designation	Immunologic Abnormality[a]	Gene Defect; Pathogenesis	Genetic Locus	Prenatal Diagnosis Options[b]
Other distinctive syndromes	Wiskott–Aldrich syndrome	Variable T, B, and Ig defects	Defect of WASP gene involved in cytoskeleton; sparse, small platelets; eczema	WASP, Xp11.23	CVS, amnio: L, G FB: CP
	Ataxia–telangiectasia	Normal	DNA repair defect in ATM gene; ataxia, progressive neurodegeneration; cancer; radiation sensitivity	ATM, 11q22-q23	CVS, amnio: L, G FB: CP
	Bloom syndrome	Normal	DNA repair defect in BLM gene; progressive neurodegeneration; cancer; radiation sensitivity	BLM, 15q26.1	CVS, amnio: L, G FB: CP
	X-linked lympho-proliferative disease	Normal	Fatal infection or immuno-compromise on Epstein–Barr virus encounter	XLP, Xq24-q26	CVS, amnio: L
	Autoimmune lympho-proliferative syndrome	Elevated $CD4^-/CD8^-$ T cells; high Ig Activated T cells	Impaired Fas-mediated apoptosis of B and T cells; lymph-adenopathy autoimmunity	TNFRSF6, 10q24; complex	CVS, amnio: G
	Immune dysregulation, polyendocrinopathy, enteropathy, X-linked IPEX		Defect of immune regulation	FOXP3, Xp11.23	Potentially CVS, amnio: G
	Autoimmune poly-endocrinopathy	Autoimmune poly-endocrinopathy, candidiasis, and ectodermal dystrophy	Defect of immune regulation	AIRE, 21q22.3 AR and AD forms	Potentially CVS, amnio: G
Phagocyte disorders	Chronic granulomatous disease (CGD)	Normal	Impaired killing of ingested organisms due to defects in four genes encoding enzymes of cytochrome oxidase system	CYBB (gp91[phox]), Xp21.1 CYBA (p22[phox]), 16q24.1 NCF1 (p47[phox]), 7q11.23 NCF2 (p67[phox]), 1q25	CVS, amnio: L, G

(continued)

651

Table 18.3. Classification of selected primary immune-deficiency diseases (continued)

Category	Designation	Immunologic Abnormality[a]	Gene Defect; Pathogenesis	Genetic Locus	Prenatal Diagnosis Options[b]
	Leukocyte adhesion type 1 deficiency (LAD1)	Normal	Defects of CD18 or other leukocyte surface proteins required for motility, adherence, and endocytosis	CD18, 21q22.3	CVS, amnio: L, G FB: CP
	Leukocyte adhesion type 2 deficiency (LAD2)	Normal	Defects of fucose glycosylation	FUCT1, 11p11.2	Unknown
	Chediak–Higashi syndrome	Normal	Defect of CHM gene causing faulty lysosomal assembly, giant cytoplasmic granules	CHS, 1q42-q44	CVS, amnio: L, G ?CP FB: CP
Complement disorders	Individual component deficiencies	Normal	C1, C2, C4, C3 deficiencies, autoimmunity and pyogenic infections; C3, C5-9 and properdin deficiencies: *Neisseria* infections	AR: chromosomes 6p, 1q, etc.; X: properdin	Unknown

[a]Ig, Immunoglobulin levels.
[b]Prenatal diagnosis options amnio = amniocyte sample; CP = cellular phenotyping (leukocyte numbers), cell surface characteristics, or in vitro function); CVS = chorionic villus sample; E = enzyme or biochemical assay; FB = fetal blood sample; FISH = fluorescence in situ hybridization; G = genotyping (i.e., specific mutation detection): L = linked polymorphic marker analysis.

female germ-line mosaicism has been documented,[17] and women have been identified whose lymphocytes had no mutation and random X inactivation, but who passed on a germ-line *IL2RG* mutation to multiple affected offspring.[17,18] As is typical of all the X-linked immunodeficiency disease genes recently identified, individual patient mutations are extremely diverse and consist primarily of changes of one to a few nucleotides; 95 different mutations were identified in a series of 136 patients studied, and further studies continue this trend.[6,19,20] The best current treatment is human lymphocyte antigen (HLA)-matched bone marrow transplantation, but most patients lack a matched related donor. Haploidentical, T-cell-depleted bone marrow transplantation has been quite successful.[2] Nevertheless, many post-transplant patients have graft-versus-host disease; many fail to make adequate antibodies and require long-term immunoglobulin replacement; and some develop autoimmune diseases due to lymphocyte dysregulation.

Gene therapy has also been piloted in X-linked SCID with success, making this the first human disease to be cured with gene therapy as the sole treatment.[21,22] The group of Alain Fischer in Paris has now treated ten infants with mutation-proven X-linked SCID by aspirating their bone marrow, enriching for stem cells, culturing the cells with activating cytokines and a retrovirus vector carrying a correct copy of the *IL2RG* cDNA, and then reinfusing the autologous cells into infants. In all but one case, the cells found their way to the bone marrow and grew and differentiated into normal, functional T lymphocytes; other hematopoietic cell lineages were also generated containing the retroviral provirus. Both T- and B-cell function improved. However, two and a half years after treatment, leukemia developed in the two youngest infants to receive gene therapy. Their leukemias were found to have been caused by insertional mutagenesis.[23] The *IL2RG* retroviral vector, when inserted in either of two locations at the 5′ region of the gene encoding the hematopoietic transcription factor LMO-2, caused inappropriate expression of LMO-2 and unrestrained clonal expansion.[24]

Prenatal diagnosis can be performed by linkage analysis or by specific mutation detection on chorionic villus samples (CVS) or amniocyte DNA.[16,25] Fetal blood sampling has also been used, as lymphocytopenia, low numbers of cells bearing the T-cell markers CD3 and CD11, and poor T-cell blastogenic responses to mitogens can be definitively demonstrated in affected fetuses by week 17 of gestation.[26] These options should be weighed against testing at birth for families who would not terminate an affected pregnancy. Regardless of whether prenatal testing is undertaken, education and counseling should emphasize early bone marrow transplantation for affected infants. Infants transplanted immediately after birth appear to have more rapid engraftment, fewer serious infections, less serious cases of graft-versus-host disease, and shorter hospitalizations than those whose transplants are delayed.[27,28]

The use of prenatal diagnosis for X-linked SCID was studied by Puck et al.,[25] who found that the great majority of families at risk for an affected pregnancy desired prenatal testing, whether or not termination of pregnancy was a consideration. In fact, parents chose to terminate the pregnancy in only two of thirteen instances of a predicted affected male fetus. To prepare for optimal treatment of an affected newborn, families and their medical providers selected bone marrow transplant centers, undertook HLA testing of family members, and even began a search for a matched, unrelated bone marrow donor. One family chose an experimental in utero bone marrow transplant, which was successful[29] (see below).

The concept of prenatal treatment for SCID is re-emerging with a new optimism. Theoretical advantages of in utero treatment include early reconstitution, a protected intrauterine environment, and the possibility of introducing normal bone marrow stem cells at the gestational age when fetal hematopoiesis is shifting from fetal liver to bone marrow. Previous attempts at human in utero bone marrow transplantation were severely compromised by technologic limitations, septic complications, and the lack of methods to remove from the graft population the mature T cells capable of reacting to fetal tissues and causing graft-versus-host reactions. In at least three patients, these difficulties have been overcome.[29–31] Fetuses affected with X-linked SCID have been infused intraperitoneally with haploidentical T-cell-depleted CD34-positive parental bone marrow cells between 17 and 20 weeks of gestation. Infants have been born with engrafted, functional T cells and have, to date, done at least as well as postnatally transplanted patients.

In 1995, the signaling pathway through γc was found to require interaction of the cytoplasmic portion of γc with a specific intracellular kinase, JAK3.[32,33] Patients of both sexes have now been found with autosomal recessive SCID immunologically identical to XSCID but caused by JAK3 protein defects. Prenatal diagnosis ruling out JAK3 SCID by mutation analysis has been performed on DNA from a CVS.[34]

Adenosine deaminase (ADA) deficiency, the first genetic defect associated with SCID, is less than half as common as X-linked SCID. ADA is found in all tissues and is important in purine metabolism. The lack of this enzyme, which is most abundant in lymphocytes, causes intracellular accumulation of toxic levels of purine intermediates, particularly deoxyadenosine.[35,36] Characteristic skeletal abnormalities of the ribs and hips are seen, along with extremely low numbers of T and B cells. Partial deficiency of ADA due to mutations that preserve some enzyme activity can cause milder forms of combined immunodeficiency presenting in childhood or even adulthood with declining T-cell numbers. Diagnosis at any age depends on the measurement of low ADA enzyme activity and high levels of circulating deoxyadenosine. More than thirty distinct mutations in the *ADA* gene have been found, making genotype–phenotype correlations possible. Although HLA-matched bone marrow transplantation is the treatment of choice for severe ADA deficiency, haploidentical T-cell-depleted transplants and enzyme replacement with ADA coupled to polyethylene glycol (PEG-ADA) have also been used successfully. In addition, gene therapy for ADA deficient SCID has also been performed and in preliminary reports appears successful. The protocol used was similar to that described above for X-linked SCID, except that the patients also received cytoreductive chemotherapy before reinfusion of their autologous gene-corrected cells.[37]

Prenatal diagnosis of ADA deficiency is facilitated by the ubiquitous expression of the enzyme; CVS and amniocyte samples have successfully yielded prenatal determinations.[38–40] However, as discussed by Hirschhorn,[38] the variable enzyme activities in carrier parents make it important to relate fetal enzyme activities to those of all available family members. ADA activity may also vary in cultured cells, depending on culture conditions. Ambiguous results from early testing could be clarified with subsequent fetal blood samples, in which red cell and lymphocyte enzyme levels can be measured, in addition to determining lymphocyte number. DNA-based prenatal diagnosis, by either linked markers or specific mutation detection, has also been accomplished.

With the discovery of disease genes for X-linked immunodeficiencies and an increasing number of autosomal forms of SCID, it is now possible to define the genetic defect at the molecular level in around 80 percent of affected patients. This is a marked contrast to the situation a decade ago, when 80 percent of patients with SCID had undetermined genetic lesions. Disease genes for several types of autosomal-recessive SCID have been recognized within the past few years. Recombinase-activating genes RAG-1 and RAG-2 were originally shown in the mouse to be required for the DNA rearrangements of T-cell-receptor and immunoglobulin genes. Defects in either of these genes cause failure of differentiation of lymphocytes because functional antigen receptors cannot be created through the normal means of assembling variable (V), diversity (D), and joining (J) domains of the antigen receptor genes of early committed lymphoid precursors. In 1996, humans with autosomal-recessive SCID with no B cells and undetectable or reduced numbers of T cells were shown to have defects in either RAG-1 or RAG-2, which are encoded by genes located adjacent to each other on chromosome 11p13.[41] There are some ethnic groups known to have an increased incidence of autosomal-recessive SCID, such as the Navajo and other Athabascan Native American populations.[42] The gene for Athabascan SCID has now been identified to be a protein involved in the DNA recombination required to generate mature T and B cell antigen receptor genes.[43] Prenatal diagnosis of the Athabascan SCID mutation has been accomplished.[44]

The recurrence risk for couples who have had an infant with SCID is assumed to be on the order of 25 percent. In the absence of specific molecular diagnostic studies, the prenatal diagnosis of SCID of unknown genotype is possible through fetal blood sampling after 17 weeks of gestation. There are available data on normal fetal blood leukocytes.[26,45–47] Potential abnormalities that can be expected in a fetus at risk can be predicted from careful analysis of the immunologic profile of the affected proband.

Purine nucleoside phosphorylase (PNP) deficiency, an extremely rare disorder, is also associated with immunodeficiency involving both T and B cells. Although severe cases may present in infancy, PNP immunodeficiency is usually more mild than SCID, coming to medical attention later in childhood. Neurologic abnormalities, including spasticity, hypotonia, and developmental delay, are prominent in PNP deficiency and may be recognized first. As with ADA, PNP is found in all tissues, including CVS cells and amniocytes. Diagnosis can be made by assay of levels of the enzyme.[48]

SCID due to autosomal recessive mutations of the gene encoding the α-chain of the receptor for interleukin-7 (*IL7RA*), have been found in a few patients, particularly those who lack T and B lymphocytes but have functional natural killer cells.[49] Another very rare human SCID disease first recognized in Mennonites in 1994 is caused by lack of a T-cell-specific signaling kinase called ZAP-70 kinase, or ζ-chain (a T-cell-receptor component) associated protein kinase. These patients have natural killer (NK) cells but no functional T cells, even though T cells with surface expression of CD4 are present.[50,51] Autosomal recessive mutations in the *ZAP-70* gene, resulting in deficient expression of ZAP-70 protein, interfere with the thymic development of CD8 T cells and antigen activation in CD4 T cells. Despite the presence of B cells and serum immunoglobulins, specific antibody responses are impaired.

Finally, major histocompatibility complex class II (MHC-II) nonexpression has been associated with moderate to severe immunodeficiency, originally classified as a form of "bare lymphocyte syndrome."[52,53] Patients present from early infancy to childhood with normal numbers of T and B cells but a preponderance of CD8 T cells, as opposed to the normal CD4/CD8 ratio of 2/1. Immunoglobulins are decreased, specific antibody production is poor, and a variety of severe bacterial and opportunistic infections can occur. Although no abnormalities of the MHC-II genes themselves have been found, three different genes regulating MHC-II expression, *CIITA* and *RFX5*, were shown in 1993 to be defective in some of the patients with this form of immunodeficiency,[54–56] and other transcription factors involved in this regulatory process are very likely to be mutated in additional patients. Although fetal blood sampling to assess fetal lymphocyte expression of

MHC-II has been used for prenatal diagnosis,[57] diagnosis of specific gene defects by linkage or specific mutation detection would be definitive and could be carried out on CVS or amniocyte DNA.

Hyper-IgM syndrome was originally thought to be a disorder of B cells because in affected patients isotypes fail to switch from IgM to IgG, IgA, or IgE. Affected patients sometimes, but not always, have very high levels of IgM, which gave the disease its name, and are incapable of secondary or booster B-cell-antibody responses. However, instances of *Candida* and *Pneumocystis* infections suggested a T-cell component to the disease. In 1993, the X-linked form of hyper-IgM syndrome was found by several groups to be caused by deficient CD40 ligand (CD40L), a receptor expressed on activated T cells.[58,59] Prenatal diagnosis has been performed on CVS DNA by means of a highly informative dinucleotide repeat polymorphism in the 3′ untranslated region of the *CD40L* gene, confirmed by specific mutation detection.[60] The binding of CD40L protein to CD40 on B cells induces B-cell proliferation, immunoglobulin isotype switching, and IL-4 production. A spectrum of X-linked and autosomal recessive diseases similar to that seen in CD40L deficiency are caused by defects in additional genes governing T-cell/B-cell interactions and B-cell isotype switching. These genes include *CD40*, *NEMO*, and a gene encoding an activation-induced cytidine deaminase (*AID*), but additional cases exist without mutations in these genes.[61] Patients are effectively treated with γ-globulin replacement therapy but do experience morbidity and are at risk for premature death.

Finally, additional well-recognized immunodeficiency syndromes exist for which the specific genetic cause is not yet fully known. DiGeorge syndrome is associated with the variable occurrence of multiple anomalies of the fetal third and fourth pharyngeal pouch structures, including thymic dysplasia or aplasia.[62] Although facial clefts, hypocalcemia due to hypoparathyroid maldevelopment, and cardiac defects may be more striking early in life, variable degrees of immunodeficiency, from mild T- and B-cell defects to autoimmune phenomena to SCID, have also been seen. Cytogenetics with fluorescence in situ hybridization (FISH) can identify small deletions or other abnormalities involving chromosome 22q11.2 in 90 percent of affected patients (see also chapter 8), and intensive studies are underway to prove that defects in one or more genes in this location that are consistently deranged in DiGeorge syndrome patients.[63–65] The transcription factor TBX1 is located in the DiGeorge critical region and when disrupted in mice causes heart defects similar to those of DiGeorge syndrome in humans,[64] but no human with a genetic lesion specifically limited to the *TBX1* gene has been found to date. Fetal sonography and echocardiography have been useful in evaluating the nonimmune aspects of this syndrome. The chromosome 22 microdeletions can be evaluated by FISH in CVS cells or amniocytes for prenatal diagnosis.[64] A minority of patients with DiGeorge sequence do not have chromosome 22 deletions but instead may have microdeletions in chromosome 10p13-p14.[66] The genetic heterogeneity of this syndrome makes study of family members a necessary part of any prenatal evaluation. Moreover, highly variable expressivity makes the interpretation of a prenatally diagnosed abnormality complex, particularly in families with both severely affected and mildly affected members.

Antibody Deficiencies

The most common complications of antibody deficiencies are recurrent sinopulmonary infections and septicemias with encapsulated bacteria. The most severe defect in this category is agammaglobulinemia, which is by far most often seen in males, frequently with an X-linked inheritance pattern. The disease gene for X-linked agammaglobulinemia

(XLA) was identified in 1993 as encoding Btk,[67,68] for Bruton tyrosine kinase, named after the discoverer of human immunodeficiency due to agammaglobulinemia. Although the precise function of Btk, an intracellular signaling tyrosine kinase, is still unknown, in patients with mutations disrupting it, B cells fail to develop from pre-B cells in the bone marrow. Diagnosis including prenatal diagnosis[69] is made by finding extremely low or absent immunoglobulins and few to no B cells; specific mutation detection or measurement of Btk kinase activity can confirm the genetic cause in patients without an X-linked family history. Lifelong γ-globulin replacement keeps many patients free of infection. However, a particularly difficult complication is the development of chronic enteroviral infection of the central nervous system. Prenatal detection of XLA was first accomplished by fetal blood enumeration of B cells,[58] but now specific mutation detection or linked markers make possible diagnosis by CVS or amniocytes in male fetuses at risk.

Additional gene defects that cause agammaglobulinemia have been found in males and females without Btk mutations. These include defects in the autosomal immunoglobulin μ heavy chain locus itself.[70] Patients have a clinical picture very similar to individuals with XLA, with complete absence of B cells, indicating that intact membrane-bound μ-chain expression is essential for B-cell maturation. Prenatal diagnosis has not been reported but is theoretically possible by DNA-based methods or fetal blood phenotype.

Other diseases characterized by antibody defects are IgA deficiency, other immunoglobulin subclass deficiencies, and common variable immunodeficiency (CVID). Although relatively common, IgA deficiency is complex in its inheritance pattern, and some relatives of patients with IgA deficiency have CVID. Some patients with no IgA are entirely without symptoms. CVID, often presenting in late childhood to adulthood, can present in many forms: hypoglobulinemia or agammaglobulinemia, subclass deficiency, or dysregulation of the immune system with autoantibodies, lymphadenopathy, splenomegaly and/or hemolytic anemia, pernicious anemia, and other autoimmune diseases. Patients with CVID, especially women, are at increased risk for neoplasms, particularly lymphomas. The incidence and significance of isolated deficiencies of IgG subclasses is not yet clear, and the genetics is not well worked out. Prenatal diagnosis is not possible at present.

PHAGOCYTE DEFICIENCIES

Patients with chronic granulomatous disease (CGD) present with lymphadenopathy, high lymphocyte counts, and recurrent infections, as listed in Table 18.1. The X-linked form of CGD, accounting for two-thirds of cases, was one of the first human diseases for which the disease gene was found by positional cloning.[71] Now, three autosomal-recessive gene defects are also recognized to cause CGD. All four genes encode proteins that are part of the oxidative killing pathway for ingested microorganisms. The disease is diagnosed by demonstration of failure of the normal respiratory burst on activation of neutrophils (see Table 18.2). Although there is no specific therapy for CGD, continuously administered antibiotics, particularly trimethoprim–sulfisoxazole, have greatly reduced the frequency of severe infections. A multicenter trial of interferon γ administration appeared to have positive results in some children by mechanisms not well understood; it is not clear which patients should be candidates for this treatment. Bone marrow transplantation can be curative if a matched donor is available, and stem-cell gene therapy trials are under development. Linkage detection and specific mutation diagnosis of fetal samples are possible.

Leukocyte adhesion deficiency (LAD) describes a very rare phagocyte defect of patients whose neutrophils fail to mobilize and migrate to sites of tissue injury. Delayed separation of the umbilical cord in infancy is followed by severe scarring skin infections, gingivitis, and systemic bacterial infections. The original gene defect associated with the majority of cases is in the gene encoding CD18, the β-chain common to several types of leukocyte surface integrin complexes composed of CD18 and various types of CD11. Recently, a second defect in the gene encoding CD11c has been associated with the LAD in conjunction with developmental and growth retardation.[72] DNA-based prenatal diagnosis is theoretically possible for families with known genotype. Fetal blood analysis for leukocyte cell surface expression of CD18 is also a potential option.

Chediak–Higashi syndrome (CHS) is an autosomal-recessive disorder characterized by giant lysosomal granules in phagocytes, melanocytes, and other cells, including even amniotic cells and chorionic villus cells.[73] Patients have hypopigmentation and recurrent pyogenic infections that do not respond well to conventional therapy. One genetic locus for CHS is a gene *LYST* that encodes a large protein of unknown function.[74] However, genetic heterogeneity has been demonstrated, and thus, prenatal diagnosis by linkage to chromosome 1q markers is not possible without having confirmed that CHS in the family is due to a chromosome 1q mutation. Prenatal diagnosis has been performed by demonstrating the abnormal granulocytes in fetal blood.[75]

COMPLEMENT DEFICIENCIES

The complement system involves more than thirty proteins encoded throughout the genome, with important clusters on chromosome 1q and within the MHC region on 6p. Because deficiencies of nearly all these proteins have been described,[76] the topic is beyond the range of this chapter. Complement deficiencies can cause increased susceptibility to infection, rheumatic disorders, or angioedema. Defects in the terminal lytic components of complement, C5 through C9, and alternative pathway components predispose patients to invasive neisserial infections. In early component defects, C1, C4, and C2, recurrent bacterial infections are seen. Prenatal testing for complement deficiencies has not been reported.

UNCLASSIFIED DEFICIENCIES

Wiskott–Aldrich syndrome (WAS) is characterized by thrombocytopenia with small dysfunctional platelets, eczema, and variable immunodeficiency. It is X-linked recessive. Patients present with petechiae or bleeding in infancy; rashes develop in the first 1–2 years of life; increased susceptibility to pneumonias, sepsis, and chronic viral infections as well as autoimmune disease are typically seen in childhood; and survivors to young adulthood have a greatly increased risk for lymphomas.[77,78] In 1994, the disease gene was identified and named *WASP* for WAS protein.[79] WASP can associate with actin in lymphoid cells and is involved in transmitting intracellular signals.[80] Some patients have a more mild phenotype, with thrombocytopenia and little or no immunodeficiency; part of this variability is due to the location and type of mutation within the *WASP* gene. The gene mutations are tracked on a centralized database.[4] HLA-matched bone marrow transplantation is the treatment of choice; treatment decisions for affected boys without a matched donor are complicated by the variable expressivity of the disease. Prenatal diagnosis can now be performed by linked marker analysis or mutation detection in fetal DNA.[81]

Ataxia–telangiectasia is a complex multiple-system disorder characterized by progressive neurologic impairment with ataxia, variable immunodeficiency, and ocular and cutaneous telangiectasias. Increased frequency of solid tumors and lymphoreticular malignancies are well documented, and patients are hypersensitive to radiation. In 1994, the disease gene *ATM* ("ataxia–telangiectasia mutated") was discovered to be a member of a family of phosphatidylinositol-3-kinase genes involved in cell-cycle control.[82] The important role of the ATM protein in DNA damage repair and lymphocyte DNA recombination helps explain the clinical features of this disease, and heterozygotes for ATM defects may be at increased risk for cancer. Prenatal diagnosis has been carried out in the past by analysis of new DNA synthesis in response to radiation of amniocytes,[83] but specific mutation diagnosis can theoretically provide more definitive information. Another DNA breakage syndrome with cancer predisposition and accompanying variable combined immunodeficiency is Bloom syndrome, for which the disease gene was also cloned in 1995.[84,85]

Another X-linked immunodeficiency disease recently assigned to a disease gene is X-linked lymphoproliferative syndrome (XLP). Affected males have no consistent immune dysfunction until they encounter Epstein–Barr virus (EBV). Most then die from severe mononucleosis, while a range of abnormalities subsequently develop in survivors, from aplastic anemia to B-cell aplasia to B-cell lymphomas. T- and NK-cell abnormalities, as well as hypogammaglobulinemia or agammaglobulinemia, have also been noted after EBV infection. When the gene was mapped to Xq25-q26, prenatal diagnosis by linkage could be performed.[86–88] Now mutations can be sought in the *SH2D1A* gene, an SH2 domain-containing adaptor protein found in lymphocytes.[89] Bone marrow transplantation has been performed presymptomatically on boys who have been determined to have inherited XLP because in retrospective series half of the initial EBV infections were fatal.

Finally, a new concept in primary immune dysfunction involves disorders of regulation of immune responses as a consequence of defective apoptosis, or programmed cell death.[90] Apoptosis of activated lymphocytes is critical to immune homeostasis and appropriate termination of physiologic immune responses. The cell-surface receptor Fas is an important mediator of lymphocyte apoptosis. Human apoptosis defects due to mutations of Fas were found in 1995 in a rare autoimmune lymphoproliferative syndrome (ALPS).[91,92] Children with ALPS have lymphadenopathy, autoimmunity, and expansion of a normally rare population of CD4⁻CD8⁻ T cells. They also have impaired T- and B-cell apoptosis in vitro. The genetics and pathogenesis of ALPS are complex and remain to be fully worked out. Cellular apoptosis defects are inherited in families with ALPS as autosomal-dominant traits, but the development of overt autoimmunity may depend on additional factors. Although not reported to date, linkage or mutation diagnosis potentially could be performed on prenatal DNA samples.

Whenever an infant is born who is known or suspected to be at risk for an inherited host defense defect, immunologic evaluation should be performed, as outlined in Table 18.2. Until the immune status of the infant is clear, he or she should be protected from exposure to infection and iatrogenic administration of potentially lethal treatments. Live vaccines should not be given to such infants until diagnostic studies have ruled out immunodeficiency. Similarly, only irradiated blood products should be given, to avoid transfusion-mediated graft-versus-host disease from transfused lymphocytes, which cannot be eliminated when patients lack functional T cells of their own.

REFERENCES

1. Stiehm ER. Immunologic disorders in infants and children, 4th ed. Philadelphia: WB Saunders, 1996.
2. Ochs HD, Smith C IE, Puck JM. Primary immunodeficiency diseases: a molecular and genetic approach. New York: Oxford University Press, 1999.

3. Committee on Primary Immunodeficiency Diseases, International Union of Immunological Societies. Primary immunodeficiency diseases: report of an IUIS Scientific Committee. Clin Exp Immunol 1999;1 (suppl):1.

4. Schwarz K, Nonoyama S, Peitsch MC, et al. WASPbase: a database of WAS- and XLT-causing mutations. Immunol Today 1996;17:496.

5. Vihinen M, Brooimans RA, Kwan S-P, et al. BTKbase: XLA mutation registry. Immunol Today 1996;17:502.

6. Puck JM, de Saint Basile G, Schwarz K, et al. IL2RGbase: a database of γc-chain defects causing human X-SCID. Immunol Today 1996;17:507.

7. Notarangelo LD, Peitsch MC, Abrahamsen TG, et al. CD40Lbase: a database of CD40L gene mutations causing X-linked hyper-IgM syndrome. Immunol Today 1996;17:511.

8. Roos D, Curnutte JT, Hossle JP et al. X-CGDbase: a database of X-CGD-causing mutations. Immunol Today 1996;17:517.

9. Pagon, RA, Covington ML. GeneTests, a directory of medical genetics laboratories. http://www.genetests. org, 2003.

10. Immune Deficiency Foundation. Immune deficiency diseases, an overview. Towson, MD: Immune Deficiency Foundation, http://www.primaryimmune.org.

11. The Jeffrey Modell Foundation, 43 West 47th Street, New York, NY 10036, http://jmfworld.com/.

12. Buckley RH, Schiff SE, Schiff RI, et al. Human severe combined immunodeficiency (SCID): genetic, phenotypic and functional diversity in 108 infants. J Pediatr 1997;130:378.

13. Noguchi M, Yi H, Rosenblatt HM, et al. Interleukin-2 receptor γ chain mutation results in X-linked severe combined immunodeficiency in humans. Cell 1993;73:147.

14. Puck JM, Deschenes SM, Porter JC, et al. The interleukin-2 receptor γ chain maps to Xq13.1 and is mutated in X-linked severe combined immunodeficiency, SCIDX1. Hum Mol Genet 1993;2:1099.

15. Puck JM, Nussbaum RL, Conley ME. Carrier detection in X-linked severe combined immunodeficiency based on patterns of X chromosome inactivation. J Clin Invest 1987;79:1395.

16. Puck JM, Krauss C, Puck SM, et al. Prenatal test for X-linked severe combined immunodeficiency by analysis of maternal X-chromosome inactivation and linkage analysis. N Engl J Med 1990;322:1063.

17. Puck JM, Pepper AE, Bédard P-M, et al. Female germline mosaicism as the origin of a unique IL-2 receptor γ-chain mutation causing X-linked severe combined immunodeficiency. J Clin Invest 1995;95:895.

18. O'Marcaigh AE, Puck JM, Pepper AE, et al. Maternal germline mosaicism for an IL2RG mutation causing X-linked SCID in a Navajo kindred. J Clin Immunol 1997;17:29.

19. Puck JM, Pepper AE, Henthorn PS, et al. Mutation analysis of IL2RG in human X-linked severe combined immunodeficiency. Blood 1997;89:1968.

20. Niemela JE, Puck JM, Fischer R, et al. Efficient detection of thirty-seven new *IL2RG* mutations in human X-linked severe combined immunodeficiency. Clin Immunol 2000;95:33.

21. Cavazzana-Calvo M, Hacein-Bey S, de Saint Basile G, et al. Gene therapy of human severe combined immunodeficiency (SCID)-X1 disease. Science 2000;288:669.

22. Hacein-Bey-Abina S, Le Deist F, Carlier F, Bouneaud C, et al. Sustained correction of X-linked severe combined immunodeficiency by ex vivo gene therapy. N Engl J Med. 2002;346:1185.

23. Hacein-Bey-Abina S, von Kalle C, Schmidt M, et al. A serious adverse event after successful gene therapy for X-linked severe combined immunodeficiency. N Engl J Med 2003; 348:255.

24. Kohn DB, Sadelain M, Glorioso JC. Occurrence of leukaemia following gene therapy of X-linked SCID. Nat Rev Cancer 2003;3:477.

25. Puck JM, Middelton LA, Pepper AE. Carrier and prenatal diagnosis of X-linked severe combined immunodeficiency: mutation detection methods and utilization. Hum Genet 1997;99:628.

26. Durandy A, Dumez Y, Griscelli C. Prenatal diagnosis of severe inherited immunodeficiencies: a five year experience. In: Vossen J, Griscelli C, eds. Progress in immunodeficiency research and therapy, vol. 2. Amsterdam: Elsevier, 1986:323.

27. Myers LA, Patel, DD, Puck JM, et al. Hematopoietic stem cell transplantation for SCID in the neonatal period leads to superior thymic output and improved survival. Blood 99:872–878, 2002.

28. Giri N, Vowels M, Ziegler JB, et al. HLA non-identical T-cell-depleted bone marrow transplantation for primary immunodeficiency diseases. Aust NZ J Med 1994;24:26.

29. Flake AW, Almeida-Porada G, Puck JM, et al. Treatment of X-linked SCID by the in utero transplantation of CD34 enriched bone marrow. N Engl J Med 1996;355:1806.

30. Wengler GS, Lanfranchi A, Frusca T, et al. In-utero transplantation of parental CD34 haematopoietic progenitor cells in a patient with X-linked severe combined immunodeficiency (SCIDXI). Lancet 1996;348: 1484.

31. Bartolome J, Porta F, Lafranchi A, et al. B cell function after haploidentical in utero bone marrow transplantation in a patient with severe combined immunodeficiency. Bone Marrow Transplant 2002; 29:625.

32. Macchi P, Villa A, Giliani S, et al. Mutations of JAK3 gene in patients with autosomal severe combined immunodeficiency (SCID). Nature 1995;377:65.

33. Russell SM, Tayebi N, Nakajima H, et al. Mutation of Jak3 in a patient with SCID: essential role of Jak3 in lymphoid development. Science 1995;270:797.

34. Schumacher RF, Mella P, Lalatta F, et al. Prenatal diagnosis of JAK3 SCID. Prenat Diagn 1999;19:653.

35. Hirschhorn R. Adenosine deaminase deficiency. Immunol Rev 1991;3:45.

36. Hershfield MS, Mitchell BS. Immunodeficiency diseases caused by adenosine deaminase deficiency and purine nucleoside phosphorylase deficiency. In: Scriver CR, Beaudet AL, Sly WS, et al., eds. The metabolic basis of inherited disease, 7th ed. New York: McGraw-Hill, 1995:1725.

37. Aiuti A, Slavin S, Aker M et al. Correction of ADA-SCID by stem cell gene therapy combined with nonmyeloablative conditioning. Science 2002;296;2410.

38. Hirschhorn R. Prenatal diagnosis of adenosine deaminase deficiency and selected other immunodeficiencies. In: Milunsky A, ed. Genetic disorders and the fetus: diagnosis, prevention, and treatment, 3rd ed. Baltimore: Johns Hopkins University Press, 1992:453.

39. Aitken DA, Gilmore DH, Frew CA, et al. Early prenatal investigation of a pregnancy at risk of adenosine deaminase deficiency using chorionic villi. J Med Genet 1986;23:52.

40. Perignon JL, Durandy A, Peter MO, et al. Prenatal diagnosis of inherited severe immunodeficiencies linked to enzyme deficiencies. J Pediatr 1987;111:595.

41. Schwarz K, Gauss G, Ludwig L, et al. RAG mutations in human B cell-negative SCID. Science 1996;274:97.

42. Jones JF, Ritenbaugh CK, Spence MA, et al. Severe combined immunodeficiency among the Navajo. I. Characterization of phenotypes, epidemiology, and population genetics. Hum Biol 1991;63:699.

43. Moshous D, Callebaut I, de Chasseval R, et al. Artemis, a novel DNA double-strand break repair/V(D)J recombination protein, is mutated in human severe combined immune deficiency. Cell 2001;105:177.

44. Li L, Zhou Y, Wang J, et al. Prenatal diagnosis and carrier detection for Athabascan severe combined immunodeficiency disease. Prenat Diagn 2002;22:763.

45. Rainaut M, Pagniez M, Hercent T, et al. Characterization of mononuclear cell subpopulations in normal fetal peripheral blood. Hum Immunol 1987;18:331.

46. Linch DC, Beverly PCL, Levinsky RJ, et al. Phenotypic analysis of fetal blood leukocytes: potential for prenatal diagnosis of immunodeficiency disorders. Prenat Diagn 1982;2:211.

47. Durandy A, Oury C, Griscelli C, et al. Prenatal testing for inherited immune deficiencies by fetal blood sampling. Prenat Diagn 1982;2:109.

48. Kleijer WJ, Hussaarts-odijk LM, Pijpers L, et al. Prenatal diagnosis of purine nucleoside phosphorylase deficiency in the first and second trimesters of pregnancy. Prenat Diagn 1989;9:401.

49. Puel A, Ziegler SF, Buckley RH et al. Defective IL7R expression in T($-$)B($+$)NK($+$) severe combined immunodeficiency. Nat Genet 1998;20;394.

50. Elder ME, Lin D, Clever J, et al. Human severe combined immunodeficiency due to a defect in ZAP-70, a T cell tyrosine kinase. Science 1994;264:1596.

51. Chan AC, Kadlecek TA, Elder ME, et al. ZAP-70 deficiency in an autosomal recessive form of severe combined immunodeficiency. Science 1994;264:1599.

52. Steimle V, Reith W, Mach B. Major histocompatibility complex class II deficiency: a disease of gene regulation. Adv Immunol 1996;61:327.

53. Klein C, Lisowska-Grospierre B, LeDeist F, et al. Major histocompatibility complex class II deficiency: clinical manifestations, immunologic features, and outcome. J Pediatr 1993;123:921.

54. Steimle V, Otten LA, Zufferey M, et al. Complementation cloning of an MHC class II transactivator mutated in hereditary MHC class II deficiency (or bare lymphocyte syndrome). Cell 1993;75:135.

55. Zhou H, Glimcher LH. Human MHC class II gene transcription directed by the carboxyl terminus of CIITA, one of the defective genes in type II MHC combined immune deficiency. Immunity 1995;2:545.

56. Durand B, Sperisen P, Emery P, et al. RFXAP, a novel subunit of the RFX DNA binding complex is mutated in MHC class II deficiency. EMBO J 1997;16:1045.

57. Durandy A, Cerf-Bensussan N, Dumez Y, et al. Prenatal diagnosis of severe combined immunodeficiency with defective synthesis of HLA molecules. Prenat Diagn 1987;7:27.

58. Notarangelo LD, Duse M, Ugazio AG. Immunodeficiency with hyper-IgM (HIM). Immunodefic Rev 1992;3:101.

59. Conley ME, Larche M, Bonagura VR, et al. Hyper-IgM syndrome associated with defective CD40-mediated B cell activation. J Clin Invest 1994;94:1404.

60. DiSanto JP, Markiewicz S, Gauchat J-F, et al. Prenatal diagnosis of X-linked hyper IgM syndrome. N Engl J Med 1994;330:969.

61. Imai K, Catalan N, Plebani A, et al. Hyper-IgM syndrome type 4 with a B lymphocyte-intrinsic selective deficiency in Ig class-switch recombination. J Clin Invest 2003;112:136.

62. Muller W, Peter HH, Kallfelz HC, et al. The DiGeorge sequence. II. Immunologic findings in partial and complete forms of the disorder. Eur J Pediatr 1989;149:96.

63. Gong W, Emanuel BS, Collins J, et al. A transcription map of the DiGeorge and velo-cardio-facial syndrome minimal critical region on 22q11. Hum Mol Genet 1996;5:789.

64. Driscoll DA, Salvin J, Sellinger B, et al. Prevalence of 22q11 microdeletions in DiGeorge and velocardiofacial syndromes: implications for genetic counseling and prenatal diagnosis. J Med Genet 1993;30:813.

65. Baldini A. DiGeorge syndrome: the use of model organisms to dissect complex genetics. Hum Mol Genet 2002;11:2363.

66. Daw SCM, Taylor C, Kraman M, et al. A common region of 10p deleted in DiGeorge and velocardiofacial syndromes. Nat Genet 1996;13:458.

67. Vetrie D, Vorechovsky I, Sideras P, et al. The gene involved in X-linked agammaglobulinaemia is a member of the *src* family of protein-tyrosine kinases. Nature 1993;361:226.

68. Tsukada S, Saffran DC, Rawlings DJ, et al. Deficient expression of a B cell cytoplasmic tyrosine kinase in human X-linked agammaglobulinemia. Cell 1993;72:279.

69. Durandy A, Griscelli C. Prenatal diagnosis of severe combined immunodeficiency and X-linked agammaglobulinemia. Birth Defects 1983;19:125.

70. Yel L, Minegishi Y, Coustan-Smith E, et al. Mutations in the μ heavy-chain gene in patients with agammaglobulinemia. N Engl J Med 1996;335:1486.

71. Orkin SH. Molecular genetics of chronic granulomatous disease. Annu Rev Immunol 1989;7:277.

72. Etzioni A. Adhesion molecular deficiencies and their clinical significance. Cell Adhesion Commun 1994;2:257.

73. Diukman R, Tanigawara S, Cowan MJ, et al. Prenatal diagnosis of Chediak–Higashi syndrome. Prenat Diagn 1992;12:877.

74. Nagle DL, Karim MA, Woolf EA, et al. Identification and mutation analysis of the complete gene for Chediak–Higashi syndrome. Nat Genet 1996;14:307.

75. Durandy A, Breton-Gorius J, Guy-Grand D, et al. Prenatal diagnosis of syndromes associating albinism and immune deficiencies (Chediak–Higashi syndrome and variant). Prenat Diagn 1993;13:13.

76. Winkelstein JA, Sullivan KE, Colten HR. Genetically determined deficiencies of complement. In: Scriver CR, Beaudet AL, Sly WS, et al., eds. Metabolic basis of inherited disease, 7th ed. New York: McGraw-Hill, 1995:3912.

77. Sullivan KE, Mullen CA, Blaese RM, et al. A multi-institutional survey of the Wiskott–Aldrich syndrome. J Pediatr 1994;125:876.

78. Sullivan KE. Genetic and clinical advances in Wiskott–Aldrich syndrome. Curr Opin Pediatr 1995;7:683.

79. Derry JM, Ochs HD, Francke U. Isolation of a novel gene mutated in Wiskott–Aldrich syndrome. Cell 1994;78:635.

80. Nonoyama S, Ochs HD. Wiskott–Aldrich syndrome. Curr Allergy Asthma Rep 2001;1:430.

81. Wengler GS, Notarangelo LD, Giliani S, et al. Mutation analysis in Wiskott Aldrich syndrome on chorionic villus DNA. Lancet 1995;346:641.

82. Savitsky K, Bar-Shira A, Gilad S, et al. A single ataxia–telangiectasia gene with a product similar to PI-3 kinase. Science 1995;268:1749.

83. Jaspers NG, Scheres JM, Dewit J, et al. Rapid diagnostic test for ataxia–telangiectasia. Lancet 1961;2: 473.

84. German J. Bloom syndrome: Aa mendelian prototype of somatic mutational disease. Medicine (Baltimore) 1993;72:393.

85. Ellis NA, Groden J, Ye TZ, et al. The Bloom's syndrome gene product is homologous to RecQ helicases. Cell 1995;83:655.

86. Skare J, Milunsky A, Byron K, et al. Mapping the X-linked lymphoproliferative syndrome. Proc Natl Acad Sci USA 1987;84:2015.

87. Skare J, Madan S, Glaser J, et al. First prenatal diagnosis of X-linked lymphoproliferative disease. Am J Med Genet 1992;44:79.

88. Schuster V, Seidenspinner S, Grimm T, et al. Molecular genetic haplotype segregation studies in three families with X-linked lymphoproliferative disease. Eur J Pediatr 1994;153:432.

89. Schuster V, Kreth HW. X-linked lymphoproliferative disease is caused by deficiency of a novel SH2 domain-containing signal transduction adaptor protein. Immunol Rev 2000;178:21.

90. Puck JM, Sneller MC. ALPS: An autoimmune human lymphoproliferative syndrome associated with abnormal lymphocyte apoptosis. Semin Immunol 1997;9:77.

91. Rieux-Laucat F, Le Deist F, Hivroz C, et al. Mutations in Fas associated with human lymphoproliferative syndrome and autoimmunity. Science 1995;268:1347.

92. Fisher GH, Rosenberg FJ, Straus SE, et al. Dominant interfering Fas gene mutations impair apoptosis in a human autoimmune lymphoproliferative syndrome. Cell 1995;81:935.

John M. Old, Ph.D., F.R.C.Path.

19

Prenatal Diagnosis of the Hemoglobinopathies

The hemoglobinopathies are a diverse group of inherited recessive disorders consisting of the structural hemoglobin variants and the thalassemias. Together, they form the most common single-gene disorder in the world population, and they are a serious public health problem in many countries. Although there is no definitive cure for the hemoglobinopathies, the methods of clinical management have improved considerably during the past few years and the life expectancy of affected individuals has been significantly increased. However, the treatment required is very expensive and is not a realistic means of controlling the disorders in many developing countries. Therefore, many countries, especially those with a high incidence of β-thalassemia, are applying an alternative method of control that involves screening the population for carriers, identifying couples at risk, and providing prenatal diagnosis.[1]

Prenatal diagnosis was first achieved in 1974 by the study of globin synthesis in fetal blood, following the development of the technique of fetal blood sampling.[2] This approach was applied for all of the hemoglobinopathies and proved very successful.[3] However, it has the disadvantage that fetal blood sampling is not possible until approximately the 18th week of pregnancy, which means a long wait for the mother and, if indicated, a relatively difficult elective abortion. It currently has been entirely replaced in most diagnostic centers by fetal DNA analysis. Prenatal diagnosis by direct mutation identification was originally developed using amniotic fluid DNA to avoid the small risk of fetal loss associated with fetal blood sampling.[4,5] However, amniocentesis is also a midtrimester procedure, and most diagnostic centers switched to the first-trimester procedure of chorionic villus sampling (CVS) soon after chorionic villus samples were shown to be a better source of fetal DNA for molecular analysis.[6] Initially, the sampling procedure was observed to carry a high risk to the fetus, but as more studies were completed, the fetal loss rate has decreased to the point at which it is lower than the risk from fetal blood sampling but 0.6 percent higher than that from amniocentesis[7] (see also discussion in chapter 5). Studies have shown that CVS performed before 10 weeks of pregnancy can cause limb-reduction defects[8]; therefore, most centers currently perform CVS at 11 weeks. This allows 1 week to obtain a prenatal diagnosis by fetal DNA analysis, which is more than enough time, because nearly every hemoglobinopathy mutation currently can be diagnosed by PCR in 1 day.

New developments in prenatal diagnosis are directed toward noninvasive fetal sampling procedures. These are the analysis of fetal cells circulating in maternal blood, the analysis of free fetal DNA in maternal plasma, and preimplantation genetic diagnosis (see also chapters 27 and 28). The first two techniques still involve the termination of pregnancy when indicated and are subject to technical problems and limited clinical application. The latter approach has the advantage that the need to terminate an affected ongoing pregnancy is eliminated, and despite being a very difficult service to organize, it has been proved technically feasible with the birth of a small number of unaffected babies. However, it is a very technically challenging, multiple-step, costly procedure and the approach is expected to supplement rather than replace CVS diagnosis.

Almost 1,000 mutant alleles have been characterized at the molecular level that result in a thalassemia phenotype or abnormal hemoglobin. The mutations are regionally specific, and in most cases, the geographic and ethnic distributions have been determined to provide the foundation of a control program by prenatal diagnosis. Numerous PCR-based techniques can be used to diagnose the globin gene mutations; the aim of this chapter is to compare and contrast these different approaches and then to describe the methods used in my laboratory in greater detail. The main requirements for methods providing molecular diagnosis of the hemoglobinopathies are speed, cost, convenience, and the ability to test for multiple mutations simultaneously. For β-thalassemia mutations, the procedures that meet these requirements are the amplification refractory mutation system (ARMS) and the reverse dot-blot hybridization system. For α-thalassemia, the technique of gap PCR is used to target specific deletion mutations. Initial studies demonstrated a certain degree of unreliability to the amplification of α-thalassemia deletions, but the primers and experimental procedures have been improved to the point at which the method can be used robustly in a multiplex format.

CLINICAL TYPES

The World Health Organization (WHO) Working Party estimated that there are more than 200 million carriers for the inherited disorders of hemoglobin (Hb) and that between 100,000 and 300,000 severely affected homozygotes or compound heterozygotes are born each year.[9] Clinically, the most important of these conditions are the α- and β-thalassemias and the Hb Lepore thalassemias, sickle cell anemia, and the compound heterozygous state for Hb E and β-thalassemia.[10] A brief account of the molecular pathology and phenotypic diversity of these disorders will be given here, but for more extensive coverage, the reader is referred to several earlier reviews.[11–13] The hematologic features of the main types of hemoglobin disorders and the method of diagnosis by DNA analysis are summarized in Table 19.1.

The Globin Genes

Hemoglobin is a tetrameric protein made up of two α-like (α or ζ) and two β-like (ϵ, γ, δ, or β) globin chains. Each globin chain is synthesized from its own globin gene located in two gene clusters, the α-like globin genes on chromosome 16 and the β-like genes on chromosome 11. The α-globin cluster includes an embryonic gene (ζ_2), two fetal/adult genes (α_1 and α_2), several pseudogenes ($\psi\zeta_1$, $\psi\alpha_1$, and $\psi\alpha_2$), and a gene of undetermined function (θ_1) arranged in the order ζ_2-$\psi\zeta_1$-$\psi\alpha_2$-$\psi\alpha_1$-α_2-α_1-θ. The β-globin cluster includes an embryonic gene (ϵ), two fetal genes ($^G\gamma$ and $^A\gamma$), two adult genes (β and δ), and a pseudogene ($\psi\beta$) in the order ϵ-$^G\gamma$-$^A\gamma$-$\psi\beta$-δ-β. Throughout development, there is a series

Table 19.1.   Phenotypes of thalassemias, sickle cell disease, and various thalassemia interactions

Type	Phenotype	DNA Diagnosis
Homozygous state		
α^0-thalassemia $(--/--)$	Hb Bart's hydrops fetalis	Gap-PCR or Southern blot
$\alpha/^+$-thalassemia $(-\alpha/-\alpha)$	No clinical problems	Gap-PCR or Southern blot
α^+-thalassemia $(\alpha^T\alpha/\alpha^T\alpha)$	Hb H disease	Gap-PCR or Southern blot
β thalassemia		
β^0 or severe β^+ mutation	Thalassemia major	PCR: ASO or ARMS
Mild β^+ mutation	Thalassemia intermedia	PCR: ASO or ARMS
$\delta\beta^0$-thalassemia	Thalassemia intermedia	Gap-PCR or Southern blot
HPFH	No clinical problems	Gap-PCR or Southern blot
Hb Lepore	Variable: intermedia to major	Gap-PCR
Hb S	Sickle cell disease	PCR: RE, ASO or ARMS
Hb C	No clinical problems	PCR: ASO or ARMS
Hb D	No clinical problems	PCR: RE, ASO or ARMS
Hb E	No clinical problems	PCR: RE, ASO or ARMS
Compound-heterozygous state		
α^0-thal/α^+-thal $(--/-\alpha)$	Hb H disease	Gap-PCR or Southern blot
α^0-thal/α^+-thal $(--/\alpha^T\alpha)$	Severe Hb H disease	Gap-PCR or Southern blot
β^0/severe β^+ thal	Thalassemia major	PCR: ASO or ARMS
Mild β^{++}/β^0 or severe β^+ thal	Variable: intermedia to major	PCR: ASO or ARMS
$\delta\beta^0/\beta^0$ or severe β^+ thal	Variable: intermedia to major	PCR or Southern blot
$\delta\beta^0$/mild β^{++} thal	Mild thalassemia intermedia	PCR or Southern blot
$\delta\beta^0$/Hb Lepore	Thalassemia intermedia	Gap-PCR or Southern blot
$\alpha\alpha\alpha/\beta^0$ or severe β^+ thal	Mild thalassemia intermedia	PCR or Southern blot
Hb Lepore/β^0 or severe β^+ thal	Thalassemia major	PCR: Gap, ASO or ARMS
Hb C/β^0 or severe β^+ thal	Variable: β-thal trait to intermedia	PCR: RE, ASO or ARMS
Hb C/mild β^{++} thal	No clinical problems	PCR: RE, ASO or ARMS
Hb D/β^0 or severe β^+ thal	No clinical problems	PCR: RE, ASO or ARMS
Hb E/β^0 or severe β^+ thal	Variable: intermedia to major	PCR: RE, ASO or ARMS
Hb O Arab/β^0 thal	Severe thalassemia intermedia	PCR: RE, ASO or ARMS
Hb S/β^0 or severe β^+ thal	Sickle cell disease	PCR: RE, ASO or ARMS
Hb S/mild β^{++} thal	Usually mild sickle cell disease	PCR: RE, ASO or ARMS
Hb S/$\delta\beta^0$-thal	Usually mild sickle cell disease	PCR: RE, Gap or Southern blot
Hb S/Hb C	Sickle cell disease, variable severity	PCR: RE, ASO or ARMS
Hb S/Hb D Punjab	Sickle cell disease	PCR: RE, ASO or ARMS
Hb S/Hb O Arab	Sickle cell disease	PCR: RE, ASO or ARMS
Hb S/HPFH	Sickle cell trait	PCR: RE, Gap or Southern blot
Hb E disorders		
Hb E + α^0-thal/α^+-thal	Similar to Hb H disease	PCR: Gap, ASO or ARMS
Hb EE + α^0-thal/α^+-thal	Severe thalassemia intermedia	PCR: Gap, ASO or ARMS
Hb EE + $\alpha^T\alpha/\alpha^T\alpha$	Mild thalassemia intermedia	PCR: Gap, ASO or ARMS

ASO = allele-specific oligonucleotide analysis; HPFH = hereditary persistence of fetal hemoglobin; RE = restriction enzyme analysis.

of coordinated switches of the production of one type of hemoglobin to another. Embryonic hemoglobin ($\alpha_2\gamma_2$-Hb Gower, $\zeta_2\gamma_2$-Hb Gower 1, and $\zeta_2\gamma_2$-Hb Portland) gives way to fetal hemoglobin ($\alpha_2\zeta_2$-Hb F), which then switches to adult hemoglobin ($\alpha_2\beta_2$-Hb A and $\alpha_2\delta_2$-Hb A$_2$). The molecular mechanisms responsible for switching on and off of the various globin genes have been the subject of intense research for many years. The phenotype of β-thalassemia or sickle cell disease in individuals with a naturally elevated level of Hb F is less severe; thus, the goal of this research is to understand and manipulate the switch in affected patients to ameliorate their disease. Several chemical agents, such as hydroxyurea and butyrate, have been shown to induce the production of Hb F.[14] Although the precise mechanism of action of these agents remains unknown, the most effective results obtained to date have been with hydroxyurea therapy in patients with sickle cell disease and sickle-β-thalassemia.[15] This is in contrast to patients with β-thalassemia, for whom the results have been disappointing, except in some patients with Hb Lepore or thalassemia intermedia who were not transfusion-dependent.[16]

α-Thalassemia

α-Thalassemia results from a deficiency of α-globin chain synthesis and can be divided into two forms: a severe form (called α_1- or α^0-thalassemia), which produces a typical thalassemic blood picture in heterozygotes, and a mild form (α_2 or α^+-thalassemia), which is almost completely "silent" in heterozygotes. Although a few types of α^+-thalassemia have been shown to result from a nondeletion type of molecular defect, the most common cause of α-thalassemia is a series of gene deletions. α^+-thalassemia results from at least six different deletions, which effectively remove one of the two α-globin genes on chromosome 16.[17] The genotype of the heterozygous state can be represented as $-\alpha/\alpha\alpha$ and that of the homozygous state as $-\alpha/-\alpha$. The clinical phenotype of the homozygous state is similar to that of α^0-thalassemia trait ($--/\alpha\alpha$ genotype), and the two conditions are best differentiated by restriction enzyme mapping. $\alpha0$-thalassemia can result from seventeen different gene deletions,[11] all of which effectively delete both α-globin genes.

Hb Bart's Hydrops Fetalis Syndrome

The most severe form of α-thalassemia is the homozygous state for α^0-thalassemia, known as Hb Bart's hydrops fetalis syndrome. This condition results from a deletion of all four globin genes, and an affected fetus cannot synthesize any α-globin to make Hb F or Hb A. Fetal blood contains only the abnormal hemoglobin Bart's (γ_4) and a small amount of Hb Portland. The resulting severe fetal anemia leads to asphyxia, hydrops fetalis, and stillbirth or neonatal death, and prenatal diagnosis is always indicated to avoid the severe toxemic complications that occur frequently in pregnancy with hydropic fetuses.

Hb H Disease

Hb H disease results from the compound heterozygous state for α^0- and α^1-thalassemia ($--/-\alpha$) or, more rarely, from the homozygous state of nondeletion α^+-thalassemia mutations affecting the dominant α_2 gene ($\alpha^T\alpha/\alpha^T\alpha$). Individuals with Hb H disease have a moderately severe hypochromic microcytic anemia and produce large amounts of Hb H (β_4) as a result of the excess β-chains in the reticulocyte. Patients may suffer from fatigue, general discomfort, and splenomegaly, but they rarely require hospitalization and lead a relatively normal life. However, there also is a more severe form of Hb H disease arising from the compound heterozygous state of α^0-thalassemia and nondeletion α^+-thalassemia ($--/\alpha^T\alpha$). Such patients seem to exhibit more severe symptoms, with a possible requirement for recurrent blood transfusions and splenectomy. Three cases of unusually severe Hb H disease associated with hydrops fetalis have been reported. In each case, the α^+-thalassemia resulted from a mutation in the α_2 gene associated with a highly unstable α-globin variant.[10] Thus, in some situations, couples at risk for this more severe form of Hb H disease have opted for prenatal diagnosis and termination of an affected fetus.[18]

β-Thalassemia

The β-thalassemias are a heterogeneous group of disorders characterized by either an absence of β-globin chain synthesis (β^0 type) or a much-reduced rate of synthesis (β^+ type). More than 170 different β-thalassemia mutations have been identified,[19] and new ones are still being characterized by sequencing of unknown samples from screening programs (an updated list can be found at http://globin.cse.psu.edu). Only seventeen mutations consist of large gene deletions, ranging from 25 bp to 67 kb; the remainder are single nucleotide changes in the β-globin gene or its flanking sequences. The mutations cause defects in transcription, RNA splicing or modification, RNA translation through a frameshift effect or the presence of a new nonsense codon, and finally some create unstable β-globin chains. They can be classified into several groups according to their phenotypic effect. Most β^0 and β^+ type of mutations are called severe mutations because either in the homozygous or compound heterozygous state they give rise to the phenotype of β-thalassemia major, a transfusion-dependent anemia from early in life.

β-Thalassemia Major

At birth, infants with β-thalassemia major are asymptomatic because of the high production of Hb F, but as this declines, affected infants present with severe anemia during the first or second year of life. Treatment is by frequent blood transfusion to maintain a hemoglobin level above 10 g/dL, coupled with iron chelation therapy to control iron overload, otherwise death results in the second or third decade from cardiac failure. This treatment does not cure β-thalassemia major, although some patients have now reached the age of 40 years in good health and have married and produced children. With the prospects for gene therapy remaining as distant as ever, the only cure for β-thalassemia for the foreseeable future is bone marrow transplantation. Although this form of treatment has proved successful when performed in young children, it is limited by the requirements of an HLA-matched sibling or relative.

β-Thalassemia Intermedia

Some β-thalassemia mutations in the homozygous state are associated with a milder clinical condition called thalassemia intermedia. Patients with thalassemia intermedia present later in life than those with thalassemia major and are capable of maintaining a hemoglobin level higher than 6 g without transfusion. Thalassemia intermedia is caused by a wide variety of genotypes, including β-thalassemia, $\delta\beta$-thalassemia, and Hb Lepore, and covers a broad clinical spectrum. Patients with a severe condition present between 2 and 6 years of age, and, although they are capable of surviving with an Hb level of 5–7 g/dL, they will not develop normally and are treated with minimal blood transfusions. At the other end of the spectrum are patients who do not become symptomatic until they reach adult life and remain transfusion-independent with Hb levels of 8–10 g/dL. However, even these milder patients tend to have iron accumulation with age, and clinical problems relating to iron overload after the third decade develop in many patients with thalassemia intermedia. Prenatal diagnosis is often requested by couples at risk of having a child with thalassemia intermedia because of the unpredictability of the phenotype.

Thalassemia intermedia may result from the moderating effect because of the coinheritance of two severe β-thalassemia mutations with either α^0-thalassemia trait or a hereditary persistence of fetal hemoglobin (HPFH) determinant, such as the partial up promoter substitution (C → T) at -158 to the $^G\gamma$ globin gene.[20] However, some individuals with β-thalassemia intermedia are simply homozygous for a mild type of β^+-thalassemia mutation. Specifically, these are IVSI-6 (T → C), CAP+1 (A → C), the transcription mutations occurring upstream of the β-globin gene in the promoter sequences at approximately -30, -90, and -105 nucleotides, and the poly (A) AATAAA → AACAAA mutation.[10] There is one exception, -29 (A → G), which has a mild phenotype in Africans but is severe in Chinese individuals, resulting in β-thalassemia major in the homozygous state.[21] This is because the mutation is associated with the -158 $^G\gamma$-globin HPFH mutation in African but not in Chinese individuals. Thus, homozygosity for these mild β^+-thalassemia mutations usually results in a very mild disorder, and prenatal diagnosis is not usually indicated.

The situation for the compound heterozygous state when one of these mild mutations is coupled with a severe mutation is less clear. Some of these individuals have a mild clinical picture, especially if it involves one of the very mild mutations, such as the "silent β-thalassemia" mutations (those associated with a normal Hb A_2 and mean corpuscular hemoglobin [MCH]). One of the most common, the mutation -101 (C → T), has been found to produce very mild clinical phenotypes in the homozygous state or in interaction with severe β-thalassemia mutations.[22] Therefore, prenatal diagnosis in at-risk couples in whom this silent allele is present should not be considered. However the position for the other silent mutations (e.g., 92 C → T, the 5′ UTR mutations, IVSII-844 C → G, +1480 C → G, and the UTR mutations) and other normal Hb A_2 mutations such as CAP+1 A → C is less clear. The unpredictability of the phenotype in compound heterozygotes for these mutations remains a diagnostic and counseling problem. Because the mutations are very uncommon, homozygotes do not exist and there is a general lack of data on cases with the coinheritance of other β-thalassemia alleles. An excellent summary of what data there are on the interactions of silent and mild alleles can be found in Weatherall and Clegg.[10]

Another genotype associated with thalassemia intermedia is the homozygous state for the Hb Lepore deletion mutation (although some such individuals have been reported to have the more severe phenotype of thalassemia major) and from the homozygous state for a couple of the very rare large deletion mutations that cause β^0-thalassemia.[23] This group of deletion mutations (which does not include the 619 bp Asian Indian deletion gene) are characterized in the heterozygous state by an unusually high Hb A_2 value.

Finally, a third class of mutations forms the other end of the spectrum of severity. These mutations are more severe than the main group of severe β^0 and β^+ mutations and produce a thalassemia intermedia phenotype in the heterozygous state, the so-called dominantly inherited inclusion body β-thalassemia.[24] The mutations all occur in exon 3 and are believed to produce a highly unstable β-globin chain, which is quickly broken down, causing overloading of the proteolytic system inside the red cell and the subsequent precipitation of free α-chains as inclusion bodies.

Hb E Disorders

Hb E (β26, Glu → Lys) is the most common abnormal hemoglobin in Southeast Asians, found at gene frequencies above 0.10 percent in some areas. Hb E heterozygotes and homozygotes are asymptomatic. Heterozygotes are clinically normal with 25–30 percent Hb E (lowered by the presence of thalassemia), and homozygotes may be mildly anemic but clinical symptoms are rare. The importance of Hb E is that it combines with different α- and β-thalassemias to a range of symptomatic disorders.[25]

Hb E-β-Thalassemia

The compound heterozygous state of Hb E and β-thalassemia, is a common disease in Thailand and parts of Southeast Asia. It results in a variable clinical picture similar to that of homozygous β-thalassemia, usually of intermediate severity. However, the clinical spectrum is heterogeneous, ranging from a condition indistinguishable from thalassemia major to a mild form of thalassemia intermedia because of the range of different β-thalassemia genes. The severest conditions are found in individuals with β^0-thalassemia, who usually have about 40–60 percent Hb F, the remainder being Hb E. Compound heterozygotes for Hb E and β^+-thalassemia have a milder disorder and produce variable amounts of Hb A.

Hb AE Bart's Disease

Hb AE Bart's disease results from the interaction of Hb H disease with heterozygous state for Hb E. The disorder is characterized by the presence of Hb A, Hb E (13–15 percent), and Hb Bart's on hemoglobin analysis. Although Hb H inclusions may sometimes be observed, Hb Bart's is usually found on electrophoresis in adults with this disorder. The clinical manifestations are similar to Hb H disease, with patients having a variable degree of anemia and splenomegaly. Two common subtypes of Hb AE Bart's disease have been observed; α^0-thalassemia/α^+-thalassemia—β^A/β^E- and α^0-thalassemia/Hb Constant Spring—β^A/β^E. The latter disorder was found to have a more severe clinical syndrome.

Hb EF Bart's Disease

Hb EF Bart's disease results from the interaction of Hb H disease with homozygous Hb E. The disorder is characterized by the presence of Hb E, Hb F, and Hb Bart's on hemoglobin analysis. Hb E constitutes approximately 80 percent, Hb F 10 percent and the Hb Bart's 10 percent. Patients with this condition have severe thalassemia intermedia, with a Hb level ranging from 6 to 10 g/dL and markedly reduced mean cell volume (MCV) and MCH values, and moderate to severe anemia. No inclusion bodies or Hb H are present, probably because the abnormal β^E-globin chains cannot form tetramers. Four genotypes for Hb EF Bart's disease have been identified: (1) Hb H disease, due to α^0/α^+-thalassemia, with homozygous Hb E; (2) Hb H disease, due to α^0-thalassemia/Hb Constant Spring, in combination with homozygous Hb E; (3) Hb H disease, due to α^0/α^+-thalassemia, with Hb E β-thalassemia; and (4) Hb H disease, due to α^0-thalassemia/Hb Constant Spring, in combination with Hb E β-thalassemia. Differentiating among these genotypes requires family studies and further investigation by DNA analysis.

Hb E/E plus $\alpha^{CS}\alpha/\alpha^{CS}\alpha$

Individuals homozygous for Hb E and homozygous Hb Constant Spring have been observed. They have mild thalassemia intermedia. Compared with homozygous Hb E alone, there were minimal red-cell changes. This may be due to the interaction of α-thalassemia with the β-thalassemia-like reduced globin synthesis of Hb E.

Sickle Cell Disease

Sickle cell disease is characterized by a lifelong hemolytic anemia, the occurrence of acute exacerbations called crises, and a variety of complications resulting from an increased propensity to infection and the deleterious effects of repeated vaso-occlusive episodes.

With active management, the proportion of patients expected to survive to 20 years of age is approximately 90 percent. The course of the illness is very variable, even within individual sibships, let alone different racial groups.

Sickle cell disease can result from a variety of different genotypes. These include the homozygous state for the sickle cell gene (sickle cell anemia), plus the compound heterozygous genotypes of Hb S with β-thalassemia, $\delta\beta$-thalassemia, Hb Lepore, Hb D Punjab, Hb O Arab, Hb C, and a few other rare abnormal hemoglobins, such as Hb C Harlem, one of six sickling variants with two amino acid substitutions.[26]

Sickle Cell Anemia

The classic picture of the homozygous state of Hb S disease is a chronic anemia, childhood susceptibility to overwhelming infections, and periodic painful or hemolytic crises. The most common cause of death in early life is infection. The mortality in childhood is believed to be approximately 1–2 percent per year in the United States and the United Kingdom; in less developed countries, such as those in Africa, the rate of infant mortality is higher. However, the clinical picture of sickle cell anemia actually is heterogeneous, with a wide range of variability in the phenotypic expression of the disease. This is due, in part, to the fact that the sickle cell mutation has arisen independently at least four times in Africa and once in Asia according to data provided by β-globin haplotype analysis.[27] The haplotypes have been assigned the name of the geographic area in which they are found most frequently. The four African haplotypes found most frequently are the Benin, Senegal, Cameroon, and the Central African Republic (CAR) or Bantu haplotype. DNA studies have shown that the sickle gene found in Mediterranean individuals is of African origin—the Benin haplotype. The fifth haplotype is the Arab-Indian haplotype, found with the Hb S gene in Saudi Arabia, Iran, and India.

Different Hb F levels are associated with homozygotes for different β-globin gene haplotypes: Cameroon (5–6 percent), Benin and Bantu (6–7 percent), Senegal (7–10 percent), and Arab-Indian (10–25 percent). Epidemiologic studies have shown that haplotypes associated with the lowest Hb F levels are associated with the most clinically severe condition, while the one with the highest, the Arab-Indian, is associated with the mildest course of the disease.[28] The other factor known to modify the disease is the coinheritance of α-thalassemia. In Africans and Indians, this is always the α^+ type. Hb SS patients homozygous for α^+-thalassemia have lower levels of Hb F, but reduced levels of hemolysis as judged by a higher hemoglobin level. Some of the variability of the disease within families could be due to different inheritance patterns of α-thalassemia.

Hb S/β-Thalassemia

In Hb S/β-thalassemia, the β-thalassemia gene interacts with the β^S-gene to increase the level of Hb S from above 50 percent to a level near that observed in Hb SS individuals. The clinical course of sickle cell β-thalassemia is very variable, ranging from a disorder identical with sickle cell anemia to a completely asymptomatic condition. The Hb concentration varies from 5 g/dL to within the normal range. The heterogeneity is mostly due to the type of β-thalassemia mutation that is coinherited. It tends to be very mild in Africans because of the likelihood of the coinheritance of one of three mild β^+ mutations commonly found in this racial group (-88, C $\rightarrow$ T; -29, A $\rightarrow$ G; CD24, T $\rightarrow$ A). However, those patients who inherit a β^0-thalassemia allele exhibit a clinical disorder very similar to sickle cell anemia. Hb S/β-thalassemia is characterized by microcytic red and target cells with occasionally sickled forms. Hemoglobin electrophoresis reveals 60–90 percent Hb S, 0–30 percent Hb A, 1–20 percent Hb F, and an increased Hb A$_2$ level above normal. The percentages of Hb S and Hb A vary depending on whether the β-thalassemia gene is β^+ or β^0 type. Coexisting α-thalassemia increases the Hb concentration, the MCV, and the MCH.

Hb S/δβ-Thalassemia

Hb S/$\delta\beta$-thalassemia is a milder form of sickle cell disease than sickle cell anemia, because the high percentage of Hb F produced by $\delta\beta$-thalassemia allele protects against sickling. Hb S/$\delta\beta$-thalassemia has been characterized in Sicilian, Italian, Greek, Arab, and African-American individuals. Patients have a mild anemia with a Hb concentration in the range of 10–12 g/dL, a significantly reduced MCH and MCV, Hb S, Hb F, and a normal or low Hb A$_2$ level.

Hb S/C Disease

Hb S/C disease is a milder version of sickle cell disease with a variable course. Most of the complications occur less frequently than in Hb SS disease. Hb C is found in parts of West Africa, where it coexists with Hb S at frequencies of up to 0.15 percent. The Hb C mutation, $\beta6$ Glu $\rightarrow$ Lys (GAG $\rightarrow$ AAG) causes a decrease in solubility of both the oxygenated and the deoxygenated forms of Hb C, resulting in the formation of crystals. In individuals homozygous for Hb C, the red cells become dehydrated and rigid, causing a hemolytic anemia, but sickling symptoms do not develop in such patients.

Hb S/D Disease

Hb S/Hb D-Punjab ($\beta121$, Glu $\rightarrow$ Gln) results in a moderately severe form of sickle cell disease. This compound heterozygous state has been observed in patients of African origin, from Central and South America, India, and in individuals with only Mediterranean or northern European ancestry. Patients have a mild to moderate hemolytic anemia (Hb of 5–10 g/dL) with sickling crises.

Hb S/Hb O-Arab Disease

Hb S/Hb O-Arab ($\beta121$, Glu $\rightarrow$ Lys) results in a severe type of sickle cell disorder. Hb S/Hb O-Arab has been observed in Arabs, Africans, Afro-Caribbeans, and African Americans. The Hb concentration varies between 6 and 10 g/dL, and the blood film is similar to that of sickle cell anemia.

Other Rare Sickle Cell Genotypes

Hb S/C-Harlem ($\beta6$ Glu $\rightarrow$ Val and $\beta73$ Asp $\rightarrow$ Asn) is a severe sickle cell disorder. Hb C-Harlem has two amino acid substitutions, the sickle cell substitution at codon 6, and one at codon 73, which makes the hemoglobin move like Hb C in electrophoresis at alkaline pH (6). In combination with Hb S it causes severe sickle cell disease.

Hb S-Antilles ($\beta6$ Glu $\rightarrow$ Val and $\beta23$ Val $\rightarrow$ Ile) has two amino acid substitutions, similar to Hb C Harlem. It is more prone to sickling than Hb S itself, and in the heterozygous state it results in a mild anemia and a moderate sickling disorder. In combination with Hb S, it is reported to produce a very severe form of sickle cell disease with a severe chronic hemolytic anemia. Compound heterozygosity for Hb C and Hb S-Antilles also produces a severe sickle cell disorder.

Hb S-Oman (β6 Glu $\rightarrow$ Val and β121 Glu $\rightarrow$ Lys) has two different phenotypes in the heterozygous state, depending on whether the patients have coinherited heterozygous or homozygous states for α-thalassemia (all patients described with Hb S-Oman have α-thalassemia). Patients with α^+-thalassemia trait have about 20 percent Hb S and a moderate sickling disorder. The blood film shows a unique form of an irreversibly sickled cell called a "Napoleon hat cell" or "yarn and knitting needle cell." In contrast, patients with Hb S-Oman trait and homozygous α^+-thalassemia have about 14 percent Hb S-Oman and are asymptomatic. The compound heterozygous state for Hb S and Hb S-Oman has been described in a few Omani patients. Patients have 25 percent Hb S and 11 percent Hb S-Oman, and the blood film shows Napoleon Hat cells. Patients have very severe disease, with an Hb level of 7 g/dL.

The interaction of Hb S with unstable β-variants may result in a mild form of sickle cell disease. Three such variants have been observed, namely, Hb Quebec-Chori, Hb Hofu, and Hb I-Toulouse. Hb S in combination with mildly unstable β-variants such as Hb Hope and Hb Siiraj can cause mild hemolysis.

CARRIER SCREENING

Community control of sickle cell anemia and thalassemia by fetal diagnosis depends on a successful population screening program.[29] Screening using hematologic methods is the first step in genetic diagnosis and normally consists of measurement of the red-cell indices, hemoglobin electrophoresis, quantitation of Hb A_2, Hb F, and Hb H, and the determination of iron status. Guidelines and a flow chart using cutoff points are followed to establish a diagnosis of a possible thalassemia phenotype.[30,31] It is important to note that such a screening program is designed to lead to a reliable presumptive diagnosis. If an unequivocal diagnosis is required, characterization methods based on DNA analysis must be used. Screening will detect most cases of β-thalassemia trait; however, there is no specific screening test for α-thalassemia trait, and this is usually made by exclusion of a raised Hb A_2 level and iron deficiency. If an abnormal hemoglobin is found by electrophoresis, again the results will give only a presumptive diagnosis of the variant.

Methods

Traditionally, a starch gel has been the medium for hemoglobin electrophoresis, but now this has been replaced by the more rapid methods of electrophoresis using cellulose acetate membrane, acid agarose, or citrate agar gel. Detailed procedures for these techniques have been published by Weatherall and Clegg.[10] However, isoelectric focusing using precast agarose gels is the method of choice, as it gives better separation of hemoglobin variants with sharper bands. It has proved useful for screening large numbers of samples, and provides better resolution and sharper bands than ordinary electrophoresis.

The Hb A_2 is estimated following its separation from Hb A using cellulose acetate electrophoresis and elution, column chromatography, or high-performance liquid chromatography (HPLC). The latter allows the rapid direct measurement of both Hb A_2 and abnormal hemoglobins on large numbers of samples. The MCH is determined together with the other red-cell indices by a standard electronic cell counter in fresh blood samples. Evaluation of blood count in samples more than 24 hours old should be treated with caution, as the red cells increase in size, leading to a falsely raised MCV (thus, the MCH is the more reliable parameter to use for diagnosis).

Reduced Red-Cell Indices with a Raised Hb A$_2$ Value

The heterozygous states for β-thalassemia are usually associated with reduced MCH values, in the 18- to 25-pg range (normal range, 26–33 pg), and reduced MCV values, in the 60- to 70-fL range and a raised Hb A$_2$ level. The red cells also have reduced osmotic fragility, which is the basis for the single-tube osmotic fragility test, and can be used as an alternative screening test if the electronic measurement of MCV is not available. Individuals found to have a low MCH (below 27 pg) are then investigated by estimating the Hb A$_2$ level. If the Hb A$_2$ level is elevated above the normal range (0–3.5 percent), then β-thalassemia trait is indicated. If the Hb A$_2$ level is unusually high (6.5–9.0 percent), then β-thalassemia trait resulting from one of the large gene deletions should be suspected.[12] The hematologic values for MCH, MCV, and Hb A$_2$ found in my laboratory for carriers of different hemoglobinopathies are listed in Table 19.2.

Reduced Red-Cell Indices with a Normal Hb A$_2$ Value

When reduced MCV and MCH levels and a normal Hb A$_2$ level (below 3.5 percent) is observed, the diagnosis may be iron deficiency, α-thalassemia, $\delta\beta$-thalassemia trait $(\epsilon\gamma\delta\beta)^0$ thalassemia trait, β-thalassemia plus δ-thalassemia trait, Hb Lepore trait, or normal Hb A$_2$ β-thalassemia trait. A raised Hb F level of 5–15 percent is indicative of $\delta\beta$-thalassemia trait. Hb Lepore (8–20 percent) can be identified by gel electrophoresis or isoelectric focusing. Normal A$_2$ β-thalassemia and α-thalassemia can be identified only by molecular analysis. The condition of β-thalassemia trait with a normal Hb A$_2$ level can be due to the coinheritance of a standard β-thalassemia mutation with a δ-thalassemia mutation,[19] or to the inheritance of a mild β^+-thalassemia allele associated with a normal or borderline Hb A$_2$ level (3.3–3.8 percent). These are listed in Table 19.3. Some, such as IVSI-6 T → C and CAP+1 A → C, are associated with reduced red-cell indices. However, some of the rarer alleles (e.g., → 92 C → T, IVSII-844 C → G, and −101 C → T) are truly silent, being associated with normal red-cell indices, and thus will not be detected by

Table 19.2. Comparison of various heterozygous conditions (average values)

Disorder/Genotype	MCH (pg)	MCV (fL)	Hb A$_2$ (%)
Normal			
$\alpha\alpha/\alpha\alpha$	30	90	2.0
$\alpha\alpha\alpha/\alpha\alpha$	29	85	2.2
α-thalassemia			
$-\alpha/\alpha\alpha$	28	85	2.4
$--/\alpha\alpha$	22	70	3.0
β^0-Thalassemia			
CD39 C → T	20	66	4.7
10.3-kb deletion	20	66	7.5
β^+-Thalassemia			
IVSI-110 G → A	21	68	4.5
IVSI-6 T → C	23	72	3.4
CAP+1 A → C	25	80	3.3
−101 C → T	28	85	3.3
β^0 trait + α^+ trait	22	70	5.7
β^0 trait + α^0 trait	26	78	6.0

CD = codon; IVS = intervening sequence.

Table 19.3. Genotypes associated with borderline Hb A$_2$ levels: a guideline of related hematologic and biosynthetic characteristics

Genotype	MCV (fL)	MCH (pg)	Hb A$_2$	α/β ratio
$\beta -101$ (C $\rightarrow$ T)	88.5 $\pm$ 7.8	30.1 $\pm$ 1.0	3.1 $\pm$ 1.0	1.3 $\pm$ 0.4
$\beta -92$ (C $\rightarrow$ T)	83.0 $\pm$ 6.0	28.3 $\pm$ 2.0	3.5 $\pm$ 0.4	1.3 $\pm$ 0.8
$\beta +33$ (C $\rightarrow$ G)	82.0 $\pm$ 9.2	27.1 $\pm$ 3.4	2.5 $\pm$ 1.4	1.3 $\pm$ 0.6
Cap+1 (A $\rightarrow$ C)	75–80	23–26	3.4–3.8	—
β IVS1-6 T $\rightarrow$ C	71.0 $\pm$ 4.0	23.1 $\pm$ 2.2	3.4 $\pm$ 0.2	1.9 $\pm$ 1.0
β IVS2-844 C $\rightarrow$ G	96.0 $\pm$ 4.0	30.3 $\pm$ 1.8	3.2 $\pm$ 0.2	1.0 $\pm$ 0.6
$\beta +1480$ (C $\rightarrow$ G)	88.3 $\pm$ 9.5	27.9 $\pm$ 6.0	2.7 $\pm$ 0.8	1.6 $\pm$ 0.4
$\alpha\alpha\alpha/\alpha\alpha$	85.5 $\pm$ 7.8	30.4 $\pm$ 5.0	2.8 $\pm$ 0.6	1.2 $\pm$ 0.4
$\delta + \beta$-thalassemia	67.6 $\pm$ 7.6	21.8 $\pm$ 3.6	3.3 $\pm$ 0.4	1.7 $\pm$ 0.6

hematologic screening. The values for the MCH, MCV, and Hb A$_2$ associated with these silent β-thalassemia alleles and genotypes associated with normal a Hb A$_2$ are summarized in Table 19.3.

Strategy for Fetal Diagnosis

In summary, the screening program used in most countries is based on the following strategy. The MCV is measured first by an electronic cell counter and then a hemolysate is prepared and examined for hemoglobin variants by starch gel or cellulose acetate electrophoresis, HPLC, or isoelectric focusing. For samples with a normal hemoglobin phenotype (AA) and a low MCV, Hb A$_2$ quantification is performed. A normal Hb A$_2$ level would usually indicate α-thalassemia unless anemia due to iron deficiency is identified. For the purpose of antenatal screening, laboratories may decide not to investigate further if the partner is found to have normal red-cell indices or not to carry any hemoglobin variant. If both partners appear to have α^0-thalassemia, β-thalassemia, or a combination that can result in a serious hemoglobinopathy, then DNA analysis is indicated. If one partner appears to have α^0-thalassemia trait and the other β-thalassemia trait, then DNA analysis should still be considered for both partners. The couple could be at risk for β-thalassemia if one has normal Hb A$_2$ β-thalassemia instead of α-thalassemia trait. Alternatively, particularly for couples of Southeast Asian origin, the couple could be at risk for Hb Bart's hydrops fetalis syndrome because the β-thalassemia trait may be masking coexisting α^0-thalassemia trait.

APPROACHES TO PRENATAL DIAGNOSIS

Prenatal Diagnosis by Fetal Blood Sampling

Prenatal diagnosis of the hemoglobinopathies was first achieved by fetal blood sampling and the estimation of the relative rates of globin chain synthesis by radiolabeling. This method, which directly measures the product of the mutant globin genes, was initiated in 1974 after the development of safe techniques for sampling fetal blood at 18–20 weeks of gestation. More than 20 centers performed prenatal diagnosis by this method, and more than 13,000 cases for hemoglobinopathies had been reported to a WHO Registry by December 1989. Overall, the program was remarkably successful, with approximately 25 percent of the fetuses being diagnosed as affected, a fetal loss rate of 3 percent, and a diagnostic error rate of 0.5 percent.[3]

Although prenatal diagnosis using fetal blood was a remarkable technical achievement, it had the disadvantages that fetal blood sampling is not possible until about the 18th week of pregnancy, possibly leading to a late elective abortion. Fetal blood sampling has now been almost entirely replaced in most diagnostic centers by mutation analysis, due to the characterization of most of the thalassemia mutations, the development of rapid DNA analysis techniques, and the introduction of CVS.

Amniotic Fluid DNA

As soon as development of the techniques for the detection of hemoglobinopathies by gene analysis began, several antenatal diagnosis centers began using fetal DNA from amniocytes.[4,32] Most prenatal diagnosis centers quickly adopted the techniques of DNA analysis, and by 1982, 175 cases of amniocyte DNA diagnosis had been reported to the WHO Registry.[33] During 1982, CVS tissue was shown to be an alternative source of fetal DNA for molecular analysis,[6] and early experience showed that chorionic villi provided relatively large amounts of DNA, allowing prenatal diagnosis in nearly all cases by the 12th week of pregnancy.[34] CVS soon replaced amniocentesis as the source of fetal DNA for prenatal diagnosis, and by December 1989, a total of 4,581 CVS diagnoses had been recorded by the WHO Registry, in comparison to 1,222 amniocyte DNA diagnoses.[3] The amniocyte DNA approach will never be entirely replaced, because it will still be necessary in cases in which a couple present themselves too late for CVS or, more rarely, where there is a failure to obtain a villus sample.

DNA can be prepared from amniotic fluid cells directly or after culturing. It takes 2–3 weeks to grow amniocytes to confluence in a 25-mL flask, but culturing has the advantage that a large amount of DNA is obtained (in our experience, the yield from such a flask has varied from 15 to 45 μg, enough DNA for all types of analyses). However, not all laboratories have the facilities for cell culture, and diagnosis can be made using DNA from noncultivated cells in most cases. Approximately 5 μg of DNA is obtained from a 15-mL amniotic fluid sample, and this is sufficient for any PCR-based method of analysis. However, for genotype analysis by Southern blotting, it is enough for only one attempt; therefore, prudently, a small portion should be set aside for culturing in case of failure. The method of DNA preparation for both cultured and noncultivated cells is essentially the same as that for chorionic villi.[35]

Chorionic Villus DNA

Both of the two main approaches to CVS, ultrasound-guided transcervical aspiration[36,37] and ultrasound-guided transabdominal sampling,[38,39] provide good-quality chorionic villus samples for fetal DNA diagnosis, and sufficient DNA normally is obtained for any method of analysis of the globin genes (see also chapter 5). For our first 200 CVS DNA diagnoses, the average yield of DNA was 46 mg; in only one instance was less than 5 mg obtained.[35]

A problem with this approach is the risk of contamination of the chorionic villus DNA with maternal DNA, which arises from the maternal decidua sometimes obtained along with the chorionic villi. However, by careful dissection and removal of the maternal decidua with the aid of a phase-contrast microscope, one can obtain pure fetal DNA samples,[40] as demonstrated by the lack of maternal DNA in chorionic villus samples by hybridization studies with an X-chromosome-specific probe. Maternal contamination can be ruled out in most cases by the presence of one maternal and one paternal allele after the amplification of highly polymorphic repeat markers.[41] A study of 161 CVS DNAs by

Southern blot analysis using the hypervariable allele probes α-globin 3' HVR and p/g3 revealed that the level of contamination from experienced centers was less than 1 percent.[42] The risk of maternal DNA contamination can be reduced to a minimum by preparing DNA from a single frond.

Fetal Cells in Maternal Blood

Fetal cells have long been known to be present in the blood of pregnant women, and they provide an attractive noninvasive approach to prenatal diagnosis provided that the fetal cells are specific for the ongoing pregnancy and a pure population of cells can be isolated for analysis. However, attempts to enrich the fetal cells using cell sorters or immunologic methods have failed to provide a population of cells pure enough for fetal DNA analysis for the detection of both the maternal and paternal mutations (see also chapter 28). The technique has been applied for the diagnosis of β-thalassemia in women whose partners carried a different thalassemia allele, as reported for the detection of a paternal Hb Lepore mutation.[43] Another approach is to identify single nucleated fetal red blood cells and use single-cell PCR to make the diagnosis. Following enrichment, nucleated fetal red blood cells have been identified by staining on a microscope slide with anti-ζ-chain antibodies and collected by micromanipulation under microscopic observation.[44] This approach has now been tried successfully for prenatal diagnosis in two pregnancies at risk for sickle cell anemia and β-thalassemia.[45] However, recent studies have shown that embryonic and fetal globins may be expressed in adult cells; thus, more specific fetal cell markers may be required for the technique to become reliable.[46]

Fetal DNA in Maternal Plasma

The analysis of fetal DNA in maternal plasma is a simpler procedure than the analysis of DNA in fetal nucleated red cells in maternal blood because no enrichment process is involved. Fetal DNA has been detected in DNA extracted from maternal plasma at 11–17 weeks of gestation and can be used for the prenatal exclusion of β-thalassemia. The technique has recently been applied for the prenatal testing of eight fetuses at risk for β-thalassemia major using allele-specific primers for the detection of the CD 41/42 (-CTTT) mutation by real time PCR.[47] The approach can only be used to detect the paternal mutation and thus is limited in that it is potentially applicable only to couples in which the paternal mutation is different to the maternal mutation.

Preimplantation Diagnosis

Preimplantation genetic diagnosis represents a state-of-the-art procedure that allows at-risk couples to have disease-free children without the need to terminate affected pregnancies. PCR-based diagnostic methods can be potentially applied for preimplantation genetic diagnosis using three types of cells: polar bodies from the oocyte/zygote stage, blastomeres from cleavage-stage embryos, and trophoectoderm cells from blastocysts (see also chapter 27).[48] A small number of centers around the world are now set up to carry out this procedure. The approach is especially useful for couples for whom religious or ethical beliefs will not permit the termination of pregnancy and for couples who have already had one or more elective abortions.

This approach is a technically challenging, multiple-step, and expensive procedure and thus is not likely to be widely used for the routine monitoring of pregnancies at risk.

The PCR protocol must be able to diagnose the required genotype in single cells reliably and accurately, and it also has to be optimized to minimize PCR failure and to avoid the problem of allele dropout. The birth of a healthy unaffected baby depends not only on an accurate diagnosis, but also on the success of each of the multiple stages of the assisted reproduction procedure. Overall, the success rate of the procedure is only 20–30 percent. Despite these obstacles, this approach has been applied for couples at risk for β-thalassemia and sickle cell anemia and has led to the birth of a small but increasing number of unaffected babies.

DNA DIAGNOSIS OF THE HEMOGLOBINOPATHIES

This section will review the various techniques of DNA analysis that are used to diagnose the hemoglobinopathies and present the methods that currently are in use in my laboratory.

α-Thalassemia

α^+-Thalassemia has been found to result from five different sizes of gene deletion, although only two are commonly encountered in practice. These are the 3.7-kb deletion $(-\alpha^{3.7})$, which has reached high frequencies in the populations of Africa, the Mediterranean area, the Middle East, the Indian subcontinent, and Melanesia, and the 4.2-kb deletion $(-\alpha^{4.2})$, which is commonly found in the Southeast Asian and Pacific populations.[49] These deletions were created by unequal crossing over between homologous sequences in the α-globin gene cluster, resulting in a chromosome with only one α-gene $(-\alpha)$ and a chromosome with three α-genes $(\alpha\alpha\alpha)$. An additional recombination event between the resulting chromosomes has given rise to a quadruplicated α-gene allele $(\alpha\alpha\alpha\alpha)$. Various nondeletion defects also have been found to cause α^+-thalassemia, and seventeen mutations have been described to date, mostly in populations from the Mediterranean area, Africa, and Southeast Asia.[49]

α^0-thalassemia results from deletions that involve both α-globin genes, and to date at least seventeen different deletions have been described.[11] The deletions that have attained high gene frequencies are found in individuals from Southeast Asia and South China $(--^{SEA})$, the Philippine Islands $(--^{FIL})$, Thailand $(--^{THAI})$, and a few Mediterranean countries, such as Greece and Cyprus $(--^{MED}$ and $-(\alpha)^{20.5})$. Although an α^0-thalassemia mutation $(--^{SA})$ has been described in Asian Indians, it is extremely uncommon, and no α^0-thalassemia deletions have been reported in individuals from sub-Saharan Africa. In Northern Europe, α-thalassemia occurs sporadically because of the lack of natural selection, and several α^0-thalassemia deletions have been reported in single British families, although one particular defect $(--^{BRIT})$ has been observed in a number of unrelated individuals living in Cheshire and Lancashire.

PCR Diagnosis

The α-thalassemia deletion alleles that can be currently diagnosed by the PCR-based technique known as gap PCR are listed in Table 19.4. These are two most common α^+-thalassemia alleles, $-\alpha^{3.7}$ and $-\alpha^{4.2}$, together with five α^0-thalassemia mutations, the $--^{MED}$, $-(\alpha)^{20.5}$, $--^{SEA}$, $--^{THAI}$, and $--^{FIL}$ alleles. Gap PCR involves the use of two primers complementary to the sense and antisense strand in the DNA regions that flank the α-thalassemia deletion.[50–52] Figure 19.1 shows the diagnosis of the $--^{MED}$ allele by this tech-

Table 19.4. Globin gene deletion mutations diagnosable by gap PCR

Disorder	Deletion	Distribution
α^0-thalassemia	$--^{SEA}$	Southeast Asia
	$--^{MED}$	Mediterranean
	$-(\alpha)^{20.5}$	Mediterranean
	$--^{FIL}$	Philippines
	$--^{THAI}$	Thailand
α^+-thalassemia	$-\alpha^{3.7}$	Worldwide
	$-\alpha^{4.2}$	Worldwide
β^0-thalassemia	290-bp deletion	Turkey, Bulgaria
	532-bp deletion	Africa
	619-bp deletion	India, Pakistan
	1393-bp deletion	Africa
	1605-bp deletion	Croatia
	3.5-kb deletion	Thailand
	10.3-kb deletion	India
	45-kb deletion	Philippines, Malaysia
$(\delta\beta)^0$ thalassemia	Hb Lepore	Mediterranean, Brazil
	Spanish	Spain
	Sicilian	Mediterranean
	Vietnamese	Vietnam
	Macedonian/Turkish	Macedonia, Turkey
$(^A\gamma\delta\beta)^0$-Thalassemia	Indian	India, Bangladesh
	Chinese	Southern China
HPFH	HPFH1 (African)	Africa
	HPFH2 (Ghanaian)	Ghana, Africa
	HPFH3 (Indian)	India

nique. Amplified product is obtained from only the deletion allele, because the distance between the two primers is too great to amplify normal DNA. The normal allele ($\alpha\alpha$) is detected by amplifying DNA sequences spanning one of the breakpoints, using a primer complementary to the deleted sequence. The primers can be multiplexed to detect more than one type of deletion per amplification reaction. We currently use a screening strategy of three amplification reactions: one for the two α^+-thalassemia alleles, one for the two Mediterranean α^0-thalassemia alleles, and one for the three Southeast Asian α^0-thalassemia alleles. Screening of carriers is targeted according to the ethnic origin of the individual, except for carriers of unknown origin, in whom all three multiplex reactions are used.

The nondeletion α^+-thalassemia mutations also may be detected by PCR, by the technique of selective amplification of the α_2-gene,[53] and then by analysis of the product for the appropriate mutation. Several of the nondeletion mutations alter a restriction enzyme site and may be analyzed for by restriction enzyme analysis, in a manner similar to that reported for the diagnosis of Hb Constant Spring by *MseI* digestion.[18] In theory, any other technique for the direct detection of point mutations, such as allele-specific oligonucleotide hybridization or allele-specific priming, may be used for the diagnosis of nondeletion α^0-thalassemia. However, no simple strategy to diagnose all the known mutations has been reported. The only published approach to date is a complex strategy involving the combined application of the indirect detection methods of denaturing gradient-gel electrophoresis (DGGE) and single-strand conformation analysis (SSCA), followed by direct DNA sequencing.[54]

Gap PCR provides a quick diagnostic test for α^0-thalassemia but requires careful application for prenatal diagnosis. Amplification of sequences in the α-globin gene

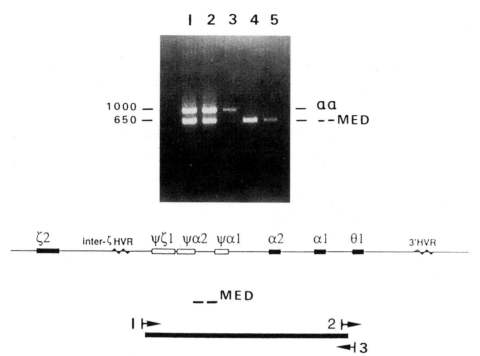

Fig. 19.1. Prenatal diagnosis of α^0-thalassemia using gap PCR to detect the $--^{MED}$ allele. The amplification products after agarose gel electrophoresis and ethidium bromide staining are shown as follows: track 1, maternal DNA; track 2, paternal DNA; track 3, normal DNA; tracks 4 and 5, different concentrations of chorionic villus DNA. A diagram shows the location of the $--^{MED}$ deletion with respect to the α-globin gene cluster, together with the positions of primers 1 and 3, which amplify $--^{MED}$ DNA to give a 650-bp product, and primers 2 and 3, which amplify only the normal allele to give a 1000-bp product.

cluster is technically more difficult than that of the β-globin gene cluster, possibly due to the higher GC content. Experience in my laboratory has shown that the first primer pairs to be published were unreliable, resulting occasionally in unpredictable reaction failure due to allele dropout. This is illustrated in Figure 19.1, in which the results for the chorionic villus DNA sample clearly give a homozygous genotype for α^0-thalassemia ($--^{MED}/--^{MED}$). However, Southern blot analysis of the same DNA sample clearly showed a heterozygous genotype ($--^{MED}/\alpha\alpha$), and a heterozygous phenotype was confirmed subsequently. However, the more recently published multiplex primers[52,53] have been found to be more robust and to give more reproducible results. As well as a redesign of the primer sequences, the addition of betaine to the reaction mixture and the use of a "hot start" amplification protocol seems to be key to the improved reliability.

Southern Blot Analysis

Southern blot analysis remains the only diagnostic test for the rare α-thalassemia deletions, and it is also used in my laboratory as a second approach for confirmation of prenatal diagnoses by gap PCR. The method also provides diagnostic information on triple and quadruple α-gene loci, which, when coinherited with β-thalassemia trait, may result in the phenotype of thalassemia intermedia.[55]

A list of the characteristic abnormal restriction fragments used in my laboratory for diagnostic purposes is presented in Table 19.5. A *Bam*HI digest hybridized to an α-globin gene probe is used to identify the single, double, triple, and quadruple α-globin gene alleles, and it provides a diagnostic test for the Mediterranean α^0-thalassemia deletion gene $-(\alpha)$.[20.5] A *Bam*HI digest hybridized to a ζ-globin gene probe provides a diagnostic test for the $--^{SEA}$ α^0-thalassemia allele and, similarly, a *Bgl*II digest hybridized to a ζ-globin gene probe provides a diagnostic test for the $--^{MED}$ allele. However, most α-thalassemia alleles are characterized by interpreting the combined results of a *Bam*HI/α-probe blot and a *Bgl*II/α-probe plot, as illustrated in Figure 19.2. This is because many of the abnormal *Bgl*II/α-probe fragments have sizes similar to those of other fragments. For example, both the $-\alpha^{3.7}$ and $\alpha\alpha\alpha$ alleles yield a 16-kb fragment; the $-\alpha^{4.2}$, $--^{SA}$, and $--^{BRIT}$ alleles yield a similar-sized fragment of 8 kb; and the $-(\alpha)^{20.5}$ and $--^{SEA}$ alleles yield fragments that can be confused with normal-sized fragments (Table 19.5). A combination of *Bam*HI and *Bgl*II digestions are used for the diagnosis of all the common α-thalassemia deletion genes except the $--^{THAI}$ and $--^{FIL}$ deletions, which require an *Sst*I digest hybridized to a DNA probe (named LO) located downstream to the ζ-globin gene.[56] For prenatal diagnosis, DNA from an affected fetus will show only the characteristic abnormal fragments and lack all of the DNA fragments produced from each parental normal chromosome (as shown in Figure 19.2). Although Southern blot analysis provides a comprehensive approach to the diagnosis of all the common α-gene deletions and rearrangements, the disadvantage of this approach is that it is a complex technique that takes 7–10 days to obtain a diagnostic result, and gap PCR is now routinely used for prenatal diagnosis of the common α^0-alassemia alleles.

Table 19.5.   The diagnosis of α-thalassemia and other alleles by Southern blotting

Allele	Restriction Enzyme/Gene Probe				
	*Bam*HI/α	*Bgl*II/α	*Bam*HI/ζ	*Bgl*II/ζ	*Sst*I/LO
$\alpha\alpha$	14	12.6	10–11.3	12.6 or 5.2	5.0
		7.4	5.9	10, 10.5, 11 or 11.3	
$\alpha\alpha\alpha$	<u>18</u>	12.6	10–11.3	12.6 or <u>16</u>	5.0
		7.4	5.9	10, 10.5, 11 or 11.3	
$\alpha\alpha\alpha\alpha$	<u>22</u>	12.6	10–11.3	12.6 or <u>20</u>	5.0
		7.4	5.9	10, 10.5, 11 or 11.3	
$-\alpha^{3.7}$	<u>10.3</u>	<u>16</u>	10–11.3	<u>16</u>	5.0
			5.9	10, 10.5, 11 or 11.3	
$-\alpha^{4.2}$	<u>9.8</u>	<u>8.0</u>	10–11.3	10, 10.5, 11 or 11.3	5.0
		7.4	5.9	<u>8.0</u>	
$-(\alpha)^{20.5}$	<u>4.0</u>	<u>10.8</u>	5.9	<u>10.8</u>	5.0
$--^{MED}$	None	None	5.9	<u>13.9</u>	5.0
$--^{SEA}$	None	None	<u>20</u>	<u>10.5</u>	5.0
			5.9		
$--^{SA}$	None	None	5.9	<u>7.0</u>	5.0
$--^{BRIT}$	None	None	5.9	<u>8.0</u>	5.0
$--^{THAI}$	None	None	None	None	<u>8.0</u>
$--^{FIL}$	None	None	None	None	<u>7.4</u>

Note: Fragment sizes are given in kilobase pairs. Characteristic abnormal fragments are underlined.

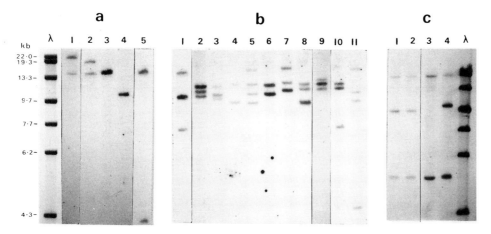

Fig. 19.2. Southern blot analysis showing the diagnosis of various α-thalassemia alleles by (a) *Bam*HI/α-probe hybridization, (b) *Bgl*II/ζ-probe hybridization, and (c) *Bam*HI/ζ-probe hybridization for the prenatal diagnosis of α^0-thalassemia. The outer two tracks show λ *Hin*dIII marker fragments. The genotypes (and band sizes in kilobase pairs) illustrated are: (a) 1: $\alpha\alpha\alpha\alpha/\alpha\alpha$ (22/14); 2: $\alpha\alpha\alpha/\alpha\alpha$ (18/14); 3: $\alpha\alpha/\alpha\alpha$ (14); 4: $-\alpha^{3.7}/\alpha^{3.7}$ (10.3); 5: $-(\alpha)^{20.5}/\alpha\alpha$ (14/4). (b) 1: $-\alpha^{3.7}/-\alpha^{4.2}$ (16/11.0/8); 2: $\alpha\alpha/\alpha\alpha$ (12.6/11.3/11.0); 3: $-(\alpha)^{20.5}/\alpha\alpha$ (12.6/11.0/10.8); 4: $\alpha\alpha/\alpha\alpha$ (12.6/10.5); 5: $-\alpha^{3.7}/\alpha\alpha$ (16/12.6/11.0/10.5); 6: $\alpha\alpha/\alpha\alpha$ (12.6/11.0); 7: $\alpha\alpha/\alpha\alpha$ (16/12.6/11.3); 8: $-^{SEA}/\alpha\alpha$ (12.6/11.3/10.5); 9: $-^{MED}/\alpha\alpha$ (13.9/12.6/11.3); 10: $-^{BRIT}/\alpha\alpha$ (12.6/11.3/8); 11: $-\alpha^{3.7}/-\alpha^{3.7}$ (16/11.0/10.5/5.5.2). (c) 1, maternal DNA: $-^{SEA}/\alpha\alpha$ (20/10/5.9); 2, paternal DNA: $-^{SEA}/\alpha\alpha$ (20/10/5.9); 3, CVS DNA: $-^{SEA}/-^{SEA}$ (20.5,9); 4, control DNA: $-^{SEA}/\alpha\alpha$ (20/11/5.9).

Note: The inter ζ-gene hypervariable region gives rise to normal DNA fragments of variable band sizes. There are four common *Bgl*II band sizes (10.0, 10.5, 11.0, and 11.3 kb), of which three are shown here. The $\psi\zeta$-gene also contains two small variable regions, which give rise to occasional variation in the size of the 12.6-kb *Bgl*II fragment (e.g., track 7). There is a polymorphic *Bgl*II site that, when present, reduces the 12.6-kb and $-\alpha^{3.7}$ 16-kb fragments to 5.2 kb (track 11).

β-Thalassemia

Although more than 170 different β-thalassemia mutations have been characterized, only about 25 occur at a frequency of 1 percent or greater and thus account for most mutations worldwide.[57] All of the mutations are regionally specific, and the spectrum of mutations has been determined. Each population has been found to have just a few of the commonly found mutations together with a larger and more variable number of rare ones.[48] The mutations can be classified broadly as being of Mediterranean, Indian, Chinese, or African origin; Table 19.6 lists the frequencies of the common mutations found in several countries from each of these four major ethnic groups. Within each ethnic group, there is still much variation in the distribution of mutations. For example, in Sardinia, the most common mutation is CD39 (C $\rightarrow$ T), which occurs at a frequency of 95 percent, whereas in Cyprus CD39 accounts for only approximately 2 percent of the mutations and the mutation IVSI-110 (G $\rightarrow$ A) is most common, at a frequency of 80 percent.[58]

The strategy for identifying β-thalassemia mutations in most diagnostic laboratories depends on knowing the spectrum of common and rare mutations in the ethnic group of the individual being screened. Usually, the common ones are analyzed first, using a PCR technique that allows the detection of multiple mutations simultaneously. This approach will identify the mutation in more than 90 percent of cases; an additional screening for the possible rare mutation will identify the defect in most of the remaining cases. Muta-

Table 19.6. The distribution of the common β-thalassemia mutations, expressed as percentage gene frequencies of the total number of thalassemia chromosomes studied

| Mutation | Mediterranean | | | India | | Chinese | | African |
	Italy	Greece	Turkey	Pakistan	India	China	Thailand	African American
−88 (C → T)					0.8			2.1
−87 (C → G)	0.4	1.8	1.2					
−30 (T → A)			2.5					
−29 (A → G)						1.9		60.3
−28 (A → G)						11.6	4.9	
CAP+1 (A → C)					1.7			
CD5 (−CT)		1.2	0.8					
CD6 (−A)	0.4	2.9	0.6					
CD8 (−AA)		0.6	7.4					
CD8/9 (+G)				28.9	12.0			
CD15 (G → A)				3.5	0.8			0.8
CD16 (−C)				1.3	1.7			
CD17 (A → T)					10.5	24.7		
CD24 (T → A)								7.9
CD39 (C → T)	40.1	17.4	3.5					
CD41/42 (−TCTT)				7.9	13.7	38.6	46.4	
CD71/72 (+A)						12.4	2.3	
IVSI-1 (G → A)	4.3	13.6	2.5					
IVSI-1 (G → T)				8.2	6.6			
IVSI-5 (G → C)				26.4		48.5	2.5	4.9
IVSI-6 (T → C)	16.3	7.4	17.4					
IVSI-110 (G → A)	29.8	43.7	41.9					
IVSII-1 (G → A)	1.1	2.1	9.7					
IVSII-654 (C → T)							15.7	8.9
IVSII-745 (C → G)	3.5	7.1	2.7					
619-bp deletion				23.3	13.3			
Others	4.1	2.2	9.7	0.5	0.9	6.8	7.9	10.6

CD = codon; IVS = intervening sequence.

tions remaining unknown after this second screening are characterized by direct DNA sequence analysis, usually after the localization of the site of the mutation by the application of a nonspecific detection method such as DGGE. Although a bewildering variety of PCR techniques have been described for the diagnosis of point mutations, most diagnostic laboratories are using one or more of the techniques described below.

Allele-Specific Oligonucleotides

The use of allele-specific oligonucleotide probes (ASOs) to hybridize to amplified DNA bound to nylon membrane in the form of dots was the first diagnostic PCR-based method to be developed. Since then it has been applied with great success, especially in populations such as the one in Sardinia with just one common mutation and a small number of rare ones.[59] The method is based on the use of two oligonucleotide probes for each mutation, one complementary to the mutant DNA sequence and the other complementary to the normal β-gene sequence at that position. The probes can be labeled with ^{32}P-labeled deoxynucleoside triphosphates, biotin, or horseradish peroxidase, but the method is limited by the need for separate hybridizations when screening for more than one mutation.

To overcome this problem, the method of reverse dot blotting has been developed, in which the roles of the oligonucleotide probe and amplified target DNA are reversed.[60] Probe pairs, complementary to the mutant and normal DNA sequences, are bound to nylon membrane in the form of dots or slots and the amplified DNA, labeled by either the use of end-labeled primers or the internal incorporation of biotinylated dUTP, is then hybridized to the filter. This procedure allows multiple mutations to be tested for in one hybridization reaction. It has been applied recently to the diagnosis of β-thalassemia mutations in Mediterraneans,[61] African Americans,[62] and Thais,[63] using a two-step procedure with one nylon strip for the common mutations and the other for the less common ones.

Primer-Specific Amplification

A number of different methods have been developed based on the principle of primer-specific amplification, which is that a perfectly matched PCR primer is much more efficient in annealing and directing primer extension than one containing one or two mismatched bases. The most widely used technique is the amplification refractory mutation system (ARMS), and its application is described in greater detail below. The technique has allowed the development of simple diagnostic strategies for the diagnosis of β-thalassemia mutations in individuals of many countries, including India, Pakistan, Thailand, Syria, Mauritius, and Sri Lanka.[63] In this method, the target DNA is amplified using a common primer and either of two allele-specific primers, one complementary to the mutation to be detected (β-thalassemia primer) and the other complementary to normal DNA at the same position in the sequence (normal primer). A second pair of primers complementary to a different part of the β-globin gene are included in the PCR to amplify a fragment simultaneously, to control the amplification step of the procedure. This quick screening method does not require any form of labeling because the amplified products are visualized simply by agarose-gel electrophoresis and ethidium bromide staining. More than one mutation may be screened for at the same time in a single PCR reaction (multiplexing), if the ARMS primers are coupled with the same common primer.[64] Fluorescence labeling of the common primer allows the sizing of the amplification products on an automated DNA fragment analyzer.[65]

If the normal and mutant ARMS primers for a specific mutation are coamplified in the same reaction, they compete with each other to amplify the target sequence. This technique is called competitive oligonucleotide priming (COP) and requires that the two ARMS primers be labeled differently. Fluorescent labels permit a diagnosis by means of a color complementation assay.[66] A variation of this method is simply to use ARMS primers that differ in length; therefore, a diagnosis can made by analysis of the different product sizes. This technique, called mutagenically separated polymerase chain reaction (MS-PCR), has been applied to the prenatal diagnosis of β-thalassemia in Taiwan.[67]

Restriction Enzyme Analysis

Approximately forty β-thalassemia mutations are known to create or abolish a restriction endonuclease site.[68] Most of these can be detected quickly by restriction endonuclease analysis of amplified DNA. The presence or absence of the enzyme site is determined from the pattern of digested fragments after agarose- or polyacrylamide-gel electrophoresis. As a screening method, this approach is limited by the small fraction of β-thalassemia mutations that affect a restriction enzyme site and because many of the restriction enzymes involved are very expensive.

Mutations that do not naturally create or abolish restriction sites may be detected by the technique of amplification-created restriction sites (ACRS). This method uses primers that are designed to insert new bases adjacent to the mutation sequence and thus to create a new restriction site allowing known mutations to be detected by restriction enzyme digestion of the PCR product.[69]

Gap PCR

Deletion mutations in the β-globin gene sequence may be detected by PCR using two primers complementary to the sense and antisense strand in the DNA regions that flank the deletion.[70] For large deletions, amplified product using flanking primers is obtained from only the deletion allele, because the distance between the two primers is too great to amplify normal DNA. In such cases, the normal allele may be detected by amplifying sequences spanning one of the breakpoints, using one primer complementary to the deleted sequence and one complementary to flanking DNA.[71] In addition to deletion β-thalassemia, Hb Lepore and a number of $\delta\beta$-thalassemia and HPFH deletion mutations can be diagnosed by this method.[72]

Unknown Mutations

A number of techniques have been applied for the detection of β-thalassemia mutations without prior knowledge of the molecular defect. The most widely used of these methods is DGGE, which allows the separation of DNA fragments differing by a single base change according to their melting properties.[73] Another approach is heteroduplex analysis using non-DGGE. Unique heteroduplex patterns can be generated for each mutation by annealing an amplified target DNA fragment with an amplified heteroduplex generator molecule, a synthetic oligonucleotide of about 130 bases in length containing deliberate sequence changes or identifiers at known mutation positions.[74] Other methods, such as mismatch cleavage (CMC), single-stranded conformational polymorphism analysis (SSCP), and protein truncation test, also are good methods of detecting unknown mutations, but they have not been applied to the hemoglobinopathies.

The above techniques simply pinpoint the presence of a mutation or DNA polymorphism in the amplified target sequence. Sequencing of the amplified product is then required to identify the localized mutation. This can now be performed very efficiently using an automated DNA sequencing machine using fluorescence detection technology. The specialized equipment required for this technique is very expensive, but as the machines become more efficient the cost will decrease and direct DNA sequencing will probably become the primary method for detecting a mutation.

Direct Detection: ARMS

The allele-specific priming technique, known as the amplification refractory mutation system (ARMS), was developed for the prenatal diagnosis of β-thalassemia in my laboratory.[75,76] For prenatal diagnosis, two primers must be designed that will generate specific amplification products: one with the mutant allele and the other with the normal sequence. The nucleotide at the 3' terminal of each primer is complementary to the base in the respective target sequence at the site of the mutation. In addition, a deliberate mismatch to the target sequence is included at the second, third, or fourth base from the 3' end. The deliberate mismatch enhances the specificity of the primer, because all 3'-terminal mismatches on their own, except for C-C, G-A, and A-A mismatches, will allow some ex-

tension of the primer and thus generate nonspecific amplification product.[77] The muta-
tion-specific ARMS primers for the most common β-thalassemia mutations and β-globin
variants are listed in Table 19.7. All are the same length (30 mers), so all can be used at
one annealing temperature (65°C), enabling screening for multiple mutations simultaneously. Primers for the specific detection of the corresponding normal allele are listed in
Table 19.8. These are required for prenatal diagnosis of cases in which both partners of
a couple at risk for β-thalassemia carry the same mutation. Each normal ARMS primer
must be tested to check that it is working correctly using DNA from an individual homozygous for the particular mutation. The list of primers in Table 19.8 is shorter than that
in Table 19.7 because of the lack of appropriate DNA controls in the laboratory.

Each ARMS primer requires a second primer to generate the allele-specific product;
in addition, two control primers must be included in the PCR reaction to generate an un-

Table 19.7. Primer sequences used for the detection of the common β-thalassemia mutations
by the allele-specific priming technique

Mutation	Oligonucleotide Sequence	Second Primer	Product Size (bp)
-88 (C → T)	TCACTTAGACCTCACCCTGTGGAGCCTCAT	A	684
-87 (C → G)	CACTTAGACCTCACCCTGTGGAGCCACCCG	A	683
-30 (T → A)	GCAGGGAGGGCAGGAGCCAGGGCTGGGGAA	A	626
-29 (A → G)	CAGGGAGGGCAGGAGCCAGGGCTGGGTATG	A	625
-28 (A → G)	AGGGAGGGCAGGAGCCAGGGCTGGGCTTAG	A	624
CAP+1 (A → G)	ATAAGTCAGGGCAGAGCCATCTATTGGTTC	A	597
CD5 ($-$CT)	TCAAACAGACACCATGGTGCACCTGAGTCG	A	528
CD6 ($-$A)	CCCACAGGGCAGTAACGGCAGACTTCTGCC	B	207
CD8 ($-$AA)	ACACCATGGTGCACCTGACTCCTGAGCAGG	A	520
CD8/9 ($+$G)	CCTTGCCCCACAGGGCAGTAACGGCACACC	B	225
CD15 (G → A)	TGAGGAGAAGTCTGCCGTTACTGCCCAGTA	A	500
CD16 ($-$C)	TCACCACCAACTTCATCCACGTTCACGTTC	B	238
CD17 (A → T)	CTCACCACCAACTTCAGCCACGTTCAGCTA	B	239
CD24 (T → A)	CTTGATACCAACCTGCCCAGGGCCTCTCCT	B	262
CD39 (C → T)	CAGATCCCCAAAGGACTCAAAGAACCTGTA	B	436
CD41/42 ($-$TCTT)	GAGTGGACAGATCCCCAAAGGACTCAACCT	B	439
CD71–72 ($+$A)	CATGGCAAGAAAGTGCTCGGTGCCTTTAAG	C	241
IVSI-1 (G → A)	TTAAACCTGTCTTGTAACCTTGATACCGAT	B	281
IVSI-1 (G → T)	TTAAACCTGTCTTGTAACCTTGATACCGAAA	B	281
IVSI-5 (G → C)	CTCCTTAAACCTGTCTTGTAACCTTGTTAG	B	285
IVSI-6 (T → C)	TCTCCTTAAACCTGTCTTGTAACCTTCATG	B	286
IVSI-110 (G → A)	ACCAGCAGCCTAAGGGTGGGAAAATAGAGT	B	419
IVSII-1 (G → A)	AAGAAAACATCAAGGGTCCCATAGACTGAT	B	634
IVSII-654 (C → T)	GAATAACAGTGATAATTTCTGGGTTAACGT*	D	829
IVSII-745 (C → G)	TCATATTGCTAATAGCAGCTACAATCGAGG*	D	738
β^SCD6 (A → T)	CCCACAGGGCAGTAACGGCAGACTTCTGCA	B	207
β^CCD6 (G → A)	CCACAGGGCAGTAACGGCAGACTTCTCGTT	B	206
β^ECD26 (G → A)	TAACCTTGATACCAACCTGCCCAGGGCGTT	B	236

Note: The above primers are coupled as indicated with primers A, B, C, or D.

A: CCCCTTCCTATGACATGAACTTAA

B: ACCTCACCCTGTGGAGCCAC

C: TTCGTCTGTTTCCCATTCTAAACT

D: GAGTCAAGGCTGAGAGATGCAGGA. The control primers used were primers D plus E: CAATGTATCATGC-
CTCTTTGCACC for all the above mutation specific ARMS primers except the two marked*, with which the $^G\gamma$-*Hind*III
RFLP primers (see Table 19.9) were used.

Table 19.8. Primer sequences used for the detection of the normal DNA sequence by the allele-specific priming technique

Mutation	Oligonucleotide Sequence	Second Primer	Product Size (bp)
−87 (C → G)	CACTTAGACCTCACCCTGTGGAGCCACCCC	A	683
CD5 (−CT)	CAAACAGACACCATGGTGCACCTGACTCCT	A	528
CD8 (−AA)	ACACCATGGTGCACCTGACTCCTGAGCAGA	A	520
CD8/9 (+G)	CCTTGCCCCACAGGGCAGTAACGGCACACT	B	225
CD15 (G → A)	TGAGGAGAAGTCTGCCGTTACTGCCCAGTA	A	500
CD39 (C → T)	TTAGGCTGCTGGTGGTCTACCCTTGGTCCC	A	299
CD41/42 (−TCTT)	GAGTGGACAGATCCCCAAAGGACTCAAAGA	B	439
IVSI-1 (G → A)	TTAAACCTGTCTTGTAACCTTGATACCCAC	B	281
IVSI-1 (G → T)	GATGAAGTTGGTGGTGAGGCCCTGGGTAGG	A	455
IVSI-5 (G → C)	CTCCTTAAACCTGTCTTGTAACCTTGTTAC	B	285
IVSI-6 (T → C)	AGTTGGTGGTGAGGCCCTGGGCAGGTTGGT	A	449
IVSI-110 (G → A)	ACCAGCAGCCTAAGGGTGGGAAAATACACC	B	419
IVSII-1 (G → A)	AAGAAAACATCAAGGGTCCCATAGACTGAC	B	634
IVSII-654 (C → T)	GAATAACAGTGATAATTTCTGGGTTAACGC	D	829
IVSII-745 (C → G)	TCATATTGCTAATAGCAGCTACAATCGAGC	D	738
β^SCD6 (A → T)	AACAGACACCATGGTGCACCTGACTCGTGA	A	527
β^ECD26 (G → A)	TAACCTTGATACCAACCTGCCCAGGGCGTC	B	236

Note: See note to Table 19.7 for details of primes A–D and control primers.

related product that indicates that the reaction mixture was set up properly and that everything is working correctly. The DNA sample is amplified with each mutant ARMS primer in a separate amplification reaction and the products visualized after electrophoresis. Figure 19.3 illustrates a screening of a sample for seven Mediterranean β-thalassemia mutations at one time. A control DNA known to carry each mutation was also amplified for comparison (even-numbered tracks). The unknown DNA sample produced an amplified product with only the IVSI-110 mutant primer (track 1). For couples of Cypriot origin, this mutation usually is screened for first because it is so common; if it is not found, all of the others are screened for simultaneously afterward. Similarly, for Asian Indian couples, the four most common mutations, IVSII-5, IVSI-1, Fr.8/9, and Fr.41/42,[78] are screened for first. The 619-bp deletion gene also is screened for in the same reaction because the control pair of primers are designed to span the deletion, and instead of a normal 861-bp fragment, a characteristic 242-bp fragment is produced.[75] Note that the DNA from an individual doubly heterozygous for the 619-bp deletion and, say, the IVSI-5 mutation will produce three bands: the 861-bp fragment from the IVSI-5 allele, an IVSI-5 specific fragment of 285 bp from the mutant IVSI-5 ARMS primer, and the 242-bp fragment.

Figure 19.4 illustrates a prenatal diagnosis for a fetus at risk for two different mutations: codon 39 and IVSI-110. A normal ARMS primer is not required in this case because the fetal DNA has to be tested with the mutant ARMS primer for each mutation. The CVS DNA in Figure 19.4 was diagnosed as β-thalassemia trait, having inherited the codon 39 mutation from the father and a normal allele from the mother.

Indirect Detection: Haplotype Analysis

Linkage analysis of restriction-fragment-length polymorphisms (RFLPs) within the β-globin gene cluster often can be used for prenatal diagnosis of β-thalassemia in the rare

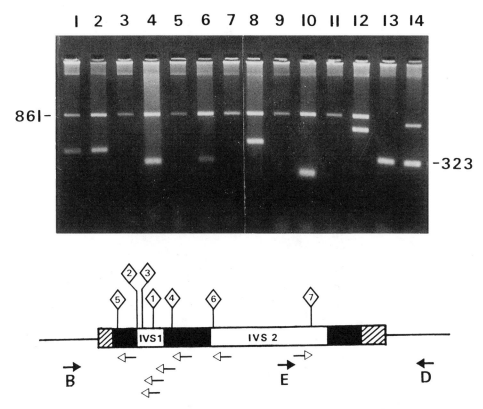

Fig. 19.3. The screening of a DNA sample for seven common Mediterranean mutations by the allele specific priming technique known as ARMS. The diagram shows the β-globin gene and the positions of the seven mutations: 1, IVSI-110; 2, IVSI-1; 3, IVSI-6; 4 codon 39; 5, codon 6; 6, IVSII-1; 7, IVSII-745. The gel shows the amplification products from DNA of a β-thalassemia heterozygote in the odd-numbered lanes, and products generated by control DNAs in the even-numbered lanes for each mutation screened for: IVSI-110, G → A (lanes 1 and 2); IVSI-1, G → A (lanes 3 and 4); IVSI-6, T → C, (lanes 5 and 6); codon 39, C → T (lanes 7 and 8); codon 6, −A, (lanes 9 and 10), IVSII-1, G → A (lanes 10 and 11), IVSII-745, C → G (lanes 13 and 14). In lanes 1–12, the control primers D and E produced an 861-bp fragment, and in lanes 13 and 14, a different pair of control primers produced a 323-bp fragment. The primers used are listed in Tables 19.5 and 19.7.

cases in which one or both of the mutations remain unidentified after screening using a direct-detection method such as ARMS. The technique also can enable the prenatal diagnosis of uncharacterized $\delta\beta$-thalassemia deletion mutations through the apparent nonmendelian inheritance of RFLPs (due to the hemizygosity created by the inheritance of deleted sequences on one chromosome). Finally, haplotype analysis may provide an alternative approach for the confirmation of a prenatal diagnosis result obtained by a direct detection method such as ARMS and, in very rare instances, has helped to reveal a possible diagnostic error.

At least eighteen RFLPs have been characterized within the β-globin gene cluster.[79] However, most of these RFLP sites are nonrandomly associated with each other; thus, they combine to produce just a handful of haplotypes.[80] In particular, they form a 5′ cluster that is 5′ to the δ gene and a 3′ cluster that extends downstream from the β-globin gene. In between is a 9-kb stretch of DNA containing a relative hot spot for meiotic recombination. The recombination between the two clusters has been calculated to be approximately 1 in 350 meioses.[81] Hybridization studies have shown that each β-thalassemia

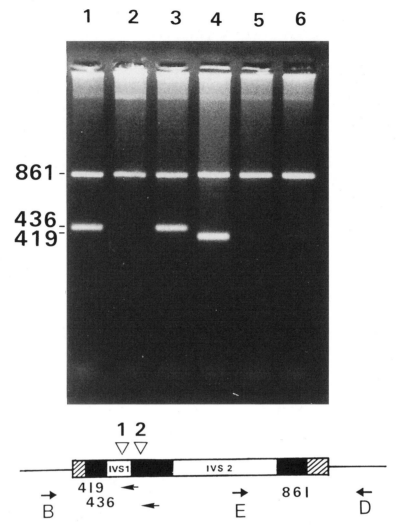

Fig. 19.4. Prenatal diagnosis of β-thalassemia by the allele-specific priming technique known as ARMS. The diagram shows the positions of the β-thalassemia mutations IVSI-110, G → A, (1) and codon 39, C → T, (2), plus the locations of the primers used to diagnose these two mutations (as specified in Table 19.5). The gel shows the amplification products using the mutant ARMS primer for codon 39 (lanes 1, 2, and 3) and for IVSI-110 (lanes 4, 5, and 6). The DNA samples were: lane 1, fetal DNA; lane 2, maternal DNA; lane 3, paternal DNA; lane 4, maternal DNA; lane 5, paternal DNA; lane 6, fetal DNA. The 436-p product is diagnostic for the codon 39 mutation and the 419-bp product for IVSI-110.

mutation is strongly associated with just one or two haplotypes,[82] probably because of their recent origin compared with the haplotypes. Thus, haplotype analysis has been used to study the origins of identical mutations found in different ethnic groups. The β-globin gene cluster haplotype normally consists of five RFLPs located in the 5' cluster (HindII/ε-gene; HindIII/^{G}γ-gene; HindIII/^{A}ψ-gene; HindII/3'øβ; and HindII/5'ψβ) and two RFLPs in the 3' cluster (AvaII/β-gene; BamHI/β-gene).[83]

All of the seven RFLPs except BamHI can be analyzed by PCR very simply and quickly.[84] Primers have been designed to span the RFLP site and produce easily identifiable fragments after electrophoresis of the digested products in an agarose gel, which usually is composed of a mixture of agarose and Nusieve agarose (1:3) to give good resolution of small fragments. The primer sequences and sizes of the fragments generated are listed in Table 19.9. The *Bam*HI RFLP is located within an L1 repetitive element, creating amplification problems and a *Hin*fI RFLP located just 3′ to the β-globin gene is used instead, because these two RFLPs have been found to exist in linkage disequilibrium.[85] Three other RFLPs are included in Table 19.9. An *Ava*II RFLP in the γβ-gene is extremely useful in haplotype analysis of Mediterranean β-thalassemia heterozygotes. The (−) allele for this RFLP is frequently found on chromosomes carrying the IVSI-110 mutation, whereas it is very rare on normal β-globin chromosomes[86] and thus is a very useful informative marker for individuals heterozygous for this mutation. The *Rsa*I RFLP located just 5′ to the β-globin gene is useful for linkage analysis because it seems to be unlinked to either the 5′ cluster or the 3′ cluster RFLPs and thus may be informative when the 5′ haplotype and the 3′ haplotype are not. Finally, the ^Gγ-*Xmn*I RFLP, created by the nondeletion HPFH C → T mutation at position −158, is included because of its use in the analysis of sickle cell gene haplotypes and in individuals with thalassemia intermedia.

If a family study is possible, we always use RFLPs for the confirmation of a prenatal diagnosis of β-thalassemia made by the direct detection of mutations using the ARMS technique. To obtain the linkage phase of informative RFLPs, one requires DNA from: (1) a normal or an affected child; (2) both sets of grandparents if no children are available; or (3) one set of grandparents if a child heterozygous for β-thalassemia is available. It is essential that one of the grandparents on each side of the family is normal with re-

Table 19.9. Oligonucleotide primers used for analysis of β-globin gene cluster RFLPs

RFLP	Primer Sequence 5′-3′	Annealing Temperature (°C)	Product Size (bp)	Absence of Site (bp)	Presence of Site (bp)
ε-*Hin*dII	TCTCTGTTTGATGACAAATTC	55	760	760	314
	AGTCATTGGTCAAGGCTGACC	55			446
^Gγ-*Xmn*I	AACTGTTGCTTTATAGGATTTT	55	650	650	450
	AGGAGCTTATTGATAACTCAGAC	55			200
^Gγ-*Hin*dIII	AGTGCTGCAAAGAAGAACAACTACC	65	323	323	235
	CTCGCATCATGGGCCAGTGAGCCTC	65			98
^Aγ-*Hin*dIII	ATGCTGCTAATGCTTCATTAC	55	635	635	327
	TCATTGTGTGATCTCTCTCAGCAG	55			308
5′ψβ-*Hin*dII	TCCTATCCATTACTGTTCCTTGAA	55	794	794	687
	ATTGTCTTATTCTAGAGACGATTT	55			107
5′ψβ-*Ava*II	TCCTATCCATTACTGTTCCTTGAA	55	794	794	442
	ATTGTCTTATTCTAGAGACGATTT	55			352
3′ψβ-*Hin*dII	GTACTCATACTTTAAGTCCTAACT	55	914	914	480
	TAAGCAAGATTATTTCTGGTCTCT	55			434
β-*Rsa*I	AGACATAATTTATTAGCATGCATG	55	1200	692	692
	CCCCTTCCTATGACATGAACTTAA	55		413	331
				100	100
					82
β-*Ava*II	GTGGTCTACCCTTGGACCCAGAGG	65	328	328	227
	TTCGTCTGTTTCCCATTCTAAACT	65			101
β-*Hin*fI	GGAGGTTAAAGTTTTGCTATGCTGTAT	55	475	320	219
	GGGCCTATGATAGGGTAAT	55		155	155
					108

spect to β-thalassemia; otherwise, the linkage phase cannot be determined. For the correct assignment, it is essential that all the individuals analyzed have been phenotyped correctly and that paternity is true. Because of the nonrandom association of the RFLPs in the 5' cluster, it is not necessary to analyze all of these RFLPs. In our laboratory, we analyze just the two *Hin*dII RFLPs in the $\gamma\beta$-gene. These two sites can identify the three most common 5' haplotypes in Caucasians ($+----$, $-++-+$, $-+-++$). We then analyze the 3' cluster RFLPs in the order *Ava*II, *Hin*fI, *Rsa*I until an informative RFLP is found. It is important to study these even if the 5' haplotype is informative for prenatal diagnosis because of the very slight change of recombination between the 5' cluster and the β-globin gene.

Informative RFLPs are found in more than 80 percent of the families studied; thus, haplotype analysis is a very useful alternative approach to provide confirmation of a diagnosis obtained by the direct detection of mutations. In our first 100 diagnoses using ARMS primers, there was only one case in which RFLP linkage analysis gave a prediction different from that obtained with the ARMS primers.[75] Fresh blood samples were obtained from all of the individuals involved in this particular case, and additional investigation revealed mislabeled DNA in the first batch of samples. Thus, a combination of the two different approaches identified one possible cause of error and misdiagnosis (switched or wrongly labeled samples). Such a strategy may help reveal other possible errors, such as maternal DNA contamination and nonpaternity.

$d\beta$-Thalassemia, Hb Lepore, and HPFH

$\delta\beta$-Thalassemia and the deletion types of HPFH are characterized by the complete absence of Hb A and Hb A_2 in homozygotes and an elevated level of Hb F in heterozygotes. Both conditions are caused by large DNA deletions involving the β-globin gene cluster affecting the β and δ genes but leaving either one or both of the γ-globin genes intact. More than fifty different deletion mutations have been identified,[87] and they can be classified into the $(\delta\beta)^0$ and $(^A\gamma\delta\beta)^0$ thalassemias, HPFH conditions, fusion chain variants, and $(\varepsilon\gamma\delta\beta)^0$ thalassemia.

$\delta\beta$-thalassemia

The $(\delta\beta)^0$ thalassemias are characterized by the Hb F consisting of both $^G\gamma$- and $^A\gamma$-globin chains, as both γ-globin genes remain intact in these conditions. Heterozygotes have normal levels of Hb A_2 and an Hb F level of 5–15 percent, which, for most mutations, is heterogeneously distributed in the red cells. There is a reduction of the non-α-globin chains compared with α-globin, and the red cells are hypochromic and microcytic. Homozygotes for this condition have thalassemia intermedia.

The $(^A\gamma\delta\beta)^0$ thalassemias are characterized by the Hb F containing only $^G\gamma$-globin chains, as the $^G\gamma$-globin gene has been deleted in these conditions. Apart from this distinction, the phenotype of the heterozygous and homozygous states are identical to those for $(\delta\beta)^0$-thalassemia.

The $(\varepsilon\gamma\delta\beta)^0$ thalassemias are conditions that result from several different long deletions that start upstream of the ε-gene and remove all of the β-globin gene cluster, or in two cases, the deletion ends between the δ- and β-genes, thus sparing the β-globin gene, but in both cases, no β-globin synthesis occurs. This is because the deletions remove the β-globin gene cluster locus control region (LCR) located 50 kb upstream of the ε-gene. In adult life, heterozygotes for this condition have a hematologic picture similar to that of β-thalassemia trait, with a normal Hb A_2 level. The homozygous condition is presumed to be incompatible with fetal survival.

Hb Lepore

Two deletions in the β-globin gene cluster create an abnormal Hb chain as a result of unequal crossing over between globin genes. Hb Lepore is a hybrid globin chain composed of δ and β gene sequences, and Hb Kenya is composed of γ and β gene sequences. Hb Lepore homozygotes have a phenotype similar to that of thalassemia major or severe thalassemia intermedia. Hb Kenya has been observed only in the heterozygous state and is similar to heterozygous HPFH, with individuals having 5–10 percent Hb F, normal red cell morphology, and balanced globin-chain synthesis.

Hereditary Persistence of Fetal Hemoglobin (HPFH)

The deletional HPFH conditions can be regarded as a type of $\delta\beta$-thalassemia in which the reduction in β-globin chain production is almost completely compensated for by the increased γ-globin chain production. Homozygous individuals have 100 percent F composed of both $^A\gamma$ and $^G\gamma$ globin chains but, in contrast to $(\delta\beta)^0$-thalassemia homozygotes, are clinically normal. Heterozygotes have an elevated Hb F level of 17–35 percent, higher than that found in $\delta\beta$-thalassemia heterozygotes, and the Hb F is distributed uniformly (pancellular) in red cells with near-normal MCH and MCV values.

Finally, there is a group of conditions called nondeletion HPFH in which heterozygous individuals have normal red cells and no clinical abnormalities and an elevated Hb F level as a result of a point mutation in the promoter region of the $^A\gamma$- or $^G\gamma$-globin gene in most cases. The percentage Hb F is variable, ranging from 1 to 3 percent in the Swiss type to 10 to 20 percent in the Greek type. The only recorded homozygotes for nondeletion HPFH are for the British type described in a single family.

PCR-based diagnosis is by gap PCR, which can now be applied, six $\delta\beta$-thalassemia, three HPFH deletion mutations and for Hb Lepore,[43] all of which have had both breakpoint sequences characterized to permit the synthesis of amplification primers.[72] These deletion mutations are listed in Table 19.4. The remaining $\delta\beta$-thalassemia and HPFH deletion mutations can be characterized only by Southern blot analysis using restriction-enzyme mapping to diagnose characteristic abnormal DNA fragments that span the breakpoint of the deletion. Selection of the right restriction-enzyme digest and gene probe depends on identifying the ethnic origin of the individual to be studied and characterization of the phenotype in the heterozygous state.

Hb S

Hb S (β Glu $\rightarrow$ Val) is caused by an A $\rightarrow$ T substitution in the second nucleotide of the sixth codon of the β-globin gene. The mutation destroys the recognition site for three restriction enzymes, Mn/I, $DdeI$, and $MstII$, the latter being the enzyme of choice for the detection of the β^S allele by Southern blot analysis[82] because it cuts infrequently around the β-globin gene, producing large DNA fragments. However, for PCR diagnosis $DdeI$ is used.[88] $DdeI$ is a frequent cutter, and several constant sites can be included in the amplified β-gene fragment to act as a control for the complete digestion of the amplified product. The primer sequences currently used in my laboratory are presented in Table 19.10. A $DdeI$ analysis of amplified DNA from a normal individual (AA), an individual with sickle cell trait (AS), and a sickle cell homozygote (SS) is shown in Figure 19.5. The β^S mutation creates a 321-bp

Table 19.10. Oligonucleotide primers for the detection of β^S, β^E, β^D Punjab, and β^0 Arab mutations as RFLPs

Mutation and Affected RE Site	Primer Sequence 5′–3′	Annealing Temperature (°C)	Product Size (bp)	Absence of Site (bp)	Presence of Site (bp)
β^SCD6 (A$_C$T) (loses *Dde*I site)	ACCTCACCCTGTGGAGCCAC	65	443	386	201
	GAGTGGACAGATCCCAAAGGACTCAAGGA	54		67	175
C^{E}CD26 (G$_C$A) loses *Mnl*I site	ACCTCACCCTGTGGAGCCAC	65	443	231	67
	GAGTGGACAGATCCCAAAGGACTCAAGGA			89	171
				56	89
				35	60
				33	35
					33
β^DPunjab CD121 (GC) (loses *Eco*RI site)	CAATGTATCATGCCTCTTTGCACC	65	861	861	552
	GAGTCAAGGCTGAGAGATGCAGGA	65	309		
β^0 Arab CD121 (G$_C$A) (loses *Eco*RI site)	CAATGTATCATGCCTCTTTGCACC	65	861	861	552
	GAGTCAAGGCTGAGAGATGCAGGA	65			309

692

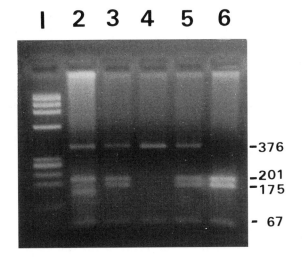

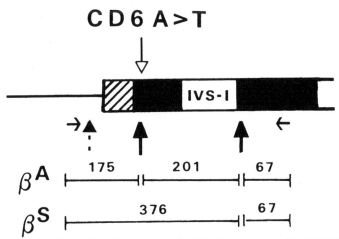

Fig. 19.5. The diagnosis of the sickle cell anemia gene by *Dde*I digestion of amplified DNA. The diagram shows the location of the two PCR primers used (as listed in Table 19.8) and the sites of the *Dde*I sites with respect to the β^S gene mutation at codon 6. The *Dde*I site 5′ to codon 6, marked by the dotted arrow, is a rare polymorphic site caused by the sequence change G → A at position −83 to the β-globin gene. When present the 175-bp fragment is cleaved to give 153-bp and 27-bp fragments as shown in lane 2. The gel shows DNA fragments from: lane 1, φX174 digested with *Hae*III; lane 2, AS individual; lane 3, fetal DNA with AS genotype; lane 4, SS individual; lane 5, AS individual; lane 6, AA individual.

fragment that is absent in the normal DNA sample. The β^S mutation can also be detected by a variety of other PCR-based techniques, such as ASO/dot blotting or the ARMS method. The primer sequences for the latter method are included in Table 19.7.

Hb C

Hb C (β6 Glu → Lys) is caused by G → A substitution in the first nucleotide of codon 6 of the β-globin gene. It is found predominantly in West Africans, and the frequency of heterozygous state has reached 28 percent in some parts of Ghana. The heterozygous state is symptomless, and the homozygous state is characterized by a variable hemolytic anemia due to the red cells' being abnormally rigid and having a shortened lifespan, but it is associated with no serious clinical disability.[10] Its importance lies in its interaction with the sickle cell gene.

The Hb C mutation also occurs inside the recognition sites for $Mn/$I, DdeI, and MstII at codon 6. However, it does not abolish the site for DdeI or MstII because the mutation affects a nonspecific nucleotide in the recognition sequence. Thus, DdeI or MstII cannot be used to detect the β^C mutation, and another method, such as allele-specific oligonucleotide hybridization to amplified DNA or the allele-specific priming technique must be used. The primer sequences used for the latter method are included in Tables 19.7 and 19.8.

Hb D-Punjab and Hb O-Arab

Hb D-Punjab (β121 Glu $\rightarrow$ Gln) and Hb O-Arab (β121 Glu $\rightarrow$ Lys) in combination with Hb S give rise to doubly heterozygous conditions that are similar in severity to homozygous sickle cell disease. Hb D-Punjab in combination with β-thalassemia trait has very little effect, and the phenotype observed is similar to that of a β-thalassemia heterozygote. In contrast, the Hb O-Arab mutation in combination with a β^0-thalassemia gene leads to a moderately severe disorder with a phenotype not dissimilar to that of Hb E thalassemia.[10]

The Hb D-Punjab and Hb O-Arab mutations abolish an EcoRI site at codon 121,[89] and their detection is carried out simply by amplification of a fragment containing the site and digesting with EcoRI. Because there are no other EcoRI sites within several kilobases of the β-globin gene, care should be taken always to run appropriate control DNA samples. The primer sequences used for this approach are listed in Table 19.10.

Hb E

Hb E results from a G $\rightarrow$ A mutation at codon 26 in the β-globin gene. This point mutation activates the cryptic splice site between codons 24 and 27, resulting in a β-thalassemia phenotype because of the production of two forms of β-globin mRNA. The normally spliced mRNA containing the β^E mutation is produced at a low level and leads to a deficiency of β^E-globin because the abnormally spliced mRNA does not produce a recognizable β-globin. The heterozygous and homozygous states for Hb E are associated with no clinical disability. The importance of Hb E lies in its interaction with β-thalassemia.

The Hb E mutation abolishes an MnlI site and may be diagnosed by PCR and restriction-enzyme analysis.[90] The primer sequences for this approach are listed in Table 19.10. However, the Hb E mutation is more commonly diagnosed by the use of ASO probes or ARMS primers, and the sequences for the latter are listed in Tables 19.7 and 19.8.

DIAGNOSTIC PITFALLS

PCR-based techniques now provide a quick and relatively simple method for the carrier detection and prenatal diagnosis of α^0-thalassemia, β-thalassemia, and sickle cell disease. The techniques have proven to be reliable and accurate as long as careful attention is given to potential diagnostic pitfalls and best practice guidelines are followed. Best practice guidelines have been prepared following a meeting of European Molecular Genetics Network (EMQN) in 2002 and can be downloaded from http://www.emqn.org/emqn.php.

Maternal DNA Contamination

The most important problem is the possible coamplification of maternal DNA sequences. With chorionic villus samples, this is avoided by the careful dissection of maternal decidua from the fetal trophoblast by microscopic dissection,[42] as shown by the experience of the Italian groups who reported no misdiagnosis in 457 first-trimester diagnoses for β-thalassemia in the Italian population using the method of dot-blot analysis.[91] Amniotic fluid cell DNA also may be contaminated with maternal DNA sequences through the contamination of an amniotic fluid sample with maternal blood. In a prenatal diagnosis program for sickle cell disease in the United States, one such misdiagnosis was reported to have occurred in a total of 500 prenatal diagnoses.[92] It is recommended that, in all diagnoses using cultured amniotic fluid cells in which the fetal genotype is determined to be identical to the maternal genotype, the diagnosis be confirmed using cultured amniocytes or by the inheritance of both maternal and paternal polymorphic markers. It is recommended as good practice to check maternal DNA contamination by polymorphism analysis using variable tandem repeat (VNTR) markers or short tandem repeat (STR) markers in all instances.

PCR Failure

Another potential source of error is the failure to amplify one of the target DNA alleles. In my own experience, this occurred once in a prenatal diagnosis of α^0-thalassemia, for which the PCR-based result was different from that obtained by Southern blot analysis because of a failure of amplification of the fetal normal α-globin gene allele. Amplification failure also may result when the hybridization of a primer or probe is compromised by an unexpected change in the target DNA sequence.[93]

Diagnostic Error Rate

It is important for clinicians to understand that direct detection methods will detect only the particular mutation screened for. A diagnostic error may occur if the fetus inherits an unsuspected mutation as a result of nonpaternity or, as happened in two prenatal diagnoses for sickle cell disease in my laboratory, when incorrect information was supplied about parental phenotypes. In both cases, the partner in question was not available for testing at the time of the prenatal diagnosis. However, such instances are very uncommon, as revealed by an audit of the accuracy of 3,254 prenatal diagnoses for the hemoglobinopathies in the United Kingdom.[94] The study revealed ten nonlaboratory errors as well as fifteen errors due to technical problems: eight diagnostic errors associated fetal blood sampling and globin chain synthesis, five errors by Southern blot analysis, and two errors with PCR techniques. The diagnostic error rate for prenatal diagnosis by PCR methods, including nonlaboratory and technical errors was calculated to be 0.41 percent, confirming it to be a more reliable method than the previous technologies of Southern blotting (0.73 percent error rate) and globin-chain synthesis (1.55 percent error rate).

In conclusion, the adoption of PCR techniques and the use of best practice guidelines has helped to minimize the misdiagnosis rate but it has not reduced it to zero and all clinicians should be aware of the slight risk of misdiagnosis and counsel couples undergoing prenatal diagnosis accordingly.

Fetal DNA Diagnosis: Guidelines for Best Practice

1. Ensure that fresh parental blood samples are obtained with the fetal sample in order to check the parental phenotypes and to provide fresh control DNA samples. In cases in which the father is not available, as often seems to happen with sickle cell prenatal diagnoses, copies of all laboratory results should be seen.
2. In such cases at risk for a sickle cell disorder, extra tests are carried out when a blood sample from the father is not available. The fetal DNA is always analyzed for β^S, β^C, and common β-thalassemia mutations in the parents' ethnic group when an AS genotype is diagnosed, to avoid an incorrect diagnosis as far as possible.
3. Ensure that the chorionic villus sample has undergone careful microscopic dissection to remove any contaminating maternal decidua.
4. Always analyze parental and appropriate control DNAs with the fetal DNA, and always repeat the fetal DNA analysis to double check the result.
5. Whenever possible, use an alternative diagnostic method to confirm the diagnosis.
6. Check for maternal DNA contamination in every case. Polymorphism analysis by PCR is used routinely to exclude error due to maternal DNA contamination or nonpaternity.
7. The fetal DNA diagnosis report should detail the types of DNA analysis used and clearly state the risk of misdiagnosis due to technical errors based on current data.

REFERENCES

1. Petrou M, Modell B. Prenatal screening for haemoglobin disorders. Prenat Diagn 1995;15:1275.
2. Kan YW, Golbus M, Trecartin R, et al. Prenatal diagnosis of homozygous β-thalassaemia. Lancet 1975;2: 790.
3. Alter BP. Antenatal diagnosis, summary of results. Ann NY Acad Sci 1990;612:237.
4. Kan YW, Dozy AM. Antenatal diagnosis of sickle-cell anemia by DNA analysis of amniotic-fluid cells. Lancet 1978;2:910.
5. Kazazian HH Jr, Philips III JA, Boehm CD, et al. Prenatal diagnosis of β-thalassaemia by amniocentesis: linkage analysis using multiple polymorphic restriction endonuclease sites. Blood 1980;56:926.
6. Old JM, Ward RHT, Petrou M, et al. First-trimester fetal diagnosis for haemoglobinopathies: three cases. Lancet 1982;2:1413.
7. Canadian Collaborative CVS-Amniocentesis Clinical Trial Group. Multicentre randomised clinical trial of chorionic villus sampling and amniocentesis. Lancet 1989;1:1.
8. Firth HV, Boyd PA, Chamberlain PF, et al. Analysis of limb reduction defects in babies exposed to chorionic villus sampling. Lancet 1994;343:1069.
9. World Health Organization. Community control of hereditary anaemias: memorandum from a WHP meeting. Bull World Health Organ 1983;61:63.
10. Weatherall DJ, Clegg JB. The thalassemia syndromes, 4th ed. Oxford: Blackwell Scientific, 2001.
11. Higgs DR. α-Thalassaemia. In: Higgs DR, Weatherall DJ, eds. Baillière's clinical haematology: international practice and research: the haemoglobinopathies. London: Baillière Tindall, 1993:117.
12. Thein SL. β-thalassaemia. In: Higgs DR, Weatherall DJ, eds. Baillière's clinical haematology: international practice and research: the haemoglobinopathies. London: Baillière Tindall, 1993:151.
13. Stamatoyannopoulos G, Nienhuis AW. Hemoglobin switching. In: Stamatoyannopoulos G, Nienhuis AW, Majerus PW, et al., eds. The molecular basis of blood diseases. Philadelphia: WB Saunders, 1994:107.
14. Rodgers GP, Steinberg MH. Pharmacologic treatment of sickle cell disease and thalassemia: the augmentation of fetal hemoglobin. In: Steinberg MH, Forget BG, Higgs DR, Nagel RL, eds. Disorders of hemoglobin: genetics, pathophysiology and clinical management. Cambridge: Cambridge University Press, 2001:1028.
15. Charache S, Terrin ML, Moore RD, et al. Effect of hydroxyurea on the frequency of painful crises in sickle cell anemia. N Engl J Med 1995;332:1317.
16. Sher GD, Ginder GD, Little J, et al. Extended therapy with intravenous arginine butyrate in patients with beta-hemoglobinopathies. N Engl J Med 1995;332:1606.

17. Higgs DR. The molecular genetics of the α globin gene family. Eur J Clin Invest 1990;20:340.

18. Ko TM, Tseng LH, Hsieh FJ, et al. Prenatal diagnosis of HbH disease due to compound heterozygosity for south-east Asian deletion and Hb Constant Spring by polymerase chain reaction. Prenat Diagn 1993;13:143.

19. Baysal E. The β- and α-thalassemia repository. Hemoglobin 1995;19:213.

20. Thein SL, Hesketh C, Wallace RB, et al. The molecular basis of thalassaemia major and thalassaemia intermedia in Asian Indians: application to prenatal diagnosis. Br J Haematol 1988;70:225.

21. Huang SZ, Wong C, Antonarakis SE, et al. The same TATA box β-thalassaemia mutation in Chinese and US blacks: another example of independent origins of mutation. Hum Genet 1986;74:152.

22. Munro S, Loudianos G, Deiana M, et al. Molecular characterisation of β-thalassaemia intermedia in patients of Italian descent and identification of three novel β-thalassaemia mutations. Blood 1991;77:1342.

23. Craig JE, Kelly SJ, Basrneston R, et al. Molecular characterisation of a novel 10.3 kb deletion causing β-thalassaemia with unusually high Hb A_2. Br J Haematol 1992;82:735.

24. Thein SL, Hesketh C, Taylor P, et al. Molecular basis for dominantly inherited inclusion body β-thalassaemia. Proc Natl Acad Sci USA 1990;87:3924.

25. Fucharoen S. Hb E disorders. In: Steinberg MH, Forget BG, Higgs DR, Nagel RL, eds. Disorders of hemoglobin: genetics, pathophysiology and clinical management. Cambridge: Cambridge University Press, 2001:1139.

26. Steinberg MH. Compound heterozygous and other sickle hemoglobinopathies. In: Steinberg MH, Forget BG, Higgs DR, Nagel RL, eds. In: Disorders of hemoglobin: genetics, pathophysiology and clinical management. Cambridge: Cambridge University Press. 2001:786.

27. Pagnier J, Mears JG, Dunda-Belkodja O, et al. Evidence of the multicentric origin of the hemoglobin S gene in Africa. Proc Natl Acad Sci USA 1984;81:1771.

28. Powars DR. β^S-gene cluster haplotypes in sickle cell anemia. Hematol Oncol Clin North Am 1991;5:475.

29. Old J. Screening and genetic diagnosis of hemoglobin disorders. Blood Rev 2003;17:43.

30. Bhavnani M, Brozovic M, Old JM, et al. Guidelines for the fetal diagnosis of globin gene disorders. J Clin Pathol 1994;47:199.

31. The Thalassaemia Working Party of the BSCH General Haematology Task Force. Guidelines for the laboratory diagnosis of hemoglobinopathies. Br J Haematol 1998;101:783.

32. Orkin SH, Alter BP, Altay C, et al. Application of endonuclease mapping to the analysis and prenatal diagnosis of the thalassaemia caused by globin gene deletion. N Engl J Med 1978;299:166.

33. Alter BP. Advances in the prenatal diagnosis of hematologic diseases. Blood 1984;64:329.

34. Old JM, Fitches A, Heath C, et al. First-trimester fetal diagnosis for haemoglobinopathy: report on 200 cases. Lancet 1986;2:763.

35. Old JM. Fetal DNA analysis. In: Davies KE, ed. Genetic analysis of the human disease: a practical approach. Oxford: IRL Press, 1986:1.

36. Rodeck CH, Nicolaides KH, Morsman JM, et al. A single-operator technique for first-trimester chorion biopsy. Lancet 1983;2:1340.

37. Ward RHT, Modell B, Petrou M, et al. A method of chorionic villi sampling in the first trimester of pregnancy under real-time ultrasonic guidance. BMJ 1983;286:1542.

38. Smidt-Jensen S, Hahnemann N, Hariri J, et al. Transabdominal chorionic villi sampling for first trimester fetal diagnosis: first 26 pregnancies followed to term. Prenat Diagn 1986;6:125.

39. Brambati B, Oldrini A, Lanzani A. First trimester diagnosis for haemoglobinopathies: report on 200 cases. Lancet 1986;2:763.

40. Elles RG, Williamson R, Niazi M, et al. Absence of maternal contamination of chorionic villi used for fetal-gene analysis. N Engl J Med 1983;308:1433.

41. Decorte R, Cuppens H, Marynen P, et al. Rapid detection of hypervariable regions by the polymerase chain reaction technique. DNA Cell Biol 1990;9:461.

42. Petrou M, Modell B, Darr A, et al. Antenatal diagnosis: how to deliver a comprehensive service in the United Kingdom. Ann NY Acad Sci 1990;612:251.

43. Camaschella C, Alfarano A, Gottardi E, et al. Prenatal diagnosis of fetal hemoglobin Lepore-Boston disease on maternal peripheral blood. Blood 1990;75:2102.

44. Sekizawa A, Watanabe A, Kimwa T, et al. Prenatal diagnosis of the fetal RhD blood type using a single fetal nucleated erythrocyte from maternal blood. Obstet Gynaecol 1996;87:501.

45. Cheung MC, Goldberg JD, Kan YW. Prenatal diagnosis of sickle cell anemia and thalassemia by analysis of fetal cells in maternal blood. Nat Genet 1996;14:264.

46. Lau ET, Kwok YK, Chui DHK, et al. Embryonic and foetal globins are expressed in adult erythroid progenitor cells and in erythroid cell cultures. Prenat Diagn 2001; 21:529.

47. Chui RW, Lau TK, Leung TN, et al. Prenatal exclusion of β-thalassaemia major by examination of maternal plasma. Lancet. 2002;360:998.
48. Kanavakis E, Traeger-Synodinos J. Preimplantation genetic diagnosis in clinical practice. J Med Genet 2002;39:6.
49. Flint J, Harding RM, Boyce AJ, et al. The population genetics of the haemoglobinopathies. In: Higgs DR, Weatherall, DJ, eds. Baillière's clinical haematology: international practice and research: the haemoglobinopathies. London: Baillière Tindall, 1993:215.
50. Dode C, Krishnamoorthy R, Lamb J, et al. Rapid analysis of $-\alpha^{3.7}$ thalassaemia and $\alpha\alpha\alpha$ anti 3.7 triplication by enzymatic amplification analysis. Br J Haematol 1992;82:105.
51. Liu YT, Old JM, Fisher CA, et al. Rapid detection of α-thalassaemia deletions and α-globin gene triplication by multiplex PCRs. Br J Haematol 1999;108;295.
52. Chong SS, Boehm CD, Higgs DR, Cutting GR. Single-tube multiplex-PCR screen for common deletional determinants of α-thalassaemia. Hemoglobin 1999;95;360.
53. Molchanova TP, Pobedimskaya DD, Postnikov YV. A simplified procedure for sequencing amplified DNA containing the α-2 or α-1 globin gene. Hemoglobin 1994;18:251.
54. Hartveld KL, Heister AJGAM, Giordano PC, et al. Rapid detection of point mutations and polymorphisms of the α-globin genes by DGGE and SSCA. Hum Mutat 1996;7:114.
55. Kulozik AE, Thein SL, Wainscoat JS, et al. Thalassaemia intermedia: interaction of the triple α-globin gene arrangement and heterozygous β-thalassaemia. Br J Haematol 1987;66:109.
56. Fischel-Ghodsian N, Vickers MA, Seip M, et al. Characterization of two deletions that remove the entire human ζ-α globin gene complex ($--$Thai and $--$Fil). Br J Haematol 1988;70:233.
57. Huisman THJ. Frequencies of common β-thalassaemia alleles among different populations: variability in clinical severity. Br J Haematol 1990;75:454.
58. Baysal E, Indrak K, Bozhurt G, et al. The β thalassaemia mutations in the population of Cyprus. Br J Haematol 1992;81:607.
59. Ristaldi MS, Pirastu M, Rosatelli C, et al. Prenatal diagnosis of β-thalassaemia in Mediterranean populations by dot blot analysis with DNA amplification and allele specific oligonucleotide probes. Prenat Diagn 1989;9:629.
60. Saiki RK, Walsh PS, Levenson CH, et al. Genetic analysis of amplified DNA with immobilized sequence-specific oligonucleotide probes. Proc Natl Acad Sci USA 1989;86:6230.
61. Maggio A, Giambona A, Cai SP, et al. Rapid and simultaneous typing of hemoglobin S, hemoglobin C and seven Mediterranean β-thalassaemia mutations by covalent reverse dot-blot analysis: application to prenatal diagnosis in Sicily. Blood 1993;81:239.
62. Sutcharitchan P, Saiki R, Huisman THJ, et al. Reverse dot-blot detection of the African-American β-thalassaemia mutations. Blood 1995;86:1580.
63. Old JM, Khan SN, Verma, et al. A multi-centre study to further define the molecular basis of β-thalassaemia in Thailand, Pakistan, Sri Lanka, Mauritius, Syria, and India, and to develop a simple molecular diagnostic strategy by amplification refractory mutation system polymerase chain reaction. Hemoglobin 2001;25:397.
64. Tan JAMA, Tay JSH, Lin LI, et al. The amplification refractory mutation system (ARMS): a rapid and direct prenatal diagnostic techniques for β-thalassaemia in Singapore. Prenat Diagn 1994;14:1077.
65. Zschocke J, Graham CA. A fluorescent multiplex ARMS method for rapid mutation analysis. Mol Cell Probes 1995;9:447.
66. Chehab FF, Kan YW. Detection of specific DNA sequence by fluorescence amplification: a color complementation assay. Proc Natl Acad Sci USA 1989;86:9178.
67. Chang JG, Lu JM, Huang JM, et al. Rapid diagnosis of β-thalassaemia by mutagenically separated polymerase chain reaction (MS-PCR) and its application to prenatal diagnosis. Br J Haematol 1995;91:602.
68. Old JM. DNA-based diagnosis of the hemoglobin disorders. In: Steinberg MH, Forget BG, Higgs DR, Nagel RL, eds. Disorders of hemoglobin: genetics, pathophysiology and clinical management. Cambridge: Cambridge University Press, 2001:941.
69. Linderman R, Hu SP, Volpato F, et al. Polymerase chain reaction (PCR) mutagenesis enabling rapid nonradioactive detection of common β-thalassaemia mutations in Mediterraneans. Br J Haematol 1991;78:100.
70. Faa V, Rosatelli MC, Sardu R, et al. A simple electrophoretic procedure for fetal diagnosis of β-thalassaemia due to short deletions. Prenat Diagn 1992;12:903.
71. Waye JS, Eng B, Hunt JA, et al. Filipino β-thalassaemia due to a large deletion: identification of the deletion endpoints and polymerase chain reaction (PCR)-based diagnosis. Hum Genet 1994;94:530.
72. Craig JE, Barnetson RA, Prior J, et al. Rapid detection of deletions causing $\delta\beta$ thalassaemia and hereditary persistence of fetal hemoglobin by enzymatic amplification. Blood 1994;83:1673.

73. Losekoot M, Fodde R, Harteveld CL, et al. Denaturing gradient gel electrophoresis and direct sequencing of PCR amplified genomic DNA: a rapid and reliable diagnostic approach to beta thalassaemia. Br J Haematol 1991;76:269.

74. Savage DA, Wood NAP, Bidwell JL, et al. Detection of β-thalassaemia mutations using DNA heteroduplex generator molecules. Br J Haematol 1995;90:564.

75. Old JM, Varawalla NY, Weatherall DJ. The rapid detection and prenatal diagnosis of β thalassaemia in the Asian Indian and Cypriot populations in the UK. Lancet 1990;336:834.

76. Old JM. Haemoglobinopathies: community clues to mutation detection. In: Elles R, ed. Methods in molecular medicine, molecular diagnosis of genetic diseases. Totowa, NJ: Humana Press, 1996:169.

77. Kwok S, Kellogg DE, McKinney N, et al. Effects of primer-template mismatches on the polymerase chain reaction: human immunodeficiency virus type I model studies. Nucleic Acids Res 1990;18:999.

78. Varawalla NY, Old JM, Weatherall DJ. Rare β-thalassaemia mutations in Asian Indians. Br J Haematol 1991;79:640.

79. Kazazian HH Jr, Boehm CD. Molecular basis and prenatal diagnosis of β-thalassaemia. Blood 1988;72:1107.

80. Antonarakis SE, Boehm CD, Diardina PJV, et al. Non-random association of polymorphic restriction sites in the β-globin gene cluster. Proc Natl Acad Sci USA 1982;79:137.

81. Chakravarti A, Buetow KH, Antonarakis SE, et al. Non-uniform recombination within the human β-globin gene cluster. Am J Hum Genet 1984;71:79.

82. Orkin SH, Little PFR, Kazazian HH Jr, et al. Improved detection of the sickle mutation by DNA analysis. N Engl J Med 1982;307:32.

83. Old JM, Petrou M, Modell B, et al. Feasibility of antenatal diagnosis of β-thalassaemia by DNA polymorphisms in Asian Indians and Cypriot populations. Br J Haematol 1984;57:255.

84. Kulozik AE, Lyons J, Kohne E, et al. Rapid and non-radioactive prenatal diagnosis of β-thalassaemia and sickle cell disease: application of the polymerase chain reaction (PCR). Br J Haematol 1988;70:455.

85. Semenza GL, Dowling CE, Kazazian HH Jr. Hinf I polymorphisms 3' to the human β globin gene detected by the polymerase chain reaction (PCR). Nucleic Acids Res 1989;17:2376.

86. Wainscoat JS, Old JM, Thein SL, et al. A new DNA polymorphism for prenatal diagnosis of β-thalassaemia in Mediterranean populations. Lancet 1984;2:1299.

87. Weatherall DJ, Clegg JB, Higgs DR, et al. The haemoglobinopathies. In: Scriver CR, Beaudet AL, Sly WS, et al., eds. The metabolic basis of inherited disease, 6th ed. New York: McGraw-Hill, 1992:2281.

88. Old JM, Thein SL, Weatherall DJ, et al. Prenatal diagnosis of the major haemoglobin disorders. Mol Biol Med 1989;6:55.

89. Trent RJ, Davis B, Wilkinson T, et al. Identification of β variant hemoglobins by DNA restriction endonuclease mapping. Hemoglobin 1984;8:443.

90. Thein SL, Lynch JR, Old JM, et al. Direct detection of haemoglobin E with *Mnl*I. J Med Genet 1987;24:110.

91. Rosatelli MC, Tuveri T, Scalas MT, et al. Molecular screening and fetal diagnosis of β-thalassaemia in the Italian population. Hum Genet 1992;89:585.

92. Wang X, Seaman C, Paik M, et al. Experience with 500 prenatal diagnoses of sickle cell diseases: the effect of gestational age on affected pregnancy outcome. Prenat Diagn 1994;14:851.

93. Chan V, Chan TPT, Lau K, et al. False non-paternity in a family for prenatal diagnosis of β-thalassaemia. Prenat Diagn 1993;13:977.

94. Old J, Petrou M, Varnavides L, et al. Accuracy of prenatal diagnosis in the UK; 25 years experience. Prenat Diagn 2000;20:986.

James C. Hyland, M.D., Ph.D., and
Leena Ala-Kokko, M.D., Ph.D.

20

Prenatal Diagnosis of Connective Tissue Disorders

The complex biology of connective tissue is reflected in the myriad types of disorders resulting from defects in its constitutive molecules. Although numerous connective tissue disorders can be traced directly to defective structural components, molecular constituents fulfill a variety of additional functions. Additional roles of connective tissue and extracellular matrix include, but are not restricted to, those involved with morphogenesis, maintenance of homeostasis, signal transduction, protection and tissue integrity.

There has been considerable advancement in defining the underlying defects in many connective tissue disorders in the past decade (see Table 20.1). This chapter will concentrate on the prenatal diagnosis of connective tissue disorders in which biochemical or molecular tests are useful. Although this chapter focuses on those connective tissue disorders for which prenatal molecular diagnosis is available, it does not focus on them exclusively.

Prenatal diagnosis of connective tissue disorders can be divided into those that are found unexpectedly on ultrasound and those in which a fetus is intentionally subjected to analysis because of a preexisting condition in a parent or previous offspring. In many instances, an accurate prenatal diagnosis of an inherited or a *de novo* condition may be achieved by biochemical or molecular means. In other instances, an accurate diagnosis based on molecular means is not available and may depend entirely on imaging studies.

Osteogenesis imperfecta (OI) and Marfan syndrome are examples of disorders representing defects in genes coding for components of connective tissue that have primarily structural functions. The chondrodysplasias represent a broad category of disorders involving the cartilage matrix. A major subset of chondrodysplasias is due to defects in the cartilage collagens type II, IX, X, and XI and cartilage oligomeric matrix protein (COMP). The phenotypic manifestations reflect the important role of cartilage in morphogenesis. Some other skeletal dysplasias are related to abnormal sulfate metabolism and represent defects in a sulfate transporter or an enzyme responsible for the activation of inorganic sulfate. Like OI and certain forms of chondrodysplasia, the heterogeneous collection of Ehlers-Danlos syndrome disorders are caused by defects in collagen genes or genes involved in posttranslational modification of collagens. In contrast, craniosynostosis and certain other skeletal dysplasias are caused by defective fibroblast growth factor receptors. Hence, these disorders reflect underlying defects in a signal transduction path-

Table 20.1. Selected inherited connective tissue disorders

Condition	Inheritance	Gene	Gene Locus	Clinical Information
Achondrogenesis II MIM 200610	AD	COL2A1	12q13–14	Lethal chondrodysplasia, shortened long bones, ossification defects
Hypochondrogenesis MIM 120140	AD	COL2A1	12q13–14	Usually lethal. Similar to but less severe than ACG II.
Spondyloepiphyseal dyplasia congenita MIM 183900	AD	COL2A1	12q13–14	Short neck, rhizomelic shortening of limbs
Spondyloepiphyseal dysplasia				
Strudwick MIM 271670	AD	COL2A1	12q13–14	Variant of SED congenita, greater metaphyseal involvement
Kniest dysplasia MIM 156550	AD	COL2A1	12q13–14	Short trunk/limbs, depressed nasal bridge, prominent eyes, hearing loss
Stickler dysplasia				
Type I MIM 108300	AD	COL2A1	12q13–14	Severe myopia, osteoarthritis, sensorineural hearing loss, cleft
Type II MIM 604841	AD	COL11A1	1p21	palate, midface hypoplasia
Type III MIM 184840	AD	COL11A2	6p21.2	Mild spondyloepiphyseal dysplasia. No eye findings.
Otospondylomega epiphyseal dysplasia (OSMED) MIM 215150	AR	COL11A2	6p21.2	Short limbs, severe hearing loss, short nonanteverted nares, midface hypoplasia, short upturned nose
Metatrophic dysplasia MIM 250600	AR	?	?	Long narrow trunk, mild limb shortening
Spondyloepiphyseal dysplasia tarda MIM 313400	X-linked	SEDL	Xp22.2	Short trunk, osteoarthritis, epiphyseal dysplasia
Schmidt metaphyseal chondrodysplasia MIM 156500	AD	COL10A1	6q21–22	Mild short stature, bowing of lower extremities, flared metaphysics
Pseudoachondroplasia MIM 177170	AD	COMP	19p12–13.1	Disproportionate short stature, short extremities with ligamentous laxity, osteoarthritis
Multiple epiphyseal dysplasia				
MIM 132400	AD	COMP	19p12–13.1	Avascular necrosis of capital femoral
	AD	COL9A1	6q12–13	epiphysis in mid-childhood. Genu
MIM 600204	AD	COL9A2	1p32.2–33	varus/valgus. Small or irregular
MIM 600969	AD	COL9A3	20q13.3	epiphysis
MIM 602109	AD	MATN–3	2p24–23	
Diastrophic dysplasia sulfate transporter dependent disorders				
Achondrogenesis 1B (ACG1B) MIM 600972	AR	DTDST	5q32–q33.1	Perinatal lethal, short trunk, neck and limbs, narrow thorax, short stubby toes, flat face.
Atelosteogenesis (A02) MIM 256050	AR	DTDST	5q32–q33.1	Usually lethal, short limbs, adducted feet, less severe features of ACG1B.

(continued)

Table 20.1. Selected inherited connective tissue disorders (continued)

Condition	Inheritance	Gene	Gene Locus	Clinical Information
Diastrophic dysplasia MIM 222600	AR	DTDST	5q32–q33.1	Slightly short trunk, more markedly shortened extremities, "hitchhiker thumb," lumbar lordosis. Thoracic kyphosis.
Recessively inherited multiple epiphyseal dysplasia MIM 226900	AR	DTDST	5q32–q33.1	Normal or mildly short stature, double-layered patella, clubfoot and/or hand deformities, joint pain.
Disorders due to fibroblast growth factor receptor mutations				
Achondroplasia MIM 100800	AD	FGFR3	4p16.3	Macrocephaly, midface hypoplasia, rhizomelic dwarfism, trident hands.
Hypochondrogenesis MIM 146000	AD	FGFR3	4p16.3	Similar to but milder than achondroplasia.
Thanatophoric dysplasia MIM 187600	AD	FGFR3	4p16.3	Neonatal lethal condition, severe rhizomelic dwarfism, profound midface hypoplasia, small thorax.
Severe achondroplasia with developmental delay and acanthosis nigricans MIM 134934.0015	AD	FGFR3	4p16.3	Short stature, midface hypoplasia, eventual mental retardation, hydrocephalus and seizures.
Pfeiffer syndrome types 1, 2, 3 MIM 1010600	AD	FGFR3 FGFR2	8p11.2 10q25–26	Craniosynostosis mainly involving coronal sutures, midface hypoplasia, ocular proptosis, arched palate, and anomalies of hands and feet. Early death types 1 and 2.
Apert syndrome MIM 101200	AD	FGFR2	10q25–26	Correlated with increased paternal age. Craniosynostosis, wide open fontanelles, asymmetric cranial base. Facial, optic, and skeletal abnormalities. Most are sporadic.
Crouzon syndrome MIM 123500	AD	FGFR2	10q24–25	Coronal or multiple suture synostosis, ocular proptosis, mild/moderate hearing loss. *De novo* associated with increased paternal age. 50% sporadic.
Crouzon syndrome with acanthosis nigricans MIM 134934–0011	AD	FGFR3	4p16.3	Rare. Female predominance. Coronal synostosis, hyperpigmentation, hyperkeratosis, melanocytic nevi.
Muenke syndrome MIM 134934	AD and sporadic	FGFR3	4p16.3	Uni or bicoronal synostosis, variable clinical presentation, midface hypoplasia, downslanting palpebral fissures and ptosis. Possible mental retardation.
Jackson–Weiss syndrome MIM 123150	AD	FGFR2	10q25.26	Craniosynostosis, midface hypoplasia, medially deviated great toes.
Saethre–Chotzen syndrome MIM 101400	AD	Twist	7p21	Wide clinical variability. Coronal, lambdoid or metopic cranio-synostosis, not seen in all patients. Mild hand and feet abnormalities.

Table 20.1. Selected inherited connective tissue disorders (continued)

Condition	Inheritance	Gene	Gene Locus	Clinical Information
Baller–Gerold syndrome MIM 218600	AD	Twist	7p21	Craniosynostosis of any or all sutures. Radial aplasia/hypoplasia. Imperforate anus.
Osteogenesis imperfecta				
Type I MIM 166200	AD	COL1A1 COL1A2 (rare)	17q21.3–22 7q21.3–22	Mild type. Normal/near normal stature. Few to numerous fractures, no deformity. Blue sclera.
Type II MIM 166210	AD	COL1A1 COL1A2	17q21.3–22 7q21.3–22	Perinatal lethal, fragile deformed extremities, small thorax and soft calvarium.
Type III MIM 259420	AD	COL1A1 COL1A2	17q21.3–22 7q21.3–22	Progressively deforming variant. Short stature, fragile bones with angular deformities. Foreshortened survival.
Type IV MIM 166220	AD	COL1A1 COL1A2	17q21.3–22 7q21.3–22	Mildly deforming variant with mild to moderate short stature. Possible in utero fractures.
Ehlers–Danlos syndrome				
Types I and II MIM 130000 MIM 130010	AD	COL5A1 COL5A2 COL1A1 COL1A2	9q34.2–34.3 2q24.3–31 17q21.3–22 7q21.3–22	Classic types. Type I: hypermobile joints, hyperextensible skin. Bowel/aorta rupture. Type II: less severe than type I
	AR	TNXA	p21.3	
Type III MIM 130020	AD	?COL5A3 ?COL3A1	19p13.2 2q24.3–q31	Hypermobile type, severe joint laxity
Type IV MIM 130050	AD	COL3A1	2q24.3–q31	Vascular type. Aneurysms, organ rupture, early death, extreme tissue fragility.
Type VI MIM 225400				
A	AR	PLOD1	1p36.2–36.3	Kyphoscoliotic types: generalized
B	AR	Unknown	Unknown	joint laxity, rupture of globe
Type VII MIM 130060				
A	AD	COL1A1	17q21.3–22	Arthrochalasis types: generalized joint
B	AD	COL1A2	7q21.3–22	hypermobility with dislocations. Kyphoscoliosis, hyperextensible skin.
Type VIIC MIM 225410	AR	Procollagen N-proteinase gene	5q23	Dermatosparactic type: severe skin fragility, herniae, premature rupture of fetal membranes.
ATP7A-dependent disorders				
Menkes disorder MIM 309400	X-linked	ATP7A	Xq12–13	Neurologic manifestations, spontaneous fractures, hypotonia, arterial rupture and connective tissue findings of occipital horn syndrome below.
Occipital horn syndrome MIM 304150	X-linked	ATP7A	Xq12–13	Milder form. Hernias, hypermobile joints, kyphoscoliosis, pectus deformities.
Marfan syndrome MIM 154700	AD	FBN1	15q21.1	Tall stature, arachnodactyly, pectus deformities, ectopia lentis, mitral-valve prolapse, aortic-root dilatation, and aneurysms.

(continued)

Table 20.1. Selected inherited connective tissue disorders (continued)

Condition	Inheritance	Gene	Gene Locus	Clinical Information
Homocystinuria MIM 236200	AR	Cystathionine β-synthetase gene	21q22.3	Ectopia lentis, myopia, osteoporosis, arachnodactyly, pectus deformities, psychiatric disorders, vascular infarction
Pseudoxanthoma elasticum MIM 177850	AR	ABCC6	16p13.1	Sagging skin, vision loss, claudication, myocardial infarction
Osteopetrosis				
Lethal in utero	AR	Unknown	Unknown	Prenatal fractures, hydrocephalus
Malignant infantile MIM 259700	AR	ATP6i	11q13	Short stature, cranial nerve dysfunction, cerebral edema cytopenias and extramedularlly hematopoiesis. Fractures.
Intermediate recessive MIM 259710	AR	CICN7 (Some cases)	16p13.3	Similar to but less severe than malignant infantile
Benign autosomal dominant MIM 166600				
Type I	AD	LRP5	11q13	Increased thickness of skull and long bones. Headaches, bone pain, cranial nerve dysfunction. Fractures not increased.
Type II	AD	CICN7	16p13.3	Skull base and pelvic sclerosis. Fractures. Cranial nerve dysfunction.
Carbonic anhydrase deficiency MIM 259730	AR	CA2	8q22	Failure to thrive. Short stature, some have fractures, blindness. Some asymptomatic.

ACG = achondrogenesis; AD = autosomal dominent; AR = autosomal recessive; LRP5 = LDL receptor-related protein 5; MIM = Mendelian Inheritance in Man; SED = spondyloepiphyseal dysplasia.

way. Pseudoxanthoma elasticum represents a connective tissue disorder due to defects in a transmembrane protein with ATPase activity that is suspected to be involved in the active transport of anions. The functional significance is the degeneration of elastic fibers in certain tissues.

DISORDERS OF BONE AND CARTILAGE

Chondrodysplasias

Chondrodysplasias is a heterogeneous group of disorders characterized by skeletal deformities and dwarfism. More than 100 clinical phenotypes have been described and range from perinatal lethal conditions to those that are mild and do not manifest for several years.[1,2] Tissues other than growing cartilage are often affected. Some prenatal cases are suspected during routine ultrasound and in some instances may be confirmed *in utero* by molecular means. Defective genes confirmed as underlying achondrogenesis and chondrodysplasias include those coding for types II, IX, X, and XI collagens, COMP, and the diastrophic dysplasia sulfate transporter.[2,3] Some related disorders due to defects in various fibroblast growth factor receptor genes are discussed below.[4]

Disorders Due to Defects in Type II Collagen, Type X Collagen, Type XI Collagen, and Cartilage Oligomeric Matrix Protein

Achondrogenesis type II and hypochondrogenesis are the most serious of the *COL2A1* collagenopathies.[2,5] Fetuses have shortened necks, ribs, and long bones. There is variable ossification of the vertebral bodies. They have large heads with soft craniums and flat faces. These two disorders are associated with prematurity and hydrops. Stillbirth or perinatal death is invariable.

Spondyloepiphyseal dysplasia congenita (SEDc) and its variant SED Strudwick characteristically present with short trunks and prominent proximal foreshortening of the extremities.[2] The neck is also short. Associated findings may include cleft palate and clubfoot, but the head is normal. They may have severe myopia, and retinal detachment can occur. Vertebral bodies are ovoid in newborns, iliac bones are short and square, and the pubic symphysis is poorly ossified. Delayed epiphyseal ossification occurs. SED Strudwick appears similar at birth but displays more metaphyseal involvement during childhood. Both disorders are caused by defects in *COL2A1*.[6–8]

Kniest dysplasia is a severe disorder also presenting with disproportionate dwarfism.[2] The trunk and limbs are short. Cleft palate, clubfoot, and inguinal hernias may also occur. Joints are enlarged, the face is flat, and coxa vara is evident. The bones of the fingers display intercarpal narrowing and long bones are dumbbell-shaped.[2] Myopia and hearing loss develop. Numerous *COL2A1* mutations have been defined.[9,10]

Stickler syndrome type I is also due to specific mutations in *COL2A1*.[2,11,12] Patients may have cleft palate, micrognathia, severe myopia with retinal detachment, and can develop sensorineural hearing loss and arthritis, but they are not short. The phenotype is not detectable *in utero*, but prenatal molecular diagnosis is available for families with confirmed *COL2A1* mutations. In contrast to Stickler syndrome type I, Stickler syndrome type II and the related Marshall syndrome are due to defects in *COL11A1*.[12,13] Finally, the nonocular form of Sticker syndrome, Stickler syndrome type III, is due to dominantly inherited defects in *COL11A2*.[14,15] Most *COL11A2* mutations cause splicing defects. These patients may exhibit mild spondyloepiphyseal dysplasia.[14] Recessively inherited *COL11A2* mutations leading to complete loss of function of *COL11A2* result in a severe phenotype. This is termed otospondylomegaepiphyseal dysplasia (OSMED).[14,16] Molecular based, prenatal diagnosis for defects in the *COL2A1, COL11A1*, and *COL11A2* is available.

Prenatal analysis of *COL10A1* is available for those families with Schmid metaphyseal chondrodysplasia, and has been reported by Milunsky et al.[17] These patients are short, with bowing of the lower extremities. They have short tubular bones with metaphyses that are flared, cup-shaped, and irregularly mineralized.[2] Coxa vara is severe. Mutations cluster in the carboxyl terminal nonhelical NC1 domain.[18,19]

Pseudoachondroplasia (PSACH) is an autosomal dominantly inherited progressive skeletal dysplasia due to mutations in *COMP*.[2] Some cases of dominantly inherited multiple epiphyseal dysplasia (MED) are caused by *COMP* mutations and others by matrilin-3 mutations *(MATN3)*.[20,21] Alternatively, other MED cases are caused by mutations in *COL9A1, COL9A2*, or *COL9A3*.[22–24] A recessive form of MED is caused by mutations in the diastrophic sulfate transporter gene and is discussed below.

COMP is a pentameric protein present in the extracellular matrix of chondrocytes and is also found in tendons and ligaments. It is a member of the thrombospondin family, and it interacts with types I, II, III, and IX collagens.[20] Type IX collagen is a member of the fibril-associated collagens with interrupted triple helices. It is believed to act as a bridge between type II collagen and other structural cartilage matrix molecules, including COMP. Matrilin-3 is a member of the oligomeric extracellular matrix protein group.[20] It is highly expressed in bone and cartilage and binds to COMP, type II collagen, and type IX collagen.

At birth, PSACH infants appear relatively unaffected.[2] They have both a normal length and head circumference. Skeletal growth decelerates between the first and second year of life. Ultimately, they develop disproportionate short stature with short extremities. Patients also have generalized ligamentous laxity except at the elbows and hips, where mobility is restricted. Additional lower extremity abnormalities lead to early osteoarthritis. The epiphyses, metaphyses, and spine are all involved.

Ultrasound is not useful for prenatal diagnosis since the skeletal abnormalities are not obvious *in utero*.[20] Clinical diagnosis can be made at birth since infants have platyspondyly.[2] Prenatal molecular diagnosis is possible. Most defined *COMP* gene mutations are clustered within exons coding for calcium binding repeats. The mutations result in amino acid substitutions or are short in-frame deletions or insertions.[20]

MED also has a delayed onset.[2] Patients with *COMP* mutations can have short stature and major disability caused by joint pain and stiffness. They typically have significant abnormalities of the capital femoral epiphyses and acetabuli. Those with CUL9A1 or COL9A2 mutations have normal or near-normal stature and significant epiphyseal abnormalities in the knees, but the hips are relatively spared. *MATN3* mutations also result in milder phenotypes than *COMP* mutations. Both the hips and the knees can be affected. Prenatal analysis of the *COL9A1, COL9A2, COL9A3*, and *MATN3* genes is offered to families with defined mutations.

Disorders Due to Defects in the Diastrophic Dysplasia Sulfate Transporter Gene

Achondrogenesis type 1B, atelosteogenesis, and related skeletal dysplasias are due to mutations in the diastrophic dysplasia sulfate transporter *(DTDST)* gene.[2,25–28] The encoded transmembrane protein is an anion exchanger and functions to transport extracellular sulfate across cell membranes. Mutations in the *DTDST* gene result in decreased intracellular chondrocyte sulfate and are manifested by decreased or absent cartilage matrix sulfated proteoglycans. The severity ranges from the lethal variants, achondrogenesis type 1B (ACG1B) and atelosteogenesis 2 (AO2), to the milder phenotypes, diastrophic dysplasia (DTD) and recessive multiple epiphyseal dysplasia (rMED).[3] This represents an arbitrary division of disorders since they actually reflect a continuum of phenotypes.

Similar to achondrogenesis type II (ACG2), ACG1B is a perinatal lethal condition.[2,3] Infants afflicted with both disorders appear phenotypically similar, although the chest is described as barrel-shaped in ACG2, and narrow in ACG1B. Another important difference is that the toes and fingers are short and stubby in ACG1B. AO2 is also a severe skeletal dysplasia. Infants have short limbs, adducted feet and a hitchhiker thumb. It is usually lethal. Tapering of the distal humerus is also observed.

DTD is a severe dysplasia that simulates achondroplasia during the first year of life. It is not usually lethal. The trunks and limbs are short, with the limbs being more foreshortened. Bilateral clubfoot, cleft palate, contractures, and hitchhiker thumbs and toes are characteristic. Patients with rMED are the least affected of those with DTDST mutations. This group of skeletal dysplasias may be first recognized on routine ultrasound and confirmed by prenatal molecular analysis of *DTDST*.

FIBROBLAST GROWTH FACTOR RECEPTOR ASSOCIATED SKELETAL DYSPLASIAS AND CRANIOSYNOSTOSIS SYNDROMES

These are caused by mutations in fibroblast growth factor receptor genes (FGFR). FGFRs function as tyrosine kinases. All mutations represent gain of function and are inherited in a dominant manner.[29]

Skeletal Dysplasias Caused by Mutations in the Fibroblast Growth Factor Receptor Gene 3 (*FGFR3*)

These include achondroplasia, hypochondroplasia, thanatophoric dysplasia, and severe achondroplasia with developmental delay and acanthosis nigricans.[29]

Achondroplasia represents the most common skeletal dysplasia in humans.[29] Patients have rhizomelic dwarfism, midface hypoplasia, and macrocephaly. Limited elbow extension and a space between the distal phalanges of the third and fourth fingers may be present. The long bones are short. Newborns are hypotonic, although this resolves, and the foramen magnum is small. The increased mortality of affected children is attributed to the foramen magnum stenosis. Homozygous or double dominant achondroplasia is a lethal condition and results from the inheritance of two copies of the defective *FGFR3*. Most cases are due to a Gly380Arg substitution.[30,31] Fewer cases are associated with Gly375Cys or Gly346Glu substitutions.[32,33]

Hypochondroplasia shares phenotypic features with achondroplasia but is milder. Affected individuals are still rhizomelic dwarfs but are not as short, and facial manifestations are not as severe. The most common defect in *FGFR3* is Lys540Asp.[34]

Thanatophoric dysplasia is usually a perinatal lethal condition.[29] Infants have severe rhizomelic dwarfism, very short ribs, and midface hypoplasia. Death is due to either respiratory compromise secondary to the small thorax or to neurologic impairment secondary to the small foramen magnum. At least two subtypes correlated with certain mutations are recognized. Type I is associated with curved tubular bones and has numerous different mutations in *FGFR3*.[35] Type II has a cloverleaf skull and straight femurs and has a specific mutation, Lys650Glu.[35]

Severe achondroplasia with developmental delay and acanthosis nigricans has recently been described. Those affected have short stature, midface hypoplasia, developmental delay, mental retardation and develop acanthosis nigricans. The have a specific *FGFR3* mutation (Lys650Met).[36]

Craniosynostosis Syndromes

The craniosynostosis syndromes are a group of disorders sharing the premature fusion of one or more sutures of the skull.[29,37] Often additional anomalies are associated. Many of these disorders are caused by defects in the *FGFR1, FGFR2,* or *FGFR3*. The craniosynostoses are autosomal dominant disorders. Most cases represent new mutations.

Patients with Pfeiffer syndrome have craniosynostosis, with broad thumbs and broad great toes that are deviated medially. Partial syndactyly can occur. Additional findings may be present. Both inherited and sporadic cases occur, with the latter having a more severe phenotype.[29] Mutations have been defined in *FGFR1* and *FGFR2*.[38–40] At least three subtypes exist. Those with type 1 have bicoronal craniosynostosis, a normal life span, and normal intelligence. These patients exhibit mutations in *FGFR1* and *FGFR2*. Type 2 patients have cloverleaf skulls, severe ocular proptosis, neurodevelopmental problems, elbow ankylosis, and foreshortened life spans. Type 3 is similar to type 2, but patients do not have cloverleaf skulls and also die young. Type 2 and type 3 have mutations restricted to *FGFR2*.[29]

Apert syndrome is a relatively severe form of craniosynostosis, with numerous organ systems being affected.[29,37] Most cases are sporadic and correlate with increased paternal age. The findings include brachycephaly, midfacial hypoplasia, broad thumbs and great toes, and partial or total syndactyly of the hands and feet. Some additional findings may include cleft palate, various structural anomalies of the central nervous system, additional limb abnormalities, vertebral fusion, and some cutaneous manifestations, including acne, hyperhidrosis, hyperkeratosis, and hypopigmentation, among others. Mental retardation may occur. Almost all cases are due to specific mutations in the *FGFR2*, Ser252Trp, and Pro253Arg.[41,42] Inherited cases are autosomal dominant.

Crouzon syndrome is the most common autosomal dominant craniosynostosis. Patients have coronal or multiple suture synostosis, maxillary hypoplasia, a prominent beaked nose, shallow orbits, and ocular proptosis.[4] One half of the cases are familial, with autosomal dominant inheritance; one half are *de novo*, and correlate with increased paternal age. Intelligence is usually normal, and brain abnormalities are rare, although progressive hydrocephalus does occur and may be associated with cerebellar herniation. Vision and hearing deficits can occur. Fusion of C2C3 is seen, but hands and feet appear normal. Numerous mutations have been identified in *FGFR2*.[40,41]

Crouzon syndrome with acanthosis nigricans is rare and is associated with a specific mutation in *FGFR3* (Ala391Glu), occurring more frequently in females.[43,44] Early-onset skin findings include hyperpigmentation, hyperkeratosis, and melanocytic nevi along with verrucous hyperplasia in flexural areas.

Patients with sporadic and familial cases of the Muenke syndrome are often misdiagnosed with another form of craniosynostosis.[37] The phenotypic presentation is very variable.[29] This syndrome is also associated with a specific *FGFR3* mutation (Pro250Arg).[45,46] The mutation rate is similar to that observed with achondroplasia. Patients can display coronal synostosis, midfacial hypoplasia, downslanting palpebral fissures, and ptosis. Bone abnormalities of the hands and feet occur. Some do not have craniosynostosis, but may have only macrocephaly or even normal-sized heads. Sensorineural hearing loss is seen in about one-third. Mental retardation can occur. Intrafamilial variation is great. Inheritance is autosomal dominant.

The Jackson–Weiss syndrome is characterized by midface hypoplasia, frontal prominence, and cutaneous syndactyly with varying degrees of medially deviated and enlarged great toes.[29] Some do not have craniofacial anomalies. Intelligence is normal. The clinical presentation is variable. This syndrome is due to a specific *FGFR2* mutation, Ala344Gly.[40,47]

Mutation analysis of the *FGFR* genes is available. With achondroplasia and hypochondroplasia, molecular based prenatal diagnosis is useful. It can determine if a fetus has inherited a predetermined mutation from an affected parent since expression of the phenotype, even in a newborn, may be subtle. In contrast, *de novo* cases of thanatophoric dysplasia can be detected by ultrasound and verified in utero with *FGFR3* analysis. Craniosynostosis may also be detected *in utero* by ultrasound. Because specific mutations in the *FGFR* genes are associated with defined disorders, an accurate diagnosis can be made.

Osteogenesis Imperfecta

Osteogenesis imperfecta (OI) is a heterogeneous disorder primarily involving bone. Inheritance is almost exclusively autosomal dominant, although some cases of germ line mosaicism and questionable autosomal recessive cases have been reported. The clinical manifestations may include fractures, blue or dark sclerae, hearing loss, bowing of the femurs, dentinogenesis imperfecta, and various other skeletal abnormalities.[48] OI is caused by defects in either *COL1A1* or *COL1A2*. These two genes encode the proα1 and proα2 chains of type I collagen.[49]

Four clinical types of OI are generally recognized.[50] Type I is the mild variant. Patients with type I OI commonly fracture the long bones, ribs, and bones of the hands. Fractures may be few or numerous. Since the fractures heal without deformity, the patients obtain a normal or near-normal stature. In most instances, OI type I is due to *COL1A1* haploinsufficiency secondary to nonsense mediated mRNA decay.[51]

Type II OI is the perinatal lethal variant.[48] Infants are often delivered prematurely and have low birth weights. As many as 60 percent die during the first day of life. They have bowed legs, beaded ribs, soft calvarium, dark sclerae, short extremities, and flexed hips. The thorax is small. Interestingly, fractures are rare as the bones are soft. The vast majority of cases represent new dominant mutations. In some families with recurrence, mosaicism has been documented. Type II OI may be detected by ultrasound during pregnancy, but may be difficult to distinguish from other skeletal dysplasias. The majority of type II OI cases result from point mutations in either *COL1A1* or *COL1A2*, leading to glycine substitutions in the triple helical regions of the proα1(I) or proα2(I) chains. Other mutations include those resulting in nonglycine substitutions, in the carboxyl-terminal portion of the molecule stop codons, splice site mutations resulting in exon skipping, and small in-frame insertions or deletions. The effects of the mutations may be manifested either through interference with procollagen chain assembly or alternatively by interference with stable triple helical formation following incorporation into procollagen.

Type III OI is known as the progressively deforming variant.[48] Fractures, short stature, and deformity may be recognized in utero. These patients have generalized osteopenia and the highest fracture rate of all OI types. This results in angular bone deformities. Severe kyphoscoliosis can develop, and the life span is foreshortened. Most cases are autosomal dominant, although rare recessively inherited cases have been seen. The dominantly inherited *COL1A1* and *COL1A2* mutations include those resulting in splice-site alterations, glycine substitutions, and single glycine deletions.

Type IV is the mildly deforming variant.[48] Fractures may also occur *in utero*. These patients are usually short, and may also develop scoliosis or kyphoscoliosis possibly compromising respiratory functions. Inheritance is exclusively autosomal dominant. Most defined *COL1A1* and *COL1A2* mutations result in glycine substitutions. Some exon skipping mutations and in-frame insertions and deletions occur.

DNA-based prenatal diagnostic testing is available for OI. The test may be applied to either suspected *de novo* cases or in families with defined preexisting mutations. Although not directly related to information contained within a prenatal diagnosis chapter, these tests are also important for cases of suspected child abuse versus OI type I.

Ehlers-Danlos Syndrome

This is a heterogeneous group of connective tissue disorders characterized by joint hypermobility, skin hyperextensibility, and tissue fragility. Patients may have additional musculoskeletal defects. About six types and several subtypes are currently recognized.[52]

Ehlers-Danlos Syndrome (EDS) Types I and II: The Classic Types

These are by far the most commonly occurring EDS types. They differ only in the degree of organ system involvement. Patients with EDS I have marked skin involvement, generalized joint hypermobility, and musculoskeletal deformities including dislocations and hypotonia. Prematurity is also characteristic. Patients with EDS I may display some of the more serious findings associated with EDS IV, including a propensity for rupture of the bowel and aorta. EDS II, also known as the mitis type, shares manifestations with EDS I, but the skin is less involved and joint laxity may be confined to hands and feet. Premature births are not increased. Patients with EDS II may remain undiagnosed.

Patients with EDS types I and II most commonly have defined mutations in either *COL5A1* or *COL5A2*.[52,53] Inheritance is almost exclusively autosomal dominant in EDS I or II. A few classic cases have been attributed to defects in *COL1A1* or *COL1A2*.[52] Rare cases have been associated with tenascin-X deficiency.[54]

Although DNA-based *COL5A1* and *COL5A2* mutation analysis is available, it has not yet been applied to prenatal diagnosis. *COL1A1* and *COL1A2* may be analyzed by the same methods applied to OI.

EDS Type III: The Hypermobility Type

These patients with generalized joint hypermobility also suffer from frequent dislocations, effusions, and precocious arthritis.[52] They often have mitral valve prolapse and velvety, hyperextensible skin. Tissue fragility is not characteristic. Candidate genes include *COL5A3* and *COL3A1*.

EDS Type IV: The Vascular Type

This is the most serious of all EDS types.[52] Patients can have spontaneous hemorrhage, aneurysms with dissection, and arteriovenous fistulas.[53,55,56] Rupture of organs, including the colon and gravid uterus, occurs. Other complications of pregnancy include an incompetent cervix, a prolapsed uterus, and fragile membranes. The skin is thin, fragile, and translucent but not hyperelastic. Wound healing is delayed. Skeletal manifestations may include slight hypermobility of the joints of the hands and feet and hip dislocation. A variety of additional complications may be seen. Although complications are rare before puberty, survival is foreshortened.

Inheritance is autosomal dominant.[52] The disorder is due to defects in type III collagen.[57,58] About 50 percent of *COL3A1* mutations are *de novo*. The majority of reported mutations are private. Genetic testing is offered for EDS type IV. DNA-based testing is usually preceded by collagen protein studies.

EDS Type VI: The Kyphoscoliotic Type

There are two subtypes, EDS VIA and EDS VIB.[52,59] Those cases characterized as EDS VIA represent the majority and display decreased activity of lysyl hydroxylase, an enzyme required for the hydroxylation of certain lysyl residues in procollagen.[52,60] Lysyl hydroxylase is encoded by the *PLOD1* gene. A number of mutations have been defined in the *PLOD1* gene in EDS VIA.[52,59,61] The hydroxylated lysines are subsequently substrates in a series of reactions resulting ultimately in the intermolecular and intramolecular cross linking of collagens. Inheritance is autosomal recessive.

Patients with EDS VI are born with hypotonia and kyphoscoliosis.[52] The kyphoscoliosis is progressive, and decreased pulmonary function often results. They have generalized joint laxity. Ocular findings may include scleral fragility, rupture of the globe, microcornea, and retinal detachment. Additional signs of tissue fragility may be manifested by premature rupture of the membranes, arterial rupture, easy bruising, and atrophic scars.[52]

Prenatal DNA-based molecular diagnosis has been accomplished in some families with defined mutations.[59]

EDS Types VIIA and VIIB: The Arthroclastic Types

Deletion or skipping of all or a portion of exon 6 in the COL1A1 or COL1A2 genes causes EDS VIIA and EDS VIIB, respectively.[52,62] Exon 6 in both genes encodes the procollagen N-propeptide cleavage site and a critical lysine residue involved in collagen cross-linking.[49,52] These patients display severe, generalized joint hypermobility with recurrent subluxations and congenital hip dislocation. Thoracolumbar scoliosis may result in short stature. The skin is thin and velvety but only moderately extensible. Muscular hypotonia can be a prominent early finding. Interestingly, a few patients have been described with features of mild OI. Inheritance is autosomal dominant.

EDS Type VIIC: The Dermatosparactic Type

EDS type VIIC is caused by a deficiency of the enzyme responsible for cleaving the procollagen N-propeptide, the N-proteinase.[52] In contrast to EDS types VIIA and VIIB, this is a recessively inherited disorder displaying severe skin involvement. Patients are born prematurely, with soft, lax, and redundant skin that is friable. Although the skin bruises and is avulsed easily, it heals readily without scarring. Additional findings include umbilical hernias and dysmorphic facial features, including micrognathia. Progressive joint laxity is also a feature.

Menkes Disease and the Occipital Horn Syndrome

These X-linked entities represent different ends of a spectrum of disorders due to defects in a common gene, ATP7A.[63–67] This gene encodes an enzyme involved with copper metabolism. The enzyme is a P-type ATPase active in the transport and sorting of copper. Depending on the metabolic state, it is either localized to the plasma membrane or to the trans-Golgi network. One function is the delivery of copper into the appropriate cellular compartment for incorporation into copper-requiring enzymes. Copper requiring enzymes are involved in a variety of metabolic reactions and are affected by defects in ATP7A.

The Occipital Horn Syndrome (OHS)

This is the milder form of ATP7A deficiency induced disorders. Patients display manifestations primarily restricted to the connective tissues and skeleton.[63] At birth, umbilical and inguinal hernias may be evident, and the skin can be wrinkled and lax. Jaundice, hypotonia and hypothermia soon develop. Motor development can be delayed. Recurrent urinary tract infections due to bladder diverticuli are common. Patients also have diarrhea. Skeletal manifestations include hypermobile joints, narrow chest, long trunk with kyphosis or scoliosis, pectus deformities, and hyperostosis of the proximal ulna and radius. Occipital exostoses and osteoporosis also develop. Vascular abnormalities including arterial aneurysms may also occur. These connective tissue manifestations are due to secondary deficiencies in lysyl oxidase activity, a copper-containing enzyme. Lysyl oxidase is required for cross linking of certain collagens and elastin. Lack of lysyl oxidase activity perturbs stable fibrillogenesis. OHS was formerly classified as EDS IX.[52]

Menkes Disease (MD)

Menkes disease represents the more severe form[63] Findings in addition to those seen in OHS include spontaneous fractures, progressive neurologic degeneration with the eventual complete retardation of psychomotor development, seizures, failure to thrive, hair changes, marked hypotonia, and dilatation and rupture of elastic arteries, including the aorta. Death usually occurs by 3 years of age. These additional manifestations seen in Menkes disease are also considered to reflect secondary deficiencies in other copper-requiring enzymes. In addition to lysyl oxidase they include deficiencies in protein concerned with cellular respiration such as cytochrome *c* oxidase, molecules involved in cellular protection against free radicals such as superoxide dismutase, and ceruloplasmin and molecules concerned with the metabolism of neurohormones or transmitters such as dopamine-β-hydroxylase and possibly peptidyl α-amidating monooxygenase. Peptidyl α-amidating monooxygenase is an enzyme involved in the posttranslational amidation of a number of essential peptide hormones and amine oxidases. Amine oxidases represent a group of enzymes found in a variety of tissues catabolizing numerous substrates, including monoamines, diamines, and polyamines. In addition, copper accumulation in certain tissues reflects its ineffective efflux.

The severe form of MD is lethal, although intermediate forms exist between it and OHS. The severity of disease is somewhat correlated with the genotype as those *ATP7A* gene mutations resulting in residual activity enzyme are in general associated with a milder phenotype.[64,65]

Biochemical tests involving the measurement of copper in chorionic villi samples are available as are copper uptake studies in cultured amniocytes. Both tests are reported to have limitations.[63] Prenatal DNA-based mutation analysis of the ATP7A gene has been developed.[64,65,68]

Marfan Syndrome and Marfan Overlap Disorders

Marfan syndrome is a serious disorder of connective tissue and is due to defects in fibrillin 1 encoded by *FBN1*.[69-72] Fibrillin 1 forms microfibrils that are in turn components of elastic fibers. The effects of defective microfibrils are manifested in numerous organ systems, including the eyes, cardiovascular system, skin, central nervous system, skeleton, lungs, and adipose tissue. The diagnostic criteria have been well defined and may include molecular findings.[73]

Patients with Marfan syndrome are long-limbed individuals with arachnodactyly. Obvious skeletal abnormalities can include pectus excavatum or carinatum, pes planus, single or multiple abnormal spinal curvatures, protrusio acetabuli, and laxity of other joints.[69] Ocular manifestations include elongation of the globe, corneal flattening, and most importantly, ectopia lentis. Findings in the cardiovascular system include mitral valve prolapse with severe regurgitation, dilatation of the valvular annulus, and redundancy of the atrioventricular valve leaflets. Arrhythmias may lead to sudden death. Dilatation of the aortic root begins *in utero* and can result in valvular regurgitation. Aortic aneurysm and the potential for dissection have possible life-threatening consequences. The rupture of apical lung blebs may lead to pneumothorax. The single central nervous system manifestation is dural ectasia. Patients may suffer from easy bruising but the most common skin manifestation is striae atrophicae.

Prenatal DNA-based *FBN1* analysis is routinely performed in those families in whom Marfan syndrome is suspected of, or having a confirmed diagnosis of Marfan syndrome.

Several additional disorders with defined defects in *FBN1* share, but do not meet, the diagnostic criteria for Marfan syndrome.[69,72,74] These disorders include familial ectopia lentis, familial aortic aneurysm, and familial aortic dissection. Some with the MASS phenotype (mitral valve prolapse, myopia, mild aortic root dilatation, striae, and mild skeletal changes) also have *FBN1* mutations.

Homocystinuria

Homocystinuria, due to defects in the enzyme cystathionine-β-synthase, may display findings that may be confused with Marfan syndrome or other connective-tissue disorders.[75] Ocular findings may include ectopia lentis, myopia, retinal detachment or degeneration, and corneal abnormalities. Reported skeletal manifestations include increased length of long bones, osteoporosis, scoliosis or kyphosis, arachnodactyly, and pectus carinatum or excavatum. In contrast to Marfan syndrome, joint mobility may be restricted. Patients may also exhibit mental retardation or have psychiatric disorders. Vascular occlusions are also common.

Inheritance is autosomal recessive. Numerous mutations have been defined in the cystathionine-β-synthetase gene (CBS).[75–78] Most mutations are private and consist of missense mutations.[76] Certain mutations are associated with specific ethnicities. Prenatal diagnosis has been accomplished by enzyme assay of cultured amniotic cells or chorionic villi.[79] Prenatal DNA-based analysis is possible in families in whom the preexisting mutations have been defined.

Pseudoxanthoma Elasticum

This is a heritable connective tissue disorder with skin, cardiovascular, and ocular manifestations.[80] The clinical findings are the result of: the progressive fragmentation and calcification of elastic fibers; the increased dermal deposition of extracellular matrix, including proteoglycan, glycosaminoglycans, fibronectin, and vitronectin; and increased production of elastic fibers in affected skin.[80–82]

The skin findings are the most apparent clinical feature, and include yellow papules or nodules that coalesce into plaques in flexural sites. The areas most often affected include the axillae, neck, antecubital and popliteal fossae, and groin. The skin eventually sags, and individuals appear prematurely aged. Ocular involvement can be serious. It is characterized by peau d'orange hyperpigmentation, angioid streaks in the fundi resulting from breaks in calcified elastic lamina of Bruch's membrane, subretinal membranes with neovascularization, retinal hemorrhages, and central vision loss.[80,81,83] Legal blindness may result. Calcification and degeneration of elastin-rich vessels also occurs. Vascular changes may lead to intermittent claudication of the lower extremities, abdominal angina due to celiac artery stenosis, gastric bleeding, and myocardial infarcts at an early age.[80,81,83] Endocardial fibroelastosis with mitral valve prolapse is also relatively common.[80]

Pseudoxanthoma is not usually evident at birth, and considerable heterogeneity exists. The disorder has been linked recently to a series of mutations in *ABCC6*.[83–88] This gene is a member of the multiple-drug resistance family and is also known as *MRP6*. *ABCC6* encodes a transmembrane transport protein with ATPase activity. Although the exact function remains unknown, evidence suggests that it may function as an active transporter of anions.[89–91] The pathophysiology remains speculative, but may be due to the accumulation of some substance secondary to failed efflux function.[83]

To date, nonsense, missense, deletions, or small and large insertions and exon-skipping mutations have been defined. Affected individuals are homozygotes or compound heterozygotes, although heterozygous carriers may be at risk for partial manifestation.[84,85] The recent identification of the defective gene permits prenatal diagnosis in families at risk and allows for genetic counseling.

Osteopetrosis

Several different forms are recognized.[92] There is an extremely rare *in utero* lethal form of osteopetrosis. Affected infants suffer fractures *in utero*. Inheritance seems to be autosomal dominant, and the disorder can be detected by ultrasound.[93]

Malignant (infantile) osteopetrosis is a separate disorder that presents during infancy.[92] Patients have restricted cranial foramina that may have an impact on the function of the cranial nerves. Basal foramina restriction can result in cerebral ischemia. Cytopenias develop due to reduced bone marrow volume. Hepatosplenomegaly reflects extramedullary hematopoiesis. Impaired drainage via the eustachian tubes or sclerosis of the middle ear bones may result in deafness. Fractures are common secondary to bone fragility. Osteomyelitis is also common. Patients are usually short with a large head and may have genu valgum. Unless the disease is successfully treated the lifespan is markedly foreshortened in this recessively inherited form of osteoporosis. Definitive treatment consists of bone marrow transplantation.

At least two separate defective genes cause the malignant infantile recessive form of osteopetrosis. In a small number of patients, the chloride channel C1C-7, is lost due to mutations in *CLCN7*.[94,95] C1C-7 mutations have also been defined in intermediate autosomal recessive osteopetrosis.[96] In a larger group with the autosomal recessive malignant variant, mutations in the *ATP6i (TCIRG1)*, encoding the α3 subunit of the vacuolar proton pump occur.[97–100] Prenatal diagnosis in the malignant recessive forms has been accomplished by ultrasound. Molecular based ATP6i prenatal diagnosis has been performed.[98,100]

Interestingly, C1C-7 gene mutations have also been documented in the benign autosomal dominant variant known as Albers-Schönberg disease (ADO II).[95] This is considered to be a common form. Clinical manifestations in ADO II include nontraumatic fractures, palsies of the cranial nerves, and osteoarthritis. The *ClCN7* mutations in the ADO II form are believed to be manifested in a dominant-negative manner, whereas those in the autosomal recessive malignant or autosomal recessive intermediate forms are believed to represent loss of function.[95]

Additional forms, including an autosomal recessive variant due to carbonic anhydrase II deficiency, are recognized. The patients with carbonic anhydrase II deficiencies do not usually have fractures, but they may be short in stature. They may have failure to thrive, developmental delays, and renal tubular acidosis. Prenatal diagnosis by molecular means in families with defined mutations is available.[92,101]

REFERENCES

1. Horton WA, Hecht JT. Chondrodysplasias: general concepts and diagnostic and management considerations. In: Royce PM, Steinmann B, eds. Connective tissue and its heritable disorders, 2nd ed. New York: Wiley-Liss, 2002:901.
2. Horton WA, Hecht JT. Chondrodysplasias: disorders of cartilage matrix proteins. In: Royce PM, Steinmann B, eds. Connective tissue and its heritable disorders, 2nd ed. New York: Wiley-Liss, 2002:909.
3. Superti-Furga A. Skeletal dysplasias related to defects in sulfate metabolism. In: Royce PM, Steinmann B, eds. Connective tissue and its heritable disorders, 2nd ed. New York: Wiley-Liss, 2002:939.

4. Francomano CA, Muenke M. Craniosynostosis syndromes and skeletal dysplasias caused by mutations in fibroblast growth factor receptor genes. In: Royce PM, Steinmann B, eds. Connective tissue and its heritable disorders, 2nd ed. New York: Wiley-Liss, 2002:961.

5. Vissing H, D'Alessio M, Lee B, et al. Glycine to serine substitutions in the triple helical domain of pro-α1(II) collagen results in a lethal perinatal form of short-limbed dwarfism. J Biol Chem 1989;264:18265.

6. Lee B, Vissing H, Ramirez F, et al. Identification of the molecular defect in a family with spondyloepiphyseal dysplasia. Science 1989;244:978.

7. Chan D, Taylor TK, Cole WG. Characterization of an arginine 789 to cysteine substitution in α1(II) collagen chains in a patient with spondyloepiphyseal dysplasia. J Biol Chem 1993;268:15238.

8. Vikkula M, Ritvaniemi P, Vuorio E, et al. A mutation in the amino terminal end of the triple helix of type II collagen causing severe osteochondrodysplasia. Genomics 1993;16:282.

9. Rimoin DI, Lachman RS. Genetic disorders of the osseous skeleton. In: Beighton P. ed. McKusick's heritable disorders of connective tissue, 5 ed. St. Louis: Mosby, 1993:557.

10. Winterpacht A, Hilbert M, Schwarze U, et al. Kniest and Stickler dysplasia phenotypes caused by collagen type II (COL2A1) defects. Nat Genet 1993;4:323.

11. Ahmad N, Ala-Kokko L, Knowlton R, et al. Stop codon in the procollagen II gene (COL2A1 in a family with the Stickler syndrome (artho-ophthalmopathy). Proc Nat Acad Sci USA 1991;88:6624.

12. Annunen S, Körkkö J, Czarny M, et al. Splicing mutations of 54-bp exons in the COL11A1 gene cause Marshall syndrome, but other mutations cause overlapping Marshall/Stickler phenotypes. Am J Hum Genet 1999;65:974.

13. Richard AJ, Yates JR, Williams R, et al. A family with Stickler syndrome type 2 has a mutation in the COL11A1 gene resulting in the substitution of glycine 97 by valine in α1(XI) collagen. Hum Mol Genet 1996;5:1339.

14. Vikkula M, Mariman E, Lui V, et al. Autosomal dominant and recessive osteochondrodysplasias associated with the COL11A2 locus. Cell 1995;80:431.

15. Sirko-Osada DA, Murray MA, Scott JA, et al. Stickler syndrome without eye involvement is caused by mutations in COL11A2, the gene encoding the α2(XI) chain of type XI collagen. J Pediatr 1998;132:368.

16. Melkoniemi M, Brunner HG, Manouvrier S, et al. Autosomal recessive disorder otospondylomegaepiphyseal dysplasia is associated with loss-of-function mutations in the COL11A2 gene. Am J Hum Genet 2000;66:368.

17. Milunsky J, Maher T, Lebo R, et al. Prenatal diagnosis for Schmid Metaphyseal chondrodysplasia in twins. Fetal Diagn Ther 1998;13:167.

18. Warman ML, Abott M, Apte SS, et al. A type X collagen mutation causes Schmid metaphyseal chondrodysplasia. Nat Genet 1993;5:79.

19. Ikegawa S, Nishimura G, Nagai T, et al. Mutations of the type X collagen gene (COL10A1) causes spondylometaphyseal dysplasia Am J Hum Genet 1998;63:1659.

20. Briggs, MD. Chapman KL. Pseudoachondroplasia and multiple epiphyseal dysplasia: mutation review, molecular interactions, and genotype to phenotype correlations. Hum Mutat 2002;19:465.

21. Briggs MD, Hoffmann SMG, King LM, et al. Pseudoachondroplasia and multiple epiphyseal dysplasia due to mutations in the cartilage oligomeric protein gene. Nat Genet 1995;10:330.

22. Czarny-Ratajczak M, Lohiniva J, Rogala, et al. A mutation in COL9A1 causes multiple epiphyseal dysplasiafurther evidence for locus heterogeneity in MED. Am J Hum Genet 2001;69:969.

23. Muragaki Y, Mariman ECM, van Beersum SEC, et al. A mutation in the gene encoding the α2 chain of the fibril-associated collagen IX, COL9A2, causes multiple epiphyseal dysplasia (EDM2) Nat Genet 1996;12:103.

24. Paassilta P, Lohiniva J, Annunen S, et al. COL9A3: a third locus for multiple epiphyseal dysplasia. Am J Hum Genet 1999;64:1036.

25. Rossi A, Superti-Furga A. Mutations in the diastrophic dysplasia sulfate transporter (DTDST) gene (SLC26A2): 22 novel mutations, mutation review, associated skeletal phenotypes and diagnostic relevance. Hum Mutat 2001;17:159.

26. Superti-Furga A, Hastbacka J, Wilcox WR, et al. Achondrogenesis IB is caused by mutations in the diastrophic dysplasia sulphate transporter gene. Nat Genet 1996;12:100.

27. Superti-Furga A, Neumann L, Riebel T, et al. Recessively inherited multiple epiphyseal dysplasia with normal stature, club foot, and double-layered patella caused by a DTDST mutation. J Med Genet 1999;36:621.

28. Hastbacka J, Kerrebrock A, Mokkala K, et al. Identification of the Finnish founder mutation for diastrophic dysplasia (DTD). Eur J Hum Genet 1999;7:664.

29. Francomano CA, Muenke M. Craniosynostosis syndromes and skeletal dysplasias caused by mutations in

fibroblast growth factor receptor genes. In: Royce PM, Steinmann B, eds. Connective tissue and its heritable disorders, 2nd ed. New York: Wiley-Liss 2002:961.

30. Shiang R, Thompson LM, Zhu YZ, et al. Mutations in the transmembrane domain of FGFR3 cause the most common genetic form of dwarfism, achondroplasia. Cell 1994;78:335.

31. Rousseau F, Bonaventure J, Legai-Mallet L, et al. Mutations in the gene encoding fibroblast growth factor receptor-3 in achondroplasia. Nature 1994;371:252.

32. Ikegawa S, Fukushima Y, Isomura, et al. Mutations of the fibroblast growth factor receptor-3 gene in one familial and six sporadic cases of achondroplasia in Japanese patients. Hum Genet 1995;96:309.

33. Superti-Furga A, Eich GU, Bucher HU, et al. A glycine-375-to-cysteine substitution in the transmembrane domain of the fibroblast growth factor receptor-3 in a newborn with achondroplasia. Eur J Pediatr 1995;95:215.

34. Bellus GA, McIntosh I, Smith EA, et al. A recurrent mutation in the tyrosine kinase domain of fibroblasts growth factor receptor-3 causes hypochondroplasia. Nat Genet 1995;10:357.

35. Tavormina PL, Shiang R, Thompson LM, et al. Thanatophoric dysplasia (types I and II) caused by distinct mutations in fibroblast growth factor receptor-3. Nat Genet 1995;9:321.

36. Tavormina PL, Bellus GA, Webster MK, et al. A novel skeletal dysplasia with developmental delay and acanthosis nigricans is caused by a Lys650Met mutation in the fibroblast growth factor receptor-3 (FGFR3) gene. Am J Hum Genet 1999;64;722.

37. Flores-Sarnat L. New insights into craniosynostosis. Semin Pediatr Neurol 2002:9;274.

38. Muenke M, Schell U, Hehr, A et al. A common mutation in the fibroblast growth factor receptor-1 gene in Pfeiffer syndrome. Nat Genet 1994;8:269.

39. Schell U, Hehr A, Feldman GJ, et al. Mutations in the FGFR1 and FGFR2 cause familial and sporadic Pfeiffer syndrome. Hum Mol Genet 1995;4:323.

40. Meyers GA, Day D, Goldberg R, et al. FGFR2 exon IIIa and IIIc mutations in Crouzon, Jackson–Weiss and Pfeiffer syndromes: evidence for missense changes, insertions and a deletion due to alternative RNA splicing. Am J Hum Genet 1996;58:491.

41. Wilkie AOM, Slaney SF, Oldridge M, et al. Apert syndrome results form localized mutations of FGFR2 and is allelic with Crouzon syndrome. Nat Genet 1995;9:165.

42. Oldridge M, Zackai EH. McDonald-McGinn DM, et al. De novo alu-element insertions in FGFR2 identify a distinct pathological basis for Apert syndrome Am J Hum Genet 1999;64:446.

43. Meyers GA, Orlow SJ, Munro IR, et al. Fibroblast growth factor receptor 3 (FGFR3) transmembrane mutation in Crouzon syndrome with acanthosis nigricans. Nat Genet 1995;11:462.

44. Superti-Furga A, Lacher ML, Steinlin M. Crouzon syndrome with acanthosis nigricans, spinal stenosis and desmo-osteoblastomas: pleiotropic effects of the FGFR3 Ala391Glu mutation. J Craniomaxillofac Surg 1996: suppl:112.

45. Bellus GA, Gaudenz K, Zackai EH, et al. Identical mutations in three different fibroblast growth factor receptor genes in autosomal dominant craniosynostosis syndromes. Nat Genet 1996;14:174.

46. Muenke M, Gripp KW, McDonald-McGinn DM, et al. A unique point mutation in the fibroblast growth factor receptor 3 gene (FGFR3) defines a new craniosynostosis syndrome. Am J Hum Genet 1997;60;555.

47. Jabs EW, Li X, Scott AF, et al. Jackson–Weiss and Crouzon syndromes are allelic with mutations in fibroblast growth factor receptor 2. Nat Genet 1994;8:275.

48. Byers PH, Cole WG. Osteogenesis Imperfecta. In: Royce PM, Steinmann B, eds. Connective tissue and its heritable disorders, 2nd ed. New York: Wiley-Liss, 2002:385.

49. Chu M-L, Prockop DJ. Collagen: Gene Structure. In: Royce PM, Steinmann B, eds. Connective tissue and its heritable disorders, 2nd ed. New York: Wiley-Liss, 2002:223.

50. Sillence D. Osteogenesis imperfecta: an expanding panorama of variants. Clin Orthop 1981;159:11.

51. Körkkö J, Ala-Kokko L, De Paepe AD, et al. Analysis of the COL1A1 and COL1A2 genes by PCR amplification and scanning by conformation-sensitive gel electrophoresis identifies only COL1A1 mutations in 15 patients with osteogenesis imperfecta type I: identification of common sequences of null allele mutations. Am J Hum Genet 1998;62:98.

52. Steinmann B, Royce PM, Superti-Furga A. The Ehlers-Danlos syndrome. In: Royce PM, Steinmann B, eds. Connective tissue and its heritable disorders, 2nd ed. New York: Wiley-Liss, 2002:431.

53. Schwarze U, Atkinson M, Hoffman GG, et al. Null alleles of the COL5A1 gene of type V collagen are a cause of classical forms of Ehlers–Danlos syndrome (types I and II). Am J Hum Genet; 2000;66:1757.

54. Schalkwijk J, Zweers MC, Steijlen PM, et al. A recessive form of the Ehlers–Danlos syndrome caused by tenascin-X- deficiency. N Engl J Med 2001;345:1167.

55. Pepin M, Schwarze U, Superti-Furga A, et al. Clinical and genetic features of Ehlers–Danlos syndrome type IV, the vascular type. N Engl J Med 2000;342:673.

56. Pepin MG, Byers PH. Ehlers–Danlos syndrome, vascular type. Gene Rev 1999 (updated 2002) www.genetests.org.
57. Schwarze U, Goldstein JA, Byers PH. Splicing defects in the COL3A1 gene: marked preference for 5′(donor) splice-site mutations in patients with exon skipping mutations and Ehlers–Danlos syndrome type IV. Am J Hum Genet 1997;61:1276.
58. Schwarze U, Schievink WI, Petty E, et al. Haploinsufficiency for one COL3A1 allele of type III procollagen results in a phenotype similar to the vascular form of Ehlers–Danlos syndrome type IV. Am J Hum Genet 2002;69:989.
59. Yeowell HN, Walker LC. Mutations in the lysyl hydroxylase 1 gene that result in enzyme deficiency and the clinical phenotype of Ehlers–Danlos syndrome type VI. Mol Genet Metab 2000;71:212.
60. Kielty CM, Grant ME. The collagen family: Structure, assembly, and organization in the extracellular matrix. In: Royce PM, Steinmann B, eds. Connective tissue and its heritable disorders, 2nd ed. New York: Wiley-Liss, 2002:159.
61. Hyland J, Ala-Kokko L, Royce PM, et al. A homozygous stop codon in the lysyl hydroxylase gene in a family with Ehlers–Danlos syndrome type VI. Nat Genet 1992;2:228.
62. Byers PH, Duvic M, Atkinson M, et al. Ehlers–Danlos syndrome type VIIA and type VIIB result from splice site-junction mutations or genomic deletions that involve exon 6 in the COL1A1 and COL1A2 genes of type I collagen. Am J Med Genet 1997;72:94.
63. Horn N, Tümer Z. Menkes disease and the occipital horn syndrome. In: Royce PM, Steinmann B. eds. Connective tissue and its heritable disorders, 2nd ed. New York: Wiley-Liss, 2002:651.
64. Gu Y-H, Kodama H, Murata Y, et al. ATP7A gene mutations in 16 patients with Menkes disease and occipital horn syndrome Am J Med Genet 2001;99:217.
65. Møller LB, Tümer Z, Lund C, et al. Similar splice-site mutations of the ATP7A gene lead to different phenotypes: classic Menkes disease or occipital horn syndrome Am J Hum Genet 2000;66:1211.
66. Dagenais SL, Adam AN, Innis JW, et al. A novel frameshift mutation in exon 23 of ATP7A (MNK) results in occipital horn syndrome and not in Menkes disease. Am J Hum Genet 2001;69:420.
67. Seidel J, Möller LB, Mentzel HJ, et al. Disturbed copper transport in humans. Part 1: mutations of the ATP7A gene lead to Menkes disease and occipital horn syndrome. Cell Mol Biol 2001;47.
68. Liu P-C, McAndrew PE, Kaler SG. Rapid and robust screening of the Menkes disease/occipital horn syndrome Gene. Genet Test 2002;6:255.
69. Pyeritz RE, Dietz HC. Marfan syndrome and other microfibrillar disorders. In: Royce PM, Steinmann B. eds. Connective tissue and its heritable disorders, 2nd ed. New York: Wiley-Liss, 2002:585.
70. Dietz HC, Cutting GR, Pyeritz RE, et al. Marfan syndrome caused by a recurrent de novo missense mutation in the fibrillin gene. Nature 1991;352:337.
71. Körkkö J, Kaitila I, Lönnqvist L, et al. Sensitivity of conformational sensitive gel electrophoresis in detecting mutations in Marfan syndrome and related conditions. J Med Genet 2002;39:34.
72. Robinson PN, Booms P, Katzke S, et al. Mutations of FBN1 and genotype–phenotype correlations in Marfan syndrome and related fibrillinopathies. Hum Mutat 2002;20:153.
73. De Paepe A, Devereux RB, Dietz HC, et al. Revised diagnostic criteria for the Marfan syndrome. Am J Med Genet 1996;62:417.
74. Milewicz DM, Urbán Z, Boyd C. Genetic disorders of the elastic fiber system. Matrix Biol 2000;19:471.
75. Skovby F, Kraus JP. The homocystinurias. In: Royce PM, Steinmann B. eds. Connective tissue and its heritable disorders, 2nd ed. New York: Wiley-Liss, 2002:627.
76. Krause JP, Janošík M, Kozich V, et al. Cystathionine β-synthase mutations in homocystinuria. Hum Mutat 1999;13:362.
77. de Franchis R, Kraus E, Kozich V, et al. Four novel mutations in the cystathionine β-synthase gene: effect of a second linked mutation on the severity of the homocystinuric phenotype. Hum Mutat 1999;13:453.
78. Gaustadnes M, Wilcken B, Oliveriusova J, et al. The molecular basis of cystathionine β. Hum Mutat 2002;20:117.
79. Fowler B, Jakobs C. Post and prenatal diagnostic methods for the homocystinurias. Eur J Pediatr 1998;157 (suppl 2):S88.
80. Nelder KH, Struk B. Pseudoxanthoma elasticum. In: Royce PM, Steinmann B eds. Connective tissue and its heritable disorders, 2nd ed. New York: Wiley-Liss, 2002:561.
81. Ohtani T, Furukawa F. Pseudoxanthoma elasticum. J Dermatol 2002;29:615.
82. Pulkkinen L, Ringpfeil, F Uitto J. Progress in heritable skin diseases: molecular bases and clinical implications. J Am Acad Dermatol 2002;47:91.
83. Ringpfeil F, Pulkkinen L, Uitto J. Molecular genetics of pseudoxanthoma elasticum. Exp Dermatol 2001;10:221.

84. Ringpfeil F, Lebwohl MG, Christiano AM, et al. Pseudoxanthoma elasticum: mutations in the MRP6 gene encoding a transmembrane ATP binding cassette (ABC) transporter. Proc Natl Acad Sci USA 2000;97:6001.

85. Le Saux O, Urban Z Tschuch C, et al. Mutations in a gene encoding an ABC transporter cause pseudoxanthoma elasticum. Nat Genet 2000;25:223.

86. Bergen AA, Plomp AS, Schuurman EJ, et al. Mutations in ABCC6 cause pseudoxanthoma elasticum. Nat Genet 2000;25:228.

87. Struck B, Cai L, Zach S, et al. Mutations of the gene encoding the transmembrane transporter protein ABCC6 cause pseudoxanthoma elasticum. J Mol Med. 2000;78:282.

88. Le Saux O, Beck K, Sachsinger C, et al. A spectrum of ABCC6 mutations is responsible for pseudoxanthoma elasticum. Am J Hum Genet 2001;69:749.

89. Ilias A, Urban Z, Seidl TL, et al. Loss of ATP-dependent transport activity in pseudoxanthoma elasticum-associated mutants of human ABCC6 (MRP6) J Biol Chem 2002;277:16860.

90. Cai J, Daoud R, Alqawi O, et al. Nucleotide binding and nucleotide hydrolysis properties of the ABC transporter MRP6 (ABCC6). Biochemistry 2002;41:8058.

91. Belinsky MG, Chen ZS, Shchaveleva I, et al. Characterization of the drug resistance and transport properties of multidrug resistance protein 6 (MRP6, ABCC6). Cancer Res 2002;62:6172.

92. Whyte M. Osteopetrosis. In: Royce PM, Steinmann B, eds. Connective tissue and its heritable disorders, 2nd ed. New York: Wiley-Liss, 2002:789.

93. El-Khazen N, Faverly D, Vamos E, et al. Lethal osteopetrosis with multiple fractures *in utero*. Am J Med Genet 1986;23:811.

94. Kornak U, Kasper D, Bosl MR, et al. Loss of CIC-7 chloride channel leads to osteopetrosis in mice and man. Cell 2001;104:205.

95. Cleiren E, Bénichou O, Van Hul EV, et al. Albers-Schönberg disease (autosomal dominant osteopetrosis type II) results form mutations in the CICN7 chloride channel gene. Hum Mol Genet 2001;10:2861.

96. Campos-Xavier AB, Saraiva JM, Ribeiro LM, et al. Chloride channel (CIC-7) mutations in intermediate autosomal recessive osteopetrosis. Hum Genet 2003;112:186.

97. Frattini A, Orchard P J, Sobacchi C, et al. Defects in TCIRG1 subunit of the vacuolar proton pump are responsible for a subset of human autosomal recessive osteopetrosis. Nat Genet 2000;25:343.

98. Sobacchi C, Frattini A, Orchard P, et al. The mutational spectrum of human malignant autosomal recessive osteopetrosis. Hum Mol Genet 2001;10:1767.

99. Michigami T, Kageyama T, Satomura K, et al. Novel mutations in the α3 subunit of vacuolar H(+)-adenosine triphosphatase in a Japanese patient with infantile malignant osteopetrosis. Bone 2002;30:436.

100. Scimeca, J-C, Quincey D, Parrinello H, et al. Novel mutations in the TCIRG1 gene encoding the a3 subunit of the vacuolar proton pump in patients affected by infantile malignant osteopetrosis. Hum Mutat 2003;21:151.

101. De Vernejoul MC, Bénichou O. Human osteopetrosis and other sclerosing disorders: recent genetic developments. Calcif Tissue Int 2001;69:1.

Aubrey Milunsky, M.B.B.Ch., D.Sc.,
F.R.C.P., F.A.C.M.G., D.C.H., and
Jacob A. Canick, Ph.D., F.A.C.B.

21

Maternal Serum Screening for Neural Tube and Other Defects

Neural tube defects (NTDs) are among the most common serious congenital defects, with an expected birth prevalence in most countries commonly put at 1 in 1000.[1] However, until the mid-1970s the birth prevalence in the United Kingdom was considerably higher, with spina bifida and anencephaly, the most common NTDs, occurring in about 4 of every 1000 births. Certain areas of Northern Ireland and Scotland had a reported birth prevalence as high as 7 to 10 per 1000 births. With the prevalence there reaching 1 percent, the development of a screening test for NTDs was a major public health priority. The discovery of the association between elevated levels of amniotic fluid (AF) and, soon afterward, maternal serum α-fetoprotein (MSAFP) and the presence of fetal NTDs in the early 1970s, and the adoption of a rational screening strategy using MSAFP has represented a major advance in our ability to identify serious fetal defects prenatally.[2]

In the years since prenatal screening was implemented on a widespread basis, a reduction in the birth prevalence of NTDs has been noted, especially in the United Kingdom. A study examining the birth prevalence in England and Wales of anencephaly and open spina bifida (SB), the two most common and serious NTDs, showed that the prevalence declined by 95 percent from the 1960s to the mid-1990s, from approximately 4 to less than 0.2 cases per 1000 births.[3] It is not possible, however, that this decline has been the result of serum screening alone, because the reduction in cases identified at midpregnancy was about half the total reduction in cases noted at term. The remainder of the decrease has been attributed to two additional reasons: the application of prenatal ultrasound as a screening tool, and an increase in the intake of folic acid as part of improved diet and through the increased use of vitamins before conception and continuing through pregnancy.

In recent years, implementation of the two newer strategies for the prevention of NTDs has markedly increased. The use of ultrasound markers has become a common alternative to serum screening in areas where second-trimester ultrasound is commonly used.[4] As for primary prevention of NTDs, while public awareness of the benefits of folic acid has been increased through effective advertising, a major thrust has been the decision by many countries, including the United States in 1996 and Canada in 1997, to require folic acid fortification of all wheat products through its addition to flour.[5,6] The impact of the new strategies on the birth prevalence of affected infants is just beginning to be assessed.

This chapter on maternal serum screening for NTDs is presented in the context of decreasing prevalence. At some point in the future, when optimal levels of folic acid are commonly consumed, the need for population-based prenatal screening for NTDs may be unnecessary. In addition, surgery for the correction of spina bifida in utero is being studied, thus far with limited success (see chapter 29).[7–9] A randomized clinical trial to determine the benefits of corrective surgery is now under way. Meanwhile, detailed and updated information on NTDs and a prenatal screening strategy that has been in effect for more than two decades remain necessary.

TYPES OF NTD

Anencephaly and the various forms of SB are the most common NTDs, and each occurs with similar prevalence. Other, less common, NTDs include exencephaly, iniencephaly, and encephalocele. Anencephaly is a lethal defect in which the cranial vault and varying amounts of brain tissue are absent. SB is associated with varying degrees of mortality and morbidity (see discussion below), depending on the size and location of the lesion and whether it is open or closed.

Approximately 85 percent of SB lesions are open, having only a membrane covering or no covering at all, while closed SB is skin-covered. The SB lesions are made up mainly of meningoceles and myeloceles or combinations thereof (myelomeningoceles). Meningoceles are herniations of the meninges, with the cord remaining in its usual position, and they constitute between 5 and 10 percent of all NTDs.[10] In contrast, myeloceles do not involve herniations, but neural tissue is exposed. Even when small, myeloceles almost invariably connote serious defects because of involvement of the cord. Myelomeningoceles, which involve both the spinal cord and the nerve roots, are associated with Arnold–Chiari malformations, in which contents of the cranial vault are displaced downward.

Women who have had a child with anencephaly may subsequently deliver a child with SB, and vice versa. However, in the vast majority of cases, the lesion is the same as the earlier one.[10,11] Fewer than 20 percent of infants with anencephaly or SB have associated malformations, whereas more than one-third of infants with encephalocele have associated malformations.[12]

PREVALENCE

NTDs are among the most common major congenital malformations in most countries. Striking variations in birth prevalence have been reported in studies done in the 1960s, 1970s, and 1980s. Extremely high rates (exceeding 8 per 1,000 births) were reported for Northern Ireland, Egypt, India, and China.[13–15]

Although large geographic and temporal variations in the frequency of NTDs are well known, a marked decrease in the prevalence of NTDs has been observed. In the United States; estimates made in the 1970s varied between 1.4 and 3.1 per 1,000 births.[16] U.S. studies in the early 1980s showed a somewhat lower prevalence, between 1.0 and 1.6 per 1,000 births for NTDs and between 0.2 and 0.8 per 1,000 births for SB, with the highest rates being found in southern Appalachia.[17,18] A 1995 report from the Centers for Disease Control and Prevention (CDC), studying the birth prevalence in 1985–1994, put the rate even lower, between 0.4 and 1.0 per 1,000 births.[19]

Nowhere has the reduction in the birth prevalence of NTDs been more dramatic than in the United Kingdom. In England and Wales, the total prevalence declined from about 3.4 per 1,000 live births and stillbirths in 1974 to just under 0.8 per 1,000 births by 1994.[20,21] A recent estimate has placed the birth prevalence by 1997 as low as 0.14 per 1,000,[3] based on data from the Office of National Statistics[22–24] and with rates adjusted for underreporting.[25] The striking reduction in the birth prevalence of open spina bifida and anencephaly in England and Wales is shown in Figure 21.1.[26]

The marked decrease in the birth prevalence is the result of a combination of primary and secondary prevention. The advent of the secondary methods of prevention, prenatal screening using MSAFP, as well as the more recent addition of ultrasound as a screening method, has been estimated to account for almost half of the decline in the United Kingdom.[20] More than half stems from primary prevention, improvement in dietary intake of folic acid, and the increased use of prenatal vitamins containing folic acid supplementation beginning in the periconceptional period.

ETIOLOGY AND PRIMARY PREVENTION

It is now known that 70 percent to perhaps as many as 85 percent of NTDs can be avoided with sufficient intake of folic acid.[27,28] This finding indicates that whatever the various causes of NTDs that have been discovered, whether genetic or environmental, many of them share a requirement for mechanisms requiring folic acid. Multiple other causes account for a minority of cases.

The heterogeneous origin of NTDs makes it important to reach a precise diagnosis for genetic counseling. The vast majority of NTDs arise as a consequence of multifactorial inheritance. Putative genetic factors (Table 21.1) as well as many environmental causal

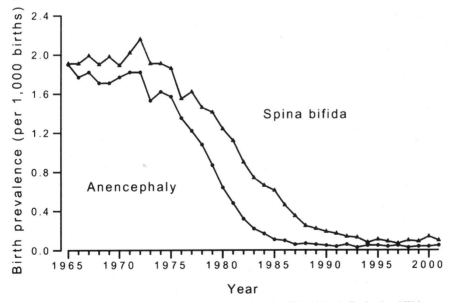

Fig. 21.1. Decline in the prevalence of anencephaly and open spina bifida births in England and Wales, 1965–2000. *Source*: Courtesy of NJ Wald, Wolfson Institute of Preventive Medicine, University of London, London, UK.

Table 21.1. Evidence for a putative causal association of genetic factors with neural tube defects

Observations Implicating Genetic Factors	Reference
Polygenic nature of most disorders	29,30
Bias in sex ratio toward higher number of females	13,31
High percentage of males in low-prevalence areas	32
Increased susceptibility if parent has HLA-DR locus	33
Increased frequency in consanguineous matings	34
Monozygotic twin concordance	12,31,32
Racial/ethnic bias in incidence	13,35
Familial recurrence pattern: affected parent: affected sibling/aunt/uncle/cousin	13
Increased incidence when there is a previous child with hydrocephaly	36
Increased incidence when there is a previous child with germ-cell tumor	37
Susceptibility of midline "developmental field"	38
Mitochondrial uncoupling gene	38a
Mutations in *PAX-3* gene	39
Abnormalities in folate and/or cobalamin metabolism	40–46a

associations (Table 21.2) have been suggested. In addition, an NTD may occur in many different syndromes (see examples in Table 21.3) and in association with chromosomal disorders (Table 21.4). The concurrence of a NTD and a chromosomal disorder may be fortuitous or may indicate the locus of a susceptibility gene.

Sever[200] and others[201] hypothesized that environmental factors were of less etiologic importance than genetic influences in a population with a low incidence rate for NTD, compared with areas or time periods with high incidence rates. In support of this hypothesis, Sever found no significant difference between rates by month of birth or conception and no significant association with maternal age or parity for anencephaly. However, he did note a significantly increased frequency with advanced maternal age for SB. Factors that support a genetic origin included a predominance of females, a higher twin concordance rate, an increased risk in siblings, a declining risk in other family members with increasing genetic distance, and the altered sex ratio in transmitting relatives.[202–204]

A cause is identifiable in 6–20 percent of NTDs[30,205,206]; most of those recognized are listed in Tables 21.2–21.4. The incidence of NTDs in liveborn infants with trisomy 18 is about 6.2 percent.[187] The reason for the increased frequency of NTDs in trisomy 18 and triploidy is unknown; their occurrence in other chromosomal defects is still possible by chance. Given the occurrence of NTDs in other chromosomal disorders (see Table 21.4), karyotyping is recommended if any additional major fetal defect is evident or when dysmorphic features are noted. Various drugs have been implicated in the etiology of NTDs. Both valproic acid[93,94,207] and carbamazepine[48] taken during the first 6 weeks of pregnancy apparently have a 2–5 percent[17,208] risk of causing SB. Clomiphene citrate to induce ovulation has been associated with NTDs by some authors but not by others.[209] It remains unclear whether the basic reasons for infertility are not more important. Questions remain about background causes in common—underlying the many apparent associations listed in Table 21.2. The major environmental maternal factors recognized include folic acid deficiency, diabetes mellitus, obesity, hyperthermia, maternal alcohol ingestion, anticonvulsant treatment, and zinc deficiency. Accumulating evidence[73,74] points to about a twofold increased risk of NTD in the offspring of obese women. Even increasing prepregnancy maternal weight, independent of folate intake, appears associated with a rising risk of NTD.[75] The effect of obesity, may at least in part, be caused by hyperinsulinemia. In a recent study of Mexican American women, hyperinsulinemia was associated with an almost twofold increase in the risk for NTD, independent of its association with maternal obesity.[210]

Folic Acid and Etiology

For more than five decades, data[56,211–214] have pointed to the likely key role of folic acid deficiency in the pathogenesis of NTDs.[45] In pregnancies with fetal NTDs, levels of serum and red blood cell folic acid and serum vitamin B_{12} have, on average, been reported to be lower than in pregnancies with normal fetuses.[215]

Red-cell folate is regarded as the better proxy for folate status, given that it reflects the folate turnover during the previous 120 days.[96] Daly et al.[40] first showed that the risk of NTD is associated with red-cell folate levels in a continuous dose–response relation-

Table 21.2.   Reported "environmental" causal associations with neural tube defects

Environmental Factors	Selected References
Aminopterin	47
Carbamazepine	48
Clomiphene citrate	49–52
Copper in drinking water	53
Efavirenz (reverse transcriptase inhibitor)	53a
Fetus interaction with residual trophoblast	54
First-trimester surgery	55
Folic acid deficiency	45,56–58
Hyperthermia	59–61,249
Industrial/agricultural exposure	62,63
Magnesium or calcium content of drinking water	64,65
Maternal alcohol ingestion	66
Maternal age <20 or >35 years	67–70
Maternal diabetes mellitus	71,72
Maternal health	68
Maternal obesity	73–75,210
Maternal weight reduction (early pregnancy)	76
Maternal zinc deficiency	77–80
Nitrates, nitrites, and magnesium salts in foods	81
Oral contraceptives	82
Parity	32
Paternal age	83
Potato blight	84
Previous spontaneous abortions/stillbirth	85,86
Season, epidemics	87
Social class/poverty/illegitimacy	67
Subfertility	88
Tea drinking	89
Thalidomide	90
Twinning	91,92
Valproic acid	93,94
Vitamin A	95
Vitamin B_{12} deficiency	96
Warfarin (Coumadin)	97

Note: Additional references in previous edition 1992.[98]

Table 21.3. Syndromes in which neural tube defects (NTDs) may be a feature

Syndrome	Type of NTD	Additional Selected Clinical Features
Acrocallosal[99]	A	Agenesis corpus callosum; mental retardation; polydactyly
Acromelic frontonasal "dysplasia"[100]	E	Agenesis corpus callosum; Dandy–Walker malformation; polydactyly; mental retardation
Amniotic bands/early amnion rupture[101]	E	Clefting; limb defects
Anophthalmia-clefting-neural tube defects[102]	SB	Clefting; eye and ear abnormalities
Anterior encephalocele[103]	E	Hydrocephalus; eye anomalies
Apert—acrocephalosyndactyly type I[104]	E	Mental retardation; craniosynostosis; agenesis corpus callosum
Boomerang dysplasia[105]	E	Short limb dwarfism; omphalocele; ossification defect
Brachydactyly type C[106]	A	Short stature; brachydactyly; phalangeal anomalies
Carpenter–Hunter[107]	E	Micromelia; polysyndactyly; fragile bones
Caudal duplication[108]	SB	Genitourinary and gastrointestinal anomalies
Caudal regression[109]	SB	Sacral, genitourinary, and anorectal anomalies
Cerebro-oculonasal[110]	E	Mental retardation; craniosynostosis; eye and nasal anomalies
CHILD[111]	SB	Limb defects; hemidysplasia; ichthyosis
Cleft lip or palate[112]	SB	Clefting; fusion of eyelids; anal atresia/stenosis
Craniomicromelic syndrome[113]	E	Craniosynostosis; short limbs; IUGR
Craniotelencephalic dysplasia[114]	E	Craniosynostosis; agenesis corpus callosum; mental retardation; microcephaly
Cranium bifidum with neural tube defects[115]	E, SB	Skull ossification defect; mental retardation; Arnold-Chiari malformation
Currarino triad[116]	SB	Anorectal and sacral anomalies; urinary reflux
Czeizel[117]	SB	Split hands and feet; obstructive urinary anomalies; diaphragmatic defect
DiGeorge[118]	SB	Mental retardation; immune deficiency; hypoparathyroidism; conotruncal cardiac defect
Disorganization-like[119]	A, SB	Tail-like protrusion; accessory limbs; hemangiomas
DK—phocomelia[120]	E	Radial defect; esophageal atresia; heart defect; anal anomaly; thrombocytopenia
Donnai/Meckel-like[121]	E	Cerebellar abnormalities; renal cysts; polydactyly
Durkin–Stamm[122]	SB	Sacral teratomas; asymmetric lower limbs; lymphomas/leukemias
Encephalocele–arthrogryposis–hypoplastic thumbs[123]	E	Arthrogryposis; hypoplastic thumbs; normal intelligence; renal dysplasia
Femoral duplication[124]	SB	Duplicated femur; imperforate anus; ambiguous genitalia; omphalocele
Fried[125]	E	Microcephaly; cleft lip; hypoplastic/absent radii
Frontofacionasal dysplasia[126]	E	Clefting; mental retardation; coloboma; eye and nasal anomalies
Frontonasal dysplasia[127]	E	Microcephaly; clefting; eye and nasal anomalies
Fullana[128]	SB	Caudal deficiency; agenesis corpus callosum; polyasplenia
Gershoni–Baruch[129]	E	Diaphragmatic agenesis; omphalocele; multiple midline and radial ray defects
Gillessen–Kaesbach[130]	SB	Microencephaly; polycystic kidneys; brachymelia; heart defects
Goldberg[131]	SB	Sacral hemangiomas; genitourinary and anorectal anomalies
Goldenhar[132]	E	Facial, ear, and vertebral anomalies; epibulbar dermoid; mental retardation

Table 21.3.   Syndromes in which neural tube defects (NTDs) may be a feature (continued)

Syndrome	Type of NTD	Additional Selected Clinical Features
Gollop[133]	SB	Ectrodactyly; split femur; hydronephrosis
Gonadal agenesis and multiple dysraphic lesions[134]	E, SB	XX-agonadism, omphalocele
Hartsfield[135]	E	Clefting; holoprosencephaly; ectrodactyly; craniosynostosis
Hegde[136]	E	Aplasia pectoralis major; limb and renal anomalies
3 H[137]	SB	Hemihypertrophy; hemihypesthesia; hemiareflexia; scoliosis
Hydrolethalus[138]	E	Hydrocephalus; osteochondrodysplasia; clefting; limb defects
Ivemark[139]	E, SB	Asplenia/polysplenia; heart defect; situs inversus
Joubert[140]	E	Dandy–Walker malformation; microphthalmia; clefting
Keutel[141]	E	Humeroradial synostosis; mental retardation; microcephaly
Klippel–Feil[142]	SB	Cervical vertebrae fusion; heart and renal anomalies; deafness
Knobloch–Layer[143]	E	Detached retina; dextrocardia; scalp defects
Kousseff[144]	SB	Conotruncal heart defects; sacral and renal anomalies
Lateral meningocele syndrome[145]	SB	Multiple lateral meningoceles, joint laxity, dysmorphic, osteosclerosis
Lehman[146]	SB	Osteosclerosis; vertebral defects
Lethal branchio-oculofacial[147]	E	Branchial cleft sinuses; eye and ear anomalies; holoprosencephaly
Limb/pelvis-hypoplasia/aplasia[148]	E, SB	Limb deficiency; thoracic dystrophy; pathologic fractures; clefting; normal intelligence
Lipomyelomeningocele—familial[149]	SB	Sacral and vertebral anomalies
Machin[150]	E	Hydrops; tracheal/laryngeal anomalies/ ear and renal anomalies
Mathias[151]	SB	Situs inversus; cardiac and splenic anomalies
Meckel–Gruber[152]	E	Mental retardation; polycystic kidneys; polydactyly
Medeira[153]	A, SB	Clefting; limb reduction; heart defect
Melanocytosis[154]	SB	Skin hyperpigmentation
Meroanencephaly[155]	A, E	Skull ossification defects; microcephaly
Morning glory[156]	E	Clefting; coloboma; optic nerve anomalies
Ochoa[157]	SB	Hydronephrosis; genitourinary and facial anomalies
Oculocerebrocutaneous[158]	E	Orbital/cerebral cysts; skin tags; focal dermal effects; mental retardation
Oculoencephalohepatorenal[159]	E	Mental retardation; ataxia; eye, cerebellar, liver, and kidney anomalies
OEIS[160]	SB	Omphalocele; bladder exstrophy; imperforate anus; spinal defects
Oral-facial-digital type II[161]	E	Clefting; deafness; polydactyly; mental retardation
Pallister–Hall[162]	E	Hypothalamic hamartoblastoma; polydactyly; imperforate anus
Patel[163]	SB	Renal agenesis; absent müllerian structures; heart defect
Phaver[164]	SB	Limb pterygia; heart, vertebral, ear, and radial defects
Porphyria, homozygous acute intermittent[165]	E	Neurovisceral dysfunction; mental retardation; skin photosensitivity
Renal-hepatic-pancreatic dysplasia[166]	E	Dandy–Walker malformation; dysplastic kidneys; hepatic fibrosis

(continued)

Table 21.3.　Syndromes in which neural tube defects (NTDs) may be a feature (continued)

Syndrome	Type of NTD	Additional Selected Clinical Features
Roberts[167]	E	Limb reduction; mental retardation; clefting; eye defects
Rogers[168]	SB	Anophthalmia/microphthalmia
Rolland–Desbuquois[169]	E	Short-limbed dwarfism; vertebral segmentation defects; clefting
Sacral agenesis[170]	SB	Sacral and vertebral defects
Sacral defects (anterior)[171]	SB	Absent sacrum; sacral teratoma/tumor
Schisis association[172]	A, E, SB	Clefting; omphalocele; diaphragmatic hernia; hypospadias
Short rib—polydactyly type II[173]	A	Structural brain anomalies; polydactyly; clefting; short ribs
Silverman[169]	E	Short-limbed dwarfism; clefting; vertebral segmentation defects
Sirenomelia[174]	A, SB	Clefting; vertebral segmentation defects; midline anomalies
Spear–Mickle[175]	SB	Scalp defect; craniostenosis
Tandon[176]	E	Clefting; colobomas; anogenital and skeletal anomalies
Tactocerebellar dysraphia[177]	E	Structural cerebellar anomalies; clefting; heart defect
Thoracoabdominal enteric duplication[178]	SB	Enteric duplication; skeletal anomalies; dextrocardia
Thrombocytopenia—absent radius[179]	SB	Thrombocytopenia; radial ray defects; heart defects; mental retardation
Velocardiofacial[180]	SB	Conotruncal heart defects; mental retardation; clefting
Waardenburg[39,181]	SB	White forelock; deafness; heterochromia iridis; dystopia canthorum
Warburg[140]	E	Hydrocephalus; agyria; eye anomalies; clefting; Dandy–Walker malformation
Weissenbacher-Zweymuller[182]	E	Skeletal dysplasia; clefting
X-linked neural tube defects[183]	A, SB	Isolated NTDs
Zimmer[184]	A	Tetra-amelia; midline anomalies

Note: A5 = anencephaly, E5 = encephalocele, SB5 = spina bifida.

ship (Figure 21.2). Table 21.5 displays the distribution of red-cell folate in cases and controls for the risk of NTD in each category. More than an eightfold difference in risk was observed between those with the lowest and those with the highest red-cell folate levels. Graphically, they demonstrated that the risk of NTD is reduced as red-cell folate levels increase well past the point at which levels would have been considered normal.

Folic acid is required for methylation reactions in cells, directly involving the biosynthesis of methionine and nucleotides and indirectly influencing the methylation of proteins, DNA, and lipids. It is by now well known that when folic acid levels are low, the levels of the precursor of methionine, homocysteine, are high. The discovery that high levels of homocysteine were associated with pregnancies affected by fetal NTDs, led researchers to investigate the enzymes central to the interactions between the folic acid and methionine pathways. Allelic variants in a number of these enzymes, in particular 5,10-

Table 21.4. Examples of neural tube defects associated with chromosomal disorders

Chromosomal Disorder	Reference
Numerical defects	
Trisomy 13	185,186
Trisomy 18	186,187
Triploidy	188,189
Trisomy 9 mosaic	190
Structural defects	
1q42–qter deletion	191
2p24–pter duplication	192,192a,193
3p duplication	193a
3q27–3qter deletion	194
4p1	186
7q32 deletion	186
11q duplication	195
13q13 deletion	186
13q22 or 31–qter deletion	196
13q33–34 deletion	196a
15q duplication	197
22q11.2 deletion	197a
Xp22.1 deletion	198
Ring chromosome 13	199
Inversion X_q	189
Balanced translocation	
t(13q14q)	189

Note: The association may well be fortuitous in most cases but may signal susceptibility gene loci in others.

methylenetetrahydrofolate reductase (MTHFR), have been found to be associated with an increased incidence of NTDs.

A common mutation (677C → T) in the *MTHFR* gene, which results in reduced enzyme activity and impaired homocysteine/folate metabolism, has been found in 5–16 percent of Caucasian cohorts studied and in 2 percent of Japanese.[41] This mutation causes mild hyperhomocysteinemia[216] and an increased risk of NTDs,[40,42] which these authors further demonstrated in a meta-analysis.[41] This mutation is thought to explain a substantial part of the elevated plasma homocysteine levels in mothers of children with NTDs. van der Put et al.[217] suggested that individuals who are homozygous for the 677C → T mutation in the *MTHFR* gene may have higher nutritional folate requirements. However, a French study[218] noted no significant difference in the distribution of this mutation in prenatally diagnosed NTDs and controls.

Although folic acid supplementation clearly reduces the risk of NTDs, the biologic mechanisms remain unclear. Low concentrations of cobalamin and folate in early-pregnancy plasma are regarded as independent risk factors for pregnancies resulting in NTDs.[96] Adams et al.[219] reviewed conflicting reports claiming abnormalities in folate metabolism by some authors without confirmation by others in such pregnancies and the fact that women with folate deficiency have not had an increased risk of having offspring with NTDs. They also reviewed evidence of both normal and abnormal cobalamin metabolism in pregnancies with NTDs. Adams et al.[219] observed increased concentrations of methyl-

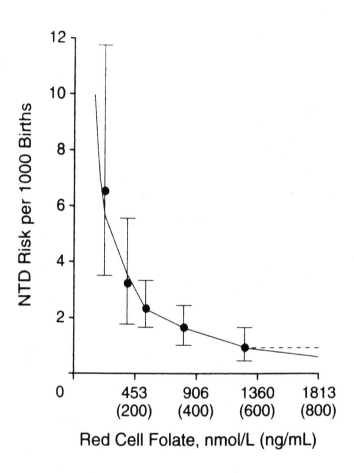

Fig. 21.2. The relationship of red-cell folate levels to the risk of neural tube defect (NTD). The solid line shows the predicted risk using logistic regression. The dotted line shows the constant risk assumed beyond a red-cell folate level of 1,292 nmol/L (570 ng/mL). The data points and error bars represent the observed risks and their 95 percent confidence intervals at the mean levels of red-cell folate. The logistic regression equation is NTD odds = exp (1.6463 − 1.2193 × ln[RCF]), where ln[RCF] is the natural log of red-cell folate measured in nanomoles per liter. If red-cell folate is measured in nanograms per milliliter, the constant in the equation becomes 0.6489, but the coefficient of 1.2193 remains the same. *Source*: Daly et al., 1995.[40]

malonic acid, a finding that would be consistent with reports of low plasma cobalamin levels in pregnancies with NTDs. The fact that differences in serum methylmalonic acid, but not cobalamin, were found apparently relates to the fact that methylmalonic acid is a more sensitive measure of cobalamin status than is serum cobalamin.[220] Although some studies have noted no difference in mean methylmalonic acid levels in pregnancies with NTDs, the increased plasma homocysteine concentrations observed[44] could possibly reflect folate and/or cobalamin deficiencies as well as abnormalities of enzymes required in folate metabolism. Indeed, nonpregnant women with a previous child with an NTD were noted to have elevated serum homocysteine levels after methionine loading. Low activity

Table 21.5. The distribution of cases and controls and the risk of NTD by red-cell folate level

Red-Cell Folate (nmol/L [ng/mL])	No. of Cases (%)	No. of Controls (%)	Risk of NTD per 1,000 Births	95% Confidence Interval
0–339 (0–149)	11 (13.1)	10 (3.8)	6.6	3.3 to 11.7
340–452 (150–199)	13 (15.5)	24 (9.0)	3.2	1.7 to 5.5
453–679 (200–299)	29 (34.5)	75 (28.2)	2.3	1.6 to 3.3
6880–905 (300–399)	20 (23.8)	77 (29.0)	1.6	1.0 to 2.4
≥906 (400)	11 (13.1)	80 (30.0)	0.8	0.4 to 1.5

Source: Daly et al., 1995.[40]

in either methionine synthase or MTHFR was commonly noted in this group.[43] Certainly a defect in methionine synthase could account for the metabolic abnormalities that lead to NTDs, and such a defect might be compensated for by increased intake of folic acid and cobalamin. Steegers-Theunissen et al.[43] noted that their abnormal results on methionine loading tests among mothers with methionine synthase abnormalities were corrected by folic acid supplementation. Other evidence implicating abnormalities in cobalamin metabolism include animal studies showing that increased cobalamin administration may be associated with increased methionine synthase activity in rats[221] and that an increased incidence of SB and congenital hydrocephalus was noted in a cobalamin-deficient rat model.[222]

Adams et al.[219] speculated that there is a convergence of evidence of abnormalities in folate and cobalamin metabolism leading to NTDs, suggesting that the cause may be related to methylation. They argued that both folate and cobalamin are involved in critical metabolic pathways providing methyl groups for the methylation of DNA—an essential process in embryogenesis.

Important insights into human NTDs have been gained from animal studies, particularly from reports on more than ten mouse mutants exhibiting various types of NTDs. The *curly-tail* mouse has been studied most extensively, the NTDs most closely resembling the human defects in location and form as well as the mode of multifactorial inheritance. Interestingly, the formation of NTDs in *curly-tail* is not reduced after folate supplementation, nor is the *MTHFR* gene defective, although plasma homocysteine levels are higher in the mutant than in control C57BL/6 mice.[223] Another interesting insight into the mechanisms involved in NTD formation is provided by the *curly-tail;* the administration of inositol can prevent NTDs in this mutant.[224,225] The mechanism is thought to involve the retinoic acid β receptor found in hindgut endoderm.

Emerging from these studies has been a closer understanding of the different mechanisms leading to failures of neural tube closure. For example, in the *splotch* mouse, abnormal migration of neural crest cells is the fault,[226] while in the *curly-tail* mice, a low proliferation rate of the cells of the gut and notochord in the region of the posterior neuropore produce a ventral curvature apparently preventing neuropore closure, with resulting SB.[227] Homozygous *splotch* mutations have decreased folate available for pyrimidine biosynthesis; supplementation with folic acid will reduce NTDs in the mutant embryos by 40 percent.[228] Mutant mice homozygous for the *Cart 1* homeobox gene mutation are born with acrania and meroanencephaly—a phenotype with striking resemblance to human NTDs.[229] *Cart 1* is a transcription factor that regulates downstream target genes and is required for forebrain mesenchyme survival. Its absence disrupts cranial neural tube morphogenesis by blocking the initiation of closure in the midbrain region. Prenatal treatment with folic acid suppressed the acrania/meroanencephaly phenotype.[229] Another knockout mouse mutant with a disrupted *AP-2* gene exhibits anencephaly, craniofacial defects, and thoracoabdominoschisis.[230] The gene-targeted mouse mutant, F52, was fortuitously observed to manifest severe NTDs not associated with other complex malformations.[231] This generated mouse mutant identifies a gene whose mutation results in isolated NTDs and is expected to be a valuable experimental model. Evidence from both mouse and human studies clearly suggests that more than one gene is involved in neural tube closure.

In addition to genetic evidence already discussed, marked sex differences are recognized according to lesion sites—low sacral lesions are more common among males than females, while the opposite is true for thoracic SB and anencephaly.[14,211] The postulate that there is a continuous, bidirectional "zipperlike" process responsible for the pattern of neural tube closure in humans[232] has been superseded by data indicating that, as in the mouse, multiple sites of anterior neural tube closure occur.[12,233,234] Golden and Chernoff[234] provided evidence for two mechanisms leading to anterior NTDs: one results from the failure of a closure and the second results from the failure of the two closures to meet. These observations provide additional insight into variations observed in the location, recurrence risk, and causes of anterior NTDs in humans. Mouse models may also contribute important information on different mechanisms for NTDs at different locations, as shown recently by Stegmann et al.[235]

Folate receptor genes that control maternal–fetal transplacental folate transport have been recognized.[236] Their expression and regulation influence cell proliferation.[237] Thus far, however, there has been no association shown between folate receptor gene defects and NTDs.[237,238,239]

For the vast majority of NTDs, environmental–genetic interaction is causal and most probably depends on dietary folate and susceptibility genes involved in homocysteine, folate, and cobalamin metabolism. The hypothesis that folic acid may have a weak abortifacient effect, accounting for selective loss of affected fetuses,[240] has been countered by the suggestion that it maintains pregnancies that would otherwise abort early enough so as not to even be recognized.[241]

For decades, multiple reports[59–61,242–244] in many mammalian species have associated hyperthermia with NTDs. Inadequate study designs yielded data in humans that were regarded as inconclusive and tenuous.[245,246] In a very carefully designed, large, broad-based, prospective study, we examined heat exposure (hot tub, sauna, electric blanket) in the first 8 weeks and fever in the first 12 weeks of pregnancy.[61] We found that women who used the hot tub in the first 8 weeks of pregnancy had a significant, 2.9 (95 percent confidence interval [CI], 1.4–6.3) relative risk of having a child with an NTD. Use of a sauna was associated with a 2.6 (95 percent CI, 0.7–10.1) relative risk, a finding that was not statistically significant. No association was noted for use of an electric blanket, an observation confirmed by others.[247] When the number of heat sources was tallied (excluding electric blanket), risk escalated with additional sources of exposure. (No data were obtained on the duration, intensity, or frequency of these heat exposures.) After exposure to two heat sources, compared with none, the relative risk of having a child with an NTD rose to 6.2 (95 percent CI, 2.2–17.2). Others have also observed an increased relative risk of NTD with fever but were unable to disentangle the confounders of infection and medication.[248,249] The mechanism by which heat exposure interferes with neural tube closure is unknown.

Analysis of the same database also focused on analysis of trace elements derived from midtrimester-collected maternal toenail clippings. We observed a clear association between elevated toenail zinc (Zn) and a fetus with a NTD.[79,80] Moreover, a linear trend was evident, relative risk increasing with escalating Zn levels. Our observations reconcile with those showing elevated hair Zn levels in mothers of children with SB.[250] It is not known whether Zn sequestration in nails or hair leaves the fetus relatively Zn-deficient or that these findings reflect a more fundamental disturbance in Zn metabolism in these mothers. Zn at physiologic concentrations enters both placental syncytiotrophoblast cells and fetal vascular endothelial cells from both protein-bound and non-protein-bound serum pools.[251] Given the extensive involvement of Zn in cellular metabolism, a role for this trace element in cells migrating to close the neural tube is highly likely.

Is There a Link between NTDs and Down Syndrome?

In the past few years, some data have linked abnormal folate metabolism with an increased risk of Down syndrome, possibly through an increase in the rate of nondisjunction. This raises the possibility that both Down syndrome and NTD prevalence can benefit from folic acid supplementation. In 1999, a study indicated that increased rate of *MTHFR* polymorphism might be associated with an increased risk of Down syndrome.[252] Two other studies have subsequently provided more evidence for that association.[253,254] Very recently, a study has examined families in the Ukraine at increased risk of Down syndrome and families in Israel at increased risk of NTDs.[255] They have found that both groups also have an increased risk for the other birth defect. They conclude that their study provides direct evidence of a link between NTDs and Down syndrome, and that folic acid supplementation might reduce the frequency of both, not just of NTDs. If these results can be confirmed, an intriguing connection between these two major types of congenital abnormalities may be a reality.

BIOLOGY OF α-FETOPROTEIN

Human α-fetoprotein (AFP) was recognized as a fetal-specific globulin in 1956,[256] and many of its physical and chemical properties have been defined.[257,258] Monoclonal antibodies have facilitated purification by immunochromatography. AFP is similar to albumin in molecular weight (about 69,000) and charge[257] but has a different primary structure and is antigenically quite distinct.[259] The primary structure of AFP is known,[259] and the gene on chromosome 4q has been cloned.[260] AFP is a glycoprotein and exists in several forms, or isoproteins, with different net charges.[257]

AFP is synthesized by the yolk sac, the gastrointestinal tract, and the liver of the fetus and is detectable as early as 29 days after conception.[261] Both the kidneys and the placenta may produce trace amounts of AFP,[261] but the fetal liver dominates AFP synthesis. The level of fetal plasma AFP peaks between 10 and 13 weeks of gestation, reaching about 3,000 μg/mL.[262] The fetal plasma concentration of AFP declines exponentially from 14 to 32 weeks and then more sharply until term (Figure 21.3). At 32 weeks of gestation, the plasma AFP concentration is about 200 μg/mL. The exponential fall in fetal plasma AFP can be attributed mainly to the dilution effect due to increasing fetal blood volume and the related decline in the amount synthesized by the fetus.[264] Synthesis of AFP decreases markedly after 32–34 weeks of gestation.

AFP enters the fetal urine and from there the amniotic fluid (AF).[262] In contrast with other proteins, the primary source of AFAFP appears to be fetal urine,[265] where the concentration is higher in AF in early but not in late pregnancy. Peak levels of AFAFP are reached between 12 and 14 weeks of gestation[266,267] and then decline by about 13 per-

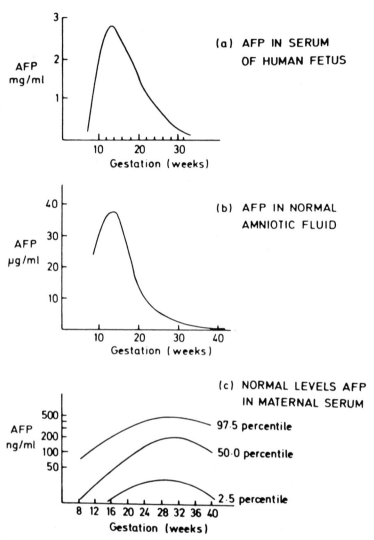

Fig. 21.3. The approximate relationship between AFP values in fetal serum (*a*), amniotic fluid (*b*), and maternal serum (*c*). *Source*: Habib, 1977.[263]

cent per week during the second trimester,[268] being almost nondetectable at term (see Figure 21.3). The concentration gradient between fetal plasma and AFAFP is about 150–200:1,[262,264] and the pattern of AFP levels in the two fetal compartments as a function of gestation is similar. The concentration gradient between fetal and maternal serum is about 50,000:1.[2] Hence, the presence of only a tiny volume of fetal blood contaminating the AF will raise the AFP level, potentially yielding a spurious result.

The AFP concentration in maternal serum or plasma during pregnancy rises above nonpregnancy levels as early as the seventh week of gestation.[269] MSAFP levels are very much lower than AFAFP levels (see Figure 21.3). The peak level of MSAFP during pregnancy occurs between 28 and 32 weeks of gestation.[270] The apparent paradoxical rise in MSAFP when AF and fetal serum levels are decreasing can be accounted for by an increasing placental permeability to fetal plasma protein with advancing gestation[271] and to increasing fetal mass and AF volume relative to a constant maternal blood volume. Transport of AFAFP contributes very little to the MSAFP compartment.[272] Hay et al.[270] noted that higher birth weights were correlated with later attainment of peak MSAFP levels and that peak levels occurred earlier in pregnancy when the fetus was female.

Newborn plasma AFP levels normally decline rapidly, with an average half-life of 5.5 days in the first 2 weeks, reaching adult levels of 1–2 ng/mL by 8 months of age.[273] AFP synthesis does not cease entirely after birth, although the concentrations in adult plasma are extremely low[274]—about 20,000 times lower than the concentrations found at birth.[264]

The function of AFP in the fetus remains unknown.[263] Because AFP has chemical and physical characteristics similar to those of albumin, it may have an osmotic role in maintaining the intravascular volume of the fetal circulation. Although AFP in the rat and mouse binds estrogens and ureterotropic activity has been described,[275] such function in the human seems unlikely.[276]

Current theory is that AFP is most probably involved in immunoregulation during pregnancy. The immune response in the mouse is suppressed by AFP.[277] Human lymphocyte transformation induced by mitogens such as phytohemagglutinin is also suppressed by human AFP.[278] Immunofluorescence studies have pointed to the presence of AFP receptors on the surface of some T-cell lymphocytes in mice. These and other data have therefore formed the basis of a suggestion that human AFP may prevent or be involved in the prevention of the immune rejection of the fetus by the mother.

Its possible functions notwithstanding, the presence of AFP during pregnancy does not appear to be necessary for the maintenance of the pregnancy or the well-being of the fetus. Severe AFP deficiency has been reported in two newborns, with no ill effects to the pregnancy or the baby.[279] In those cases, the second-trimester AFAFP levels were both less than 0.5 ng/mL. In another case, a maternal serum AFP of 0.00 multiples of the median (MoM) was reported on triple marker screening, and was associated with a finding of trisomy 21.[280] The authors cautioned that although congenital absence of AFP is not thought to be associated with adverse obstetrical or fetal outcome, very low or undetectable MSAFP levels should still be considered in screening for Down syndrome. Recently, in a report of almost 840,000 pregnancies undergoing routine prenatal screening, undetectable levels of maternal serum AFP (defined as <2 mg/mL) were found in eight pregnancies (1 in 105,000).[281]

MSAFP SCREENING

Early studies of MSAFP were fully reviewed previously.[282–284] MSAFP was first observed in the circulation during pregnancy in 1970, and soon after, it was noted to be elevated in normal pregnancy. Even higher levels were then found in association with threatened abortion and fetal death. In 1972, Hino et al.[285] first reported high MSAFP with anencephaly. Confirmation of this observation came first in the third trimester, and soon after, in the second trimester, setting the stage for eventual MSAFP screening of all women.

Experience with MSAFP Screening

MSAFP screening for NTDs, at least in the United States, became a standard of expected obstetric care in 1985. Extensive experience with screening between 1973 and 1986 was reviewed by Milunsky[282,283] and others.[2,286–288] The first major study was the U.K. Collaborative Study,[289] which included 18,684 singleton and 163 twin pregnancies without

NTDs and 381 singleton pregnancies with fetal NTDs (146 with anencephaly, 142 with SB, and 13 with encephalocele). This study established realistic expectations for detection rates of open NTDs and defined 16–18 weeks of pregnancy as the most efficient screening period. Use of 2.0 or 2.5 MoM as upper-limit cutoff points yielded detection rates at that time of 70–85 percent for open SB and 95 percent for anencephaly and false-positive rates of 2–5 percent. The distribution of MSAFP values in unaffected pregnancies and those with open NTDs, ventral wall defects, and Down syndrome (DS) are shown in Figure 21.4. The calculated odds of a woman bearing a child with an NTD varies with the incidence of NTDs and the chosen upper limit of normal MSAFP (Table 21.6).

With the advent of multiple-marker screening, the question has been studied of whether the additional markers, besides MSAFP, would be useful in screening for SB and anencephaly.[292–294] In SB, none of the additional markers is abnormal. However, in anencephaly, unconjugated estriol (uE3) is very low (0.2 MoM, on average). In contrast, hCG or inhibin A levels, on average, are not different from unaffected. This is because uE3 is synthesized by the placenta from precursors supplied by the fetal adrenal cortex, and the fetal adrenal is hypofunctional in anencephaly, because of a lack of ACTH stimulation caused by the lack of corticotropin-releasing hormone signaling from the small or absent

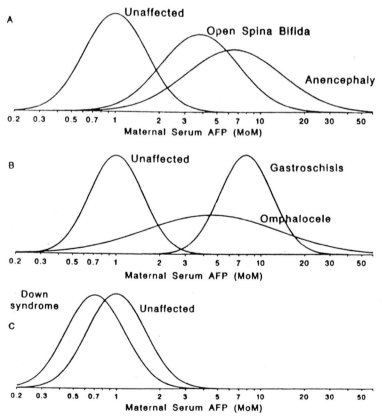

Fig. 21.4. The distribution of maternal serum α-fetoprotein values, expressed as MoM in singleton pregnancies. *A,* Unaffected, open spina bifida, and anencephalic pregnancies at 16–18 weeks of gestation. *B,* Unaffected, omphalocele, and gastroschisis pregnancies. *C,* Fetal Down syndrome and unaffected pregnancies. *Source*: Knight, 1991.[290]

Table 21.6. The odds of individual women with particular serum AFP levels at 16–18 weeks of gestation having a fetus with open spina bifida

	Odds at Given Birth Incidence[a]	
Serum AFP (MoM)	1 per 1,000	2 per 1,000
2.0	1:800	1:400
2.5	1:290	1:140
3.0	1:120	1:59
3.5	1:53	1:27
4.0	1:26	1:13
4.5	1:14	1:7
5.0	1:7	1:4

Source: Data from Fourth Report of the U.K. Collaborative Study on Alpha-Fetoprotein in Relation to Neural Tube Defects 1982.[291]
Note: Multiple pregnancies have been excluded by ultrasonography.
[a]In the absence of antenatal diagnosis and selective abortion.

hypothalamus. Although the observation of very low uE3 in the presence of elevated AFP is indicative of anencephaly, it is also indicative of recent fetal death. The diagnostic power of ultrasound is all that is needed to definitively identify anencephaly after a finding of elevated MSAFP.

Encephaloceles are NTDs that are protrusions of meninges through a skull defect, usually occipital or frontal in location. Typically, they are skin covered, do not leak, and hence are rarely detected by MSAFP screening. In a report of eleven cases, nine had normal MSAFP values and one (with an omphalocele) had a raised level, as did one other without a recognizable reason.[295]

Given the rise of approximately 15 percent per week in MSAFP values through the second trimester,[290,296] the use of medians at each gestational week had been recommended.[289] This method also allowed for interlaboratory differences and facilitated comparative studies. The median was preferred to the mean because it is less influenced by occasional outlying values and because AFP values at any time during the screening period are log-normally distributed. Therefore, the mean overestimates the center of a distribution of AFP concentrations, while the median provides a more stable and more correct estimate of the central value.

Current practice is to use day-specific rather than week-specific medians to calculate a woman's MoM value. The rationale for day-specific medians is that given that AFP levels are constantly rising during the period when screening is done, once an equation for the association between median AFP level and gestational age is calculated, each woman who is screened will, on average, have a more precise calculation of her individual AFP MoM by using her day-specific rather than week-specific median. It stands to reason that a woman who is dated at 16 weeks 0 days and another woman who is dated at 16 weeks 6 days would each have a closer estimate of her MoM when a median AFP level specific for that same day of pregnancy is used rather than a single median for the entire week. Although day-specific medians should be used for the benefit of the individual and require no extra effort for the screening program, on a population basis, screening performance is not measurably improved (Cuckle HS, personal communication).

Determination of the predictive values and relative risk associated with either high or low MSAFP values is important. We prospectively assessed the sensitivity, specificity,

Table 21.7. The sensitivity, specificity, and predictive values for selected pregnancy outcomes after the detection of abnormal MSAFP values

MSAFP and Frequency Outcome	Sensitivity (%)	Specificity (%)	Predictive Value	
			Positive (%)	Negative (%)
Elevated MSAFP values				
Spina bifida	90.9	96.0	1.9	99.99
Anencephaly	100.0	96.0	1.7	100.0
Other NTDs	50.0	95.9	0.4	99.98
Other major congenital defects	16.7	96.0	2.5	99.5
Fetal death	25.5	96.0	2.6	99.7
Neonatal death	16.7	96.0	0.9	99.8
Newborn complications	13.2	96.1	5.5	98.5
Oligohydramnics	12.5	96.0	1.3	99.6
Abruptio placentae	11.3	96.0	1.7	99.4
Pre-eclamptic toxemia	8.9	96.0	3.6	98.4
Maternal hyperthyroidism	10.0	96.0	0.2	99.9
Low birth weight	14.4	96.2	8.1	8.0
Low MSAFP values				
Chromosomal defect	39.1	96.5	2.0	99.9
Fetal death	10.9	96.5	1.1	99.7

Source: Milunsky et al., 1989.[297]

overall predictive values, and relative risk of NTD and other congenital defects[297] (Tables 21.7 and 21.8). Among 13,486 women with singleton pregnancies, 3.9 percent had high and 3.4 percent had low MSAFP values. The expected high relative risk for NTDs was 224. For low MSAFP, chromosomal defects (relative risk [RR], 11.6) and fetal death (RR, 3.3) were the only significant observations. High MSAFP predicted the detection of 100 percent and 90.9 percent of anencephaly and of SB, respectively (see Table 21.7). A progressive increase in the incidence of fetal defects[298] and subsequent pregnancy complications[299] occur as MSAFP rises; in one study, the anomaly rate rose from 3.4 percent at 2.5 MoM to 40.3 percent at >7.0 MoM[300] (Figure 21.5).

Practical Aspects of MSAFP Screening

The MSAFP screening approach accepted by most major centers can be summarized as follows. Blood sampling is recommended, optimally at 16 weeks, but no earlier than 15 weeks and no later than 20 completed weeks. The optimal detection efficiency of NTDs was shown[289] to be during 16–18 weeks of gestation. Both the variance of MSAFP according to gestational weeks related to assay imprecision as well as within-individual fluctuation have been considered, and no practical value was determined in performing a repeat MSAFP assay on either the same or a second sample taken up to 1 month later.[291]

The ultrasound study requested after detection of an elevated MSAFP level aims primarily at determination of an accurate gestational age, diagnosis of multiple pregnancy, and detection of structural fetal/placental defects. If the pregnancy stage provided by the patient's menstrual dates is confirmed by the ultrasound study and no defects have been visualized, genetic counseling to discuss the diagnostic options that are available should be offered as soon as possible. Although an amniocentesis was the primary diagnostic recommendation for many years, more recently patients have been given the option of tar-

Table 21.8. Pregnancy outcome according to the level of MSAFP

Pregnancy Outcome	Total Number	MSAFP							
		Normal		High		Low[a]		High or Low[a]	
		N	%	N	%	N	%	N	%
Neural tube defects	21	2	0.0	19	3.6	0		19	1.9
Chromosomal defects	20	14	0.1	0		6	1.3	6	0.6
Other major congenital defects	82	65	0.5	13	2.5[b]	4	0.9[c]	17	1.7
All major defects combined[d]	123	81	0.6	32	6.0	10	2.2	42	4.2
Fetal death	54	38	0.3	11	2.1	5	1.1	16	1.6
Stillbirth	48	45	0.4	1	0.2	2	0.4	3	0.3
Neonatal death	24	19	0.1	4	0.8	1	0.2	5	0.5
All other losses combined[d]	126	102	0.8	16	3.0	8	1.7	24	2.4
Premature rupture of membranes	350	315	2.5	25	4.7	10	2.2	35	3.5
Oligohydramnios	39	34	0.3	3	0.6	2	0.4	5	0.5
Abruptio placentae	74	66	0.5	6	1.1	2	0.4	8	0.8
Toxemia	209	182	1.5	18	3.4	9	2.0	27	2.7
Polyhydramnios	19	18	0.1	1	0.2	0		1	0.1
Other major pregnancy complications combined[d]	691	615	4.9	53	10.0	23	5.0	76	7.7
Newborn complications	157	132	1.1	18	3.4	7	1.5	25	2.5
Other pregnancy complications	384	352	2.8	20	3.8	12	2.6	32	3.2
Maternal illness	310	295	2.4	6	1.1	9	2.0	15	1.5
Other minor congenital defects	29	29	0.2	0		0		0	
None of the above	11,666	10,899	87.2	385	72.6	392	85.0	777	78.4
All pregnancies	13,486	12,495		530		461		991	

Source: Milunsky et al., 1992[296]

Note: Data are arranged in hierarchical order so that each case is covered only once.

[a] Low MSAFP value.

[b] Gastrochisis (3 cases); renal agenesis (2 cases); multiple anomalies (2 cases); urinary tract obstruction (1 case); imperforate anus, cloaca, and malformed bowel (1 case); tetralogy of Fallot (1 case); congenital toxoplasmosis (1 case); cystic hygroma (1 case); absent bladder and cystic kidneys (1 case).

[c] Multiple anomalies (1 case); endocardial fibroclastosis (1 case); hydrocephalus (1 case); branchial fistula (1 case).

[d] Subtotals, nonhierarchical.

737

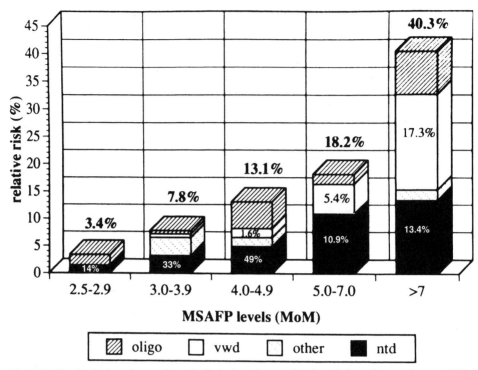

Fig. 21.5. The distribution of anomalies and oligohydramnios as a function of elevated maternal serum AFP (MSAFP). Oligo = oligohydramnios; other = subchorionic bleeding, intra-abdominal echogenicity, hydronephrosis, echogenic bowel, dilated kidney, heart defect; VWD = ventral-wall defect.
Source: Reichler et al., 1994.[300]

geted (level II) ultrasound as an alternative. However, women should be fully informed of the full sequence of possible testing. In our experience, even the very best ultrasonographers may miss SB, especially in the L5–S2 region, making amniocentesis a firm recommendation if the ultrasound is negative and the high MSAFP remains unexplained.[301–303] The relative performance of ultrasound and amniocentesis is discussed in a later section (see also chapters 21 and 23).

Most laboratories use an upper-limit cutoff of the normal range equivalent to ≥ 2.0 or ≥ 2.5 MoM. Clearly, the selection of a specific cutoff level reflects a compromise between missing open NTDs and performing unnecessary amniocenteses on pregnancies with normal fetuses. The actual odds that a woman will carry a fetus with open SB have been calculated as a function of the level of MSAFP (see Table 21.6). These odds relate to pregnancies with a single fetus; note that a correction in the gestational age through the use of ultrasound would change the odds that a fetus will be affected.

Assay Considerations

Almost all laboratories use either a radioimmunoassay or an enzyme immunoassay to measure MSAFP and AFAFP, and immunoassays from dried blood specimens have been successful.[304] In recent years there has been a major shift from assays done manually to assays on automated platforms, having rapid throughput and exhibiting improved precision. This improvement in assay methods has led to a reappraisal of the distribution characteristics of MSAFP and its performance in screening for open NTDs. It is now estimated that when more precise AFP assays are used, the false-positive rate in screening for anencephaly and open SB is reduced from 2.0 to 0.8 percent and the detection rate is increased from 81 to 83 percent.[305]

All laboratories are expected to establish their own normal ranges. Continuous quality control is necessary in the performance of screening and diagnostic assays.[306] Guidelines have been issued by the American Society of Human Genetics[307,308] and the Canadian Society of Clinical Chemists,[309] and regulations have been promulgated by the College of American Pathologists. This college operates nationwide external proficiency testing in the United States, an essential element in population-based screening programs. In addition, some states restrict screening to only one or a few approved laboratories or require that their own proficiency testing program be followed. Lessons learned from the debacle of uncontrolled newborn screening for phenylketonuria led to this important approach.

FACTORS THAT INFLUENCE THE INTERPRETATION OF MSAFP

The distribution of MSAFP values in a population of pregnant women is governed by a range of factors. Wald has estimated the impact of many of these factors on the variance of MSAFP at any given point in gestation.[26] He has found that about half the variance is caused by differences between the pregnancies themselves. Another 17 percent is caused by fluctuations in MSAFP within a pregnancy, and about 14 percent is due to assay error. Half of the remaining 18 percent is caused by errors in dating the pregnancy, which leaves less than 10 percent contributed by other factors, such as maternal weight, maternal race, and diabetic status.

Gestational Age

Accurate assessment of gestational age and the method of dating has a major impact on MSAFP screening. Optimal detection rates are between 16 and 18 weeks, and screening is best confined to 15–20 weeks. Assignment of gestational age is most commonly done by self-reporting by the patient of the first day of her last menstrual period (LMP) or by sonographic measurement of the fetus. The most commonly applied ultrasound dating methods are first-trimester crown-to-rump length (CRL), usually measured beginning at about 7 weeks, and second-trimester measurement of biparietal diameter (BPD), femur length, abdominal circumference, or a composite of the second-trimester measures.

Gestational dating by ultrasound measurement has been shown to improve the performance of screening for NTDs for two reasons. First, ultrasound estimation of gestational age is, on a population basis, more accurate than a woman's recollection of her LMP.[310–312] Certainly, many women have regular menstrual cycles and have very accurate recall of their LMP, but as many as 40 percent of LMP dates are unreliable,[310,313] leading to a broadened distribution of AFP MoM values. This difference alone will lead to better screening performance, because the distributions of AFP MoM values for a screened population will be tighter when the population is dated by ultrasound than when it is dated by LMP.

Second, ultrasound dating by second-trimester BPD will markedly improve screening for open SB because it will tend to underestimate the gestation of an affected fetus, thus leading to a lower AFP median being used to calculate the AFP MoM. The result is to artificially increase the AFP MoM in affected pregnancies, enhancing the chances that such pregnancies will have an AFP MoM above the screening cutoff.[314] The reason for a smaller BPD in open SB pregnancy is the occurrence in almost cases of an Arnold–Chiari

II malformation, involving movement of the cranial vault contents down the neural tube, leading to the formation of a smaller calvarium, and consequently to a small BPD measurement. The average decrease in the apparent gestation in a pregnancy affected by SB and dated by BPD is 16 days, which leads to a marked improvement in performance, estimated to be 11 percentage points (79 percent in LMP-dated pregnancies and 90 percent in BPD-dated pregnancies, both for a 5 percent false-positive rate).[314]

Maternal Weight

MSAFP concentrations vary according to maternal weight.[315] The heavier the woman, the lower the MSAFP level, as a result of dilution of AFP in a larger blood volume. Adjustment of the MSAFP value for maternal weight increases the detection rate for open SB[316] and is especially important when screening for chromosome defects (see also chapter 22). Dividing the observed MoM by the expected MoM for a given weight enables adjustment for differences in weight. Adams et al.[317] described a detailed method for computing risks based on MSAFP values and known variables. Correction for weight up to 250 lb significantly increased the rate of elevated MSAFP results, suggesting overcorrection.[186] These authors recommended linear correction of MSAFP up to 200 lb only, with those weighing more still being adjusted for this weight only. In contrast, Wald et al. found that an equation comparing maternal weight to the log of the MoM is valid to weights up to about 260 lb.[311,318] Published weight equations may not be optimal for some screening programs because of differences in the mean weight of the population being tested. Neveux et al.,[319] using a reciprocal-linear equation to describe the association between maternal weight and MoM value, recommended that screening laboratories calculate their own weight-correction formulas, based on data from their own population, and monitor the mean maternal weight periodically, updating the formulas when necessary. It is clear, that when done properly, adjustment of the MoM value according to maternal weight will reduce the variability of the AFP MoM distribution.[311]

Maternal-weight MSAFP adjustment is also important because of the convincing finding of increased risk of NTDs in obese mothers.[73–75,320–322] Obese mothers have an approximately twofold increased risk compared with women of average weight. In addition, obese mothers have an increased risk of another birth defect identified because of elevated MSAFP, fetal omphalocele,[73,320] although this is apparently not true for the other major ventral wall defect, gastroschisis.[320] Without appropriate maternal weight adjustment of the MSAFP MoM, those with the highest risk would have the lowest average MoM values, and therefore, the lowest screening performance.

Maternal Age

The frequency of NTDs has a U-shaped distribution for maternal age. However, no correction has been considered necessary for NTD screening.

Maternal Ethnicity

Black women have 10–15 percent higher MSAFP levels than nonblacks,[35,323,324] requiring automatic adjustments in any formula used to interpret an MSAFP result. This step is especially important, given the lower incidence of NTDs among blacks.[325]

MSAFP levels are lower in Oriental women than in whites—6 percent lower in one study.[326] Thus far, these lower values have not been regarded as significant enough to require adjustments for MSAFP interpretation. Hispanic women have lower MSAFP values than Caucasians,[35] suggesting that women at risk for NTDs might be missed when screening cutoffs for Caucasians are used. In a small study of 3,046 Hispanic and 15,154 Caucasian women, the percentage of Hispanic women with elevated MSAFP was not significantly different from that of Caucasians.[35] Adjustment of medians for NTD screening was not recommended (see also chapter 22). Ultimately, the use of ethnic-group-specific medians[233,326] should yield better risk assessment data.

Maternal Insulin-Dependent Diabetes Mellitus

MSAFP levels in pregnant women with insulin-dependent diabetes mellitus (IDDM) beginning at or before conception have been reported to be about 20 percent lower than in nondiabetic women during the second trimester,[72,327–329] and, for the past 25 years, adjustments have been made in MSAFP interpretation, unless a normal range for IDDM has been established. There is increasing evidence, however, that this effect may no longer be found, most likely because pregnant women with IDDM are now kept in much tighter glycemic control than in years past.[330–333] Programs that are adjusting MSAFP levels in cases of IDDM should continue doing so until the evidence has been further confirmed and studied. Regardless of its effect on MSAFP levels, IDDM is associated with a much higher frequency of NTDs (10-fold in our study,[72] 3.5-fold in others[334]) in the offspring of these patients, which must be noted when the risk of IDDM after screening is calculated.

The reason for lower MSAFP values in IDDM remains unclear. Relative intrauterine growth restriction in IDDM probably occurs consistently through the end of the second trimester, resulting in diminished synthesis, secretion, excretion, or transport of AFP. First-trimester ultrasound studies in IDDM pregnancies showed that the fetuses were, on average, smaller than normal, with about one-third having even more marked fetal growth restriction.[335]

Given the twofold to fourfold increase in the frequency of all malformations in the offspring of women with IDDM,[336] all such patients should undergo a level II ultrasound study. In one study of 393 women with IDDM who had both MSAFP and ultrasound, 32 had defects at delivery that were detected through both MSAFP screening and ultrasound.[337] No malformations missed by ultrasound were detected by MSAFP screening.

In this context, a salutary and surprising rate of fetal aneuploidy (13.2 percent) was reported among fifty-three pregnancies with NTDs,[300] supporting AF chromosome study in all cases (see also Table 21.4.)

Multiple Pregnancy

A level II ultrasound study is recommended at around 16 weeks of gestation in all multiple pregnancies, given the increased frequency of fetal defects. The concentration of MSAFP is proportional to the number of fetuses.[338] Hence, the upper-limit cutoff in twin pregnancy is twice that for singletons, usually 4.0 or 5.0 MoM. For six triplet and three quadruplet pregnancies, the average MSAFP level was, respectively, three and five times greater than in singleton pregnancies.[339] In our prospective study,[297] we noted that 53 percent of twin pregnancies had MSAFP values ≥ 2.0 MoM. Both we and others[338] have noted an ominous prognosis in twin pregnancy when MSAFP levels exceeded 5 MoM for singleton pregnancies. Ghosh et al.[338] observed that 59 percent of such cases ended in fetal death, stillbirth, or a fetus papyraceous in one twin. In eleven of their cases in which twins were discordant for NTDs, the MSAFP value exceeded 5 MoM. One curious and

Table 21.9. The detection rate, false-positive rate, and odds of being affected by anencephaly or open spina bifida, given a positive result (OAPR) for twin pregnancies, according to the level of AFP (assuming a singleton birth prevalence of 1 per 1,000 births for each defect, in the absence of antenatal diagnosis and selective abortion)

AFP Level (MoM)	Detection Rate		OAPR		
	Anencephaly	Open Spina Bifida	False-Positive Rate	Anencephaly	Open Spina Bifida
≥2.0	100%	96%	4%	1:200	1:210
≥2.5	99	89	30	1:130	1:150
≥3.0	98	80	19	1:85	1:100
≥3.5	96	69	12	1:55	1:76
≥4.0	93	58	7.8	1:37	1:59
≥4.5	89	48	5.0	1:25	1:46
≥5.0	83	39	3.3	1:17	1:37
≥5.5	77	31	2.2	1:13	1:31
≥6.0	70	25	1.4	1:8.8	1:25

Source: Cuckle et al., 1990.[343]

Note: Derived from Gaussian distribution of $\log_{10}$ AFP, using the means and standard deviations specified in Cuckle et al., 1990.[343]

MoM = multiple of the normal median for singletons at the same gestation and laboratory.

Table 21.10. The odds of being affected by anencephaly or spina bifida for individual twin pregnancies, according to the level of AFP (assuming a singleton birth prevalence of 1 per 1,000 births for each defect in the absence of antenatal diagnosis and selective abortion)

AFP Level (MoM)	Anencephaly	Open Spina Bifida
2.0	1:48,000	1:1,700
2.2	1:23,000	1:1,200
2.4	1:12,000	1:830
2.6	1:6,900	1:620
2.8	1:4,100	1:470
3.0	1:2,600	1:370
3.2	1:1,700	1:300
3.4	1:1,100	1:240
3.6	1:760	1:200
3.8	1:540	1:170
4.0	1:390	1:140
4.2	1:290	1:120
4.4	1:220	1:110
4.6	1:170	1:93
4.8	1:130	1:82
5.0	1:100	1:73
5.2	1:82	1:65
5.4	1:66	1:58
5.6	1:54	1:53
5.8	1:44	1:48
6.0	1:37	1:44

Source: Cuckle et al., 1990.[343]

Note: Derived from Gaussian distributions of $\log_{10}$ AFP using the means and standard deviations specified in Cuckle et al., 1990.[343]

MoM = multiple of the normal median for singletons at the same gestation and laboratory.

yet unexplained observation is that MSAFP in monozygous twin pregnancies is higher than in dizygous twin pregnancies.[340] Brock et al.[341] found that in twin pregnancies, low MSAFP levels provided an early signal of growth restriction and high values warned of possible premature delivery. Redford and Whitfield[342] found a 40 percent perinatal mortality in twin pregnancy when MSAFP values were ≥4.0 MoM.

Cuckle et al.[343] studied MSAFP in 46 discordant twin pregnancies with open NTD and 169 unaffected twins between 13 and 24 weeks of gestation. Using a 5.0 MoM cutoff level, their estimated detection rate was 83 percent for anencephaly but only 39 percent for open SB (Table 21.9). They calculated the odds of being affected by an open NTD for individual twin pregnancies (Table 21.10) according to the MSAFP level. For example, at an incidence rate of 3 SB infants per 1,000 births, an MSAFP level of 5.0 MoM yielded odds of 1 in 73. When MSAFP values are ≥5.0 MoM after sonography, we advocate amniocentesis for AFAFP and acetylcholinesterase (AChE) studies.

Fetal Sex and MSAFP

MSAFP values are, on average, higher when the fetus is male,[344,345] and the effect is most pronounced at levels of 1.5 MoM and higher.[26,346] However, adjustments of MSAFP values for fetal sex are unnecessary.

Raised MSAFP in Sequential Pregnancies

Wald and Cuckle[347] studied MSAFP in 1,717 women between 16 and 21 weeks of gestation in each of two pregnancies, neither with a fetus affected by an NTD. Women with high MSAFP values (≥2.5 MoM) in the first pregnancy had raised values in 6.8 percent of the second pregnancies. In contrast, among women with normal MSAFP values in the first pregnancy, only 1.9 percent had raised AFP in the second. Although this difference was statistically highly significant, the effect was too small to be of practical value.

Maternal Smoking

No significant effect of smoking on MSAFP has been detected.[348,349]

MSAFP AND ADVERSE PREGNANCY OUTCOME

Maternal serum screening introduces a "noisy" system into physicians' offices, requiring constant attention, response, documentation, and, most important, time expenditure to address the indisputable new anxieties.[350] Data on MSAFP screening antedated multiple analyte use (see also chapter 22) and provided additional insight in non-NTD pregnancies. Unexplained elevated MSAFP values with normal AFAFP denote a probable breach in the integrity of the fetoplacental interface due to either or both placental or membrane pathology.[351–354] In our prospective study of such cases, significant observations included undetectable major congenital defects (RR, 4.7) excluding NTDs, fetal deaths (RR, 8.1), neonatal death (RR, 4.7), low birth weight (RR, 4.0), oligohydramnios (RR, 3.4), and abruptio placentae (RR, 3.0). Either high or low MSAFP values (see Table 21.8) were found in 34.2 percent of all major congenital defects, 19.1 percent of all stillbirths or fetal-neonatal deaths, 15.9 percent of serious newborn complications, and 11.0 percent of major pregnancy complications. The probabilities of specific pregnancy outcomes related to MSAFP values are listed in Table 21.8.

A summary of reports on MSAFP and adverse pregnancy outcome covering 225,000 pregnancies is shown in Table 21.11.[355] Ample evidence of placental pathology (Table

Table 21.11. Studies evaluating the relation of unexplained elevations of MSAFP and poor pregnancy outcome

Author (References)	Location (year)	Pregnancies Screened	MoM cutoff	LBW risk	IUGR risk	Premature delivery risk	Abruption risk	IUFD risk	Perinatal death	Pre-eclampsia
Brock et al.	Scotland (1977, 1979)	15,481	2.3	2.5×				+	+	+
Wald et al.	England (1977, 1980)	3,194	3	4.7×		5.8×			3.5×	
		4,198								
Macri	New York (1978)	6,031	2	2×						
Gordon et al.	England (1978)	1,055	2			3.5×			4.5×	9.5×
Smith	England (1980)	1,500	2	+	+	+				+
Evans and Stokes	Wales (1984)	2,913	2	3×					8×	
Burton et al.	North Carolina (1983, 1988)	42,037	2.5	2×			+	8×	10×	
Persson et al.	Sweden (1983)	10,147	2.3	2.8×		2×	10×		3×	
Haddow et al.	Maine (1983)	3,636	2	3.6×		2×				
Purdie et al.	Scotland (1983)	7,223	2.5	2.5×			20×			
Fuhrmann and Weitzel	West Germany (1985)	50,000	2.5	3.5×				8.6×		
Williamson et al.	Iowa (1986)	1,161		poor outcomes						
Robinson et al.	California (1989)	35,787	2	3.5×						
Ghosh et al.	Hong Kong	9,838	2	+						
Schnittger and Kjessler	Sweden (1984)	18,037	2	+			+		+	
Hamilton et al.	Scotland (1985)	10,885	2.5	103	2×	>10×	3×		8×	
Doran et al.	Ontario (1987)	8,140	2	63				+		
Milunsky et al.	Massachusetts (1989)	13,486	2	43			3×	8×	+	2.3×

Source: Katz et al., 1990[355]

Note: IUFD = intrauterine fetal demise, IUGR = intrauterine growth retardation, LBW = low birth weight, MoM = multiple of the median, + = increased risk but unquantified.

744

21.12) is consistent with this hypothesis. There is a 20–58 percent likelihood of adverse pregnancy outcome in women with an unexplained raised MSAFP level[355,397] (see also chapter 22 for multiple analyte screening). Hyperechogenic fetal bowel (see also chapter 23) in association with an elevated MSAFP level is also associated with subsequent pregnancy complications, including intrauterine growth restriction and fetal/neonatal death.[398] One study focused on 556 women with high MSAFP levels who had normal sonograms and amniocentesis results. The risk of adverse pregnancy outcome rose from 19 to 29 percent and up to 70 percent when their MSAFP levels were 2.5–2.9, 3.0–5.0, and ≥5.0 MoM, respectively.[399] Moreover, and especially worrisome, are our observations[13] and those of others[352] showing that after an elevated MSAFP, normal AFAFP, no detectable AChE, and normal ultrasound, a risk approximating 4 percent may remain for the fetus having a serious congenital defect (e.g., hydrocephalus, cardiac defect, limb-reduction defect). Associated placental pathology is the likely mechanism for the raised MSAFP.

A number of major obstetric complications in association with elevated MSAFP are recognized (see Table 21.12) and some need further consideration.

Fetal Death

In 1965, Tatarinov[400] first noted high MSAFP after fetal death. We found a relative risk of 8.1 (95 percent CI 4.8–13,4),[297] and others[401] found a range of relative risk rising from 2.4 to 10.4 with escalating levels of MSAFP for fetal death. Threatened spontaneous abortion has also long been associated with elevated MSAFP levels.[362] These authors showed that women with high MSAFP had a tenfold greater likelihood of miscarrying than those with normal values. In women with low MSAFP values, we found a relative risk of 3.3 for fetal death.[297]

Low Birth Weight

There is a highly significant association between elevated MSAFP and subsequent low birth weight.[375] We found a relative risk of 4.0 (95 percent CI, 3.0–5.3) for this association,[297] while others[402] have pointed out that the risk of having a low-birth-weight infant increases as the MSAFP rises. Placental pathology is the likely reason for this association.

Miscellaneous Pregnancy Complications

Pathologic processes that interfere with placental integrity are likely to be associated with elevated MSAFP. It is no surprise, then, that we found statistically significant relative risks for specific pregnancy complications (see Tables 21.7 and 21.8). Fetal loss is very likely if oligohydramnios is associated with a raised MSAFP.[98,352,403] Prudence would dictate continuing careful surveillance of all women with high MSAFP (after normal ultrasonographic and amniocentesis results), with special attention in the third trimester and to labor, delivery, and the neonatal period.

Fetomaternal hemorrhage may occur without vaginal bleeding and may be signaled by a raised MSAFP level.[370] Both transabdominal and transcervical CVS may cause fetomaternal bleeding (see also chapter 5) with elevations in MSAFP, reported in one study in 18 percent and 5 percent, respectively.[404] MSAFP levels were higher after transabdominal procedures and were also associated with a subsequent increased fetal loss rate. Because fetomaternal bleeding may follow amniocentesis (see also chapter 2) in 7–15 percent of cases, evaluation of MSAFP should be done before any tap. Cordocentesis fre-

Table 21.12.   The complications of pregnancy that may be associated with elevated
MSAFP in the second trimester of pregnancy

Complication	Reference
Fetal	
Abdominal pregnancy	356,357
Ectopic pregnancy	358
Fetal death	352,359
Multiple pregnancy	342
Oligohydramnios[a]	297,352
Polyhydramnios[a]	297
Pregnancy reduction	360
Rh disease	361
Stillbirth	355
Threatened abortion	362
Placental	
Abruptio placentae[a]	297
Chorioamnionitis (includes chronic villitis)[a]	363
Choriocarcinoma[a]	364,365
Chorionic villus sampling (CVS)	366,367
Cordocentesis	368
Cytomegalovirus infection (villitis)	369
Fetomaternal hemorrhage	370
HELLP syndrome	371
Hydatidiform mole	372–374
Intrauterine growth retardation[a]	297
Low birth weight[a]	297,375
Maternal herpes infection with fetal liver necrosis	258
Parvovirus (B19) infection	376
Placental growth impairment	358
Placenta previa[a]	297,377
Placenta accreta, increta and percreta	378
Placental chorangioma (hemangioma)	379–382
Placental vascular lesions (including sonolucency,	
hemorrhage, thrombosis, infarction)[a]	363,367,368,383–386
Postamniocentesis	387
Pre-eclamptic toxemia[a]	297,388,389
Premature rupture of membranes[a]	297
Thrombophilias	390
Triploidy (with hydropic placental degeneration,	
[may also be spina bifida])	391–393
Umbilical cord hemangioma	394
Uterus-separate/bicornuate/unicornuate	395
Vaginal bleeding	396

Note: Additional references in previous editions 1973, 1979, 1992, and 1998.[98,283,284,609]
[a]Occurring in the second or third trimester but possibly preceded by second-trimester elevation in
MSAFP.

quently results in fetomaternal hemorrhage, and in one study, MSAFP was elevated in 30
percent after the procedure.[405]

The majority of pregnancies with extremely high MSAFP values (>8 MoM) are associated with major structural fetal defects or fetal death before 20 weeks of gestation.
Killam et al.[406] analyzed 44 such patients from among 40,676 screened pregnancies. A
putative cause was determined in 82 percent at the initial ultrasound—primarily fetal defects, fetal death, or placental abnormality. Among pregnancies with a liveborn infant, 88
percent had at least one obstetrical complication. Congenital malformations such as sep-
tate, unicornuate, and bicornuate uteri may be associated with "unexplained" MSAFP el-

evations.[395] These patients are at increased risk for subsequent complications of pregnancy such as placental abruption, uterine rupture, and retained placenta.

OTHER CAUSES OF ELEVATED MSAFP LEVELS

Ventral Wall, Congenital Nephrosis, and Other Disorders

Certain fetal defects, as well as disorders that may affect either mother or fetus, may be associated with an elevated MSAFP level (Tables 21.13 and 21.14). Some of these maternal disorders may confound routine MSAFP screening. Etiologic overlap may also occur, exemplified by fetal disorders that have associated placental defects. A major Scottish study showed that MSAFP was elevated in 89 percent of fetuses with omphalocele and in 100 percent of those with gastroschisis.[426]

Congenital nephrosis is an autosomal recessive disorder caused by mutation of the *NPHS1* gene which codes for nephrin, a cell-adhesion protein in the glomerulus. It is most common in Finland (about 1 in 8,000 livebirths) and among those of Scandinavian extraction, but cases have been diagnosed throughout the world, with enriched prevalence noted in Malta and among Pennsylvania Mennonites.[443,444] Although more than sixty mutations in the *NPHS1* gene have been reported, a single mutation (121delCT) is found in 78 percent of Finnish cases.[445] Mean survival approximates 8 months; renal transplantation is the only effective treatment.[446,447] Congenital nephrosis is almost invariably associated with markedly elevated AFAFP and MSAFP values.[258,448] In a recent study of

Table 21.13. Fetal defects that may be associated with elevated MSAFP in the second trimester of pregnancy

Defect	Reference
Acardiac twin fetus	98,374,407
Aplasia cutis congenita	408
Arteriovenous fistula (intracranial)	409
Congenital nephrosis	258,382,410
Cystic adenomatoid malformation (lung)	380–382,411
Epidermolysis bullosa	412,413
Esophageal atresia	414
Fetal disorders with elevated AFAFP	(See Table 21.21)
Fetal hypothyroidism	415
Hydrocephalus	374
Limb-reduction defect	352,374
Multiple acyl-CoA dehydrogenase deficiency	416
NTD (anencephaly; spina bifida; encephalocele; iniencephaly; exencephaly)	98,106,417
Polycystic kidney disease	374,418
Renal agenesis	374,419
Renal cysts	420
Roberts–SC phocomelia syndrome	421
Sex chromosome aneuploidy (includes XXY;XXYY;XO)	98,422
Simpson–Golabi–Behmel syndrome	423
Triploidy (with spina bifida or placental degeneration)	391–393
Trisomy 8	424,425
Ventral wall defects (omphalocele/exomphalos; gastroschisis; body stalk defect; thoracoabdominal wall defect)	98,156,374,426

Note: Additional references in 1992 edition.[98]

Table 21.14. Disorders associated with elevated serum AFP
in infants and nonpregnant women

Disorder	Reference
Infants	
Ataxia telangiectasia	427
Cystic fibrosis (mostly negative reports)	428
Congenital hypothyroidism	415
Congenital nephrosis	371,382
Indian childhood cirrhosis	429
Neonatal hepatitis	430
Polycystic kidney disease	374,418
Severe neonatal illness	431
Tyrosinosis	432
Teratoma	433,434
Beckwith-Wiedemann syndrome	435
Women (nonpregnant)	
Gastrointestinal cancer	436
Germ cell tumors (includes ovarian: Sertoli-Leydig)	437,438
Hepatic cancer	439
Hereditary persistence of AFP	440,441
Viral hepatitis	442

pregnancies with affected and carrier fetuses[449] (Figure 21.6), the median AFP levels in affected pregnancies were very high (8.3 MoM in maternal serum and 33 MoM in AF). A potential confounder to prenatal diagnosis of congenital nephrosis using AFAFP was the finding in the same study that pregnancies with carrier fetuses also had elevated median MSAFP and AFAFP levels in the second trimester (3.2 MoM in maternal serum and 8.9 MoM in AF). Although the AFP levels were, on average, lower in carrier pregnancies, the overlap between AFP levels in carrier and case pregnancies was high. Kestila and Jarvela[445] suggest that serial measurement of AFAFP will differentiate between carriers of and those affected with the disease; AFAFP in affected fetuses will remain elevated while AFAFP in carrier fetuses will decrease over time. Another potential pitfall is overestimating gestational age and finding a normal AFAFP in an affected fetus. Even with accurate gestational age assessment, neither the AFAFP nor the MSAFP levels may exceed >2.5 MoM. Amniocentesis repeated at 18 weeks (or later if necessary) may reveal a marked elevation in AFP values as was noted in one illustrative case.[450–452]

Hyperechoic fetal kidneys, which may nor may not also be enlarged with calyceal dilation,[453] serve as another nonspecific indicator of possible congenital nephrosis. These sonar observations together with placental enlargement may be seen in the third trimester[454] (see also chapters 23 and 24).

Fetal teratomas are not usually malignant and may be amenable to surgery soon after birth. Fortuitous diagnosis is the rule through routine ultrasound or elevated AFAFP (see below). In ten cases of fetal sacrococcygeal teratoma, MSAFP values were not significantly elevated.[455]

Mild *benign fetal obstructive uropathy* may be associated with raised MSAFP levels.[456] These authors examined sixty-one consecutive patients with elevated MSAFP and eighty others with normal values. Ultrasonographers were blinded to the MSAFP results. Among male fetuses, 33 percent had pyelectasis, compared with only 5 percent of controls. Among female fetuses, pyelectasis was seen in 16 percent of high-MSAFP cases

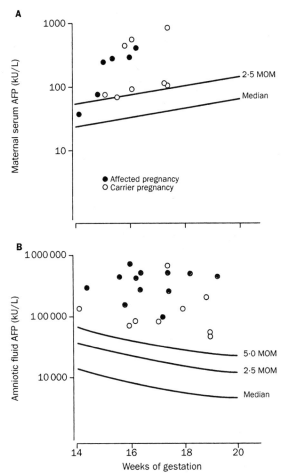

Fig. 21.6. MSAFP and AFAFP levels in pregnancies in which the fetus was affected with (closed circles) or a carrier for (open circles) congenital nephrosis (Finnish type). *Source*: Patrakka et al., 2002.[449] Reprinted with permission from Elsevier.

and in no controls. Fetal proteinuria seems unlikely, but associated placental pathology may explain these observations.

Acardiac Twin

Pregnancy termination of an apparently normal fetus after the discovery of elevated MSAFP and AFAFP with normal results on ultrasound is rare. One potential pitfall, which may occur despite a diligent ultrasonographic search, is the presence of a subjacent dead acardiac twin.

Hereditary persistence of AFP is a rare autosomal dominant disorder without apparent clinical effects[440,441] that may first be discovered in a healthy woman through routine MSAFP screening. This disorder requires consideration when:

1. MSAFP values are raised, AFAFP is normal, and high-resolution ultrasound reveals no placental or fetal defects;

2. MSAFP values remain elevated through *and after* pregnancy;
3. A previous pregnancy with unexplained MSAFP elevation also resulted in a normal child; inferential diagnosis is clinched if a healthy maternal sibling, parent, or previous child has raised MSAFP values (when not pregnant); a mutation at a regulatory locus for AFP has been described.[457]

MANAGEMENT PROTOCOL FOR UNEXPLAINED ELEVATED MSAFP VALUES

After the detection of an elevated MSAFP level, demonstration of no abnormality on a level II ultrasound, and the finding of a normal AFAFP, AChE, and fetal karyotype, further and continuing attention is necessary. Ample data, presented above, document the increased risk of adverse pregnancy outcome and probable residual risk of undetected fetal malformation (see also chapter 22 for risks using multiple analytes). A prudent management protocol for these patients would include:

1. Genetic counseling, not only to explain the laboratory and ultrasonographic findings and limitations, but also to evaluate the family pedigree for potential causes or associations.
2. Serial level II ultrasound at 16, 19, and 23 weeks of gestation (selective abortion is difficult to obtain after 24 weeks), especially for fetal growth, intracranial anatomy, complete limb and digit evaluation, and AF volume.
3. Fetal echocardiogram at 20–23 weeks, given the approximate 1 percent frequency of congenital cardiac defects, and their occurrence in patients with elevated MSAFP.[317,399]
4. A Kleihauer–Betke test for Rh-negative women, to determine fetomaternal bleeding, to establish a cause for the high MSAFP, and to prevent Rh sensitization.
5. Viral titers in maternal sera, when infections (e.g., cytomegalovirus, parvovirus) are suspected, and specific viral DNA analysis of AF cells (see chapter 30).
6. Lupus anticoagulant, antiphospholipid,[458] and factor V Leiden DNA[390,459] studies in women with previous vascular thromboses or unexplained fetal death.
7. Third-trimester ultrasound (perhaps best between 28 and 32 weeks) for fetal growth, anatomy, and AF volume.
8. Late third-trimester fetal movement counts, nonstress tests, and biophysical profiles.

Although cost–benefit studies of the preceding or similar protocols have yet to be done, the outline presented would reflect prudent care and attention to a pregnancy that is clearly at appreciably higher risk than normal.

AMNIOCENTESIS OR ULTRASOUND FOR ELEVATED MSAFP LEVELS

AF studies for both AFP and AChE result in a detection rate of 95 to 98 percent for open NTDs and a false-positive rate of 0.4 percent in women with elevated MSAFP levels.[460,461] Advances in high-resolution ultrasound have raised detection rates closer to those achieved by AF studies preceded by MSAFP screening. Notwithstanding this progress, small anterior encephaloceles and SB can be missed, and oligohydramnios, maternal habitus, and fetal position may prevent accurate ultrasonographic assessment[98,462] (see also chapter 23).

Studies that include detection and false-positive rates for NTDs were assessed[463] after the claim[464] that high-resolution ultrasound might suffice for NTD diagnosis, rather than dependence on amniocentesis. For anencephaly and SB, the data show overall detection rates of 100 percent and 88 percent, respectively, and a false-positive rate of 1.2 percent. A majority of these studies were completed before the recognition of intracranial signs of SB (see also chapter 23). The data of Nadel et al.[464] yielded a 100 percent sensitivity for detection of NTD in their small series. However, ascertainment and selection bias may have confounded these conclusions.[465]

In a series of 257 pregnancies with elevated MSAFP, 16 fetal defects were detected by AFAFP and AChE study, 4 (25 percent) of which had been missed by ultrasound.[301] In a subsequent paper,[419] these authors, adding to this experience, reported on 36 defective fetuses among 331 women with elevated MSAFP. Six (16.7 percent) fetuses with defects were missed by ultrasound. Despite the authors' 83 percent sensitivity by ultrasound, they calculated a >1 percent risk of fetal defects when the MSAFP value was >3 MoM and concluded that amniocentesis should be offered routinely when MSAFP elevation is found. In another similar study[466] of 681 women with elevated MSAFP, 13 (1.9 percent) fetal defects were detected by amniocentesis study and were missed by ultrasound. In a series of 313 women undergoing amniocentesis for elevated MSAFP levels, Barth et al.[467] missed one of four chromosome defects on ultrasound. Early gestational age, small defects, and technical failure were implicated as causes of misdiagnosis. In another study, a risk of chromosomal abnormality in nonselected patients mostly younger than 35 years of age with elevated MSAFP and a normal ultrasound report was close to background expectations (0.6 percent).[468]

Complementary use of high-resolution ultrasound and amniocentesis after the discovery of an elevated MSAFP remains the safest policy, with SB detection rates exceeding 95 percent with rare false-positive results, plus detection of a few mostly unexpected chromosomal abnormalities. Given the strong trend toward ultrasound follow-up alone, because it poses no risks to the mother or fetus, a reasonable option following a confirmed elevated MSAFP result would first involve a detailed ultrasound examination. If a clear diagnosis of SB or other open fetal defects is apparent, amniocentesis is not required. However, if ultrasound does not reveal an open fetal defect or if the findings are equivocal, the patient should be offered amniocentesis to increase the likelihood that, if a defect is indeed present, it will be found.

MSAFP VERSUS ULTRASOUND SCREENING

The efficacy and impact of MSAFP screening for NTDs is well documented.[98,469] A policy of screening all pregnancies for NTDs using high-resolution ultrasound assumes safety of ultrasound; high predictive values, sensitivity, and specificity; availability of the necessary number of skilled and trained individuals; availability of good equipment; and demonstration of cost effectiveness. In general, while harmful effects have not been observed among those born after exposure to ultrasound in utero,[470] reservations about the aforementioned items lead to a lack of support for routine ultrasound scanning[471] (see also chapters 22 and 23).

These cautions are reasonable even with the identification of two ultrasound markers in the brain and cranium in most fetuses with SB. These markers are the so-called fruit signs, the "lemon" sign, in which the front cranial vault is puckered in on the corners, and the "banana" sign, in which the cerebellar hemispheres are often seen as a bow or banana shape. Both fruit signs are a result of the Arnold–Chiari malformation caused by SB, the pulling down of the brain stem and the cerebellum through the foramen magnum. In an analysis of the published data, Wald and coauthors found that the performance of the two fruit signs in screening rivaled screening with MSAFP.[26,472] In thirteen studies on the lemon sign and eight on the banana sign, the compiled SB detection rates were 86 percent and 93 percent and the false-positive rates were 0.23 percent and 0.05 percent, respectively. However, the authors caution that the results are not likely to be nearly as good in clinical practice, given that the published studies were almost all done on women known to be at high risk of SB. In addition, we have as yet no indication that screening a low-risk general pregnant population by sonographers in the offices of primary care providers will be able to approach the performance of researchers in dedicated, academic ultrasound centers.

MSAFP SCREENING: POLICY GUIDELINES

Laboratory guidelines on MSAFP screening for NTDs were published by the National Committee for Clinical Laboratory Standards (NCCLS) in 1997.[473] The policy for screening for chromosome defects is discussed in chapter 22.

MSAFP SCREENING FOR NTDS BEFORE 14 WEEKS

There is no recognized correlation between MSAFP and AFAFP values in the first trimester. Experience thus far indicates no likely benefit of early screening for NTDs. One brief report noted normal MSAFP levels at 11–12 weeks in two fetuses with acrania and one with SB.[474] In a prospective set of first-trimester studies of twelve cases with SB and three with anencephaly, only one SB case yielded an elevated MSAFP value at 14 weeks.[475] Neither unconjugated estriol nor intact β-human chorionic gonadotropin (β-hCG) were effective indicators of NTDs in this study. Another prospective study of nineteen NTD cases also showed that first-trimester MSAFP screening was of no value, with the median value in the NTD pregnancies only 1.2 MoM.[476]

Although first-trimester screening with MSAFP is not appropriate, some laboratories have lowered the NTD screening window from 15 to 14 weeks of gestation. The impetus for this is that screening for Down syndrome using triple markers is acceptable at 14 weeks; thus, it would be efficient to screen for NTDs at the same time.[477] However, data from the original multicenter study on MSAFP as a screening test for NTDs, the U.K. Collaborative Study of 1977, clearly showed that screening performance at 14 weeks was inferior to screening from 15 weeks on.[289] The estimate from the data in that study is that the detection rate at 14 weeks is no more than 50 percent, using an MoM cutoff of 2.5 MoM, clearly inferior to the 80 percent or higher attainable beginning at 15 or 16 weeks of pregnancy.

AMNIOTIC FLUID AFP

Brock and Sutcliffe[478] first observed elevated AFAFP concentrations when the fetus had an open NTD. The slight overlap in values between affected and unaffected pregnancies was recognized early on.[268] These data indicated that the optimal time for amniocentesis for AFP assay, resulting in the least overlap, was 16–18 weeks. To achieve similar false-positives rates for each gestational week, that study concluded that it was necessary to increase the upper-limit cutoff level as pregnancy advanced (Table 21.15). It was also noted that the risk of open SB varies, depending on the concentration of AFAFP, the reason for the amniocentesis, and the background prevalence of open SB (Table 21.16). Table 21.16 also reflects the odds for open SB if MSAFP as well as AFAFP elevations are known.

Units Used in Reporting AFAFP Results

AFAFP levels decrease logarithmically, at a rate of about 15 percent per week, during the period of 15–22 gestational weeks in which they are used in prenatal diagnosis. For this reason and because of variability of AFP values from assay to assay, as in screening with MSAFP, the reported AFAFP value is normalized in some way. As with MSAFP, the MoM is the normalizing unit most commonly used in reporting AFAFP results. The MoM cut-offs often used in AFAFP testing are 2.0 and 2.5. However, until about 15 years ago, it was not uncommon to report AFAFP results as the number of standard deviations (SDs) above (or below) the mean level for each week of gestation, with a cutoff of +5.0 SD

Table 21.15. AFAFP: the detection rate for open neural tube defects and the false-positive rate

Gestation (Completed Weeks)	AFP Cutoff Level (MoM)	Detection Rate		Crude False-Positive Rate (All Non-NTD Singletons) (%)
		Anencephaly (%)	Open Spina Bifida (%)	
13–15	2.5	100 (21/21)	96 (22/23)	0.7 (24/3,279)
16–18	3.0	99 (96/97)	99 (73/74)	0.7 (58/7,858)
19–21	3.5	99 (69/70)	95 (20/21)	1.0 (15/1,561)
22–24	4.0	94 (32/34)	100 (5/5)	1.5 (6/407)
13–24	as above	98.2 (218/222)	97.6 (120/123)	0.79[a] (103/13,105)

Source: Adapted from Second Report of the U.K. Collaborative Study on Alpha-Fetoprotein in Relation to Neural Tube Defects 1979.[268]

Note: Numbers of pregnancies are shown in parentheses.

[a]The "practical" false-positive rate (excluding miscarriages and serious malformations) was 0.48 percent (61/12,804).

Table 21.16. The odds of having a fetus with open SB (compared with a viable fetus without a serious malformation) before and after a positive AFAFP test at 16–18 weeks of gestation, according to the prevalence of open SB and the reason for the amniocentesis

Prevalence of Open Spinal Bifida[a]	Before Reason for Amniocentesis	AFAFP Test	Odds of Having a Fetus with Open SB after AFAFP Level Found to Be a Cutoff Level			
			3.0 MoM	3.5 MoM	4.0 MoM	4.5 MoM
1 per 1,000	Serum AFP $2.53median[b]	1:2	9:1	16:1	17:1	26:1
	Previous infant with NTD	1:100	2:1	4:1	4:1	7:1
	Other	1:1000	1:4	1:2	1:2	2:3
2 per 1,000	Serum AFP $2.53median[b]	1:13	18:1	32:1	35:1	52:1
	Previous infant with NTD	1:50	5:1	8:1	9:1	14:1
	Other	1:500	1:2	1:1	1:1	3:2
3 per 1,000	Serum AFP $2.53median[b]	1:9	26:1	46:1	50:1	75:1
	Previous infant with NTD	1:33	7:1	13:1	14:1	20:1
	Other	1:333	2:3	1:1	3:2	2:1

Source: Adapted from Second Report of the U.K. Collaborative Study on Alpha-Fetoprotein in Relation to Neural Tube Defects 1979.[268]

[a]In the absence of antenatal diagnosis and selective abortion.

[b]At 16–18 weeks of gestation, based on a single serum AFP test, followed by the use of ultrasound to correct gestational age; if patients with raised levels are tested twice and the average value is used, the odds ratios are increased by about one-third.

units or more considered clearly elevated, and +3.0–4.9 SD units considered borderline elevated. The SD method of reporting, similar to that commonly used in clinical chemistry, was phased out in favor of the more stable and better understood MoM unit, already being used in reporting MSAFP results. In both cases, the reference data for AFAFP are gestational-age-specific. In the case of the MoM, the reference data are completed week-specific median values, and in the case of SDs above the mean, the reference data are completed week-specific mean values.

Experience with AFAFP Assays

AFAFP assays have long been routine, and extensive series have been reported[263,268,273–278,478–483] and reviewed.[98] Tabulated summary data of our first 100,000 cases noted in the previous edition[98] indicated a recurrence rate for a NTD after the birth of a previously affected child as 1.4 percent. Because some samples sent from other states included parents with SB occulta, no reliable recurrence risks could be given for an affected parent. The risk of recurrence after the birth of two previous children with NTDs was 5.9 percent. Routine assays of AF obtained largely because of advanced maternal age yielded an NTD rate of 1 per 492 cases studied. This figure is considerably higher than expected, given that these represent only cases with no family history. Among the 499 NTDs that occurred in the first 100,000 cases studied, 29 (5.8 percent) were closed lesions associated with a normal AFAFP. The 317 other congenital defects diagnosed reflect only those with an elevated AFAFP.

Among the 100,000 cases, only 779 (0.78 percent) had an elevated (≥5 SD) AFAFP at ≤24 weeks of pregnancy. The outcomes of these 779 pregnancies (Table 21.17) showed that almost 66.9 percent had NTDs or other serious congenital defects. Fetal blood admixture was considered the reason for the elevated AFP in 10.5 percent of cases, while

Table 21.17. Pregnancy outcome in 100,000 consecutive cases after the detection of elevated AFAFP at 24 weeks of gestation

Outcome	AFAFP ≥ 5 SD (%)	AFAFP 3 to <5 SD (%)
Malformation		
NTD	355[a] (45.6)	15[b] (7.7)
Other defects	166[c] (21.3)	11[d] (5.6)
Normal outcome		
Fetal blood positive	82 (10.5)	59 (30.3)
Fetal blood not tested	25 (3.2)	51 (26.2)
Fetal blood negative	44 (5.6)	47 (24.1)
Elective abortion (normal fetus)	10 (1.3)	
Fetal death	97 (12.5)	11 (5.6)
Stillbirth	1 (0.5)	
Total	779 (0.78)	195 (0.2)

[a]Anencephaly (154), spina bifida (175), encephalocele (17), iniencephaly (2), exencephaly (1), Meckel syndrome (6).
[b]Spina bifida (14), Meckel syndrome (1).
[c]Chromosomal defects (35) include trisomies 21, 18, 13, and 8; 45,X; 4,X/46,XX, 47,XXY; ventral-wall defects (82); cystic hygroma (8); congenital nephrosis (3); miscellaneous defects: multiple anomalies (4); prune belly syndrome (3); amniotic band syndrome (4); dead twin (3); hydrops fetalis (5); hydronephrosis (2); sacrococcygeal teratoma (2); nasopharyngeal teratoma (2); acardiac fetus (1); persistent fetal circulation (1); inborn error unspecified (1); microcephaly (1); Noonan syndrome (1); nuchal cyst (1); hamartoma (1); skin lesions with resorbed twin (1); chorangioma (1); ascites (1); hydrocephaly (1); short umbilical cord (1).
[d]Chromosomal defects (6); omphalocele (4), multiple anomalies (1).

no clear explanation other than probable undetectable fetal blood admixture obtained in another 3.2 percent of cases.

AFAFP and Acetylcholinesterase from Early Amniocentesis Fluid

Normal values for AFAFP for 11–14 weeks of gestation have been determined.[267,484,485] Thus far, the sensitivity and predictive value of NTD detection between 11 and 13 weeks has not been documented. Burton et al.[486] found AChE activity in five of ninety-three (5.4 percent) AF samples drawn between 11 and 14 weeks of gestation. All five cases were falsely positive (no leaking lesion), and several weeks later, amniocentesis samples in four of the five were AChE-negative. Another small study suggested AChE reliability after the twelfth week.[487] Despite the correct diagnoses of NTD at 10 and 11 weeks, there is still no reliable basis for recommending amniocentesis for prenatal diagnosis of NTDs between 11 and 13 weeks, especially considering that early amniocentesis is no longer recommended, primarily because of the increased risk of fetal talipes equinovarus associated with the procedure[488] (see chapter 2).

False-Positive and False-Negative Rates

The practical false-positive rate[268] describes how frequently a viable normal fetus would be terminated because of a single false-positive AFAFP result (Table 21.18). Of our 779 cases with AFP $\geq$5 SD, in 10 (1.3 percent), there was elective abortion of a normal fetus (see Table 21.17) before AChE assays were in use, and during our early experience, 2 cases could not be explained even after autopsy, including examination of the placenta and electron microscopy of the kidneys.[479,494] Two others were unwanted pregnancies, terminations having been done even before second samples were reported as normal AFAFP. In one pregnancy, a dead twin was the likely explanation of the elevated AFAFP in the other sac, but ultrasound study was insufficient to reassure the parents, who elected to abort. No further elective abortion of a normal fetus has occurred after our AFP assays in the last 80,000 of these 100,000 cases, in which AChE assay and high-resolution ul-

Table 21.18.　Practical false-positive rates after AFAFP assays to detect neural tube defects

Reference	No. of Pregnancies (%)	False-Positive Rate After One Amniocentesis (%)	False-Positive Rate After Two Amniocenteses (%)
Second Report of the U.K. Collaborative Study[268]	13,490	0.48	0.2[a]
Milunsky[479]	20,000	—	0.06
Crandall and Matsumoto[480]	34,000	—	0.9[b]
Aitken et al.[489]	3,244	1.8	0.4[b]
A. Milunsky, unpublished and cumulative data (1992)[98]	100,000	—	0.01[b]
Loft et al.[490]	9,964	0.23[b]	—
Guibaud et al.[491]	18,000	0.05[b]	—
Crandall and Chua[492]	7,440	0.1	—
Sepulveda et al.[493]	1,737	0.4	—

[a]Estimated.
[b]Using AChE assays.

Table 21.19. The efficiency of detection of neural tube defects using qualitative gel AChE and elevated AFP (24 weeks of gestation)

Pregnancy Outcome	Author's Series		Published Series		Combined Series (total)	
	Number of Pregnancies	AChE Positive (%)	Number of Pregnancies	AChE Positive (%)	Number of Pregnancies	AChE Positive (%)
Anencephaly/exencephaly/ iniencephaly	121[a]	121 (100) 121 (119,1,1)	638	636 (99.7)	759	757 (99.7)
Open spina bifida	169[b]	167 (98.9)	483	481 (99.6)	652	648 (99.4)
Encephalocele	24	13 (92.9)	11	11 (100)	35	24 (68.6)
Omphalocele/gastroschisis/ open ventral wall defect	101	45 (44.6)	102	69 (67.7)	203	114 (56.2)
Cystic hygroma	16	12 (75.0)	11	7 (63.3)	27	19 (70.4)
Meckel syndrome	0[c]	5 (83.3)	1	1 (100)	7	6 (85.7)
Other serious defects	61	31[d] (50.8)	34	7 (20.6)	95	38 (40.0)
Congenital nephrosis	3	0 (0)	1	0 (0)	4	0 (0)
Fetal death	43	28 (65.1)	96	47 (50.0)	139	75 (54.0)
Apparently normal fetus— elective abortion	10[c]	2 (20.0)	3	2 (66.7)	13	4 (30.8)
Apparently normal newborn	378	32 (8.5)	235	15 (6.4)	613	47 (7.7)
Total cases with elevated AFP	922	456 (49.5)	1,612	1,276	2,534	1,732
Normal AFP and normal child	820	9 (1.1)	5,363	10 (0.2)	6,183	24 (0.4)

[a]Two additional cases had normal AFP but were AChE-positive.

[b]One additional case had normal AFP but was AChE-positive.

[c]One additional case had normal AFP but was AChE-positive.

[d]Nasopharyngeal teratoma (2), sacrococcygeal teratoma (2), amniotic band syndrome (2), trisomy 18 (3), trisomy 13 (1), 45XO (1), multiple congenital abnormalities (3), hydrocephaly and multiple fractures (1), hydrocephaly (very bloody) (1), microcephaly—brain hernation (1), dead twin (3), acardiac fetus (1), skin lesions and incomplete twinning (1), ascites (2), hydrops fetalis (4), hydrocele (1), elective abortion—dilation and evacuation, no fetus (2).

trasound have been used as adjunctive tests. Therefore, our cumulative practical false-positive rate (see Table 21.18) using ≥3 SD above the mean for AFP was 10 per 100,000 (0.01 percent), which is unchanged with AChE (Table 21.19). In this entire experience, no satisfactory explanation was possible for two of the aborted fetuses, both of which were studied about 20 years ago.

Our experience with no elective abortion of a normal fetus in more than 80,000 cases suggests a true false-positive rate (using AFP, AChE, and ultrasound) of 0.002 percent.

Assays for AFAFP in our routine prenatal diagnosis cases show that about 1 in 183 (0.6 percent) has a leaking fetal defect. The AFAFP was elevated between 3 and 5 SD above the mean in 15 pregnancies ≥24 weeks with NTDs (see Table 21.17). Fourteen fetuses had SB and one had Meckel syndrome; all were positive for AChE. Only 15 of 370 NTDs (4.1 percent) had AFP values between 3 and 5 SD above the mean. Because a few cases of open SB have been reported with AFAFP values between 2 and 3 SD above the mean, we assay samples for AChE from all patients with values ≥2 SD above the mean or ≥2 MoM or with a family history. From overall experience, about 4.7 percent of all NTDs appear "closed" during the second trimester (Table 21.20). This figure constitutes the expected false-negative rate.

In both our studies[10] and the U.K. Collaborative Study,[268] raised AFAFP between 16 and 18 weeks that was associated with open SB yielded occasional infants at birth with closed SB. Brock[483] summarized how both the calculated false-positive and false-nega-

Table 21.20. Selected studies showing the frequency of closed NTDs among all NTDs detected prenatally and at birth

Reference	Total NTDs	Closed NTDs (%)
Second Report of the U.K. Collaborative Study[268]	385	29 (7.5)
Wyvill et al.[495]	61	1 (1.6)
Aitken et al. (prospective)[489]	177	7 (4.0)
Milunsky[479] and unpublished data	499	29 (5.8)
Total studied	1,121	66 (4.7)

tive rates vary according to the actual cutoff points used. Rarely, SB or an encephalocele may be present when the AFAFP is within the normal range and yet AChE is detected. Aitken et al.[489] noted one such case with SB among 171 NTDs studied prospectively. We had one closed SB case with a normal AFAFP before the AChE assay was available. Retrospective analysis yielded a positive AChE result. Almost all false-positive AFAFP and AChE assay results are due to fetal blood admixture. Fetal serum rather than red blood cells appears to be the main source of AChE that enters both cerebrospinal fluid and AF.[496] Fetal blood contamination yielding a false-positive AChE result is due to an erythrocyte concentration exceeding 60×10^6 cells/mL.[497]

The severity of SB cannot be inferred from the concentration of AFP. Because of the closure of an NTD and/or decreasing fetal serum AFP levels, assays for AFP at >24 weeks of gestation may yield normal AFP results. In twenty such cases (two of anencephaly, eighteen of SB), we noted that all probably had normal AFAFP values but were nevertheless AChE-positive. AF assays for NTDs suspected in the third trimester should therefore focus on AChE and not AFP.

In a karyotypic study of fetuses with isolated NTDS, seven of forty-three (16.3 percent) had a chromosomal abnormality, compared with an expected 0.3 percent based solely on maternal age.[189] Although not all of these determined cytogenetic anomalies were clinically significant, the authors pointed to a significant increase of karyotypic abnormalities in fetuses with isolated NTDs and recommended genetic studies in all such cases.

In a summary of fourteen studies, the median AFAFP value in fetal Down syndrome was found to be 0.69 MoM.[498,499] Other markers—unconjugated estriol, total human chorionic gonadotropin (hCG), and free β-hCG—used in serum screening for Down syndrome, had medians of about 0.5, 1.7, and 2.10, respectively,[498,500] similar to their values in maternal serum.

Sensitivity, Specificity, and Predictive Value

A sensitivity of 98 percent for open NTDs[268] can be expected, using AFAFP alone, and rising to >99 percent when AChE is also used.[98] Fetal blood contamination will lower sensitivity and cannot be corrected for reliability. A specificity of >99 percent for *open* NTD is achievable. Predictive values will vary with the prevalence of NTD, family history, and cutoff level used. AFAFP ≥ 2.0 and ≥ 2.5 MoM yielded risks for *open* NTD of 24–41 percent and 41–63 percent, respectively.[268,479,501]

Multiple Pregnancy

Given the increased risk of malformations, including NTDs among twins[12,502] and speculation about the role of the twinning process in the etiology of NTDs,[91,92,503] special care is needed in the evaluation for structural defects (see also chapters 23 and 24). For non-identical twins or triplets discordant for open NTDs or fetal death, we and others[504,505] have repeatedly observed elevated AFAFP and AChE presence in the sac of the affected fetus and normal results in the unaffected twin. There have been occasional exceptions in which dizygous twins discordant for NTDs or fetal death have had elevated AFAFP and AChE presence in both sacs, as also noted by others.[506–508]

Causes of Elevated AFAFP in the Absence of NTDs

A raised AFAFP without the concomitant presence of AChE poses increased risks for that pregnancy.[509] Elevated AFAFP is found in many leaking fetal defects (Table 21.21); the value of the observation is confounded only by fetal blood admixture. Because fetal blood may be present in association with some defects, a level II ultrasound would be recommended in all cases with unexplained elevated AFAFP.

In normal pregnancy, AFP reaches the AF mostly by fetal urination.[541] Any fetal skin defects, including NTDs and omphalocele, allow the egress of serum containing AFP into the AF, leading to a quantitative increase in its concentration.[542] Other defects causing fetal proteinuria (e.g., congenital nephrosis) could also result in a raised AFP level. Heinonen et al.[410] reported an elevated AFAFP after a high MSAFP level in forty-three of forty-four pregnancies with fetal congenital nephrosis. The range of AFAFP levels were 5.1–43.5 MoM; the sensitivity was 100 percent and the specificity was 99 percent. The one missed case resulted from a normal MSAFP screen. Unexplained high AFAFP levels that are AChE-negative may decrease appreciably at a second amniocentesis 2 weeks later if the fetus is likely to be normal or rise if congenital nephrosis or another serious defect is present. Disorders interfering with swallowing or digestion (e.g., esophageal or duodenal atresia) might diminish the turnover of AFP or through regurgitation of biliary secretions raise the AFAFP concentration. Although fetal renal agenesis could be expected to involve low or absent AFAFP values, we and others[543] have found normal concentrations.

Cystic hygromas, which may be found particularly in association with Turner or Down syndrome (among others), may also occur in the absence of any chromosome abnormality (see also chapter 23). A review of 142 cases detected by ultrasound showed 58 percent with Turner syndrome, 28 percent with various chromosomal defects, and 22 percent with normal karyotypes.[544] Moreover, elevated AFAFP, with or without positive AChE in such cases, may well be due to direct aspiration of cystic fluid[515] rather than transudation of fetal serum.[545] Cystic hygromas may resolve and, with normal karyotypes, may result in normal neonatal survival.[515] Nevertheless, initial detection should be followed by detailed sonographic evaluation of the entire fetus, karyotype, and family history.[546]

Elevated AFAFP levels in association with omphalocele or open ventral-wall defects occur in at least 67 percent of cases. The use of densitometric analysis of AF to distinguish such lesions from NTDs[547] has been superseded by high-resolution ultrasound study.

When fetal blood contamination has been clearly excluded as the reason for a raised AFP level, our data and those of others[480] are similar, in that there is about a two-thirds risk that the fetus has either an NTD or another serious congenital defect. Raised MSAFP and AFAFP values were observed in the case of a fetus with a small pilonidal sinus.[528] The significance of the association is doubtful. Equally doubtful is the reported association with hydrocele, in which high AFAFP and AChE were detected,[548] given the later development of hydrocele. Not all cases of fetal sacrococcygeal teratoma have raised

Table 21.21.   Fetal conditions that may be associated with elevated AFAFP and/or AChE

Likely Mechanism	Condition	Reference
Leakage through skin	NTDs—anencephaly, spina bifida, encephalocele, exencephaly, iniencephaly	98,478
	Anterior abdominal wall defect—omphalocele, gastroschisis, abdominothoracic defect, body-stalk abnormality	494,510–512
	Exstrophy of bladder (cloaca)	513,514
	Epidermolysis bullosa	412,413
	Aplasia cutis congenita	512
	Chromosomal defects—trisomies 21, 18, 13, 8; 45X, 45X/46XX, 47XXY (see also Table 21.4)	98
	Cystic hygroma (see text)	479,480,515
	Nuchal cyst	516
	Prune belly syndrome	517
	Median palatoschisis	518
	Scalp defect (see chromosome defects)	
	Amniotic band syndrome	519
	Fetal death (autolysis)	481,520
	Twin with cotwin death	521
	Acardiac twin fetus	494
	Meckel syndrome	98
	Fetus, papyraceous	522,523
	Hydrops/fetal ascites	494,523,524
	Lymphangiectasia	525
	Bladder neck-obstruction (massive distention and death)	526
	Urethra absent	527
	Rhesus hemolytic disease (see also hydrops)	361
	? Pilonidal sinus	528
	Sacrococcygeal teratoma	480,529,530
	Hamartoma (see Table 21.17)	98
Urinary tract leakage	Congenital nephrosis	98,479,531
	Denys–Drash syndrome	532
	Hydronephrosis	479,531,533
	Polycystic kidney disease[a]	418
Leakage of placental origin	Fetal blood in amniotic fluid	98,360
	Hydatidiform mole	372–374
	Umbilical cord hemangioma	534
Leakage of pulmonary origin	Cystic adenomatoid malformation of lung	382,411
? Reduced intestinal AFP clearance or leakage	Pharyngeal teratoma	519
	Esophageal atresia	535
	Duodenal atresia	512,536
	Annular pancreas	537
	Intestinal atresia	480,494,531,538
Unknown site of "leakage"	Multiple congenital defects	98,479,539
	Hydrocephalus	520,540
	Dandy–Walker malformation	519
	Tracheoesophageal fistula	519
	Herpes virus infection (maternal) with fetal liver necrosis	518
	Noonan syndrome (see Table 21.17)	98
	Tetralogy of Fallot	520

Note: Additional references in previous editions 1979, 1986, 1992, and 1998.[98,283,284,609]
[a]No AChE detected.

AFAFP or are AChE-positive.[549] No significant association between AFAFP levels and fetal or neonatal death, preterm delivery, or low birth weight was noted in one study.[485]

Elevated AFAFP and Sonography

Highly skilled and superbly equipped experts in obstetrical ultrasound occasionally miss an NTD, despite being apprised about an elevated AFAFP level and the presence of AChE. Small sacral NTDs are the lesions that are mostly commonly missed. However, other cryptic defects may be present (see Table 21.21). Given the precision of the assay for AFP, patient reassurance that all is well in the face of an unremarkable targeted ultrasound study when AFAFP is elevated (with or without the presence of AChE in a noncentrifuged sample free of fetal blood) is unwarranted. In one series of 263 fetuses with high AFAFP and a normal sonogram, 11 (4.2 percent) had closed central nervous system defects (hydrocephalus in 5, Dandy–Walker malformation in 2), 2 had congenital nephrosis, 1 had tracheoesophageal fistula, and 1 had a small omphalocele.[519]

Meckel Syndrome

The prenatal detection of Meckel syndrome may be difficult. Only five of our seven cases had an AFAFP ≥5 SD above the mean. An additional case had a normal AFP but was positive for AFAChE. AChE was positive in five of six cases assayed. Chemke et al.[550] described a fetus with this syndrome, with high AFAFP without an NTD, postulating excessive synthesis of AFP by the polycystic kidneys. Whatever the origin of AFP or AChE in this syndrome, caution should attend every effort at prenatal diagnosis for this autosomal recessive disorder.

Johnson and Holzwarth[551] reviewed published experience of thirty-two cases and added three of their own. They again emphasized the variability of the clinical expression of Meckel syndrome. In an overall analysis of seventy-nine cases unrelated to prenatal diagnosis, they noted that 57 percent had combined encephalocele, polycystic kidneys, and polydactyly; 16 percent had encephalocele and polycystic kidneys; and 15 percent had polycystic kidneys and polydactyly. Only 3 percent had encephalocele and polydactyly. Most disturbing was the report by Seller[547] that 9 percent had only one of these abnormalities. Elsewhere, one of two affected siblings had only urethral atresia and preaxial polydactyly.[552] Patients at risk should understand the pleiotropic nature of this gene and should not be lulled into reassurance given a high probability of a correct diagnosis by ultrasound between 11 and 14 weeks of gestation.[553]

Problems and Pitfalls

Aspiration of Urine

In our experience, maternal urine is inadvertently aspirated at amniocentesis in about 1 in 2,000 cases. Most often, this occurs because patients have been requested to have a full bladder for the preceding ultrasound study. For ultrasonically guided amniocentesis, some prefer to keep the bladder distended during the procedure. A sample submitted as AF is usually first suspected as being urine when no AFP is detected on assay. It would seem judicious for obstetricians performing amniocenteses to drop some AF immediately on aspiration onto one of the many types of test strips available that allow for the determination of pH, protein, and sugar, to obviate the problem. Duncan[554] suggested the useful routine of testing the urine voided immediately before amniocentesis and keeping the test strip alongside another on which a few drops of AF are placed for comparison. The aspiration of maternal urine instead of AF had led, at least in two cases, to a failure to detect anencephaly and open SB.[555,556]

Brown or Green AF

A 1.6 percent frequency of discolored AF obtained during the second trimester has been noted previously.[283] When brown AF was associated with an elevated AFP, an untoward outcome of pregnancy was extremely likely (93.6 percent). The experience of Seller[557] was very similar. In contrast, brown AF in the second trimester not associated with an elevated AFP does not seem to augur ill for the pregnancy.[558] An earlier intrauterine bleed with resulting blood breakdown products is the likely cause for the discolored AF.

Green AF shown by spectrophotometric scanning is usually due to meconium. An incidence rate of 1.7 percent in midtrimester AF was reported by Allen,[559] with an associated mortality rate of 5.1 percent. AF meconium reflects a characteristic layering effect on ultrasound.[560]

AMNIOTIC FLUID ACHE

The assay for neuronal-derived AChE[561] is a critical adjunct in the prenatal diagnosis of open NTDs.[460,513] The most common assay is polyacrylamide-gel electrophoresis (PAGE),[562] in which AChE can be distinguished from nonspecific cholinesterase on the basis of mobility in such gels. AChE appears as a faster second migrating band, which can be suppressed by the addition of a specific inhibitor (BW284C51). Normal AF has a single, slow-moving band of nonspecific cholinesterase.

Loft[460] compared PAGE, an immunoassay using a monoclonal antibody, to AChE and to a spectrophotometric assay. Although the third was found to be completely unsuitable, almost identical performance in clear AF was obtained for the first two. When fetal blood was present in the AF, the immunoassay was clearly less satisfactory than PAGE, yielding a higher false-positive rate. Better visualization of AChE bands in PAGE has been claimed by using dark-field illumination.[538]

Experience with AFAChE

Extensive clinical use of AChE for prenatal diagnosis of NTDs followed the initial major study. Loft,[460] in a review of twenty combined studies, noted detection rates of 98.6, 95.5, and 95.2 percent for anencephaly, for all SB, and for encephalocele, respectively. These rates are compared with those in the second collaborative study report[268] and with our own experience (see Table 21.19). However, case selection differed slightly among some studies, in that AFAFP was considered elevated variably between 2.5 and 3 SD above the mean or at $\geq$2.5 MoM. Despite this variation, the overall detection efficiency for anencephaly and for SB was 99.7 and 99.4 percent, respectively. Only 68.6 percent of encephaloceles leaked. Although many reports make distinctions between detection rates for open versus closed SB, the clinician counseling a patient before amniocentesis needs to know the overall detection and practical false-positive rates (see Tables 21.18 and 21.19).

Precise interpretation of a PAGE for AFAChE assay depends on gestational age. False-positive rates from AF samples at $\geq$12 weeks of gestation have ranged from 4.3 to 33.3 percent.[487,492,563,564] False-positive AFAChE rates between 13 and 24 weeks of gestation in the period 1979–1984 were up to 1.8 percent (see Table 21.18). More recently, rates in clear AF samples have been ≤0.22 percent (see Table 21.18).

Given the clear risk of false-positive AChE results before 15 weeks,[564,565] high-resolution ultrasound (serially if needed) and occasionally a second amniocentesis about 2 weeks later is recommended. Increased false-positive and false-negative rates have also been noted after 24 weeks.[460] False-negative AFAChE may also occur rarely with open NTDs.[566–568] After fetal death, an AChE band is frequently seen in the gel and can sometimes be distinguished from the pattern seen with open NTDs.[569,570] The vast majority of disorders associated with elevated AFAFP (see Table 21.21) may also have detectable AChE activity. Some open lesions close later in pregnancy and a few have normal AFAFP and no detectable AChE. The ever-possible confounding with fetal blood admixture is now usually resolved by high-resolution ultrasound (see also chapter 23). Sepulveda et al.[493] retrospectively audited 1,737 consecutive AF samples that they obtained for chromosome studies and that included assays for AFP and AChE. In 25 cases elevated AFAFP and/or positive AChE was observed. High-resolution ultrasonography correctly identified all 18 fetuses with defects and associated elevated AFAFP and/or positive ACHE. In the remaining 7 fetuses, no anomalies were detected and all appeared normal after birth (a false-positive rate of 0.4 percent). These authors suggested that these biochemical assays would not be cost effective in centers where high-resolution ultrasonography is done before amniocentesis. Despite their conclusion, they presented no evidence concerning their cost–benefit claims.

In combined series, ventral abdominal-wall defects without distinguishing omphalocele from gastroschisis were detected in 56.2 percent of cases using AFAFP and AChE (see Table 21.19). The presence of AChE in these cases, as in other leaking lesions, probably reflects transudation of fetal plasma.[571,572] For ventral-wall defects, AChE secretion from intestinal nerve plexuses and butyrylcholinesterase secretion from intestinal muscle cells may explain the positive PAGE results.[573,574] Usually, high AChE and low butyrylcholinesterase activities characterize AFs from open NTDs; the opposite usually occurs in open ventral-wall defects. Both PAGE assays[575] and monoclonal immunoassays[460] can assist in distinguishing open NTDs from ventral abdominal-wall defects by densitometric demonstration of a denser pseudocholinesterase band in the latter.[572,576,577] However, it is more appropriate to select ultrasound study immediately if an elevated AFAFP with or without positive AChE is found, given the need for a precise diagnosis and distinction between gastroschisis and omphalocele (see also chapter 23). Between 25 and 33 percent of fetuses with omphalocele have other associated defects, including subsequent mental retardation, compared with about 10–36 percent (mainly gut atresias) in those with gastroschisis.[98,578]

An abnormal karyotype is frequent with omphalocele, 20–22 percent in two studies,[578] but as high as 54 percent in another,[579] probably reflecting ascertainment bias, with more complex cases being referred. Prognosis for survival depends primarily on the presence of other anomalies, ranging from 7 percent to almost 100 percent.[578] Mode of delivery seems not to have affected survival rates.[578] In contrast, gastroschisis is not typically associated with an abnormal karyotype, and survival, while highly likely, is predicated on other factors (e.g., prematurity, sepsis, and associated intestinal atresias).[578]

Cases in which borderline AFAFP values are found to be positive for AChE and fetal blood admixture require high-resolution ultrasound, serially if necessary. Decisions should be made on the ultrasonographic findings; referral to nomograms[580] is useful only when ultrasound facilities are not available.

Table 21.22. The odds of having a fetus with open SB after positive AFP and AChE tests

Birth Incidence of SB	Before Reason for Amniocentesis	Odds of Fetus with SB	
		After AChE	Positive AChE
1 per 1,000	Raised maternal serum AFP	9:1	144:1
	Previous infant with NTD	2:1	32:1
	Other	1:4	4:1
2 per 1,000	Raised maternal serum AFP	18:1	288:1
	Previous infant with NTD	5:1	80:1
	Other	1:2	8:1
3 per 1,000	Raised maternal serum AFP	26:1	416:1
	Previous infant with NTD	7:1	112:1
	Other	2:3	16:1

Source: After Collaborative Acetylcholinesterase Study 1981.[566]

Among 6,183 normal children born after AFAFP was found to be normal, 24 (0.4 percent) in combined series (see Table 21.19) were AFAChE-positive.[494,566,581–584] In another study[575] of 1,300 AFs, faint AChE bands were identified in 9 (0.7 percent), none of which was associated with congenital defects. Fetal blood in the AF may well explain even some of these, the AChE source being fetal serum.[538]

The Collaborative AChE Study[566] showed that a woman with an elevated AFAFP who was AChE-positive had a much greater likelihood of carrying a fetus with a serious leaking fetal defect (Table 21.22). In a report of two fetuses with esophageal atresia, inexplicable AChE-positive AF in the face of normal AFAFP was noted.[538] One other fetus affected by tracheoesophageal fistula was AFAChE-negative.

Advantages and Disadvantages of the AChE Assay

Although the AChE assay is also nonspecific, it has a major advantage over AFP in not being dependent on gestational age, at least in the second trimester. Its greater sensitivity than AFP is offset by the need for a second assay with an inhibitor, the use of which is not free of risk to laboratory personnel. It is also less efficient and more expensive than the AFP assay.

In addition to the problem of fetal blood contamination, at least two other pitfalls have been encountered. An error resulting in a positive AChE may occur when fetal calf serum is mistakenly introduced into the AF in the process of isolating AF cells. The bovine AChE will then be indistinguishable from the human enzyme. A second error involves old or mishandled AF, in which AChE derives from red blood cells, thereby leading to a false-positive result. The use of the predictive-value positive concept has been recommended, especially when borderline results are obtained.[585] The advent of AChE and of widely available level II ultrasound has markedly decreased the need for such a risk calculation.

RECOMMENDATIONS FOR PRENATAL DIAGNOSIS OF NTDS USING AFAFP AND ACHE ASSAYS

1. Couples with an increased risk of having a child with an NTD should be offered (or referred for) genetic counseling and amniocentesis.
2. AF from patients at increased risk should be assayed for both AFP and AChE.

3. AChE assays should be done on all AF samples with AFP values ≥ 2 MoM (some centers use ≥ 1.85 MoM).
4. MSAFP screening should not be relied on to exclude a fetal NTD.
5. Accurate ultrasonic fetal age assessment is mandatory immediately preceding amniocentesis because the AFAFP level steadily decreases through the second trimester.
6. Level II ultrasound is recommended for every woman with an increased risk of having a child with an NTD.
7. Both ultrasound and amniocentesis should be offered at 15–16 weeks of gestation.
8. A 1-mL aliquot of AF is best placed directly into a small tube at the time of amniocentesis, specifically for AFP and AChE assay of a noncentrifuged sample.
9. Obstetricians should discard the first 1–2 mL of AF if the sample contains fresh blood, to minimize problems in the interpretation of the AFP and AChE assays.
10. To exclude the possibility that urine has been obtained inadvertently, one or two drops of AF should be placed on a urine testing strip at the time of amniocentesis.
11. If fetal blood is present in the AF and is associated with an elevated AFP level and a normal sonogram, then a second amniocentesis is recommended in about 10 days.
12. Every AF sample obtained for any reason should be assayed for AFP.
13. Every laboratory receiving AF must first have established a normal range of AFP per gestational week and be able to provide accurate and reliable results, including MoMs or the number of SDs above the mean.
14. Fetal hemoglobin should be assayed or fetal red cells should be counted in all samples in which the AFP concentration exceeds the upper-limit cutoff.
15. A clear written policy should exist, showing the AFP level at which an AChE assay is automatically done.
16. If the AFAFP value is raised above the upper-limit cutoff (usually ≥ 2 MoMs), corroborative evidence should be sought before any decision is made to terminate a pregnancy. If ultrasound studies reveal no fetal abnormalities, and the karyotype is normal, a second amniocentesis should be performed in about 10 days, even if the first sample is also AChE-positive. This process should also assist in avoiding any sample mix-up.
17. *Direct* and *rapid* communication from the laboratory to the physician and from the physician to the patient should take place if any abnormal assay result is found.
18. Genetic counseling should be urged for all couples when a fetal defect is found or suspected or if laboratory results require further explanation.
19. No pregnancy should be terminated after the observation of an unexplained elevated AFAFP with or without the presence of AChE, without the couple's full understanding of the possibility that a fetus without apparent anatomic or other abnormality might be aborted.
20. In cases in which only AFAFP values have been high and AChE has been negative, and after parents have elected to abort the pregnancy, careful preparations should be made to obtain fetal kidney tissue for electron microscopy, aimed at determining a diagnosis of congenital nephrosis. It is unacceptable, and indeed negligent, when faced with a potential 25 percent risk of recurrence, to omit

proper preparations for light and electron microscopy of the kidneys to diagnose this fatal disorder. Characteristic findings are marked dilatation of proximal tubular lumina and Bowman's spaces and fusion of foot processes of the podocytes of the renal glomeruli.[586] Couples who do not receive this thoughtful care and attention will be denied the opportunity of knowing whether they have a 25 percent risk in a subsequent pregnancy and whether they need to consider other options (such as artificial insemination by donor).

21. Renal tissue studies would be unnecessary if DNA analysis of amniotic fluid cells yields definitive mutations in the nephrin gene.[97]

22. When necessary, fetal tissue should be stored frozen ($-70°$F), in anticipation of DNA mutation analysis of the congenital nephrosis gene,[97] for diagnosis and subsequent prenatal diagnosis.

OTHER TECHNIQUES TO DETECT NTDS

The complementary use of AFAFP and AChE, combined with ultrasonography, yields an extremely high degree of accuracy. Any new test challenging the first two biochemical assays would have to exceed their demonstrated complementary value. In particular, any new technique would have distinct advantages if it could achieve specificity, avoid variation with gestational age, render the effects of maternal or fetal blood contamination of AF irrelevant, and avoid significant overlap between the normal and abnormal ranges. Thus far, these strictures seem to impose too great a challenge for any approach attempting to replace the established tests. In fact, as noted in earlier reviews[98,284] evaluations for α_2-macroglobulin, β-lipoprotein, β-trace protein, fibrinogen degradation products, glucose, albumin, group-specific component, total protein, brain-specific protein S-100, 5-hydroxyindoleacetic acid, rapidly adherent AF cells, concanavalin A binding, glial fibrillary acidic protein, synaptosomal D2 protein, and various amino acids, have all been unsuccessful.

PRIMARY PREVENTION OF NTDS

Genetic Counseling

Given the heterogeneous etiology of NTDs (see Tables 21.1–21.4), great care should be exercised in providing genetic counseling (see also chapter 1). Primary prevention of NTDs through risk counseling, however, is extremely limited because about 95 percent of such offspring are delivered by women without a previously affected child.

The recurrence risk for first-degree relatives of probands with NTDs of polygenic origin usually parallels the population incidence.[587] Nevertheless, many confounding factors exist in assessing recurrence risks. These include a worldwide decline in the incidence of NTDs[588] (see discussion below), ethnic differences, and time and space variations. Hence, the range of risk figures in Table 21.23 provides some guidance but will require revision (especially the U.K. figures) to account for the declining incidence and the wide use of folic acid supplements. Recurrence risks for NTDs due to known causes (see Tables 21.2–21.4) will relate directly to such etiology.

It is not possible to derive specific risk figures that are uniformly applicable worldwide. Etiologic heterogeneity,[63] use of folic acid, and known racial, ethnic, geographic, maternal age, and other factors confound any such effort. All counselors would agree that prenatal studies be recommended to women who have had one or more affected progeny.

Table 21.23. The risks of neural tube defect (NTD) according to family history

Family History	Risk of NTD			Reference		
	United States	United Kingdom	Canada	United States	United Kingdom	Canada
One previous child with NTD	1.4–3.2	4.6–5.2	2.4–6.0	479,480,587,589,590	13,591,592	10,593,694
Two previous children with NTD	6.4	10–20	4.8	479	589,595,596	594
Three previous children with NTD		21–25			595	593
Affected parent and one sibling with NTD	see text	3	4.5		595	
Affected parent and one sibling with NTD		13			596	
All first cousins	0.26	0–0.6		590		13
All maternal first cousins			0.9			593
All paternal first cousins			0.5			593
Affected maternal nephew/niece	0.99		0.6–1.3	597		10
One child with multiple vertebral anomalies		3–7				598
One child with spinal dysraphism		4			599	
One sibling and a second-degree relative affected		9			595	
One sibling and a third-degree relative affected		7			595	

A similar consensus would lead to amniocentesis for the siblings of women who have affected offspring. Because the risks of the siblings of a male who sired a child with an NTD for also having an affected child are higher than background, amniocentesis should be seriously considered in such cases. A similar situation applies to the first cousins of both parents of an affected child. All these family members should be offered genetic counseling and should be apprised of their risks and options. In very experienced centers, MSAFP screening and targeted ultrasound studies in these family members are likely to be efficacious.

Other variations require consideration. Congenital vertebral anomalies may involve single or multiple vertebrae and may affect any portion of each bone. Wynne-Davies[598] concluded from both genetic and epidemiologic evidence that multiple vertebral anomalies in the absence of SB were causally related to the NTDs. She estimated that after the birth of a child with multiple vertebral anomalies, the recurrence risk is 2–3 percent, while that for an NTD is 3–7 percent. Prenatal studies are therefore clearly recommended in these women at risk.

Spinal dysraphism—a disorder in which the conus medullaris is tethered and possibly associated with various anomalies of the cord, vertebrae, or overlying skin[600,601]— was also observed to have etiologic associations with NTDs.[599] Spinal dysraphism in one child also provides a clear indication for prenatal studies in subsequent pregnancies.

Whether adults with SB occulta have an increased risk of bearing progeny with NTD remains unsettled. Critical questions of an epidemiologic nature (e.g., ascertainment bias, variations in diagnostic interpretation, age ranges, number of cases) can be leveled at most available studies.[98,602] A reasonably safe policy in these cases is the offer of MSAFP screening with targeted ultrasound study. The recognition that open and occult SB may occur as autosomal dominant disorders in Mormon[95] and perhaps some other families should give rise to caution in counseling.

Some authors have maintained that the siblings of children born with multiple malformations including an NTD have higher risks for both NTDs and congenital defects in general.[206] However, Hunter[10] found that the presence or absence of an additional malformation did not influence the familial nature of NTDs. Whether there is an increased frequency of NTDs in the siblings of children with esophageal atresia, with or without tracheoesophageal fistula, remains uncertain. Fraser and Nussbaum[603] found 1 NTD among 141 siblings in a highly selected group, a criticism that has been applied to data resulting in similar conclusions. The most useful data from Sweden[604] and Canada[605] do not show an increase in NTDs in the siblings of those with esophageal atresia.

Toriello and Higgins[590] showed a high degree of concordance for the type of NTD among affected sibling pairs. Their findings supported probable heterogeneity for open SB based on the level of the defect. Moreover, they observed that virtually all associated anomalies were midline defects. A significant association between NTDs and cleft lip/palate has also been noted by others.[590,606] Hunter et al.[607] concluded that nonvertebral malformations were more commonly associated with SB involving thoracic (27.2 percent) than lumbar (12 percent), cervical (16.7 percent), or sacral (12.5 percent) vertebrae.

Hall et al.[608] reported that apparently unrelated congenital defects occurred more often among probands with craniorachischisis (62 percent), encephalocele (30 percent), or multiple NTDs (25 percent) than among those with anencephaly (14.7 percent) or SB (10.1 percent). The level of the spinal lesion may also relate to etiology and familial risk. These authors observed NTDs in 7.8 percent of siblings of probands with high SB, but in only 0.7 percent with low lesions. Others[63] have made similar observations. NTDs were seen in 2.2 percent of the siblings of anencephalic probands and in none of the siblings of probands with craniorachischisis, encephalocele, or multiple NTDs.

Nutritional Supplementation

Data implicating a dietary deficiency, probably folate deficiency, in the pathogenesis of NTDs have been published repeatedly over the past five decades.[45,609] Only one flawed study reported no association.[610]

In 1989, we published results of the first prospective, broadly based, large (22,776 women) midtrimester study, which examined the relation of multivitamin (with and without folic acid) intake and the risk of NTDs.[57] The prevalence of NTDs was 3.5 per 1,000 among women who never used multivitamins before or after conception or who used multivitamins before conception only. The prevalence of NTDs for women who used folic-acid-containing multivitamins during the first 6 weeks of pregnancy was significantly lower: 0.9 per 1,000.[57] We concluded that multivitamins with folic acid taken when planning pregnancy and for the first 6 weeks after conception provided about 70 percent protection against NTDs. An additional important observation was the strikingly higher prevalence of NTDs in women with a positive family history who did not take supplements (13.0 of 1,000), compared with those with a family history who did (3.5 of 1,000).

In 1991, the U.K. Medical Research Council (MRC) multicountry, randomized, double-blind intervention trial was published.[58] The study aimed to determine whether supplementation with folic acid or a mixture of seven other vitamins taken at about the time of conception could prevent a recurrence of NTDs. Analysis of 1,195 women who had at least one previous affected offspring and for whom pregnancy outcomes were known, revealed a 72 percent protective effect (RR, 0.28; 95 percent CI, 0.12B0.71). Although a large daily dose (4 mg) of folic acid was used, no harmful effect was noted. Much lower effective doses (0.36 mg daily) were used by Smithells et al.[56] and were recorded by us.[57] Subsequently, a major Hungarian double-blind, randomized intervention trial based on preventing the occurrence of NTDs clearly demonstrated the efficacy of periconceptional folic acid supplementation.[611] The authors used multivitamins containing 0.4–0.8 mg folic acid taken at least 1 month before and 3 months after conception. In their nonsupplemented group, the NTD rate was 6 in 2,104, while no case occurred among the 2,052 women who took supplements.

The reason that some 30 percent of cases of NTD occur despite folic acid supplementation is unclear, as is the reported reduced efficacy of folic acid supplementation in Hispanic women.[612] Lessons from experiments with *curly-tail* mice suggest that this folate resistance might be overcome by dietary supplementation with the B-complex vitamin myoinositol.[613] Apparently, myoinositol treatment stimulates protein kinase C activity and upregulates retinoic acid receptor-β expression, thereby reducing delay in closure of the posterior neuropore.

The weight of the evidence supporting periconceptional folic acid supplementation for all women for the purpose of avoiding NTDs led to a call for public health policy. Consequently, the Centers for Disease Control and Prevention (CDC) in the United States issued clear recommendations, on September 12, 1992, that all women of childbearing age who are capable of becoming pregnant take 0.4 mg/day of folic acid daily.[614] An expert advisory group in the United Kingdom made a similar recommendation,[615] including 4–5 mg/day of folic acid for women who had previously had an affected child. The difficulties—economic, educational, and personal—of successful implementation of this recommendation were recognized, and an alternative policy of fortification of grain products with folic acid was approved by the U.S. Food and Drug Administration in 1996.[5] However, the level that was set (140 μg/100 g of grain product) is considerably less than the target amount because it will, on average, raise the folic acid intake only by about 100 μg per day.[616] Hesitation in implementing an optimal food fortification policy has revolved around the safety issue.[617] The lower-than-optimal amount of folic acid in fortified flour was chosen because that level would avoid ingestion by nontargeted consumers of more than 1,000 μg of folic acid per day.

The prime concern is the "masking" of cobalamin deficiency by folic acid, precipitating the neurologic complications of pernicious anemia. Certain medications (e.g., methotrexate, some anticonvulsants, some sulfa drugs) may be less effective for patients taking folic acid. Claims that seizure frequency increased in epileptics taking 5 mg of folic acid three times per day for 1–3 years[618] were not supported by the results of other studies, including those that were double-blind and randomized.[619,620] Other concerns for which data are weak relate to potential folate neurotoxicity, reduced zinc absorption, hypersensitivity to folic acid, and increased susceptibility to malaria.[617] In contrast, possible advantages of food fortification with folic acid include a decrease in cardiovascular disease (associated with reduced homocysteine) and in the frequency of cervical and colorectal cancer.[621] Mills recently questioned how much folic acid is enough.[622] Although many are reluctant to advocate for higher folic acid intake, Wald et al.,[28] in a recent analysis, argued that even the widely recommended 400 μg per day dose is far from optimal for prevention. By analyzing thirteen studies in which folic acid intake was correlated with serum folate levels, they demonstrate that daily intake of 5 mg is optimal, and would reduce the risk of NTD by about 85 percent.[28]

As of early 2003, thirty-nine countries, including twenty-one in the Western hemisphere, fifteen in Asia and the Middle East, and two in Africa, are fortifying or are about to fortify grain with folic acid (Wald N: personal communication). Only one European country, the Ukraine, is among those that fortify. It is disappointing that the United Kingdom, where one of the definitive studies linking folic acid sufficiency to prevention of NTDs, has not yet implemented fortification of grain. This, in spite of the following strong statement issued by a governmental advisory committee: "On scientific, medical and public health grounds, the committee concluded that universal folic acid fortification of flour at 240 μg/100 g in food products would have a significant effect in preventing NTD-affected conceptions and births without resulting in unacceptably high intakes in any group in the population."[623]

Claims have also been made about the efficacy of periconceptional multivitamin use and the prevention of other congenital defects (e.g., conotruncal and other cardiac defects, cleft lip/palate, and urinary tract).[624–628] Confirmation of such claims is needed in additional prospective studies. Because the DiGeorge/velocardiofacial syndrome occurs with typical conotruncal cardiac defects in up to 90 percent of cases, exclusion of these diagnoses by fluorescence in situ hybridization studies is necessary before claims can be credible. Reductions in the frequency of other congenital defects were not observed in our prospective study[51] or in the U.K. Medical Research Council trial.[629]

Further Evidence of a Decline in the NTD Birth Prevalence

During the past few years, two important large-scale studies have documented the changing livebirth prevalence of babies with NTDs. The CDC reported that the prevalence of

NTDs in the United States between 1996 and 2001 declined by 23 percent (24 percent for SB and 21 percent for anencephaly) among approximately 3.5 million livebirths per year during this period.[630] The prevalence decreased from 2.5 to 2.0 per 10,000 during this period. The report included all states except Maryland, New Mexico, and New York. The authors commented that these declines have occurred coincident with the introduction of folic acid fortification of flour in the United States. Another study done in northern China, in an area with a high rate of NTDs, and in southern China, in an area with a low rate of NTDs, examined changes in the birth prevalence of NTDs between 1993 and 1995 among 130,000 women who took folic acid (400 μg per day) at any time before or during pregnancy and 118,000 who had not taken folic acid.[631] The prevalence in the high risk area declined by almost 79 percent (from 4.8 to 1.0 per 1000) and in the low-risk region, the prevalence declined by 40 percent (from 1.0 to 0.6 per 1000). These studies provide strong evidence that dietary folic acid supplementation can reduce the prevalence of NTDs.

Patient and Family Considerations

In developed countries, the use of obstetrical ultrasound and maternal serum screening has made the unexpected birth of a child with anencephaly a relatively rare event. When prenatal diagnosis has not been made, almost all anencephalics are stillborn or die within hours or days of birth.[632] Occasionally, such an infant may survive many months, more especially when parents insist on extreme life-prolonging measures. Serious morbidity and mortality complicate the lives of those children surviving with SB, their outlook depending on the severity of the lesion, its location, and the nature and expertise of the treatment provided. The degrees of handicap among survivors with SB were assessed in studies published 20–25 years ago.[633–640]

There is a paucity of more recent long-term outcome studies for SB. Results of 2 major cohorts followed for 20–25 years and up to 38 years are respectively summarized in Table 21.24.[641–642a] The first study of 117 children born with open SB, first assessed at 16–20 years of age, noted that only 8 (7 percent) had little or no disability, while 25 (21 percent) had died within their first year, a total of 48 (41 percent) having died by 16 years of age. Among the 69 (59 percent) who survived to age 16 years, 60 had been shunted for hydrocephalus, 2 of whom became blind as a consequence. Mental retardation was noted in 22 (19 percent), seizures in 12 (17 percent), 52 (44 percent) with incontinence, and 35 (30 percent) being wheelchair-dependent. Lifelong continuous care was required by 33 (28 percent). At 25-year follow-up, some 48 percent had died. In a further follow-up of these patients between 32–38 years, 54 percent had died.[642b] Among 54 survivors, 46 (85 percent) had had a shunt, 39 (72 percent) had an IQ $\geq$80, and only 11 (20 percent) were fully continent.

In the second study spanning 20–25 years of 118 children born with SB, about 71 (60 percent) had survived with 19 patients lost to follow-up. The range of complications seen in the first study is, as expected, reflected in the later study, with some notable improvement in the degree of morbidity. However, the high frequency (86 percent) of shunting required for the treatment of hydrocephalus is the same in both studies. In the second study, 41 percent of the shunted study population had two to three shunt revisions. Residual fecal incontinence at 25 years (between 8 and 16 percent) and the urinary incontinence (albeit well managed by self-catheterization in most) remained troublesome problems. Being wheelchair-bound, mentally handicapped, and requiring lifelong contin-

Table 21.24. Selected complications in two original cohorts of 117 and 118 patients with SB with an extended followup (%) 641–642b

	Original Cohort (%)	Survivors 16 years (%)	Survivors Mean Age 25 years (%)	Survivors Mean Age 35 years (%) (32–38 years)	Original Cohort	Deceased[b]	Survivors 20–25 years
Number with SB	117	69 (59)	61 (52)	54	118[a]	28 (24)	71 (60)
Died by age 1 year	25 (21)						
Died by age 16 years	48 (41)						
Died by age 25 years	5 (48)						
Hydrocephalus and shunt		60 (87)	52 (85)	46 (85)		24 (86)	61 (86)
Visual defect (blind)		2[b] (6)	27 (44)	2 (3.7)			12 (17)
Mental retardation [IQ < 80]		22 (32)	18 (30)				16 (23)
Epilepsy		32 (17)	14 (23)				
Urinary incontinence		52 (75)	45 (74)				60 (85)c
Wheelchair-dependent		35 (51)	41 (67)	7 (13)			29 (41)
Lifelong continuous care		33 (48)	33 (54)	20 (37)			13 (18)
Chronic pressure sores		32 (46)	19 (31)	30 (55.6)			
Unsatisfactory urinary incontinence control		19 (28)	14 (23)				15[3]
Hypertension on treatment		—	9 (15)				
Depression on treatment		—	4 (7)				
Obesity		23 (33)	16 (26)	30 (55.6)			
Fecal incontinence		24 (30)	5 (3)				11 (16)
High school							26 (36)
College							35 (49)
Special education							26 (37)
Employed				13 (241)			33 (45)
Sclerosis							25 (49)
Tethered cord							23 (32)
Latex allergy							23 (32)
Cervical decompression/tracheostomy/and/or gastrostomy						19 (68)	11 (16)
Respiratory support				2 (3.7)			

[a] blind = 2.

[b] 19 patients lost to followup.

[c] All maintained on clean intermittent catheterization of their bladders, 90% doing their own.

uous care have remained serious issues. On the positive side, 49 percent achieved university entrance and 45 percent were employed. Thirty-two percent required surgery for a tethered cord and a remarkable 32 percent developed latex allergy, 6 of the 23 affected patients experiencing severe, life-threatening anaphylactic reactions. Latex sensitization is now recognized as a significant problem in children with SB.[643]

Many factors have an impact on survival for those born with open SB,[644] and reported survival rates vary significantly. In Glasgow, Scotland, 71 percent survived to 5 years, whereas in the Atlanta region, cumulative survival was calculated to reach 84 percent.[645,646] Although there is clear evidence of improving survival rates,[646] death rates continue to climb through early adulthood; the two most common causes of death are unrecognized shunt malfunction and renal failure. End-stage renal failure in twenty-five patients with spina bifida after hemodialysis and renal transplantation yielded 5-year survival rates around 80 percent.[646]

Life expectancy surveys based on the enormous experience (904 patients with SB) of the Seattle group suggested 50 years for those with hydrocephalus treated between 1957 and 1974.[647] Unfortunately, follow-up data are incomplete.

The moral, ethical, and medicolegal[98,648–652] aspects of care of the defective newborn have been thoroughly debated. The effects of having a child with SB on a marriage have also been repeatedly studied.[653] The 10-year longitudinal study by Tew et al.[654] demonstrated clear deterioration in the marital relationships of families who had at least one child with a major NTD, including a divorce rate twice that of the general population. Although other studies have drawn similar conclusions concerning marital disharmony, not unexpectedly, some have noted little or no negative effect of having severely affected children in these families.[655] Perhaps the least attention has been devoted to the degree of suffering and quality of life of the affected children, especially those most severely affected, who died before reaching their 10th birthday.[656,657] Minimal attention has been paid to the long-range effects of a severely myelodysplastic child on his or her siblings. Shurtleff and Lamers's[658] observation of the remarkable rate of abandonment by the parents of children with SB is both poignant and telling, and one that has implications for the affected child and the unaffected siblings.

REFERENCES

1. Connor M, Ferguson-Smith MA. Essential medical genetics, 5th ed. Oxford: Blackwell Science, 1997.
2. Wald NJ, Cuckle HS. Open neural tube defects. In: Wald NJ, ed. Antenatal and neonatal screening. Oxford: Oxford University Press, 1984:25.
3. Morris JK, Wald NJ. Quantifying the decline in the birth prevalence of neural tube defects in England and Wales. J Med Screen 1999;6:182.
4. Hay S, McLean E. The timing and content of routine obstetric ultrasound in the United Kingdom. 1994 Survey on behalf of the Royal College of Radiographers. London: RCOG, 1994.
5. Food and Drug Administration. Food standards: amendment of standards of identity for enriching grain products to require addition of folic acid. Fed Regist 1996;61:8781.
6. Food and Drug Regulations (1066) Amendments, Health Canada. www.hc-sc.gc.ca/food-aliment/ns-sc/ne-en/ng-qn/e_1066eng01.html.
7. Tulipan N, Bruner JP. Myelomeningocele repair in utero: a report of three cases. Pediatr Neurosurg 1998;28:177.
8. Adzick NS, Sutton LN, Cromblehome TM, et al. Successful fetal surgery for spina bifida. Lancet 1998;352:1675.
9. Mazzola CA, Albright AL, Sutton LN, et al. Dermoid inclusion cysts and early spinal cord tethering after fetal surgery for myelomeningocele. N Engl J Med 2002;347:256.
10. Hunter AGW. Neural tube defects in Eastern Ontario and Western Quebec: demography and family data. Am J Med Genet 1984;19:45.

11. Drainer E, May HM, Tolmie JL. Do familial neural tube defects breed true? J Med Genet 1991;28:605.
12. Kallen B, Cocchi G, Knudsen LB, et al. International study of sex ratio and twinning of neural tube defects. Teratology 1994;50:322.
13. Elwood JM, Elwood JH. Epidemiology of anencephalus and spina bifida. Oxford: Oxford University Press, 1980.
14. Verma IC. High frequency of neural-tube defects in North India. Lancet 1978;1:879.
15. Carter CO. Genetics of common malformations. In: Gairdner D, Hull D, eds. Recent advances in paediatrics. London: Churchill Livingstone, 1971:527.
16. Holmes LB, Driscoll SG, Atkins L. Etiologic heterogeneity of neural-tube defects. N Engl J Med 1976;294:365.
17. Sever LE, Sanders M, Monsen R. An epidemiologic study of neural tube defects in Los Angeles County. II. Etiologic factors in an area with low prevalence at birth. Teratology 1982;25:323.
18. Jorde LB, Fineman RM, Martin RA. Epidemiology of neural tube defects in Utah, 1940–1979. Am J Epidemiol 1984;119:487.
19. Surveillance for anencephaly and spina bifida and the importance of prenatal diagnosis. United States, 1985–1994. MMWR 44:1–13.
20. Murphy M, Seagroatt V, Hey K, et al. Neural tube defects, 1974–1994: down but not out. Arch Dis Child 1996;75:F133.
21. Cuckle HS, Wald N. The impact of screening for neural tube defects in England and Wales. Prenat Diagn 1987;7:91.
22. Rogers SC, Weatherall JAC. Anencephalus, spina bifida and congenital hydrocephalus. England and Wales 1964–1972. (Office of Population Censuses and Surveys. Studies on Medical and Population Subjects No 32). London: HMSO, 1976.
23. Office of National Statistics (1996). Congenital malformation statistics 1993 (notifications) (Series M B 3, no. 9). London: HMSO, 1996.
24. Office of National Statistics (1998). Congenital anomaly statistics 1995 and 1996 (notifications) (Series M B 3, no. 11). London: The Stationery Office, 1998.
25. Rankin J, Glinianaia S, Brown R, et al. The changing prevalence of neural tube defects: a population-based study in the north of England, 1984–96. Northern Congenital Abnormality Survey Steering Group. Paidiatr Perinat Epidemiol 2000;14:104.
26. Wald N. Neural tube defects. In: Wald N, Leck I, eds., Antenatal and neonatal screening, 2nd ed. Oxford: Oxford University Press, 2000:61.
27. Medical Research Council Vitamin Study Research Group. Prevention of neural tube defects: Results of the Medical Research Council Vitamin Study. Lancet 1991;228:131.
28. Wald NJ, Law MR, Morris JK, Wald DS. Quantifying the effect of folic acid. Lancet 2001;358:2069.
29. Carter CO. Genetics of common malformations. In: Gairdner D, Hull D, eds. Recent advances in paediatrics. London: Churchill Livingstone, 1971:527.
30. Holmes LB, Driscoll SG, Atkins L. Etiologic heterogeneity of neural-tube defects. N Engl J Med 1976;294:365.
31. Leck I. Epidemiological clues to the causation of neural tube defects. In: Dobbins J, ed. Prevention of spina bifida and other neural tube defects. New York: Academic Press, 1983:155.
32. Sever LE. An epidemiologic study of NTDs in Los Angeles County. I. Prevalence at birth based on multiple sources of case ascertainment. Teratology 1982;25:315.
33. Schacter B, Weitkamp LR, Johnson EW. Parental HLA compatibility, fetal wastage and neural tube defects: Evidence for a T/t-like locus in humans. Am J Med Genet 1984;36:1082.
34. Naderi S. Congenital abnormalities in newborns of consanguineous and nonconsanguineous parents. Obstet Gynecol 1979;53:195.
35. Crandall BF, Lebhertz TB, Schroth PC, et al. Alpha-fetoprotein concentrations in maternal serum: Relation to race and body weight. Clin Chem 1983;29:531.
36. Cohen T, Stern E, Rosenmann A. Sib risk of neural tube defect: is prenatal diagnosis indicated in pregnancies following the birth of a hydrocephalic child? J Med Genet 1979;16:14.
37. Birch JM. Anencephaly in stillborn siblings of children with germ cell tumor. Lancet 1980;1:1257.
38. Opitz JM, Gilbert EF. CNS anomalies and the midline as a "developmental field." Am J Med Genet 1982;12:443.
38a. Volcik KA, Shaw GM, Zhu H, et al. Risk factors for neural tube defects: associations between uncoupling protein 2 polymorphisms and spina bifida. Birth Defects Res Part A Clin Mol Teratol 2003;67:158.
39. Baldwin CT, Hoth CF, Amos JA, et al. An exonic mutation in the HuP2 paired domain gene causes Waardenburg's syndrome. Nature 1992;355:637.

40. Daly LE, Kirke PN, Molloy A, et al. Folate levels and neural tube defects. JAMA 1995;274:1698.

41. van der Put NMJ, Eskes TKAB, et al. Is the common 677C → T mutation in the methylenetetrahydro-folate reductase gene a risk factor for neural tube defects? A meta-analysis. Q J Med 1997;90:111.

42. Whitehead AS, Gallagher P, Mills JL, et al. A genetic defect in 5,10 methylenetetrahydrofolate reductase in neural tube defects. Q J Med 1995;88:763.

43. Steegers-Theunissen R, Boers G, Trijbels FJ, et al. Neural-tube defects and derangement of homocys-teine metabolism. N Engl J Med 1991;324:199.

44. Mills JL, McPartlin JM, Kirke PN, et al. Homocysteine metabolism in pregnancies complicated by neural tube defects. Lancet 1995;345:149.

45. Butterworth CE Jr, Bendich A. Folic acid and the prevention of birth defects. Annu Rev Nutr 1996;16:73.

46. Steegers-Theunissen RP, Boers GH, Blom HJ. Neural tube defects and elevated homocysteine levels in amniotic fluid. Am J Obstet Gynecol 1995;172:1436.

46a. Wald NJ, Hackshaw AK, Stone R, et al. Blood folic acid and vitamin B12 in relation to neural tube de-fects. Br J Obstet Gynaecol 1996;103:319.

47. Thiersch JB. Therapeutic abortions with a folic acid antagonist, 4-aminopteroylglutamic acid (4-amino P.G.A.) administered by the oral route. Am J Obstet Gynecol 1952;63:1928.

48. Rosa FW. Spina bifida in infants of women treated with carbamazepine during pregnancy. N Engl J Med 1991;324:6.

49. Cornel MC, Ten Kate LP, TeMeerman GJ. Ovulation induction, in vitro fertilisation, and neural tube de-fects. Lancet 1989;2:1530.

50. Lancaster PAL. Congenital malformations after in vitro fertilisation. Lancet 1987;2:1392.

51. Volsett SE. Ovulation induction and neural tube defects. Lancet 1990;1:178.

52. Milunsky A, Derby LE, Jick H. Ovulation induction and neural tube defects. Teratology 1990;42:467.

53. Wald NJ, Hambridge M. Maternal serum copper concentration and neural tube defects. Lancet 1977;2:560.

53a. De Santis M, Carducci B, De Santis L, et al. Periconceptional exposure to efavirenz and neural tube de-fects. Arch Intern Med 2002;162:355.

54. Durkin MV, Kaveggia EG, Pendleton E, et al. Sequential fetus-fetus interaction and CNS defects. Lancet 1976;2:43.

55. Källén B, Mazze RI. Neural tube defects and first trimester operations. Teratology 1990;41:717.

56. Smithells RW, Sheppard S, Schorah CJ, et al. Possible prevention of neural tube defects by periconcep-tional vitamin supplementation. Lancet 1980;1:339.

57. Milunsky A, Jick H, Jick SS, et al. Multivitamin/folic acid supplementation in the earliest weeks of preg-nancy reduces the prevalence of neural tube defects. JAMA 1989;262:2847.

58. Medical Research Council Vitamin Study Research Group. Prevention of neural tube defects: results of the Medical Research Council Vitamin Study. Lancet 1991;228:131.

59. Miller P, Smith DW, Shepard TH. Maternal hyperthermia as a possible cause of anencephaly. Lancet 1978;1:519.

60. Shiota K. Neural tube defects and maternal hyperthermia in early pregnancy: Epidemiology in a human embryo population. Am J Med Genet 1982;12:281.

61. Milunsky A, Ulcickas M, Rothman K. Maternal heat exposure and neural tube defects. JAMA 1992;268:882.

62. Brender JD, Suarez L. Paternal occupation and anencephaly. Am J Epidemiol 1990;131:517.

63. Blatter BM, Lafeber AB, Peters PWJ, et al. Heterogeneity of spina bifida. Teratology 1997;55:224.

64. Fedrick J. Anencephalus and the local water supply. Nature 1970;227:176.

65. Elwood JM. Anencephalus and drinking water composition. Am J Epidemiol 1978;105:460.

66. Friedman JM. Can maternal alcohol ingestion cause neural tube defects? J Pediatr 1982;101:221.

67. Edwards JH. Congenital malformations of the central nervous system in Scotland. Br J Prev Soc Med 1958;12:115.

68. McDonald AD. Maternal health and congenital defect: A prospective investigation. N Engl J Med 1985;258:767.

69. Fedrick J. Anencephalus in Scotland, 1961–1972. Br J Prev Soc Med 1976;30:132.

70. Janerich DT. Maternal age and spina bifida: Longitudinal versus cross-sectional analysis. Am J Epidemiol 1973;96:389.

71. Kucera J. Rate and type of congenital anomalies among offspring of diabetic women. J Reprod Med 1971;7:61.

72. Milunsky A, Alpert E, Kitzmiller J, et al. Prenatal diagnosis of neural tube defects. VIII. The importance of serum alpha-fetoprotein screening in diabetic women. Am J Obstet Gynecol 1982;142:1030.

73. Waller DK, Mills JL, Simpson JL, et al. Are obese women at higher risk for producing malformed offspring? Am J Obstet Gynecol 1994;170:541.

74. Shaw GM, Velie EM, Schaffer D. Risk of neural tube defect: affected pregnancies among obese women. JAMA 1996;275:1093.

75. Prentice A, Goldberg G. Maternal obesity increases congenital malformations. Nutr Rev 1996;54:146.

76. Robert E, Francannet C, Shaw G. Neural tube defects and maternal weight reduction in early pregnancy. Reprod Toxicol 1995;9:57.

77. Cavdar AO, Arcasey A, Bayce T, et al. Zinc deficiency and anencephaly in Turkey. Teratology 1980;22:141.

78. Buamah PK, Russell M, Bates G, et al. Maternal zinc status: a determination of central nervous system malformation. Br J Obstet Gynaecol 1984;91:788.

79. Milunsky A, Morris JS, Ulcickas M, et al. Maternal toenail zinc (Zn) elevations and fetal neural tube defects (NTDs). Am J Hum Genet 1990;47:A282.

80. Milunsky A, Morris JS, Jick H, et al. Maternal zinc and fetal neural tube defects. Teratology 46:1992;341.

81. Knox EG. Anencephalus and dietary intakes. Br J Prev Soc Med 1972;26:219.

82. Cuckle HS, Wald NJ. Evidence against oral contraceptives as a cause of neural tube defects. Br J Obstet Gynaecol 1982;89:547.

83. McIntosh GC, Olshan AF, Baird PA. Paternal age and the risk of birth defects in offspring. Epidemiology 1995;6:282.

84. Renwick JH. Hypothesis: Anencephaly and spina bifida are usually preventable by avoidance of a specific but unidentified substance present in certain potato tubers. Br J Obstet Gynaecol 1972;26:67.

85. Cuckle HS. Recurrence risk of neural tube defects following a miscarriage. Prenat Diagn 1983;3:287.

86. Carmi R, Gohar J, Meizner I, et al. Spontaneous abortion: high risk factor for neural tube defects in subsequent pregnancy. Am J Med Genet 1994;51:93.

87. Dallaire L, Melancon S, Potier M, et al. Date of conception and prevention of neural tube defects. Clin Genet 1984;26:304.

88. Barrett C, Hakim C. Anencephaly, ovulation stimulation, subfertility and illegitimacy. Lancet 1973;2:916.

89. Fedrick J. Anencephalus and maternal tea drinking: evidence for a possible association. Proc R Soc Med 1974;67:356.

90. Wilson JS, Vallance-Owen J. Congenital deformities and insulin antagonism. Lancet 1966;2:940.

91. Riccardi VM, Bergman CA. Anencephaly with incomplete twinning (diprosopus). Teratology 1977;16:137.

92. Windham GC, Sever LE. Neural tube defects among twin births. Am J Hum Genet 1982;34:988.

93. Robert E, Guibaud P. Maternal valproic acid and congenital neural tube defects. Lancet 1982;2:937.

94. Guibaud S, Robert E, Simplot A, et al. Prenatal diagnosis of spina bifida aperta after first-trimester valproate exposure. Prenat Diagn 1993;13:772.

95. Fineman RM, Jorde LB, Martin RA, et al. Spinal dysraphia as an autosomal dominant defect in 4 families. Am J Med Genet 1982;12:457.

96. Kirke PN, Molloy AM, Daly LE, et al. Maternal plasma folate and vitamin B_{12} are independent risk factors for neural tube defects. Q J Med 1993;86:703.

97. Olsen AS, Georgescu A, Johnson S, et al. Assembly of a 1-Mb restriction-mapped cosmid contig spanning the candidate region for Finnish congenital nephrosis: (NPHS1) in 19q13.1. Genomics 1996;34:223.

98. Milunsky A, ed. Genetic disorders and the fetus: Diagnosis, prevention, and treatment, 3rd ed. Baltimore: Johns Hopkins University Press, 1992.

99. Gelman-Kohan Z, Antonelli J, Ankori-Cohen H, et al. Further delineation of the acrocallosal syndrome. Eur J Pediatr 1991;150:797.

100. Verloes A, Gillerot Y, Walczak E, et al. Acromelic frontonasal "dysplasia": further delineation of a subtype with brain malformation and polydactyly (Toriello syndrome). Am J Med Genet 1992;42:180.

101. Cusi V, Antich J, Vela A, et al. Neural tube defect and amniotic band sequence. Genet Couns 1993;4:203.

102. Fryns JP, Legius E, Moerman P, et al. Apparently new "anophthalmia-plus" syndrome in sibs. Am J Med Genet 1995;58:113.

103. Suwanwela C, Suwanwela N. A morphological classification of sincipital encephalomeningoceles. Neurosurgery 1972;36:201.

104. Cohen MM Jr, Kreiborg S. The central nervous system in the Apert syndrome. Am J Med Genet 1990;35:36.

105. Canki-Klain N, Stanescu V, Stanescu R, et al. Lethal short limb dwarfism with dysmorphic face, omphalocele and severe ossification defect: Piepkorn syndrome or severe "boomerang dysplasia." Ann Genet (Paris) 1992;35:129.

106. Stagiannis KD, Sepulveda W, Fusi L, et al. Exencephaly in autosomal dominant brachydactyly syndrome. Prenat Diagn 1995;15:70.

107. Carpenter BF, Hunter AGW. Micromelia, polysyndactyly, multiple malformations, and fragile bones in a stillborn child. J Med Genet 1982;19:311.

108. Dominguez R, Rott J, Castillo M, et al. Caudal duplication syndrome. Am J Dis Child 1993;147:1048.

109. Towfighi J, Housman C. Spinal cord abnormalities in caudal regression syndrome. Acta Neuropathol 1991;81:458.

110. Richieri-Costa A, Guuion-Almeida ML. Mental retardation, structural anomalies of the central nervous system, anophthalmia and abnormal nares: a new MCA/MR syndrome of unknown cause. Am J Med Genet 1993;47:702.

111. Christiansen JV, Petersen HO, Sogaard H. The CHILD syndrome: congenital hemidysplasia with ichthyosiform erythroderma and limb defects: a case report. Acta Derm Venereol 1984;64:165.

112. Kazarian E, Goldstein P. Ankyloblepharon filiforme adnatum with hydrocephalus, meningomyelocele and imperforate anus. Am J Ophthalmol 1977;84:355.

113. Barr M Jr, Heidelberger KP, Comstock CH. Craniomicromelic syndrome: a newly recognized lethal condition with craniosynostosis, distinct facial anomalies, short limbs, and intrauterine growth retardation. Am J Med Genet 1995;58:348.

114. Hughes HE, Harwood-Nash DC, Becker LE. Craniotelencephalic dysplasia in sisters: further delineation of a possible syndrome. Am J Med Genet 1983;14:557.

115. Anegawa S, Hayashi T, Torigoe R, et al. Meningomyelocele associated with cranium bifidum: rare coexistence of two major malformations. Childs Nerv Syst 1993;9:278.

116. Thomas M, Halaby FA, Hirschauer JS. Hereditary occurrence of anterior sacral meningocele: report of ten cases. Spine 1987;12:351.

117. Czeizel A, Losonci A. Split hand, obstructive urinary anomalies and spina bifida or diaphragmatic defect syndrome with autosomal dominant inheritance. Hum Genet 1987;77:203.

118. Nickel RE, Pillers D-AM, Merkens M, et al. Velo-cardio-facial syndrome and DiGeorge sequence with meningomyelocele and deletions of the 22q11 region. Am J Med Genet 1994;52:445.

119. Miyamoto T, Hagari S, Mihara M, et al. Tail-like protrusion on the nape with cervical spina bifida. Arch Dermatol 1993;129:918.

120. Froster-Iskenius U, Meinecke P. Encephalocele, radial defects, cardiac, gastrointestinal, anal, and renal anomalies: a new multiple congenital anomaly (MCA) syndrome? Clin Dysmorphol 1992;1:37.

121. Donnai D. Unknown case: stillborn white male: 30 weeks (MG 2746). Proc Gr Genet Center 1988;7:64.

122. Durkin-Stamm MV, Gilbert EF, et al. An unusual dysplasia-malformation-cancer syndrome in two patients. Am J Med Genet 1978;1:279.

123. Podder S, Shepherd RC, Shillito P, et al. A cognitively normal boy with meningoencephalocele, arthrogryposis and hypoplastic thumbs. Clin Dysmorphol 1995;4:70.

124. Balog B, Skinner SR. Case report: unilateral duplication of the femur associated with myelomeningocele. J Pediatr Orthop 1984;4:488.

125. Fried K, Mundel G, Rief A, et al. A Meckel-like syndrome? Clin Genet 1974;5:46.

126. Gollop TR, Kiota MM, Martins RMM, et al. Frontofacionasal dysplasia: evidence for autosomal recessive inheritance. Am J Med Genet 1984;19:301.

127. Grubben C, Fryns JP, deZegher F, et al. Anterior basal encephalocele in the median cleft face syndrome: comments on nosology and treatment. Genet Couns 1990;38:103.

128. Rodriguez JI, Palacios J, Omenaca F, et al. Polyasplenia, caudal deficiency, and agenesis of the corpus callosum. Am J Med Genet 1991;38:99.

129. Bird LM, Newbury RO, Ruiz-Velasco R, et al. Recurrence of diaphragmatic agenesis associated with multiple midline defects: evidence for an autosomal gene regulating the midline. Am J Med Genet 1994;53:33.

130. Gillessen-Kaesbach G, Meinecke P, Garret C, et al. New autosomal recessive lethal disorder with polycystic kidneys type Potter I, characteristic face, microcephaly, brachymelia, and congenital heart defects. Am J Med Genet 1993;45:511.

131. Goldberg NS, Hebert AA, Esterly NB. Sacral hemangiomas and multiple congenital abnormalities. Arch Dermatol 1986;122:684.

132. Aleksic S, Budzilovich G, Greco MA, et al. Intracranial lipomas, hydrocephalus and other CNS anomalies in oculoauriculo-vertebral dysplasia (Goldenhar–Gorlin syndrome). Childs Brain 1984;11:285.

133. Kohn G, El Shawwa R, Grunebaum M. Aplasia of the tibia with bifurcation of the femur and ectrodactyly: evidence for an autosomal recessive type. Am J Med Genet 1989;33:172.

134. Kennerknecht I, Mattfeldt T, Paulus W, et al. XX-agonadism in a fetus with multiple dysraphic lesions: a new syndrome. Am J Med Genet 1997;70:413.

135. Young ID, Zuccollo JM, Barrow M, et al. Holoprosencephaly, telecanthus and ectrodactyly: a second case. Clin Dysmorphol 1992;1:47.

136. Hegde HR, Leung AKC. Aplasia of pectoralis major muscle and renal anomalies. Am J Med Genet 1989;32:109.

137. Nudleman K, Andermann E, Andermann F, et al. The hemi 3 syndrome: hemihypertrophy, hemihypaesthesia, hemireflexia and scoliosis. Brain 1984;107:533.

138. Sharma AK, Phadke S, Chandra K, et al. Overlap between Majewski and hydrolethalus syndromes: a report of two cases. Am J Med Genet 1992;43:949.

139. Pantke OA, Gorlin RJ, Burke BA. Polysplenia syndrome with skeletal and central nervous system anomalies. BDOAS 1975;11:252.

140. Nishimaki S, Yoda H, Seki K, et al. A case of Dandy–Walker malformation associated with occipital meningocele, microphthalmia, and cleft palate. Pediatr Radiol 1990;20:608.

141. Keutel J, Kindermann I, Mockel H. Eine wahrscheinlich autosomal rezessiv vererbte skeletmissbildung mit humeroradialsynostose. Humangenetik 1970;9:43.

142. Cochrane DD, Haslam RHA, Myles ST. Cervical neuroschisis and meningocoele manque in type I (no neck) Klippel–Feil syndrome. Pediatr Neurosurg 1991;16:174.

143. Sertie AL, Quimby M, Moreira ES, et al. A gene which causes severe ocular alterations and occipital encephalocele (Knobloch syndrome) is mapped to 21q22.3. Hum Mol Genet 1996;5:843.

144. Kousseff BG. Sacral meningocele with conotruncal heart defects: a possible autosomal recessive trait. Pediatrics 1984;74:395.

145. Gripp KW, Scott CI, Hughes HE, et al. Lateral meningocele syndrome: three new patients and review of the literature. Am J Med Genet 1997;70:229.

146. Lehman RAW, Stears JC, Wesenberg RL, et al. Familial osteosclerosis with abnormalities of the nervous system and meninges. J Pediatr 1977;90:49.

147. Hing AV, Torack R, Dowton SB. A lethal syndrome resembling branchio-oculo-facial syndrome. Clin Genet 1992;41:74.

148. Raas-Rothschild A, Goodman RM, Meyer S, et al. Pathological features and prenatal diagnosis in the newly-recognised limb/pelvis-hypoplasia/aplasia syndrome. J Med Genet 1988;25:687.

149. Seeds JW, Jones FD. Lipomyelomeningocele: prenatal diagnosis and management. Obstet Gynecol 1986;67:34S.

150. Machin GA, Popkin JS, Zachs D, et al. Fetus with asymmetric parietal encephalocele, and hydrops secondary to laryngeal atresia. Am J Med Genet 1987;3 (suppl):311.

151. Mathias RS, Lacro RV, Jones KL. X-linked laterality sequence: situs inversus, complex cardiac defects, splenic defects. Am J Med Genet 1987;28:111.

152. Sugiura Y, Suzuki Y, Kobayashi M. The Meckel syndrome: report of two Japanese sibs and a review of literature. Am J Med Genet 1996;67:312.

153. Medeira A, Dennis N, Donnai D. Anencephaly with spinal dysraphism, cleft lip and palate and limb reduction defects. Clin Dysmorphol 1994;3:270.

154. Schwartz RA, Cohen-Addad N, Lambert MW, et al. Congenital melanocytosis with myelomeningocele and hydrocephalus. Cutis 1986;37:37.

155. Isada NB, Qureshi F, Jacques SM, et al. Meroanencephaly: Pathology and prenatal diagnosis. Fetal Diagn Ther 1993;8:423.

156. Caprioli J, Lesser RL. Basal encephalocele and morning glory syndrome. Br J Ophthalmol 1983;67:349.

157. Elejalde BR. Genetic and diagnostic considerations in three families with abnormalities of facial expression and congenital urinary obstruction: "the Ochoa syndrome." Am J Med Genet 1979;3:97.

158. Ferguson JW, Hutchison HT, Rouse BM. Ocular, cerebral and cutaneous malformations: confirmation of an association. Clin Genet 1984;25:464.

159. Lewis SME, Roberts EA, Marcon MA, et al. Joubert syndrome with congenital hepatic fibrosis: an entity in the spectrum of oculo-encephalo-hepato-renal disorders. Am J Med Genet 1994;52:419.

160. Cohen AR. The mermaid malformation: cloacal exstrophy and occult spinal dysraphism. Neurosurgery 1991;28:834.

161. Reardon W, Harbord MG, Hall-Craggs MA, et al. Central nervous system malformations in Mohr's syndrome. J Med Genet 1989;26:659.

162. Finnigan DP, Clarren SK, Haas JE. Extending the Pallister–Hall syndrome to include other central nervous system malformations. Am J Med Genet 1991;40:395.

163. Patel R-RA, Bixler D. Renal agenesis with meningomyelocele and absence of Mullerian structures. Am J Med Genet 1988;29:441.

164. Powell CM, Chandra RS, Saal HM. PHAVER syndrome: an autosomal recessive syndrome of limb ptery-

gia, congenital heart anomalies, vertebral defects, ear anomalies, and radial defects. Am J Med Genet 1993;47:807.

165. Llewellyn DH, Smyth SJ, Elder GH, et al. Homozygous acute intermittent porphyria: compound heterozygosity for adjacent base transitions in the same codon of the porphobilinogen deaminase gene. Hum Genet 1992;89:97.

166. Walpole IR, Goldblatt J, Hockey A, et al. Dandy–Walker malformation (variant), cystic dysplastic kidneys, and hepatic fibrosis: a distinct entity or Meckel syndrome? Am J Med Genet 1991;39:294.

167. Van Den Berg DJ, Francke U. Roberts syndrome: a review of 100 cases and a new rating system for severity. Am J Med Genet 1993;47:1104.

168. Rogers RC. Unknown case: SN (GGC-8217) 23 month old white male. Proc Gr Genet Center 1988;7:55.

169. Aleck KA, Grix A, Clericuzio C, et al. Dyssegmental dysplasias: clinical, radiographic, and morphologic evidence of heterogeneity. Am J Med Genet 1987;27:295.

170. Fellous M, Boue J, Malbrunot C, et al. A five-generation family with sacral agenesis and spina bifida: possible similarities with the mouse T-locus. Am J Med Genet 1982;12:465.

171. Cohn J, Bay-Nielsen E. Hereditary defect of the sacrum and coccyx with anterior sacral meningocele. Acta Paediatr Scand 1969;58:268.

172. Martínez-Frías ML. Spina bifida and hypospadias: a non random association or an X-linked recessive condition? Am J Med Genet 1994;52:5.

173. Martínez-Frías ML, Bermejo E, Urioste M, et al. Short rib-polydactyly syndrome (SRPS) with anencephaly and other central nervous system anomalies: a new type of SRPS or a more severe expression of a known SRPS entity? Am J Med Genet 1993;47:782.

174. Rodríguez JI, Palacios J, Razquin S. Sirenomelia and anencephaly. Am J Med Genet 1991;39:25.

175. Spear SL, Mickle JP. Simultaneous cutis aplasia congenita of the scalp and cranial stenosis. Plast Reconstr Surg 1983;71:413.

176. Tandon RK, Burke JP, Strachan IM. Clefting syndrome with typical and atypical irido-retinochoroidal colobomatous defects. J Pediatr Ophthalmol Strabismus 1994;31:120.

177. Smith MT, Huntington HW. Inverse cerebellum and occipital encephalocele: a dorsal fusion defect uniting the Arnold–Chiari and Dandy–Walker spectrum. Neurology 1977;27:246.

178. Wolf YG, Merlob P, Horev G, et al. Thoraco-abdominal enteric duplication with meningocele, skeletal anomalies and dextrocardia. Eur J Pediatr 1990;149:786.

179. Hedberg VA, Lipton JM. Thrombocytopenia with absent radii: a review of 100 cases. Am J Pediatr Hematol Oncol 1988;10:51.

180. Driscoll DA, Spinner NB, Budarf ML, et al. Deletions and microdeletions of 22q11.2 in velo-cardio-facial syndrome. Am J Med Genet 1992;44:261.

181. Chatkupt S, Chatkupt S, Johnson WG. Waardenburg syndrome and myelomeningocele in a family. J Med Genet 1993;30:83.

182. Chemke J, Carmi R, Galil A, et al. Weissenbacher-Zweymuller syndrome: a distinct autosomal recessive skeletal dysplasia. Am J Med Genet 1992;43:989.

183. Baraitser M, Burn J. Neural tube defects as an X-linked condition. Am J Med Genet 1984;17:383.

184. Rodriguez JI, Rodriguez-Peralto JL, Muro M, et al. Anencephaly and limb deficiencies. Am J Med Genet 1992;44:66.

185. Taylor AI. Autosomal trisomy syndromes: a detailed study of 27 cases of Edward's syndrome and 27 cases of Patau's syndrome. J Med Genet 1968;5:227.

186. Drugan A, Dvorin E, Johnson MP, et al. The inadequacy of the current correction for maternal weight in maternal serum alpha-fetoprotein interpretation. Obstet Gynecol 1989;74:698.

187. Flannery DB, Kahler SG. Neural tube defects in trisomy 18. Prenat Diagn 1986;6:97.

188. Simpson JL, Dische R, Morillo-Cucci G, et al. Triploidy (69,XXY) in a liveborn infant. Ann Genet (Paris) 1972;15:103.

189. Harmon JP, Hiett AK, Palmer CG, et al. Prenatal ultrasound detection of isolated neural tube defects: Is cytogenetic evaluation warranted? Obstet Gynecol 1995;86:595.

190. Haslam RHA, Broske SP, Moore CM, et al. Trisomy 9 mosaicism with multiple congenital anomalies. J Med Genet 1973;10:180.

191. Tolkendorf E, Hinkel E, Gabriel A, et al. A new case of deletion 1q42 syndrome. Clin Genet 1989;35:289.

192. Singer N, Gersen S. The value of chromosome analysis in cases of neural tube defects: a case of anencephaly associated with fetal dup(2)(p24-pter). Prenat Diagn 1987;7:567.

192a. Doray B, Favre R, Gasser B, et al. Recurrent neural tube defects associated with partial trisomy 2p22-pter: report of two siblings and review of the literature. Genet Couns 2003;14:165.

193. Winsor SHM, McGrath MJ, Khalifa M, et al. A report of recurrent anencephaly with trisomy 2p23-2pter:

additional evidence for the involvement of 2p24 in neural tube development and evaluation of the role for cytogenetic analysis. Prenat Diagn 1997;17:665.

193a. Kennedy D, Silver MM, Winsor EJ, et al. Inverted duplication of the distal short arm of chromosome 3 associated with lobar holoprosencephaly and lumbosacral meningomyelocele. Am J Med Genet 2000;91:167.

194. Jokiaho I, Salo I, Niem KM, et al. Deletion 3q27—3qter in an infant with mild dysmorphism, parietal meningocele, and neonatal miliaria rubra-like lesions. Hum Genet 1989;83:302.

195. Bader PI, Heney SM, Munsick RA, et al. Brief clinical report: neural tube defects in dup(11q). Am J Med Genet 1984;19:5.

196. Tranebjaerg L, Nielsen KB, Tommerup N, et al. Interstitional deletion 13q: further delineation of the syndrome by clinical and high-resolution chromosome analysis of five patients. Am J Med Genet 1988;29:739.

196a. Luo J, Balkin N, Stewart JF, et al. Neural tube defects and the 13q deletion syndrome: evidence for a critical region in 13q33-34. Am J Med Genet 2000;91:227.

197. Lacro RV, Jone KL, Mascarello JT, et al. Duplication of distal 15q: Report of five new cases from two different translocation kindreds. Am J Med Genet 1987;26:719.

198. Plaja A, Vendrell T, Sarret E, et al. Terminal deletion of Xp in a dysmorphic anencephalic fetus. Prenat Diagn 1994;14:410.

199. Schmid W, Muhlethaler JP, Briner J, et al. Ring chromosome 13 in a polymalformed anencephalic. Humangenetik 1975;27:63.

200. Sever LE. An epidemiologic study of NTDs in Los Angeles County. I. Prevalence at birth based on multiple sources of case ascertainment. Teratology 1982;25:315.

201. Borman GG, Smith AH, Howard JK. Risk factors in the prevalence of anencephalus and spina bifida in New Zealand. Teratology 1986;33:221.

202. Byrne J, Cama A, Reilly M, et al. Multigeneration maternal transmission in Italian families with neural tube defects. Am J Med Genet 1996;66:303.

203. Elwood JM, Little J, Elwood JH. Epidemiology and control of neural tube defects. Oxford: Oxford University Press, 1992.

204. McManus S. Neural tube defects: Identification of "high-risk" women. Ir Med J 1987;80:166.

205. Khoury MF, Erickson JD, James LM. Etiologic heterogeneity of neural tube defects. II. Clues from family studies. Am J Hum Genet 1982;34:980.

206. Martin RA, Fineman RM, Jorde LB. Phenotypic heterogeneity in neural tube defects: a clue to causal heterogeneity. Am J Med Genet 1983;16:519.

207. Cotariu D, Zaidman JL. Developmental toxicity of valproic acid. Life Sci 1991;48: 1341.

208. Jones KL. Smith's recognizable patterns of human malformation, 5th ed. Philadelphia: WB Saunders, 1997:566.

209. Werler MM, Louik C, Shapiro S, et al. Ovulation induction and risk of neural tube defects. Lancet 1994;344:445.

210. Hendricks KA, Nuno OM, Suarez L, et al. Effects of hyperinsulinemia and obesity on risk of neural tube defects among Mexican Americans. Epidemiology 2001;12:630.

211. Hibbard ED, Smithells RW. Folic acid metabolism and human embryopathy. Lancet 1965;1:1254.

212. Smithells RW, Neven NC, Seller MJ, et al. Further experience of vitamin supplementation for prevention of NTD recurrences. Lancet 1983;1:1027.

213. Laurence KM, James N, Miller MH, et al. Double-blind randomised controlled trial of folated treatment before conception to prevent recurrence of neural-tube defects. BMJ 1981;282:1509.

214. Mulinare J, Cordero JF, Erickson JD, et al. Periconceptional use of multivitamins and the occurrence of neural tube defects. JAMA 1988;260:3141.

215. Wald NJ, Hackshaw AK, Stone R, et al. Blood folic acid and vitamin B_{12} in relation to neural tube defects. Br J Obstet Gynaecol 1996;103:319.

216. Kluijtmans LAJ, van den Heuvel LPW, Boers GHJ, et al. Molecular genetic analysis in mild hyperhomocysteinemia: a common mutation in the methylenetetrahydrofolate reductase gene is genetic risk factor for cardiovascular disease. Am J Hum Genet 1996;58:35.

217. van der Put NMJ, van den Heuvel LP, Streegers-Theunissen RPM, et al. Decreased methylenetetrahydrofolate reductase activity due to the $677C \rightarrow T$ mutation in families with spina bifida offspring. J Mol Med 1996;74:691.

218. Mornet E, Muller F, Lenvoisé-Furet A, et al. Screening of the C677T mutation on the methylenetetrahydrofolate reductase gene in French patients with neural tube defects. Hum Genet 1997;100:512.

219. Adams MJ Jr, Khoury MJ, Scanlon KS, et al. Elevated midtrimester serum methylmalonic acid levels as a risk factor for neural tube defects. Teratology 1995;51:311.

220. Lindenbaum J, Savage DG, Stabler SP, et al. Diagnosis of cobalamin deficiency. II. Relative sensitivities of serum cobalamin, methylmalonic acid, and total homocysteine concentrations. Am J Hematol 1990;34:99.

221. Stabler SP, Brass EP, Marcell PD, et al. Inhibition of rat cobalamin-dependent enzyme activity by cobalamin analogues. J Clin Invest 1991;74:1422.

222. Woodard JC. Study of one-carbon metabolism in neonatal vitamin B_{12}-deficient rats. J Nutr 1969;98:139.

223. Tran P, Hiou-Tim F, Frosst P, et al. The curly-tail (ct) mouse, an animal model of neural tube defects, displays altered homocysteine metabolism without folate responsiveness or a defect in MTHFR. Mol Genet Metab 2002;76:297.

224. Seller MJ. Vitamins, folic acid and the cause and prevention of neural tube defects. Ciba Found Symp 1994;181:161.

225. Greene NDE, Copp AJ. Inositol prevents folate-resistant neural tube defects in the mouse. Nat Med 1997;3:60.

226. Goulding M, Paquette A. Pax genes and neural tube defects in the mouse. In Bock G, Marsh J, eds. Neural tube defects. Ciba Foundation Symposium 181. Chichester: John Wiley, 1994:103.

227. Copp AJ, Brook FA, Roberts HJ. A cell-type-specific abnormality of cell proliferation in mutant (curly tail) mouse embryos developing spinal neural tube defects. Development 1988;104:285.

228. Fleming A, Copp AJ. Embryonic folate metabolism and mouse neural tube defects. Science 1998;280:2107.

229. Zhao Q, Begringer RR, de Crombrugghe B. Prenatal folic acid treatment suppresses acrania and meroanencephaly in mice mutant for the Cart1 homeobox gene. Nat Genet 1996;13:275.

230. Zhang J, Hagopian-Donaldson S, Serbedzija G, et al. Neural tube, skeletal and body wall defects in mice lacking transcription factor AP-2. Nature 1996;381:238.

231. Wu M, Chen DF, Sasoaka T, et al. Neural tube defects and abnormal brain development in F52-deficient mice. Proc Natl Acad Sci USA 1996;93:2110.

232. Seller MJ. Neural tube defects and sex ratios. Am J Med Genet 1987;26:699.

233. Van Allen MI, Kalousek DK, Chernoff GF, et al. Evidence for multisite closure of the neural tube in humans. Am J Med Genet 1993;47:723.

234. Golden JA, Chernoff GF. Multiple sites of anterior neural tube closure in humans: evidence from anterior neural tube defects (anencephaly). Pediatrics 1995;95:506.

235. Stegmann K, Boecker J, Richter B, et al. A screen for mutations in human homologs of mice exencephaly genes Tcfap2a and Msx2 in patients with neural tube defects. Teratology 2001;13:169.

236. Antony AC. Folate receptors. Annu Rev Nutr 1996;16:501.

237. Rosenquist TH, Finnell RH. Genes, folate and homocysteine in embryonic development. Proc Nutr Soc 2001;60:53.

238. Heil SG, van der Put NM, Trijbels FJ, et al. Molecular genetic analysis of human folate receptors in neural tube defects. Eur J Hum Genet 1999;7:393–396.

239. O'Leary VB, Mills JL, Kirke PN, et al. Analysis of the human folate receptor beta gene for an association with neural tube defects. Mol Genet Metab 2003;79:129.

240. Hook EB, Czeizel AE. Can terathanasia explain the protective effect of folic-acid supplementation on birth defects? Lancet 1997;350:513.

241. Hall JG. Terathanasia, folic acid and birth defects. Lancet 1997;350:1322.

242. Smith DW, Clarren SK, Harvey MAS. Hyperthermia as a possible teratogenic agent. J Pediatr 1978;92:878.

243. Layde PM, Edmonds LD, Erickson JD. Maternal fever and neural tube defects. Teratology 1980;21:105.

244. Fisher NL, Smith DW. Occipital encephalocele and early gestational hyperthermia. Pediatrics 1981; 68:480.

245. Editorial. Hyperthermia and the neural tube. Lancet 1978;2:560.

246. Editorial. Is hyperthermia a teratogen? BMJ 1978;2:1586.

247. Dlugosz L, Vena J, Byers T, et al. Congenital defects and electric bed heating in New York State: a register-based case-control study. Am J Epidemiol 1992;135:1000.

248. Lynberg MC, Khoury MJ, Lu X, et al. Maternal flu, fever, and the risk of neural tube defects: a population-based case-control study. Am J Epidemiol 1994;140:244.

249. Chamber CD, Johnson KA, Dick LM, et al. Maternal fever and birth outcome: a prospective study. Teratology 1998;58:251.

250. Bergmann KE, Makosch E, Tews KH. Abnormalities of hair zinc concentration in mothers of newborn infants with spina bifida. Am J Clin Nutr 1980;33:2145.

251. Bax CMR, Bloxam DL. Two major pathways of zinc(II) acquisition by human placental syncytiotrophoblast. J Cell Physiol 1995;164:546.

252. James SJ, Pogribna M, Pobribny IP, et al. Abnormal folate metabolism and mutation in the methyl-enetetrahydrofolate reductase gene may be maternal risk factors for Down syndrome. Am J Clin Nutr 1999;70:495.

253. Al-Gazali LI, Padmanabhan R, Melnyk S, et al. Abnormal folate metabolism and genetic polymorphism of the folate pathway in a child with Down syndrome and neural tube defect. Am J Med Genet 2001;103:128.

254. O'Leary VB, Parle-McDermott A, Molloy AM, et al. MTRR and MTHFR polymorphism: link to Down syndrome? Am J Med Genet 2002;107:151.

255. Barkai G, Arbuzova S, Berkenstadt M, et al. Frequency of Down's syndrome and neural-tube defects in the same family. Lancet 2003;361:1331.

256. Bergstrand CG, Czar B. Demonstration of a new protein fraction in serum from the human fetus. Scand J Clin Lab Invest 1956;8:174.

257. Alpert E, Drysdale JW, Isselbacher KJ, et al. Human AFP: isolation, characterization and demonstration of microheterogeneity. J Biol Chem 1972;247:3792.

258. Seppälä M. Immunologic detection of alpha-fetoprotein as a marker of fetal pathology. Clin Obstet Gynecol 1977;20:737.

259. Morinaga T, Sakai M, Wegmann T, et al. Primary structures of human alpha-fetoprotein and its mRNA. Proc Natl Acad Sci USA 1983;80:4604.

260. Gibbs PE, Zielinski R, Boyd C, et al. Structure, polymorphism, and novel repeated DNA elements revealed by a complete sequence of the human alpha-fetoprotein gene. Biochemistry 1987;26;1332.

261. Gitlin D, Perricelli A, Gitlin GM. Synthesis of alpha-fetoprotein by liver, yolk sac, and gastrointestinal tract of the human conceptus. Cancer Res 1972;32:979.

262. Gitlin D, Boesman M. Serum alpha-fetoprotein, albumin, and gamma-G-globulin in the human conceptus. J Clin Invest 1966;45:1826.

263. Habib ZA. Maternal serum alpha-fetoprotein: its value in antenatal diagnosis of genetic disease and in obstetrical-gynaecological care. Acta Obstet Gynecol Scand 1977;61 (suppl):1.

264. Gitlin D. Normal biology of alpha-fetoprotein. In: Hirai H, Alpert E, eds. Carcinofetal proteins: biology and chemistry. New York: New York Academy of Sciences, 1975:7.

265. Seppälä M, Rouslahti E. Alpha-fetoprotein in amniotic fluid: an index of gestational age. Am J Obstet Gynecol 1972;114:595.

266. Brock DJH, Scrimgeour JB, Nelson MM. Amniotic fluid alpha-fetoprotein measurements in the early prenatal diagnosis of central nervous system disorders. Clin Genet 1975;7:163.

267. Jorgensen FS, Sundberg K, Loft AGR, et al. Alpha-fetoprotein and acetylcholinesterase activity in first- and early second-trimester amniotic fluid. Prenat Diagn 1995;15:621.

268. Second Report of the U.K. Collaborative Study on Alpha-Fetoprotein in Relation to Neural Tube Defects. Amniotic fluid alpha-fetoprotein measurement in antenatal diagnosis of anencephaly and open spina bifida in early pregnancy. Lancet 1979;2:652.

269. Seppälä M, Rouslahti E. Alpha-fetoprotein. In: Keller PJ, ed. Contributions to gynecology and obstetrics. Basel: Karger, 1976:143.

270. Hay DM, Forrester PI, Hancock RL, et al. Maternal serum alpha-fetoprotein in normal pregnancy. Br J Obstet Gynaecol 1976;83:534.

271. Brock DJH. Feto-specific proteins in prenatal diagnosis. Mol Aspects Med 1980;3:433.

272. Los FJ, DeBruijn HWA, van Beek Calkoen-Carpay T, et al. AFP transport across the fetal membranes in the human. Prenat Diagn 1984;5:277.

273. Wu JT, Book L, Sudar K. Serum alpha-fetoprotein (AFP) levels in normal infants. Pediatr Res 1981;15:50.

274. Nishi S, Hirai H. Radioimmunoassay of alpha-fetoprotein in hematoma, other liver diseases and pregnancy. GANN Monogr Cancer Res 1973;14:79.

275. Mizejewski GJ, Vonnegut M, Jacobson HI. Studies of the intrinsic antiuterotropic activity of murine alpha-fetoprotein. J Int Soc Oncodev Biol Med 1986;7:19.

276. Alpert E. Human alpha-fetoprotein (AFP): Developmental biology and clinical significance. In: Popper H, Schaffner F, eds. Progress in liver diseases. New York: Grune & Stratton, 1976.

277. Murgita RA, Tomasi TB. Suppression of the immune response by AFP. J Exp Med 1975;141:269.

278. Dattwyler RJ, Murgita R, Tomasi TB. Binding of alpha-fetoprotein to murine T cells. Nature 1975;256:656.

279. Greenberg F, Faucett A, Rose E, et al. Congenital deficiency of α-fetoprotein. Am J Obstet Gynecol 1992;167:509.

280. Sher C, Shohat M. Congenital deficiency of AFP and Down syndrome screening. Prenat Diagn 1997;17:884.

281. Muller F, Dreux S, Sault C, Galland A, et al. Very low alpha-fetoprotein in Down syndrome maternal serum screening. Prenat Diagn 2003;23:584–587.

282. Milunsky A. The prenatal diagnosis of hereditary disorders. Springfield, Ill.: Charles C Thomas, 1973.

283. Milunsky A. Genetic disorders and the fetus: diagnosis, prevention and treatment. New York: Plenum Press, 1979.

284. Milunsky A. Genetic disorders and the fetus: Diagnosis, prevention and treatment, 2nd ed. New York: Plenum Press, 1986.

285. Hino M, Koki Y, Nishi S. Alpha-fetoprotein in pregnant women. Igakuno Ayumi 1972:512.

286. Ferguson-Smith MA. The reduction of neural tube defects by maternal serum alpha-fetoprotein screening. Br Med Bull 1983;39:365.

287. Schnittger A, Kjessler B. Alpha-fetoprotein screening in obstetric practice. Acta Obstet Gynecol Scand 1984;119 (suppl):1.

288. Furhmann W, Weitzel HK. Maternal serum alpha-fetoprotein screening for neural tube defects: report of a combined study in Germany and short overview on screening in populations with low birth prevalence of NTD. Hum Genet 1985;69:47.

289. Wald NJ, Cuckle H, Brock, DJH, et al. Maternal serum alpha-fetoprotein measurement in antenatal screening for anencephaly and spina bifida in early pregnancy: report of the UK Collaborative Study on Alpha-Fetoprotein in Relation to Neural-Tube Defects. Lancet 1977;1:1323.

290. Knight GJ. Maternal serum α-fetoprotein screening. In: Hommes FA, ed. Techniques in diagnostic human biochemical genetics: a laboratory manual. New York: Wiley-Liss, 1991:491.

291. Fourth Report of the U.K. Collaborative Study on Alpha-Fetoprotein in Relation to Neural Tube Defects. Estimating an individual's risk of having a fetus with open spina bifida and the value of repeat alpha-fetoprotein testing. J Epidemiol Commun Health 1982;36:87.

292. Canick JA, Knight GJ, Palomaki GE, et al. Second trimester levels of maternal serum unconjugated estriol and human chorionic gonadotropin in pregnancies affected by anencephaly and open spina bifida. Prenat Diagn 1990;10:733.

293. Lambert-Messerlian GM, Palomaki GE, Canick, JA. Second trimester levels of maternal serum inhibin A in pregnancies affected by fetal neural tube defects. Prenat Diagn 2000;20:680.

294. Yaron Y, Hamby DD, O'Brien JE, et al. Combination of elevated maternal serum alpha-fetoprotein (MSAFP) and low estriol is highly predictive of anencephaly. Am J Med Genet 1998;75:297.

295. Wininger SJ, Donnenfeld AE. Syndromes identified in fetuses with prenatally diagnosed cephaloceles. Prenat Diagn 1994;14:839.

296. Knight GK, Palomaki GE. Maternal serum alpha-fetoprotein and the detection of open neural tube defects. In: Elias S, Simpson JL, eds., Maternal serum screening. New York: Churchill Livingstone, 1992: 41–58.

297. Milunsky A, Jick SS, Bruell CL, et al. Predictive values, relative risks, and overall benefits of high and low maternal serum α-fetoprotein screening in singleton pregnancies: new epidemiologic data. Am J Obstet Gynecol 1989;161:291.

298. Crandall B, Robinson L, Grau P. Risks associated with an elevated maternal serum α-fetoprotein level. Am J Obstet Gynecol 1991;165:581.

299. Larson JM, Pretorius DH, Budorick NE, et al. Value of maternal serum α-fetoprotein levels of 5.0 MoM or greater and prenatal sonography in predicting fetal outcome. Radiology 1993;189:77.

300. Reichler A, Hume Jr RF, Drugan A, et al. Risk of anomalies as a function of level of elevated maternal serum α-fetoprotein. Am J Obstet Gynecol 1994;171:1052.

301. Drugan A, Zador IE, Evans MI, et al. A normal ultrasound does not obviate the need for amniocentesis in patients with elevated serum alpha-fetoprotein. Obstet Gynecol 1988;72:627.

302. Richards DS, Seeds JW, Cefalo RC, et al. Elevated maternal serum alpha-fetoprotein with normal ultrasound: is amniocentesis always appropriate? A review of 26,089 screened patients. Obstet Gynecol 1988;71:203.

303. Candenas M, Villa R, Collar RF, et al. Maternal serum alpha-fetoprotein screening for neural tube defects. Acta Obstet Gynecol Scand 1995;74:266.

304. Verloes A, Schoos R, Koulischer L. Non-radioactive assay of AFP, hCG, and uE3 from dried blood specimens: a low-cost alternative for maternal screening for trisomy 21. Prenat Diagn 1992;12:1073.

305. Wald NJ, Hackshaw AK, George LM. Assay precision of serum α-fetoprotein in antenatal screening for neural tube defects and Down's syndrome. J Med Screen 2000;7:74.

306. Ellis AR. Antenatal screening for Down's syndrome: Can we do better? Ann Clin Biochem 1993;30:421.

307. American College of Obstetricians and Gynecologists, Committee on Obstetric Practice. Committee Opinion. Washington, DC: American College of Obstetricians and Gynecologists, 1994:141.

308. American College of Obstetricians and Gynecologists. Educational Bulletin 228. Washington, DC: American College of Obstetricians and Gynecologists, 1996.

309. Canadian Task Force on the Periodic Health Examination. Periodic health examination, 1994 update. 3. Primary and secondary prevention of neural tube defects. Can Med Assoc J 1994;151:159.

310. Geirsson RT. Ultrasound instead of last menstrual period as the basis of gestational age assignment. Ultrasound Obstet Gynecol 1991;1:212.

311. Wald NJ, Cuckle HS, Densem JW, et al. Maternal serum screening for Down's syndrome: the effect of routine ultrasound scan determination of gestational age and adjustment for maternal weight. Br J Obstet Gynaecol 1992;99:144.

312. Benn PA, Borgida A, Horne D, et al. Down syndrome and neural tube defect screening: the value of using gestational age by ultrasonography. Am J Obstet Gynecol 1997;176:1056.

313. Rahim RR, Cuckle HS, Sehmi IK, et al. Compromise ultrasound dating policy in maternal serum screening for Down syndrome. Prenat Diagn 2002;22:1181.

314. Wald N, Cuckle H, Boreham J, et al. Small biparietal diameter of fetuses with spina bifida: implications for antenatal screening. Br J Obstet Gynaecol 1980;87:219.

315. Wald NJ, Cuckle HS, Boreham J, et al. The effect of maternal weight on maternal serum alpha-fetoprotein levels. Br J Obstet Gynaecol 1981;88:1094.

316. Johnson AM, Palomaki GE, Haddow JE. Maternal serum alpha-fetoprotein levels in pregnancies among black and white women with fetal open spina bifida: a United States collaborative study. Am J Obstet Gynecol 1990;162:328.

317. Adams MF, Windham GC, Greenberg F, et al. Clinical interpretation of maternal serum alpha-fetoprotein concentrations. Am J Obstet Gynecol 1984;148:241.

318. Watt HC, Wald NJ. Alternative methods of maternal weight adjustment in maternal serum screening for Down syndrome and neural tube defects. Prenat Diagn 1998;18:842.

319. Neveux LM, Palomaki GE, Larrivee DA, et al. Refinements in managing maternal weight adjustment for interpreting prenatal screening results. Prenat Diagn 1996;16:1115.

320. Watkins ML, Scanlon KS, Mulinare J, et al. Is maternal obesity a risk factor for anencephaly and spina bifida? Epidemiology 1996;7:507.

321. Kallen K. Maternal smoking, body mass index, and neural tube defects. Am J Epidemiol 1998;147:1103.

322. Watkins ML, Rasmussen SA, Honein MA, et al. Maternal obesity and risk for birth defects. Pediatrics 2003;111:1152.

323. Johnson AM. Racial differences in maternal serum screening. In: Mizejewski JG, Porter IH, eds. Alpha-fetoprotein and congenital disorders. New York: Academic Press, 1985:183.

324. Benn PA, Clive JM, Collins R. Medians for second-trimester maternal serum α-fetoprotein, human chorionic gonadotropin, and unconjugated estriol: differences between races or ethnic groups. Clin Chem 1997;43:333.

325. Greenberg F, James LM, Oakley GP. Estimates of birth prevalence rates of spina bifida in the United States from computer-generated maps. Am J Obstet Gynecol 1983;145:570.

326. O'Brien JE, Drugan A, Chervenak FA, et al. Maternal serum alpha-fetoprotein screening: the need to use race specific medians in Asians. Fetal Diagn Ther 1993;8:367.

327. Wald NJ, Cuckle HS, Borcham J, et al. Maternal serum alpha-fetoprotein and diabetes mellitus. Br J Obstet Gynaecol 1979;86:101.

328. Greene MF, Haddow JE, Palomaki GE, et al. Maternal serum alpha-fetoprotein levels in diabetic pregnancies. Lancet 1988;8606:345.

329. Braunstein GD, Mills JL, Reed GF, et al. Comparison of serum placental protein hormone levels in diabetic and normal pregnancy. J Clin Endocrinol Metab 1989;68:3.

330. Baumgarten A, Reece EA, Davis N, et al. A reassessment of maternal serum alpha-fetoprotein in diabetic pregnancy. Eur J Obstet Reprod Biol 1988;28:289.

331. Baumgarten A, Robinson J. Prospective study of inverse relationship between maternal glycosylated hemoglobin and serum alpha-fetoprotein concentrations in pregnant women with diabetes. Am J Obstet Gynecol 1988;159:77.

332. Martin AO, Dempsey LM, Minogue J, et al. Maternal serum alpha-fetoprotein levels in pregnancies complicated by diabetes: implication for screening programs. Am J Obstet Gynecol 1990;163:1209.

333. Sancken U, Bartels I. Biochemical screening for chromosomal disorders and neural tube defects (NTD): is adjustment of maternal alpha-fetoprotein (AFP) still appropriate in insulin-dependent diabetes mellitus (IDDM)? Prenat Diagn 2001;21:383.

334. Wald NJ, Cuckle HS. Recent advances in screening for neural tube defects and Down's syndrome. Ballieres Clin Obstet Gynaecol 1987;1:649.

335. Pedersen JF, Molsted-Pedersen L. Early growth retardation in diabetic pregnancy. BMJ 1979;1:18.

336. Bennet PH, Webner C, Miller M. Congenital anomalies and the diabetic pregnancy. In: Pregnancy metabolism, diabetes and the fetus. Ciba Foundation Symposium 63. Amsterdam: Excerpta Medica, 1979.

337. Greene MF, Benacerraf BR. Prenatal diagnosis in diabetic gravidas: utility of ultrasound and maternal serum alpha-fetoprotein screening. Obstet Gynecol 1991;77:5.

338. Ghosh A, Woo JSK, Rawlinson HA, et al. Prognostic significance of raised serum alpha-fetoprotein levels in twin pregnancies. Br J Obstet Gynaecol 1982;89:817.

339. Wald NJ, Cuckle H, Stirrat G. Maternal serum alpha-fetoprotein levels in triplet and quadruplet pregnancy. Br J Obstet Gynaecol 1978;85:124.

340. Wald NJ, Cuckle HS, Peck S, et al. Maternal serum alpha-fetoprotein in relation to zygosity. BMJ 1979;1:445.

341. Brock DJH, Barron L, Watt M, et al. The relation between maternal plasma alpha-fetoprotein and birth weight in twin pregnancies. Br J Obstet Gynaecol 1979;86:710.

342. Redford DHA, Whitfield CR. Maternal serum alpha-fetoprotein in twin pregnancies uncomplicated by neural tube defect. Am J Obstet Gynecol 1985;152:550.

343. Cuckle HS, Wald N, Stevenson JD, et al. Maternal serum alpha-fetoprotein screening for open neural tube defects in twin pregnancies. Prenat Diagn 1990;10:71.

344. Sowers SG, Reish RL, Burton BK. Fetal sex-related differences in maternal serum alpha-fetoprotein during the second trimester of pregnancy. Am J Obstet Gynecol 1983;146:786.

345. Szabo M, Veress L, Munnich A, et al. Maternal age-dependent and sex-related changes in gestational serum alpha-fetoprotein. Fetal Diagn Ther 1995;10:368.

346. Petrikovsky B. Maternal serum alpha fetoprotein concentration and fetal sex. Prenat Diagn 1989;9:449.

347. Wald NJ, Cuckle HS. Raised maternal serum alpha-fetoprotein levels in subsequent pregnancies. Lancet 1981;1:1103.

348. Haddow JE, Palomaki G, Kloza EM, et al. Does smoking influence serum alpha-fetoprotein levels in midtrimester pregnancies? Br J Obstet Gynaecol 1984;91:1188.

349. Canick JA, Barbieri RL. The effect of smoking on hormone levels in vivo and steroid hormone biosynthesis in vitro. In: Wald N, Baron J, eds. Smoking and hormone-related disorders. Oxford: Oxford University Press, 1990:208.

350. Evans MI, Bottoms SF, Carlucci T, et al. Determinants of altered anxiety after abnormal maternal serum alpha-fetoprotein screening. Am J Obstet Gynecol 1988;159:15.

351. Los FJ, Beekhuis JR, Marrink J, et al. Origin of raised maternal serum alpha-fetoprotein levels in second-trimester oligohydramnios. Prenat Diagn 1992;12:39.

352. Dyer SN, Burton BK, Nelson LH. Elevated maternal serum α-fetoprotein levels and oligohydramnios: poor prognosis for pregnancy outcome. Am J Obstet Gynecol 1987;157:336.

353. Richards DS, Seeds JW, Katz VL, et al. Elevated maternal serum alpha-fetoprotein with oligohydramnios: ultrasound evaluation and outcome. Obstet Gynecol 1988;72:337.

354. Kelly RB, Nyberg DA, Mack LA, et al. Sonography of placental abnormalities and oligohydramnios in women with elevated alpha-fetoprotein levels: comparison with control subjects. AJR Am J Roentgenol 1989;153:815.

355. Katz VL, Chescheir NC, Cefalo RC. Unexplained elevations of maternal serum alpha-fetoprotein. Obstet Gynecol Surv 1990;45:719.

356. Tromans PM, Coulson R, Lobb MO, et al. Abdominal pregnancy associated with extremely elevated serum alpha-fetoprotein: case report. Br J Obstet Gynaecol 1984;91:296.

357. Bombard AT, Nakagawa S, Runowicz CD, et al. Early detection of abdominal pregnancy by maternal serum AFP+ screening. Prenat Diagn 1994;14:1155.

358. Barret RJ, Harper MA, Marshall RB. Tuboovarian pregnancy associated with elevated maternal serum alpha-fetoprotein: a case report. J Reprod Med 1990;35:277.

359. Seppälä M, Ruoslahti E. Alpha-fetoprotein in maternal serum: a new marker for detection of fetal distress and intrauterine death. Am J Obstet Gynecol 1973;115:48.

360. Milunsky A. The prevention of genetic disease and mental retardation. Philadelphia: WB Saunders, 1975.

361. Seppälä M, Ruoslahti E. Alpha-fetoprotein in Rh-immunized pregnancies. Obstet Gynecol 1973;42:701.

362. Garoff L, Seppälä M. Prediction of fetal outcome in threatened abortion by maternal serum placental lactogen and alpha-fetoprotein. Am J Obstet Gynecol 1975;121:257.

363. Salafia CM, Silberman L, Herrera NE, et al. Placental pathology at term associated with elevated midtrimester maternal serum alpha-fetoprotein concentration. Am J Obstet Gynecol 1988;158:1064.

364. Milunsky A, Alpert E, Yeransian J, et al. Normal serum alpha-fetoprotein levels during mid-pregnancy. N Engl J Med 1981;304:974.

365. Ollendorff DA, Goldberg JM, Abu-Jawdeh GM, et al. Markedly elevated maternal serum alpha-fetoprotein associated with a normal fetus and choriocarcinoma of the placenta. Obstet Gynecol 1990;76:494.

366. Blakemore KJ, Baumgarten A, Schoenfeld-DiMaio M, et al. Rise in maternal serum alpha-fetoprotein

concentration after chorionic villus sampling and the possibility of isoimmunization. Am J Obstet Gynecol 1986;155:988.

367. Fuhrmann W, Altland K, Kohler A, et al. Feto-maternal transfusion after chorionic villus sampling: Evaluation by maternal serum alpha-fetoprotein measurement. Hum Genet 1988;78:83.

368. Weiner C, Grant S, Hudson J, et al. Effect of diagnostic and therapeutic cordocentesis on maternal serum alpha-fetoprotein concentration. Am J Obstet Gynecol 1989;161:706.

369. Katz VL, Cefalo RC, McCune BK, et al. Elevated second trimester maternal serum alpha-fetoprotein and cytomegalovirus infection. Obstet Gynecol 1986;68:580.

370. Lele A, Carmody P, Hurd M, et al. Fetomaternal bleeding following diagnostic amniocentesis. Obstet Gynecol 1982;60:64.

371. Morssink LP, Heringa MP, Beekhuis JR, et al. The HELLP syndrome: its association with unexplained elevation of MSAFP and MShCG in the second trimester. Prenat Diagn 1977;17:601.

372. Smith D, Picker RH, Saunders D, et al. Hydatidiform mole with co-existent viable fetus detected by routine AFP screening. BMJ 1980;280:1213.

373. Toftager-Larsen K, Lund Petersen P, Norgaard-Pedersen B. Maternal serum alpha-fetoprotein in the diagnosis of hydatidiform mole. Dan Med Bull 1981;28:123.

374. Milunsky A, Alpert E. Results and benefits of a maternal serum alpha-fetoprotein screening program. JAMA 1984;252:1438.

375. Brock DJH, Barron L, Jelen P, et al. Maternal serum alpha-fetoprotein measurements as an early indicator of low birth weight. Lancet 1977;2:5.

376. Carrington D, Whittle MJ, Gibson AAM, et al. Maternal serum alpha-fetoprotein: a marker for fetal aplastic crisis during intrauterine human parvovirus infection. Lancet 1987;1:433.

377. Koontz W, Seeds J, Adams N, et al. Elevated maternal serum alpha-fetoprotein, second trimester oligohydramnios, and pregnancy outcome. Obstet Gynecol 1983;62:301.

378. Zelop C, Nadel A, Frigoletto FD, et al. Placenta accreta/percreta/increta: a cause of elevated maternal serum alpha-fetoprotein. Obstet Gynecol 1991;80:693.

379. Schnittger A, Liedgren S, Radberg C, et al. Raised maternal serum and amniotic fluid alpha-fetoprotein levels associated with a placental haemangioma. Br J Obstet Gynaecol 1980;87:824.

380. Nelson LH, Bensen J, Burton BK. Outcomes in patients with unusually high maternal serum alpha-fetoprotein levels. Am J Obstet Gynecol 1987;157:572.

381. Thomas RL, Blakemore KJ. Evaluation of elevations in maternal serum alpha-fetoprotein: a review. Obstet Gynecol Surv 1990;45:269.

382. Albright SG, Katz VL. Alpha-fetoprotein findings in a case of cystic adenomatoid malformation of the lung. Clin Genet 1989;35:75.

383. Boyd PA, Keeling JW. Raised maternal serum alpha-fetoprotein in the absence of fetal abnormality: placental findings: a quantitative morphometric study. Prenat Diagn 1986;6:369.

384. Katz VL, Bowes WA Jr, Sierkh AE. Maternal floor infarction of the placenta associated with elevated second trimester serum alpha-fetoprotein. Am J Perinatol 1987;4:225.

385. Fleischer AC, Kurtz AB, Wapner RJ, et al. Elevated alpha-fetoprotein and a normal fetal sonogram: association with placental abnormalities. Am J Roentgenol 1988;150:881.

386. Jauniaux E, Gibb D, Moscoso G, et al. Ultrasonographic diagnosis of a large placental intervillous thrombosis associated with elevated maternal serum alpha-fetoprotein level. Am J Obstet Gynecol 1990;163:1558.

387. Lachman E, Hingley SM, Bates G, et al. Detection and measurement of fetomaternal haemorrhage: serum alpha-fetoprotein and the Kleihauer technique. Br Med J 1977;1:1377.

388. Walters N, Lao T, Smith V. Alpha-fetoprotein elevation and proteinuric pre-eclampsia. Br J Obstet Gynaecol 1985;92:341.

389. Khalil FK, Bonnet M, Guibaud S, et al. Alpha-fetoprotein levels in placenta, maternal, and cord blood in normal and pathologic pregnancy. Obstet Gynecol 1979;54:117.

390. Ochshorn Y, Kupferminc MJ, Eldor A, et al. Second-trimester maternal serum alpha-fetoprotein (MSAFP) is elevated in women with adverse pregnancy outcome associated with inherited thrombophilias. Prenat Diagn 2001;21:658.

391. O'Brien WF, Knuppel RA, Kousseff B, et al. Elevated maternal serum alpha-fetoprotein in triploidy. Obstet Gynecol 1988;71:994.

392. Pircon RA, Towers CV, Porto M, et al. Maternal serum alpha-fetoprotein and fetal triploidy. Prenat Diagn 1989;9:701.

393. Freeman SB, Priest JH, MacMahon WC, et al. Prenatal ascertainment of triploidy by maternal serum alpha-fetoprotein screening. Prenat Diagn 1989;9:339.

394. Jauniaux E, Moscoso G, Chitty L, et al. An angiomyxoma involving the whole length of the umbilical cord. J Ultrasound Med 1988;9:419.

395. Heinonen S, Ryynanen M, Kirkinen P, et al. Uterine malformation: a cause of elevated maternal serum alpha-fetoprotein concentrations. Prenat Diagn 1996;16:635.

396. Haddow JE, Knight GJ, Kloza EM, et al. Alpha-fetoprotein, vaginal bleeding and pregnancy risk. Br J Obstet Gynaecol 1986;93:589.

397. Brazerol WF, Grover S, Donnenfeld AE. Unexplained elevated maternal serum α-fetoprotein levels and perinatal outcome in an urban clinic population. Am J Obstet Gynecol 1994;171.

398. Achiron R, Seidman DS, Horowitz A, et al. Hyperechogenic fetal bowel and elevated serum alpha-fetoprotein: a poor fetal prognosis. Obstet Gynecol 1996;88:368.

399. Simpson JL, Elias S, Morgan CD, et al. Does unexplained second-trimester (15 to 20 weeks' gestation) maternal serum alpha-fetoprotein elevation presage adverse perinatal outcome? Am J Obstet Gynecol 1991;3:8.

400. Tatarinov YS. Content of embryo-specific alpha-globulin in the blood serum of human fetus, newborn and adult man in primary care of the liver. Vopr Med Khim 1965;11:20.

401. Waller DK, Lustig LS, Cunningham GC, et al. Second-trimester maternal serum alpha-fetoprotein levels and the risk of subsequent fetal death. N Engl J Med 1991;325:6.

402. Wald NJ, Cuckle HS, Boreham J. Maternal serum AFP levels and birth weight. Br J Obstet Gynaecol 1980;87:860.

403. Stirrat GM, Gouch JD, Bullock S, et al. Raised maternal serum AFP, oligohydramnios and poor fetal outcome. Br J Obstet Gynaecol 1981;88:231.

404. Smidt-Jensen S, Philip J, Zachary JM, et al. Implications of maternal serum alpha-fetoprotein elevation caused by transabdominal and transcervical CVS. Prenat Diagn 1994;14:35.

405. van Selm M, Kanhai HHH, van Loon AJ. Detection of fetomaternal haemorrhage associated with cordocentesis using serum α-fetoprotein and the Kleihauer technique. Prenat Diagn 1995;15:313.

406. Killam WP, Miller RC, Seeds JW. Extremely high maternal serum alpha-fetoprotein levels at second-trimester screening. Obstet Gynecol 1991;78:257.

407. Hamilton MPR, Abdalla HI, Whitfield CR. Significance of raised maternal serum alpha-fetoprotein in singleton pregnancies with normally formed fetuses. Obstet Gynecol 1985;54:465.

408. Cruikshank SH, Granados JL. Increased amniotic acetylcholinesterase activity with a fetus papyraceous and aplasia cutis congenita. Obstet Gynecol 1988;71:1997.

409. Mizejewski GJ, Polansky S, Mondragon-Tiu FA, et al. Combined use of alpha-fetoprotein and ultrasound in the prenatal diagnosis of arteriovenous fistula in the brain. Obstet Gynecol 1987;70:452.

410. Heinonen S, Ryynanen M, Kirkinen P, et al. Prenatal screening for congenital nephrosis in East Finland: results and impact on the birth prevalence of the disease. Prenat Diagn 1996;16:207.

411. Petit P, Bossens M, Thomas D, et al. Type III congenital cystic adenomatoid malformation of the lung: another cause of elevated alpha fetoprotein? Clin Genet 1987;32:172.

412. Yacoub T, Campbell CA, Gordon YB, et al. Maternal serum alpha-fetoprotein in epidermolysis bullosa simplex. BMJ 1979;1:307.

413. Bick DP, Balkite EA, Baumgarten A, et al. The association of congenital skin disorders with acetylcholinesterase in amniotic fluid. Prenat Diagn 1987;7:543.

414. Chodirker BN, Chudley AE, MacDonald KM, et al. MSAFP levels and oesophageal atresia. Prenat Diagn 1994;14:1086.

415. Ben-Neriah Z, Yagel S, Zelikoviz B, et al. Increased maternal serum alpha-fetoprotein in congenital hypothyroidism. Lancet 1991;337:437.

416. Chisholm CA, Vavalidis F, Lovell MA, et al. Prenatal diagnosis of multiple acyl-CoA dehydrogenase deficiency: association with elevated alpha-fetoprotein and cystic renal changes. Prenat Diagn 2001;21:856.

417. Brock DJH, Bolton AE, Monaghan JM. Prenatal diagnosis of anencephaly through maternal serum alpha-fetoprotein measurement. Lancet 1973;2:293.

418. Townsend RR, Goldstein MD, Filly RA, et al. Sonographic identification of autosomal recessive polycystic kidney disease associated with increased maternal serum/amniotic fluid alpha-fetoprotein. Obstet Gynecol 1988;71:1008.

419. Schell DL, Drugan A, Brindley BA, et al. Combined ultrasonography and amniocentesis for pregnant women with elevated serum alpha-fetoprotein: revising the risk estimate. J Reprod Med 1990;35:543.

420. Scott RJ, Goodburn SF. Potter's syndrome in the second trimester: prenatal screening and pathological findings in 60 cases of oligohydramnios sequence. Prenat Diagn 1995;15:519.

421. Gruber A, Rabinerson D, Kaplan B, et al. Prenatal diagnosis of Roberts syndrome. Prenat Diagn 1994;14:511.

422. Fejgin M, Zeitune M, Amiel A, et al. Elevated maternal serum alpha-fetoprotein level and sex chromosome aneuploidy. Prenat Diagn 1990;10:413.

423. Hughes-Benzie RM, Tolmie JL, McNay M, et al. Simpson–Golabi–Behmel syndrome: disproportionate fetal overgrowth and elevated maternal serum alpha-fetoprotein. Prenat Diagn 1994;14:313.

424. Schneider M, Klein-Vogler U, Tomiuk J, et al. Pitfall: Amniocentesis fails to detect mosaic trisomy 8 in a male newborn. Prenat Diagn 1994;14:651.

425. Miller R, Stephan MJ, Hume RJ, et al. Extreme elevation of maternal serum alpha-fetoprotein associated with mosaic trisomy 8 in a liveborn. Fetal Diagn Ther 2001;16:120.

426. Morrow RJ, Whittle MJ, McNay MB, et al. Prenatal diagnosis and management of anterior abdominal wall defects in the West of Scotland. Prenat Diagn 1993;13:111.

427. Waldman TA, McIntire KR. Serum alpha-fetoprotein levels in patients with ataxia telangiectasia. Lancet 1972;2:1112.

428. Norgaard-Pedersen B, Axelsen NH. Alpha-fetoprotein-like activity in sera from patients with malignant and nonmalignant disease and healthy individuals. Clin Chim Acta 1976;71:343.

429. Agarwal SS, Mehta SK, Bajpai PC. Alpha-fetoprotein in Indian childhood cirrhosis. Lancet 1974;2:175.

430. Andres JM, Lilly FR, Altman RP, et al. Alpha$_1$-fetoprotein in neonatal hepatobiliary disease. J Pediatr 1977;91:217.

431. Ainbender E, Brown E, Kierney C, et al. Clinical applications of alpha-fetoprotein determinations. In: Crandall BF, Brazier MAB, eds. Prevention of neural tube defects: the role of alpha-fetoprotein. New York: Academic Press, 1978:169.

432. Belanger L, Belanger M, Prive L, et al. Tyrosinemie hereditaire et alpha-l-foetoproteimie. Pathol Biol 1973;21:449.

433. Oi S, Tamaki N, Kondo T, et al. Massive congenital intracranial teratoma diagnosed in utero. Childs Nerv Syst 1990;6:459.

434. Smart PJ, Schwarz C, Kelsey A. Ultrasonographic and biochemical abnormalities associated with the prenatal diagnosis of epignathus. Prenat Diagn 1990;10:327.

435. Pavanello L, Rizzoni G, Andreetta B, et al. α-Fetoprotein in Wiedemann–Beckwith syndrome. J Pediatr 1986;109:392.

436. McIntire KR, Waldmann TA, Go VLW, et al. Simultaneous radioimmunoassay for carcinoembryonic antigen and alpha-fetoprotein in neoplasms of the gastrointestinal tract. Ann Clin Lab Sci 1974;4:104.

437. Talerman A, Haije WG. Alpha-fetoprotein and germ cell tumors: a possible role of yolk sac tumor production of alpha-fetoprotein. Cancer 1974;34:1722.

438. Mann WJ, Chumas J, Rosenwaks Z, et al. Elevated serum alpha-fetoprotein associated with Sertoli–Leydig cell tumors of the ovary. Obstet Gynecol 1986;67:141.

439. Heyward WL, Bender TR, Kilkenny S, et al. Early detection of primary hepatocellular carcinoma by screening for alpha-fetoprotein in high-risk families. Lancet 1983;2:1161.

440. Ferguson-Smith MA, Yates JRW, Kelly D, et al. Hereditary persistence of alpha-fetoprotein: a new autosomal dominance trait identified in antenatal screening programme for spina bifida. Cytogenet Cell Genet 1985;40:628.

441. Greenberg F, Rose E, Alpert E. Hereditary persistence of alpha-fetoprotein. Gastroenterology 1990; 98:1083.

442. Ruoslahti E, Seppälä M, Rasanen JA, et al. Alpha-fetoprotein and hepatitis B antigen in acute hepatitis and primary cancer of the liver. Scand J Gastroenterol 1973;8:197.

443. Koziell A, Grech V, Hussain S, et al. Genotype/phenotype correlations of NPHS1 and NPHS2 mutations in nephritic syndrome advocate a functional inter-relationship in glomerular filtration. Hum Mol 2002;11:379.

444. Bolk S, Puffenberger EG, Hudson J, et al. Elevated frequency and allelic heterozygosity of congenital nephritic syndrome, Finnish type, in the old order Mennonites. Am J Hum Genet 1999;65:1785.

445. Kestila A, Jarvela I. Prenatal diagnosis of congenital nephrotic syndrome (CNF, NPHS1). Prenat Diagn 2003;23:323.

446. Mahan JD, Mauer SM, Sibley RK, et al. Congenital nephrotic syndrome: evolution of medical management and results of renal transplantation. J Pediatr 1984;105:549.

447. Holmberg C, Jalanko H, Koskimies O, et al. Renal transplantation in small children with congenital nephrotic syndrome of the Finnish type. Transplant Proc 1991;23:1378.

448. Ryyanen M, Seppälä M, Kuusela P, et al. Antenatal screening for congenital nephrosis in Finland by maternal serum alpha-fetoprotein. Br J Obstet Gynaecol 1983;90:437.

449. Patrakka J, Martin P, Salonen R, et al. Proteinuria and prenatal diagnosis of congenital nephrosis in fetal carriers of nephrin gene mutations. Lancet 2002;359:1575.

450. Schneller M, Braga SE, Moser H, et al. Congenital nephrotic syndrome: clinico-pathological heterogeneity and prenatal diagnosis. Clin Nephrol 1983;19:243.

451. Suren A, Grone JH, Kallerhoff M, et al. Prenatal diagnosis of congenital nephrosis of the Finish type (CNF) in the second trimester. Int J Gynaecol Obstet 1993;41:165.

452. Morris J, Ellwood D, Kennedy D, et al. Amniotic alpha-fetoprotein in the prenatal diagnosis of congenital nephrotic syndrome of the Finnish type. Prenat Diagn 1995;15:482.

453. Santalaya J, Farolan M, Czapar G, et al. Clinical and pathological findings in two siblings with congenital nephrotic syndrome. Fetal Diagn Ther 1994;9:170.

454. Moore B, Pretorius D, Scioscia A, et al. Sonographic findings in a fetus with congenital nephrotic syndrome of the Finnish type. J Ultrasound Med 1992;11:113.

455. Kirkinen P, Heinonen S, Vanamo K, et al. Maternal serum alpha-fetoprotein and epithelial tumour marker concentrations are not increased by fetal sacrococcygeal teratoma. Prenat Diagn 1997;17:47.

456. Petrikovsky BM, Nardi DA, Rodis JF, et al. Elevated maternal serum alpha-fetoprotein and mild fetal uropathy. Obstet Gynecol 1991;78:262.

457. McVey JH, Michaelides K, Hansen LP, et al. A G → A substitution in an HNF I binding site in the human alpha-fetoprotein gene is associated with hereditary persistence of alpha-fetoprotein (HPAFO). Hum Mol Genet 1993;2:379.

458. Silver RM, Draper ML, Byrne JB, et al. Unexplained elevations of maternal serum alpha-fetoprotein in women with antiphospholipid antibodies: a harbinger of fetal death. Obstet Gynecol 1994;83:150.

459. Preston FE, Rosendaal FR, Walker ID, et al. Increased fetal loss in women with heritable thrombophilia. Lancet 1996;348:913.

460. Loft AGR. Determination of amniotic fluid acetylcholinesterase activity in the antenatal diagnosis of foetal malformations: the first ten years. J Clin Chem Clin Biochem 1990;28:893.

461. Wald N, Cuckle H, Nanchahal K. Amniotic fluid acetylcholinesterase measurement in the prenatal diagnosis of open neural tube defects: second report of the Collaborative Acetylcholinesterase Study. Prenat Diagn 1989;9:813.

462. Nyberg DA, Mahony BS, Pretorius DH. Diagnostic ultrasound of fetal anomalies: text and atlas. Chicago: Year Book, 1990.

463. Wald NJ, Cuckle HS, Haddow JE, et al. Sensitivity of ultrasound in detecting spina bifida. N Engl J Med 1991;324:769.

464. Nadel AS, Green JK, Holmes LB, et al. Absence of need for amniocentesis in patients with elevated levels of maternal serum alpha-fetoprotein and normal ultrasonographic examinations. N Engl J Med 1990;323:557.

465. Hersey DW. Sensitivity of ultrasound in detecting spina bifida. N Engl J Med 1991;324:771.

466. Lindfors KK, Gorczyca DP, Hanson FW, et al. The roles of ultrasonography and amniocentesis in evaluation of elevated maternal serum alpha-fetoprotein. Am J Obstet Gynecol 1991;164:1571.

467. Barth WH Jr, Frigoletto FD Jr, Krauss CM, et al. Ultrasound detection of fetal aneuploidy in patients with elevated maternal serum alpha-fetoprotein. Obstet Gynecol 1991;77:897.

468. Megerian G, Godmilow L, Donnenfeld AE. Ultrasound-adjusted risk and spectrum of fetal chromosomal abnormality in women with elevated maternal serum alpha-fetoprotein. Obstet Gynecol 1955;85:952.

469. Cuckle HS, Wald NJ, Nanchahal K, et al. Repeat maternal serum alpha-fetoprotein testing in antenatal screening programmes for Down's syndrome. Br J Obstet Gynaecol 1989;96:52.

470. American College of Obstetricians and Gynecologists. Ultrasonography in pregnancy. Technical bulletin no. 187. Washington, DC: American College of Obstetricians and Gynecologists, 1993.

471. National Institute of Child Health and Development. Consensus Development Report. Washington, DC: Government Printing Office, 1980.

472. Wald N, Kennard A, Donnenfeld A, et al. Ultrasound scanning for congenital abnormalities. In: Wald N, Leck I, eds., Antenatal and neonatal screening, 2nd ed. Oxford: Oxford University Press, 2000:441.

473. Assessing the quality of systems for alpha-fetoprotein (AFP) assays used in prenatal screening and diagnosis of neural tube defects; approved guidelines. NCCLS document I/LA17-A. Wayne, PA: NCCLS. 1997.

474. Shalev E, Zalel Y, Dan U, et al. Maternal serum α-fetoprotein in the first trimester cannot predict neural tube defects. Prenat Diagn 1992;12:309.

475. Aitken DA, McCaw G, Crossley JA, et al. First-trimester biochemical screening for fetal chromosome abnormalities and neural tube defects. Prenat Diagn 1993;13:681.

476. Wald NJ, Hackshaw A, Stone R, et al. Serum alpha-fetoprotein and neural tube defects in the first trimester of pregnancy. Prenat Diagn 1993;13:1047.

477. Wald NJ, Watt HC, Haddow JE, et al. Screening for Down syndrome at 14 weeks of pregnancy. Prenat Diagn 1998;18:291.

478. Brock DJH, Sutcliffe RG. Alpha-fetoprotein in the antenatal diagnosis of anencephaly and spina bifida. Lancet 1972;2:197.

479. Milunsky A. Prenatal detection of neural tube defects. VI. Experience with 20,000 pregnancies. JAMA 1980;244:2731.

480. Crandall BF, Matsumoto M. Routine amniotic fluid alpha-fetoprotein measurement in 34,000 pregnancies. Am J Obstet Gynecol 1984;149:744.

481. Milunsky A, Alpert E. The value of alpha-fetoprotein in the prenatal diagnosis of neural tube defects. J Pediatr 1974;84:889.

482. Blatter BM, Lafeber AB, Peters PWJ, et al. Prenatal diagnosis of neural tube defects. I. Problems and pitfalls: analysis of 2,495 cases using the alpha-fetoprotein assay. Obstet Gynecol 1976;48:1.

483. Brock DJH. The use of amniotic fluid AFP action limits in diagnosing open neural tube defects. Prenat Diagn 1981;1:11.

484. Crandall BF, Hanson FW, Tenannt F, et al. Alpha-fetoprotein levels in amniotic fluid between 11 and 15 weeks. Am J Obstet Gynecol 1989;160:1204.

485. Brumfield CG, Cloud GA, Davis RO, et al. The relationship between maternal serum and amniotic fluid alpha-fetoprotein in women undergoing early amniocentesis. Am J Obstet Gynecol 1990;163:903.

486. Burton BK, Nelson LH, Pettenati JM. False-positive acetylcholinesterase with early amniocentesis. Obstet Gynecol 1989;74:607.

487. Muller F, Oury JF, Boue A. First-trimester amniotic fluid acetylcholinesterase electrophoresis. Prenat Diagn 1989;9:173.

488. Canadian Early and Mid-Trimester Amniocentesis Trial (CEMAT) Group. Randomized trial to assess the safety and fetal outcome of early and midtrimester amniocentesis. Lancet 1998;351:242.

489. Aitken DA, Morrison NM, Ferguson-Smith MA. Predictive value of amniotic acetylcholinesterase analysis in the diagnosis of fetal abnormalities in 3700 pregnancies. Prenat Diagn 1984;4:329.

490. Loft AGR, Larsen SO, Norgaard-Pedersen B. A comparison of amniotic fluid alpha-fetoprotein and acetylcholinesterase in the prenatal diagnosis of open neural tube defects and anterior abdominal wall defects. Prenat Diagn 1993;13:93.

491. Guibaud S, Simplot A, Guibaud L. "Faint-positive" or "false-positive" amniotic fluid acetylcholinesterase: a diagnostic dilemma. Prenat Diagn 1995;15:388.

492. Crandall BF, Chua C. Detecting neural tube defects by amniocentesis between 11 and 15 weeks' gestation. Prenat Diagn 1993;15:339.

493. Sepulveda W, Donaldson A, Johnson RD, et al. Are routine alpha-fetoprotein and acetylcholinesterase determinations still necessary at second-trimester amniocentesis? Impact of high-resolution ultrasonography. Obstet Gynecol 1995;85:107.

494. Milunsky A, Alpert E. Prenatal diagnosis of neural tube defects. II. Problems and pitfalls: analysis of false positive and false negative alpha-fetoprotein results. Obstet Gynecol 1976;48:6.

495. Wyvill PC, Hullin DA, Elder GH, et al. A prospective study of amniotic fluid cholinesterase: comparison of quantitative methods for the detection of open neural tube defects. Prenat Diagn 1984;4:319.

496. Cole KJ, Seller MJ. A gel electrophoresis of maternal and fetal serum cholinesterase from normal pregnancies and those affected by neural tube defects. Clin Chim Acta 1982;119:1.

497. Barlow RD, Cuckle HS, Wald NJ. False positive gel-acetylcholinesterase results in blood-stained amniotic fluids. Br J Obstet Gynaecol 1982;94:821.

498. Spencer K. Between-pregnancy biological variability of maternal serum alpha-fetoprotein and free beta hCG: implications for Down syndrome screening in subsequent pregnancies. Prenat Diagn 1997;17:31.

499. Zeitune M, Aitken DA, Graham GW, et al. Amniotic fluid alpha-fetoprotein, gamma-glutamyltranspeptidase, and autosomal trisomies. Prenat Diagn 1989;9:559.

500. Cuckle HS, Wald NJ, Densem JW, et al. Second trimester amniotic fluid oestriol, dehydroepiandrosterone sulphate, and human chorionic gonadotrophin levels in Down's syndrome. Br J Obstet Gynaecol 1991;98:1160.

501. Crandall BF, Matsumoto M. Ultrasound and biochemical tests for the prenatal detection of NTDs and other abnormalities. In: Sarti D, ed. Diagnostic ultrasound: text and cases. Chicago: Year Book, 1987:901.

502. Myrianthopoulos NC. Congenital malformations in twins: epidemiologic survey. Birth Defects Orig Artic Ser 1975;11:1.

503. Knox EG. Twins and neural tube defects. Br J Prev Soc Med 1974;28:73.

504. Stiller RJ, Lockwood CJ, Belanger K, et al. Amniotic fluid alpha-fetoprotein concentrations in twin gestations: dependence on placental membrane anatomy. Am J Obstet Gynecol 1988;158:1088.

505. Schnatterly P, Hogge WA. Alpha fetoprotein and acetylcholinesterase levels in twins discordant for neural tube defects: dependence on type of fetal membranes. Am J Med Genet 1989;32:146.

506. Holbrook RH Jr, Krovoza AM, Schelley S, et al. Biamnial elevated alpha-fetoprotein and positive acetyl-cholinesterase in twins, one with anencephaly. Prenat Diagn 1987;7:653.

507. Selbing A, Larsson L. Acetylcholinesterase activity in amniotic fluid of normal and anencephalic fetus in diamniotic twin pregnancy. Acta Obstet Gynecol Scand 1986;65:93.

508. Johnson VP, Vidgoff J, Wilson N, et al. Alpha-fetoprotein and acetylcholinesterase in twins discordant for neural tube defect. Prenat Diagn 1989;9:831.

509. Crandall BF, Matsumoto M. Risks associated with an elevated amniotic fluid α-fetoprotein level. Am J Med Genet 1991;39:64.

510. Nevin NC, Armstrong MJ. Raised alpha-fetoprotein levels in amniotic fluid and maternal serum in a triplet pregnancy in which one fetus had an omphalocele. Br J Obstet Gynaecol 1975;82:826.

511. De Bruijn HW, Huisjes HJ. Omphalocele and raised alphafetoprotein in amniotic fluid. Lancet 1975;1:525.

512. Leschot NJ, Treffers PE. Elevated amniotic fluid alpha-fetoprotein without neural-tube defects. Lancet 1975;2:1141.

513. Brock DJH, Hayward C. Gel electrophoresis of amniotic fluid acetylcholinesterase as an aid to the pre-natal diagnosis of fetal defects. Clin Chim Acta 1980;108:135.

514. Gosden C, Brock DJH. Prenatal diagnosis of exstrophy of the cloaca. Am J Med Genet 1981;8:95.

515. Sorokin Y, Johnson MP, Drugan A, et al. Amniotic fluid alpha-fetoprotein levels in the differential diag-nosis of cystic hygroma. Fetal Ther 1989;4:178.

516. Seppälä M, Aula P, Rapola J, et al. Congenital nephrotic syndrome: prenatal diagnosis and genetic coun-seling by estimation of amniotic fluid and maternal serum alpha-fetoprotein. Lancet 1976;2:123.

517. Pescia G, Cruz JM, Weihs D. Prenatal diagnosis of prune-belly syndrome by means of raised maternal AFP levels. J Genet Hum 1982;30:271.

518. Seppälä M. The use of alpha fetoprotein in prenatal diagnosis. Int J Gynaecol Obstet 1976;14:308.

519. Robbin M, Filly RA, Fell S, et al. Elevated levels of amniotic fluid α-fetoprotein: sonographic evalua-tion. Radiology 1993;188:165.

520. Seppälä M. Fetal pathophysiology of human alpha-fetoprotein. Ann N Y Acad Sci 1975;259:59.

521. Streit JA, Penick GD, Williamson RA, et al. Prolonged elevation of alpha-fetoprotein and detectable acetylcholinesterase after death of an anomalous twin fetus. Prenat Diagn 1989;9:1.

522. Cruikshank SH, Granados JL. Increased amniotic acetylcholinesterase activity with a fetus papyraceous and aplasia cutis congenita. Obstet Gynecol 1988;71:997.

523. Winsor EJT, Brown BSJ, Luther ER, et al. Deceased cotwin as a cause of false positive amniotic fluid AFP and AChE. Prenat Diagn 1987;7:485.

524. Crandall BF, Kasha W, Matsumoto M. Prenatal diagnosis of neural tube defects: experience with acetyl-cholinesterase gel electrophoresis. Am J Med Genet 1982;12:361.

525. Holzgreve W, Rempen A, Beller FK. Fetal lymphangiectasia: another cause for a positive amniotic fluid acetylcholinesterase test. Arch Gynaecol 1986;239:123.

526. Vinson PC, Goldenberg RL, Davis RO, et al. Fetal bladder-neck obstruction and elevated amniotic-fluid alpha-fetoprotein. N Engl J Med 1977;297:1351.

527. Nevin NC, Ritchie A, McKeown F, et al. Raised alpha-fetoprotein levels in amniotic fluid and maternal serum associated with distension of fetal bladder caused by absence of urethra. J Med Genet 1978;15:61.

528. Jandial V, Thom H, Gibson J. Raised alpha-fetoprotein levels associated with minor congenital defect. BMJ 1976;3:22.

529. Schmid W, Muhlethaler JP. High amniotic fluid alpha-1-fetoprotein in a case of fetal sacrococcygeal ter-atoma. Humangenetik 1975;26:353.

530. Hecht F, Hecht BK, O'Keeffe D. Sacrococcygeal teratoma: prenatal diagnosis with elevated alpha-feto-protein and acetylcholinesterase in amniotic fluid. Prenat Diagn 1982;2:229.

531. Guibaud S, Simplot A, Bonnet M, et al. Acetylcholinesterase du liquide amniotique application au diag-nostic prenatal des defauts de fermeture du tube neural. Il Test qualitatif. J Genet Hum 1982;30:119.

532. Devriendt K, van den Berghe K, Moerman P, et al. Elevated maternal serum and amniotic fluid alpha-fetoprotein levels in the Denys–Drash syndrome. Prenat Diagn 1996;16:455.

533. Guibaud S, Simplot A, Bonnet-Capela M. Difficulties in interpretation of AChE gel results in third trimester pregnancies. Prenat Diagn 1985;5:303.

534. Resta RG, Luthy DA, Mahony BS. Umbilical cord hemangioma associated with extremely high alpha-fetoprotein levels. Obstet Gynecol 1988;72:488.

535. Seppälä M, Laes E, Harvo-Naponen M. Elevated amniotic alpha-fetoprotein in congenital oesophageal atresia. J Obstet Gynaecol Br Commonw 1974;81:827.

536. Weinberg AG, Milunsky A, Harrod MJ. Elevated amniotic fluid alpha-fetoprotein and duodenal atresia. Lancet 1975;2:496.

537. Ainbender E, Hirschhorn K. Routine alpha-fetoprotein studies in amniotic fluid. Lancet 1976;1:597.

538. Holzgreve W, Golbus MS. Amniotic fluid acetylcholinesterase as a prenatal diagnostic marker for upper gastrointestinal atresias. Am J Obstet Gynecol 1983;147:837.

539. Leschot NJ, Heyting C, Schaik MV, et al. Amniotic fluid gel acetylcholinesterase determination in prenatal diagnosis: dark field illumination as a method for improving the detection of precipitation bands. Prenat Diagn 1985;5:237.

540. Mehta S, Spencer K. Antenatal diagnosis of neural tube defects using a coated bead immunoassay for acetylcholinesterase in amniotic fluid. Ann Clin Biochem 1988;25:569.

541. Seppälä M, Ruoslahti E. Alpha-fetoprotein in normal and pregnancy sera. Lancet 1972;1:375.

542. Brock DJH. Mechanisms by which amniotic-fluid alpha-fetoprotein may be increased in fetal abnormalities. Lancet 1976;2:345.

543. Seller MJ, Berry AC. Amniotic-fluid alpha-fetoprotein and fetal renal agenesis. Lancet 1978;1:660.

544. Cohen MM, Schwartz S, Schwarz MF, et al. Antenatal detection of cystic hygroma. Obstet Gynecol Surv 1989;44:481.

545. Sutherland GR, Holt D, Rogers JG. Amniotic-fluid alpha-fetoprotein in Turner syndrome. Lancet 1977;1:649.

546. Chervenak FA, Isaacson G, Blakemore KJ, et al. Fetal cystic hygroma. N Engl J Med 1983;309:822.

547. Seller MJ. Phenotypic variation in Meckel syndrome. Clin Genet 1981;20:74.

548. Verp MS, Milunsky A, Simpson F, et al. Elevated alpha-fetoprotein and acetylcholinesterase associated with hydrocele. Am J Med Genet 1984;19:651.

549. Brock DJH, Richmond DH, Liston WA. Normal second-trimester amniotic fluid alpha-fetoprotein and acetylcholinesterase associated with fetal sacrococcygeal teratoma. Prenat Diagn 1983;3:343.

550. Chemke J, Miskin A, Rav-Acha Z, et al. Prenatal diagnosis of Meckel syndrome: alpha-fetoprotein and beta-trace protein in amniotic fluid. Clin Genet 1977;11:2.

551. Johnson VP, Holzwarth DR. Prenatal diagnosis of Meckel syndrome: case reports and literature review. Am J Med Genet 1984;18:699.

552. Wright C, Healicon R, English C, et al. Meckel syndrome: what are the minimum diagnostic criteria? J Med Genet 1994;31:482.

553. Sepulveda W, Sebire NJ, Souka A, et al. Diagnosis of the Meckel–Gruber syndrome at eleven to fourteen weeks' gestation. Am J Obstet Gynecol 1997;176:316.

554. Duncan SLB. Antenatal misdiagnosis of neural-tube defects. Lancet 1975;2:709.

555. Field B, Kerr C. Antenatal diagnosis of neural-tube defects. Lancet 1975;2:324.

556. Brock DJH. Biochemical and cytological methods in the diagnosis of neural tube defects. In: Steinberg AG, Bearn AG, Motulsky AG, et al., eds. Progress in medical genetics. Philadelphia: WB Saunders, 1977:1.

557. Seller MJ. Amniotic fluid alpha-fetoprotein and Turner's syndrome. Lancet 1977;1:995.

558. Hankins GD, Rowe J, Quirk JG, et al. Significance of brown and/or green amniotic fluid at the time of second trimester genetic amniocentesis. Obstet Gynecol 1984;64:353.

559. Allen R. The significance of meconium in mid-trimester genetic amniocentesis. Am J Obstet Gynecol 1985;152:413.

560. Benacerraf BR, Gatter MA, Ginsburgh F. Ultrasound diagnosis of meconium-stained amniotic fluid. Am J Obstet Gynecol 1984;149:570.

561. Chubb IW, Pilowsky PM, Springell HJ, et al. Acetylcholinesterase in human amniotic fluid: an index of fetal neural development? Lancet 1979;1:688.

562. Smith AD, Wald NJ, Cuckle HS, et al. Amniotic-fluid acetylcholinesterase as a possible diagnostic test for neural-tube defects in early pregnancy. Lancet 1979;1:685.

563. Drugan A, Syner FN, Belsky R, et al. Amniotic fluid acetylcholinesterase: implications of an inconclusive result. Am J Obstet Gynecol 1988;159:469.

564. Campbell J, Cass P, Wathen N, et al. First-trimester amniotic fluid and extraembryonic coelomic fluid acetylcholinesterase electrophoresis. Prenat Diagn 1992;12:609.

565. Drugan A, Syner FN, Greb A, et al. Amniotic fluid alpha-fetoprotein and acetylcholinesterase in early genetic amniocentesis. Obstet Gynecol 1988;72:35.

566. Collaborative Acetylcholinesterase Study. Amniotic fluid acetylcholinesterase electrophoresis as a secondary test in the diagnosis of anencephaly and open spina bifida in early pregnancy. Lancet 1981;1:321.

567. Brock DJH, Barron L, van Heyningen V. Prenatal diagnosis of neural tube defects with a monoclonal antibody specific for acetylcholinesterase. Lancet 1985;1:5.

568. Boogert A, Aarnoudse JG, De Bruijn HWA, et al. False-negative amniotic fluid acetylcholinesterase in a case of meningo-encephalocele. Prenat Diagn 1989;9:133.

569. Voigtländer T, Friedl W, Cremer M, et al. Quantitative and qualitative assay of amniotic-fluid acetyl-cholinesterase in the prenatal diagnosis of neural tube defects. Hum Genet 1981;59:227.

570. Coombes EJ, Wood PJ, Spencer K, et al. Improved discrimination in the detection of neural tube defects: five biochemical tests compared. Clin Chim Acta 1982;122:249.

571. Dale G, Archibald A, Bonham JR, et al. Diagnosis of neural tube defects by estimation of amniotic fluid acetylcholinesterase. Br J Obstet Gynaecol 1981;88:120.

572. Burton BK. Positive amniotic fluid acetylcholinesterase: distinguishing between open spina bifida and ventral wall defects. Am J Obstet Gynaecol 1986;155:984.

573. Appleyard ME, Smith AD. In vitro release of acetylcholinesterase from Auerbach's plexus of guinea-pig ileum. Br J Pharmacol 1982;92:530P.

574. Appleyard ME, Smith AD. Secretion of acetylcholinesterase and butyrylcholinesterase from the guinea-pig isolated ileum. Br J Pharmacol 1989;97:490.

575. Goldfine C, Haddow J, Hudson G, et al. Densitometry as an aid in amniotic fluid gel acetylcholinesterase analysis. Am J Obstet Gynecol 1983;145:317.

576. Peat D, Brock DJH. Quantitative estimation of the density ratios of cholinesterase bands in human amniotic fluids. Clin Chim Acta 1984;138:319.

577. Kelly JC, Petrocik E, Wassman ER. Amniotic fluid acetylcholinesterase ratios in prenatal diagnosis of fetal abnormalities. Am J Obstet Gynecol 1989;161:703.

578. Heydanus R, Raats MAM, Los FJ, et al. Prenatal diagnosis of fetal abdominal wall defects: a retrospective analysis of 44 cases. Prenat Diagn 1996;16:411.

579. Gilbert WM, Nicolaides KH. Fetal omphalocele: associated malformations and chromosomal defects. Obstet Gynecol 1987;70:633.

580. Wald NJ, Cuckle HS. Nomogram for estimating an individual's risk of having a fetus with open spina bifida. Br J Obstet Gynaecol 1982;89:598.

581. Milunsky A, Sapirstein VS. Prenatal diagnosis of open neural tube defects using the amniotic fluid acetyl-cholinesterase assay. Obstet Gynecol 1982;59:1.

582. Crandall BF, Kasha W, Matsumoto M. Prenatal diagnosis of neural tube defects: experiences with acetyl-cholinesterase gel electrophoresis. Am J Med Genet 1982;12:361.

583. Read AP, Fennell S, Donnai D, et al. Amniotic fluid acetylcholinesterase: a retrospective and prospective study of the qualitative method. Br J Obstet Gynaecol 1982;89:111.

584. Barlow RD, Cuckle HS, Wald NJ. False positive gel-acetylcholinesterase results in blood-stained amniotic fluids. Br J Obstet Gynaecol 1982;89:821.

585. Sheffield LJ, Sackett DL, Goldsmith CM, et al. A clinical approach to the use of predictive values in the prenatal diagnosis of NTDs. Am J Obstet Gynecol 1983;145:319.

586. Rapola J. Renal pathology of fetal congenital nephrosis. Acta Pathol Microbiol Scand [A] 1981;89:63.

587. Janerich DT, Piper J. Shifting genetic patterns in anencephaly and spina bifida. J Med Genet 1978;15:101.

588. Elwood JM, Mousseau G. Geographical, secular and ethnic influences in anencephalus. J Chronic Dis 1978;31:483.

589. Carter CO, Roberts JA. The risk of recurrence after two children with central nervous-system malformations. Lancet 1967;1:306.

590. Toriello H, Higgins JV. Occurrence of neural tube defects among first-, second-, and third-degree relatives of probands: results of a United States study. Am J Med Genet 1983;15:601.

591. Carter CO, David PA, Laurence KM. A family study of major central nervous system malformations in South Wales. J Med Genet 1968;5:81.

592. Owens JR, Simpkin JM, Garris F. Recurrence rates for neural tube defects. Lancet 1985;1:12.

593. Lippman-Hand A, Fraser FC, Cushman Biddle CJ. Indications for prenatal diagnosis in relatives of patients with neural tube defects. Obstet Gynecol 1978;51:72.

594. McBride ML. Sibling risks of anencephaly and spina bifida in British Columbia. Am J Med Genet 1979;3:377.

595. Smith C. Implications of antenatal diagnosis. In: Emery AEH, ed. Antenatal diagnosis of genetic disease. London: Churchill Livingstone, 1973:137.

596. Nevin NC, Johnston WP. Risk of recurrence after two children with central nervous system malformations in an area of high incidence. J Med Genet 1980;17:87.

597. Zackai EG, Spielman RS, Mellman WJ, et al. The risk of neural tube defects to first cousins of affected individuals. In: Crandall BF, Brazier MAB, eds. Prevention of neural tube defects: the role of alpha-fetoprotein. New York: Academic Press, 1978:99.

598. Wynne-Davies R. Congenital vertebral anomalies: aetiology and relationship to spina bifida cystica. J Med Genet 1975;12:280.

599. Carter CO, Evans KA, Till K. Spinal dysraphism: genetic relation to neural tube malformations. J Med Genet 1976;13:343.
600. James CCM, Lassman LP. Spinal dysraphism: Spina bifida occulta. New York: Appleton-Century-Crofts, 1972.
601. Anderson FM. Occult spinal dysraphism: a series of 73 cases. Pediatrics 1975;55:826.
602. Field B, Kerr C. Offspring of parents with spina bifida occulta. Lancet 1975;2:1257.
603. Fraser FC, Nussbaum E. Neural tube defects in children with tracheo-oesophageal dysraphism. Lancet 1980;2:807.
604. Windham GC, Bjerkedal T. Malformation frequencies in sibs of atresia cases. Lancet 1982;2:816.
605. Baird PA, MacDonald EC. Siblings of children with tracheoesophageal dysraphism. Can Med Assoc J 1981;125:1083.
606. Martin RA, Fineman RM, Jorde LB. Phenotypic heterogeneity in neural tube defects: a clue to causal heterogeneity. Am J Med Genet 1983;16:519.
607. Hunter AGW, Cleveland RH, Blickman JG, et al. A study of level of lesion, associated malformations and sib occurrence risks in spina bifida. Teratology 1996;54:213.
608. Hall JG, Friedman JM, Kenna BA, et al. Clinical, genetic, and epidemiological factors in neural tube defects. Am J Hum Genet 1988;43:827.
609. Milunsky A, ed. Genetic disorders and the fetus: diagnosis, prevention, and treatment, 4th ed. Baltimore: Johns Hopkins University Press, 1998.
610. Mills JL, Rhoads GG, Simpson JL, et al. The absence of a relation between the periconceptional use of vitamins and neural-tube defects. N Engl J Med 1989;321:430.
611. Czeizel AE, Dudas I. Prevention of the first occurrence of neural-tube defects by periconceptional vitamin supplementation. N Engl J Med 1992;327:1832.
612. Shaw GM, Schaffer D, Velie EM, et al. Periconceptional vitamin use, dietary folate, and the occurrence of neural tube defects. Epidemiology 1995;6:219.
613. Green ND. Inositol prevents folate-resistant neural tube defects in the mouse. Nat Med 1997;3:60.
614. Centers for Disease Control. Recommendations for the use of folic acid to reduce the number of cases of spina bifida and other neural tube defects. Morb Mortal Wkly Rep 1992;41:1.
615. Tucker KL, Mahnken B, Wilson PWF, et al. Folic acid fortification of the food supply. JAMA 1996;276:1879.
616. Centers for Disease Control and Prevention and Prevention Working Group on Folic Acid. Position paper on folic acid food fortification and the prevention of spina bifida and anencephaly (SBA). Atlanta: Centers for Disease Control and Prevention, 1993.
617. Campbell NRC. How safe are folic acid supplements? Arch Intern Med 1996;156:1638.
618. Reynolds EH, Wales MB. Effects of folic acid on the mental state and fit-frequency of drug-treated epileptic patients. Lancet 1967;1:1086.
619. Norris JW, Pratt RF. A controlled study of folic acid in epilepsy. Neurology 1971;21:659.
620. Brown RS, DiStanislao PT, Beaver WT, et al. The administration of folic acid to institutionalized epileptic adults with phenytoin-induced gingival hyperplasia: a double-blind, randomized, placebo-controlled, parallel study. Oral Surg Oral Med Oral Pathol Oral Radiol Endod 1991;71:565.
621. Beresford SAA. How do we get enough folic acid to prevent some neural tube defects? Am J Public Health 1994;84:348.
622. Mills JL. Fortification of foods with folic acid: how much is enough? N Engl J Med 2000;342:1442.
623. Department of Health. Folic acid and the prevention of disease. Report on Health and Social Subjects No. 50. Report of the Committee on Medical Aspects of Food and Nutrition Policy. London: Stationery Office, 2000.
624. Czeizel AE. Prevention of congenital abnormalities by periconceptional multivitamin supplementation. BMJ 1993;306:1645.
625. Shaw GM, Lammer EJ, Wasserman CR, et al. Risks of orofacial clefts in children born to women using multivitamins containing folic acid periconceptionally. Lancet 1995;346:393.
626. Li De-K, Daling JR, Mueller BA, et al. Periconceptional multivitamin use in relation to the risk of congenital urinary tract anomalies. Epidemiology 1995;6:212.
627. Botto LD, Khoury MJ, Mulinare J, et al. Periconceptional multivitamin use and the occurrence of conotruncal heart defects: results from a population-based, case-control study. Pediatrics 1996;98:911.
628. Czeizel AE, Toth M, Rockenbauer M. Population-based case control study of folic acid supplementation during pregnancy. Teratology 1996;53:345.
629. Medical Research Council Vitamin Study Research Group. Prevention of neural tube defects: Results of the Medical Research Council Vitamin Study. Lancet 1991;338:131.

630. Mathews TJ, Honein MA, Erickson JD. Spina bifida and anencephaly prevalence—United States, 1991–2001. MMWR Recomm Rep 2002;51(RR-13):9–11.

631. Berry RJ, Li Z, Erickson JD, et al. Prevention of neural-tube defects with folic acid in China. N Engl J Med 1999;341:1485.

632. Kalucy M, Bower C, Stanley F, et al. Survival of infants with neural tube defects in Western Australia 1966–1990. Paediatr Perinatol Epidemiol 1994;8:334.

633. Hagard S, Carter F, Milne RG. Screening for spina bifida cystica: a cost–benefit analysis. Br J Prev Soc Med 1976;30:40.

634. McLaughlin J, Shurtleff D, Laners J, et al. Influence of prognosis on decisions regarding the care of newborns with myelodysplasia. N Engl J Med 1985;312:1589.

635. Adams MM, Greenberg F, Khoury MJ, et al. Survival of infants with spina bifida. Am J Dis Child 1985;139:514.

636. Althouse R, Wald NJ. Survival and handicap of infants with spina bifida. Arch Dis Child 1980;55:845.

637. Charney E, Weller S, Sutton L, et al. Management of the newborn with myelomeningocele: time for a decision making process. Pediatrics 1985;75:58.

638. Gross R. Newborns with myelodysplasia: the rest of the story. N Engl J Med 1985;312:1632.

639. Castree B, Walker J. The young adult with spina bifida. BMJ 1981;283:1040.

640. Laurence KM, Beresford A. Degree of physical handicap, education, and occupation of 51 adults with spina bifida. Br J Prev Soc Med 1976;30:197.

641. Hunt GM. Open spina bifida: outcome for a complete cohort treated unselectively and followed into adulthood. Dev Med Child Neurol 1990;32:108.

642. Hunt GM, Poulton A. Open spina bifida: a complete cohort reviewed 25 years after closure. Dev Med Child Neurol 1995;37:19.

642a. Bowman RM, McLone DG, Grant JA, et al. Spina bifida outcome: a 25-year prospective. Pediatr Neurosurg 2001;34:114.

642b. Hunt GM, Oakeshoff P. Outcome in people with open spina bifida at age 35: prospective community based cohort study. BMJ 2003;326:1365.

643. Pires G, Morais-Almeida M, Gaspar A, et al. Risk factors for latex sensitization in children with spina bifida. Allergol Immunopathol (Madr). 2002;30:5.

644. Bamforth SJ, Baird PA. Spina bifida and hydrocephalus: a population study over a 35-year period. Am J Hum Genet 1989;44:225.

645. Dastgiri S, Gilmour WH, Stone DH. Survival of children born with congenital anomalies. Arch Dis Child 2003;88:391.

646. Patrick GM, Mahony JF, Disney AP. The prognosis for end-stage renal failure in spinal cord injury and spina bifida: Australia and New Zealand. Austr NZ J Med 1994;24:36.

647. Dillon CM, Davis BE, Duguay S, et al. Longevity of patients born with myelomeningocele. Eur J Pediatr Surg 2000;10:33.

648. Duffs RS, Campbell AGM. Moral and ethical dilemmas in the special-care nursery. N Engl J Med 1979;289:890.

649. Hayden PW, Shurtleff DB, Broy AB. Custody of the myelodysplastic child: implications for selection for early treatment. Pediatrics 1974;53:254.

650. Venes JL, Juttenlocher PR, Paxson CL Jr, et al. Management of the infant with unmanageable disease. N Engl J Med 1974;290:518.

651. Robertson JA. Discretionary non-treatment of defective newborns. In: Milunsky A, Annas GJ, eds. Genetics and the law. New York: Plenum Press, 1976:451.

652. Burt RA. Authorizing death for anomalous newborns: ten years later. In: Milunsky A, Annas GJ, eds. Genetics and the law, vol. III. New York: Plenum Press, 1985:259.

653. Hare EH, Laurence KM, Payne H, et al. Spina bifida and family stress. BMJ 1966;2:757.

654. Tew BJ, Payne H, Laurence KM. Must a family with a handicapped child be a handicapped family? Dev Med Child Neurol 1974;16:95.

655. Li HR, Borjeson M-C, Lagerkvist B, et al. Children with myelomeningocele: The impact of disability on family dynamics and social conditions: A Nordic study. Dev Med Child Neurol 1994;36:1000.

656. Tew BJ, Laurence KM. The effects of admission to hospital and surgery on children with spina bifida. Hydrocephalus Spina Bifida 1976;37 (suppl):119.

657. Herskowitz J, Marks AN. The spina bifida patient as a person. Dev Med Child Neurol 1977;19:413.

658. Shurtleff DB, Lamers J. Clinical considerations in the treatment of myelodysplasia. In: Crandall BF, Brazier MAB, eds. Prevention of neural tube defects: the role of alpha-fetoprotein. New York: Academic Press, 1978:103.

Howard S. Cuckle, B.A., M.Sc., D.Phil., and
Svetlana Arbuzova, M.D., Ph.D., D.Med.Sc.

22

Multimarker Maternal Serum Screening for Chromosomal Abnormalities

In the past, antenatal screening for chromosomal abnormalities was a simple matter of noting the maternal age and referring for invasive prenatal diagnosis those regarded by local policy or national convention as having advanced reproductive age. Similarly, a history of aneuploidy in a previous child or even a family history was generally regarded as sufficient grounds for prenatal diagnosis. But the discovery in the early 1980s that second-trimester maternal serum α-fetoprotein (AFP) levels were reduced on average in pregnancies affected by fetal aneuploidy has led to a sea change in clinical practice. Routine screening, based on testing maternal serum for multiple markers together with the determination of one or more ultrasound markers, can now obtain a fourfold to fivefold increase in the proportion of affected pregnancies detected antenatally. However, the screening strategies needed to achieve this benefit are complex, involve statistical manipulation, and are expressed in unfamiliar terms. In this chapter we attempt to clarify such screening by revealing step by step the underlying principles and explaining the terminology as well as demonstrating the relative efficiency of different strategies.

CHROMOSOMAL ABNORMALITIES

Aneuploidy is a common event in pregnancy, with a wide spectrum of medical consequences from the lethal to the completely benign. Most affected embryos abort spontaneously early in the first trimester; many of them even before there are clinical signs of pregnancy. Those that survive into the second trimester also experience high late intrauterine mortality and increased risk of infant death. Viability and clinical outcome vary according to the genotype. This chapter will concentrate on the more common forms of aneuploidy that are sufficiently viable to survive to term in relatively large numbers and are amenable to screening.

By far the most frequent of these is Down syndrome (DS), with a birth prevalence in the absence of prenatal diagnosis and elective abortion, of 1–2 per 1,000 births in developed countries. Consequently, it is considered first and more extensively than Edwards and Patau syndromes, which have about one-tenth and one-twentieth the birth prevalence, respectively, and the sex chromosome aneuploidies, which are common but relatively benign.

SCREENING AND PRENATAL DIAGNOSIS

There is a fundamental difference between screening and diagnostic tests, despite the fact that the same terms are used to describe their results: "true positive," "false positive," "true negative," and "false negative." The aim of screening is limited to the identification from among apparently healthy individuals of those at a high enough risk of a specific disease to warrant further investigation. In the context of chromosomal abnormalities, these investigations involve invasive procedures with some risk—chorionic villus sampling (CVS), amniocentesis, and occasionally percutaneous umbilical cord sampling—to obtain material for prenatal diagnosis. Thus, screening does not aim to make a diagnosis, but rather by prior selection to limit the use of unnecessary and risky diagnostic procedures, and curtail costs.

In the past, prenatal diagnosis for chromosomal abnormality was largely restricted to women of advanced maternal age or those with a previously affected child. Today, screening tests based on multiple markers are provided to all women. The principal markers are continuous variables whose distribution of values is higher or lower on average in affected pregnancies. Typically, screening markers have considerable overlap in the distribution of results between affected and unaffected individuals. In contrast, the distribution of values for a variable used in diagnosis would have virtually no overlap. The potential utility for screening for a given marker depends on the extent of separation between the two distributions. This can be expressed as the absolute difference between the distribution means divided by the average standard deviation for the two distributions, a form of Mahalinobis distance. (The Mahalinobis distance of a value v is $(v - m)/s$, where m and s are the distribution mean and standard deviation. In this chapter we use the term to refer to $|m_a - m_u|/((s_a + s_u)/2)$, where m_a, m_u, s_a, and s_u are the affected and unaffected means and standard deviations.)

For continuous variables, the choice of a cutoff level that determines whether a value is positive or negative is arbitrary because there is no intrinsic division between the distributions. The choice will be influenced by the perceived relative importance of the detection rate (DR), the proportion of affected pregnancies referred for prenatal diagnosis, and the false-positive rate (FPR), the proportion of unaffected pregnancies referred. Although the DR and FPR are a function of the marker itself, the positive predictive value (PPV), the chance of being affected given that the result is positive, is also dependent on the prior risk in those screened. So published PPVs from case–control studies or estimated when screening a high-risk population are not generally applicable.

PRINCIPAL MARKERS

There are more than fifty maternal blood, maternal urine, or ultrasound markers of DS, but just seven are widely used in routine multimarker screening: maternal serum human chorionic gonadotropin (hCG), the free-β subunit of hCG, α-fetoprotein (AFP), unconjugated estriol (uE$_3$), inhibin A, pregnancy-associated plasma protein (PAPP)-A, and ultrasound nuchal translucency (NT). An eighth marker, ultrasound nuchal skin fold (NF), while widely measured, is not often incorporated into screening programs. There are benefits of doing so, and NF should be considered one of the principle markers. The so-called soft ultrasound markers determined at the time of the late second trimester anomaly scan ("genetic sonogram") are not generally used in the program. Soft ultrasound markers are discussed further in chapter 23.

Maternal serum AFP was the first analyte to be used in DS screening after the observation that levels were reduced on average in pregnancies with chromosomal abnormalities in general[1] and DS in particular,[2] in both the first and second trimesters. Umbilical cord serum and amniotic fluid AFP levels are also lower than normal. The biology of AFP is discussed in chapter 21. The reason for the decreased AFP is unknown, but in the second trimester it may reflect hepatic immaturity. Histologic study has revealed undervascularization of the placentas of fetuses with various chromosomal defects, possibly representing placental immaturity with arrested or delayed angiogenesis.[3] In the first trimester, AFP is predominantly of fetal yolk sac origin.

Maternal serum hCG[4] and free β-hCG[5] levels are increased on average in DS pregnancies; the latter in both the first and second trimesters, although the extent of increase is greater as pregnancy progresses. Gonadotropins are glycoproteins with epitopes on the protein surface. hCG is a 39.5-kD glycoprotein made up of two nonidentical α- and β-subunits that exist either free or bound to each other. Free α-hCG levels are also increased in DS, but the marker is not widely used in screening. Although the reason for increased hCG is unknown, placental immaturity in the fetus with DS is likely. Six different genes code for the β-subunit of hCG, but only one α-subunit gene is known thus far. Not all the factors involved in hCG secretion are known, but cyclic adenosine monophosphate (cAMP), prolactin, corticosteroids, and gonadoliberin influence release, while polyamines, estradiol, and progesterone inhibit release.

Total maternal urinary estriol excretion in the third trimester of DS pregnancies is lower than in unaffected pregnancies,[6] and subsequently the level of maternal serum uE_3 was also found to be lower than average[7] in both the first and second trimesters. In the fetus with DS there is adrenal hypoplasia, and the adrenal cortex produces dehydroepiandrosterone sulfate (DHEAS), which the fetal liver hydroxylates. The newly formed product, 16α-hydroxy-DHEAS, is formed in the fetal liver by hydroxylation of DHEAS and transported to the placenta, where it undergoes desulfation and aromatization into estriol.

Inhibin levels have been shown to be increased in DS pregnancies, using assays that detect all species[8] and those specific for inhibin A.[9] These increases are not as marked before 13 weeks of gestation as they are later. Inhibin is a dimer of 32 kD with an α-subunit and one of two similar but distinguishable β-subunits. Of two mature forms, dimeric inhibin A and inhibin B, only the former is present in pregnancy sera. Inhibin is considered to have a role in the regulation of gonadotropin biosynthesis and secretion, ovarian and placental steroidogenesis, and oocyte maturation. Inhibin is regarded as a member of the transforming growth factor β superfamily and is characterized by its ability to suppress follicle-stimulating hormone secretion.

PAPP-A levels are reduced in first-trimester DS pregnancies,[10] but this reduction is less prominent as pregnancy progresses and there is little or no effect by the second trimester. PAPP-A is a 750 kDa α_2 mobile glycoprotein containing sixteen atoms of zinc and having a high affinity for heparin. In maternal serum, PAPP-A is complexed with the proform of eosinophil major basic protein. The reason for the low levels in Down syndrome is not known but it is likely to be connected with placental insufficiency and may be the same mechanism that leads to low levels in nonviable pregnancies.

NT is increased in DS pregnancies,[11] but there is a narrow window at 11–13 weeks (crown-to-rump length, 45–85 mm) when subcutaneous edema can readily be measured in the fetal neck. NT is visualized in the sagittal section used for crown-to-rump length, and it is recommended that a standardized technique be adopted for measurement.[12] The reasons for the increased edema in DS are not known, but the most plausible explanations are altered composition of the cellular matrix,[13] abnormal or delayed development of the lymphatic system, and cardiac insufficiency.

NF can be measured only in the second trimester, and is increased in DS pregnancies.[14] A thick nuchal pad is a phenotypic feature of DS and is seen in most affected newborns. NF is visualized in the same transverse section used for biparietal diameter measurement. Although the same mechanism is likely to cause both the increased NT and increased NF in DS pregnancies, there is no correlation between the two markers within any pregnancy.[15]

ALLOWING FOR GESTATION

All eight markers are continuous variables whose levels in unaffected pregnancies change with gestation. For the serum markers this is allowed for by the use of multiples of the gestation specific median (MoMs) for unaffected pregnancies. Most ultrasound studies of NT or NF have not allowed for gestation at all, but increasingly NT is being reported either in MoMs or deviations from the gestation-specific median. The best results are obtained when the unaffected medians are calculated to the day of gestation using regression curves. For NT some practitioners use center- or operator-specific curves.[16]

Meta-analysis of all the published literature is the most reliable way to estimate, for each marker, the relative increase or decrease on average in DS pregnancies and the extent of separation between affected and unaffected distributions. In our analysis, the average MoM was derived from two large published meta-analyses: second-trimester hCG, free β-hCG, uE$_3$, and AFP[17]; and first-trimester uE$_3$ and AFP.[18] As the mean PAPP-A MoM for DS decreased steadily throughout the first trimester, a meta-analysis-derived regression curve was used to estimate the gestation-specific mean[17] and similarly for free β-hCG.[19] For second-trimester inhibin A the meta-analysis of ten studies[20] was used, updated to include three more recent retrospective studies,[21–23] and at 13 weeks used the mean of cases obtained from a graph in the publication[24–27] or from the authors[28] and a single published series.[29] For NT, we carried out a meta-analysis using the eleven studies in which MoMs either were reported or could be derived from a figure or table in the publication.[29–39] In five of the studies the results were acted on clinically and so are subject to "viability" bias that will skew the results upward. This bias arises because a proportion of those with high NT levels and termination of pregnancy would have been destined to miscarry, whereas nonviable DS pregnancies with normal levels will not be known to the investigators. The results of one prospective intervention study, the massive multicenter Fetal Medicine Foundation study,[40] have been used to allow for this statistically and estimated that the skew increases the mean by 11 percent.[32] In the current meta-analysis, we applied this factor to the five intervention studies before taking the weighted average of all eleven. We combined in a meta-analysis the four studies in which NF values in MoMs were either reported or could be derived from a figure in the publication.[41–44] The sources of data used to estimate the standard deviations needed for the Mahalinobis distance are specified in "Likelihood Ratios" below.

Table 22.1 shows the average MoM for each marker together with the Mahalinobis distance, based on these meta-analyses. The values are shown only for gestations in which there is a potentially useful separation between the affected and unaffected distributions. As a guide, maternal age, which is a poor DS screening variable, has a Mahalinobis distance of about 1, and AFP when used to screen for spina bifida has a value of about 2.4.

NT is by far the single best individual marker. Among the serum markers, PAPP-A is the most discriminatory, but the Mahalinobis distance declines rapidly with increasing gestation. Free β-hCG is more discriminatory at 14–18 weeks than at 10–13 weeks, al-

Table 22.1.   Mean level in Down syndrome (DS) for each maternal serum marker according to gestation, and the Mahalinobis distance

Marker	Gestation (weeks)	DS Cases	MoM	Mahalinobis Distance
NT	11–13	703	2.03	1.84
PAPP-A	10		0.39	1.25
	11	249	0.48	1.04
	12		0.62	0.73
	13		0.72	0.52
Free β-hCG	10		1.74	0.85
	11	480	1.91	1.02
	12		2.05	1.15
	13		2.16	1.26
	14–18	477	2.30	1.25
hCG	14–18	850	2.02	1.15
Inhibin A	13	49	1.99	1.36
	14–18	603	1.85	1.10
AFP	10–13	542	0.79	0.50
	14–18	1,140	0.73	0.89
uE_3	10–13	226	0.74	0.60
	14–18	613	0.73	0.90
NF	14–24	234	1.45	1.05

though there is a gradual change in Mahalinobis distance between 10 and 18 weeks. At 14–18 weeks of gestation hCG is less discriminatory than free β-hCG, and before 13 weeks it is a poor marker. At 14–18 weeks, inhibin A has a discriminatory power comparable to that of hCG, and although in the first trimester generally it too is a weak marker, at 13 weeks it is more discriminatory than PAPP-A. AFP and uE_3 are not very discriminatory markers but perform a little better when measured in the second trimester than in the first. NF is less discriminatory than NT but is comparable with the second-trimester serum markers.

RISK SCREENING

Statistically, the optimal way of interpreting the multimarker profile is to estimate the risk of DS from the marker levels.[45] This is done by modifying the prior risk, that attained before testing, by a factor known as the "likelihood ratio," derived from the marker profile and comparing the posterior risk with a fixed cutoff risk. If the risk is greater than the cutoff, the result is regarded as positive, otherwise it is negative. This approach will yield a higher detection rate for a given false-positive rate than any other method of test interpretation. It also provides a way of encapsulating the result for the purposes of counseling. The method is optimal even if a single marker is used and whether the marker is physical or biochemical.

The prior risk of DS, based on maternal age and family history, can be expressed as a probability, say p, or a rate of 1 in $1/p$ and needs to be converted into an odds of $p:(1 - p)$. The posterior risk is calculated by multiplying the left-hand side of the odds by the likelihood ratio from the marker profile (x) and the result reexpressed as the rate of 1 in $1 + (1 - p)/px$ or the probability $px/[1 + p(x - 1)]$. The prior risk can be related to the chance of having a term pregnancy with the disorder or the chance of the fetus being affected at the time of testing. Insofar as the aim of screening is to reduce birth prevalence, the former is the most appropriate. But screening is also about providing women with information on which to base an informed choice about prenatal diagnosis, and it can be argued that the latter is more relevant.

This calculation assumes that the marker levels and age are independent determinants of risk and that the marker levels are unrelated to the probability of intrauterine survival. There is no strong evidence against these assumptions, although extreme values of some of the biochemical and ultrasound markers are associated with increased fetal losses for unaffected pregnancies.

Age-Specific Risk at Term

The best available estimate is obtained by meta-analysis of published birth prevalence rates for individual years of age that were carried out before prenatal diagnosis became common. Four meta-analyses have been published based on eleven different maternal-age-specific birth prevalence series. The studies differed in the number of series included, the method of pooling series, the type of regression equation and the extent to which the maternal age range was restricted.

In the first, all eight series published at that time were included, with a total of 4,000–5,000 DS and more than 5 million unaffected births.[46] For each year of age, data were pooled by taking the average birth prevalence rate across the series weighted by the number of births. A three-parameter additive-exponential regression equation was used of the form $y = a + \exp(b + cx)$, where y is prevalence and x is age. A single regression was performed over the entire age range. In the second study, the same eight series were included, but a separate analysis was carried out for the two series that the authors regarded to be most complete.[47] Pooling was by summation of the birth prevalence numerators and denominators. Two different additive-exponential regression equations were used, the linear equation above and a five-parameter version with a cubic exponential component. The maternal age range was restricted in four ways: 15–49, 20–49, 15–45, 20–45, The third study included four series comprising the two "most complete" series above, extended by more recent data, and two newer series.[48] A separate analysis was carried out after excluding one of the new series. Pooling was by summation. Three-, five-, and six-parameter additive-exponential regression equations were used, the latter having a quartic exponential component. There was no age restriction. The last study included nine series, six of the original eight, with the updated recent data, the two additional series used in the third study, and an additional new series.[49] A separate analysis was carried out after excluding one of the original series. Pooling is by the use of a weighting factor that estimates the proportional underascertainment in each series. The regression analysis simultaneously estimates the curve parameters and this proportion. A three-parameter logistic regression equation is used of the form $y = a + (1 - a)/[1 + \exp(-b - cx)]$, where a is between 0 and 1. There was no age restriction.

There is little practical difference between the nineteen regression curves published in the different meta-analyses over the 15–45-year age range. The real differences emerge at older ages: for example at age 50 the risks range from 1 in 5 to 1 in 18. There is no simple way of deciding which of the curves is the most accurate because the age-specific rates differ between the component series of the meta-analyses, partly because of underascertainment and possibly because of real underlying differences between the populations.

Recently, another curve has been published using data on about 11,000 cases from the U.K. National Down Syndrome Cytogenetic Register (NDSCR), a very complete national database.[50] The estimates differ from those obtained by previous meta-analyses: significantly higher at ages 36–41 and considerably lower after age 45. These discrepancies may be due to the fact that 45 percent of NDSCR cases were diagnosed prenatally and 82 percent of these ended in termination of pregnancy, whereas the previous series were collected before antenatal screening and prenatal diagnosis became widespread. To estimate birth prevalence it was necessary to allow for intrauterine survival following prenatal diagnosis, and the authors used the same survival rate at all ages and indications for prenatal diagnosis. Although there is no direct evidence that survival rates are dependent on the marker profile, extreme levels of all the markers have been reported in nonviable unaffected pregnancies. Because the average marker profile of screening detected cases varies with age, this may have led to bias.[51]

Risk at the Time of the Test

Some screening programs report the risk of DS at the time of the test rather than the risk of a term affected pregnancy. This can be calculated from the intrauterine survival rates of DS from the first and second trimesters, say, p_1 and p_2. The relative risk in the first trimester, second trimester, and at birth is $1/p_1:1/p_2:1$. Studies of prenatal diagnosis are used to estimate fetal loss rates, either by comparing the observed number of cases with that expected from birth prevalence, given the maternal age distribution, or by follow-up of individuals declining termination of pregnancy, using direct or actuarial survival analysis. Published prevalence studies include 341 DS cases diagnosed at chorionic villus sampling and 1,159 at amniocentesis.[52] There are three published follow-up series, including 110 cases diagnosed at amniocentesis[53] and a series of 126 cases from the NDSCR, which has been analyzed according to the gestational age at prenatal diagnosis.[54] However, the Register study is biased because some miscarriages may have occurred in women who did intend to terminate their pregnancies, thus inflating the rates. An actuarial survival analysis of the Register data has now been carried out[55] that overcomes the bias and is more data efficient, since all cases contribute to the estimate, not just those in which termination was refused.

Actual and potential heterogeneity between the various studies precludes a grand meta-analysis to estimate the fetal loss rates. But an informal synthesis has been carried out and reached the conclusion that about one-half of DS pregnancies are lost after first-trimester CVS and one-quarter after midtrimester amniocentesis.[56]

It is also possible to calculate risks at individual weeks of gestation. A formula derived from a large prenatal diagnosis series can be used to estimate the survival rate for 8 to 20 weeks of 58, 61, 64, 67, 70, 72, 75, 77, 79, 80, 82, 83, and 85 percent.[57] Another approach is regression, taking the first-trimester survival to be based on cases diagnosed by CVS at 10 weeks on average and the second trimester by amniocentesis at 17 weeks, and assigning a survival rate of 100 percent at 40 weeks. A quadratic formula, $0.114 + 0.0507x - 0.000714x^2$ (x = completed weeks) has a good fit and yields rates of: 47, 51, 54, 58, 62, 65, 68, 71, 74, 77, 80, 82, and 84 percent.

These calculations assume that fetal loss rates do not vary with maternal age. However, the studies used to calculate the overall rates are based largely on women aged over 35, so this cannot be readily examined. Because the fetal loss rate in general increases markedly with maternal age,[58] it is likely that this will also happen in DS pregnancies.

LIKELIHOOD RATIOS

All eight markers follow an approximately log gaussian distribution over most of their range. In this situation, the likelihood ratio (LR) for a single marker is calculated by the ratio of the heights of the two overlapping distributions at the specific level. Beyond the normal range, it is standard practice to use the LR at the end of the range. The distributions are determined by the mean level in DS and the matrix of variances (standard deviation squared) in both DS and unaffected pregnancies. The method is the same for more than one marker except that the heights of multivariate log gaussian distributions are used. These are dependent, in addition, on the matrix of covariances between markers within DS and unaffected pregnancies.

The variance–covariance matrices are best derived by meta-analysis. The most accurate results are obtained, where possible, by tailoring the matrices to the population being tested. Briefly, this involves using meta-analyses to derive the difference in variance–covariance matrix between DS and unaffected pregnancies. Then the latter is added to the matrix for unaffected pregnancies in the local population. In the current analysis we derived an unaffected matrix from 29,516 women screened in Leeds: 11,019 having serum markers measured at 10–13 weeks, 18,497 at 14–18 weeks, and 5,177 having NT and center-specific MoMs. The standard deviation was estimated by the 10th to 90th centile range on a log scale divided by 2.563, and the covariance was estimated by excluding outliers exceeding 3 standard deviations from the mean. Separate variance–covariance matrices for the serum markers were derived for each week of gestation from 10 to 13. For matrices other than inhibin the corresponding difference between the serum matrices was derived from published meta-analyses.[17,18] For inhibin at 14–18 weeks, the difference in variance between DS and unaffected pregnancies was derived by carrying out a meta-analysis of twelve second-trimester studies: ten cited by Lam and Tang,[20] together with two others.[21,29] Most of these studies did not include enough data to estimate the difference in covariance, so the correlation coefficients were estimated directly by taking the weighted average between studies. For inhibin at 13 weeks, a single study was used.[29] For NT, the difference in variance between DS and unaffected pregnancies was derived from the weighted average in seven studies[29,32,33,35,37–39]; no covariance with serum markers was assumed. The correlation coefficients between PAPP-A at 10–13 weeks and serum markers at 14–18 weeks could not be tailored and were estimated directly from five studies.[29,59–62] For NF, the standard deviations were estimated directly from three of the studies[41,43,44]; no covariance with serum markers was assumed except for second-trimester hCG or free β-hCG in DS pregnancies since two of the studies found an association[43,44] and the correlation coefficient was estimated directly.

In this chapter we use a single set of parameters, but in practice two sets are needed for the serum markers. The variance–covariance matrices are different in women whose gestational age is based on menstrual dates and those in whom ultrasound biometry has been used. Although an individual scan estimate of gestation has wide confidence limits, on average, scanning is the more precise method and leads to a reduction in variance. In contrast, the mean marker profile should not differ according to the dating method. Infants with DS are growth restricted at term,[63] but early biometric measures other than long bone measurements do not appear to be altered in early pregnancy. An international multicenter collaborative study has investigated possible bias in the two main biometric measures of gestation, crown-to-rump length and biparietal diameter.[64] In 55 case–control sets using the former and 146 for the latter, the median difference in measurements was zero for both measures.

MODELING PERFORMANCE

Two widely used methods of estimating DS screening detection and false-positive rates are numerical integration and Monte-Carlo stimulation. Numerical integration uses the theoretical log gaussian distributions of each marker in DS and unaffected pregnancies.[45] The theoretical range is divided into a number of equal sections thus forming a "grid" in multidimensional space. The Gaussian distributions are then used to calculate for each section (square for two markers, cube for three, etc.): the proportion of DS and unaffected pregnancies in the section and the LR. It is then a matter of applying these values to a specified maternal population. At each maternal age, the number of DS and unaffected pregnancies is estimated from the age-specific risk curve. The distributions of DS risks are then calculated from the grid values. Monte-Carlo stimulation also uses the Gaussian distributions, but instead of rigid summation over a fixed grid it uses a random sample of points in multidimensional space to simulate the outcome of a population being screened.

The model predicted detection and false-positive rates are highly dependent on the maternal population specified, usually a national population whose maternal age structure has been published. An alternative is to standardize for age by using a standard female population and a set of age-specific fertility rates[65] or simply to use a Gaussian distribution of maternal ages.[66] We use the latter in this analysis with a mean age of 27 and a standard deviation of 5.5 years. Whichever method is used, the comparison of performance *between* strategies is reasonably robust regardless of the population specified.

When assessing the relative benefits of different strategies, it is best either to fix the false-positive rate (say, 5 percent or 1 percent) and compare the detection rates or to fix the detection rate (say, 75 percent or 85 percent) and compare the false-positive rates. However, when changing strategy it would be confusing to alter the cutoff risk in order to maintain the DR or FPR as before. So in practice it is common to retain the cutoff (say 1 in 200, 250, or 300 at term) and allow both DR and FPR to vary. In this chapter, performance is presented using all three methods.

MULTIMARKER STRATEGIES

It has become common to refer to certain combinations or markers by a shorthand: "double," "triple," "quadruple," "combined," "integrated," "integrated serum," or "comprehensive" tests. Although this may be convenient, it can be misleading and restrictive. The ordinal implies that the screening efficiency of the triple is necessarily better than the double and worse than the quadruple. And then there is an implication of uniqueness. Thus, the triple has become solely usable for the particular second-trimester combination of three markers for which it was first coined. Other three-marker combinations also have high screening potential, or indeed the same combination, but performed in the first trimester they cannot be called triple tests, and this may restrict their use. Similarly, all the marker combinations involve the integration of multiple information and the integrated test is not special in this regard.

In this chapter we eschew these shorthands and either specify the specific combinations explicitly or use more general descriptive terms. Four types of policy option that combine two methods, such as serum testing and ultrasound, are considered when the methods are performed: at the same time ("concurrent"); at different times ("sequential") with results not reported until all are complete ("nondisclosure"); intermediate results reported as they are ready ("stepwise"); or a hybrid of immediate and delayed reporting dependent on the result ("contingent").

MODEL PREDICTIONS

Serum Screening Alone

Most experience with serum screening is in the second trimester, when it became a natural extension to established AFP screening programs for NTDs. Maternal serum AFP screening for spina bifida is most efficient at 16–18 weeks of gestation (see chapter 21). In the second trimester most centers use a two- or three-marker combination of either hCG or free β-hCG and AFP, with or without uE_3. A small number of centers have extended this to a fourth marker: neutrophil alkaline phosphatase and free α-hCG have been tried and abandoned, whereas inhibin A is now more firmly established.

Table 22.2 shows the model-predicted detection and false-positive rates for two to four combinations used at 14–18 weeks of gestation. For a fixed 5 percent false-positive rate, the detection rate ranges from 58.0 to 71.7 percent. Substitution of free β-hCG for hCG increases detection by over 3 percent; extending the two-marker free β-hCG and AFP combination with the addition of uE_3 increases detection by over 4 percent and inhibin as a fourth marker increases it by an additional 6 percent. For a fixed 75 percent detection rate, these incremental changes lead to a more than halving of the false-positive rate.

Table 22.3 shows the estimated detection and false-positive rates for two- and four-marker combinations at 10–13 weeks of gestation. For a 5 percent false-positive rate the range of detection rates is 56.4 to 71.4 percent, similar to second-trimester serum screening. With the commonly used two-marker combination of PAPP-A and free β-hCG, the detection rate varies according to week of gestation, with the best results at 10 weeks; however, the addition of uE_3 and AFP reduces these differences. At 13 weeks, substitution of inhibin for PAPP-A does not have a marked effect on detection.

Ultrasound Alone

With NT alone, at 11–13 weeks the model-predicted detection rate for a 5 percent false-positive rate is 76.1 percent (at 1 percent it is 64.5 percent). For an 85 percent detection

Table 22.2. Screening with two to four maternal serum markers at 14–18 weeks of gestation

Combination	Cutoff Risk (at Term)									
	DR for FPR		FPR for DR		1 in 200		1 in 250		1 in 300	
	1%	5%	75%	85%	DR	FPR	DR	FPR	DR	FPR
hCG and AFP	35.9	58.0	14.5	27.0	54.2	3.9	58.2	5.1	61.4	6.3
+uE_3	41.7	62.7	12.1	24.3	57.4	3.5	60.9	4.6	63.8	5.6
+uE_3 and inhibin	49.0	68.5	8.3	18.3	63.1	3.3	66.1	4.2	68.6	5.0
Free β-hCG and AFP	37.0	61.4	11.4	21.5	58.2	4.2	62.4	5.4	65.6	6.5
+uE_3	43.8	66.1	9.2	18.7	61.4	3.6	65.1	4.7	68.0	5.7
+uE_3 and inhibin	51.5	71.7	6.5	14.5	66.0	3.2	69.2	4.1	71.8	5.0

DR = detection rate; FPR = false-positive rate.

Table 22.3.   Maternal serum screening with two or four markers at 10–13 weeks of gestation

Combination	DR for FPR 1%	DR for FPR 5%	FPR for DR 75%	FPR for DR 85%	1 in 200 DR	1 in 200 FPR	1 in 250 DR	1 in 250 FPR	1 in 300 DR	1 in 300 FPR
10 weeks										
PAPP-A and free β	39.6	63.7	10.1	19.5	59.0	3.7	63.1	4.8	66.3	5.9
+AFP and uE$_3$	48.4	71.4	6.4	13.4	64.9	3.2	68.4	4.1	71.3	4.9
11 weeks										
PAPP-A and free β	36.0	59.6	12.5	23.1	55.8	4.0	60.1	5.2	63.4	6.3
+AFP and uE$_3$	47.0	69.6	7.3	15.2	63.8	3.3	67.3	4.3	70.2	5.2
12 weeks										
PAPP-A and free β	33.6	56.8	14.2	25.4	53.6	4.1	58.1	5.4	61.7	6.7
+AFP and uE$_3$	50.0	70.9	6.8	14.5	65.3	3.3	68.5	4.2	71.1	5.1
13 weeks										
PAPP-A and free β	34.4	58.0	13.4	24.1	54.9	4.2	59.5	5.5	63.1	6.8
+AFP and uE$_3$	49.4	71.0	6.6	13.8	65.9	3.5	69.1	4.4	71.8	5.3
Inhibin and free β	31.1	56.3	13.4	23.0	55.5	4.8	60.4	6.2	64.2	7.6
+AFP and uE$_3$	48.8	70.8	6.7	13.7	65.9	3.6	69.5	4.6	72.4	5.6

DR = detection rate; FPR = false-positive rate.

rate, the false-positive rate is 15.4 percent (at 75 percent it is 4.4 percent). The detection and false-positive rates for a cutoff risk at term of 1 in 200 are 68.7 percent and 1.9 percent; for 1 in 250 they are 70.6 percent and 2.4 percent; for 1 in 300, 72.2 percent and 3.0 percent. Hence, ultrasound NT has a model predicted efficiency similar to that of four-marker serum screening at 11 weeks and 14–18 weeks, but less than at 10 weeks.

With NF alone, at 14–22 weeks the rates are for a 5 percent false-positive rate is 57.6 percent (at 1 percent it is 42.0 percent). For an 85 percent detection rate, the false-positive rate is 38.8 percent (at 75 percent it is 19.7 percent). The detection and false-positive rates for a cutoff risk at term of 1 in 200 are 50.6 percent and 1.7 percent; for 1 in 250 they are 53.4 percent and 3.5 percent; for 1 in 300, 55.9 percent and 4.4 percent.

Concurrent Serum and Ultrasound Screening

There is an important practical constraint influencing the design of concurrent strategies, namely, that the results of a scan can be reported to the patient immediately, whereas a serum result usually will not be available for a number of days. The reason for the delay is that biochemical assays are normally done in batches, which, to avoid unnecessary expense include about 50–100 samples. However, techniques have been developed recently that allow single samples to be tested economically, with results available in an hour. This means that if the test equipment is installed close to the ultrasound unit, combined serum and ultrasound results can be reported together. Concurrent screening can also be performed without such equipment provided a blood sample is obtained a few days before the scheduled scan appointment and arrangements made to ensure that the serum MoMs are available for risk calculation as soon as the NT or NF are measured.

Table 22.4 shows the effect of adding concurrent NT to the first-trimester serum combinations in Table 22.3. For a 5 percent false-positive rate the detection rate increases to 85.8 to 90.5 percent. With two serum markers the best results are at 10 weeks of gestation, although there is a 2 percent difference between gestations. With four serum markers, the gestational differences disappear almost entirely. Because NF is a weaker marker than NT, the effect of adding concurrent NF to second-trimester serum combinations, shown in Table 22.5, is not as great. For a 5 percent false-positive rate, the detection rate ranges from 72.3 to 81.9 percent, a narrower difference between the combinations than those shown in Table 22.2.

Nondisclosure Sequential Screening: Serum and Ultrasound

Combining an NT scan with a second-trimester serum sample yields results similar to those of concurrent first-trimester screening. Table 22.6 shows that for a 5 percent false-positive rate the detection rate ranges from 82.1 to 90.5 percent. For the widespread second-trimester free β-hCG and AFP combination, the sequential screening detection rate is 87.2 percent, almost as high as for concurrent PAPP-A and free β-hCG at 10 weeks of gestation. First-

Table 22.4. First-trimester concurrent screening: two or four maternal serum markers at 10–13 weeks of gestation and NT at 11–13 weeks of gestation

| | Cutoff Risk (at Term) | | | | | | | | | |
| | DR for FPR | | FPR for DR | | 1 in 200 | | 1 in 250 | | 1 in 300 | |
Serum	1%	5%	75%	85%	DR	FPR	DR	FPR	DR	FPR
10 weeks										
PAPP-A and free β	76.8	88.0	0.8	3.2	80.2	1.6	81.8	2.1	83.1	2.5
+AFP and uE$_3$	80.2	90.5	0.5	2.0	82.6	1.4	84.0	1.8	85.2	2.1
11 weeks										
PAPP-A and free β	75.2	86.6	1.0	4.0	79.2	1.8	80.8	2.2	82.1	2.6
+AFP and uE$_3$	79.5	89.9	0.6	2.3	82.2	1.5	83.7	1.9	84.9	2.2
12 weeks										
PAPP-A and free β	74.3	85.8	1.1	4.5	78.5	1.8	80.1	2.3	81.5	2.7
+AFP and uE$_3$	80.7	90.4	0.6	2.0	83.3	1.5	84.7	1.9	85.8	2.2
13 weeks										
PAPP-A and free β	74.7	86.1	1.1	4.3	78.9	1.8	80.5	2.3	81.8	2.7
+AFP and uE$_3$	80.6	90.5	0.6	2.0	83.4	1.5	84.8	1.9	85.8	2.3
Inhibin and free β	73.8	85.8	1.2	4.5	78.6	1.9	80.4	2.4	81.8	2.9
+AFP and uE$_3$	80.5	90.4	0.6	2.0	83.4	1.6	84.7	1.9	85.8	2.3

DR = detection rate; FPR = false-positive rate.

Table 22.5. Second-trimester concurrent screening: two to four maternal serum markers and NF scanning at 14–18 weeks of gestation

| | Cutoff Risk (at Term) | | | | | | | | | |
| | DR for FPR | | FPR for DR | | 1 in 200 | | 1 in 250 | | 1 in 300 | |
Serum	1%	5%	75%	85%	DR	FPR	DR	FPR	DR	FPR
hCG and AFP	56.2	72.3	6.4	16.1	65.6	2.6	70.3	4.1	72.0	4.9
+uE$_3$	60.3	75.5	4.8	13.2	68.6	2.5	70.8	3.1	72.7	3.8
+uE$_3$ and inhibin	65.8	80.2	2.8	8.7	73.3	2.3	75.3	2.9	78.3	4.1
Free β-hCG and AFP	57.2	73.9	5.5	13.5	67.1	2.7	69.8	3.5	73.9	5.0
+uE$_3$	61.8	77.4	4.0	10.9	70.3	2.5	72.6	3.1	74.6	3.8
+uE$_3$ and inhibin	67.6	81.9	2.3	7.2	74.9	2.3	76.9	2.8	78.5	3.4

DR = detection rate; FPR = false-positive rate.

trimester serum testing followed by second-trimester NF is more effective than concurrent second-trimester screening, with a detection rate range of 74.7 to 83.3 percent (Table 22.7).

Nondisclosure Sequential Screening: Two Serum Samples

Table 22.8 shows the performance of three to five serum marker policies using first-trimester PAPP-A and three different second-trimester combinations. Because the efficiency of PAPP-A decreases with gestation, the detection rates for all combinations are much higher when it is measured at 10 weeks. If testing is always done at this optimal time, the detection rate for a 5 percent false-positive rate is 73.7 to 80.6 percent. This represents a 9 percent increase in detection compared with testing a single sample for four markers at either 10 or 14–18 weeks of gestation.

Table 22.6. Nondisclosure sequential screening: NT at 11–13 weeks of gestation and two to four maternal serum markers at 14–18 weeks of gestation

	Cutoff Risk (at Term)									
	DR for FPR		FPR for DR		1 in 200		1 in 250		1 in 300	
Serum	1%	5%	75%	85%	DR	FPR	DR	FPR	DR	FPR
hCG and AFP	70.1	82.1	2.0	7.3	74.8	1.9	76.5	2.4	77.9	2.9
+uE$_3$	76.9	87.2	0.8	3.5	80.2	1.7	81.7	2.1	82.9	2.5
+uE$_3$ and inhibin	79.9	89.3	0.6	2.4	82.5	1.6	83.8	1.9	84.9	2.3
Free β-hCG and AFP	75.7	87.2	0.9	3.7	79.8	1.8	81.4	2.2	82.8	2.7
+uE$_3$	78.2	88.7	0.6	2.8	81.4	1.6	83.0	2.1	84.1	2.4
+uE$_3$ and inhibin	81.1	90.5	0.6	1.9	83.6	1.5	84.9	1.9	85.9	2.2

DR = detection rate; FPR = false-positive rate.

Table 22.7. Nondisclosure sequential screening: two or four maternal serum markers at 10–13 weeks of gestation and NF scanning at 14–18 weeks of gestation

	Cutoff Risk (at Term)									
	DR for FPR		FPR for DR		1 in 200		1 in 250		1 in 300	
Serum	1%	5%	75%	85%	DR	FPR	DR	FPR	DR	FPR
10 weeks										
PAPP-A and free β	61.2	78.7	3.6	9.1	71.3	2.5	73.9	3.2	75.9	3.9
+AFP and uE$_3$	66.9	83.3	2.2	6.0	75.1	2.2	77.3	2.7	79.2	3.3
11 weeks										
PAPP-A and free β	58.7	76.3	4.6	11.1	69.5	2.7	72.1	3.4	74.3	4.2
+AFP and uE$_3$	65.9	82.1	2.4	6.8	74.5	2.3	76.7	2.9	78.6	3.5
12 weeks										
PAPP-A and free β	57.1	74.7	5.1	12.5	68.1	2.8	70.9	3.6	73.0	4.3
+AFP and uE$_3$	67.9	83.0	2.1	6.3	75.8	2.3	77.9	2.9	79.6	3.4
13 weeks										
PAPP-A and free β	57.7	75.5	4.8	11.8	68.9	2.8	71.6	3.6	73.8	4.3
+AFP and uE$_3$	67.5	83.1	2.2	6.2	76.0	2.4	78.1	3.0	79.8	3.5
Inhibin and free β	56.0	74.7	5.1	11.8	68.8	3.1	71.7	3.9	74.0	4.7
+AFP and uE$_3$	67.5	83.1	2.2	6.2	76.0	2.4	78.2	3.0	80.0	3.6

DR = detection rate; FPR = false-positive rate.

Table 22.8. Nondisclosure sequential screening: PAPP-A at 10–13 weeks of gestation and two to four maternal serum markers 14–18 weeks of gestation

14–18 Week Serum Markers	Cutoff Risk (at Term)									
	DR for FPR		FPR for DR		1 in 200		1 in 250		1 in 300	
	1%	5%	75%	85%	DR	FPR	DR	FPR	DR	FPR
PAPP-A at 10 weeks										
Free β-hCG and AFP	54.9	73.7	5.6	13.4	67.5	3.0	70.3	3.8	72.5	4.5
+uE$_3$	57.5	75.4	4.9	12.2	69.0	2.8	71.5	3.6	73.6	4.3
+uE$_3$ and inhibin	64.3	80.6	2.9	7.9	73.9	2.6	76.1	3.2	78.0	3.8
PAPP-A at 11 weeks										
Free β-hCG and AFP	51.7	70.9	7.0	15.8	65.1	3.2	68.1	4.0	70.4	4.8
+uE$_3$	54.6	72.9	6.0	14.3	66.7	3.0	69.5	3.7	71.8	4.5
+uE$_3$ and inhibin	61.7	78.8	3.5	9.2	72.2	2.7	74.7	3.4	76.5	4.0
PAPP-A at 12 weeks										
Free β-hCG and AFP	47.0	67.2	8.9	18.6	62.0	3.4	65.3	4.3	67.9	5.3
+uE$_3$	50.7	70.0	7.4	16.5	64.2	3.2	67.2	4.0	69.7	4.9
+uE$_3$ and inhibin	58.3	76.5	4.4	10.8	70.3	2.9	72.9	3.7	75.0	4.4
PAPP-A at 13 weeks										
Free β-hCG and AFP	44.2	65.2	9.8	19.6	60.4	3.6	64.0	3.6	66.9	5.6
+uE$_3$	48.4	68.6	8.1	17.2	63.1	3.3	66.2	4.2	69.0	5.2
+uE$_3$ and inhibin	56.4	75.6	4.8	11.2	69.6	3.1	72.5	3.9	74.7	4.6

DR = detection rate; FPR = false-positive rate.

Nondisclosure Sequential Screening: Two Sera and Ultrasound

With the addition of NT to two serum sample strategies, there is a smaller detection rate differential according to when PAPP-A is tested (Table 22.9). At the optimal 10-week gestation, the detection rate for a 5 percent false-positive rate is 93.5 percent if four second-trimester markers are used, 3 percent higher than for concurrent first-trimester screening with four markers. For a 1 percent false-positive rate the detection rate is 6 percent higher. If PAPP-A is tested at 13 weeks, the improvement in detection is less than half that at 10 weeks.

It is important to note that this extra detection accrues, not from an additional sample but from the use of five instead of four serum markers. Several new markers are currently being developed, and it is possible that in the future a similar detection rate could be achieved by concurrent screening. This would only require a fifth marker with a Mahalinobis distance of about 1.

The addition of NF to two serum sample strategies substantially increases detection compared with concurrent second-trimester screening with four markers (Table 22.10). When PAPP-A is tested at 13 weeks, the detection rate for a 5 percent false-positive rate is increased by about 6 percent; for 1 percent false-positives the increase is 8 percent. At 10 weeks the increases are 2 percent and 3 percent, respectively.

Stepwise Sequential Screening

With sequential combinations involving long waiting times for reporting results, it is difficult for the professional not to act on intermediate findings that would by themselves be screen-positive. This is particularly so for NT, for which stepwise rather than nondisclosure sequential screening is likely to be the norm, if not the official policy.

Table 22.9. Nondisclosure sequential screening: PAPP-A at 10–13 weeks of gestation, NT at 11–13 weeks of gestation, and two to four maternal serum markers at 14–18 weeks of gestation

14–18 Week Serum Markers	Cutoff Risk (at Term)									
	DR for FPR		FPR for DR		1 in 200		1 in 250		1 in 300	
	1%	5%	75%	85%	DR	FPR	DR	FPR	DR	FPR
PAPP-A at 10 weeks										
Free β-hCG and AFP	82.4	91.1	0.5	1.6	84.4	1.4	85.5	1.7	86.4	2.0
+uE$_3$	83.3	91.6	0.5	1.4	84.9	1.3	86.0	1.7	86.9	2.0
+uE$_3$ and inhibin	86.2	93.5	0.5	0.8	87.1	1.2	88.1	1.5	89.0	1.8
PAPP-A at 11 weeks										
Free β-hCG and AFP	81.0	90.2	0.6	2.0	83.3	1.5	84.6	1.8	85.6	2.2
+uE$_3$	82.1	90.8	0.5	1.7	84.0	1.4	85.2	1.7	86.2	2.1
+uE$_3$ and inhibin	85.1	92.8	0.5	1.0	86.4	1.3	87.5	1.6	88.3	1.9
PAPP-A at 12 weeks										
Free β-hCG and AFP	79.2	89.1	0.6	2.5	82.1	1.6	83.5	2.0	84.5	2.3
+uE$_3$	80.6	89.9	0.6	2.1	83.0	1.5	84.3	1.9	85.3	2.2
+uE$_3$ and inhibin	83.8	92.1	0.6	1.2	85.5	1.4	86.7	1.7	87.6	2.0
PAPP-A at 13 weeks										
Free β-hCG and AFP	78.2	88.5	0.6	2.8	81.4	1.6	82.9	2.0	84.0	2.4
+uE$_3$	79.8	89.5	0.6	2.3	82.5	1.5	83.8	1.9	84.9	2.3
+uE$_3$ and inhibin	83.1	91.8	0.6	1.4	85.1	1.4	86.3	1.8	87.3	2.1

DR = detection rate; FPR = false-positive rate.

Table 22.10. Nondisclosure sequential screening: PAPP-A at 10–13 weeks of gestation: two to four maternal serum markers and NF at 14–18 weeks of gestation

14–18 Week Serum Markers	Cutoff Risk (at Term)									
	DR for FPR		FPR for DR		1 in 200		1 in 250		1 in 300	
	1%	5%	75%	85%	DR	FPR	DR	FPR	DR	FPR
PAPP-A at 10 weeks										
Free β-hCG and AFP	68.6	82.5	2.1	6.8	75.2	2.2	77.2	2.7	78.8	3.3
uE$_3$	70.5	83.5	1.8	6.0	76.3	2.0	78.1	2.6	79.6	3.1
+uE$_3$ and inhibin	75.9	87.6	0.9	3.4	80.5	1.9	82.1	2.3	83.4	2.7
PAPP-A at 11 weeks										
Free β-hCG and AFP	66.5	80.8	2.6	8.1	73.6	2.2	75.8	2.8	77.3	3.4
+uE$_3$	68.7	82.2	2.1	7.1	75.0	2.1	76.9	2.7	78.4	3.2
+uE$_3$ and inhibin	74.1	86.3	1.1	4.2	79.3	2.0	80.9	2.4	82.3	2.9
PAPP-A at 12 weeks										
Free β-hCG and AFP	63.4	78.3	3.5	10.2	71.2	2.4	73.6	3.0	75.4	3.7
+uE$_3$	66.0	80.1	2.8	8.8	73.0	2.2	75.0	2.8	76.7	3.4
+uE$_3$ and inhibin	71.8	84.8	1.5	5.1	77.8	2.1	79.6	2.6	81.0	3.1
PAPP-A at 13 weeks										
Free β-hCG and AFP	61.7	77.0	4.1	11.3	70.0	2.4	72.4	3.1	74.4	3.8
+uE$_3$	64.8	79.4	3.1	9.3	72.3	2.3	74.5	2.9	76.2	3.5
+uE$_3$ and inhibin	70.7	84.3	1.7	5.5	77.3	2.2	79.1	2.7	80.6	3.2

DR = detection rate; FPR = false-positive rate.

Table 22.11. Stepwise screening with NT followed by maternal serum free β-hCG, AFP, and uE_3, according to cutoff

Strategy	Cutoff (at Term)	Detection Rate (%)	False-positive Rate (%)
Stepwise	1 in 200	84.0	3.1
Nondisclosure		84.0	2.4
		85.6	3.1
Stepwise	1 in 250	86.0	4.8
Nondisclosure		86.0	3.3
		88.4	4.8
Stepwise	1 in 300	86.7	5.3
Nondisclosure		86.7	3.6
		89.1	5.3

To exemplify this, we consider a stepwise sequential policy, whereby NT is acted on if the risk is above the cutoff and a second-trimester serum test is carried out only in women with negative results. Table 22.11 shows that this will increase the false-positive rate for the same detection rate in comparison with nondisclosure screening. Moreover, for that many false-positives, nondisclosure screening would achieve a much higher detection rate.

In some centers, stepwise screening is carried out by default because the provision of ultrasound NT screening and second-trimester serum screening services are by different units. Moreover, this uncoordinated approach often leads to erroneous risk calculation when the NT is not taken into account when interpreting the serum result.

Contingent Screening

There is little likelihood of a very low risk result based on first-trimester screening becoming screen-positive when second-trimester tests are done. This line of reasoning might suggest a type of contingent screening whereby a stepwise policy is adopted, except that only those with borderline risks have second-trimester tests. However, the loss of efficiency is even greater than for stepwise screening. Table 22.12 exemplifies this, with the same markers as Table 22.11 and a 1 in 250 cutoff. Even when as many as one-fifth are in the borderline zone the loss of detection is substantial.

Prospective Intervention Studies

In general, statistical modeling may be a useful technique for comparing competing policy options, but models rest on many assumptions and need to be validated. In the current context there are two questions to be addressed: How reliable are the model-predicted DR and FPR values? and How accurate are the individual risk estimates? There are sufficient published results to show that both aspects of modeling are robust, but two problems need to be considered before this can be demonstrated.

First, the observed detection rate in DS screening intervention studies is necessarily an overestimate of the true rate because of the nonviability bias described above in relation to mean NT estimation. One unbiased estimate is derived from the observed numbers of DS cases: screen detected terminated (n_1) or not (n_2), missed by screening but terminated subsequently (n_3) or born (n_4); using the formula $(n_1 * p + n_2)/(n_1 * p + n_2 + n_3 * p + n_4)$, where p is the intrauterine survival rate for DS at the time of prenatal di-

Table 22.12. Contingent screening with NT followed by maternal serum free β-hCG, AFP, and uE$_3$ and 1 in 250 cutoff, according to borderline

Strategy	Borderline Risk (at Term)	Needing Serum (%)	Detection Rate (%)	False-positive Rate (%)
Contingent	1 in 250–500	2.7	76.7	4.2
Nondisclosure			76.7	0.6
			89.5	4.2
Contingent	1 in 250–1000	8.2	79.1	4.3
Nondisclosure			79.1	0.7
			89.6	4.3
Contingent	1 in 250–1500	13.5	80.6	4.4
Nondisclosure			80.6	0.9
			89.8	4.4
Contingent	1 in 250–2000	19.7	82.2	4.5
Nondisclosure			82.2	1.2
			89.9	4.5

agnosis. Another approach is to calculate the expected number of DS births, given the maternal age distribution of screened women, e, and use the formula $1 - (n_2 + n_4)/e$.

Second, the confidence limits on a DR estimate in even the largest intervention study will be quite large, and meta-analysis of all published studies would seem to be the best option. Although screening protocols differ markedly in terms of marker combination, cutoff, and maternal age distribution, pooling the results, with suitable adjustment for viability bias, is a guide to actual performance. Nevertheless detailed comparisons, say between centers using two markers and those using three, are probably precluded.

In Table 22.2 there are twenty-five large second-trimester serum studies using combinations that can be analyzed.[67–74] The results for a total of 1,324,000 screened women, including 1,691 observed with DS, yield an observed detection rate of 72 percent, equivalent to 66 percent after allowance for bias, and a false-positive rate of 6.2 percent. In thirteen of the studies, information on the uptake of screening was also given, and the overall uptake rate was 81 percent. In twenty-two studies the proportion of those with screen-positive results who went on to have prenatal diagnosis was also given, and it was 77 percent overall. However, it was not always clear if those who did not have the procedure refused the offer or had a revision of risk following ultrasound examination.

Of the many studies using NT without serum markers, only five expressed the results in terms of risk.[40,75–78] The combined results include a total of 141,000 screened women, of whom 631 were observed to have a DS infant. This yielded an observed detection rate of 84 percent, equivalent to 72 percent after allowance for bias, and a false-positive rate of 8.9 percent. There have so far been five studies with concurrent serum markers[79–83]: 41,000 women, 173 DS, 90 percent observed and 82 percent unbiased detection rate, with a 6.1 percent false-positive rate.

In nine studies the results were published in such a way that the accuracy of individual risk estimation could be assessed as well as overall performance.[40,84–91] These studies broke down the results into groups according to the estimated risk used on the test report. For each group, the average risk was given together with the observed DS prevalence, adjusted for viability bias. They all found that the estimated risk was close to the observed value.

ADDITIONAL MARKERS

First-trimester NT and second-trimester NF measurements are not made in isolation. Particularly in the second trimester, the scan may also reveal a marker in the ears, nose, hands, heart, long bones, kidneys, brain, or bowel. To incorporate them into risk screening, LRs would be needed in addition to some measure of association with the existing markers.

Unlike with ultrasound, the extension of biochemical screening to include less discriminatory markers is restricted by financial considerations. Therefore, although it may be reasonable to consider the benefits of adding a fifth biochemical marker to concurrent screening strategies, this is unlikely to happen unless a large incremental gain in detection or reduction in the false-positive rate is predicted.

Nasal Bone

This is the most promising additional marker at present. Four nonintervention prospective studies have found that absence of the nasal bone (NB) on ultrasound examination at 11–13 weeks is a highly discriminating DS marker.[92–95] In the first study, carried out in women about to have prenatal diagnosis because of positive NT screening, the DR was 73 percent (43 of 59) and FPR 0.5 percent (3 of 603).[92] This series was later extended, and the rates in the new cases were 69 percent (50 of 72) and 0.4 percent (1 of 248), respectively.[93] In the other studies, the rates were: 60 percent (3 of 5) and 0.6 percent (1 of 175)[94]; 70 percent (19 of 27), and 0.6 percent (34 of 5,525).[95] Combining the four studies, absence of NB is associated with a 120-fold LR, and presence reduces risk 3.4-fold.

Table 22.13 shows that there is a substantial increase in detection as a consequence of adding NB to three policies involving NT: PAPP-A at 10 weeks with four serum markers at 14–18 weeks, concurrent first-trimester screening at 10 weeks, and NT alone. The benefits of concurrent serum testing over ultrasound screening alone are still large: 4–7 percent, depending on the false-positive rate. But the benefits of sequential over concurrent screening are reduced to 1–2 percent.

The modeling assumes that NB is uncorrelated with NT or the serum markers. Because of the study design this cannot be verified directly, but in the DS pregnancies, the median NT was similar for those with and those without NB, so a general correlation is unlikely. A correlation between NB and the serum markers is unlikely because NT is not correlated with them. If a correlation is eventually found, this can be incorporated into

Table 22.13.   Addition of ultrasound NB determination* to the four best policies

Markers (weeks)	Nasal Bone	DR for FPR		
		0.5%	1%	5%
PAPP-A (10); NT (11–13); free β, AFP, uE$_3$, inhibin (14–18)	No	82.6	86.2	93.5
	Yes	93.3	95.0	97.9
PAPP-A, free β, AFP, uE$_3$ (10); NT (11–13)	No	75.4	80.2	90.5
	Yes	90.5	93.0	96.9
NT alone (11–13)	No	59.7	64.5	76.1
	Yes	82.9	87.8	92.7
Free β, AFP, uE$_3$, inhibin, NF (14–18)	No	61.9	67.6	81.9
	Yes	79.4	83.8	92.2

DR = detection rate; FPR = false-positive rate.
*With NT at 11–13 weeks for NB absence; with NF at 14–18 weeks for hypoplasia.

the model, but experience with other markers shows that the detection rate is not particularly sensitive to such correlations.

NB measurement rather than absence per se may also be a marker, but not until the second trimester. In a first-trimester series of seventy-nine cases, fifty-four of which had absent nasal bone, the remaining twenty-five had normal NB length.[96] However, there have been three reports of reduced NB length later in pregnancy. A case report of three DS pregnancies has been described in which two had absent NB and the third had nasal size below the normal 2.5th centile.[97] In a preamniocentesis series at 15–22 weeks of gestation, nasal hypoplasia, defined as absence or length under 2.5 mm, was found in 62 percent (21 of 34) of cases and 1.2 percent (12 of 982) of unaffected pregnancies.[98] In a series of women referred to a tertiary ultrasound center at 15–20 weeks, 38 percent (6 of 16) cases had absent NB and all of the remainder had a high BPD/NB ratio.[99] Among the 223 unaffected pregnancies, one had absent NB and 22 percent had a high ratio. More information is needed on the distribution of NB length, preferably in MoMs before the efficiency of the marker can be modeled. However, simply using the results from the second study to determine likelihood ratios for those with and without hypoplasia shows that a large increase in detection can be expected (see Table 22.13).

Long Bones

The short stature associated with children with Down syndrome is reflected in utero by smaller-than-average long bones measured by ultrasound. There have been proposals to incorporate into serum screening protocols either humerus length (HL)[100] or femur length (FL), HL, and NF.[44] Some studies report FL and HL results in MoMs, but many use the transformation biparietal diameter (BPD)/FL or BPD/HL, which change with gestation and so themselves need to by expressed in MoMs.

There are five papers from which FL or FL/BPD in MoMs can be derived,[44,101–105] yielding an overall mean of 0.94 MoM and Mahalinobis distance 0.80. No correlations with NF or serum markers can be assumed until the small correlations with uE_3 in DS and with AFP in unaffected pregnancies can be confirmed.[44] Modeling predicts that the detection rate for fixed false-positive rates when FL is added to NF and four marker serum screening is under 2 percent: 83.4 percent for a 5 percent false-positive rate and 69.3 percent for 1 percent.

There is a high degree of correlation between FL and HL, and one modeling exercise estimated that incorporating them both into the protocol increased detection by under 1 percent.[44]

Ductus Venosus Doppler

In one study, both color Doppler examination and NT measurement were carried out in 18 DS and 343 unaffected pregnancies.[106] Using NT alone, with a 95th centile cutoff, the observed detection rate was 89 percent (16 of 18) with a false-positive rate of 4.7 percent (16 of 343). Using Doppler alone, considering the result positive if there was absent or reverse flow, the detection and false-positive rates were 100 percent (18 of 18) and 2.0 percent (7 of 343). This does suggest a potential benefit, but there is evidence of correlation with NT.[107] There was abnormal atrial contraction velocity in 70 percent of 34 pregnancies with chromosomal abnormalities and NT above the 95th centile, 30 percent of 119 with raised NT and normal karyotype, and just 1 percent of 174 with NT under the 95th centile.

Pregnancy-Specific Glycoprotein (SP)-1

Maternal serum SP-1 levels are on average reduced in the first trimester and increased in the second. The average level in a total of 111 published cases at 10–14 weeks of gestation is 0.81 MoM and in 379 at 15–22 weeks 1.47 MoM.[108] The use of SP-1 as a fifth first-trimester serum marker would increase the detection rate by only about 1 percent, whereas in the second trimester there would be a 2–4 percent increase.[109] The first-trimester results would probably be better if samples were taken earlier than 11 weeks of gestation because there is a tendency for the average level in DS pregnancies to become closer to 1 MoM as the first trimester advances.

Urinary hCG Species

There are several markers of DS in maternal urine. Although there is the additional complication of standardizing for concentration, as determined by the creatinine level, some of them have screening potential, and a combination of urine and serum screening could be considered.

The urine marker that has been most studied so far is the β-core fragment of hCG, its major metabolic product. In the second trimester of pregnancy the mean based on a meta-analysis of seven studies,[110] extended to include two additional studies,[29,111] is 3.70 MoM with a Mahalinobis distance of 1.51. Levels are also raised in the first trimester, but to a much lesser extent. Other urinary hCG species, intact hCG, free β-hCG, and hyperglycosylated hCG, also known as invasive trophoblast antigen or ITA, are also elevated on average in affected pregnancies, while maternal urine total estrogen and total estriol levels are reduced.

When all the hCG species are measured in the same samples, ITA appears to be the most discriminatory.[29] A preamniocentesis study estimated the screening efficiency of combining second-trimester serum AFP, uE$_3$, and hCG with urinary ITA and β-core hCG plus ultrasound NT, HL, and anomalies.[112] Among 568 women, 17 of whom had fetuses with DS, the detection rate for 5 percent false-positives was 94 percent. Another study estimated that for an 85 percent detection rate, the false-positive rate of first- and second-trimester serum combinations with and without NT would be reduced by about one-third if urinary ITA is also measured.[29]

However, caution is needed in interpreting urine results because there is significant heterogeneity between the published studies, probably because of differences in assay method, study design, and the integrity of urine samples during transport and storage. Maternal serum ITA is also a marker of DS,[113] but more studies are needed before it can be considered as a simpler and more reliable alternative to urinary ITA.

Fetal Cells

It is now well established that there is fetal DNA circulation in the maternal blood in most pregnancies (see chapter 28). This can be demonstrated using PCR to amplify Y-chromosome-specific sequences when the fetus is male. In principle, the DNA could be used to diagnose DS, and several techniques are being developed to do this. The methodologic problem is to extract sufficient fetal DNA while minimizing maternal DNA contamination. The methods tried so far are expensive and not sufficiently reliable to compete with biochemical or ultrasound screening, but this may change.

INDIVIDUAL PERFORMANCE

The DR and FPR figures in Tables 22.2 to 22.13 predict screening performance for the population as a whole. This is important for public health planners, who need to know the best or at least the most cost-effective strategy. But for pretest counseling, the individual woman needs to know the DR and FPR specific for her age, and since the prior risk increases with age, it necessarily follows that for any risk cutoff, both the DR and FPR will also increase. Table 22.14 shows the values for five maternal ages and four policies. The effect of maternal age is less for the more efficient screening policies because it is an increasingly minor variable in the risk calculation.

There are two identifiable subgroups of women, those with twins and those with a previous affected pregnancy, whose age-specific DR and FPR will be substantially different from Table 22.14. There are also subgroups whose screening performance will be

Table 22.14. Screening efficacy for four policies at five selected maternal ages

Markers (weeks of gestation)	Maternal Age									
	25		30		35		40		45	
	DR	FPR	DR	FPR	DR	FPR	DR	FPR	DR	FPR
Cutoff 1 in 200[a]										
PAPP-A (10); NT (11–13); free β, AFP, uE$_3$, inhibin (14–18)	82.6	0.7	84.8	1.1	88.9	2.4	93.7	7.1	97.3	19.9
PAPP-A, free β, AFP, uE$_3$ (10), NT (11–13)	76.2	0.8	79.0	1.2	85.3	3.0	92.3	9.0	97.1	24.8
Free β, AFP, uE$_3$, inhibin, NF (14–18)	65.8	1.3	69.7	1.9	78.4	4.9	88.7	15.1	96.7	43.9
Free β, AFP, uE$_3$, inhibin (14–18)	51.7	1.6	59.4	3.0	71.8	7.2	87.4	23.0	96.9	56.6
Cutoff 1 in 250										
PAPP-A (10); NT (11–13); free β, AFP, uE$_3$, inhibin (14–18)	83.7	0.9	85.9	1.4	89.9	3.0	94.4	8.3	97.8	23.3
PAPP-A, free β, AFP, uE$_3$ (10); NT (11–13)	77.9	1.1	80.6	1.5	86.6	3.6	93.2	10.6	97.6	28.6
Free β, AFP, uE$_3$, inhibin, NF (14–18)	67.8	1.6	72.0	2.5	80.1	5.9	90.3	18.4	97.5	50.4
Free β, AFP, uE$_3$, inhibin (14–18)	55.6	2.2	61.5	3.5	74.6	8.8	89.1	26.4	97.8	63.7
Cutoff 1 in 300										
PAPP-A (10); NT (11–13); free β, AFP, uE$_3$, inhibin (14–18)	84.9	1.1	86.8	1.6	90.7	3.5	95.0	9.7	98.0	26.0
PAPP-A, free β, AFP, uE$_3$ (10); NT (11–13)	79.0	1.2	81.9	1.8	87.7	4.3	93.9	12.0	98.0	32.6
Free β, AFP, uE$_3$, inhibin, NF (14–18)	69.9	2.0	73.5	2.9	81.8	7.0	91.6	21.6	98.1	56.3
Free β, AFP, uE$_3$, inhibin (14–18)	59.5	3.0	64.2	4.2	77.2	10.7	91.1	31.2	98.4	69.2

DR = detection rate; FPR = false-positive rate.
[a]At term.

altered unless special care is taken with the interpretation of their test, including those who have undergone assisted reproduction, with certain maternal disorders, those who have had a previous false-positive screening result, smokers, and those from certain ethnic minorities.

Twins

In spontaneous pregnancies the rate of twinning increases with age, and depending on the maternal age distribution and the extent of assisted reproduction in the population, some 1–2 percent of pregnancies are twins. The interpretation of a DS screening test in twins differs from singletons, and at all ages the screening efficiency is lower.

Despite the presence of two fetuses, the risk of an affected pregnancy appears to be the same as in singletons. The birth prevalence of DS can be estimated by meta-analysis of five cohort studies, including 106 DS twins.[114,115] The estimate is only 3 percent higher than the prevalence in singletons. None of the studies were stratified for maternal age, and the chance of having a twin increases with age. Therefore, the observed small increase in the crude DS prevalence rate among twins implies a reduction in the age-specific prevalence. However, until there is a more precise estimate of these rates, it is reasonable to assume that the prior term risk for twins does not differ from that of singletons. There are no data on the prior risk during pregnancy.

In unaffected twin pregnancies, the average serum marker level is increased about twofold, whereas the other distribution parameters appear to be the same as in singletons. In one meta-analysis the values for AFP, uE_3, hCG, and free β-hCG are 2.26, 1.68, 2.06, and 2.07 MoM, respectively.[116] There is only one study of inhibin A in twins with a median of 1.99 MoM,[117] and combining three studies of PAPP-A, the average is 1.96 MoM.[118–120] The marker distribution parameters in twins in whom one or both of the fetuses has DS cannot be estimated directly because there are insufficient published data. An indirect method has been described that assumes that each fetus contributes the expected amount for an affected or an unaffected singleton and that the same deviation from expectation seen in unaffected twins also applies.[116] The average NT level in twins appeared to be similar to that in singletons,[121–123] and the same is assumed for NF.

When NT is used alone, each fetus is treated like a separate singleton, except that the prior risk to each fetus is half the age-specific risk in singletons. The practice is to use the CRL for each fetus to calculate its own gestation for using MoMs. When biochemistry alone is used, a reasonable approximation of risk can be derived from the discordant parameters because affected concordance is infrequent: 12 percent (9 of 75) in one series.[124] Alternatively, the weighted average of concordant and discordant LRs can be used, although the concordance rate is likely to alter with age. Although for NT it might be best to calculate fetus-specific gestations, with biochemistry it makes sense to use the larger of the two CRLs to estimate overall gestation if MoMs are to be used.

When both NT and biochemistry are available, risk can be calculated separately for each fetus or an overall risk that at least one fetus is affected can be calculated. The latter can be calculated from the sum of the two individual NT LRs multiplied by the biochemistry LR, taking account of zygosity. The ultrasound "lambda" sign, caused by invasion of the intertwin membrane by chorionic villi, can be determined at the NT scan and will accurately estimate zygosity.[125]

Table 22.15 shows the age-specific DR and FPR for different screening strategies in twins, based on the proportion of twins in the United States. Whites that are monozygous:

Table 22.15. Twin pregnancy: screening efficiency for four policies at five selected maternal ages

| Markers (weeks) | Maternal Age | | | | | | | | | |
| | 25 | | 30 | | 35 | | 40 | | 45 | |
	DR	FPR	DR	FPR	DR	FPR	DR	FPR	DR	FPR
Cutoff 1 in 200[a]										
PAPP-A (10); NT (11–13); free β, AFP, uE$_3$, inhibin (14–18)	66.1	0.7	71.3	1.2	78.7	3.3	87.2	9.8	95.7	38.1
PAPP-A, free β, AFP, uE$_3$ (10); NT (11–13)	65.9	0.8	69.4	1.4	76.9	3.6	84.9	10.7	95.6	45.1
Free β, AFP, uE$_3$, inhibin, NF (14–18)	47.8	0.9	52.4	1.7	62.8	4.8	81.0	21.2	98.0	80.6
Free β, AFP, uE$_3$, inhibin (14–18)	17.4	0.6	21.9	1.3	39.9	6.0	81.2	40.6	99.4	94.5
Cutoff 1 in 250										
PAPP-A (10); NT (11–13); free β, AFP, uE$_3$, inhibin (14–18)	70.1	0.9	73.3	1.5	80.6	4.2	88.5	11.8	96.7	46.2
PAPP-A, free β, AFP, uE$_3$ (10); NT (11–13)	68.3	1.1	71.7	1.8	78.5	4.4	86.9	14.0	96.6	52.8
Free β, AFP, uE$_3$, inhibin, NF (14–18)	50.8	1.3	55.2	2.2	65.8	6.2	84.1	27.0	99.0	88.6
Free β, AFP, uE$_3$, inhibin (14–18)	20.0	1.0	25.4	1.9	46.5	8.5	86.6	50.9	99.6	96.9
Cutoff 1 in 300										
PAPP-A (10); NT (11–13); free β, AFP, uE$_3$, inhibin (14–18)	71.8	1.2	75.0	1.9	82.0	5.0	89.7	14.0	97.5	53.4
PAPP-A, free β, AFP, uE$_3$ (10); NT (11–13)	69.9	1.4	73.7	2.3	79.6	5.1	88.3	17.1	97.5	59.7
Free β, AFP, uE$_3$, inhibin, NF (14–18)	52.9	1.7	57.2	2.7	68.2	7.5	86.9	33.1	99.5	93.0
Free β, AFP, uE$_3$, inhibin (14–18)	22.8	1.4	28.9	2.6	53.8	12.5	89.9	58.8	99.7	97.9

DR = detection rate; FPR = false-positive rate.
[a]At term.

16 percent, 13 percent, 10 percent, 9.7 percent, and 5.5 percent at ages 25, 30, 35, 40, and 45, respectively.[126] For all policies, screening efficiency is much lower in twins than in singletons and is extremely low for policies that do not involve NT or NF.

Previous Affected Pregnancy

Women who have had a DS pregnancy are at increased risk of recurrence. Some will consider the risk sufficiently high to warrant invasive prenatal diagnosis without screening. Others will want to have their risk assessed by screening before making this decision.

In a small proportion of cases there will be a parental structural chromosome rearrangement, and the recurrence risk can be quite high, depending on the specific parental genotype. The most frequent is a heterozygous Robertsonian balanced translocation, and for female carriers the risk is great enough to dwarf the age-specific risk at most ages. For example, among 185 amniocenteses in such women, 15 percent of fetuses had a translocation.[127] In contrast, male carriers of a balanced translocation do not appear to have a high risk; all seventy amniotic fluid samples in the same study had a normal karyotype.

If a woman has had a previous pregnancy with DS and the additional chromosome 21 was not inherited, there is still an increased risk of recurrence. There are three available estimates of excess risk. In an unpublished study of more than 2,500 women who had first-trimester invasive prenatal diagnosis, the excess risk compared with the maternal-age specific expected risk was 0.75 percent (Nicolaides K, personal communication). In a meta-analysis of second-trimester amniocentesis results in 4,953 pregnancies, the excess was 0.54 percent.[128] A meta-analysis of 433 livebirths had 5 recurrences, an excess risk of 0.52 percent.[129] The weighted average of these rates, allowing for fetal losses, is 0.77 percent in the first trimester, 0.54 percent in the second, and 0.42 percent at term and can be added to the age-specific risk expressed as a probability. The recurrence risk is relatively large for young women, but by the age of about 40 it is not materially different from the risk in women without a family history.

Table 22.16 shows the model-predicted detection and false-positive rates for women with a previous DS pregnancy. As expected, for all screening policies both rates will be higher than for singletons, and the difference in efficiency according to maternal age will be reduced.

There is evidence that some mothers of infants with DS have abnormal folate and methyl metabolism, as well as mutations in folate genes,[129a] features in common with neural tube defects (NTDs). A relatively high DS risk might be expected in women who are at increased risk for NTDs. In a study of 493 such families, 445 with a history of NTD and 48 with isolated hydrocephalus, there were a total of 11 DS cases among 1,492 at-risk pregnancies, compared with 1.87 expected on the basis of maternal age.[130] On the basis of this series, the age-specific risk is increased 5.9-fold in families with NTD. This is consistent with the observation in the same study of 7 NTDs among 1,847 pregnancies in 516 families at high risk of DS, compared with 1.37 expected (see discussion in chapter 6).

Assisted Reproduction

When a nonspontaneous pregnancy has been achieved in a subfertile couple, often after a long waiting period and with some difficulty, there is additional reason to avoid the hazards of invasive prenatal diagnosis. Such couples need to have the maximum number of markers tested in order to produce the best available DS risk.

There is no reason to believe that the age-specific risk of DS is higher in pregnancies conceived by in vitro fertilization (IVF) than for spontaneous pregnancies. The DS prevalence in the combined data from four age-matched or age-standardized studies is 0.23 percent.[131–134] The average for the controls, weighted according to the number of cases, was 0.21 percent naturally conceived pregnancies. Similarly, the results from three large series of pregnancies achieved by intracytoplasmic sperm injection (ICSI) are consistent with no increased risk (however, see also chapter 7). Among 1,244 women who had undergone prenatal diagnosis after ICSI, the risk was 0.32 percent (four cases), compared with the expected rate of 0.23 percent for women aged 33, the average in this series.[135] In one total series of 1,003 infants born after ICSI the rate was 0.10 percent (one case), compared with 0.13 percent (7 of 5,446) in a conventional IVF series collected in the same country.[136] And in a series of 643 women, of whom 158 had prenatal diagnosis, the rate was 0.47 percent (three cases), compared with an expected rate of 0.17 percent for their age and gestation.[137]

Table 22.16. Previous DS pregnancy: screening efficiency for four policies at five selected maternal ages

| | Maternal Age | | | | | | | | | |
| | 25 | | 30 | | 35 | | 40 | | 45 | |
Markers (weeks)	DR	FPR	DR	FPR	DR	FPR	DR	FPR	DR	FPR
Cutoff 1 in 200[a]										
PAPP-A (10); NT (11–13); free β, AFP, uE$_3$, inhibin (14–18)	91.6	4.3	91.8	4.5	92.9	5.7	94.9	9.5	97.6	21.6
PAPP-A, free β, AFP, uE$_3$ (10); NT (11–13)	89.1	5.3	89.5	5.6	91.0	7.2	93.8	11.9	97.3	26.6
Free β, AFP, uE$_3$, inhibin, NF (14–18)	84.0	9.0	84.6	9.6	86.8	12.2	91.5	21.3	97.1	47.1
Free β, AFP, uE$_3$, inhibin (14–18)	80.3	13.4	81.6	14.7	84.2	18.0	91.0	31.1	97.5	60.6
Cutoff 1 in 250										
PAPP-A (10); NT (11–13); free β, AFP, uE$_3$, inhibin (14–18)	92.5	5.3	92.7	5.6	93.6	6.9	95.6	11.5	97.9	25.0
PAPP-A, free β, AFP, uE$_3$ (10); NT (11–13)	90.4	6.6	90.8	7.1	92.1	8.7	94.8	14.4	97.8	31.0
Free β, AFP, uE$_3$, inhibin, NF (14–18)	85.9	11.0	86.4	11.7	88.2	14.4	92.9	25.3	97.9	54.1
Free β, AFP, uE$_3$, inhibin (14–18)	83.2	16.6	83.8	17.5	86.3	21.2	92.3	34.7	98.2	67.4
Cutoff 1 in 300										
PAPP-A (10); NT (11–13); free β, AFP, uE$_3$, inhibin (14–18)	93.2	6.2	93.4	6.5	94.2	7.9	96.1	13.2	98.2	27.7
PAPP-A, free β, AFP, uE$_3$ (10); NT (11–13)	91.4	7.7	91.8	8.2	92.8	9.8	95.4	16.7	98.2	34.5
Free β, AFP, uE$_3$, inhibin, NF (14–18)	87.3	12.9	87.8	13.6	89.7	17.1	93.9	23.9	98.3	59.1
Free β, AFP, uE$_3$, inhibin (14–18)	84.9	19.0	85.9	20.5	88.4	25.0	93.9	40.4	98.5	70.9

DR = detection rate; FPR = false-positive rate.
[a]At term.

When calculating the age-specific risk of Down syndrome in pregnancies achieved by IVF, whether conventional or using ICSI, care is needed with regard to the maternal age. If a donor egg was used, the maternal age at term is calculated from the age of the donor at the time of sampling plus 266 days, the time from conception to term. A similar calculation is done if the woman's own egg was used and it was frozen after sampling. These calculations assume (1) that risk relates to the age of the donor rather than the recipient and that storage has no effect on risk, and (2) that the couple have been shown to have normal karyotypes.

On average, first- and second-trimester hCG and free β-hCG levels are raised in pregnancies conceived by IVF, ICSI, or other forms of assisted reproduction such as intrauterine insemination or after ovulation induction alone. In the combined results of 16 series[138–153] the overall mean value was 1.12 MoM. However, there is considerable heterogeneity between the series, possibly because of the method of gestational assessment, the cause of infertility, or the type of therapy—for example, whether the oocytes are donated or obtained from the patient, frozen or fresh.

Maternal Diseases

The maternal serum marker profile is altered in women with insulin-dependent diabetes, and although the effect is relatively small, most screening programs adjust the levels accordingly before estimating an individual's risk. One approach is to divide the observed MoM by the average value in diabetic women: for AFP, uE_3, and hCG based on meta-analysis,[108] for inhibin on the mean of two studies,[154,155] or a single study for PAPP-A.[156] It is generally assumed that the prior DS risk is not altered, although there is some evidence of increased aneuploidy risk in women with gestational diabetes.[157–159]

High hCG and free β-hCG levels have been reported in women who had had a renal transplant[160,161] or were in end-stage renal failure and on dialysis[162] when they were screened. One of the transplant studies[81] found a strong positive correlation between free β-hCG and serum creatinine, and from a table in the publication it can be estimated that the expected hCG MoM is 0.0125 times creatinine raised to the power 1.070, which might be used to adjust the level.

Previous False-Positive Result

The chance of having a false-positive result is increased among those who have had a false-positive result in a previous pregnancy. Maternal age alone will necessarily produce a correlation in risks between pregnancies, but the phenomenon is also due to a degree of consistency in marker levels between pregnancies to the same woman. Positive correlations have been found for AFP,[163–167] hCG,[164,165,167] free β-hCG,[166,168] uE_3,[164,167] and PAPP-A.[168] There have been two studies of NT: one found no effect,[168] and while the second reported a significant correlation, the results were not expressed in MoMs.[169] Tables have been published for use in counseling women about the relative increase in the positive rate given a previous screen-positive result.[164,166,168] The relative increase declines with age, since in older women age per se becomes a dominant reason for a positive result. Also the relative increase is lower for combinations using NT because this marker is not correlated between pregnancies.

Smoking

In the second trimester, both hCG and free β-hCG levels are reduced on average in smokers with a median of 0.79 MoM in ten studies combined.[170–179] In the first trimester, free β-hCG levels may not be reduced, but PAPP-A levels are, and to a similar extent as in second-trimester hCG.[180,181] Inhibin levels appear to be increased to an even greater extent than both these markers,[176,179,182] but levels are not materially altered in the other serum markers[108] or NT.[183]

Several studies have reported that smoking is less common in the mothers of infants with DS. However, smoking habits are subject to strong birth cohort effects, so it is important to take full account of maternal age. Most of the data come from age-matched case–control studies or where age was adjusted for in the analysis but the method of age adjustment in some studies was based on broad age bands, and this may not be adequate. This was demonstrated in one study, which found a relative risk of 0.87 with broad age grouping, 0.89 adjusting for additional variables, and 1.00 when age adjustment, together with the additional variables, was in single-year bands.[184] The latest overview on this topic concludes that there is no difference in risk.[179]

Ethnicity

In women of Afro-Caribbean origin, on average AFP and hCG are increased, with medians of 1.15 and 1.18 MoM, respectively, in one meta-analysis,[108] whereas uE_3 levels are unaltered. In the only studies reported so far, the median inhibin A was 0.92 MoM,[185] median PAPP-A was 1.57 MoM,[186] and median NT, 0.98 MoM.[187] The marker profile may also differ in women of South Asian origin, albeit to a smaller extent,[108,187] and from the Far East.[188–190] These differences do not matter in ethnically homogeneous populations, but some centers that serve an ethnically mixed population allow for this in risk calculation. Those with large enough minorities can use MoMs with ethnic-specific medians, otherwise an ethnic multiplication factor can be used to adjust ordinary MoMs.

There are many individual reports of relatively high or low birth prevalence in different ethnic groups. A meta-analysis using data from countries with reliable systems for collecting information on maternal ages found that two groups had some evidence for rates greater than those in Europeans[191]: those of Mexican and Central American origin in California (standardized indices, 1.19 and 1.30 in two studies) and Jews of Asian or African origin in Israel (1.27). The standardized indices were markedly reduced in some populations, including three studies in Africans, but the authors conclude that this is likely to be due to incomplete ascertainment.

Other Factors

All the serum markers used in DS screening demonstrate a negative correlation between the level, expressed in MoMs, and maternal weight. This is usually explained in terms of dilution. A fixed mass of chemical produced in the fetoplacental unit is diluted by a variable volume in the maternal unit. But this cannot be the only factor involved, because the extent of correlation differs between the markers. The correlation is almost twice as great for PAPP-A than for AFP or hCG; inhibin has a weaker correlation than these two, and for uE_3 there is hardly any association at all, particularly in the first trimester. It is standard practice to adjust all serum marker levels for maternal weight, dividing the observed MoM by the expected value for the weight derived by regression. The best regression formula is the inverse regression curve[192]; although a log-linear curve does not differ markedly from the inverse curve for most women,[193] it considerably underadjusts for weight in light women and overadjusts in those at the higher end of the weight range. NT levels are not related to maternal weight.[33] Adjustment for this factor does not introduce any bias because the average maternal weight is similar in DS and unaffected pregnancies.[194]

Several other factors are known to be associated with one or more markers, but they are not used to formally adjust levels. This is because the association is weak or the factor is subjective or impractical to assess. There is a weak association between most markers and gravidity or parity (for review, see Wald et al.[108]). Vaginal bleeding can lead to a high AFP level, presumably because of fetomaternal transfusion, and is associated with increased DS risk.[195] However, it is an extremely variable and subjective factor ranging from "spotting," which is very common in early pregnancy, to threatened abortion. Throughout pregnancy, maternal serum hCG levels are higher in pregnancies in which the fetus is female. Gender has not hitherto been taken into account when interpreting screening results, but this may change now that it can be determined with reasonable accuracy by ultrasound.[196]

EDWARDS SYNDROME

Many centers have extended their multiple marker screening program for DS to include Edwards syndrome (trisomy 18). This involves calculating the risk of both disorders from the maternal age and marker profile using a multivariate Gaussian model.[197–200]

The maternal-age-specific risk of trisomy 18 can be taken to be a fixed fraction of the corresponding DS risk: 1 of 10 at term, 1 of 4.5 at midtrimester, and 1 of 3 in late first trimester. These fractions are obtained by the incidence ratio in six series of routinely karyotyped neonates,[201] five large amniocentesis series,[202] a further multicenter study,[203] and five large chorionic villus sampling series.[204]

The mean maternal serum level in Edwards syndrome for serum AFP, uE_3, hCG or free β-hCG, inhibin, and PAPP-A are 0.68, 0.44, 0.31, 0.81, and 0.14 MoM, respectively, based on two published meta-analyses[197,205] extended to include more recent data.[198,206–216] There is no obvious difference in mean levels between hCG and free β-hCG and for all markers between trimesters. The median NT in two prospective studies was 3.27 MoM[205] and 3.21 MoM[217] (subsequently reanalyzed[218]). Allowing for viability bias, which is even stronger than for DS, as the incidence ratio shows, the best estimate of the mean is 2.77 MoM. The standard deviations and most of the correlation coefficients can be derived from the weighted mean of those in one of the meta-analyses[197] and eight other series;[198,205,206,208–210,214,216] the remainder can be assumed to be the same as in unaffected pregnancies. The distribution of NF appears to be similar in Edwards syndrome and DS,[219] so the same parameters can be used for both.

A large proportion of cases of Edwards syndrome are detected as a result of a positive DS screening test. Table 22.17 shows the estimated detection rates for four DS screening policies, together with the rates when DS screening is extended to include explicit Edwards syndrome screening. The Edwards syndrome detection rate is particularly high in the first trimester, even without explicit screening, because most cases are associated with raised NT. Second-trimester screening cannot achieve such high detection even with explicit screening.

Table 22.17. Edwards syndrome detection rate for a given false-positive rate[a] with four policies, according to Down syndrome cutoff

Markers (weeks)	Down Syndrome Cutoff[b]	Edwards Syndrome False-Positive Rate			
		None	0.1%	0.2%	0.3%
PAPP-A (10); NT (11–13); free β, AFP, uE_3,	1 in 200	81.2	*	*	89.7
inhibin (14–18)	1 in 250	82.1	*	*	90.0
	1 in 300	82.9	*	*	95.8
PAPP-A, free β, AFP, uE_3 (10); NT (11–13)	1 in 200	85.0	91.2	94.0	95.1
	1 in 250	86.0	91.9	94.4	95.4
	1 in 300	86.7	92.4	94.6	95.5
Free β, AFP, uE_3, inhibin, NF (14–18)	1 in 200	51.3	79.0	81.7	82.9
	1 in 250	53.6	79.6	82.1	83.6
	1 in 300	55.6	80.1	82.8	84.2
Free β, AFP, uE_3, inhibin (14–18)	1 in 200	36.0	68.3	72.0	74.0
	1 in 250	39.0	69.2	72.8	74.6
	1 in 300	41.6	71.0	73.9	75.5

[a]In addition to that for Down syndrome screening alone.
[b]At term.
*Estimate unreliable.

OTHER ABNORMALITIES

Some centers interpret tests with low risk of DS, Edwards syndrome, or NTD results as screen-positive when one or more of the markers has an extremely high or low value. Although there are many fetal conditions with abnormal marker profiles, on average they are rare, and most pregnancies with extreme results are normal. For example, no abnormalities were found in twelve with hCG over 10 MoM[220] and two were found in seventy-nine with PAPP-A over 5 MoM.[221] However, some marker combinations do select a very high risk group with decidedly adverse pregnancy outcome, including fetal/neonatal loss, low birth weight, intrauterine growth restriction, and various congenital defects.[221a,221b] These patients warrant further investigation and surveillance.

It has been suggested that first-trimester aneuploidy screening be extended to include Patau syndrome (trisomy 13) as well as DS and Edwards syndrome.[222] In the second trimester, uE_3 levels are reduced[223] and preliminary results indicate that inhibin is increased,[208] but the marker profile is more extreme in the first trimester, with extremely high NT coupled with very low free beta-hCG and AFP.[224] The proposed algorithm uses one set of parameters to calculate the combined risk of Edwards or Patau syndrome. Model predictions are that 95 percent can be detected for a 0.3 percent false-positive rate. The disorder, with a prevalence about one-half of Edwards syndrome, is generally lethal.

Other common aneuploidies have abnormal marker profiles, and although an explicit risk screening has not been suggested, they are often detected as part of DS and Edwards syndrome screening or NTD screening. In triploidy there are two distinct types of second-trimester marker profile: (1) grossly elevated AFP, hCG, and inhibin with low to normal uE_3 and (2) very low hCG, uE_3 and inhibin with low to normal AFP.[225] The same distinction has now been observed in the first trimester; also, with type 1, NT is increased while with type 2, PAPP-A is extremely reduced.[226] There are also two distinct patterns for Turner syndrome with and without hydrops; both types have reduced uE_3, but hCG levels are increased with hydropic disease and reduced when there is no hydrops.[227,228] On average PAPP-A levels are low and NT levels are very high.[229] There are case reports and small series[229] in which the marker profile was abnormal with certain fetal sex chromosome abnormalities. However, the results are subject to strong bias, because the cases were generally diagnosed by studies occasioned by abnormal screening results. Because sex chromosome disorders are mostly undetected and hence underreported at birth, those with normal profiles would be unrecognized. Similarly, viability bias distorts case reports of marker profiles in lethal chromosomal disorders.

Smith–Lemli–Opitz (SLO) syndrome is a rare autosomal recessive disorder leading to moderate to severe mental retardation. There is reduced fetal production of cholesterol, an estriol precursor, and in a series of thirty-three cases the median maternal serum uE_3 level was 0.23 MoM.[230] Placental sulfatase deficiency is a relatively common X-linked disorder leading to abnormal estriol biosynthesis and extremely low maternal serum uE_3 levels. For example, in one series of nine pregnancies with low or absent second-trimester maternal serum uE_3 levels, six were found to have a complete and one a partial deletion of the steroid sulfatase deficiency gene.[231] Placental sulfatase deficiency is generally a mild condition, although occasionally there is mental retardation, and prenatally diagnosed cases are not usually terminated.

Cornelia de Lange syndrome (CdLS) is a fetal abnormality characterized by mental retardation and severe limb reduction. In a series of eighteen second-trimester pregnancies the median maternal serum PAPP-A level was 0.21 MoM; free β-hCG and inhibin levels were also reduced with medians of 0.67 and 0.62 MoM, respectively.[232] There have also been four case reports of increased NT or cystic hygroma.[233–236]

Several studies have reported increased NT in pregnancies with major cardiac abnormality.[237–246] From some of the studies it is possible to derive an observed detection rate: 61 percent,[243] 40–56 percent,[241] 51 percent,[246] 27–36 percent,[244] 11 percent,[242] and 12–15 percent.[245] These differences may reflect referral, ascertainment, and viability biases. Moreover, the studies used a variety of NT cutoff levels[247] (see also chapter 23).

In the first-trimester hydatidiform mole, ectopic pregnancy and impending or actual fetal loss is a frequent finding in women with extremely low PAPP-A levels.[248–250] In the second trimester this occurs, albeit to a lesser extent, with low uE_3.[251,252]

PLANNING A PROGRAM

There is now a wide range of possible DS screening strategies and detailed policies. The tables in this chapter can serve as a guide to health planners as to the relative efficiency of the competing approaches. However, although efficiency is important, other determinants of choice include the financial and human costs, as well as organizational matters.

Until recently, the most common practice was two or three serum marker screenings in the second trimester, but as we have shown, a much greater detection rate can be achieved by other policies, particularly those involving NT. This is widely accepted by planners, and the only factor limiting a rapid shift in practice toward concurrent serum and NT screening in the first trimester is lack of adequate ultrasound facilities and experience with CVS. In places where only a gradual change is possible it would be logical to begin by screening twin pregnancies, women who have had a previous DS pregnancy and those having assisted conception.

A systematic review of economic evaluations of antenatal screening included ten studies of DS screening, seven using biochemistry and two based solely on the anomaly scan.[253] The reviewers concluded that serum screening was cost effective but pointed out that the incremental cost of adding additional markers rather than the average cost was not generally reported, and this was critical for health planners. First-trimester screening was not considered by the papers reviewed, but this has been assessed in five subsequent publications.[254–258] Two of them calculated incremental costs and concluded that a change from second-trimester three-marker screening to first-trimester screening would be cost effective.[255,257] However, unit costs vary in different localities,[259] and health care systems and planners wishing to use the published calculations of incremental costs may need to substitute their own unit costs. Moreover, some analyses use unrealistic detection rates, and those from the latest meta-analysis could be substituted.

The human advantages of first-trimester screening are obvious: earlier reassurance, and if termination of pregnancy is necessary, it can be completed before fetal movements are felt. The early termination of DS pregnancies that are destined to miscarry anyway is also an advantage because it prevents a late miscarriage and yields information on recurrence risk, both empirical and in some cases following the consequent discovery of a parental balanced translocation.

Termination of pregnancy is safer in the first trimester than later in pregnancy[260] (see chapter 26) and with sufficient experience CVS is no more hazardous than amniocentesis (see chapter 5). The most up-to-date Cochrane Review included 9,000 pregnancies from three large randomized trials, and the fetal loss rate was one-third higher for CVS.[261] However, a subsequent National Institutes of Health randomized trial of almost 4,000 women found an absolute increase of just 0.26 percent.[262,263] Furthermore the Review took no account of nonrandomized studies such as the WHO-sponsored Registry, which after the first 139,000 procedures registered concluded that "chorionic villus sampling is a safe procedure with an associated fetal loss rate comparable to that of amniocentesis."[264]

Planners cannot consider DS screening in isolation. For example, in some health care settings with limited ultrasound facilities, it may be necessary to choose between universal NT scanning at 11–13 weeks and anomaly scanning at 18–20 weeks. Some may have to choose between serum testing for DS at 10–13 weeks and AFP testing at 16–18 weeks. But either anomaly scanning or AFP testing is needed in order to screen for NTDs. Those wishing to introduce universal NT scanning together with concurrent serum testing while retaining the second serum sample may wish to consider sequential nondisclosure screening because of the detection advantage. However, the extra detection is relatively small, and when experience is gained with NB scanning it will diminish, and there are serious practical difficulties.

The biggest problem is the extended period of several weeks between initiating the process and its completion, and the consequent anxiety. Some women will find this unacceptable and would rather have a test with a slightly lower detection rate; others will take the opposite view. So far there is no published information on relative uptake in studies in which women have been given an informed choice. The long wait also puts pressure on clinicians to disclose intermediate results, effectively leading to stepwise screening. Although stepwise sequential screening is less efficient, it does overcome some of the waiting problems and allows early prenatal diagnosis for most affected pregnancies. However, this must be weighed against the additional anxiety generated by false reassurance, when a screen-negative result on one method changes to screen-positive on the next.

CONCLUSION

Since multimarker serum screening for DS was first introduced, there has been a steady increase in the detection rate, in relatively small increments, as new markers have been added. The incorporation of ultrasound markers has continued and accelerated the process as well as raising the level of complexity. Today, detection rates in excess of 90 percent are achievable and at a lower false-positive rate than in the past. The rate of progress shows no signs of abating.

REFERENCES

1. Merkatz IR, Nitowsky HM, Macri JN, et al. An association between low maternal serum alpha-fetoprotein and fetal chromosome abnormalities. Am J Obstet Gynecol 1984;148:886.
2. Cuckle HS, Wald NJ, Lindenbaum RH. Maternal serum alpha-fetoprotein measurement: A screening test for Down syndrome. Lancet 1984;1:926.
3. Kuhlmann RS, Werner AL, Abramowicz J, et al. Placental histology in fetuses between 18 and 23 weeks' gestation with abnormal karyotype. Am J Obstet Gynecol 1990;163:1264.
4. Bogart MH, Pandian MR, Jones OW. Abnormal maternal serum chorionic gonadotropin levels in pregnancies with fetal chromosome abnormalities. Prenat Diagn 1987;7:623.
5. Macri JN, Kasturi RV, Krantz DA, et al. Maternal serum Down syndrome screening: free beta-protein is a more effective marker than human chorionic gonadotropin. Am J Obstet Gynecol 1990;163:1248.
6. Jorgensen PI, Trolle D. Low urinary oestriol excretion during pregnancy in women giving birth to infants with Down's syndrome. Lancet 1972;2:782.
7. Canick JA, Knight GJ, Palomaki GE, et al. Low second trimester maternal serum unconjugated oestriol in pregnancies with Down's syndrome. Br J Obstet Gynaecol 1988;95:330.
8. Van Lith JM, Pratt JJ, Beekhuis JR, et al. Second-trimester maternal serum immunoreactive inhibin as a marker for fetal Down's syndrome. Prenat Diagn 1992;12:801.

9. Wallace EM, Grant VE, Swanston IA, et al. Evaluation of maternal serum dimeric inhibin A as a first-trimester marker of Down's syndrome. Prenat Diagn 1995;15:359.

10. Brambati B, Lanzani A, Tului L. Ultrasound and biochemical assessment of first trimester pregnancy. In Chapman, M, Grudzinskas G, Chard T, eds. The embryo: normal and abnormal development and growth. New York: Springer-Verlag, 1991:181.

11. Nicolaides KH, Azar G, Byrne D, et al. Fetal nuchal translucency: ultrasound screening for chromosomal defects in first trimester of pregnancy. BMJ 1992;304:867.

12. Snijders RJ, Thom EA, Zachary JM, et al. First-trimester trisomy screening: nuchal translucency measurement training and quality assurance to correct and unify technique. Ultrasound Obstet Gynecol 2002;19:353.

13. von Kaisenberg CS, Krenn V, Ludwig M, et al. Morphological classification of nuchal skin in human fetuses with trisomy 21, 18, and 13 at 12–18 weeks and in a trisomy 16 mouse. Anat Embryol 1998;197:105.

14. Benacerraf BR, Barss VA, Laboda LA. A sonographic sign for the detection in the second trimester of the fetus with Down's syndrome. Am J Obstet Gynecol 1985;151:1078.

15. Salomon LJ, Bernard JP, Taupin P, et al. Relationship between nuchal translucency at 11–14 weeks and nuchal fold at 20–24 weeks of gestation. Ultrasound Obstet Gynecol 2001;18:636.

16. Logghe H, Cuckle H, Sehmi I. Centre-specific ultrasound nuchal translucency medians needed for Down's syndrome screening. Prenat Diagn 2003;23:389.

17. Cuckle HS. Improved parameters for risk estimation in Down's syndrome screening. Prenat Diagn 1995;15:1057.

18. Cuckle HS, van Lith JMM. Appropriate biochemical parameters in first trimester screening for Down's syndrome. Prenat Diagn 1999;19:505.

19. Spencer K, Crossley JA, Aitken DA, et al. Temporal changes in maternal serum biochemical markers of trisomy 21 across the first and second trimester of pregnancy. Ann Clin Biochem 2002;39:567.

20. Lam YH, Tang MHY. Second-trimester maternal serum inhibin-A screening for fetal Down's syndrome in Asian women. Prenat Diagn 1999;19:463.

21. Renier MA, Vereecken A, van Herck E, et al. Second trimester maternal dimeric inhibin-A in the multiple-marker screening test for Down's syndrome. Hum Reprod 1998;13:744.

22. Yoshida K, Kuwabara Y, Tanaka T, et al. Dimeric inhibin A as a fourth marker for Down's syndrome maternal serum screening in native Japanese women. J Obstet Gynaecol Res 2000;26:171.

23. Debieve F, Bouckaert A, Hubinont C, et al. Multiple screening for fetal Down's syndrome with the classic triple test, dimeric inhibin A and ultrasound. Gynecol Obstet Invest 2000;49:221.

24. Wallace EM, Swanston IA, Groome NP. Evaluation of maternal serum dimeric inhibin A as a first trimester marker of Down's syndrome. Prenat Diagn 1995;15:359.

25. Aitken DA, Wallace EM, Crossley JA, et al. Dimeric inhibin A as a marker for Down's syndrome and trisomy 18 pregnancies at 7–18 weeks gestation. N Engl J Med 1996;334:1231.

26. Wald NJ, Densem JW, George L, et al. Prenatal screening for Down's syndrome using inhibin A as a serum marker. Prenat Diagn 1996;16:143.

27. Spencer K. Inhibin-A levels in Down syndrome pregnancies. Prenat Diagn 2001;21:441.

28. Cuckle HS, Holding S, Jones R, et al. Combining inhibin A with existing second-trimester markers in maternal serum screening for Down's syndrome. Prenat Diagn 1996;16:1095.

29. Wald NJ, Rodeck C, Hackshaw AK, et al. First and second trimester antenatal screening for Down's syndrome: the results of the Serum, Urine and Ultrasound Screening Study (SURUSS). Health Technol Assess 2003;7:1.

30. Scott F, Boogert A, Sinosich M, et al. Establishment and application of a normal range for nuchal translucency across the first trimester. Prenat Diagn 1996;16:629.

31. Biagiotti R, Periti E, Brizzi L, et al. Comparison between two methods of standardization for gestational age differences in fetal nuchal translucency measurement in first-trimester screening for trisomy 21. Ultrasound Obstet Gynecol 1997;9:248.

32. Nicolaides KH, Snijders RJ, Cuckle HS. Correct estimation of parameters for ultrasound nuchal translucency screening. Prenat Diagn 1998;18:519.

33. de Graaf IM, Prjkrt E, Bilardo CM, et al. Early pregnancy screening for fetal aneuploidy with serum markers and nuchal translucency. Prenat Diagn 1999;19:458.

34. Spencer K, Spencer CE, Power M, et al. One stop clinic for assessment of risk for fetal anomalies: a report of the first year of prospective screening for chromosomal anomalies in the first trimester. Br J Obstet Gynaecol 2000;107:1271.

35. Krantz DA, Hallahan TW, Orlando F, et al. First-trimester Down syndrome screening using dried blood biochemistry and nuchal translucency. Obstet Gynecol 2000;96:207.

36. Zoppi MA, Ibba RM, Floris M, et al. Fetal nuchal translucency screening in 12495 pregnancies in Sardinia. Ultrasound Obstet Gynecol 2001;18:649.

37. Crossley JA, Aitken DA, Cameron AD, et al. Combined ultrasound and biochemical screening for Down's syndrome in the first trimester: a Scottish multicentre study. Br J Obstet Gynaecol 2002;109:667.

38. Lam YH, Lee CP, Sin SY, et al. Comparison and integration of first trimester fetal nuchal translucency and second trimester maternal serum screening for fetal Down syndrome. Prenat Diagn 2002;22:730.

39. Herman A, Dreazen E, Herman AM, et al. Bedside estimation of Down syndrome risk during first-trimester ultrasound screening. Ultrasound Obstet Gynecol 2002;20:468.

40. Snijders RJM, Noble P, Sebire N, et al. UK multicentre project on assessment of risk of trisomy 21 by maternal age and fetal nuchal-translucency thickness at 10–14 weeks of gestation. Lancet 1998;352:343.

41. Locatelli A, Piccoli MG, Vergani P, et al. Critical appraisal of the use of nuchal fold thickness measurements for the prediction of Down syndrome. Am J Obstet Gynecol 2000;182:192.

42. Bahado-Singh RO, Oz U, Hsu CD, et al. Ratio of nuchal thickness to humerus length for Down syndrome detection. Am J Obstet Gynecol 2001;184:1284.

43. Souter VL, Nyberg DA, El-Bastawissi A, et al. Correlation of ultrasound findings and biochemical markers in the second trimester of pregnancy in fetuses with trisomy 21. Prenat Diagn 2002;22:175.

44. Benn PA, Kaminsky LM, Ying J, et al. Combined second-trimester biochemical and ultrasound screening for Down syndrome. Obstet Gynecol 2002;100:1168.

45. Royston P, Thompson SG. Model-based screening by risk with application to Down's syndrome. Stat Med 1992;11:257.

46. Cuckle HS, Wald NJ, Thompson SG. Estimating a woman's risk of having a pregnancy associated with Down's syndrome using her age and serum alpha-fetoprotein level. Br J Obstet Gynaecol 1987;94:387.

47. Hecht CA, Hook EB. The imprecision in rates of Down syndrome by 1-year maternal age intervals: a critical analysis of rates used in biochemical screening. Prenat Diagn 1994; 14:729.

48. Hecht CA, Hook EB. Rates of Down syndrome at livebirth by one-year maternal age intervals in studies with apparent close to complete ascertainment in populations of European origin: a proposed rate schedule for use in biochemical screening. Am J Med Genet 1996;62:376.

49. Bray I, Wright DE, Davies CJ, et al. Joint estimation of Down syndrome risk and ascertainment rates: a meta-analysis of nine published data sets. Prenat Diagn 1998;18:9.

50. Morris JK, Mutton D, Alberman E. Revised estimates of the maternal age specific live birth prevalence of Down's syndrome. J Med Screen 2002;9:2.

51. Cuckle H. Potential biases in Down syndrome birth prevalence estimation. J Med Screen 2002;9:192.

52. Bray IC, Wright DE. Estimating the spontaneous loss of Down syndrome fetuses between the time of chorionic villus sampling and livebirth. Prenat Diagn 1998;18:1045.

53. Hook EB, Topol BB, Cross PK. The natural history of cytogenetically abnormal fetuses detected at midtrimester amniocentesis which are not terminated electively: new data and estimates of the excess and relative risk of late fetal death associated with 47,+21 and some other abnormal karyotypes. Am J Hum Genet 1989;45:855.

54. Hook EB, Mutton DE, Ide R, et al. The natural history of Down syndrome conceptuses diagnosed prenatally that are not electively terminated. Am J Hum Genet 1995;57:875.

55. Morris JK, Wald NJ, Watt HC. Fetal loss in Down syndrome pregnancies. Prenat Diagn 1999;19:142.

56. Cuckle H. Down syndrome fetal loss rate in early pregnancy. Prenat Diagn 1999;19:1177.

57. Snijders RJ, Sundberg K, Holzgreve W, et al. Maternal age- and gestation-specific risk for trisomy 21. Ultrasound Obstet Gynecol 1999;13:167.

58. Nybo Andersen AM, Wohlfahrt J, Christens P, et al. Maternal age and fetal loss: population based register linkage study. BMJ 2000;320:1708.

59. Campogrande M, Viora E, Errante G, et al. Correlations between first and second trimester markers for Down's syndrome screening. J Med Screen 2001;8:163.

60. Maymon R, Bergman M, Segal S, et al. Sequential first and second trimester screening tests: correlation of the markers' levels in normal versus Down syndrome affected pregnancies. Prenat Diagn 2001;21:1175.

61. Spencer K, Liao AW, Ong CY, et al. Maternal serum levels of dimeric inhibin A in pregnancies affected by trisomy 21 in the first trimester. Prenat Diagn 2001;21:441.

62. Cuckle HS, Sehmi IK, Jones RG. Correlation between maternal serum PAPP-A and inhibin. Prenat Diagn 2002;22:161.

63. Khoury MJ, Erickson JD, Cordero JF, et al. Congenital malformations and intrauterine growth retardation: a population study. Pediatrics 1988;82;83.

64. Wald NJ, Smith D, Kennard A, et al. Biparietal diameter and crown-rump length in fetuses with Down's syndrome: implications for antenatal serum screening for Down's syndrome. Br J Obstet Gynaecol 1993;100:430.

65. van der Veen WJ, Beekhuis JR, Cornel MC, et al. A demographic approach to the assessment of Down syndrome screening performance. Prenat Diagn 1997;17:17.

66. Cuckle H, Aitken D, Spencer K, et al. Age-standardisation for monitoring performance in Down's syndrome screening programmes. Xxxxx, in press.

67. Cuckle H. Established markers in second trimester maternal serum. Early Hum Dev 1996;47: suppl:27.

68. Cuckle H. Integrating Down's syndrome screening. Curr Opin Obstet Gynaecol 2001;13:175.

69. Beaman JM, Goldie DJ. Second trimester screening for Down's syndrome: 7 years experience. J Med Screen 2001;8:128.

70. Salonen R, Turpeinen U, Kurki L, et al. Maternal serum screening for Down's syndrome on population basis. Acta Obstet Gynecol Scand 1997;76:817.

71. Ford C, Moore AJ, Jordan PA, et al. The value of screening for Down's syndrome in a socioeconomically deprived area with a high ethnic population. Br J Obstet Gynaecol 1998;105:855.

72. Chao AS, Chung CL, Wu CD, et al. Second trimester maternal serum screening using alpha fetoprotein, free beta human chorionic gonadotropin and maternal age specific risk: result of chromosomal abnormalities detected in screen positive for Down syndrome in an Asian population. Acta Obstet Gynecol Scand 1999;78:393.

73. Muller F, Forestier F, Dingeon B; ABA Study Group. Second trimester trisomy 21 maternal serum marker screening: results of a countrywide study of 854,902 patients. Prenat Diagn 2002;22:925.

74. Wald NJ, Huttly WJ, Hackshaw AK. Antenatal screening for Down's syndrome with the quadruple test. Lancet 2003;361:835.

75. Thilaganathan B, Slack A, Wathen NC. Effect of first-trimester nuchal translucency on second-trimester maternal serum biochemical screening for Down's syndrome. Ultrasound Obstet Gynecol 1997;10:261.

76. Brizot ML, Carvalho MH, Liao AW, et al. First-trimester screening for chromosomal abnormalities by fetal nuchal translucency in a Brazilian population. Ultrasound Obstet Gynecol 2001;18:652.

77. Gasiorek-Wiens A, Tercanli S, Kozlowski P, et al. Screening for trisomy 21 by fetal nuchal translucency and maternal age: a multicenter project in Germany, Austria and Switzerland. Ultrasound Obstet Gynecol 2001;18:645.

78. Zoppi MA, Ibba RM, Floris M, et al. Fetal nuchal translucency screening in 12495 pregnancies in Sardinia. Ultrasound Obstet Gynecol 2001;18:649.

79. Krantz DA, Hallahan TW, Orlandi F, et al. First-trimester Down syndrome screening using dried blood biochemistry and nuchal translucency. Obstet Gynecol 2000;96:207.

80. Schuchter K, Hafner E, Stangi G, et al. The first trimester "combined test" for the detection of Down syndrome pregnancies in 4939 unselected pregnancies. Prenat Diagn 2002;22:211.

81. von Kaisenberg CS, Gasiorek-Wiens A, Bielicki M, et al. Screening for trisomy 21 by maternal age, fetal nuchal translucency and maternal serum biochemistry at 11–14 weeks: a German multicenter study. J Matern Fetal Neonat Med 2002;12:89.

82. Bindra R, Heath V, Uao A, et al. One-stop clinic for assessment of risk for trisomy 21 at 11–14 weeks: a prospective study of 15030 pregnancies. Ultrasound Obstet Gynecol 2002;20:219.

83. Spencer K, Spencer CE, Power M, et al. Screening for chromosomal abnormalities in the first trimester using ultrasound and maternal serum biochemistry in one-stop clinic: a review of three years prospective experience. Br Obstet Gynaecol 2003;110:281.

84. Wald NJ, Hackshaw AK, Huttly W, et al. Empirical validation of risk screening for Down's syndrome. J Med Screen 1996;3:185.

85. Canick JA, Rish S. The accuracy of assigned risks in maternal serum screening. Prenat Diagn 1998;18:413.

86. Onda T, Tanaka T, Takeda O, et al. Agreement between predicted risk and prevalence of Down syndrome in second-trimester triple-marker screening in Japan. Prenat Diagn 1998;18:956.

87. Spencer K. Accuracy of Down's syndrome risks produced in a prenatal screening program. Ann Clin Biochem 1999;36:101.

88. Wald NJ, Huttly WJ. Validation of risk estimation using the quadruple test in prenatal screening for Down syndrome. Prenat Diagn 1999;19:1083.

89. Spencer K. Accuracy of Down syndrome risks produced in a first-trimester screening programme incorporating fetal nuchal translucency thickness and maternal serum biochemistry. Prenat Diagn 2002;22:244.

90. Prefumo F, Thilaganathan B. Agreement between predicted risk and prevalence of Down syndrome in first trimester nuchal translucency screening. Prenat Diagn 2002;22:917.

91. Meier C, Huang T, Wyatt PR, et al. Accuracy of expected risk of Down syndrome using the second-trimester triple test. Clin Chem 2002;48:653.

92. Cicero S, Curcio P, Papageorghiou A, et al. Absence of nasal bone in fetuses with trisomy 21 at 11–14 weeks of gestation: an observational study. Lancet 2001;358:1665.

93. Cicero S, Bindra R, Rembouskos G, et al. Integrated ultrasound and biochemical screening for trisomy 21 using fetal nuchal translucency, absent fetal nasal bone, free beta-hCG and PAPP-A at 11 to 14 weeks. Prenat Diagn 2003;23:306.

94. Otaño L, Aiello H, Igarzabal L, et al. Association between first trimester absence of fetal nasal bone on ultrasound and Down syndrome. Prenat Diagn 2002;22:930.

95. Zoppi MA, Ibba RM, Axiana C, et al. Absence of fetal nasal bone and aneuploidies at first-trimester nuchal translucency screening in unselected pregnancies. Prenat Diagn 2003;23:496.

96. Cicero S, Bindra R, Rembouskos G, et al. Fetal nasal bone length in chromosomally normal and abnormal fetuses at 11–14 weeks of gestation. J Matern Fetal Neonat Med 2002;11:400.

97. Sonek JD, Nicolaides KH. Prenatal ultrasonographic diagnosis of nasal bone abnormalities in three fetuses with Down syndrome. Am J Obstet Gynecol 2002;186:139.

98. Cicero S, Sonek JD, McKenna DS, et al. Nasal bone hypoplasia in trisomy 21 at 15–22 weeks' gestation. Ultrasound Obstet Gynecol 2003;21:15.

99. Bromley B, Lieberman E, Shipp TD, et al. Fetal nose bone length: a marker for Down syndrome in the second trimester. J Ultrasound Med 2002;21:1387.

100. Bahado-Singh RO, Oz AU, Kovanci E, et al. New Down syndrome screening algorithm: ultrasonographic biometry and multiple serum markers combined with maternal age. Am J Obstet Gynecol 1998;179:1627.

101. Benacerraf BR, Gelman R, Frigoletto FD Jr. Sonographic identification of second-trimester fetuses with Down's syndrome. N Engl J Med. 1987;317:1371.

102. Cuckle HS, Wald NJ, Quinn J, et al. Ultrasound fetal femur length measurement in the screening for Down syndrome. Br J Obstet Gynaecol 1989;96:1373.

103. Rotmensch S, Luo JS, Liberati M, et al. Fetal humeral length to detect Down syndrome. Am J Obstet Gynecol 1992;166:1330.

104. Owen J, Wenstrom KD, Hardin JM, et al. The utility of fetal biometry as an adjunct to the multiple-marker screening test for Down syndrome. Am J Obstet Gynecol 1994;171:1041.

105. Vergani P, Locatelli A, Piccoli MG, et al. Critical reappraisal of the utility of sonographic fetal femur length in the prediction of trisomy 21. Prenat Diagn 2000;20:210.

106. Murta CG, Moron AF, Avila MA, et al. Application of ductus venosus Doppler velocimetry for the detection of fetal aneuploidy in the first trimester of pregnancy. Fetal Diagn Ther 2002;17:308.

107. Zoppi MA, Putzolu M, Ibba RM, et al. First-trimester ductus venosus velocimetry in relation to nuchal translucency thickness and fetal karyotype. Fetal Diagn Ther 2002;17:52.

108. Wald NJ, Kennard A, Hackshaw A, et al. Antenatal screening for Down's syndrome. Health Technol Assess 1998;2:1.

109. Cuckle H. Impact of improved screening efficiency on the future role of non-invasive testing. In: Hahn S, Holzgreve W, eds. Fetal cells and fetal DNA in maternal blood. Basel, Switzerland: S Karger, 2001:124.

110. Cuckle HS, Canick JA, Kellner LH. Collaborative study of maternal urine β-core human chorionic gonadotrophin screening for Down syndrome. Prenat Diagn 1999;19:911.

111. Hsu J-J, Spencer K, Aitken DA, et al. Urinary free beta hCG. beta core fragment and total oestriol as markers of Down syndrome in the second trimester of pregnancy. Prenat Diagn 1999;19:146.

112. Bahado-Singh R, Shahabi S, Karaca M, et al. The comprehensive midtrimester test: high-sensitivity Down syndrome test. Am J Obstet Gynecol 2002;186:803.

113. Spencer K, Talbot JA, Abushoufa RA. Maternal serum hyperglycosylated human chorionic gonadotrophin (HhCG) in the first trimester of pregnancies affected by Down syndrome, using a sialic acid-specific lectin immunoassay. Prenat Diagn 2002;22:656.

114. Wald NJ, Cuckle HS. Recent advances in screening for neural tube defects and Down's syndrome. In: Rodeck CH, ed. Fetal diagnosis of genetic defects. Baillière's Clinical Obstetrics and Gynaecology, vol. 1. London: Baillière Tindall, 1987:649.

115. Doyle PE, Beral V, Botting B, et al. Congenital malformations in twins in England and Wales. J Epidemiol Community Health 1990;45:43.

116. Cuckle H. Down's syndrome screening in twins. J Med Screen 1998;5:3.

117. Watt HC, Wald NJ, George L. Maternal serum inhibin-A levels in twin pregnancies: implications for screening for Down's syndrome. Prenat Diagn 1996;16:927.

118. Spencer K. Screening for trisomy 21 in twin pregnancies in the first trimester using free beta-hCG and PAPP-A, combined with fetal nuchal translucency thickness. Prenat Diagn 2000;20:91.

119. Niemimaa M, Suonpaa M, Heinonen S, et al. Maternal serum human chorionic gonadotrophin and pregnancy-associated plasma protein A in twin pregnancies in the first trimester. Prenat Diagn 2002;22:183.

120. Spencer K, Nicolaides KH. Screening for trisomy 21 in twins using first trimester ultrasound and mater-

nal serum biochemistry in a one-stop clinic: a review of three years experience. Br J Obstet Gynaecol 2003;110:276.

121. Sebire NJ, Snijders RJ, Hughes K, et al. Screening for trisomy 21 in twin pregnancies by maternal age and fetal nuchal translucency thickness at 10–14 weeks of gestation. Br J Obstet Gynaecol 1996;103:999.

122. Maymon R, Dreazen E, Rozinsky S, et al. Comparison of nuchal translucency measurement and second-trimester triple serum screening in twin versus singleton pregnancies. Prenat Diagn 1999;19:727.

123. Spencer K. Screening for trisomy 21 in twin pregnancies in the first trimester using free beta-hCG and PAPP-A, combined with fetal nuchal translucency thickness. Prenat Diagn 2000;20:91.

124. Mutton D, Alberman E, Hook EB. Cytogenetic and epidemiological findings in Down syndrome, England and Wales 1989 to 1993. National Down Syndrome Cytogenetic Register and the Association of Clinical Cytogeneticists. J Med Genet 1996;33:387.

125. Stenhouse E, Hardwick C, Maharaj S, et al. Chorionicity determination in twin pregnancies: how accurate are we? Ultrasound Obstet Gynecol 2002;19:350.

126. Meyers C, Adam R, Dungan J, et al. Aneuploidy in twin gestations: when is maternal age advanced? Obstet Gynecol 1997;89:248.

127. Boué A, Gallano P. A collaborative study of the segregation of inherited chromosome arrangements in 1356 prenatal diagnoses. Prenat Diagn 1984;4:45.

128. Arbuzova S, Cuckle H, Mueller R, et al. Familial Down syndrome: evidence supporting cytoplasmic inheritance. Clin Genet 2001;60:456.

129. Hook EBH. In: Brock DJH, Rodeck CH & Ferguson-Smith MA, eds. Prenatal diagnosis and screening. Edinburgh: Churchill Livingstone, 1992:351.

129a. James SJ, Pogribna M, Pigribny IP, et al. Abnormal folate metabolism and mutation in the methylenetetrahydrofolate reductase gene may be maternal risk factors for Down syndrome. Am J Clin Nutr 1999;70:495.

130. Barkai G, Arbuzova S, Berkenstadt M, et al. Frequency of Down's syndrome and neural-tube defects in the same family. Lancet 2003;361:1331.

131. Bergh T, Ericson A, Hillensjo T, et al. Deliveries and children born after in-vitro fertilisation in Sweden 1982–95: a retrospective cohort study. Lancet 1999;354:1579.

132. Ericson A, Kallen B. Congenital malformations in infants born after IVF: a population-based study. Hum Reprod 2001;16:504.

133. Westergaard HB, Johansen AM, Erb K, et al. Danish National In-Vitro Fertilization Registry 1994 and 1995: a controlled study of births, malformations and cytogenetic findings. Hum Reprod 1999;14:1896.

134. Koivurova S, Hartikainen AL, Gissler M, et al. Neonatal outcome and congenital malformations in children born after in-vitro fertilization. Hum Reprod 2002;17:1391.

135. Bonduelle M, Van Assche E, Joris H, et al. Prenatal testing in ICSI pregnancies: incidence of chromosomal abnormalities in 1586 karyotypes and relation to sperm parameters. Hum Reprod 2002;17:2600.

136. Wennerholm UB, Bergh C, Hamberger L, et al. Obstetric outcome of pregnancies following ICSI, classified according to sperm origin and quality. Hum Reprod 2000;15:1189.

137. Loft A, Petersen K, Erb K, et al. A Danish national cohort of 730 infants born after intracytoplasmic sperm injection (ICSI) 1994–1997. Hum Reprod 1999;14:2143.

138. Barkai G, Goldman B, Ries L, et al. Down's syndrome screening marker levels following assisted reproduction. Prenat Diagn 1996;16:1111.

139. Ribbert LS, Kornman LH, De-Wolf BT, et al. Maternal serum screening for fetal Down syndrome in IVF pregnancies. Prenat Diagn 1996;16:35.

140. Heinonen S, Ryynanen M, Kirkinen P, et al. Effect of in vitro fertilization on human chorionic gonadotropin serum concentrations and Down's syndrome screening. Fertil Steril 1996;66:398.

141. Frishman GN, Canick JA, Hogan JW, et al. Serum triple-marker screening in in vitro fertilization and naturally conceived pregnancies. Obstet Gynecol 1997;90:98.

142. Lam YH, Yeung WSB, Tang MHY, et al. Maternal serum alpha-fetoprotein and human chorionic gonadotrophin in pregnancies conceived after intracytoplasmic sperm injection and conventional in vitro fertilization. Hum Reprod 1999;14:2120.

143. Hsu TY, Hsu CY, Ou JJ, et al. Maternal serum screening for Down syndrome in pregnancies conceived by intra-uterine insemination. Prenat Diagn 1999;19:1012.

144. Wald N, White N, Morris JK, et al. Serum markers for Down's syndrome in women who have had in vitro fertilisation: implications for antenatal screening. Br J Obstet Gynaecol 1999;106:1304.

145. Maymon R, Shulman A. Comparison of triple serum screening and pregnancy outcome in oocyte donation versus IVF pregnancies. Hum Reprod 2001;16:691.

146. Bar-Hava I, Yitzhak M, Krissi H, et al. Triple-test screening in in vitro fertilization pregnancies. J Assist Reprod Genet 2001;18:226.

147. Räty R, Virtanen A, Koskinen P, et al. Maternal serum beta-hCG levels in screening for Down syndrome are higher in singleton pregnancies achieved with ovulation induction and intrauterine insemination than in spontaneous singleton pregnancies. Fertil Steril 2001;76:1075.

148. Wøjdeman KR, Larsen SO, Shalmi A, et al. First trimester screening for Down syndrome and assisted reproduction: no basis for concern. Prenat Diagn 2001;21:563.

149. Liao AW, Heath V, Kametas N, et al. First-trimester screening for trisomy 21 in singleton pregnancies achieved by assisted reproduction. Hum Reprod 2001;16:1501.

150. Niemimaa M, Heinonen S, Seppälä M, et al. First-trimester screening for Down's syndrome in in vitro fertilization pregnancies. Fertil Steril 2001;76:1282.

151. Perheentupa A, Ruokonen AA, Tuomivaara L, et al. Maternal serum β-HCG and α-fetoprotein concentrations in singleton pregnancies following assisted reproduction. Hum Reprod 2002; 17:794.

152. Räty R, Virtanen A, Koskinen P, et al. Serum free β-hCG and alpha-fetoprotein levels in IVF, ICSI and frozen embryo transfer pregnancies in maternal mid-trimester serum screening for Down's syndrome. Hum Reprod 2002;17:481.

153. Maymon R, Shulman A. Serial first- and second-trimester Down's syndrome screening tests among IVF-versus naturally-conceived singletons. Hum Reprod 2002;17:1081.

154. Wald NJ, Watt HC, George L. Maternal serum inhibin-A in pregnancies with insulin-dependent diabetes mellitus: implications for screening for Down's syndrome. Prenat Diagn 1996;16:923.

155. Wallace EM, Crossley JA, Ritoe SC, et al. Maternal serum inhibin-A in pregnancies complicated by insulin dependent diabetes mellitus. Br J Obstet Gynaecol 1997;104:946.

156. Pedersen JF, Sorensen S, Molsted-Pedersen L. Serum levels of human placental lactogen, pregnancy-associated plasma protein A and endometrial secretory protein PP14 in first trimester of diabetic pregnancy. Acta Obstet Gynecol Scand 1998;77:155.

157. Narchi H, Kulaylat N. High incidence of Down's syndrome in infants of diabetic mothers. Arch Dis Child 1997;77:242.

158. Pelz J, Kunze J. Down's syndrome in infants of diabetic mothers. Arch Dis Child 1998;79:199.

159. Moore LL, Bradlee ML, Singer MR, et al. Chromosomal anomalies among the offspring of women with gestational diabetes. Am J Epidemiol 2002;155:719.

160. Cararach V, Casals E, Martinez S, et al. Abnormal renal function as a cause of false-positive biochemical screening for Down's syndrome. Lancet 1997;350:1295.

161. Karidas CN, Michailidis GD, Spencer K, et al. Biochemical screening for Down syndrome in pregnancies following renal transplantation. Prenat Diagn 2002;22:226.

162. Cheng PJ, Liu CM, Chang SD, et al. Elevated second-trimester maternal serum hCG in patients undergoing haemodialysis. Prenat Diagn 1999;19:955.

163. Wald NJ, Cuckle HS. Raised maternal serum alpha-fetoprotein levels in subsequent pregnancies. Lancet 1981;1:1103.

164. Holding S, Cuckle HS. Maternal serum screening for Downs syndrome taking account of the result in a previous pregnancy. Prenat Diagn 1994;14:321.

165. Dar H, Merksamer R, Berdichevsky D, et al. Maternal serum markers levels in consecutive pregnancies: a possible genetic predisposition to abnormal levels. Am J Med Genet 1996;61:154.

166. Spencer K. Between-pregnancy biological variability of maternal serum alpha-fetoprotein and free beta hCG: implications for Down syndrome screening in subsequent pregnancies. Prenat Diagn 1997;17:39.

167. Wax JR, Lopes AM, Benn PA, et al. Unexplained elevated midtrimester maternal serum levels of alpha fetoprotein, human chorionic gonadotropin, or low unconjugated estriol: recurrence risk and association with adverse perinatal outcome. J Matern Fetal Med 2000;9:161.

168. Spencer K. Between pregnancy biological variability of first trimester markers of Down syndrome: implications for screening in subsequent pregnancies. Prenat Diagn 2001;21:445.

169. Maymon R, Padoa A, Dreazen E, et al. Nuchal translucency measurements in consecutive normal pregnancies: is there a predisposition to increased levels? Prenat Diagn 2002;22:759.

170. Bernstein L, Pike MC, Lobo RA, et al. Cigarette smoking in pregnancy results in marked decrease in maternal hCG and oestradiol levels. Br J Obstet Gynaecol. 1989;96:92.

171. Cuckle H, Wald N, Densem J, et al. The effect of smoking in pregnancy on maternal serum alpha-fetoprotein, unconjugated oestriol, human chorionic gonadotrophin, progesterone and dehydroepiandrosterone sulphate levels. Brit J Obstet Gynaecol 1990;97:272.

172. Bartels I, Hoppe-Sievert B, Bockel B, et al. Adjustment formulae for maternal serum alpha-fetoprotein,

human chorionic gonadotropin, and unconjugated oestriol to maternal weight and smoking. Prenat Diagn 1993;13:123.

173. Palomaki GE, Knight GJ, Haddow JE, et al, Wald NJ, Kennard A. Cigarette smoking and levels of maternal serum alpha-fetoprotein, unconjugated estriol, and hCG: impact on Down syndrome screening. Obstet Gynecol 1993;81:675.

174. Spencer K. The influence of smoking on maternal serum AFP and free beta hCG levels and the impact on screening for Down syndrome. Prenat Diagn 1998;18:225.

175. Hafner E, Stangl G, Rosen A, et al. Influence of cigarette-smoking on the result of the triple test. Gynecol Obstet Invest 1999;47:188.

176. Ferriman EL, Sehmi IK, Jones R, et al. The effect of smoking in pregnancy on maternal serum inhibin A levels. Prenat Diagn 1999;19:372.

177. Tislaric D, Brajenovic-Milic B, Ristic S, et al. The influence of smoking and parity on serum markers for Down's syndrome screening. Fetal Diagn Ther 2002;17:17.

178. Crossley JA, Aitken DA, Waugh SM, et al. Maternal smoking: age distribution, levels of alpha-fetoprotein and human chorionic gonadotrophin, and effect on detection of Down syndrome pregnancies in second-trimester screening. Prenat Diagn 2002;22:247.

179. Rudnicka AR, Wald NJ, Huttly W, et al. Influence of maternal smoking on the birth prevalence of Down syndrome and on second trimester screening performance. Prenat Diagn 2002;22:893.

180. Spencer K. The influence of smoking on maternal serum PAPP-A and free beta hCG levels in the first trimester of pregnancy. Prenat Diagn 1999;19:1065.

181. De Graaf IM, Cuckle HS, Pajkrt E, et al. Co-variables in first trimester maternal serum screening. Prenat Diagn 2000;20:186.

182. Renier MA, Vereecken A, Van Herck E, et al. Second trimester maternal dimeric inhibin-A in the multiple-marker screening test for Down's syndrome. Hum Reprod 1998;13:744.

183. Spencer K, Ong CY, Liao AW, et al. First trimester markers of trisomy 21 and the influence of maternal cigarette smoking status. Prenat Diagn 2000;20:852.

184. Chen C-L, Gilbert TJ, Daling JR. Maternal smoking and Down syndrome: the confounding effect of maternal age. Am J Epidemiol 1999;149:442.

185. Spencer K, Ong CY, Liao AW, et al. The influence of ethnic origin on first trimester biochemical markers of chromosomal abnormalities. Prenat Diagn 2000;20:491.

186. Watt HC, Wald NJ, Smith D, et al. Effect of allowing for ethnic group in prenatal screening for Down's syndrome. Prenat Diagn 1996;16:691.

187. Thilaganathan B, Khare M, Williams B, et al. Influence of ethnic origin on nuchal translucency screening for Down's syndrome. Ultrasound Obstet Gynecol 1998;12:112.

188. Onda T, Kitagawa M, Takeda O, et al. Triple marker screening in native Japanese women. Prenat Diagn 1996;16:713.

189. Tompkinson DG, Cunningham GC. Race-specific median MSAFP values by gestational age. Am J Hum Genet 1992;51 (suppl): A272.

190. Ferriman EL, Sehmi IK, Jones RG, et al. Serum Screening in a Japanese Population. Prenat Diagn 2000;20:437.

191. Carothers AD, Hecht CA, Hook EB. International variation in reported livebirth prevalence rates of Down syndrome, adjusted for maternal age. J Med Genet 1999;36:386.

192. Neveux LM, Palomaki GE, Larrivee DA, et al. Refinements in managing maternal weight adjustment for interpreting maternal screening results. Prenat Diagn 1996;16:1115.

193. Watt HC, Wald NJ. Alternative methods of maternal weight adjustment in maternal serum screening for Down syndrome and neural tube defects. Prenat Diagn 1998;18:842.

194. Wald NJ, Cuckle HS. Recent advances in screening for neural tube defects and Down's syndrome. In: Rodeck CH, ed. Fetal diagnosis of genetic defects, Baillière's clinical obstetrics and gynaecology, vol.1(3). London: Baillière Tindall, 1987:649.

195. Cuckle H, van Oudgaarden ED, Mason G, et al. Taking account of vaginal bleeding in screening for Down's syndrome. Br J Obstet Gynaecol 1994;101:948.

196. Meagher S, Davison G. Early second-trimester determination of fetal gender by ultrasound. Ultrasound Obstet Gynecol 1996;8:322.

197. Barkai G, Goldman B, Ries L, et al. Expanding multiple marker screening for Down's syndrome to include Edward's syndrome. Prenat Diagn 1993;13:843.

198. Palomaki GE, Haddow JE, Knight GJ, et al. Risk-based prenatal screening for trisomy 21 using alpha-fetoprotein, unconjugated oestriol and human chorionic gonadotropin. Prenat Diagn 1995;13:843.

199. Benn PA, Leo MV, Rodis JF, et al. Maternal serum screening for fetal trisomy 18: a comparison of fixed cutoff and patient-specific risk protocols. Obstet Gynecol 1999;93:707.

200. Benn PA, Ying J, Beazoglou T, et al. Estimates for the sensitivity and false-positive rates for second trimester serum screening for Down syndrome and trisomy 18 with adjustment for cross-identification and double-positive results. Prenat Diagn 2001;21:46.

201. Hook EB, Hammerton JL. The frequency of chromosome abnormalities detected in consecutive newborn studies; differences between studies; results by sex and severity of phenotypic involvement. In Hook EB, Porter IH, eds. Population cytogenetics: studies in humans. New York: Academic Press, 1977:63.

202. Hook EB, Cross PK, Regal RR. The frequency of 47,+21, 47,+18, and 47+13 at the uppermost extremes of maternal ages: results on 56,094 fetuses studied prenatally and comparisons with data on livebirths. Hum Genet 1984;68:211.

203. Hook EB, Mutton DE, Ide R, et al. The natural history of Down syndrome conceptuses diagnosed prenatally that are not electively terminated. Am J Hum Genet 1995;57:875.

204. Cuckle H. Down syndrome fetal loss rate in early pregnancy. Prenat Diagn 1999;19:1177.

205. Tul N, Spencer K, Noble P, et al. Screening for trisomy 18 by fetal nuchal translucency and maternal serum free beta-hCG and PAPP-A at 10–14 weeks of gestation. Prenat Diagn 1999;19:1035.

206. Spencer K, Mallard AS, Coombes EJ, et al. Prenatal screening for trisomy 18 with free beta human chorionic gonadotrophin as a marker. BMJ 1993;307:1455.

207. Cuckle HS, Sehmi IK, Jones R. Inhibin A and non-Down's syndrome aneuploidy. Prenat Diagn 1999;19:787.

208. Biagiotti R, Cariati E, Brizzi L, et al. Maternal serum screening for trisomy 18 in the first trimester of pregnancy. Prenat Diagn 1998;18:907.

209. Spencer K, Crossley JA, Green K, et al. Second trimester levels of pregnancy associated plasma protein-A in cases of trisomy 18. Prenat Diagn 1999;19:1127.

210. Bersinger NA, Leporrier N, Herrou M, et al. Maternal serum pregnancy-associated plasma protein A (PAPP-A) but not pregnancy-specific beta 1-glycoprotein (SP1) is a useful second-trimester marker for fetal trisomy 18. Prenat Diagn 1999;19:537.

211. de Graaf IM, Prjkrt E, Bilardo CM, et al. Early pregnancy screening for fetal aneuploidy with serum markers and nuchal translucency. Prenat Diagn 1999;19:458.

212. Kennedy DM, Edwards VM, Worthington DJ. Maternal serum screening for trisomy 18: assessing different statistical models to optimize detection rates. Prenat Diagn 2000;20:676.

213. Spencer K, Heath V, Flack N, et al. First trimester maternal serum AFP and total hCG in aneuploidies other than trisomy 21. Prenat Diagn 2000;20:635.

214. Spencer K, Liao AW, Ong CY, et al. Maternal serum activin A and inhibin A in trisomy 18 pregnancies at 10–14 weeks. Prenat Diagn 2001;21:571.

215. Ochshorn Y, Kupferminc MJ, Wolman I, et al. First trimester PAPP-A in the detection of non-Down syndrome aneuploidy. Prenat Diagn 2001;21:547.

216. Muller F, Sault C, Lemay C, et al. Second trimester two-step trisomy 18 screening using maternal serum markers. Prenat Diagn 2002;22:605.

217. Sherod C, Sebire NJ, Soares W, et al. Prenatal diagnosis of trisomy 18 at the 10–14-week ultrasound scan. Ultrasound Obstet Gynecol 1997;10:387.

218. Wald NJ, Hackshaw AK, Watt H. Nuchal translucency and trisomy 18. Prenat Diagn 1999;19:995.

219. Borrell A, Costa D, Martinez JM, et al. Criteria for fetal nuchal thickness cutoff: a re-evaluation. Prenat Diagn 1997;17:23.

220. Blundell G, Ashby JP, Martin C, et al. Clinical follow-up of high mid-trimester maternal serum intact human chorionic gonadotrophin concentrations in singleton pregnancies. Prenat Diagn 1999;19:219.

221. Cuckle H, Arbuzova S, Spencer K, et al. Frequency and clinical consequences of extremely high maternal serum PAPP-A levels. Prenat Diagn 2003;23:385.

221a. Milunsky A, Nebiolo L. Maternal serum triple analyte screening and adverse pregnancy outcome. Fetal Diagn Ther 1996;11:249.

221b. Milunsky A. Multianalyte maternal serum screening for chromosomal defects. In: Milunsky A, ed. Genetic disorders and the fetus: diagnosis, prevention, and treatment, 4th ed. Baltimore: Johns Hopkins University Press, 1998.

222. Spencer K, Nicolaides KH. A first trimester trisomy 13/trisomy 18 risk algorithm combining fetal nuchal translucency thickness, maternal serum free beta-hCG and PAPP-A. Prenat Diagn 2002;22:877.

223. Saller DN Jr, Canick JA, Blitzer MG, et al. Second-trimester maternal serum analyte levels associated with fetal trisomy 13. Prenat Diagn 1999;19:813.

224. Spencer K, Ong C, Skentou H, et al. Screening for trisomy 13 by fetal nuchal translucency and mater-
     nal serum free beta-hCG and PAPP-A at 10–14 weeks of gestation. Prenat Diagn 2000;20:411.
225. Benn PA, Gainey A, Ingardia CJ, et al. Second trimester maternal serum analytes in triploid pregnancies:
     correlation with phenotype and sex chromosome complement. Prenat Diagn 2001;21:680.
226. Spencer K, Liao AW, Skentou H, et al. Screening for triploidy by fetal nuchal translucency and maternal
     serum free beta-hCG and PAPP-A at 10–14 weeks of gestation. Prenat Diagn 2000;20:495.
227. Saller DN Jr, Canick JA, Schwartz S, et al. Multiple-marker screening in pregnancies with hydropic and
     nonhydropic Turner syndrome. Am J Obstet Gynecol 1992;167:1021.
228. Lambert-Messerlian GM, Saller DN Jr, Tumber MB, et al. Second-trimester maternal serum inhibin A
     levels in fetal trisomy 18 and Turner syndrome with and without hydrops. Prenat Diagn 1998;18:1061.
229. Spencer K, Tul N, Nicolaides KH. Maternal serum free beta-hCG and PAPP-A in fetal sex chromosome
     defects in the first trimester. Prenat Diagn 2000;20:390.
230. Bradley LA, Palomaki GE, Knight GJ, et al. Levels of unconjugated estriol and other maternal serum
     markers in pregnancies with Smith–Lemli–Opitz (RSH) syndrome fetuses. Am J Med Genet 1999;82:355.
231. Kashork CD, Sutton VR, Fonda Allen JS, et al. Low or absent unconjugated estriol in pregnancy: an in-
     dicator for steroid sulfatase deficiency detectable by fluorescence in situ hybridization and biochemical
     analysis. Prenat Diagn 2002;22:1028.
232. Aitken DA, Irelland M, Berry E, et al. Second-trimester pregnancy associated plasma protein-A levels
     are reduced in Cornelia de Lange syndrome pregnancies. Prenat Diagn 1999;15:1035.
233. Bruner JP, Hsia YE. Prenatal findings in Brachmann–de Lange syndrome. Obstet Gynecol 1990;76:966.
234. Drolshagen LF, Durmon G, Berumen M, et al. Prenatal ultrasonographic appearance of "Cornelia de
     Lange" syndrome. J Clin Ultrasound 1992;20:470.
235. Sekimoto H, Osada H, Kimura H, et al. Prenatal findings in Brachmann–de Lange syndrome. Arch Gy-
     necol Obstet 2000;263:182.
236. Huang WH, Porto M. Abnormal first-trimester fetal nuchal translucency and Cornelia de Lange syndrome.
     Obstet Gynecol 2002;99:956.
237. Gembruch U, Knopfle G, Bald R, et al. Early diagnosis of fetal congenital heart disease by transvaginal
     echocardiography. Ultrasound Obstet Gynecol 1993;3:310.
238. Achiron R, Rotstein Z, Lipitz S, et al. First-trimester diagnosis of fetal congenital heart disease by trans-
     vaginal ultrasonography. Obstet Gynecol 1994;84:69.
239. Montenegro N, Matias A, Areias JC, et al. Increased fetal nuchal translucency: possible involvement of
     early cardiac failure. Ultrasound Obstet Gynecol 1997;10:265.
240. Von Kaisenberg CS, Huggon I, Hyett JA, et al. Cardiac gene expression of GATA-4 transcription factor
     in human trisomy 21 fetuses with increased nuchal translucency. Prenat Diagn 1998;18:267.
241. Hyett J, Perdu M, Sharland G, et al. Using fetal nuchal translucency to screen for major congenital car-
     diac defects at 10–14 weeks of gestation: population based cohort study. BMJ 1999;318:81.
242. Schwarzler P, Carvalho JS, Senat MV, et al. Screening for fetal aneuploidies and fetal cardiac abnormal-
     ities by nuchal translucency thickness measurement at 10–14 weeks of gestation as part of routine ante-
     natal care in an unselected population. Br J Obstet Gynaecol 1999;106:1029.
243. Simpson JM, Sharland GK. Nuchal translucency and congenital heart defects: heart failure or not? Ul-
     trasound Obstet Gynecol 2000;16:30.
244. Michailidis GD, Economides DL. Nuchal translucency measurement and pregnancy outcome in kary-
     otypically normal fetuses. Ultrasound Obstet Gynecol 2001;17:102.
245. Mavrides E, Cobian-Sanchez F, Tekay A, et al. Limitations of using first-trimester nuchal translucency
     measurement in routine screening for major congenital heart defects. Ultrasound Obstet Gynecol
     2001;17:106.
246. Orvos H, Wayda K, Kozinszky Z, et al. Increased nuchal translucency and congenital heart defects in eu-
     ploid fetuses: the Szeged experience. Eur J Obstet Gynecol Reprod Biol 2002;101:124.
247. Hyett JA. Increased nuchal translucency in fetuses with a normal karyotype. Prenat Diagn 2002;22:864.
248. Cuckle HS, Sehmi IK, Jones R, et al. Low maternal serum PAPP-A and fetal viability. Prenat Diagn
     1999;19:788.
249. Ong CY, Liao AW, Spencer K, et al. First trimester maternal serum free beta human chorionic go-
     nadotrophin and pregnancy associated plasma protein A as predictors of pregnancy complications. Br J
     Obstet Gynaecol 2000;107:1265.
250. Yaron Y, Heifetz S, Ochshorn Y, et al. Decreased first trimester PAPP-A is a predictor of adverse preg-
     nancy outcome. Prenat Diagn 2002;22:778.
251. Benn PA, Craffey A, Horne D, et al. Elevated maternal serum alpha-fetoprotein with low unconjugated
     estriol and the risk for lethal perinatal outcome. J Matern Fetal Med 2000;9:165.

252. Cuckle HS, Densem JW, Wald NJ. Detection of hydatidiform mole in maternal serum screening programmes for Down's syndrome. Br J Obstet Gynaecol 1992;99:495.

253. Petrou S, Henderson J, Roberts T, et al. Recent economic evaluations of antenatal screening: a systematic review and critique. J Med Screen 2000;7:59.

254. Vintzileos AM, Ananth CV, Smulian JC, et al. Cost-benefit analysis of prenatal diagnosis for Down syndrome using the British or the American approach. Obstet Gynecol 2000;95:577.

255. Gilbert RE, Augood C, Gupta R, et al. Screening for Down's syndrome: effects, safety, and cost effectiveness of first and second trimester strategies. BMJ 2001;323:423.

256. Caughey AB, Kuppermann M, Norton ME, et al. Nuchal translucency and first trimester biochemical markers for down syndrome screening: a cost-effectiveness analysis. Am J Obstet Gynecol 2002;187:1239.

257. Christiansen M, Olesen Larsen S. An increase in cost-effectiveness of first trimester maternal screening programmes for fetal chromosome anomalies is obtained by contingent testing. Prenat Diagn 2002;22:482.

258. Cusick W, Buchanan P, Hallahan TW, et al. Combined first-trimester versus second-trimester serum screening for Down syndrome: a cost analysis. Am J Obstet Gynecol 2003;188:745.

259. Roberts T, Henderson J, Mugford M, et al. Antenatal ultrasound screening for fetal abnormalities: a systematic review of studies of cost and cost effectiveness. Br J Obstet Gynaecol 2002;109:44.

260. Lawson HW, Frye A, Atrash HK, et al. Abortion mortality, United States, 1972–1987. Am J Obstet Gynecol 1994;171:1365.

261. Alfirevic Z, Gosden CM, Neilson JP. Chorionic villus sampling versus amniocentesis for prenatal diagnosis. The Cochrane Library, Issue 4, 2002. Oxford: Update Software.

262. Rhoads GG, Jackson LG, Schlesselman SE, et al. The safety and efficacy of chorionic villus sampling for early prenatal diagnosis of cytogenetic abnormalities. N Engl J Med 1989;320:609.

263. Jackson LG, Zachary JM, Fowler SE, et al. A randomized comparison of transcervical and transabdominal chorionic-villus sampling. The U.S. National Institute of Child Health and Human Development Chorionic-Villus Sampling and Amniocentesis Study Group. N Engl J Med 1992;327:594.

264. Kuliev A, Jackson L, Froster U, et al. Chorionic villus sampling safety. Report of World Health Organization/EURO meeting in association with the Seventh International Conference on Early Prenatal Diagnosis of Genetic Diseases, Tel-Aviv, Israel, May 21, 1994. Am J Obstet Gynecol 1996;174:807.

Yves G. Ville, M.D., Kypros H. Nicolaides, M.B.B.S., $\qquad$ 23
M.R.C.O.G., and Stuart Campbell, M.B.B.S., F.R.C.O.G.

Prenatal Diagnosis of Fetal Malformations by Ultrasound

Ultrasound is the key to the prenatal diagnosis of most fetal malformations. This safe prenatal investigation is offered mostly to pregnant women at the optimal gestations of 11–14 weeks and 20–24 weeks. It allows an examination of the external and internal anatomy of the fetus and the detection of not only major malformations but also of subtle markers of chromosomal abnormalities and genetic syndromes.

The first fetal malformation to be detected antenatally by ultrasonography leading to the termination of pregnancy for medical indication was anencephaly.[1] Subsequently, thousands of reports have appeared in the scientific literature describing the diagnosis of an ever-expanding range of fetal structural and functional abnormalities. This chapter provides an overview of the prenatal diagnosis of some of these defects and their associated abnormalities. Special emphasis is placed on the diagnosis of fetal abnormalities during the first trimester of pregnancy. Indeed, improvement of the techniques and wider access to ultrasound examination for pregnant women have moved the challenge of prenatal diagnosis of fetal abnormalities, especially chromosomal disorders, to the first trimester. The new developments of an old technique, fetoscopy, which has recently been rediscovered because of the miniaturization of the instruments and the development of endoscopic fetal surgery, will also be highlighted.

Routine ultrasound screening of the whole population has the potential advantage of detecting most major fetal malformations. For this reason, the Royal College of Obstetricians and Gynaecologists in Great Britain recommended that (1) more facilities for high-quality ultrasound machines and for training of personnel be provided to all obstetric departments, and (2) all pregnant women be offered a proper ultrasound scan at approximately 20 weeks of gestation for fetal biometry but also for a systematic search for major and minor defects.[2]

The usefulness of screening low-risk populations by ultrasound has been challenged.[3] Six large series examined the value of a detailed ultrasound examination before 24 weeks of gestation in populations in which the incidence of major abnormalities ranged from 1.4 to 2.5 percent.[3-8] Authors reported heterogeneous ranges of sensitivity and positive predictive values (17–71 percent and 75–98 percent, respectively), but excellent specificity and negative predictive values (99.9 percent and 98–99.5 percent, respectively). However, more skeptical opinions about the value and the cost effectiveness of ultrasound screening for fetal abnormalities have been posited.[3] Unfortunately, this large study of 15,151 women focused on a selected low-risk population (representative of 37 percent of the general population) and reported a lower rate of detection than most of the other studies; the power of this analysis was also too low to make conclusions about many secondary outcomes (e.g., perinatal mortality and morbidity, survival rate if a major anomaly is present, termination of pregnancy for major fetal abnormalities). Studies in which a detailed second-trimester scan was conducted at 20–22 weeks of gestation seem to report a higher detection rate than those in which this was done earlier; another factor to take into account is also probably the minimal standard required for fetal cardiac examination when this is included in the routine scan: a four-chamber view alone is likely to be less accurate than a combined view of the short axis of the heart and imaging of the crossing of the great arteries. The usefulness and cost effectiveness of prenatal ultrasound are likely to depend on the standards required for prenatal care and the competence of the operators and therefore reflect to a great extent a social choice rather than technical limitations.

COMMON DEFECTS AMENABLE TO PRENATAL DIAGNOSIS

Craniospinal Defects

Neural Tube Defects

Incidence and prevalence,[9] etiology,[10] morbidity and mortality,[11] and prevention[12] are fully discussed in chapter 21.

Ultrasonographically, the diagnosis of anencephaly can be made as early as 12 weeks of gestation. When the cephalic pole of the fetus is situated deeply in the pelvis, transvaginal rather than transabdominal sonography can be used. Absence of the cranial vault and cerebral hemispheres are constant findings. However, the facial bones and brainstem and portions of the occipital bones and midbrain are usually present. Associated spinal lesions are found in up to 50 percent of cases. Encephaloceles are recognized as cranial defects with herniated fluid-filled or brain-filled cysts. They are most commonly found in an occipital location (70–75 percent of cases), but alternative sites include the frontoethmoidal and parietal regions. Associated abnormalities include hydrocephaly, Dandy-Walker malformation, and Meckel syndrome. The prognosis for encephaloceles is inversely related to the amount of herniated cerebral tissue.[13]

For the diagnosis of spina bifida SB,[14] each neural arch from the cervical to the sacral region must be examined transversely, longitudinally, and in a frontal plane. In the transverse scan, the normal neural arch appears as a closed circle with an intact skin covering, whereas in SB, the arch is U-shaped and there is an associated bulging meningocele or myelomeningocele. The extent of the defect and any associated kyphoscoliosis are best assessed in the longitudinal and frontal scans. The prognosis for the lesion is assessed by applying the same criteria as those used by Lorber[15] postnatally. However, limb movements may appear to be normal even with major lumbosacral lesions and are therefore of no prognostic significance.

The ultrasonographic diagnosis of fetal open spina bifida (OSB) has been greatly enhanced by the recognition of associated abnormalities in the skull and brain.[16,17] These abnormalities include cerebral ventriculomegaly, microcephaly, frontal bone scalloping (lemon sign; Figure 23.1), and obliteration of the cisterna magna with either an "absent" cerebellum or abnormal anterior curvature of the cerebellar hemispheres (banana sign; see

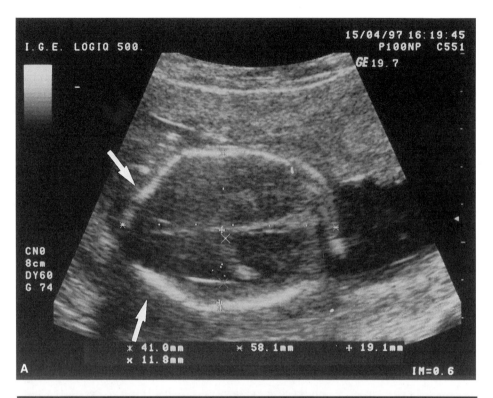

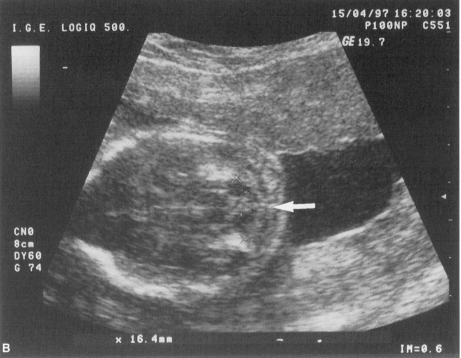

Fig. 23.1. Transverse section of the fetal head (*A*) at the level of the septum cavum pellucidum, demonstrating the "lemon" sign (scalloping of the frontal bones), and suboccipital bregmatic view (*B*), demonstrating the "banana" sign (anterior curvature of the cerebellar hemispheres and obliteration of the cisterna magna), in a 21-week fetus with OSB (arrow), visible on a frontal plane (*C*).

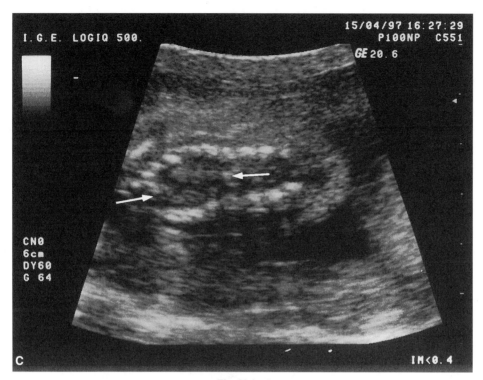

Fig. 23.1. *C*

Figure 23.1). Nyberg et al.[17] suggested that the presence of a lemon sign is related to gestational age. Among their fifty cases with OSB, they noted a lemon sign in 89 percent of the 27 fetuses examined before 24 weeks, in 50 percent of the 16 fetuses examined between 24 and 34 weeks, and in none of the seven fetuses examined after 35 weeks.

Van den Hof et al.[18] evaluated the incidence and diagnostic accuracy of the lemon and cerebellar ultrasonic markers, as well as head size and ventriculomegaly in their study of 1,561 patients at high risk for fetal neural tube defects. In the 130 fetuses with OSB, there was a relationship between gestational age and the presence of each of these markers (Table 23.1). The lemon sign was present in 98 percent of fetuses at ≤24 weeks of gestation but in only 13 percent of those at >24 weeks of gestation. Cerebellar abnormalities were present in 95 percent of fetuses irrespective of gestation; however, the cerebellar abnormality at ≤24 weeks of gestation was predominantly the banana sign (72 percent), whereas at gestations >24 weeks, it was cerebellar "absence" (81 percent). Both growth retardation and cerebral ventriculomegaly significantly worsened with gestation, while the head circumference remained disproportionately small throughout gestation.

These easily recognizable alterations in skull and brain morphology are often more readily attainable than detailed spinal views. Indeed, Van den Hof et al.[18] reported that in several of their cases with very obvious cranial and cerebellar signs, the ultrasonographic demonstration of the spinal lesion was possible only after a prolonged and diligent search by experienced operators. It was especially reassuring that all sacral tip lesions were consistently accompanied by these ultrasound markers. In contrast, the only case with a totally normal skull and brain was one with an extensive lumbar defect that was readily

Table 23.1. Ultrasound findings in 130 fetuses with OSB in relation to gestational age

	Gestation (Weeks)	
Feature	≤24 weeks (n = 107)	>24 weeks (n = 23)
Lemon-shaped skull	105 (98%)	3 (13%)
Abnormal cerebellum	103 (96%)	21 (91%)
Banana-shaped	74 (69%)	4 (17%)
Absent	29 (27%)	17 (74%)
Va/H: >97.5th centile	61 (57%)	18 (78%)
Vp/H: >97.5th centile	79 (74%)	19 (83%)
HC: <2.5th centile	20 (19%)	10 (43%)
AC: <2.5th centile	8 (7%)	9 (39%)

AC = abdominal circumference; H = hemisphere; HC = head circumference; Va = anterior cerebral ventricle; Vp = posterior cerebral ventricle.

visible on spinal views. Similarly, in the study of Nyberg et al.,[17] the three cases of OSB with a normal-shaped skull at <24 weeks of gestation, also had lumbar lesions.

In routine ultrasound scanning of pregnant women, demonstration of fetal cranial and cerebellar markers identifies a group at high risk of OSB. Even for gestations >24 weeks, when the lemon sign is no longer useful, cerebellar signs, cerebral ventriculomegaly, and relative microcephaly are often present. Patients with suspected fetal cranial and cerebellar signs as well as those with raised maternal serum α-fetoprotein (AFP), antifolate medications, or a history of NTDs should be referred to experienced ultrasonographers, who can make a confident diagnosis of OSB by a diligent examination of the fetal spine. Present data indicate that in such patients, if an ultrasound examination of the fetal spine, cranium, and cerebellum appear to be normal, the chance of an undetected spinal lesion must be extremely low. Hence, amniocentesis for the measurement of AFP and acetylcholinesterase must be carefully considered because the procedure-related risk of fetal death even in the hands of experienced operators could reach 1 percent.[19] (See also chapter 2.)

The assumption that spinal dysraphism leads to progressive neurologic deficit only after birth has prompted investigators to assess the effectiveness of in utero closure of NTDs in the prevention of handicap (see chapter 29). Similar defects artificially induced in monkey fetuses have been successfully closed using a paste containing allogenic crushed bone particles.[20]

Hydrocephalus

Congenital hydrocephalus, with an incidence of 5–25 per 10,000 births,[21] may result from chromosomal and genetic abnormalities, intrauterine hemorrhage, or congenital infection, although many cases have as yet no recognized cause. Burton[22] found that for male siblings of male patients with congenital aqueductal stenosis, the risk of recurrence is 12 percent, suggesting that up to 25 percent of cases of aqueductal obstruction in males may be inherited as an X-linked recessive disorder. In other cases, the risk of recurrence varies according to cause. The outlook in cases of congenital hydrocephalus is poor, with high fetal wastage or perinatal death due mainly to the associated anomalies. Severe mental retardation is common among the survivors.[23]

Fetal hydrocephalus is diagnosed sonographically, from 16 weeks of gestation, by the demonstration of abnormally dilated lateral cerebral ventricles.[24] Certainly before 24 weeks and particularly in cases of associated SB, the biparietal diameter and head circumference may be small rather than large for gestation. A transverse axial scan of the fetal head at the level of the cavum septum pellucidum will demonstrate the lateral borders of the anterior horns, the medial and lateral borders of the posterior horns of the lateral ventricles, the choroid plexuses, the third ventricle, and the Sylvian fissure. In hydrocephalus, the ratio of the anterior and/or posterior horn of the lateral ventricle to that of the cerebral hemisphere is above the 95th centile of the appropriate reference range for gestation. The level of the obstruction is defined by examining the aqueduct of Sylvius and the third and fourth ventricles.

Fetal lateral cerebral ventriculomegaly is associated with a high incidence of morphologic and chromosomal defects (Table 23.2).[25-34] SB is found in 28–67 percent of the cases, and conversely, ventriculomegaly is present in approximately 75 percent of fetuses with SB.[18] Although there are several reports on antenatally diagnosed ventriculomegaly, they cannot be considered appropriate for defining the natural history of the condition, because in the vast majority of cases, the cause of fetal death was iatrogenic (Table 23.2). Nevertheless, both fetal or perinatal death and neurologic development in survivors are strongly related to the presence of other malformations and chromosomal defects. Although mild ventriculomegaly is associated with a good prognosis, it is also the group with the highest incidence of chromosomal abnormalities.[29]

Earlier experimental studies[35] and clinical efforts were only partly successful.[23,35-37] More recent surgical approaches are discussed in chapter 29.

Ventriculoamniotic shunting has been abandoned and the currently available data do not allow definite conclusions concerning its efficacy. Nevertheless, it is certain that many of the cases treated in the early 1980s were inappropriate, because they even included fetuses with holoprosencephaly and porencephalic cysts. It is possible that shunting is beneficial provided that (1) all intracerebral and extracerebral malformations and chromosomal defects are excluded, and (2) serial ultrasound scans demonstrate progressive lateral cerebral ventriculomegaly.

Table 23.2. Summary of reports on antenatally diagnosed hydrocephalus, providing data on the presence of additional defects, incidence of chromosomal abnormalities (where possible, only for cases without holoprosencephaly), and survival rate

| Author | Cases | Additional Defects | | | Chromosomally Abnormal | Alive |
		Total	HE	NTD		
Chervenak et al.[25]	53	44 (83%)	—	15 (28%)	4/?	28%
Cochrane et al.[26]	41	32 (78%)	3 (7%)	15 (37%)	1/?	34%
Pretorius et al.[32]	40	28 (70%)	1 (3%)	13 (33%)	2/7 (29%)	15%
Pilu et al.[31]	30	9 (30%)	—	—	3/30 (10%)	?
Serlo et al.[33]	38	32 (84%)	1 (3%)	—	4/?	26%
Nyberg et al.[30]	61	51 (84%)	13 (21%)	23 (38%)	2/21 (10%)	16%
Vintzileos et al.[34]	20	16 (70%)	1 (5%)	6 (30%)	2/19 (11%)	45%
Hudgins et al.[28]	47	35 (74%)	15 (32%)	—	1/47 (2%)	40%
Drugan et al.[27]	43	31 (72%)	3 (7%)	18 (42%)	5/19 (26%)	44%
Nicolaides et al.[29]	267	209 (78%)	—	184 (67%)	12/64 (19%)	9%

HE = holoprosencephaly; NTD = neural tube defect.

Hydranencephaly

Congenital absence of the cerebral hemispheres with preservation of the midbrain and cerebellum may result from widespread vascular occlusion in the distribution of the internal carotid arteries, prolonged severe hydrocephalus, an overwhelming infection such as toxoplasmosis or cytomegalovirus, or defects in embryogenesis. The condition is generally not inherited and is usually incompatible with survival beyond early infancy.

Ultrasonographically, the complete absence of echoes from the anterior and middle fossae distinguishes hydranencephaly from severe hydrocephalus in which a thin rim of remaining cortex and the midline echo can always be identified.

Holoprosencephaly

Holoprosencephaly, with an incidence of 0.6–1.9 per 10,000 births,[38] encompasses a heterogeneous group of cerebral malformations resulting from either failure or incomplete cleavage of the forebrain. Although in many cases the cause is a chromosomal abnormality or a monogenic disorder, in many cases the cause is unknown. The risk of recurrence in cases of primary trisomy is approximately 1 percent. In the group without chromosomal defects, the presence of associated malformations may lead to the diagnosis of a syndrome with a known mode of inheritance. In others, parental consanguinity or a history of affected siblings would suggest a genetic, probably autosomal recessive inheritance. For sporadic, nonchromosomal holoprosencephaly, an empirical recurrence risk of 6 percent has been derived.[39]

Prenatal diagnosis by ultrasonography is based on the demonstration of a single dilated midline ventricle replacing the two lateral ventricles or partial segmentation of the ventricles in the standard transverse view of the fetal head for measurement of the biparietal diameter. Although some authors have suggested that confident diagnosis requires the additional demonstration of facial abnormalities, such as hypotelorism, facial cleft, or proboscis, these are not always present. Reports on antenatally diagnosed holoprosencephaly have established a high association with facial and other malformations as well as chromosomal defects (Table 23.3).[40–43]

Microcephaly

Microcephaly, with a birth incidence of approximately 1 per 10,000, is commonly found in the presence of other brain abnormalities, such as encephalocele or holoprosencephaly, chromosomal defects, or genetic syndromes. Other etiologic factors include fetal hypoxia,

Table 23.3. Summary of major series on antenatally diagnosed holoprosencephaly, providing data on the presence of additional defects and incidence of chromosomal abnormalities at well as outcome

Author	Cases	Additional Defects		Chromosomally Abnormal	Outcome		
		Facial	Extrafacial		Alive	PND	TOP
Filly et al.[42]	5	—	—	1 (20%)	—	4	1
Nyberg et al.[43]	7	—	1 (14%)	4 (57%)	—	7	—
Chervenak et al.[41]	14	3 (21%)	4 (29%)	6 (43%)	2	7	5
Berry et al.[40]	38	14 (37%)	21 (55%)	11 (29%)	2	7	29

PND = perinatal death; TOP = termination of pregnancy.

intrauterine infection, and exposure to radiation or other teratogens, including the anticoagulant warfarin. Prognosis depends on the underlying cause, but in approximately 90 percent of the cases, there is severe mental retardation.[44]

Prenatal diagnosis by sonography is based on the demonstration of a decrease in the
head-to-abdomen circumference ratio[45] and the associated abnormal intracranial pathology. When the intracranial anatomy is normal, the condition is defined by a biparietal diameter >3 SD below the mean. In milder cases, demonstration of a progressive decrease
in the head circumference until it falls below the fifth centile, in the presence of normal
growth in the abdominal circumference, is necessary. This difference may not become apparent before 26 weeks of gestation.

Choroid Plexus Cysts

The choroid plexuses are easily visualized from 9 weeks of gestation, when they occupy
almost the entire hemispheres. Thereafter, and until 24 weeks of gestation, there is a rapid
decrease in the size of both the choroid plexus and the lateral cerebral ventricle in relation to the hemisphere. Choroid plexus cysts (Figure 23.2), which are often bilateral, are
found in 0.2–2.3 percent of fetuses at 16–18 weeks of gestation,[46] but in more than 90
percent of cases they resolve by 26–28 weeks. Although they are usually of no pathologic
significance, they are associated with an increased risk for chromosomal abnormalities,
mainly trisomy 18 and trisomy 21. (See also "Ultrasonographically Detectable Markers
of Fetal Chromosomal Defects" on page 869.)

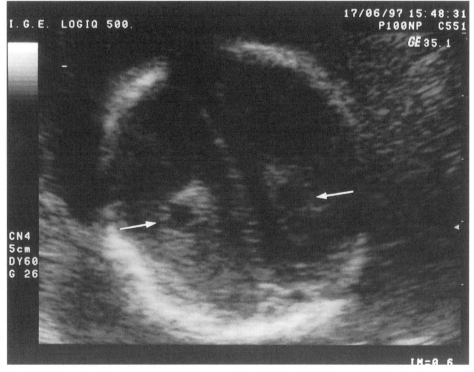

Fig. 23.2. Coronal section of the fetal head, demonstrating bilateral choroid plexus cysts (arrows).

Dandy–Walker Malformation

The Dandy–Walker malformation is a nonspecific marker of chromosomal abnormalities, genetic syndromes, congenital infection, or teratogens.[47] In general, the associated mortality rate is high and mental development among survivors is poor.

Ultrasonographically, the contents of the posterior fossa are visualized through a transverse suboccipitobregmatic section of the fetal head. In the Dandy–Walker malformation, there is cystic dilatation of the fourth ventricle with partial or complete agenesis of the vermis; in more than 50 percent of the cases, there is associated hydrocephalus.[48]

Cardiovascular Defects

Gross structural abnormalities of the heart or of major blood vessels that could actually or potentially affect the proper functioning of the heart are found in 8 per 1,000 livebirths and in 27 per 1,000 stillbirths.[49] The cause of heart defects is heterogeneous and probably depends on the interplay of multiple genetic and environmental factors.[50] Environmental factors that have been implicated in the causation of cardiac defects include maternal diabetes mellitus or collagen disease, exposure to drugs such as lithium, and viral infections such as rubella. Specific mutant gene defects and chromosomal abnormalities account for less than 5 percent of the patients. When a previous sibling has had congenital heart defect, in the absence of a known genetic syndrome, the risk of recurrence is 1–4 percent. In general, this is highest for left-to-right shunts and endocardial fibroelastosis and lowest for right-to-left shunts and outflow obstructions. When a parent is affected, the risk for the offspring is up to 17 percent.[51]

Findings commonly associated with cardiac defects include dysrhythmias, hydrops, chromosomal abnormalities, and multisystem malformations. Extracardiac defects, particularly craniospinal, gastrointestinal, and renal, are found in approximately one-third of the cases. Although some of the cardiac defects resolve spontaneously (e.g., ventricular septal defect) and others are easily correctable (e.g., patent ductus), major structural abnormalities are either inoperable (e.g., hypoplastic left heart) or carry high operative risks (e.g., truncus arteriosus).

Cardiac defects are the most common congenital abnormalities (see chapter 1). About half are either lethal or require surgery, and half are asymptomatic. The first two groups are referred to as critical. Specialist echocardiography at around 20 weeks of gestation can identify the majority of critical cardiac defects, but the major challenge in prenatal diagnosis is to identify the high-risk group for referral to specialist centers. Currently, screening is based on examination of the four-chamber view of the heart at the 20-week scan, but this identifies only about 25 percent of the critical cardiac defects.[52]

The heart occupies approximately one-third of the thorax, and in this view, the normal ventricles, atria, atrioventricular valves, ventricular and atrial septae, foramen ovale flap, and pulmonary venous connections can be identified. Copel et al.[53] reported that 96 percent of ultrasonographically detectable fetal cardiac defects demonstrate some abnormalities in this view. Angulation of the transducer from the four-chamber view is necessary for the demonstration of the normal aortic and pulmonary arterial origins from the left and right ventricles, respectively, and for the diagnosis of great arterial malalignment.[52,54]

Real-time directed M-mode echocardiography improves the accuracy of the cross-sectional scan in the diagnosis of cardiac defects and provides additional information on cardiac geometry and function.[52–54] This method is particularly useful in the diagnosis and evaluation of dysrhythmias and the monitoring of in utero antiarrhythmic therapy. In the presence of an arrhythmia, particularly complete heart block, an underlying cardiac defect should be sought, because this may be present in 20–25 percent of the cases.[55,56] When a fetal abnormality is suspected, pulsed Doppler studies for measurement of blood velocity across the valves are helpful in the assessment of fetal cardiac function[57] (see also chapter 24).

Echocardiography has been successfully applied to the prenatal assessment of the fetal cardiac function and structure[52–59] and has led to the diagnosis of most cardiac abnormalities. However, the majority of published reports refer to the prenatal diagnosis of moderate to major defects in high-risk populations. Because currently only the more severe types of heart defects are usually diagnosed antenatally, they are associated with higher mortality than those diagnosed after birth. Thus, Crawford et al.[60] reported that the mortality rate for antenatally diagnosed defects was 83 percent, compared with only 19 percent for those that were missed on prenatal sonography.

With improved expertise and equipment, basic echocardiography for the examination of the four-chamber view, the connection of the great arteries, and the detection of dysrhythmias should be incorporated in the routine ultrasound screening programs for all pregnancies. Suspected anomalies can then be referred to specialized centers for further elucidation of the problem.

Pulmonary Abnormalities

Cystic Adenomatoid Malformation of the Lung

Cystic adenomatoid malformation of the lung is a rare congenital abnormality of unknown cause.[61] There is a broad spectrum of clinical presentations. Some infants present in the first week of life with severe, and often fatal, respiratory insufficiency. Smaller lesions are often asymptomatic until late childhood, and they are easily corrected by excision of the affected pulmonary segment or lobe.

Prenatal diagnosis is based on the ultrasonographic or magnetic resonance imaging (see chapter 25) of a hyperechogenic pulmonary tumor that is either solid (microcystic) or cystic. Polyhydramnios is a common feature, and this may be a consequence of decreased fetal swallowing of amniotic fluid due to esophageal compression or increased fluid production by the abnormal lung tissue. When there is compression of the heart and major blood vessels in the thorax, fetal hydrops develops. Prognostic features for poor outcome include microcystic disease, major lung compression causing pulmonary hypoplasia, and development of hydrops fetalis irrespective of the type of the lesion. Adzick[62] examined eighteen of their cases and reviewed another seventeen from the literature. In fourteen of the fifteen cases with microcystic disease, the fetuses were hydropic, and they all died either before or after birth; the one nonhydropic fetus survived. In contrast, sixteen of the twenty-two cases with macrocystic disease were nonhydropic and all but one survived; none of the six cases with hydrops survived.

Large intrathoracic cyst causing major mediastinal shift and associated hydrops can be effectively treated by the insertion of thoracoamniotic shunts[63,64] (see chapter 29). This condition is also the most gratifying experience of open fetal surgery, and Adzick et al. reported that five of seven operated fetuses survived without pulmonary hypoplasia.[65]

Diaphragmatic Hernia

Diaphragmatic hernia is found in 2–5 per 10,000 births, and approximately 30 percent of the infants are stillborn.[66] Associated lethal nonpulmonary malformations are found in

95 percent of the stillbirths and in up to 60 percent of those that die within 24 hours of delivery. Craniospinal defects, including the otherwise rare iniencephaly, and cardiac anomalies predominate.[67] Furthermore, although isolated diaphragmatic hernia is an anatomically simple defect that is easily correctable, the mortality rate for infants in whom respiratory distress develops, requiring operative repair within the first 24 hours of life remains at 50–80 percent.[68] By contrast, the survival for infants in whom symptoms develop after the first 24 hours of life is nearly 100 percent.[69,70] The main cause of death is hypoxemia due to pulmonary hypertension resulting from the abnormal development of the pulmonary vascular bed. Although this is not extensively documented, the more widespread use of high-frequency oxygenation might further improve these results.

Prenatally, the diaphragm is imaged by ultrasonography or magnetic resonance (see chapter 25) as an echo-free space between the thorax and abdomen. Congenital diaphragmatic hernia, which results from failure of closure of the posterolateral pleuroperitoneal fold at 8–9 weeks of gestation, can be diagnosed by the demonstration of stomach and intestines (90 percent of the cases) or liver (50 percent) in the thorax and the associated mediastinal shift to the opposite side. Polyhydramnios, ascites, and other malformations are often present.

Extensive animal studies have suggested that pulmonary hypoplasia and hypertension due to intrathoracic compression are reversible by in utero surgical repair[71] (see also chapters 24 and 29). However, such therapy is likely to have limited success in the human because the bronchial tree is fully developed by the 16th week of gestation.[72–76] Early surgical approaches achieved mixed results,[73] but novel techniques (chapter 29) show greater promise.[74–76] Our experience using the PLUG (Plug the Lung Until it Grows) technique (see chapter 29) now exceeds seventeen cases, most done under local or regional anesthesia. At this stage we also remove the balloon before birth, so that EXIT procedures become unnecessary. The survival rate for babies with LCDH who were operated on between 26 and 28 weeks was 50 percent, while in the control group of eligible patients who declined fetoscopic endoluminal tracheal occlusion (FETO), it was 0 percent. There were no maternal complications, and fetal morbidity so far is no more than expected in this population (reflux, one patch revision). The minimally invasive nature of the procedure makes it more acceptable, particularly in a European setting, where open fetal surgery has not gained acceptance. We now propose a formal trial to evaluate this procedure.[77]

Hydrops Fetalis

Hydrops fetalis, with an incidence of 3–10 per 10,000 births, is characterized by generalized skin edema and pericardial, pleural, or ascitic effusions. This is a nonspecific finding in a wide variety of fetal and maternal disorders, including hematologic, chromosomal, cardiovascular, renal, pulmonary, gastrointestinal, hepatic, and metabolic abnormalities, congenital infection, neoplasms, and malformations of the placenta or umbilical cord.[78–82] With the widespread introduction of immunoprophylaxis and the successful treatment of rhesus disease by fetal blood transfusions, non-rhesus causes have become responsible for at least 75 percent of the cases and make a greater contribution to perinatal mortality. Although in many instances the underlying cause may be determined by maternal antibody and infection screening, fetal ultrasound scanning including echocardiography and Doppler studies, and fetal blood sampling, quite often the abnormality remains unexplained even after expert postmortem examination.

Although isolated ascites, in both fetuses and neonates, may be transitory,[83] the spontaneous resolution of hydrops has not been reported and the prognosis for this condition, irrespective of the underlying pathology, is extremely poor, with reported mortality rates of 80–95 percent.

Pleural Effusions

Fetal pleural effusions (Figure 23.3) may be an isolated finding or they may occur in association with generalized edema and ascites. Irrespective of the underlying cause, infants affected by pleural effusions usually present in the neonatal period with severe, and often fatal, respiratory insufficiency. This is either a direct result of pulmonary compression caused by the effusions or is due to pulmonary hypoplasia secondary to chronic intrathoracic compression. The overall mortality of neonates with pleural effusions is 25 percent, with a range from 15 percent in infants with isolated pleural effusions to 95 percent in those with gross hydrops. Longaker et al.[84] reported that the mortality rate in cases of antenatally diagnosed chylothorax was 53 percent.

Isolated pleural effusions in the fetus either may resolve spontaneously or can be treated effectively after birth. Nevertheless, in some cases, severe and chronic compression of the fetal lungs can result in pulmonary hypoplasia and neonatal death. In others, mediastinal compression leads to the development of hydrops and polyhydramnios, which are associated with a high risk of premature delivery and perinatal death.[84–86] Attempts at prenatal therapy by repeated thoracocenteses for drainage of pleural effusions have been generally unsuccessful in reversing the hydropic state, because the fluid reaccumulates within 24–48 hours of drainage.[87]

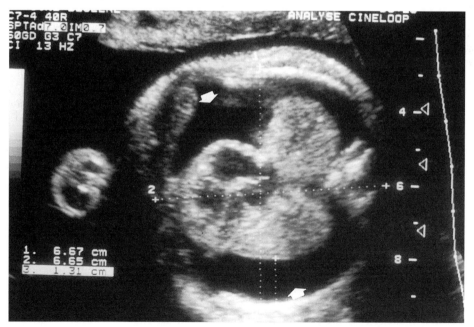

Fig. 23.3. Bilateral moderate pleural effusion on a transverse plane of the fetal thorax (arrow).

Interval insertion shunt to delivery

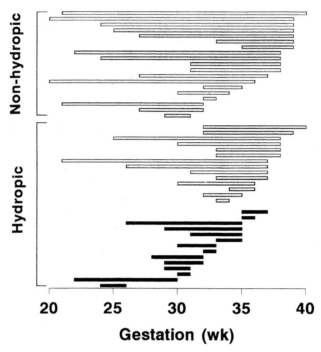

Fig. 23.4. Thoracoamniotic shunting in forty-seven fetuses with pericardial effusion ($n = 1$), cystic adenomatoid malformation ($n = 3$), or pleural effusion ($n = 43$); in thirty cases, there was generalized edema. The horizontal lines connect the gestation at shunting with the gestation at delivery. In the nonhydropic group, all nineteen infants survived. In the hydropic group, fourteen survived (light shading) and fourteen died (dark shading). Although the mean gestation at shunting was similar, the time between shunting and delivery in hydropic fetuses that died was shorter, presumably because in this group, the shunting did not prevent the worsening of hydrops and/or the development of polyhydramnios.

A more promising approach is long-term drainage by the insertion of thoracoamniotic shunts (Figure 23.4).[88,89] This is useful both for diagnosis and treatment. First, the diagnosis of an underlying cardiac abnormality or other intrathoracic lesion may become apparent only after effective decompression and return of the mediastinum to its normal position. Second, it can reverse fetal hydrops, resolve polyhydramnios and thereby reduce the risk of preterm delivery, and may prevent pulmonary hypoplasia. Third, it may be useful in the prenatal diagnosis of pulmonary hypoplasia because in such cases the lungs often fail to expand after shunting. Third, it may help distinguish between hydrops due to primary accumulation of pleural effusions, in which case the ascites and skin edema may resolve after shunting, and other causes of hydrops, such as infection, in which drainage of the effusions does not prevent worsening of the hydrops.

Abdominal Wall Defects

The normal anterior abdominal wall and umbilicus can be readily identified from 13 to 14 weeks of gestation. Normal development depends on the fusion of four ectomesodermic folds (cephalic, caudal, and two lateral).

Omphalocele (Exomphalos)

Omphalocele, with an incidence of 1–3 per 10,000 live births,[90,90a] results from failure of normal embryonic regression of the midgut from the umbilical stalk into the abdominal coelom between the 5th and the 10th week of gestation. The abdominal contents, including intestines and liver or spleen covered by a sac of parietal peritoneum and amnion, are herniated into the base of the umbilical cord. Less often, there is an associated failure in the cephalic embryonic fold resulting in the pentalogy of Cantrell (upper midline omphalocele, anterior diaphragmatic hernia, sternal cleft, ectopia cordis, and intracardiac defects) or failure of the caudal fold, in which case the omphalocele may be associated with exstrophy of the bladder or cloaca, imperforate anus, colonic atresia, and sacral vertebral defects.[91] The Beckwith–Wiedemann syndrome is the association of omphalocele, macrosomia, organomegaly, and macroglossia.[92]

The majority of cases are sporadic and the recurrence risk is usually thought to be <1 percent. However, in some cases, there may be an X-linked or autosomal dominant pattern of inheritance.[92a,92b] Beckwith–Wiedemann syndrome is usually sporadic, and the result of an autosomal dominant mutation in chromosome 11p15 or due to uniparental disomy.[93] Omphalocele is a correctable malformation[94] in which survival depends primarily on whether or not other malformations or chromosomal defects are present.[95] For isolated lesions, survival rates of more than 90 percent are reported in the pediatric literature.[96–99,102] The mortality is much higher with cephalic fold defects than with lateral and caudal defects.

The diagnosis of omphalocele is based on the demonstration of the midline anterior abdominal wall defect, the herniated sac with its visceral contents, and the umbilical cord insertion at the apex of the sac. Ultrasonographic examination should be directed toward defining the extent of the lesion and excluding other malformations.

Gastroschisis

In gastroschisis, with an incidence of 0.3–2 per 10,000 births,[90a,101,102] the primary body folds and the umbilical ring develop normally, and evisceration of the intestine occurs through a small abdominal wall defect located just lateral and usually to the right of an intact umbilical cord. The loops of intestine lie uncovered in the amniotic fluid and become thickened, edematous, and matted. Associated chromosomal abnormalities are rare, but other malformations are found in up to 53 percent of the cases.[90a,102a] The vast majority of cases are thought to be sporadic, although there are examples of familial gastroschisis, suggesting the possibility of an autosomal dominant mode of inheritance, with variable expressivity.[101] Postoperative survival ranged from 70 to 95 percent,[97,102] but more recently was reported as 12.5 percent.[102a]

Prenatal diagnosis is based on the demonstration of the normally situated umbilicus and the herniated loops of intestine, which are free-floating and widely separated. Although raised maternal serum AFP levels may lead to the possible detection of up to 77 percent of such fetuses[101] (see also chapter 21), a far greater percentage are likely to be detected by routine ultrasonography.

Body Stalk Anomaly

This fatal condition, with a birth incidence of 1 in 14,000,[102] results from a developmental failure of the cephalic, caudal, and lateral body folds. It is an anterior abdominal wall defect with absence of the umbilicus and umbilical cord and fusion of the placenta to the herniated viscera. The abdominal contents lie outside the abdominal cavity, the sac covered by placenta and amnion, and there is associated severe kyphoscoliosis.

Prenatal diagnosis is made after visualization of an anterior abdominal wall defect attaching the fetus to the placenta or uterine wall. Neural tube defects, gastrointestinal and genitourinary anomalies, and abnormalities of the pericardium, heart, liver, and lungs are often present.[102]

Bladder Exstrophy and Cloacal Exstrophy

Bladder exstrophy is a defect of the caudal fold of the anterior abdominal wall; a small defect may cause epispadias alone, while a large defect leads to exposure of the posterior bladder wall. In cloacal exstrophy, both the urinary and gastrointestinal tracts are involved. An early mesodermal defect at about 29 days of development has three consequences: (1) failure of cloacal septation, the cloaca persisting with the ureters, ileum, and hindgut opening into it; (2) the cloacal membrane breaks down, leading to exstrophy of the cloaca, failure of fusion of the pubic rami, and often omphalocele; (3) herniation of a dilated spinal cord into abnormal vertebrae in the lumbosacral region. Exstrophy of the cloaca and bladder exstrophy are thought to be due to two different expressions of a primary polytopic developmental field defect.[102b]

The incidence of bladder exstrophy is 1 per 30,000–40,000 births and is twice as common in males as in females.[102b] Cloacal exstrophy is extremely rare, with a birth incidence of 1 per 200,000.[102b,103,104] The recurrence risk is approximately 1 percent; the chance of an affected parent having an affected offspring is 1 in 70.[105] Cloacal exstrophy leads to sterility; therefore, although a genetic inheritance is possible, it is more likely to be a sporadic problem.

With aggressive reconstructive bladder, bowel, and genital surgery, survival is more than 80 percent. Although it has been suggested that gender reassignment to female should occur, psychologic follow-ups of such patients suggest that both males and females with this condition are capable of a normal lifestyle with normal intelligence, although some form of urinary tract diversion is required for all. Furthermore, both sexes have been reported to be fertile after surgery.[106]

Prenatally, the diagnosis should be considered when the bladder cannot be seen on the scan. The presence of omphalocele is a risk factor. Renal abnormalities are found in up to 60 percent of cases of cloacal exstrophy, including renal agenesis, hydronephrosis, and multicystic dysplasia. Omphalocele is seen in more than 80 percent of cases, and more rarely, cardiac and other gastrointestinal defects are present.

Gastrointestinal Tract Defects

Sonographically, the fetal stomach is visible from 9 weeks of gestation as a sonolucent cystic structure in the upper left quadrant of the abdomen. This is a consistent finding and, in a review of more than 9,000 fetal scans, the stomach was seen in 99 percent of the cases.[107] The bowel is normally uniformly echogenic until the third trimester, when prominent meconium-filled loops of large bowel are commonly seen. The liver comprises most of the upper abdomen, and the left lobe is greater in size than the right lobe because of its greater supply of oxygenated blood. The gallbladder is seen as an ovoid cystic structure to the right and below the intrahepatic portion of the umbilical vein. The spleen may also be visualized in a transverse plane posterior and to the left of the fetal stomach.

Esophageal Atresia

The incidence of esophageal atresia is 2–12 per 10,000 births, and in 90 percent of the cases, there is an associated tracheoesophageal (T-E) fistula.[108] Rarely, esophageal atresia is transmitted as an autosomal dominant disorder.[108a] Both conditions result from failure of the primitive foregut to divide into the anterior trachea and posterior esophagus, which normally occurs during the 4th week of gestation. Associated major abnormalities, mainly cardiac, are found in 50–70 percent of the infants,[109] and the fistula may be seen as part of the VATER association (vertebral and ventricular septal defects, anal atresia, T-E fistula, renal anomalies, radial dysplasia, and single umbilical artery). Survival is primarily dependent on birth weight and the presence of other anomalies. Thus, for babies with an isolated T-E fistula weighing more than 2.5 kg, when an early diagnosis is made avoiding reflux and aspiration pneumonitis, postoperative survival is at least 95 percent.[110]

Prenatally, the diagnosis of esophageal atresia is suspected when, in the presence of polyhydramnios, repeated ultrasonographic examinations fail to demonstrate the fetal stomach.[111,112] If there is an associated fistula, the stomach will fill, suggesting that only 10 percent of cases of esophageal atresia may be amenable to prenatal diagnosis. Furthermore, gastric secretions may be sufficient to distend the stomach and make it visible. The differential diagnosis for the combination of absent stomach and polyhydramnios includes intrathoracic compression, by conditions such as diaphragmatic hernia, and musculoskeletal anomalies causing inability of the fetus to swallow.

Duodenal Atresia

Duodenal atresia or stenosis has an incidence of 1 in 10,000 live births. In most cases, the condition is sporadic, although a familial inheritance has been suggested by an autosomal recessive pattern in some families.[113] At 5 weeks of embryonic life, the lumen of the duodenum is obliterated by proliferating epithelium. The patency of the lumen is usually restored by the 11th week, and failure of vacuolization may lead to stenosis or atresia. More than 50 percent of fetuses with duodenal atresia have associated abnormalities, including trisomy 21 and skeletal defects (vertebral and rib anomalies, sacral agenesis, radial abnormalities, and talipes), gastrointestinal abnormalities (esophageal atresia/tracheoesophageal fistula, intestinal malrotation, Meckel diverticulum, and anorectal atresia), cardiovascular malformations (endocardial cushion defects and ventricular septal defects), and renal defects.[113,113a] The overall mortality of this condition has been reported as 7–36 percent, and this is mainly due to the associated abnormalities.[113,113a,113b] Duodenal obstruction is a more serious disorder than previously believed, with an increased mortality rate even when the karyotype is normal.[113a]

Prenatal diagnosis is based on the demonstration of the characteristic "double bubble" appearance of the dilated stomach and proximal duodenum, commonly associated with polyhydramnios. However, obstruction due to a central web may result in only a "single bubble," representing the fluid-filled stomach.[114] The most important feature is that the stomach bubble crosses the midline. Continuity of the duodenum with the stomach should be demonstrated to differentiate a distended duodenum from other cystic masses, including choledochal or hepatic cysts. Although the characteristic double bubble can be seen as early as 20 weeks, it is usually not diagnosed until 26–28 weeks, suggesting that the fetus is unable to swallow a volume of amniotic fluid sufficient for bowel dilatation to occur before the end of the second trimester.

Bowel Obstruction

Small bowel atresias and stenosis occur in 2–3 per 10,000 births. The most common sites are the distal ileum (36 percent), proximal jejunum (31 percent), distal jejunum (20 percent), and proximal ileum (13 percent). Intestinal obstruction at any level may lead to proximal bowel dilatation and, on rare occasions, even to perforation. Intestinal atresias are more common than stenosis, they are usually multiple, and they are thought to result from vascular accidents during development. Although the condition is usually sporadic, in multiple intestinal atresia, familial cases have been described.[115] In a combined series of 589 infants with a total jejunoileal atresia, additional abnormalities were found in 44 percent of cases, and they included malrotation of the bowel, imperforate anus, meconium peritonitis, omphalocele, or gastroschisis in 20 percent of the infants; cardiovascular or chromosomal anomalies were found in 7 percent of cases.[113] Anorectal atresia, with an incidence of 2 per 10,000 live births, results from abnormal division of the cloaca during the 9th week of development. Associated defects such as genitourinary, vertebral, cardiovascular, and gastrointestinal anomalies, are found in 70–90 percent of the cases. Infants with bowel obstruction typically present in the early neonatal period with symptoms of vomiting and abdominal distention. The prognosis is related to the gestational age at delivery, the presence of associated abnormalities, and the site of obstruction.

Ultrasonographically, jejunal and ileal obstructions are imaged as multiple fluid-filled loops of bowel in the abdomen. The abdomen is usually distended, and active peristalsis may be observed. If bowel perforation occurs, transient ascites, meconium peritonitis, and meconium pseudocysts may ensue.[114] Polyhydramnios is usually present, especially with proximal obstructions. Similar bowel appearances and polyhydramnios may be found in fetuses with Hirschsprung disease, the megacystis–microcolon–intestinal hypoperistalsis syndrome, and congenital chloride diarrhea. Occasionally, calcified intraluminal meconium in the fetal pelvis may be seen; this suggests a diagnosis of anorectal atresia. When considering a diagnosis of small-bowel obstruction, care should be taken to exclude renal tract abnormalities and other intra-abdominal cysts such as mesenteric, ovarian, or duplication cysts.

Meconium Peritonitis

Intrauterine perforation of the bowel may lead to a local sterile chemical peritonitis, with the development of a dense calcified mass of fibrous tissue sealing off the perforation. Bowel perforation usually occurs proximal to some form of obstruction, although this cannot always be demonstrated. Intestinal stenosis or atresia and meconium ileus account for 65 percent of the cases. Other causes include volvulus and Meckel diverticulum. Meconium ileus is the impaction of abnormally thick and sticky meconium in the distal ileum; in the majority of cases, this is due to cystic fibrosis (CF). Meconium peritonitis is associated with a more than 50 percent mortality in the neonatal period.[116]

The diagnosis should be considered if the fetal bowel is observed to be dilated or whenever an area of fetal intra-abdominal hyperechogenicity is detected. The likelihood of perforation is increased if a thin rim of ascites is also demonstrated. The differential diagnosis of hyperechogenic bowel includes (1) intra-amniotic hemorrhage, (2) early ascites, (3) fetal hypoxia, (4) meconium peritonitis, and (5) cystic fibrosis and chromosomal abnormality (see below). Therefore, when other causes of bowel hyperechogenicity are not obvious, chromosome analysis and DNA studies for CF are indicated (see also chapter 15). In this condition, hyperechogenic bowel can be a transient ultrasound feature and this should be discussed during counseling.[117]

Hyperechogenic Bowel

Hyperechogenicity of the fetal bowel is defined as bowel of similar or greater echogenicity than surrounding bone,[117] and has been noted in up to 1.5 percent of second-trimester fetuses.[117a] Hyperechogenic bowel has been observed with chromosomal abnormalities,[118] CF,[118a] α-thalassemia,[118b] and cytomegalovirus and toxoplasmosis infections (see chapters 6 and 30). A prospective collaborative study of 641 fetuses with hyperechogenic bowel and a demonstrated CF mutation yielded a 3.1 percent risk of CF.[118c] A similar smaller study (175 fetuses) recorded a 2.9 percent risk.[118d] These authors also noted that in all cases in their series of CF and aneuploidy, echogenicity was multifocal. When hyperechogenicity was associated with bowel dilatation, the risk of CF was 17 percent, and even higher (25 percent), if the gallbladder was absent.

Hepatosplenomegaly

The fetal liver and spleen can be measured by ultrasonography.[119,120] Causes of hepatosplenomegaly include immune and nonimmune hydrops, congenital infection, and metabolic disorders, and it is seen in Beckwith–Wiedemann and Zellweger syndromes. Hepatic enlargement may also be caused by hemangioma, which is usually hypoechogenic, or hepatoblastoma, in which there are areas of calcification. Hepatic calcification can also be caused by intrauterine infections (see chapter 30).

Abdominal Cysts

Abdominal cystic masses are frequent findings at ultrasound examination. Renal tract anomalies or dilated bowel are the most common explanations, although cystic structures may arise from the biliary tree, ovaries, mesentery, or uterus. The correct diagnosis of these abnormalities may not be possible by ultrasound examination, but the most likely diagnosis is usually suggested by the position of the cyst, its relationship with other structures, and the normality of other organs.

Choledochal cysts are uncommon and their cause is unknown. Early diagnosis and removal of the cyst may avoid the development of biliary cirrhosis, portal hypertension, calculi formation, or adenocarcinoma. In a series of 1,433 patients with congenital choledochal cyst, the operative mortality was 10 percent.[119] Prenatally, the diagnosis may be made ultrasonographically by the demonstration of a cyst in the upper right side of the fetal abdomen.[120–122] The differential diagnosis includes enteric duplication cyst, liver cysts, situs inversus, or duodenal atresia. The absence of polyhydramnios or peristalsis may help differentiate the condition from bowel disorders.

Ovarian cysts are common; they may be found in up to one-third of newborns at autopsy, although they are usually small and asymptomatic.[123] Fetal ovarian cysts are hormone-sensitive and tend to occur more frequently in diabetic or rhesus-isoimmunized mothers as a result of placental hyperplasia. The majority of cysts are benign and resolve spontaneously in the neonatal period. Potential complications include development of ascites, torsion, infarction, or rupture. Prenatally, the cysts are usually unilateral and unilocular, although if the cyst undergoes torsion or hemorrhage, the appearance is complex or solid. There is no associated polyhydramnios as in bowel obstruction. Obstetric management should not be changed unless an enormous or rapidly enlarging cyst is detected, in which case prenatal aspiration may be considered.

A difficult differential diagnosis is posed by hydrometrocolpos, which also presents as a cystic or solid mass arising from the pelvis of a female fetus.[124] Other genitourinary or gastrointestinal anomalies are common and include renal agenesis, polycystic kidneys, esophageal atresia, duodenal atresia, and imperforate anus.[123,124] Most cases are sporadic, although a few cases are genetic, such as the autosomal recessive McKusick–Kaufman syndrome with hydrometrocolpos, polydactyly, and congenital heart disease.

Mesenteric or omental cysts may represent obstructed lymphatic drainage or lymphatic hamartomas. The fluid contents may be serous, chylous, or hemorrhagic.[125] Postnatal management is conservative, and surgery is reserved for cases with symptoms of bowel obstruction or acute abdominal pain following torsion or hemorrhage into a cyst. Complete excision of cysts may not be possible because of the proximity of major blood vessels, and in up to 22 percent of cases, there is recurrence after surgery.[125] Although malignant change in mesenteric cysts has been described, this is rare. Antenatally, the diagnosis is suggested by the finding of a multiseptate or unilocular, usually midline, cystic lesion of variable size; a solid appearance may be secondary to hemorrhage. Antenatal aspiration may be considered in cases of massive cysts resulting in thoracic compression.

Kidneys and Urinary Tract

The kidneys, located below the level of the stomach, on either side, and anterior to the spine, are visible by ultrasonography as early as 9 weeks of gestation.[126] Both the renal length and circumference increase with gestation, but the ratio of renal to abdominal circumference remains approximately 30 percent throughout pregnancy.[127] The normal ureters are rarely seen in the absence of distal obstruction or reflux. The fetal bladder can be visualized from the first trimester; changes in volume over time help to differentiate it from other cystic pelvic structures.

Urinary tract anomalies occur in approximately 2–3 per 1,000 pregnancies.

Renal Agenesis

Bilateral renal agenesis is reported in 1–3 per 10,000 births, while unilateral disease is much more common (20 per 10,000 births).[128,129] Renal agenesis is the consequence of failure of differentiation of the metanephric blastema during the 25th–28th day of development, and both ureters and kidneys and renal arteries are absent.[130] Although it may be secondary to a chromosomal abnormality or part of a genetic syndrome, such as Fraser syndrome, more commonly it is an isolated finding. In nonsyndromic cases, the risk of recurrence is approximately 3 percent. However, 13 percent of first-degree relatives of affected infants have unilateral renal agenesis themselves, and in these families, the risk of recurrence is increased.[131]

Antenatally, the condition is suspected by the combination of oligohydramnios and empty fetal bladder from as early as 13–14 weeks.[132] Examination of the renal areas is often hampered by the "crumpled" position adopted by these fetuses, and care should be taken to avoid the mistaken diagnosis of perirenal fat and large fetal adrenals for the absent kidneys. Romero et al.[133] reported cases of renal agenesis diagnosed by ultrasound, while at autopsy, the kidneys were actually present. To distinguish renal agenesis from growth restriction as the cause of oligohydramnios, the ultrasonographic examination should perhaps be preceded by the intra-amniotic instillation of normal saline. However, Doppler is now proving to be an effective noninvasive technique for this distinction. If growth restriction due to uteroplacental insufficiency is severe enough to be associated with oligohydramnios, Doppler studies of the uteroplacental and fetal circulations would be suggestive of severe fetal hypoxemia. In contrast, in renal agenesis, Doppler results are usually normal.

Prenatal diagnosis of unilateral renal agenesis is difficult because there are no major features, such as oligohydramnios/empty bladder, to alert the ultrasonographer to the fact that one of the kidneys is absent.

Pelvic Kidney

A pelvic kidney is found in approximately 1 in 1,200 autopsies. Antenatally, the diagnosis is suspected when the ultrasonographer fails to visualize the kidneys in the usual anatomical sites in the presence of normal amniotic fluid volume and fetal bladder.[134] The diagnosis can easily be missed because, as in renal agenesis, the adrenal glands can be mistaken for kidneys. They are also associated with an increased risk of cardiovascular, skeletal, and gastrointestinal defects.

Congenital Nephrotic Syndrome

Congenital nephrotic syndrome or Finnish nephropathy has a frequency of 1 in 8,000–10,000 births in Finland[135] (see also chapter 21). Prenatally, diagnosis of this autosomal recessive disease is suspected in cases with enlarged kidneys and increased volume of amniotic fluid, when there is elevated maternal serum and amniotic fluid AFP level in the absence of detectable acetylcholinesterase in the amniotic fluid. Diagnosis can now be achieved by DNA diagnostics (see chapter 10).

Infantile Polycystic Kidney Disease (Potter Type I)

The incidence of Potter type I renal dysplasia is approximately 2 per 100,000 births. It may occur sporadically, but it is more commonly inherited as an autosomal recessive condition. The disease has a wide spectrum of renal and hepatic involvement and, in its severe forms, it is uniformly fatal. It has been subdivided into perinatal, neonatal, infantile, and juvenile types on the basis of the age of onset of the clinical presentation and the degree of renal tubular involvement.[136] Although recurrences tend to be group-specific, we have seen one family in which the four subdivisions were each represented in the four affected infants.

Prenatal diagnosis is confined to the types with earlier onset (perinatal and probably the neonatal types) and is based on the demonstration of bilaterally enlarged and homogeneously hyperechogenic kidneys. There is often associated oligohydramnios, but this is not invariably so. However, these sonographic appearances may not become apparent before 24 weeks of gestation; therefore, serial scans should be performed for exclusion of the diagnosis.[129,137,138]

Multicystic Dysplastic Kidneys (Potter Type II)

The condition, which is generally sporadic, is thought to be a consequence of either developmental failure of the mesonephric blastema to form nephrons or early obstruction due to urethral or ureteric atresia. The collecting tubules become cystic and the diameter of the cysts determines the size of the kidneys, which may be enlarged or small. Ultrasonographically, the former are recognized as large multicystic and the latter are recognized as shrunken irregular and hyperechogenic. The disorder can be bilateral, unilateral, or segmental; if bilateral, there is associated oligohydramnios and the bladder is either distended or "absent." Exploration of the renal fossa in some cases revealed no renal artery, renal vein, ureter, or cysts, suggesting that renal agenesis and dysplastic kidneys may be different ends of a spectrum of renal malformation. This is further supported by the finding that in 11–14 percent of cases with multicystic kidneys, there is contralateral renal agenesis.[139]

There is still controversy regarding the postnatal management of patients with multicystic dysplasia; some urologists advocate prophylactic nephrectomy and others adopt a conservative approach. The parents and family should also be scanned to exclude autosomal dominant branchio-otorenal syndrome.[131]

Potter Type III Renal Dysplasia

Potter type III renal dysplasia is characterized by markedly enlarged irregular kidneys with innumerable cysts of variable sizes interspread among normal or compressed renal parenchyma. It is the common morphologic expression of autosomal dominant adult polycystic kidney disease (APKD) and of other mendelian disorders such as tuberous sclerosis, Jeune syndrome, Sturge–Weber syndrome, Zellweger syndrome, Laurence–Moon–Biedl syndrome, and Meckel–Gruber syndrome. Both kidneys are generally equally enlarged and only rarely is one involved so slightly that it remains of normal size. One-third of the cases have cysts in the liver, pancreas, spleen, or lungs, and one-fifth are found to have cerebral aneurysms.[140]

Adult Polycystic Kidney Disease

One in 1,000 people carry a mutant gene for APKD. APKD is usually asymptomatic until the third or fourth decade of life, and although histologic evidence of the disease is likely to be present from intrauterine life, the age of onset of gross morphologic changes that are potentially detectable by ultrasonography is uncertain. Rarely, however, kidneys that are anatomically similar may cause death in infancy or early childhood and the condition has been designated as "adult variety occurring in infancy."

Prenatal diagnosis by ultrasonography is confined to a few case reports, and the kidneys have been described as enlarged and hyperechogenic with or without multiple cysts. Unlike infantile polycystic kidneys, in which there is a loss of the corticomedullary junction, in APKD there is accentuation of this junction.[141] The amniotic fluid volume is either normal or reduced. The kidney size is usually smaller than the infant polycystic kidneys. The clinical course of children diagnosed antenatally is not yet certain.

Those counseling parents whose infants are affected with APKD should emphasize that the prenatal demonstration of sonographically normal kidneys does not necessarily exclude the possibility of developing polycystic kidneys in adult life. Moreover, there is a need to determine whether the APKD is type I, II, or III by DNA linkage analysis or mutation detection. Prenatal diagnosis can now be made from chorionic villus sampling or amniotic fluid cells by DNA analysis[142] (see also chapter 10).

Obstructive Uropathies

The term *obstructive uropathy* encompasses a wide variety of pathologic conditions characterized by dilatation of part or all of the urinary tract. When the obstruction is complete and occurs early in fetal life, renal hypoplasia (deficiency in total nephron population) and dysplasia (Potter type II; formation of abnormal nephrons and mesenchymal stroma) ensue. On the other hand, when intermittent obstruction allows for normal renal development or when it occurs during the second half of pregnancy, hydronephrosis will result, and the severity of the renal damage will depend on the degree and duration of the obstruction. Dilatation of fetal urinary tract frequently, but not absolutely, signifies obstruction.[143–145] Conversely, a fetus with obstruction may not have any urinary tract dilatation.[146]

Hydronephrosis accounts for 87 percent of fetal renal anomalies,[147] and the incidence is 1–5 per 1,000 births. Mild hydronephrosis is thought to be significant if the antero-posterior diameter of the pelvis is >4 mm at 16–20 weeks, >5 mm at 20–30 weeks, and >7 mm at 30–40 weeks.[145,148] Transient hydronephrosis may be due to relaxation of smooth muscle of the urinary tract by the high levels of circulating maternal hormones or maternal–fetal overhydration.[149] However, if the renal pelvis measures more than 10 mm with a pelvis-to-kidney diameter ratio of more than 50 percent with rounded calyces, the disease is usually progressive.[150] Similarly, during the first 24 hours of life, there may be transient disappearance of mild and moderate hydronephrosis due to relative dehydration and decreased glomerular filtration rate. Therefore, postnatal assessment of the baby should be delayed until 48 hours after birth.

Ureteropelvic junction obstruction is usually sporadic, and although in some cases there is an anatomic cause, such as ureteral valves, in most instances the underlying cause is thought to be functional. In 70–90 percent of cases, the condition is unilateral.[150] Prenatal diagnosis is based on the demonstration of hydronephrosis in the absence of dilated ureters and bladder. Occasionally, perinephric urinomas and urinary ascites may be present. Postnatally, renal function is assessed by serial isotope imaging studies, and if there is deterioration, pyeloplasty is performed. However, the majority of infants have moderate or good function and can be treated conservatively.[151]

Ureterovesical junction obstruction is characterized by hydronephrosis and hydroureter in the presence of a normal bladder. The causes are diverse, including ureteric stricture or atresia, retrocaval ureter, vascular obstruction, valves, diverticulum, ureterocele, and vesicoureteral reflux.[152] Ureteroceles are usually found in association with duplication of the collecting system. In ureteral duplication, the upper pole moiety characteristically obstructs and the lower one refluxes. The dilated upper pole may enlarge to displace the nondilated lower pole inferiorly and laterally.

Vesicoureteric reflux is suspected when intermittent dilatation of the upper urinary tract over a short period is seen on ultrasound scanning. Occasionally, in massive vesicoureteric reflux without obstruction, the bladder appears persistently dilated because it empties but rapidly refills with refluxed urine.[153] Primary megaureter can be distinguished from ureterovesical junction obstruction by the absence of significant hydronephrosis.

Urethral Obstruction

Urethral obstruction can be caused by urethral agenesis, persistence of the cloaca, urethral stricture, or posterior urethral valves. Posterior urethral valves occur only in males and are the commonest cause of bladder outlet obstruction.[129] The condition is sporadic and is found in 1–2 per 10,000 boys.[154] With posterior urethral valves, there is usually incomplete or intermittent obstruction of the urethra, resulting in an enlarged and hypertrophied bladder with varying degrees of hydroureters, hydronephrosis, a spectrum of renal hypoplasia and dysplasia, oligohydramnios, and pulmonary hypoplasia. In some cases, there is associated urinary ascites from rupture of the bladder or transudation of urine into the peritoneal cavity.

Megacystis–microcolon–intestinal hypoperistalsis syndrome is a rare condition of uncertain cause that also presents with dilated bladder, ureters, and pelvicalyceal system, but in the absence of urinary tract obstruction.[155] The fetuses are usually female, and the amniotic fluid volume is normal or increased. There is associated shortening and dilatation of the proximal small bowel, and microcolon with absent or ineffective peristalsis. In approximately 7 percent of cases, there is omphalocele.[155] The disease is usually fatal, caused by bowel and renal dysfunction.

In fetal lamb, ureteric ligation during the first half of gestation results in dysplastic kidneys, whereas in the second half of pregnancy, ureteric ligation is associated with the development of hydronephrosis but preservation of renal architecture.[156] Harrison et al.[157,158] showed that ligation of the urethra and urachus in fetal lambs at 95–105 days of gestation causes severe hydronephrosis and pulmonary hypoplasia. Decompression of the obstructed fetuses by suprapubic cystostomy at 120 days of gestation improves survival. Furthermore, with decompression, there is significant resolution of the urinary tract dilatation and the newborns have less respiratory difficulty (see also chapter 29). Glick et al.[159] demonstrated that ureteric ligation at 65 days of gestation produces renal dysplasia and that subsequent decompression before term prevents renal dysplasia and produces reversible postobstructive changes. At term, the degree of pathologic changes seen in the obstructed and then decompressed kidneys was proportional to the length of time the obstruction existed.

Encouraged by the results of these animal studies, and on the assumption that unrelieved obstruction causes progressive renal and pulmonary damage, several investigators have performed in utero decompression of the urinary tract in the human, either by open surgical diversion[160] or by the ultrasound-guided insertion of suprapubic vesicoamniotic catheters[161,162] (see full discussion in chapter 29).

The most common underlying pathology was posterior urethral valves, which had a survival of 74 percent. This compares favorably with the reported mortality of 45 percent in untreated posterior urethral valves.[163] However, Reuss et al.[164] reported that eight of nine fetuses with posterior urethral valves who had no antenatal intervention survived. This technique carries a significant fetal/neonatal morbidity; indeed, vesicoamniotic shunts become obstructed or displaced in up to 25 percent of cases,[165] requiring additional interventions to replace the shunt, with their attendant complications, such as preterm labor and delivery and chorioamnionitis. Less common complications include abdominal wall defect.

These problems could potentially be avoided by intrauterine surgery aiming at curing the malformation (posterior urethral valves in utero). The experience in humans is mainly that of one team.[166]

The feasibility of fetal cystoscopy in humans was assessed in a population of thirteen fetuses referred for sonographic suspicion of lower obstructive uropathy and serial vesicocenteses were performed for urine biochemistry. This was possible in eleven of thirteen cases at 20 (16–28) weeks. Small fiberoptics could be introduced through an 18-gauge needle. The bladder mucosa was characterized (trabeculation, edema, hemorrhage), and dilatation of the ureteral orifices was performed. The urethra was successfully cannulated in three of eleven cases; four did not meet the criteria and three decided to terminate the pregnancy.

These results fail to demonstrate conclusively that in utero intervention improves renal or pulmonary function beyond what can be achieved by postnatal surgery. However, they expose the need for (1) the investigation of these fetuses with the aim of excluding associated nonrenal abnormalities, and (2) the development of reliable criteria for the prenatal diagnosis of irreversible renal and pulmonary damage. The limited experience in human fetal surgery and the potential technical and developmental problems that arise from en-doscopic fetal surgery of posterior urethral valves make it necessary to work on an ani-mal model before any further therapeutic attempt in the human fetus.

In the antenatal evaluation of obstructive uropathy, the ultrasonographic finding of multicystic kidneys is associated with renal dysplasia. In hydronephrosis, both the degree of pelvicalyceal dilatation and the volume of amniotic fluid are poor predictors of out-come; urodochocentesis or pyelocentesis with measurement of sodium, calcium, urea, and creatinine provides useful information for more accurate counseling of the parents. Fur-thermore, fetal urinary biochemistry provides a rational basis for selecting patients who may benefit from vesicoamniotic shunting or other intrauterine urinary diversion proce-dures and allows evaluation of the possible effectiveness of such therapeutic interventions. Poor fetal renal function can be inferred from high urinary sodium and calcium levels and from low urea and creatinine (Figure 23.5).[167,168]

Serial measurements of the fetal urine biochemical parameters are likely to lead to a more objective assessment of the fetal renal function and should ideally be undertaken before any definite decision has been made about the management of the pregnancy.[169]

Skeletal Dysplasias

There is a wide range of rare skeletal dyplasias, each with a specific mode of inheritance, genotype, phenotype, recurrence risk, and implications for neonatal survival and quality of life.[170,171] (See chapter 20 for full discussion.) Gene discovery (see chapter 20) has made accurate prenatal diagnosis a reality. The incidental discovery of a skeletal dyspla-sia on routine ultrasound screening in a pregnancy not known to be at risk for a specific syndrome necessitates a systematic examination to arrive at the correct diagnosis. All limbs

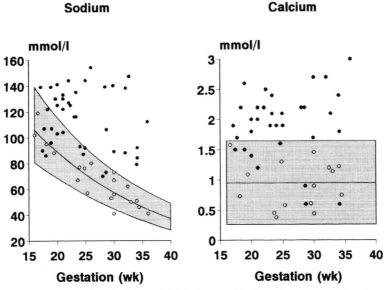

Fig. 23.5. Urinary sodium (left) and calcium (right) in fetuses with obstructive uropathy, plotted on the ap-propriate reference ranges (mean, 95th and 5th centiles) with gestation. In twenty cases, the fetuses survived and/or did not have any evidence of renal dysplasia (open circles); the remaining forty fetuses died and/or there was histologic evidence of renal dysplasia (closed circles).

must be evaluated for length, shape, mineralization, and movement, and associated abnormalities in other systems, particularly the head, thorax, and spine, should be sought (Table 23.4). A putative diagnosis may then allow definitive confirmation via mutation analysis.

The majority of bones of the appendicular system can be imaged in the early second trimester, and several nomograms relating the length of long bones to menstrual age or biparietal diameter have been published.[172,173] The severe limb reductions associated with osteogenesis imperfecta type II, achondrogenesis, and thanatophoric, diastrophic, and chondroectodermal dysplasias can be detected by a single measurement at 16–18 weeks of gestation (Figure 23.6). In the case of achondroplasia, however, the diagnosis may not become obvious until 22–24 weeks; therefore, serial measurements are necessary. Mutation analysis may be indicated if there is uncertainty (see chapter 10). Homozygous achondroplasia, which is usually lethal, manifests abnormally short limbs earlier than the heterozygous form. Syndromes vary in the degree of severity to which the proximal (rhizomelic dwarfism, e.g., achondroplasia) or distal (mesomelic dwarfism, e.g., chondroectodermal dysplasia) long bones are affected. The femur, however, is abnormally short even in mesomelic dwarfism; therefore, in our routine fetal abnormality screening, we tend to confine limb measurement to the femur. When dealing with pregnancies at risk for a skeletal dysplasia, both segments of all limbs are measured.

A minor degree of lateral curvature of the femur is commonly seen in normal fetuses. Pronounced bowing, however, is observed in association with campomelic dysplasia, thanatophoric dwarfism, autosomal dominant osteogenesis imperfecta, achondrogenesis, and hypophosphatasia. In the latter, fractures and callus formation may also be detected.[174] Reduced echogenicity of bones, suggestive of hypomineralization, is seen in disorders such as hypophosphatasia, osteogenesis imperfecta, and achondrogenesis. The virtual absence of ossification of the spine, characteristic of achondrogenesis, may lead to the erroneous diagnosis of complete spinal agenesis. Similarly, the pronounced clarity with which the cerebral ventricles are imaged, as a result of the poorly mineralized globular cranium in

Table 23.4. Limb-reduction deformities: associated abnormalities

Feature	Example
Cranium	
Megalocephaly	Achondroplasia
Brachcephaly	Achondrogenesis
Prominent forehead	Thanatophoric dysplasia
Microcephaly	Chondrodysplasia punctata
Chest	
Short, barrel-shaped	Achondrogenesis
Long, narrow	Asphyxiating thoracic dystrophy
Narrow, pear-shaped	Thanatophoric dwarfism
Rib fractures	Osteogenesis imperfecta
Spine	
Lumbar lordosis	Achondroplasia
Scoliosis	Diastrophic dwarfism
Flattened vertebrae	Thanatophoric dwarfism
Unossified bodies	Achondrogenesis

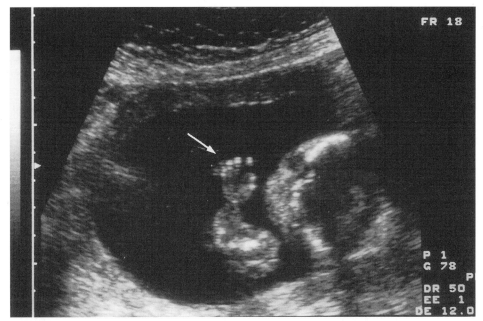

Fig. 23.6. Ultrasonographic picture of the arm, forearm, and hand (arrow) of a fetus with a lethal skeletal dysplasia at 15 weeks.

cases of hypophosphatasia, may result in the misdiagnosis of hydrocephalus. Care must be exercised, however, because lesser degrees of hypomineralization may not be detectable.

Isolated limb-reduction deformities such as amelia (complete absence of extremities), acheiria (absence of the hand), phocomelia (seal limb), or aplasia–hypoplasia of the radius or ulna are often inherited as part of a genetic syndrome (Holt–Oram syndrome, Fanconi pancytopenia, thrombocytopenia with absent radii syndrome) and are readily diagnosable by ultrasonography in an at-risk fetus. Other causes of focal limb loss include the amniotic band syndrome, thalidomide exposure, and caudal regression syndrome.

Ultrasonography can aid in the diagnosis of conditions characterized by limitation of flexion or extension of the limbs such as arthrogryposis and multiple pterygium syndrome. Fetal fingers and toes can be seen and, with meticulous examination, abnormalities of numbers, shape, movement, and attitudes can be recognized.

Abnormalities of the Amniotic Fluid Volume

Ultrasonographically, the diagnosis of polyhydramnios or oligohydramnios is made when there is excessive or virtual absence of echo-free spaces around the fetus.

Polyhydramnios

The incidence of polyhydramnios is 1–3 percent using the definition of a vertical deepest pool (VDP) of at least 8 cm.[175,176] Severe polyhydramnios defined by a VDP >15 cm represents 5 percent of all cases and is most often associated with other fetal abnormalities.

Polyhydramnios is often associated with maternal diabetes, monozygotic twin pregnancies, and fetal malformations. The rate of reported abnormalities varies with the criteria used for the diagnosis of polyhydramnios, and they may be detected in up to 50 percent of cases.[175–177] Craniospinal defects (such as anencephaly), facial tumors, gastrointestinal obstruction, compressive pulmonary disorders (such as pleural effusions or asphyxiating thoracic dystrophy), and arthrogryposis produce polyhydramnios by interfering with fetal swallowing. Maternal diabetes mellitus or fetal diabetes insipidus causes fetal polyuria. In most of these conditions, the polyhydramnios develops in the late second or the third trimester. Acute polyhydramnios at 18–24 weeks is seen mainly in association with twin-to-twin transfusion syndrome. Testing for maternal diabetes, detailed sonographic examination for anomalies, and fetal karyotyping should constitute the cornerstones of the diagnostic protocol in the investigation of these cases.

The aim is to reduce the risk of very premature delivery and the maternal discomfort that often accompanies severe polyhydramnios. Treatment will obviously depend on the diagnosis, and will include better glycemic control of maternal diabetes mellitus, antiarrhythmic medication for fetal hydrops due to dysrhythmias, and thoracoamniotic shunting for fetal pulmonary cysts or pleural effusions. For the other cases, polyhydramnios may be treated by repeated amniocenteses every few days and drainage of large volumes of amniotic fluid. However, the procedure itself may precipitate premature labor. An alternative and effective method of treatment is the administration of indomethacin to the mother.[178] However, this drug may cause fetal ductal constriction, and close monitoring by serial fetal echocardiographic studies is necessary.

In twin-to-twin transfusion syndrome, development of acute polyhydramnios before 28 weeks of gestation is associated with a high perinatal mortality rate, primarily due to spontaneous abortion or very premature delivery of growth retarded or hydropic babies. This subject is analyzed in detail below.

Oligohydramnios

Oligohydramnios in the second trimester is usually the result of preterm premature rupture of the membranes, urinary tract malformations, and uteroplacental insufficiency, and it is associated with a high perinatal mortality. Although diligent ultrasonographic search for fetal malformations is essential, it should be emphasized that, in the absence of the "acoustic window" normally provided by the amniotic fluid and the "undesirable" postures often adopted by these fetuses, confident exclusion of a fetal malformation may be impossible. Nevertheless, in cases of preterm prelabor rupture of the membranes, detailed questioning of the mother may reveal a history of chronic leakage of amniotic fluid. Furthermore, in uteroplacental insufficiency, Doppler blood flow studies will often demonstrate the characteristically high impedance to flow in the placental circulation and redistribution of the fetal circulation in favor of the brain at the expense of the viscera.[179] In the remaining cases, intra-amniotic instillation of normal saline may help improve ultrasonographic examination and lead to the diagnosis of fetal abnormalities such as renal agenesis. Fetal blood sampling for diagnosis of chromosomal abnormalities, fetal infection, and fetal hypoxia provides additional information in the prenatal evaluation of these cases.

DETECTION OF ABNORMALITIES IN THE FIRST TRIMESTER OF PREGNANCY

Ultrasonography

When fetal development is not a limiting factor, most abnormalities detectable in the second trimester can be described at 12–14 weeks of gestation. We will describe the most common abnormalities amenable to an early diagnosis as a result of a routine examination performed at 10–14 weeks. Many of the abnormalities described below have been diagnosed when a detailed scan has been performed after the finding of an unusual aspect of the fetal nuchal area. The nuchal translucency represents the fluidlike collection in the subcutaneous tissue at the back of the fetal neck that is present during the first trimester (Figure 23.7). Nuchal translucency can be measured successfully by transabdominal ultrasound examination in about 95 percent of cases; in the others, it is necessary to perform vaginal sonography.[180]

Anencephaly

In anencephaly, the primary defect is absence of the cranial vault (Figure 23.8), with subsequent disruption of the cerebral cortex.[181] Prenatal ultrasonographic diagnosis of anencephaly during the second and third trimesters is based on the demonstration of absent cranial vault and cerebral hemispheres. During the first trimester, anencephaly presents with acrania and varying degrees of cerebral degeneration. In normal fetuses, mineralization of the skull, and therefore hyperechogenicity in comparison to the underlying tissues, occurs at around the 10th week of gestation.[182]

In a multicenter study involving 55,237 pregnancies at 10–14 weeks of gestation, there were forty-seven fetuses with anencephaly (prevalence, about 1 in 1,200).[183] During the first phase of the study, 34,830 fetuses were examined, and in eight of the thirty-one (25.8 percent) with anencephaly, the diagnosis was not made at the 10–14 week scan. Following the audit, 20,407 fetuses were examined, and in all sixteen with anencephaly, the diagnosis was made at the 10–14-week scan. These findings demonstrate that anen-

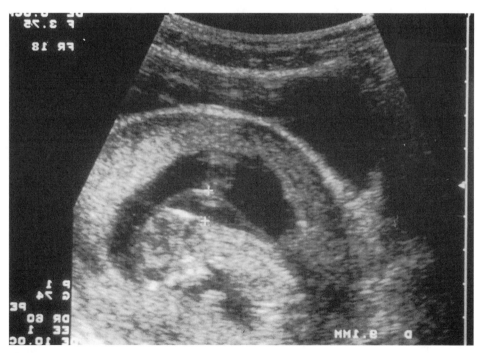

Fig. 23.7. Ultrasonographic picture demonstrating subcutaneous nuchal translucency (between the calipers). In some cases, the translucency extends over a wide area of the fetus but is most prominent behind the neck.

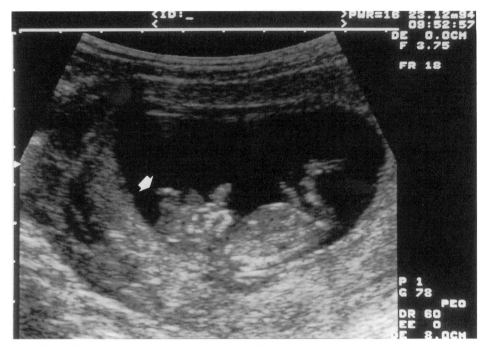

Fig. 23.8. Sagittal view of a 12-week fetus with exencephaly (arrow).

cephaly can be reliably diagnosed at the routine 10–14-week ultrasound scan, provided the specific sonographic features are searched for and recognized.

Cardiac Defects

In a study involving pathologic examination of the heart and great arteries after surgical termination of pregnancy in 112 chromosomally abnormal fetuses identified by nuchal translucency (NT) screening, the majority had abnormalities of the heart and great arteries.[184] The most common cardiac lesion seen in trisomy 21 fetuses was an atrioventricular or ventricular septal defect. Trisomy 18 was associated with ventricular septal defects and/or polyvalvular abnormalities. In trisomy 13, there were atrioventricular or ventricular septal defects, valvular abnormalities, and narrowing of either the isthmus or truncus arteriosus. Turner syndrome was associated with severe narrowing of the whole aortic arch. In all four groups of chromosomally abnormal fetuses, the aortic isthmus was significantly narrower than in normal fetuses and the degree of narrowing was significantly greater in fetuses with high NT thickness. It is postulated that narrowing of the aortic isthmus may be the basis of increased NT thickness in all four chromosomal abnormalities.

In a study of 1,389 chromosomally normal fetuses with increased nuchal translucency at 10–14 weeks of gestation, the prevalence of major cardiac defects (diagnosed either by postmortem examination following termination of pregnancy, intrauterine death, or neonatal death or by clinical examination and appropriate investigation of livebirths) was 17 per 1,000.[184] The prevalence of cardiac defects increased with NT thickness.[185] Two fetal echocardiographic studies at 10–16 weeks of gestation reported that sixteen of the twenty fetuses with cardiac defects had abnormal collection of nuchal fluid.[186,187]

Erratum

Figure 23.8, on page 864, was erroneously duplicated as figure 23.9, on page 865. Figure 23.9 should be as follows:

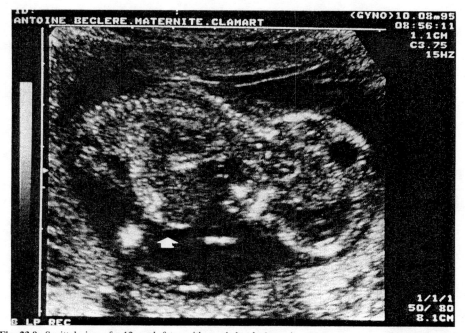

Fig. 23.9. Sagittal view of a 12-week fetus with omphalocele (arrow).

Chromosomally normal fetuses with increased NT thickness, particularly more than 3.5 mm, should be rescanned at 16 and 20 weeks, and special attention should be given to the examination of the heart and great arteries.

Omphalocele (Exomphalos)

Ultrasound studies examining the association between fetal abnormalities and chromosomal defects often fail to take into account the maternal age and gestational age distribution of their population and inevitably report a wide range of results; the reported frequency of chromosomal defects in fetuses with omphalocele varies from 10 to 66 percent (see also chapters 6 and 21).

Omphalocele, or herniation of abdominal viscera into the base of the umbilical cord, can be diagnosed at any gestation if liver is involved. In cases in which only bowel is involved, it is essential that the minimum crown-to-rump length (CRL) of 45 mm is considered; otherwise, this can be mistaken for the physiologic herniation of bowel (Figure 23.9).

In a study involving 15,726 singleton pregnancies at 11–14 weeks of gestation, the data were used to calculate both the prevalence of omphalocele and the risk of associated chromosomal defects, mainly trisomy 18, at different stages of pregnancy.[188] The estimated prevalence of omphalocele in a population with the maternal age distribution of all deliveries in England and Wales, which is very similar to that of the United States (median age, 28 years), is 7.4 per 10,000 at 12 weeks of gestation, and this decreases to 3.5 at 20 weeks and 2.9 in livebirths. Similarly, the estimated frequency of chromosomal defects in fetuses with omphalocele decreases from 40 percent at 12 weeks of gestation to 28 percent at 20 weeks and 15 percent in livebirths. These findings are not surprising, because omphalocele is a common feature of chromosomal defects that are associated with a high rate of intrauterine lethality.

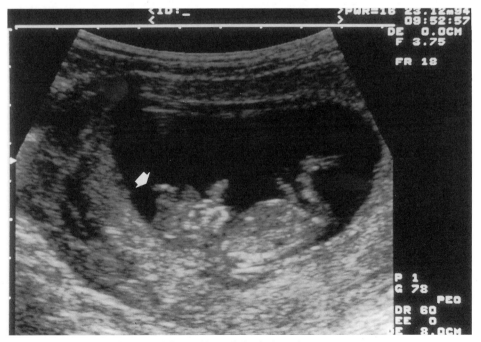

Fig. 23.9. Sagittal view of a 12-week fetus with omphalocele (arrow).

Megacystis

The fetal bladder is visible in only 50 percent of fetuses at 10 weeks but in nearly all cases if the CRL is more than 67 mm.[126,189,190] At 10–14 weeks of gestation, the longitudinal diameter of the fetal bladder (BL) increases with gestation to a maximum of 6 mm or BL-to-CRL ratio of 10 percent.

In a study of 24,492 singleton pregnancies, there was megacystis in 15 cases (prevalence of about 1 in 1,600).[190] In three of the fifteen cases with megacystis, there were chromosomal abnormalities. In the chromosomally normal group, there were seven cases with spontaneous resolution, whereas in four cases, there was progression to severe obstructive uropathy (Figure 23.10). The BL was 8–12 mm in the seven cases with resolution and in one of the four with progressive megacystis; in the other three with progressive obstruction, the BL was >16 mm. Therefore, severe megacystis (BL, >16 mm) evolves into severe second-trimester oligohydramnios and renal dysplasia. With mild to moderate megacystis (BL, 8–12), usually but not invariably, there is spontaneous resolution.

Other Abnormalities and Genetic Syndromes

In the vast majority of fetuses with increased NT and normal karyotype, the translucency resolves and the babies are normal. However, in some cases, increased NT may be associated with an underlying abnormality, such as cardiac defect, diaphragmatic hernia, skeletal dysplasia, renal defect, obstructive uropathy, or omphalocele. In some cases, especially those with NT >3.5 mm, the babies may have a rare genetic syndrome such as Jarcho–Levin syndrome or Smith–Lemli–Opitz syndrome.[191] The prevalence of these syndromes is less than

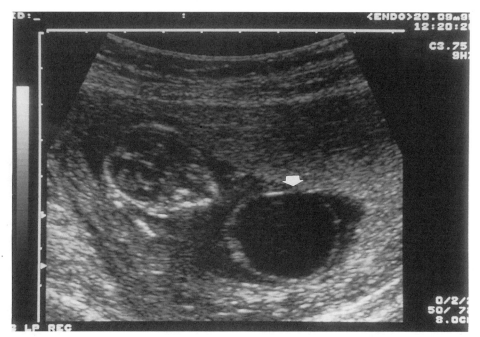

Fig. 23.10. Frontal view of a 12-week fetus with megacystis (arrow) that proved to be related to prune-belly syndrome.

1 per 20,000, and it is impossible at present to know what percentage of affected fetuses actually have increased NT at 10–14 weeks. It is therefore important that centers participating in the multicenter study have good documentation of all pregnancy outcomes so that we can identify as quickly as possible which genetic syndromes are associated with increased NT.

If the NT at 10–14 weeks is >3.5 mm and fetal karyotype is normal, a very detailed scan should be carried out at 20 weeks and attention should be given to the detection of not only major defects but also small dysmorphic features.

Genetic syndromes reported in association with increased NT include the following:

- arthrogryposis or multiple pterygium syndrome[192]
- amnion disruption sequence
- Noonan syndrome
- Jarcho–Levin syndrome
- Smith–Lemli–Opitz syndrome
- Stickler syndrome
- various skeletal dysplasias.

Fetoscopy/Embryoscopy

Direct visualization of the embryo and the fetus can be achieved by embryoscopy and fetoscopy, respectively. Both techniques rely on the visualization of the conceptus through an optical device made of lenses or fiberoptics. These were considered vital tools for prenatal diagnosis in the 1970s and early 1980s but became obsolete with improving ultrasound technology in the late 1980s.

Embryoscopy is historically the oldest technique for visualizing the embryo and is best used for genetic syndromes known to be expressed in the same families by constant external fetal structural abnormalities (e.g., Ellis–van Creveld, Smith–Lemli–Opitz, DOOR syndrome, Apert, Rothmund–Thomson, Baller–Gerold).[193] The procedure can be performed only before 10 weeks when the extracoelomic space disappears, ideally at 9 weeks of gestation. A 1.5- to 2-mm-diameter rigid endoscope is introduced via the cervix through the still thick villus chorion and is put in contact with the amnion; the embryo is examined through this translucent membrane. The risk of miscarriage is around 12.5 percent.[193]

When the parents can bear delaying the diagnosis until 12–14 weeks, first-trimester ultrasound examination can suspect or even diagnose most of these conditions. However, complete examination of the fetal anatomy by ultrasound is very unlikely, and lethal or complex anomalies as well as isolated structural defects can be associated with other abnormalities that may not be recognized by ultrasound examination. One option is to wait for a detailed ultrasound examination in the second trimester, but this is rarely welcomed by the parents, whose anxiety calls for rapid and complete fetal evaluation, especially when termination of the pregnancy is an option.

Confirmation of prenatally diagnosed anomalies is critical for effective counseling. However, when termination of the pregnancy is requested in the first trimester, some patients will decline the burden of a mutilator induced by prostaglandins, and dilatation-aspiration techniques seriously limit postmortem examination.

Further development and refinement of this technology have allowed direct visualization of the fetus with a fiberoptics endoscope that could be directed in the amniotic cavity through a 19- to 20-gauge needle.[194] Precise assessment of the fetal anatomy should be carried out before evacuation, and transabdominal fetoscopy is another option. Various

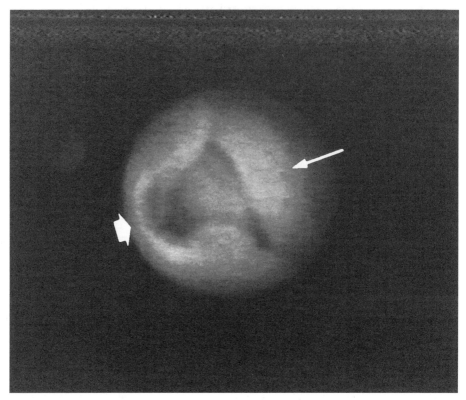

Fig. 23.11. Fetoscopic diagnosis of cleft lip (thick arrow) at 12 weeks, as opposed to the normal lower lip (thin arrow), using a 1-mm endoscope through a 1.3-mm needle.

anomalies such as facial clefts (Figure 23.11), encephalocele, and Smith–Lemli–Opitz and Meckel–Gruber syndromes have been diagnosed with this technique.[195]

There are several concerns regarding the use of this new method of investigation.

1. Care should be taken in diagnosing fetal anomaly in the first trimester. Fetoscopy offers an incomplete evaluation of the external fetal anatomy and must be carried out under ultrasound control.
2. Human data on the safety of fetoscopic white light for the developing retina are still limited.
3. The risk of abortion following the procedure is at present unknown. Before the development of high-resolution ultrasonography, transabdominal fetoscopy was carried out with more invasive instruments and was associated with a fetal loss rate of 4–8 percent. The procedure-related risk of miscarriage for the present technique is probably not much greater than that of early amniocentesis (see discussion in chapter 2). Our endoscope[195] is passed through an 18-gauge needle and adds an extra minute to the procedure of amniocentesis, which can be performed at the same time. Fetoscopy should therefore not add much to the background risk of amniocentesis performed at the same gestational age. However, this remains to be demonstrated, and patients should be counseled accordingly, especially if this technique finds widespread application in early fetal diagnosis and therapy.

ULTRASONOGRAPHICALLY DETECTABLE MARKERS OF FETAL CHROMOSOMAL DEFECTS

The methods of screening to identify the high-risk group are maternal age, ultrasound findings at 11–14 weeks and/or in the second trimester and maternal serum biochemical testing at 11–14 weeks and/or in the second trimester. To calculate the individual risk, it is necessary to take into account the background risk (which depends on maternal age and gestational age) and multiply this by a series of factors, which depend on the results of ultrasound findings and maternal serum biochemical tests carried out during the course of the pregnancy. Every time a test is carried out, the background risk is multiplied by the test factor to calculate a new risk, which then becomes the background risk for the next test. This process is called "sequential screening."[196]

In 1866, Langdon Down reported that the skin of individuals with trisomy 21 appears to be too large for their body.[197] In the 1990s, it was realized that this excess skin can be visualized by ultrasonography as increased NT in the third month of intrauterine life.[198]

Ultrasonographic Detection of Chromosomal Markers in the First Trimester of Pregnancy

Fetal Nuchal Translucency

Measurement of the fluidlike collection in the subcutaneous tissue at the back of the fetal neck, NT, which is present only during the first trimester, can be achieved by transabdominal or transvaginal examination (see Figure 23.7). The technical requirements to obtain reliable and repeatable measurements are as follows:

- The equipment must be of good quality and the average time allocated for each fetal scan should be at least 10 minutes. A good sagittal section of the fetus, as for measurement of fetal CRL, should be obtained. The magnification should be such that the fetus occupies at least three-fourths of the image.
- Care must be taken to distinguish between fetal skin and amnion because, at this point in gestation, both structures appear as thin membrane. This is achieved by waiting for spontaneous fetal movement away from the amniotic membrane; alternatively, the fetus is bounced off the amnion by asking the mother to cough and/or by tapping the maternal abdomen. When NT is difficult to measure or seems to be unusually thick (>2.5 mm), color Doppler examination is a useful tool to rule out the presence of a nuchal cord.
- The maximum thickness of the subcutaneous translucency between the skin and the soft tissue overlying the cervical spine should be measured. During the scan, more than one measurement must be taken and the maximum one should be recorded.

Fetal NT thickness increases with CRL; therefore, in determining whether a given NT thickness is increased, it is essential to take gestation into account. In a fetus with a given CRL, every NT measurement represents a factor that is multiplied by the background risk to calculate a new risk.[199] The larger the NT, the higher the multiplying factor becomes and therefore the higher the new risk. In contrast, the smaller the NT measurement, the smaller the multiplying factor becomes and therefore the lower the new risk.[200]

There are numerous prospective studies examining the implementation of NT measurement in screening for trisomy 21 (Table 23.5).[200–213] Although different cutoffs were used for identifying the screen-positive group, with consequent differences in the false-positive and detection rates, they all reported high detection rates. The combined results on a total of 174,473 pregnancies, including 728 with trisomy 21, demonstrated a detection rate of 77 percent for a false positive rate of 4.7 percent.

Trisomy 21 is associated with increased maternal age, increased fetal NT thickness, increased maternal serum free β-hCG and decreased serum pregnancy associated plasma protein-A (PAPP-A) concentration. We have previously estimated that the most effective method of screening for trisomy 21 would be by a combination of maternal age, fetal NT and serum biochemistry at 11–14 weeks of gestation (Table 23.6). (See also full discussion in chapter 22.) It was predicted that for a false-positive rate of 5 percent the detection rate of trisomy 21 by this method would be about 90 percent, which is superior to the 30 percent achieved by maternal age alone, the 65 percent by maternal age and second-trimester serum biochemistry and the 75 percent by maternal age and first-trimester fetal NT.[214–216] Pregnancy outcome, including karyotype results or the birth of a phenotypically normal baby, was obtained from 14,383 consecutive cases managed with this

Table 23.5. Studies examining the implementation of fetal nuchal translucency (NT) screening

Study	Gestation No.	Weeks	Cutoff	FPR	DR Trisomy 21
Pandya et al.[200a]	1,763	10–14	NT $\geq$ 2.5mm	3.6%	3 of 4 (75%)
Szabo et al.[200b]	3,380	9–12	NT $\geq$ 3.0mm	1.6%	28 of 31 (90%)
Taipale et al.[201]	6,939	10–14	NT $\geq$ 3.0mm	0.8%	4 of 6 (67%)
Hafner et al.[202]	4,371	10–14	NT $\geq$ 2.5mm	1.7%	4 of 7 (57%)
Pajkrt et al.[203]	1,547	10–14	NT $\geq$ 3.0mm	2.2%	6 of 9 (67%)
Snijders et al.[200]	96,127	10–14	NT $\geq$ 95th centile	4.4%	234 of 327 (72%)
Economides et al.[204]	2,281	11–14	NT $\geq$ 99th centile	0.4%	6 of 8 (75%)
Schwarzler et al.[205]	4,523	10–14	NT > 2.5mm	2.7%	8 of 12 (67%)
Theodoropoulos et al.[206]	3,550	10–14	NT $\geq$ 95th centile	2.3%	10 of 11 (91%)
Zoppi et al.[207,207a]	12,311	10–14	NT $\geq$ 95th centile	5.0%	52 of 64 (81%)
Gasiorek-Wiens et al.[208]	23,805	10–14	NT $\geq$ 95th centile	8.0%	174 of 210 (83%)
Brizot et al.[209]	2,996	10–14	NT $\geq$ 95th centile	5.3%	7 of 10 (70%)
Audibert et al.[210]	4,130	10–14	NT $\geq$ 95th centile	4.3%	9 of 12 (75%)
Wayda et al.[211]	6,750	10–12	NT $\geq$ 2.5mm	4.3%	17 of 17 (100%)

Source: Adapted from Nicolaides, 2003.[199]
FPR = false-positive rate; DR = detection rate.

Table 23.6. Detection rate for trisomy 21 and false positive rate of screening tests

Screening Test	Detection Rate	False Positive Rate
Maternal age (MA)	30% (or 50%)	5% (or 15%)
MA + serum β-hCG and PAPP-A at 11–14 weeks	60%	5%
MA + fetal nuchal translucency (NT) at 11–14 weeks	75% (or 70%)	5% (or 2%)
MA + fetal NT and nasal bone (NB) at 11–14 weeks	90%	5%
MA + fetal NT and serum β-hCG and PAPP-A at 11–14 weeks	90% (or 80%)	5% (or 2%)
MA + fetal NT and NB and serum β-hCG and PAPP-A at 11–14 weeks	97% (or 95%)	5% (or 2%)
MA + serum biochemistry at 15–18 weeks	60–70%	5%
Ultrasound for fetal defects and markers at 16–23 weeks	75%	10–15%

Source: Adapted from Nicolaides, 2003.[199]

protocol.[217] The median maternal age of these cases was 34 (range, 15–49) years and in 6,768 (47.1 percent) the age was 35 years or greater. The median gestation at screening was 12 (range, 11–14) weeks and the median fetal CRL was 64 (range, 45–84) mm. The estimated risk for trisomy 21 based on maternal age, fetal NT and maternal serum free β-hCG and PAPP-A was 1 in 300 or greater in 6.8 percent (967 of 14,240) normal pregnancies, in 91.5 percent (75 of 82) of those with trisomy 21 and in 88.5 percent (54 of 61) of those with other chromosomal defects. For a fixed false-positive rate of 5 percent the respective detection rates of screening for trisomy 21 by maternal age alone, maternal age and serum free β-hCG and PAPP-A, maternal age and fetal NT, and by maternal age, fetal NT and maternal serum biochemistry were 30.5 percent, 59.8 percent, 79.3 percent, and 90.2 percent, respectively.

Consequently, with this method of screening and invasive testing for all screen-positive pregnancies, one chromosomally normal fetus will die for every 18 abnormal fetuses that are detected. Alternatively, health care planners may recommend that the minimum detection rate should be 60 percent, which can be achieved with screening by fetal NT and serum biochemistry at 11–14 weeks at a false-positive rate of less than 1 percent and a risk cutoff for invasive testing of one in nine. In this case, one chromosomally normal fetus will die for every 213 abnormal fetuses that are detected. In these calculations it is assumed that the doctors performing CVS are appropriately trained, in which case the procedure-related risk of miscarriage would be 1 percent, which is the same as for second-trimester amniocentesis.

In counseling women, an alternative approach is to accept that decisions made by health care planners based on arbitrary equations of the burdens of miscarriage to those of the birth of a chromosomally abnormal baby are contrary to the basic principle of informed consent. Our responsibility is to assess the risk of a pregnancy being affected using the most accurate method and to allow the parents to decide for themselves for or against invasive testing. This provides evidence that currently the most effective method of screening for chromosomal defects is that provided by a combination of maternal age, fetal NT, and maternal serum free β-hCG and PAPP-A at 11–14 weeks and supports the view that the time has come for a total shift to first-trimester screening (see also chapter 22).

With the advent of rapid immunoassays, it has become possible to provide pretest counseling, biochemical testing of the mother, ultrasound examination of the fetus and posttest counseling of a combined risk estimate, all within a 1-hour visit to a multidisciplinary one-stop clinic for assessment of risk (OSCAR) for fetal anomalies.[218]

Fetal Nasal Bone

At 11–14 weeks of gestation the nasal bone is not visible by ultrasonographic examination in about 60–70 percent of fetuses with trisomy 21 and in less than 1 percent of chromosomally normal fetuses.[219] This may become a powerful adjunct to other methods of screening, especially in the first trimester, once training and reproducibility questions can be addressed appropriately for screening in the general population in centers using NT screening.

Phenotypic Expression of Fetal Aneuploidies in the Second Trimester

In the first trimester, a common feature of many chromosomal defects is increased NT thickness. In later pregnancy each chromosomal defect has its own syndromic pattern of abnormalities. Fetal *trisomy 21* is associated with a tendency to brachycephaly, mild ventriculomegaly, nasal hypoplasia, nuchal edema (or increased nuchal fold thickness), cardiac defects, mainly atrioventricular septal defects, duodenal atresia and echogenic bowel, mild hydronephrosis, shortening of the femur and more so of the humerus, sandal gap, clinodactyly and midphalanx hypoplasia of the fifth finger. *Trisomy 18* is associated with a strawberry-shaped head, choroid plexus cysts, absent corpus callosum, enlarged cisterna magna, facial cleft, micrognathia, nuchal edema, heart defects, diaphragmatic hernia, esophageal atresia, exomphalos, usually with bowel only in the sac, single umbilical artery, renal defects, echogenic bowel, myelomeningocele, growth restriction and shortening of the limbs, radial aplasia, overlapping fingers and talipes or rocker-bottom feet. In *trisomy 13* common defects include holoprosencephaly and associated facial abnormalities, microcephaly, cardiac and renal abnormalities with often enlarged and echogenic kidneys, exomphalos, and postaxial polydactyly. *Triploidy,* in which the extra set of chromosomes is paternally derived, is associated with a molar placenta; pregnancy rarely persists beyond 20 weeks. When there is a double maternal chromosome contribution, the pregnancy may persist into the third trimester. The placenta is of normal consistency but thin, and the fetus demonstrates severe asymmetrical growth restriction. Commonly there is mild ventriculomegaly, micrognathia, cardiac abnormalities, myelomeningocele, syndactyly, and "hitch-hiker" toe deformity. The lethal type of *Turner syndrome* presents with large nuchal cystic hygromata, generalized edema, mild pleural effusions and ascites, cardiac abnormalities, and horseshoe kidney, which are suspected by the ultrasonographic appearance of bilateral mild hydronephrosis.

The Incidence of Abnormalities in Common Chromosomal Defects

The incidence of various abnormalities detected by ultrasound examination during the second and third trimesters in fetuses with trisomies 21, 18, and 13; triploidy; and Turner syndrome is shown in Table 23.7. For example, in trisomy 21, the most commonly found abnormalities are nuchal edema, mild hydronephrosis, relative shortening of the femur, and cardiac abnormality.

The combined data from Nyberg et al. and Bromley et al. are summarized in Table 23.7.[220,221] The incidence of each marker in trisomy 21 pregnancies can be divided by their incidence in chromosomally normal pregnancies to derive the appropriate likelihood ratio Table 23.8. For example, an intracardiac echogenic focus is found in 28.2 percent of trisomy 21 fetuses and in 4.4 percent chromosomally normal fetuses, resulting in a positive likelihood ratio of 6.41 (28.2 of 4.4) and a negative likelihood ratio of 0.75 (71.8 of 95.6). Consequently, the finding of an echogenic focus increases the background risk by a factor of 6.41, but at the same time absence of this marker should reduce the risk by 25 percent. The same logic applies to each one of the six markers in Table 23.7. Thus, in a 25-year-old woman undergoing an ultrasound scan at 20 weeks of gestation, the background risk is about 1 in 1,000. If the scan demonstrates an intracardiac echogenic focus, but the nuchal fold is not increased, the humerus and femur are not short and there is no hydronephrosis, hyperechogenic bowel, or major defect; the combined likelihood ratio should be 1.1 ($6.41 \times 0.67 \times 0.68 \times 0.62 \times 0.85 \times 0.87 \times 0.79$), and consequently her risk remains at about 1 in 1,000. The same is true if the only abnormal finding is mild hydronephrosis, which has a combined likelihood ratio of 1.0 ($6.77 \times 0.67 \times 0.68 \times 0.62 \times 0.75 \times 0.87 \times 0.79$). In contrast, if the fetus is found to have both an intracardiac echogenic focus and mild hydronephrosis but no other defects, the combined likelihood ratio should be 8.42 ($6.41 \times 6.77 \times 0.67 \times 0.68 \times 0.62 \times 0.87 \times 0.79$) and consequently the risk is increased from 1 in 1,000 to 1 in 119.

Table 23.7. Incidence of ultrasound abnormalities in 461 fetuses with chromosomal defects examined at the Harris Birthright Research Centre for Fetal Medicine

	Chromosomal Defect				
	Trisomy				
Fetal Abnormality	21 (%; $n = 155$)	18 (%; $n = 137$)	13 (%; $n = 54$)	Triploidy (%; $n = 50$)	Turner (%; $n = 65$)
Skull/brain					
Strawberry-shaped head	—	54	—	—	—
Brachycephaly	15	29	26	10	32
Microcephaly	—	1	24	—	5
Ventriculomegaly	16	14	9	18	2
Holoprosencephaly	—	3	39	—	—
Choroid plexus cysts	8	47	2	—	—
Absent corpus callosum	—	7	—	—	—
Posterior fossa cyst	1	10	15	6	—
Enlarged cisterna magna	7	16	25	—	—
Face/neck					
Facial cleft	1	10	39	2	—
Micrognathia	1	53	9	44	—
Nuchal edema	38	5	22	4	6
Cystic hygromata	1	2	—	—	88
Chest					
Diaphragmatic hernia	—	10	6	2	—
Cardiac abnormality	26	52	43	16	48
Abdomen					
Omphalocele	—	31	17	2	—
Duodenal atresia	8	—	2	—	—
Absent stomach	3	20	2	2	—
Mild hydronephrosis	30	16	37	4	8
Other renal abnormalities	7	12	24	6	6
Other					
Hydrops	20	4	7	2	80
Small for gestational age	20	74	61	100	55
Relatively short femur	28	25	9	60	59
Abnormal hands/feet	25	72	52	76	2
Talipes	3	30	11	8	—

Prefumo et al.[222] scanned 7,686 normal singleton pregnancies and determined that first-trimester NT is associated with isolated cardiac echogenic foci. They concluded that risk calculations for trisomy 21 based on NT should not use cardiac foci as an independent marker.[222] In estimating the risk in a pregnancy with a marker, it is logical to take into account the results of previous screening tests. For example, in a 39-year-old woman at 20 weeks of gestation (background risk for trisomy 21 of about 1 in 100), who had a 11–14-week assessment by fetal NT and serum free β-hCG and PAPP-A that resulted in a tenfold reduction in risk (to about 1 in 1,000) after the diagnosis of a short femur but no other abnormal findings at the 20-week scan (likelihood ratio of 1.6, see Table 23.8), the estimated new risk is 1 in 625.

Notwithstanding the foregoing discussion, a meta-analysis by Smith-Bindman et al.[222a] evaluated the use of second-trimester ultrasound markers to detect fetal Down syndrome. They analyzed fifty-six papers encompassing 1,930 fetuses with Down syndrome

Table 23.8. Incidence of major and minor defects or markers in the second-trimester scan in trisomy 21 and chromosomally normal fetuses in the combined data of two major series[220,221]

	T21	Normal	Positive LR	Negative LR	LR for Isolated Marker
Nuchal fold	107/319 (33.5%)	59/9331 (0.6%)	53.05 (39.37–71.26)	0.67 (0.61–0.72)	9.8
Short humerus	102/305 (33.4%)	136/9254 (1.5%)	22.76 (18.04–28.56)	0.68 (0.62–0.73)	4.1
Short femur	132/319 (41.4%)	486/9331 (5.2%)	7.94 (6.77–9.25)	0.62 (0.56–0.67)	1.6
Hydronephrosis	56/319 (17.6%)	242/9331 (2.6%)	6.77 (5.16–8.80)	0.85 (5.16–8.80)	1.0
Echogenic focus	75/266 (28.2%)	401/9119 (4.4%)	6.41 (5.15–7.90)	0.75 (0.69–0.80)	1.1
Echogenic bowel	39/293 (13.3%)	58/9227 (0.6%)	21.17 (14.34–31.06)	0.87 (0.83–0.91)	3.0
Major defect	75/350 (2.4%)	61/9384 (0.65%)	32.96 (23.90–43.28)	0.79 (0.74–0.83)	5.2

Source: Adapted from Nicolaides, 2003.[199]

Note: From these data, the positive and negative likelihood ratios (with 95% confidence interval) for each marker can be calculated. In the last column is the likelihood ratio for each marker found in isolation.

LR = likelihood ratio.

and 13,0365 unaffected fetuses. In their determination of sensitivity, specificity, and positive and negative likelihood ratios, they assessed the following markers: choroid plexus cyst, thickened nuchal fold, echogenic intracardiac focus, echogenic bowel, renal pyelectasis, and humeral and femoral shortening. Their main conclusion was that individual markers alone were inefficient in discriminating between fetuses with and without Down syndrome, and hence should not be used as indicators for amniocentesis except when associated with other structural abnormalities.

Fetal Abnormalities with Chromosomal Defects

Brain Abnormalities

Ventriculomegaly. In 14 published series on fetal ventriculomegaly,[25–28,31,223–228] the mean incidence of chromosomal defects was 13 percent; the incidence was 2 percent for fetuses with no other detectable abnormalities and 17 percent for those with additional abnormalities. The most common chromosomal defects were trisomies 21, 18, and 13 and triploidy.

Holoprosencephaly. In the published studies[40–43,227,229,230] on fetal holoprosencephaly, the mean incidence of chromosomal defects among ninety-three cases was 33 percent; the incidence was 4 percent for fetuses with apparently isolated holoprosencephaly and 39 percent for those with additional abnormalities. The commonest chromosomal defects were trisomies 13 and 18.

Microcephaly. In a series of 2,086 fetuses that were karyotyped because of fetal malformations or growth retardation, the diagnosis of microcephaly was made if the head circumference was below the 5th centile and the ratio of head circumference to femur length was below the 2.5th centile.[227] There were 52 cases of microcephaly, and 8 (15 percent) of these had chromosomal defects. Eydoux et al.[231] reported chromosomal defects in 5 (25 percent) of 20 cases. In the combined data from these two series, twelve of the thirteen chromosomally abnormal fetuses had additional abnormalities, and the most common chromosomal defect was trisomy 13. Others have emphasized the heterogeneity, variability, and complexities involved in the prenatal detection of microcephaly.[231a] These authors found microcephaly with chromosomal abnormality in 23.3 percent of 30 cases.

Choroid Plexus Cysts. (See Figure 23.2.) Several reports[222,222a227,230,232–253] have documented an association between choroid plexus cysts and chromosomal defects, particularly trisomy 18 (13 percent). The mean incidence of chromosomal defects in the various published series was 8 percent, with an incidence of 1 percent for apparently isolated lesions and 54 percent for those with additional abnormalities.

In a meta-analysis of 13 prospective studies encompassing 24,6545 second-trimester cases, including 1,346 fetuses with isolated choroid plexus cysts, Yoder et al.[253a] noted that 7 had trisomy 18 and 5 had trisomy 21. The likelihood of trisomy 18 was 13.8-fold greater than the a priori risk in fetuses with isolated choroid plexus cysts. The likelihood of trisomy 21 was not significantly increased. A subsequent meta-analysis of eight prospective trials aimed to determine the incidence of trisomy 18 in women <35 years of age with isolated fetal choroid plexus cysts.[253b] This study of 10,6732 women included 1,235 such cases, an incidence of 1.2 percent. No cases of trisomy 18 were observed, the authors concluding that amniocentesis was not warranted when an *isolated* choroid plexus cyst is observed. A salutary observation of a false-positive rate ranging from 3.9–15.7 percent was noted by DeVore,[253c] depending on which ultrasound markers were used to determine fetal trisomy 18.

Snijders et al.[252] suggested that because the incidence of chromosomal defects is associated with maternal age, it is possible that the wide range in the reported incidence of chromosomal defect is the mere consequence of differences in the maternal age distribution of the populations examined in the various studies. Issues of ascertainment bias and completeness of follow-up also need consideration. If the choroid plexus cysts are apparently isolated, then the maternal-age-related risk for trisomy 18 is increased by a factor of 1.5.

Absent Corpus Callosum. Three studies with a total of seventeen fetuses with absent corpus callosum reported trisomy 13 in one fetus who had additional malformations.[254–256] We diagnosed absence of the corpus callosum in 7 percent of 137 fetuses with trisomy 18.

Short Frontal Lobe. Trisomy 21 is associated with brachycephaly, which is thought to be due to reduced growth of the frontal lobe. Frontothalamic distance is measured from the inner table of the frontal bone to the posterior thalamus. Bahado-Singh et al.[257] reported that in 19 fetuses with trisomy 21 at 16–21 weeks of gestation, the frontothalamic distance to biparietal diameter ratio was significantly lower than in 125 normal controls; in 21 percent of fetuses with trisomy 21, the ratio was below the 5th centile. These findings await confirmation from further studies.

Posterior Fossa Abnormalities. In the combined data from five series[48,226,229,238,259] on a total of 101 fetuses with enlarged posterior fossa, the mean incidence of chromosomal defects, mainly trisomy 18, was 44 percent.

Abnormal Shape of the Head

Strawberry-Shaped Skull. Some fetuses with trisomy 18 have a characteristic shape of the head that is best seen in the suboccipitobregmatic view. There is flattening of the occiput and narrowing of the frontal part of the head. The most likely explanation for the narrow frontal region is hypoplasia of the face and frontal cerebral lobes. Similarly, flattening of the occiput may be due to hypoplasia of the hindbrain. In a series of 54 fetuses with a strawberry-shaped head, they all had additional malformations and 44 (81 percent) had chromosomal defects.[260] A strawberry-shaped skull is a subjective marker rather than a measurable feature.

Brachycephaly. Brachycephaly is a well-recognized feature of children with Down syndrome. However, two prenatal ultrasonographic studies have found no difference in the mean cephalic index (biparietal to occipitofrontal diameter ratio) between 25 second-trimester fetuses with trisomy 21 and 325 normal controls.[261] In our series of 451 fetuses with chromosomal defects, the mean cephalic index was increased, but in the majority of cases, the index was below the 97.5th centile; brachycephaly was observed in 15 percent of fetuses with trisomy 21, 28 percent of those with trisomy 18 or 13, 10 percent of those with triploidy, and 32 percent of those with Turner syndrome.

Facial Abnormalities. Facial cleft and other facial abnormalities are common features of certain chromosomal defects. These abnormalities are usually detected by careful examination of the face after the diagnosis of other fetal abnormalities and/or growth retardation.

Facial Cleft. Postnatally, chromosomal defects are found in less than 1 percent of babies with facial cleft.[262] However, in seven prenatal series reporting on a total of 118 fetuses,[229,263–268] 40 percent had chromosomal defects, most commonly trisomies 13 and 18; in all fetuses with chromosomal defects, there were additional abnormalities.

The high incidence of chromosomal defects and other abnormalities in the prenatal studies indicates that the populations examined were preselected. Presumably, in the majority of cases detailed, ultrasound examination leading to the diagnosis of facial clefting was performed in referral centers because routine scanning had demonstrated the presence of a variety of extrafacial defects.

Micrognathia. In two studies reporting on sixty-five cases in which micrognathia was diagnosed antenatally, all fetuses had additional malformations and/or growth retardation. The incidence of chromosomal defects was 62 percent and the commonest was trisomy 18.[266,267] Conversely, we diagnosed micrognathia in 53 percent of fetuses with trisomy 18 and 44 percent of those with triploidy, while postmortem studies have demonstrated micrognathia to be present in more than 80 percent of these fetuses.[269] This suggests that at present only severe micrognathia is amenable to prenatal diagnosis.

Ocular and Nasal Abnormalities. Eye abnormalities, such as hypotelorism and cyclopia, and nasal defects, such as nasal aplasia or hypoplasia, single nostril, or proboscis are often seen in the presence of holoprosencephaly, and they are associated with trisomies 13 and 18.[266] Although all chromosomally abnormal fetuses with holoprosencephaly have extracraniofacial abnormalities, the risk for chromosomal defects increases if facial defects are also present.[40]

Macroglossia. Postnatally, macroglossia and a flat profile are common features of trisomy 21. Antenatally, these abnormalities are rarely diagnosed unless other features of trisomy 21 are found. In a series of 69 fetuses with trisomy 21, macroglossia was diagnosed in 10 percent of those examined at <28 weeks and 20 percent of those diagnosed at <28 weeks.[266] It is possible that with advancing gestation there is progressive enlargement and/or protrusion of the tongue to account for the higher incidence of macroglossia at term.

Small Ears. Chromosomally abnormal infants often have small ears. Three prenatal ultrasonographic studies have confirmed that the ear length of fetuses with chromosomal defects is decreased.[270–272]

Neck Abnormalities

Nuchal Cystic Hygromata. Nuchal cystic hygromata are developmental abnormalities of the lymphatic system. Although they are rarely seen postnatally, they are found in 0.5 percent of spontaneously aborted fetuses.[273] Prenatal diagnosis by ultrasonography is based on the demonstration of a bilateral, septated, cystic structure located in the occipitocervical region. This condition should be distinguished from nuchal edema, which has a high association with trisomies, or unilateral cervical cysts, which are usually detected in the third trimester and have a good prognosis after postnatal surgery.

Reports on antenatally diagnosed cystic hygromata[200,223,226,228–230,255–270,274–289b] have established an association with hydrops fetalis in 40–100 percent of the cases, congenital heart defects in 0–92 percent of the cases, and chromosomal defects in 46–90 percent of the fetuses; the most common being Turner syndrome. Survival, either as a result of the natural history or because of termination of pregnancy, is less than 5 percent.

Azar et al.[272] suggested that the wide range in the reported incidence of hydrops fetalis, cardiac defects, and both the presence and types of chromosomal defects may be a consequence of differences in the diagnostic criteria for cystic hygromata used in the various reports. In their study, which examined only fetuses with septated, cervical, dorsal hygromata, 75 percent had chromosomal defects; Turner syndrome accounted for 94 percent. In a fetus with cystic hygromata, the risk for Turner syndrome is increased if the mother is young, if there is a fetal cardiac defect, and if the ratio of head circumference to femur length is increased. Unlike with most other abnormalities, in cystic hygromata, the incidence of chromosomal defects is high, even for apparently isolated hygromata. The two most likely explanations for this finding are (1) the limited number of reported cases, and (2) the most common chromosomal defect is Turner syndrome, in which the associated coarctation of the aorta can be difficult to diagnose antenatally.

Benacerraf et al.[290,291] noted the association between increased soft-tissue thickening on the posterior aspect of the neck and trisomy 21. In a series of 1,704 consecutive amniocenteses at 15–20 weeks of gestation in which there were 11 fetuses with trisomy 21, 45 percent of the trisomic fetuses and 0.06 percent of the normal fetuses had nuchal thickness more than 5 mm. Similarly, Lynch et al.,[292] who retrospectively examined the sonograms of nine pairs of discordant twins, found increased nuchal thickening in five of the nine fetuses with trisomy 21 but in none of the normal co-twins. However, Perella et al.[293] retrospectively examined the sonograms of 14 fetuses with trisomy 21 and 128 normal controls and found increased nuchal thickening in only 21 percent of the trisomic fetuses and in 9 percent of the normals. Similarly, Nyberg et al.[294] reviewed the sonographic findings of 68 consecutive fetuses with trisomy 21 at 14–24 weeks of gestation and found increased nuchal thickening in only 5 (7 percent). In the Smith-Bindman et al. meta-analysis discussed above,[222a] the authors observed that despite a seventeenfold increased risk of Down syndrome when a thickened nuchal fold was seen, the overall sensitivity of this ultrasound marker was too low for it to be a practical screening test for Down syndrome. A multicenter study evaluating the utility of the "genetic sonogram" concluded with a sensitivity of 46.5 percent for Down syndrome diagnosis in the 176 trisomy 21 cases.[294a] In this eight-center series, combined ultrasound markers yielded a diagnostic sensitivity of 71.6 percent.

Nicolaides et al.[295] considered nuchal edema to be present if in the midsagittal plane of the neck there was subcutaneous edema (at least 7 mm) that produced a characteristic tremor on ballottement of the fetal head. This was distinguished from nuchal cystic hygromata and hydrops fetalis, in which there was generalized edema. In a series of 144 fetuses with nuchal edema, 37 percent had chromosomal defects, mainly trisomy 21, but also other trisomies, deletions or translocations, triploidy, and Turner syndrome.[266] Furthermore, the chromosomally normal fetuses had a very poor prognosis because in many cases there was an underlying skeletal dysplasia, genetic syndrome, or cardiac defect. In a total of 371 cases in nine reports[266,273,296–303] on fetal nuchal thickening, 33 percent had chromosomal defects (18 percent if isolated) and the commonest was trisomy 21. The most likely explanation for the high incidence of chromosomal defects, even for apparently isolated nuchal edema, is that the most common defect is trisomy 21, in which the associated abnormalities are usually subtle.[294–303]

Hydrops Fetalis. In a review of the literature up to 1989, 303 chromosomal defects were noted in 16 percent of 600 fetuses with nonimmune hydrops; the most common being trisomy 21 and Turner syndrome, found in 38 percent and 35 percent of the cases, respectively. In our series of 214 fetuses with non-rhesus hydrops (excluding those with cystic hygromata, mentioned above), 12 percent had chromosomal defects, mainly trisomy 21. In a series of 51 stillborn fetuses, 12 percent had a chromosomal abnormality.[303a]

Thoracic Abnormalities

Diaphragmatic Hernia. In seven prenatal series[230,266,287,304–307] reporting on a total of 173 fetuses with diaphragmatic hernia, 18 percent had chromosomal defects, most commonly trisomy 18; the incidence was 2 percent for those with apparently isolated diaphragmatic hernia and 39 percent for those with multiple additional abnormalities. Diaphragmatic hernia in association with other anomalies yielded a chromosomal abnormality in 16 of 17 cases in a series of 201 fetuses and babies.[307a]

Cardiac Abnormalities. Nora and Nora[50] reported that heart defects are found in more than 99 percent of fetuses with trisomy 18, in 90 percent of those with trisomy 13, in 50 percent of those with trisomy 21, in 40–50 percent of those with deletions or partial trisomies involving chromosomes 4, 5, 8, 9, 13, 14, 18, or 22, and in 35 percent of those with 45,XO.

Prenatal studies of ultrasonographically detectable fetal cardiac abnormalities[50,266,308–311] have reported chromosomal defects in 28 percent of 829 cases. The most common defects were trisomies 21, 18, and 13 and Turner syndrome. Chromosomal defects were found in 16 percent of cases with apparently isolated heart defects and in 65 percent of those with additional abnormalities. There are two possible explanations for the high incidence of chromosomal defects, even for apparently isolated cardiac abnormalities. First, the defect involved is trisomy 21, in which associated abnormalities are subtle, and second, the results are mainly due to one study in which other abnormalities may have been missed.

Echogenic foci or "golf balls" within the ventricles of the fetal heart.[312,313] are observed in routine second-trimester scans in 0.5–1.2 percent, and their size varies from 1 to 6 mm. Histologic studies have shown these foci to be due to mineralization within a papillary muscle.[314] Follow-up studies of fetuses with echogenic foci have demonstrated normal ventricular function and competent atrioventricular valves.[313] Echogenic foci in association with multiple other abnormalities frequently signal the presence of a chromosomal abnormality.[314] Intracardiac echogenic foci increase the risk of Down syndrome fivefold to sevenfold.[312]

Gastrointestinal Tract Abnormalities

Esophageal Atresia. Postnatally, chromosomal defects were reported in 3–4 percent of neonates with esophageal atresia.[115,314,315] In a prenatal series of 20 fetuses with no visible stomach and the presumptive diagnosis of esophageal atresia, 85 percent had trisomy 18, and in all cases there were additional abnormalities.[316] The most likely explanation for the very high incidence in chromosomal defects found prenatally, compared with that after birth, is that fetuses with trisomy 18 often die in utero or are born at previable stages of gestation, due to the polyhydramnios; unlike chromosomally normal fetuses, in trisomy 18, esophageal atresia is not usually associated with tracheoesophageal fistula. In addition, as with facial defects, in the majority of fetuses with esophageal atresia, the diagnosis was made by detailed ultrasound examination after the detection of other abnormalities or growth retardation at routine scanning.

Duodenal Atresia. Postnatally, trisomy 21 is found in 20–30 percent of cases of duodenal atresia.[110] In prenatal series, the mean incidence of chromosomal defects was 38 percent among 44 cases when isolated and up to 64 percent when multiple abnormalities were present.[223,229,230,288,316]

Bowel Obstruction. In a series of twenty-four fetuses with dilated bowel (including fourteen cases of small and six cases of large bowel obstruction and four cases of megacystis–microcolon–intestinal hypoperistalsis syndrome or myotonia dystrophica), the karyotype was normal in all but one case, in which the fetus had multiple other abnormalities.[316]

Echogenic Bowel. In six series reporting on hyperechogenic bowel, 20 percent had chromosomal defects, mainly trisomy 21. Bromley et al.[317] estimated that 12.5 percent of fetuses with trisomy 21 have hyperechogenic bowel, that in 41 percent of these the echogenic bowel may be the only ultrasound finding, and that the risk of Down syndrome in fetuses with isolated hyperechogenic bowel is 1.4 percent. In the Harris Birthright Research Centre for Fetal Medicine, hyperechogenic bowel was observed in 280 fetuses, and this was most commonly associated with placental insufficiency and intrauterine growth restriction; chromosomal defects were found only in fetuses with additional, often multiple, abnormalities. In a prospective French collaborative study with known outcome in 655 fetuses, hyperechogenic bowel was observed in 2.5 percent of those with Down syndrome and a 1 percent risk of other severe chromosomal anomalies.[117a] Isolated hyperechogenicity was observed in eleven of seventeen Down syndrome fetuses, in contrast to none in the smaller series quoted earlier.[118c]

Abdominal Cysts. Abdominal cysts include ovarian (see Fig. 23.9), mesenteric, adrenal, and hepatic cysts. In a series of twenty-seven fetuses with abdominal cysts, the karyotype was normal in twenty-six cases; in one fetus with multiple adrenal cysts and hepatosplenomegaly due to the Beckwith–Wiedemann syndrome, the karyotype was 46XX/46XX, dup(11p).[316]

Anterior Abdominal Wall Abnormalities

Omphalocele. In liveborn infants with omphalocele, the incidence of chromosomal defects, mainly trisomies 18 and 13, is approximately 10 percent, whereas in antenatal series, the reported incidence is about 36 percent.[223,230–232,307,316–332] The karyotype is more likely to be abnormal if the omphalocele is associated with additional abnormalities (46 percent compared with 8 percent for apparently isolated omphalocele). Furthermore, the incidence of chromosomal abnormalities is higher when the omphalocele sac contains only bowel than in cases in which the liver is included.

Gastroschisis. In four reports on a total of sixty-three fetuses with gastroschisis, there were no chromosomal defects.[230,316,329,330,332]

Urinary Tract Abnormalities. In 15 series[223,230–232,282,283,316,327,331–338] on 145 cases, the overall incidence of associated chromosomal abnormalities varied from 2 percent (mainly for isolated mild pyelectasis) to 33 percent; the mean incidence for isolated abnormalities was 3 percent, and the incidence for those with additional abnormalities was 24 percent. Renal anomalies detected prenatally in association with multiple fetal anomalies and chromosomal defects, result in a high mortality—76 percent in one series of 41 cases.[338a] In particular, oligohydramnios increased the risk of death.

In the largest series, renal abnormalities were classified as (1) mild hydronephrosis, in which only the renal pelvices are dilated and both the bladder and amniotic fluid volume are normal; (2) moderate to severe hydronephrosis, with varying degrees of pelvic–calyceal dilatation; (3) multicystic dysplasia, with multiple noncommunicating cysts of variable size and irregular hyperechogenic stroma; and (4) renal agenesis.[339] The overall incidence of chromosomal defects was 12 percent, and the most common were trisomies 21, 18, and 13. The pattern of chromosomal defects, and consequently that of associated malformations, was related to the different types of renal abnormalities. The risk for chromosomal defects was similar for fetuses with unilateral or bilateral involvement, different types of renal abnormalities, urethral or ureteric obstruction, and oligohydramnios or normal/reduced amniotic fluid volume. However, the incidence of chromosomal defects in females was almost double (18 percent) that in males (10 percent).

Skeletal Abnormalities

Short Femur. Benacerraf et al.[290] reported that if the ratio of the actual femur length to the expected length, based on the biparietal diameter, was ≤0.91, the sensitivity and specificity for detecting fetuses with trisomy 21 at 15–21 weeks of gestation was 68 percent and 98 percent, respectively. Subsequent studies have confirmed that trisomy 21 is associated with relative shortening of the femur, but the sensitivity and specificity of this test were lower than those in the original report. In an additional five studies involving a total of seventy-seven fetuses with trisomy 21, there was no significant difference in the ratio of mean biparietal diameter to femur length and/or the measured-to-expected femur ratio from that of normal controls.[261,292,340–342] However, although no significant difference in femur length in trisomy 21 was observed between black, Hispanic, and white groups, the fetal femoral length was shorter in the Asian group studied.[321]

In a series of 155 fetuses with trisomy 21 diagnosed in the Harris Birthright Research Centre for Fetal Medicine, there was relative shortening of the femur, demonstrated by a ratio of head circumference to femur length above the 97.5th centile, in 28 percent of the cases. In fetuses with trisomy 18, trisomy 13, triploidy, and Turner syndrome, the incidences of relative shortening of the femur were 25, 9, 60, and 59 percent, respectively.

Short Humerus. In a postmortem study of fetuses with Down syndrome, FitzSimmons et al.[343] reported that shortening of the long bones of the upper extremity was more pronounced than that of the lower extremity. Four prenatal ultrasonographic studies at 15–22 weeks of gestation have confirmed that in trisomy 21 there is relative shortening of the humerus, but they produced conflicting results regarding the value of this feature in screening for trisomies,[343–347] as discussed above.[222a]

Malformations of the Extremities. Characteristic abnormalities in the extremities are commonly found in a wide range of chromosomal defects, and the detection of abnormal hands or feet at the routine ultrasound examination should stimulate the search for other markers of chromosomal defects. Syndactyly is associated with triploidy, clinodactyly, and sandal gap with trisomy 21; polydactyly is associated with trisomy 13; and overlapping fingers, rocker-bottom feet, and talipes are associated with trisomy 18.

Talipes. Talipes equinovarus or calcaneovarus is a common abnormality, found in 1–2 per 1,000 live births. In the majority of cases, the cause is uncertain, but in some families, an autosomal recessive mode of inheritance has been described.

In 243 fetuses with talipes examined at the Harris Birthright Research Centre for Fetal Medicine, only 22 percent had isolated talipes. In the others, the talipes was associated with (1) chromosomal defects, (2) neural tube or brain abnormalities, (3) oligohydramnios due to renal abnormalities or preterm prelabor amniorrhexis, (4) skeletal dysplasias such as osteogenesis imperfecta, or (5) arthrogryposis, in which, in addition to the talipes, there was fixed flexion or extension deformity of all major joints.

In three series on a total of 127 cases of antenatally diagnosed talipes equinovarus, 33 percent had chromosomal defects, mainly trisomy 18.[226,249,348–349] All fetuses with chromosomal defects had multiple abnormalities.

Intrauterine Growth Restriction (IUGR). Although low birth weight is a common feature of many chromosomal defects, the incidence of chromosomal defects in small- for-gestational-age neonates is less than 1–2 percent.[350–352] However, data derived from postnatal studies underestimate the association between chromosomal defects and growth restriction, because many pregnancies with chromosomally abnormal fetuses result in spontaneous abortion or intrauterine death. Furthermore, because the degree of IUGR is generally more severe in the more lethal types of chromosomal defects, in antenatally diagnosed, early-onset, severe IUGR, the types of chromosomal defects are different from those recognized at birth.

In two prenatal series reporting on a total of 621 growth-restricted fetuses, the incidence of chromosomal defects was 19 percent (4 percent if isolated to 38 percent if associated with other abnormalities).[230,353]

Snijders et al.[353] examined findings in 458 fetuses with an abdominal circumference and subsequently birth weight below the 5th centile for gestation. The commonest chromosomal defects were triploidy and trisomy 18. The characteristic Swiss-cheese appearance of a molar placenta was found in only 17 percent of fetuses with triploidy; in the others, the placenta looked normal and the main feature was severe asymmetrical growth retardation. The triploidies were most commonly encountered in the second trimester, while the aneuploidies, deletions, and translocations were found in the third-trimester group of fetuses. These findings suggest that triploidy is associated with the most severe form of early-onset growth retardation and that most affected fetuses die before the third trimester.

The highest incidence of chromosomal defects was found in cases in which, in addition to the growth retardation, there were fetal structural abnormalities, in cases in which the amniotic fluid volume was normal or increased, and in the group with normal waveforms from both uterine and umbilical arteries.

These findings demonstrate that IUGR due to chromosomal defects presents differently from IUGR due to placental insufficiency. The latter is characterized by increased impedance to flow in the uterine and/or umbilical arteries, with consequent fetal hypoxemia, redistribution in the fetal circulation, impaired renal perfusion, and reduced urine production and amniotic fluid volume.

It is generally assumed that fetal causes of IUGR, such as chromosomal defects, are associated with early-onset, symmetrical impairment in growth of all parts of the body. In contrast, placental insufficiency is associated with late-onset, asymmetrical impairment in growth, primarily affecting the abdomen and sparing the head and femur. However, the study of Snijders et al.[353] demonstrated that relative shortening of the femur is found in both the chromosomally normal and abnormal fetuses.

Fetuses with triploidy have severe, early-onset, asymmetrical IUGR (increased head-to-abdomen circumference ratio), whereas fetuses with chromosomal defects other than triploidy are symmetrically growth restricted before 30 weeks, but the ones diagnosed after this gestation are usually asymmetrically growth-retarded.

Because in normal pregnancy the head-to-abdomen circumference ratio decreases with gestation, it could be postulated that chromosomal defects interfere with the developmental clock that controls the switch from preferential growth of the head to growth of the abdomen.

MULTIPLE PREGNANCIES

During the past 20 years, both the average maternal age and the use of assisted reproduction techniques have increased, with a concomitant increase in the number of multiple pregnancies at increased risk for chromosomal defects. In multiple pregnancies compared with singletons, prenatal diagnosis is complicated because:

- effective methods of screening, such as maternal serum biochemistry, are not as efficacious;
- the techniques of invasive testing may provide uncertain results or may be associated with higher risks of miscarriage; and
- fetuses may be discordant for an abnormality, in which case one of the options for the subsequent management of the pregnancy is selective feticide.

At 10–14 weeks, the prevalence of twins is about 2 percent. About 80 percent are dichorionic and 20 percent are monochorionic. All monochorionic twins are monozygotic, and about 90 percent of dichorionic twins are dizygotic and 10 percent monozygotic.

Zygosity and Chorionicity

About two-thirds of twins are dizygotic (nonidentical). They result from the fertilization of two separate eggs. There are two placentas (dichorionic) and these can be either adjacent to each other or on opposite sides of the uterus. When they are next to each other, the intertwin membrane is thick, and at the junction with the placenta, there is a lambda sign (a triangular piece of placental extension). The one-third of twins who are monozygotic, start as one cell mass that splits into two at some stage during the first 13 days after fertilization. In about one-third of cases, splitting occurs within the first three days after fertilization, and in these cases, there are two separate placentas (dichorionic with a lambda sign). When splitting occurs after day 3, there are common blood vessels joining the two placentas, which therefore act as if they were one (monochorionic). In these cases, the intertwin membrane is thin, and at the junction with the placenta, there is no lambda sign.[354,355]

Risk of Fetal Loss in Multiple Pregnancies[356]

In singleton pregnancies,

- the risk of fetal death between 12 and 24 weeks is about 0.5 percent.
- the risk of intrauterine death after 24 weeks and neonatal death is about 0.5 percent.

In dichorionic twin pregnancies,

- the risk of fetal death between 12 and 24 weeks is about 2 percent.
- the risk of intrauterine death after 24 weeks and neonatal death is about 2 percent.

In monochorionic twin pregnancies,

- the risk of fetal death between 12 and 24 weeks is about 12 percent.
- the risk of intrauterine death after 24 weeks and neonatal death is about 4 percent.
- the intertwin difference in CRL and birth weight is the same as in dichorionic twins.

In triplet pregnancies managed expectantly,

- the risk of fetal death between 12 and 24 weeks is about 3 percent.
- the risk of intrauterine death after 24 weeks and neonatal death is about 6 percent.
- the chance of a pregnancy ending with at least one survivor is about 95 percent.
- the chance of a survivor being disabled is about 2 percent.

In triplet pregnancies iatrogenically reduced to twins,

- the risk of fetal death between 12 and 24 weeks is about 8 percent.
- the risk of intrauterine death after 24 weeks and neonatal death is about 3 percent.
- the chance of a pregnancy ending with at least one survivor is about 91 percent.
- the chance of a survivor being disabled is about 0.5 percent.

Nuchal Translucency Screening in Twins[357]

An ultrasound study involving 448 twin pregnancies at 10–14 weeks demonstrated that NT screening is equally effective in identifying trisomic fetuses in twins and in singletons. In twins, it is imperative that the chorionicity is first determined and then the CRL and NT are measured for each fetus. As with singleton pregnancies, increased NT may also be a marker of cardiac or other defects. In monochorionic twins, increased NT may also be a marker of twin-to-twin transfusion.

In dichorionic twins, the NT is measured in each fetus and this is combined with maternal age to calculate the risk for trisomies in each fetus. If the risk of at least one of the fetuses is more than 1 in 50, then chorionic villus sampling (CVS) should be considered. If the risk is less, then amniocentesis is preferable.

In monochorionic twins (always identical), at present, the calculation of risk for trisomies is based on the combination of maternal age and the NT of the fetus with the highest measurement. If the parents choose invasive testing, only one placenta or amniotic sac needs to be sampled.

The Choice between Amniocentesis and CVS[358]

Amniocentesis at 16 weeks can be carried out through a single uterine entry, and both twins can be sampled by the same needle, which is advanced through the intertwin membrane. The risk of miscarriage is about 1 percent, which is similar to that in singletons (see full discussion in chapter 2).

There is a need for selection of the appropriate diagnostic technique, depending on the likelihood for selective feticide. If the risk is high, CVS should be the technique of choice; otherwise, amniocentesis is preferable. The only way to determine risks is by NT screening.

Discordancy for Abnormalities

When one fetus is normal and the other has abnormalities such as anencephaly, spina bifida, cardiac defects, or omphalocele, it is equally possible that the fetuses are identical or nonidentical. If the abnormality is lethal, it is best to manage such pregnancies expectantly. If the abnormality is serious but not lethal, selective feticide can be considered. In dichorionic twins, intracardiac potassium chloride (KCl) can be used, but in monochorionic twins, occlusion of the umbilical cord is necessary (see chapter 2).

Discordancy for Intrauterine Growth Restriction

When one fetus is normally grown and the other is growth retarded, it is three times as likely that the pregnancy is dichorionic as monochorionic. If the IUGR fetus shows signs of distress and the pregnancy is more than 30 weeks, it is best to undertake delivery. If the pregnancy is less than 32 weeks, the management depends on chorionicity. Dichorionic twins with a dying IUGR fetus at less than 32 weeks can be managed expectantly. Monochorionic twins with a dying IUGR fetus at 26–32 weeks should be delivered; before 26 weeks, selective feticide by cord occlusion should be considered.

Twin-to-Twin Transfusion Syndrome

Monochorionic twin pregnancies presenting during the second trimester with severe twin-to-twin transfusion syndrome are associated with a high risk of miscarriage, perinatal death, and chronic handicap in survivors.[359–364] Although survival can be improved by serial amniodrainage, there is a persistent risk of serious chronic handicap in 15–50 percent of the survivors.[365–367a] A more recent development in the management of this condition is the use of fetoscopy and laser coagulation to interrupt the placental vascular communications between the twins, which may constitute the underlying mechanism of the syndrome. Irrespective of the vascular nature of the anastomoses or their depth within the placenta, their afferent and efferent branches are superficial.[368,369] Although the intertwin membrane does not necessarily overlie these common cotyledons, the systematic coagulation of all crossing vessels should inevitably include the branches of these anastomoses. This treatment approach may lead to survival of at least one of the twins in about 70 percent of pregnancies.[370]

In a study of 26 multiple pregnancies, laser ablation resulted in 53 percent of the fetuses surviving, with 96 percent developing normally at a mean age of 35.8 months.[370a] In contrast with endoscopic surgery, in which survival both with time and in different centers remains stable at 55 percent for fetuses and more than 70 percent for pregnancies with at least one survivor, with the alternative method of treatment, serial amniodrainage, there are marked differences in reported results from different series. As reported by Saunders et al.,[362] in series before 1991, the survival was 30–40 percent, whereas in the past 6 years, using apparently the same technique, the survival improved up to 83 percent.[364] Thus, three centers in five different papers[365,371–373] have reported that in 53 pregnancies treated with serial amniocentesis and in 14 managed with watchful waiting, the fetal survival rates were 76 percent and 36 percent, respectively, suggesting that the condition was milder than in previous studies. Also of importance, the largest series included six dichorionic pregnancies.[371–373] In a multicenter study of stage-based treatment, neonatal survival in the serial amniocentesis group was 66.7 percent, in contrast with the laser ablation group (83.2 percent).[373a]

The perinatal morbidity is also an important issue. In 4 percent of our survivors, neurologic handicap is likely to develop. Pinette et al.[364] reported that 36 percent of the survivors in a population treated by serial amniocentesis had cerebral palsy. Bajoria et al.[365] noted the presence of porencephalic cyst in 29 percent of the survivors (4 of 14) and cardiac dysfunction in another 4 survivors. Trespidi et al.[366] reported a severe handicap rate of 15 percent in the surviving twins (4 of 26) when managed similarly.[367] The main underlying mechanism of perinatal handicap in twin-to-twin transfusion syndrome is thought to be an acute hemodynamic imbalance between the twins, following a hypotensive period or fetal death, leading to an acute and significant transfer of blood from the normotensive to the hypotensive or dead fetus. This continues until the transfusing twin's mean arterial pressure equals the transfused twin's systemic filling pressure. A randomized controlled intention-to-treat trial was conducted in six centers in Europe and in the United States from January 1999 through to September 2002.[374] Patients were eligible if the diagnosis of severe twin-to-twin transfusion syndrome (TTTS) was established before 26+0 weeks of gestation. The interim analysis performed after 142 inclusions, showed a statistically significant benefit in the laser group for survival of at least one infant (76.4 percent vs. 51.4 percent) (relative risk = 1.49 [1.14–1.93], $p = 0.002$) and the decision to stop the recruitment was taken. A significantly higher gestational age at delivery was observed in the laser group as well as a higher mean birth weight. The occurrence of periventricular leukomalacia was significantly lower in the laser group, and the likelihood of severe morbidity in the survivor of a single fetal death was five times higher in the amniodrainage group. Endoscopic laser coagulation of chorionic plate vascular anastomoses can therefore be considered a more effective first-line treatment of severe TTTS than serial amniodrainage.

Acardiac Twins

Acardiac twins or twin reversed arterial perfusion (TRAP) sequence is the most extreme manifestation of twin-to-twin transfusion syndrome and is found in approximately 1 percent of monozygotic twin pregnancies in the second and third trimesters.[375] The underlying mechanism is thought to be disruption of normal vascular perfusion and development of the acardiac twin due to an umbilical artery-to-artery anastomosis with the normal twin. The outcome for the normal twin is not uniformly poor. Moore et al.[376] reported that it depends on the weight of the acardiac fetus: when the weights of the twins were compared and the donor's weight was >70 percent, 50–70 percent, and <50 percent, the risk for congestive heart failure in the donor was 100 percent, 70 percent, and 8 percent, respectively; the overall mortality is nevertheless around 50 percent. However, these data are not applicable in the first and early second trimesters, and although the disorder is asymptomatic at this early gestational age, the normal twin is likely to develop well-described complications later on, such as polyhydramnios and subsequent miscarriage or preterm delivery, heart failure, and intrauterine death or severe disability. Later in pregnancy, prenatal treatment has been attempted by serial amniodrainage or the administration of indomethacin to the mother[376,377] (see also chapter 2).

Invasive approaches have concentrated on occlusion of its umbilical cord. Endoscopic cord ligation[377] can be used. However, this has been recognized as a high risk factor for preterm prelabor rupture of the amniotic membranes.[378] Another technique for arresting flow in the umbilical cord vessels of the acardiac twin is endoscopic laser coagulation.[379] The main limitation of the technique seems to be the size and water content of the Wharton jelly to prevent laser coagulation after 20 weeks. Because of the failure of laser coagulation of the cord at later gestational ages, bipolar forceps have also been used successfully. Purpose-designed devices of ≤3 mm as well as adapted cannulas and trocars are available. These procedures can be performed with one port under ultrasound guidance within the sac of the target fetus and may require amnioinfusion to precede the procedure. In an initial series of ten cases, Deprest et al. reported that two patients had PPROM and underwent a termination. The other eight patients delivered at a mean gestational age of 35 weeks (i.e., more than 15 weeks after the procedure).[380] Nicolini et al.[381] reported on their experience in seventeen cases). The survival rate was 81 percent (thirteen of sixteen survivors; one patient underwent termination of pregnancy because of an abnormality diagnosed later on). There was one fetal hemorrhage because of cord perforation, which can occur if too much energy is applied. Monopolar coagulation, has also been used. At early gestational ages, the needle is inserted into the fetus, but later in gestation the umbilical cord is also targeted. Published experience so far includes eleven cases of TRAP sequence.[382] Two procedures failed at the first attempt (18 percent), but in both cases reintervention was successful. The total survival rate was 73 percent (eight of eleven). The risk of failure may be increased at later gestational ages.

Currently, it is not possible to say what the optimal method is for selective feticide in TRAP or in other discordant monochorionic pregnancies for fetal anomalies. Different techniques are applicable at different gestational ages and for different indications.

REFERENCES

1. Campbell S, Johnstone FD, Holt EM, et al. Anencephaly: Early ultrasonic diagnosis and active management. Lancet 1972;2:1226.
2. Royal College of Obstetricians and Gynaecologists Study Group. The antenatal diagnosis of fetal abnormalities. In: Drive GO, Donnai D, eds. Proceedings of the Eighteenth Study Group of the Royal College of Obstetricians and Gynaecologists. London: Springer Verlag, 1991.
3. Ewingman BG, Crane JP, Frigoletto FD, et al. Effect of prenatal ultrasound screening on perinatal outcome. N Engl J Med 1993;329:821.
4. Waldenstrom U, Axelsson O, Nilsson S, et al. Effects of routine one-stage ultrasound screening in pregnancy: a randomized controlled trial. Lancet 1988;8611:585.
5. Saari-Kempainen A, Karjalainen O, Ylostalo P, et al. Ultrasound screening and perinatal mortality: controlled trial of systematic one-stage screening in pregnancy. Lancet 1990;336:387.
6. Levi S, Crouzet P, Schaaps JP, et al. Ultrasound screening for fetal malformations. Lancet 1989;8639:678.
7. Chitty LS, Hunt GH, Moore J, et al. Effectiveness of routine ultrasonography in detecting fetal structural abnormalities in a low risk population. BMJ 1991;303:1165.
8. Shirley I, Bottomley F, Robinson VP, et al. Routine radiographer screening for fetal abnormalities by ultrasound in an unselected low-risk population. Br J Radiol 1992,65:564.
9. Alberman E. Epidemiology of neural tube defects. In: Jordan JA, Symonds EM, eds. The diagnosis and management of neural tube defects. London: Royal College of Obstetricians and Gynaecologists, 1978:1.

10. Holmes LB, Driscoll SG, Atkins L. Etiologic heterogeneity of neural tube defects. N Engl J Med 1976;294:365.

11. Nelson MD Jr, Bracchi N, Naidich TP, et al. The natural history of repaired myelomeningocele. Radiographics 1988;8:695.

12. Wald NJ, Bower C. Folic acid, pernicious anemia, and prevention of neural tube defects. Lancet 1994;343:307.

13. Lorber J. The prognosis of occipital encephalocele. Dev Med Child Neurol 1967;13:75.

14. Campbell S, Pryse-Davies J, Coltard TM, et al. Ultrasound in the diagnosis of spina bifida. Lancet 1975;1:1065.

15. Lorber J. Results of treatment of myelomeningocele: an analysis of 524 unselected cases, with special reference to possible selection for treatment. Dev Med Child Neurol 1971;13:279.

16. Nicolaides KH, Gabbe SG, Guidetti R, et al. Ultrasound screening for spina bifida: cranial and cerebellar signs. Lancet 1986;ii:72.

17. Nyberg DA, Mack LA, Hirch J, et al. Abnormalities of fetal cranial contour in sonographic detection of spina bifida: evaluation of the lemon sign. Radiology 1988;167:387.

18. Van den Hof MC, Nicolaides KH, Campbell J, et al. Evaluation of the lemon and banana signs in one hundred thirty fetuses with open spina bifida. Am J Obstet Gynecol 1990;162:322.

19. Tabor A, Madsen M, Obel EB, et al. Randomized controlled trial of genetic amniocentesis in 4604 low risk women. Lancet 1986;1:1287.

20. Michejda M. Antenatal treatment of neural tube defects In: Kurjak A, ed. The fetus as a patient. New York: Elsevier Science Publishers, 1985:131.

21. Stein SC, Feldman JG, Apjel S, et al. The epidemiology of congenital hydrocephalus: a study in Brooklyn NY, 1968 to 1976. Childs Brain 1981;8:253.

22. Burton BK. Recurrence risk of congenital hydrocephalus. Clin Genet 1979;16:47.

23. McCullough DC, Balzer-Martin LA. Current prognosis in overt neonatal hydrocephalus. J Neurosurg 1982;57:378.

24. Campbell S. Early prenatal diagnosis of neural tube defects by ultrasound. Clin Obstet Gynecol 1977;20:351.

25. Chervenak FA, Berkowitz RL, Tortora M, et al. The management of fetal hydrocephalus. Am J Obstet Gynecol 1985;151:933.

26. Cochrane DD, Myles ST, Nimrod C, et al. Intrauterine hydrocephalus and ventriculomegaly: associated abnormalities and fetal outcome. Can J Neurol Sci 1984;12:51.

27. Drugan A, Krause B, Canady A, et al. The natural history of prenatally diagnosed cerebral ventriculomegaly. JAMA 1989;261:1785.

28. Hudgins RJ, Edwards MSB, Goldstein R, et al. Natural history of fetal ventriculomegaly. Pediatrics 1988;82:692.

29. Nicolaides KH, Berry S, Snijders RJM, et al. Fetal lateral cerebral ventriculomegaly: associated malformations and chromosomal defects. Fetal Diagn Ther 1990;5:5.

30. Nyberg DA, Mack LA, Hirsch J, et al. Fetal hydrocephalus: sonographic detection and clinical significance of associated anomalies. Radiology 1987;163:187.

31. Pilu G, Rizzo N, Orsini LF, et al. Antenatal recognition of cerebral anomalies. Ultrasound Med Biol 1986;12:319.

32. Pretorius DH, Davis K, Manco-Johnson ML, et al. Clinical course of fetal hydrocephalus: 40 cases. AJR Am J Roentgenol 1985;144:827.

33. Serlo W, Kirkinen P, Jouppila P, et al. Prognostic signs of fetal hydrocephalus. Childs Nerv Syst 1986;2:93.

34. Vintzileos AM, Campbell WA, Weinbaum PJ, et al. Perinatal management and outcome of fetal ventriculomegaly. Obstet Gynecol 1987;69:5.

35. Michejda M, Hodgen GD. In utero diagnosis and treatment of non-human primate fetal skeletal anomalies. I. Hydrocephalus. JAMA 1981;246:1093.

36. Foltz EL, Shurtleff DB. Five year comparative study of hydrocephalus in children with and without operations (113 cases). J Neurosurg 1963;20:1064.

37. Clewell WH, Johnson ML, Meier PR. A surgical approach to the treatment of fetal hydrocephalus. N Engl J Med 1982;306:1320.

38. Saunders ES, Shortland D, Dunn PM. What is the incidence of holoprosencephaly? J Med Genet 1984;21:21.

39. Cohen MM. Perspectives on holoprosencephaly: Part I. Epidemiology, genetics and syndromology. Teratology 1989;40:211.

40. Berry SM, Gosden CM, Snijders RJM, et al. Fetal holoprosencephaly: associated malformations and chromosomal defects. Fetal Diagn Ther 1990;5:92.

41. Chervenak FA, Isaacson G, Hobbins JC, et al. Diagnosis and management of fetal holoprosencephaly. Obstet Gynecol 1985;66:322.

42. Filly RA, Chin DH, Callen PW. Alobar holoprosencephaly: ultrasonographic prenatal diagnosis. Radiology 1984;151:455.

43. Nyberg DA, Mack LA, Bronstein A, et al. Holoprosencephaly: prenatal sonographic diagnosis. AJR Am J Roentgenol 1987;149:1051.

44. Martin H. Microcephaly and mental retardation. Am J Dis Child 1970;119:128.

45. Campbell S, Thoms A. Ultrasound measurement of fetal head to abdomen circumference in the assessment of growth retardation. Br J Obstet Gynaecol 1977;84:165.

46. Gabrielli S, Reece AR, Pilu G, et al. The significance of prenatally diagnosed choroid plexus cysts. Am J Obstet Gynecol 1989;160:1207.

47. Murray J, Johnson J, Bird T. Dandy–Walker malformation: Etiologic heterogeneity and empiric recurrence. Clin Genet 1985;28:272.

48. Nyberg DA, Cyr DR, Mack LA, et al. The Dandy–Walker malformation: prenatal sonographic diagnosis and its clinical significance. J Ultrasound Med 1988;7:65.

49. Hoffman JIE, Christianson R. Congenital heart disease in a cohort of 19,502 births with long-term follow-up. Am J Cardiol 1978;42:641.

50. Nora JJ, Nora AH. The evolution of specific genetic and environmental counseling in congenital heart disease. Circulation 1978;57:205.

51. Whittemore R, Hobbins JC, Engle MA. Pregnancy and its outcome in women with and without surgical treatment of congenital heart disease. Am J Cardiol 1982;50:641.

52. Tegnander E, Eik-Ness SH, Johansen OJ, et al. Prenatal detection of heart defects at the routine fetal examination at 18 weeks in a non-selected population. Ultrasound Obstet Gynecol 1995;5:372.

53. Copel JA, Pilu G, Green J, et al. Fetal echocardiographic screening for congenital heart disease: the importance of the four chamber view. Am J Obstet Gynecol 1987;157:648.

54. Allan LD, Tynan MJ, Campbell S, et al. Echocardiographic and anatomical correlates in the fetus. Br Heart J 1980;44:444.

55. Kleinman CS, Donnerstein RL, Jaffe CC, et al. Fetal echocardiography: a tool for evaluation of in utero cardiac arrhythmias and monitoring of in utero therapy: analysis of 71 patients. Am J Cardiol 1983;51:237.

56. Stewart PA, Tonge HM, Wladimiroff JW. Arrhythmia and structural abnormalities of the fetal heart. Br Heart J 1983;50:550.

57. Allan LD, Chita SK, Al-Ghazali W, et al. Doppler echocardiographic evaluation of the normal fetal heart. Br Heart J 1987;57:528.

58. Kleinman C, Donnerstein R, DeVore G, et al. Fetal echocardiography for evaluation of in utero congestive heart failure. N Engl J Med 1982;306:568.

59. Wladimiroff JW, Stewart PA, Tonge HM. The role of diagnostic ultrasound in the study of fetal cardiac abnormalities. Ultrasound Med Biol 1984;10:457.

60. Crawford DC, Chita SK, Allan LD. Prenatal detection of congenital heart disease: factors affecting obstetric management and survival. Am J Obstet Gynecol 1988;159:352.

61. Stocker JT, Madewell JE, Drake RM. Congenital cystic malformation of the lung: classification and morphological spectrum. Hum Pathol 1977;8:155.

62. Adzick NS. The fetus with cystic adenomatoid malformation. In: Harrison MR, Golbus MS, Filly RA, eds. The unborn patient: prenatal diagnosis and treatment. Philadelphia: WB Saunders, 1991:320.

63. Nicolaides KH, Blott MJ, Greenough A. Chronic drainage of fetal pulmonary cyst. Lancet 1987;2:618.

64. Clark SL, Vitale DJ, Minton SD, et al. Successful fetal therapy for cystic adenomatoid malformation associated with second trimester hydrops. Am J Obstet Gynecol 1987;157:294.

65. Adzick NS, Harrison MR, Flake AW, et al. Fetal surgery for cystic adenomatoid malformation of the lung. J Pediatr Surg 1993;28:1411.

66. Harrison MR, Bjordal RI, Landmark F. Congenital diaphragmatic hernia: the hidden mortality. J Pediatr Surg 1979;13:227.

67. Puri P, Gorman F. Lethal nonpulmonary anomalies associated with congenital diaphragmatic hernia: implications for intrauterine surgery. J Pediatr Surg 1984;19:29.

68. Hansen J, Jones S, Burrington J, et al. The decreasing incidence of pneumothorax and improving survival in infants with congenital diaphragmatic hernia. J Pediatr Surg 1984;19:385.

69. Wiener ES. Congenital posterolateral diaphragmatic hernia: new dimensions in management. J Pediatr Surg 1982;12:149.

70. Marshall A, Sumner E. Improved prognosis in congenital diaphragmatic hernia: experience of 62 cases over 2 year period. J R Soc Med 1982;75:607.

71. Harrison MR, Bressack MA, Churg AM, et al. Correction of congenital diaphragmatic hernia in utero II. Simulated correction permits fetal lung growth with survival at birth. Surgery 1980;88:260.

72. Reid LM. Lung growth in health and disease. Br J Dis Chest 1984;78:105.

73. Harrison MR, Adzick NS, Longaker MT, et al. Successful repair in utero of a fetal diaphragmatic hernia after removal of herniated viscera from the left thorax. N Engl J Med 1990;322:1582.

74. Harrison MR, Adzick NS, Flake AW, et al. Correction of diaphragmatic hernia in utero. IV. Hard-earned lessons. J Pediatr Surg 1993;28:1411.

75. Harrison MR, Adzick NS, Flake AW, et al. The CDH two-step a dance of necessity. J Pediatr Surg 1993:28:813.

76. Harrison MR, Adzick NS, Flake AW, et al. Correction of congenital diaphragmatic hernia in utero. VIII. Response of hypoplastic lungs to tracheal occlusion. J Pediatr Surg 1996;31:1339.

77. Deprest J, Van Schoubroeck D, Lewi L, et al. Percutaneous fetoscopic endoluminal tracheal occlusion (FETO) for severe congenital diaphragmatic hernia. J Perinat Med 2003; suppl I.

78. Holzgreve W, Holzgreve B, Cruz JR. Non-immune hydrops fetalis: diagnosis and management. Semin Perinatol 1985;9:52.

79. Hutchison AA, Drew JH, Yu VYH, et al. Non-immunologic hydrops fetalis: a review of 61 cases. Obstet Gynecol 1982;59:347.

80. Keeling JW, Gough DJ, Iliff PJ. The pathology of non-rhesus hydrops. Diagn Histopathol 1983;6:89.

81. Warsoff SL, Nicolaides KH, Rodeck CH. Immune and non-immune hydrops. Clin Obstet Gynecol 1986;29:533.

82. Andersen HM, Drew JH, Beischer NA, et al. Non-immune hydrops fetalis: changing contribution to perinatal mortality. Br J Obstet Gynaecol 1983;90:636.

83. Platt LD, Collea JV, Joseph DM. Transitory fetal ascites: an ultrasound diagnosis. Am J Obstet Gynecol 1978;132:906.

84. Longaker MT, Laberge J-M, Dansereau J, et al. Primary fetal hydrothorax: natural history and management. J Pediatr Surg 1989;24:573.

85. Benacerraf BR, Frigoletto FD, Wilson M. Successful midtrimester thoracocentesis with analysis of the lymphocyte population in the pleural effusion. Am J Obstet Gynecol 1986;155:398.

86. Pijpers L, Reuss A, Stewart PA, et al. Noninvasive management of isolated bilateral fetal hydrothorax. Am J Obstet Gynecol 1989;161:330.

87. Landy HJ, Daly V, Heyl PS, et al. Fetal thoracocentesis with unsuccessful outcome. J Clin Ultrasound 1990;18:50.

88. Blott M, Nicolaides KH, Greenough A. Pleuroamniotic shunting for decompression of fetal pleural effusions. Obstet Gynecol 1988;71:798.

89. Rodeck CH, Fisk NM, Fraser DI, et al. Long-term in utero drainage of fetal hydrothorax. N Engl J Med 1988;319:1135.

90. Carpenter MW, Curci MR, Dibbens AW. Perinatal management of ventral wall defects. Obstet Gynecol 1984;64:646.

90a. Stoll C, Alembik Y, Dott B, et al. Risk factors in congenital abdominal wall defects (omphalocele and gastroschisis): a study in a series of 265,858 consecutive births. Ann Genet 2001;44:201.

91. Cantrell JR, Haller JA, Ravitch MM. A syndrome of congenital defects involving the abdominal wall, sternum, diaphragm, pericardium, and heart. Surg Gynecol Obstet 1958;27:602.

92. Li M, Squire JA, Weksberg R. Molecular genetics of Wiedemann–Beckwith syndrome. Am J Med Genet 1988;79:253.

92a. Kanagawa SL, Begleiter ML, Ostlie DJ, et al. Omphalocele in three generations with autosomal dominant transmission. J Med Genet 2002;39:184.

92b. Pryde PG, Greb A, Isada NB, et al. Familial omphalocele: considerations in genetic counseling. Am J Med Genet 1991;44:624.

93. Eggermann T, Zerres K, Eggermann K, et al. Uniparental disomy: clinical indications for testing in growth retardation. Eur J Pediatr 2002;161:305.

94. Grosfield JL, Dawes L, Weber TR. Congenital abdominal wall defects: current management and survival. Surg Clin North Am 1981;61:1037.

95. Hasan S, Hermansen MC. The prenatal diagnosis of ventral abdominal wall defects. Am J Obstet Gynecol 1986;155:842.

96. Kirk EP, Wah RM. Obstetric management of the fetus with omphalocele or gastroschisis. Am J Obstet Gynecol 1983;146:512.

97. Kohn MK, Shi EC. Gastroschisis and exomphalos: recent trends and factors influencing survival. Aust N Z J Surg 1990;60:199.

98. Lafferty PM, Emmerson HJ, Fleming PJ, et al. Anterior abdominal wall defects. Arch Dis Child 1989;64:1029.

99. Larsson LI, Kullendorff CM. Late surgical problems in children born with abdominal wall defects. Ann Chir Gynaecol 1990;79:23.

100. Mabo R, Mann L, Ferguson-Smith MA, et al. Prenatal assessment of anterior abdominal wall defects and their prognosis. Prenat Diagn 1984;4:427.

101. Mayer T, Black R, Matlak ME, et al. Gastroschisis and omphalocele: an eight year review. Ann Surg 1980;192:783.

102. Baird PA, MacDonald EC. An epidemiologic study of congenital malformations of the anterior abdominal wall in more than half a million consecutive live births. Am J Hum Genet 1981;33:470.

102a. Durfee SM, Downard CD, Benson CB, et al. Postnatal outcome of fetuses with the prenatal diagnosis of gastroschisis. J Ultrasound Med 2002;21:269.

102b. Martinez-Frias ML, Bermejo E, Rodriguez-Pinilla E, et al. Exstrophy of the cloaca and exstrophy of the bladder: two different expression of a primary developmental field defect. Am J Med Genet 2001;99:261.

103. Graivier L. Exstrophy of the cloaca. Am J Surg 1968;34:387.

104. Jeffs RD, Lepor H. Management of the exstrophy-epispadias complex and urachal anomalies. In: Walsh PC, ed. Campbell's urology, 5th ed. Philadelphia: WB Saunders, 1986:1882.

105. Shapiro E, Lepor H, Jeffs RD. The inheritance of the exstrophy epispadias complex. J Urol 1984;132:308.

106. Howell C, Caldamone A, Snyder H, et al. Optimal management of cloacal exstrophy. J Paediatr Surg 1983;18:365.

107. Manning FA. Ultrasound in prenatal diagnosis. In: Creasy RK, Resnik R, eds. Maternal fetal medicine: principles and practice. Philadelphia: WB Saunders, 1984:203.

108. Holder TM, Ashcraft KW. Developments in the care of patients with esophageal atresia and tracheoesophageal fistula. Surg Clin North Am 1981;61:1051.

108a. Celli J, van Beusekom E, Hennekam RC, et al. Familial syndromic esophageal atresia maps to 2p23–p24. Am J Hum Genet 2000;66:436.

109. German JC, Mahour GH, Wooley MM. Esophageal atresia and associated anomalies. J Pediatr Surg 1976;11:299.

110. Randolph JG, Altman RP, Anderson KD. Selective surgical management based upon the clinical status in infants with esophageal atresia. J Thorac Cardiovasc Surg 1977;74:335.

111. Farrant P. The antenatal detection of oesophageal atresia by ultrasound. Br J Radiol 1980;53:1202.

112. Zemlyn M. Prenatal detection of esophageal atresia. J Clin Ultrasound 1981;9:453.

113. Touloukian RJ. Intestinal atresia. Clin Perinatol 1978;5:3.

113a. Brantberg A, Blaas HG, Salvesen KA, et al. Fetal duodenal obstructions: increased risk of prenatal sudden death. Ultrasound Obstet Gynecol 2002;20:439.

113b. Bailey PV, Tracy TF Jr, Connors RH, et al. Congenital duodenal obstruction: a 32-year review. J Pediatr Surg 1993;28:92.

114. Zimmerman HB. Prenatal demonstration of gastric and duodenal obstruction by ultrasound. J Assoc Can Radiol 1978;29:138.

115. Dickson JAS. Apple peel small bowel: an uncommon variant of duodenal and jejunal atresia. J Pediatr Surg 1970;5:595.

116. Blumenthal DH, Rushovich AM, Williams RK, et al. Prenatal sonographic findings of meconium peritonitis with pathological correlations. J Clin Ultrasound 1982;10:350.

117. Stringer MD, Thornton JG, Mason GC. Hyperechogenic fetal bowel. Arch Dis Child 1996;74:F1.

117a. Simon-Bouy B, Muller F; French Collaborative Group. Hyperechogenic fetal bowel and Down syndrome: results of a French collaborative study based on 680 prospective cases. Prenat Diagn 2002;22:189.

118. Hill LM, Fries J, Hecker J, et al. Second trimester echogenic small bowel: an increased risk for perinatal outcome. Prenat Diagn 1994;14:845.

118a. Bosco AF, Norton ME, Lieberman E. Predicting the risk of cystic fibrosis with echogenic fetal bowel and one cystic fibrosis mutation. Obstet Gynecol 1999;94:1020.

118b. Lam YH, Tang MH, Lee CP, et al. Echogenic bowel in fetuses with homozygous alpha-thalassemia-1 in the first and second trimester. Ultrasound Obstet Gynecol 1999;14:180.

118c. Muller F, Simon-Bouy B, Girodon E, et al. Predicting the risk of cystic fibrosis with abnormal ultrasound sings of fetal bowel: results of a French molecular collaborative study based on 641 prospective cases. Am J Med Genet 2002;110:109.

118d. Al-Kouatly HB, Chasen St, Streltzoff J, et al. The clinical significance of fetal echogenic bowel. Am J Obstet Gynecol 2001;185;1035.

119. Schmidt W, Yarkoni S, Jeanty P, et al. Sonographic measurements of the fetal spleen: clinical implications. J Ultrasound Med 1985;4:667.

120. Vintzileos AM, Neckles S, Campbell WA, et al. Fetal ultrasound measurements during normal pregnancy. Obstet Gynecol 1985;66:477.

121. Yamaguchi M. Congenital choledochal cyst: analysis of 1,433 patients in the Japanese literature. Am J Surg 1980;140:653.

122. Elrad H, Mayden KL, Ahart S, et al. Prenatal ultrasound diagnosis of choledochal cyst. J Ultrasound Med 1985;4:553.

123. Carlson DH, Griscom NT. Ovarian cysts in the newborn. Am J Radiol 1972;116:664.

124. Davis GH, Wapner RJ, Kurtz AB, et al. Antenatal diagnosis of hydrometrocolpos by ultrasound examination. J Ultrasound Med 1984;3:371.

125. Kurtz RJ, Heimann TM, Holt J, et al. Mesenteric and retroperitoneal cysts. Ann Surg 1986;203:109.

126. Green JJ, Hobbins JC. Abdominal ultrasound examination of the first trimester fetus. Am J Obstet Gynecol 1988;159:165.

127. Grannum P, Bracken M, Silverman R, et al. Assessment of fetal kidney size in normal gestation by comparison of ratio of kidney circumference to abdominal circumference. Am J Obstet Gynecol 1980;136:249.

128. Campbell M. Embryology and anomalies of urogenital tract. In: Campbell M, ed. Clinical pediatric urology. Philadelphia: WB Saunders, 1951:169.

129. Crane JP. Renal abnormalities. In: Sabagha RE, ed. Diagnostic ultrasound applied to obstetrics and gynecology. Philadelphia: JB Lippincott, 1987:386.

130. Potter EL. Bilateral absence of ureters and kidneys: a report of 50 cases. Obstet Gynecol 1965;25:3.

131. Roodhooft AM, Birnholz JC, Holmes LB. Familial nature of congenital absence and severe dysgenesis of both kidneys. N Engl J Med 1984;310:1341.

132. Gray DL, Crane JP. Prenatal diagnosis of urinary tract malformation. Pediatr Nephrol 1988;2:326.

133. Romero R, Cullen M, Grannum P, et al. Antenatal diagnosis of renal anomalies with ultrasound. III. Bilateral renal agenesis. Am J Obstet Gynecol 1985;151:38.

134. Hill LM, Peterson CS. Antenatal diagnosis of fetal pelvic kidneys. J Ultrasound Med 1987;6:393.

135. Norio R, Nevanlinna HR, Perheentupa J. Hereditary diseases in Finland: rare flora in rare soil. Ann Clin Res 1973;5:109.

136. Blyth H, Ockenden BG. Polycystic disease of kidneys and liver presenting in childhood. J Med Genet 1971;8:257.

137. Romero R, Cullen M, Jeanty P, et al. The diagnosis of congenital renal anomalies with ultrasound. Am J Obstet Gynecol 1984;150:259.

138. Zerres K, Hansmann M, Mallman R, et al. Autosomal recessive polycystic kidney disease: problems of prenatal diagnosis. Prenat Diagn 1988;8:215.

139. Kleiner B, Filly RA, Mack L, et al. Multicystic dysplastic kidney: observations on the contralateral disease in the fetal population. Radiology 1986;161:27.

140. Hartnett M, Bennett W. Extrarenal manifestations of cystic kidney disease. In: Gardner KD, ed. Cystic diseases of the kidneys. New York: Wiley, 1976:201.

141. McHugo JM, Shafi MI, Rowlands D, et al. Prenatal diagnosis of adult polycystic kidney disease. Br J Radiol 1988;61:1072.

142. Pretorius DH, Lee ME, Manco-Johnson ML, et al. Diagnosis of autosomal dominant polycystic kidney disease in utero and in the young infant. J Ultrasound Med 1987;6:249.

143. Blane CE, Koff SA, Bowerman RA, et al. Nonobstructive hydronephrosis: Sonographic recognition and therapeutic implications. Radiology 1983;147:95.

144. Glazer GM, Filly RA, Callen PW. The varied sonographic appearance of the urinary tract in the fetus and newborn with urethral obstruction. Radiology 1982;144:563.

145. Grignon A, Filion R, Filiatrault D, et al. Urinary tract dilatation in utero: classification and clinical applications. Radiology 1986;160:645.

146. Mahony BS, Callen PW, Filly RA. Fetal urethral obstruction: US evaluation. Radiology 1985;157:221.

147. Mandell J, Blyth BR, Peters CA, et al. Structural genitourinary defects detected in utero. Radiology 1991;178,193.

148. Benacerraf BR, Mandell J, Estroff JA, et al. Fetal pyelectasis: a possible association with Down syndrome. Obstet Gynecol 1990;976:59.

149. Hoddick WK, Filly RA, Mahony BS, et al. Minimal fetal renal pyelectasis. J Ultrasound Med 1985;4:85.

150. Kleiner B, Callen PW, Filly RA. Sonographic analysis of the fetus with ureteropelvic junction obstruction. AJR Am J Roentgenol 1987;148:359.

151. Thomas DFM. Urological diagnosis in utero. Arch Dis Child 1984;59:913.

152. Caione P, Zaccara A, Capozza N, et al. How prenatal ultrasound can affect the treatment of ureterocele in neonates and children. Eur Urol 1989;16:195.

153. King LR. Posterior urethra. In: Kelalis PP, King LR, Belman AB, eds. Clinical pediatric urology. Philadelphia: WB Saunders, 1985:527.

154. Reuss A, Wladimiroff JW, Niermeijer MF. Antenatal diagnosis of renal tract anomalies by ultrasound. Pediatr Nephrol 1987;1:546.

155. Vintzileos AM, Eisenfeld LI, Herson VC, et al. Megacystis–microcolon–intestinal hypoperistalsis syndrome: prenatal sonographic findings and review of the literature. Am J Perinatol 1986;3:297.

156. Beck AD. The effect of intrauterine urinary obstruction upon the development of the fetal kidney. J Urol 1971;105:784.

157. Harrison MR, Ross N, Noall R, et al. Correction of congenital hydronephrosis in utero. I. The model: fetal urethral obstruction produces hydronephrosis and pulmonary hypoplasia in fetal lambs. J Pediatr Surg 1983;18:247.

158. Nakayama DK, Glick PL, Harrison MR, et al. Experimental pulmonary hypoplasia due to oligohydramnios and its reversal by relieving thoracic compression. J Pediatr Surg 1983;18:347.

159. Glick PL, Harrison MR, Noall RA, et al. Correction of congenital hydronephrosis in utero. III. Early midtrimester ureteral obstruction produces renal dysplasia. J Pediatr Surg 1983;18:681.

160. Harrison MR, Golbus MS, Filly RA, et al. Fetal surgery for congenital hydronephrosis. N Engl J Med 1982;54:32.

161. Berkowitz RL, Glickmann MG, Smith GJW, et al. Fetal urinary tract obstruction: what is the role of surgical intervention in utero? Am J Obstet Gynecol 1982;144:367.

162. Rodeck CH, Nicolaides KH. Ultrasound guided invasive procedures in obstetrics. Clin Obstet Gynaecol 1983:10:515.

163. Nakayama DK, Harrison MR, deLorimer AA. Prognosis of posterior urethral valves presenting at birth. J Pediatr Surg 1986;21:43.

164. Reuss A, Wladimiroff JW, Stewart PA, et al. Non-invasive management of fetal obstructive uropathy. Lancet 1988;2:949.

165. Elder JS, Duckett JW, Snyder HM. Intervention for fetal obstructive uropathy: has it been effective? Lancet 1987;2:1007.

166. Quintero RA, Hume R, Smith C, et al. Percutaneous fetal cystoscopy and endoscopic fulguration of posterior urethral valves. Am J Obstet Gynecol 1995;172:206.

167. Elder JS, O'Grady JP, Ashmead G, et al. Evaluation of fetal renal function: unreliability of fetal urinary electrolytes. J Urol 1990;144:574.

168. Nicolaides KH, Cheng HH, Snijders RS, et al. Fetal urine biochemistry in the assessment of obstructive uropathy. Am J Obstet Gynecol 1992,166:932.

169. Johnson MP, Bukowski TP, Reitleman C, et al. In utero surgical treatment of fetal obstructive uropathy: a new comprehensive approach to identify appropriate candidates for vesicoamniotic shunt therapy. Am J Obstet Gynecol 1994;170:1770.

170. Jones KL. Smith's recognizable patterns of human malformation. 4th ed. London: WB Saunders, 1988.

171. Stevenson RE, Hall JG, Goodman RM. Human malformations and related anomalies. New York: Oxford University Press, 1993.

172. Jeanty P, Kirkpatrick C, Dramaix-Wilmet M, et al. Ultrasonic evaluation of fetal limb growth. Part I. Radiology 1981;140:165.

173. Jeanty P, Dramaix-Wilmet M, van Kertem J, et al. Ultrasonic evaluation of fetal limb growth: Part II. Radiology 1982;143:751.

174. Rumack CM, Johnson ML, Zunkel D. Antenatal diagnosis of osteogenesis imperfecta. Clin Diagn Ultrasound 1981;8:210.

175. Chamberlain PF, Manning FA, Morrison I, et al. Ultrasound evaluation of amniotic fluid volume. II. The relationship of increased amniotic fluid volume to perinatal outcome. Am J Obstet Gynecol 1984;150:250.

176. Barkin SZ, Pretorius DH, Becket MK, et al. Severe polyhydramnios: Incidence of anomalies. Am J Radiol 1987;148:155.

177. Hill LM, Breckle R, Thomas M, et al. Polyhydramnios: ultrasonically detected prevalence and neonatal outcome. Obstet Gynecol 1987;69:21.

178. Cabrol D, Landesman R, Muller, et al. Treatment of polyhydramnios with prostaglandin synthetase inhibitor (indomethacin). Am J Obstet Gynecol 1987;157:422.

179. Bilardo CM, Nicolaides KH, Campbell S. Doppler measurements of fetal and uteroplacental circulations: relationship with umbilical venous blood gases measured at cordocentesis. Am J Obstet Gynecol 1990;162:115.

180. Nicolaides KH, Azar G, Byrne D, et al. Fetal nuchal translucency: Ultrasound screening for chromosomal defects in first trimester of pregnancy. BMJ 1992;304:867.

181. Wilkins-Haug L, Freedman W. Progression of exencephaly to anencephaly in the human fetus: an ultrasound perspective. Prenat Diagn 1991;11:227.

182. Green JJ, Hobbins JC. Abdominal ultrasound examination of the first trimester fetus. Am J Obstet Gynecol 1988;159:165.

183. Johnson SP, Sebire NJ, Snijders RJM, et al. Ultrasound screening for anencephaly at 10–14 weeks of gestation. Ultrasound Obstet Gynecol 1997;9:16.

184. Hyett JA, Moscoso G, Papanagiotou G, et al. Abnormalities of the heart and great arteries in first trimester chromosomally normal fetuses with increased nuchal translucency thickness at 11–13 weeks of gestation. Ultrasound Obstet Gynecol 1996;7;245.

185. Noscos G, Nicolaides K. First trimester nuchal translucency and cardiac septal defects in fetuses with trisomy 21. Am J Obstet Gynecol 1995;172:1911.

186. Achiron R, Rotstein Z, Lipitz S, et al. First-trimester diagnosis of fetal congenital heart disease by transvaginal ultrasonography. Obstet Gynecol 1994;84:69.

187. Gembruch U, Knopfle G, Bald R, et al. Early diagnosis of fetal congenital heart disease by transvaginal echocardiography. Ultrasound Obstet Gynecol 1993;3:310.

188. Snijders RJ, Sebire NJ, Souka A, et al. Fetal exomphalos and chromosomal defects: relationship to maternal age and gestation. Ultrasound Obstet Gynecol 1995;6:250.

189. Braithwaite JM, Armstrong MA, Economides DL. Assessment of fetal anatomy at 12 to 13 weeks of gestation by transabdominal and transvaginal sonography. Br J Obstet Gynaecol 1996;103:82.

190. Sebire NJ, Von Kaisenberg C, Rubio C, et al. Fetal megacystis at 10–14 weeks of gestation. Ultrasound Obstet Gynecol 1996;8:387.

191. Ville Y. Nuchal translucency in the first trimester of pregnancy: ten years on and still a pain in the neck? Ultrasound Obstet Gynecol 2001,18:5.

192. Hyett J, Noble P, Sebire NJ, et al. Lethal congenital arthrogryposis presents with increased nuchal translucency at 10–14 weeks of gestation. Ultrasound Obstet Gynecol 1997;9:310.

193. Dumez Y, Oury JF, Duchatel F. Embryoscopy and congenital malformations. In: Proceedings of the international conference on chorionic villus sampling and early prenatal diagnosis. Athens: International Meeting on CVS. Xxxxxx: Xxxxx, 1988.

194. Pennouhat GH, Thebault Y, Ville Y, et al. First trimester transabdominal fetoscopy. Lancet 1992;340:429.

195. Ville Y, Bernard JP, Doumerc S, et al. Transabdominal fetoscopy in fetal anomalies diagnosed by ultrasound in the first trimester of pregnancy. Ultrasound Obstet Gynecol 1996;8:11.

196. Snijders RJM, Nicolaides KH. Assessment of risks. In: Xxxxx XX, ed. Ultrasound markers for fetal chromosomal defects. Carnforth, UK: Parthenon Publishing, 1996:63.

197. Down LJ. Observations on an ethnic classification of idiots. London: London Hospital, 1866;3:259.

198. Nicolaides KH, Azar G, Byrne D, et al. Fetal nuchal translucency: ultrasound screening for chromosomal defects in first trimester of pregnancy. BMJ 1992;304:867.

199. Nicolaides KH. Screening for chromosomal defects. Ultrasound Obstet Gynecol 2003,4:313.

200. Snijders RJM, Noble P, Sebire N, et al. UK multicentre project on assessment of risk of trisomy 21 by maternal age and fetal nuchal translucency thickness at 10–14 weeks of gestation. Lancet 1998;351:343.

200a. Pandya PP, Snijders RJ, Johnson SP, et al. Screening for fetal trisomies by maternal age and fetal nuchal translucency thickness at 10 to 14 weeks of gestation. Br J Obstet Gynaecol 1995;102:957.

200b. Szabo J, Gellen J, Szemere G. First-trimester ultrasound screening for fetal aneuploidies in women over 35 and under 35 years of age. Ultrasound Obstet Gynecol 1995;5:161.

201. Taipale P, Hiilesmaa V, Salonen R, et al. Increased nuchal translucency as a marker for fetal chromosomal defects. N Engl J Med 1997;337:1654.

202. Hafner E, Schuchter K, Liebhart E, et al. Results of routine fetal nuchal translucency measurement at 10–13 weeks in 4,233 unselected pregnant women. Prenat Diagn 1998;18:29.

203. Pajkrt E, van Lith JMM, Mol BWJ, et al. Screening for Down's syndrome by fetal nuchal translucency measurement in a general obstetric population. Ultrasound Obstet Gynecol 1998;12:163.

204. Economides DL, Whitlow BJ, Kadir R, et al. First trimester sonographic detection of chromosomal abnormalities in an unselected population. Br J Obstet Gynaecol 1998; 105:58.

205. Schwarzler P, Carvalho JS, Senat MV, et al. Screening for fetal aneuploidies and fetal cardiac abnormalities by nuchal translucency thickness measurement at 10–14 weeks of gestation as part of routine antenatal care in an unselected population. Br J Obstet Gynaecol 1999;106:1029.

206. Theodoropoulos P, Lolis D, Papageorgiou C, et al. Evaluation of first-trimester screening by fetal nuchal translucency and maternal age. Prenat Diagn 1998;18:133.

207. Zoppi MA, Ibba RM, Floris M, et al. Fetal nuchal translucency screening in 12 495 pregnancies in Sardinia. Ultrasound Obstet Gynecol 2001; 18: 649.

207a. Zoppi MA, Ibba RM, Putzolu M, et al. Assessment of risk for chromosomal abnormalities at 10–14 weeks of gestation by nuchal translucency and maternal age in 5,210 fetuses at a single centre. Fetal Diagn Ther 2000;15:170.

208. Gasiorek-Wiens A, Tercanli S, Kozlowski P, et al. Screening for trisomy 21 by fetal nuchal translucency and maternal age: a multicenter project in Germany, Austria and Switzerland. Ultrasound Obstet Gynecol 2001;18:645.

209. Brizot ML, Carvalho MHB, Liao AW, et al. First-trimester screening for chromosomal abnormalities by fetal nuchal translucency in a Brazilian population. Ultrasound Obstet Gynecol 2001;18:652.

210. Audibert F, Dommergues M, Benattar C, et al. Screening for Down syndrome using first-trimester ultrasound and second-trimester maternal serum markers in a low-risk population: a prospective longitudinal study. Ultrasound Obstet Gynecol 2001;18:26.

211. Wayda K, Kereszturi A, Orvos H, et al. Four years experience of first-trimester nuchal translucency screening for fetal aneuploidies with increasing regional availability. Acta Obstet Gynecol Scand 2001;80:1104.

212. Brizot ML, Snijders RJM, Bersinger NA, et al. Maternal serum pregnancy associated placental protein A and fetal nuchal translucency thickness for the prediction of fetal trisomies in early pregnancy. Obstet Gynecol 1994;84:918.

213. Brizot ML, Snijders RJM, Butler J, et al. Maternal serum hCG and fetal nuchal translucency thickness for the prediction of fetal trisomies in the first trimester of pregnancy. Br J Obstet Gynaecol 1995;102:1227.

214. Spencer K, Souter V, Tul N, et al. A screening program for trisomy 21 at 10–14 weeks using fetal nuchal translucency, maternal serum free β-human chorionic gonadotropin and pregnancy associated plasma protein-A. Ultrasound Obstet Gynecol 1999;13:231.

215. Snijders RJM, Noble P, Sebire N, et al. UK multicentre project on assessment of risk for trisomy 21 by maternal age and fetal nuchal translucency thickness at 10–14 weeks of gestation. Lancet 1999;18:519.

216. Wald NJ, Kennard A, Hackshaw A, et al. Antenatal screening for Down's syndrome. Health Technol Assess 1998;2:1.

217. Bird LM, Dixson B, Masser-Frye D, et al. Choroid plexus cysts in the mid-trimester fetus-practical application suggests superiority of an individualized risk method of counseling for trisomy 18. Prenat Diagn 2002;22:792.

218. Spencer K, Spencer CE, Power M, et al. One stop clinic for assessment of risk for fetal anomalies: a report of the first year of prospective screening for chromosomal anomalies in the first trimester. Br J Obstet Gynaecol 2000;107:1271.

219. Cicero S, Curcio P, Papageorghiou A, et al. Absence of nasal bone in fetuses with trisomy 21 at 11–14 weeks of gestation: an observational study. Lancet 2001:358:1665.

220. Nyberg DA, Souter VL, El-Bastawissi A, et al. Isolated sonographic markers for detection of fetal Down syndrome in the second trimester of pregnancy. J Ultrasound Med 2001;20:1053.

221. Bromley B, Lieberman E, Shipp TD, et al. The genetic sonogram: a method of risk assessment for Down syndrome in the second trimester. J Ultrasound Med 2002;21:1087.

222. Prefumo F, Presti F, Thilaganathan B, et al. Association between increased nuchal translucency and second trimester cardiac echogenic foci. Obstet Gynecol 2003;101:899.

222a. Smith-Bindman R, Hosmer W, Feldstein VA, et al. Second-trimester ultrasound to detect fetuses with Down syndrome. JAMA 2001;285:1044.

223. Rizzo N, Pitalis MC, Pilu G, et al. Prenatal karyotyping in malformed fetuses. Prenat Diagn 1990;10:17.

224. Bromley B, Frigoletto FD, Benacerraf BR. Mild fetal lateral cerebral ventriculomegaly: clinical course and outcome. Am J Obstet Gynecol 1991;164:863.

225. Anhoury P, Andre M, Droulle P, et al. Dilatation des ventricules cerebraux decouverte in utero: a propos de 85 cas. J Gynecol Obstet Biol Reprod 1991;20:191.

226. Blumfield CG, Davis RO, Hauth JC, et al. Management of prenatally detected nonlethal fetal anomalies: is a karyotype of benefit? Am J Obstet Perinatol 1991;8:255.

227. Nicolaides KH, Snijders RJM, Gosden CM, et al. Ultrasound markers of chromosomal abnormalities. Lancet 1992;340:704.

228. Holzgreve W, Feiel R, Louwen F, et al. Prenatal diagnosis and management of fetal hydrocephaly and lissencephaly. Child Nerv Syst 1993;9:408.

229. Hsieh FJ, Ko TM, Tseng LH, et al. Prenatal cytogenetic diagnosis in amniocentesis. J Formos Med Assoc 1992;91:276.

230. Wilson RD, Chitayat D, McGillivray BC. Fetal ultrasound abnormalities: correlation with fetal karyotype, autopsy findings, and postnatal outcome: five-year prospective study. Am J Med Genet 1992;44:586.

231. Eydoux P, Choiset A, Le Porrier N, et al. Chromosomal prenatal diagnosis: study of 936 cases of intrauterine abnormalities after ultrasound assessment. Prenat Diagn 1989;9:255.

231a. Den Hollander NS, Wessels MW, Los FJ, et al. Congenital microcephaly detected by prenatal ultrasound: genetic aspects and clinical significance. Ultrasound Obstet Gynecol 2000;15:282.

232. Nicolaides KH, Rodeck CH, Gosden CM. Rapid karyotyping in non-lethal fetal malformations. Lancet 1986;i:283.

233. Ricketts NEM, Lowe EM, Patel NB. Prenatal diagnosis of choroid plexus cysts. Lancet 1987;1:213.

234. Chitkara U, Cogswell C, Norton K, et al. Choroid plexus cysts in the fetus: a benign anatomic variant or pathologic entity? Report of 41 cases and review of the literature. Obstet Gynecol 1989;72:185.

235. Clark SL, DeVore GR, Sabey PL. Prenatal diagnosis of the fetal choroid plexus. Obstet Gynecol 1989;72:585.

236. Daniel A, Athayde N, Ogle R, et al. Prospective ranking of the sonographic markers for aneuploidy: data of 2143 prenatal cytogenetic diagnoses referred for abnormalities on ultrasound. Aust N Z J Obstet Gynaecol 2003;43:16.

237. DeRoo TR, Harris RD, Sargent SK, et al. Fetal choroid plexus cysts: prevalence, clinical significance and sonographic appearance. AJR Am J Roentgenol 1988;151:1179.

238. Chan L, Hixson JL, Laifer SA, et al. A sonographic and karyotypic study of second trimester fetal choroid plexus cysts. Obstet Gynecol 1989;73:703.

239. Hertzberg BS, Kay HH, Bowie JD. Fetal choroid plexus lesions: relationship of antenatal sonographic appearance to clinical outcome. J Ultrasound Med 1989;8:77.

240. Ostlere SJ, Irving HC, Lilford RJ. A prospective study of the incidence and significance of fetal choroid plexus cysts. Prenat Diagn 1989;9:205.

241. Thorpe-Beeston JG, Gosden CM, Nicolaides KH. Choroid plexus cysts and chromosomal defects. Br J Radiol 1990;63:783.

241a. Achiron R, Barkai G, Katznelson MBN, et al. Fetal lateral ventricle choroid plexus cysts: The dilemma of amniocentesis. Obstet Gynecol 1991;78:815.

242. Chinn DH, Miller EI, Worthy LM, et al. Sonographically detected fetal choroid plexus cysts: frequency and association with aneuploidy. J Ultrasound Med 1991;10:255.

243. Platt LD, Carlson DE, Medearis AL, et al. Fetal choroid plexus cysts in the second trimester of pregnancy: a cause of concern. Am J Obstet Gynecol 1991;164:1652.

244. Twining P, Zuccollo J, Clewes J, et al. Fetal choroid plexus cysts: a prospective study and review of the literature. Br J Radiol 1991b;64:98.

245. Zerres K, Schuler H, Gembruch U, et al. Chromosomal findings in fetuses with prenatally diagnosed cysts of the choroid plexus. Hum Genet 1992;89:301.

246. Nadel AS, Bromley BS, Frigoletto FD Jr, et al. Isolated choroid plexus cysts in the second-trimester fetus: Is amniocentesis really indicated? Radiology 1992;185:545.

247. Perpignano MC, Cohen HL, Klein VR, et al. Fetal choroid plexus cysts: beware the smaller cyst. Radiology 1992;182:715.

248. Howard RJ, Tuck SM, Long J, et al. The significance of choroid plexus cysts in fetuses at 18–20 weeks: an indication for amniocentesis? Prenat Diagn 1992;12:685.

249. Oettinger M, Odeh M, Korenblum R, et al. Antenatal diagnosis of choroid plexus cyst: suggested management. Obstet Gynecol Surv 1993;48:635.

250. Porto M, Murata Y, Warneke LA, et al. Fetal choroid plexus cysts: an independent risk factor for chromosomal anomalies. J Clin Ultrasound 1993;21:103.

251. Nava S, Godmilow L, Reeser S, et al. Significance of sonographically detected second trimester choroid plexus cysts: a series of 211 cases and a review of the literature. Ultrasound Obstet Gynecol 1994;4:448.

252. Snijders RJM, Shawwa L, Nicolaides KH. Fetal choroid plexus cysts and trisomy 18: assessment of risk based on ultrasound findings and maternal age. Prenat Diagn 1994;14:1119.

253. Walkinshaw S, Pilling D, Spriggs A. Isolated choroid plexus cysts: the need for routine offer of karyotyping. Prenat Diagn 1994;14:663.

253a. Yoder PR, Sabbacha RE, Gross SJ, et al. The second-trimester fetus with isolated choroid plexus cysts: a meta-analysis of risk of trisomies 18 and 21. Obstet Gynecol 1999;93:869.

253b. Demasio K, Canterino J, Ananth C, et al. Isolated choroid plexus cyst in low-risk women less than 35 years old. Am J Obstet Gynecol 2002;187:1246.

253c. DeVore GR. Second trimester ultrasonography may identify 77 to 97% of fetuses with trisomy 18. J Ultrasound Med 2000;19:565.

254. Comstock C, Culp D, Gonzalez J, et al. Agenesis of the corpus callosum in the fetus: Its evolution and significance. J Ultrasound Med 1985;4:613.

255. Lockwood CJ, Ghidini A, Aggarwal R, et al. Antenatal diagnosis of partial agenesis of the corpus callosum: a benign cause of ventriculomegaly. Am J Obstet Gynecol 1988;159:184.

256. Vergani P, Ghidini A, Strobelt N, et al. Prognostic indicators in the prenatal diagnosis of agenesis of corpus callosum. Am J Obstet Gynecol 1994;170:753.

257. Bahado-Singh RO, Wyse L, Dorr MA, et al. Fetuses with Down syndrome have disproportionately shortened frontal lobe dimensions on ultrasonogram examination. Am J Obstet Gynecol 1992:167:1009.

258. Watson WJ, Katz VL, Chescheir NC, et al. The cisterna magna in second-trimester fetuses with abnormal karyotypes. Obstet Gynecol 1992;79:723.

259. Estroff JA, Scott MR, Benacerraf BR. Dandy–Walker variant: prenatal sonographic features and clinical outcome. Radiology 1992;185:755.

260. Nicolaides KH, Salvesen D, Snijders RJM, et al. Strawberry shaped skull: associated malformations and chromosomal defects. Fetal Diagn Ther 1992;7:132.

261. Shah YG, Eckl CJ, Stinson SK, et al. Biparietal diameter/femur length ratio, cephalic index, and femur length measurements: not reliable screening techniques for Down syndrome. Obstet Gynecol 1990;75:186.

262. Pashayan HM. What else to look for in a child born with a cleft of the lip or palate. Cleft Palate J 1983;20:54.

263. Saltzman DH, Benacerraf BR, Frigoletto FD. Diagnosis and management of fetal facial clefts. Am J Obstet Gynecol 1986;155:377.

264. Hsieh FJ, Lee CN, Wu CC, et al. Antenatal ultrasonic findings of craniofacial malformations. J Formos Med Assoc 1991;90:551.

265. Benacerraf BR, Muliken JB. Fetal cleft lip and palate: sonographic diagnosis and postnatal outcome. Plast Reconstr Surg 1993;92:1045.

266. Nicolaides KH, Salvesen D, Snijders RJM, et al. Facial defects: associated malformations and chromosomal defects. Fetal Diagn Ther 1993,8:1.

267. Turner GM, Twining P. The facial profile in the diagnosis of fetal abnormalities. Clin Radiol 1993;47:389.

268. Bronshtein M, Blumenfeld I, Kohn J, et al. Detection of cleft lip by early second-trimester transvaginal sonography. Obstet Gynecol 1994;84:73.

269. Benacerraf BR, Frigoletto FD, Green MF. Abnormal facial features and extremities in human trisomy syndromes: prenatal US appearance. Radiology 1986;159:243.

270. Birnholz JC, Farrell EE. Fetal ear length. Pediatrics 1988;81:555.

271. Lettieri L, Rodis JF, Vintzileos AM, et al. Ear length in second-trimester aneuploid fetuses. Obstet Gynecol 1993;81:57.

272. Azar G, Snijders RJM, Gosden CM, et al. Fetal nuchal cystic hygromata: associated malformations and chromosomal defects. Fetal Diagn Ther 1991;6:46.

273. Byrne J, Blanc W, Warburton D, et al. The significance of cystic hygroma in fetuses. Hum Pathol 1984;15:61.

274. Chervenak FA, Isaacson G, Blakemore KJ, et al. Fetal cystic hygroma: cause and natural history. N Engl J Med 1983;309:822.

275. Newman DE, Cooperberg PI. Genetics of sonographically detected intrauterine fetal cystic hygromas. Can Med Assoc J 1984;35:77.

276. Redford DHA, Mcnay MB, Fergusson-Smith ME, et al. Aneuploidy and cystic hygroma detectable by ultrasound. Prenat Diagn 1984;4:377.

277. Marchese C, Savin E, Dragone E, et al. Cystic hygroma: prenatal diagnosis and genetic counseling. Prenat Diagn 1985;5:221.

278. Pearce MJ, Griffin D, Campbell S. The differential prenatal diagnosis of cystic hygromata and encephalocele by ultrasound examination. J Clin Ultrasound 1985;13:317.

279. Nicolaides KH, Rodeck CH, Lange I, et al. Fetoscopy in the assessment of unexplained fetal hydrops. Br J Obstet Gynaecol 1985;92:671.

280. Carr RF, Ochs RH, Ritter DA, et al. Fetal cystic hygroma and Turner's syndrome. Am J Dis Child 1986;140:580.

281. Palmer CG, Miles JH, Howard-Peebles PN, et al. Fetal karyotype following ascertainment of fetal anomalies by ultrasound. Prenat Diagn 1987;7:551.

282. Hegge FN, Prescott GH, Watson PT. Sonography at the time of genetic amniocentesis to screen for fetal malformations. Obstet Gynecol 1988;71:522.

283. Abramowicz JS, Warsof SL, Doyle DL, et al. Congenital cystic hygroma of the neck diagnosed prenatally: outcome with normal and abnormal karyotype. Prenat Diagn 1989;9:321.

284. Miyabara S, Sugihara H, Maehara N, et al. Significance of cardiovascular malformations in cystic hygroma: a new interpretation of the pathogenesis. Am J Med Genet 1989;34:489.

285. Tannirandorn Y, Nicolini U, Nicolaidis P, et al. Fetal cystic hygromata: insights gained from fetal blood sampling. Prenat Diagn 1990;10:189.

286. MacLeod AM, McHugo MB. Prenatal diagnosis of nuchal cystic hygroma. Br J Radiol 1991;64:802.

287. Bernard P, Chabaud JJ, Le Guern H, et al. Hygroma kystiques du cou: diagnostic antenatal, facteurs pronostiques, conduite a tenir: a propos de 42 cas. J Gynecol Obstet Biol Reprod 1991;20:487.

288. Gagnon S, Fraser W, Fouquette B, et al. Nature and frequency of chromosomal abnormalities in pregnancies with abnormal ultrasound findings: an analysis of 117 cases with review of the literature. Prenat Diagn 1992;12:9.

289. Ville Y, Borghi E, Pons JC, et al. Fetal karyotype from cystic hygroma fluid. Prenat Diagn 1992;12:139.

289a. Gallagher PG, Mahoney MJ, Gosche JR. Cystic hygroma in the fetus and newborn. Semin Perinatol 1999;23:341.

289b. Fujita Y, Satoh S, Nakayama H, et al. In utero evaluation and the long-term prognosis of living infants with cystic hygroma. Fetal Diagn Ther 2001;16:402.

290. Benacerraf BR, Barss VA, Laboda LA. A sonographic sign for the detection in the second trimester of the fetus with Down's syndrome. Am J Obstet Gynecol 1985;151:1078.

291. Benacerraf BR, Gelman R, Frigoletto FD. Sonographic identification of second trimester fetuses with Down's syndrome. N Engl J Med 1987;317:1371.

292. Lynch L, Berkowitz GS, Chitkara U, et al. Ultrasound detection of Down syndrome: is it really possible? Obstet Gynecol 1989;73:267.

293. Perella R, Duerinckx AJ, Grant EG, et al. Second trimester sonographic diagnosis of Down syndrome: role of femur length shortening and nuchal-fold thickening. AJR Am J Roentgenol 1988;151:981.

294. Nyberg DA, Mack LA, Hirsch J, et al. Fetal hydrocephalus: sonographic detection and clinical significance of associated anomalies. Radiology 1987;163:187.

294a. Hobbins JC, Lezotte DC, Persutte WH, et al. An 8-center study to evaluate the utility of mid-term genetic sonograms among high-risk pregnancies. J Ultrasound Med 2003;22:33.

295. Nicolaides KH, Azar G, Snijders RJM, et al. Fetal nuchal edema: associated malformations and chromosomal defects. Fetal Diagn Ther 1992;7:123.

296. Toi A, Simpson GF, Filly RA. Ultrasonically evident fetal nuchal skin thickening: is it specific for Down syndrome? Am J Obstet Gynecol 1987;156:150.

297. Crane J, Gray D. Sonographically measured nuchal skinfold thickness as a screening tool for Down syndrome: results of a prospective clinical trial. Obstet Gynecol 1991;77:553.

298. Kirk JS, Comstock CH, Fassnacht MA, et al. Routine measurement of nuchal thickness in the second trimester. J Matern Fetal Med 1992;1:82.

299. Benacerraf BR, Laboda LA, Frigoletto FD. Thickened nuchal fold in fetuses not at risk for aneuploidy. Radiology 1992;184:239.

300. DeVore GR, Alfi O. The association between an abnormal nuchal skin fold, trisomy 21 and ultrasound abnormalities identified during the second trimester of pregnancy. Ultrasound Obstet Gynecol 1993;3:387.

301. Donnenfeld AE, Carlson DE, Palomaki GE, et al. Prospective multicenter study of second-trimester nuchal skinfold thickness in unaffected and Down syndrome pregnancies. Obstet Gynecol 1994;84:844.

302. Watson WJ, Miller RC, Menard MK, et al. Ultrasonographic measurement of fetal nuchal skin to screen for chromosomal abnormalities. Am J Obstet Gynecol 1994;170:583.

303. Jauniaux E, Maldergem LV, Munter CD, et al. Nonimmune hydrops fetalis associated with genetic abnormalities. Obstet Gynecol 1990;75:568.

303a. Rodriguez MM, Chaves F, Romanguera RL, et al. Value of autopsy in nonimmune hydrops fetalis: series of 51 stillborn fetuses. Pediatr Dev Pathol 2002;5:365.

304. Benacerraf BR, Adzick NS. Fetal diaphragmatic hernia: Ultrasound diagnosis and clinical outcome in 19 cases. Am J Obstet Gynecol 1987;156:573.

305. Thorpe-Beeston G, Gosden CM, Nicolaides KH. Congenital diaphragmatic hernia: associated malformations and chromosomal defects. Fetal Ther 1989;4:21.

306. Sharland GK, Lockhart SM, Heward AJ, et al. Prognosis in fetal diaphragmatic hernia. Am J Obstet Gynecol 1992;166:9.

307. Witters I, Legius E, Moerman P, et al. Associated malformations and chromosomal anomalies in 42 cases of prenatally diagnosed diaphragmatic hernia. Am J Med Genet 2001;103:278.

307a. Dillon E, Renwick M, Wright C. Congenital diaphragmatic herniation: antenatal detection and outcome. Br J Radiol 2000;73:360.

308. Allan LD, Sharland GK, Chita SK, et al. Chromosomal anomalies in fetal congenital heart disease. Ultrasound Obstet Gynecol 1991;1:8.

309. Blake DM, Copel JA, Kleinman CS. Hypoplastic left heart syndrome: prenatal diagnosis, clinical profile, and management. Am J Obstet Gynecol 1991;165:529.

310. Smythe JF, Copel JA, Kleinman CS. Outcome of prenatally detected cardiac malformations. Am J Cardiol 1992;69:1471.

311. Paladini D, Calabro R, Palmieri S, et al. Prenatal diagnosis of congenital heart disease and fetal karyotyping. Obstet Gynecol 1993;81:679.

312. Sotiriadis A, Makrydimas G, Ionnidis JP. Diagnostic performance of intracardiac echogenic foci for Down syndrome: a meta-analysis. Obstet Gynecol 2003;101:1009.

313. How HY, Villafane J, Parihus RR, et al. Small hyperechoic foci of the fetal cardiac ventricle: a benign sonographic finding? Ultrasound Obstet Gynecol 1994;4:205.

314. Brown DL, Roberts DJ, Miller WA. Left ventricular echogenic focus in the fetal heart: pathologic correlation. J Ultrasound Med 1994;13:613.

315. Louhimo I, Lindahl H. Esophageal atresia: primary results of 500 consecutively treated patients. J Pediatr Surg 1983;18:217.

316. Nicolaides KH, Snijders RJM, Cheng H, et al. Fetal abdominal wall and gastrointestinal tract defects: associated malformations and chromosomal defects. Fetal Diagn Ther 1992;7:102.

317. Bromley B, Doubilet P, Frigoletto FD, et al. Is fetal hyperechoic bowel on second-trimester sonogram an indication for amniocentesis? Obstet Gynecol 1994;83:647.

318. Dicke JM, Crane JP. Sonographically detected fetal bowel: significance and implications for pregnancy management. Obstet Gynecol 1992;80:778.

319. Scioscia AL, Pretorius DH, Budorick NE, et al. Second trimester echogenic bowel and chromosomal abnormalities. Am J Obstet Gynecol 1992;167:889.

320. Nyberg DA, Dubinsky TD, Resta RG, et al. Echogenic fetal bowel during the second trimester: clinical importance. Radiology 1993;188:527.

321. Nakayama DK, Harrison MK, Gross BH, et al. Management of the fetus with an abdominal wall defect. J Pediatr Surg 1984;19:408.

322. Gilbert WM, Nicolaides KH. Fetal omphalocele: associated malformations and chromosomal defects. Obstet Gynecol 1987;70:633.

323. Sermer M, Benzie RJ, Pitson L, et al. Prenatal diagnosis and management of congenital defects of the anterior abdominal wall. Am J Obstet Gynecol 1987;156:308.

324. Hughes M, Nyberg DH, Mack LH, et al. Fetal omphalocele: prenatal US detection of concurrent anomalies and other predictors of outcome. Radiology 1989;173:371.

325. Nyberg DA, Fitzsimmons J, Mack LH, et al. Chromosomal abnormalities in fetuses with omphalocele: significance of omphalocele contents. J Ultrasound Med 1989;8:299.

326. Benacerraf BR, Saltzman DH, Estroff JH, et al. Abnormal karyotype of fetuses with omphalocele: prediction based on omphalocele contents. Obstet Gynecol 1990;75:317.

327. Holzgreve W, Miny P, Gerlach B, et al. Benefits of placental biopsies for rapid karyotyping in the second and third trimesters (late chorionic villus sampling) in high-risk pregnancies. Am J Obstet Gynecol 1990;162:1188.

328. Getachew MM, Goldstein RB, Edge V, et al. Correlation between omphalocele contents and karyotypic abnormalities: sonographic study in 37 cases. Am J Roentgenol 1991;158:133.

329. Rezai K, Holzgreve W, Schloo R, et al. Pranatale chromosomenbefunde bei sonographisch auffalligen feten. Geburtshilfe Frauenheilkd 1991;51:211.

330. Van Geijn EJ, van Vugt, Sollie JE, et al. Ultrasonographic diagnosis and perinatal management of fetal abdominal wall defects. Fetal Diagn Ther 1991;6:2.

331. Sotiriadis A, Makrydimas G, Ionnidis JP. Diagnostic performance of intracardiac echogenic foci for Down syndrome: a meta-analysis. Obstet Gynecol 2003;101:1009.

332. Morrow RJ, Whittle MJ, McNay MB, et al. Prenatal diagnosis and management of anterior abdominal wall defects in the west of Scotland. Prenat Diagn 1993;13:111.

333. Corteville JE, Dicke JM, Crane JP. Fetal pyelectasis and Down syndrome: is genetic amniocentesis warranted? Obstet Gynecol 1992;79:770.

334. Blumfield CG, Davis RO, Joseph DB, et al. Fetal obstructive uropathies: importance of chromosomal abnormalities and associated anomalies to perinatal outcome. J Reprod Med 1991;36:662.

335. Stoll C, Alembik Y, Roth MP, et al. Risk factors in internal urinary system malformations. Pediatr Nephrol 1990;4:319.

336. Shah DM, Roussis P, Ulm J, et al. Cordocentesis for rapid karyotyping. Am J Obstet Gynecol 1990b;162:1548.

337. Benacerraf BR, Mandell J, Estroff JA, et al. Fetal pyelectasis: a possible association with Down syndrome. Obstet Gynecol 1990;76:58.

338. Reuss A, Wladimiroff JW, Stewart PA, et al. Non-invasive management of fetal obstructive uropathy. Lancet 1988;ii:949.

338a. Oliveira EA, Cabral AC, Pereira AK, et al. Outcome of fetal urinary tract anomalies associated with multiple malformations and chromosomal abnormalities. Prenat Diagn 2001;21:129.

339. Nicolaides KH, Cheng H, Snijders RJM, et al. Fetal renal defects: associated malformations and chromosomal defects. Fetal Diagn Ther 1992;7:1.

340. Kovac CM, Brown JA, Apodaca CC, et al. Maternal ethnicity and variation of fetal femur length calculations when screening for Down syndrome. J Ultrasound Med 2002;21:719.

341. LaFollette L, Filly RA, Anderson R, et al. Fetal femur length to detect trisomy 21: a reappraisal. J Ultrasound Med 1989;8:657.

342. Twining P, Whalley DR, Lewin E, et al. Is a short femur length a useful ultrasound marker for Down's syndrome? Br J Radiol 1991;64:990.

343. FitzSimmons J, Droste S, Shepard TH, et al. Long bone growth in fetuses with Down syndrome. Am J Obstet Gynecol 1989;161:1174.

344. Biagiotti R, Periti E, Cariati E. Humerus and femur length in fetuses with Down syndrome. Prenat Diagn 1994;14:429.

345. Benacerraf BR, Neuberg D, Frigoletto FD. Humeral shortening in second trimester fetuses with Down syndrome. Obstet Gynecol 1991;77:223.

346. Rotmensch S, Luo JS, Liberati M, et al. Fetal humeral length to detect Down syndrome. Am J Obstet Gynecol 1992;166:1330.

347. Rodis JF, Vintzileos AM, Fleming AD, et al. Comparison of humerus length with femur length in fetuses with Down syndrome. Am J Obstet Gynecol 1991;165:1051.

348. Jeanty P, Romero R, d'Alton M, et al. In utero sonographic detection of hand and foot deformities. J Ultrasound Med 1985;4:595.

349. Benacerraf BR. Antenatal sonographic diagnosis of congenital clubfoot: a possible indication for amniocentesis. J Clin Ultrasound 1986;14:703.

350. Ounsted M, Moar V, Scott A. Perinatal morbidity and mortality in small-for-dates babies: the relative importance of some maternal factors. Early Hum Dev 1981;5:367.

351. Khoury MJ, Erickson JD, Cordero JF, et al. Congenital malformations and intrauterine growth retardation: a population study. Pediatrics 1988;82:163.

352. Chen ATL, Chan YK, Falek A. The effects of chromosomal abnormalities on birth weight in man. Hum Hered 1972:209.

353. Snijders RJM, Sherrod C, Gosden CM, et al. Severe fetal growth retardation: associated malformations and chromosomal abnormalities. Fetal Diagn Ther 1993;168:547.

354. Benirschke K, Kim CK. Multiple pregnancy. N Engl J Med 1973,288:1276.

355. Bessis R, Papiernik E. Echographic imagery of amniotic membranes in twin pregnancies. In: Gedda L, Parisi P, eds. Twin research 3: twin biology and multiple pregnancy. New York: Alan R. Liss, 1990:183.

356. Sebire NJ, Snijders RJ, Hughes K, et al. The hidden mortality of monochorionic twin pregnancies. Br J Obstet Gyn1ecol 1997;104:1203.

357. Sebire NJ, Snijders RJM, Hughes K, et al. Screening for trisomy 21 in twin pregnancies by maternal age and fetal nuchal translucency thickness at 10–14 weeks of gestation. Br J Obstet Gynaecol 1996;103:999.

358. Sebire NJ, Noble PL, Psarra A, et al. Fetal karyotyping in twin pregnancies: selection of technique by measurement of fetal nuchal translucency. Br J Obstet Gynaecol 1996;103:887.

359. Weir PE, Ratten GJ, Beischer NA. Acute polyhydramnios: a complication of monozygous twin pregnancy. Br J Obstet Gynaecol 1979;86:849.

360. Larroche JC, Droulle P, Delezoide AL, et al. Brain damage in monozygous twins. Biol Neonate 1990;57:261.

361. Gonsoulin W, Moise KJ Jr, Kirshon B, et al. Outcome of twin-twin transfusion diagnosed before 28 weeks of gestation. Obstet Gynecol 1990;75:214.

362. Saunders NJ, Snijders RJM, Nicolaides KH. Therapeutic amniocentesis in twin–twin transfusion syndrome appearing in the second trimester of pregnancy. Am J Obstet Gynecol 1992;166:820.

363. Machin GA, Still K. The twin-twin transfusion syndrome: vascular anatomy of monochorionic placentas and their clinical outcomes. In: Keith LG, Papiernik E, Keith DM, et al., eds. Multiple pregnancy: epidemiology, gestation and perinatal outcome. New York: Parthenon, 1995:367.

364. Pinette MG, Pan Y, Pinette SG, et al. Treatment of twin-twin transfusion syndrome. Obstet Gynecol 1993;82:841.
365. Bajoria R, Wigglesworth J, Fisk NM. Angioarchitecture of monochorionic placentas in relation to the twin-twin transfusion syndrome. Am J Obstet Gynecol 1995;172:856.
366. Trespidi L, Boschetto C, Caravelli E, et al. Serial amniocentesis in the management of twin-twin transfusion syndrome: when is it valuable? Fetal Diagn Ther 1997;12:15.
367. De Lia JE, Cruikshank DP, Keye WR Jr. Fetoscopic neodymium:YAG laser occlusion of placental vessels in severe twin-twin transfusion syndrome. Obstet Gynecol 1990;75:1046.
367a. Ropacka M, Markwitz W, Blickstein I. Treatment options for the twin-twin transfusion syndrome: a review. Twin Res 2002;5:507.
368. Ville Y, Hecher K, Ogg D, et al. Successful outcome after Nd:YAG laser separation of chorioangiopagus-twins under sonoendoscopic control. Ultrasound Obstet Gynecol 1992;2:429.
369. Ville Y, Hyett J, Hecher K, et al. Preliminary experience with endoscopic laser surgery for severe twin-twin transfusion syndrome. N Engl J Med 1995;332:224.
370. Mahony BS, Petty CN, Nyberg DA, et al. The stuck twin phenomenon: ultrasonographic findings, pregnancy outcome and management with serial amniocentesis. Am J Obstet Gynecol 1990;163:1513.
370a. DeLia JE, Kuhlmann RS, Harstad TW, et al. Fetoscopic laser ablation of placental vessels in severe previable twin-twin transfusion syndrome. Am J Obstet Gynecol 1995;172:1202.
371. Urig MA, Clewell WH, Elliott JP. Twin–twin transfusion syndrome. Am J Obstet Gynecol 1990;163:1522.
372. Elliott JP, Urig MA, Clewell WH. Aggressive therapeutic amniocentesis for treatment of twin–twin transfusion syndrome. Obstet Gynecol 1991;77:537.
373. Reisner DP, Mahony BS, Petty CN, et al. Stuck twin syndrome: outcome in thirty-seven consecutive cases. Am J Obstet Gynecol 1993;169:991.
373a. Quintero RA, Dickinson JE, Morales WJ, et al. Stage-based treatment of twin–twin transfusion syndrome. Am J Obstet Gynecol 2003;188:1333.
374. Ville Y. Data presented at the 19th meeting of the International Fetal Medicine and Surgery Society, 27–30 April 2003, Zermatt, Switzerland. 2003.
375. Van Allen MI, Smith DW, Shepard TH. Twin reversed arterial perfusion sequence: study of 14 pregnancies with acardius. Semin Perinatol 1983;7:285.
376. Moore TR, Gale S, Benirshke G. Perinatal outcome of forty-nine pregnancies complicated by acardiac twining. Am J Obstet Gynecol 1990;163:907.
377. Ash K, Harman CR, Gritter H. TRAP sequence, successful outcome with indomethacin treatment. Obstet Gynecol 1990;76:960.
378. Deprest JA, Evrard VA, Van Schouebroeck D, et al. Endoscopic cord ligation in selective feticide. Lancet 1996;348:890.
379. Ville Y, Hyett J, Vandenbussche FPA, et al. Endoscopic laser coagulation of umbilical cord vessels in twin reversed arterial perfusion sequence. Ultrasound Obstet Gynecol 1994;4:396.
380. Deprest J, Audibert F, Van Schoubroeck D, et al. Bipolar cord coagulation of the umbilical cord in complicated monochorionic twin pregnancy. Am J Obstet Gynecol 2000; 182:340.
381. Nicolini U, Poblete A, Boschetto C, et al. Complicated monochorionic twin pregnancies: experience with bipolar cord coagulation. Am J Obstet Gynecol 2000; 185:703.
382. Holmes A, Jauniaux E, Rodeck C. Monopolar thermocoagulation in acardiac twinning. Br J Obstet Gynaecol 2001;108:1000.

J. W. Wladimiroff, M.D., Ph.D., F.R.C.O.G.   # 24

Prenatal Diagnosis and Management of Abnormal Fetal Development in the Third Trimester of Pregnancy

This chapter focuses on the impact of diagnostic ultrasound on third-trimester pregnancies. Inevitably, a choice had to be made. Most of third-trimester pathology relates to intrauterine growth restriction (IUGR), premature labor due to premature rupture of membranes with associated risk of lethal fetal pulmonary hypoplasia, and fetal congenital malformations. Ultrasound technology is still improving, with three-dimensional, and in the near future four-dimensional, ultrasound (including movements of the fetus) being applied in obstetric care. On the other hand, magnetic resonance imaging (MRI) is becoming increasingly helpful in identifying the exact nature of a range of fetal abnormalities (see chapter 25). Diagnostic ultrasound is instrumental in the safe performance of a range of invasive procedures from chorionic villus sampling (CVS) and amniocentesis to fetal invasive therapy and surgery; the latter is still in its infancy. Doppler technology plays a major part in our understanding of fetal circulatory redistribution in fetal growth restriction, in which ductus venosus velocity waveform changes are closely associated with less-favorable fetal outcomes. Other pathologic disorders include nonimmune fetal hydrops and twin-to-twin transfusion syndrome. Diagnosis, prognosis, and management of the most prevalent malformations will be presented, with emphasis on fetal heart, diaphragm, renal outflow tract, and central nervous system. These aspects of third-trimester ultrasonography will be highlighted in this chapter.

INVASIVE DIAGNOSTIC PROCEDURES

Traditional third-trimester invasive diagnostic procedures are represented by amniocentesis, late placental biopsy, and in some instances cordocentesis. Other procedures include fetal skin sampling for the antenatal diagnosis of inherited skin diseases. Third-trimester amniocentesis is mainly performed for fetal karyotyping. Rapid aneuploidy detection can now be achieved through nonradioactive (e.g., fluorescence) in-situ hybridization (FISH), which allows the detection of specific DNA sequences in morphologically preserved chromosomes, cells, and tissues[1–3] (see chapter 8). FISH permits the rapid (2 days) detection of the most common aneuploidies (13, 18, 21, X, and Y), which comprise most of the chromosomal aberrations causing birth defects in liveborn infants. This greatly contributes to the efficiency of counseling couples about the obstetric management in case of a sonographically established fetal anomaly.[1] FISH as a stand-alone technique requires smaller amounts of amniotic fluid (AF) than for classic cytogenetic analysis.[2] With the introduction of comparative genomic hybridization techniques it has become possible to perform cytogenetic studies in fetal material following fetal death and detect small deletions at both central and telomere level.[4]

Cordocentesis allows direct access to fetal blood and the circulation. This has lead to valuable information on fetal oxygenation, fetal erythrocyte isoimmunization, alloimmune thrombocytopenia, intrauterine fetal infection, coagulation factor deficiencies, hemoglobinopathies, immunologic deficiencies, nonimmune hydrops fetalis, and diagnosis of twin-to-twin transfusion syndrome. Cordocentesis also permits rapid (48–72 hr) fetal karyotyping. The procedure may cause complications, especially when performed in high-risk pregnancies, with reported rates ranging from 0.6 to 2.8 percent[5] (see chapter 2). Direct fetal blood analysis in erythrocyte isoimmunization demonstrated a correlation between fetal bilirubin levels and fetal hemolytic disease. The addition of fetal bilirubin for anemia risk assessment was therefore advocated.[6] A promising noninvasive technique is the Doppler recording of peak-systolic velocities in the fetal middle cerebral artery, which are raised in fetal anemia.[7,8]

Human parvovirus B19 causes fetal nonimmune hydrops and death. This virus can be detected in fetal blood by the polymerase chain reaction (PCR) technique.[9] Intravascular transfusion therapy in these fetuses suffering from anemia has been shown to be effective. Cordocentesis also has been instrumental in providing information on fetal biochemistry and acid–base status in the presence of uteroplacental insufficiency. Measurement of hemoglobin, lactate concentration, oxygen content, pH, and blood gas levels is helpful in determining which fetuses are hypoxic and acidemic.[10] IUGR is associated with markedly lower concentrations of most amino acids, notably the branched-chain amino acids.[11] Cordocentesis is an essential part of the diagnostic workup in nonimmune hydrops. Umbilical venous pressure measurements are used to establish the underlying cause of fetal hydrops. Elevated venous pressure is associated with increased cardiothoracic ratios.[12] Platelet transfusions under ultrasound guidance have been successful in the antenatal management of fetal thrombocytopenia.[13] Other invasive sampling methods include fetal skin biopsy through fetoscopy.[14] Risks of fetoscopy include leakage of AF via the vagina, infection, prematurity, and maternal, fetal, and placental injuries. A limited number of skin disorders with an autosomal dominant (e.g., bullous congenital ichthyosiform erythroderma) or autosomal recessive inheritance pattern (harlequin ichthyosis, Sjögren–Larsson syndrome, epidermolysis bullosa lethalis, epidermolysis bullosa dystrophica, anhidrotic ectodermal dysplasia, and nonbullous ichthyosiform erythroderma) have been diagnosed. With the rapid advances in DNA analysis, it is likely that more skin disorders will become detectable.

THE SMALL-FOR-GESTATIONAL-AGE FETUS

Regulation of fetal growth starts before pregnancy.[15] IUGR leading to the fetus becoming small for gestation represents a heterogeneous group of conditions that results in the failure of the fetus to achieve its genetic potential for growth before birth.[16] Newborns with a low birth weight for gestational age are at great risk for fetal distress,[17] impaired neurologic development,[18] and diabetes and hypertension in adult life.[19]

Detection of the small-for-gestational-age (SGA) fetus is based on sonographic measurement of the fetal upper abdominal circumference, provided that menstrual dates are certain, or early sonographic determination from fetal crown-rump length or fetal biparietal diameter for fetal dating has been made. The fetal upper abdominal circumference is the best single antenatal predictor of fetal weight.[20] A proportion of SGA fetuses will be small as a consequence of chromosomal disorders, structural abnormalities, or infectious disorders. A detailed anomaly scan is, therefore, one of the first steps in the diagnostic process.[20]

Causes and Associated Factors

A high prevalence of maternal thrombophilia has been demonstrated in IUGR due to utero-placental insufficiency with raised frequencies for factor V Leiden mutation, prothrombin gene mutation, and protein S mutation.[21] SGA is associated not only with pregnancy-induced hypertension or chronic renal disease but also with a range of other abnormal situations or conditions, such as maternal smoking, use of illegal drugs (e.g., cocaine, heroin, or marijuana), placental mosaicism, and certain fetal structural anomalies. The third trimester of pregnancy is a critical time of exposure to maternal smoking.[22] Long-term effects of smoking during pregnancy have been highlighted in a study of IUGR in smokers,[23] demonstrating impaired neurologic development at 12–16 months after allowing for the effect of gestational age at delivery, birth weight, social factors, and oxygenation at cordocentesis.

CONFINED PLACENTAL MOSAICISM

After the introduction of CVS, it became evident that approximately 1–2 percent of diploid fetuses are supported by placentas with a different and often mosaic chromosomal constitution.[24] This confined placental mosaicism (CPM) may give rise to an increased incidence of IUGR[25] and fetal loss,[26] although this association has not been confirmed in other series.[27] It has been postulated that one of the reasons for the adverse pregnancy outcome is a failure of placental function resulting from a high proportion of poorly functioning trisomic cells in the placenta.[24] Specific chromosomes, presumably those carrying imprinted growth-related or placental function genes, may be implicated in impaired pregnancy progress in the event of imbalance.[25] Particularly, chromosomes 7[28] and 4[29] are involved in fetal development. One of the mechanisms responsible for adverse pregnancy outcome in cases of CPM may be uniparental disomy.[30] This involves the presence of a chromosome pair derived solely from one parent in a diploid offspring. Particularly, maternal uniparental disomy for chromosome 16 has been associated with severe IUGR.[31]

Maternal Drug Dependency and Fetal Development

The use of illicit drugs by pregnant women is still increasing, with an estimated 5 million women of childbearing age using these drugs on a regular basis.[32] The impact of these substances on infants is considerable. Cocaine and heroin are the most frequently used drugs. Exposure to cocaine during the period of organogenesis can result in major structural malformations such as defects of the central nervous system,[33] cardiovascular defects,[34] and renal[35] as well as skeletal defects,[36,37] the latter resulting from vascular insults or interruptions at specific critical periods during development. The possible significance of such claims must be considered against the confounding environmental effects, multiple-drug use with synergistic/additive effects, family history, maternal illnesses, and genetic predisposition. Maternal drug use has also been associated with a raised incidence of premature labor and reduced fetal birth weight.[38] Cocaine produces a vasoconstriction in the uterine and placental vasculature as a result of cocaine's ability to increase blood catecholamine levels and the sensitivity of the uterine vasculature to norepinephrine and epinephrine.[39] Other maternal dependencies include alcohol abuse resulting in the fetal alcohol syndrome and other alcohol effects in children characterized by compromised growth, health, and behavioral and cognitive ability.[40,41]

Fetal Blood Sampling

Data from direct sampling of fetal blood by cordocentesis or from the umbilical cord at delivery have greatly enhanced our understanding of a range of factors playing a part in normal and abnormal fetal growth. For instance, epidermal growth factor may have an important role in placental growth and function.[42] Raised fetal adenosine as well as leptin concentrations have been established in the umbilical vein of SGA fetuses.[43,44] Because an inverse relationship exists between adenosine concentrations and fetal breathing movements, elevated adenosine levels may be associated with reduced oxygen consumption. Higher levels of atrial natriuretic factor (ANF) have been demonstrated in SGA fetuses, probably in response to atrial distention from increased placental vascular resistance or hypoxic heart failure.[45] Also, raised levels of vasoactive intestinal protein (VIP) have been reported in SGA fetuses.[46] The same authors showed a significant correlation between fetal arterial Doppler measurements and VIP levels, particularly the cerebral arterial circulation. Insulin growth factor is raised in the SGA fetus, which may indicate a terminal process in the fetal adaptation to placental failure.[47]

Management of the SGA Fetus

Identification of a subset of SGA fetuses at risk of increased mortality or morbidity remains a substantial challenge in daily obstetric care. Sonographic assessment of AF volume, placental maturity, and fetal weight in a low-risk antenatal population at 30–32 and 36–37 weeks of gestation may reduce the risk of a growth-restricted infant, but it does not affect the rate of admission to a neonatal unit.[48] Studies of SGA fetuses and their outcome are now dominated by Doppler measurements.[49] Uterine artery Doppler measurements have been advocated mainly as a predictor of preeclampsia and IUGR during the second trimester of pregnancy. However, also in growth-restricted fetuses delivered at 34 weeks or later, the presence of uterine artery Doppler waveforms is associated with a fourfold increased risk of adverse neonatal outcome.[50] The most characteristic changes occur in the umbilical artery and descending aorta with a reduction or even loss or reversal of end-diastolic velocities reflecting increased fetoplacental downstream impedance.[51,52] As a result, Doppler resistance indices such as the pulsatility index and resistance index are raised. Abnormal umbilical artery flow velocities are nearly always associated with high lactate levels, hypoxemia, hypercapnia, and even acidemia.[53,54] As the index rises, both the severity of the growth restriction and fetal hypoxemia increase.[18] However, no index changes were found in the fetal renal arteries.[55] Examination of cardiac and venous blood flow in association with arterial blood flow redistribution in advanced hypoxemia and acidemia add to the process of Doppler fetal surveillance.[56] It has been demonstrated that similar to observations in fetal lambs, fetal SGA may be associated not only with sparing of the brain[57] but also with a decrease in vascular resistance and increase in blood flow to the adrenal gland[58] and coronary arteries.[59] Resistance indices in the peripheral pulmonary arteries are raised in SGA fetuses, probably because of hypoxemic pulmonary vasoconstriction[60] and secondary morphologic alterations of the vessel wall with thickening of the muscular component of peripheral lung vessels.[61] Increased resistance has been established in the fetal mesenteric artery, which may be a late sign of fetal hemodynamic redistribution and is frequently related to necrotizing enterocolitis in the newborn.[62]

At the cardiac level, increased right ventricular afterload as a result of high impedance to flow in the fetoplacental arteries is associated with reduced left ventricular afterload due to cardiac and cerebral vasodilatation. This leads to redistribution of cardiac output in favor of the left ventricle.[63] With advancing fetal hypoxemia, combined cardiac output will decrease,[64] which is also suggested by reduced flow velocities in the cardiac outflow tract.[52] This process of myocardial dysfunction is reflected in changes on the venous side of the circulation.[65] The raised right ventricular afterload, right ventricular end-diastolic pressure, and central venous pressure will lead to a reduction in forward flow to the right atrium, as shown by Doppler studies on the venous side of the fetal circulation.[54,66] Initially, increased late diastolic reverse flow coincident with atrial contraction can be observed. With progressing fetal compromise, this extends to other venous vessels, such as the ductus venosus and umbilical vein, the latter transforming from a flat into a pulsatile flow pattern.[67] Abnormal venous flow patterns are almost always associated with a combination of fetal hypoxemia and acidemia.[54,66] Changes in diastolic ductus venosus flow velocities and a double pulsation in the umbilical vein are closely related to perinatal mortality.[68]

Surveillance of the SGA fetus by Doppler sonography is based on the detection of a progressive decline of the fetal condition. The Doppler changes presented here reflect arterial impedance changes expressing centralization of the fetal circulation with brain, adrenal and coronary "sparing" as an adaptive mechanism. Earlier studies suggest that routine use of umbilical artery velocimetry has no effect on gestational age at delivery, the rates of either induction of labor or cesarean section, neonatal care, or medium-care admissions.[69] Major differences regarding study design makes a simple meta-analysis a dubious undertaking.[70] In the presence of hemodynamic redistribution and a nonreassuring, nonreactive, nonstress test, Doppler assessment of the ductus venosus correlates with adverse perinatal outcome. In this clinical situation, there is no benefit of the contraction stress test in terms of prediction.[71] In another study, ductus venosus pulsatile index and short-term variation in fetal heart rate were shown to be important indicators for the optimal timing of delivery before 32 weeks of gestation.[72]

The further improvement in high-resolution ultrasound equipment has created renewed interest in fetal volume flow measurements. Barbera et al.[73] found a good correlation between sonographic volume measurements in the human umbilical vein and venous volume measurements in the fetal lamb. In our center, a tenfold increase in umbilical venous volume flow, but a significant reduction in umbilical venous volume flow when standardized for fetal weight was found in normal human pregnancies during the second half of gestation[74] (Figures 24.1 and 24.2). Reduced (≥ 2 SD) umbilical venous volume flow was established in the vast majority of a subset of growth-restricted fetuses with a birth weight below the fifth centile for weight of gestation[74] (Figures 24.1 and 24.2). In the presence of fetal growth restriction, an inverse relationship was found between brain to liver volume ratio as measured by three-dimensional ultrasound and umbilical venous volume flow standardized for fetal weight.[75] Volume flow measurements in the umbilical vein and ductus venosus reveal that in the human fetus, the averaged fraction shunted through the ductus venosus was 28–32 percent at 18–20 weeks and decreased to 22 percent at 25 weeks

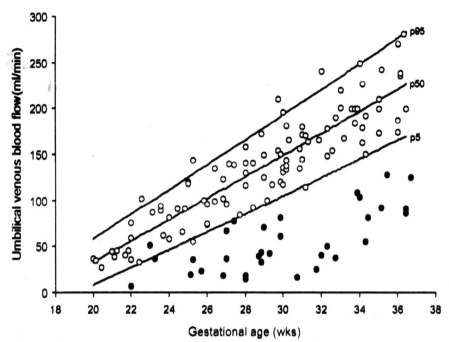

Fig. 24.1. Umbilical venous volume flow (ml/min) during the second half of pregnancy. The open circles represent normal fetal development; the closed circles represent fetal growth restriction. *Source:* Boito et al., 2002.[74] Reproduced by permission of *Ultrasound Obstetrics and Gynecology.*

and to 18 percent at 31 weeks of gestation.[76] It was suggested that in the human fetus a higher proportion of umbilical blood is directed to the liver and less shunted through the ductus venosus than was previously established in animal experimental work.[76] Also, in the fetal descending aorta reduced volume has been documented in the presence of IUGR.[77]

INSULIN-DEPENDENT DIABETES MELLITUS

Sonographic examination of the patient with insulin-dependent diabetes mellitus (IDDM) comprises a detailed fetal anomaly scan to rule out fetal abnormalities, a fetal biometry scan to establish fetal growth and size, and assessment of the amount of AF. Congenital malformations account for 30–60 percent of the perinatal mortality in diabetic pregnancy. Strict metabolic control starting before conception resulted in a decrease in the rate of malformations in these infants, the frequency being 0.8 percent, as opposed to 7.5 percent when strict metabolic control was initiated after the 8th week of pregnancy.[78] The teratogenic effect that diabetes obviously has early in gestation focuses on the fetal cardiovascular, skeletal, urogenital, and neural tube systems. Serial measurements of fetal upper abdominal circumference should lead to early detection of macrosomia, which is associated with increased rates of cesarean section and perinatal mortality and morbidity. Management based on maternal glycemic criteria has been compared with management based on relaxed glycemic criteria and fetal upper abdominal circumference measurements in order to select women for insulin treatment of gestational diabetes mellitus with fasting hyperglycemia. The latter management strategy identified pregnancies at low risk for macrosomia and resulted in the avoidance of insulin therapy in 38 percent of women without increasing rates

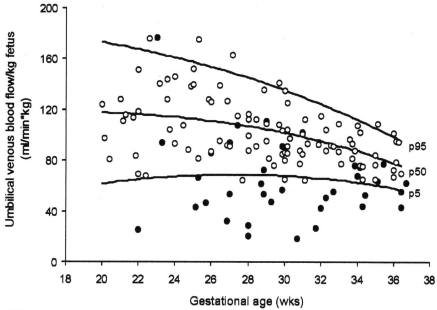

Fig. 24.2. Umbilical venous volume flow standardized for fetal weight (ml/min/kg) during the second half of pregnancy. The open circles represent normal fetal development; the closed circles represent fetal growth restriction (<5th centile). The umbilical artery pulsatility index was significantly raised in the subset of growth-restricted fetuses with flow volume data below the normal range. *Source:* Boito et al., 2002.[74] Reproduced by permission of *Ultrasound Obstetrics and Gynecology.*

of neonatal morbidity.[79] Another report demonstrated that a fetal upper abdominal circumference measurement at 28 weeks of gestation was needed to direct metabolic therapy because insulin administration introduced after 32 weeks had a poor effect on fetal growth.[80] Sonographic measurement of the fetal upper abdominal circumference was considered less useful by Landon,[81] who pointed out the limitations and potential inaccuracy of current sonographic methods to detect the large-for-gestational-age fetus of a diabetic mother.

AMNIOTIC FLUID VOLUME

AF is essential for the normal development of the fetal respiratory, gastrointestinal, and urinary tracts; the musculoskeletal system; and fetal growth.[82] Various processes contribute to the formation and removal of AF (i.e., fetal micturition,[83] tracheal secretions,[84] the transfer between AF and fetal blood perfusing the fetal surface of the placenta, and the exchange of fluid across the fetal membranes between AF and maternal blood)[85,86] (see also chapter 3). Removal of AF results mainly from fetal swallowing.[87] During the third trimester of pregnancy, AF volume averages 700–800 mL, decreasing thereafter. Approximately 1,000 mL of fluid flows in and out of the amniotic compartment daily.[85]

Various methods for estimating AF volume have been proposed, of which the single vertical pocket,[88] two-diameter pocket,[89] and AF index (AFI)[90] are the most often applied.

Oligohydramnios

Assessment of the presence or absence of oligohydramnios constitutes an integral part of the fetal evaluation. The causes for the presence of oligohydramnios include fetal malformations with emphasis on the urinary tract system, premature rupture of membranes, and placental insufficiency.[91] The AFI and single deepest (vertical) pocket are currently used to identify oligohydramnios but are poor predictors. Only the single deepest pocket measurement is predictive of a compromised fetus (umbilical artery pH) and has been correlated with perinatal mortality.[92] When studying survival rates in the presence of oligohydramnios, the gestational age should be taken into account. Shipp et al.[93] found a very different survival rate in fetuses diagnosed with severe oligohydramnios in the second versus the third trimester of pregnancy, the perinatal mortality being higher in the early gestational age period. The most severe form of oligohydramnios is associated with poor fetal outcome and increased risk of pulmonary hypoplasia. An eightfold increase in perinatal mortality has been reported in severe oligohydramnios compared with moderate oligohydramnios.[94] Similar results were demonstrated by Chamberlain et al.[95] Anhydramnios is uniformly lethal, because it is usually associated with severe bilateral renal pathology or triploidy and will inevitably result in severe lung hypoplasia.

IUGR is one of the most common complications associated with severe oligohydramnios.[96] Golan et al.[96] reported a 24 percent incidence of IUGR in 145 pregnancies complicated by second- or third-trimester oligohydramnios. A similar proportion (20.5 percent) was found by Shipp et al.[93] The same authors found that premature rupture of membranes represented one-third of second-trimester cases of oligohydramnios, as opposed to only 3 percent of those in the third trimester. Hadi et al.[97] found a similar large discrepancy, with survival rates of 6.7 percent and 98 percent, respectively. A considerable difference in outcome was also established for anomalies during the second and third trimester of pregnancy: 1.5 percent versus 41 percent.[93] This difference in survival rate may be partly due to the fact that most fetuses with Potter syndrome were detected before 24 weeks of gestation and that a number of malformations established after 30 weeks were not renal in origin.[93]

Polyhydramnios

The volume of AF varies with daily changes regulated by complex interactions between the maternal, fetal, and placental compartments.[86] The incidence of polyhydramnios has been reported as ranging from 0.2 percent to 1.9 percent.[98] Ultrasonographic quantitation of AF volume by means of the AFI has been shown to be reproducible in detecting polyhydramnios.[99] Perinatal morbidity and mortality are increased in the presence of polyhydramnios.[95] The etiology of polyhydramnios involves both fetal and maternal disorders (i.e., maternal diabetes mellitus, isoimmunization, fetal structural and chromosomal anomalies, multiple gestation, and idiopathic origin). Ben-Chetrit et al.[100] reported a 19.2 percent incidence of fetal anomalies: 39 percent were gastrointestinal defects, 26 percent were nervous system defects, and 22 percent were urinary tract anomalies. The incidence of chromosomal abnormalities in the presence of polyhydramnios varies between 3.2 percent[101] and 12 percent.[102,103] Dashe et al.[104] reported an anomaly detection rate in pregnancies with polyhydramnios of nearly 80 percent, irrespective of the degree of AF increase. The residual anomaly risk after normal sonographic evaluation was 2 percent or lower when hydramnios was mild or moderate and 11 percent if severe. This wide variation is mainly determined by the sonographic detection of associated structural anomalies. Barnhard et al.[105] emphasized that the finding of polyhydramnios on routine ultrasonography requires additional evaluation. In the presence of polyhydramnios associated with a suspected fetal anomaly or IUGR, the patient should undergo cytogenetic evaluation by

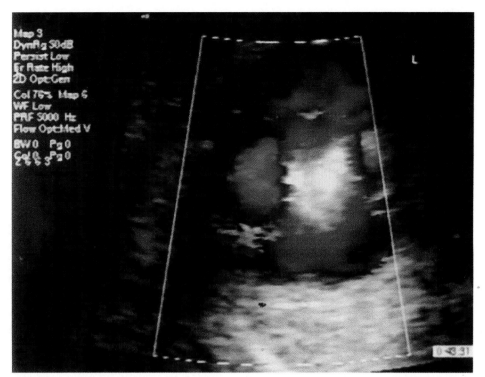

Fig. 24.3. Atrioventricular septal defect characterized by a single atrium and large ventricular septal defect resulting in a single flow pattern demonstrating turbulence. Source: By permission of M. Wessels.

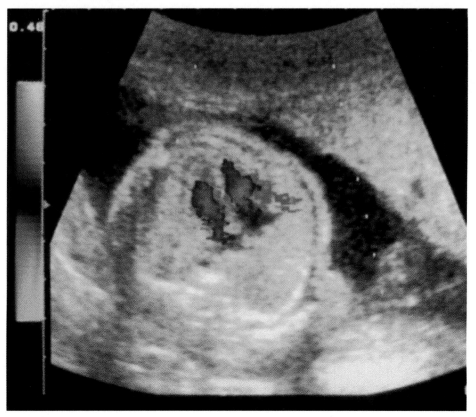

Fig. 24.4. Normal blood flow through the left and right heart at 26 weeks of gestation (four-chamber view).

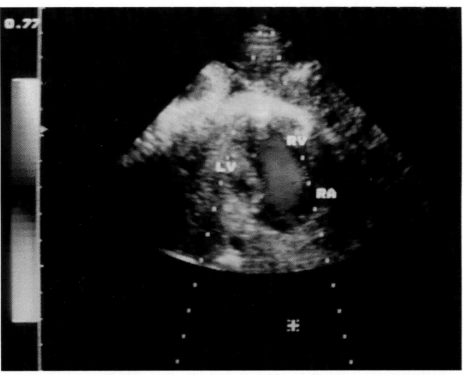

Fig. 24.5. Hypoplastic left heart syndrome. Blood flow is restricted to the right heart at 27 weeks of gestation (four-chamber view). LV = left ventricle; RV = right ventricle; RA = right atrium.

means of amniocentesis (FISH) or cordocentesis. An incomplete or difficult ultrasono-graphic evaluation is also an indication for fetal karyotype determination. However, under normal anatomic circumstances, there is no need to do all this. Polyhydramnios alone is not an absolute indication for invasive genetic evaluation.[105] The preterm delivery rate in polyhydramnios is higher than that in the normal population, with premature deliveries in approximately 14 percent of patients with unexplained polyhydramnios, 28 percent of patients with insulin-dependent diabetes, and 37 percent of pregnancies with fetal malformations.[106] Thus, the underlying cause of polyhydramnios is a major factor in determining when delivery will occur. In some instances, polyhydramnios will resolve before delivery. In this subset, there is a significantly higher prevalence of glucose intolerance and fetal macrosomia than in patients with normal pregnancies.[107]

SONOGRAPHIC ASSESSMENT OF FETAL LUNG HYPOPLASIA

Normal lung growth refers to an increase in cell number and seems to be influenced primarily by physical factors such as intrauterine and intrathoracic space, lung liquid volume and pressure, and breathing movements. Several mechanisms have been put forward to explain the association between oligohydramnios and pulmonary hypoplasia. First, there may be decreased space for lung growth because of compression of the uterine wall on the fetal chest and abdomen. Second, restriction of fetal breathing movements may occur because of prolonged thoracic compression. Fetal breathing movements may stimulate lung growth by intermittently distending the lungs with fluid aspirated into the trachea.[108] However, as shown in some animal experiments, it seems unlikely that inhibition of fetal breathing is the predominant cause of oligohydramnios-related pulmonary hypoplasia. Third, there is increased efflux of lung liquid from the intrapulmonary space to the amniotic space, resulting in a decrease of intrapulmonary pressure.[109] This highlights the importance of the presence of intrapulmonary fluid and of a normal balance of volume and pressure in the developing fetal lung.

Oligohydramnios may increase lung fluid loss by compression of the lungs, with consequent decreased lung volume within the potential airways, thus leading to pulmonary hypoplasia. Another important physical factor that can interfere with fetal lung growth is the intrathoracic cavity. A smaller-than-normal intrathoracic space may be responsible for the development of fetal pulmonary hypoplasia.[108] Conditions that can be named in this respect are congenital diaphragmatic hernia, fetal hydrops, tumors of the thorax, including adenomatoid malformations and skeletal anomalies deforming the thoracic cage.[110] Paralysis of the diaphragm may, apart from limiting the intrathoracic space, interfere with fetal breathing movements, and this may have an additional negative effect on fetal lung growth.[111] Finally, normal pulmonary arterial flow during the canalicular and alveolar stages of fetal lung development appears to be essential for normal lung growth.[112] Ligation of the left pulmonary artery during the late canalicular stage of lung development in fetal sheep creates pulmonary hypoplasia with significantly reduced lung weight and lung volume.

Pulmonary hypoplasia, either unilateral or bilateral, is a poorly defined condition of incomplete development of the lung, so it fails to reach adult size.[113] This defective development is due to a decrease in the number of lung cells, airways, and alveola, with a resulting decrease in organ size and weight.[114] Because growth of the pulmonary blood vessels parallels development of the airways, it is not surprising that disturbance of the pulmonary vascular bed coincides with pulmonary hypoplasia. A decrease in total size of the pulmonary vascular bed, a decrease in the number of vessels per unit of lung tissue and increased pulmonary arterial smooth muscle have been described.[115]

The reported incidence of pulmonary hypoplasia in the general population ranges from 9 to 11 per 10,000 livebirths and is 14 per 10,000 of all births.[116] Perinatal mortality is high, approximately 70 percent in most series.[117] Premature rupture of the membranes (PROM) is a common obstetric problem that occurs in approximately 10 percent of all pregnancies.[118] The reported incidence of pulmonary hypoplasia due to oligohydramnios based on chronic amniotic leakage varies between 8 and 26 percent, of which 55–100 percent was lethal.[119]

Prenatal Prediction of Pulmonary Hypoplasia

An accurate prenatal test for detecting pulmonary hypoplasia is highly desirable from the obstetrician's point of view, because of the high perinatal mortality rate. Because the prediction of the nonlethal forms of pulmonary hypoplasia will not drastically change obstetric management, the reliable prenatal prediction of the lethal form might alter obstetric management. A number of methods have been proposed.

Whereas some authors revealed that persistent severe oligohydramnios is an independent significant predictor of lung hypoplasia,[117] others imply that this is codependent with gestational age at the time of PROM, and thus does not predict pulmonary hypoplasia when evaluated alone.[120] Data on the predictive value of the presence or absence of fetal breathing movements are still contradictory. Blott et al.[121] showed a sensitivity and predictive value of the absence of fetal breathing for pulmonary hypoplasia up to 100 percent. Nevertheless, there are also reports that fail to determine any correlation between the absence of fetal breathing movements and pulmonary hypoplasia.[117] Fisk et al.[122] demonstrated that restitution of AF volume in human pregnancies complicated by severe oligohydramnios does not acutely alter the incidence of fetal breathing movements, suggesting that impairment of fetal breathing is not the mechanism for oligohydramnios-related pulmonary hypoplasia.

Biometric indices such as fetal–thoracic circumference measurements and thoracic circumference to abdominal circumference ratio have been shown to have a low sensitivity and accuracy in the prediction of lethal pulmonary hypoplasia. A recent study by Laudy et al.[123] demonstrated that it is now possible to obtain reliable data on fetal lung volume using three-dimensional ultrasound. Normal values have been established demonstrating an approximately sevenfold rise in fetal lung volume during the second half of pregnancy.[124] The applicability of three-dimensional ultrasonography in the prediction of lung hypoplasia still needs to be determined.

To establish the validity of fetal pulmonary artery Doppler velocimetry in the prediction of lethal pulmonary hypoplasia, two questions need to be answered. First, can hemodynamic changes be expected in the presence of lung hypoplasia? Postmortem studies have demonstrated increased pulmonary vascular muscularization in hypoplastic lungs. This may result in elevated pulmonary vascular resistance and reduced pulmonary artery compliance. Second, will hemodynamic changes be reflected in pulmonary artery Doppler flow velocity waveform recordings, in the presence of pulmonary hypoplasia? Hemodynamic changes in the pulmonary vascular bed associated with pulmonary hypoplasia should have a bearing on pulmonary blood flow and may, therefore, result in changes in pulmonary artery Doppler flow velocity waveforms.[123] It was demonstrated that Doppler velocimetry detects changes in blood flow velocity waveforms from the proximal and middle arterial branches of the fetal pulmonary circulation in the presence of pulmonary hypoplasia. The best prediction was achieved by combining clinical, biometric, and Doppler parameters. Doppler velocimetry of the arterial pulmonary circulation alone fails to be the single and ultimate prenatal test in the prediction of lung hypoplasia.[123,124] In a recent report[125] it was suggested that the acceleration time/ejection time ratio of either right or left pulmonary artery is an accurate parameter for predicting the subsequent development of pulmonary hypoplasia and clinical outcomes, with a positive and negative predictive value of 100 percent.

It can be concluded that various ultrasound techniques have been introduced in an attempt to reliably predict fetal lung hypoplasia. So far, not a single test has met 100 percent accuracy, which is needed to arrive at a responsible clinical decision. A combination of tests may ultimately provide the best diagnostic option.

NONIMMUNE FETAL HYDROPS

Fetal hydrops is characterized by excessive accumulation of extracellular fluid, resulting in cardiac and pleural effusion, ascites, and skin edema. Often there is polyhydramnios. Nonimmune fetal hydrops has to be distinguished from fetal hydrops because of maternal alloimmunization against fetal red-cell antigens. The incidence ranges from 1 in 1,500 to 1 in 3,800 births.[126] Nonimmune fetal hydrops can be reliably diagnosed by ultrasound and may be secondary to a range of causes such as infections, fetal structural anomalies (whether or not associated with mainly structural chromosomal abnormalities), fetal tumors, hematologic disorders, or metabolic diseases (lysosomal storage diseases). Common infectious agents associated with nonimmune fetal hydrops are cytomegalovirus, adenovirus, and parvovirus (B19).[127] In case of parvovirus infection, destruction of fetal erythrocytes will lead to anemia (see chapter 30).

A host of fetal anomalies is associated with nonimmune fetal hydrops, among which are cystic hygroma, lung anomalies (congenital cystic adenomatoid malformations, diaphragmatic hernia), cardiovascular, gastrointestinal, and skeletal anomalies (thanatophoric dysplasia, asphyxiating thoracic dysplasia, and osteogenesis imperfecta).[128] Fetal cardiovascular anomalies, including cardiac rhythm disturbances resulting in congestive heart failure, represent 25–35 percent of all cases of nonimmune fetal hydrops. Placental chorioangiomas, neuroblastomas, and tuberous sclerosis are fetal tumors associated with nonimmune fetal hydrops.[128] Hematologic disorders include fetal hemorrhage, hemoglobinopathies, and hemolysis, which through producing fetal anemia are associated with nonimmune fetal hydrops. Hemoglobinopathies often have a high recurrence risk, as is the case in autosomal recessive α-thalassemia (see chapter 19) in Mediterranean populations, whereas fetal glucose-phosphate dehydrogenase is transmitted as an X-linked recessive disorder among Greeks and Africans.[128]

The diagnosis and management of nonimmune fetal hydrops very much depends on the actual cause of this condition. A detailed ultrasound scan, including fetus, placenta and AF volume, should detect a considerable number of fetal anomalies. Cordocentesis is needed to obtain valuable information on the fetal chromosome pattern, blood count, infections, and metabolic disorders. The latter represents 2–3 percent of all cases of nonimmune fetal hydrops. Maternal screening includes Coombs test for red-cell isoimmunization, the Kleihauer–Betke test for establishing fetomaternal hemorrhage, and IgG and IgM antibody titers, which need to be checked for infectious diseases. Diagnosis of fetal α-thalassemia is made by means of DNA-analysis (see chapter 19).

Fetal outcome in the presence of nonimmune fetal hydrops is poor, with a mortality rate between 50 and 98 percent.[129] Treatment methods are still limited. Fetal anemia should be remedied by erythrocyte transfusions and fetal cardiac rhythm disturbances by antiarrhythmic drugs. Symptomatic treatment consists of drainage of hydrothorax and/or ascites. Fetal surgical intervention has been carried out in a number of anomalies causing fetal hydrops, such as congenital adenomatoid malformation and sacrococcygeal teratoma[130] (see chapters 29 and 25). Delivery is nearly always premature, but is determined by gestational age, the severity and nature of the underlying cause of nonimmune fetal hydrops, the success of treatment and fetal growth and condition. In a case of perinatal death, autopsy is essential in an attempt to elucidate the cause of a particular case of fetal hydrops.[131]

THE TWIN-TO-TWIN TRANSFUSION SYNDROME

The twin-to-twin transfusion syndrome (TTTS) is characterized by the presence of oligohydramnios in one sac and polyhydramnios in the other in a monochorionic–diamniotic twin pregnancy. Oligohydramnios is defined by a maximum vertical fluid pocket of less than 2 cm and polyhydramnios by a maximum vertical fluid pocket of more than 8 cm. TTTS complicates 10 to 15 percent of monochorionic twin pregnancies,[132] and it accounts for up to 17 percent of perinatal deaths in twins.[132]

TTTS develops from a net unbalanced flow of blood between two monochorionic fetuses through placental vascular communications.[133] Placental anastomoses are superficial or deep. Superficial anastomoses are bidirectional, either arterioarterial or venovenous.[134] In contrast, deep anastomoses (arteriovenous) represent a shared cotyledon, in which the arterial supply is derived from one twin, and the venous drainage is to the other; they are unidirectional, and this may result in unequal distribution of flow.[132] Doppler studies have shown that arterioarterial anastomoses are present in the vast majority of uncomplicated monochorionic pregnancies, but are rarely present in TTTS.[135] This suggests that bidirectional arterioarterial anastomoses compensate for hemodynamic imbalance caused by unidirectional arteriovenous anastomoses.[136] Quintero et al.[137] indicated that TTTS follows a certain time course characterized by progressive development of renal failure in the donor twin, abnormal Doppler findings, congestive heart failure with hydrops and ultimately fetal death.

There is still controversy regarding the most effective treatment of TTTS (see chapters 2 and 29). Expectant management of TTTS will result in almost 100 percent perinatal mortality.[138] Therapeutic measures include serial amniocentesis, laser therapy, and umbilical cord occlusion. The objective of serial amniocentesis is to reduce the amount of fluid in the sac of the recipient twin and thus reduce the risk of preterm labor and delivery.[139] The number of repeat procedures is determined by the rate of reaccumulation of liquor in the gestational sac of the recipient twin. The success rate is 66 percent (chance of survival of at least one twin). The objective of the laser therapy is to eliminate any and all blood exchange between the fetuses.[140–142] Quintero et al.[143] presented a precise and reproducible technique (selective laser photocoagulation of communicating vessels), allowing distinction between communicating vessels and normal individually perfused areas of the placenta. This approach was associated with an 85 percent success rate as defined by a survival of at least one fetus and a 3–5 percent risk of cerebral palsy. Accurate identification of arteriovenous anastomoses would minimize damage of adjacent nonanastomotic vasculature. Accurate identification of arteriovenous anastomosis would permit less invasive methods of ablation, such as by embolization, interstitial laser, or focused ultrasound.[135]

Thus far, Doppler ultrasound has not provided accurate targeting of the anastomoses responsible for TTTS. Doppler ultrasound does provide information on hemodynamic changes following laser therapy. Gratacos et al.[144] described a progressive improvement of signs of right cardiac overload in the recipient twin, while the donor twin experienced a substantial increase in umbilical venous volume flow. Two prospective nonrandomized clinical trials have demonstrated laser therapy to be superior to serial amniocentesis.[141,145] Both studies have been criticized for their inclusion criteria and ultrasound standards. A randomized control trial is awaited. The objective of umbilical cord occlusion is to prevent blood exchange between the fetuses at the umbilical cord level of one of the twins. This means ligation of the cord under endoscopic or ultrasound guidance[146,147] or by applying bipolar electrocautery.[148] A success rate of 76 percent was established. A less attractive solution to TTTS is the iatrogenic disruption of the membrane dividing the two cavities. It involves repeated piercing of the dividing membrane, allowing liquor from the recipient to enter the sac of the donor. It seems that the success rates of different treatment methods ought to be reviewed in relation to the disease stage of TTTS.

Although TTTS is considered to be a complication almost unique to monochorionic twins, some reports have described TTTS associated with dichorionic twin placentae.[149] The presence of functional interfetal vascular anastomosis has been confirmed in this rare condition.

DETECTION AND MANAGEMENT OF FETAL ANOMALIES IN THE THIRD TRIMESTER OF PREGNANCY

This discussion is focused on the role of ultrasound in detecting fetal anomalies, the management of such pregnancies and the available treatment methods. A more detailed appraisal of a selection of common major malformations follows. Screening for fetal anomalies is now done mostly during the early second trimester of pregnancy. In the third trimester, sonographic examinations for fetal anomalies are performed mostly in pregnancies at risk, due for example to an abnormal antenatal finding such as IUGR, abnormal AF volume, or fetal cardiac arrhythmia. Maternal disorders, including insulin-dependent diabetes mellitus, epilepsy with anticonvulsant drugs, and autoimmune disease also merit screening.

Indication-Based Ultrasound Examination

Perinatal mortality is now in the range of 8–9 per 1,000 births in industrialized countries. The improvement reflects predominantly enhanced intrapartum and neonatal care. IUGR, preterm delivery, and fetal anomalies are still major determinants of perinatal mortality and morbidity. Thus, the prevention and early detection of congenital anomalies have become important parts of maternal health care.

About 2–3 percent of newborns have detectable congenital structural anomalies (see chapter 1). Major fetal anomalies are associated with preterm delivery, increased perinatal morbidity and mortality, unwarranted obstetric surgery, and prolonged postnatal hospitalization, all of which exact emotional, social, and financial hardships on the families involved and on society as a whole. Prenatal detection of a malformed fetus allows the woman a range of options, varying from pregnancy termination to possible intrauterine treatment and adjustment of obstetric management. The latter involves the immediate availability of sophisticated neonatal care of the structurally abnormal infant. The potential advantage of prenatal diagnosis of a major but nonlethal fetal malformation is adjustment of the timing, mode, and geographic location of the delivery. Forewarned, the parents can avert the delivery of a child in a hospital that is ill prepared to care for the problem. Indication-based ultrasound investigations apply to selective (levels 2 and 3) ultrasound imaging, targeted at women with increased risk of fetal structural anomalies. They entail a more detailed examination of fetal morphology and physiologic function than the screening-based scan. One or several organ systems, depending on the indication, are subjected to scrupulous sonographic investigation. For instance, an indication-based scan of the fetal heart includes not only the visualization of the four-chamber view but also the ventriculoarterial outflow, the venous inflow, the aortic arch, and the ductus arteriosus.

Risk Factors Found during Pregnancy

Diagnostic investigations for suspected fetal pathology are based on abnormal obstetric findings, which may become manifest only during the late second and third trimesters of pregnancy, such as polyhydramnios, oligohydramnios, severe IUGR, preterm labor, and fetal cardiac arrhythmias. Women with pregnancies thus affected are often referred to tertiary centers for diagnostic evaluation by means of detailed ultrasonography and invasive prenatal diagnosis if indicated. The prevalence of fetal structural anomalies in this category is approximately 35–40 percent.[150] In an estimated 20 percent of cases, more than one organ system is involved. This is often based on the presence of a particular syndrome or chromosomal abnormality.[150] In advanced pregnancies, swift information on the fetal chromosome pattern is essential for optimal obstetric management.

The overall sensitivity of an indication-based fetal anomaly scan is 85–95 percent. This is explained mainly by the higher level of scanning expertise in referral centers, better knowledge of genetic syndromes, the availability of superior ultrasound equipment, and the presence of pediatric specialists for consultation. Nevertheless, even in experienced hands, the reported sensitivity of a detailed cardiac scan remains somewhat lower (i.e., 70–80 percent).

FETAL CARDIAC DEFECTS

Congenital heart disease constitutes an important proportion of all major congenital malformations, which are present in 2–3 percent of neonates[151] (see chapter 1). The estimated birth prevalence of cardiac malformations is 8 in 1,000.[152] Approximately half of the cases of congenital heart disease have only minor consequences or can easily be corrected surgically. Yet, more than 20 percent of prenatal deaths and 45 percent of infant deaths due to congenital malformations are related to cardiovascular anomalies.[153,154] At present, the cause of congenital heart disease is, to a large extent, unknown. Approximately 90 percent of the cases are of multifactorial origin (e.g., resulting from an interaction between genetic constitution and environmental influences without further etiologic specification).[155] Congenital heart disease has proven to be accessible to prenatal detection in many cases.[156–158]

Cardiovascular anomalies are strongly associated with other anomalies or chromosomal aberrations.[159] The overall risk for aneuploidy in a fetus with congenital heart disease is approximately 30 percent.[160] Recently, it was shown that chromosomal microdeletions in 7q and 22q are responsible for certain cardiac syndromes[161] (e.g., Williams–Beuren syndrome, DiGeorge syndrome) (see chapters 1 and 8). A recent study indicated that second- and third-trimester in utero diagnosis of Down syndrome has a poor outcome when associated with congenital heart disease and/or IUGR.[162] The following sections will deal with the fetal cardiac examination, prenatal sonographic diagnosis of a selection of cardiac anomalies and fetal outcome.

The Cardiac Examination

Examination of the fetal heart requires high-quality scanning expertise, even more so than for other fetal organ structures. The integration of the four-chamber view alone into the standard examination in fifteen centers in the Rotterdam region achieved a detection rate for heart defects of only 4–5 percent.[163] To improve detection rates, visualization of the great vessels should be added to the four-chamber view.[164] This applies in particular to anomalies such as transposition of the great arteries, tetralogy of Fallot, truncus arteriosus communis and double-outlet right ventricle. Color Doppler may aid in the detection of ventricular septal defects and atrioventricular valve regurgitation. The ideal time for performing a fetal cardiac examination is around 20 weeks of gestation.[165] For markedly increased risks of congenital heart disease, as in the case of increased nuchal translucency or a family history of congenital heart disease, an initial scan to exclude major malformations should be performed by expert sonographers as early as 12–14 weeks of gestation.[165] Yagel et al.[166] established a 64 percent detection rate at 13–16 weeks, which increased to 81 percent when a second examination was added at 20–22 weeks. This rate was similar to the subset examined at only 20–22 weeks, resulting in a detection rate of 78 percent. The detection rate for small isolated septal defects is relatively poor.[167] Chaoui and Ewing[168] proposed three standard cross-sectional views to be included in the fetal cardiac scan: the four-chamber, the five-chamber (includes the ascending aorta), and the three-vessel view (includes the pulmonary trunk, aortic arch, aortic isthmus, and superior vena cava).

Color Doppler evaluation of systole and diastole is an integral component of the standard examination. Other aspects that should be included in the fetal heart scan are[169]: (1) the cardiothoracic ratio (normal, 0.33) to exclude cardiomegaly; (2) cardiac position to exclude mediastinal shift of a normal heart due to pressure effects of conditions such as diaphragmatic hernia, cystic adenomatoid malformation of the lung, pleural effusion or unilateral lung hypoplasia, and disorders of embryonic laterality determination resulting in abnormal atrial situs (isomerism and mirror-image arrangement); and (3) pericardial effusion ($\geq$2 mm) such as in heart failure and a wide range of chromosomal abnormalities, genetic syndromes, metabolic diseases, and certain congenital infections.

Some controversy still exists around the clinical significance of so-called echogenic foci within the fetal heart (see chapter 23). They are almost always seen in the left ventricle, within a papillary muscle. Echogenic intracardiac foci are generally thought to be a variant of normal,[170] although a recent report[171] suggested that the presence of echogenic intracardiac foci in a population otherwise at low risk for aneuploidy seems to warrant the performance of fetal chromosome analysis. For three-dimensional visualization of the fetal heart, see "Advances in Imaging Technology" below.

Cardiac function has been studied mainly in relation to IUGR (see also "Fetal Growth Restriction" below). Fetal hypoxemia may impair myocardial contractility, resulting in reduced ventricular filling properties with a lower E/A ratio at atrioventricular valve level,[172] lower peak velocities in the ascending aorta and main pulmonary artery,[173] increased aortic and decreased pulmonary acceleration time,[174] and a relative increase of left cardiac output associated with decreased right cardiac output.[175] IUGR has also been associated with a reduced isovolumic relaxation time.[176] A new approach to the evaluation of fetal cardiac function is the Doppler myocardial performance index,[177] which is calculated as ICT + IRT/ET (ICT and IRT represent isovolumic contraction and relaxation time; ET represents ejection time).

Diagnosis of Selected Cardiac Anomalies

Septal Defects and Outflow Obstructions

Ventricular septal defects (VSD) represent the most common form of congenital heart disease, with an estimated incidence of 0.38 per 1,000 livebirths.[178] They are classified into perimembranous inlet or trabecular or outlet defects, depending on their location in the septum. On ultrasound examination, there is a dropout of echoes at the level of the intraventricular septum on a four-chamber view. VSDs are not associated with hemodynamic compromise in utero. Atrial septal defects are situated close to the endocardial cushion (so-called ostium primum defect) or in the area of the foramen ovale (ostium secundum defect). The latter defects are mostly isolated but may be part of a syndrome such as the Holt–Oram syndrome.[179] Because the foramen ovale is patent during intrauterine life, atrial septal defects are not associated with cardiac compromise. The incidence of atrioventricular septal defects is 0.12 per 1,000 livebirths.[178] In the complete form, there is fusion of the mitral and tricuspid valves into one large atrioventricular valve, which is often incompetent, as expressed by systolic regurgitation from the ventricles into the atria and resulting in congestive heart failure[180] (Figure 24.3). Color-coded Doppler ultrasound can be helpful in identifying the regurgitant jet. Atrioventricular septal defects are often associated with chromosomal anomalies, such as trisomy 18 and trisomy 21 or cardiosplenic syndromes.[181]

Aortic and Pulmonary Stenosis; Aortic Arch Anomalies

Pulmonary stenosis is usually of the valvar type, leading to a pressure buildup in the right ventricle, with subsequent muscular hypertrophy.[182] Congestive heart failure is rare. Aortic stenosis is observed in 0.04 per 1,000 livebirths[178]; its most common form is the valvar type. Prenatal diagnosis of valvar aortic stenosis is determined by Doppler ultrasound identification of poststenotic turbulence.[182] In severe forms of aortic stenosis, left ventricular overload, together with subendocardial ischemia, may lead to intrauterine impairment of cardiac function.[182]

Coarctation of the aortic arch is characterized by a local narrowing of the juxtaductal arch, usually between the left subclavian artery and the ductus arteriosus.[182] The incidence is 0.18 per 1,000 livebirths. The abnormality is suspected on the basis of ventricular size discrepancy in the four-chamber view.[183] The most sensitive diagnostic feature is the presence of transverse aortic arch and isthmus narrowing.[183]

Hypoplastic Left Heart

The hypoplastic left heart is characterized by a small left ventricle and mitral and/or aortic atresia[184] (Figures 24.4 and 24.5). The incidence of this anomaly is 0.16 per 1,000 livebirths.[178] Depending on the degree of left ventricular hypoplasia, the final diagnosis may depend on the demonstration of hypoplasia of the ascending aorta and atresia of the aortic valve.[182] Color-coded Doppler flow will be useful in that it displays retrograde blood flow within the ascending aorta and aortic arch.[182]

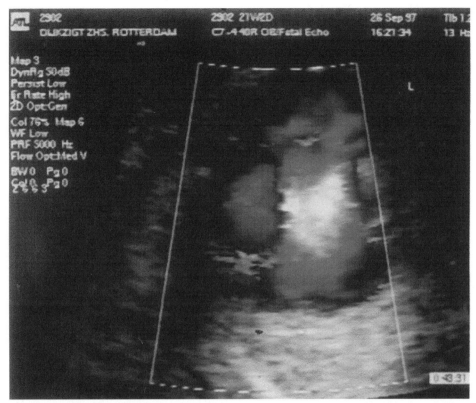

Fig. 24.3. Atrioventricular septal defect characterized by a single atrium and large ventricular septal defect resulting in a single flow pattern demonstrating turbulence. *Source:* By permission of M. Wessels, Eramus University Medical School.[84]

Conotruncal Malformations

Accurate visualization of ventricular–arterial connections is essential for a correct diagnosis of conotruncal malformations. Long-axis views of both ventricles allow optimal visualization of the outflow tracts and origin of the great arteries.[185] Conotruncal malformations include double-outlet right ventricle, transposition of the great arteries, tetralogy of Fallot, and truncus arteriosus.

In double-outlet right ventricle (DORV), the aortic and pulmonary valves arise either completely or nearly completely from the right ventricle. The prevalence is 0.03 per 1,000 livebirths.[178] On ultrasound examination, features of DORV are alignment of the two vessels totally or predominantly from the right ventricle.[185] DORV may be associated with extracardiac anomalies or abnormal karyotypes. Cardiac compromise is unlikely.

In transposition of the great arteries, the aorta arises from the right ventricle and is situated anterior and to the left of the pulmonary artery, which is connected to the left ventricle that lies posteriorly and medially.[185] The prevalence is 0.2 per 1,000 livebirths.[178] In the presence of complete transposition of the great arteries, which is one of the most difficult cardiac anomalies to establish prenatally, the two great arteries do not cross but arise parallel from the base of the heart.[185] Cardiac failure will not occur during intrauterine life. Associated defects such as ventricular septal defects or pulmonary stenosis may be present.

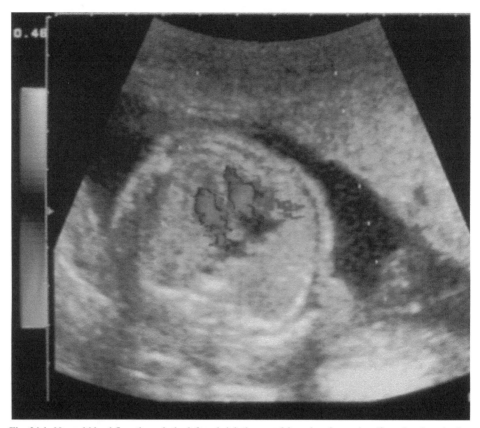

Fig. 24.4. Normal blood flow through the left and right heart at 26 weeks of gestation (four-chamber view).

Tetralogy of Fallot is characterized by malalignment, ventricular septal defect with anterior displacement of the infundibular septum, subpulmonary narrowing, and overriding aortic root.[185] Biometric measurement of the aortic and pulmonary artery diameter will reveal a relatively large ascending aortic diameter. Depending on the degree of pulmonary artery obstruction, color-coded Doppler ultrasound may demonstrate absence of forward flow or even reverse flow. However, this will not lead to cardiac compromise during fetal life.

Truncus arteriosus is presented by a single arterial vessel, originating from the heart and overriding the ventricular septum. Prenatal ultrasound will demonstrate a single semilunar valve overriding the ventricular septal defect and a direct continuity existing between one or two pulmonary arteries and the single arterial trunk. There is often thickening of the semilunar valve and incompetence of the truncal valve.[185]

Fetal Outcome

More than 50 percent of ventriculoseptal defects located in the perimembranous or muscular septum will close spontaneously, usually during the first year of life. Some close during intrauterine life. Defects in the inlet or outlet septum require surgical repair.[186] Infants with an isolated atrioventricular septal defect will remain asymptomatic for a few

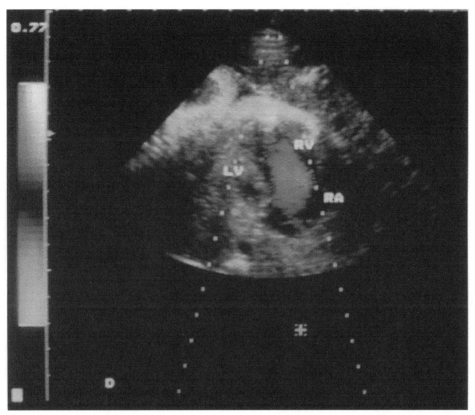

Fig. 24.5. Hypoplastic left heart syndrome. Blood flow is restricted to the right heart at 27 weeks of gestation (four-chamber view). LV = left ventricle; RV = right ventricle; RA = right atrium.

weeks, but signs of congestive heart failure will develop soon thereafter. Survival after atrioventricular septal defect repair is high, exceeding 90 percent.[187] Surgical options are now available for aortic stenosis. However, the survival rate in this subset of congenital heart disease is limited, with a survival rate of 37.5 percent reported by Allan et al.[188] In the subset of conotruncal anomalies, data compilation by Shi-Joon Yoo et al.[189] from prenatal studies by Allan et al.[190] and Palladini et al.[191] shows a survival rate (excluding termination of pregnancy) of 90 percent for tetralogy of Fallot, 70 percent for complete transposition, 77 percent for DORV, but only 25 percent for truncus arteriosus communis. The outcome of hypoplastic left heart syndrome is still limited. Of interest is that morbidity and mortality are significantly reduced when the diagnosis is made before birth (100 percent survival as opposed to 66 percent when diagnosed postnatally).[192,193] Postnatal management consists of prostaglandin administration to maintain patency of the ductus arteriosus followed by the Norwood procedure or primary cardiac transplantation.[194] Also, the antenatal diagnosis of coarctation of the aorta has resulted in reduced mortality and improved preoperative hemodynamic stability compared with postnatal diagnosis.[195] Both collapse and death were more common in the postnatally diagnosed group. There was echocardiographic evidence of ductal patency in the antenatally diagnosed infants. Increased respiratory rate was associated with postnatal presentation.

DISTURBANCES OF CARDIAC RHYTHM

Fetal heart rate patterns play an important role in the assessment of the fetal condition and, therefore, in obstetric management. Treatment methods have been introduced to normalize heart rate. Success rates depend on the nature and duration of the tachycardia, the presence or absence of hydrops, gestational age, and the degree of placental perfusion.

Methods of Recording Fetal Heart Rate and Rhythm

An abnormal heart rate and/or an abnormal heart rhythm usually is first noted through the ordinary stethoscope. More sophisticated recording techniques are available for detailed analysis of fetal heart rhythm: simultaneous M-mode recording of atrial and ventricular activity[196] and Doppler velocimetry at atrioventricular and outflow-tract level (ascending aorta, pulmonary artery), yielding information on intracardiac flow patterns relative to the preceding mechanical events during the cardiac cycle. Venous flow velocity recording in the inferior vena cava will help in establishing increased late diastolic venous retrograde flow as a sign of cardiac compromise due to a particular disturbance of cardiac rate or rhythm. Doppler waveform recording in the inferior vena cava and ductus venosus may also be helpful in monitoring the effectiveness of antiarrhythmic agents.[197] Enhancing the Doppler sample volume to cover both inflow (mitral valve) and outflow (ascending aorta), simultaneous recording of flow velocity waveforms at inflow and outflow level will be feasible, allowing calculation of isovolumetric contraction and relaxation time next to filling and ejection time and thus providing more detailed information on fetal systolic and diastolic cardiac function.[198] It is essential that structural cardiac anomalies be excluded before embarking on any kind of antiarrhythmic treatment.

Supraventricular Ectopic Rhythms

The most prevalent fetal cardiac rhythm disturbance is supraventricular ectopic rhythms. They may occur very early during diastole (i.e., during the refractory period of the atrioventricular conduction system), resulting in absent conduction into the ventricle and therefore no ventricular response. Resetting of the atrial pacemaker will result in a longer than normal pause between ventricular ejections.[199] Doppler velocimetry will demonstrate passive E-wave filling after ventricular systole, with the early A-wave being more or less superimposed on the E-wave.[199] The postextrasystolic peak is more pronounced because of increased diastolic ventricular preload during the prolonged diastolic filling period (Frank–Starling mechanism).[200] Supraventricular ectopic rhythms occurring later in diastole may be conducted into the ventricle, resulting in a diminished stroke volume, due to the shortened diastole. In our Rotterdam series of 292 cases of supraventricular ectopic rhythms less than 1 percent developed into sustained tachycardia; the underlying mechanism usually involved accessory conduction pathways at the level of the atrioventricular junction.[201]

Fetal Tachyarrhythmias

Fetal tachyarrhythmias, with an incidence of 4–6 per 1,000 livebirths, is a relatively rare disorder, which may result in nonimmune hydrops and ultimately fetal death. Sinus tachycardia (1:1 atrioventricular relationship) may be caused by β-mimetics such as ritodrine, fetal distress, intrauterine infection, or fetal hyperthyroidism. Ventricular tachycardia is extremely rare. Supraventricular tachycardia[199] is mostly of a reciprocating or atrioventricular re-entrant cause. A circular movement of electrical impulses is initiated by an extrasystole, which is conducted slowly through the atrioventricular node to the ventricle and then re-enters the atrial tissue through an accessory conduction pathway outside the atrioventricular node. The rate of this type of supraventricular tachycardia is usually 240–260 bpm. Less common are atrial flutter and, in particular, atrial fibrillation. Atrial flutter[199] results from a circular re-entrant movement of the electrical energy within the atria. Heart rate usually varies between 400 and 480 bpm. Varying degrees of atrioventricular block may be seen, from 2:1 to complete dissociation of atrial and ventricular activity. In our experience, atrioventricular rate relationships under these circumstances can be best determined from simultaneous M-mode recordings of atrial and ventricular activity. Supraventricular tachycardia may result in fetal hydrops. Although it is not clear why hydrops develops in some fetuses and not in others, factors such as venous hydrostatic pressure and serum oncotic pressure play a role.[199] Hydrops is likely to occur at heart rates above 240 bpm. Copel and Kleinman[199] reported congenital heart disease in 5 of 19 cases (25 percent) of atrial flutter/fibrillation. Supraventricular tachycardia (SVT) may be related to cardiac tumors or atrial septal aneurysm,[202] fetal myocarditis, or preexcitation syndrome.[203]

The objective of intrauterine treatment of fetal tachycardias is to restore normal heart rate and rhythm. The need for antiarrhythmic treatment in the presence of fetal tachycardia is determined by a number of factors, such as gestational age, the nature and duration of the tachycardia, and the absence or presence of fetal hydrops. Although a previable fetus with sustained fetal tachycardia needs treatment, a fetus at term should be delivered with the view of optimal antiarrhythmic treatment immediately after birth. In cases of short periods of tachycardia, close monitoring of the fetus for early signs of fetal hydrops should suffice. However, in our experience, sustained fetal tachycardia with or without fetal hydrops should be treated. There must be a thorough understanding of the underlying nature of the tachycardia and the potential electrophysiologic effect of the given antiarrhythmic agent.[204] One should also be aware of potential side effects and possible interactions between antiarrhythmic agents. This dictates a close cooperation between various disciplines, such as the obstetrician, pediatric cardiologist, adult cardiologist, and pharmacologist. Traditionally, treatment of the fetus is carried out transplacentally via the mother. Some centers have resorted to direct treatment of the fetus through cordocentesis.[204] The advantage of direct access to the fetal circulation, which allows rapid determination of drug concentrations and therefore effective treatment schedules, must be offset against the risks of repeated invasive procedures (i.e., cordocentesis). Vagal stimulation maneuvers have been proposed by some.[205]

Digoxin has been the drug of choice for treatment of SVT.[199,201,206] It is administered to the mother and reaches the fetus transplacentally. In the presence of fetal hydrops, placental transfer is diminished and, therefore, may result in treatment failure. A digoxin-like immunoreactive substance has been shown to be present in pregnant women as well as in the fetal circulation, particularly in the presence of fetal hydrops.[199,207] This may interfere with maternal serum determinations of digoxin levels during antiarrhythmic treatment. In our own laboratory, digoxin treatment starts with a loading dose of 1.0 mg divided over 12 hours followed by an oral maintenance dose of 0.75 mg daily. Maternal serum digoxin levels of 1.5–2.5 ng/mL are the aim. When digoxin fails to restore normal sinus rhythm, several other drugs have been used, such as propranolol, quinidine, procainamide (type IA antiarrhythmic agents), verapamil, and amiodarone (type III agent) given either to the mother or directly to the fetus.[202,208] Amiodarone may express considerable side effects, including interference with normal fetal thyroid function[209] and myocardial development.[210] However, only recently Jouannic et al.[211] proposed the use of amiodarone as a second-line therapy. The same group demonstrated that the response to prenatal therapy may be poorer in cases presenting with tricuspid regurgitation.[212] Verapamil, which is a calcium antagonist, may result in bradycardia and hypotension, especially in the neonate and infant. Therefore, in our opinion, the use of verapamil should be avoided in fetal SVT, as others have suggested.[213]

Flecainide, a type IC agent, has gained popularity, despite adverse effects noted in adults after myocardial infarction.[214–216] In some centers, flecainide has been the drug of first choice.[217–219] The type I antiarrhythmic agents quinidine, and procainamide have been shown to be effective in the treatment of fetal tachycardias.[160,201] However, toxic side effects of these agents have been observed in the mother.[220] Adenosine has been shown to be effective in breaking SVTs involving the atrioventricular node as a limb of the circuit.[205,221] However, its very short half-life makes it unsuitable as a prophylactic agent.[201,222] Another drug that has been successful in the treatment of fetal supraventricular tachycardia is sotalol. This is a drug with both beta-blocking and type III antiarrhythmic properties.[223,224] No serious side effects either to the mother or fetus have been reported.[225] New recording techniques such as fetal magnetocardiography[226] have provided insights into the initiation and termination of re-entrant fetal supraventricular fetal arrhythmia.

Fetal Bradyarrhythmias

A fetal bradyarrhythmia is traditionally defined as a heart rate below 100 bpm. Sinus bradycardia is characterized by 1:1 atrioventricular concordance. Sustained sinus bradycardia may occur in fetal distress, sinus node dysfunction as seen in maternal hypothermia,[227] and long-QT syndrome.[228] Sonographic examination of the fetal heart usually reveals normal cardiac anatomy and normal fetal condition, as expressed by good fetal movement.

Complete heart block is associated with structural cardiac anomalies in approximately half of all fetuses. Visceral heterotaxy with left atrial isomerism and atrioventricular discordance are the most common findings.[199] Nonimmune hydrops may develop, resulting in poor fetal outcome. Maternal autoantibodies (anti-SSA and anti-SSB) may be responsible for fetal heart block associated with structurally normal hearts. These antibodies have a strong affinity for the fetal cardiac conduction system and may also bind cardiac myocytes, resulting in myocarditis.[229]

Treatment of fetal heart block has generally been problematic. However, in fetuses with early signs of cardiac failure or particularly slow ventricular escape rhythm, treatment may be beneficial. Fetal drug therapy has been aimed at three different features of the bradyarrhythmia: cardiac failure, autoimmune inflammation, and slow heart rate.[230] Cardiac failure in the hydropic fetus with heart block has been treated with digoxin and furosemide either transplacentally[231] or directly in the umbilical vein.[232]

Plasmapheresis and corticosteroids have been advocated in the treatment of second-degree heart block early in the course of the disease to prevent the progression of myocarditis and to assist in the return to normal sinus rhythm. Some promising results have been reported.[233] Administration of sympathomimetic drugs such as terbutaline[234] and albuterol[235] to raise fetal heart rate has been advocated for the treatment of fetal complete heart block. Still experimental is prenatal ventricular pacing. Fetal lamb studies have demonstrated that ventricular pacing can be successful.[236,237]

FETAL DIAPHRAGMATIC HERNIA

The diaphragm is a dome-shaped musculotendinous septum between the thoracic and abdominal cavity and consists of a central aponeurotic segment and a peripheral muscular part. The embryologic development ends around the 8th week of conception and consists of the fusion of four different components (i.e., ventrally from the septum transversum (mesoderm), which fuses with the pleuroperitoneal membranes, with the dorsal foregut mesentery, and laterally with muscular components of the thoracic wall). The last areas to close are the posterolaterally situated foramina (Bochdalek), which are sealed by the pleuroperitoneal membranes. The normal diaphragm allows the passage of organs, vessels, and nerves from the thoracic into the abdominal cavity. The normal fetal diaphragm can be observed discretely as a smooth hypoechoic line between the fetal lungs and the liver or spleen.

Congenital diaphragmatic hernia is characterized by protrusion of abdominal viscera into the thoracic cavity through a diaphragmatic defect. Consequently, lung development may be impaired and may even result in pulmonary hypoplasia. Surfactant deficiency does not seem to contribute to the pathophysiology of congenital diaphragmatic hernia.[238] Either delayed fusion of the four diaphragmatic components or a primary diaphragmatic defect with secondary migration of abdominal organs into the thoracic cavity is hypothesized to cause this defect. Almost all hernias occur through the posterolaterally located Bochdalek foramina, which characteristically involves the left side (75 percent). Foramen of Morgagni hernias occur in the anteromedial retrosternal part of the diaphragm as a result of maldevelopment of the septum transversum. Eventration of the diaphragm is characterized by herniated viscera that are covered by a sac composed of abdominal peritoneal layers and components of the congenitally weak diaphragm; although this anomaly is not a hernia in the strict sense, it may have the same dramatic effects on fetal lung development as a true diaphragmatic hernia. In more than half of all cases of congenital diaphragmatic hernia, associated structural or chromosomal abnormalities have been found.[239]

The typical sonographic findings of diaphragmatic hernia are mediastinal shift caused by the herniated viscera and the visualization of abdominal organs in the thoracic cavity. Polyhydramnios, which is thought to result from gastrointestinal obstruction, is common and is frequently the indication for the initial ultrasound examination.[240] The differential diagnosis of fetal diaphragmatic hernia includes cystic adenomatoid malformation of the lung, bronchogenic cysts, and bronchopulmonary sequestration. The prognosis of diaphragmatic hernia diagnosed in utero is poor and depends largely on the associated structural and chromosomal anomalies and the degree of the secondary pulmonary hypoplasia. Contradictory findings have been reported concerning the role of prenatal magnetic resonance (MR) lung volumetry in predicting the outcome in fetuses with congenital diaphragmatic hernia (see chapter 25). While Paek et al.[241] and Mahieu-Caputo et al.[242] considered MR lung volumetry a good predictor, this was not supported by Walsh et al.[243] who found the presence of liver herniation and the volume of the liver within the chest as reflected by the liver/diaphragm ratio to be helpful in predicting fetal outcome. Others have suggested fetal pulmonary artery size,[244] the fetal lung diameter[245] and lung diameter/thoracic circumference ratio to be helpful.[246] Congenital heart disease constitutes the majority of associated anomalies. The incidence of an abnormal karyotype is 10.5 percent but rises to 20 percent when only fetuses with multiple anomalies were included. Poly-hydramnios occurs in about 75 percent.[247] A systematic review of thirty-five studies re-porting data for congenital diaphragmatic hernia between 1985 and 1998[248] showed a median overall mortality rate of 58 percent for infants diagnosed in utero, 48 percent if born alive, and 33 percent postoperatively. Diagnosis before 25 weeks of gestation is not always a bad prognostic sign, with a median mortality of 60 percent. Outcome was worse for fetuses with additional anomalies (median mortality, 93 percent). The most significant cause of mortality in infants with congenital diaphragmatic hernia is not pulmonary hy-pertension but iatrogenic injury to their hypoplastic lungs.[249]

Open fetal surgery for congenital diaphragmatic hernia has been suggested as a strat-egy for salvaging selected fetuses at high risk for pulmonary hypoplasia (see chapter 29). However, the results of these techniques have been disappointing, because hysterotomy induces premature labor and because reduction of the herniated liver from the thorax into the fetal abdomen is associated with fetal death.[250] This seems to be related to the fact that the liver does not simply rotate up into the chest through a diaphragmatic defect but more likely develops in the chest, along with its abnormal vascular anatomy.[251] Newer in utero techniques include endoscopic temporary occlusion of the trachea.[252] Further ad-vances in perinatal treatment include administration of antenatal corticosteroids for stim-ulating lung development.[253]

OBSTRUCTIVE UROPATHY

Fetal obstructive uropathies involve a heterogeneous group of developmental abnormali-ties that result in partial or complete obstruction of urinary outflow at any level of the uri-nary tract. Sonographic dilatation of any part of the fetal urinary tract is, therefore, highly suggestive of an obstructive uropathy, although this will not always be true. From a clin-ical point of view, obstructive uropathies can be divided into high-level (ureter) and low-level (urethra) obstructions. Sonographic detection of high-level obstructions consists of the demonstration of a dilated fetal renal pelvis (hydronephrosis) and/or ureter. Low-level obstructions can be recognized through visualization of a dilated fetal bladder and prox-imal urinary tract. Occasionally, a dilated urethra can be demonstrated.

Hydronephrosis is characterized by a persistent excess fluid collection within the renal pelvis. Congenital hydronephrosis is most commonly caused by an obstruction of the pelvic–ureteric junction (PUJ) and results from an intrinsic narrowing at the junction be-tween the ureter and the renal pelvis. This narrowing may be due to high ureteral inser-tion, anomalous vessels, crossing bands, abnormal muscle thickness, valves, stricture, or ischemia.[254] Anatomical causes for PUJ are found in only a minority of patients. In most instances, a functional PUJ is suspected (i.e., the junction is patent to passage of a probe). Other causes of congenital hydronephrosis include obstruction of the vesicoureteric junc-tion (VUJ) causing vesicoureteric reflux (VUR). Antenatal renal dilatation occurs infre-quently in the presence of VUR, and when it does, the fetus will probably be male.[255] Despite the reported association of hydronephrosis and trisomy 21, the presence of iso-lated pyelectasis does not warrant fetal karyotyping, because the risk of trisomy 21 is less than 1 in 340.[256] Mild transient hydronephrosis without evidence of renal-tract anomalies after birth has been described,[257] possibly as a reflection of the normal physiologic changes in the size of the pyelum, as has also been reported in neonates. Fetal hydronephrosis seems to be overdiagnosed. Sherer[258] proposed that the largest anteroposterior renal pelvic measurements should be between 8 and 10 mm during the second trimester of pregnancy and >10 mm during the third trimester of pregnancy.

Several authors have reported on the criteria regarding the severity and prognosis of hydronephrosis (see chapter 29).[259–261] The degree and presence of hydronephrosis may depend on fetal bladder filling.[262] Oligohydramnios can be the result of inadequate passage of urine or severely impaired renal function. The degree of dilatation does not always correlate with the severity of the obstruction. This can be explained by secondary pressure-related renal dysplasia with decreased urinary production or by rupture of any part of the urinary tract, resulting in decompression of the renal pelvis. Also, pelvic–ureteric atresia may be present. The prognosis of obstructive uropathy depends on the localization, severity, and duration of obstruction.[263] Dilatation above the level of obstruction with an increase of pressure inside the urinary system possibly results in structural and functional changes within the kidney.[264] A reliable sonographic diagnosis of secondary renal dysplasia is not always possible. Of interest is the finding of an increased recurrence risk rate of 67 percent of fetal hydronephrosis in subsequent pregnancies.[265] Mothers of fetuses displaying hydronephrosis have a relative risk of 6.1 of having another affected child in a subsequent pregnancy.[265] Approximately 10–30 percent of prenatal cases of hydronephrosis are diagnosed as VUR neonatally.[266]

Infravesical or urethral-level obstructions produce a broad spectrum of sonographic features antenatally. The most prominent sign is a persistent distended fetal bladder (megacystis); occasionally, a dilated proximal urethra (keyhole sign) and a secondary compensatory hypertrophied bladder wall may be identified. As a result of VUR, secondary bilateral dilatation of the fetal ureter and renal pelvis can also be observed. Causes for urethral-level obstructions include posterior urethral valves (PUVs), urethral stenosis or agenesis, and a persistent cloaca. PUVs occur only in males and are the single most common cause of fetal bladder obstruction. Also, males are more commonly affected with urethral stenosis. Secondary to the infravesical obstruction, bladder decompression through development of a paranephric pseudocyst may occur with secondary urinary ascites formation through leakage of this urinoma or through transmural leakage across the bladder wall.[267] Distention of the fetal bladder and proximal urinary tract is associated with the prune belly syndrome, which is characterized by abdominal wall muscle deficiency, dilatation of the urinary tract, and cryptorchidism; the vast majority are males. In females, lower urinary tract obstruction may be related to urethral agenesis, the megacystis–microcolon–intestinal hypoperistalsis syndrome, a usually lethal autosomal recessive trait characterized by a dilated unobstructed lower urinary tract in the absence of oligohydramnios[268] and cloacal persistence.[269]

Congenital low-level obstructive uropathy is associated with poor perinatal outcome.[270] Affected fetuses are at risk for oligohydramnios-induced pulmonary hypoplasia or renal failure. Because the association between ultrasound findings and fetal renal function is poor, analysis of fetal urine biochemistry was expected to improve the selection of cases amenable to antenatal treatment[271] (see chapter 29). Ideally, fetuses with irreversible renal damage, with other abnormalities, and with abnormal karyotypes should be excluded. Urinary constituents change with gestational age due to renal maturation. High fetal urinary concentrations of sodium and calcium were found to be the best predictors of renal failure.[272] In 1993, elevated levels of β_2-microglobulin were added.[273] New markers for fetal renal damage include increased fetal urinary insulin-like growth factor 1 (IUGF-1) and binding protein 3 (IUGFBP-3).[274] However, single measurements of any of these variables are unlikely to be reliable predictors of irreversible renal damage.[275] More than 90 percent of obstructive urologic lesions do not need treatment until after birth.[276] About 20 percent of abnormalities evident in utero are not present after birth.[277]

Antenatal treatment may improve postnatal renal and pulmonary function. Minimum invasive nephroamniotic or vesicoamniotic stenting is the preferred method of treatment. Vesicoamniotic stenting effectively reverses oligohydramnios. However, its ability to achieve sustainable good renal function in infancy is variable.[278] For instance, pulmonary function cannot be assured with restoration of AF.[278] Amnioinfusion may play a role in the uterine evaluation and treatment of fetal obstructive uropathy, but the risks of chorioamnionitis, premature rupture of membranes, and premature labor are significant.[279] Recently, others have once again stressed that greater standardization of patient selection, diagnosis, treatment, and outcome measurement is of paramount importance to allow an accurate assessment of the efficacy and proper role of fetal therapy.[258] In the past, poor patient selection has led to futile attempts to intervene in hopeless cases, while fetuses who would have done well, even without intervention, may have been put at unnecessary risk by operative procedures. Although multiple studies with animal models have shown the benefits of midgestational intervention, no data seem to be available from randomized control trials to compare survival and postnatal renal function with and without vesicoamniotic shunt replacement.[280]

THE FETAL CENTRAL NERVOUS SYSTEM

The ultrasonic features of most central nervous system (CNS) structures are well documented. Transvaginal sonography has further refined the imaging of the normal developing CNS. Transvaginal scanning of the fetal brain can be carried out if the fetus is in the vertex position. Using this approach, coronal, sagittal, and parasagittal sections of the developing brain can be obtained.[281,282] The midcoronal section is of particular importance, because it not only contains parts of the lateral ventricles but also displays essential midline structures such as the corpus callosum and cavum septi pellucidi. The latter is situated between the anterior horn and below the corpus callosum in the midline.[283] Although coronal and sagittal plains can be more easily obtained by transvaginal than by transabdominal approach, the former technique has limitations with respect to applicability. Some issues regarding transabdominal sonography of the fetal CNS deserve special attention regarding their clinical significance and outlook such as hydrocephaly, choroid plexus cyst, and spina bifida. Some CNS anomalies have a genetic basis.

Hydrocephaly

Hydrocephaly is characterized by a dilatation of the cerebral ventricles as a result of an increased amount of cerebrospinal fluid with an accompanying increase in intraventricular pressure and subsequently an increase in fetal head size.[284] Hydrocephaly may develop in isolation (0.4–0.9 in 1000 livebirths) but is more often associated with brainstem, cerebellar, and/or spinal defects (0.5–3 in 1000 livebirths).[284] Based on the communication between the cerebral ventricles and the subarachnoid space, hydrocephaly may be classified as noncommunicating or communicating.[284] The diagnosis can be made either from determination of the ratio of lateral ventricle to hemisphere[285] or by measurement of the lateral ventricular atrium.[286] A high ratio of lateral ventricle to hemisphere is significantly correlated with a poor psychomotor development.[287,288] Other observations that may lead to the diagnosis of hydrocephaly are dangling of the choroid plexus[289] or increased distance (>3 mm) between the choroid plexus and the medial wall of the lateral ventricle at the level of the atrium.[290] Fetal outcome in hydrocephaly is very much determined by the presence or absence of associated anomalies. Ventricular dilatation may be caused by different fetal abnormalities such as Chiari II malformation, aqueductal stenosis, Dandy–Walker malformation, intracranial masses, dysgenesis of the corpus callosum, and encephalocele.[291] Chiari II or Arnold–Chiari malformation is one of the most common causes of congenital hydrocephaly. The Arnold–Chiari malformation consists of a number of combinations of brainstem and cerebellar malformations. Usually there is associated ventriculomegaly and spinal defects (meningocele or meningomyelocele).[292] The bony posterior fossa is extremely small. The medulla and even the pons may also be displaced downward into the cervical spinal canal.[291] From the effacement of the cisterna magna[293] to the banana-shaped cerebellum or even absent cerebellum[294] these abnormal findings are almost always associated with ventriculomegaly and a spinal defect at lumbosacral level. D'Addario et al.[291] measured the so-called gestational-age-independent clivus–supraocciput angle representing the shape of the posterior fossa. A cutoff value below which a Chiari malformation can be suspected is 72 degrees.

Fetal outcome in hydrocephaly is very much determined by the presence or absence of associated anomalies. In most published series, more than one-half to two-thirds of all fetuses displayed structural and/or chromosomal anomalies in addition to hydrocephaly, resulting in perinatal death in the majority of cases.[287,295–297] Outcome appears to be better in isolated mild cerebral ventriculomegaly (ventricular atrial diameter, 10–15 mm). In a retrospective analysis of twenty-two cases, four infants displayed developmental delay at an average follow-up of 28 months.[298] Unilateral fetal ventriculomegaly is usually an isolated finding; when mild and stable, it has little measurable effect on developmental outcome.[299,300] In general, an appropriate prognosis of hydrocephaly can be given only after careful imaging of intracerebral and extracerebral anatomy as well as fetal karyotyping and TORCH (toxoplasmosis, rubella, cytomegalovirus, herpes simplex) analysis. Obstetric management is determined by the gestational age at diagnosis, the severity of the hydrocephaly or size of the fetal head, and the presence of additional anomalies. Options may include termination of pregnancy, cesarean section delivery, or vaginal delivery. Ventriculoamniotic shunt placement has proven to be unsuccessful. With increasing concern about fetuses experiencing pain, cephalocentesis is gradually being abandoned.

Choroid Plexus Cysts

The choroid plexus cyst has a uniform echogenic appearance and is located primarily in the lateral ventricles, the majority disappear by 24–25 weeks of gestation.[301] Choroid plexus cysts are usually not significant but may be associated with trisomies 18 and 21[302] (see chapter 23). Careful scanning of the entire fetus should determine other structural anomalies indicative of chromosomal or other disorders.

Agenesis of the Corpus Callosum

The corpus callosum is one of three bundles of fibers that connect the two cerebral hemispheres while forming the floor of the interhemispheric fissure and the roof of the third ventricle and the frontal horns.[303] The entire corpus callosum may be absent, or more often, there may be partial agenesis. The corpus callosum cannot be directly demonstrated on the traditional axial scan. However, indirect signs include lateral displacement of the medial walls of the anterior horns, upward displacement of the third ventricle, and enlargement of the posterior horns and atria.[303] Prenatally, it may be impossible to differentiate between the complete and incomplete forms of corpus callosum agenesis. The prognosis is not determined by how much of the corpus callosum is absent.

Spina Bifida

Spina bifida (SB) is one of the most common severe congenital defects of the central nervous system. The prevalence depends on ethnic, racial, and socioeconomic backgrounds[304] (see chapters 1 and 21). The morbidity and mortality rates are high[305] and are discussed in detail in chapter 1. Despite improvement in surgical management of SB in recent decades, resulting in improved life expectancy, no improvement in the degree of durability or quality of life of affected individuals has been shown.[306] In the United States in 1999, the lifelong costs for an individual born with SB was estimated to be about $300,000.[307] Parents faced with a diagnosis of SB and having the option to decide on the future of the pregnancy, mostly opt for termination of pregnancy. Mansfield et al.[308] reported a termination rate associated with prenatally diagnosed SB of between 20 and 100 percent, with an average of 64 percent. In a Dutch study[309] the termination rate was as high as 92 percent. In the same study, there was a striking difference in survival rate among newborns in which the condition was known prenatally (28 percent) or only after birth (79 percent). This was determined by the fact that those detected prenatally, even those diagnosed late in pregnancy, include the most severe cases, presenting with hydrocephaly, breech presentation, or polyhydramnios.

FETAL THERAPY

Over the years, some interesting developments have taken place in the treatment of fetal abnormalities (see chapter 29). Improvement in sonographic resolution, Doppler, and three-dimensional ultrasound techniques has led to better indications for closed (endoscopic) and open surgical procedures. Endoscopic treatment methods will be discussed mainly in the separate presentations on fetal anomalies, when appropriate. A distinction should be made between obstetric endoscopy and endoscopic fetal surgery.[310] The first involves surgical interventions on the placenta, umbilical cord, and fetal membranes such as yttrium–aluminum–garnet (YAG) laser coagulation of placental vessels in case of TTTS and cord occlusion in monochorionic pregnancy. The second type addresses some rare fetal conditions requiring in utero surgery (diaphragmatic hernia). Experience in fetal anomaly scanning built up over the past 20–25 years, as well as animal experimental work, has provided a better understanding of the natural history of a range of fetal anomalies. Moreover, surgical, anesthetic, and tocolytic methods for hysterotomy and fetal surgery were developed in nonhuman primates.[130] Central to any open surgical procedure on the fetus is that the advantages to the affected fetus should clearly be weighed against the procedure-related risks to the mother and fetus. Fetal surgery demands a multidisciplinary approach that includes obstetricians, neonatologists, pediatric surgeons, and geneticists as well as a dedicated infrastructure. Only a few centers in the United States are currently involved in this kind of pioneering work.

Open fetal surgical procedures have been carried out on a limited scale for obstructive uropathy, congenital diaphragmatic hernia, cystic adenomatoid malformations, sacrococcygeal teratoma, and SB[130,311–315] (see chapter 29). In a recent overview of in utero fetal surgery,[130] some success was reported in closing meningomyeloceles at the lumbosacral level and removing a fetal sacrococcygeal teratoma. It is suggested that surgical repair of this defect is preferably performed at 20–25 weeks of gestation, applying either a clear film of hyaluronic acid to the exposed spinal cord or using artificial covering in case of dura deficiency.[130]

A review of the medical records from 1981 to 1999 by Holmes et al.[315] revealed that fetal intervention for posterior urethral valves carries a considerable risk to the fetus. The long-term outcomes indicate that intervention may not change the prognosis of renal function. The same authors stated that fetal surgery for obstructive uropathy should be performed only for the carefully selected patient who has severe oligohydramnios and "normal"-appearing kidneys.

Less successful so far has also been the repair of a diaphragmatic hernia (see chapter 29). This type of anomaly may lead to pulmonary hypoplasia. Conditions for surgical repair of a diaphragmatic hernia introduced by the Philadelphia team included large-volume liver herniation, a lung–heart circumference ratio of less than 0.9, indicative of severe compression of the contralateral right lung; no associated anomalies, and a normal fetal karyotype.[130] The open hysterotomy approach for congenital diaphragmatic hernia has failed so far. Endoscopic tracheal occlusion appears to be more promising.[130,252]

ADVANCES IN IMAGING TECHNOLOGY

Progress is being made in the further technical improvement of three-dimensional (3D) and lately four-dimensional (4D) ultrasound and its application in normal and abnormal fetal development. Another technique, which is making inroads into fetal imaging, is MRI.

3D/4D Ultrasonography

The introduction of 3D ultrasonography has provided the perinatologist with new possibilities for displaying fetal anatomy as well as storage and processing of imaging data. Several rendering modes are available. The multiplanar mode enables tomographic examination of stored volumes in various small steps. The surface mode allows 3D reconstruction of well-defined regions of interest, such as cleft lip or cleft palate (Figures 24.6 and 24.7) and limb defects.[316] Detailed information has been collected on the shape and contents of the brain cavities.[317] The transparent mode is used mainly for depicting the fetal skeleton, such as ribs or spine.[318] The position of the long bones can be established in more detail in relation to the feet and hands and the hands in relation to the fingers.[319] Doppler-related 3D fetal echocardiography is a promising new method. Because it derives from a complex assembly of sequentials acquired in 2D images to allow visualization of both the heart and great vessels, this approach has some important limitations.[320]

A fourth mode includes color Doppler in conjunction with the transparent mode for the 3D visualization of the fetal vascular system. 3D ultrasound is also used for volume measurements such as fetal heart volume to determine impending fetal cardiac failure, fetal liver volume (Figure 24.8), fetal brain volume, and upper arm and fetal thigh volume in relation to fetal growth. A tenfold increase in normal fetal lung volume[124,321] and a tenfold increase in normal fetal liver volume[322] and in fetal brain volume[323] has been established during the second half of pregnancy. Also, fetal liver vascularization has been determined using 3D power Doppler ultrasound and quantitative 3D power Doppler histogram analysis. A significant gestational-age-related increase was established for the fetal vascularization index, flow index, and vascularization–flow index.[324] A disadvantage of 3D ultrasonography is the time spent on building up an image. With the introduction of

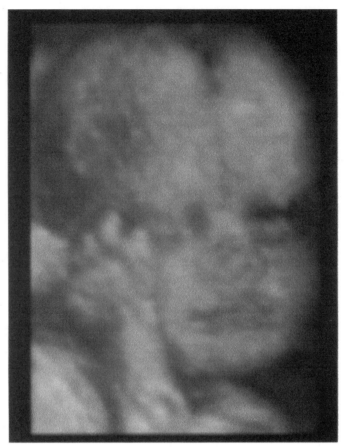

Fig. 24.6. Frontal view of a normal fetal face obtained by 3D ultrasound at 27 weeks of gestation. *Source:* Reproduced by permission of Dr. N. Roelfsema, Erasmus University Medical School.[84]

4D ultrasound, a nearly simultaneous visualization of fetal movements and depiction of the fetal surface can be obtained. This would be of particular interest in assessing cardiac volume changes with the view of determining cardiac output. However, further improvement of frame rate and image resolution is needed.

Magnetic Resonance Imaging

Under circumstances of obesity or oligohydramnios, ultrasound findings may be inconclusive. Here, MRI could be a valuable tool in the evaluation of fetal abnormalities. Until recently, the application in fetal diagnosis was very limited because of the acquisition times of several minutes in the presence of fetal movements. However, lately the development of ultrafast magnetic resonance imaging sequences has provided an acceptable solution to the problems of fetal movements.[325] MRI examinations are performed mainly to study abnormal anatomy of the central nervous system and spine,[326,327] but also other structures such as the face and neck, liver, and lungs have been clearly identified[328–330] (see chapter 25). It should be emphasized that ultrasound is still the primary imaging technique for the detection of fetal anomalies.

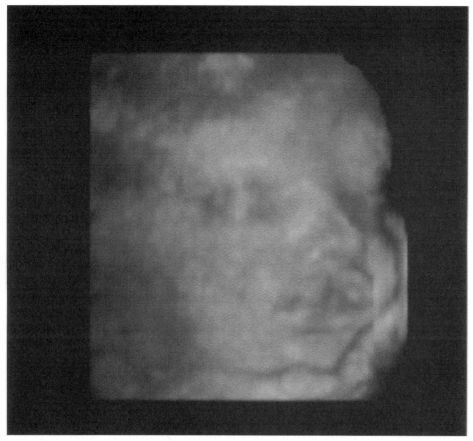

Fig. 24.7. Frontal view of a fetal face with a facial cleft obtained by 3D ultrasound at 33 weeks of gestation. *Source:* Reproduced by permission of Dr. N. Roelfsema, Erasmus University Medical School.[84]

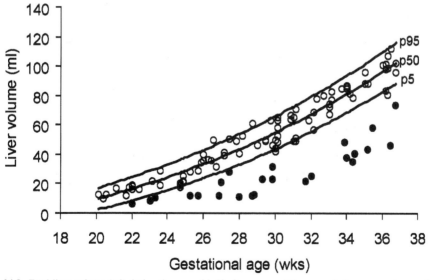

Fig. 24.8. Fetal liver volume (ml) during the second half of pregnancy. The open circles represent normal fetal development; the closed circles represent fetal growth restriction. *Source:* Boito et al. 2002.[322] Reproduced by permission of *Radiology*.

ACKNOWLEDGMENT

I wish to thank my secretary, Mrs. Sylvia Sollie-Breur, for checking the layout and typing of the manuscript.

REFERENCES

1. Whiteman DAH, Klinger K. Efficiency of rapid in situ hybridization methods for prenatal diagnosis of chromosome abnormalities causing birth defects. Am J Hum Genet 1991;49:A1279.
2. Philip J, Bryndorf T, Christensen B. Prenatal aneuploidy detection in interphase cells by fluorescence in situ hybridization (FISH). Prenat Diagn 1994;4:1203.
3. Gersen SL, Carelli MP, Klinger KW, et al. Rapid prenatal diagnosis of 14 cases of triploidy using FISH with multiple probes. Prenat Diagn 1995;15:1.
4. Veltman JA, Schoenmakers EF, Eussen BH, et al. High-throughput analysis of subtelomeric chromosome rearrangements by use of array-based comparative genomic hybridization. Am J Hum Genet 2002;70:1269.
5. Ghidini A, Sepulveda W, Lockwood CJ, et al. Complications of fetal blood sampling. Am J Obstet Gynecol 1993;168:1339.
6. Weiner CP. Human fetal bilirubin levels and fetal hemolytic disease. Am J Obstet Gynecol 1992;166:1449.
7. Mari G, Detti L, Oz U, et al. Accurate prediction of fetal hemoglobin by Doppler ultrasonography. Obstet Gynecol 2000;99:589.
8. Divakaran TG, Waugh J, Clark TJ, et al. Noninvasive techniques to detect fetal anemia due to red blood cell alloimmunization: a systematic review. Obstet Gynecol 2001;98:509.
9. Kovacs BW, Carlson DE, Sharbahrami B, et al. Prenatal diagnosis of human parvovirus B19 in nonimmune hydrops fetalis by polymerase chain reaction. Am J Obstet Gynecol 1992;167:461.
10. Pardi G, Cetin I, Marconi AM, et al. Diagnostic value of blood sampling in fetuses with growth retardation. N Engl J Med 1993;328:692.
11. Cetin I, Marconi AM, Corbetta C, et al. Fetal amino acids in normal pregnancies and in pregnancies complicated by intrauterine growth retardation. Early Hum Dev 1992;29:183.
12. Johnson P, Sharland G, Allan LD, et al. Umbilical venous pressure in nonimmune hydrops fetalis: correlation with cardiac size. Am J Obstet Gynecol 1992;167:1309.
13. Saino S, Teramo K, Kekomaki R. Prenatal treatment of severe fetomaternal alloimmune thrombocytopenia. Transfus Med 1999;9:321.
14. Elias S. Use of fetoscopy for the prenatal diagnosis of hereditary skin disorders. Curr Probl Dermatol 1987;16:1.
15. Robinson JS, Moore VM, Owens JA, et al. Origins of fetal growth restriction. Eur J Obstet Gynecol Reprod Biol 2000;92:13.
16. Holmes RP, Soothill PW. Intra-uterine growth retardation. Curr Opin Obstet Gynecol 1996;8:148.
17. Sanderson DA, Wilcox MA, Johnson IR. The individualised birthweight ratio: a new method of identifying intrauterine growth retardation. Br J Obstet Gynaecol 1994;101:310.
18. Scherjon SA, Smolders-de Haas H, Kok JH, et al. The brain-sparing effect: antenatal cerebral Doppler findings in relation to neurologic outcome in very preterm infants. Am J Obstet Gynecol 1993;169:169.
19. Barker DJP, Gluckman PD, Godfrey KM, et al. Fetal nutrition and cardiovascular disease in adult life. Lancet 1993;341:938.
20. Smith GC, McNay MB, Fleming JE. The relation between fetal abdominal circumference and birthweight: findings in 3512 pregnancies. Br J Obstet Gynaecol 1997;104:186.
21. Kupferminc MJ, Many A, Bar-Am A et al. Mid-trimester severe intrauterine growth restriction is associated with a high prevalence of thrombophilia. Br J Obstet Gynaecol 2002;109:1373.
22. Higgins S. Smoking in pregnancy. Curr Opin Obstet Gynecol 2002;14:145.
23. Soothill PW, Ajayi RA, Campbell S. Fetal oxygenation at cordocentesis, maternal smoking and childhood neuro-development. Eur J Obstet Gynecol Reprod Biol 1995;59:21.
24. Kalousek DK. Current topic: Confined placental mosaicism and intrauterine fetal development. Placenta 1994;15:219.
25. Wolstenholme J, Rooney DE, Davison EV. Confined placental mosaicism, IUGR and adverse pregnancy outcome: a controlled retrospective U.K. collaborative survey. Prenat Diagn 1994;14:345.
26. Wapner RJ, Simpson JL, Golbus MS, et al. Chorionic mosaicism: association with fetal loss but not with adverse perinatal outcome. Prenat Diagn 1992;12:347.
27. Roland B, Lynch L, Berkowitz G, et al. Confined placental mosaicism in CVS and pregnancy outcome. Prenat Diagn 1994;14:589.

28. Reddy NS, Blakemore KL, Stetten G, et al. The significance of trisomy 7 mosaicism in chorionic villus cultures. Prenat Diagn 1990;10:417.

29. Kalousek DK, Langlois S, Barrett IJ, et al. Uniparental disomy for chromosome 16 in humans. Am J Hum Genet 1993;52:8.

30. Engel E. Uniparental disomy, isodisomy and imprinting: probable effects in man and strategies for their detection. Am J Med Genet 1993;40:670.

31. Vaughan J, Zehra A, Bower S, et al. Human maternal uniparental disomy for chromosome 16 and fetal development. Prenat Diagn 1994;14:751.

32. U.S. General Accounting Office. Drug exposed infants. Washington, DC: Government Printing Office, 1990. GAO/HRD publication no. 90–138.

33. Kesrouani A, Fallet C, Vuillard E, et al. Pathologic and laboratory correlation in microcephaly associated with prenatal cocaine exposure. Early Hum Dev 2001;63:79.

34. Hoyme HE, Jones KL, Dixon SD, et al. Prenatal cocaine exposure and fetal vascular disruption. Pediatrics 1990;85:743.

35. Mitra SC, Seshan SV, Salcedo JR, et al. Maternal cocaine abuse and fetal renal arteries: a morphometric study. Pediatr Nephrol 2000;14:315.

36. Van den Anker JN, Cohen-Overbeek TE, Wladimiroff JW, et al. Prenatal diagnosis of limb-reduction defects due to maternal cocaine use. Lancet 1991;338;1332.

37. Esmer MC, Rodriguez-Soto G, Carrasco-Daza D, et al. Cloverleaf skull and multiple congenital anomalies in a girl exposed to cocaine in utero: case report and review of the literature. Childs Nerv Syst 2000;16:176.

38. Hadeed AJ, Siegel SR. Maternal cocaine use during pregnancy: effect on the newborn infant. Pediatrics 1989;84:205.

39. Plessinger MA, Woods JR Jr. Maternal, placental, and fetal pathophysiology of cocaine exposure during pregnancy. Clin Obstet Gynecol 1993;36:267.

40. Hannigan JH, Armant DR. Alcohol in pregnancy and neonatal outcome. Semin Neonatol 2000;5:243.

41. Eustace LW, Kang DH, Coombs D. Fetal alcohol syndrome: a growing concern for health care professionals. J Obstet Gynecol Neonatal Nurs 2003;32:215.

42. Gabriel R, Alsat E, Evain-Brion D. Alterations of epidermal growth factor receptor in placental membranes of smokers: relationship with intrauterine growth retardation. Am J Obstet Gynecol 1994;170:1238.

43. Yoneyama Y, Shin S, Iwasaki T, et al. Relationship between plasma adenosine concentration and breathing movements in growth-retarded fetuses. Am J Obstet Gynecol 1994;171:701.

44. Cetin I, Morpurgo PS, Radaelli T, et al. Fetal plasma leptin concentrations: relationship with different intrauterine growth patterns from 19 weeks to term. Pediatr Res 2000;48:646.

45. Ville Y, Proudler A, Abbas A, et al. Atrial natriuretic factor concentration in normal, growth retarded, anemic, and hydropic fetuses. Am J Obstet Gynecol 1994;171:777.

46. Rizzo G, Montuschi P, Capponi A, et al. Blood levels of vasoactive intestinal polypeptide in normal and growth retarded fetuses: relationship with acid-base and haemodynamic status. Early Hum Dev 1995;41:69.

47. Bocconi L, Mauro F, Maddalena SE, et al. Insulinlike growth factor 1 in controls and growth-retarded fetuses. Fetal Diagn Ther 1998;13:192.

48. McKenna D, Tharmaratnam S, Mahsud S, et al. A randomized trial using ultrasound to identify the high-risk fetus in a low-risk population. Obstet Gynecol 2003;101:626.

49. Gagnon R, Van den Hof M, Bly S, et al. The use of fetal Doppler in obstetrics. J Obstet Gynaecol Can 2003;25:601.

50. Vergani P, Roncaglia N, Andreotti C, et al. Prognostic value of uterine artery Doppler velocimetry in growth-restricted fetuses delivered near term. Am J Obstet Gynecol 2002;187:932.

51. Trudinger BJ, Giles WB, Cook CM, et al. Fetal umbilical artery flow velocity waveforms and placental resistance: clinical significance. Br J Obstet Gynaecol 1985;92:23.

52. Groenenberg IAL, Wladimiroff JW, Hop WCJ. Fetal cardiac and peripheral arterial flow velocity waveforms in intrauterine growth retardation. Circulation 1989;80:1711.

53. Farine D, Kelly EN, Ryan G, et al. Absent and reversed umbilical artery end-diastolic velocity. In: Copel JA, Reed KL, eds. Doppler ultrasound in obstetrics and gynecology. New York: Raven, 1995:187.

54. Hecher K, Campbell S, Doyle P, et al. Assessment of fetal compromise by Doppler ultrasound investigation of the fetal circulation. Circulation 1995;91:129.

55. Stigter RH, Mulder EJH, Bruinse HW, et al. Doppler studies on the fetal renal artery in the severely growth-restricted fetus. Ultrasound Obstet Gynecol 2001;18:141.

56. Gembruch U. Assessment of the fetal circulatory state in uteroplacental insufficiency by Doppler ultrasound: which vessels are the most practicable? Ultrasound Obstet Gynecol 1996;8:77.

57. Wladimiroff JW, Tonge HM, Stewart PA. Doppler ultrasound assessment of cerebral blood flow in the human fetus. Br J Obstet Gynaecol 1986;93:471.

58. Mari G, Uerpairojkit B, Abuhamad AZ, et al. Adrenal artery velocity waveforms in the appropriate and small-for-gestational-age fetus. Ultrasound Obstet Gynecol 1996;8:82.

59. Baschat AA, Gembruch U. Evaluation of the fetal coronary circulation. Ultrasound Obstet Gynecol 2002;20:405.

60. Morin FC III, Weiss KT. Response of the fetal circulation to stress. In: Polin RA, Fox WW, eds. Fetal and neonatal physiology. Philadelphia: WB Saunders, 1992:620.

61. Haworth SG. Development of the pulmonary circulation: Morphological aspects. In: Polin RA, Fox WW, eds. Fetal and neonatal physiology. Philadelphia: WB Saunders, 1992:667.

62. Korszun P, Dubiel M, Breborowicz G, et al. Fetal superior mesenteric artery blood flow velocimetry in normal and high-risk pregnancy. J Perinat Med 2002;30:235.

63. Rizzo G, Arduini D, Romanini C. Doppler echocardiographic assessment of fetal cardiac function. Ultrasound Obstet Gynecol 1992;2:434.

64. Rizzo G, Capponi A, Rinaldo D, et al. Ventricular ejection force in growth-retarded fetuses. Ultrasound Obstet Gynecol 1995;5:247.

65. Makikallio K, Vuolteenaho O, Jouppila P, et al. Ultrasonographic and biochemical markers of human fetal cardiac dysfunction in placental insufficiency. Circulation 2002;105:2058.

66. Reed KL, Chaffin DG, Anderson CF. Umbilical venous Doppler velocity pulsations and inferior vena cava pressure elevation in fetal lambs. Obstet Gynecol 1996;87:617.

67. Baschat AA, Gembruch U, Reiss I, et al. Relationship between arterial and venous Doppler and perinatal outcome in fetal growth restriction. Ultrasound Obstet Gynecol 2000;16:407.

68. Hofstaetter C, Gudmundsson S, Hansmann M. Venous Doppler velocimetry in the surveillance of severely compromised fetuses. Ultrasound Obstet Gynecol 2002;20:233.

69. Whittle MJ, Hanretty KP, Primrose MH, et al. Screening for the compromised fetus: a randomized trial of umbilical artery velocimetry in unselected pregnancies. Am J Obstet Gynecol 1994;170:555.

70. Westergaard HB, Langhoff-Roos J, Lingman G, et al. A critical appraisal of the use of umbilical artery Doppler ultrasound in high-risk pregnancies: use of meta-analyses in evidence-based obstetrics. Ultrasound Obstet Gynecol 2001;17:466.

71. Figueras F, Martinez JM, Puerto B, et al. Contraction stress test versus ductus venosus Doppler evaluation for the prediction of adverse perinatal outcome in growth-restricted fetuses with non-reassuring non-stress test. Ultrasound Obstet Gynecol 2003;21:250.

72. Hecher K, Bilardo CM, Stigter RH, et al. Monitoring of fetuses with intrauterine growth restriction: a longitudinal study. Ultrasound Obstet Gynecol 2001;18:564.

73. Barbera A, Galan HL, Ferrazzi E, et al. Relationship of umbilical vein blood flow to growth parameters in the human fetus. Am J Obstet Gynecol 1999;181:174.

74. Boito S, Struijk PC, Ursem NT, et al. Umbilical venous volume flow in the normally developing and growth-restricted fetus. Ultrasound Obstet Gynecol 2002;19:344.

75. Boito S, Struijk PC, Ursem NT, et al. Fetal brain/liver volume ratio and umbilical volume flow parameters relative to normal and abnormal human development. Ultrasound Obstet Gynecol 2003;21:256.

76. Kiserud T, Rasmussen S, Skulstad S. Blood flow and the degree of shunting through the ductus venosus in the human fetus. Am J Obstet Gynecol 2000;182:147.

77. Gardiner H, Brodszki J, Eriksson A, et al. Volume blood flow estimation in the normal and growth-restricted fetus. Ultrasound Med Biol 2002;28:1107.

78. Fuhrmann K, Reiher H, Semmler K, et al. Prevention of congenital malformations in infants of insulin-dependent diabetic mothers. Diabetes Care 1983;6:219.

79. Kjos SL, Schaefer-Graf U, Sardesi S, et al. A randomized controlled trial using glycemic plus fetal ultrasound parameters versus glycemic parameters to determine insulin therapy in gestational diabetes with fasting hyperglycemia. Diabetes Care 2001;24:1904.

80. Rossi G, Somigliana E, Moschetta M, et al. Adequate timing of fetal ultrasound to guide metabolic therapy in mild gestational diabetes mellitus: results from a randomized study. Acta Obstet Gynecol Scand 2000;79:649.

81. Landon MB. Prenatal diagnosis of macrosomia in pregnancy complicated by diabetes mellitus. J Matern Fetal Med 2000;9:52.

82. Brace RA. Physiology of amniotic fluid volume regulation. Clin Obstet Gynecol 1997;40:280.

83. Wladimiroff JW, Campbell S. Fetal urine production rates in normal and complicated pregnancy. Lancet 1974;1:151.

84. Mann SE, Nijland MJ, Ross MG. Mathematic modelling of human amniotic fluid dynamics. Am J Obstet Gynecol 1996175:937.
85. Gilbert WM, Brace RA. Amniotic fluid volume and normal flows to and from the amniotic cavity. Semin Perinatol 1993;17:150.
86. Ross MG, Nijland MJ. Fetal swallowing: relation to amniotic fluid regulation. Clin Obstet Gynecol 1997;40:352.
87. Sherer DM, Langer O. Oligohydramnios: use and misuse in clinical management. Ultrasound Obstet Gynecol 2001;18:411.
88. Manning FA, Hill LM, Platt LD. Qualitative amniotic fluid volume determination by ultrasound: antepartum detection of intrauterine growth retardation. Am J Obstet Gynecol 1981;139:254.
89. Magann EF, Nolan TE, Hess LW, et al. Measurement of amniotic fluid volume: accuracy of ultrasonography techniques. Am J Obstet Gynecol 1992;167:1533.
90. Rutherford SE, Phelan JP, Smith CV, et al. The four-quadrant assessment of amniotic fluid volume: an adjunct to antepartum fetal heart rate testing. Obstet Gynecol 1987;70:353.
91. Mercer LJ, Brown LG. Fetal outcome with oligohydramnios in the second trimester. Obstet Gynecol 1986;67:840.
92. Magann EF, Chauhan SP, Bofill JA, et al. Comparability of the amniotic fluid index and single deepest pocket measurements in clinical practice. Aust NZ J Obstet Gynaecol 2003;43:75.
93. Shipp TD, Bromley B, Pauker S, et al. Outcome of singleton pregnancies with severe oligohydramnios in the second and third trimesters. Ultrasound Obstet Gynecol 1996;7:108.
94. Moore TR, Longo J, Leopold GR, et al. The reliability and predictive value of an amniotic fluid scoring system in severe second-trimester oligohydramnios. Obstet Gynecol 1989;73:739.
95. Chamberlain PF, Manning FA, Morrison I, et al. Ultrasound evaluation of amniotic fluid volume. II. The relationship of increased amniotic fluid volumes to perinatal outcome. Am J Obstet Gynecol 1984;150:250.
96. Golan A, Lin G, Evron S. Oligohydramnios: maternal complications and fetal outcome in 145 cases. Gynecol Obstet Invest 1994;37:91.
97. Hadi HA, Hodson CA, Strickland D. Premature rupture of the membranes between 20 and 25 weeks' gestation: role of amniotic fluid volume in perinatal outcome. Am J Obstet Gynecol 1994;170:1139.
98. Phelan JP, Martin GI. Polyhydramnios: fetal and neonatal implications. Clin Perinatol 1989;16:987.
99. Croom CS, Bainias BB, Ramos-Santo E. Do semiquantitative amniotic fluid indexes reflect actual volume? Am J Obstet Gynecol 1992;167:995.
100. Ben-Chetrit A, Hochner-Celnikier D, Ron M, et al. Hydramnios in the third trimester of pregnancy: a change in the distribution of accompanying fetal anomalies as a result of early ultrasonographic prenatal diagnosis. Am J Obstet Gynecol 1990;612:1344.
101. Brady K, Polzin WJ, Kopelman JN, et al. Risk of chromosomal abnormalities in patients with idiopathic polyhydramnios. Obstet Gynecol 1992;79:234.
102. Carlson DE, Platt LD, Medearis AL, et al. Quantifiable polyhydramnios: diagnosis and management. Obstet Gynecol 1990;75:989.
103. Zahn CM, Hankins GDV, Yeomans ER. Karyotypic abnormalities and hydramnios: role of amniocentesis. J Reprod Med 1993;38:559.
104. Dashe JS, McIntire DD, Ramus RM et al. Hydramnios: anomaly prevalence and sonographic detection. Obstet Gynecol 2002;100:134.
105. Barnhard Y, Bar-Hava I, Divon MY. Is polyhydramnios in an ultrasonographically normal fetus an indication for genetic evaluation? Am J Obstet Gynecol 1995;173:1523.
106. Many A, Lazebnik N, Hill LM. The underlying cause of polyhydramnios determines prematurity. Prenat Diagn 1996;16:55.
107. Hill LM, Lazebnik N, Many A, et al. Resolving polyhydramnios: clinical significance and subsequent neonatal outcome. Ultrasound Obstet Gynecol 1995;6:421.
108. Kitterman JA. Fetal lung development. J Dev Physiol 1984;6:67.
109. DiFiore JW, Wilson JM. Lung development. Semin Pediatr Surg 1994;3:221.
110. Sherer DM, Davis JM, Woods JR. Pulmonary hypoplasia: a review. Obstet Gynecol Surv 1990;45:792.
111. Liggins GC. Growth of the fetal lung. J Dev Physiol 1984;6:237.
112. Pringle KC. Human fetal lung development and related animal models. Clin Obstet Gynecol 1986;29:502.
113. Page DV, Stocker JT. Anomalies associated with pulmonary hypoplasia. Am Rev Respir Dis 1982;125:216.
114. Thurlbeck WM. Prematurity and the developing lung. Clin Perinatol 1992;19:497.
115. Levin DL. Morphologic analysis of the pulmonary vascular bed in congenital left-sided diaphragmatic hernia. J Pediatr 1978;92:805.

116. Moessinger AC, Santiago A, Paneth NS, et al. Time-trends in necropsy prevalence and birth prevalence of lung hypoplasia. Paediatr Perinat Epidemiol 1989;3:421.

117. Kilbride HW, Yeast J, Thibeault DW. Defining limits of survival: lethal pulmonary hypoplasia after premature rupture of membranes. Am J Obstet Gynecol 1996;175:675.

118. Rudd EG. Premature rupture of the membranes: a review. J Reprod Med 1985;30:843.

119. McIntosh N, Harrison A. Prolonged premature rupture of membranes in the preterm infant: a 7 year study. Eur J Obstet Gynecol Reprod Biol 1994;57:1.

120. Lauria MR, Gonik, Romero R. Pulmonary hypoplasia: pathogenesis, diagnosis and antenatal prediction. Obstet Gynecol 1995;86:466.

121. Blott M, Greenough A, Nicolaides KH, et al. The ultrasonography assessment of the fetal thorax and fetal breathing movements in the prediction of pulmonary hypoplasia. Early Hum Dev 1990;21:143.

122. Fisk NM, Talbert DG, Nicolini U, et al. Fetal breathing movements in oligohydramnios are not increased by amnioinfusion. Br J Obstet Gynaecol 1992;99:464.

123. Laudy JAM, Tibboel D, Robben SGF, et al. Prenatal prediction of fetal pulmonary hypoplasia: clinical biometric and Doppler velocity correlates. Pediatrics 2002;109:259.

124. Laudy JA, Janssen MM, Struyk PC, et al. Three-dimensional ultrasonography of normal fetal lung volume: a preliminary study. Ultrasound Obstet Gynecol 1998;11:13.

125. Fuke S, Kanzaki T, Mu J, et al. Antenatal prediction of pulmonary hypoplasia by acceleration time/ejection time ratio of fetal pulmonary arteries by Doppler blood flow velocimetry. Am J Obstet Gynecol 2003;188:228.

126. Watson J, Campbell S. Antenatal evaluation and management in nonimmune hydrops fetalis. Obstet Gynecol 1986;67:589.

127. Jordan JA, Huff D, DeLoia JA. Placental cellular immune response in women infected with human parvovirus B19 during pregnancy. Clin Diagn Lab Immunol 2001;8:288.

128. Winn HN. Non-immune fetal hydrops. In: The fetus as a patient. Chervenak FA, Kurjak A, Papp Z, eds. New York: Parthenon, 2002:229.

129. Castillo R, Devoe L, Hadi H, et al. Pleural effusions and pulmonary hypoplasia. Am J Obstet Gynecol 1987;157:1252.

130. Coleman BG, Adzick S, Crombleholme TM, et al. Fetal therapy: state of the art. J Ultrasound Med 2002;21:1257.

131. Santolaya J, Alley D, Jaffe R, et al. Antenatal classification of hydrops fetalis. Obstet Gynecol 1992;79:256.

132. Denbow ML, Cox P, Talbert D, Fisk NM. Colour Doppler energy insonation of placental vasculature in monochorionic twins: absent arterio-arterial anastomoses in association with twin-to-twin transfusion syndrome. Br J Obstet Gynaecol 1998;105:760.

133. Quintero R, Quintero L, Bornick P, et al. The donor-recipient (D-R score): in vivo endoscopic evidence to support the hypothesis of a net transfer of blood from donor to recipient in twin-twin transfusion syndrome. Prenat Neonat Med 2000;5:84.

134. Fisk N. The scientific basis of feto-fetal transfusion syndrome and its treatment. In: Ward R, Whittle M, eds. Multiple pregnancy. London: RCOG Press, 1995:235.

135. Denbow ML, Cox P, Taylor M, et al. Placental angioarchitecture in monochorionic twin pregnancies: relationship to growth, feto-fetal transfusion syndrome, and pregnancy outcome. Am J Obstet Gynecol 2000;182:417.

136. Taylor MJO, Talbert DG, Fisk NM. Mapping the monochorionic equator: the new frontier. Ultrasound Obstet Gynecol 1999;14:372.

137. Quintero R, Morales W, Allen M, et al. Staging of twin-twin transfusion syndrome. J Perinatol 1999;19:550.

138. Weir P, Ratten G, Beischner N. Acute polyhydramnios: a complication of monozygous twin pregnancy. Br J Obstet Gynaecol 1979;86:849.

139. Elliott JP, Sawyer AT, Radin TG, et al. Large-volume therapeutic amniocentesis in the treatment of hydramnios. Obstet Gynecol 1994;84:1025.

140. Ville Y, Hecher K, Gagnon A, et al. Endoscopic laser coagulation in the management of severe twin-to-twin transfusion syndrome. Br J Obstet Gynaecol 1998;105:446.

141. Hecher K, Plath H, Bregenzer R, et al. Endoscopic laser surgery versus serial amniocentesis in the treatment of severe twin-twin transfusion syndrome. Am J Obstet Gynecol 1999;180:717.

142. Quintero RA, Comas C, Bornick PW, et al. Selective versus non-selective laser photocoagulation of placental vessels in twin-twin transfusion syndrome. Ultrasound Obstet Gynecol 2000;16:230.

143. Quintero R, Quintero L, Morales W, et al. Amniotic fluid pressures in severe twin-twin transfusion syndrome. Prenat Neonat Med 1998;3:607.

144. Gratacos E, Van Schoubroeck D, Carreras E, et al. Impact of laser coagulation in severe twin-twin trans-

fusion syndrome on fetal Doppler indices and venous blood flow volume. Ultrasound Obstet Gynecol 2002;20:125.

145. Ville Y, Hyett J, Hecher K, et al. Management of severe twin-twin transfusion: amniodrainage compared to endoscopic surgery (abstract). Ultrasound Obstet Gynecol 1994;4:130.

146. Lemery D, Vanlieferinghen P, Gasq M, et al. Fetal umbilical cord ligation under ultrasound guidance. Ultrasound Obstet Gynecol 1994;4:399.

147. Quintero R, Romero R, Reich H, et al. In utero percutaneous umbilical cord ligation in the management of complicated monochorionic multiple gestations. Ultrasound Obstet Gynecol 1996;8:16.

148. Deprest JA, Audibert F, Van Schoubroeck D, et al. Bipolar coagulation of the umbilical cord in complicated monochorionic twin pregnancy. Am J Obstet Gynecol 2000;182:240.

149. King AD, Soothill PW, Montemagno R. Twin to twin transfusion in a dichorionic pregnancy without the oligohydramnios-polyhydramnios sequence. Br J Obstet Gynaecol 1995;102:334.

150. Wladimiroff JW. Routine ultrasonography for the detection of fetal structural anomalies. In: Wildschut HIJ, Weiner CP, Peter TJ, eds. When to screen in obstetrics and gynaecology. London: WB Saunders, 1996:108.

151. Cornel MC, De Wall HEK, Haveman TM, et al. Birth prevalence of congenital anomalies in the Northern Netherlands. Ned Tijdschr Geneeskd 1991;135:2032.

152. Campbell M. Incidence of cardiac malformations at birth and later, and neonatal mortality. Br Heart J 1973;35:189.

153. Young ID, Clarke M. Lethal malformations and perinatal mortality: a 10 year review with comparison of ethnic differences. BMJ 1987;295:89.

154. Keith JD. Prevalence, incidence and epidemiology. In: Keith JD, Row RD, Vlad P, eds. Heart disease in infancy and childhood. New York: MacMillan Publishing, 1978:3.

155. Nora JJ, Hart-Nora A. The genetic contribution to congenital heart diseases. In: Nora JJ, Takao A, eds. Congenital heart disease: causes and processes. Mount Kisko, NY: Futura Publishing, 1984:3.

156. Allan LD, Crawford DC, Anderson RH, et al. Echocardiographic and anatomical correlations in fetal congenital heart disease. Br Heart J 1984;52:542.

157. Copel JA, Pilu G, Green J, et al. Fetal echocardiographic screening for congenital heart disease: the importance of the four-chamber view. Am J Obstet Gynecol 1987;157:648.

158. Cullen S, Sharland GK, Allan LD, et al. Potential impact of population screening for prenatal diagnosis of congenital heart disease. Arch Dis Child 1992;67:775.

159. Wladimiroff JW, Stewart PA, Sachs ES, et al. Prenatal diagnosis and management of congenital heart defects: significance of associated fetal anomalies and prenatal chromosome studies. Am J Med Genet 1985;21:285.

160. Wladimiroff JW, Stewart PA. Treatment of fetal arrhythmias. Br J Hosp Med 1985;34:134.

161. Zerres K, Rudnik-Schöneborn S. Genetic counseling in families with congenital heart defects. In: Yagel S, Silverman NH, Gembruch U, eds. Fetal cardiology. London: Martin Dunitz-Taylor & Francis Group, 2003:520.

162. Wessels MW, Los FJ, Frohn-Mulder IM, et al. Poor outcome in Down syndrome fetuses with cardiac anomalies or growth retardation. Am J Med Genet 2003;116A:147.

163. Buskens E, Stewart PA, Hess J, et al. Efficacy of fetal echocardiography and yield by risk category. Obstet Gynecol 1996;87:423.

164. Chaoui R. The four-chamber view: four reasons why it seems to fail in screening for cardiac abnormalities and suggestions to improve detection rate. Ultrasound Obstet Gynecol 2003;22:3.

165. Allan LD. Cardiac anatomy screening: what is the best time for screening in pregnancy? Curr Opin Obstet Gynecol 2003;15:143.

166. Yagel S, Achiron R. First and early second trimester of fetal heart screening. In: Yagel S, Silverman NH, Gembruch U, eds. Fetal cardiology. London: Martin Dunitz-Taylor & Francis Group, 2003:160.

167. Wong SF, Chan FY, Cincotta RB, et al. Factors influencing the prenatal detection of structural congenital heart diseases. Ultrasound Obstet Gynecol 2003;21:19.

168. Chaoui R, McEwing R. Three cross-sectional planes for fetal color Doppler echocardiography. Ultrasound Obstet Gynecol 2003;21:81.

169. Huggon IC. Practical guide to fetal echocardiography. Prenat Neonat Med 2001;6:38.

170. Petrikovsky B, Klein V, Herrara M. Prenatal diagnosis of intra-atrial cardiac echogenic foci. Prenat Diagn 1998;18:968.

171. Wax JR, Cartin A, Pinette MG, et al. Sonographic grading of fetal intracardiac echogenic foci in a population at low risk of aneuploidy. J Clin Ultrasound 2003;31:31.

172. Rizzo G, Arduini D, Romanini C, et al. Doppler echocardiographic assessment of atrioventricular velocity waveforms in normal and small for gestational age fetuses. Br J Obstet Gynaecol 1988;95:65.

173. Groenenberg IAL, Hop WCJ, Wladimiroff JW. Doppler flow velocity waveforms in the fetal cardiac out-flow tract: reproducibility of waveform recording and analysis. Ultrasound Med Biol 1991;17:583.

174. Rizzo G, Arduini D, Romanini C, et al. Doppler echocardiographic evaluation of time to peak velocity in aorta and pulmonary artery of small for gestational age fetuses. Br J Obstet Gynaecol 1990;97:603.

175. Al Ghazali W, Chita SK, Chapman MG, et al. Evidence of redistribution of cardiac output in asymmetrical growth retardation. Br J Obstet Gynaecol 1989;96:697.

176. Tsyvian PB, Malkin K, Wladimiroff JW. Assessment of mitral A-wave transit time to cardiac outflow tract and isovolumic relaxation time of the left ventricle in the appropriate and small-for-gestational age human fetus. Ultrasound Med Biol 1997;23:187.

177. Friedman D, Buyon J, Kim M, et al. Fetal cardiac function assessed by Doppler myocardial performance index (Tei Index). Ultrasound Obstet Gynecol 2003;21:33.

178. Fyler DC, Buckley LP, Hellenbrand WE, et al. Report of the New England Regional Cardiac Program. Pediatrics 1980;65:375.

179. Brons JT, Van Geijn HP, Wladimiroff JW, et al. Prenatal ultrasound diagnosis of the Holt Oram syndrome. Prenat Diagn 1988;8:175.

180. Kleinman CS, Donnerstein RL, DeVore GR, et al. Fetal echocardiography for evaluation of in utero congestive heart failure: a technique for study of nonimmune fetal hydrops. N Engl J Med 1982;306:568.

181. Machado MV, Crawford DC, Anderson RH, et al. Atrioventricular septal defect in prenatal life. Br Heart J 1988;59:352.

182. Jeanty P, Prandstraller A, Perolo A, et al. Prenatal diagnosis of congenital heart disease: septal defects and outflow obstructions. In: Wladimiroff JW, Pilu G, eds. Ultrasound and the fetal heart. London: Parthenon, 1996:47.

183. Hornberger LK, Sahn DJ, Kleinman CS, et al. Antenatal diagnosis of coarctation of the aorta: a multicenter experience. J Am Coll Cardiol 1994;23:417.

184. Silverman NH, Enderlein MA, Golbus MS. Ultrasonic recognition of the aortic valve atresia in utero. Am J Cardiol 1984;53:391.

185. Prandstraller D, Pilu G, Perolo A, et al. Prenatal diagnosis of conotruncal malformations. In: Wladimiroff JW, Pilu G, eds. Ultrasound and the fetal heart. New York: Parthenon, 1996:61.

186. Masuda M, Kado H, Kajihara N, et al. Early and late results of total correction of congenital cardiac anomalies in infancy. Jpn J Thorac Cardiovasc Surg 2001;49:497.

187. Birk E, Silverman NH. Intracardiac shunt malformations. In: Yagel S, Silverman NH, Gembruch U, eds. Fetal cardiology. London: Martin Dunitz-Taylor & Francis Group, 2003:201.

188. Allan LD, Apfel HD, Printz BF. Outcome after prenatal diagnosis of the hypoplastic left heart syndrome. Heart 1998;79:371.

189. Shi-Joon Yoo, Hornberger LK, Smallhorn JF. Ventricular outflow tract anomalies. In: Yagel S, Silverman NH, Gembruch U, eds. Fetal cardiology. London: Martin Dunitz-Taylor & Francis Group, 2003:223.

190. Allan LD, Sharland GB, Milburn A, et al. Prospective diagnosis of 1,006 consecutive cases of congenital heart disease in the fetus. J Am Coll Cardiol 1994;23:1452.

191. Paladini D, Rustico M, Todros T, et al. Conotruncal anomalies in prenatal life. Ultrasound Obstet Gynecol 1996;8:241.

192. Tworetzky W, McElhinney DB, Reddy VM, et al. Improved outcome after fetal diagnosis of hypoplastic left heart syndrome. Circulation 2001;103:1269.

193. Mahle WT, Clancy RR, McGaurn SP, et al. Impact of prenatal diagnosis on survival and neurologic morbidity in neonates with the hypoplastic left heart syndrome. Pediatrics 2001;107:1277.

194. Parry AJ, Hanley FL. Prospects for fetal cardiac surgery. In: Yagel S, Silverman NH, Gembruch U, eds. Fetal cardiology. London: Martin Dunitz-Taylor & Francis Group, 2003;485.

195. Franklin O, Burch M, Manning N, et al. Prenatal diagnosis of coarctation of the aorta improves survival and reduces morbidity. Heart 2002;87:67.

196. Allan LD, Anderson RH, Sullivan ID, et al. Evaluation of fetal arrhythmias by echocardiography. Br Heart J 1983;50:240.

197. Gembruch U, Krapp M, Germer U, et al. Venous Doppler in the sonographic surveillance of fetuses with supraventricular tachycardia. Eur J Obstet Gynecol Reprod Biol 1999;84:187.

198. Splunder van IP, Wladimiroff JW. Cardiac functional changes in the human fetus in the late first and early second trimesters. Ultrasound Obstet Gynecol 1996;7:411.

199. Copel JA, Kleinman CS. Fetal arrhythmias. In: Wladimiroff JW, Pilu G, eds. Ultrasound and the fetal heart. New York: Parthenon, 1996:93.

200. Reed KL, Sahn DJ, Marx GR, et al. Cardiac Doppler flows during fetal arrhythmias: physiologic consequences. Obstet Gynecol 1987;70:1.

201. Kleinman CS, Copel JA. Electrophysiological principles and fetal antiarrhythmic therapy. Ultrasound Obstet Gynecol 1991;1:286.

202. Jouppila P, Mäkäräinen L, Räsänen J, et al. Aggressive direct treatment of a fetus with supraventricular tachycardia and hydrops fetalis. Ultrasound Obstet Gynecol 1993;3:279.

203. Ko JK, Deal BJ, Strasburger JF, et al. Supraventricular tachycardia mechanisms and their age distribution in pediatric patients. Am J Cardiol 1992;69:1028.

204. Hansmann M, Gembruch U, Bald R, et al. Fetal tachyarrhythmias: transplacental and direct treatment of the fetus: a report of 60 cases. Ultrasound Obstet Gynecol 1991;1:162.

205. Gowda RM, Khan IA, Mehta NJ, et al. Cardiac arrhythmias in pregnancy: clinical and therapeutic considerations. Int J Cardiol 2003;88:129.

206. Ebenroth ES, Cordes TM, Darragh RK. Second-line treatment of fetal supraventricular tachycardia using flecainide acetate. Pediatr Cardiol 2001;22:483.

207. Younis JS, Granat M. Insufficient transplacental digoxin transfer in severe hydrops fetalis. Am J Obstet Gynecol 1987;157:1268.

208. Azancot-Benisty A, Jacqz-Aigrain E, Guirgis NM, et al. Clinical pharmacological study of fetal supraventricular tachyarrhythmias. J Pediatr 1992;121:608.

209. Laurent M, Betremieux P, Biron P, et al. Neonatal hypothyroidism after treatment by amiodarone during pregnancy. Am J Cardiol 1987;60:942.

210. Nag AC, Lee ML, Shepard D. Effect of amiodarone on the expression of myosin isoforms and cellular growth of cardiac muscle cells in culture. Circ Res 1990;67:51.

211. Jouannic JM, Delahaye S, Fermont L, et al. Fetal supraventricular tachycardia: a role for amiodarone as second-line therapy? Prenat Diagn 2003;23:152.

212. Jouannic JM, Le Bidois J, Fermont L, et al. Prenatal ultrasound may predict fetal response to therapy in non-hydropic fetuses with supraventricular tachycardia. Fetal Diagn Ther 2002;17:120.

213. Garson A. Medicolegal problems in the management of cardiac arrhythmias in children. Pediatrics 1987;79:84.

214. Cardiac Arrhythmia Suppression Trial Investigators. Preliminary report: effect of encainide and flecainide on mortality in a randomized trial of arrhythmia suppression after myocardial infarction. N Engl J Med 1989;321:406.

215. Fish FA, Gillette PC, Woodrow-Benson D. Proarrhythmia, cardiac arrest and death in young patients receiving encainide and flecainide. J Am Coll Cardiol 1991;18:356.

216. Allan LD, Chita SK, Sharland GK, et al. Flecainide in the treatment of fetal tachycardias. Br Heart J 1991;65:46.

217. Frohn-Mulder IME, Stewart PA, Witsenburg M, et al. The efficacy of flecainide versus digoxin in the management of fetal supraventricular tachycardia. Prenat Diagn 1995;15:1297.

218. Krapp M, Baschat AA, Gembruch U, et al. Flecainide in the intrauterine treatment of fetal supraventricular tachycardia. Ultrasound Obstet Gynecol 2002;19:158.

219. Nakata M, Anno K, Matsumori LT, et al. Successful treatment of supraventricular tachycardia exhibiting hydrops fetalis with flecainide acetate: a case report. Fetal Diagn Ther 2003;18:83.

220. Ward RM. Maternal drug therapy for fetal disorders. Semin Perinatol 1992;16:12.

221. Meijboom EJ, Van Engelen AD, Van de Beek EW, et al. Fetal arrhythmias. Curr Opin Cardiol 1994;9:97.

222. Harrison JK, Greenfield RA, Wharton JM. Acute termination of supraventricular tachycardia by adenosine during pregnancy. Am Heart J 1992;123:1386.

223. Meden H, Neeb U. Transplazentare kardioversion bei fetaler supraventrikularer tachycardie mit sotalol. Z Geburtshilfe Perinatol 1990;194:182.

224. Oudijk MA, Ruskamp JM, Ambachtsheer BE, et al. Drug treatment of fetal tachycardias. Paediatr Drugs 2002;4:49.

225. Wagner X, Jouglard J, Moulin M, et al. Coadministration of flecainide acetate and sotalol during pregnancy: lack of teratogenic effects, passage across the placenta, and excretion in human breast milk. Am J Heart J 1990;119:700.

226. Wakai RT, Strasburger JF, Li Z, et al. Magnetocardiographic rhythm patterns at initiation and termination of fetal supraventricular tachycardia. Circulation 2003;107:307.

227. Aboud E, Neales K. The effect of maternal hypothermia on the fetal heart rate. Int J Gynecol Obstet 1999;66:163.

228. Donofrio MT, Gullquist SD, O'Connell NG, et al. Fetal presentation of congenital long QT syndrome. Pediatr Cardiol 1999;20:441.

229. Horsfall AC, Venables PJW, Taylor PV, et al. Ro and La antigens and maternal autoantibody idiotype in the surface of myocardial fibres in congenital heart block. J Autoimmun 1991;4:165.

230. Schmidt KG. Fetal bradyarrhythmia. In: Yagel S, Silverman NH, Gembruch U, eds. Fetal cardiology. London: Martin Dunitz-Taylor & Francis Group, 2003;346.
231. Harris JP, Alexson CG, Manning JA et al. Medical therapy for the hydropic fetus with congenital complete atrioventricular block. Am J Perinat 1993;10:217.
232. Anandakumar C, Biswas A, Chew SLS, et al. Direct fetal therapy for hydrops secondary to congenital atrioventricular heart block. Obstet Gynecol 1996;87:835.
233. Copel JA, Buyon JP, Kleinman CS. Successful in utero treatment of fetal heart block. Am J Obstet Gynecol 1995;173:1384.
234. Bergman B, Bokström H, Borga O, et al. Transfer of terbutaline across the human placenta in late pregnancy. Eur J Respir Dis 1984;65 (suppl 134):81.
235. Groves AM, Allan LD, Rosenthal E. Therapeutic trial of sympathomimetics in three cases of complete heart block in the fetus. Circulation 1995;92:3394.
236. Kikuchi Y, Shiraishi H, Igarashi H, et al. Cardiac pacing in fetal lambs: intrauterine transvenous cardiac pacing for the treatment of complete atrioventricular block. PACE 1995;18:417.
237. Liddicoat JR, Klein JR, Reddy M, et al. Hemodynamic effects of chronic prenatal ventricular pacing for the treatment of complete atrioventricular block. Circulation 1997;96:1025.
238. Sullivan KM, Hawgood S, Flake AW, et al. Amniotic fluid phospholipid analysis in the fetus with congenital diaphragmatic hernia. J Pediatr Surg 1994;29:1020.
239. Puri P, Gorman F. Lethal non-pulmonary anomalies associated with congenital diaphragmatic hernia: implications for early intrauterine surgery. J Pediatr Surg 1984;19:29.
240. Harrison MR, Langer JC, Adzick NS, et al. Correction of congenital diaphragmatic hernia in utero. V. Initial experience. J Pediatr Surg 1990;25:47.
241. Paek BW, Coakley FV, Lu Y, et al. Congenial diaphragmatic hernia: prenatal evaluation with lung volumetry: preliminary experience. Radiology 2001;220:63.
242. Mahieu-Caputo D, Sonigo P, Dommergues M, et al. Fetal lung volume measurement by magnetic resonance imaging in congenital diaphragmatic hernia. BJOG 2001;108:863.
243. Walsh DS, Hubbard AM, Olutoye OO, et al. Assessment of fetal lung volumes and liver herniation with magnetic resonance imaging in congenital diaphragmatic hernia. Am J Obstet Gynecol 2000;183:1067.
244. Sokol J, Bohn D, Lacro RV, et al. Fetal pulmonary artery diameters and their association with lung hypoplasia and postnatal outcome in congenital diaphragmatic hernia. Am J Obstet Gynecol 2002;186:1085.
245. Laudy JAM, Van Gucht M, Van Dooren MF, et al. Congenital diaphragmatic hernia: an evaluation of the prognostic value of the lung-to-head ratio and other prenatal parameters. Prenat Diagn 2003;23:634.
246. Bahlmann F, Merz E, Hallermann C, et al. Congenital diaphragmatic hernia: ultrasonic measurement of fetal lungs to predict pulmonary hypoplasia. Ultrasound Obstet Gynecol 1999;14:162.
247. Manni M, Heydanus R, Den Hollander NS, et al. Prenatal diagnosis of congenital diaphragmatic hernia: a retrospective analysis of 28 cases. Prenat Diagn 1994;14:187.
248. Beresford MW, Shaw NJ. Outcome of congenital diaphragmatic hernia. Pediatr Pulmonol 2000;30:249.
249. Langham MR Jr, Kays DW, Beierle EA, et al. Twenty years of progress in congenital diaphragmatic hernia at the University of Florida. Am Surg 2003;69:45.
250. Ford WD. Fetal intervention for congenital diaphragmatic hernia. Fetal Diagn Ther 1994;9:398.
251. MacGillivray TE, Jennings RW, Rudolph AM, et al. Vascular changes with in utero correction of diaphragmatic hernia. J Pediatr Surg 1994;29:992.
252. Harrison MR, Albanese CT, Hawgood SB, et al. Fetoscopic temporary tracheal occlusion by means of detachable balloon for congenital diaphragmatic hernia. Am J Obstet Gynecol 2001;185:730.
253. Smith NP, Jesudason EC, Losty PD. Congenital diaphragmatic hernia. Paediatr Respir Rev 2002;3:339.
254. Elder JS. Antenatal hydronephrosis: fetal and neonatal management. Pediatr Urol 1997;44:1299.
255. Scott JE, Renwick M. Antenatal renal pelvic measurements: what do they mean? BJU Int 2001;87:376.
256. Thompson MO, Thilaganathan B. Effect of screening for Down syndrome on the significance of isolated fetal hydronephrosis. Br J Obstet Gynaecol 1998;19:347.
257. Morin L, Cendron M, Crombleholme TM, et al. Minimal hydronephrosis in the fetus: clinical significance and implications for management. J Urol 1996;155:2047.
258. Sherer DM. Is fetal hydronephrosis overdiagnosed? Ultrasound Obstet Gynecol 2000;16:601.
259. Grignon A, Filion R, Filiatrault D, et al. Urinary tract dilatation in utero: classification and clinical applications. Radiology 1986;160:645.
260. Scott JE, Wright B, Wilson B, et al. Measuring the fetal kidney with ultrasonography. Br J Urol 1995;76:769.
261. Ouzounian JG, Castro MA, Fresquez M, et al. Prognostic significance of antenatally detected fetal pyelectasis. Ultrasound Obstet Gynecol 1996;7:424.

262. Petrikofsky BM, Cuomo MI, Schneider EP, et al. Isolated fetal hydronephrosis: beware the effect of bladder filling. Prenat Diagn 1995;15:827.

263. Nicolini U, Vaughan JI, Fisk NM, et al. Cystic lesions of the fetal kidneys: diagnosis and prediction of postnatal function by fetal urine biochemistry. J Pediatr Surg 1992;27:1451.

264. Harrison MR, Filly RA. The fetus with obstructive uropathy: Pathophysiology, natural history, selection, and treatment. In: Harrison MR, Golbus MS, Filly RA, eds. The unborn patient, 2nd ed. Philadelphia: WB Saunders, 1990:329.

265. Degani S, Leibovitz Z, Shapiro I, et al. Fetal pyelectasis in consecutive pregnancies: a possible genetic predisposition. Ultrasound Obstet Gynecol 1997;10:9.

266. Herndon CD, McKenna PH, Kolon TF, et al. A multicenter outcomes analysis of patients with neonatal reflux presenting with prenatal hydronephrosis. J Urol 1999;162:1203.

267. Hecher K, Henning K, Spernol R, et al. Spontaneous remission of urinary tract obstruction and ascites in a fetus with posterior urethral valves. Ultrasound Obstet Gynecol 1991;1:426.

268. Carlsson SA, Hokegard KH, Mattson LA. Megacystis-microcolon-intestinal hypoperistalsis syndrome: antenatal appearance in two cases. Acta Obstet Gynecol Scand 1992;71:645.

269. Bartholomew TH, Gonzales ET. Urologic management in cloacal dysgenesis. Urology 1978;11:549.

270. Reuss AR, Stewart PA, Wladimiroff JW, et al. Non-invasive management of fetal obstructive uropathy. Lancet 1988;2:949.

271. Nicolini U. Prenatal diagnosis and fetal therapy. Curr Opin Obstet Gynecol 1993;5:50.

272. Nicolaides KH, Cheng HH, Snijers RJ, et al. Fetal urine biochemistry in the assessment of obstructive uropathy. Am J Obstet Gynecol 1992;166:932.

273. Lipitz S, Ryan G, Samuell C, et al. Fetal urine analysis for the assessment of renal function in obstructive uropathy. Am J Obstet Gynecol 1993;168:174.

274. Bussieres L, Labore K, Souberbielle JC, et al. Fetal urinary insulin-like growth factor 1 and binding protein 3 in bilateral obstructive uropathies. Prenat Diagn 1995;15:1047.

275. Spitzer A. The current approach to the assessment of fetal renal function: fact or fiction? Pediatr Nephrol 1996;10:230.

276. Housley HT, Harrison MR. Fetal urinary tract abnormalities: natural history, pathophysiology, and treatment. Urol Clin North Am 1998;25:63.

277. Ebel KD. Uroradiology in the fetus and newborn: diagnosis and follow-up of congenital obstruction of the urinary tract. Pediatr Radiol 1998;28:630.

278. McLorie G, Farhat W, Khoury A, et al. Outcome analysis of vesicoamniotic shunting in a comprehensive population. J Urol 2001;166:1036.

279. Feldman B, Hassan S, Kramer RL, et al. Amnioinfusion in the evaluation of fetal obstructive uropathy: the effect of antibiotic prophylaxis on complication rates. Fetal Diagn Ther 1999;14:172.

280. Walsh DS, Johnson MP. Fetal interventions for obstructive uropathy. Semin Perinatol 1999;23:484.

281. Blaas HG, Eik-Nes SH, Berg S, et al. In-vivo three-dimensional ultrasound reconstructions of embryos and early fetuses. Lancet 1998;352:1182.

282. Pooh RK, Pooh KH. The assessment of fetal brain morphology and circulation by transvaginal three-dimensional sonography and power Doppler. J Perinat Med 2002;30:48.

283. Monteagudo A, Timor-Tritsch IE, Moomjy M. Nomograms of the fetal lateral ventricles using transvaginal sonography. J Ultrasound Med 1993;5:265.

284. Monteagudo A, Timor-Tritsch IE. Fetal neurosonography of congenital brain anomalies. In: Timor-Tritsch IE, Monteagudo A, Cohen HL, eds. Ultrasonography of the prenatal and neonatal brain, 2nd ed. New York: McGraw Hill, 2001.

285. Jeanty P, Dramaix-Wilmet M, Delbeke D, et al. Ultrasonic evaluation of fetal ventricular growth. Neuroradiology 1981;21:127.

286. Cardozo JD, Goldstein RB, Filly RA. Exclusion of fetal ventriculomegaly with a single measurement of the width of the lateral ventricular atrium. Radiology 1988;169:711.

287. Den Hollander NS, Vinkesteijn A, Schmitz-van Splunder IP, et al. Prenatally diagnosed fetal ventriculomegaly: prognosis and outcome. Prenat Diagn 1998;18:557.

288. Futagi Y, Suzuki Y, Toribe Y, et al. Neurodevelopmental outcome in children with fetal hydrocephalus. Pediatr Neurol 2002;27:111.

289. Cardozo JD, Filly RA, Podarsky AE. The dangling choroid plexus: a sonographic observation of value in excluding ventriculomegaly. Am J Radiol 1988;151:767.

290. Mahony BS, Nyberg DA, Hirsch JH, et al. Mild idiopathic lateral cerebral ventricular dilatation in utero: sonographic evaluation. Radiology 1988;169:715.

291. D'Addario V, Pinto V, Del Bianco A, et al. The clivus-supraocciput angle: a useful measurement to eval- uate the shape and size of the fetal posterior fossa and to diagnose Chiari II malformation. Ultrasound Ob- stet Gynecol 2001;18:146.

292. Gilbert-Barness E, ed. Potter's pathology of the fetus and infant, vol. 2. St. Louis: Mosby Year Book, 1997.

293. Goldstein RB, Podrasky AE, Filly RA, et al. Effacement of the fetal cisterna magna in association with myelomeningocele. Radiology 1989;172:409.

294. Nicolaides KH, Campbell S, Gabbe SG, et al. Ultrasound screening for spina bifida: cranial and cerebel- lar signs. Lancet 1986;2:72.

295. Drugan A, Krause B, Canady A, et al. The natural history of prenatally diagnosed cerebral ventriculomegaly. JAMA 1989;261:1785.

296. Bromley B, Frigoletto FD, Benacerraf BR. Mild fetal lateral cerebral ventriculomegaly: clinical course and outcome. Am J Obstet Gynecol 1991;163:863.

297. Durfee SM, Kim FM, Benson CB. Postnatal outcome of fetuses with the prenatal diagnosis of asymmet- ric hydrocephalus. J Ultrasound Med 2001;20:179.

298. Mercier A, Eurin D, Mercier PY, et al. Isolated mild fetal cerebral ventriculomegaly: a retrospective analy- sis of 26 cases. Prenat Diagn 2001;21:589.

299. Pilu G, Falco P, Gabrielli S, et al. The clinical significance of fetal isolated cerebral borderline ventricu- lomegaly: report of 31 cases and review of the literature. Ultrasound Obstet Gynecol 1999;14:320.

300. Kinzler WL, Smulian JC, McLean DA, et al. Outcome of prenatally diagnosed mild unilateral cerebral ventriculomegaly. J Ultrasound Med 2001;20:257.

301. Chudleigh P, Pearce JM, Campbell S. The prenatal diagnosis of transient cysts of the fetal choroid plexus. Prenat Diagn 1984;4:135.

302. Porto M, Murata Y, Warneke G, et al. Fetal choroid plexus cysts: an independent risk factor for chromo- somal anomalies. J Clin Ultrasound 1993;21:103.

303. Comstock CH, Chervenak FA. Transabdominal sonography of the fetal forebrain. In: Chervenak FA, Kur- jak A, Comstock CH, eds. Ultrasound and the fetal brain. New York: Parthenon, 1995:43.

304. International Centre for Birth Defects, EUROCAT. World Atlas of Birth Defects. Geneva: World Health Organization, 1998;20.

305. Hunt GM, Poulton A. Open spina bifida: a complete cohort reviewed 25 years after closure. Dev Med Child Neurol 1995;37:19.

306. Date I, Yagyu Y, Asari S, et al. Long-term outcome in surgically treated spina bifida cystica. Surg Neurol 1993;40:471.

307. Botto LD, Moore CA, Khoury MJ, et al. Neural-tube defects. N Engl J Med 1999;341:1509.

308. Mansfield C, Hopfer S, Marteau TM. Termination rates after prenatal diagnosis of Down syndrome, spina bifida, anencephaly, and Turner and Klinefelter syndromes: a systematic literature review. European Con- certed Action: DADA (Decision-making After the Diagnosis of a fetal Abnormality). Prenat Diagn 1999;19:808.

309. Olde Scholtenhuis MAG, Cohen-Overbeek TE, Offringa M, et al. Audit of prenatal and postnatal diagno- sis of isolated open spina bifida in three university hospitals in The Netherlands. Ultrasound Obstet Gy- necol 2003;21:48.

310. Gratacos E, Deprest J. Current experience with fetoscopy and the Eurofoetus registry for fetoscopic pro- cedures. Eur J Obstet Gynecol Reprod Biol 2000;92:151.

311. Crombleholme TM, Harrison MR, Langer JC, et al. Early experience with open fetal surgery for congen- ital hydronephrosis. J Pediatr Surg 1988;23:1114.

312. Harrison MR, Adzick NS, Longaker MT, et al. Successful repair in utero of a fetal diaphragmatic hernia after removal of herniated viscera from seventh left thorax. N Engl J Med 1990;322:1582.

313. Adzick NS, Harrison MR, Flake AW, et al. Fetal surgery for cystic adenomatoid malformation of the lung. J Pediatr Surg 1993;28:806.

314. Sydorak RM, Albanese CT. Minimal access techniques for fetal surgery. World J Surg 2003;27:95.

315. Holmes N, Harrison MR, Baskin LS. Fetal surgery for posterior urethral valves: long-term postnatal out- comes. Pediatrics 2001;108:E7.

316. Merz E, Miric-Tesanic D, Welter C. Value of the electronic scalpel (cut-mode) in the evaluation of the fetal face. Ultrasound Obstet Gynaecol 2000;16:564.

317. Benoit B, Tomislav H, Kurjak A, et al. Three-dimensional sonoembryology. J Perinat Med 2002;30:63.

318. Schild RL, Wallney T, Fimmers R, et al. Fetal lumbar spine volumetry by three-dimensional ultrasound. Ultrasound Obstet Gynecol 1999;13:335.

319. Kos M, Hafner T, Funduk-Kurjak B, et al. Limb deformities and three-dimensional ultrasound. J Perinat Med 2002;30:40.

320. Meyer-Wittkof M, Cooper S, Vaughan J, et al. Three-dimensional (3D) echocardiographic analysis of congenital heart disease in the fetus: comparison with cross-sectional (2D) fetal echocardiography. Ultrasound Obstet Gynecol 2001;17:485.

321. Chang CH, Yu CH, Chang FM, et al. Volumetric assessment of normal fetal lungs using three-dimensional ultrasound. Ultrasound Med Biol 2003;29:935.

322. Boito S, Laudy JAM, Struijk PC, et al. Three-dimensional assessment of liver volume, head circumference and abdominal circumference in healthy and growth-restricted fetuses. Radiology 2002;223:661.

323. Roelfsema N, Hop WCJ, Boito SME, et al. Three-dimensional sonographic measurement of normal fetal brain volume during the second half of pregnancy. Am J Obstet Gynecol 2003, in press.

324. Chang CH, Yu CH, Ko HC, et al. Assessment of normal fetal liver blood flow using quantitative three-dimensional power Doppler ultrasound. Ultrasound Med Biol 2003;29:943.

325. Martin C. Magnetic resonance imaging in perinatal medicine. In: Controversies in perinatal medicine. Carrera JM, Chervenak FA, Kurjak A, eds. New York: Parthenon, 2003:175.

326. Vimercati A, Greco P, Vera L, et al. The diagnostic role of "in utero" magnetic resonance imaging. J Perinat Med 1999;27:303.

327. Kojima K, Suzuki Y, Miyajima S, et al. Antenatal evaluation of an encephalocele in a dizygotic twin pregnancy using fast magnetic resonance imaging. Fetal Diagn Ther 2003;18:289.

328. Amin R, Nicolaidis P, Kawashima A, et al. Normal anatomy of the fetus at MR imaging. Radiographics 1999;19:S201.

329. Robert Y, Cuilleret V, Vaast P, et al. Prenatal thoracic MR imaging. Arch Pediatr 2003;10:340.

330. Hata N, Wada T, Chiba T, et al. Three-dimensional volume rendering of fetal MR images for diagnosis of congenital cystic adenomatoid malformation. Acad Radiol 2003;10:309.

Anne M. Hubbard, M.D. **25**

Prenatal Magnetic Resonance Imaging for Fetal Abnormalities

The use of magnetic resonance imaging (MRI) in the evaluation of the fetus was enhanced with the introduction of ultrafast scans developed for adult abdominal imaging.[1] In the 1990s, faster imaging sequences were developed including half-Fourier, single shot turbo spin-echo (HASTE), and echo-planar imaging (EPI).[2] These sequences acquire a single slice in less than 400 msec and decrease the artifacts caused by fetal motion. Maternal sedation or fetal paralysis is not required to obtain diagnostic images.

Ultrafast MRI produces detailed and reproducible images of fetal anatomy.[3–6] MRI is most useful in the evaluation of abnormalities of the fetal brain, neck, chest, and abdomen. The extremities are not well evaluated with MRI because of motion. In addition, evaluation of the fetus before 18 weeks of gestation is difficult because of the small size of the fetus.

Safety is always the first consideration when evaluating the fetus. To date, no known harmful effects to the developing human fetus have been documented using clinical scanners at field strengths of 1.5 Tesla or less. However, safety has not been proven. Animal studies have been performed looking at the effects of radiofrequency (RF) fields on fetal development.[7] Even at high levels above maximum permissible human guidelines, consistent morphologic abnormalities have not been identified.[7] Evaluation of health care workers employed in MRI showed no increased incidence of fetal anomalies or spontaneous abortion compared with controls.[8] In utero exposure to echo-planar imaging has not been shown to have any effect on fetal growth.[9] One follow-up study of children who were imaged in utero showed no increased occurrence of disease.[10]

Heating secondary to RF deposition is a major safety concern with MRI. One study evaluated heating affects of MRI with HASTE imaging in a pregnant pig model.[11] Although no heating occurred in the fetal tissues or the amniotic fluid, animal models may not be adequate to evaluate human RF and heating. RF deposition is related to the size, shape, and position of the patient, and animals and people bear few similarities in these respects.

Contrast agents are not used in pregnant patients because gadolinium crosses the placenta. The toxicity of gadolinium to the human fetus is not known, although toxicity has been demonstrated in animal studies, with increased incidence of fetal death and abnormalities.[12]

CENTRAL NERVOUS SYSTEM

Ultrasound (US) is the primary screening method for evaluation of the fetus. However, there are pitfalls in the evaluation of the fetal brain and spine with US.[13] The brain's appearance on US is based on the ability to obtain specific images of the cerebrum, cerebellum, and spine. Maternal obesity, oligohydramnios, or a suboptimal fetal position may result in inadequate US images. MRI is less affected by these factors. As a result, MRI changed the diagnosis and management of 40 to 45 percent of fetuses with central nervous system (CNS) abnormalities suspected on prior sonography.[14–16]

MRI's significant impact on the evaluation of the fetal brain has provided more specific information about normal development. For instance, myelination of the fetal brain can be evaluated in vivo. MRI reveals changes in the developing brain due to neuronal migration, gyral formation, and myelination. In vitro MRI shows specific patterns of growth that correlate with anatomic developments based on pathologic specimens.[17] At 16–20 weeks, the cerebral surface is relatively smooth, with minimal infolding of the sylvian fissures (Figure 25.1). With progressive brain maturation, increased sulcation is clearly depicted with MRI.[18,19] The appearance of specific sulci can be used as an indicator of

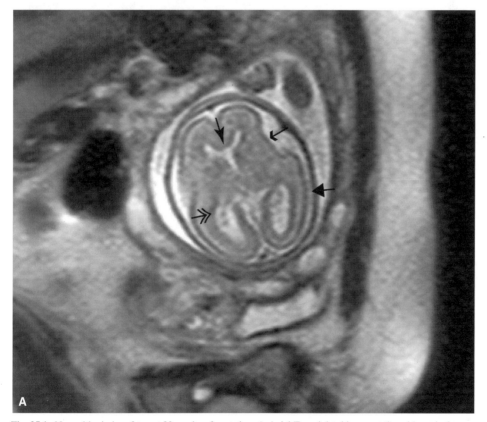

Fig. 25.1. Normal brain in a fetus at 22 weeks of gestation. *A*, Axial T$_2$-weighted image at the midventricular level shows smooth cortical surfaces with minimal infolding of the sylvian fissures (small arrow). There are three discrete parenchymal zones; the periventricular (double arrow), cortical (arrowhead with tail), and intermediate zone. The corpus callosum is present with anterior connection white matter fibers (curved arrowhead with tail). (See Fig. 25.1B on page 946)

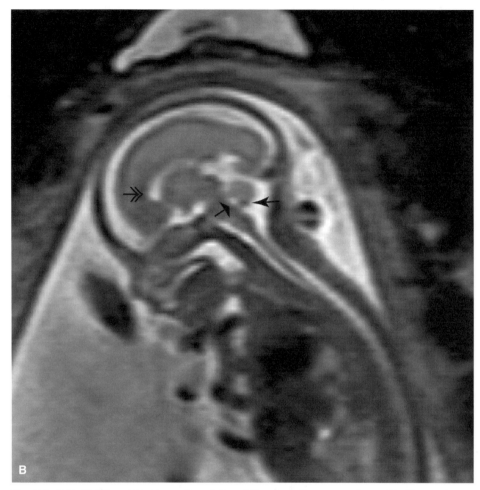

Fig. 25.1. *B*, Sagittal T$_2$-weighted image through the midline shows the corpus callosum (double arrow), fourth ventricle (broad arrow), and cerebellum (curved arrowhead with tail).

fetal maturity.[20] The in utero MRI visualization of specific sulci lags 2 to 3 weeks behind the visualization on fetal pathologic specimens.[21] A multilayered pattern of parenchyma corresponding to cellular migration has been shown with MRI (Figure 25.2). Normal migration of the parenchymal layers, gray matter, early myelination of the internal capsule and optic radiations have been shown in the second and third trimesters in vivo. MRI depicts signal changes corresponding to both increased cellularity and the maturing myelination.[22] The fast imaging with steady-state free precession technique (TruFISP) has been used to evaluate brain maturation. HASTE and TruFISP have been reported to provide comparable image quality in the second trimester, when there is little myelination. Myelination in the third trimester is better revealed with TruFISP imaging as hypointense bands.[23]

Abnormalities of neuronal migration were previously thought to be rare. However, they are present in more than 20 percent of postnatal MRI diagnoses of CNS anomalies[24]

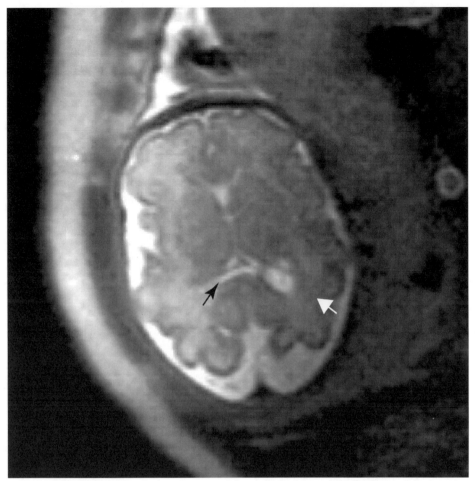

Fig. 25.2. Normal brain in a fetus at 32 weeks of gestation. Axial T_2-weighted image through the midventricular level (black arrow) shows increased sulcation of the cortex and increasing complexity of the intermediate zone (white arrow).

(Figure 25.3). Abnormalities of neuronal migration may be isolated or present in association with other cerebral anomalies. MRI visualized areas of heterotopic brain in 54 percent of third-trimester fetuses with a postnatal diagnosis of a migrational disorder. Third-trimester MRI demonstrated 80 percent of lissencephaly, 73 percent of polymicrogyria, and 100 percent of schizencephaly.[25] Polymicrogyria, the presence of an increased number of small gyri, has been documented in utero.[14,24] Polymicrogyria may result from injury to normal cellular interactions at the external limiting membrane, the pial–glial barrier. Most findings indicate that ischemia is the most common form of injury.[24,25]

Schizencephaly is a neuronal migration anomaly characterized by gray-matter-lined clefts extending from the ventricle to the cortical surface. The lips of the clefts may be fused or separate (Figure 25.4). Prognosis is related to the amount of cortex involved, and the cause may be genetic or ischemic. This defect is better visualized and characterized with MRI than with US.[26]

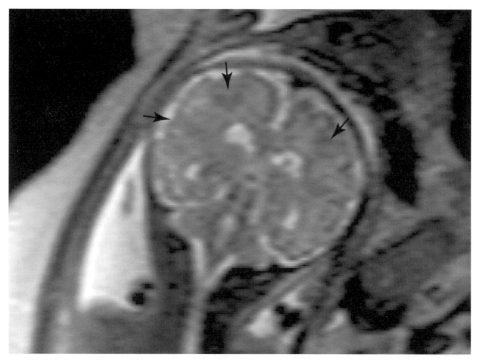

Fig. 25.3. Heterotopic gray matter in a fetus at 33 weeks of gestation. Coronal T$_2$-weighted image shows multiple low-signal-intensity lesions (arrows) in the subcortical area.

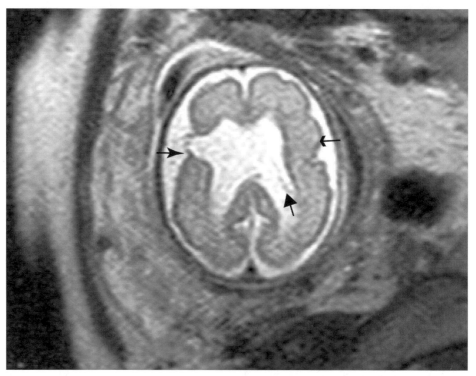

Fig. 25.4. Schizencephaly in a fetus at 26 weeks of gestation. Axial T$_2$-weighted image shows a large gray matter lined cleft (curved arrowhead with tail) in the right parietal lobe. There is ventriculomegaly (arrowhead with tail). There is abnormal and asymmetric sulcation (small arrow) of the brain.

Ventriculomegaly is the most common referral for MRI evaluation of the fetal CNS. The criterion for determination of enlargement of the ventricles on US is an atrial measurement greater than 10 mm in width on the transverse image of the brain. However, this represents 3 SD from the mean. A recent study showed that the mean atrial ventricular size on US was 6.4 ± 1.2 mm.[27] The mean ventricular size on MRI has been demonstrated to be 6.5 mm and is independent of gestational age.[28] Mild to moderate enlargement of the ventricles is frequently associated with other anomalies.[29] Outcomes of fetal hydrocephalus subsequently reveal normal intelligence in only 50 to 60 percent of cases. Associated CNS abnormalities have been diagnosed in 84 percent of fetuses with hydrocephalus. In cases with severe, rapidly progressing hydrocephalus, there is invariably poor postnatal outcome[30] (Figure 25.5). MRI is more accurate than US in determining the cause of ventriculomegaly and identifying associated CNS anomalies.[14]

Genetic counseling after the detection of mild fetal ventriculomegaly has been difficult. There are no large long-term follow-up studies that document outcome. One study reviewed twenty-six cases of mild ventriculomegaly, with atria 10 to 15 mm on US. There

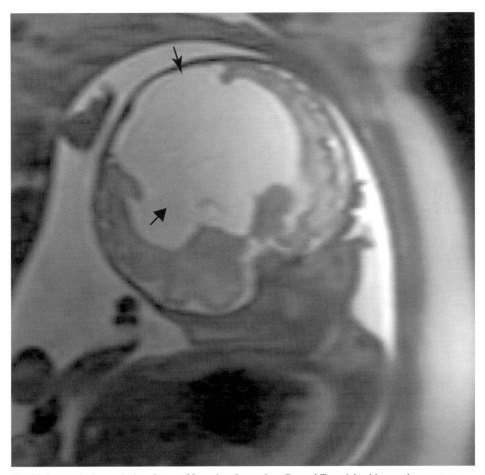

Fig. 25.5. Ventriculomegaly in a fetus at 32 weeks of gestation. Coronal T_2-weighted image shows severe ventricular (large arrow) dilation with loss of cortex (arrowhead with tail) over the parietal convexities. The destruction may be secondary to ischemia or pressure necrosis.

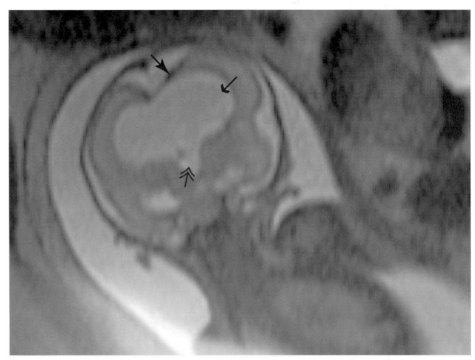

Fig. 25.6. Aqueductal stenosis in a fetus at 25 weeks of gestation. Coronal T_2-weighted image shows dilation of the lateral (small arrow) and the third (double arrow) ventricles. There is thinning of the parietal cortex (curved arrowhead with tail).

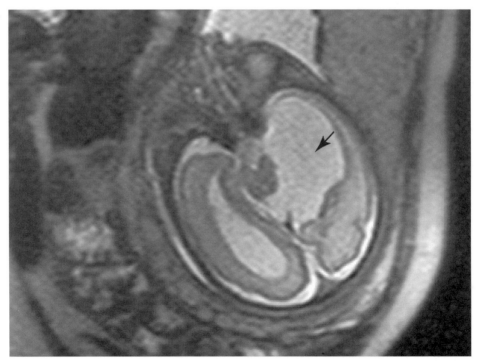

Fig. 25.7. Porencephaly in a fetus at 32 weeks of gestation. Axial T_2-weighted image through the lateral ventricles shows asymmetric ventricular size with focal dilation of the right temporal horn (arrow) and thinning of the overlying cortex.

was no developmental delay at 2 years of age in fetuses that had regressive ventriculomegaly. Developmental delay occurred in 15 percent of cases in which nonregressive ventriculomegaly developed at any time during gestation. When fetal ventriculomegaly developed in the third trimester, 50 percent subsequently had developmental delay. Late-onset ventriculomegaly has an even worse prognosis.[31]

The MR findings of congenital aqueductal stenosis are dilation of the lateral and third ventricles and a normal-sized fourth ventricle (Figure 25.6). There is usually obliteration of the subarachnoid space.[14] Ventriculomegaly may be due to ischemic or infectious events that cause cerebral atrophy. There may be unilateral or bilateral enlargement of the lateral ventricles with associated porencephaly[32] (Figure 25.7). Frequently, there is enlargement of the extra-axial spaces with cerebral atrophy. With postischemic or postinflamma-tory changes in the brain, there may also be irregularity of the ventricular surfaces (Figure 25.8).

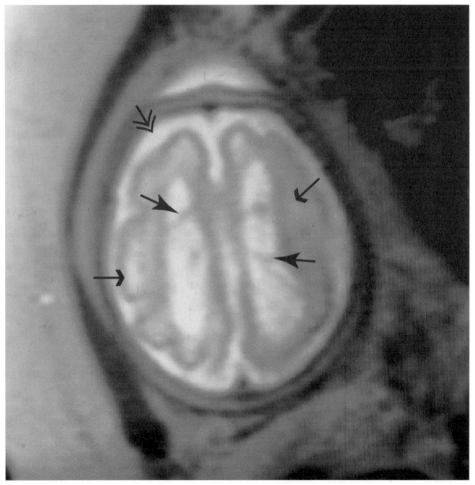

Fig. 25.8. Encephalomalacia in a fetus at 31 weeks of gestation. Axial T_2-weighted through the ventricles shows mild ventriculomegaly with septation (curved arrowheads with tail) in the ventricles. There is enlargement of the extra-axial space (double arrow) consistent with atrophy. The parenchyma has areas of heterogeneous high signal intensity consistent with leukoencephalomalacia (small arrows).

The frequency of in utero cerebral ischemic injuries is not known. In one study, 14 percent of perinatal deaths were associated with ischemic changes.[33] Ischemic injury to the brain has a variable appearance. The morphology depends on the area affected and the time between the insult and imaging.[34] The MRI findings include ventricular dilation, microcephaly, hydranencephaly, porencephaly, multicystic encephalomalacia, capsular ischemia, periventricular leukoencephalomalacia with cyst formation, and corpus callosum and cerebral atrophy. MRI is superior to US in demonstrating all of these changes (Figure 25.9). The possibility of detecting acute hypoxic–ischemic brain lesions by prenatal MRI or US is low. In a few cases, prenatal diffusion-weighted MRI has been used to detect acute cerebral ischemic lesions, demonstrating a decrease of the average apparent diffusion coefficient.[35]

Abnormalities of the corpus callosum are often diagnosed on prenatal imaging. There may be complete or partial absence of the corpus callosum. The normal corpus

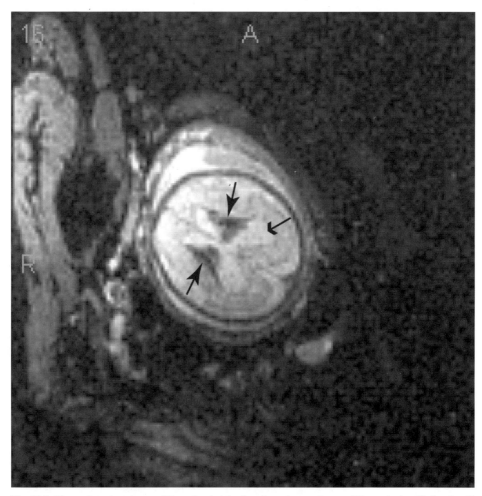

Fig. 25.9. Hemorrhage in a fetus at 29 weeks. Axial echo-planar image shows mild ventricular dilation (small arrow). There are areas of very low signal intensity (curved arrowheads with tail) in the periventricular zone and choroid plexus consistent with hemorrhage.

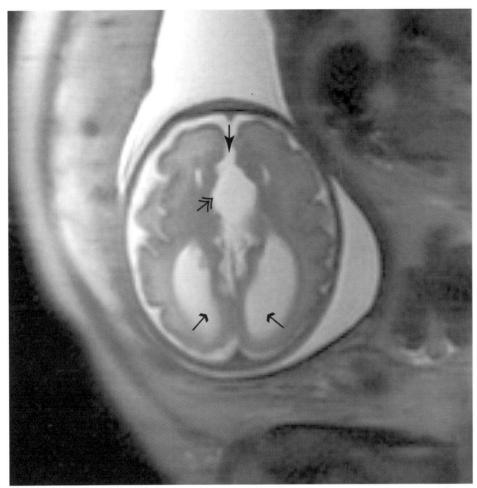

Fig. 25.10. Agenesis of the corpus callosum in a fetus at 33 weeks of gestation. Axial T_2-weighted image shows absence of fibers (curved arrowhead with tail) crossing the midline. There is widening of the inter-hemispheric fissure (double arrow) with cystic dilation of the roof of the third ventricle and mild colpocephaly with dilation of the occipital horns (small arrows).

callosum is well developed by 20 weeks, so major abnormalities of the corpus callosum should be present on prenatal MRI (Figure 25.10). MR reveals associated CNS abnormalities in 60 percent of patients with callosal abnormalities.[25] The complete absence of the corpus callosum appears the same on both MRI and US. The images reveal an increased separation of the bodies of the lateral ventricles and upward displacement of the third ventricle, with or without an associated interhemispheric cyst,[25] and there is a lack of connecting white-matter fibers between the cerebral hemispheres. Partial absence of the corpus callosum may be difficult to diagnose with US, while the lack of development of the posterior corpus callosum or thinning is shown with MRI. Arachnoid cysts occur in the midline in the area of the roof of the third ventricle and may be misinterpreted as agenesis of the corpus callosum. MRI can differentiate these abnormalities.

Holoprosencephaly is a malformation of the prosencephalon with a failure of normal midline cleavage that is frequently associated with incomplete midface development. The severe forms, semilobar and alobar holoprosencephaly, are easily diagnosed with a monoventricle and obvious fusion of the cerebral hemispheres (Figure 25.11). MRI is most helpful to distinguish the lobar form of holoprosencephaly from other causes of ventriculomegaly.[25,36] In lobar holoprosencephaly, there is a falx, some separation of the cerebral hemispheres, and partial fusion of the thalami and rostral portion of the brain.

Although the vein of Galen malformation is uncommon, it is the most common cerebral vascular malformation diagnosed prenatally. Using MRI, the large vein is easy to identify, and congestive heart failure may also be evident since it is frequently present. Ventriculomegaly may be present secondary to obstruction of the third ventricle or cere-

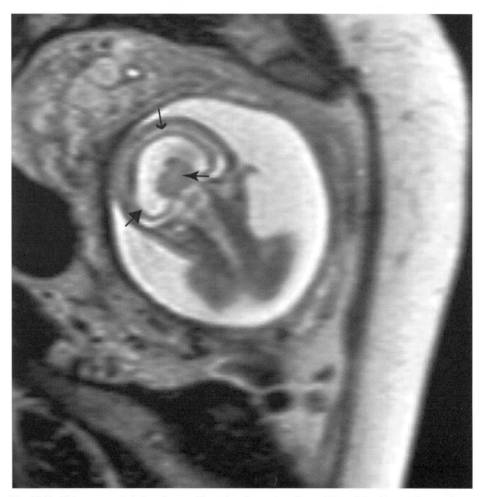

Fig. 25.11. Holoprosencephaly in a fetus at 22 weeks of gestation. Coronal T_2-weighted image shows a large monoventricle (large arrow) with no division of the cerebral cortex (small arrow) in the midline. The thalami are fused (curved arrowhead with tail).

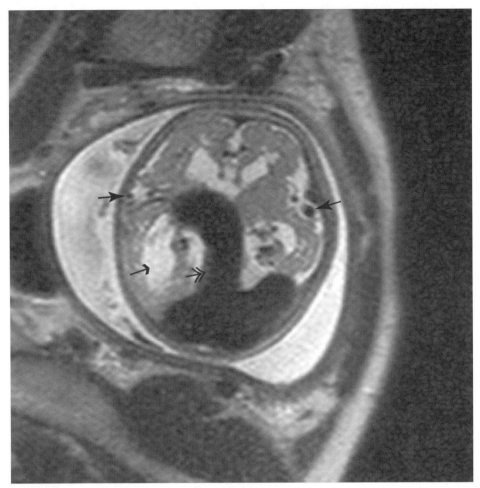

Fig. 25.12. Vein of Galen malformation in a fetus at 34 weeks of gestation. Axial T$_2$-weighted image shows severe dilation of the straight sinus, vein of Galen (double arrow), and multiple areas of low signal intensity representing collateral vessels (curved arrowhead with tail). There is ventriculomegaly (small arrow).

bral atrophy. A midline mass of low-signal intensity is seen in the area of the straight sinus and vein of Galen on both T$_1$- and T$_2$-weighted images secondary to flow within the dilated vessels[37] (Figure 25.12). On US this may be confused with other masses if Doppler is not performed.

Tuberous sclerosis (TS) is an autosomal dominant disorder that affects the brain, heart, skin, kidneys, and other organs (Figure 25.13). It may result in mild or severe mental retardation and seizures. Prenatal imaging diagnosis is based on detecting cardiac rhabdomyomas that can be shown in the mid–second trimester. The diagnostic accuracy increases with increasing numbers of cardiac rhabdomyomas.[38] Approximately 50 percent of patients with a postnatal diagnosis of TS have cardiac rhabdomyomas; however, most of these are not present on US at 20 weeks of gestation. MRI provides better definition of the periventricular region than US. Subependymal tubers, which have been demon-

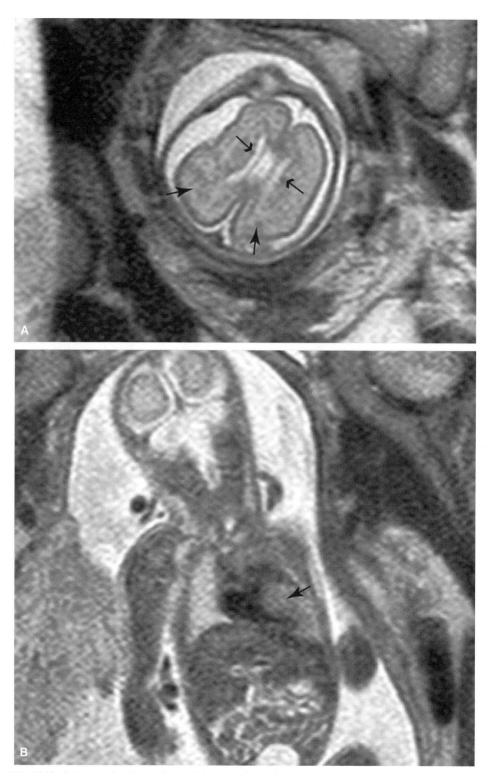

Fig. 25.13. Tuberous sclerosis in a fetus at 24 weeks of gestation. *A*, Axial T$_2$-weighted image of the brain shows heterotopic gray matter (curved arrowhead with tail) in the subcortical area and a small periventricular nodule (small arrow). *B*, Coronal T$_2$-weighted image of the chest shows a large intermediate signal intensity rhabdomyoma (arrow) of the left ventricular wall.

strated in the brain at 21 weeks, are low-signal on T_2-weighted images and high-signal on T_1-weighted images. The lesion may appear as a defect in the contour of the ventricular wall. Heterotopic brain may be identified in the subcortical region. Hamartomas may not be evident since they may not develop in the brain until after birth.[38]

MRI is also useful in diagnosing fetal brain tumors. Brain tumors are uncommon in childhood; to date, the prenatal diagnosis of tumors has been anecdotal. However, tumor characteristics, size, and location can be shown with MRI[39,40] (Figure 25.14).

MR provides superior images to reveal abnormalities of the posterior fossa, which often have a poor prognosis.[41] Mega cisterna magna, Dandy–Walker malformation and Dandy–Walker variant represent a spectrum of developmental abnormalities. Mega cisterna magna has an intact cerebellar vermis and fourth ventricle with an enlarged posterior fossa cerebrospinal fluid space (Figure 25.15). Dandy–Walker malformation is agenesis of the inferior vermis, cystic dilation of the fourth ventricle communicating with

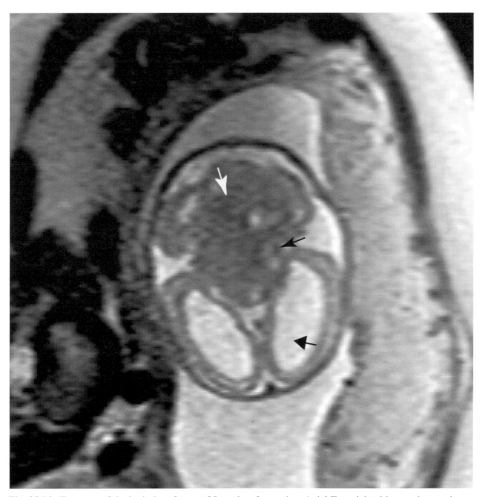

Fig. 25.14. Teratoma of the brain in a fetus at 25 weeks of gestation. Axial T_2-weighted image shows a large heterogeneous solid mass (curved arrowheads with tail) at the base of the brain. There is associated ventriculomegaly (large arrow).

the cisterna magna, and enlargement of the posterior fossa with upward displacement of the tentorium.[25] Supratentorial malformations are present in 68 percent of Dandy–Walker malformations, and hydrocephalus usually develops after birth (Figure 25.16). Dandy–Walker variant consists of hypoplasia of the inferior cerebellar vermis, with cystic dilation of the fourth ventricle, but without enlargement of the posterior fossa. Compared with US, MRI better shows the posterior fossa, specifically the vermis, fourth ventricle, and associated abnormalities[42] (Figure 25.17).

Various abnormalities of the brain are associated with spinal dysraphism, and, again, imaging technologies are useful in their diagnosis. The posterior fossa MR findings in Chiari II malformation include a small, cone-shaped posterior fossa, obliteration of the fourth ventricle, and downward herniation of the cerebellar tonsils.[14] Ventriculomegaly may also be present. Open spina bifida can be diagnosed with MRI and US. MRI shows a cystic lesion usually in the lumbosacral spine with widening of the lamina (Figure 25.18).

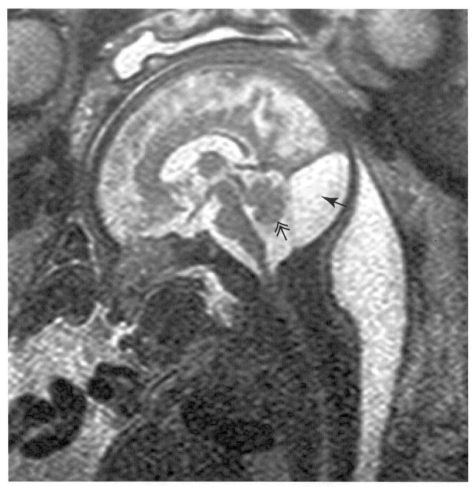

Fig. 25.15. Mega cisterna magna in a fetus at 33 weeks of gestation. Sagittal T_2-weighted image though the midline shows an intact inferior cerebellar vermis (double arrow) and normal fourth ventricle. The cerebral spinal fluid space of the posterior fossa is enlarged (curved arrowhead with tail) with elevation of the tentorium.

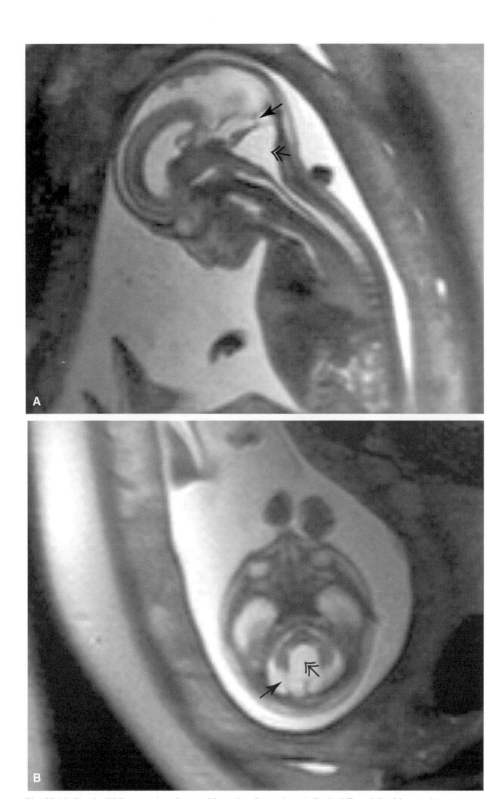

Fig. 25.16. Dandy–Walker cyst in a fetus at 22 weeks of gestation. *A*, Sagittal T$_2$-weighted image shows agenesis of the inferior cerebellar vermis and a large cisterna magna (double arrow). There is a small remnant of the superior vermis (curved arrowhead with tail). *B*, Axial T$_2$-weighted image shows inferior vermian agenesis (curved arrowhead with tail). The dilated fourth ventricle (double arrow) communicates with the cisterna magna.

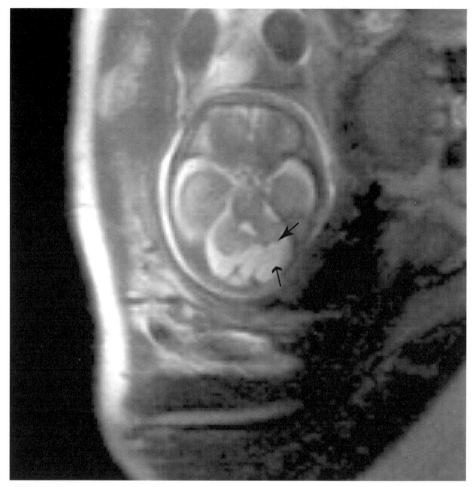

Fig. 25.17. Posterior fossa arachnoid cyst in a fetus at 34 weeks of gestation. Axial T_2-weighted image shows compression of the cerebellar hemisphere (curved arrowhead with tail) by a cyst (small arrow). The fourth ventricle is normal.

Simple meningocele or neural elements within the sac may be present.[43] Both MRI and US can determine the level of dysraphism. In one study, US was found to be more accurate in determining the defect level and evaluating small sacral lesions.[44]

MRI is also useful as a follow-up tool after in utero fetal surgery to repair meningomyelocele (MMC).[45] Following in utero surgery, MRI shows the improvement in hindbrain herniation with reaccumulation of cerebrospinal fluid within the posterior fossa.[45] Short-term follow-up of patients treated with in utero repair of MMC showed a decreased incidence of postnatal ventricular shunt placement in the first year of life: 91 percent in patients with postnatal closure of MMC compared with 59 percent following in utero closure of MMC.[46]

Although sacrococcygeal tumors (SCTs) may be diagnosed in utero[47] using either MRI or US, MRI does have some advantages. SCTs arise from the coccyx, are usually benign and are classified according to the amount of extrapelvic or intrapelvic tumor[48] (Figure 25.19). (The classification is important to the surgeon in predicting if the tumor

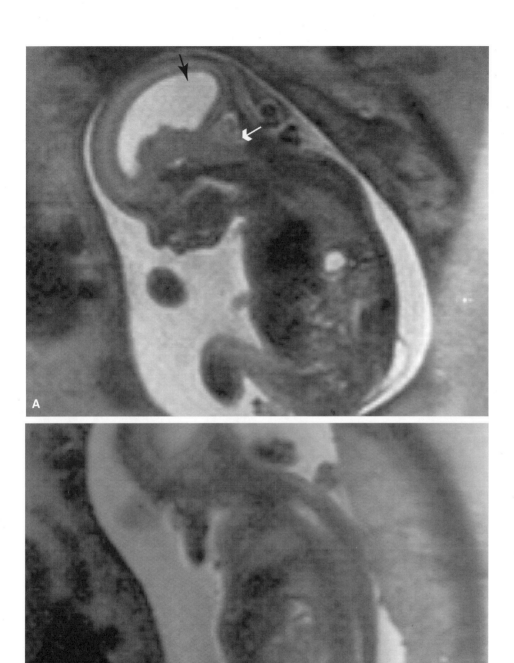

Fig. 25.18. Myelomeningocele in a fetus at 22 weeks of gestation. *A,* Sagittal T_2-weighted image shows mild ventriculomegaly (curved arrowhead with tail) with a small cone-shaped posterior fossa and downward herniation of the cerebellar tonsils (white arrow) consistent with Chiari II malformation. *B,* Sagittal T_2-weighted image through the lower spine shows a moderate sized thecal sac (curved arrowhead with tail) beginning in the midlumbar spine (small arrow).

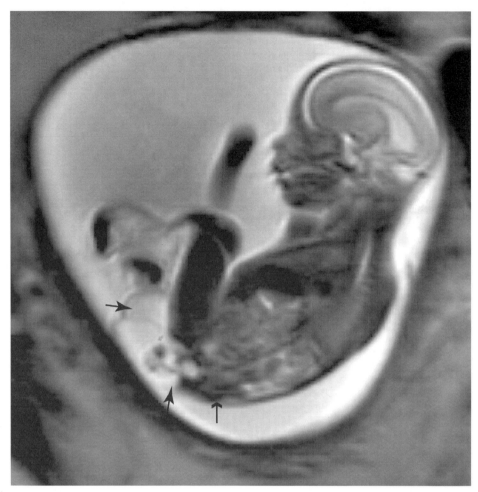

Fig. 25.19. Sacrococcygeal teratoma in a fetus at 21 weeks of gestation. Sagittal T_2-weighted image shows a multicystic mass (curved arrowheads with tail) arising from coccyx (small arrow) with no intrapelvic extension.

can be resected.) SCTs may be cystic and/or solid (Figure 25.20) and are frequently associated with polyhydramnios. The larger the solid component the more likely the lesion will have increased vascularity, which may lead to hydrops and subsequent fetal demise. Doppler US demonstrates increased flow in the fetal aorta and inferior vena cava and increased fetal cardiac output. Poor outcome has been related to the degree of increased vascularity of solid lesions and not the size of the tumor.[49] MRI correlates well with US in evaluating the size of the tumor as well as solid versus cystic components. However, MRI better defines intraspinal and intrapelvic extension of the tumor[50] and also differentiates tumors that are predominantly cystic from sacral meningomyelocele.

In fetuses with hydrops, SCTs have been successfully removed in utero with resolution of the hydrops. Surgery may also be performed immediately after delivery.[51] Thus, accurate knowledge of the extension of the tumor into the pelvis, displacement of the urinary bladder, and position of the rectum is important for adequate surgical planning before or at birth. MRI is able to depict this information accurately.

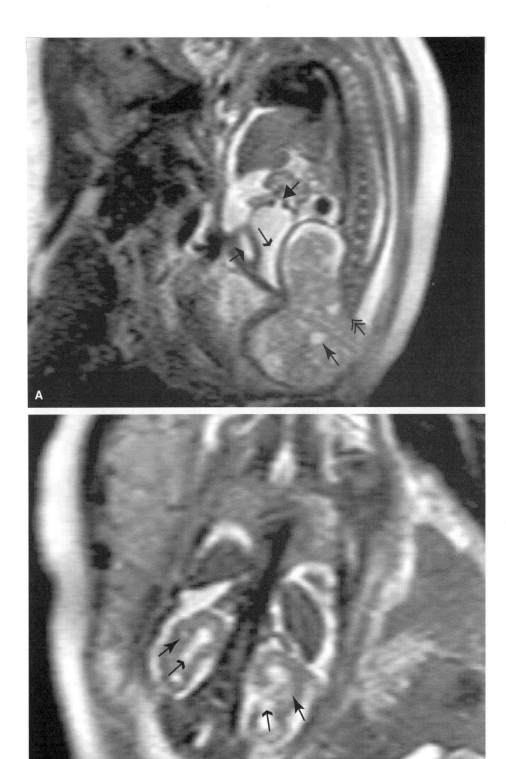

Fig. 25.20. Sacrococcygeal teratoma in a fetus at 29 weeks of gestation. *A,* Sagittal T$_2$-weighted image shows a large, mixed solid and cystic mass (curved arrowhead with tail) arising from the tip of the spine (double arrow). There is intrapelvic extension of the tumor with superior displacement of the urinary bladder (broad arrow). There is a dilated vagina (small arrow) and cervical os (large arrow). There is moderate ascites. *B,* Coronal T$_2$-weighted image shows oligohydramnios. There is dilation of the renal pelves (small arrows) with small cysts in the renal cortices (curved arrowheads with tail) consistent with dysplasia.

963

NECK

Fetal neck masses are uncommon but are important to identify since they may cause life-threatening airway obstruction at birth. The most common neck masses are cystic hygromas, teratomas, and goiters. These lesions can be identified with prenatal US; however, MRI is used for further characterization of the lesion and delivery planning.[52]

A cystic hygroma is a congenital failure of normal cannulation of the lymphatic system.[53] Lesions occurring in the posterior nuchal region early in the second trimester are frequently associated with hydrops and chromosomal abnormalities including trisomy 18, Turner syndrome, and trisomy 21. Lymphangiomas of the anterior neck area are usually isolated abnormalities that may result in morbidity when they largely infiltrate tissue planes or surround the airway and neurovascular structures.[53] There may also be extension into the chest[52] (Figure 25.21). Lymphangiomas have a multilocular appearance on MRI with fluid–fluid levels shown on T_2-weighted images. Hemorrhage may be present.

Teratoma of the neck usually occurs in the midline,[54] and although they are benign, large teratomas may cause hypoplasia of the facial bones. On MRI, these tumors are solid and cystic[52,55] (Figure 25.22). Calcifications are frequently present in teratomas and are easily identified with US but difficult to show with MRI.

Congenital high airway obstruction syndrome (CHAOS) is a syndrome with high fetal mortality that is characterized by complete or partial obstruction of the fetal airway, preventing the egress of alveolar fluid from the lungs.[56] Causes include laryngotracheal atresia, laryngeal web, and laryngeal cyst (Figure 25.23). The prenatal presentation is large fluid-filled lungs that are echogenic on US with eversion of the diaphragm and dilation of the tracheobronchial tree. The echogenic lungs may be misdiagnosed as bilateral congenital cystic adenomatoid malformation (CCAM), although this condition is rare. There is usually hydrops with skin and scalp edema and ascites due to compression of the heart and obstruction of venous return. The lungs will be large, homogeneous, and very high in signal intensity on T_2-weighted sequences.[57] The dilated tracheobronchial tree is hyperintense on T_2-weighted imaging, thus establishing its fluid content, the diagnosis, and the level of the obstruction.

It is now possible to deliver a fetus with a large neck mass or other abnormality associated with ventilation compromise while maintaining umbilical and placental circulation to the fetus using the EXIT (ex utero intrapartum treatment) procedure.[58,59] Imaging technologies are crucial to facilitating this procedure since it poses significant risks to both the mother and fetus. Hysterotomy is performed under deep maternal anesthesia to relax the uterine musculature and delay placental–uterine separation.[60] This allows 40 to 50 minutes of continued perfusion of the fetus to establish an airway, vascular access, and possible removal of the mass. The technique has been successful in maintaining oxygenation of the baby.[61] However, deep anesthesia can cause maternal bleeding with the risk of hysterectomy or death. Consequently, as much information as possible is needed about the anatomy of the mass and its relationship to the airway and great vessels to plan delivery and potential immediate surgery.[52,58] MRI can provide this crucial information.

CHEST

The most important determinant of fetal survival after birth is adequate development of the lungs. The bronchi and bronchioles are developed by 16 to 20 weeks of gestational age, with the appearance of a significant number of alveolar ducts and blood vessels by 16 to 24 weeks of gestation. The normal fetal lung on T_2-weighted images is homoge-

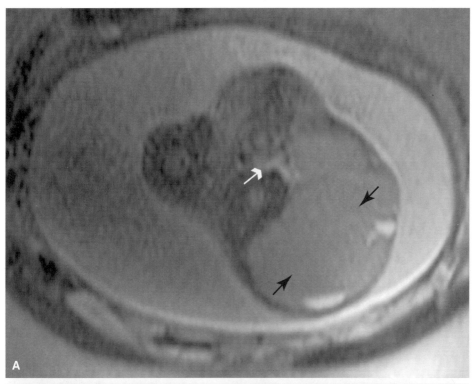

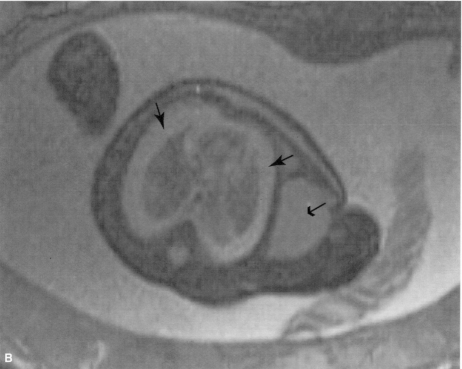

Fig. 25.21. Lymphangioma of the neck in a fetus at 36 weeks of gestation. *A*, Axial T$_2$-weighted image shows a large multicystic mass (black arrows) in the left neck with extension into the left upper chest. There is significant displacement of the trachea (white arrow). *B*, Axial T$_2$-weighted image through the chest reveals a septated cystic mass (small arrow) involving the left lateral chest wall. There are large bilateral effusions (curved arrowheads with tail) that were chylous on aspiration.

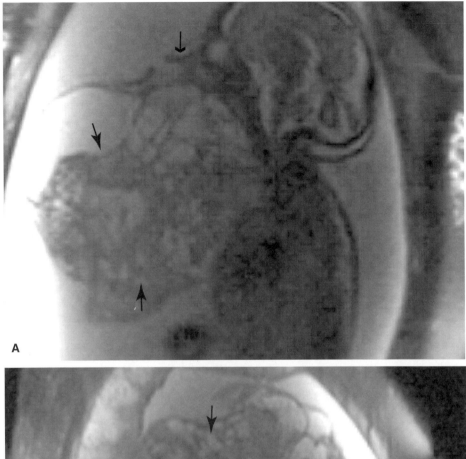

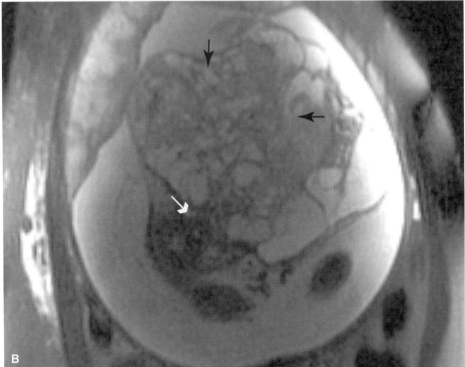

Fig. 25.22. Cervical teratoma in a fetus at 30 weeks of gestation. *A,* Sagittal T$_2$-weighted image shows a large mixed-signal-intensity, solid and cystic mass (curved arrowhead with tail) in the anterior neck with obliteration of the oropharynx (small arrow) and distortion of the facial bones (arrowhead). There is severe polyhydramnios. *B,* Axial T$_2$-weighted image shows severe displacement and compression of the trachea (white arrow) at the thoracic inlet by the mass (curved arrowheads with tail).

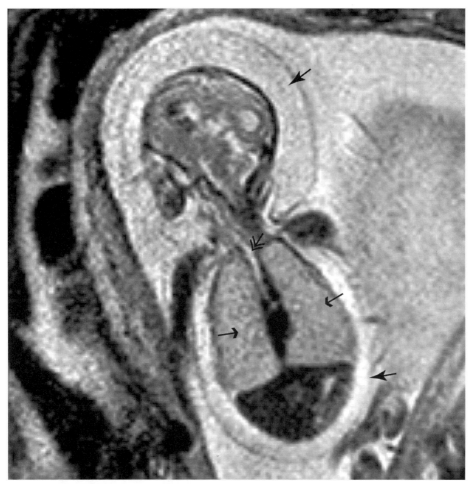

Fig. 25.23. Congenital high airway obstruction syndrome in a fetus at 22 weeks of gestation. Coronal T$_2$-weighted image shows bilateral, severely enlarged high-signal-intensity lungs (small arrows) with eversion of the diaphragm. The trachea (double arrow) is dilated below the atretic larynx. There is severe skin and scalp edema (curved arrowhead with tail), consistent with hydrops.

neous, with intermediate- to high-signal intensity relative to muscle. The signal intensity of the lungs increases with maturation, secondary to increasing numbers of alveoli and production of alveolar fluid.[57] The best imaging predictor of lung maturity has been comparison of the US-measured circumference of the fetal chest to gestational age and the femur length.[62] However, these measurements are inaccurate if there is an intrathoracic mass. Normal lung volumes have been documented with echo-planar MRI and have been shown to increase exponentially with increasing gestational age.[63] Another, larger, study using fast spin-echo T$_2$-weighted images showed that the normal fetal lung volume increased with age as a power curve and that the spread of values increased with age.[64] The MRI lung volumes were 10 percent less than volumes obtained on pathologic specimens. Fetal lungs have also been shown to have progressive decrease in T$_1$ signal and increase in T$_2$ signal intensity with growth.[65] Relaxation time measurements may provide additional information about the normal and abnormal development of the lungs in utero. Studies are now being done to see if lung volumes may be predictive of survival in pulmonary hypoplasia[66] (see Figure 25.26). However, the main determinant of pulmonary hypoplasia is probably the underdevelopment of the pulmonary arteries, and reliable visualization of the small pulmonary vessels is not currently possible with US and MRI.[67]

The most common masses within the fetal chest are CCAM, bronchopulmonary sequestration (BPS), fetal hydrothorax, and congenital diaphragmatic hernia (CDH), and MRI can be useful in their identification. CCAM is a multicystic mass of pulmonary tissue with an abnormal proliferation of bronchiolar structures that connects to the normal bronchial tree. CCAM differs from normal lung by an increase in cell proliferation and a decrease in apoptosis.[68] The vascular supply is from the pulmonary artery and drains via the pulmonary veins. CCAM may arise in any segment or lobe of the lung and occasionally involves multiple lobes.

On prenatal MRI, the appearance of CCAM depends on whether they are microcystic or macrocystic.[57] Type 1 or microcystic lesions are hyperintense on T_2-weighted images compared with the normal lung and relatively homogeneous (Figure 25.24). With increasing numbers of microcysts or macrocysts, discrete cysts can be revealed on MRI

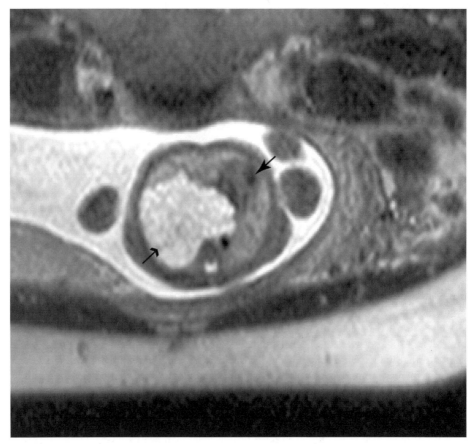

Fig. 25.24. Congenital cystic adenomatoid malformation of the lung in a fetus at 24 weeks of gestation. Axial T_2-weighted image shows a large, homogeneous high-signal-intensity mass (small arrow) in the right lower lobe that crosses the midline with displacement and compression of the heart (curved arrowhead with tail).

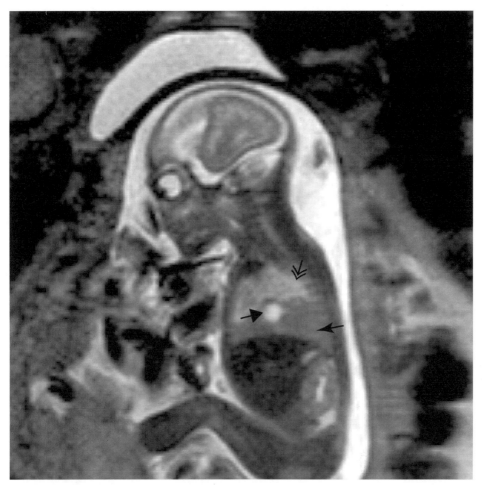

Fig. 25.25. Congenital cystic adenomatoid malformation in a fetus at 23 weeks of gestation. Sagittal T$_2$-weighted image shows a high-signal-intensity mass (double arrow) in the upper lobe with one prominent cyst (large arrow). Note the difference in the signal intensity of the mass compared to the normal lung (curved arrowhead with tail).

(Figure 25.25). MRI demonstrates normal compressed lung tissue better than US, which is important in determining resectability. The natural history of CCAM is variable. The tumor may enlarge, or CCAM may decrease in size or involute in 15 to 30 percent of cases on US. However, this may be misleading. In one study of infants with prenatal involution of a CCAM, twenty-two of twenty-three had postnatal CT scans that showed lung cysts or focal lobar hyperinflation.[69]

Hydrops may be present with large CCAM due to obstruction of systemic venous return. Hydrops may occur in up to 40 percent of fetuses with CCAM. Lesions with large cysts have a high incidence of hydrops. Large tumors associated with hydrops and a dominant cyst may be treated with thoracoamniotic shunting. In utero removal of a CCAM with hydrops in a fetus less than 32 weeks of gestation yields a 60 percent survival rate.[70] After 32 weeks of gestation the fetus can be delivered and the tumor removed.

A BPS is a mass of nonfunctioning pulmonary tissue that lacks connection to the tracheobronchial tree. BPS detected prenatally is usually extralobar. Extralobar sequestrations receive blood supply from a systemic artery. Although most common in the posterior segment of the left lower lobe, they may occur in any segment or lobe.[71] Fifty percent of BPSs are atypical and associated with other anomalies, including CDH, anomalous pulmonary venous drainage, pulmonary hypoplasia with scimitar syndrome, bronchogenic cyst, bronchial esophageal connection, and horseshoe lung. Pulmonary sequestrations are a subgroup of lung lesion with a favorable prognosis.[72] Hydrops is uncommon, unless there is an associated pleural effusion.[73] On T_2-weighted images, there is a wedge-shaped area of very high, homogeneous signal intensity[57,74] (Figure 25.26). Prenatal US better demonstrates anomalous systemic vessels because of the ability to perform real-time vascular imaging with color flow.

BPS may occur in the upper abdomen and be confused with an adrenal neuroblastoma. Although BPS in the chest is usually solid and homogeneous, in the upper abdomen it is usually cystic.[75]

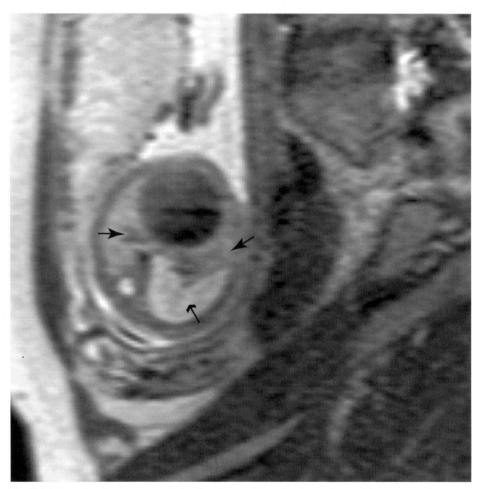

Fig. 25.26. Bronchopulmonary sequestration in a fetus at 26 weeks of gestation. Axial T_2-weighted image shows a well-defined homogeneous wedge-shaped mass (arrowhead) in the left lower lobe that is of higher signal intensity compared to the normal lung (arrows).

Multiple chest lesions may be found simultaneously. Although chest lesions such as CCAM, PBS, and bronchogenic cyst were once thought of as distinct lesions, there is significant overlap in their pathologic occurrence, suggesting a similar embryologic development (Figure 25.27). The most common lesion is a hybrid that has the pathologic characteristics of a CCAM and BPS.[76] Lesions consisting of BPS, CCAM, and bronchogenic cyst have been described with US and MRI[77,78] (Figures 25.28 and 25.29).

CDH represents a failure of formation of the diaphragmatic leaflets, occurring most commonly in the posterior aspect of the left diaphragm. CDH is present on the left in 88 percent, on the right in 10 percent, and bilaterally in 2 percent. Survival rates in fetuses with CDH range from 40 to 90 percent, with no significant improvement over the past 20 years.[79] Survival is related to the degree of pulmonary hypoplasia associated with the CDH. The best prenatal predictor of outcome remains the lung-to-head circumference ratio (LHR) as revealed by US.[80] Fetuses with an LHR greater than 1.4 have a favorable outcome, while those with a ratio of less than 1.0 rarely survive. There is a correlation between the lung volume determined on MRI and both fetal outcome and the US-determined

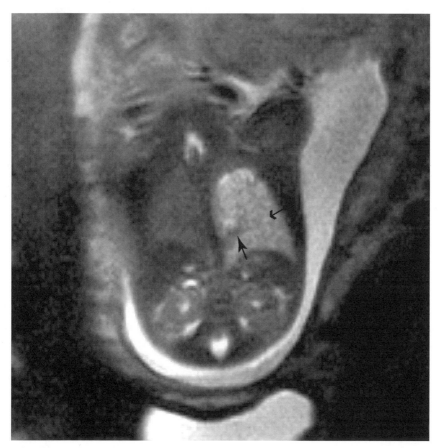

Fig. 25.27. Hybrid lesion with imaging findings of congenital cystic adenomatoid malformation and bronchopulmonary sequestration in a fetus at 23 weeks of gestation. Coronal T_2-weighted image shows a heterogeneous, high-signal-intensity mass (small arrow) containing cysts in the left lower lobe. A large feeding vessel (curved arrowhead with tail) arises from the aorta.

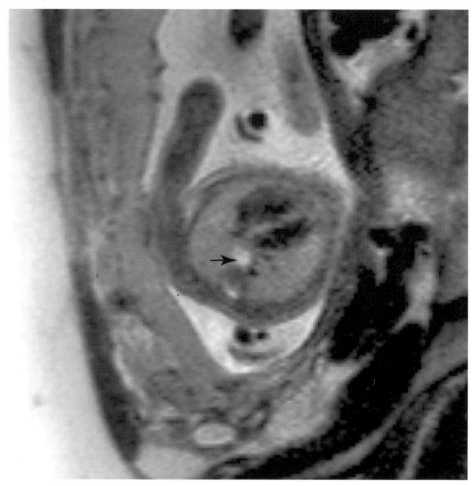

Fig. 25.28. Bronchogenic cyst in a fetus at 24 weeks of gestation. Axial T_2-weighted image shows a small discrete high-signal-intensity mass (arrow) just inferior to the carina and anterior to the spine.

LHR in fetuses with isolated left CDH when it was adjusted for gestational age at delivery and birth weight.[81] In a study at our institution it was the percentage of liver that herniated into the chest—and not the calculated fetal lung volume—that correlated with outcome in fetuses with CDH.[82] Herniation of liver into the chest in a patient with CDH has been shown to be associated with a worse prognosis, with a survival rate of less than 50 percent. Antenatal branch pulmonary artery (PA) size correlates with postmortem lung weight. In fetuses with CDH, a larger contralateral PA, significant size discrepancy of branch PA, and larger main PA diameter correlated with postnatal death and respiratory morbidity. Progressive ipsilateral PA hypoplasia suggested progressive in utero lung hypoplasia.[83]

On US, CDH is diagnosed by demonstrating a shift of the heart away from the midline and an area of increased echogenicity at the chest base.[84] Careful evaluation of the position of the stomach is important. Uncertainty in the early diagnosis of CDH that presents as an echogenic chest mass is still described.[85] In one study of patients with post-

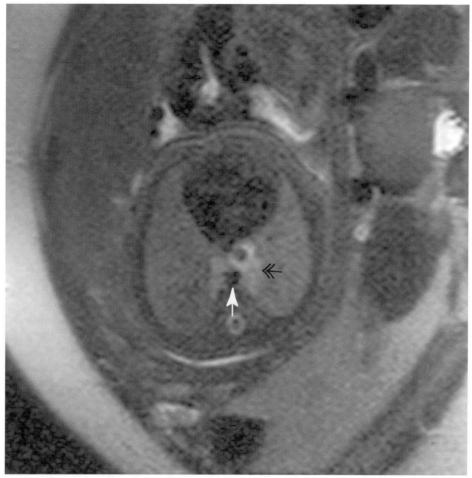

Fig. 25.29. Duplication cyst of the esophagus in a fetus at 31 weeks of gestation. Axial T_2-weighted image shows a well-defined high-signal-intensity mass (double arrow) anterior to the aorta (white arrow) and spine at the area of the gastroesophageal junction.

natal repair of CDH, the diagnosis had not been established on prenatal US in 50 percent of fetuses.[86] Evaluating the position of the liver on US may be difficult, as the echotexture of the liver and lung is similar. US depends on demonstrating the position of the portal and hepatic veins above or below the diaphragm to predict herniation of the liver into the chest.[87] With MRI there is direct visualization of the position of the liver[88] (Figure 25.30). On T_1-weighted images, the liver is high-signal-intensity and conspicuous, adjacent to the low-signal-intensity lungs. The position of the liver relative to the diaphragm is easily determined. On T_2-weighted images, the liver is low-signal-intensity and isointense to muscle. MRI has been shown to be more sensitive than US for detecting thoracic liver herniation.[89] Meconium-filled bowel is hyperintense on T_1-weighted images, making the position of the bowel easy to determine. MRI is most helpful in evaluation of right CDH, which is more frequently confused with CCAM, than left CDH since the stomach remains in the left upper abdomen.[89] Right CDH usually contains liver and bowel.

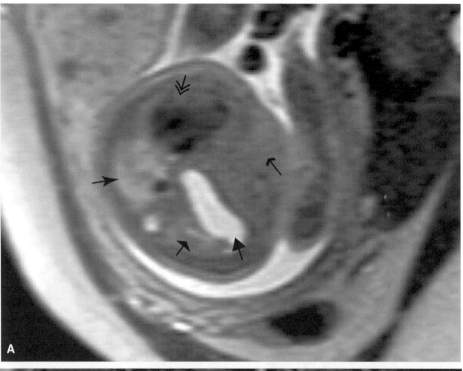

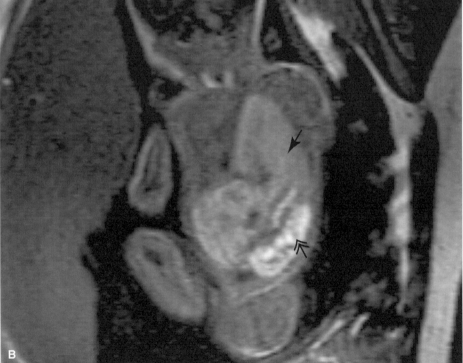

Fig. 25.30. Congenital diaphragmatic hernia in a fetus at 25 weeks of gestation. *A*, Axial T₂-weighted image shows displacement of the heart (double arrow) to the right with herniation of bowel (broad arrow), stomach (large arrow), and liver (small arrow) into the left chest. There is a small amount of the right lung tissue present (curved arrowhead with tail). *B*, Coronal T₁-weighted image shows the left lobe of liver (curved arrowhead with tail) extending into the chest. Meconium (double arrow) is seen in the bowel.

The diagnosis of bilateral CDH is easily missed on US.[90] Signs include anterior displacement of the heart with minimal lateral shift.[91] The diagnosis is readily made on MRI by showing liver in the right chest and bowel in the left chest. The prenatal recognition of bilateral CDH is important, as there is a significant increased incidence of chromosome abnormalities and syndromes compared with unilateral CDH.[92]

Intrauterine therapy has been performed at some institutions using tracheal occlusion to promote lung growth.[93] Criteria for being included in this therapy was herniation of liver into the chest and lung volumes that fell into a poor prognostic category. Tracheal occlusion resulted in significant lung growth in a subset of fetuses with severe CDH, but survival remained poor because of abnormalities in pulmonary function and prematurity.[94]

Eventration of the diaphragm is uncommon but may be confused with CDH. MRI can be helpful in differentiation because of accurate detection and localization of the bowel, diaphragm, and lung.[95] This differentiation is important since the outcome of eventration is significantly better than CDH.

MRI is also useful for evaluating atypical chest masses.[57] A foregut cyst on MRI is a fluid-filled cyst with high, homogeneous T_2 signal intensity.[96] The cyst may be large, and there is a connection to vertebrae and associated vertebral anomalies (Figure 25.31).

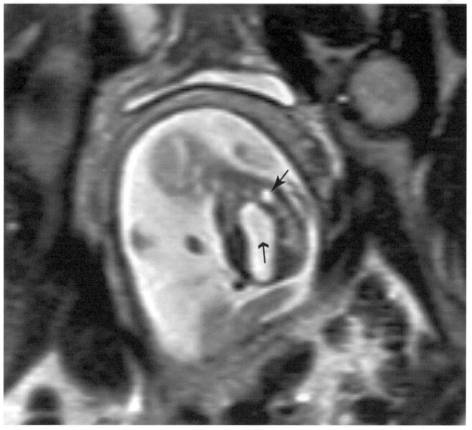

Fig. 25.31. Neurenteric cyst in a fetus at 19 weeks of gestation. Sagittal T_2-weighted image shows a large cyst (small arrow) in the chest and abdomen connecting to a defect in the spine with kyphosis and focal dilation of the dural sac (curved arrowhead with tail).

Anterior mediastinal masses are uncommon in utero. Fetal mediastinal teratoma has rarely been reported.[97] On US, these are complex cystic and solid masses. Because they are unusual lesions, they may be misdiagnosed as a CCAM. MRI demonstrates the anatomy of the trachea and great vessels in the thoracic inlet, superior mediastinum, and the normal lung. Lymphangiomas, which may occur anywhere in the body, are more likely to violate tissue planes. They appear as complex cystic masses (Figure 25.32).

ABDOMEN

The fetal liver is visualized on prenatal MRI, being very high in signal intensity on T_1-weighted images (see Figure 25.30) and low to intermediate in signal on T_2-weighted images.[59] Physiologic changes have been demonstrated within the fetal liver using echo-

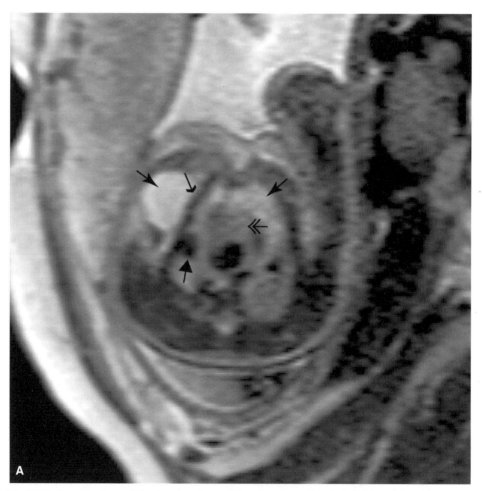

Fig. 25.32. Lymphangioma of the chest in a fetus at 29 weeks of gestation. *A*, Axial T_2-weighted image shows a high-signal-intensity cystic mass (curved arrowhead with tail) in the right anterior chest wall. There is a large mass in the anterior mediastinum (curved arrowhead with tail) that surrounds the thymus (double arrow) and the superior vena cava (broad arrow). The rib (small arrow) is thin and irregular.

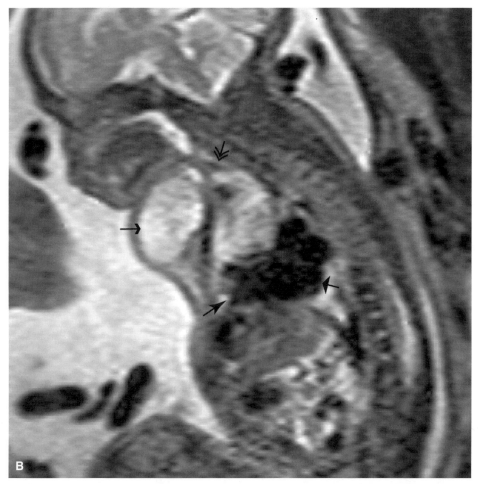

Fig. 25.32. *B,* Sagittal T$_2$-weighted image shows a mass (small arrow) on the anterior chest wall. The intrathoracic component extends from the thoracic inlet (double arrow) to the diaphragm (curved arrowhead with tail) with posterior displacement of the heart (broad arrow).

planar imaging (EPI).[98] Iron causes lower signal intensity on EPI and T$_2$-weighted images due to susceptibility effects. In early fetal life, the majority of erythropoiesis occurs in the liver. There is a large change in the distribution of erythropoiesis between 20 and 26 weeks of gestation. Changes in liver signal intensity are present throughout fetal life, which points to MRI's potential use in early noninvasive physiologic assessment of the fetus. Changes in T$_2$ measurements of the fetal liver have been documented following maternal oxygenation based on the blood oxygenation level dependence (BOLD) of the MRI signal.[99] This technique may help evaluate placental insufficiency.

Abdominal masses can be detected with prenatal MRI.[100] Tumors of the liver are rare in the fetus, but include hemangioendotheliomas, hepatoblastomas, and hamartomas. Hemangioendotheliomas are mixed in intensity, depending on the size of the vascular pools and the degree of fibrosis. Hepatomegaly is usually present. Hamartomas are typically irregular cystic masses that may have calcifications. Hepatomegaly may also be seen with hydrops, infection, anemia, metabolic abnormalities, and Beckwith–Wiedemann syndrome.

Meconium-filled bowel is visualized on prenatal MRI as high-signal intensity meconium-filled tubular structures on T_1-weighted images[57] (see Figure 25.30). If meconium is not seen, an anomaly of the bowel should be suspected, such as atresia or perforation. On T_2-weighted images the stomach and proximal bowel are high in signal. MRI helps differentiate abnormalities such as bowel obstruction from cystic abdominal masses.[101] MRI can also determine the site of bowel atresia[102] (Figure 25.33).

Neuroblastoma is one of the more common solid childhood tumors arising from undifferentiated neural tissue in the adrenal medulla or sympathetic ganglia.[103] Neuroblastic nodules are present in the adrenal glands of 100 percent of fetuses aborted in the second trimester and in 2 percent of neonatal autopsies, and they represent a normal embryologic

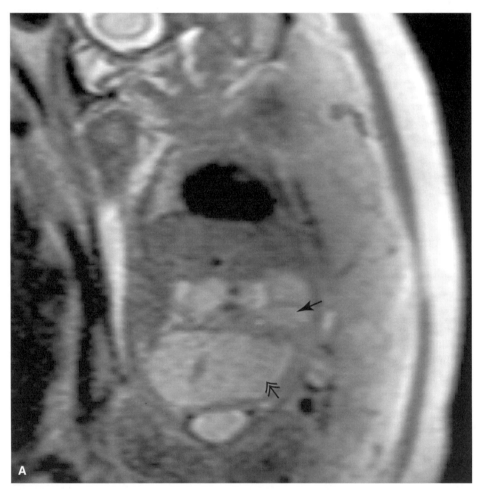

Fig. 25.33. Meconium ileus in a fetus at 31 weeks of gestation. *A*, Coronal T_2-weighted image shows a severely dilated (double arrow) loop of bowel and multiple other less dilated loops of bowel (curved arrowhead with tail).

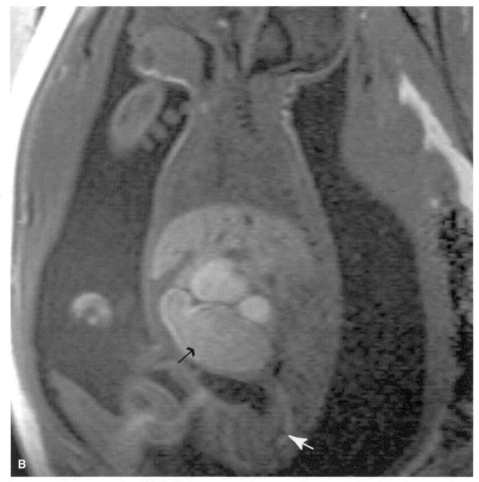

Fig. 25.33. *B,* Sagittal T_1-weighted shows the severely dilated loop of bowel (small arrow) is high-signal-intensity-containing meconium. There are multiple other dilated loops. The descending colon and rectum (white arrow) contain meconium, but are very small, consistent with a microcolon.

structure that regresses or differentiates with maturation. The incidence of postnatal clinical neuroblastoma is only 1 in 10,000 to 30,000. Adrenal cysts are also present in fetal neuroblastomas that are uncommon in postnatal neuroblastoma. Cysts may be a variant of the normal development of the fetal adrenal gland.

Congenital renal masses are rare, but mesoblastic nephroma has been diagnosed in utero.[103] These are predominantly solid masses. This or any abdominal mass may be associated with polyhydramnios secondary to compression of the bowel.

Fetal renal anomalies are often associated with oligohydramnios and can make the performance of US difficult.[104] MRI is not as affected by diminished amniotic fluid. The normal fetal kidney is intermediate in signal intensity on T_2-weighted images and higher than surrounding muscle. The T_2 signal intensity of the cortex is slightly lower than the medulla. The renal pelves and bladder are high-signal-intensity on T_2-weighted images. Normal ureters are not visualized.

Renal anomalies are increasingly detected with US because of significant improvements in technology. It is estimated that 1 in 1,000 fetuses have renal anomaly.[105] The mortality after antenatal detection of fetal uropathy is 20 to 50 percent.[106] Associated anomalies have been found in 50 percent of fetuses[105,106] (Figures 25.34 and 25.35).

With uropathy due to lower urinary tract obstruction (LUTO), the urinary bladder is dilated and thick-walled (Figure 25.36). MRI is equal to US in the accuracy of identifying a LUTO but is no better at differentiating the three main causes: posterior urethral valves, urethral atresia, and prune belly syndrome. With progressive obstruction of the bladder there is dilation of the renal collecting systems. Renal dysplastic changes occur with progressive dilation of the renal tubules and may progress to cortical cyst.[107] Renal dysplastic changes are seen as heterogeneous areas of increased cortical T_2 signal inten-

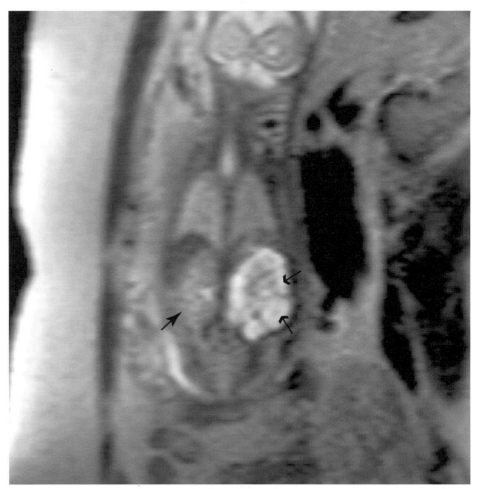

Fig. 25.34. Multicystic dysplastic kidney in a fetus at 22 weeks of gestation. Coronal T_2-weighted image shows multiple discrete cysts in the left kidney (small arrows) without identifiable normal renal parenchyma. The normal right kidney (curved arrowhead with tail) is intermediate in signal intensity.

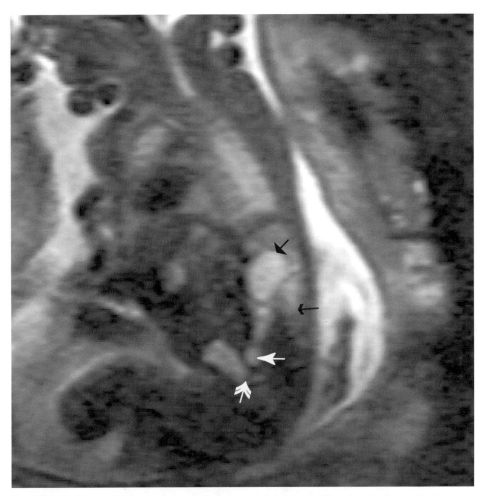

Fig. 25.35. Duplex renal collecting system with ureterocele in a fetus at 28 weeks of gestation. Sagittal T$_2$-weighted image shows dilation of the upper pole renal collecting system (broad arrow) with dilation of the ureter (curved arrowhead with tail) down to the bladder. The lower pole of the kidney is normal (small arrow). There is a small ureterocele (double arrow).

sity and cysts. In cases of questionable increased echogenicity on US, MRI can help determine whether abnormalities are dysplastic changes or normal cortical variants. The presence of renal dysplasia associated with a urinary tract obstruction is a poor prognostic sign and associated with decreased renal function. If dysplastic changes are present prenatally, intervention is usually not indicated. In a fetus with no sign of renal dysplasia, favorable urine electrolytes and β-macroglobulins, vesicoamniotic shunting can be offered. Trials of in utero antegrade fetoscopy are being performed in order to diagnosis LUTO and ablate posterior valves.[108]

MRI is most helpful in defining the anatomy of complex renal anomalies, such as bladder exstrophy and cloacal anomalies (Figure 25.37). The ability to define the bowel and the urinary tract helps distinguish these from other forms of LUTO.

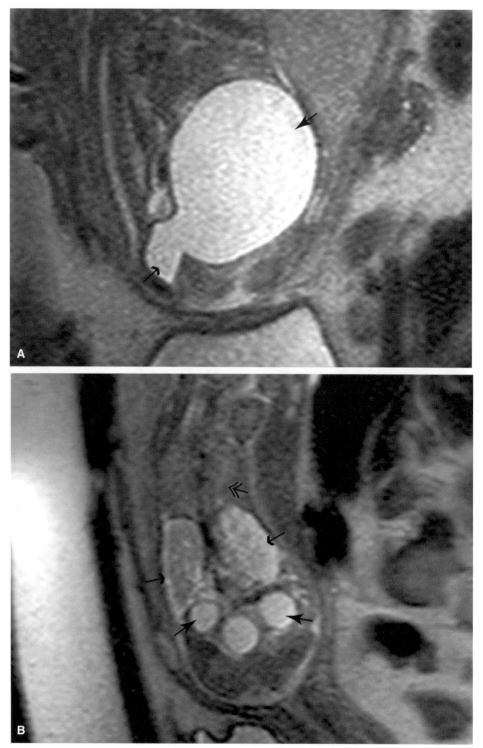

Fig. 25.36. Lower-urinary-tract obstruction in a fetus at 20 weeks of gestation. *A*, Sagittal T$_2$-weighted image shows marked enlargement of the urinary bladder (curved arrowhead with tail) with thickening of the bladder wall and dilation of the posterior urethra (small arrow). There is oligohydramnios. *B*, Coronal T$_2$-weighted image shows dilated ureters (curved arrowheads with tail) and severe cortical dysplasia with numerous small renal cortical cysts (small arrows). The lungs (double arrow) are small with decreased signal intensity for this gestational age.

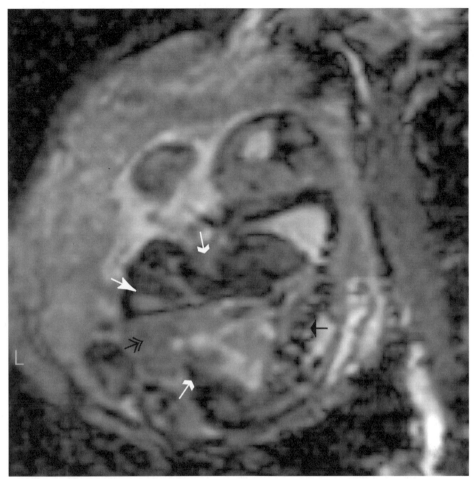

Fig. 25.37. Omphalocele with cloacal exstrophy in a fetus at 22 weeks of gestation. Sagittal echo-planar image shows lack of fluid in the urinary bladder with a defect (small arrow) in the anterior abdominal wall extending from the chest to the pelvis. There is herniation of liver (curved arrowhead with tail) and bowel (double arrow) through the abdominal wall defect. A defect below the umbilicus is consistent with bladder or cloacal exstrophy. There is scoliosis with vertebral body abnormalities (broad white arrows).

CONCLUSION

MRI technology continues to improve and will provide faster imaging and higher resolution. At present, MRI is an adjunct to a prenatal US. Fetal MRI has been shown to provide significant additional information that affects the accuracy of diagnosis, prenatal counseling, management, prenatal intervention, and delivery planning.

REFERENCES

1. Weinreb J, Lowe T, Cohen J, et al. Human fetal anatomy: MR imaging. Radiology 1985;157:715.
2. Semelka R, Kelekis N, Thomasson D, et al. HASTE MR imaging: description of technique and preliminary results in the abdomen. J Magn Reson Imaging 1996;6:698.
3. Johnson I, Stehling M, Blamire A, et al. Study of internal structures of the human fetus in utero by echo planar magnetic resonance imaging. Am J Obstet Gynecol 1990;63:601.

4. Quinn T, Hubbard A, Adzick N. Prenatal magnetic resonance imaging enhances fetal diagnosis. J Pediatr Surg 1998;33:553.
5. Yamashita Y, Namimoto T, Abe Y, et al. MR imaging of the fetus by a HASTE sequence. AJR Am J Roentgenol 1997;168:513.
6. Levine D, Barnes P, Sher S, et al. Fetal fast MR imaging: reproducibility, technical quality, and conspicuity of anatomy. Radiology 1998;206:549.
7. O'Connor M. Intrauterine effects in animals exposed to radiofrequency and microwave fields. Teratology 1999;59:287.
8. Kanal E, Gillen J, Evans J, et al. Survey of reproductive health among female MR workers. Radiology 1993;187:395.
9. Myers C, Duncan K, Gowland P, et al. Failure to detect intrauterine growth restriction following in utero exposure to MRI. Br J Radiol 1998;71:549.
10. Baker P, Johnson I, Harvey P, et al. A three-year follow-up of children imaged in utero with echo-planar magnetic resonance. Am J Obstet Gynecol 1994;170:32.
11. Levine D, Zuo C, Faro CB, et al. Potential heating effect in the gravid uterus during MR HASTE imaging. J Magn Reson Imaging 2001;13:856.
12. Okuda Y, Sagami F, Tirone P, et al. Reproductive and developmental toxicity study of gadobenate dimeglumine formulation. Study of embryo-fetal toxicity in rabbits by intravenous administration. J Toxicol Sci 1999;1:79.
13. Hertzberg B, Kliewer M, Bowie J. Sonographic evaluation of fetal CNS: technical and interpretive pitfalls. AJR 1999;172:523.
14. Levine D, Barnes P, Madsen J, et al. Central nervous system abnormalities, assessed with prenatal magnetic resonance imaging. Obstet Gynecol 1999;94:1011.
15. Simon E, Goldstein R, Coakley F, et al. Fast MR imaging of fetal CNS anomalies in utero. AJNR 2000;21:1688.
16. Twickler D, Magee K, Caire J, et al. Second-opinion magnetic resonance imaging for suspected fetal central nervous system abnormalities. Am J Obstet Gynecol 2003;188:492.
17. Brisse H, Fallet C, Sebag G, et al. Supratentorial parenchyma in the developing fetal brain: in vitro MR study with histologic comparison. AJNR 1997;8:1491.
18. Garel C, Chantrel E, Brisse H, et al. Fetal cerebral cortex: normal gestational landmarks identified using prenatal MR imaging. AJNR 2001;22:184.
19. Lan M, Yamashita Y, Tang T, et al. Normal fetal brain development: MR imaging with a half-fourier rapid acquisition with relaxation enhancement sequence. Radiology 2000;15:205.
20. Naidich T, Grant J, Altman N, et al. The developing cerebral surfaces. Preliminary report on the patterns of sulcal and gyral maturation: anatomy, ultrasound and magnetic resonance imaging. Neuroimaging Clin North Am 1994;4:201.
21. Girard N, Raybaud C, Ponce M, et al. In vivo MR study of brain maturation in normal fetuses. AJNR 1995;16:407.
22. Levine D, Barnes P. Cortical maturation in normal and abnormal fetuses as assessed with prenatal MR imaging. Radiology 1999;210:751.
23. Chung H, Chen C, Zimmerman R, et al. T_2-weighted fast MR imaging with True FISP versus HASTE: comparative efficacy in the evaluation of normal fetal brain maturation. AJR Am J Roentgenol 2000;175:1375.
24. Barkovich A, Rowley H, Bollen A, et al. Correlation of prenatal events with the development of polymicrogyria. AJNR 1995;16:822.
25. Sonigo P, Rypens F, Carteret M, et al. MR imaging of fetal cerebral anomalies. Pediatr Radiol 1998;28:212.
26. Denis D, Maugey-Laulom, Carles D, et al. Prenatal diagnosis of schizencephaly by fetal magnetic resonance imaging. Fetal Diagn Ther 2001;16:354.
27. Almog B, Gamzu R, Achiron R, et al. Fetal lateral ventricular width: what should be its upper limit? A prospective cohort study and reanalysis of the current and previous data. J Ultrasound Med 2003;22:39.
28. Twickler DM, Reichel T, McIntire DD, et al. Fetal central nervous system ventricle and cisterna magna measurements by magnetic resonance imaging. Am J Obstet Gynecol 2002;187:927.
29. Nyberg D, Mack L, Hirsch J, et al. Fetal hydrocephalus: sonographic detection and clinical significance of associated anomalies. Radiology 1987;163:187.
30. Oi S, Honda Y, Hidaka M, Sato O, et al. Intrauterine high-resolution magnetic resonance imaging in fetal hydrocephalus and prenatal estimation of postnatal outcomes with "perspective classification." J Neurosurg 1998;88:685.
31. Mercier A, Eurin D, Mercier PY, et al. Isolated mild fetal cerebral ventriculomegaly: a retrospective analysis of 26 cases. Prenat Diagn 2001;21:589.

32. Toma P, Lucigrai G, Ravegnani M, et al. Hydrocephalus and porencephaly: prenatal diagnosis by ultrasonography and MR imaging. Comput Assist Tomogr 1990;14:843.

33. Low JA, Killen H, Derrick EJ. The clinical diagnosis of asphyxia responsible for brain damage in the human fetus. Am J Obstet Gynecol 1992;167:11.

34. de Laveaucoupet J, Audipert F, Guis F, et al. Fetal magnetic resonance imaging (MRI) of ischemic/hemorrhagic brain injury. Prenat Diagn 2001;21:729.

35. Baldoli C, Righini A, Parazzini C, et al. Demonstration of acute ischemic lesions in the fetal brain by diffusion magnetic resonance imaging. Ann Neurol 2002;52:243.

36. Toma P, Costa A, Magnano G, et al. Holoprosencephaly: prenatal diagnosis by sonography and magnetic resonance imaging. Prenat Diagn 1990;10:429.

37. Martinez-Lage J, Santos JG, Poza M, et al. Prenatal magnetic resonance imaging detection of a vein of Galen aneurysm. Childs Nerv Syst 1993;9:377.

38. Levine D, Barnes P, Korf B, et al. Tuberous sclerosis in the fetus: second-trimester diagnosis of subependymal tubers with ultrafast MR imaging. AJR Am J Roentgenol 2000;175:1067.

39. Diguet A, Laquerriere A, Eurin D, et al. Fetal capillary haemangioblastoma: an exceptional tumour: a review of the literature. Prenat Diagn. 2002;22:979.

40. Mazouni C, Porcu-Buisson G, Girard N, et al. Intrauterine brain teratoma: a case report of imaging (US, MRI) with neuropathologic correlations. Prenat Diagn 2003;23:104.

41. Ecker J, Shipp T, Bromley B, et al. The sonographic diagnosis of Dandy–Walker and Dandy–Walker variant: associated findings and outcomes. Prenat Diagn 2000;20:328.

42. Stazzone M, Hubbard A, Bilaniuk L, et al. Ultrafast MR imaging of the normal posterior fossa in fetuses. AJR Am J Roentgenol 2000;175:835.

43. Nakahara T, Uozumi T, Monden S, et al. Prenatal diagnosis of open spina bifida by MRI and ultrasonography. Brain Dev 1993;15:75.

44. Mangels KJ, Tulipan N, Tsao LY, et al. Fetal MRI in the evaluation of intrauterine myelomeningocele. Pediatr Neurosurg 2000;32:123.

45. Sutton L, Adzick N, Bilaniuk L, et al. Improvement in hindbrain herniation demonstrated by serial fetal MRI following fetal surgery for myelomeningocele. JAMA 1999;282:1626.

46. Brunner J, Tulipan N, Paschall R, et al. Fetal surgery for myelomeningocele and the incidence of shunt-dependent hydrocephalus. JAMA 1999;282:1819.

47. Kirkinen P, Partanen K, Merikanto J, et al. Ultrasonic and magnetic resonance imaging of fetal sacrococcygeal teratoma. Acta Obstet Gynecol Scand 1997;76:917.

48. Altman RP, Randolph JG, Lilly JR. Sacrococcygeal teratoma: American Academy of Pediatric Surgical Section Survey. J Pediatr Surg 1974;9:389.

49. Westerburg B, Feldstein V, Sandberg P, et al. Sonographic prognostic factors in fetuses with sacrococcygeal teratoma. J Pediatr Surg 2000;35:322.

50. Avni FE, Guibaud L, Robert Y, et al. MR imaging of fetal sacrococcygeal teratoma: diagnosis and assessment. AJR Am J Roentgenol 2002;78:179.

51. Kitano Y, Flake AW, Crombleholme TM, et al. Open fetal surgery for life-threatening fetal malformations. Semin Perinatol 1999;23:448.

52. Hubbard AM, Crombleholme T, Adzick NS. Prenatal MRI evaluation of giant neck masses in preparation for fetal EXIT procedure. Am J Perinatol 1998;15:253.

53. Chervenak F, Issacson G, Blakemore K, et al. Fetal cystic hygroma: cause and natural history. N Engl J Med 1983;109:822.

54. Azizkhan R, Haase G, Applebaum H. Diagnosis, management, and outcome of cervicofacial teratomas in neonates: a Childrens Cancer Group study. J Pediatr Surg 1995;30:312.

55. Tsuda H, Matsumoto M, Yamamoto K, et al. Usefulness of ultrasonography and magnetic resonance imaging for prenatal diagnosis of fetal teratoma of the neck. J Clin Ultrasound 1996;4:217.

56. Kalache KD, Chaoui R, Tennstedt C, et al: Prenatal diagnosis of laryngeal atresia in two cases of congenital high airway obstruction syndrome (CHAOS). Prenat Diagn 1997;17:577.

57. Hubbard AM, Adzick NS, Crombleholme TM, et al. Congenital chest lesions: diagnosis and characterization with prenatal MR imaging. Radiology 1999;212:43.

58. Liechty K, Crombleholme TM, Flake A, et al. Intrapartum airway management for giant fetal neck masses: the EXIT (ex utero intrapartum treatment) procedure. Am J Obstet Gynecol 1997;177:870.

59. Hirose S, Sydorak RM, Tsao K, et al. Spectrum of intrapartum management strategies for giant fetal cervical teratoma. J Pediatr Surg 2003;38:446.

60. Mychaliska G, Bealer J, Graf J, et al. Operating on placental support: the ex utero intrapartum treatment (EXIT) procedure. J Pediatr Surg 1997;32:227.

61. Bouchard S, Johnson MP, Flake AW, et al. The EXIT procedure: experience and outcome in 31 cases. J Pediatr Surg 2002;37:418.

62. Ohlsson A, Fong K, Rose T, et al. Prenatal ultrasonic prediction of autopsy-proven pulmonary hypoplasia. Am J Perinatol 1992;9:334.

63. Duncan K, Gowland P, Moore R, et al. Assessment of fetal lung growth in utero with echo planar MR imaging. Radiology 1999;210:197.

64. Rypens F, Metens T, Rocourt N, et al. Fetal lung volume: estimation at MR imaging-initial results. Radiology 2001;219:236.

65. Duncan K, Gowland P, Freeman A, et al. The changes in magnetic resonance properties of the fetal lungs: a first result and a potential tool for the non-invasive in utero demonstration of fetal lung maturation. Br J Obstet Gynaecol 1999;106:122.

66. Coakley F, Lopoo J, Lu Y, et al. Normal and hypoplastic fetal lungs: volumetric assessment with prenatal single-shot rapid acquisition with relaxation enhancement MR imaging. Radiology 2000;216:107.

67. Fuke S, Kanzaki T, Mu J, et al. Antenatal prediction of pulmonary hypoplasia by acceleration time/ejection time ratio of fetal pulmonary arteries by Doppler blood flow velocimetry. Am J Obstet Gynecol 2003;188:228.

68. Cass DL, Quinn TM, Yang EY, et al. Increased cell proliferation and decreased apoptosis characterize congenital cystic adenomatoid malformation of the lung. J Pediatr Surg 1998;33:1043.

69. Blau H, Barak A, Karmazyn B, et al. Postnatal management of resolving fetal lung lesions. Pediatrics 2002;109:105.

70. Adzick NS, Harrison MR, Crombleholme TM, et al. Fetal lung lesions: management and outcome. Am J Obstet Gynecol 1998;179:884.

71. John PR, Beasley SW, Mayne V. Pulmonary sequestration and related congenital disorders. Pediatr Radiol 1989;20:4.

72. Bratu I, Flageole H, Chen MF, et al The multiple facets of pulmonary sequestration. J Pediatr Surg 2001;36:784.

73. Lopoo JB, Goldstein RB, Lipshutz GS, et al. Fetal pulmonary sequestration: a favorable congenital lung lesion. Obstet Gynecol 1999;94:567.

74. Dhingsa R, Coakley FV, Albanese CT, et al. Prenatal sonography and MR imaging of pulmonary sequestration. AJR Am J Roentgenol 2003;180:433.

75. Pumberger W, Moroder W, Weisbauer P. Intraabdominal extralobar pulmonary sequestration exhibiting cystic adenomatoid malformation: prenatal diagnosis and characterization of a left suprarenal mass in the newborn. Abdom Imaging 2001;26:28.

76. Cass DL, Crombleholme TM, Howell LJ, et al. Cystic lung lesions with systemic arterial blood supply: a hybrid of congenital cystic adenomatoid malformation and bronchopulmonary sequestration. J Pediatr Surg 1997;7:986.

77. Kim KW, Kim W, Cheon J, et al. Complex bronchopulmonary foregut malformation: extralobar pulmonary sequestration associated with a duplication cyst of mixed bronchogenic and esophageal type. Pediatr Radiol 2001;31:265.

78. MacKenzie TC, Guttenberg ME, Nisenbaum HL, et al. A fetal lung lesion consisting of bronchogenic cyst, bronchopulmonary sequestration, and congenital cystic adenomatoid malformation: the missing link? Fetal Diagn Ther 2001;16:193.

79. Harrison M, Adzick N, Estes J, et al. A prospective study of the outcome of fetuses with diaphragmatic hernia. JAMA 1994;271:382.

80. Sbragia L, Paek B, Filly R, et al. Congenital diaphragmatic hernia without herniation of the liver: does the lung-to-head ration predict survival? J Ultrasound Med 2000;19:845.

81. Paek BW, Coakley FV, Lu Y, et al. Congenital diaphragmatic hernia: prenatal evaluation with MR lung volumetry: preliminary experience. Radiology 2001;220:63.

82. Walsh DS, Hubbard AM, Olutoye OO, et al. Assessment of fetal lung volumes and liver herniation with magnetic resonance imaging in congenital diaphragmatic hernia. Am J Obstet Gynecol 2000;183:1067.

83. Sokol J, Bohn D, Lacro RV, et al. Fetal pulmonary artery diameters and their association with lung hypoplasia and postnatal outcome in congenital diaphragmatic hernia. Am J Obstet Gynecol 2002;186:1085.

84. Chinn D, Filly R, Callen P, et al. Congenital diaphragmatic hernia diagnosed prenatally by ultrasound. Radiology 1983;148:119.

85. Vettraino IM, Lee W, Comstock CH. The evolving appearance of a congenital diaphragmatic hernia. J Ultrasound Med 2002;21:85.

86. Lewis DA, Reickert C, Bowerman R, et al. Prenatal ultrasonography frequently fails to diagnose congenital diaphragmatic hernia. J Pediatr Surg 1997;32:352.

87. Bootstaylor B, Filly R, Harrison M, et al. Prenatal sonographic predictors of liver herniation in congenital diaphragmatic hernia. J Ultrasound Med 1995;14:515.

88. Hubbard A, Adzick N, Crombleholme T, et al. Left-sided congenital diaphragmatic hernia: value of prenatal MR imaging in preparation for fetal surgery. Radiology 1997;203:636.

89. Hubbard AM, Crombleholme T, Adzick N, et al. Prenatal MRI of congenital diaphragmatic hernia. Am J Perinatol 1999;16:407.

90. Paek B, Danzer E, Machin G, et al. Prenatal diagnosis of bilateral diaphragmatic hernia: diagnostic pitfalls. J Ultrasound Med 2000;19:495.

91. Song MS, Yoo SJ, Smallhorn JF, et al. Bilateral congenital diaphragmatic hernia: diagnostic clues at fetal sonography. Ultrasound Obstet Gynecol 2001;17:255.

92. The Congenital Diaphragmatic Hernia Study Group. Bilateral congenital diaphragmatic hernia. J Pediatr Surg 2003;38:522.

93. Hendrick M, Estes J, Sullivan K, et al. Plug the lung until it grows (PLUG): a new method to treat congenital diaphragmatic hernia in utero. J Pediatr Surg 1994;29:612.

94. Flake AW, Crombleholme TM, Johnson MP, et al. Treatment of severe congenital diaphragmatic hernia by fetal tracheal occlusion: clinical experience with fifteen cases. Am J Obstet Gynecol 2000;183:1059.

95. Tsukahara Y, Ohno Y, Itakura A, et al. Prenatal diagnosis of congenital diaphragmatic eventration by magnetic resonance imaging. Am J Perinatol 2001;18:241.

96. Gulrajani M, David K, Sy W, et al. Prenatal diagnosis of a neuroenteric cyst by magnetic resonance imaging. Am J Perinatol 1993;18:304.

97. Wang RM, Shih JC, Ko TM. Prenatal sonographic depiction of fetal mediastinal immature teratoma. J Ultrasound Med 2000;19:289.

98. Duncan K, Baker P, Gowland P, et al. Demonstration of changes in fetal liver erythropoiesis using echoplanar magnetic resonance imaging. Am J Physiol 1997;273:965.

99. Semple SI, Wallis F, Haggarty P, et al. The measurement of fetal liver T2* in utero before and after maternal oxygen breathing: progress toward a non-invasive measurement of fetal oxygenation and placental function. Magn Reson Imaging 2001;19:921.

100. Toma P, Lucigrai G, Dodero P, et al. Prenatal detection of abdominal mass by MR imaging performed while the fetus is immobilized with pancuronium bromide. AJR Am J Roentgenol 1990;154:1049.

101. Saguintaah M, Couture A, Veyrac C, et al. MRI of the fetal gastrointestinal tract. Pediatr Radiol. 2002;32:395.

102. Benachi A, Nigo P, Jouannic JM, et al. Determination of anatomical location of an antenatal intestinal occlusion by magnetic resonance imaging. Ultrasound Obstet Gynecol 2001;18:163.

103. Garmel SH, Crombleholme TM, Semple JP, et al. Prenatal diagnosis and management of fetal tumors. Semin Perinatol 1994;18;350.

104. Levine D, Goldstein H, Callen P, et al. The effect of oligohydramnios on detection of fetal anomalies with sonography. AJR Am J Roentgenol 1997;168:1609.

105. Estes J, Harrison M. Fetal obstructive uropathy. Semin Pediatr Surg 1993;2:129.

106. Cusick E, Didier F, Droulle P, et al. Mortality after an antenatal diagnosis of fetal uropathy. J Pediatr Surg 1995;30:463.

107. Lazebnick N, Bellinger M, Ferguson J, et al. Insights into the pathogenesis and natural history of fetuses with multicystic dysplastic kidney disease. Prenat Diagn 1999;9:418.

108. Johnson M, Bukowski T, Reitleman C, et al. In utero surgical treatment of fetal obstructive uropathy: a new comprehensive approach to identify appropriate candidates for vesicoamniotic shunt therapy. Am J Obstet Gynecol 1994;170:1770.

Lee P. Shulman, M.D., Sherman Elias, M.D., F.A.C.O.G., F.A.C.M.G., F.A.C.S., and Joe Leigh Simpson, M.D., F.A.C.O.G., F.A.C.M.G, F.R.C.O.G.

26

Induced Abortion for Genetic Indications: Techniques and Complications

Women who undergo prenatal genetic screening or diagnosis during the first and second trimesters and are found to be carrying fetuses with abnormalities may choose to continue or to terminate their pregnancies. Most women found to be carrying fetuses with autosomal trisomies and severe structural abnormalities ultimately choose to terminate their pregnancies, although this is less true for sex chromosome polysomy.[1–3] Studies in Europe[4] and Canada[5] have demonstrated that the expansion of prenatal diagnosis and the decision to terminate abnormal fetuses has made for a considerable reduction in infant mortality rates. Indeed, the study by van der Pal-de Bruin et al. demonstrated that differences in the practice of prenatal screening and diagnosis and termination of pregnancies characterized by congenital anomalies contributed to the reductions in overall perinatal mortality rates observed in various European regions.[4]

Many safe techniques for terminating pregnancies during the first and second trimesters are available; the decision concerning which technique to use is based primarily on fetal gestational age and the experience of the obstetrician and, in some situations, the wishes of the woman. This chapter focuses on the techniques, complications, and risks of abortion performed during the first and second trimesters of pregnancy. Readers desiring more surgically oriented descriptions of the various techniques of pregnancy termination should seek other sources.[6–9]

FIRST-TRIMESTER TECHNIQUES

The expanding use of techniques such as chorionic villus sampling (CVS) and first-trimester endovaginal ultrasonography now enable many women to undergo safe and reliable first-trimester prenatal screening and diagnosis. Detecting fetal disorders in the first trimester permits women to undergo first-trimester pregnancy termination, a procedure that is safer and less emotionally traumatic than termination performed during the second trimester.

Suction Curettage

Suction curettage remains the most common method for pregnancy termination in the United States.[10,11] The procedure is usually performed between 7 and 13 weeks of gestation and does not require hospitalization, except in high-risk cases (e.g., a patient with a bleeding disorder or severe maternal cardiovascular disease).

Technique

Determination of gestational age must be performed before suction curettage. If pelvic examination demonstrates uterine size to be appreciably different from the reported gestational age, ultrasound should be used to determine the correct fetal number and gestational age. Our group and some others routinely obtain an ultrasound examination before all termination procedures to assess fetal number and gestational age. This practice has demonstrably reduced the frequency of failed evacuation procedures in the first trimester and eliminated the performance of termination procedures in advanced-gestational-age pregnancies. Similarly, Goldstein et al.[12] found that preprocedure ultrasound and postprocedure examination of products of conception considerably decreased procedure-related morbidity.

Suction curettage for first-trimester pregnancy termination usually requires cervical dilation. The endocervical canal can be manually dilated using instruments having progressively increasing diameters (e.g., Pratt dilators, Hegar dilators). Alternatively, synthetic dilators (e.g., Dilapan [polyacrylonitrile], Lamicel [magnesium sulfate sponge]) or the seaweed *Laminaria japonicum* are often used. These osmotic dilators serve to dilate the endocervical canal by absorbing cervical moisture. This uptake in water and the resulting expansion of the dilator produces both a softening of the cervix and dilation of the endocervical canal to two to three times the original diameter. Schulz et al.[13] showed that procedures using *L. japonicum* resulted in a fivefold reduction in cervical lacerations compared with manual dilation; however, optimal results with *L. japonicum* require several hours, whereas manual techniques can be applied for immediate dilation. Our clinical experience indicates similar dilating efficiency between Lamicel and *L. japonicum*, with Lamicel tents resulting in adequate dilation in a shorter interval (4–6 hours) than laminaria tents (12–14 hours). Hern[14] reported that although Laminaria and Dilapan demonstrated similar efficacy for cervical dilation, the Dilapan dilator was more likely to disintegrate, retract, or present minor problems associated with poor dilation (e.g., dilator stuck in cervical canal).

Endogenous prostaglandins released as a result of cervical manipulation and dilation may also cause cervical softening; indeed, administration of certain prostaglandin analogs are known to result in cervical softening[15] and make for a more facile cervical dilation. Oral misoprostol (a prostaglandin E_1 analog) appears effective and safe for facilitating cervical dilation before first-trimester suction curettage.[16] More recently, others[17] also showed that vaginal and oral misoprostol provided safe and effective preoperative dilation. MacIsaac et al.[18] demonstrated that vaginal misoprostol (400 mg) was superior to oral misoprostol (400 mg) with regard to mean dilation and caused less discomfort than laminaria tents in a randomized trial of women undergoing surgical abortion. Antiprogesterone compounds such as mifepristone (RU486) have also been shown to be effective in softening the cervix and facilitating cervical dilation.[19] Carbonne et al.[20] compared vaginal gemeprost (a prostaglandin E_1 analog) with oral mifepristone and found that although both products reduced the time for cervical dilation before first-trimester suction curettage, cervical dilation was easier with a 48-hr regimen of oral mifepristone than with vaginal gemeprost. Indeed, the efficacy of mifepristone for cervical ripening before first-trimester uterine evacuation has been demonstrated by a study sponsored by the World Health Organization.[21] Platz-Christensen et al.[22] found mifepristone to be equal to misoprostol for cervical ripening and dilation before first-trimester pregnancy termination, with misoprostol being less expensive and easier to administer than mifepristone. Regardless of the mechanical or chemical technique used, cervical softening can be accomplished before dilation and will facilitate the dilation procedure, shorten the overall operative time, and reduce the morbidity associated with the procedure.[23]

If manual dilation is required to dilate the cervix, placement of a paracervical block is appropriate before the procedure; xylocaine without epinephrine is one agent commonly used. If synthetic dilators or *L. japonicum* are used, a paracervical block can be deferred until their removal. Some operators add synthetic vasopressin (Pitressin) or other vasoactive substances to the injectable anesthetic,[24] although the safety and efficacy of this practice are undetermined. Vasovagal syncope, or "cervical shock," can occur after administration of a paracervical block. Although the patient may appear to have had a seizure, vasovagal syncope is self-limited and is differentiated from seizure activity by bradycardia, rapid recovery, and a lack of postictal state. Use of atropine in the administered anesthetic agent can prevent vasovagal syncope in women who have demonstrated such activity in the past.[7]

Once endocervical dilation has been achieved, a suction curette (without suction having been started) is inserted into the uterine cavity. The choice of suction curette size is dependent on gestational age. The size of the suction curette usually equals the gestational age (in weeks) of the pregnancy. For example, a number 9 suction curette (9-mm diameter) would be used to evacuate a 9-week-size uterus. Transparent polyethylene tubing is connected to the curette once the curette is within the uterine cavity. In turn, the other end of the tubing is connected to the collection vessel. Suction is then applied using an aspiration device (e.g., Model VH-II Aspiration Machine, Berkeley Bio-Medical Engineering, Inc, Berkeley, CA). The curette is rotated on its axis with little motion along the longitudinal axis of insertion, aspirating uterine contents. When no additional tissue can be aspirated, the curette is withdrawn, with suction being maintained. A metal curette can be used to verify that all products of conception have been removed; however, experienced clinicians will frequently not perform sharp curettage after suction curettage because too vigorous curettage can markedly increase the risk for postabortion intrauterine adhesion formation. When performed, the sharp metal curette used for this purpose should be the largest curette that easily passes into the uterus. If products remain within the cavity after sharp curettage, suction curettage is repeated.

After the procedure, patients are monitored for 30 minutes for hemorrhage or changes in vital signs. Women who are Rh-negative and unsensitized receive 300 μg of Rh-immune globulin. Prophylactic antibiotics are effective in preventing infection.[25,26] We usually prescribe a 5-day regimen of tetracycline or doxycycline. Methylergonovine maleate (Methergine) is effective for decreasing the risk of postabortion bleeding from uterine atony and helps prevent development of hematometra[27] (see below). Accordingly, patients are given a five-dose regimen of 0.2 mg methylergonovine maleate to be taken orally every 4 hr, beginning immediately after completion of the procedure. In all cases, products of conception should be examined carefully by the clinician to assess completion of the procedure and gross placental or fetal abnormalities.[12]

Morbidity

First-trimester suction curettage remains a safe and effective method for pregnancy termination.[28] In a series of 170,000 consecutive suction curettage procedures performed between 5 and 14 weeks of gestation, Hakim-Elahi et al.[29] reported that only 1 in 1,405 cases (0.07 percent) required hospitalization because of incomplete abortion, sepsis, uterine perforation, hemorrhage, inability to complete the procedure, or combined (intrauterine and tubal) pregnancy. Minor complications such as mild infection, incomplete abortion requiring repeat suction, cervical stenosis or laceration, or convulsive seizure resulting from the administration of local anesthetic occurred in 1 of 118 cases (0.84 percent) in the same series. More recent data confirm the safety reported in earlier studies[30-32] and report comparable safety in programs located in historically underserved areas of the world.[33-35]

It may be a surprise to the non-obstetrician–gynecologist that complication rates for suction curettage performed before the 7th week are higher than for procedures done between weeks 8 and 10.[10,36] Presumably, this reflects difficulty in completing uterine evacuation as a result of the small size of the conceptus at this stage of pregnancy, a problem frequently encountered with menstrual extraction (see below). Conversely, suction curettage performed after the 13th week is technically more difficult and results in a higher rate of complications because of the larger size of the conceptus. Also, first-trimester suction curettage procedures performed in an outpatient setting result in low rates of morbidity and mortality, comparable to procedures performed within a hospital setting.[10]

Recent reviews of pregnancy outcomes in Danish women who had undergone surgical abortions found an increased risk of subsequent preterm and postterm deliveries.[37] There was no increased risk for any pregnancy-related complication compared with those of similar parity and age among those women.[38]

Immediate Complications

Complications resulting from suction curettage can be either immediate or delayed. Immediate complications include hemorrhage and uterine perforation. Postabortion hemorrhage usually results from cervical laceration, uterine perforation, or uterine atony. The risk of cervical laceration can be decreased by either careful manual dilation or by use of cervical osmotic dilators (e.g., *Laminaria*, Lamicel).[39] The location of uterine perforation, a complication more significant in the pregnant than in the nonpregnant state, determines the amount of bleeding and, hence, expression of symptoms. A fundal perforation may go undetected because there is likely to be neither excess bleeding nor other symptoms. However, a lateral uterine perforation may lacerate the uterine artery or uterine vein, resulting in immediate and profuse bleeding per vagina. A broad ligament hematoma may also develop as a result of a lateral perforation and present as a delayed complication manifest by diffuse lower abdominal pain, pelvic mass, or maternal fever. Use of general anesthesia has been associated with an increased risk for cervical laceration and uterine perforation,[40] as well as uterine atony. However, Hakim-Elahi et al.[29] found no increase in morbidity in women undergoing suction curettage with general anesthesia using methohexital.

Immediate postoperative pain without overt bleeding per vagina may indicate development of hematometra. Hematometra (also known as uterine distention syndrome or postabortion syndrome) usually presents with dull, aching lower abdominal pain, possibly accompanied by tachycardia, diaphoresis, or nausea. The onset is usually within the first hour after completion of the procedure. Pelvic examination reveals a large globular uterus that is tense and tender. Treatment requires immediate uterine evacuation, allowing the uterus to contract to a normal postprocedure size. Administration of intramuscu-lar methylergonovine maleate (Methergine, 0.2 mg) is then given to ensure continued con-traction of the uterus.

Overall, hemorrhage, cervical laceration, and uterine perforation occurred in 1.1 per-cent of 42,598 suction curettage procedures performed at 8 weeks of gestation.[27] These complications were even less frequent (0.06 percent) in another series of 170,000 con-secutive cases.[29] The marked difference in complication rates between the two studies may reflect operator experience. Tietze and Lewit[36] published their report at a time when legal abortion was just beginning to become available in the United States; relatively few physicians were experienced in suction curettage. Hakim-Elahi et al.[29] described the on-going experience of three large Planned Parenthood abortion clinics in New York City from 1971 (when abortion became legal in the state of New York) through 1987; most of the procedures were performed by experienced obstetricians.

Delayed Complications

Delayed complications of suction curettage may be defined as those occurring more than 72 hours after the procedure. These occur in 1–2 percent of cases and include fever, in-fection, hemorrhage, and retained products of conception (usually occurring in combina-tion).[29,36] Retained products of conception may present as postabortion bleeding, fever, midline pelvic mass, or pelvic–abdominal pain. Ultrasound can be helpful in arriving at a diagnosis for delayed postabortion complications; however, any evidence of retained products of conception (e.g., enlarged uterus) should prompt the physician to repeat the suction curettage.

Many delayed complications should, in theory, be preventable. Careful examination of the tissue obtained by suction curettage should detect an unsuccessful termination of a singleton pregnancy due to either an ectopic pregnancy or technical difficulties in com-pletely evacuating the uterus. Failure to obtain chorionic villi necessitates an ultrasound examination; if an intrauterine pregnancy is visualized, ultrasonography can be used to assist in locating the products of conception for suction curettage. Women with suspected ectopic pregnancies should be carefully monitored with serial human chorionic go-nadotropin (hCG) levels. Although surgical interventions (e.g., salpingectomy, salpingos-tomy) have traditionally been used to treat ectopic pregnancies, nonsurgical regimens using methotrexate are now commonly used.[41,42]

Mortality

First-trimester suction curettage has the lowest maternal mortality rate of any surgical method of pregnancy termination.[28] The reported death rate is far less than the national maternal mortality rate of 9 per 100,000 live births.[7,29,43] Hakim-Elahi et al.[29] reported no maternal deaths in 170,000 consecutive first-trimester suction curettage procedures. The above-cited studies, as well as studies by other investigators,[30–32] all indicate that first-trimester suction curettage is the safest method for surgical pregnancy termination (Table 26.1); second-trimester techniques of dilation and evacuation, intra-amniotic in-stillation of abortifacients, and hysterotomy or hysterectomy all carry higher mortality rates (Table 26.2). Despite the differences in morbidity and mortality in first- and second-trimester procedures, mortality rates after the *Roe v. Wade* U.S. Supreme Court ruling le-galizing abortion were considerably lower for all induced abortion compared with other types (e.g., spontaneous) of abortion.[44]

Table 26.1.   Mortality rates associated with first-trimester suction curettage

Study	Years of Study	Number of Deaths	Number of Cases
Nathanson[30]	1970–1971	0	26,000
Hodgson and Portmann[31]	1972–1973	0	10,453
Hodgson[32]	1972–1973	0	20,248
Atrash et al.[43]	1972–1982	0.8*	100,000*
Hakim-Elahi et al.[29]	1971–1987	0	170,000

*Mortality rate calculated from Centers for Disease Control Annual Abortion Surveillance Reports.

Table 26.2.   Death rate from legal abortion in the United States, 1972–1982

Procedure	Gestational Age (Weeks)						
	≤8	9–10	11–12	13–15	16–20	≥21	Total
Suction curettage	0.5	1.0	1.8	NA	NA	NA	0.8
D and E	NA	NA	NA	3.6	9.5	10.4	5.1
Instillation	NA	NA	NA	5.0	10.9	11.7	10.1
Hysterectomy/hysterotomy	NA	48.2	33.1	62.6	80.9	115.1	44.8
Total	0.5	1.1	1.8	4.3	11.1	11.8	1.6

Source: Adapted from Atrash et al., 1987,[43] Table II.

Note: Death rate is the number of maternal deaths per 100,000 procedures.

Menstrual Extraction

Pregnancy interruption of very early pregnancies (i.e., before about 42 days after the last menses) can be achieved by so-called menstrual extraction (also known as menstrual regulation or minisuction curettage). Developed in the early 1970s,[45,46] this procedure can be performed in the physician's office with minimal equipment.

Menstrual extraction is optimally performed within 2 weeks of a "missed" period. The procedure should not be performed later than 7 weeks of gestation because this increases the risk for incomplete abortion, infection, and hemorrhage.[6] Due to the gestational age constraints, this technique is usually not applicable for genetic pregnancy terminations. Medical methods (see below) will probably replace menstrual extraction for the termination of early pregnancies, although early gestational procedures such as menstrual extraction will likely remain popular in regions of the world that may not be able to afford or effectively manage medical protocols for pregnancy termination.

Technique

A narrow cannula (e.g., Karman cannula) is guided through the undilated endocervical canal into the uterine cavity. Minimal cervical dilation may be necessary if the cannula cannot be easily passed into the uterine cavity. A 30- or 50-mL syringe is then attached to the Luer-lock end of the cannula and products of conception are aspirated by multiple (15–20) rapid withdrawals of the syringe plunger to 30- or 50-mL negative pressure (depending on syringe size). After aspiration, the catheter is removed under continuous maximum negative pressure.

Aspirated contents are then placed in a Petri dish containing a small amount of sterile water or saline to examine the aspirate for chorionic villi. Absence of chorionic villi may indicate incomplete abortion or ectopic pregnancy; appropriate diagnostic measures (e.g., ultrasound, serum progesterone, serial hCG assays) should then be initiated. Use of prophylactic antibiotics should be considered. Rh-immune globulin should be administered to all unsensitized Rh-negative patients.

Morbidity and Mortality

In the 1980s, the unfavorable experience with menstrual extraction led most obstetrician–gynecologists in the United States to abandon this procedure. Because menstrual extraction is performed so soon after a missed menstrual period, one problem was that the procedure was unwittingly performed on many nonpregnant women (27–59 percent).[47,48] However, great improvements in pregnancy detection tests would surely now decrease the number of procedures being performed on nonpregnant women to negligible levels. The sensitivity of commonly available pregnancy tests now permits accurate pregnancy detection before a missed period.[49]

Another problem was that failure rates from incomplete abortion or a continuing viable pregnancy were 10–11 percent.[10,45,46] Moreover, operative complications (e.g., infection, hemorrhage, uterine perforation) were similar to first-trimester suction curettage[32] (see above). Thus, many of the potential advantages of menstrual extraction over first-trimester suction curettage were negated. Nonetheless, the procedure is still performed, primarily in underdeveloped nations and by some obstetricians in the United States; it is also used in some regions where abortion is unavailable for economic or political reasons.[10]

Manual Vacuum Aspiration (MVA)

Meyer[50] reported on the transition from the aforementioned menstrual extraction to manual vacuum aspiration. In this report, the use of pregnancy tests, pathology evaluation, and diagnostic assessment in cases of failure to obtain products of conception were detailed in a successful in-office use of manual vacuum aspiration for early pregnancy termination. MVA is performed in a somewhat different fashion from menstrual extraction and is facilitated with current pregnancy diagnostic methods.

As with suction curettage (see below), assessment of gestational age and maternal anatomic findings that could complicate the procedure are determined before starting the procedure. MVA is usually performed in the office and, unlike menstrual extraction, may involve minimal dilation (osmotic dilators, active dilators, prostaglandin) before insertion of a curette. Once inserted, the curette is attached to a manual aspirator and several aspirations are performed until the operator determines that the uterus is emptied. Tissue obtained at the time of aspiration is sent to the pathology laboratory for confirmation of products of conception. The procedure is usually performed from 6 to 10 completed weeks of gestation.[51,52] A recent review[53] found no differences regarding efficacy and safety of MVA and dilation and curettage (suction curettage); cost and time to completion were considerably reduced in the MVA procedures.

Although most first-trimester termination procedures for fetal abnormalities will be performed after 10 completed weeks, this procedure holds great promise for its safety, efficacy, and cost effectiveness, thus allowing women carrying fetuses with demonstrable problems detected early in pregnancy to choose a procedure best suited to their wishes and needs.

RU486 (Mifepristone)

Progesterone plays an integral role in implantation and in early development of the conceptus; its deficiency is associated with pregnancy loss.[54] Predictably, progesterone antagonists are effective in interrupting early pregnancies, which are dependent on progesterone for normal development and maintenance. This offers a nonsurgical method for early pregnancy interruption.

The most commonly used antiprogesterone analog for early pregnancy interruption is RU486, or mifepristone. RU486 has high affinity for progesterone receptors, blocking normal progesterone binding and function. This compound has been shown to be an effective and safe abortifacient in early gestation. In a series of 100 very early pregnancies (within 10 days of a missed period), RU486 was effective in causing complete abortion in 85 of the 100 women.[55] Baird et al.[56] showed that a single oral dose (400–600 mg) of RU486 induced bleeding per vagina in most patients; however, the frequency of incomplete abortion in women using *only* a single dose of RU486 was approximately 20 percent. On the other hand, use of a prostaglandin analog (gemeprost suppository per vagina or sulprostone intramuscular injection) as an adjunct to RU486 resulted in complete abortion (without need for further surgical evacuation) in 95 of 100 women whose pregnancies were 42 days or less after their last menstrual period.[56] Similar success rates were reported by others.[57–62] Misoprostol, a prostaglandin E_1 analog, is also effective as a co-inductor of first-trimester abortion. Vaginal misoprostol appears far more effective and better tolerated than oral misoprostol for the induction of first-trimester abortion with mifepristone.[63]

The optimal drug dosages for the combination of RU486 and prostaglandin analogs and the most efficacious time during pregnancy for these drugs to be administered have not yet been determined. Initial studies using systemic prostaglandin analogs alone for first-trimester pregnancy interruption demonstrated that complete abortion could be induced in approximately 90 percent of cases. This was the case provided that systemic prostaglandin analogs were administered before 8 weeks of gestation (i.e., 56 days of amenorrhea or 42 days of gestation). However, patients given these prostaglandin analogs reported a high frequency of gastrointestinal side effects, including nausea, vomiting, and diarrhea, thereby limiting the usefulness of systemic prostaglandins alone as an effective first-trimester abortifacient.[64–66] A single 600-mg oral dose of RU486 followed 36–48 hours later by either 1 mg gemeprost (intravaginal suppository) or intramuscular sulprostone (0.25, 0.375, or 0.5 mg; all three doses with similar rates of complete abortion) resulted in complete abortion in 96 percent of 2,115 women who were amenorrheic for 49 days or less.[67] The mean time of expulsion of products of conception after administration of the prostaglandin analog was shortest in patients receiving 0.5 mg sulprostone (4.5 hr) and longest in women receiving gemeprost (22.7 hr).

A World Health Organization (WHO)[68] multicenter comparison demonstrated that a single 600-mg oral dose of RU486 and a five-dose regimen (25 mg every 12 hr for five doses), both followed by 1 mg gemeprost after the initiation of the regimens, were equally effective in causing complete abortion (92.0 percent for the single-dose regimen and 93.4 percent for the five-dose regimen). This study demonstrated a lack of dose–response relationship for RU486 (at the doses studied); indeed, several regimens using low single or multiple doses of mifepristone and various prostaglandin analogs have been shown to have similar efficacy and salutary side effect profiles.[69,70]

As with menstrual extraction, RU486 is not, at present, a method being offered to most women considering pregnancy termination for fetal abnormality. However, advances in prenatal genetic screening and diagnosis may eventually make nonsurgical methods of early pregnancy termination applicable to the diagnosis of certain fetal abnormalities.

Morbidity and Mortality

Most women (90–95 percent) treated with RU486 and prostaglandin analogs report transient abdominal cramping.[68,71] Other side effects include nausea, vomiting, diarrhea, breast tenderness, and bleeding per vagina that is heavier than normal menses. In the WHO study[68] these minor complications occurred in similar frequencies in both the single-dose study group and the five-dose study group. More serious complications (e.g., heavy bleeding, infection) are rare. No deaths resulting from the administration of RU486, with or without prostaglandin analogs, were reported in the WHO study[68] or in any of the cited studies.

Of considerable interest to clinicians who care for women considering pregnancy after an abnormal prenatal diagnostic test is recent evidence that medical protocols may be applicable to women considering pregnancy termination up to 12 weeks of gestation. A regimen of mifespristone followed 48 hours later by a course of vaginal gemeprost resulted in complete abortion in twenty-four of twenty-five women with twenty-three of the twenty-four successful cases requiring no more than two gemeprost vaginal pessaries.[72] The sole failure underwent surgical evacuation because of heavy bleeding. In a different study, a regimen of mifepristone followed 36 to 48 hours later by repeated doses of misoprostol was successful in 458 of 483 (94.8 percent) cases.[73]

Other Systemic Abortifacients

Drugs and substances used for indications other than abortion can also act as systemic abortifacients. Prostaglandin analogs, currently used for nonabortion indications, have been used without medical approbation in areas where legal abortions are either not available or prohibitively expensive. For example, Coelho et al.[74] from Brazil described using misoprostol, a readily available prostaglandin E_1 analog commonly prescribed for the treatment of peptic ulcer disease and gastritis resulting from chronic nonsteroidal anti-inflammatory drug use. Misoprostol also causes uterine contractions and thus has become a popular abortifacient in Brazil, where abortion is illegal. However, misoprostol has been shown to be effective when used in combination with mifepristone (see above). Misoprostol used alone as an abortifacient may not be as effective as mifepristone but will result in complete abortion in almost two-thirds of cases.[75,76] However, a recent study[77] shows that a high-dose regimen of oral misoprostol was highly effective in causing complete abortion, with 91 percent of women having a complete second-trimester abortion within 24 hours. Another prostaglandin E_1 analog, gemeprost, has also been shown to have similar efficacy when used alone as an abortifacient,[78] although it also has been shown to be an effective co-inductor of uterine evacuation when used with mifepristone.

Another systemic abortifacient that is being used with increasing frequency is methotrexate. With the continuing lack of FDA approval for mifepristone and the extensive use of methotrexate to treat ectopic pregnancy,[41,42] methotrexate is now being used in combination with prostaglandin analogs to induce early pregnancy termination. Although initial studies suggest the efficacy of methotrexate combination regimens to be slightly less than mifepristone combination regimens, high rates of completed terminations can be obtained when methotrexate is used with misoprostol or gemeprost.[79,80]

SECOND-TRIMESTER TECHNIQUES

Despite increasing use of first-trimester CVS, early amniocentesis, and endovaginal ultrasonography, the majority of prenatal diagnostic testing is still performed in the late first and second trimesters. Thus, the necessity for second-trimester genetic pregnancy terminations remains. Second-trimester pregnancy termination procedures carry morbidity and mortality rates higher than first-trimester techniques.

Dilation and Evacuation

In the United States, dilation and evacuation (D and E) is the most common technique used for second-trimester pregnancy termination.[11] D and E has the lowest mortality rate of all second-trimester pregnancy termination procedures (see Table 26.2) and morbidity rates comparable to or lower than other second-trimester techniques.[7,81] In addition, a recent study[82] found no adverse impact on future childbearing after a second-trimester D and E if preoperative cervical dilation was achieved by the use of Laminaria. Women undergoing D and E do not usually require hospitalization, unlike those who undergo labor-induction techniques; D and E is therefore less expensive than labor-induction techniques.[83] The psychologic benefits of a rapid outpatient method have also been documented. Kaltreider et al.[84] reported that thirty patients undergoing D and E experienced less postoperative pain, anger, and depression than twenty women undergoing labor-induction methods. In addition, D and E requires less time to complete than labor-induction methods.[85]

Although D and E is the most commonly used technique for second-trimester pregnancy termination, labor-induction methods (e.g., systemic prostaglandins) are still the most commonly used for genetic pregnancy termination. Indeed, an informal survey of the seven prenatal diagnostic centers involved in the U.S. Collaborative Chorionic Villus Sampling Study[86] showed that six of the seven centers participating in the study used labor-induction methods (primarily vaginal prostaglandin suppositories) for second-trimester genetic terminations.

Why is D and E not commonly performed for second-trimester genetic pregnancy terminations? There are several potential reasons. One is that not all obstetrician–gynecologists are trained or are willing to perform this procedure. However, most large medical centers now have personnel trained in this procedure. Obstetrician–gynecologists who perform second-trimester D and E require special training and ongoing experience; lower rates of morbidity and mortality are achieved only when D and E is performed by such physicians.[87]

A second rationale for not using D and E for pregnancy terminations performed for genetic indications is concern about the ability to confirm the genetic diagnosis. Our group has reported considerable success in confirming abnormal prenatal diagnoses by pathologic, cytogenetic, or DNA analyses of products of conception obtained by D and E.[88–90] Specifically, we confirmed prenatal diagnoses in 114 consecutive pregnancies terminated after diagnosis of fetal abnormalities.[90] A fetal cytogenetic complement from products of conception was obtained in all but 1 of 114 cases studied. In addition, ultrasound-directed retrieval of selected organs confirmed prenatal ultrasound diagnoses of fetal structural abnormalities in 13 cases. More recently, others[91] were able to obtain a cytogenetic result on approximately 99 percent of their cases of D and E. Diagnostic confirmation is thus possible following D and E in the majority of cases; confirmation of fetal cytogenetic abnormalities should be possible in almost all cases, whereas the diagnosis of structural abnormalities will rely on not only the expertise of the clinician but also on the expertise of the pathologist and geneticist who evaluate the particular abnormal pregnancy. However, detection of associated structural defects in cases characterized by multiple anomalies will likely require pathologic evaluation of an intact fetus to have the best chance to identify a syndrome and thus provide the most accurate counseling for future pregnancies.

Technique

As with first-trimester pregnancy termination, assessment of gestational age must be performed before second-trimester abortion procedures. In almost all cases of second-trimester genetic termination, ultrasound has been performed before the decision to terminate the procedure. Second-trimester D and E invariably requires dilation of the cervix. Although careful manual dilation usually allows sufficient cervical dilation to allow uterine evacuation in most cases, this technique carries increased risk for cervical laceration, hemorrhage, and unsuccessful uterine evacuation.[13] The preferred technique uses cervical dilators that gradually expand within the endocervical canal as a result of absorbing moisture from the cervix (see above). Many obstetricians use Laminaria tents made from the seaweed *L. japonicum* for second-trimester D and E procedures. Proper use of Laminaria tents requires leaving them in place for 12–18 hours to achieve optimal cervical dilation, usually necessitating a 2-day procedure. Alternatively, synthetic dilating devices (e.g., Lamicel, Dilapan) achieve safe and optimal dilation within 6–8 hours and enable the entire procedure to be completed within 1 day.

General anesthesia should be avoided, if possible, because it increases maternal morbidity and mortality.[92] A paracervical block is administered before uterine evacuation. Some obstetrician–gynecologists add small amounts of vasopressin or other vasoactive substances to the xylocaine, apparently resulting in significantly less intraoperative blood loss.[24] Occasionally patients experience vasovagal syncope following administration of the paracervical block (see above); this usually resolves quickly. Certain maternal cardiac disorders (e.g., cardiac arrhythmias) may be relative contraindications to paracervical analgesia. In addition, we begin all patients on prophylactic antibiotics at the time of cervical dilation, and antiemetic and antianxiety medications are provided as needed.

Products of conception are evacuated using instruments specifically designed to extract intrauterine contents at this stage of gestation. We prefer either Sopher or Bierer forceps; other available ovum forceps are also listed in Table 26.3. Concurrent ultrasonography is also helpful in facilitating uterine evacuation,[93,94] especially when extracting intact specific fetal parts are necessary to confirm prenatal diagnoses.[89,90] Although ultrasound guidance is not essential for safe and successful uterine evacuation, we find that it often

Table 26.3. Ovum forceps used for second-trimester dilation and evacuation

Barrett
Bierer
Clemetson
Forester
Kelly placental forceps
Moore
Peterson
Sanger
Sopher
Van Lith

facilitates the evacuation procedure, particularly in problematic cases such as when patients have severe uterine anteversion or anteflexion.

After the products of conception have been evacuated, suction curettage is performed to remove any remaining tissue. As with first-trimester procedures, the obstetrician–gynecologist must examine the specimen to verify that all products of conception have been removed. For terminations performed because of fetal anatomic abnormalities, products of conception should also be examined and labeled by individuals with expertise in dysmorphology before preparing specimens for pathologic and other confirmatory laboratory analyses. Of course, the confirmatory analyses selected (e.g., cytogenetic, DNA, enzymatic) will depend on the specific prenatal diagnosis.

After D and E, we observe patients for excessive vaginal bleeding or changes in vital signs. Patients are instructed to expect some lower abdominal cramping, vaginal bleeding (similar to menstrual flow in volume), and possibly low-grade fever. Severe manifestations of these signs and symptoms may presage serious complications and require immediate evaluation by a physician. To prevent uterine atony, intramuscular methylergonovine maleate (0.2 mg) is given immediately on completion of the procedure, followed by an oral regimen of 0.2 mg methylergonovine maleate every 4 hours for five doses. Rh-immune globulin (300 μg) is administered to unsensitized Rh-negative patients. We also personally contact patients by telephone 24–48 hours after the procedure and arrange postoperative visits no later than 10 days to 2 weeks later.

Morbidity

When performed by an experienced obstetrician–gynecologist,[87] D and E carries significantly lower morbidity rates than do methods requiring labor induction or surgical procedures (i.e., hysterotomy, hysterectomy).[43,95–98] Kafrissen et al.[97] compared the safety of 9,572 D and E procedures with 2,805 instillation procedures using an instillate composed of prostaglandin F2α and urea. All procedures were performed between 13 and 24 weeks of gestation. Serious complications (fever >38°C, hemorrhage requiring blood transfusion or performance of unintended surgery as result of an abortion-related incident) occurred in 0.49 percent of patients undergoing D and E procedures compared with 1.03 percent of patients undergoing prostaglandin/urea procedures. Of all complications evaluated, only uterine perforation occurred more frequently in the D and E group. Among women undergoing abortions through the 15th menstrual week, Robins and Surrago[96] found that 400 patients undergoing D and E had a lower frequency of complications (i.e., blood loss requiring transfusion, cervical laceration, retained products of conception, fever, vomiting, and diarrhea) than 112 patients undergoing labor induction abortions by intravaginal prostaglandin suppositories.

Peterson et al.[99] reported that the rate of unplanned hospitalizations resulting from D and E at 13 weeks was 0.6 percent, but was 1.4 percent at 20–21 weeks. However, others[100] found that D and E procedures performed from 18 to 22 weeks were characterized by low complication rates of less than 1 percent. Thus, D and E performed *later* in the second trimester results in morbidity rates no greater, and possibly less than, labor-induction techniques. Nonetheless, the other substantive advantages of D and E (e.g., outpatient procedure, less expensive to perform) make this technique more advantageous compared with other second-trimester techniques (i.e., systemic or intra-amniotic abortifacients, hysterotomy, or hysterectomy).

A major complication of D and E is uterine perforation. The severity of signs and symptoms depends on the location of the uterine perforation. Lateral perforations involving laceration of the uterine artery or vein are most dangerous because of the possibility of profuse hemorrhage. However, the use of concurrent ultrasound guidance may reduce the incidence of uterine perforation.[93,94] Other causes of hemorrhage include cervical or vaginal laceration, uterine atony, retained products of conception, or coagulopathy (apparently secondary to release of tissue thromboplastin into the maternal venous system during D and E). Although ultrasound-directed uterine evacuation, postoperative methylergonovine maleate, and careful inspection of products of conception will reduce the incidence of intraoperative and postoperative hemorrhage, complications will invariably occur. Operators must be prepared to administer necessary resuscitation maneuvers needed to stabilize such patients and to subsequently manage their complications.

Infection is another serious complication that may occur after D and E. Antibiotic prophylaxis is effective in decreasing febrile morbidity in both first- and second-trimester uterine evacuation procedures.[25,26] Frequently, postoperative infection is the result of retained products of conception. If there is any evidence of retained products of conception, suction curettage should be performed to evacuate the uterus. Ultrasonography may be particularly useful in evaluating and treating such patients.

Mortality

Overall, D and E is the safest technique for second-trimester pregnancy termination. D and E is as safe for the woman as having a normal pregnancy and delivery,[101] a statement that cannot be made about other techniques of second-trimester pregnancy termination. The Joint Program for the Study of Abortion (JPSA III) showed D and E to be associated with the lowest maternal death to case ratio compared with instillation techniques or hysterotomy/hysterectomy (see Tables 26.2 and 26.4).[43,98] Maternal mortality rates associated with D and E procedures increase with the gestational age at which the procedure is performed and become similar to that of instillation procedures later in the second trimester (i.e., >16 weeks of gestation) (see Table 26.4).[98] In addition to safety, the other benefits of D and E procedures (e.g., low cost, shorter time to complete abortion, less psychologic stress for the woman) make D and E the preferred method for almost all second-trimester pregnancy terminations.

Systemic Abortifacients

The primary advantage of systemic abortifacients is ease of use. Their noninvasive application does not require surgical expertise; therefore, they can be easily used by non-

Table 26.4. Mortality rates of second-trimester pregnancy-termination procedures

Procedure	Gestational Age at Time of Abortion (Weeks)			
	13–15	16–20	≥21	Total Rate
D and E	3.2	9.2	12.0	4.9
All instillation*	5.5	12.0	13.3	9.6
Saline	1.7	15.2	12.9	11.6
Prostaglandin F2α	12.1	6.0	14.2	6.4
Hysterotomy/hysterectomy	64.9	84.5	123.0	47.8

Source: Adapted from Grimes and Schulz, 1985.[98]
Note: All mortality rates are deaths per 100,000 cases.
*Refers to all instillation procedures, irrespective of agent(s) used.

obstetrician–gynecologists. However, clinicians who perform second-trimester pregnancy terminations with systemic abortifacients must be ready to provide surgical care should there be a failed induction, retained products of conception, or if such techniques result in the very rare but life-threatening complication of uterine rupture.[102]

The most commonly used systemic abortifacients for second-trimester pregnancy termination are prostaglandin analogs that stimulate uterine contractions and result in the expulsion of the products of conception. However, antiprogesterones such as RU486 have been shown to facilitate and expedite second-trimester pregnancy termination performed by use of systemic abortifacients,[103–105] although their use alone in such cases has been shown to yield poor results, with incomplete expulsion of the products of conception.[69]

The most frequently used prostaglandin analog in the United States is prostaglandin E_2 (PGE_2; dinoprostone) in suppository (20 mg) form. The suppository is placed intravaginally on a regular schedule (usually every 3–4 hours until delivery), either directly into the posterior fornix of the vagina or held in place with a diaphragm. Intramuscular injections of 15-methyl prostaglandin F2α are also used for second-trimester pregnancy termination; however, this abortifacient is no longer marketed in the United States. More recently, several groups have reported the use of misoprostol for first- and second-trimester pregnancy terminations. In the second trimester, pregnancy terminations using misoprostol are performed with a 200-μg intravaginal tablet that is repeated every 12 hours until completion. One study found no effect with regard to procedure efficacy when misoprostol was provided in oral form.[106] However, Jain and Mishell[107] showed that the rate of successful abortion was 81 percent with dinoprostone and 89 percent with misoprostol, with similar times to completion. The main advantage of misoprostol over dinoprostone is a more salutary side-effect profile, with considerably fewer gastrointestinal effects and less hyperpyrexia. Other studies[108,109] demonstrated that prostaglandin E_1 analogs are as effective as prostaglandin E_2 analogs for inducing second-trimester pregnancy termination, but with considerably fewer and less severe side effects; these findings are comparable to a recent report[77] showing a 91 percent success rate for second-trimester pregnancy termination using a high-dose misoprostol protocol. Finally, Autry et al.[81] found the use of misoprostol to be the safest method for medical induction for second-trimester pregnancy termination.

Surrago and Robins[110] reported that the mean time from drug administration to abortion was 13.4 hours using 20-mg prostaglandin E_2 vaginal suppositories (one every 3 hours); 90 percent of women aborted within 24 hours. Robins and Mann[111] reported that the mean time from drug administration to abortion was 16 hours using 15-methyl prostaglandin F2α (250 μg intramuscular every 2 hours), with 80 percent of women completing the abortion after 24 hours. A more recent study[112] found intravaginal PGE_2 to be a more effective and a more rapid abortifacient than intramuscular 15-methyl prostaglandin F2α. Concurrent intravenous oxytocin augmentation is used in some centers, although it is unclear whether this significantly decreases the interval to expulsion.[110] Owen and Hauth[113] found that concurrent oxytocin expedited pregnancy termination when vaginal PGE_2 suppositories were used. Pretreatment with Laminaria or synthetic dilators definitely shortens the time to abortion, thereby reducing the amount of prostaglandin administered and, accordingly, the side effects experienced.[114,115]

Systemic abortifacients result in an intact abortus, which, in some cases, may be necessary for diagnostic confirmation. However, in our experience (see above), D and E usually provides tissues adequate for most diagnostic confirmations.[88–90] This is true even in cases of structural anomalies, and certainly for cytogenetic studies. Thus, we believe there

is little or no diagnostic or obstetric advantage in inducing labor by systemic abortifacients compared with using D and E, except for situations in which personnel trained in
D and E are not available.

Morbidity and Mortality

Maternal systemic effects of PGE$_2$ vaginal suppositories include nausea, vomiting, diarrhea, hypotension, and tachycardia. Surrago and Robins[110] reported vomiting in 37 percent and diarrhea in 31 percent of 112 patients undergoing pregnancy termination by PGE$_2$
vaginal suppositories; 29 percent of the women had fever >38°C during the termination
procedure. Gastrointestinal side effects are more common when intramuscular 15-methyl
prostaglandin F2α is used: 83 percent reported vomiting and 71 percent had diarrhea in
another series.[111] However, Jain and Mishell[107] reported significantly fewer side effects
with misoprostol, with efficacy similar to that of dinoprostone.

Because of the relatively high incidence of incomplete abortion, complications such
as blood loss requiring transfusion and sepsis can occur after the administration of systemic prostaglandins. Although systemic prostaglandins are relatively safe and easy to use,
maternal mortality can still occur as a result of failure to recognize complications in a
timely fashion or from intraoperative complications (e.g., uterine perforation, hemorrhage)
secondary to surgical procedures required for incomplete abortions.

Intra-amniotic Abortifacients

The instillation of intra-amniotic abortifacients is another method of second-trimester pregnancy termination that has been used since the 1960s. However, intra-amniotic instillation of abortifacient agents such as saline, prostaglandin F2α, 15-methyl prostaglandin
F2α, and urea have now largely been replaced by the considerably safer and more facile
techniques of D and E and labor induction using systemic abortifacients [43,84,97,98,116–119]
(see Tables 26.2 and 26.4). Another disadvantage of instillation techniques for terminations for genetic indications is that some agents (e.g., saline, urea) result in tissue necrosis, thereby compromising many confirmatory tests. Finally, the reduced number of
instillation procedures performed in the United States, Europe, and the rest of the world
over the past two decades has left few clinicians with sufficient expertise to perform such
procedures.

Hysterotomy/Hysterectomy

Although commonly used as methods of abortion in the late 1960s and early 1970s, hysterotomy and hysterectomy have essentially been abandoned because of high rates of maternal morbidity and mortality[120] (see Table 26.1). Hysterotomy refers to the removal of
the fetus through an incision in the uterus, whereas hysterectomy refers to the removal of
the pregnancy by removing both the uterus and the fetus as a single unit. When performed
in the second trimester, both procedures require an abdominal incision and extensive surgical manipulation. These procedures result in the highest rates of morbidity and mortality among abortion procedures (see Tables 26.2 and 26.4). However, there is bias in these
data in that these procedures were usually performed on very ill patients who would not
be able to tolerate 20–30 hours of labor. Such patients would be expected to have higher
complication rates irrespective of the method used to terminate the pregnancy.

Hysterotomy is warranted only in situations in which systemic or intra-amniotic methods of termination have failed and no trained personnel experienced in performing D and E are available. Hysterectomy may be justified in very rare instances when the need for termination is accompanied by uterine pathology (e.g., cancer). We have not encountered such a need in over 25 years of offering prenatal diagnostic services.

Counseling Patients about Second-Trimester Procedures

How should patients be counseled concerning second-trimester pregnancy termination procedures? If alternatives exist, that will primarily depend on the wishes of the patient, the fetal diagnosis, and the potential need for further pathologic assessment. With regard to safety, we believe that D and E is the method of choice if trained personnel are available and if the pregnancy is ≤17 weeks of gestation. Geneticists should be aware that evaluation of products of conception obtained by D and E is reliable for confirming most prenatal diagnoses.

The optimal procedure for terminating pregnancies in the second half of the second trimester (>17 weeks of gestation) is less clear. D and E carries similar morbidity and mortality rates as systemic abortifacient procedures when performed at this stage of pregnancy, although Schneider et al.[100] found that D and E was as safe as induction methods when performed between 18 and 22 weeks. Other benefits of D and E (e.g., rapidity of procedure, lower costs, improved psychologic well-being) lead us to consider D and E to be the preferred method for second-trimester pregnancy termination after 17 weeks of gestation, except when an intact fetus is needed for diagnostic confirmation.

Few data exist concerning the safety of even later pregnancy termination procedures (>20 weeks of gestation). Many states preclude pregnancy termination after 24 weeks of gestation except to save the life of the mother. If necessary, however, either intra-amniotic agents or systemic prostaglandins should be used because the size of the conceptus at this stage of pregnancy makes routine D and E technically problematic. Ongoing federal legislation in the United States may have further negative implications for performing D and E in the later portion of the second trimester.[121,122]

SELECTIVE ABORTION AND FETAL REDUCTION IN MULTIPLE GESTATIONS

Improved ultrasound technology and invasive prenatal diagnostic procedures (e.g., amniocentesis, CVS) have enabled earlier and more accurate detection of fetal abnormalities in multiple gestations (see also chapters 2, 5, and 23). Occasionally, this leads to the dilemma of detecting discordance in a multiple gestation involving normal and abnormal fetuses. In such cases, selective abortion is used, with the objective of causing death of the abnormal fetus(es) with continued gestation of the normal fetus(es). Advances in assisted reproductive technologies also have led to an increased incidence of multiple gestation, particularly as result of ovulation induction.[123]

Pregnancies with three or more fetuses have significantly higher spontaneous abortion rates than singleton or twin pregnancies,[124,125] and infants of multiple birth have significantly higher morbidity and mortality rates than singletons.[126] A variation of selective abortion applied to multifetal pregnancies (i.e., three or more fetuses) is to arbitrarily "reduce" the number of fetuses (usually to two or three) to reduce the risks of mortality and morbidity of the remaining fetuses. In this section, we discuss the surgical aspects of selective abortion and fetal reduction. Detailed ethical analyses of such decisions are provided elsewhere,[127–129] and in chapter 32.

Second-Trimester Selective Abortion

Selective abortion of abnormal fetuses was initially performed in the second trimester. Aberg et al.[130] reported the birth of a normal infant at 33 weeks after selective termination at 20 weeks of gestation of a co-twin affected with Hurler syndrome. Selective termination in this case was performed by fetal exsanguination by ultrasound-directed needle cardiac puncture. In the second report of a successful selective birth, Beck et al.[131] used hysterotomy at 22 weeks of gestation to remove an abnormal twin. Subsequent successes were also reported by Rodeck et al.,[132] who used fetoscopic-guided air embolization into the umbilical vein to selectively abort abnormal fetuses. Antsaklis et al.[133] used a fetoscopic-guided intracardiac injection of calcium gluconate. However, most centers that currently offer selective feticide use intracardiac injection of potassium chloride (KCl).[134,135]

Technique

Most centers in the United States that perform second-trimester selective abortion currently use the intracardiac KCl injection technique. Detailed descriptions of the other techniques are discussed elsewhere.[136]

Ultrasound is required to locate and identify the normal and abnormal fetuses. In the case of a fetus with a structural abnormality, ultrasonographic visualization of the fetal defect at the time of selective abortion is sufficient. However, for cases in which fetuses have diagnosed abnormalities with no discriminating ultrasonographic findings (e.g., a fetus with Duchenne muscular dystrophy diagnosed by DNA analysis of amniotic fluid cells), careful documentation of fetal positions at the time of amniocentesis is necessary for determining the normal and abnormal fetuses at the time of selective abortion.

An ultrasound examination is initially performed to confirm fetal number, viability, gestational age, placental location, and positions of the normal and abnormal fetuses. Choice of needle insertion site is based on ultrasound determination of the easiest access to the fetus(es) to be terminated. Before needle insertion, the patient may be premedicated for sedation and to decrease fetal movements (e.g., intravenous meperidine, 50 mg; prochlorperazine, 10 mg; and diazepam, 5–10 mg) and to inhibit uterine contractions (ritodrine hydrochloride, 3 mg).[137] Under continuous ultrasound guidance and through an aseptic field, a 20- or 22-gauge needle is inserted transabdominally into the amniotic sac of the abnormal fetus. The needle stylet is removed and a 5-mL syringe is attached to the hub of the needle to withdraw amniotic fluid for confirmatory studies (if applicable). The tip of the needle is then passed into the fetal thorax and heart. Correct placement of the needle is confirmed by observation of negative pressure within the 5-ml syringe. Sterile KCl (2 mEq/mL) is injected in 2- mL increments until asystole is ultrasonographically demonstrated[136]; in the series reported by Golbus et al.,[136] the volume of KCl needed to cause asystole ranged from 2 to 7 mL. Intracardiac instillation of KCl may not always result in permanent asystole of the affected fetus; several instillations may be required to complete the procedure. The overall incidence of multiple instillations has not been determined, although most procedures are apparently completed after a single instillation.[136,137]

After the procedure, ultrasound examination should be repeated every 30 minutes for 1 to 2 hours to verify absence of fetal heart activity. If fetal heart activity is still present, the procedure must be repeated. Unsensitized Rh-negative patients should receive Rh-immune globulin. The benefit of prophylactic antibiotics is as yet undetermined. Golbus et al.[136] administered antibiotic prophylaxis for selected cases requiring a greater degree of manipulation. Chitkara et al.[137] gave all patients intravenous antibiotic prophylaxis (ce-

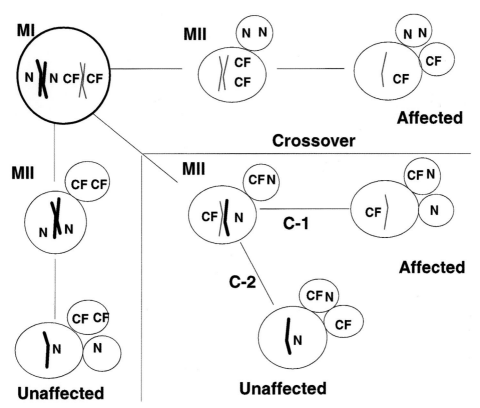

Fig. 27.1. The scheme demonstrating the principle of preimplantation genetic analysis by sequential DNA analysis of the first and second polar body, using the CF locus as an example.

Fluorescent In Situ Hybridization, Trisomy 21 Identification

Chromosome 21 - red, Chromosome 18 - green

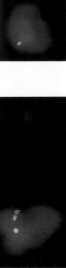

2nd Polar Body Chromatin

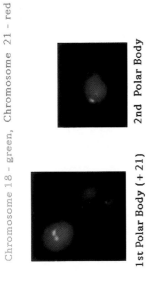

1st Polar Body Chromatin

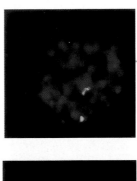

Embryo Nucleus, Trisomy 21

Fig. 27.3. Patterns of signals in an oocyte with trisomy 21, revealed by testing of both first and second polar bodies by FISH, using chromosome 18 and 21 specific probes. Normally, the first polar body should have two signals for chromosome 18 (two green dots) and two for chromosome 21 (two red dots), whereas only a single red or green dot should be seen in the second polar body. However, the second polar body shows no red signal instead of one for chromosome 21 (only a green dot for chromosome 18 is seen), demonstrating the result of nondisjunction of chromosome 21 in the second meiotic division, leading to trisomy 21 in the embryo, as shown by follow-up blastomere FISH analysis confirming the polar body diagnosis.

Fluorescent In Situ Hybridization, Monosomy 21 Identification

Chromosome 18 - green, Chromosome 21 - red

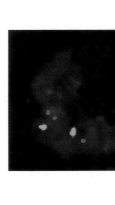

2nd Polar Body

1st Polar Body (+ 21)

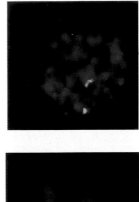

Blastomere Nuclei , Monosomy 21

Fig. 27.2. Patterns of signals in the oocyte with monosomy 21, revealed by testing of both first and second polar bodies by FISH, using chromosome 18 and 21 specific probes. Normally, the first polar body should have two signals for chromosome 18 (two green dots) and two for chromosome 21 (two red dots), whereas only a single red or green dot should be seen in the second polar body. However, the first polar body shows three signals instead of two for chromosomes 21 (three red dots), demonstrating the result of chromatid 21 malsegregation in the first meiotic division and normal segregation of chromosome 18 (two green dots). Follow-up blastomere FISH analysis in the resulting embryo confirmed the diagnosis of monosomy 21.

fazolin sodium, 1 g) before selective abortion. Serial ultrasound examinations should be scheduled to monitor the surviving fetus(es).

Morbidity and Mortality

Selective pregnancy reduction carries several predictable risks: inadvertent loss of remaining fetuses, premature labor, premature delivery, disseminated intravascular coagulopathy, infection, and psychologic problems.[127] Pregnancy loss rates in women undergoing selective abortion have ranged widely. Golbus et al.[136] reported the outcomes of eighteen patients undergoing selective abortions in twin pregnancies during the second trimester by one of the following methods: intracardiac KCl ($n = 7$), cardiac puncture—air embolus ($n = 7$), hysterotomy ($n = 2$), fetal exsanguination ($n = 1$), and cardiac tamponade using intracardiac saline ($n = 1$). Fourteen women were delivered of normal infants and four women lost their entire pregnancy. All four complete pregnancy losses involved monochorionic twins. Transabdominal intracardiac instillation of KCl was considered to be the procedure of choice because of its ease of performance.[136]

Chitkara et al.[137] reported a series of seventeen second-trimester twin selective abortions in which a co-twin was found to have a cytogenetic or structural abnormality. Intracardiac instillation of KCl was used in ten cases—fetal exsanguination and air embolus (two); air embolus and saline intracardiac injection (two); air embolus and fetal exsanguination (two). Exsanguination and saline intracardiac injection was used in one case. In each of the first six consecutive cases, the entire pregnancy was lost; however, in the last eleven cases (ten of which were performed by intracardiac instillation of KCl), all women were delivered of healthy infants. More recently, assessments of centers with considerable overall experience indicates a procedure-related pregnancy loss rate of approximately 5 percent.[134,138,139,140] To date, no reported cases of second-trimester selective abortion have resulted in maternal mortality. Greater experience using KCl has demonstrated a decreasing morbidity with second-trimester selective reduction.[141]

First-Trimester Fetal Reduction

First-trimester fetal reduction is most commonly used to reduce the number of fetuses in multifetal pregnancies (three or more fetuses) to decrease the risk of preterm delivery. CVS and endovaginal ultrasonography have permitted detection of fetal abnormalities in the first trimester, making this technique applicable for selective abortion of abnormal fetuses. Counseling women carrying a multifetal gestation with one or more affected fetuses should be nondirective and include the fetal and maternal implications of selective reduction and pregnancy continuation.[142] Mulcahy et al.[143] first reported the selective termination of a male co-twin at risk for hemophilia A; fetal sex was determined by CVS, and selective abortion was performed.

Technique

Most centers in the United States currently use transabdominal intracardiac instillation of KCl to cause fetal death.[144–147] The technique for first-trimester transabdominal intracardiac instillation of KCl is the same as the technique used for second-trimester intracardiac instillation of KCl (see above), except that only 1–2 mEq KCl are usually needed to cause asystole.[142,143] The postoperative protocol is essentially the same for both second- and first-trimester procedures, although confirmation of fetal asystole can be accomplished in 15–30 minutes after the procedure.

Timor-Tritsch et al.[148] reported the successful use of "transvaginal puncture" for first-trimester reduction with salutary outcomes similar to those for transabdominal procedures. This transvaginal approach may be the only option available if this approach provides the only access to the abnormal fetus(es).

The optimal gestational age to perform selective pregnancy reduction remains uncertain. Those who perform transabdominal procedures generally advocate 10–11 weeks,[128,143,145,146] whereas those who use a transcervical aspiration approach recommend performing selective reduction at 6–9 weeks of gestation.[147]

First-trimester fetal reduction precludes subsequent second-trimester maternal serum AFP (MSAFP) screening and amniotic fluid AFP (AFAFP) analysis. Grau et al.[149] reviewed MSAFP and AFAFP analyses of forty women who underwent fetal reduction procedures at approximately 12 weeks of gestation. Twenty-one of the twenty-two women (95.5 percent) who elected to undergo MSAFP screening during the second trimester were found to have elevated MSAFP levels. Among fifty-three amniotic fluid specimens analyzed from the women carrying multiple gestations and obtained during the second trimester, thirteen (24.5 percent) were found to have abnormally elevated AFAFP levels (>2.0 MoM), and one specimen (1.9 percent) was positive for acetylcholinesterase. None of the abnormal MSAFP or AFAFP levels or the single case with a positive acetylcholinesterase were associated with fetal abnormalities. Our group[150] studied the effect of first-trimester reduction procedures on the maternal serum analytes AFP, unconjugated estriol, and hCG. We confirmed the elevation of second-trimester MSAFP levels and found that levels of hCG and unconjugated estriol appear to be unaltered. As such, MSAFP screening and AFAFP analysis after selective abortion does not provide useful clinical information regarding the presence of fetal neural tube defects or other structural defects associated with elevated AFP levels. The efficacy of multianalyte screening for fetal chromosome abnormalities in these cases remains undetermined.

Morbidity and Mortality

As with second-trimester selective abortion, fetal reduction may result in inadvertent loss of remaining fetuses, premature labor, premature delivery, disseminated intravascular coagulopathy, infection, and psychologic problems.[127] Multiple instillations may also be required to achieve asystole.

Tabsh[147] reported that none of the forty women undergoing selective fetal reduction by intracardiac instillation of KCl lost the entire pregnancy. Evans et al.[128] reported that five of twenty-two patients (22.7 percent) lost their entire pregnancy. Lynch et al.[144] reported that in eighty-five cases of fetal reduction by transabdominal intracardiac instillation of KCl, forty-five women were delivered of viable infants, thirty-two pregnancies were ongoing, and only eight women (9.4 percent) had lost their entire pregnancy. Hemorrhage, maternal infection, premature rupture of the membranes, and premature labor and delivery have predictably occurred, although the frequency of these complications is surprisingly low.[151–154] Although disseminated intravascular coagulopathy (DIC) is recognized as occurring in cases of spontaneous fetal death in multiple gestations,[155] DIC has thus far not been reported in women undergoing selective fetal reduction. Maternal mortality has not been reported.

Recent reports of collaborative studies of clinical outcomes of multifetal reduction for a variety of indications demonstrate considerable improvement in overall pregnancy loss rates. Most studies report an approximately 5 percent risk of pregnancy loss, with lower loss rates being associated with experienced operators[156] and the number of fetuses being reduced.[141,142] Antsaklis et al.[133] noted that second-trimester selective abortion has a risk of pregnancy loss (8.3 percent) comparable to procedures performed in the first trimester (5.6 percent; *p* not significant), a similar finding echoed by others[139] (4.3 percent pregnancy loss in the first trimester and 4.0 percent in the second trimester; *p* not significant). Monochorionic multifetal pregnancy is a contraindication to first-trimester selective reduction. The reported rate of pregnancy loss in cases of monochorionic multifetal pregnancies approaches 100 percent.[136,146]

We and others routinely offer CVS before multifetal reduction. In more than seventy-five cases we have had no pregnancy losses or an inaccurate diagnostic outcome. Eddleman et al. reported a 1.4 percent pregnancy loss rate in and a "probable" 1.2 percent karyotypic inaccuracy rate among 73 women who underwent CVS for 165 fetuses before multifetal reduction. However, other groups report successful prenatal diagnosis following multifetal reduction.[157–159] Regardless of the beliefs of clinicians as to the "best" approach to prenatal diagnosis and fetal reduction, it appears that the outcomes of both protocols appear similar. A small percentage of cases will not permit a particular approach to prenatal diagnosis because of technical or anatomic considerations. However, for the majority of cases in which prereduction CVS or postreduction amniocentesis are feasible, patient choice should play a central role in determining which approach to use for women desiring prenatal diagnosis and multifetal reduction.

REFERENCES

1. Verp MS, Bombard AT, Simpson JL, et al. Parental decision following prenatal diagnosis of fetal chromosome abnormality. Am J Med Genet 1988;29:613.
2. Grevengood C, Shulman LP, Dungan JS, et al. Severity of abnormality influences decision to terminate pregnancies affected with fetal neural tube defects. Fetal Diagn Ther 1994;9:273.
3. Zlotogora J. Parental decisions to abort or continue a pregnancy with an abnormal finding after an invasive prenatal test. Prenat Diagn 2002;22:1102.
4. Van der Pal-de Bruin KM, Graafmans W, Biermans MC, et al. The influence of prenatal screening and termination of pregnancy on perinatal mortality rates. Prenat Diagn 2002;22:966.
5. Liu S, Joseph KS, Kramer MS. Relationship of prenatal diagnosis and pregnancy termination to overall infant mortality in Canada. JAMA 2002;287:1561.
6. Hern WM. First and second trimester abortion techniques. In: Leventhal JM, ed. Current problems in obstetrics and gynecology. Chicago: Year Book Medical Publishers, 1983:5.
7. Stubblefield PG. Pregnancy termination. In: Gabbe SG, Niebyl JR, Simpson JL, eds. Obstetrics: normal and problem pregnancies. New York: Churchill Livingstone, 1991:1303.
8. Shulman LP, Ling FW. Surgical termination of pregnancy. In: Mann WJ, Stovall TG, eds. Gynecologic surgery. New York: Churchill Livingstone, 1996:795.
9. Shulman LP, Lipscomb GH, Ling FW. Management of abnormal pregnancies. In: Paul, M, Lichtenberg, S, Borgatta L, Grimes D Stubblefield P, eds. A clinician's guide to medical and surgical abortion. New York: Churchill Livingstone, 1999:482.
10. Castodot RG. Pregnancy termination: techniques, risks and complications and their management. Fertil Steril 1986;45:5.
11. American College of Obstetricians and Gynecologists. Methods of midtrimester abortion. ACOG Technical Bulletin 109. Washington, DC: American College of Obstetricians and Gynecologists, 1987.
12. Goldstein SR, Danon M, Watson C. An updated protocol for abortion surveillance with ultrasound and immediate pathology. Obstet Gynecol 1994;83:797.
13. Schulz KF, Grimes DA, Cates W Jr, et al. Measures to prevent cervical laceration during suction curettage abortion. Lancet 1983;1:1182.
14. Hern WM. Laminaria versus Dilapan osmotic cervical dilators for outpatient dilation and evacuation abortion: randomized cohort comparison of 1,001 patients. Am J Obstet Gynecol 1994;171:1324.
15. Uldberg N, Ulmsten U. The physiology of cervical ripening and cervical dilatation and the effect of abortifacient drugs. Bailliere Clin Obstet Gynecol 1990;4:263.

16. Ngai SW, Tang OS, Lao T, et al. Oral misoprostol versus placebo for cervical dilatation before vacuum aspiration in first trimester pregnancy. Hum Reprod 1995;10:1220.

17. Singh K, Fong YF. Preparation of the cervix for surgical termination of pregnancy in the first trimester. Hum Reprod Update 2000;6:442.

18. MacIsaac L, Grossman D, Balisteri E, et al. A randomized controlled trial of laminaria, oral misoprostol and vaginal misoprostol before abortion. Obstet Gynecol 1999;93:766.

19. Lefebvre Y, Proulx L, Elie R, et al. The effects of RU-486 on cervical ripening: clinical studies. Am J Obstet Gynecol 1990;162:61.

20. Carbonne B, Brennand JE, Maria B, et al. Effects of gemeprost and mifepristone on the mechanical properties of the cervix prior to first trimester termination of pregnancy. Br J Obstet Gynaecol 1995;102:553.

21. World Health Organization. Cervical ripening with mifepristone (RU486) in late first trimester abortion. World Health Organization Task Force on Postovulatory Methods of Fertility Regulation. Contraception 1994;50:461.

22. Platz-Christensen JJ, Nielsen S, Hamberger L. Is misoprostol the choice for induced cervical ripening in early pregnancy termination? Acta Scand Obstet Gynecol 95;74:809.

23. Darney PD, Dorwand K. Cervical dilation before first-trimester elective abortion: a controlled comparison of meteneprost, laminaria and hypan. Obstet Gynecol 1987;70:397.

24. Koplik L. Personal communication, 1990.

25. Burnhill MS, Armstead JW. Reducing the morbidity of vacuum aspiration abortion. Int J Gynaecol Obstet 1978;16:204.

26. Levallois P, Rioux JE. Prophylactic antibiotics for suction curettage abortion: results of a clinical controlled trial. Am J Obstet Gynecol 1988;158:100.

27. Sands RX, Burnhill MS, Hakim-Elahi E. Post-abortal uterine atony. Obstet Gynecol 1974;43:595.

28. Blumenthal PD. Abortion: Epidemiology, safety and technique. Curr Opin Obstet Gynecol 1992;4:506.

29. Hakim-Elahi E, Tovell HMM, Burnhill MS. Complications of first-trimester abortion: a report of 170,000 cases. Obstet Gynecol 1990;76:129.

30. Nathanson BN. Ambulatory abortion: experience with 26,000 cases (July 1, 1970 to August 1, 1971). N Engl J Med 1972;286:403.

31. Hodgson JE, Portmann KC. Complications of 10,453 consecutive first-trimester abortions: a prospective study. Am J Obstet Gynecol 1974;120:802.

32. Hodgson JE. Major complications of 20,248 consecutive first trimester abortions: problems of fragmented care. Adv Plann Parent 1975;9:52.

33. Korejo R, Noorani KJ, Bhutta S. Sociocultural determinants of induced abortions. J Coll Physicians Surg Pak 2003;13:260.

34. Hollander D. Although abortion is highly restricted in Cameroon, it is not uncommon among young urban women. Int Fam Plan Perspect 2003;29:49.

35. Talukder SI, Haque A. Frequency of abortion in different seasons and age groups. Mymensingh Med J 2003;12:8.

36. Tietze C, Lewit S. Joint Program for the Study of Abortion (JPSA): early medical complications of legal abortion. Stud Fam Plann 1972;3:97.

37. Zhou W, Sorensen HT, Olsen J. Induced abortion and subsequent pregnancy duration. Obstet Gynecol 1999;94:948.

38. Zhou W, Olsen J. Are complications after an induced abortion associated with reproductive failures in a subsequent pregnancy? Acta Obstet Gynecol Scand 2003;82,177.

39. Atienza MF, Burkman RT, King TM. Forces associated with cervical dilatation at suction abortion: qualitative and quantitative data in studies completed with a force-sensing instrument. In: Naftolin F, Stubblefield PG, eds. Dilatation of the uterine cervix. New York: Raven Press, 1980:343.

40. Peterson HB, Grimes DA, Cates W Jr, et al. Comparative risk of death from induced abortion at ≤12 weeks' gestation performed with local versus general anesthesia. Am J Obstet Gynecol 1981;141:763.

41. Stovall TG, Ling FW, Carson SA, et al. Nonsurgical diagnosis and treatment of tubal pregnancy. Fertil Steril 1990;54:537.

42. Lipscomb GH, Meyer NL, Flynn DE, et al. Oral methotrexate for treatment of ectopic pregnancy. Am J Obstet Gynecol 2002;186:1192.

43. Atrash HK, MacKay T, Binkin NJ, et al. Legal abortion mortality in the United States, 1972–1982. Am J Obstet Gynecol 1987;156:605.

44. Smargisso DM, Lester D. Mortality from abortion after Roe vs. Wade. Psychol Rep 2002;91:780.

45. Goldsmith S, Margolis AJ. Aspiration abortion without cervical dilatation. Am J Obstet Gynecol 1971;110:580.

46. Karman H, Potts M. Very early abortion using a syringe as a vacuum source. Lancet 1972;1:1051.

47. Atienza MF, Burkman RT, King TM, et al. Menstrual extraction. Am J Obstet Gynecol 1975;121:490.

48. Hodgson JE. A reassessment of menstrual regulation. Stud Fam Plann 1977;8:263.

49. Speroff L, Glass RH, Kase NG. Clinical gynecologic endocrinology and infertility. Baltimore: Williams & Wilkins, 2002:281.

50. Meyer JH Jr. Early office termination of pregnancy by soft cannula vacuum aspiration. Am J Obstet Gynecol 1983;147:202.

51. Creinin MD. Randomized comparison of efficacy, acceptability and cost of medical versus surgical abortion. Contraception 2000:62:117.

52. Dean G, Cardenas L, Darney P, et al. Acceptability of manual versus electric aspiration for first trimester abortion: a randomized trial. Contraception 2003;67:201.

53. Kulier R, Fekih A, Hofmeyr GJ, et al. Surgical methods for first trimester termination of pregnancy. Cochrane Database Syst Rev 2001;4:CD002900.

54. Tho PT, Byrd JR, McDonough PG. Etiologies and subsequent reproductive performance of 100 couples with recurrent abortion. Fertil Steril 1978;32:389.

55. Couzinet B, Le Strat N, Ulmann A, et al. Termination of early pregnancy by the progesterone antagonist RU 486 (mifepristone). N Engl J Med 1986;315:1565.

56. Baird DT, Rodger M, Cameron IT, et al. Prostaglandins and antigestagens for the interruption of early pregnancy. J Reprod Fertil Suppl 1988;36:173.

57. Maria B, Stampf F. Termination of early pregnancy using mifepristone in combination with prostaglandin analogs. Acta Obstet Gynecol Scand Suppl 1989;149:31.

58. Swahn ML, Bygdeman M. Termination of early pregnancy with RU 486 (mifepristone) in combination with a prostaglandin analogue (sulprostone). Acta Obstet Gynecol Scand 1989;68:293.

59. Ulmann A, Dubois C. Clinical trials with RU 486 (mifepristone): an update. Acta Obstet Gynecol Scand Suppl 1989;149:9.

60. United Kingdom Multicentre Trial. The efficacy and tolerance of mifepristone and prostaglandin in first trimester termination of pregnancy. Br J Obstet Gynaecol 1990;97:480.

61. Ashok PW, Templeton A, Wagaarachchi PT, et al. Factors affecting the outcome of early medical abortion: a review of 4,132 consecutive cases. Br J Obstet Gynaecol 2002;109:1281.

62. Creinin MD, Potter C, Holovanisin M, et al. Mifepristone and misoprostol and methotrexate/misoprostol in clinical practice for abortion. Am J Obstet Gynecol 2003;188:664.

63. el-Refaey H, Rajasekar D, Abdalla M, et al. Induction of abortion with mifepristone (RU486) and oral or vaginal misoprostol. N Engl J Med 1995;332:983.

64. Bygdeman M, Breune K, Christensen N, et al. A comparison of two stable prostaglandin E analogues for termination of early pregnancy and for cervical dilatation. Contraception 1980;22:471.

65. Smith SK, Baird DT. The use of 16,16-dimethyl-trans-Delta sub 2-PGE sub 1 methyl ester (ONO 802) vaginal suppositories for the termination of early pregnancy: a comparative study. Br J Obstet Gynaecol 1980;87:712.

66. Csapo AI, Peskin EG, Pulkkinen M, et al. "Menstrual induction" with sulprostone. Prostaglandins 1982;24:657.

67. Silvestre L, Dubois C, Renault M, et al. Voluntary interruption of pregnancy with mifepristone (RU 486) and a prostaglandin analogue: a large-scale French experience. N Engl J Med 1990;322:645.

68. World Health Organization. Pregnancy termination with mifepristone and gemeprost: a multicenter comparison between repeated doses and a single dose of mifepristone. Fertil Steril 1991;56:32.

69. Bygdeman M, Swahn ML, Gemzell-Danielsson K, et al. The use of progesterone antagonists in combination with prostaglandin for termination of pregnancy. Hum Reprod 1994;9S:121.

70. Jing X, Weng L. [A study on the optimal regimen of mifepristone with prostaglandin for termination of early pregnancy.] Chung Hua Fu Chan Chih 1995;30:38.

71. Rodger MW, Baird DT. Induction of therapeutic abortion in early pregnancy with mifepristone in combination with prostaglandin pessary. Lancet 1987;2:1415.

72. Vyjayanthi S, Piskorowskyj N. Medical termination of pregnancy at 9–12 weeks of gestation. J Obstet Gynaecol 2002;22:669.

73. Hamoda H, Ashok PW, Flett GM, et al. Medical abortion at 64 to 91 days of gestation: a review of 483 consecutive cases. Am J Obstet Gynecol 2003;188:1315.

74. Coelho HLL, Misago C, da Fonseca WVC, et al. Selling abortifacients over the counter in Fortaleza, Brazil. Lancet 1991;338:247.

75. Bugalho A, Faundes A, Jamisse L, et al. Evaluation of the effectiveness of vaginal misoprostol to induce first-trimester abortion. Contraception 1996;53:244.

76. Koopersmith TB, Mishell DR Jr. The use of misoprostol for termination of early pregnancy. Contraception 1996;53:238.

77. Ramin KD, Ogburn PL, Danilenko DR, et al. High-dose oral misoprostol for mid-trimester pregnancy interruption. Gynecol Obstet Invest 2002;54:176.

78. Norman JE, Thong KJ, Rodger MW, et al. Medical abortion in women of less than or equal to 56 days amenorrhea: a comparison between gemeprost (a PGE1 analogue) alone and mifepristone and gemeprost. Br J Obstet Gynaecol 1992;99:601.

79. Creinin MD, Vittinghoff E, Galbraith S, et al. A randomized trial comparing misoprostol three and seven days after methotrexate for early abortion. Am J Obstet Gynecol 1995;173:1578.

80. Medical Letter. Methotrexate and misoprostol for abortion. Med Lett Drugs Ther 1996;38:39.

81. Autry AM, Hayes EC, Jaobson GF, et al. A comparison of medical induction and dilation and evacuation for second-trimester abortion. Am J Obstet Gynecol 2002;187:393.

82. Kalish RB, Chasen ST, Rosenzweig LB, et al. Impact of midtrimester dilation and evacuation on subsequent pregnancy outcome. Am J Obstet Gynecol 2002;187:882.

83. Crist T, Williams P, Lee SH, et al. Midtrimester pregnancy termination: a study of the cost effectiveness of dilatation and evacuation in a free-standing facility. North Carolina Med J 1983;44:549.

84. Kaltreider NB, Goldsmith S, Margolis AJ. The impact of midtrimester abortion techniques on patients and staff. Am J Obstet Gynecol 1979;135:235.

85. Grimes DA, Hulka JF, McCutchen ME. Midtrimester abortion by dilatation and evacuation versus intraamniotic instillation of prostaglandin F2α: a randomized clinical trial. Am J Obstet Gynecol 1980;137:785.

86. Rhoads GG, Jackson LG, Schlesselman SE, et al. The safety and efficacy of chorionic villus sampling for early prenatal diagnosis of cytogenetic abnormalities. N Engl J Med 1989;320:609.

87. Cates W, Schulz KF, Grimes DA, et al. Dilatation and evacuation procedures and second-trimester abortions: the role of physician skill and hospital setting. JAMA 1982;248:559.

88. Shulman LP, Ling FW, Meyers CM, et al. Dilatation and evacuation is a preferable method for midtrimester genetic termination of pregnancy. Prenat Diagn 1989;9:47.

89. Shulman LP, Ling FW, Meyers CM, et al. Dilation and evacuation for second trimester genetic pregnancy termination. Obstet Gynecol 1990;75:1037.

90. Shulman LP, Ling FW, Meyers CM, et al. Dilation and evacuation for second-trimester genetic pregnancy termination: update on a reliable and preferable method. Am J Gynecol Health 1991;5:30.

91. Bernick BA, Ufberg DD, Nemiroff R, et al. Success rate of cytogenetic analysis at the time of second trimester dilation and evacuation. Am J Obstet Gynecol 1998;179:957.

92. Stubblefield PG. Midtrimester abortion by curettage procedures: an overview. In: Hodgson JE, ed. Abortion and sterilization: medical and social aspects. San Diego: Academic Press, 1981:277.

93. Hornstein MD, Osathanondh R, Birnholz JC, et al. Ultrasound guidance for selected dilatation and evacuation procedures. J Reprod Med 1986;31:947.

94. Darney PD, Sweet RL. Routine intraoperative ultrasonography for second trimester abortion reduces incidence of uterine perforation. J Ultrasound Med 1989;8:71.

95. Robins J, Surrago EJ. Early midtrimester pregnancy termination: a comparison of dilatation and evacuation and prostaglandin-induced abortion. Obstet Gynecol 1982;48:216.

96. Robins J, Surrago EJ. Early midtrimester pregnancy termination: a comparison of dilatation and evacuation and intravaginal prostaglandin F2α. J Reprod Med 1982;27:415.

97. Kafrissen ME, Schulz KF, Grimes DA, et al. Midtrimester abortion: intraamniotic instillation of hyperosmolar urea and prostaglandin F2-alpha vs. dilatation and evacuation. JAMA 1984;251:916.

98. Grimes DA, Schulz KF. Morbidity and mortality from second-trimester abortions. J Reprod Med 1985;30:505.

99. Peterson WF, Berry FN, Grace MR, et al. Second-trimester abortion by dilatation and evacuation: an analysis of 11,747 cases. Obstet Gynecol 1983;62:185.

100. Schneider D, Halperin R, Langer R, et al. Abortion at 18–22 weeks by laminaria dilation and evacuation. Obstet Gynecol 1996;88:412.

101. Rovinsky JJ. Abortion on demand. Mt Sinai J Med 1984;51:12.

102. Zieger W, Leveringhaus A, Pilch H, et al. [Uterine rupture during induced abortion with prostaglandins in the second trimester.] Geburtshilfe Frauenheilkd 1995;55:592.

103. Gottlieb C, Bygdeman M. The use of antiprogestin (RU486) for termination of second trimester pregnancy. Acta Obstet Gynecol Scand 1991;70:199.

104. el-Refaey H, Templeton A. Induction of abortion in the second trimester by a combination of misoprostol and mifepristone: a randomized comparison between two misoprostol regimens. Hum Reprod 1995b;10:475.

105. Thong KJ, Lynch P, Baird DT. A randomised study of two doses of gemeprost in combination with mifepristone for induction of abortion in the second trimester of pregnancy. Contraception 1996;54:97.

106. Wong KS, Ngai CS, Chan KS, et al. Termination of second trimester pregnancy with gemeprost and misoprostol: a randomized double-blind placebo-controlled trial. Contraception 1996;54:23.

107. Jain JK, Mishell DR Jr. A comparison of intravaginal misoprostol with prostaglandin E_2 for termination of second-trimester pregnancy. N Engl J Med 1994;331:290.

108. Thong KJ, Baird DT. Induction of second trimester abortion with mifepristone and gemeprost. Br J Obstet Gynaecol 1993;100:758.

109. Ho PC, Chan YF, Lau W. Misoprostol is as effective as gemeprost in termination of second trimester pregnancy when combined with mifepristone: a randomised comparative trial. Contraception 1996;53:281.

110. Surrago EJ, Robins J. Midtrimester pregnancy termination by intravaginal administration of prostaglandin E_2. Contraception 1982;26:285.

111. Robins J, Mann LI. Second generation prostaglandins: Midtrimester pregnancy termination by intramuscular injection of a 15-methyl analog of prostaglandin $F2\alpha$. Fertil Steril 1976;27:104.

112. Borgida AF, Rodis JF, Hanlon W, et al. Second trimester abortion by intramuscular 15-methyl-prostaglandin $F2\alpha$ or intravaginal prostaglandin E_2 suppositories: a randomized trial. Obstet Gynecol 1995;85:697.

113. Owen J, Hauth JC. Concentrated oxytocin plus low-dose prostaglandin E_2 compared with prostaglandin E_2 vaginal suppositories for second trimester pregnancy termination. Obstet Gynecol 1996;88:110.

114. Stubblefield PG, Naftolin F, Frigoletto FD, et al. *Laminaria* augmentation of intraamniotic $PGF2\alpha$ for midtrimester pregnancy termination. Prostaglandins 1975;10:413.

115. Stubblefield PG, Naftolin F, Lee EY, et al. Combination therapy for midtrimester abortion: *Laminaria* and analogues of prostaglandin. Contraception 1976;13:723.

116. Corson SL, Bolognese RJ. Intra-amniotic prostaglandin $F2\alpha$ as a mid-trimester abortifacient: effect of oxytocin and laminaria. J Reprod Med 1975;14:47.

117. Herabutya Y, Prasertsawat P. Mid-trimester abortion using hypertonic saline or prostaglandin E_2 gel: an analysis of efficacy and complications. J Med Assoc Thai 1994;77:148.

118. Binkin NJ, Schulz KF, Grimes DA, et al. Urea-prostaglandin versus hypertonic saline for instillation abortion. Am J Obstet Gynecol 1983;146:947.

119. Grimes DA, Schulz KF, Cates W Jr, et al. The safety of midtrimester abortion. In: Keith LG, Kent DR, Berger GS, et al., eds. The safety of fertility control. New York: Springer-Verlag, 1979:198.

120. DeCherney AH, Schwarz RH, Drobney H. Infection as a complication of therapeutic abortion. Pa Med 1972;12:49.

121. Vause S, Sands J, Johnston TA, et al. Could some fetocides be avoided by more prompt referral after diagnosis of fetal abnormality? J Obstet Gynecol 2002;22:243.

122. Senat MV, Fischer C, Ville Y. Funipuncture for fetocide in later termination of regency. Prenat Diagn 2002;22:354.

123. Schinker JC, Yarkoni S, Granat M. Multiple pregnancies following induction of ovulation. Fertil Steril 1981;35:105.

124. Bronsteen RA, Evans MI. Multiple gestation. In: Fetal diagnosis and therapy: science, ethics and the law. Philadelphia: Lippincott Harper, 1989:242.

125. Smith-Levitin M, Kowalik A, Birnholz J, et al. Selective reduction of multifetal pregnancies to twins improves outcome over nonreduced triplet gestations. Am J Obstet Gynecol 1996;175:878.

126. Kiely JL. The epidemiology of perinatal mortality in multiple births. Bull N Y Acad Med 1990;66:618.

127. Elias S, Annas G. Reproductive genetics and the law. Chicago: Year Book Medical, 1987:124.

128. Evans MI, May M, Drugan A, et al. Selective termination: clinical experience and residual risks. Am J Obstet Gynecol 1990;162:1568.

129. Berkowitz RL, Lynch L. Selective reduction: an unfortunate misnomer. Obstet Gynecol 1990;75:873.

130. Aberg A, Miterian F, Cantz M, et al. Cardiac puncture of fetus with Hurler's disease avoiding abortion of unaffected co-twin. Lancet 1978;2:990.

131. Beck L, Terinde R, Dolffe M. Zwillingsschwangerschaft mit freier Trisomie 21 eines Kindes. Sectio parva mit Entfernung des kranken und spätere Gebert des gesunden Kindes. Gerburtshilfe Fraunheikd 1980;40:397.

132. Rodeck CH, Mibashan J, Abramowicz J, et al. Selective feticide of the affected twin by fetoscopic air embolism. Prenat Diagn 1982;2:189.

133. Antsaklis A, Politis J, Karagiannopoulos C, et al. Selective survival of only the healthy fetus following prenatal diagnosis of thalassaemia major in binovular twin gestation. Prenat Diagn 1984;4:289.

134. Eddleman KA, Stone JL, Lynch L, et al. Selective termination of anomalous fetuses in multifetal pregnancies: two hundred cases at a single center. Am J Obstet Gynecol 2002;187:1168.

135. Rochon M, Stone J. Invasive procedures in multiple gestations. Curr Opin Obstet Gynecol 2003;15:167.

136. Golbus MS, Cunningham N, Goldberg JD, et al. Selective termination of multiple gestations. Am J Med Genet 1988;31, 339.

137. Chitkara U, Berkowitz RL, Wilkins IA, et al. Selective second-trimester termination of the anomalous fetus in twin pregnancies. Obstet Gynecol 1989;73:690.

138. Evans MI, Goldberg JD, Horenstein J, et al. Selective termination for structural, chromosomal, and mendelian anomalies: international experience. Am J Obstet Gynecol 1999;181:893.

139. Lipitz S, Shulman A, Achiron R, et al. A comparative study of multifetal pregnancy reduction from triplets to twins in the first versus early second trimesters after detailed fetal screening. Ultrasound Obstet Gynecol 2001;18:35.

140. Stone J, Eddleman K, Lynch L, et al. A single center experience with 1,000 consecutive cases of multifetal pregnancy reduction. Am J Obstet Gynecol 2002;187:1163.

141. Evans MI, Krivchenia EL, Gelber SE, et al. Selective reduction. Clin Perinatol 2003;30:103.

142. Lipitz S, Mashiach S, Seidman DS. Multifetal pregnancy reduction: the case for non-directive patient counseling. Hum Reprod 1994;9:1978.

143. Mulcahy M, Robernar B, Reid SE. Chorion biopsy, cytogenetic analysis and selective termination in a twin pregnancy at risk of haemophilia. Lancet 1984;2:866.

144. Lynch L, Berkowitz RL, Chitkara U, et al. First-trimester transabdominal multifetal pregnancy reduction: a report of 85 cases. Obstet Gynecol 1990;75:735.

145. Berkowitz RL, Lynch L, Chitkara U, et al. Selective reduction of multifetal pregnancies in the first trimester. N Engl J Med 1988;318:1043.

146. Wapner RJ, Davis GH, Johnson A, et al. Selective reduction of multifetal pregnancies. Lancet 1990;335:90.

147. Tabsh KMA. Transabdominal multifetal pregnancy reduction: report of 40 cases. Obstet Gynecol 1990;75:739.

148. Timor-Tritsch IE, Peisner DB, Monteagudo A, et al. Multifetal pregnancy reduction by transvaginal puncture: evaluation of the technique used in 134 cases. Am J Obstet Gynecol 1993;168:799.

149. Grau P, Robinson L, Tabsh K, et al. Elevated maternal serum alpha-fetoprotein and amniotic fluid alpha-fetoprotein after multifetal pregnancy reduction. Obstet Gynecol 1990;76:1042.

150. Shulman LP, Phillips OP, Cervetti TA. Maternal serum analyte levels after first-trimester multifetal pregnancy reduction. Am J Obstet Gynecol 1996;174:1072.

151. Evans MI, Dommergues M, Wapner RJ, et al. Efficacy of transabdominal pregnancy reduction: collaborative experience among the world's largest centers. Obstet Gynecol 1993;82:61.

152. Evans MI, Dommergues M, Timor-Tritsch I, et al. Transabdominal versus transvaginal multifetal pregnancy reduction: International collaborative experience of more than one thousand cases. Am J Obstet Gynecol 1994;170:902.

153. Evans MI, Dommergues M, Wapner RJ, et al. International, collaborative experience of 1,789 patients having multifetal pregnancy reduction: a plateauing of risks and outcomes. J Soc Gynecol Invest 1996;3:23.

154. Berkowitz RL, Lynch L, Stone J, et al. The current status of multifetal pregnancy reduction. Am J Obstet Gynecol 1996;174:1265.

155. Romero R, Duffy TP, Berkowitz RL, et al. Prolongation of a preterm pregnancy complicated by death of a single twin in utero and disseminated intravascular coagulation. N Engl J Med 1989;310:772.

156. Evans MI, Berkowitz RL, Wapner RJ, et al. Improvement in outcomes of multifetal pregnancy reduction with increased experience. Am J Obstet Gynecol 2001;184:97.

157. Eddleman KA, Stone JL, Lynch L, et al. Chorionic villus sampling before multifetal pregnancy reduction. Am J Obstet Gynecol 2000;183:1078.

158. MacLean LK, Evans MI, Carpenter RJ Jr., et al. Genetic amniocentesis following multifetal pregnancy reduction does not increase the risk of pregnancy loss. Prenat Diagn 1998;18:186–88.

159. Baker CL, Feldman B, Shalhoub AG, et al. Demographic factors for utilization of invasive genetic testing after multifetal pregnancy reduction. Fetal Diagn Ther 2003;18:140.

Yury Verlinsky, Ph.D., and Anver Kuliev, M.D., Ph.D.

27

Preimplantation Genetic Diagnosis

Couples at high risk for having offspring with inherited diseases may benefit from new methods for diagnosing genetic disease during the earliest stages of development of the human zygote and embryo before implantation. The development of preimplantation genetic diagnosis (PGD) techniques makes it possible to overcome the most sensitive issue in the avoidance of genetic disease—abortion. Termination of pregnancy is not acceptable for some populations or ethnic groups and may create a negative reaction to genetic disease programs. Therefore, PGD provides an option for women at high risk who would find this approach ethically more acceptable.

Developments in PGD[1–4] have shown that the methods for detecting most genetic conditions after implantation could be applied to gametes and preimplantation embryos, using the same criteria as for prenatal diagnosis for the identification of individuals and couples at genetic risk. In addition, most recently PGD has appeared to be applicable to conditions that have never been considered as indications for prenatal diagnosis.[5–7]

PGD seems to be a natural evolution of the genetic disease-prevention technology, from a period with limited genetic counseling and no prenatal diagnosis or treatment to a point when all options, including PGD, are available.[8] For example, when treatment and information on recurrence risk was introduced, many couples either refrained from reproduction or terminated their pregnancies. The impact of PGD on the existing policies for the prevention of genetic disease is obvious from the increasing use of PGD for the avoidance of unnecessary termination of many wanted pregnancies.

APPROACHES FOR PREIMPLANTATION GENETIC DIAGNOSIS

When prenatal genetic diagnosis was considered in perspective, in 1984, the World Health Organization (WHO) emphasized the relevance of developing earlier approaches for genetic analysis with the possibility of diagnosis before implantation.[9,10] The following possibilities for PGD were mentioned: genetic analysis of the first or second polar bodies and embryo biopsy at the cleavage or blastocyst stage.[10,11] However, the realization of some of these approaches became possible only after introduction of the polymerase chain reaction (PCR)[12] and the success in micromanipulation and embryo biopsy.

The attempts for PGD were undertaken in mammalian embryos more than 15 years ago,[13–18] when it was demonstrated that material could be removed from mammalian preimplantation embryos and analyzed successfully without destroying the viability of the embryo in in vitro fertilization (IVF). PGD of human genetic disease was first demonstrated by Handyside et al.[19] for X-linked diseases and by Verlinsky et al.[20] for autosomal recessive diseases. More than 1,000 children without detectable birth defects have already been born following these procedures,[21–25] demonstrating that PGD can be performed safely in humans. Two main approaches for genetic diagnosis before implantation have emerged: PGD based on biopsy of gametes using polar bodies and PGD based on embryo biopsy at the cleavage stage. The review of the developments of preconception and preimplantation genetic diagnosis and the existing problems in the possible wider application of these early approaches to clinical practice are presented below.

Polar Body Sampling

Biopsy of gametes opened an intriguing possibility of preconception diagnosis of inherited diseases, because genetic analysis of biopsied gamete material made it realistic to select gametes containing an unaffected allele for fertilization and subsequent transfer.[26] In this way, not only the selective abortion of an affected fetus but also fertilization involving affected gametes may be avoided as an option for couples at risk for conceiving a genetically abnormal fetus.

1. Although preconception genetic diagnosis could be achieved by genotyping either oocytes or sperm, the latter approach is not realistic at present. Despite extensive studies, claims to have successfully separated X and Y spermatozoa have not been confirmed by use of this method in the prevention of X-linked disorders. However, with the application of flow cytometric sperm sorting, studies of possible DNA-based X-enriched sperm separation have been renewed, resulting in a few unaffected pregnancies and births.[27] No method exists to retain the viability of sperm after genotype analysis, although PCR permits genotyping individual human sperm.[28,29] Development of methods of culturing the primary spermatocytes and spermatogonia followed by genetic analysis of maturated spermatides is theoretically possible, but this still remains a subject for future research, such as in the framework of the current attempts for gaploidization.[31] (Tesarik J, Mendoza C. 2003 Somatic cell haploidization: an update. *Reproductive BioMedicine Online*, **6**, 60–65.) Most recently the technique of sperm duplication has been introduced, which may allow to test the duplicate of the sperm before using its copy for ICSI.[31a]

The only approach for preconception diagnosis at present, therefore, seems to be genotyping oocytes, based on micromanipulation, biopsy, and subsequent genetic analysis. It is possible to obtain the genotype of an oocyte by direct analysis, but this analysis destroys the oocyte. To be useful in clinical practice, the requirement for any genetic test is that it not destroy or affect the viability of the oocyte. So far, attempts for noninvasive genotyping of the oocyte or pre-embryo before transfer based on the study of the materials secreted into culture media have not been promising.[31–35] An approach to predict successful pregnancy by the analysis of spare embryos also is not practical, because it provides a possible explanation for the outcome of pregnancy only retrospectively.[36] To evaluate the quality of oocytes before insemination, a noninvasive approach for testing the oocyte has been developed, based on removing the first and second polar body using micromanipulation techniques and performing genetic analysis of polar-body DNA.[4,20,26] The polar-body approach was used by Monk and Holding[37] for testing the possibility of amplification of β-globin sequences in the mouse. In the absence of crossover, the first polar body will be homozygous for the allele not contained in the oocyte and second polar body. However, the first-polar-body approach will not predict the eventual genotype of the oocytes, if crossover occurs, because the primary oocyte in this case will be heterozygous for the abnormal gene. The frequency of crossover will vary with the distance between the locus and the centromere, approaching as much as 50 percent for telomeric genes, for which the first polar body approach would be of only limited value, unless the oocytes can be tested further. Therefore, the analysis of the second polar body is needed to detect hemizygous normal oocytes resulting after the second meiotic division. In fact, the present experience shows that the most accurate diagnosis can be achieved in cases in which the first polar body is heterozygous, so that the detection of the normal or mutant gene in the second polar body predicts the opposite mutant or normal genotype of the resulting maternal contribution to the embryo after fertilization.[4]

To study a possible detrimental effect of the procedure, micromanipulated oocytes were followed and evaluated at different stages of development.[3,38] No significant decrease was observed in the fertilization rate for oocytes after polar-body removal; the percentage of embryos entering cleavage was the same in oocytes subjected to the procedure and in the control oocytes. Also, there was no increase in the percentage of polyspermic embryos in the micromanipulated oocytes. No long-term effect was observed by culturing the affected (micromanipulated) embryos to blastocyst stage; the proportion of embryos reaching this stage was similar to that known for nonmicromanipulated oocytes. A follow-up study of the viability of the sampled oocytes through implantation and postimplantation development also suggests no detrimental effect of polar-body removal. In this study, the first polar body was removed in the framework of assisted fertilization or clinical trial on polar-body preimplantation diagnosis of age-related aneuploidies (see below). The absence of any deleterious effect of polar-body removal on fertilization, preimplantation, and, possibly, postimplantation development makes it possible to consider the polar-body approach to be a nondestructive test for genotyping the oocytes before fertilization and implantation.

In another study, to assess the effect of the second polar-body sampling on the viability and the developmental potential of the resulting embryo, 343 biopsied and 445 non-biopsied mouse embryos were compared for the percentage of embryos reaching the blastocyst stage.[39] More than 70 percent of biopsied embryos formed morphologically normal blastocysts, which was not statistically different from approximately 80 percent in the control group. There was no difference in the cell count of blastocysts obtained from biopsied and control groups either, suggesting that the sampling of the second polar body does not have a significant effect on preimplantation development. This is in agreement with anticipation, based on the fact that the first and the second polar bodies are extruded from the developing oocyte during meiosis and are not required for successful fertilization and normal embryonic development.

Blastomere Biopsy

Despite clear advantages, the polar-body approach does not provide diagnosis of the paternal alleles and the gender of the embryo and therefore cannot be used to avoid the transfer of male embryos in cases of the X-linked disorders, unless specific diagnosis can be done on oocytes using the polar-body approach (see below). The fact that the genotype of the oocyte is inferred from the genotype of the polar body, rather than determined directly, is another weakness. In the above situations, blastomere biopsy becomes an important complement to the polar-body diagnosis.

The embryo biopsy is performed at the four- to eight-cell stage; the microtools used for embryo biopsy are the same as for the polar-body removal, except for minor modifications.[4] As noted above, preimplantation diagnosis by blastomere biopsy was first demonstrated for X-linked disorders and performed for gender determination of human embryos.[19] Eight couples known to be at risk for transmitting various X-linked diseases participated in this first clinical trial, including those at risk for X-linked mental retardation, Lesch–Nyhan syndrome, adrenoleukodystrophy, retinitis pigmentosa, hereditary sensory motor neuron disease type II, and Duchenne muscular dystrophy. Embryo biopsy was performed on day 3, at the six- to ten-cell stage, and one to three blastomeres were removed from each cleaving embryo. Y-chromosome-specific sequence was amplified from the biopsied cells for gender determination while corresponding biopsied embryos were returned to culture and those diagnosed as females were transferred to achieve a pregnancy. As a result, five women became pregnant: three after one treatment cycle, one after two treatment cycles, and one after three treatment cycles. Ten of twenty-two biopsied embryos transferred implanted, suggesting a 45 percent implantation rate per embryo transferred. From ten embryos implanted, seven developed to the fetal heart stage; chorionic villus sampling (CVS) confirmed six embryos, and one was misdiagnosed. The pregnancy with a misdiagnosed singleton male was terminated, and the other six females all have been born free of genetic disorders.

One of the important observations of the study was an exceptionally high success rate in achieving pregnancies after blastomere biopsy, which seemed to be twice as high as that in the best IVF programs. In fact, the study of the viability of the biopsied pre-embryos did not reveal any detrimental effect of the above procedures: more than 70 percent of the manipulated embryos reached blastocyst stage, with no significant reduction in cell number and energy substances (glucose and pyruvate) uptake.[40]

PGD at the cleavage stage has become a method of choice in most centers and has been applied in approximately 3,000 cycles, resulting in the birth of hundreds of children free from genetic disorders.[22–25] Nevertheless, there are still many problems to be resolved, including the possibility of misdiagnosis due to the high rate of allele dropout and the high frequency of mosaicism at the cleavage stage (see below).

Blastocyst Biopsy

Blastocyst biopsy was first reported as a possibility for PGD in rabbits by Gardner and Edwards[41] and seems to be the most realistic option among other not yet realized but possible approaches for PGD in humans. As in the human blastocyst, the number of cells increases up to more than 100, when as many as 10–30 cells from IVF embryos can be biopsied. Another advantage of this approach is that trophectoderm cells are biopsied without affecting the inner cell mass, from which the embryo is derived. As feasibility of the use of the technique will obviously depend on the possible detrimental effect of the manipulations, the viability of biopsied blastocysts in vitro was studied, using morphologic criteria and the patterns of hCG secretion. Because there is no information on the development of nonmanipulated embryos in vitro for comparison, thirty-six nonmanipulated human embryos from day 3 to day 14 were also investigated. Hatching was observed in 38.5 percent of blastocysts; hCG was detected first on day 8, peaked at day 10, and was still detectable in some blastocysts at day 14.[42] For the individual blastocysts, the pattern of hCG secretion correlated with the assessment of morphology.[43]

An elegant method for trophectoderm biopsy, described by Muggleton-Harris et al.,[44] avoids the problem of cell stickiness at that stage. Human blastocysts were available at day 5 or day 6 of in vitro culture and thus were fully expanded, although in practice, it would be preferable to use day 4 or day 5 blastocysts. The blastocysts were treated with acid Tyrode solution to remove the sperm and thin the zona but not to take the zona off entirely. Without slitting the zona, two siliclad-coated glass microneedles were used to manipulate the blastocyst in small drops of medium. Although one microneedle held the blastocyst in place, the other was inserted through the zona and the trophectoderm cells from the opposite pole were pulled through the zona. One or two serial biopsies of two to five cells can be taken from different areas of the human blastocyst trophectoderm, or up to fifteen cells from the mouse blastocyst, without affecting the viability.

Initially, blastocyst biopsy could be introduced only through uterine lavage because the proportion of embryos that reaches this stage in IVF programs was very low.[45,46] However, with the present tendency of the day 5 (blastocyst) transfer, the blastocyst biopsy may have important clinical implications. Despite the obvious potential advantage of blastocyst biopsy, there has not been many reported attempts to use this approach for PGD of human genetic diseases. A lavage clinical cycle performed at the Baylor Center for Hemophilia A, although the embryo was male and could not be transferred,[47] and a few successful PGD cycles were performed for translocations, resulting in ongoing pregnancies.[47a] The ongoing research on the development of blastocyst biopsy in experimental animals and humans will make it possible to consider the usefulness of blastocyst biopsy not only as an alternative approach for PGD but also for confirmation of preconception or blastomere genetic analysis as well as a backup procedure if these approaches fail.

PREIMPLANTATION GENETIC ANALYSIS

Initially, PGD was justified only for high-risk pregnancies. Maternal age was not expected to be an indication for such early diagnosis, not only because PGD of chromosomal disease had not been established, but also because advanced maternal age was considered to be a contraindication to PGD. However, the development and improvement of the methods for sampling and genetic analysis of oocytes and preimplantation embryos has made it possible to initiate the application of PGD for the prevention of genetic and chromosomal disorders. In addition, PGD is becoming useful as a tool in assisted reproduction technologies, especially for improving the effectiveness of IVF in patients of advanced maternal age. As a result, most clinical cycles currently have been performed for preimplantation testing of age-related aneuploidies.[21–25]

Single-Gene Disorders

DNA analysis for preconception and preimplantation diagnosis has become realistic, with the application of PCR, which makes it possible to amplify minute quantities of DNA obtained from a single cell.[12,19,20] Because this increases the chance of DNA contamination in PGD, specially designed decontamination procedures were applied at the initial stages, which were based on the elimination of double-stranded DNA sequences.[48–50] In addition, the possible sources of contamination were also excluded carefully, such as the embryology reagents, water, salt solutions, oligonucleotides, Taq polymerase, and other PCR reagents.[50] It has been suggested that all reagents be tested for contamination and their ability to amplify DNA before their use in preconception and preimplantation diagnostic procedures so that decontamination procedures could be applied to eliminate low-level DNA contamination.

One of the important sources of contamination in preimplantation diagnosis is cellular contamination, such as cumulus cells, spermatozoa, or cell fragments, which might be amplified simultaneously with polar bodies or blastomeres, creating the possibility for erroneous diagnosis. Because potential misdiagnosis of PGD at the cleavage stage may be caused by sperm DNA contamination, it is currently a routine IVF practice to perform cleavage-stage PGD for single-gene defects following microsurgical fertilization by intracytoplasmic sperm injection.

The other important problem is to avoid misdiagnosis caused by the preferential amplification or failure of allele-specific amplification, referred to as allele dropout (ADO), which may happen in single-cell genetic analysis, so this was initially studied for each gene locus in question before PGD was undertaken. As much as 8 percent of allele dropout was observed in PCR analysis of the first polar bodies, reaching over 20 percent in blastomeres.[51] False-negative diagnoses have been observed using PGD for X-linked disorders, myotonic dystrophy, fragile X syndrome and cystic fibrosis (CF).[3,21,22,52] To ensure that the allele dropout does not lead to misdiagnosis, a multiplex PCR is introduced, which involves a simultaneous detection of the mutant allele and linked polymorphic markers.[4,51,53,54] A set of polymorphic markers are studied in patients in preparation for preimplantation diagnosis, to ensure their informativeness in each particular family. Accordingly, the more polymorphic markers are available, the more accurate the diagnosis might be. For example, for preimplantation diagnosis of the β-globin gene, two polymorphic markers (short tandem repeats [STRs] at 59 and HUMTHO1) were used, which were shown to be strongly linked to the β-globin gene.[4,54] In addition, STRs in different chromosomes are amplified simultaneously, to be able to sort out a possible contamination with sperm DNA or maternal follicular cells.[54]

A system of multiplex PCR involving two separate regions of the CF gene (mainly ΔF508 in exon 10 and a region in intron 6 containing a tightly linked polymorphism to the ΔF508 mutation) was developed to minimize the potential misdiagnosis in PGD of CF.[4] The initial PCR reaction contains two pairs of outside primers. After the first round of PCR, two separate aliquots are amplified using the inside primers specific for each side. Embryos are transferred only when both the polymorphic site and the mutation agree. This dual amplification allows the detection of ADO and prevents transfer of misdiagnosed affected embryos. According to the currently collected data, each additional linked marker allows detection of up to a half of potential ADO, with almost up to 100 percent detection rate with three closely linked markers.[4,53]

As mentioned above, one of the major indications for preimplantation diagnosis in most centers was the risk of X-linked disease. Initially, this was performed using cleavage-stage biopsy and DNA amplification of Y-specific and then both X- and Y-specific sequences by PCR.[19,55,56] Later, fluorescence in situ hybridization (FISH) with X- and Y-chromosome-specific probes was used.[57-59] In addition, the use of a chromosome-18-specific probe in combination with X and Y probes seemed to be useful to minimize misdiagnosis due to mosaicism and ploidy assessment.[60] Hundreds of clinical cycles were performed for X-linked disorders by gender determination, resulting in the birth of many unaffected children.[21,22] Misdiagnosis may occur when DNA amplification is used at the cleavage stage.[51] Consequently preimplantation sex determination is currently performed by FISH in most centers.

More than 1,000 PGD cycles overall have been carried out for the detection of single-gene defects, resulting in more than 200 births of children free from specific genetic conditions.[21-23] The CF ΔF508 mutation has been the major indication for PGD of single-gene defects. However, at least 4 misdiagnoses were reported in these cases, all performed at the cleavage stage PGD for couples in which parents were carriers of different mutations of the gene tested. The list of genetic disorders for which cleavage stage

PGD and polar-body analysis has been done is presented in Table 27.1, and involved the development of a specific strategy based on extensive preliminary studies.

Of these clinical cycles, preconception genetic diagnosis of single-gene disorders based on the sequential first- and second-polar-body analysis was performed in approximately 300 cycles for different genetic conditions (see Figure 27.1).[4,24,25] For cases in

Table 27.1. Genetic disorders for which PGD was performed*

α_1-Antitrypsin
Adenomatous polyposis coli
Adenosine deaminase deficiency
Alport disease
Alzheimer disease (early-onset)
Charcot—Marie–Tooth disease 1A and 1B
Citrullinemia
Cystic fibrosis
Duchenne muscular dystrophy
Ectodermal dysplasia (PKP1)
Epidermolysis bullosa
Familial dysautonomia
Fanconi anemia A and C
Fragile X syndrome
Gaucher disease
Hemophilia A
Hemophilia B
Holoprosencephaly (SSH)
Huntington disease
Hurler syndrome
Hypophosphatasia
Kell I group genotyping
Lesch–Nyhan syndrome
Long-chain 3-hydroxyacyl-CoA dehydrogenase deficiency
Lowe syndrome
Machado–Joseph disease (SCA III)
Marfan syndrome
Medium-chain acyl–CoA dehydrogenase deficiency
Multiple epiphyseal dysplasia
Myotonic muscular dystrophy
Myotubular myotonic dystrophy
Neurofibromatosis I and II
Niemann–Pick disease
Ornithine transcarbamylase deficiency
p53 Oncogene mutations
Phenylketonuria
Polycystic kidney disease types 1 and 2
Retinitis pigmentosa
Rhesus (RhD) incompatibility
Sickle cell disease
Spinocerebellar ataxia
Tay–Sachs disease
Thalassemias
Von Hippel–Lindau disease
Wiskott–Aldrich syndrome
X-linked hydrocephalus

*The list presently contains approximately 200 genetic conditions, for which PGD has been performed.

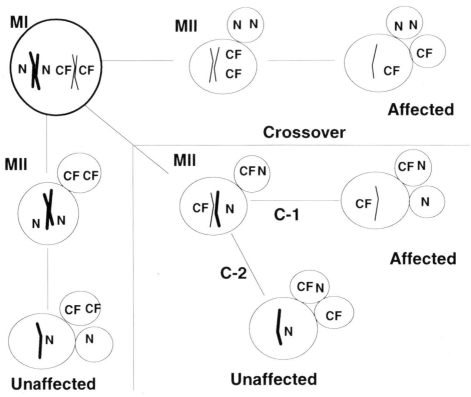

Fig. 27.1. The scheme demonstrating the principle of preimplantation genetic analysis by sequential DNA analysis of the first and second polar body, using the CF locus as an example. (See color insert.)

which diagnosis of oocytes was not informative or abnormal, the resulting embryos were followed by blastomere biopsy to investigate the reliability of the polar-body diagnosis. The data showed that although preconception evaluation of the genotype of the oocyte was extrapolated from the diagnosis of the first and second polar body, there have been no misdiagnoses. For example, there is no need for further information about embryos, in which the first polar bodies were found to be heterozygous and the second polar body hemizygous for the abnormal gene.[4]

The sequential first- and second-polar-body analysis appeared also to be useful for specific diagnosis in the X-linked disorders, because PGD by gender determination leads to discarding 50 percent of unaffected male embryos. This was applied to eight couples at risk for having children with X-linked genetic disorders, including hemophilia B, fragile X syndrome, myotubular myotonic dystrophy, ornithine transcarbamylase deficiency and X-linked hydrocephalus.[61] Overall, thirteen PGD cycles were performed, resulting in the detection of embryos with a predicted mutation-free maternal contribution, which were transferred back to the patients in all cycles, yielding four clinical pregnancies, which resulted in the births of three healthy children and one affected child.

The list for PGD of single-gene disorders currently includes late-onset disorders with genetic predisposition, which have never been indications for prenatal diagnosis. Applied first for Li–Fraumeni syndrome, determined by p53 tumor suppressor gene mutations,[62] PGD was then offered to couples at risk for other cancers, including familial adenomatous polyposis, Von Hippel–Lindau syndrome, retinoblastoma,[63] neurofibromatosis type I and II[64] and familial posterior fossa brain tumor. Overall, twenty PGD cycles were performed, resulting in the preselection and transfer of forty mutation-free embryos, which have yielded five unaffected clinical pregnancies and four healthy children born thus far.[6] Despite the controversy of PGD use for the late-onset disorders, the data demonstrate the usefulness of this approach as the only acceptable option for at-risk couples who wish to avoid the birth of children with inherited predisposition to cancer and subsequently have a healthy child of their own.

The other unexpected application of PGD was for the autosomal dominant presenile form of dementia due to Alzheimer disease (AD).[7] The results demonstrated feasibility of PGD for early-onset AD, providing a nontraditional option for patients, who may wish to avoid the transmission of the mutant gene to their future children.

Preimplantation HLA matching has recently emerged as a tool for the preselection of a potential donor progeny for bone marrow transplantation.[5] This was first applied to Fanconi anemia (FA), in which the preselection and transfer of unaffected embryos with an HLA match for the affected sibling yielded a clinical pregnancy. The subsequent birth of a healthy carrier of the FA gene, whose cord blood was transplanted to the affected sibling, resulted in a successful hematopoietic reconstitution. The method has currently been applied for HLA genotyping in eighteen cycles (five for thalassemia, six for FA, one for Wiskott–Aldrich syndrome, and six for leukemia) from eleven couples overall, involving the testing of 197 embryos including specific gene analyses, and of 86 embryos for HLA typing only. This resulted in the preselection of 37 (19 percent) HLA matched embryos, including 21 (17.5 percent) in combination with preselection of unaffected embryos, following mutation testing, and 16 (22 percent) not involving mutation analysis. These HLA-matched embryos have been transferred back to patients, resulting in five clinical pregnancies and the birth of five HLA-matched children.[23]

The most recent application of PGD for the Sonic Hedgehog mutation causing holoprosencephaly provides a practical option also for a large group of couples at risk for having children with congenital malformations.[65]

Chromosomal Disorders

Published data on cytogenetic analysis of unfertilized oocytes from IVF programs[3,66] demonstrate a great potential for preimplantation diagnosis of chromosomal disorders. The theoretical rate of chromosomally abnormal embryos at fertilization is approximately 40 percent, taking into account both the rate of aneuploidies in oocytes and sperm and fertilization-related abnormalities.[66,67] As can be expected from the mouse data,[67,68] most embryos with these chromosomal abnormalities, although compatible with cleavage, will be lost during implantation. An additional loss of chromosomally abnormal embryos is realized after implantation, which is clinically recognized as spontaneous abortion; more than half of spontaneous abortions are caused by chromosomal abnormalities. As a result of this selection against chromosomal abnormalities before and after implantation, only 0.65 percent of newborns have chromosomal disorders, most of which lead to serious disability and early death (see also chapter 6).

A wide range in the frequency of chromosomal aneuploidy in human oocytes has been reported (from as low as 17 percent to as high as 70 percent), but most of these studies have been performed on poor-quality oocytes left over after the failure of IVF attempts. The major problem with all available cytogenetic data concerning human oocytes is that they have been obtained on the analysis of meiotic chromosomes, which in many cases were not appropriate for evaluation of the exact number of chromosomes and for detecting structural chromosomal abnormalities. Suppose that hypohaploidy found in oocytes was artificially induced by spreading techniques. The hypohaploid chromosome sets might then be ignored and the frequency of the chromosomal abnormalities would be calculated by doubling the number of hyperhaploid oocytes. This assumption ignores all possible cases of chromatid malsegregation and/or chromosome lagging, is inconsistent with a nonrandom chromosome disjunction hypothesis, and contradicts the results of our observation that even with high-quality preparations prepared from mouse oocytes with special precautions and by the best spreading technique, the rate of hypohaploidy is always higher than the rate of hyperhaploidy.[70] To improve the cytogenetic analysis of unfertilized oocytes, an approach for turning a meiotic chromosome set into mitotic chromosomes was introduced, using parthenogenetic activation of human oocytes by puromycin, a protein inhibitor that can activate oocytes not only at the second but even at the first meiotic metaphase.[71] From seventy-eight human unfertilized oocytes treated by puromycin, seventy were activated parthenogenetically, with the possibility of cytogenetic investigation of mitotic chromosomes in forty-six oocytes. The appropriate quality of the chromosomal preparations made it possible to identify a number of aneuploid oocytes, including clear hypohaploid chromosome sets, suggesting the need for reconsideration of the existing strategy for the evaluation of the frequency of chromosomal aberrations in oocytes.

An attempt at a noninvasive cytogenetic analysis of oocytes was undertaken by Modlinsky and McLaren,[72] who performed visualization of the chromosomes of the second polar body of the mouse by transplanting the polar body into a fertilized egg. In some cases, the transplanted polar body transformed in a presumably haploid group of mitotic chromosomes; however, the success rate was very low, and even when the chromosomes were visualized, they were not suitable for karyotyping. Later, the possibility of predicting the karyotype of the oocytes using the first and second polar bodies was explored in the mouse model using the same and other approaches.[3,73,74] The data showed that both the first- and second-polar-body chromosomes may be visualized and considered for a possible preimplantation prediction of the karyotype of the oocyte. Cytogenetic investigation of the first polar body may have important practical implications because more than 80 percent of all chromosomal nondisjunctions originate from malsegregation at maternal meiosis I.[75] On the other hand, the visualization of chromosomes of the second polar body will make it possible to evaluate the result of nondisjunction at the second meiotic division. No data were available regarding the possibility for visualization of chromosomes of the first polar body, except for a discouraging observation long ago that, in some instances, the disintegrating chromosomes in the first polar body may be recognized as nonseparated chromatid pairs, degenerating to the point of fragmentation after extrusion.[76] According to our observations, immediately after extrusion, the first-polar-body chromosomes are uncountable if analyzed. The individual chromosomes of the first polar body become recognizable and countable only after 2–3 hr of in vitro culture and during the next 2–3 hr, with degeneration following 6–7 hr after extrusion.[70] These observations suggest that cytogenetic investigation of the first polar body may be feasible, but the period during which the analysis can be performed is very short.

Various approaches were tested in the attempt to visualize the second-polar-body chromosomes. One approach involved electrofusion of the mouse second polar body with intact and/or enucleated mouse zygotes. Thirty-four percent of second-polar-body nuclei were transformed into the metaphase plate, although 40 percent of them had chromosomal aberrations. The same results were obtained by electrofusion of the second polar body with a foreign one-cell mouse embryo; the proportion of metaphase plates reached 65 percent when the recipient one-cell-stage mouse embryo was enucleated. However, more than one-third of the metaphase plates had chromosomal aberrations; the increase in their frequency was related to the age of polar bodies used for the fusion experiments.[74]

The other approach involved the treatment of one-cell-stage mouse embryos with okadaic acid (a specific inhibitor of phosphates 1 and 2A), leading to visualization of chromosomes in the nucleus of the second polar body.[77] Of 215 polar bodies treated by okadaic acid, analyzable second-polar-body chromosomes were present in 173 (80 percent). The visualized chromosomes of the second polar body were unichromatid G1 premature condensed chromosomes of good quality, suitable for differential staining.

2. Most recently, nuclear transfer techniques have been used to convert interphase nuclei of the second polar bodies or blastomeres into metaphase chromosomes, which appeared to be of practical value in PGD for translocations.[4] Progress has been achieved also in using microarray technology and comparative genome hybridization, but their practical implications for PGD are still limited.[23,24,77a]

The introduction of FISH analysis has facilitated analysis of polar bodies and blastomeres in interphase, enabling the detection and avoidance of the age-related risk for Down syndrome in older women undergoing IVF. To investigate whether polar-body cytogenetic analysis using the FISH technique may predict the karyotype of the corresponding oocytes, an extensive study was done on the human oocytes that had remained unfertilized 1–2 days after insemination in an IVF program.[78] The first polar bodies were removed from these oocytes by micromanipulation and analyzed simultaneously with their corresponding oocytes, using directly labeled fluorescent α-satellite DNA probes that hybridize specifically with the centromeric region of the human X or chromosome 18 (Vysis, Naperville, IL). Fluorescent signals were seen as two red dots in chromatids of the X chromosomes and two green dots in chromatids of chromosome 18 in the second meiotic metaphase (MII). Identical specific signals (the paired dots) were found in the remnants of the first polar body (IPB), even in fragmented chromatin masses. In the series of 130 oocytes, in which the number of X chromosomes and chromosome 18 specific signals were analyzable both in MII and in the IPB, five nondisjunction events were detected. In one oocyte, there was a chromosome 18 nondisjunction (four signals in MII and no signal in IPB), in two oocytes chromatid 18 nondisjunction (three signals in MII, one in IPB) and in two oocytes the X-chromatid malsegregation (three signals in MII, one in IPB) was found. A similar study was undertaken with simultaneous application of probes for chromosomes X, Y, 18, and 13/21 or X, Y, 18, and 16.[79] The data clearly showed that the polar-body FISH analysis can be useful for cytogenetic analysis of human oocytes for detection of chromosome and chromatid nondisjunction at the meiotic division.

Based on these data, the first- and second-polar-body FISH analysis using chromosome-specific probes for chromosomes 13, 16, 18, 21, and 22 (Vysis, Downers Grove, IL) was offered to IVF patients of advanced maternal age, who have a considerably low pregnancy rate compared with younger patients.[80–82] At present, 1,297 PGD cycles were performed from the IVF patients of average age of 38.5 years, using FISH analysis of 6,733 oocytes. A total of 3,509 (52 percent) aneuploid oocytes were detected, originating comparably from the first and second meiotic divisions. Overall, meiotic division errors were observed in 41.8 percent oocytes in meiosis I (see Figure 27.2), 30.7 percent in meiosis II (see Figure 27.3), and 27.6 percent in both. In a total of 45.1 percent of the abnormal oocytes with complex

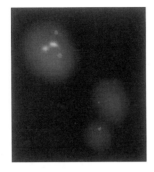
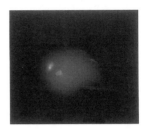

1st Polar Body (+ 21)   2nd Polar Body

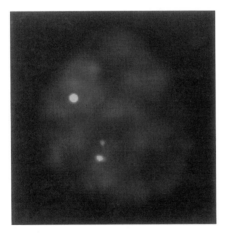
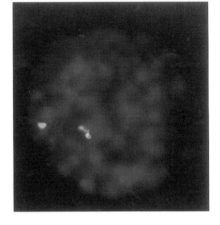

Blastomere Nuclei, Monosomy 21

Fig. 27.2. Patterns of signals in the oocyte with monosomy 21, revealed by testing of both first and second polar bodies by FISH, using chromosome-18- and chromosome-21-specific probes. Normally, the first polar body should have two signals for chromosome 18 (two green dots) and two for chromosome 21 (two red dots), whereas only a single red or green dot should be seen in the second polar body. However, the first polar body shows three signals instead of two for chromosome 21 (three red dots), demonstrating the result of chromatid 21 malsegregation in the first meiotic division and normal segregation of chromosome 18 (two green dots). Follow-up blastomere FISH analysis in the resulting embryo confirmed the diagnosis of monosomy 21. (See color insert.)

errors, the same chromosome in both meiotic divisions was involved in 21.5 percent of cases, while different chromosomes were observed in 78.5 percent of oocytes. Of 3,224 detected aneuploidy-free zygotes, 2,587 were transferred in 1,100 treatment cycles (2.35 embryos per transfer), resulting in 241 (21.9 percent) clinical pregnancies and 176 healthy children born, suggesting a positive clinical outcome following aneuploidy testing of oocytes in a group of IVF patients of average age of 38.5 years (see Table 27.2).

3. The above overall rates of nuclear abnormalities in oocytes are comparable to those detected in preimplantation embryos in PGD for aneuploidies at the cleavage stage,

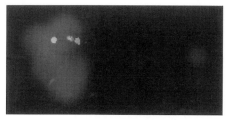

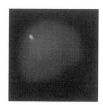

1st Polar Body Chromatin   2nd Polar Body Chromatin

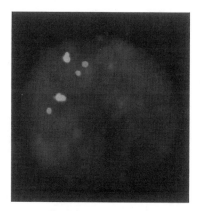

Embryo Nucleus

Fig. 27.3. Patterns of signals in an oocyte with trisomy 21, revealed by testing of both first and second polar bodies by FISH, using chromosome-18- and chromosome-21-specific probes. Normally, the first polar body should have two signals for chromosome 18 (two green dots) and two for chromosome 21 (two red dots), whereas only a single red or green dot should be seen in the second polar body. However, the second polar body shows no red signal instead of one for chromosome 21 (only a green dot for chromosome 18 is seen), demonstrating the result of nondisjunction of chromosome 21 in the second meiotic division, leading to trisomy 21 in the embryo, as shown by follow-up blastomere FISH analysis confirming the polar body diagnosis. (See color insert.)

taking into consideration additional fertilization-related abnormalities and paternally derived meiotic errors, which could also have been detected at this stage. In approximately the same size of PGD cycles performed for aneuploidy at the cleavage stage by the Saint Barnabas and SISMER centers, the proportion of embryos with chromosomal abnormalities was as high as 60 percent.[83,84] However, the types of anomalies in oocytes and the embryos were significantly different, which is at-

Table 27.2. Clinical outcome of transfers of selected trisomy-free embryos after preimplantation polar body FISH analysis (average maternal age, 38.5 years)

Total Cycles	Normal Oocytes	Total Oocytes Transferred	No. of Transfers	No. of Pregnancies	No. of Children Born
1297	3224	2587	1100	241	176

tributable mainly to a high frequency of mosaicism, comprising approximately a half of the chromosomal abnormalities at the cleavage stage. The overall experience of PGD for chromosomal disorders is currently close to 4,000 cases, confirming the positive impact on the clinical outcome.[23,24,83,84–86] The need to further quantify its impact in randomized controlled studies remains, and these are currently in progress. It is obvious, however, that the improvement of the outcome of PGD may be expected only when the number of embryos biopsied is equal to or higher than the number of embryos expected to be replaced without PGD.[83] The clinical impact of aneuploidy testing, in terms of the improved pregnancy and implantation rates, as well the improved outcome of pregnancies through the reduction of spontaneous abortions, has been further confirmed not only for IVF patients of advanced maternal age, but also for other poor prognosis patients, including those with repeated IVF failures, repeated spontaneous abortions, and altered karyotypes.[84]

Because there are no morphologic criteria for identification of chromosomally normal oocytes and embryos, a blind selection of oocytes for transfer may lead to the transfer of embryos from abnormal oocytes and, accordingly, to a possible discard of actually normal embryos, resulting in numerous failed attempts by infertile couples of advanced maternal age before they may become pregnant. The development of an accurate preimplantation cytogenetic diagnosis will make it possible not only to prevent chromosomal disorders before pregnancy but also to enable the avoidance of fertilization and pregnancy failures determined by chromosomal abnormalities. The presented data further support the clinical usefulness of PGD for assisted reproduction, as more than half of the preimplantation embryos are chromosomally abnormal from the outset, and should not be transferred to IVF patients of advanced maternal age.

Therefore, the further improvement of IVF efficiency will be unrealistic without the preselection of aneuploidy-free oocytes and embryos. The current tendency of limiting the number of transferred embryos to only two, and even to only one in the blastocyst transfer, aims to avoid the complications of multiple pregnancies. The preselection of chromosomally normal embryos will soon become a standard IVF practice, since it is pointless to transfer untested embryos, more than 50 percent of which are aneuploid, thereby compromising the outcome of IVF in a traditional setting. Meanwhile, the information on the availability of such an option should be provided at least to IVF patients who have a poor prognosis, so they could have the opportunity of improving their chances to become pregnant and avoiding the establishment of pregnancy destined to be lost due to chromosomal aneuploidy. The clinical outcome is currently available in approximately 700 clinical pregnancies resulting from the PGD for aneuploidies, supporting the above-mentioned observations of the positive impact on the implantation and pregnancy rates and the improvement of the pregnancy outcomes.

PGD is valuable for the carriers of balanced translocations, who have an extremely poor chance of having an unaffected pregnancy. More than 400 clinical cycles have been performed at present, resulting in at least one hundred clinical pregnancies and births of unaffected children. The data are in agreement with previous reports suggesting a considerable reduction in the spontaneous abortion rate in PGD patients with balanced translocations.[83,87,88]

ETHICAL AND LEGAL ISSUES

Considerations on ethical and legal issues are evolving, along with the evolution of the technology for the control of genetic diseases, and have become one of the key subjects in discussing the acceptability of preconception and preimplantation diagnosis of genetic disorders. Ethical and legal issues would determine, to a considerable extent, whether these new approaches will be promoted to become an integral part of preventive genetics services or will be waived on ethical grounds.[8,89] PGD could be regarded as an ethically acceptable procedure in the context of a general objective of genetic service, which, according to the WHO, is to help genetically disadvantaged people live and reproduce as normally and as responsibly as possible.[9] Because it is heavily based on IVF, it also is relevant to mention that IVF is considered to be ethically acceptable in many countries.[90–93] However, complex ethical and legal issues are confronted differently in various countries.[94] For example, in Germany, the future of PGD will depend on an Embryo Protection Law, which has been in effect since 1991.[95] This law is very strict and prohibitive for embryo research. However, it prohibits only destructive research that impairs chances of the embryo of up to the eight-cell stage to become a human being. In fact, blastomere biopsy after this stage, as well as blastocyst biopsy, may be possible without any conflict with the law, because, together with CVS, such embryo biopsies are considered beneficial, allowing decisions to be made before replacement. Therefore, there may be no conflict that would prohibit the establishment of PGD in Germany if it is done either before the pronucleate or after the eight-cell stage. However, this must be done for diagnostic purposes only, not for research. Even in the case of tripronucleate embryos, only observation is permitted, not experimentation. In contrast, in France, there seems to be no law at all concerning either PGD or embryo research. However, the National Ethical Committee attitude toward PGD is influenced by the fact that the diagnosis is based on genetic analysis of only one or a few cells and that all male embryos after gender determination are discarded, half of them being completely normal. Another concern is that PGD increases the need for IVF, which is provided in France free of charge. Finally, prenatal diagnosis, also provided free of charge, was enough to avoid genetic disorder, so the provision of PGD was considered to be an additional prenatal test, without taking into account the suffering caused by selective abortions after prenatal diagnosis.

In some countries, such as Belgium, the decision for embryo research and PGD rests completely with institutional review boards, so there is no problem with the development of the technique and its implementation into clinical practice. In other countries, such as the Netherlands, PGD will be governed by the law on medical experiments, which contains a section on embryo research. It prohibits "cloning," but probably will not ban PGD research because it provides an alternative to prenatal diagnosis and abortion of genetically affected fetuses. In England, PGD, as well as the practice of IVF and research involving human embryos, is regulated through a statutory body, the Human Fertilization and Embryology Authority and the Fertilization and Embryology Act (1990), allowing research on human embryos up to 14 days of development under an appropriate license. In Spain, although a 1988 law regulating human embryo research forbade the fertilization of human oocytes for any purpose other than human procreation, it permited research on embryos within 14 days of preimplantation development under the supervision of the national health and scientific authorities.[96] Therefore, this law did not conflict with the development of research in preimplantation genetics and its application to assisted reproduction practices.

In the United States and Australia, the legal status of PGD and the community attitudes are different even in various states. For example, in the six states of Australia, only three have laws governing IVF and embryo research. In Victoria, embryo research is prohibited, except for approved experiments, although this law does not actually affect PGD because IVF is allowed for infertile couples, and PGD also can be justified as the procedure for avoiding the risk of transmitting genetic disease to affected children. In Western Australia, PGD cannot be done because of the Experimentation Law, whereas in South Australia, it is possible unless destructive to an implantable human embryo.

In the United States, the issue of embryo research is closely associated with the debates on abortion or cloning, and there has been no government system for regulating reproductive research projects. Because there is no ethical advisory board (EAB) that is legally given responsibility for reviewing such research proposals, federal funding for human embryo research has not been available. In addition, a wide variation of policy positions exists among different states, mainly being compromised over consideration of the question of when human life begins. However, despite existing differences in current legal restrictions in this field, selection of pre-embryos on genetic grounds may be ethically acceptable based on the fact that the goal of avoiding the birth of offspring with severe genetic handicaps is part of the constitutional rights of procreative liberty.[97] President Clinton signed into effect the National Institutes of Health Revitalization Act of 1993, lifting the requirement (45 CFR 46.204.d) for a federal-level EAB review for IVF research and leaving consideration for clinical research related to IVF to individual institutional review boards. The U.S. Congress document states that none of the federal funds may be used for research in which a human embryo or embryos are destroyed, discarded, or knowingly subjected to risk of injury or death greater than allowed for research on fetuses in utero.[98]

In Canada, recent legislation to regulate assisted human reproduction technologies has been introduced, entitled an "Act Respecting Assisted Human Reproduction," which allows PGD for medical reasons, but excludes identifying sex of an embryo for social purposes.[99]

Important ethical issues have recently been raised with increasing use of PGD for preimplantation gender determination for social reasons,[100–102] late-onset disorders with genetic predisposion,[6,7,102,103] and preimplantation HLA typing to produce an HLA-compatible donor for treating a family member with fatal bone marrow disease or cancer, requiring a stem-cell transplantation.[5,98,104] Although there is no actual difference in the application of PGD for the latter conditions, the controversy can be explained by the fact that in traditional prenatal diagnosis if the fetus was found to carry the gene predisposing to a late-onset disorder or to be HLA unmatched, a couple would have to make an extremely difficult decision about pregnancy termination, which could hardly be justified by such a finding. Alternatively, PGD technology allows genetic testing of human eggs and embryos before pregnancy is established, making it totally realistic to establish only HLA-matched or potentially normal pregnancies without genetic predisposition to late-onset disorders.

Notwithstanding the foregoing considerations, PGD is now becoming an established clinical option in reproductive medicine and is applied using separate consent forms and research protocols approved by institutional ethics committees. The number of apparently healthy children born after PGD has passed its first thousand, showing that there is no evidence of any incurred adverse effect. However, these protocols would still require confirmatory CVS or amniocentesis and a follow-up monitoring of its safety and accuracy. Although PGD will help solve some of the longstanding ethical problems, such as the abortion issue (which will be avoided as a result of this new approach), other issues could become a serious obstacle, particularly those related to "designer babies." These considerations are highly relevant to the subject of PGD, as well as to any other new methods as we proceed with further development of appropriate technology for controlling genetic disability.

CONCLUSION

Although the introduction of first-trimester prenatal diagnosis by CVS has considerably improved the possibility for the avoidance of genetic diseases, a selective abortion is an issue in the case of an affected fetus. PGD has been initiated to provide the option of avoiding the birth of an affected child without the need for abortion as an obligatory component in the prevention program. This chapter describes these important developments with the emphasis on addressing the problems of implementation of PGD into clinical practice.

Currently, PGD has been applied clinically in at least fifty centers around the world. More than 1,000 unaffected children have already been born after PGD in more than 5,000 clinical cycles performed for single-gene and chromosomal disorders. Two approaches for PGD have been mainly used: polar-body removal and blastomere biopsy. Both of these approaches became possible due to the progress in micromanipulation and biopsy and in genetic analysis of single cells by PCR. The use of both of these approaches has already demonstrated the feasibility of preimplantation diagnosis of genetic and chromosomal disorders and also the improvement of the reliability and safety of this new technique in assisted reproduction. The indications for PGD have been expanded beyond those used in prenatal diagnosis to include couples at high risk for having a child with a genetic disorder (in the face of antipathy toward elective abortion), IVF patients of advanced maternal age, couples at risk for producing offspring with late-onset genetic disorders, and preimplantation HLA matching. Because of the high frequency of chromosomal abnormalities in early pregnancy, the introduction of preimplantation cytogenetic analysis will not only make it possible to avoid the risk of age-related aneuploidies, but will also considerably improve the embryo recovery and pregnancy outcome following PGD and will improve the effectiveness of IVF programs in general. Finally, PGD is of great benefit for couples carrying balanced translocations, reducing the risk of spontaneous abortion fourfold As demonstrated, the ethical considerations in the introduction of this new technology are of great importance because PGD may contribute considerably to the development of more ethically acceptable approaches for the prevention and avoidance of genetic disorders, obviating the need for a selective abortion.

REFERENCES

1. Verlinsky Y, Kuliev AM. Preimplantation genetics. New York: Plenum Press, 1991.
2. Edwards RG. Preconception and preimplantation diagnosis of genetic diseases. Cambridge, UK: Cambridge University Press, 1993.
3. Verlinsky Y, Kuliev AM. Preimplantation diagnosis of genetic diseases: a new technique for assisted reproduction. New York: Wiley-Liss, 1993.
4. Verlinsky Y, Kuliev AM. Atlas of preimplantation genetic diagnosis, New York: Parthenon, 2000.
5. Verlinsky Y, Rechitsky S, Schoolcraft W, et al. Preimplantation diagnosis for Fanconi anemia combined with HLA matching. JAMA 2001;285:3130.
6. Rechitsky S, Verlinsky O, Chistokhina A. et al. Preimplantation genetic diagnosis for cancer predisposition. Reprod Biomed Online 2002;5:148.
7. Verlinsky Y, Rechitsky S, Verlinsky O, et al. Preimplantation diagnosis for early onset Alzheimer disease caused by V717L mutation. JAMA 2002;287:1038.
8. Kuliev AM, Modell B. Ethical issues in the control of genetic diseases. In: Verlinsky Y, Kuliev AM, eds. Preimplantation genetics. New York: Plenum Press, 1991:233.
9. World Health Organization. Perspectives of fetal diagnosis of congenital diseases. WHO unpublished document HMG/Serono/84.4. Geneva: World Health Organization, 1984.
10. Kuliev A, Modell B, Galjaard H. Perspectives in fetal diagnosis of congenital disorders. Arns Serono Symposia, Rome, 1985.

11. McLaren A. Prenatal diagnosis before implantation: opportunities and problems. Prenat Diagn 1985;5:85.

12. Saiki R, Scharf S, Faloona F, et al. Enzymatic amplification of beta-globin genomic sequences and restriction site analysis for diagnosis of sickle cell anemia. Science 1985;230:1350.

13. Leonard M, Kirszenbaum M, Cotinot C, et al. Sexing bovine embryos using a Y chromosome specific probe. Theriogenology 1987;27:248.

14. Monk M, Handyside AH. Sexing of preimplantation mouse embryos by measurement of X-linked gene dosage in single blastomere. J Reprod Fertil 1988;82:365.

15. Monk M, Muggleton-Harris AL, Rawling E, et al. Preimplantation diagnosis of HPRT-deficient male mice and carrier female mouse embryo by trophectoderm biopsy. Hum Reprod 1988;3:377.

16. Summers PM, Campbell JM, Miller MW. Normal in-vivo development of marmoset monkey embryos after trophectoderm biopsy. Hum Reprod 1988;3:389.

17. Gordon JW, Gang I. Use of zona drilling for safe and effective biopsy of murine oocytes and embryos. Biol Reprod 1990;42:869.

18. Handyside AH, Pattison JK, Penketh RJA, et al. Biopsy of human preimplantation embryos and sexing by DNA amplification. Lancet 1989;1:347.

19. Handyside AH, Kontogiani EH, Hardy K, et al. Pregnancies from biopsied human preimplantation embryos sexed by Y-specific DNA amplification. Nature 1990,344:768.

20. Verlinsky Y, Ginsberg N, Lifchez A, et al. Analysis of the first polar body: preconception genetic diagnosis. Hum Reprod 1990;5:826.

21. International Working Group on Preimplantation Genetics 2001. Preimplantation genetic diagnosis: experience of three thousand clinical cycles. Report of the 11th Annual Meeting International Working Group on Preimplantation Genetics, in conjunction with the 10th International Congress of Human Genetics, Vienna, May 15, 2001. Reprod Biomed Online 2001;3:49.

22. ESHRE Preimplantation Genetic Diagnosis Consortium. Data Collection III, May 2002. Hum Reprod 2002;17:233.

23. Kuliev A, Verlinsky Y. Thirteen years experience of preimplantation diagnosis: Report of Fifth International Symposium on Preimplantation Genetics. Reprod Biomed Online 2003;8:229–235..

24. Wells D, Levy B. Cytogenetics in reproductive medicine: the contribution of comparative genomic hybridization (CGH). Bioessays 2003;25:289.

25. Verlinsky Y, Cohen J, Munne S., et al. The first thousand babies born after preimplantation genetic diagnosis JAMA 2003 (in press).

26. Kuliev A, Rechitsky S, Verlinsky O, et al. Preembryonic diagnosis for sickle cell disease. Mol Cell Endocrinol 2001; 183:S19.

27. Levinson G, Keyvanfar K, Wu JC, et al. DNA-based X-enriched sperm separation as an adjunct to preimplantation genetic testing for the prevention of X-linked disease. Hum Reprod 1995;10:970.

28. Li H, Gyllensten UB, Cui X, et al. Amplification and analysis of DNA sequences in single human sperm and diploid cells. Nature 1988;335:414.

29. Arnheim N, Li H, Ciu X, et al. Single sperm PCR analysis: Implications for preimplantation diagnosis. In: Verlinsky Y, Kuliev AM, eds. Preimplantation genetics. New York: Plenum Press, 1991;121.

30. Lacham- Kaplan O, Daniels R, Trounson A. Fertilization of mouse oocytes using somatic cells as male germ cells. Reprod Biomed Online 2001;3:205.

31. Leese HJ, Hooper MAK, Edwards RG, et al. Uptake of pyruvate by early human embryos determined by a non-invasive technique. Hum Reprod 1986;1:181.

31a. Willadsen S, Munne S, Schmmel T, Cohen J 2003 Applications of nuclear sperm duplication. Fifth International Symposium on Preimplantation Genetics, 5–7, June, Antalya, Turkey: 35.

32. Leese HJ. Analysis of embryos by non-invasive methods. Hum Reprod 1987;2:37.

33. Wales RG, Whittingham DG, Hardy K, et al. Metabolism of glucose by human embryos. J Reprod Fertil 1987;79:289.

34. Hardy K, Hooper MAK, Handyside AH, et al. Non-invasive measurement of glucose and pyruvate uptake by individual human oocytes and preimplantation embryos. Hum Reprod 1989;4:188.

35. Adinolfi M, Polani PE. Prenatal diagnosis of genetic disorders in preimplantation embryos: Invasive and non-invasive approaches. Hum Genet 1989;83:16.

36. Zenzes MT, Wang P, Casper RF. Chromosome status of untransferred (spare) embryos and probability of pregnancy after in-vitro fertilisation. Lancet 1992;340:391.

37. Monk M, Holding C. Amplification of beta-haemoglobin sequence in individual human oocytes and polar bodies. Lancet 1990; 335:985.

38. Verlinsky Y, Rechitsky S, Evsikov S, et al. Preconception and preimplantation diagnosis for cystic fibrosis. Prenat Diagn 1992;12:103.

39. Kaplan B, Wolf G, Kovalinskaya L, et al. Viability of embryos following second polar body removal in a mouse model. Assist Reprod Genet 1995;12:747.
40. Hardy K, Handyside AH, Winston RML. The human blastocyst: cell number, death and allocation during late preimplantation development in vitro. Development 1989;107:597.
41. Gardner RL, Edwards RG. Control of the sex ratio at full term in the rabbit by transferring sexed blastocysts. Nature 1968;218:346.
42. Dokras A, Sargent IK, Ross C, et al. Trophectoderm biopsy in human blastocyst. Hum Reprod 1990;5:821.
43. Dokras A, Sargent IK, Ross C, et al. The human blastocyst: Morphology and human chorionic gonadotrophin secretion in vitro. Hum Reprod 1991;6:1143.
44. Muggleton-Harris AL, Glazier AM, Pickering S, et al. Genetic diagnosis using PCR and FISH analysis of biopsied cells from both the cleavage and blastocyst stages of individual cultured human preimplantation embryos. Hum Reprod 1995;10:183.
45. Dawson KJ, Rutherford AJ, Winston NJ, et al. Human blastocyst transfer: is it a feasible proposition? Hum Reprod 1988;145:44.
46. Bolton VN, Wren ME, Parsons JH. Pregnancies following in vitro fertilization and transfer of human blastocysts. Fertil Steril 1991;55:83.
47. Verlinsky Y, Munne S, Simpson JL, et al. Current status of preimplantation diagnosis. J Assist Reprod Genet 1997;1:72.
47a. McArthur S, Marshall J, Wright D, de Boer K 2003 Fifth International Symposium on Preimplantation Genetics, 5–7 June, Antalya, Turkey. P. 33.
48. Porter-Jordan K, Garrett C. Source of contamination in polymerase chain reaction assay. Lancet 1990;19:1220.
49. Bianchi DW, Flint AF, Pizzimenti MF, et al. Isolation of fetal DNA from nucleated erythrocytes in maternal blood. Proc Natl Acad Sci USA 1990;87:3279.
50. Strom CM, Rechitsky S. DNA analysis of polar bodies and preembryos. In: Verlinsky Y, Kuliev AM, eds. Preimplantation diagnosis of genetic diseases: a new technique in assisted reproduction. New York: Wiley-Liss, 1993:69.
51. Rechitsky S, Strom C, Verlinsky O, et al. Allele drop out in polar bodies and blastomeres. J Assist Reprod Genet 1998; 15:253.
52. Handyside AH, Delhanty JDA. Cleavage stage biopsy of human embryos and diagnosis of X-linked recessive disease. In: Edwards RG, ed. Preconception and preimplantation diagnosis of human genetic disease. Cambridge, UK: Cambridge University Press, 1993:239.
53. Rechitsky S, Verlinsky O, Strom C, et al. Experience with single-cell PCR in preimplantation genetic diagnosis: how to avoid pitfalls. In: Hahn S, Holzgreve W, editors. Fetal cells in maternal blood: new developments for a new millennium. 11th Fetal Cell Workshop, Basel: Karger, 2000:8.
54. Kuliev A, Rechitsky S, Verlinsky O, et al. Birth of healthy children after preimplantation diagnosis of thalassemias. J Assist Reprod Genet 1999,16:184.
55. Grifo JA, Tang YX, Cohen J, et al. Ongoing pregnancy in a hemophilia carrier by embryo biopsy and simultaneous amplification of X and Y chromosome specific DNA from a single blastomere. JAMA 1992;6:727.
56. Verlinsky Y, Handyside A, Grifo J, et al. Preimplantation diagnosis of genetic and chromosomal disorders. J Assist Reprod Genet 1994;11:236.
57. Griffin DK, Wilton LJ, Handyside AH, et al. Diagnosis of sex in preimplantation embryos by fluorescent in situ hybridization. Hum Genet 1992;89:18.
58. Munné S, Weier HUG, Stein J, et al. A fast and efficient method for simultaneous X and Y in situ hybridization of human blastomeres. J Assist Reprod Genet 1993;10:82.
59. Delhanty JDA, Griffin DK, Handyside AH, et al. Detection of aneuploidy and chromosomal mosaicism in human embryos during preimplantation sex determination by fluorescent in situ hybridisation (FISH). Hum Mol Genet 1993;2:1183.
60. Munné S, Grifo J, Cohen J, et al. Chromosome abnormalities in human arrested preimplantation embryos: a multiple-probe FISH study. Am J Hum Genet 1994;55:150.
61. Verlinsky Y, Rechitsky, Ivakhnenko V, et al. Polar body based PGD for X-linked disorders. Reprod Biomed Online 2001;4:36.
62. Verlinsky Y, Rechitsky S, Verlinsky O, et al. Preimplantation diagnosis for p53 tumor suppressor gene mutations. Reprod Biomed Online 2001;2:102.
63. Girardet A, Hamamah S, Anahory T, et al. First preimplantation genetic diagnosis of hereditary retinoblastoma using informative microsatellite markers. Mol Hum Reprod 2003;9:111.
64. Verlinsky Y, Rechitsky, Verlinsky O, et al. Preimplantation diagnosis for neurofibromatosis. Reprod Biomed Online 2002;4:218.

65. Verlinsky Y, Rechitsky S, Verlinsky O, et al . Preimplantation diagnosis for sonic hedgehog mutation causing familial holoprosencephaly. N Eng J Med 2003;348:1449–54.

66. Plachot M. Chromosomal abnormalities in oocytes. Mol Cell Endocrinol 2001;183:S59.

67. Martin RH, Spriggs E, Rademaker AW. Multicolour fluorescence in situ hybridization analysis of aneuploidy and diploidy frequencies in 225,846 sperm from ten normal men. Biol Reprod 1996;54:394.

68. Gropp A. Chromosomal animal model of human disease: fetal trisomy and development failure. In: Berry
L, Poswillo DE, eds. Teratology. Berlin: Springer-Verlag, 1975:17.

69. Epstein CJ. Mouse monosomies and trisomies as experimental systems for studying mammalian aneuploidy. Trends Genet 1985;1:129.

70. Dyban A, De Sutter P, Verlinsky Y. Preimplantation cytogenetic analysis. In: Verlinsky Y, Kuliev AM, eds.
Preimplantation diagnosis of genetic diseases: a new technique in assisted reproduction. New York: Wiley-
Liss, 1993:93.

71. De Sutter P, Dozortsev D, Cieslak J, et al. Parthenogenetic activation of human oocytes by puromycin. J
Assist Reprod Genet 1992;9:328.

72. Modlinsky J, McLaren A. A method for visualizing the chromosomes of the second polar body of the
mouse egg. J Embryol Exp Morphol 1980;60:97.

73. Dyban AP, De Sutter P, Dozortsev D, et al. Visualization of second polar body chromosomes in fertilized
and artificially activated mouse oocytes treated with okadaic acid. J Assist Reprod Genet 1992;9:572.

74. Verlinsky Y, Dozortsev D, Evsikov S. Visualization and cytogenetic analysis of second polar body chromosomes following its fusion with one-cell mouse embryo. J Assist Reprod Genet 1994;11:123.

75. Antonarakis SE, Petersen MB, McInnis MG, et al. The meiotic stage of nondisjunction in trisomy 21: determination by using DNA polymorphisms. Am J Hum Genet 1992;50:544.

76. Rodman TC. Chromosomes of the first polar body in mammalian meiosis. Exp Cell Res 1971;68:205.

77. Dyban A, De Sutter P, Verlinsky Y. Okadaic acid induces premature chromosome condensation reflecting
the cell cycle progression in one cell stage mouse embryos. Mol Reprod Dev 1993; 34:403.

77a. Wilton L, Voullaire L, Sargent RM, Williamson R, McBain J 2003 Preimplantation diagnosis of aneuploidy
using comparative genomic hybridization. *Fertil Steril* **80**, 860–868.

78. Dyban A, Fredine M, Severova E, et al. Detection of aneuploidy in human oocytes and corresponding first
polar bodies by FISH. J Assist Reprod Genet 1995;13:72.

79. Munné S, Dailey T, Sultan KM, et al. The use of first polar bodies for preimplantation diagnosis of aneuploidy. Hum Reprod 1995;10:1014.

80. Verlinsky Y, Cieslak J, Freidine M, et al. Polar body diagnosis of common aneuploidies by FISH. J Assist
Reprod Genet 1996;13:157.

81. Verlinsky Y, Cieslak J, Ivakhnenko V, et al. Birth of healthy children following preimplantation diagnosis
of common aneuploidies by polar FISH analysis. Fertil Steril 1996,66:126.

82. Kuliev A, Cieslak J, Illkewitch Y, et al. Chromosomal abnormalities in a series of 6733 human oocytes in
preimplantation diagnosis of age-related aneuploidies. Reprod Biomed Online 2003;6:54.

83. Munne S. Preimplantation genetic diagnosis of numerical and structural chromosome abnormalities. Reprod Biomed Online 2002;4:183.

84. Gianaroli L, Magli MC, Ferraretti AP, et al. Preimplantation diagnosis for aneuploidies in patients undergoing in vitro fertilization with poor prognosis: identification of the categories for which it should be proposed. Fertil Steril 1999;72:837.

85. Munne S, Magli C, Cohen J, et al. Positive outcome after preimplantation diagnosis of aneuploidy in human
embryos. Hum Reprod 1999;14:2191.

86. Munne S, Sandalinas M, Escudero T, et al. 2003 Improved implantation after preimplantation genetic diagnosis of aneuploidy. *Reproductive BioMedicine Online* **7**, 91–97.

87. Munné S, Sandalinas M, Escudero T, et al. Outcome of preimplantation genetic diagnosis of translocations. Fertil Steril 2000;73:1209.

88. Verlinsky Y, Cieslak J, Evsikov S, et al. Nuclear transfer for full karyotyping and preimplantation diagnosis for translocations. Reprod Biomed Online 2002;5:303.

89. Ethics Committee of the American Fertility Society. Ethics and the new reproductive technologies. Fertil
Steril 1990;53 (suppl 2):5.

90. Walters L. Ethics and new reproductive technologies: an international review of committee statements.
Hastings Cent Rep 1987;17(3).

91. Milunsky A. Ethical and selected medical aspects of preimplantation genetic diagnosis. In: Verlinsky Y,
Kuliev AM, eds. Preimplantation genetics. New York: Plenum Press, 1991:245.

92. Cohen J, Hotz RL. Human embryo research: ethics and recent progress. Curr Opin Obstet Gynecol 1991;3:678.
93. Burn J, Strachan T. Human embryo use in developmental research. Nat Genet 1995;11:3.
94. Verlinsky Y, Handyside AH, Simpson JL. Current progress in preimplantation genetic diagnosis. J Assist Reprod Genet 1993;10:353.
95. Schreiber HL. The legal situation regarding assisted reproduction in Germany. Reprod Biomed Online 2003;6:8.
96. Pienado JA, Russell SE. The Spanish Care governing assisted reproduction techniques: a summary. Hum Reprod 1990;5:634.
97. Robertson J. Extending preimplantation genetic diagnosis: the ethical debate. Ethical issues in new uses of preimplantation genetic diagnosis. Hum Reprod 2003; 18:465–471.
98. Marshal E. Embryologists dismayed by sanctions against geneticist. Science 1997;275:472.
99. Gali RP, Woodside JL. Proposed Canadian legislation to regulate reproductive technologies and related research. Reprod Biomed Online 2003;6:114.
100. Kilani Z, Haj Hassan L. Sex selection and preimplantation genetic diagnosis at the Farah Hospital. Reprod Biomed Online 2002;4:8.
101. Malpani A, Malpani A, Modi D. The use of preimplantation genetic diagnosis in sex selection for family balancing in India. Reprod Biomed Online 2001;4:16.
102. Edwards RG. Social and ethical issues of PGD, cloning and gene therapy. Reprod Biomed Online 2003; 6 (in press).
103. Towner D, Loewy RS. Ethics of preimplantation diagnosis for a woman destined to develop early-onset Alzheimer disease. JAMA 2002;287:1038.
104. Damewood MD. Ethical implications of a new application of preimplantation diagnosis. JAMA 2001;285:3143.

Diana W. Bianchi, M.D.

28

Prenatal Diagnosis through the Analysis of Fetal Cells and Cell-Free Nucleic Acids in the Maternal Circulation

Noninvasive prenatal diagnosis, through the analysis of intact fetal cells and cell-free fetal nucleic acids in maternal blood, has the potential to revolutionize prenatal medicine. Previously, the focus of research efforts in this area was on the physical separation and genetic analysis of intact fetal cells circulating in maternal blood. The international study sponsored by the National Institute of Child Health and Human Development (the "NIFTY Trial")[1] on this topic will soon conclude that while fetal cells are present in the maternal circulation, there is not a robust and reliable enough method currently available to isolate them for widespread clinical applications.[2] Intriguingly, however, recent data from a variety of laboratories, suggest that in abnormal pregnancies there is an increase in the bidirectional trafficking of both cells and nucleic acids between the pregnant woman and her fetus.[3] These abnormalities can potentially be exploited to permit noninvasive diagnosis of conditions as diverse as preeclampsia and fetal aneuploidy. Furthermore, there is increasing evidence that fetal stem and progenitor cells persist in the maternal body following pregnancy. These retained fetal cells may have an important impact on subsequent maternal health.[4]

INTACT FETAL CELLS

A Brief History

Clinical studies of maternal–fetal blood group antigen incompatibility showed that both fetal erythrocytes and fetal platelets enter into the maternal circulation during pregnancy.[5] Placental-derived trophoblast sprouts were documented in maternal blood sampled from both the uterine vein at hysterotomy[6] and from the maternal lungs at autopsy.[7] With the exception of trophoblasts, however, fetal cells isolated from maternal blood cannot be identified on the basis of morphology alone. In 1969, Walknowska and colleagues cultured peripheral blood lymphocytes from thirty pregnant women and screened hundreds of maternal metaphases to find an occasional 46,XY karyotype.[8] Male cells were detected in twenty-one of thirty pregnant women; nineteen of these twenty-one women gave birth to a male infant. Of the nine women who did not have evidence of the Y chromosome present, six gave birth to females. Cells with a 46,XY karyotype were detected as early as 14 weeks of gestation. The proportion of 46,XY mitoses present in the nineteen pregnancies with male fetuses ranged from 0.2 to 1.5 percent. Although these initial studies were conducted before the development of fluorescent chromosome banding techniques, subsequent work using quinacrine to detect interphase Y chromatin yielded similar results.[9]

Fetal Cell Types

Trophoblast

Trophoblast sprouts are attractive candidates for fetal-cell isolation due to their unique morphology and intimate contact with maternal blood.[10] They are formed very early in gestation and migrate actively into the maternal side of the placenta. The process of trophoblast invasion induces a transformation of the maternal spiral arteries, which results in partial loss of their muscular layer and a generalized increase in diameter.[11] Two types of trophoblasts invade maternal tissue: the *interstitial* trophoblasts, which are in direct contact with maternal decidua and myometrium, and the *endovascular* trophoblasts, which are located in the lumen of the spiral arteries. The endovascular trophoblasts are the subtype that enter the maternal circulation in two distinct phases.[11] The first phase peaks in the middle of the first trimester and results in transformation of the maternal decidual arteries. The second phase peaks around 11–12 weeks of gestation and transforms the spiral arteries. Despite this, many investigators have had difficulty isolating them from the circulation of normal pregnant women, which may be because of the effective clearance of these "foreign bodies" as they enter the maternal pulmonary circulation. This contrasts with the reports of trophoblast detection in blood samples recovered from the inferior vena cava, uterine vein, and peripheral circulation of women with pregnancy-induced hypertension.[12–14] As early as 1893, Schmorl described the frequent presence of trophoblasts in the lungs of pregnant women who died from eclampsia.[7] However, Douglas et al. demonstrated syncytiotrophoblasts in the circulating blood of pregnant women from 18 weeks of gestation until term and concluded that this migration of trophoblasts was a normal process in pregnancy.[6]

One difficulty with the isolation of trophoblasts from maternal blood is the relative lack of suitable and specific monoclonal antibodies to facilitate their isolation.[15,16] One monoclonal antibody, H315, was initially described as specific for the recognition of trophoblast cell surface antigens.[17] In a study of mononuclear cell suspensions obtained from forty-six pregnant women at different points in gestation, three types of cells stained with the H315 monoclonal antibody.[18] Small (<5 μm) anucleate cells were detected in 33 percent of maternal samples at a frequency of 3 per 1,000. Medium-sized (7 μm) cells were detected in 50 percent of the women, at a frequency of 8 per 1,000, independent of the timing in pregnancy. Finally, large polynucleated cells (on the order of 12–14 μm) were present in 80 percent of the maternal samples, at a frequency of 1–4 per 1,000. The control samples included five nonpregnant women and three men, half of whom had cells that reacted with the H315 antibody at a frequency of 1 per 1,000. Subsequently it was shown by Bertero et al.[19] that DNA polymorphisms present in the H315-positive cells isolated from maternal blood were identical to the maternal pattern and different from the fetal pattern, indicating that the purified cells were not fetal in origin. Covone et al.[20] also failed to detect Y chromosomal DNA in H315-positive cells isolated from maternal blood in pregnancies bearing males. They concluded that the H315 antigen was adsorbed onto maternal leukocytes and that this antibody was not useful for prenatal diagnosis.

The search for a truly trophoblast-specific reagent led Mueller et al. to test 6,800 candidate antibodies.[21] Two monoclonal antibodies, FD0161G and FD066Q, were identified that define a single trophoblast membrane surface protein. Three other antibodies (FD0338P, FD078P, and FD093P) recognize different epitopes on another trophoblast cell surface antigen. The antibodies FD066Q and FD0338P were used to isolate trophoblast cells from thirteen pregnant women who were mostly in their first trimester. The physical separation of candidate fetal cells was accomplished with the use of antibody-conjugated magnetic beads. The PCR was performed to amplify and detect Y-chromosomal DNA. In eight of thirteen samples, amplified male DNA was detected. A correct prediction of fetal sex was made in twelve of thirteen cases. In one case, male DNA was detected, but the fetus was shown to be female. Durrant et al. also described a monoclonal antibody, known as 340, that recognizes a cell surface antigen expressed on both syncytiotrophoblasts and cytotrophoblasts.[22] Van Wijk et al. used a two-step procedure to enrich for the presence of trophoblast.[23] Their technique consisted of a multiple-density gradient centrifugation step, followed by maternal white-cell depletion of CDw50-positive cells. In thirty-six pregnancies studied between 6 and 15 weeks of gestation, fetal gender was determined correctly by PCR in thirteen of fifteen male fetuses and twenty of twenty-one female fetuses, for an overall accuracy of 91.7 percent. Although this study did not conclusively prove that trophoblasts were present in maternal blood it did show that fetal DNA could be detected in the cellular fraction of cells that have the same density characteristics as trophoblast.

More direct evidence of trophoblast circulation came from studies using nonradioactive in situ hybridization for the *achaete scute complex like 2* (*ASCL2*) gene that is expressed by extravillus trophoblast. Van Wijk et al.[24] identified one *ASCL2*-positive cell per milliliter of maternal blood. Unfortunately, this group experienced technical difficulties when trying to combine RNA hybridization with fluorescence in situ hybridization (FISH), which led to a high degree of false-positive staining with *ASCL2*. Subsequently, this group also used monoclonal antibody to HLA-G antigens that are specifically expressed in extravillus and endovascular trophoblast, and showed that HLA-G-positive XY trophoblasts circulate within the blood of pregnant women.[25] Karyotypically abnormal HLA-G-positive trophoblasts were also detected in the blood of a pregnant woman whose fetus had Down syndrome[25] and another woman with a partial mole.[26]

Leukocytes

In 1979, Herzenberg et al. described the use of the fluorescence-activated cell sorter (FACS) to physically separate fetal from maternal cells on the basis of cell surface antigen characteristics.[27] In a study of 138 pregnant women and their spouses, human lymphocyte antigen (HLA)-A2 was used as a detection marker for fetal cells.[28] Only blood from women who tested negative for HLA-A2, with spouses who were positive for HLA-A2 was flow-sorted. At the time of initial screening (15–16 weeks of gestation), fetal sex and HLA type were unknown. The mononuclear cells were isolated from peripheral blood by Ficoll–Hypaque density-gradient centrifugation and stained with monoclonal antibody against HLA-A2. Cells that bound antibody were sorted onto microscope slides and stained with quinacrine dye. The presumed fetal cells were analyzed for the presence of interphase Y chromatin. There was a highly significant correlation between the detection of the Y body in sorted cells and the presence of both male sex and HLA-A2 at birth ($p = 0.0000058$).[28] This study provided convincing evidence that fetal lymphocytes circulated in maternal blood as early as 15 weeks of gestation.

The separation of fetal lymphocytes from maternal blood by anti-HLA antibodies has two major challenges. For one, the tremendous polymorphism at the HLA loci makes antibody selection difficult. In addition, nonpaternity becomes a variable if fetal-cell isolation is based on paternal HLA loci alone. Separation strategies involving lymphocytes are further complicated by the fact that fetal lymphocyte cell surfaces are not inherently different from their maternal counterparts. Finally, several groups, including our own, have described the curious phenomenon of persistence of fetal lymphocytes in maternal blood for as long as decades postpartum.[29–32] The relative longevity of lymphocytes creates difficulties in establishing certainty that isolated cells derive from the current pregnancy. For this reason, many investigators are not actively pursuing isolation of fetal lymphocytes for genetic diagnosis of the current pregnancy.

The presence of fetal granulocytes in the maternal circulation has been studied infrequently. In 1975, Zilliacus and co-workers[33] estimated that fetal granulocytes comprised 0.02–0.04 percent of mononuclear cell samples obtained from nineteen pregnant women in their second and third trimesters. Wessman et al. used nonradioactive in situ hybridization techniques and density-gradient centrifugation to demonstrate that 0.26 percent of maternal mononuclear cells hybridized to a Y-chromosome probe.[34] These cells had a morphology consistent with the appearance of granulocytes. These results were surprising and seemed to indicate that either a large number of fetal granulocytes circulate within maternal blood or that nonspecific hybridization to the DNA probe had occurred. In over a decade since this study was published, other investigators have not replicated this finding.

Nucleated Erythrocytes

The passage of fetal erythrocytes into the maternal circulation was originally documented in 1957 by Creger and Steele.[35] To determine the cause of erythroblastosis fetalis, they studied twenty-three pregnant women who were ABO blood group A, and they compared those who had infants with blood group O to those who had infants with blood group A. They counted the cells that did not agglutinate with anti-A serum in maternal blood samples, as a means of estimating the number of blood group O (fetal) cells present. On average, the mothers who gave birth to infants with blood group O had significantly greater numbers of unagglutinated cells than the mothers of infants with blood group A. The counts were greatly decreased at the 6-week postpartum visit. This was interpreted as demonstrating a "flow" of erythrocytes from fetus to mother during pregnancy. Other investigators quantified the number of fetal erythrocytes in maternal blood, using the Kleihauer–Betke acid-elution technique.[36,37] In 1984, Medearis et al.[38] used the FACS to detect Rh-positive blood group (D) erythrocytes in blood samples obtained after vaginal delivery in Rh(D)-negative primigravidas. All of the sixteen postpartum women had significant numbers of circulating Rh-positive cells. The results corresponded to a fetal hemorrhage of 28–564 μL into the mother's blood.[38] It is not known, however, whether the hemorrhage occurred antenatally or as a consequence of labor and delivery.

Because most pregnancies are blood-group-compatible, we have concentrated our fetal-cell-isolation efforts on nucleated erythrocytes. Our initial hypothesis was that blood-group-compatible fetal erythrocytes, in small numbers, would circulate in the mother, un-challenged by her immune system.[39] Nucleated erythrocytes represent a good target-cell population for fetal-cell sorting experiments because they are unlikely to circulate in the peripheral blood of a normal adult. They are, however, present in significant numbers in the blood of early fetuses. Nucleated erythrocytes (NRBCs), by definition, contain a nucleus and have a full complement of nuclear genes. Because NRBCs are nearly completely differentiated and have a lifespan of approximately 3 months, isolated NRBCs are likely to derive from the ongoing pregnancy being studied. Finally, there are 1,000-fold more red cells than white cells available for analysis after fetomaternal transfusion.

In 1990, my colleagues and I described the use of murine monoclonal antibody directed against the transferrin receptor antigen (CD71) to identify NRBCs in the peripheral blood of pregnant women.[39] CD71 was selected because erythroblasts have been shown to express this antigen on their cell surfaces from the burst-forming units, erythroid stage, including nuclear extrusion (reticulocyte).[40] The CD71 antigen is not unique to NRBCs; it is found on any cell incorporating iron, such as activated lymphocytes, tumor cells, and trophoblast sprouts. The samples from the pregnant women revealed the consistent presence of a small but well-demarcated CD71-positive population. In each case, the CD71-positive cells were sorted onto microscope slides for morphology and detection of fetal hemoglobin using the Kleihauer–Betke technique. In pregnant women, the CD71-positive sorted cells were predominantly reticulocytes; NRBCs containing fetal hemoglobin, monocytes, lymphocytes, and erythrocytes containing adult hemoglobin were also seen. These data were interpreted as demonstrating that, with enrichment by flow sorting, NRBCs could be isolated from the blood of pregnant women. Subsequently, the circulation of fetal NRBCs has been confirmed by many different experimental methods.[41–45]

Although many investigators presume that NRBCs in maternal blood are exclusively fetal, the work of Gänshirt et al. showed that significant numbers of NRBCs in the blood of pregnant women are maternal.[46] The numbers remain fairly constant during gestation and are unrelated to invasive procedures and the number of prior pregnancies. Significantly increased numbers of both fetal and maternal NRBCs have been observed in the circulation of pregnant women with preeclampsia.[47]

Mesenchymal Cells

More recently, a novel population of cells, mesenchymal stem/progenitor cells (MSCs), were identified in first-trimester fetal blood, liver, and bone marrow.[48] MSCs derived from fetal blood can be cultured and differentiated into fat, bone, and cartilage. O'Donoghue et al.[49] developed optimal protocols to enrich for fetal MSCs in maternal blood samples. Using artificial mixtures, they successfully cultured one male fetal MSC in as many 25 million adult female nucleated cells. Using posttermination samples as a biologic model in which an increased fetomaternal hemorrhage would be expected,[50] they were able to detect male fetal MSC in only one of twenty samples. Thus, the frequency of fetal MSCs in the blood of pregnant women appears to be quite low. This likely precludes their clinical use in noninvasive prenatal diagnosis, but it suggests that they may have long-ranging effects on maternal health.

Frequency of Fetal Cells in Maternal Blood

The fetal-cell literature is replete with promising small studies that advocate for a particular cell type or method of isolation. Yet, fifteen years after the development of sophisticated isolation methods and the advent of sensitive molecular techniques to detect fetal genes or chromosomes, fetal cells in maternal blood have not entered the mainstream of prenatal diagnosis. Why is this? The major limitation appears to be the generally low number of fetal cells found in most maternal samples, which has been demonstrated in four key studies using different techniques.

Using FISH analysis, Hamada et al. looked for male cells in unsorted maternal blood samples; fetal cells were identified by their nuclear hybridization to a Y-chromosome-specific probe.[51] The frequency of Y-positive cells increased as gestation progressed, from less than 1 in 10^5 during the first trimester to 1 in 10^4 at term. These workers screened as many as 144,000 nuclei per pregnant woman to find evidence of a single male cell. More recently, Krabchi et al. examined second-trimester blood samples from twelve pregnant women known to be carrying male fetuses.[52] They examined the entire 3 mL maternal blood sample using the same methanol:glacial acetic acid (Carnoy fixative) solution used in routine cytogenetic studies. No other enrichment methods were used. Fetal XY nuclei were reproducibly detected at a concentration of two to six nuclei per milliliter of maternal whole blood. Although these studies conclusively show the presence of fetal cells in maternal blood, the approaches used are clearly impractical for routine clinical diagnosis; either an automated imaging system must be used or some enrichment of the proportion of fetal cells present in a maternal sample must precede cytogenetic analysis.

As an alternative way of measuring the number of fetal cells present in maternal blood independent of cell type and minimizing sample processing, we developed a method of quantitative PCR.[53] In an early version of quantitative PCR, we measured the number of male fetal cells present by performing PCR amplification of Y-chromosome-specific sequences and compared the amount of [^{32}P]deoxyribonucleoside triphosphate incorporated into sample amplification products with standard curves generated from known DNA concentrations.

In a subsequent study, we examined 230 midtrimester maternal blood samples.[54] Of these, 199 women carried fetuses with a normal karyotype and 31 carried aneuploid fetuses. Results of radioactive PCR amplification of the Y-chromosome sequence and phosphorimage analysis were calculated to determine the number of male fetal cell equivalents in 16 mL of maternal whole blood. In samples obtained from the 90 pregnant women carrying 46,XY fetuses, the mean number of cells detected was 19 (range, 0.1–91), or approximately 1 fetal cell per milliliter of maternal blood. Remarkably, the results obtained when the fetus was 47,XY,+21 were elevated sixfold, or a mean of 110 fetal cells in 16 mL of maternal blood. The increased number of fetal cells detected when the fetus was aneuploid was highly significant ($p = 0.001$). This study was the first to suggest that fetomaternal cell trafficking was affected by karyotype, and therefore, fetal-cell isolation from maternal blood should be easier and more accurate for aneuploid fetuses.

With the advent of the sensitive technique of real-time kinetic PCR amplification, in 2001 Ariga et al. analyzed serial blood samples every 2–4 weeks from twenty pregnant women carrying male fetuses throughout their pregnancies.[55] Two of the twenty women studied had evidence of male DNA as early as 7 weeks of gestation. All women studied had evidence of male DNA in their circulation by the third trimester of pregnancy. This group calculated that there were 2–40 fetal cells per milliliter of maternal whole blood.

In summary, these four studies performed in different laboratories in different parts of the world provide conclusive evidence that fetal cells are present in maternal blood. The estimated numbers of fetal cells per milliliter of maternal blood provided by the authors of the various studies are remarkably similar. They indicate that the expected number of fetal cells (except, perhaps in the setting of aneuploidy or following termination of pregnancy) is low, and that enrichment methods are needed to detect them.

Methods of Fetal-Cell Enrichment and Analysis

Given the relative rarity of fetal cells in maternal blood, some form of fetal-cell enrichment appears necessary to permit genetic analysis. Two approaches are possible: "positive" selection of fetal cells or of cells that possess characteristics of immature or fetal cells; and "negative" depletion of unwanted maternal cells. Some groups combine both strategies. An initial enrichment step facilitates the removal of many maternal cells, including non-nucleated erythrocytes and lymphocytes. This usually is performed through density-gradient centrifugation or through the use of red-cell lytic buffers. This is further complicated by the fact that fetal cells in maternal blood are in a variety of developmental stages; some of them are also undergoing apoptosis.[56] Subsequent "purification" can be performed by any of the methods listed in Table 28.1.[57–60] Magnetic-activated cell sorting (MACS) has been used for depletion and positive selection, both individually and sequentially.

Currently, there is no clearly superior laboratory technique for fetal-cell isolation. Each method has its benefits and limitations with respect to fetal-cell recovery, cost, ease of separation, and time required for separation. Important concepts are yield (actual number of fetal cells recovered) and purity (percentage of fetal cells relative to maternal cells in the enriched sample). Methods that result in high yield may have low purity, and vice versa.

A key aspect of fetal-cell isolation is the choice of marker, which generally refers to the cell-surface or cytoplasmic protein that identifies the cells as fetal or maternal in origin. The only fetal markers that are unique to fetal cells are the embryonic globins, zeta and epsilon, which generally target only cells produced during the first trimester.[61–63] With regard to fetal nucleated erythrocytes, antibodies to the transferrin receptor (CD71),[39,43,46] thrombospondin receptor (CD36),[64] and glycophorin A (GPA)[42] are all effective in recognizing fetal cells. However, they also identify immature maternal red cells, resulting in low purity. We have advocated for the use of antibody to gamma globin, which can be used in flow-sorting protocols or on slides as a fetal-cell identifier (Figure 28.1).[65,66]

Antibodies to trophoblast markers, such as the nonclassical antigen, HLA-G,[11] show promise, but have yet to be validated in large clinical trials. Antibodies to common leukocyte antigens, such as CD45, as well as specific leukocyte subsets, have been used to deplete maternal mononuclear cells.

Table 28.1.   Cell-separation techniques used in the isolation of fetal cells

Selective lysis of adult erythrocytes
Density-gradient centrifugation
Agglutination/centrifugation of erythrocytes (RosetteSep)[57]
Fluorescence-activated cell sorting (FACS)
Magnetic-activated cell sorting (MACS)
Ferrofluids/magnetic separation
Immunomagnetic beads
Avidin–biotin columns
Charged flow separation[58]
Micromanipulation[59]
Size filtration[60]

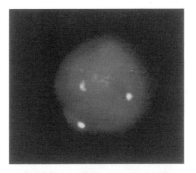

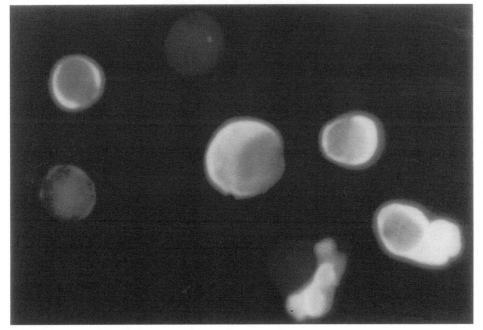

Fig. 28.1. Fetal cells isolated from a woman carrying a fetus with triploidy (69,XXX). *Upper panel*, three copies of the X chromosome in a sorted fetal cell. *Lower panel*, many sorted cells that contain fetal hemoglobin. Fetal cells are larger than maternal cells and have a high nuclear:cytoplasmic ratio. *Source*: Courtesy of Dr. Yun-Ling Zheng.

Clinical Applications: Aneuploidy Detection and the NIFTY Trial

Over the past decade, the development of molecular cytogenetic techniques has had a strong influence on this field, permitting cytogenetic diagnosis on rare nondividing cells. FISH analysis using chromosome-specific probes on isolated fetal cells can be performed to predict gender and diagnose aneuploidy. Initially, a variety of case reports demonstrated that FISH detection of fetal cells was feasible.[41,67–71] These reports were followed by larger case series, such as those by Gänshirt-Ahlert et al.[72] and Simpson and Elias.[73] In the latter reference, the authors summarized their experience with sixty-nine maternal blood samples obtained both before and after a diagnosis of fetal aneuploidy by first-trimester chorionic villus sampling (CVS) or second-trimester amniocentesis.[73] Fetal NRBCs were flow-sorted using antibodies to CD71 and GPA; enriched samples served as templates for

FISH analysis. The probes used in this study included a repetitive sequence on the X chromosome, centromeric alphoid repeat sequence from the Y chromosome, and material from the long arms of chromosomes 18 and 21. Although they did not calculate sensitivity and specificity of clinical diagnosis because of changes in laboratory protocols, what was striking about their data was the increased percentage of fetal cells detected when the fetus was aneuploid (average, 19.6 percent of cells; range, 0–74 percent). This group successfully diagnosed fetal Klinefelter syndrome (47,XXY), trisomy 18, and trisomy 21.

Because the feasibility of FISH diagnosis using fetal cells isolated from maternal blood was demonstrated, the National Institute of Child Health and Human Development (NICHD) funded a prospective, multicenter clinical study from 1994 to 2003 known as the "NIFTY trial."[1] The purpose of this study was to compare the accuracy of noninvasive fetal aneuploidy detection by FISH using fetal cells in maternal blood to conventional prenatal metaphase cytogenetic diagnosis by CVS or amniocentesis. After the first 5 years of the study, an interim analysis of the data was performed. The interim results of this largest study of fetal cells to date, in which 2,744 fully processed blood samples were obtained before an invasive procedure, are now published.[2] Of the study subjects, 1,292 carried singleton male fetuses. One of the major limitations of this study was that multiple processing protocols were used. The data showed that target fetal cell recovery and detection were better using MACS than FACS. In male fetuses, using blinded FISH analysis, at least one (presumptive fetal) cell with both X and Y chromosome signals was seen in 41.4 percent of cases (95 percent confidence interval, 37.4–45.5 percent). There was a higher than expected false-positive rate of gender detection of 11.1 percent, due primarily to the use of indirectly labeled FISH probes at one site. Importantly, the sensitivity of detection of at least one fetal cell was significantly higher (74.4 percent confidence interval, 76.0–99.0 percent) and the false-positive rate was lower (0.6–4.1 percent) when the fetus was aneuploid. These results validate the speculation in earlier studies that there is increased fetomaternal trafficking in cases of aneuploidy, and demonstrate that it should be easier to find fetal cells in the maternal circulation when the fetus is chromosomally abnormal.

Future Directions

Taking into account the results of the NIFTY trial as well as the other studies described here, it is apparent that technologic advances are needed before fetal-cell analysis can be used clinically for screening or diagnosis. Research efforts are focusing on novel separation strategies (such as microfluidics and laser-capture microdissection) and novel antibodies to identify fetal cells. An important advance will be in the area of automated imaging, in which maternal blood samples can be processed minimally (reducing the possibility for fetal-cell loss) and placed on multiple slides that can be scanned for the presence of fetal chromosomal or cytoplasmic markers. The "low purity" approach taken by Krabchi and co-workers[52] required an enormous amount of human time at the microscope. Automated imaging has the potential to significantly reduce that time, while simultaneously maximizing the potential for fetal-cell retention and diagnosis.

CELL-FREE FETAL NUCLEIC ACIDS

A new aspect of research in this area involves the discovery that large amounts of cell-free DNA and RNA circulate within the blood of pregnant women. These nucleic acids are likely derived from apoptotic cells and are amplifiable, permitting multiple prenatal diagnostic applications.

History

Mandel and Metais, working as early as 1947 (before Watson and Crick), precipitated and measured DNA from the plasma and serum of healthy and sick people.[74] The next major advances in this field occurred in plants. Stroun and Anker[75,76] were studying the development of the plant tumor, crown gall, which is caused by bacterial DNA that translocates into plant cells. These tumors undergo metastasis, which is remarkable, because plant cells do not circulate, because they are trapped by a cell wall that contains cellulose. They hypothesized that cell-free DNA was able to traverse the cell walls to circulate within the plant, and that this DNA was responsible for the metastases.

Subsequently, in 1977, Leon et al.[77] reported that minute quantities of DNA are present in the serum of normal individuals (mean, 13 ± 3 ng/mL) and that increased quantities circulate in cancer patients (mean, 280 ng/mL). In 1996, the detection of tumor-specific DNA sequences in the plasma of serum and cancer patients brought great excitement and attention.[78,79] Suddenly an intellectual bridge was created between the studies of plant cancer and human disease. Characteristics of tumor DNA, such as decreased strand stability, the presence of specific oncogenes, tumor-suppressor genes, microsatellite alterations, and point mutations of the *ras* genes, were shown to be present in DNA extracted from the plasma of cancer patients.[80] The results obtained in many different cancers suggested that plasma DNA might be a suitable target for the development of non-invasive diagnostic, prognostic, and follow-up tests.[77]

Working in a cancer center in Hong Kong, and aware of the similarities between the aggressively growing fetoplacental unit and a tumor, Lo et al.[81] initially asked the question whether fetal DNA is present in the plasma and serum of pregnant women. Using PCR amplification of Y-specific DNA sequences and agarose-gel electrophoresis, they were able to detect fetal DNA in most plasma/serum samples of pregnant women bearing male fetuses. The development of real-time PCR techniques, using the $5'$ to $3'$ exonuclease activity of Taq polymerase, enabled these authors eventually to use a quantitative approach to measure the concentration of fetal DNA in maternal plasma.[82] The concentration of the ubiquitously present β-globin gene was used as a measure of the total amount of extracted DNA in maternal plasma/serum samples. The absolute concentration of fetal DNA in maternal plasma was similar to that in maternal serum. The main difference between plasma and serum was the presence of a larger quantity of background maternal DNA in serum (released from the clot) compared with plasma.[83] In this study, the high concentrations of fetal DNA in plasma/serum allowed for the detection of fetal *SRY* genes in maternal plasma or serum from every pregnant woman carrying a male fetus ($n = 12$). The data demonstrated an overall increase in fetal DNA concentration as gestation advanced, with a remarkable sharp increase during the last 8 weeks of pregnancy.

The turnover of circulating fetal DNA was subsequently studied by investigating the clearance of circulating fetal DNA after delivery.[84] Most of the women studied (seven of eight) had undetectable levels of circulating fetal DNA by 2 hours postpartum. The mean half-life for fetal DNA was estimated to be 16.3 minutes (range, 4–30). Assuming there are no abrupt changes in circulating fetal DNA clearance associated with delivery, the authors speculated that to maintain a steady state, fetal DNA must be continuously liberated in large quantities into maternal circulation. The tissue source of this DNA is unknown, but it is hypothesized to be predominantly derived from the placenta. Lo et al.'s calculations suggested that fetal DNA is liberated at a mean rate of 2.24×10^4 copies/min into the maternal circulation. The rapid turnover implies that fetal DNA measurement provides an almost real-time picture of fetal DNA production and clearance, and, thus, may be useful for monitoring fetomaternal events with rapid dynamics.

Clinical Applications of Fetal DNA Measurement in Maternal Plasma and Serum

The clinical applications of this technique have primarily centered on the quantitation of fetal DNA sequences and the detection of uniquely fetal gene sequences.[85] To date, a major limitation of the quantitation work is that it has been restricted to the genetic analysis of male fetuses, because they possess a Y chromosome, which the pregnant woman lacks. Thus, Y-chromosome-specific DNA sequences of fetal origin may be easily and accurately detected in the maternal plasma.[86] However, the beauty of using fetal nucleic acid measurement in maternal plasma and serum is that it is useful for the prenatal diagnosis of aneuploidy as well as a variety of different nongenetic complications of pregnancy. For example, there is a fivefold increase in the amount of fetal DNA in samples obtained from women with preeclampsia (381 genome-equivalents [GE]/mL, compared with 76 GE/mL in maternal plasma).[87–91] Furthermore, there appears to be a biphasic elevation of fetal DNA in the circulation of women in whom preeclampsia will ultimately develop. Using a case–control series of archived serum samples from the Calcium Prevention of Preeclampsia (CPEP) study, Levine et al.[92] showed that there is a statistically significant increase in circulating cell-free fetal DNA in cases (women who will manifest symptoms of preeclampsia) that is detectable as early as 17 weeks of gestation (Figure 28.2). A second phase of DNA elevation occurs in cases approximately 3 weeks before the develop-

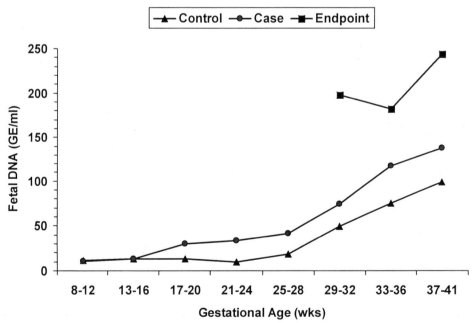

Fig. 28.2. Presymptomatic cell-free fetal DNA measurements in women in whom preeclampsia ultimately developed (cases) and those who did not (controls) in a subset of women studied in the Calcium Prevention of Preeclampsia trial. The end-point specimens were collected after the development of clinical symptoms. The data show that cell-free fetal DNA elevation occurs long before the development of hypertension and proteinuria. *Source*: Courtesy of Richard Levine, M.D.

ment of hypertension and proteinuria. As a result of these studies, there is great interest in using the measurement of cell-free fetal DNA as a predictive marker for the development of preeclampsia and as an indication of when to begin treatment.

Increased levels of cell-free fetal DNA in maternal serum may also indicate a risk for preterm delivery. In normal pregnancies, sequential measurements of fetal DNA in the serum/plasma of pregnant women demonstrate a gradual increase as gestation advances, increasing sharply after 32 weeks of gestation.[82] This sharp rise may reflect changes occurring at the maternofetal interface of the placenta.[93] In cases of preterm labor, Leung et al.[94] provided data to support the hypothesis that an increase in maternal plasma fetal DNA concentration may herald impending delivery. Studying only women carrying male fetuses, this group found significantly higher fetal DNA concentrations in women ($n =$ 20) who had spontaneous preterm deliveries between 26 and 34 weeks of gestation. Moreover, lower concentrations of fetal DNA were associated with successful tocolytic therapy. These results led to the interesting concept of a screening test that may help to differentiate true preterm labor and preterm labor that can be successfully treated by tocolytic therapy.

The quantity of circulating male fetal DNA is also affected by fetal karyotype. Studying intact fetal cells, my colleagues and I initially observed a sixfold elevation of DNA in maternal blood samples taken from fetuses with trisomy 21[54] and questioned whether a parallel increase would also be observed using fetal DNA in maternal plasma. In a collaborating study between the Chinese University of Hong Kong and our own group, the median circulating fetal DNA concentrations in second-trimester samples from women in one center carrying trisomy 21 ($n = 7$) and euploid male fetuses ($n = 19$) were 46.0 GE/mL and 23.3 GE/mL, respectively.[95] The corresponding numbers at the second center were 48.2 GE/mL for trisomy 21 pregnancies ($n = 6$) and 16.3 GE/mL for euploid male pregnancies ($n = 18$). Overall, there appears to be about twice as much fetal DNA circulating in the pregnant woman when the fetus has trisomy 21. Other groups have either validated[96,97] or have been unable to show[98] that maternal serum fetal DNA levels are elevated when the fetus has trisomy 21. Using a blinded case–control approach with archived serum samples originally obtained for routine second trimester maternal serum screening, Wataganara et al.[99] demonstrated that fetal DNA levels were elevated in the sera of women carrying fetuses with trisomy 13 but not trisomy 18. A major limitation of the quantitative approach for the detection of fetal aneuploidy is that the current basis of detection uses gene sequences from the Y chromosome and is therefore limited to male fetuses. However, in a model system, Farina et al. investigated the potential performance of male cell-free fetal DNA as a screening marker for Down syndrome.[100] They showed that cell-free fetal DNA was independent of estriol, α-fetoprotein, inhibin A, and β-hCG, and adding its measurement to the standard second-trimester maternal quadruple screen increased the rate of Down syndrome detection from 81 to 86 percent, with a false-positive rate of 5 percent.

Another clinical application in which detection of uniquely fetal gene sequences has been used is in the noninvasive diagnosis of fetal rhesus D (Rh(D)) status. Knowledge of fetal Rh(D) genotype is useful for the management of Rh(D)-sensitized pregnant women whose partners are heterozygous for the Rh(D) gene because no further diagnostic or therapeutic procedures are necessary if the fetus is Rh(D)-negative. To date, the feasibility of fetal Rh(D) genotyping from maternal plasma and serum has been reported in several studies.[101–105] The real-time quantitative PCR system has been successfully used to determine fetal Rh(D) status from plasma samples of Rh(D)-negative pregnant women. In the samples obtained from women in their second- or third-trimester of pregnancy, the results of Rh(D) PCR analyses of maternal plasma DNA were completely concordant with the results of serologic analysis, except that there were two false-negative results in the first trimester.[101] The technique of analyzing fetal DNA from maternal plasma is at present reproducible enough to become a routine diagnostic test for the noninvasive prenatal diagnosis of fetal Rh(D) genotype in Europe.[106] This approach may allow restriction of immunoprophylaxis to only Rh(D)-negative women who carry an Rh(D)-positive fetus. This is important, because the supply of Rh(D) immune globulin is limited.

Attempts have been made to detect fetal DNA in maternal plasma independently of gender, but most reports have used specific translocations or polymorphisms that are only applicable in individual families. Chen et al.[107] reported the detection of a paternally inherited fetal aneuploidy (3p trisomy and 7q36 deletion) that resulted from a paternal t(3;7) reciprocal translocation. Myotonic dystrophy is an autosomal dominant disorder associated with the expansion of an unstable CTG trinucleotide repeat in the 3' untranslated region of the DM kinase gene. In one study, paternally derived expanded alleles were detected in maternal plasma DNA.[108] In another study, achondroplasia was suspected in a fetus with short limbs. DNA was extracted from maternal plasma, and a segment of the fibroblast growth factor receptor gene 3 was amplified. A diagnostic G-to-A transition was demonstrated at position 1138 using restriction-enzyme analysis of amplified products.[109] These studies indicate the feasibility of clinical studies using maternal plasma DNA analysis, but they do not provide a widely applicable method of fetal DNA quantitation for female fetuses.

Clinical Applications of Cell-Free RNA in Maternal Plasma and Serum

The development of real-time quantitative reverse transcription-PCR (RT-PCR) assays for specific gene transcripts[110] and the demonstration of tumor-derived RNA sequences in the plasma and serum of cancer patients[111,112] were key advances in the detection of cell-free RNA in peripheral blood. Again, cancer diagnostics led the way to applications in prenatal diagnosis. Tumor-associated RNA targets detected in peripheral blood include mRNA of the tyrosinase gene,[113] telomerase components,[110,114] and Epstein–Barr viral RNA.[115] The detection of circulating mRNA sequences was unexpected because of the known lability of RNA and the presence of ribonuclease in plasma. It is currently thought, on the basis of an in vitro model[116] and filtration experiments,[117] that mRNA is protected from degradation because it is circulating within apoptotic bodies. Evidence obtained from human promyelocytic leukemic HL-60 cells undergoing spontaneous or drug-induced apoptosis suggests that DNA and RNA are packaged into separate apoptotic bodies for degradation.[118]

Poon and colleagues[119] first demonstrated that fetal ZFY mRNA sequences could be detected in the maternal plasma of 22 percent of women in early pregnancy and 63 percent of women in later pregnancy. This work was performed using a two-step RT-PCR assay that was difficult to replicate. Recently, a very important paper was published that demonstrated that mRNA in peripheral blood is remarkably stable.[120] Using real-time RT-PCR this group analyzed the effects of two variables on RNA concentration in sixty-five peripheral blood specimens: time delay in processing of blood and freezing and thawing of plasma and serum. In addition, the stability or lability of cell-free RNA when added to plasma was investigated. The results showed that plasma RNA was stable in EDTA blood stored at 4°C for as long as 24 hr, but that centrifuged clotted blood must be processed within 6 hr. A single freeze/thaw cycle produced no significant effect on the recovery of RNA from plasma and serum. In contrast, >99 percent of *added* cell-free RNA could not be detected or amplified in plasma after only 15 sec. This data implies that mRNA is protected in the circulation by its likely association with particles, and suggests that fetal or placental mRNA sequences may be detected in maternal serum or plasma samples if processed appropriately. This group has also amplified transcripts from two placental-specific genes, hCG and human placental lactogen.[121] They recently addressed an initial clinical application for cell-free RNA in the prenatal diagnosis of preeclampsia by amplifying mRNA of the corticotropin-releasing hormone (CRH) locus.[122] Plasma CRH mRNA concentrations were greatly elevated in third trimester pregnant women with a clinical diagnosis of preeclampsia.

FETAL CELL MICROCHIMERISM

History

The possible persistence of fetal cells in maternal blood after delivery was initially a concern because of the potential for diagnostic error arising from the genetic analysis of cells originating from a prior pregnancy. This may eventually turn out to be the most biologically significant aspect of the study of circulating fetal cells in maternal blood during pregnancy. The existence of male lymphocytes in maternal blood was demonstrated 1–5 years after the delivery of a male infant.[29,30] Using PCR amplification of Y-chromosome-specific sequences, results have been inconsistent. Some investigators have failed to find evidence of fetal cells in maternal blood after delivery,[123] whereas others have detected them for only a few months.[124,125] Most of these groups, however, amplified DNA extracted from whole maternal blood, and they did not use any technique of fetal cell enrichment or purification. It is entirely possible that the methods used were not sensitive enough to detect very small subpopulations of fetal cells.

An alternative approach is to define and then physically separate unique subsets of maternal mononuclear cells to identify the cell surface characteristics of fetal cells that persist and proliferate. In one report, we studied eight women who were not currently pregnant but who had previously given birth to a male infant between 6 months and 27 years earlier.[31] We flow-sorted cells that bound monoclonal antibody to cell surface antigens present on B lymphocytes (CD19+, CD23+), T lymphocytes (CD3+, CD4+, CD5+), and hematopoietic stem and progenitor cells (CD34+, CD38+). In the absence of PCR contamination, the presence of a Y-chromosome sequence was evidence of continued circulation of male cells. Remarkably, six of the eight women studied had male DNA detected in their flow-sorted CD34+ CD38+ cells, even 27 years after delivery.[31] That pregnancy might induce a state of physiologic microchimerism was an unexpected observation. Evans et al. also found long-term evidence of circulating fetal CD3+, CD14+, CD19+, and CD56/16+ in the peripheral blood of 33 percent (16 of 48) healthy postpartum women and 60 percent (12 of 20) women with scleroderma.[32] Furthermore, HLA compatibility was not a requirement for the development of persistent fetal-cell microchimerism.

The discovery of the long-term persistence of the CD34+,CD38+ fetal progenitor cells and the CD4+ cells highlighted the need to better understand the long-term consequences of pregnancy on maternal health.[126] There are currently two alternative hypotheses under investigation: that fetal cells may participate in a graft-versus-host reaction, and account for the higher incidence of autoimmune disease in women; and that fetal cells acquired naturally via pregnancy and delivery constitute a novel population of stem cells that may repair diseased or injured maternal tissue. Although it is beyond the main focus of this chapter, this is an exciting and rapidly evolving area of inquiry, and a brief summary will be given here.

Do Persistent Fetal Cells Cause Maternal Disease?

Nelson hypothesized that the disorder scleroderma develops as a consequence of fetal (graft) versus maternal (host) disease.[127] Emerging evidence indicates the presence of unusually high numbers of male (presumed fetal) cells in the peripheral blood of women afflicted with severe scleroderma.[128] Persisting fetal cells have been shown in the both the peripheral blood[129,130] and tissues[131,132] of women with systemic sclerosis. Scaletti et al. demonstrated proof of concept that the fetal cells could react against maternal histocompatibility antigens.[133] This group obtained skin biopsies from women with scleroderma, and cultured male CD4+ lymphocytes from them. Similarly, an association has been shown between the presence of male (presumed fetal) cells and autoimmune thyroid disorders.[134,135]

Do Persistent Fetal Cells Repair Injured Maternal Tissue?

In our laboratory, we have found evidence of fetal-cell microchimerism in association with nonautoimmune diseases such as thyroid adenomas,[134] ovarian cancer, and hepatitis C.[136] There is good evidence that fetal CD34+ cells persist in maternal blood for decades following pregnancy.[31,137] This led to the hypothesis that fetal stem and/or progenitor cells may serve as an additional source of stem cells that would be available to participate in the maternal response to tissue injury. Although we do not know if fetal stem cells have an advantage over maternal stem cells, we do have evidence that fetal cells in maternal tissue have the capability of differentiating into epithelial or hepatic cells.[138]

SUMMARY AND RECOMMENDATIONS

Since the previous edition of this textbook, there have been many exciting and unexpected advances in prenatal diagnosis by the analysis of fetal cells and nucleic acids in maternal blood. It is clear that the biology of pregnancy affects the development of the placenta, and that in turn affects fetomaternal transfer of cells and nucleic acids. It is fortunate for clinical applications that there is increased fetomaternal trafficking in many abnormal fetal conditions. However, to become part of routine prenatal screening for Down syndrome, major technical advances are needed to isolate and analyze rare fetal cells. In contrast, some applications for the measurement and/or detection of cell-free fetal DNA in maternal plasma and serum are already in clinical use. These include fetal gender and rhesus D genotype diagnosis. As groups move away from Y-chromosome sequence measurement and toward analysis of specific fetal gene expression using cell-free mRNA, clinical applications will develop that are equally relevant for female and male fetuses. Finally, the demonstration of the long-term persistence and differentiation capabilities of fetal stem cells in the mother has enormous biologic significance. What started out as a "simple" effort to provide noninvasive cytogenetic diagnosis may end up explaining why women live longer than men.

REFERENCES

1. de la Cruz F, Shifrin H, Elias S, et al. Prenatal diagnosis by use of fetal cells isolated from maternal blood. Am J Obstet Gynecol 1995;173:1354.

2. Bianchi DW, Simpson JL, Jackson LG, et al. Fetal gender and aneuploidy detection using fetal cells in maternal blood: analysis of NIFTY data. National Institute of Child Health and Development Fetal Cell Isolation Study. Prenat Diagn 2002;22:609.

3. Bianchi DW, Lo YM. Fetomaternal cellular and plasma DNA trafficking: the Yin and the Yang. Ann NY Acad Sci 2001;945:119.

4. Khosrotehrani K, Bianchi DW. Fetal cell microchimerism: helpful or harmful to the parous woman? Curr Opin Obstet Gynecol 2003;15:195.

5. Schröder J. Transplacental passage of blood cells. J Med Genet 1975;12:230.

6. Douglas GW, Thomas L, Carr M, et al. Trophoblast in the circulating blood during pregnancy. Am J Obstet Gynecol 1959;78:960.

7. Schmorl G. Pathogisch-anatomische untersuchungen uber puerperaleklampsie. Leipzig: Vogel, 1893.

8. Walknowska J, Conte FA, Grumbach MM. Practical and theoretical implication of fetal/maternal lymphocyte transfer. Lancet 1969;1:1119.

9. Grosset L, Barrelet V, Odartchenko N. Antenatal fetal sex determination from maternal blood during early pregnancy. Am J Obstet Gynecol 1974;120:60.

10. Hawes CS, Suskin HA, Petropoulos A, et al. A morphologic study of trophoblast isolated from peripheral blood of pregnant women. Am J Obstet Gynecol 1994;170:1297.

11. Oudejans CBM, Tjoa ML, Westerman BA, et al. Circulating trophoblast in maternal blood. Prenat Diagn 2003;111.

12. Chua S, Wilkins T, Sargent I, et al. Trophoblast deportation in pre-eclamptic pregnancy. Br J Obstet Gynaecol 1991;98:973.

13. Yeoh SC, Sargent I, Redman C. Fetal cells in maternal blood and their use in non-invasive prenatal diagnosis. Prog Obstet Gynaecol 1992;4:51.

14. Sargent IL, Johansen M, Chua S, et al. Clinical experience: Isolating trophoblasts from maternal blood. Ann NY Acad Sci 1994;731:154.

15. Tse DB, Anderson P, Goldbard S, et al. Characterization of trophoblast reactive monoclonal antibodies by flow cytometry and their application for fetal cell isolation. Ann NY Acad Sci 1994;731:162.

16. Yagel S, Shpan P, Dushnik M, et al. Trophoblasts circulating in maternal blood as candidates for prenatal genetic evaluation. Hum Reprod 1994;9:1184.

17. Bulmer JN, Billington WD, Johnson PM. Immunohistologic identification of trophoblast populations in early human pregnancy with the use of monoclonal antibodies. Am J Obstet Gynecol 1984;148:19.

18. Covone AE, Johnson PM, Mutton D, et al. Trophoblast cells in peripheral blood from pregnant women. Lancet 1984;2:841.

19. Bertero MT, Camaschella C, Serra A, et al. Circulating "trophoblast" cells in pregnancy have maternal genetic markers. Prenat Diagn 1988;8:588.

20. Covone AE, Kozman R, Johnson PM, et al. Analysis of peripheral maternal blood samples for the presence of placental-derived cells using Y-specific probes and McAb H315. Prenat Diagn 1988;5:591.

21. Mueller UW, Hawes CS, Wright AE, et al. Isolation of fetal trophoblast cells from peripheral blood of pregnant women. Lancet 1990;336:197.

22. Durrant LG, McDowall KM, Holmes RA, et al. Screening of monoclonal antibodies for isolation of trophoblasts from maternal blood for prenatal diagnosis. Prenat Diagn 1994;14:131.

23. Van Wijk IJ, van Vugt JMG, Mulders MAM, et al. Enrichment of fetal trophoblast cells from the maternal peripheral blood followed by detection of fetal deoxyribonucleic acid with a nested X/Y polymerase chain reaction. Am J Obstet Gynecol 1996;174:871.

24. Van Wijk IJ, Van Vugt JMG, Konst AAM, et al. Identification of HASH2-positive extravillus trophoblast cells in the peripheral blood of pregnant women. Trophoblast Res 1998;11:23.

25. Van Wijk IJ, Griffioen S, Tjoa ML, et al. HLA-G expression in trophoblast cells circulating in maternal peripheral blood during early pregnancy. Am J Obstet Gynecol 2001;184:991.

26. Van Wijk IJ, de Hoon AC, Mulders MAM, et al. Identification of triploid trophoblast cells in peripheral blood of a woman with partial hydatidiform molar pregnancy. Prenat Diagn 2001;21:1142.

27. Herzenberg LA, Bianchi DW, Schroder J, et al. Fetal cells in the blood of pregnant women: detection and enrichment by fluorescence-activated cell sorting. Proc Natl Acad Sci USA 1979;76:1453.

28. Iverson GM, Bianchi DW, Cann HM, et al. Detection and isolation of fetal cells from maternal blood using the fluorescence-activated cell sorter (FACS). Prenat Diagn 1981;1:61.

29. Schröder J, Tiilikainen A, de la Chapelle A. Fetal leukocytes in the maternal circulation after delivery. I. Cytological aspects. Transplantation 1974;17:346.

30. Ciaranfi A, Curchod A, Odartchenko N. Survie de lymphocytes foetaux dans le sang maternal postpartum. Schweiz Med Wochenschr 1977;107:134.

31. Bianchi DW, Zickwolf GK, Weil GJ, et al. Male fetal progenitor cells persist in maternal blood for as long as 27 years postpartum. Proc Natl Acad Sci USA 1996;93:705.

32. Evans PC, Lambert N, Maoloney S, et al. Long-term fetal microchimerism in peripheral blood mononuclear cell subsets in healthy women and women with scleroderma. Blood 1999;93:2033.

33. Zilliacus R, de la Chapelle A, Schröder J, et al. Transplacental passage of foetal blood cells. Scand J Haematol 1975;15:333.

34. Wessman M, Ylinen K, Knuutila S. Fetal granulocytes in maternal venous blood detected by in situ hybridization. Prenat Diagn 1992;12:993.

35. Creger WP, Steele MR. Human fetomaternal passage of erythrocytes. N Engl J Med 1957;256:158.

36. Cohen F, Zuelzer WW. Transplacental passage and postnatal survival of fetal erythrocytes in heterospecific pregnancies. Blood 1967;30:796.

37. Zipursky A, Hull A, White FD, et al. Foetal erythrocytes in the maternal circulation. Lancet 1959;1:451.

38. Medearis AL, Hensleigh PA, Parks DR, et al. Detection of fetal erythrocytes in the maternal blood post partum with the fluorescence-activated cell sorter. Am J Obstet Gynecol 1984;148:290.

39. Bianchi DW, Flint AF, Pizzimenti MF, et al. Isolation of fetal DNA from nucleated erythrocytes in maternal blood. Proc Natl Acad Sci USA 1990;87:3279.

40. Loken MR, Shah VO, Dattilio KL, et al. Flow cytometric analysis of human bone marrow. I. Normal erythroid development. Blood 1987;69:255.

41. Price JO, Elias S, Wachtel SS, et al. Prenatal diagnosis using fetal cells isolated from maternal blood by multiparameter flow cytometry. Am J Obstet Gynecol 1991;165:1731.

42. Wachtel S, Elias S, Price J, et al. Fetal cells in the maternal circulation: isolation by multiparameter flow cytometry and confirmation by polymerase chain reaction. Hum Reprod 1991;6:1466.

43. Gänshirt-Ahlert D, Burschyk M, Garritsen HS, et al. Magnetic cell sorting and the transferrin receptor as potential means of prenatal diagnosis from maternal blood. Am J Obstet Gynecol 1992;166:1350.

44. Holzgreve W, Garritsen HSP, Gänshirt-Ahlert D. Fetal cells in the maternal circulation. J Reprod Med 1992;37:410.

45. Bianchi DW, Stewart JE, Garber MF, et al. Possible effect of gestational age on the detection of fetal nucleated erythrocytes in maternal blood. Prenat Diagn 1991;11:523.

46. Gänshirt D, Smeets FW, Dohr A, et al. Enrichment of fetal nucleated red blood cells from the maternal circulation for prenatal diagnosis: experiences with triple density gradient and MACS based on more than 600 cases. Fetal Diagn Ther 1998;13:276.

47. Holzgreve W, Ghezzi F, DiNaro E, et al. Disturbed feto-maternal cell traffic in preeclampsia. Obstet Gynecol 1998;91:669.

48. Campagnoli C, Roberts IA, Kumar S, et al. Identification of mesenchymal stem/progenitor cells in human first-trimester fetal blood, liver and bone marrow. Blood 2001;98:2396.

49. O'Donoghue K, Choolani M, Chan J, et al. Identification of fetal mesenchymal stem cells in maternal blood implications for non-invasive prenatal diagnosis. Mol Hum Reprod 2003;9:497.

50. Bianchi DW, Farina A, Weber W, et al. Significant fetal-maternal hemorrhage after termination of pregnancy: implications for development of fetal cell microchimerism. Am J Obstet Gynecol 2001;184:703.

51. Hamada H, Ariami T, Kubo T, et al. Fetal nucleated cells in maternal peripheral blood: frequency and relationship to gestational age. Hum Genet 1993;91:427.

52. Krabchi K, Gros-Louis F, Yan J, et al. Quantification of all fetal nucleated cells in maternal blood between the 18th and 22nd week of pregnancy using molecular cytogenetic techniques. Clin Genet 2001;60:145.

53. Bianchi DW, Shuber AP, DeMaria M, et al. Fetal cells in maternal blood: determination of purity and yield by quantitative polymerase chain reaction. Am J Obstet Gynecol 1994;171:922.

54. Bianchi DW, Williams JW, Sullivan LM, et al. PCR quantitation of fetal cells in maternal blood in normal and aneuploid pregnancies. Am J Hum Genet 1997;61:822.

55. Ariga H, Ohto H, Busch MP, et al. Kinetics of fetal cellular and cell-free DNA in the maternal circulation during and after pregnancy: implications for non-invasive prenatal diagnosis. Transfusion 2001;41:1524.

56. Sekizawa A, Samura O, Zhen DK, et al. Apoptosis in fetal nucleated erythrocytes circulating in maternal blood. Prenat Diagn 2000;20:886.

57. Bischoff FZ, Marquez-Do DA, Martinez DI, et al. Intact fetal cell isolation from maternal blood: improved isolation using a simple whole blood progenitor cell enrichment approach (RosetteSep). Clin Genet 2003;63:483.

58. Wachtel SS, Sammons D, Manley M, et al. Fetal cells in maternal blood: recovery by charge flow separation. Hum Genet 1996;98:162.
59. Takabayashi H, Kuwabara S, Ukita T, et al. Development of non-invasive fetal DNA diagnosis from maternal blood. Prenat Diagn 1995;15:74.
60. Vona G, Beroud C, Benachi A, et al. Enrichment, immunomorphological, and genetic characterization of fetal cells circulating in maternal blood. Am J Pathol 2002;160:51.
61. Mesker WE, Ouwerkerk-van Velzen MC, Oosterwijk JC, et al. Two-colour immunocytochemical staining of gamma (gamma) and epsilon (epsilon) type haemoglobin in fetal red cells. Prenat Diagn 1998;18:1131.
62. Choolani M, O'Donnell H, Campagnoli C, et al. Simultaneous fetal cell identification and diagnosis by epsilon-globin chain immunophenotyping and chromosomal fluorescence in situ hybridization. Blood 2001;98:554.
63. Choolani M, O'Donoghue K, Talbert D, et al. Characterization of first trimester fetal erythroblasts for non-invasive prenatal diagnosis. Mol Hum Reprod 2003;9:227.
64. Bianchi DW, Zickwolf GK, Yih MC, et al. Erythroid-specific antibodies enhance detection of fetal nucleated erythrocytes in maternal blood. Prenat Diagn 1993;3:293.
65. DeMaria MA, Zheng Y-L, Zhen D, et al. Improved fetal nucleated erythrocyte sorting purity using intracellular antifetal hemoglobin and Hoechst 33342. Cytometry 1996;25:37.
66. Zheng YL, DeMaria M, Zhen DK, et al. Flow sorting of fetal erythroblasts using intracytoplasmic antifetal haemoglobin: preliminary observations on maternal samples. Prenat Diagn 1995;15:897.
67. Bianchi DW, Mahr A, Zickwolf GK, et al. Detection of fetal cells with 47,XY,+21 karyotype in maternal peripheral blood. Hum Genet 1992;90:368.
68. Cacheux V, Milesi-Fluet C, Tachdijian G, et al. Detection of 47,XYY trophoblast fetal cells in maternal blood by fluorescence in situ hybridization after using immunomagnetic lymphocyte depletion and flow cytometry sorting. Fetal Diagn Ther 1992;7:190.
69. Zheng YL, Craigo SD, Price CM, et al. Demonstration of spontaneously dividing male fetal cells in maternal blood by negative magnetic cell sorting and FISH. Prenat Diagn 1995;15:573.
70. Bischoff FZ, Lewis DE, Simpson JL, et al. Detection of low-grade mosaicism in fetal cells isolated from maternal blood. Prenat Diagn 1995;15:1182.
71. Elias S, Price J, Dockter M, et al. First trimester prenatal diagnosis of trisomy 21 in fetal cells from maternal blood. Lancet 1992;340:1033.
72. Gänshirt-Ahlert D, Borjesson-Stoll R, Burschyk M, et al. Detection of fetal trisomies 21 and 18 from maternal blood using triple gradient and magnetic cell sorting. Am J Reprod Immunol 1993;30:194.
73. Simpson JL, Elias S. Isolating fetal cells from maternal blood: advances in prenatal diagnosis through molecular technology. JAMA 1993;270:2357.
74. Mandel P, Metais P. Les acides nucleiques du plasma sanguin chez l'homme. C.R. Acad Sci Paris 1948;142:241.
75. Stroun M, Anker P, Maurice P, Gaban PB. Circulating nucleic acids in higher organisms. Int Rev Cytol 1977;51:1.
76. Stroun M, Maurice P, Vasioukhin V, Lyautey J, Lederrey C, Lefort F, Rossier A, Chen XQ, Anker P. The origin and mechanism of circulating DNA. NY Acad Sci 2000;906:161.
77. Leon SA, Shapiro B, Sklaroff DM, et al. Free DNA serum of cancer patients and the effect of therapy. Cancer Res 1977; 37:646.
78. Chen XQ, Stroun M, Magnenat JL, Nicod LP, Kurt AM, Lyautey J, et al. Microsatellite alterations in plasma DNA of small cell lung cancer patients. Nat Med 1996;2:1033.
79. Nawroz H, Koch W, Anker P, Stroun M, Sidransky D. Microsatellite alterations in serum DNA of head and neck cancer patients. Nat Med 1996;2:1035.
80. Anker P, Mulcahy H, Chen XQ, Stroun M. Detection of circulating tumour DNA in the blood (plasma/serum) of cancer patients. Cancer Metastasis Rev 1999;18:65.
81. Lo YMD, Corbetta N, Chamberlain PF, et al. Presence of fetal DNA in maternal plasma and serum. Lancet 1997;350:485.
82. Lo YMD, Tein MSC, Lau TK, et al. Quantitative analysis of fetal DNA in maternal plasma and serum: implications for noninvasive prenatal diagnosis. Am J Hum Genet 1998; 62:768.
83. Lee TH, Montalvo L, Chrebtow V, et al. Quantitation of genomic DNA in plasma and serum samples: higher concentrations of genomic DNA found in serum than in plasma. Transfusion 2001;4:276.
84. Lo YMD, Zhang J, Leung TN, et al. Rapid clearance of fetal DNA from maternal plasma. Am J Hum Genet 1999;64:218.
85. Pertl B, Bianchi DW. Fetal DNA in maternal plasma: emerging clinical applications. Obstet Gynecol 2001;98:483.

86. Costa JM, Benachi A, Gautier E, et al. First-trimester fetal sex determination in maternal serum using real-time PCR. Prenat Diagn 2001;21:1070.

87. Lo YMD, Leung TN, Tein MSC, et al. Quantitative abnormalities of fetal DNA in maternal plasma in pre-eclampsia. Clin Chem 1999;45:184.

88. Holzgreve W, Ghezzi F, Di Naro E, et al. Disturbed fetomaternal cell traffic in preeclampsia. Obstet Gynecol 1998;91:669.

89. Holzgreve W, Hahn S. Novel molecular biological approaches for the diagnosis of preeclampsia. Clin Chem 1999;45:451.

90. Zhong XY, Laivuori H, Livingston JC, et al. Elevation of both maternal and fetal extracellular circulating deoxyribonucleic acid concentrations in the plasma of pregnant women with preeclampsia Am J Obstet Gynecol 2001;184:414.

91. Swinkels DW, de Kok JB, Hendriks JC, et al. Hemolysis, elevated liver enzymes and low platelet count (HELLP) syndrome as a complication of preeclampsia in pregnant women increases the amount of cell-free fetal and maternal DNA in maternal plasma and serum. Clin Chem 2002;48:650.

92. Levine RJ, Qian C, LeShane ES, et al. Two stage elevation of cell-free fetal DNA in maternal sera before onset of preeclampsia. Am J Obstet Gynecol 2004, in press.

93. Bianchi DW. Fetal DNA in maternal plasma: The plot thickens and the placental barrier thins. Am J Hum Genet 1998;62:763.

94. Leung TN, Zhang J, Lau TK, et al. Maternal plasma fetal DNA as a marker for preterm labour. Lancet 1998;352:1904.

95. Lo YMD, Lau TK, Zhang J, et al. Increased fetal DNA concentrations in the plasma of pregnant women carrying fetuses with trisomy 21. Clin Chem 1999;45:1747.

96. Zhong XY, Burk MR, Troeger C, et al. Fetal DNA in maternal plasma is elevated in pregnancies with aneuploid fetuses. Prenat Diagn 2000;20:795.

97. Lee T, LeShane ES, Messerlian GM, et al. Down syndrome and cell-free fetal DNA in archived maternal serum. Am J Obstet Gynecol 2002;187:1217.

98. Ohashi Y, Miharu N, Honda H, et al. Quantitation of fetal DNA in maternal serum in normal and aneuploid pregnancies. Hum Genet 2001;108:123.

99. Wataganara T, LeShane ES, Farina A, et al. Maternal serum cell-free fetal DNA levels are increased in cases trisomy 13 but not trisomy 18. Hum Genet 2003;112:204.

100. Farina A, LeShane ES, Lambert-Messerlian GM, et al. Evaluation of cell-free fetal DNA as a second trimester maternal serum marker of Down syndrome pregnancy. Clin Chem 2003;49:239.

101. Lo YMD, Hjelm NM, Fidler C, et al. Prenatal diagnosis of fetal Rh(D) status by molecular analysis of maternal plasma. N Engl J Med 1998;339:1734.

102. Faas BHW, Beuling EA, Christiaens GCML, et al. Detection of fetal Rh(D)-specific sequences in maternal plasma. Lancet 1998;352:1196.

103. Bischoff FZ, Nguyen DD, Marquez-Do D, et al. Noninvasive determination of fetal Rh(D) status using fetal DNA in maternal serum and PCR. J Soc Gynecol Invest 1999;6:64.

104. Zhong XY, Holzgreve W, Hahn S. Detection of fetal Rhesus D and sex using fetal DNA from maternal plasma by multiplex polymerase chain reaction. Br J Obstet Gynaecol 2000;107:766.

105. Costa JM, Giovangrandi Y, Ernault P, et al. Fetal RHD genotyping in maternal serum during the first trimester of pregnancy. Br J Haematol 2002;119:255.

106. Finning KM, Martin PG, Soothill PW, et al. Prediction of fetal D status from maternal plasma: introduction of a new noninvasive fetal *RHD* genotyping service. Transfusion 2002;42:1079.

107. Chen CP, Chern SR, Wang W. Fetal DNA in maternal plasma: the prenatal detection of a paternally inherited fetal aneuploidy. Prenat Diagn 2000;20:353.

108. Amicucci P, Gennarelli M, Novelli G, et al. Prenatal diagnosis of myotonic dystrophy using fetal DNA obtained from maternal plasma. Clin Chem 2000;46:301.

109. Saito H, Sekizawa A, Morimoto T, et al. Prenatal DNA diagnosis from maternal plasma in the case of fetal achondroplasia. Lancet 2000;356:1170.

110. Dasi F, Lledo S, Garcia-Granero E, et al. Real-time quantification in plasma of human telomerase reverse-transcriptase (hTERT) mRNA: a simple blood test to monitor disease in cancer patients. Lab Invest 2001;81:767.

111. Wong IHN, Chan AT, Johnson PJ. Quantitative analysis of circulating tumor cells in peripheral blood of osteosarcoma patients using osteoblast-specific mRNA markers: a pilot study. Clin Cancer Res 2000;6:2183.

112. Silva JM, Dominguez G, Silva J, et al. detection of epithelial messenger RNA in the plasma of breast cancer patients is associated with poor prognosis tumor characteristics. Clin Cancer Res 2001;7:2821.

113. Kopreski MS, Benko FA, Kwak LW, et al. Detection of tumor messenger RNA in the serum of patients with malignant melanoma. Clin Cancer Res 1999;5:1961.

114. Chen XQ, Bonnefoi H, Pelte MF, et al. Telomerase mRNA as a detection marker in the serum of breast cancer patients. Clin Cancer Res 2000;6:3823.

115. Lo KW, Lo YMD, Leung SF, et al. Analysis of cell-free Epstein–Barr virus associated RNA in the plasma of patients with nasopharyngeal carcinoma. Clin Chem 1999;45:1292.

116. Hasselmann DO, Rappl G, Tilgen W, et al. Extracellular tyrosinase mRNA within apoptotic bodies is protected from degradation in human serum. Clin Chem 2001;47:1488.

117. Ng EKO, Tsui NBY, Lam NYL, et al. Presence of filterable and nonfilterable mRNA in the plasma of cancer patients and healthy individuals. Clin Chem 2002;48:1212.

118. Halicka HD, Bedner E, Darzynkiewicz Z. Segregation of RNA and separate packaging of DNA and RNA in apoptotic bodies during apoptosis. Exp Cell Res 2000;260:248.

119. Poon LLM, Leung TN, Lau TK, et al. Presence of fetal RNA in maternal plasma. Clin Chem 2000; 46:1832.

120. Tsui NB, Ng EK, Lo YM. Stability of endogenous and added RNA in blood specimens, serum, and plasma. Clin Chem 2002;48:1647.

121. Ng EK, Tsui NB, Lau TK, et al. mRNA of placental origin is readily detectable in maternal plasma. Proc Natl Acad Sci USA 2003;100:4748.

122. Ng EK, Leung TN, Tsui NB, et al. The concentration of circulating corticotrophin-releasing hormone mRNA in maternal plasma is increased in preeclampsia. Clin Chem 2003;49:727.

123. Lo YMD, Patel P, Baigent CN, et al. Prenatal sex determination from maternal peripheral blood using the polymerase chain reaction. Hum Genet 1993;90:483.

124. Hsieh TT, Pao CC, Hor JJ, et al. Presence of fetal cells in maternal circulation after delivery. Hum Genet 1993;92:204.

125. Hamada H, Arinami T, Hamaguchi H, et al. Fetal nucleated cells in maternal peripheral blood after delivery. Am J Obstet Gynecol 1994;170:1188.

126. Bianchi, DW. Fetomaternal cell trafficking: a new cause of disease? Am J Med Genet 2000; 91:22.

127. Nelson JL. Viewpoint. Maternal-fetal immunology and autoimmune disease: is some autoimmune disease auto-allo or all-autoimmune? Arthritis Rheum 1996;39:191.

128. Nelson JL, Furst DE, Maloney S, et al. Microchimerism and HLA-compatible relationships of pregnancy in scleroderma. Lancet 1998;351:559.

129. Artlett CM, Cox LA, Ramos RC, et al. Increased microchimeric CD4+ T lymphocytes in peripheral blood from women with systemic sclerosis. Clin Immunol 2002; 103:303.

130. Lambert NC, Lo YM, Erickson TD, et al. Male microchimerism in healthy women and women with scleroderma: cells or circulating DNA? A quantitative answer. Blood 2002; 100:2845.

131. Johnson KL, Nelson JL, Furst DE, et al. Fetal cell microchimerism in tissue from multiple sites in women with systemic sclerosis. Arthritis Rheum 2001;44:1848.

132. Artlett CM, Smith JB, Jimenez SA. Identification of fetal DNA and cells in skin lesions from women with systemic sclerosis. N Engl J Med 1988; 338:1186.

133. Scaletti C, Vultaggio A, Bonifacio S, et al. Th2-oriented profile of male offspring T cells present in women with systemic sclerosis and reactive with maternal major histocompatibility complex antigens. Arthritis Rheum 2002; 46:445.

134. Srivasta B, Srivatsa S, Johnson KL. Microchimerism of presumed fetal origin in thyroid specimens from women: a case-control study. Lancet 2001; 358:2034.

135. Klintschar M, Schwaiger P, Mannweiler S, et al. Evidence of fetal microchimerism in Hashimoto's thyroiditis. J Clin Endocrinol Metab 2001; 86:2494.

136. Johnson KL, Samura O, Nelson JL, et al. Significant fetal cell microchimerism in a nontransfused woman with hepatitis C: evidence of long-term survival and expansion. Hepatology 2002;36:1295.

137. Adams KM, Lambert NC, Heimfeld S, et al. Male DNA in female donor apheresis and CD34-enriched products. Blood 2003, 102:3845.

138. Khosrotehrani K, Johnson KL, Cha, et al. Pregnancy-associated fetal progenitor/stem cells (PAPCs) differentiate into epithelial cells and hepatocytes in maternal organs. Am J Hum Genet 2003;73S:622.

Diana L. Farmer, M.D., Hanmin Lee, M.D.,
Michael R. Harrison, M.D., and
Kerilyn K. Nobuhara, M.D.

29

Fetal Therapy

While the majority of prenatally diagnosed disorders are best managed by treatment after birth, a few highly select diseases with predictable devastating developmental consequences may benefit from fetal therapy.[1] Fetal therapy is perhaps the best example of a multidisciplinary enterprise, in which success depends on the coordinated collaboration and participation of principals from multiple fields of expertise: pediatric surgery, obstetrics, perinatology, genetics, anesthesiology, echocardiography, social work, nursing, and bioethics.[1,2] Although these health care providers do not routinely work closely together, in the setting of fetal intervention their creative interface and combined talents are orchestrated beautifully to provide comprehensive maternal–fetal care that has begun to blur the distinction of fetal therapy, generally falling into the confines of either one of three categories—medical, genetic, or surgical.[1-3]

ETHICAL CONSIDERATIONS

A fundamental and longstanding challenge in fetal therapy has been to maintain a balance between risks to both the pregnant woman and fetus against potential benefit to *only* the fetus.[4-6] The woman carrying a fetus with a diagnosed anomaly is essentially an "innocent bystander" in such therapies, as her involvement entails only risk, including impairment to her future fertility potential. Generally speaking, a major and potentially lifesaving fetal intervention is deemed warranted if maternal risks can be minimized and good fetal outcome ensured. If hysterotomy and, thus, its attendant lifelong risk for uterine rupture can be avoided, then a more minor improvement in fetal outcome may be acceptable. Most centers performing fetal surgery have instituted oversight committees, with members from varied disciplines who are not involved in the fetal procedures, to act in an advisory and quality assurance role. These committees are responsible for reviewing, usually at monthly intervals, all fetal evaluations and surgical procedures performed at their institution, regardless of whether or not an adverse event occurred. However, this relatively nascent field remains largely self-regulated through the ongoing commitment of the clinicians and researchers involved. At the most recent International Fetal Medicine and Surgery Society meeting, the membership proposed guidelines that include rigorous nondirective informed consent processes, as well as minimal requirements for standards of care, post-intervention follow-up, and registry data collection.

SURGICAL THERAPY

Surgical intervention to correct an anatomic defect in an unborn human fetus has been performed for more than two decades in the United States, starting in the early 1980s, with the investigators at the University of California, San Francisco, as the acknowledged pioneers of this enterprise. Since the field's early development, the framework for offering fetal intervention has adhered to and continues to adhere to demanding standards. That is, a logical and rigorous sequence of events must occur before any operation is attempted on a human fetus at any given institution[7]: (1) the developmental pathophysiology of the potentially lethal correctable lesion must be studied in animal model(s); (2) the natural history of the disease must be documented in human fetuses via serial ultrasound observation; (3) selection criteria for intervention is delineated; and (4) the anesthetic, tocolytic, and surgical techniques for hysterotomy and fetal surgery must be developed and/or refined. Over the ensuing 20 years the investment in basic and clinical research encompassed in this framework has benefited an increasing number of fetal patients and has spurred continued research into the normal and abnormal development of the fetus and the implications for therapy.

In the past decade, fetal surgery has experienced tremendous change. Medical and lay communities alike have become more familiar and accepting of in utero surgical therapy. Research, development, improvements, and implementation of fetal procedures have become international endeavors, with nearly a dozen centers worldwide offering surgical intervention. Third-party payers have acknowledged the crossover of fetal surgical procedures from the experimental realm to that of recognized options for therapy by authorizing reimbursement for the majority of these operations. More significant is that, until recently, only fetuses with mortal defects were considered candidates for prenatal correction. Now, a certain comfort level within the enterprise must be inferred from the fact that fetal surgical procedures are being performed for nonlethal conditions. Despite the rather explosive application of fetal surgery, the enterprise remains fragile in terms of dealing with several lingering ethical issues, primarily, the question of risk versus benefit posed to both mother and fetus, and issues of safety and efficacy that remain unproven for many of the procedures.

Maternal Risks

The viability of fetal surgery as a treatment approach is predicated first and foremost on a responsibility to the pregnant woman and her family, because she, along with her unborn child, is a patient in this setting.[6] Invasive fetal therapy evolved in a logical manner with the initial and paramount challenge being that of maternal safety. Thus, the first technical issue addressed was how to safely open and close the gravid uterus such that bleeding and membrane separation were prevented and a water-tight closure was attained. That problem was solved by using an absorbable stapling device and special back-biting retractors for the uterine edges,[8,9] closing the uterus in two layers with absorbable sutures, and supplementing the seal with fibrin glue. Early on in the research, all aspects of fetal surgery (e.g., anesthesia, monitoring, surgical procedure, etc.) were tested in the most rigorous animal model, the nonhuman primate, whose anatomy and physiology during pregnancy quite closely resemble that of human pregnancy.[10,11]

In open fetal surgery, the site of hysterotomy depends on the position of the fetus and the placenta, but excludes the lower uterine segment (which is not fully developed in the second trimester). Thus, delivery after fetal surgery and all future pregnancies must be by cesarean section to avoid the risk of uterine scar dehiscence during labor. Clearly, an advantage of fetoscopic surgery versus open procedures has been that future deliveries can be vaginal. Fortunately, the ability to carry and deliver subsequent pregnancies does not appear to be jeopardized by fetal surgery. Farrell et al. surveyed seventy women who underwent fetal surgery, and found that, of the forty-five respondents, thirty-five attempted subsequent pregnancies. Thirty-two were successful, resulting in thirty-one livebirths. Two women had a preoperative history of infertility failed to conceive.[12]

To date, there have been no reported maternal deaths as a result of open fetal surgery, but at least one death has been associated with a percutaneous fetal intervention. Operative morbidity is rare, but maternal transfusions and serious infections have occurred. A more daunting problem has been maternal morbidity related to preterm labor and side effects of tocolytic therapy, especially the pulmonary edema associated with high doses.[13–15] Although reversible, this complication emphasizes the need for close maternal monitoring. Fetoscopic procedures appear to incite less uterine irritability compared with open fetal surgery; thus, preterm labor has been seen less frequently.[16]

Fetal Surgical Techniques

The development of open and minimal-access fetal surgical techniques continues to evolve, as clinical necessity motivates constant innovation to improve the feasibility and safety for the fetus and the mother. Today, however, operative techniques for opening and closing the gravid uterus, monitoring of the fetus intraoperatively, and maintaining fetal homeostasis are relatively standardized.[8,9] For example, anesthesia of the mother and her baby, established with halogenated agents, provides profound uterine relaxation.[9,17] In addition, an epidural catheter is inserted to enhance postoperative pain control. In the operating room, the mother is positioned in left lateral decubitus position to avoid inferior vena caval compression by the gravid uterus, and is continuously monitored using standard techniques, including pulse oximetry, a blood pressure cuff, large-bore intravenous catheters, measurement of urine output, and EKG. Pulse oximetry, radiotelemetry, and, most reliably, intraoperative ultrasound provide adequate assessment of fetal heart rate, temperature, intra-amniotic pressure, and other parameters such as pH and tissue oxygenation. The two principal routes of fetal access are discussed below.

Open Fetal Surgery[18,19]

The timing of open fetal surgery depends on the malformation being treated and the pathophysiologic course dictated by that disorder. In general, small size, tissue integrity, and accurate early diagnosis are significant limiting factors at less than 18 weeks of gestation, while beyond 30 weeks of gestation, a high risk of premature rupture of the membranes and preterm labor are associated with manipulations on the uterus, in which case, it is then more reasonable to deliver the fetus and treat the malformation with standard postnatal care. For these reasons, open fetal procedures have been performed between 18 and 30 weeks of gestation.

Open fetal surgery is performed through a maternal hysterotomy. After a low abdominal transverse incision exposes the uterus, fetal position and placental location are identified with intraoperative ultrasound. An anterior or posterior hysterotomy is then performed using the absorbable uterine stapler device that provides hemostasis and seals the membranes to the myometrium.[18] The appropriate fetal part is then exposed and the fetus is given an intramuscularly administered narcotic and paralytic agent. Warm lactated Ringer solution is continuously infused around the fetus and open uterus to maintain fetal body temperature. For fetal monitoring, a sterile pulse oximeter can be used, and a radiotelemetric device is sometimes implanted submuscularly (usually on the chest wall).[20] After repair of the defect, the fetus is returned to the womb and amniotic fluid is restored with warm saline containing an antibiotic such as nafcillin. The uterine incision is closed with in two layers, and fibrin glue is used to help seal the uterine incision.

Minimal Access Fetal Surgery—Fetoscopy[20,21]

Although fetoscopic techniques for direct optical visualization of the fetus are not new, modifications to existing postnatal endoscopic techniques and development of new fetoscopic instruments not only make the procedures safer, more reliable, quicker, and hence more commonplace, but they have also paved the way for minimal access fetal surgery. One advantage of fetoscopy is to preserve fetal homeostasis by protecting the intrauterine physiologic milieu. This strategy avoids the morbidity associated with uterine incision (e.g., preterm labor, postoperative bleeding, and the necessity for cesarean delivery[21]). In the near future, many applications of open fetal surgery will be modified to be performed fetoscopically.

Briefly, for fetoscopic procedures, the mother is placed in a modified lithotomy position. Anesthetic techniques, tocolytic therapy, and maternal monitoring are used as described above. Preoperative and intraoperative sonography maps the positions of the placenta and the fetus and guides trocar placement. A low transverse abdominal incision may be necessary to expose the uterus, which must be delivered from the maternal abdomen if the placenta is anterior. Trocars are placed under ultrasound guidance to avoid injury to the placenta. Continuous irrigation using a pump irrigation system via the sheath of the hysteroscope optimizes visibility (Figure 29.1). This system maintains a constant intrauterine fluid volume, avoids the risk of air embolus with gas distention of the uterus, ensures a continuously washed operative field, improves visibility by exchanging the cloudy amniotic fluid with lactated Ringer solution, and keeps the fetus warm. One of the difficult obstacles of fetoscopy is manipulating the fetus into the correct position and keeping it there for the duration of the procedure. This frequently frustrating problem is best illustrated by the development of fetoscopic tracheal occlusion to treat congenital diaphragmatic hernia (CDH), in which a chin stitch was used to keep the fetal neck exposed by extending the head. At the end of the procedure, amniotic fluid volume is assessed by sonography and optimized. Antibiotics are infused, the trocars are withdrawn and the puncture site is closed with an absorbable suture and fibrin glue.

The ex Utero Intrapartum Treatment Procedure

The ex utero intrapartum treatment, or EXIT, procedure was originally developed to reverse temporary tracheal occlusion in patients who had undergone fetal surgery for severe CDH. In a select group of fetuses with CDH, tracheal occlusion is used to obstruct the normal egress of fetal lung fluid and to stimulate lung expansion and growth. With the airway obstructed, airway management at birth is critical. The solution is to arrange delivery in such a way that the occlusion could be removed and the airway secured while the baby remained on placental support (Figure 29.2). While the uterus is kept relaxed and with the uteroplacental blood flow intact, the fetus can remain on a maternal "heart–lung machine" while the airway is secured. Although the technique of tracheal occlusion remains under study in clinical trials, EXIT procedures have been shown to be useful for management of other causes of fetal airway obstruction, such as neck and mouth teratomas and large cystic hygromas.

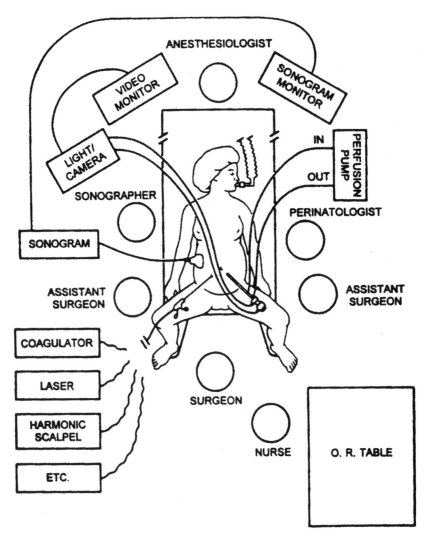

Fig. 29.1. The operating room setup for fetoscopic surgery includes two monitors at the head of the table: one for the fetoscopic picture and the other for the real-time ultrasound image. A multidisciplinary team approach, including surgeons, sonographer, anesthesiologist, perinatologist, nurse, and perfusionist is required for fetoscopic surgery.

Anatomic Defects Amenable to Fetal Surgery[19]

As stated above, the principles developed in the 1980s that underlie the clinical application of fetal surgery remain largely unchanged. Rigorous groundwork has been accomplished for a number of anomalies that are amenable to fetal surgical intervention.

Congenital Diaphragmatic Hernia[22]

CDH occurs in 1 in 2,400 births.[23] It is a defect in the diaphragmatic musculature that allows bowel to herniate into the chest cavity. In turn, compression of the lung by the bowel leads to pulmonary hypoplasia. With compressive forces limiting growth, the pulmonary

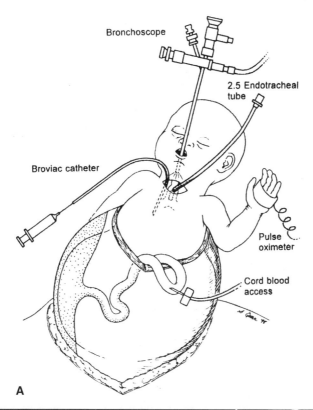

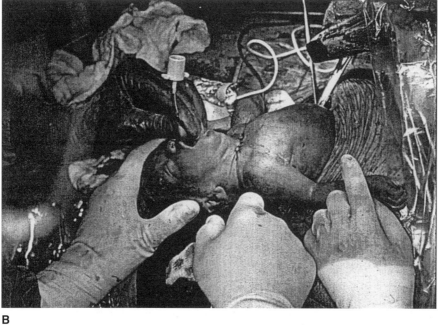

Fig. 29.2. *A,* Schematic drawing of a fetus with laryngeal atresia and congenital high airway obstruction syndrome (CHAOS) undergoing tracheostomy with a 2.5-French endotracheal tube using the EXIT strategy. *B,* EXIT procedure for a fetus at 31 weeks of gestation.

vascular bed is hypoplastic, resulting in pulmonary hypertension, and on delivery, the persistence of the fetal circulation. If these patients survive aggressive resuscitation they often require circulatory support on extracorporeal membrane oxygenation (ECMO) and extended intensive care.

Short- and long-term outcomes for treated fetuses vary due to time of diagnosis, size of the hernia, and location of treatment (see discussion in chapter 25). Survival remains poor for the most severely affected neonates as a result of their crippled pulmonary status. Tertiary referral centers with ECMO report a 70–76 percent survival rate,[24] but this mortality may be misleading because it excludes fetuses who die in utero and/or those who could not be resuscitated and supported on ECMO and died very shortly after birth.[25]

To promote lung growth and reverse the effects of potentially lethal pulmonary hypoplasia, strategies for in utero treatment have been the focus of research and development over the past two decades.[26,27] The evolution in techniques and overall treatment strategy for fetal CDH mirrors a global trend in fetal surgery. There has been a transition from open hysterotomy to minimally invasive "fetoscopic" repair, a move away from recapitulation of the postnatal repair to a direct assault on the fetal pathophysiologic defect,[20,21] and the conduct of proper randomized controlled trials,[28] rather than reliance and inference based on anecdotal case reports, to test new methods.[29]

Significant research in the natural history of this defect has defined a clinical spectrum of severity, such that fetuses with CDH are now routinely stratified into risk groups based on gestational age at diagnosis, an estimation of lung size (i.e., the lung-to-head ratio), and on the presence or absence of liver herniation (so-called liver up or liver down, respectively)[30] (see also chapter 25). These three factors are important prognostic indicators. One retrospective study demonstrated 93 percent survival in patients with liver down, compared with 43 percent survival in those with liver up.[2] The lung-to-head ratio (LHR) is calculated from ultrasound measurements of the right lung volume and the fetal head circumference obtained at 24–26 weeks of gestation. An LHR less than 1.0 is almost universally fatal, whereas a measure greater than 1.4 is associated with no mortality. An LHR from 1.0 to 1.4 has a mortality of 60 percent.[31,32]

A decade has passed since the first successful open fetal surgery for severe CDH was performed at the University of California, San Francisco.[33] The procedure involved complete anatomic repair of the diaphragmatic defect after a maternal hysterotomy and partial removal of the fetus. Although complete repair before birth was feasible, it did not improve outcome over controls. This approach has since been abandoned.[34]

Though the initial results of the in utero therapy for CDH were disappointing, further research as well as an experiment of nature (congenital tracheal atresia) led to an exciting realization: fetal tracheal occlusion can correct the pulmonary hypoplasia associated with CDH.[26,27] Normally, the fetal lung produces a continuous flow of lung fluid that exits through the trachea into the amniotic fluid. Experimentally, external drainage of fetal lung fluid retards lung growth, resulting in pulmonary hypoplasia. In contrast, tracheal obstruction accelerates lung growth resulting in pulmonary hyperplasia. Wilson et al.[26] created a fetal lamb model and showed that tracheal occlusion could prevent pulmonary hypoplasia and accelerate lung growth. Hedrick further confirmed these findings and noted that with the lung growth came some reduction of the viscera back into the abdominal cavity.[27] One detrimental effect of tracheal occlusion has been identified as a decrease in the number of type II pneumocytes and thus a decrease in the surfactant production of occluded lungs.[35–38]

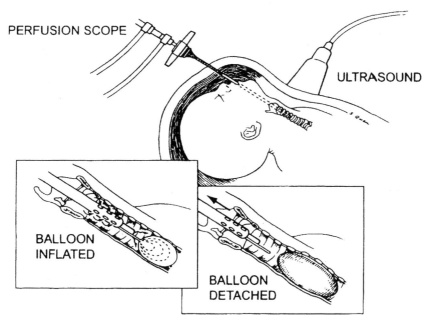

Fig. 29.3. One method for treating severe congenital diaphragmatic hernia in utero uses a detachable balloon to occlude the fetal trachea. Under sonographic and endoscopic guidance, the fetal trachea is cannulated with the telescope. After inflation, the balloon is detached 2 cm proximally to the carina (inset).

Armed with this basic research background, techniques of in utero tracheal occlusion were developed.

The fetoscopic approach now uses small scopes and video equipment, for detachable balloon placement by fetal bronchoscopy (Figure 29.3). An obvious major advantage of fetoscopic surgery was the lack of maternal hysterotomy and its associated morbidity. In a pilot study, survival for severely affected fetuses was 75 percent, compared with 40–50 percent for historic controls. The safety and efficacy of fetoscopic temporary tracheal occlusion to treat severe CDH has been tested in an NIH-sponsored trial, with the results to be published shortly. In Europe, researchers are investigating reversible in utero temporary tracheal occlusion that would allow delivery at a family's home center.

For the subset of CDH fetuses with the worst prognosis (diagnosis made at <24 weeks of gestation; liver up; LHR, <1.4), temporary occlusion of the fetal trachea accomplished without hysterotomy offers promise for improved outcomes. The future of this type of therapy depends on the enthusiastic and responsible participation of fetal surgeons to better define the limits of our capabilities, refine our technical skills, and overcome the limitations of preterm labor.[39]

Obstructive Uropathy

Obstructive uropathy occurs in 1 in 1,000 livebirths.[40] Unilateral urinary obstruction (e.g., ureteropelvic junction obstruction) has a good prognosis and usually does not require fetal intervention. Fetuses with bilateral obstruction, principally male fetuses with posterior urethral valves (PUV), are potential candidates for prenatal intervention based on the degree and duration of the obstruction.[41-43] Newborns with partial bilateral obstruction may have only mild and reversible hydronephrosis. However, children born at term with a high-grade obstruction may already have advanced hydronephrosis and renal dysplasia that is incompatible with life. The outcome of patients with urinary-tract obstruction is principally dependent on the development of oligohydramnios. Fetuses with oligohydramnios identified in the early second trimester have a mortality rate in excess of 90 percent.[44,45]

Fetuses with PUV have been salvaged by drainage of the obstructed urinary system and restoration of amniotic fluid (AF) to normal levels, initially accomplished by open fetal surgery with vesicoamniotic shunting, and now done worldwide via insertion of percutaneously placed vesicoamniotic shunts in a clinical office-based setting. Careful patient selection and timing are necessary to avoid salvaging fetuses whose lungs are functional but who go on to die from renal failure.[43] The true efficacy of this procedure is unknown because a clinical trial was never performed and the international registry is no longer active.

Prenatal ultrasound diagnosis is very accurate in the detection of fetal hydronephrosis and in determining the level of the urinary obstruction. When sonography demonstrates bilateral hydronephrosis, the initial assessment of fetal renal function is the determination of the quantity of AF. Because the majority of AF in middle and late pregnancy is the product of fetal urination, the presence of a normal AF volume implies the production and excretion of urine by at least one functioning kidney. Decreasing AF volume on serial ultrasound examinations in the setting of bilateral hydronephrosis is usually an indicator of deteriorating renal function. Renal function can then be assessed in two ways: by the appearance of the renal parenchyma on ultrasound and by the laboratory analysis of urine via bladder aspiration. The presence of cortical cysts or increased echogenicity is highly predictive of renal dysplasia; the absence of these findings, however, does not preclude it.[45] Direct sampling of the fetal urine provides critical information about fetal renal function. Normal fetal urinary chemistry includes a urinary sodium less than 100 mEq/dL, chloride less than 90 mEq/dL, osmolarity less than 200 mOsm/L, and β_2-microglobulin less than 4 mg/dL.[42,43] Values greater than these indicate that the fetal kidney is unable to resorb these molecules and predicts poor postnatal renal function. Three successive bladder aspirations must be performed, each separated by at least 24 hours. The first one empties stagnant bladder urine, the second empties the urine that was stagnant in the collecting system, and the third is most reflective of kidney function.

A dilemma in the management of fetuses with hydronephrosis is how to select fetuses with dilated urinary tracts that have a problem so severe that renal and pulmonary function may be compromised at birth, and yet have renal function that is preserved enough to profit from prenatal intervention. Only fetuses who present with (or develop) oligohydramnios with normal renal function (via urine electrolytes and protein), are less than 30 weeks of gestation, and have no associated anomalies are considered for prenatal intervention.[42,43]

The aim of prenatal intervention is to bypass or directly treat the obstruction. If the urinary tract is adequately drained, restoration of AF will enhance fetal lung growth and abrogate any further renal function deterioration. Methods of urinary-tract decompression include percutaneous vesicoamniotic shunt placement, fetoscopic vesicostomy, open vesicostomy, and fetoscopic fulguration of posterior urethral valves. Currently, the most widely used and accepted means of treating bladder outlet obstruction is by percutaneous insertion of a double-J vesicoamniotic shunt.

The outcomes of fetuses treated by this technique have been variable. Recent reports[42,43,46] confirm that persistent oligohydramnios is the best predictor of prognosis and that there must be strict selection criteria, including the presence of "normal"-appearing kidneys on ultrasound.

Congenital Cystic Adenomatoid Malformation (CCAM)

CCAM is a space-occupying congenital cystic lesion of the lung (see chapter 25) that may grow and induce hydrops by causing mediastinal shift and compromise of venous return to the heart. The presentation of hydrops is associated with a mortality rate approaching 100 percent.[47,48] The majority of fetuses diagnosed with a lung mass are found to have a CCAM that either undergoes spontaneous resolution or is best managed with close surveillance and treatment after birth.[49] A small subset of fetuses with large lung lesions will become hydropic, rapidly deteriorate, and die in utero. For this subset of fetuses, open fetal surgical resection of the lung mass, involving maternal hysterotomy, fetal thoracotomy, and ligation and resection of the mass has proven successful. The most comprehensive report to date describes over sixteen fetuses who have undergone fetal intervention, with a survival rate of >60 percent.[50]

Sacrococcygeal Teratoma[51]

Fetal sacrococcygeal teratoma is a tumor arising from the presacral space, which may grow to massive proportions and, as with CCAM, in some fetuses, induces high-output failure from tumor vascular steal[52] (see chapter 25). Maternal hysterotomy and resection of the tumor can save these rare fetuses. Recently, percutaneous radiofrequency ablation has been used to effectively stop blood flow to the tumor in four fetuses, two of whom survived, although adjacent soft-tissue injury was seen in both cases.[53]

Twin-to-Twin Transfusion Syndrome

Twin-to-twin transfusion syndrome (TTTS) is the most common and devastating complication of monochorionic twin pregnancies in which placental vascular connections result in one twin "stealing" the blood supply to the other twin, ultimately resulting in the death of both twins.[54] Wide variation in the manifestations of TTTS, including the gestational age at presentation and acuteness of onset, has been observed, and it has been theorized that the range in clinical manifestations relates to the number, size, and type of intertwin vascular connections within the shared placenta. TTTS is associated with a high risk of miscarriage, perinatal death, and subsequent handicap in survivors. It is a progressive disorder, with reported fetal mortality greater than 80 percent, if left untreated. Some cases of TTTS respond to serial, large-volume amniocenteses of the polyhydramniotic sac; a 50–60 percent survival rate has been reported with this technique.[55–57] Several authors advocate laser photocoagulation of the placental vascular anastomoses as a more direct, definitive therapy that targets active vessels, while others elect to coagulate all vessels seen crossing the intertwin septum, thereby effectively dividing the circulations.[58–60] Randomized controlled trials are under way in both Europe and the United States to compare fetoscopic laser ablation of abnormal placental vessels to amnioreduction to treat this disorder.

Myelomeningocele (MMC)

Although spina bifida (MMC) is not a fatal lesion, it is undeniably devastating (see chapter 1). Prenatal MMC treatment has brought substantial focus on this once relatively small

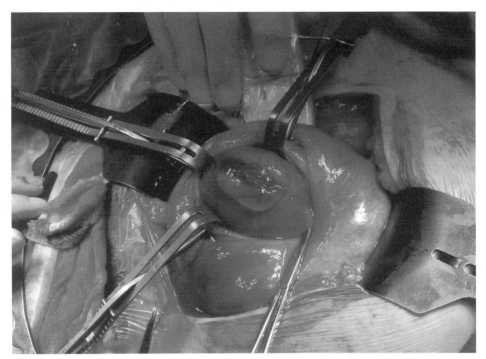

Fig. 29.4. *Left,* Exposure of the unrepaired fetal myelomeningocele sac through the hysterotomy.

field of fetal surgery. To date, over 100 women and their unborn fetuses have undergone in utero surgery to repair the spinal defect[61,62] (Figure 29.4). No fetus has been cured of the disease. From published reports and informal surveys, it appears that most fetuses show no significant improvement in their level of paralysis compared to that seen after optimal postnatal care.[63,64] However, as many as one-third of the fetuses may have improvement in the Chiari malformation, thus decreasing the need for ventriculoperitoneal shunting.[65–68] On the other hand, significant maternal and fetal complications have been associated with the surgery, including uterine rupture, maternal bleeding, fetal death, and prematurity.[69] In addition, long-term outcome for these patients is largely unknown, because follow-up for most of these fetuses has been poor. Many women elect pregnancy termination, and others chose natural birth and postnatal care for their affected offspring. For women who wish to consider treatment before birth, an NIH-sponsored multicenter randomized controlled trial of fetal MMC surgery is underway. The results of this trial are critical to establish both the safety and efficacy of this procedure before its becoming widely disseminated.

MEDICAL THERAPY

Congenital Adrenal Hyperplasia (CAH)

CAH is the first inherited inborn error of metabolism treated in utero (see full discussion in chapter 16). Prenatal therapy to prevent virilization must be begun before the determination of gender or disease status.[70–73] The general approach has been to pharmacologically suppress the fetal adrenal by giving the mother dexamethasone.[70–74]

The fundamental principles guiding efforts to prevent masculinization of the affected female fetus are logically extended to other medical fetal therapies. The concepts of a thorough informed consent procedure, thorough documentation of progress, and high-risk obstetric management have generally been followed by investigators in these fields.

Methylmalonic Acidemia

Methylmalonic acidemia is related to a functional vitamin B_{12} deficiency (see also chapter 13). Coenzymatically active vitamin B_{12} is required for the conversion of methylmalonyl–coenzyme A to succinyl$_{12}$coenzyme A. Genetically determined causes for methylmalonic acidemia include defects in methylmalonyl$_{12}$coenzyme A mutase or in the metabolism of vitamin B_{12} to the coenzymatically active form, adenosylcobalamin, by the converting enzyme. Some patients respond to large-dose B_{12} therapy, which can enhance the amount of the active holoenzyme (mutase apoenzyme plus adenosylcobalamin). There are at least five complementation groups in this enzymatic classification. Ampola and colleagues[75] were the first to attempt prenatal diagnosis and treatment of a B_{12}-responsive variant of methylmalonic acidemia. The diagnosis was made posthumously by chemical analysis of blood and urine of the proband, who died of severe acidosis and dehydration at 3 months of age. At 19 weeks of gestation, an amniocentesis was performed to make the prenatal diagnosis in a subsequent pregnancy. Elevation of methylmalonic acid content was documented in the cell-free amniotic fluid. Cultured amniocytes had defective propionate oxidation, undetectable levels of adenosylcobalamin, and normal succinate oxidation and methylmalonyl–coenzyme A mutase activity in the presence of added adenosylcobalamin. These studies established the diagnosis of methylmalonic acidemia due to deficiency synthesis of adenosylcobalamin. Maternal methylmalonyl aciduria was determined at 23 weeks of gestation, which confirmed the diagnosis. The maternal methylmalonic aciduria is known to be associated with fetal methylmalonic acidemia and not to be present in maternal heterozygotes carrying a normal fetus. The maternal urine values offer an excellent monitoring tool for fetal therapy.

Cyanocobalamin (10 mg/day) was administered orally to the mother in divided doses. A slight reduction in maternal urinary methylmalonic acid excretion was achieved, with only a marginal increase in maternal serum B_{12} levels. Therefore, at 34 weeks of gestation, 5 mg/day of cyanocobalamin administered as an intramuscular injection was initiated. The maternal serum B_{12} level rose sixfold above normal, and the maternal urinary excretion of methylmalonic acid progressively decreased to slightly above normal by delivery. Amniotic fluid methylmalonic acid levels were three to four times the normal mean level, despite prenatal treatment. Postnatally, the diagnosis of methylmalonic acidemia was confirmed. The newborn suffered no acute neonatal complications and had an extremely high serum level of vitamin B_{12}. In this case, the prenatal therapy certainly improved the fetal biochemistry and secondarily improved the maternal biochemistry. Whether there was any significant clinical benefit to this fetus cannot be sufficiently ascertained. Nyhan[76] suggested that an increased frequency of minor anomalies may be associated with untreated fetal methylmalonic acidemia. Thus, very early or perhaps even prophylactic treatment with vitamin B_{12} before prenatal diagnosis for the at-risk fetus may be indicated for the optimal therapy of B_{12}-responsive methylmalonic acidemia. It seems likely that reduction of the fetal burden of methylmalonic acidemia should have a developmental benefit and could reduce the neonatal risk. However, this remains speculative.

Evans and colleagues followed a dose–response vitamin B_{12} regimen in the treatment of methylmalonic acidemia and showed a need for an increasingly higher dose as the pregnancy progressed.[77] To maintain plasma and urinary methylmalonic acid within the normal range, vitamin B_{12} doses needed to be increased sevenfold from the first to the second trimester.

Multiple Carboxylase Deficiency

Biotin-responsive multiple carboxylase deficiency is an inborn error of metabolism in which the mitochondrial biotin-dependent enzymes, pyruvate carboxylase, propionyl–coenzyme A carboxylase, and β-methylcrotonyl coenzyme A carboxylase have diminished activity. Affected patients present as newborns or in early childhood with dermatitis, severe metabolic acidosis, and a characteristic pattern of organic acid excretion in their urine.[78] Metabolism in patients and in cells cultured in vitro can be restored toward normal levels by biotin supplementation. Such therapy has been used for fetuses affected with this severe disorder of metabolism. Roth and colleagues[79] treated a fetus without the benefit of prenatal diagnosis in a case in which two siblings had died from multiple carboxylase deficiency. The first sibling died at 3 days of age; in the second sibling, the diagnosis was made posthumously during the neonatal period. Because of the severe neonatal manifestations and the relative harmlessness of biotin, oral administration of this compound was given to the mother at a dose of 10 mg/day. No untoward effects were noted, and the maternal urinary biotin excretion increased 100-fold. Dizygotic twins were subsequently delivered at term. Cord blood and urinary organic acid profiles were normal. Cord blood biotin concentrations were fourfold and sevenfold greater than normal. Both neonatal courses were unremarkable. Cultured fibroblasts of twin B had virtually complete deficiency of all three carboxylase activities, while twin A was normal.

Packman and colleagues[80] also reported successful prenatal therapy for a fetus at risk for multiple carboxylase deficiency. These reports provide compelling evidence that biotin administration effectively prevents neonatal complications in certain patients with biotin-responsive multiple carboxylase deficiency. No toxicity has been observed. Further experience with vitamin-responsive disorders will be useful in the determination of the optimal mode and dose interval for fetal therapy.

Menkes Kinky-Hair Syndrome

Hurley and Bell[81] investigated possible deleterious effects of prenatal copper administration in mice with the recessive mutant "crinkled" gene. This is speculated to be the mouse homolog of Menkes syndrome in the human. Dietary supplementation of copper sulfate partially ameliorated the effects of the crinkled gene in the offspring. Copper nitrilotriacetate appeared to be superior to copper sulfate in increasing postnatal survival and body copper content of the mutant offspring of heterozygotes. Postnatal supplementation was not effective.

These studies may lead to insights relevant to prenatal treatment in Menkes syndrome, a sex-linked disorder characterized by progressive degeneration of neurologic function in infants. Menkes syndrome can be diagnosed in utero by demonstrating abnormally increased copper uptake in cultured amniocytes incubated in a high-copper medium,[81] but direct mutation analysis will be preferable. Menkes syndrome, like the mouse homolog, has proven refractory to postnatal copper therapy; it is conceivable that prenatal therapy may be of benefit.[82]

Future Developments

Vitamin therapy has been used in the two vitamin-responsive genetic errors of metabolism noted above. A significant number of other vitamin-responsive defects are known (see chapters 13 and 17). The in utero treatment approach would seem to be a possibility for these conditions, especially those with neonatal manifestations. We speculate that in addition to these disorders, there may be genetic defects for which prenatal vitamin E administration may be justifiable. Postnatally, vitamin E administration prevents abnormalities of leukocyte function and improves shortened red-cell survival in glutathione synthetase deficiency. Because grossly lowered intracellular glutathione levels in this mutant state seem to predispose to oxidant-mediated cellular damage, it might be desirable to consider prenatal antioxidant therapy with vitamin E. Most patients with glutathione synthetase deficiency have neurologic impairment, which can be progressive. Future studies may confirm this speculation.

In abetalipoproteinemia, which is associated with very low serum vitamin E levels, progressive and fatal neurologic impairment develops. High-dose vitamin E supplementation can slow or prevent these neurologic changes. Prenatal treatment might therefore be justifiable on an experimental basis. However, at present, it is not known when this damage begins and, therefore, when in utero treatment should be initiated.

Gene Therapy

Genetic approaches to fetal therapy using preimplantation injection of DNA into the male pronucleus of an in vitro fertilized embryo have been successful in ewes but are not likely to be used in the near future in humans. This subject has been reviewed extensively elsewhere.[83]

An alternative approach has been the use of hematopoietic stem-cell therapy, which has been successful in the prenatal treatment of X-linked severe combined immunodeficiency disorder (SCID).

Hematopoietic stem cell therapy for the treatment of congenital disease has tremendous theoretical appeal. The replacement of defective cells with normal cells during specific periods of organ development and cellular ontogeny may have significant advantages over postnatal transplantation. Regulatory events during fetal development may favor the normal incorporation of transplanted cells and their proliferation. Early in gestation, immunologic barriers that are prohibitive to postnatal cellular therapy may not exist. Finally, successful prenatal cellular therapy could prevent prenatal and completely preempt postnatal complications of the disease. Several opportunities for prenatal cellular therapy exist that need to be explored experimentally and, when appropriate, clinically. Cells that may be transplanted to treat specific target diseases include the hematopoietic stem cell (HSC), central nervous system (DNS) "stem cell," hepatocytes, myoblasts or fibroblasts, and vascular endothelial cells. The rationale for transplantation may be replacement of a defective cell lineage with normal cells, as in the treatment of immunodeficiency diseases by prenatal hematopoietic stem-cell transplantation, or the replacement of a deficient enzyme or factor by normal or genetically engineered cells, as in the treatment of inborn errors of metabolism by CNS stem cells, or hemophilia by hepatocytes. In addition, prenatal tolerance induction in preparation for postnatal cellular or organ transplantation may be a useful approach.

Prenatal Hematopoietic Stem Cell Transplantation

The engraftment and clonal proliferation of a relatively small number of normal HSCs can sustain normal hematopoiesis for a lifetime. This observation provides the compelling rationale for bone marrow transplantation (BMT) and is now supported by thousands of long-term survivors of BMT, who otherwise would have died from hematological disease. Realization of the full potential of BMT, however, continues to be limited by a critical shortage of immunologically compatible donor cells, the inability to control the recipient or donor immune response, and the requirement for recipient myeloablation to achieve engraftment. The price of human leukocyte antigen (HLA) mismatch remains high: the greater the mismatch, the higher the incidence of graft failure, graft-versus-host disease (GVHD), and delayed immunologic reconstitution. Current methods of myeloablation have high morbidity and mortality rates. In combination, these problems remain prohibitive for most patients who might benefit from BMT. A theoretically attractive alternative, which potentially can address many of the limitations of BMT, is in utero transplantation of HSC. This approach is potentially applicable to any congenital hematopoietic disease that can be diagnosed prenatally and can be cured or improved by engraftment of normal HSCs.

Rationale for in Utero Transplantation

The rationale for in utero transplantation is to take advantage of the window of opportunity created by normal ontogeny. There is a period, before population of the bone marrow and before thymic processing of self-antigen, when the fetus theoretically should be receptive to engraftment of foreign HSC without rejection and without the need for myeloablation. In the human fetus, the ideal window would appear to be before 14 weeks of gestation, before release of differentiated T lymphocytes into the circulation, and while the bone marrow is just beginning to develop sites for hematopoiesis. It certainly may extend beyond that in immunodeficiency states, particularly when T-cell development is abnormal. During this time, presentation of foreign antigen by thymic dendritic cells theoretically should result in clonal deletion of reactive T cells during the negative selection phase of thymic processing. Recent advances in prenatal diagnosis have made possible the diagnosis of a large number of congenital diseases during the first trimester. Technical advances in fetal intervention make transplantation feasible by 10–2 weeks of gestation. The ontologic window of opportunity falls well within these diagnostic and technical constraints, making application of this approach a realistic possibility.

Because of the unique fetal environment, prenatal HSC transplantation could theoretically avoid many of the current limitations of postnatal BMT. There would be no requirement for HLA matching, resulting in expansion of the donor pool. Transplanted cells would not be rejected, and space would be available in the bone marrow, eliminating the need for toxic immunosuppressive and myeloablative drugs. The mother's uterus is the ultimate sterile isolation chamber, eliminating the high risk and costly 2–4 months of isolation required after postnatal BMT and before immunologic reconstitution. Finally, prenatal transplantation would preempt the clinical manifestations of the disease, avoiding the recurrent infections, multiple transfusions, growth retardation, and other complications that cause immeasurable suffering for the patient and often compromise postnatal treatment.

Source of Donor Cells

The source of donor cells may be critical to the success of engraftment. The most obvious advantage of the use of fetal cells is the minimal number of mature T cells in fetal-liver-derived populations before 14 weeks of gestation. This alleviates any concern about GVHD and avoids the necessity of T-cell depletion, which detrimentally influences engraftment.

Although there may be important homing, proliferative, and developmental advantages to the use of fetal cells, there are practical and ethical advantages to the use of cord blood or postnatal HSC sources. There are legitimate ethical concerns regarding the use of fetal tissue for transplantation that must be addressed. In addition, fetal tissue obtained by the usual methods has a high degree of microbial contamination.[13] The transplantation of transmissible viral, fungal, or bacterial disease could have disastrous consequences for the recipient fetus or mother. Although the fetal liver is a rich source of HSCs, small size limits total cell yield, and currently, the specific donor cells are not renewable. In contrast, the use of adult-derived cells would allow a renewable, relatively infection-free, ethically acceptable source of donor cells. One appealing strategy would be tolerance induction by the in utero transplantation of highly purified adult bone marrow HSC from a living related donor, followed by single or multiple postnatal "booster" injections.

DISEASES AMENABLE TO PRENATAL TREATMENT

Generally speaking, any disease that can be diagnosed early in gestation, that is improved by BMT, and for which postnatal treatment is unsatisfactory is a target. Some diseases are far more likely to be treated successfully by prenatal transplantation than others. The list can be divided into three general categories: hemoglobinopathies, immunodeficiency disorders, and inborn errors of metabolism. Each of the diseases has unique considerations for treatment, and each may respond differently. Of particular relevance to the prenatal approach, in which experimental levels of engraftment have been relatively low, is that in many of the target diseases, engrafted normal cells would be predicted to have a significant survival advantage over diseased cells. This would have the clinical effect of amplification of the level of engraftment in the peripheral circulation. In addition, even with minimal levels of engraftment, specific tolerance for donor antigen should be induced, allowing additional cells from the same donor to be given to the tolerant recipient after birth.

Hemoglobinopathies

The sickle cell anemia and thalassemia syndromes make up the largest patient groups potentially treatable by prenatal stem-cell transplantation. Both groups can be diagnosed in the first trimester. Both have been cured by postnatal BMT, but BMT is not recommended routinely because of its prohibitive morbidity and mortality rates and the relative success of modern medical management. In both diseases, the success of BMT is indirectly related to the morbidity of the disease, that is, the younger the patient, the fewer transfusions received, and the less organ compromise from iron overload, the better the results. With both diseases, the primary questions relevant to prenatal transplantation are: (1) What levels of normal peripheral cell expression are necessary to alleviate clinical disease? and (2) Can adequate levels of donor cell engraftment be achieved by in utero HSC transplantation? At present, only indirect evidence exists to answer these questions.

In sickle cell disease (SCD), the pathophysiology is directly related to the concentration of hemoglobin S (HbS) within red cells, which results in marked rheologic abnormality, including hyperviscosity, cellular adherence, and sickling, with a result of vaso-occlusion and tissue ischemia. In examining the in vitro relationships between hematocrit (HCT) and viscosity using mixtures of sickle and normal red blood cells (RBCs), Schmalzer et al.[84] observed that the primary determinant of viscosity is the sickle HCT (fraction of RBCs that contain HbS). Adverse effects of HCT on viscosity were seen at a sickle HCT level in the low 20s. Oxygen delivery, as gauged by the maximal point on the HCT versus viscosity curve, was markedly improved by exchanging normal for sickle RBCs (even when the total HCT was held constant). The clinical correlate of this in vitro information is chronic exchange transfusion therapy, which is indicated after cerebrovascular accidents in SCD. Maintenance of the proportion of HbS below 30 percent reduces the risk of recurrent stroke from 60 to 90 percent to less than 10 percent. The maximal HbS that effectively prevents stroke is unknown, but a transfusion regimen maintaining an HbS of 50 percent was found to be effective in preventing recurrent stroke in a small study group of SCD.

The clinical manifestations of thalassemia are secondary to hypoxia related to severe anemia and ineffective erythropoiesis. It is now standard therapy to transfuse patients with thalassemia major from an early age, which suppresses endogenous erythropoiesis and maintains oxygen delivery. When instituted at an early age, this effectively prevents the bone marrow expansion and secondary bony changes as well as the hemodynamic and cardiac manifestations of the disease. The necessary normal hemoglobin (Hb) level required is controversial, but good results have been achieved with maintenance of a Hb of 9 g/dL.

Although these levels of normal Hb are higher than have been achieved experimentally (30 percent donor Hb is maximal), there would be a significant survival advantage of normal cells in both diseases. In SCD, erythrocytes have a circulating half-life of 10–20 days (normal half-life, ~120 days) before destruction. In thalassemia, most cells (80 percent) never leave the bone marrow and also have shortened survival in the periphery. Therefore, engraftment of even a few normal stem cells could result in significantly amplified levels of peripheral-donor-cell expression.

Immunodeficiency Diseases

These represent an extremely heterogeneous group of diseases (see chapter 18 for full discussion) that differ in their likelihood of cure by achievement of hematopoietic chimerism. Once again, the most likely to benefit from even low levels of donor-cell engraftment are diseases in which a survival benefit exists for normal cells. The best example of this situation is SCID. Several different molecular causes of SCID have been identified, with approximately two-thirds of cases being of X-linked recessive inheritance (X-SCID). The genetic basis of X-SCID has been defined recently[85] as a mutation of the gene encoding the common -y chain (-yc), which is a common component of several members of the cytokine receptor superfamily, including those for interleukin-2 (IL-2), IL-4, IL-7, IL-9, IL-15, and possibly IL-13. Children affected with X-SCID, therefore, have simultaneous inactivation of multiple cytokine systems, resulting in a block in thymic T-cell development and diminished T-cell response. B cells, although present in normal or even increased numbers, are dysfunctional, either because of the lack of helper T-cell function or because of an intrinsic defect in B-cell maturation. Another form of SCID is secondary to adenosine deaminase (ADA) deficiency. Clinical experience with HLA-matched sibling bone marrow or fetal liver or thymus transplantation generally has been successful without myeloablative therapy, which suggests that the lymphoid progeny of relatively few engrafted normal HSCs have a selective growth advantage in vivo over genetically defective cells.[86] The competitive advantage of nonaffected cells in X-SCID is best supported by the discovery of skewed X-inactivation in female carriers.[87] Only T cells containing the normal X chromosome are present in the circulation. Evidence that ADA production confers a survival advantage derives from the early experience with gene therapy for ADA-deficiency SCID. ADA-gene-corrected autologous T cells have persisted for prolonged periods despite discontinuation of the T-cell infusions. Transfer of ADA-gene-corrected cells versus uncorrected cells from the same SCID patient into an immunodeficient BNX mouse results in survival of the corrected cells and death of the uncorrected cells, confirming a survival advantage for ADA-producing cells, even when there is normal ADA production in the surrounding environment. Unfortunately, other diseases, such as chronic granulomatous disease, would not be expected to provide a competitive advantage for donor cells. Nevertheless, in all these conditions, even a partial reconstitution of the defective cell or component would ameliorate at least partially the clinical manifestations of the disease and should result in donor-specific tolerance. If higher levels of engraftment are needed, additional HSC transplants from the same donor could be performed after birth without fear of rejection.

We successfully treated a fetus with X-SCID in a family in which a previously afflicted child died at 7 months of age. Diagnosis by chorionic villus sampling in the second pregnancy showed another affected male. For this couple, abortion was not an option. After lengthy informed consent, paternal bone marrow was harvested, T cells were depleted, and the cells were injected intraperitoneally into the fetus beginning at about 16 weeks of gestation. Subsequent injections were performed at 17 and 18 weeks. The baby presently shows a split chimerism; all of the infant's T cells were those of the father and most of the infant's B cells were his own. He has achieved normal milestones and immune progress through 3 years of age.[88] Other cases have been recently tried, using higher T-cell concentrations, that have ended in fetal demise.[89] Many details remain to be worked out.

Biochemical Genetic Storage Disorders

An even more heterogeneous group of diseases, the lysosomal enzyme deficiency disorders, result in the accumulation of substrates such as gangliosides, mucopolysaccharides, glycogen, or sphingolipids. Depending on the specific enzyme abnormality and the compounds that accumulate, specific patterns of tissue damage and organ failure occur. These include CNS deterioration, growth failure, dysostosis multiplex and joint disability, hepatosplenomegaly, myocardial or cardiac disease, upper airway obstruction, pulmonary infiltration, corneal clouding, and hearing loss (see chapters 11 and 12). The potential efficacy of prenatal HSC transplantation for the treatment of these diseases must be considered on an individual disease basis. The purpose of BMT in these diseases is to provide HSC-derived mononuclear cells that can repopulate various organs in the body, including the liver (Kupffer cells), skin (Langerhans cells), lung (alveolar macrophages), spleen (macrophages), lymph nodes, tonsils, and brain (microglia). Patients who have been corrected by postnatal BMT, such as Gaucher disease or Maroteaux–Lamy syndrome (minimal CNS involvement), are certainly reasonable candidates for prenatal treatment. In many cases, postnatal BMT has corrected the peripheral manifestations of the disease and has arrested the neurologic deterioration but has not reversed neurologic injury that is present in disorders such as metachromatic leukodystrophy and Hurler syndrome. In these cases, the neurologic injury may begin well before birth. Postnatal maturation of the blood–brain barrier restricts access to the CNS of transplanted cells or the deficient enzyme. These considerations suggest that prenatal treatment may be necessary for a cure. The primary question is whether donor HSC-derived microglial elements would populate the CNS, providing the necessary metabolic correction within the blood–brain barrier. In my opinion, these represent the least likely group of diseases to benefit from in utero HSC transplantation.

CONCLUSION

Although still not available for many disorders, there are an increasing number of congenital and genetic abnormalities for which in utero treatment is possible and, in some cases, now routine. Advances in surgical, medical, and genetic therapies have progressed at different paces for different disorders, but there is great hope and enthusiasm that progress will continue to expand the number of disorders for which therapy can be effective.[90]

REFERENCES

1. Harrison MR. Fetal surgery: Trials, tribulations and turf. J Pediatr Surg 2003;38:275.
2. Evans ML, Harrison MR, Flake AW. Fetal therapy. Best Pract Res Clin Obstet Gyneaecol 2002;16:671.
3. Harrison MR, Evans MI, Adzick NS, et al., eds. The unborn patient: the art and science of fetal therapy, 3rd ed. Philadelphia: WB Saunders, 2001.
4. Chervenak FA, McCullough LB, Skupski D, et al. Ethical issues in the management of pregnancies complicated by fetal anomalies. Obstet Gynecol Surv 2003;58:473.
5. Lyerly AD, Cefalo RC, Socol M, et al. Attitudes of maternal-fetal specialists concerning maternal-fetal surgery. Am J Obstet Gynecol 2001;185:1052.
6. Lyerly AD, Gates EA, Cefalo RC, et al. Toward the ethical evaluation and use of maternal-fetal surgery. Obstet Gynecol. 2001;98:689.
7. Harrison, MR, Filly RA, Golbus MS, et al. Fetal treatment 1982. N Engl J Med 1982;307:1651.
8. Harrison MR, Anderson J, Rosen MA, et al. Fetal surgery in the primate. I. Anesthetic, surgical and tocolytic management to maximize fetal-neonatal survival. J Pediatr Surg 1982;17:115.
9. Adzick NS, Harrison MR, Glick PL, et al. Fetal surgery in the primate. III. Maternal outcome after fetal surgery. J Pediatr Surg 1986;21:477.
10. Brans YW, Kuehl TJ. Nonhuman primates in perinatal research. New York: Wiley, 1988.
11. Nakayama DK, Harrison MR, Seron-Ferre M, et al. Fetal surgery in the primate. II. Uterine electromyographic response to operative procedures and pharmacologic agents. J Pediatr Surg 1984;19:333.
12. Farrell JA, Albanese CT, Jennings RW, et al. Maternal fertility is not affected by fetal surgery. Fetal Diagn Ther 1999;14:190.
13. DiFederico EM, Burlingame JM, Kilpatrick SJ, et al. Pulmonary edema in obstetric patients is rapidly resolved except in the presence of infection or of nitroglycerin tocolysis after open fetal surgery. Am J Obstet Gynecol 1998;179;925.
14. Hamel H, Bonniaud P, Baudouin N, et al. Pulmonary edema and tocolysis with beta agonists. Rev Mal Respir 2002;19:241.
15. DiFederico EM, Harrison M, Matthay MA. Pulmonary edema in a woman following fetal surgery. Chest 1996;109:1114.
16. Noah MM, Norton ME, Sandberg P, et al. Short-term maternal outcomes that are associated with the EXIT procedure, as compared with cesarean delivery. Am J Obstet Gynecol 2002;186:773.
17. Cauldwell CB, Rosen MA, Jennings RW. Anesthesia and monitoring for fetal intervention. In: Harrison MR, Evans MI, Adzick NS, et al., eds. The unborn patient: the art and science of fetal therapy, 3rd ed. Philadelphia: WB Saunders, 2001:149.
18. Harrison MR and Adzick NS. Open fetal surgical techniques. In: Harrison MR, Evans MI, Adzick NS, et al. (eds): The unborn patient: the art and science of fetal therapy, 3rd ed. Philadelphia: WB Saunders, 2001:247.
19. Kitano Y, Flake AW, Crombleholme TM, et al. Open fetal surgery for life-threatening fetal malformations. Semin Perinatol 1999;23:448.
20. Albanese CT, Harrison MR. Surgical treatment for fetal disease: the state of the art. Ann NY Acad Sci 1998;847:74.
21. Sydorak RM, Albanese CT. Minimal access techniques for fetal surgery. World J Surg 2003;27:95.
22. Jennings RW, Adzick NS, Longaker MT, et al. New techniques in fetal surgery. J Pediatr Surg 1992;27:1329.

23. Butler N, Claireaux AE. Congenital diaphragmatic hernia as a cause of perinatal mortality. Lancet 1962;1:659.
24. Adzick NS, Harrison MR., Glick PL, et al. Diaphragmatic hernia in the fetus: prenatal diagnosis and outcome in 94 cases. J Pediatr Surg 1985;20:357.
25. Harrison MR, Bjordal RI, Langmark F, et al. Congenital diaphragmatic hernia: the hidden mortality. J Pediatr Surg 1978;13:227.
26. Wilson JM, DiFiore JW, Peters CA. Experimental fetal tracheal ligation prevents the pulmonary hypoplasia associated with fetal nephrectomy: possible application for CDH. J Pediatr Surg 1993;28:1433.
27. Hedrick MH, Estes JM, Sullivan KM, et al. Plug the lung until it grows (PLUG): a new method to treat congenital diaphragmatic hernia in utero. J Pediatr Surg 1994;29:612.
28. Harrison MR, Sydorak RM, Farrell JA, et al. Fetoscopic temporary tracheal occlusion for congenital diaphragmatic hernia: prelude to a randomized, controlled trial. J Pediatr Surg 2003;38:1012.
29. Harrison MR, Albanese CT, Hawgood SB, et al. Fetoscopic temporary tracheal occlusion by means of detachable balloon for congenital diaphragmatic hernia. Am J Obstet Gynecol 2001;185:730.
30. Metkus AP, Filly RA, Stringer MD, et al. Sonographic predictors of survival in fetal diaphragmatic hernia. J Pediatr Surg 1996;31:148.
31. Lipshutz GS, Albanese CT, Feldstein VA, et al. Prospective analysis of lung-to-head ratio predicts survival for patients with prenatally diagnosed congenital diaphragmatic hernia. J Pediatr Surg 1997;32:1634.
32. Keller RL, Glidden DV, Paek BW, et al. The lung-to-head ratio and fetoscopic temporary tracheal occlusion: prediction of survival in severe left congenital diaphragmatic hernia. Ultrasound Obstet Gynecol 2003;21;244.
33. Harrison MR, Adzick NS, Longaker MT, et al. Successful repair in utero of a fetal diaphragmatic hernia after removal of herniated viscera from the left thorax. N Engl J Med 1990;323:1279.
34. Harrison MR, Adzick NS, Bullard KM, et al. Correction of congenital diaphragmatic hernia in utero VII: a prospective trial. J Pediatr Surg 1997;32:1637.
35. Bin Saddiq W, Piedboeuf B, Laberge JM, et al. The effects of tracheal occlusion and release on type II pneumocytes in fetal lambs. J Pediatr Surg 1997;32:834.
36. Yoshizawa J, Chapin CJ, Sbragia L, et al. Tracheal occlusion stimulates cell cycle progression and type I cell differentiation in lungs of fetal rats. Am J Physiol Lung Cell Mol Physiol. 2003;285:L344.
37. Bullard KM, Sonne J, Hawgood S, et al. Tracheal ligation increases cell proliferation but decreases surfactant protein in fetal murine lungs in vitro. J Pediatr Surg 1997;32:207; discussion 211–13.
38. Flageole H, Evrard VA, Piedboeuf B, et al. The plug-unplug sequence: an important step to achieve type II pneumocyte maturation in the fetal lamb model. J Pediatr Surg 1998;33:299.
39. Dennes WJB and Bennett PR. Preterm labor: The Achilles heel of fetal intervention. In: Harrison MR, Evans MI, Adzick NS, et al., eds. The unborn patient: the art and science of fetal therapy, 3rd ed. Philadelphia: WB Saunders, 2001:171.
40. Johnson MP. Fetal obstructive uropathy. In: Harrison MR, Evans MI, Adzick NS, et al., eds. The unborn patient: the art and science of fetal therapy, 3rd ed. Philadelphia: WB Saunders, 2001:259.
41. Freedman AL, Johnson MP, Gonzalez R. Fetal therapy for obstructive uropathy: past, present, future? Pediatr Nephrol 2000;14:167.
42. Johnson MP, Bukowski TP, Reitleman C, et al. In utero surgical treatment of fetal obstructive uropathy: a new comprehensive approach to identify appropriate candidates for vesicoamniotic shunt therapy. Am J Obstet Gynecol 1994;170:1770.
43. Crombleholme TM, Harrison MR, Golbus MS, et al. Fetal intervention in obstructive uropathy: prognostic indicators and efficacy of intervention. Am J Obstet Gynecol 1990;162:1239.
44. Brophy MM, Austin PF, Yan Y, et al. Vesicoureteral reflux and clinical outcomes in infants with prenatally detected hydronephrosis. J Urol 2002;168:1716.
45. Estroff JA, Mandell J, Benacerraf BR. Increased rental parenchymal echogenicity in the fetus: importance and clinical outcome. Radiology 1991;181:135.
46. Freedman AL, Johnson MP, Smith CA, et al. Long-term outcome in children after antenatal intervention for obstructive uropathies. Lancet 1999;354:374.
47. Miller JA, Corteville JE, Langer JC. Congenital cystic adenomatoid malformation in the fetus: natural history and predictors of outcome. J Pediatr Surg 1996;31:805.
48. Adzick NS, Harrison MR, Glick PL. et al. Fetal cystic adenomatoid malformation: prenatal diagnosis and natural history. J Pediatr Surg 1985;20:483.
49. Adzick NS, Harrison MR, Crombleholme TM, et al. Fetal lung lesions: management and outcome. Am J Obstet Gynecol 1998;179:884.

50. De Santis M, Masini L, Noia G, et al. Congenital cystic adenomatoid malformation of the lung: antenatal ultrasound findings and fetal-neonatal outcome: fifteen years of experience. Fetal Diagn Ther 2000;15:246.

51. Flake AW. Fetal sacrococcygeal teratoma. Semin Pediatr Surg 1993;2:113.

52. Langer JC, Harrison MR, Schmidt KG, et al. Fetal hydrops and death from sacrococcygeal teratoma: rationale for fetal surgery. Am J. Obstet Gynecol 1989;160:1145.

53. Paek BW, Jennings RW, Harrison MR, et al. Radiofrequency ablation of human fetal sacrococcygeal teratoma. Am J Obstet Gynecol 2001;184:503.

54. Farmer DL and Hirose S. Fetal intervention for complications of monochorionic twinning. World J Surg 2003;27:103.

55. Trespidi L, Boschetto C, Caravelli E, et al. Serial amniocenteses in the management of twin-twin transfusion syndrome: when is it valuable? Fetal Diagn Ther 1997;12:15.

56. Elliott JP, Urig MA, Clewell WH. Aggressive therapeutic amniocentesis for treatment of twin-twin transfusion syndrome. Obstet Gynecol 1991;77:537.

57. Abdel-Fattah SA, Carroll SG, Kyle PM, et al. Amnioreduction: how much to drain? Fetal Diagn Ther 1999;14:279.

58. De Lia JE, Kuhlmann RS, Harstad TW, et al. Fetoscopic laser ablation of placental vessels in severe previable twin-twin transfusion syndrome. Am J Obstet Gynecol 1995;172;1202.

59. Quintero RA, Morales WJ, Mendoza G, et al. Selective photocoagulation of placental vessels in twin-twin transfusion syndrome: evolution of a surgical technique. Obstet Gynecol Surv 1998;53:S97.

60. Quintero RA, Comas C, Bornick PW, et al. Selective versus non-selective laser photocoagulation of placental vessels in twin-to-twin transfusion syndrome. Ultrasound Obstet Gynecol 2000;16:230.

61. Sutton LN, Adzick NS, Bilaniuk LT, et al. Improvement in hindbrain herniation demonstrated by serial fetal magnetic resonance imaging following fetal surgery for myelomeningocele. JAMA 1999;282:1826.

62. Burner JP, Tulipan N, Paschall RL, et al. Fetal surgery for myelomeningocele and the incidence of shunt-dependent hydrocephalus. JAMA 1999;282:1819.

63. Tulipan N, Hernanz-Schulman M, Lowe LH, et al. Intrauterine myelomeningocele repair reverses preexisting hindbrain herniation. Pediatr Neurosurg 1999;31:137.

64. Tubbs RS, Chambers MR, Smyth MD, et al. Late gestational intrauterine myelomeningocele repair does not improve lower extremity function. Pediatr Neurosurg 2003;38:128.

65. Tulipan N, Hernanz-Schulman M, Bruner JP. Reduced hindbrain herniation after intrauterine myelomeningocele repair: a report of four cases. Pediatr Neurosurg 1998;29:274.

66. Tulipan N. Sutton LN, Bruner JP, et al. The effect of intrauterine myelomeningocele repair on the incidence of shunt-dependent hydrocephalus. Pediatr Neurosurg 2003;38:27.

67. Holmes NM, Nguyen HT, Harrison MR, et al. Fetal intervention for myelomeningocele: effect on postnatal bladder function. J Urol 2001;166:2383.

68. Walsh DS, Adzick NS, Sutton LN, et al. The rationale for in utero repair of myelomeningocele. Fetal Diagn Ther 2001;16:312.

69. Flake AW. Prenatal intervention: ethnical considerations for life-threatening and non-life-threatening anomalies. Semin Pediatr Surg 2001;10:212.

70. Evans, MI, Chrousos GP, Mann DL, et al. Pharmacologic suppression of the fetal adrenal gland in utero: attempted prevention of abnormal, external genital masculinization in suspected congenital adrenal hyperplasia. JAMA 1985;253:1015.

71. David M, Forrest M. Prenatal treatment of congenital adrenal hyperplasia resulting from 21-hydroxylase deficiency. J Pediatr 1984;105:799.

72. Pang S, Pollack MS, Marshall RN, et al. Prenatal treatment of congenital adrenal hyperplasia due to 21-hydroxylase deficiency. N Engl J Med 1990;322:111.

73. Forrest MG, David M. Prevention of sexual ambiguity in children with 21-hydroxylase deficiency by treatment in utero. Pediatr 1992;47:351.

74. Miller WL. Genetics, diagnosis and management of 21-hydroxylase deficiency. J Clin Endocrinol Metab 1994;78:241.

75. Ampola MG, Mahoney MJ, Nakamura E. Prenatal therapy of a patient with vitamin B_{12} responsive methylmalonic acidemia. N. Engl J Med 1975;293:313.

76. Nyhan WL. Prenatal treatment of methylmalonic acidemia. N Engl J Med 1975;293:353.

77. Evans MI, Duquette DA, Rinaldo P. et al. Modulation of B_{12} dosage and response in fetal treatment of methylmalonic aciduria (MMA): titration of treatment dose to serum and urine MMA. Fetal Diagn Ther 1997;12:21.

78. Scriver C, Beaudet A, Valle D. The metabolic basis of inherited disease, 7th ed. New York: McGraw-Hill, 1994.

79. Roth KS, Yang W, Allen L. Prenatal administration of biotin: biotin responsive multiple carboxylase deficiency. Pediatr Res 1982;16:126.

80. Packman S, Cowan MJ, Golbus MS. Prenatal treatment of biotin responsive multiple carboxylase deficiency. Lancet 1982;1:1425.

81. Hurley LS, Bell LT. Genetic influence on response to dietary manganese deficiency in mice. J Nutr 1974;104:133.

82. Stevenson RE, Hall JG, Goodman RM. Human malformations and related anomalies. New York: Oxford University Press, 1993.

83. Yaron Y, Kramer R, Johnson MP, et al. Gene therapy: is the future here yet? Obstet Gynecol Clin North Am 1997;24:179.

84. Schmalzer EA, Lee JO, Brown AK, el al. Viscosity of mixtures of sickle and normal red cells at varying hematocrit levels: Implications for transfusion. Transfusion 1987;27:228.

85. Noguchi M, Yi H, Rosenblatt HM, et al. Interleukin-2 receptor gamma chain mutation results in X-linked severe combined immunodeficiency in humans. Cell 1993;73:147.

86. Buckley RH, Schiff SE, Schiff RI, et al. Haploidentical bone marrow stem cell transplantation in human severe combined immunodeficiency. Semin Hematol 1993;30–92.

87. Puck JM, Stewart CC, Nussbaum RL. Maximum-likelihood analysis of human T-cell X chromosome inactivation patterns: normal women versus carriers of X-linked severe combined immunodeficiency. Am J Hum Genet 1992;50:742.

88. Flake AW, Puck JM, Almieda-Porada G, et al. Successful in utero correction of X-linked recessive severe combined immunodeficiency (X-SCID): fetal intraperitoneal transplantation of CD34 enriched paternal bone marrow cells (EPPBMC). N Engl J Med 1996;335:1806.

89. Blakemore K, Bambach B, Moser H, et al. Engraftment following in utero bone marrow transplantation for globoid cell leukodystrophy. Am J Obstet Gynecol 1996;174:312.

90. Flake AW. Surgery in the human fetus: the future. J Physiol (Lond) 2003;547:45.

Fernand Daffos, M.D., François Jacquemard, M.D.,
Véronique Mirlesse, M.D., Stéphane Romand, M.D.,
and Philippe Thulliez, M.D.

30

Prenatal Diagnosis of Fetal Infection

Viral infection of the embryo or fetus via hematogenous transplacental spread may result in death and resorption of the embryo, abortion and stillbirth of the fetus, prematurity, intrauterine growth restriction, and developmental anomalies. Fortunately, despite the frequency of fetal infection (see below), the vast majority of infected newborns are not affected. Some, however, may manifest the consequences of infection in utero only months to years later (e.g., deafness, chorioretinitis).

The discussion in this brief chapter focuses on the most common infections that clearly cause fetal anomalies (toxoplasmosis, cytomegalovirus, varicella, rubella, and parvovirus) and are also detectable by DNA studies. For further in-depth study, other sources and reviews are available.[1–14]

PRENATAL DIAGNOSIS OF FETAL TOXOPLASMOSIS

Since 1985, prenatal diagnosis of congenital toxoplasmosis has been reliably performed in women with suspected or confirmed *Toxoplasma* infection acquired during pregnancy.[15] Availability of prenatal diagnosis has profoundly changed the management of fetal infection before birth through the use of specific algorithms for decisions regarding prenatal treatment or termination of pregnancy, which previously were mostly on the sole basis of maternal infection. Consequently, termination of pregnancy for maternal infection with *Toxoplasma gondii* has now become unusual, thanks to prenatal diagnosis along with the possibility of treatment of the infected fetus in utero via the mother, with the combination regimen of pyrimethamine and sulfonamides.[16] These major advances in the field of diagnosis and therapy has facilitated a change in the indications for medical termination of pregnancy for toxoplasmosis almost exclusively for cases with severe lesions detected by ultrasonography.

Since the early 1990s, the introduction of polymerase chain reaction (PCR) techniques applied to amniotic fluid (AF) cells represented a major breakthrough for a more accurate, safe, simple, and rapid result of prenatal diagnosis compared with previously used techniques requiring both amniocentesis and fetal blood sampling.

Indications for Prenatal Diagnosis

Prenatal diagnosis could be recommended for all women with proven or highly suspected *Toxoplasma* primary infection during pregnancy. Because of a low rate and lack of specificity of clinical signs, a diagnosis of *Toxoplasma* infection is best established by systematic serologic screening of nonimmune pregnant women. This screening allows an accurate and early diagnosis of maternal infection but is recommended on a systematic basis only in France and Austria. Clinical signs are present in less than 40 percent of women and are often neglected and nonspecific: asthenia, low-grade fever, myalgia, and lymphadenopathy.[17]

Given the limited but significant risk of fetal loss associated with cordocentesis or amniocentesis, prenatal diagnosis should be restricted to only proven or highly suspected cases of maternal primary infection. In addition, the risk of maternal–fetal transmission of *T. gondii* as well as severity of fetal infection varies according to the gestational age at the time of maternal infection and should be considered before a decision is made about prenatal diagnosis. It should be kept in mind that the most severe consequences of fetal infection are most frequently observed in the rare cases of early maternal–fetal transmission, whereas a large majority (85 percent) of infants appear normal at birth as a result of late, but more frequent vertical transmission.[17] A recent collaborative study precisely estimated that the risk of maternal–fetal transmission is low (<10 percent) before 13 weeks but sharply increases for infections acquired later (40 percent at 26 weeks and >80 percent just before delivery).[18] Thus, prenatal diagnosis is questionable for periconceptional infections because in these cases, the risk of fetal loss following amniocentesis (approximately 0.5 percent) is equivalent to or higher than the risk of congenital toxoplasmosis.[19] Conversely, in cases of late maternal infection during the third trimester or for those occurring a few days before expected delivery, the estimated risk of fetal infection is so high that a presumptive curative treatment combining pyrimethamine plus sulfonamides (see below) without prenatal diagnosis must be considered.[20]

Prenatal Diagnosis with the Use of the PCR Test

Following initial promising results in experimental studies, Grover et al. first reported on the accuracy and usefulness of PCR for direct detection of *T. gondii* DNA in AF.[21,22] In this study, PCR targeting a portion of the thirtyfold repeated B1 sequence gene of *T. gondii* was more sensitive than mouse inoculation or tissue culture; it detected *T. gondii* in eight of ten AF samples of cases with proven congenital infection. Other promising results were obtained with PCR detection of several DNA targets of *T. gondii*, including the single copy gene of surface protein P30[23,24] or a 100-fold repeated sequence of 18s ribosomal DNA.[25] For the first time, a simple method of prenatal diagnosis based on AF analysis enabled reliable results to be obtained within a short period (24 hr). Moreover, fetal blood sampling, which carries a higher risk of fetal loss[26] than amniocentesis would no longer be necessary. However, in these initial studies, sporadic false-positive reactions occurred and optimal sensitivity was not achieved. Although most laboratories now use the B1 protein gene as the most relevant and reliable target in routine practice, the PCR technique, because of its widespread use is far from being standardized and its sensitivity and specificity may vary greatly between laboratories.[27] Thus, the diagnostic value of PCR on AF largely depends on the experience and technical ability within each laboratory.

More recently, Antsaklis et al.,[28] in a study of ninety-three women with *T. gondii* seroconversion during pregnancy, reported on the efficacy of PCR for prenatal diagnosis of fetal infection. Eighteen pregnancies (19.4 percent) showed evidence of fetal infection. Of the twelve subjected to PCR, ten (83.3 percent) were positive. When PCR analysis was combined with mouse inoculation with AF, a prenatal detection rate of 94.4 percent was achieved.

Specificity of Prenatal Diagnosis with PCR

In our experience as well as in other reference centers for prenatal diagnosis, a positive PCR denotes fetal infection, as long as no contamination has occurred during testing, because all positive prenatal diagnoses are confirmed either by conventional methods or by subsequent autopsy findings or serologic postnatal follow-up.[19,29] However, important variations in specificity of PCR between different laboratories were identified in two recent interlaboratory comparison studies of artificial AF samples without *T. gondii* or spiked with known amounts of *T. gondii* DNA or whole tachyzoites.[27,30] All laboratories were known to perform PCR methods with a high level of sensitivity. Nevertheless, in each study, two of five and four of fifteen evaluated laboratories found one or more control samples to be falsely positive. These discrepancies could be related to the choice of relevant primers, but also to specific in-house developed procedures of the reaction as well as with preanalytical treatment of the clinical sample, which may differ in many ways. However, no particular PCR protocol could be clearly related with a higher risk of false-positive results, although laboratories using nested PCR seemed to have a higher rate of false-positive tests. It must be emphasized that in five of six false-positive results, uracil–DNA–glycosylase was not used to prevent carryover contamination of samples. These investigations also highlighted contamination risks associated with handling steps. Real-time PCR instruments have recently emerged as a significant breakthrough in the reliability of PCR assays because reaction tubes no longer need to be opened after amplification steps, thus avoiding the main source of potential contamination by amplicons from previous reactions.[31]

Because a decision-making process currently relies almost exclusively on the result of PCR analysis of AF, it is of utmost importance that specificity and positive predictive value of prenatal diagnosis using PCR be optimized to prevent any unnecessary potentially toxic treatment or termination of pregnancy. Thus, given the important rate of false-positive results found in some laboratories, some authors strongly recommend that PCR alone should not be used for the prenatal diagnosis of congenital infection.[27] In this view, mouse inoculation with AF could be considered as an additional method to overcome some possible important variations in quality of testing with PCR. Besides, this latter method allows the isolation and preservation of *T. gondii* strains. However, PCR on AF has proved far more sensitive than any other diagnostic test, and in a number of cases a positive PCR can be the only method to demonstrate a fetal infection in otherwise asymptomatic children.

Sensitivity of Prenatal Diagnosis with PCR

Differences in Sensitivity in Relation to the Techniques Used. A number of studies have demonstrated the reliability and higher sensitivity of PCR compared with conventional methods.[17] In 1994 Hohlfeld et al. reported a significant improvement in B1-PCR reliability with the addition of an internal positive control to monitor sensitivity of PCR reaction to avoid false-negative results.[19] This study reported a PCR sensitivity of 97.4 percent (and a negative predictive value of 99.7 percent), compared with an overall sensitivity of parasitologic tests ranging from 64 percent to 72 percent. Finally, these results have demonstrated that a reliable PCR test performed on AF could be considered as a complete alternative to other conventional methods. A recently developed real-time PCR assay targeting a newly described 529-bp 300-fold repeated genomic fragment of *T. gondii* demonstrated a 10- to 100-fold higher sensitivity by quantitative PCR in AF, as compared with the 35-fold repeated B1 gene.[32,33] This newly characterized genomic target likely represents an improvement of sensitivity of prenatal diagnosis with PCR assays.

Nevertheless, significant variations in sensitivity between investigators have also been demonstrated by Pelloux et al.[27] using artificial AF samples spiked with tachyzoîtes of *T. gondii*. Among fifteen European laboratories involved in prenatal diagnosis, nine were able to detect a single parasite, whereas two found no *Toxoplasma* in any of the eight positive aliquots. Again, no clear link with specific PCR procedures was found to explain such important discrepancies, but it also appeared that sensitivity of PCR for prenatal diagnosis should also include preanalytical steps, including timing of sampling and preparation of AF sample for PCR analysis. Because replication of *T. gondii* is intracellular, PCR tests performed in pellets of fetal cells likely achieve higher sensitivity than on whole AF samples but also carry a higher risk of PCR inhibitors. In some reports, a rather low sensitivity could be explained by an amniocentesis performed too soon after maternal infection (before detection of specific IgG) or too early during gestation.[34] Previous studies have documented the possibility of delayed transplacental transfer of parasites, hence it is recommended that amniocentesis be done at least 4 weeks after the estimated date of maternal infection to optimize the rate of DNA recovery from AF.[19,29] On the other hand, reliability of PCR before 18 weeks of gestation has not been evaluated and should not be recommended because of the low fetal cell concentration in AF.

The current recommendations for an accurate prenatal diagnosis of congenital toxoplasmosis are summarized in Table 30.1.

Differences in Sensitivity in Relation to the Selection of Cases. In a number of cases, differences between investigators in PCR sensitivity are likely to be explained not only

Table 30.1. Recommendations for prenatal diagnosis of congenital toxoplasmosis

Indication	Maternal primary *Toxoplasma* infection during pregnancy
Amniocentesis	>18th week of pregnancy
	>4 weeks after maternal infection
	AF sample = 10 to 20 mL
Technique	PCR on AF
	+
	Mouse inoculation with AF
PCR	Target: B1 gene or 529-bp multicopy genomic fragment
	DNA extraction
	Monitoring of sensitivity (internal control)
	Prevention of contamination (uracil–DNA–glycosylase)
Delay of result	PCR = 24 hr
	Mouse inoculation = 3 to 6 weeks

by a lack of a technical standard but also by major differences in the selection and definition of cases of congenital infection. So far, in most studies, performances of PCR have been assessed comparatively with conventional prenatal diagnostic methods, without taking into account the definitive status of infants with negative prenatal diagnosis, which can be determined only after birth and during subsequent long-term follow-up of the child.[19,35] Therefore, the sensitivity and negative predictive values of PCR on AF may be overestimated, because a significant number of offspring are lost to follow-up after birth. A recent prospective study conducted in 270 cases of maternal seroconversion with prenatal diagnosis and long-term follow-up after birth revealed an overall sensitivity of B1-targeted PCR of only 64 percent (95 percent confidence interval [CI], 53–75 percent) and a negative predictive value of 88 percent (95 percent CI, 84–92 percent).[29] Moreover, this study also demonstrated that sensitivity of PCR was linked to the gestational age at maternal infection and performed optimally for maternal infection occurring during the second trimester. A diminished sensitivity of PCR was observed for maternal infection occurring after 30 weeks, possibly resulting from low parasite concentrations, as shown by recent studies using quantitative PCR in AF samples.[36] Therefore, given the high rate of maternal–fetal transmission during the third trimester, these results may raise the question of a presumptive specific anti-*Toxoplasma* treatment (Table 30.2) without amniocentesis in case of maternal infection occurring late during pregnancy.[20]

Therapeutic Options

Positive Prenatal Diagnosis

A positive PCR in AF denotes fetal infection. The severity of congenital toxoplasmosis depends on gestational age at seroconversion: early fetal infections most likely result in fetal death or serious sequelae (ventriculomegaly associated with cerebral calcifications and chorioretinitis), whereas almost all fetuses infected during the third trimester are asymptomatic at birth.[17] Hence, in cases of fetal infection, proven by PCR analysis, in association with abnormal findings at ultrasound monitoring, a decision for medical termination should be considered, given the poor prognosis of congenital symptomatic infection. On the other hand, a specific antiparasitic treatment combining pyrimethamine and sulfonamide should be offered to otherwise infected fetuses without signs[16] (Table 30.2). The treatment regimen is administered orally via the mother and is designed to prevent and reduce infectious sequelae, due to its synergistic activity against *T. gondii*.[37] A more difficult situation could be encountered for early fetal infections (<20 weeks) with no ultrasonographic signs and for which both therapeutic options (termination vs medical treatment) could be discussed. A recent study identified quantitative real-time PCR in AF as a promising prognostic marker of fetal infection and could be of value for therapeutic decisions in case of early acquired fetal infection without signs of abnormality.[36]

Table 30.2. Prenatal treatment

Indication	Drug	Dose	Duration
Positive PCR in AF or	Pyrimethamine	50 mg/day	
Late maternal infection	Sulfadiazine	1.5 g × 2/day	Until delivery
	Folinic acid	50 mg /week	

Negative Prenatal Diagnosis

A negative PCR in AF cannot completely rule out congenital infection, due to either a delayed transplacental transmission after amniocentesis or a low *T. gondii* concentration, below the detection threshold of PCR assays. Therefore, in cases of negative prenatal diagnosis, careful ultrasonographic monitoring should be recommended to detect some rare cases of delayed symptomatic infections.[19,29] After delivery, a placental examination should be performed together with a serologic follow-up of the child, to rule out congenital infection.

CONCLUSION

Direct detection of *Toxoplasma* DNA in AF PCR is currently viewed as the most sensitive, specific, safe, and rapid method for diagnosis of fetal infection. As far as a PCR method is considered totally specific for *Toxoplasma* infection, it reliably represents a complete alternative to other conventional methods of prenatal diagnosis. However, because the risk of amniocentesis is not negligible, this procedure should be offered only to pregnant women with serologically proven or highly suspected primary infection.

PRENATAL DIAGNOSIS OF FETAL CYTOMEGALOVIRUS INFECTION

Cytomegalovirus (CMV) is the largest virus of the herpesviridae family. Like all herpesviruses (herpes simplex types I and II, herpesvirus varicella, Epstein–Barr virus, human herpes viridae VI, VII, and VIII), it undergoes latency and reactivation.

CMV is the most common infectious agent known to be transmitted from the mother to the fetus during pregnancy and is the major viral cause of congenital infections.[38] Leading to global damage of the brain, CMV infection is also the major cause of infectious congenital deafness and of sensorineural sequelae. Sensorineural hearing loss contributes to the educational deficit of these children, many of them requiring long-term care and special educational support.

Thus, there is a medical need for reducing disease attributed to congenital CMV infection, by prevention of maternal infection, prenatal diagnosis of infected fetuses, attempts at treatment with an effective therapy during pregnancy and after birth, and vaccine development.

CMV occurs in 0.3 to 2 percent of all livebirths. The estimated number of infants with congenital infection born annually in the United States, United Kingdom, and France are shown in Table 30.3.

Table 30.3. Annual public health impact of congenital CMV

	United States[39]	United Kingdom[39]	France[40]
No. of live births	4,000,000	700,000	750,000
No. with congenital infection	40,000 (1%)	2,100 (0.3%)	7,500 (1%)
No. with CMV disease	2,800 (7%)	147 (7%)	750 (10%)
No. with fatal disease	336 (12%)	18 (12%)	75 (10%)
No. with sequelae	2,218 (79%)	116 (80%)	480 (64%)
No. asymptomatic	37,200 (93%)	1,953 (93%)	6,750 (90%)
No. with sequelae	5,580 (15%)	293 (15%)	675 (10%)
Total no. damaged	8,134 (20%)	427 (20%)	1,230 (16%)

In Europe, the prevalence of antibody to CMV in childbearing women is around 60 percent, whereas it is higher for populations of low socioeconomic status, presumably a reflection of factors such as crowding, sexual practices, and increasing exposure to infants.[41] The risk of contamination is very important for seronegative women in contact with children or immunocompromised patients with massive viral excretion. In populations with high seropositivity rates, the risk of transmission is most important for seronegative people. In day care centers, the incidence of primary infection is fourfold to tenfold higher than in the general population.[42]

According to low or high socioeconomic status, the risk of primary maternal infection is about three times higher among the higher-income susceptible women (45 percent), compared with 15 percent in the lower-income group. In both groups, transmission to the fetus occurred in about 30–40 percent of cases. More than 10–15 percent of congenitally infected neonates are symptomatic at birth, and 85 to 90 percent are asymptomatic congenitally infected newborns. Among the asymptomatic newborns, sequelae developed in about 10 percent, while about 90 percent of infants that were asymptomatic at birth developed normally.[43]

Pathogenesis of Congenital Infection

When primary maternal infection occurs, the virus can be transmitted to the fetus by infected maternal lymphocytes. The maternal immune response begins proximate to virus transmissions, whereas in the case of recurrent infection, virus transmission occurs in the presence of both humoral and cell-mediated immune responses.

CMV is excreted in urine, saliva, cervix, oropharyngeal secretions, semen, blood and transplanted organs, and milk. The spread of infection appears to require close or intimate contacts with infected secretions. Women of childbearing age usually acquire CMV from their children, who became infected in day care centers. The higher risk of seroconversion is for parents with a child attending day care, shedding CMV in saliva and urine. Transfer of virus occurs after contact with diapers or oral secretions, and urine on hands, particularly with a child who is in day care. CMV has been shown to retain infectivity for hours on plastic surfaces and has been isolated from toys and surfaces in day care centers.

Transmission of the virus is often preventable because it is most often transmitted through infected body fluids that come in contact with hands and then are absorbed through the nose or mouth of a susceptible person. Therefore, care should be taken when handling children and items such as diapers. Simple hand washing with soap and water is effective in removing the virus from the hands.[39] The risks appear to be almost exclusively associated with women who previously have not been infected with CMV and who are having their first infection with the virus during pregnancy. There appears to be little risk of CMV-related complications for women who have been infected at least 6 months before conception. For this group, which makes up 50–80 percent of the women of childbearing age, the rate of newborn CMV infection is 1 percent, and these infants appear to have no significant illness or abnormalities.

After primary maternal infection, CMV persists for life in the host tissues. It can be both a silent companion, and a potential killer if infection is transmitted to the fetus during pregnancy. Primary CMV infection during pregnancy poses the greatest fetal risk because the antiviral immune response begins proximate to the transmission to the fetus due to maternal viremia through the placenta, whereas in recurrent infection, virus transmission occurs in the presence of both humoral and cell-mediated immune responses. The mechanism of CMV transmission to the fetus is not well known. Fetal contamination occurs 2 or 3 weeks after maternal viremia. Replication of the virus in the fetus requires 2 or 3 weeks before the appearance of fetal viremia, followed by excretion in the urine. Thus, presence of the virus in AF can be diagnosed only 5 or 6 weeks after maternal primary infection.

Generalized CMV disease is almost always the result of primary maternal infection. Many women (1–4 percent) acquire CMV during pregnancy, but only 30–40 percent transmit the virus to their fetuses. From those infected fetuses, clinically apparent infection occurs in less than 15 percent of the infected newborns.[43] Congenital infections may also result from recurrences of infection, either reactivation of infection, or reinfection with the same or a different strain of CMV during pregnancy. The rate of vertical transmission was found to be 0.2–2 percent in previously seropositive mothers undergoing recurrent infection during pregnancy.

Severe damage after recurrent maternal infection is clearly uncommon. Intrauterine infection results from maternal viremia, with subsequent placental infection, and hematogenous dissemination to the fetus. Fetal infection is more virulent in the first half of gestation. Excretion of CMV into urine and saliva persists for years. Infants with symptomatic congenital CMV infection excrete larger amounts of virus in the first few months of life than do those with asymptomatic infection. Naturally acquired perinatal CMV infections result from exposure to infected maternal genital secretions at birth or to breast milk during the first months of life. Exposure to CMV in the maternal genital tract has resulted in a 30–50 percent rate of perinatal infection. The transmission from mother to infant via breast milk occurs in 30–70 percent if nursing lasts for more than 1 month.

Diagnosis of viral reactivations and reinfections[44,45] is very difficult to accomplish during pregnancy. Observation of congenital infection in mothers who were defined as immune against CMV at least 1 year before pregnancy attests to the reality of reactivations or reinfections. The prognosis for such infections is usually better than after primary infection. The reason remains unclear; perhaps passive transplacental transfer of maternal IgG increases fetal defenses against CMV infection. Information about the outcome of pregnancies complicated by CMV infection acquired shortly before or around the date of conception is difficult to establish. Periconceptional infections carry a low risk of fetal contamination. When the onset of infection is well documented at least 3 months before infection, parents can be reassured and counseled to continue their pregnancy without resorting to antenatal testing unless required by parental anxiety. On the other hand, the option of prenatal diagnosis should be offered if recent infection (periconceptional or early postconceptional) is suspected. The observation that about 20 percent of immunocompetent subjects with primary infection are still virus-positive at 6 months after onset, and the consideration that such viremia is a marker of potential infectivity, suggests that waiting at least 6 months before initiation of pregnancy is reasonable.

Clinical Maternal Manifestations

Primary infection acquired during pregnancy is described as asymptomatic in about 90 percent of cases. When present, signs and symptoms are often so slight that they escape the memory of the majority of patients. The most commonly recognized clinical manifestations are mild and nonspecific: fatigue, malaise, headache, low-grade fever, myalgia and lymphadenopathy, hepatomegaly, and splenomegaly.

A careful medical interview is useful because symptoms can be recalled, allowing quite precise dating of the onset of infection. A slight increase in serum levels of liver enzymes is also frequently observed, because clinical manifestation of asthenia often lead to laboratory tests. In our experience, mild symptoms and/or liver function abnormalities can frequently be observed if the pregnant woman is carefully questioned.

Pathology

CMV can cause a multisystem disease in which all major organs are involved. Invasion of the central nervous system is the most important consequence of fetal infection with CMV. The infection can be described as focal encephalitis, vasculitis, and periependymitis.

Acute encephalitis leads to cell necrosis, gliosis, and calcification. Vasculitis leads to lower brain perfusion and sclerosis. Meningoencephalitis is frequently associated. Calcifications resulting from brain necrosis can be located anywhere in the brain, not only in the periventricular location. Microcephaly results from direct cell necrosis and lowered brain perfusion resulting from vasculitis. Anomalies of cell migration (resulting in heterotopias) and brain gyration (resulting in polymicrogyria) have also been described. Hydrocephaly is rarely important, resulting from periaqueductal involvement. Usually mild hydrocephaly results from the rarefaction of brain tissues with enlargement of pericerebral spaces.

Viral inclusion-bearing cells and viral antigen-containing cells can also be found within structures of the inner ear, including the organ of Corti, and the cochlea. Furthermore, involvement of the eye, including chorioretinitis, optic neuritis, cataract formation, and microphthalmos, have been demonstrated. CMV has been isolated from fluid of the anterior chamber of the eye.

Involvement of the liver is common in congenital CMV infections. Hepatomegaly, elevated levels of serum transaminases and direct hyperbilirubinemia are frequently seen in infants with symptomatic congenital infections. Hematologic abnormalities, including thrombocytopenia, anemia, and extramedullary hematopoiesis, are common in symptomatically infected infants. These abnormalities usually resolve during the first year of life.

Congenital Infection

Symptomatic Infection[46]

The severity of infection in the fetus depends on the gestational age at the time of transmission of virus; the manifestations vary according to both of the following patterns: Approximately 10 percent of the infants with congenital CMV infections have signs and symptoms at birth, which indicate possible infection. Half of them present generalized infectious disease characterized by clinical manifestations reflected by multiple organ involvement, in particular the reticuloendothelial and central nervous systems, with or without ocular and auditory damage.

The most common manifestations are growth retardation, prematurity, petechiae, jaundice, hepatosplenomegaly, microcephaly, lethargy, hypotonia, elevated transaminases, thrombocytopenia, hemolysis, and increased cerebrospinal fluid proteins. Among the most severely affected infants, mortality may be as high as 30 percent. Sensorineural deafness is the most common handicap caused by congenital CMV infection. CMV is considered to be one of the most important causes of deafness in childhood. The frequency and severity are worse in patients with symptomatic infection than in patients with subclinical infection. The sensorineural hearing loss is bilateral in nearly one-third of the cases and the severity (loss of 50 to 100 db) can produce serious difficulties with verbal communication and learning. Deafness can develop or become more severe after the first year of life, and although in most cases the deterioration occurs during the first 2–3 years of life; documented cases of onset at 6 years have been reported.

The likelihood of survival with normal intellect and hearing after severe symptomatic infection is small, as most infants develop various degrees of mental retardation, seizures, deafness, and chorioretinitis, leading finally to disorders of language, learning, and hearing.

Psychomotor retardation, usually combined with microcephaly and other neurologic complications, is very frequent, associated with sensorineural hearing loss, and ocular lesions, and poor intellectual prognosis.[39,47] If transplacental transmission occurs early, that is if the mother has acquired infection early, and if there has been a short delay before the viruses spread from the placenta to the fetus, a progressive disease can occur in nearly 10 percent of cases. This may result in fetal death in utero and spontaneous abortion, or in delivery of a live child with signs of central nervous system involvement including microcephaly, hydrocephalus, meningoencephalitis, intracranial calcifications, deafness, and chorioretinitis. Signs of generalized infection may also be present, including hepatosplenomegaly, jaundice, rash, anemia and thrombocytopenia, myocarditis, pericarditis, and pleural effusion. Repetition of ultrasound is mandatory to detect subtle signs of infection. Repeatedly normal scans give a good probability that the fetus is infected but will be asymptomatic. But the signs can be so slight that they usually cannot be diagnosed if the status of the fetus (infected or not) remains unknown (i.e., when prenatal diagnosis has not been performed).

If the transmission of CMV to the fetus occurs later, either because of late acquisition of infection by the mother or because of delayed spreading of viruses to the fetus, the congenital infection can be subclinical at birth but may evolve months or years after birth and result in sensorineural hearing loss, chorioretinitis, and mental retardation. It must be emphasized that ultrasound signs of brain involvement can be difficult to diagnose for nonspecialized ultrasonologists and that brain lesions are very difficult to diagnose during normal ultrasound survey of the pregnancy. Only very careful examination is likely to identify the alterations of cephalic growth measurements and other brain signs of CMV infection.

Asymptomatic Infection

Nearly 90 percent of congenitally infected infants have no early clinical manifestations, and although their long-term outcome is much better, severe deafness can develop in 10 percent, and more rarely other complications, including microcephaly, spastic diplegia, mental retardation, and chorioretinitis. Probably these offspring would have been identified as mildly symptomatic (i.e., with viremia, hepatitis, mild thrombocytopenia). This emphasizes the difficulty in distinguishing between asymptomatic and symptomatic neonatal CMV infection. Minor signs, such as failure to thrive, hepatosplenomegaly, jaundice, and others, can go unrecognized, and if recognized they do not usually lead to the diagnosis of congenital CMV infection. Moreover, psychomotor retardation, neurologic dysfunction, hearing loss, and chorioretinitis may take years to identify.

Serology

Diagnosis of primary infection can be achieved in two circumstances:

1. The presence of maternal clinical manifestations already described, leading to the serologic diagnosis.

2. Screening for seroconversion on a seronegative mother, usually when there is a risk of contamination (e.g., parents of infants in day care centers, workers in day care centers).

Mothers should receive information to make informed choices about further testing.[47] Appropriate information should be provided stepwise: In the presence of IgM, information is given about the possibility of a false-positive result, persistent IgM, cross-reactive IgM due to other viral infections, the possibility of preconceptional infection assessed by the avidity index, and the risk of primary infection. The risk concerning primary infection should be detailed only when the diagnosis is certain. In this situation, the different issues (i.e., fetal infection or not—symptomatic and asymptomatic congenital infection—risk of a false-positive result after amniocentesis, and the role of ultrasound survey) are explained.

If gestational time allows for the option of amniocentesis, a choice is given between serial ultrasound scans (usually each month) and prenatal diagnosis. If the fetus is infected, fetal blood sampling to establish the prognosis of the infected fetus is proposed, and ultrasound scans are repeatedly done every 2 weeks to detect any fetal growth or brain abnormalities.

Options for the termination of pregnancy (according to the local laws) are also discussed in the case of symptomatic infection with ultrasound abnormalities, with a high risk of fetal sequelae. Determination of maternal status should be done as early as possible at the beginning of pregnancy, or before if possible. If there is no virus-specific IgG in the serum, the pregnant woman is seronegative. Adequate counseling can be done in an attempt to prevent primary infection during pregnancy. If IgG and IgM are positive, primary infection can be suspected because it is consistently associated with a virus-specific IgM antibody response. Nevertheless, the presence of specific IgM is not sufficient to diagnose CMV primary infection.[48] In this situation, IgG avidity assay can help to identify recent infection. This assay is based on the observation that virus-specific IgG of low avidity is produced during the first months after primary infection, whereas a maturation process leads to the production of IgG of higher avidity. The presence of high IgM levels and a low IgG avidity index (<30 percent) are highly suggestive of a recent (<3 months) primary infection. On the other hand, when the avidity index is high (>80 percent), it is highly suggestive that primary infection occurred >3 months before. It is of major importance that serologic testing can be done as early as possible during pregnancy, because after 3 months, even a high-avidity index does not exclude infection during pregnancy. An intermediate index (>30 percent and <80 percent) may be a reliable indicator of a preconception infection if the first assay was done in the first month of pregnancy. When the avidity index is low, the rate of fetal infection (25 percent) is quite similar to the rate after primary infection during the first trimester. In some situations, adequate interview of the mother helps to identify the date of infection, and minor clinical signs (fever, cough, myalgia) can be identified.

Determination of viremia by PCR in maternal lymphocytes, and urine culture, provides reliable estimates of the exact date of maternal infection, as the risk of recent maternal infection is very low when the avidity index is intermediate, and maternal blood PCR and urine cultures are negative during the first 2 months of pregnancy.[47] Sometimes, a low rate of IgM can be observed even though specific IgG values are negative: this situation can be encountered when maternal infection begins. A new assay is mandatory 3 weeks later to confirm the primary infection. Nonspecific, elevated IgM from other viral stimulation can also be observed. Another possibility is the appearance of specific IgG after passive immunization against the D gene.

Determination of Virus and Viral Products in Maternal Blood[47,49]

The demonstration of maternal viremia can help to identify recent infection at the beginning of pregnancy when serologic tests are unable to distinguish between preconception and postconception infection. Before amniocentesis, detection of maternal viremia is mandatory, as any contamination of the AF by maternal blood can lead to a false-positive prenatal diagnosis result.

Several methods have been developed to identify and quantify CMV in maternal blood:

- Conventional methods using human fibroblast cultures facilitate diagnosis by immunofluorescence or immunoperoxidase techniques within 72 hr. Study of cytopathic effect requires 3 weeks.
- Determination of antigenemia (i.e., number of pp65-positive peripheral blood leukocytes).
- Hybridization techniques of CMV DNA with specific probes and detection with isotopic or immunologic methods.
- Detection and quantification of CMV DNA by PCR in whole blood or in maternal leukocytes, which is the most common method used to detect and quantify CMV in maternal blood.

Diagnosis of Congenital Infection in the Fetus

Major clinical indications for prenatal diagnosis are documented primary CMV infections in the mothers and ultrasonographic signs that occur in fetal CMV infection (intrauterine growth restriction [IUGR], ascites, hyperechogenic fetal bowel, central nervous system abnormalities). CMV isolation from AF is the reference method for prenatal diagnosis, because of its high sensitivity and specificity.[50,51]

If done at least 6 weeks after maternal infection, and not before 22 weeks of gestation, both PCR and cultures have an excellent sensitivity and absolute specificity. Nevertheless, care must be taken to use both techniques simultaneously to prevent false diagnoses, mainly due to a short delay between maternal infection and sampling. Moreover, some fetal contamination can occur after amniocentesis, usually leading to fewer effects than when contracted just after maternal infection. The difference in sensitivity between sampling before and after 22 weeks is significant. Quantification of viral load in AF by PCR shows that the viral load always increases during pregnancy when the fetus is infected. Hence, prognostication based on the viral load in AF is problematic, because some results show a correlation between very low quantification and a good outcome, very high quantification an even worse outcome.[47]

Fetal blood sampling under ultrasound guidance allows examination of fetal blood, for both the determination of specific IgM and the quantification of viral load.[47,49,50,52] Nonspecific signs of fetal infection include thrombocytopenia, elevated liver enzymes, erythroblastosis, and anemia. Such signs may be good predictors of adverse fetal outcome if associated with ultrasonographic abnormalities and IUGR.

Fetal autopsy can be practiced in two situations. Intrauterine fetal death with suspected fetal infection (retrospective diagnosis of primary maternal infection, or ultrasound abnormalities known to be frequently associated with CMV fetal disease): the visualization of inclusion-bearing cells in placental and fetal tissues establishes a diagnosis and the cause of death. When termination of pregnancy is required in a case of symptomatic infection, autopsy is needed to confirm the viral infection.

In all cases of maternal primary infection, neonatal evaluation for viral infection is recommended despite a negative prenatal diagnosis result. Even if primary infection had been suspected or ascertained, neonatal evaluation is necessary. When clinical signs known to be found in congenital CMV infection are present, urine must be tested for evidence of virus. Tests for saliva remain to be evaluated. The gold standard is the isolation by culture or PCR from urine in the 10 first days of life, to exclude neonatal infections contracted during delivery or following breast-feeding. Both PCR and culture should be done in these situations. Universal screening of neonates remains controversial. Both PCR and culture must be done in all cases of suspected or proved maternal infection. The cost would be prohibitive. Further simplifications could be investigated: diagnosis with PCR on saliva, and diagnosis with PCR using dried blood spots on filter paper, as already done for some for genetic and metabolic disorders.

Ultrasonographic Signs

Ultrasonographic abnormalities known to be found frequently in fetal CMV infection can be evident: hydrops, microcephaly, ascites, severe IUGR with oligohydramnios and brain abnormalities, hepatosplenomegaly with ascites and liver calcifications. In some other cases, ultrasound signs can be more difficult to identify: late appearance of mild IUGR, nonspecific thickness of the placenta, mild hydrocephaly with brain abnormalities such as periventricular calcifications, and decrease in expected cranial size.

Consequences of fetal infection should be evaluated serially by ultrasound examinations during pregnancy. The most characteristic alteration is the decrease of the growth of cephalic circumference, associated with intracranial periventricular densities, enlargement of of pericerebral spaces, germinative cysts, and perivascular densities of thalamic arteries. Necrotic brain tissue may later calcify and become visible on ultrasound. Obstruction of the aqueduct of Sylvius leads to the rapid enlargement of the third and lateral ventricles, usually progressive during a short period (1 or 2 weeks). Obstruction of the foramen of Monro can lead to unilateral hydrocephalus, but the signs are much less frequent than for toxoplasmosis.

Microcephaly associated with mild hydrocephaly and calcification is usually diagnosed during the third trimester. The chronology of the appearance of signs of brain involvement is now well known. Early diagnosis is difficult, but it can be suspected with careful and serial examination of the brain aimed at determining a decrease in fetal head growth, periventricular hyperechogenicity, and ventricular dilatation. These signs may not be detected during routine ultrasound scans. When diagnosed in known infected fetuses (i.e., after positive result of prenatal diagnosis), they indicate a poor prognosis for impaired neural development.

Brain abnormalities are the most common signs that can be seen in cases of symptomatic fetal infection, especially when infection has occurred during the first half of pregnancy.[53-56] Serial ultrasound scans are of critical importance during pregnancy. When prenatal diagnosis has been negative, the risk of delayed transplacental passage is low, but ultrasound scans should be performed monthly, seeking subtle signs of fetal infection. When these signs are present, repetition of amniocentesis should be discussed.

Decreased head growth is the most important and early sign of brain involvement. Growth curves of the fetus must be established in order to detect the onset of IUGR. After primary maternal CMV infection, fetuses must be monitored each month. When the fetus is infected, ultrasound scans are recommended every 2 weeks. Mild cerebral ventricular dilatation, usually bilateral and symmetrical, is rarely due to aqueduct obstruction, but rather to severe neuronal cell loss (lowered blood perfusion due to impairment of brain arteries), necrosis, and sclerosis. Compression of the aqueduct of Sylvius occurs first in the occipital region before involving the entire lateral ventricles. Its evolution may be very rapid, over a period of a few days, and is associated with a poor prognosis.

Cerebral ventricular dilatation can be present at the time of prenatal diagnosis or appear shortly thereafter in case of infections in the first half of pregnancy. Serial ultrasound examinations are then indicated even if the ultrasound scan showed no evidence of abnormality at the date of amniocentesis. The absence of cerebral ventricular dilatation is not necessarily a good prognostic sign, as major brain lesions can be seen without involvement of the aqueduct of Sylvius.

Intracranial densities are more frequently observed than ventricular dilatation, with frequent periventricular location. They can be associated with the other signs of brain involvement:

- Mild hydrocephaly, "ex vacuo," not caused by compression but by neuronal cell loss.
- Perivascular densities of thalamic arteries
- Germinative cysts
- Enlargement of pericerebral spaces

Ultrasound examination of the fetal brain should be systematically done not only in the axial plane but also in the coronal, sagittal, and parasagittal planes through the anterior fontanel, which can be accessed and subsequently used as an acoustic window. If the fetus is in a vertex presentation, imaging the fetal brain with high-frequency transvaginal probes results in high-quality images. Improvement of the quality of the ultrasound probes and standardization of the planes and sections lead to more accurate diagnosis of "subtle signs" during pregnancy and obtain images comparable to those obtained after birth by high-frequency probes through the anterior fontanel. These densities cannot be seen with magnetic resonance imaging (MRI). After birth, computed tomography (CT) allows accurate neuroanatomic localization and count of intracranial calcifications.

Hyperechogenic fetal bowel is also an ultrasonographic marker of fetal infection (toxoplasmosis as well as CMV). This sign can be encountered in two situations:

1. Evidence at the time of amniocentesis of hyperechogenic fetal bowel leads to prenatal diagnosis studies not only for CMV but also for toxoplasmosis, cystic fibrosis, and chromosomal abnormalities.
2. Appearance during the follow-up of a presumed noninfected fetus (prenatal diagnosis already performed and negative) of hyperechogenic bowel: this situation can be a marker of fetal infection, and a second amniocentesis should be discussed.

Other ultrasonographic signs correspond to placental inflammation, hepatic involvement, and effusions, showing that fetal CMV infection is a multisystem disease. Some signs may be transient. The placenta is often enlarged with a "frosted glass" appearance. Enlargement of the liver and liver densities are often observed when there is hepatic enzyme elevation on fetal blood sampling. Examination should also include a search for ascites, pleural effusion, and pericardial effusion. Ultrasound monitoring is not sufficient for a definitive diagnosis of fetal infection because signs are not pathognomonic of CMV infection.

Most infected fetuses are not severely damaged and cannot be identified, although their risk of late complications (mental retardation, severe deafness, chorioretinitis) is not uncommon.

Forming a Prognosis

Fetal CMV disease seems to be preferentially associated with infection occurring in the first half of pregnancy. Correlation of high levels of viral load and appearance of CMV disease have been reported in immunocompromised patients. However, the clinical significance of CMV viral load in the AF and fetal blood of infected fetuses remains difficult to establish, as viral DNA accumulates in AF instead of being cleared. In contrast, low levels of DNA (<10.2 genome-equivalents/mL) are more likely associated with asymptomatic fetuses than high levels, whereas some fetuses with high levels in AF may have a good outcome. Variables such as gestational age at maternal infection, time of intrauterine infection, and timing of prenatal diagnosis must be considered. A high viral load in AF is likely to indicate a severely damaged fetus. In asymptomatic disease, low viral levels clearly indicate a small probability of fetal disease.

Determination of biochemical and hematologic parameters as well as the viral load in fetal blood enables a more accurate prediction of the extent of newborn involvement. Cranial ultrasonographic findings[54,55] also influence the prognosis and include:

- Decrease of the growth curve of the head
- Calcifications, not only periventricular but in any location[57]
- Calcifications of the thalamic arteries
- Germinal cysts (nonspecific), under ependyma
- Appearance of ventricular dilatation

Observation of isolated signs (such as single subependymal calcification or isolated germinal cyst) is not usually corelated with severe brain impairment and microcephaly. Nevertheless, association is correlated with worse prognosis. Many infants may be born with unrecognized microcephaly and generalized disease, because routine third-trimester scans not detailed enough to identify these signs. Moreover, some fetuses can present signs of acute hypoxia with IUGR and be delivered (by cesarean section) before the diagnosis of fetal infection could be established.

When IUGR is diagnosed during pregnancy, prenatal studies for CMV infection, as well as for chromosomes, are indicated (see chapI have no pimpossible to verifieossibility to verifieter 6). Occurrence of IUGR during the survey of a known infected fetus requires further studies that include:

- Detailed ultrasonographic scans to identify signs of brain involvement
- Fetal blood sampling to check hematologic and biochemical parameters, and determination of the viral load

When IUGR is associated with other ultrasonographic and biologic signs of symptomatic fetal infection, there is a high probability of a severely damaged fetus. If no abnormality is found, another cause of IUFR must be considered, and a careful survey is necessary. In utero MRI of the fetal brain would then also be valuable (see chapter 25).

Some abnormalities are not incompatible with a good fetal outcome:

- Isolated brain abnormalities
- Isolated hepatomegaly
- Isolated hyperechogenic small bowel

However, the occurrence of these signs can also indicate disseminated fetal infection; therefore, fetal blood sampling and brain MRI are required to ascertain the normality of other parameters. In utero MRI is a reliable tool for brain investigation in cases of CMV fetal infection: it can confirm microcephaly, ventricular dilatation, and enlargement of pericerebral spaces (see also chapter 25). Identification of abnormalities in the cerebral gyri (e.g., polymicrogyria, pachygyria) and impaired neuronal migration (nodular heterotopias) can be done only by MRI, not by ultrasound. Discordance between detailed ultrasound scans and MRI is uncommon, but in some cases of uncertainty regarding brain involvement, MRI provides precise information about brain involvement.

Treatment of Congenital Infection

Treatment regimens will vary according to the circumstances[58]:

1. To prevent maternal primary infection. Maternal vaccination, when achieved, would be the ideal tool to immunize childbearing women. An immediate goal would be to prevent maternal infection through hygiene counseling (avoid contact with saliva, urine, diapers of infants, especially in day care centers).
2. To prevent fetal transmission of the virus, treatment should in theory be given just after primary infection, before the supposed transmission to the fetus. Diminishing the maternal viral load would probably reduce the rate of fetal transmission and perhaps the viral load transmitted to the fetus.
3. Prenatal treatment of infected fetuses would require antiviral drug therapy without maternal or fetal toxicity.

Ganciclovir has been available for several years for the treatment of life-threatening CMV disease in immunocompromised patients. The high degree of hematologic toxicity and its potential teratogenic effects have contraindicated use during pregnancy.[59] The digestive absorption rate is low; thus, intravenous treatment is required. Anecdotal treatments by cord or via AF administration have been discouraging, although fetal viremia decreased after treatment. Improving bioavailability could permit better digestive absorption by the mother, but toxicity limits use before the third trimester. However, fetal infection and development of clinical manifestations usually occur earlier.

Postnatal ganciclovir administration has been used for the treatment of infected symptomatic neonates,[60] with intravenous administration for 6 weeks. Although the viral load decreased during treatment, it has been difficult to conclude that treatment of such infected neonates with a high probability of neurologic sequelae improved the clinical outcome. Clinical trials with valacyclovir should be easier to conduct during pregnancy because of lower toxicity. Valacyclovir, the hydrochloride salt of the L-valine ester of acyclovir is well absorbed by the gastrointestinal tract, avoiding digestive degradation, and is rapidly converted into acyclovir by first-pass hydrolysis in the liver.[61] Bioavailability of acyclovir after the oral administration of valacyclovir is three to five times higher than that obtained after the oral administration of acyclovir.[62] The excretion of acyclovir is renal. Valacyclovir 8 g/day is more efficient than acyclovir 4 g/day in both herpes and CMV[63] infection in patients infected with the human immunodeficiency virus, and has few side effects. In these patients, Valacyclovir produces CMV viral load reduction from baseline to 1.3 logs, and a decrease in visceral complications.[64] This decrease raises expectations of a significant reduction of fetal infection rates when administered after maternal infection, and a reduction of fetal disease. (Trials should answer whether treatment should be given to all infected fetuses or only to symptomatic fetuses with ultrasonographic or biologic abnormalities.)

Vaccination

Because fetal CMV infection is the major cause of congenital infection resulting in mental retardation, active immunoprophylaxis (i.e., vaccination) seems to be the best tool to resolve this major health problem. Because this congenital disease is overwhelming and due to primary maternal infection, the ultimate goal is to develop a vaccine that can be administered to seronegative women of childbearing age to prevent the occurrence of the initial infection during pregnancy. Immunization against CMV before pregnancy reduces the rate of fetal infection from 40 percent to 2 percent and reduces the rate and gravity of sequelae.

Over the past 30 years, attempts to develop an Herpes CMV vaccine have been directed at five major strategic approaches:

1. Live attenuated vaccines
2. Recombinant virus vaccines
3. Subunit vaccines
4. Peptide vaccines
5. DNA vaccines

First attempts are difficult to evaluate; furthermore, two major problems are the basis for great concern: (1) persistence in the body of the vaccine virus strain as a latent virus that periodically reactivates, and (2) CMV may be oncogenic in vivo.[39,47]

Prevention

Most countries have developed prevention programs aiming to prevent maternal infection during pregnancy, because the routes of transmission and the high-risk populations are well known. Efficacy of prevention is difficult to establish, because of the need for large population studies and the risk of relapse while following recommendations. Adler et al.[65] reported effective prevention of CMV primary infection among pregnant seronegative mothers in contact with their first infant excreting CMV, giving recommendations about personal hygiene.

At a time when pregnant women can find information on the Internet, physicians should be aware of the National Center for Infectious Diseases Internet site (United States) on CMV (http://www.cdc.gov/ncidod/diseases/cmv.htm), which indicates:

Recommendations for pregnant women with regard to CMV infection:

- Throughout the pregnancy, practice good personal hygiene, especially hand-washing with soap and water, after contact with diapers or oral secretions (particularly with a child who is in day care).
- Women in whom a mononucleosislike illness develops during pregnancy should be evaluated for CMV infection and counseled about the possible risks to the unborn child.
- Laboratory testing for antibody to CMV can be performed to determine if a woman has already had CMV infection.
- Recovery of CMV from the cervix or urine of women at or before the time of delivery does not warrant a caesarean section.

- The demonstrated benefits of breast-feeding outweigh the minimal risk of acquiring CMV from the breast-feeding mother.
- There is no need to either screen for CMV or exclude CMV-excreting children from schools or institutions because the virus is frequently found in many healthy children and adults.

Recommendations for individuals providing care for infants and children:

- Female employees should be educated concerning CMV, its transmission, and hygienic practices, such as hand-washing, which minimize the risk of infection.
- Susceptible nonpregnant women working with infants and children should not routinely be transferred to other work situations.
- Pregnant women working with infants and children should be informed of the risk of acquiring CMV infection and the possible effects on the unborn child.

Routine laboratory testing for CMV antibody in female workers is not recommended, but can be performed to determine their immune status

Screening for Congenital CMV Infection

Several attitudes must be considered toward screening of congenital CMV infections:

- Identification of seronegative mothers before or at the beginning of pregnancy
- Screening for maternal primary infection
- Prenatal diagnosis of infected fetuses following identification of maternal primary infection
- Identification of infected neonates

To our knowledge, routine screening of pregnant women has never been recommended by any health authority, in any country. However, most obstetricians offer pregnant women tests if an infection is suspected or exposure has occurred.[66] Reliable assays are available to determine maternal CMV immune status. Seronegative pregnant women can be informed about preventive measures. Efficacy of these measures is difficult to prove in large populations, but they can be effective individually. Prenatal diagnosis appears to be very beneficial in reducing the number of terminated pregnancies. When the fetus is shown not to be infected, pregnancy termination can be avoided. If the fetus is infected, determination of prognostic factors enables identification of fetuses who will likely have an adverse outcome. Termination of pregnancy may then be offered, according to the law of the country, and trials of in utero therapy may also be initiated. Appropriate patient information requires that women of childbearing age be informed about CMV disease and the opportunity for screening.[67] Failure to provide such information is unethical, and legally risky. In our opinion, identification of seronegative mothers before or at the beginning of pregnancy, especially for mothers with a first child in a day care center, appears to be appropriate from a medical, legal, and ethical point of view.

PRENATAL DIAGNOSIS OF FETAL VARICELLA INFECTION

Varicella during pregnancy can be responsible for three very different types of complication. Severe maternal disease includes acute pneumonia, can be life threatening to the mother, and should be recognized promptly. Neonatal varicella comes as a complication of maternal infection occurring immediately before delivery. The focus here is on fetal infection during the first half of pregnancy that leads to the congenital varicella syndrome in the most severe form, as well as an isolated immune response, or zoster during the first year of life.

Since 1991, PCR assays for detection of (VZV) DNA in AF and fetal tissues have been widely used as a valuable tool for the diagnosis of fetal infections.

Virologic Bases[68]

VZV belongs to the group of alpha herpes viridae with a linear double-strand DNA molecule consisting of approximately 125,000 base pairs. Computer analysis of the sequence predicted the presence of approximately 70 open reading frames. The genome is similar to other alpha herpes viruses with a significant collinearity with the herpes simplex virus type 1 (HSV-1). VZV DNA is enclosed in a nucleocapsid.

The virus is fragile, is rapidly destroyed by heat, and loses its infectivity after being frozen. After contact with the host, the incubation period lasts for 14–15 days, with two phases of viremia. The virus is thought to replicate in the local lymphoid tissues and then spread to reticuloendothelial cells during the first viremia. The replication in the liver and spleen precedes the second viremia and the appearance of the vesicular rash. After the primary infection, the virus remains in latency mostly in sensory nerve tissue. Reactivation leads to zoster in healthy patients or to general disease among patients with immunodeficiency.

Epidemiology

Most women already have acquired immunity for VZV before pregnancy (90 percent of adult women in the United States[69] and 94.8 percent in Germany[70]). The incidence of varicella during pregnancy is correlated with the frequency of nonimmune women at a childbearing age and to their risk of exposure. The risk is higher for migrant populations, among whom seropositivity is lower. The global rate of varicella during pregnancy is estimated at between 0.7 and 2–3 in 1,000.[71]

Clinical Aspects of Maternal Infection

The typical skin rash includes a general progression of the lesions through macular, papular, vesicular, and pustular stages. Skin lesions appear on the trunk, face, scalp, and extremities. Lesions of all stages of development are present at the same time. The lesions usually heal without permanent scarring unless secondary bacterial infection occurs. The rash is often severe. No new lesion should appear after day 7.

The most common severe complication in pregnant women is pneumonia. It usually develops within 1 week of the rash and might progress rapidly to hypoxia and respiratory failure. The evolution might be life threatening in the absence of prompt diagnosis and treatment.

Consequences for the Pregnancy and the Fetus

No significant increase of spontaneous abortion, stillbirth, and prematurity has been described after varicella during pregnancy. Fetal infection resulting from varicella during pregnancy can lead to various consequences according to the term of maternal infection and the susceptibility of the fetus. Intrauterine varicella infection can also occur without clinical sequelae at any stage of pregnancy.

The congenital varicella syndrome is the most severe consequence of fetal infection and was first described as an association between congenital anomalies in the newborn and varicella infection in early pregnancy.[72] The child born after a maternal rash at 8 weeks of gestation had associated hypotrophy, foot malposition, skin lesions, hydrocephaly, cortical atrophy, cerebellar atrophy, and optic nerve atrophy.

Many cases of congenital varicella syndrome have been described over the years in association with varicella during the first 24 weeks of pregnancy. Cases have occurred mainly during the first 20 weeks of pregnancy, although it has been described up to 27 weeks. Many anomalies have been related to the infection:

- Intrauterine growth restriction
- Neurologic involvement with hydrocephaly, microcephaly, cortical or cerebellar atrophy
- Pathologic examinations have revealed focal necrosis and parenchymal cysts
- Autonomic nervous system involvement has led to neurologic impairment of bladder function, phrenic nerve paralysis, and Horner syndrome
- Peripheral nerve lesions have resulted in limb deformities
- Ocular lesions cover a wide range of anomalies, including chorioretinitis, cataract, optic nerve atrophy, and microphthalmia
- Skin lesions are frequent and can range from small scars to large acute scars
- Polyvisceral damage can lead to hepatitis, intestinal fibrosis, or hydronephrosis

The frequencies of the most common features are presented in Table 30.4.

Before the recent developments of molecular biology, proof of fetal infection was difficult to obtain, as viral culture has a high rate of false-negative results[73] and fetal blood IgM antibodies are very inconstant.[74]

VZV DNA detection in AF, fetal blood, or tissues in cases showing typical signs of intrauterine varicella infection by ultrasound or postnatal examination proved the link between maternal varicella during pregnancy and the congenital varicella syndrome. PCR has become an essential diagnostic tool for diagnosis.[75–77]

Pathogenesis of Fetal Infection

The precise mechanism of infection with VZV in utero is not known. Transplacental transmission probably takes place during the viremic phase before the maternal rash. Manifestations of the congenital varicella syndrome suggest an association between initial fetal infection with visceral lesions and lesions due to in utero zoster in multiple sites following a short latency period.[78] This could explain the wide range of in utero lesions as well

Table 30.4. Congenital varicella syndrome: clinical features and their relative frequency

Main Anomaly (n = 25)	Total No. of Infants (%)
Skin: dermatomal cicatricial skin lesions, contractures	18 (72)
Skeleton: limb hypoplasia associated with reduction deformities	18 (72)
Eye: microphthalmia, chorioretinitis, cataract, Horner syndrome	11 (44)
Central nervous system: microcephaly, brain atrophy, paralysis, convulsions, encephalitis	
Other organ defects (e.g., gastrointestinal, genitourinary)	5 (20)
Multiorgan involvement (hemorrhagic rash and dystrophy)	6 (24)
Death postpartum or later	9 (36)

Source: Data from Enders and Miller, 2000.[70]

as the occurrence of postnatal zoster. The clinical manifestations range from severe multisystem involvement to dermatomal skin scarring as the only defect at birth.[79] About 1 percent of fetuses will have no immediate consequences of in utero infection but will present with zoster during the first year of life.

Diagnosis of Fetal Infection

Technologic advances in obstetrical ultrasound and molecular biology have greatly simplified the prenatal diagnosis of fetal infection in cases of varicella rash during the first part of pregnancy. Ultrasound can identify severe anomalies in infected fetuses

- Fetal growth restriction
- Hyperechogenic bowel or lungs or liver
- Malposition of the limbs or contractures
- Microcephaly, ventricular dilatation, or microphthalmia

Some of these images are transitory (bowel hyperechogenicity); others cannot be detected by ultrasound alone (e.g., skin lesions); others (e.g., phrenic-nerve paralysis) can eventually be detected if infection in the fetus is suspected.

VZV DNA testing on AF by PCR assay taken at least 4 weeks after skin healing, is the most sensitive technique for the detection of fetal infection. Primers have been described that amplify different regions of the VZV genome.[75] Whether on fetal tissues,[76] AF,[73] or fetal blood,[80] PCR assay has become the reference tool for the diagnosis of fetal infection.

The possibility of persistent VZV viral load in maternal peripheral cells is well known. The risk of AF contamination by maternal blood during amniocentesis could lead to a false-positive result. After a short series controlling the duration of positive VZV PCR on maternal lymphocytes (our data), we now always control for negative maternal peripheral blood VZV DNA before any invasive procedure and wait for it to become negative before performing the amniocentesis.

Frequency of Transmission

Most studies concerning the evaluation of the frequency of maternal fetal transmission of VZV during the first half of pregnancy conclude that there is about a 1 percent risk of severe lesions after a typical maternal rash.[70] The largest series reported included 1,373 women who had a typical rash during pregnancy. The rate of transmission was estimated on postnatal findings.[74] The only large series relying on prenatal diagnosis by PCR analysis on AF was published by our team[73] in 1997. This study concerned 107 women who presented with a typical skin rash before 24 weeks of gestation. The transmission rate of maternal infection was 8.4 percent, with 2.8 percent occurrence of congenital varicella syndrome and 3.8 percent postnatal zoster. Since 1997, our counseling policy for women who have had varicella during the first 24 weeks of pregnancy is to propose prenatal diagnosis on AF even in absence of ultrasound anomalies.

Although amniocentesis has a small risk for the pregnancy (see chapter 2), valuable information can be obtained. More than 90 percent of patients can be reassured when VZV DNA is not detected and a normal ultrasound survey has been documented. In the case of a positive result, a high-resolution ultrasound survey can provide a high degree of reassurance. In these cases, MRI studies are suggested and may reveal cerebral or ocular anomalies. It is essential to keep in mind that a positive PCR result in AF is not always predictive of fetal anomalies.

Since 1997, more than 300 new prenatal diagnostic cases of VZV infection by PCR on AF after maternal infection during the first 24 weeks of gestation have been added to the series of Mouly, totaling more than 410 cases (our data). The general transmission rate was 5.1 percent (21 of 410) with 1 percent (3 of 21) being extremely severe cases of congenital varicella syndrome. In this series of 21 infected fetuses, 1 of 3[74] presented with some kind of damage (including skin lesions, Horner syndrome, and parasympathetic lesion of the lower limbs). We believe that the information of a possible mild lesion can be important to pregnant women, and may help practitioners to organize an optimal survey of the pregnancy and perinatal care.

Treatment and Prevention

The vaccination against VZV uses the Oka strain, which is a live attenuated strain, developed by M. Takahashi.[81] It is now widely used in Japan and has been recommended in the United States since 1995 for nonimmune children over 1 year old. The immunogenicity and efficacy of the vaccine in healthy children has been demonstrated in blinded, placebo-controlled studies. Its administration is contraindicated in pregnant women or immunodeficient patients. In countries where the vaccination is not systematic, it could be given to nonimmune women or exposed health care workers before conception.[81]

Specific γ-globulins (varicella–zoster immune globulin [VZIG]) have been proved to prevent severe disease in an immunocompromised host. The timing of administration should not exceed 72 hr after exposure. Various countries recommend their administration after exposure during pregnancy, in nonimmune women.[74] The dose recommended for an adult is 625 units. By preventing the occurrence of maternal illness, VZIG could therefore limit fetal risk. In France, we do not have easy access to VZIG, which makes it difficult to obtain in such a short period.

Antiviral agents have shown to be efficient in the treatment of varicella. Acyclovir and its prodrug valacyclovir have been widely used in cases of severe maternal disease and in cases of perinatal varicella in pregnant women. The absence of known toxicity on the Glaxo registration has led the International Herpes Medical Forum to recommend the use of acyclovir during pregnancy to limit the occurrence of severe infection in women.

Pregnant women with varicella infection should be treated with oral acyclovir (800 mg five times daily for 7 days) at any time of gestation.[82] The same plasma level of acyclovir can be obtained after 1 g of valacyclovir given orally, three times a day.

A number of reports suggest that acyclovir given 7 days following exposure, but not at the time of exposure, will prevent clinical varicella in most of the recipients.[83] However this is not a general recommendation, because the experience involves a small number of patients. In a case of varicella during pregnancy, this early treatment should be considered, as it might also reduce the risk of maternal–fetal transmission.

Maternal–fetal transfer of acyclovir and valacyclovir is excellent, but further studies are needed to explore whether therapeutic fetal levels can be achieved via the mother.

CONCLUSION

In countries that do not have access to systematic vaccination, the occurrence of varicella during pregnancy remains a fairly frequent event. Fetal infection not always detectable by ultrasound may lead to fetal death. The high specificity of PCR is a major tool for prenatal diagnosis, although it needs an invasive procedure and experienced team to assess reliability and to limit complications. There are few large prospective series, which would be essential if treatment could be offered after diagnosis of fetal infection.

PRENATAL DIAGNOSIS OF CONGENITAL RUBELLA

Rubella infection during pregnancy rarely occurs in countries where specific vaccination is compulsory. In France, in 2000, there were 53 cases of primary rubella infection during pregnancy (about 7 in 100,000 pregnancies), and the number of neonates affected with congenital rubella was 1 in 100,000 livebirths. However, in countries where vaccination is optional, maternal rubella remains a problem.

Risk of Fetal Infection

The risk of congenital rubella occurs classically after maternal primary infection before the 16th week of gestation. When maternal infection occurs after this period, there is no need for prenatal diagnosis, because the risk of fetal malformation due to the virus is nil and the risk of neurologic problems is very infrequent. Nevertheless, diagnostic studies of infected neonates should be done at birth, to avoid the infection of other seronegative mothers or infants in the maternity ward, because viral excretion is very high at birth in infected neonates.

There are some reports of documented maternal reinfection with rubella virus leading to fetal infection and congenital rubella.

The major determinant of fetal outcome is the stage of the gestation at the time of the maternal infection. Fetal infection occurs at the time of maternal viremia (which starts 7 days before the infection and stops classically 1 or 2 days after the rash). The rubella virus has been found in chorionic villi taken by chorionic villus sampling and in products of conception, but this is not frequent.[84] The risk of transplacental passage of the virus reaches a maximum at the beginning and at the end of the pregnancy. Table 30.5 shows the frequency of fetal infection according to the stage of the gestation.

Studies by Miller[85] can be compared with the results that we published, which were based on in vivo prenatal diagnosis cases.[86] Since that time, we have an experience of 143 cases of prenatal diagnosis of congenital rubella on fetal blood sampling; 66 maternal seroconversions occurred before 12 weeks of amenorrhea. In this group, the percentage of fetal contamination was 57 percent. There was one false-negative diagnosis at the beginning of this series due to fetal blood sampling performed too early (before 22 weeks, at a time when some infected fetuses are not able to synthesize IgM). In 77 cases, maternal infection was between 13 and 18 weeks. Thirty-four fetuses (44 percent) were in-

Table 30.5. Fetal infection with rubella virus according to the stage of gestation

Weeks of Gestation	% of Fetal Infection (from Miller et al.[85])	% of Fetal Infection (from Daffos et al.[86])
0–2	—	35
4–6	—	57
7–12	—	66
12–18	58	67
19–20	39	—
21–24	34	—
25–32	30	—
33–38	60	—
>38	100	—

fected. Twenty mothers decided to continue the pregnancy and 3 of these neonates had severe deafness diagnosed after birth.

Definition of Maternal Infection

Primary maternal infection is defined as certain if, during a pregnancy in which an earlier serology was negative or unknown, and at least two of the following criteria are present:

1. Documented rubella exposure or typical clinical rash
2. Seroconversion of rubella antibodies
3. Significant rubella IgM antibodies

Maternal reinfection is considered certain when a proven previous serology was positive (confirmed on two tests) and when a significant increase of rubella antibodies occurs. In this situation, measurement of the rubella antibody titers further complements the diagnostic effort.

In cases of reinfection, affected fetuses are usually found only when mothers had a reappearance of IgM. It is clear that rubella vaccination during pregnancy does not lead to fetal abnormalities.

Prenatal Diagnosis of Fetal Infection

Prenatal diagnosis is feasible by using fetal blood taken by cordocentesis after 22 weeks of gestation,[86] provided that maternal infection occurred during the first 18 weeks of pregnancy. Infection is detected by the presence of specific fetal IgM. This procedure requires the ability to prevent even the slightest contamination of the fetal blood by maternal blood, to avoid false-positive diagnosis of fetal infection (presence of specific IgM of maternal origin). In addition, the presence of an acid-labile interferon-α in fetal blood seems a very specific indicator of fetal contamination. Diagnosis can also be inferred by the presence of a nonspecific biologic syndrome associating erythroblastosis, anemia, and thrombocytopenia, with increases in fetal γ-glutamyl transferase and lactate dehydrogenase.

Recent developments raise the possibility of direct detection of rubella virus RNA by hybridization to fetal tissue such as chorionic villi,[87] AF cells, or fetal blood.[88] The technique used for the detection of rubella virus RNA is a reverse transcription (RT)-PCR. The construction of a synthetic RNA molecule has also been proposed for use as an internal control for amplification in the first step of an RT-nested PCR assay for RNA virus detection as well as for semiquantitation of RNA in samples[89] to be studied. The sensitivity of these techniques is still under investigation. They would, however, allow an earlier and easier prenatal diagnosis on AF. Meanwhile, a negative prenatal diagnosis using these procedures must be confirmed on fetal blood taken at 22 weeks of gestation.

CONCLUSION

During the past 10 years, there has been a very important decrease in maternal rubella seroconversions during pregnancy. But some women, because of inadequate care (lack of vaccination after the first pregnancy and exposure during the second pregnancy by infection from the first child) still give birth to infected neonates. Therefore, it appears that the best way to avoid congenital rubella is to interrupt the transmission of the virus by vaccinating all children. Combination of this strategy with screening of all women preconceptionally or as early as possible in the beginning of pregnancy, along with prenatal diagnosis and medical termination of infected fetuses, would lead to a drastic reduction in the prevalence of affected neonates.

PRENATAL DIAGNOSIS OF HUMAN PARVOVIRUS B19 INFECTION

Infection with parvovirus B19 occurs usually during short outbreaks of erythema infectiosum in winter and spring in temperate climates. The rate of seropositivity is about 40–60 percent in Western Europe. The greatest risk of transmission occurs in the prodromal phase, before the onset of the rash. Hence, avoiding persons with an established rash or exclusion of infected children from school or day care centers is not specifically recommended by the Centers for Disease Control and Prevention. Teachers, health care workers, and day care workers seem to be at increased risk for acquiring parvovirus B19 infection.

The majority of maternal infections with parvovirus B19 during pregnancy are probably asymptomatic or, at least, not clinically recognized. The risk for a susceptible pregnant woman contracting the disease during an outbreak bas been estimated to be about 1.4 percent, and almost 85 percent of women acquiring acute parvovirus B19 infection will deliver healthy newborns. Other infants will die in utero in the absence of treatment by intrauterine transfusion, the efficacy of which depends on the gravity of the initial disease).[90]

The only way to diagnose all maternal infections is to practice universal screening. However, treatment of pregnant women with proven acute parvovirus B19 infection remains controversial. Assessment of the fetus by weekly ultrasound is recommended for 4–6 weeks (time of the majority of diagnoses of hydrops), although hydrops has been reported up to 12 weeks after maternal infection. Given the rarity of the disease and the occurrence of seasonal outbreaks, universal screening is not recommended, but can be reserved for pregnant women with a greater risk of infection. Parvovirus B19 can result in a fetal aplastic crisis with severe fetal anemia.

Most often, prenatal diagnosis of fetal parvovirus B19 infection is considered under two different circumstances:

1. Clinical and/or serologic evidence of maternal infection
2. Nonimmune fetal hydrops (with or without ascites) on ultrasound during pregnancy

In these two situations, prenatal diagnosis of fetal infection is easily performed by detection of the virus by PCR on AF or/and fetal blood. In the first situation, in which the virus is present in the fetal compartment, the objective will be to anticipate the risk of severe fetal anemia with hydrops or in utero death. The percentage risk of transplacental passage of the virus is not clearly known, but may approximate 30 percent, and the interval between maternal infection and fetal hydrops is variable from 8 to 20 weeks.[91] A weekly follow-up of serum α-fetoprotein levels in maternal blood may be useful for the detection and prediction of severe fetal anemia,[92] along with regular ultrasound studies.

In the second circumstance with hydrops, fetal blood sampling facilitates confirmation of the degree of fetal anemia, the degree and the stage of the aplastic crisis (erythroblast count[93]), and the need for in utero fetal transfusion. No fetal transfusion is needed when there is fetal anemia, as long as there is an erythroblastosis, which indicates that the aplastic crisis is over. Furthermore, it is not necessary to repeat fetal transfusions because the aplastic crises do not persist for a long period and usually occur at the time of fetal infection. In some very severe cases, hydrops is also due to fetal myocarditis and cardiac insufficiency, which can be detected by ultrasound. In this situation, even after urgent in utero transfusion the hydrops persists and leads to fetal death.

REFERENCES

1. Remington JS and Klein JO. Infectious diseases of the fetus and newborn infant, 5th ed. Philadelphia: W.B. Saunders, 2001.
2. Montoya JG. Laboratory diagnosis of Toxoplasma gondii infection and toxoplasmosis. J Infect Dis 2002;185 (suppl 1):S73.
3. Pelloux H, Fricker-Hidalgo H, Pons JC, et al. [Congenital toxoplasmosis: prevention in the pregnant woman and management of the neonate]. Arch Pediatr 2002;9:206.
4. Bastien P. Molecular diagnosis of toxoplasmosis. Trans R Soc Trop Med Hyg 2002;96 (suppl 1):S205.
5. Hill D, Dubey JP. Toxoplasma gondii: transmission, diagnosis and prevention. Clin Microbiol Infect 2002;8:634.
6. Pass RF, Burke RL. Development of cytomegalovirus vaccines: prospects for prevention of congenital CMV infection. Semin Pediatr Infect Dis 2002;13:196.
7. Revello MG, Gerna G. Diagnosis and management of human cytomegalovirus infection in the mother, fetus, and newborn infant. Clin Microbiol Rev 2002;15:680.
8. Griffiths PD. Strategies to prevent CMV infection in the neonate. Semin Neonatol 2002;7:293.
9. Webster WS. Teratogen update: congenital rubella. Teratology 1998;58:13.
10. Forrest JM, Turnbull FM, Sholler GF, et al. Gregg's congenital rubella patients 60 years later. Med J Aust 2002;177:664.
11. Plotkin SA. Rubella eradication. Vaccine 2001;19:3311.
12. Brown KE. Haematological consequences of parvovirus B19 infection. Baillieres Best Pract Res Clin Haematol 2000;13:245.
13. Heegaard ED, Brown KE. Human parvovirus B19. Clin Microbiol Rev 2002;15:485.
14. Nunoue T, Kusuhara K, Hara T. Human fetal infection with parvovirus B19: maternal infection time in gestation, viral persistence and fetal prognosis. Pediatr Infect Dis J 2002;21:1133.
15. Desmonts G, Daffos F, Forestier F, et al. Prenatal diagnosis of congenital toxoplasmosis. Lancet 1985;1:500.
16. Couvreur J, Thulliez P, Daffos F, et al. Foetopathie toxoplasmique: traitement in utero par l'association pyrimethamine-sulfamides. Arch Fr Pediatr 1991;48:397.
17. Remington JS, McLeod R, Desmonts G, et al. Toxoplasmosis. In: Klein JO, Remington JS, editors. Infectious diseases of the fetus and newborn infant, 5th ed. Philadelphia: W.B. Saunders, 2001:140.
18. Dunn D, Wallon M, Peyron F, et al. Mother-to-child transmission of toxoplasmosis: risk estimates for clinical counselling. Lancet 1999;353:1829.
19. Hohlfeld P, Daffos F, Costa JM, et al. Prenatal diagnosis of congenital toxoplasmosis with a polymerase chain reaction test on amniotic fluid. N Engl J Med 1994;331:695.
20. Berrebi A, Kobuch WE, Bessières MH et al. Termination of pregnancy for maternal toxoplasmosis. Lancet 1994;344:36.
21. Burg JL, Grover CM, Pouletty P, et al. Direct and sensitive detection of a pathogenic protozoan, Toxoplasma gondii by polymerase chain reaction. J Clin Microbiol 1989;27:1787.
22. Grover CM, Thulliez P, Remington JS, et al. Rapid prenatal diagnosis of congenital Toxoplasma infection by using polymerase chain reaction on amniotic fluid. J Clin Microbiol 1990;28:2297.
23. Dupuy-Camet J, Lavareda de Souza S, Bougnoux ME, et al. Preventing congenital toxoplasmosis. Lancet 1990;2:1017.
24. Savva D, Morris JC, Johnson JD, et al. Polymerase chain reaction for detection of Toxoplasma gondii. J Med Microbiol 1990;32:25.
25. Cazenave J, Forestier F, Bessières MH, et al. Contribution of a new PCR assay to the prenatal diagnosis of congenital toxoplasmosis. Prenat Diagn 1992;12:119.
26. Ghidini A, Sepulveda W, Lockwood CJ, et al. Complications of fetal blood sampling. Am J Obstet Gynecol 1993;168:1339.
27. Pelloux H, Guy E, Angelici MC, et al. A second European collaborative study on polymerase chain reaction for Toxoplasma gondii, involving 15 teams. FEMS Microbiol Lett 1998;165:231.
28. Antsaklis A, Daskalakis G, Papantoniou N, et al. Prenatal diagnosis of congenital toxoplasmosis. Prenat Diagn 2002;22:1107.
29. Romand S, Wallon M, Franck J, et al. Prenatal diagnosis using polymerase chain reaction on amniotic fluid for congenital toxoplasmosis. Obstet Gynecol 2001;97:296.

30. Guy EC, Pelloux H, Lappalainen M, et al. Interlaboratory comparison of polymerase chain reaction for the detection of *Toxoplasma gondii* DNA added to samples of amniotic fluids. Eur J Clin Microbiol Infect Dis 1996;15:836.

31. Costa JM, Pautas C, Ernault P, et al. Real-time PCR for diagnosis and follow-up of Toxoplasma reactivation after allogeneic stem cell transplantation using fluorescence resonance energy transfer hybridization probes. J Clin Microbiol 2000;38:2929.

32. Homan WL, Vercammen M, De Braekeleer J, et al. Identification of a 200- to 300-fold repetitive 529 bp DNA fragment in Toxoplasma gondii, and its use for diagnostic and quantitative PCR. Int J Parasitol 2000;30:69.

33. Reischl U, Bretagne S, Kruger D, et al. Comparison of two DNA targets for the diagnosis of toxoplasmosis by real-time PCR using fluorescence resonance energy transfer hybridization probes. BMC Infect Dis 2003;3:7.

34. Jenum PA, Stray-Pedersen B, Melby KK, et al. Incidence of *Toxoplasma gondii* infection in 35940 pregnant women in Norway and pregnancy outcome for infected women. J Clin Microbiol 1998;36:2900.

35. Gratzl R, Hayde M, Kohlhauser C, et al. Follow-up of infants with congenital toxoplasmosis detected by polymerase chain reaction analysis of amniotic fluid. Eur J Clin Microbiol Infect Dis 1998;17:853.

36. Romand S, Chosson M, Franck J, et al. Usefulness of quantitative PCR in amniotic fluid as early prognostic marker of fetal infection with *Toxoplasma gondii*. Am J Obstet Gynecol, in press.

37. Derouin F, Chastang C. In vitro effects of folate inhibitors on Toxoplasma gondii. Antimicrob Agents Chemother 1989;33:1753.

38. Weller TH. The cytomegaloviruses: ubiquitous agents with protean clinical manifestations. N Engl J Med 1971;285:203.

39. Stagno S. Cytomegalovirus. In Remington J, Klein JO, Eds. Infectious diseases of the fetus and newborn infant, 4th ed. Philadelphia: W.B. Saunders, 1995.

40. Collinet F, Subtil D, Puech F. Problèmes posés par le dépistage du CMV chez la femme enceinte. Paris: Collège National des Gynécologues Obstétriciens, Vigot Ed, 2002.

41. Gaytant MA, Steegers E, Semmekrot BA, et al. Congenital cytomegalovirus infection: review of the epidemiology and outcome. Obstet Gynecol Surv 2002;57:245.

42. Ranger-Rogez, Venot C, Aubard Y, et al. Cytomegalovirus. In: Denis F, eds. Les virus transmissibles de la mère à l'enfant. John Libbey Eurotext, 1999.

43. Fowler K, Stagno S, Pass RF. The outcome of congenital cytomegalovirus infection in relation to maternal antibody status. New Engl J Med 1992;326:663.

44. Boppana SB, Rivera LB, Fowler KB, et al. Intrauterine transmission of cytomegalovirus to infants of women with preconceptional immunity. N Engl J Med 2002;344:1366.

45. Nigro G, Mazzocco M, Anceschi MM, et al. Prenatal diagnosis of fetal cytomegalovirus infection after primary or recurrent maternal infection. Obstet Gynecol 1999;94:6:909.

46. Boppana S, Pass RF, Britt, WS et al. Symptomatic congenital cytomegalovirus infection: neonatal morbidity and mortality. Pediatr Infect Dis J 1992;11:93.

47. Revello MG, Gerna G. Diagnosis and management of human cytomegalovirus infection in the mother, fetus, and newborn infant. Clin Microbiol Rev 2002;15:680.

48. Grangeot-Keros L, Mayaux MJ, Lebon P, et al. Value of cytomegalovirus (CMV) IgG avidity index for the diagnosis of primary CMV infection in pregnant women. J Infect Dis 1998;178:599.

49. Revello MG, Zavattoni M, Furione M, et al. Quantification of human cytomegalovirus fluid of mothers of congenitally infected fetuses. J Clin Microbiol 1999;37:3350.

50. Lynch L, Daffos F, Emanuel D, et al. Prenatal diagnosis of fetal cytomegalovirus infection. Obstet Gynecol 1991;165:714.

51. Gouarin S, Palmer P, Cointe D, et al. HCMV infection: a collaborative and comparative study of virus detection in amniotic fluid by culture and by PCR. J Clin Virol 2001;21:47.

52. Revello MG, Zavattoni M, Sarasini A. Prenatal diagnostic and prognostic value of human cytomegalovirus load and IgM antibody response in blood of congenitally infected fetuses. J Infect Dis 1999;180:1320.

53. Jay V, Otsubo H, Hwang P, et al. Coexistence of hemimegalencephaly and chronic encephalitis: detection of CMV by the polymerase chain reaction. Childs Nerv Syst 1997;13:35.

54. Barkovich AJ, Lindan CE. Congenital cytomegalovirus infection of the brain: imaging analysis and embryologic considerations. AJNR 1994;15:703.

55. Steinlin MI, Nadal D, Eich GF, et al. Late intrauterine cytomegalovirus infection: clinical and neuroimaging findings. Pediatr Neurol 1996;15:249.

56. Malinger G, Lev D, Zahalka N, et al. Fetal cytomegalovirus infection of the brain: the spectrum of sonographic findings. Am J Neuroradiol 2003;24:28.

57. Koga Y, Mizumoto M, Matsumoto Y, et al. Prenatal diagnosis of fetal intracranial calcifications. Am J Obstet Gynecol 1990;163:1543.
58. Ward RM. Drug therapy of the fetus. J Clin Pharmacol 1993;33:780.
59. Whitley RJ, Cloud G, Gruber W, et al. Ganciclovir treatment of symptomatic congenital cytomegalovirus infection: results of a stage 2 study. National Institute of Allergy and Infectious Diseases Collaborative Group. J Infect Dis 1997;175:1080.
60. Nigro G, Scholz H, Bartmann U, et al. Ganciclovir therapy for symptomatic congenital cytomegalovirus infection in infants: a two regimen experience. J Pediatr 1994;124:318.
61. Bell AR. Valacyclovir update. Adv Exp Med Biol 1999; 458:149.
62. Frenkel LM, Brown ZA, Bryson YJ, et al. Pharmacokinetics of acyclovir in the term human pregnancy and neonate. Am J Obstet Gynecol 1991;164:569.
63. Emery VC, Sabin C, Feinberg JE, et al. Quantitative effects of valacyclovir on the replication of cytomegalovirus (CMV) in persons with advanced human immunodeficiency virus disease: baseline CMV load dictates time to disease and survival. J Infect Dis 1999;180:695.
64. Lowance D, Neumayer H-H, Legendre C, et al. Valacyclovir reduces the incidence of cytomegalovirus disease and acute rejection in renal allograft recipients. N Engl J Med 1999;340:1462.
65. Adler SP, Finney JW, Manganello AM, et al. Prevention of child-to-mother transmission of cytomegalovirus by changing behaviours: a randomized controlled trial. Pediatr Infect Dis J 1996;15:240.
66. Hagay ZJ, Biran G, Ornoy A, et al. Congenital cytomegalovirus infection: a long-standing problem still seeking a solution. Am J Obstet Gynecol 1996;174:241.
67. Ville Y. The megalovirus. Ultrasound Obstet Gynecol 1998;12:151.
68. Ruyechan WT, Hay J. DNA replication. In: Arvin AM, Gershon AA, eds. Varicella–zoster virus. Cambridge, UK: Cambridge University Press, 2000.
69. Seward J, Galil K, Wharton M. Epidemiology of varicella. In: Arvin AM, Gershon AA, eds. Varicella–zoster virus. Cambridge, UK: Cambridge University Press, 2000.
70. Enders G, Miller E. Varicella and herpes zoster in pregnancy and the newborn. In: Arvin AM, Gershon AA, eds. Varicella–zoster virus. Cambridge, UK: Cambridge University Press, 2000.
71. Fairley CK, Miller E. Varicella zoster virus epidemiology: a changing scene? J Infect Dis 1996;174 (suppl 3):S314.
72. Laforet EG, Lynch CL. Multiple congenital defects following maternal varicella: report of a case. N Engl J Med 1947;236:534.
73. Mouly F, Mirlesse V, Meritet JF, et al. Prenatal diagnosis of fetal varicella–zoster virus infection with polymerase chain reaction of amniotic fluid in 107 cases. Am J Obstet Gynecol 1997:177;894.
74. Enders G, Miller E, Cradock-Watson J, et al. Consequences of varicella and herpes zoster in pregnancy: a prospective study of 1739 cases. Lancet 1994;343:1547.
75. Puchhammer-Stöckl E, Kunz C, Wagner G, et al. Detection of varicella zoster virus (VZV) DNA in fetal tissues by polymerase chain reaction. J Perinat Med 1994;22:65.
76. Pons J, Rozenberg F, Imbert M, et al. Prenatal diagnosis of second trimester congenital varicella syndrome. Prenat Diagn 1992;11:975.
77. Sauerbrei A. Varicella zoster virus infections in pregnancy. Intervirology 1998:41:191.
78. Higa K, Dan K, Manabe H. Varicella zoster virus infections during pregnancy: hypothesis concerning the mechanisms of congenital malformations. Obstet Gynecol 1987;69:214.
79. Birthistle K, Carrington D. Fetal varicella syndrome: a reappraisal of the literature. J Infect 1998;36:25.
80. Harger JH, Ernest JM, Thurnau GR, et al. Frequency of congenital varicella syndrome in a prospective cohort of 347 pregnant women. Obstet Gynecol 2002;100:260.
81. Takahashi M, Plotkin SA. Development of the Oka vaccine. In: Arvin AM, Gershon AA, eds. Varicella–zoster virus. Cambridge, UK: Cambridge University Press, 2000.
82. Whitley RJ. Treatment of Varicella. In: Arvin AM, Gershon AA, eds. Varicella–zoster virus. Cambridge, UK: Cambridge University Press, 2000.
83. Asano Y, Yoshikawa T, Suga S, et al. Post exposure prophylaxis of varicella in family contact by oral acyclovir. Pediatrics 1993;92:219.
84. Enders G, Nickerl-Pacher U, Cradock-Watson JE. Outcome of confirmed periconceptional maternal rubella. Lancet 1988;1:1445.
85. Miller E, Cradock-Watson JE, Pollock TM. Consequences of confirmed maternal rubella at successive stages of pregnancy. Lancet 1982;2:781–86.
86. Daffos F, Forestier F, Grangeoit-Keros L, et al. Prenatal diagnosis of congenital rubella. Lancet 1984;1:162.
87. Terry GM, Ho-Terry L, Warren RC, et al. First trimester prenatal diagnosis of congenital rubella: a laboratory investigation. Br Med J (Clin Res Ed) 1986;292:930.

88. Tang JW, Aarons E, Hesketh LM, et al Prenatal diagnosis of congenital rubella infection in the second trimester of pregnancy. Prenat Diagn 2003;23:509.

89. Revello MG, Baldanti F, Sarasini A, et al. Prenatal diagnosis of rubella virus infection by direct detection and semiquantitation of viral RNA in clinical samples by reverse transcription-PCR. J Clin Microbiol 1997;35:708.

90. Rodis JF, Quinn DL, Gary GW Jr, et al. Management and outcomes of pregnancies complicated by human B19 parvovirus infection: a prospective study. Am J Obstet Gynecol 1990;163:1168.

91. Nunoue T, Kusuhara K, Hara T. Human fetal infection with parvovirus B19: maternal infection time in gestation, viral persistence and fetal prognosis. Pediatr Infect Dis J 2002;21:1133.

92. Carrington D, Gilmore DH, Whittle MJ, et al. Maternal serum alpha-fetoprotein: a marker of fetal aplastic crisis during intrauterine human parvovirus infection. Lancet 1987;1:433.

93. Forestier F, Tissot JD, Vial Y, et al. Haematological parameters of parvovirus B19 infection in 13 fetuses with hydrops foetalis. Br J Haematol 1999;104:925.

Mary Z. Pelias, Ph.D., J.D.

31

Medicolegal Aspects of Prenatal Diagnosis

Since the early 1970s, medical malpractice suits for "wrongful birth" and "wrongful life" have established a serious legal risk for health care professionals whose patients are at risk for having children with predictable mental or physical defects. Medical professionals and persons in the allied health professions have been held accountable for their failure to keep abreast of new technologic developments and for failure to act on knowledge of an increased risk that the offspring of their patients will have hereditary or environmentally induced defects. Early attempts to predict birth defects were limited to indirect examination of the fetus by stethoscope or by x-rays and to calculating genetic, or mendelian, risks and other statistical probabilities. More recently, however, the expansion of technology in prenatal diagnosis has allowed direct examination of the fetus by fetoscopy, ultrasonic and magnetic resonance imaging, and indirect determination of fetal status by amniocentesis, chorionic villus sampling, and fetal tissue sampling. This explosion of knowledge has dramatically increased the physician's obligation to keep patients fully informed about their reproductive options.

This chapter is intended not as legal advice, but as a review of the important principles in the torts of wrongful birth and wrongful life, with a view to informing practitioners in reproductive medicine about their risk of medical malpractice allegations. Although the growth of case law now precludes a summary of all cases that have been settled or have reached the appellate courts, a review of the salient issues and significant cases will outline the type of professional conduct that is likely to be construed by the courts as substandard. Because this discussion is only an introduction to this specialized area of medical malpractice, any health care professional who has questions or doubts about a specific situation should consult an attorney on an individual basis.

GENERAL CONCEPTS OF MEDICAL MALPRACTICE

Torts are civil wrongs that occur between private parties. Tort law is broadly divided into intentional wrongdoing and negligent wrongdoing. Suits in medical malpractice are usually brought under a theory of negligence, a concept that has a much broader meaning in the law than the common meaning of neglect. Fundamental to an action in medical malpractice is a legally recognized relationship between the two parties. This relationship is technically one of implied contract, and it gives rise to the duties owed by the parties to each other. To establish a clear case of medical negligence in a court of law, the plaintiff/health care consumer must prove that the defendant/health care provider owed a duty to the plaintiff to meet a professional standard of care, that the duty was breached, and that the breach of duty was the proximate cause of legally cognizable injury to the plaintiff. The plaintiff asks that money damages be awarded as compensation for the injury. These damages may be "general" damages for physical and emotional pain and suffering, or "special" damages for economic losses, including medical expenses, lost wages, and the costs of rearing the child. Occasionally, when the conduct of a defendant has been grossly negligent or egregious, a court may permit consideration of "punitive" damages in addition to general and special damages.

After the plaintiff's allegations have been filed and served, the defendant/health care provider prepares an appropriate rebuttal. The defenses may include an assertion that the plaintiff's claims have no basis in the law or that the plaintiff's claims have been extinguished under the statute of limitations. The defendant also may directly deny some or all of the allegations. Other defenses may include lack of a duty owed, lack of proximate cause between the breach and injury, or impossibility of measuring damages.

If the case goes to trial, both parties are responsible for presenting their evidence to the court. The standard of care to which the health care provider is held is most often established by the testimonial evidence of expert witnesses, who usually are other physicians and health care providers. Such witnesses are called by both the plaintiff and the defendant to strengthen their respective assertions. Testimonial evidence may be elicited from other witnesses as well, and any pertinent tangible evidence, such as copies of medical records, may be submitted for consideration. Finally, the judge or jury, the "trier of fact," considers and renders its decision, or verdict. Although the immediate objective of going to court is to win a case, the ultimate goal of submitting disputes to a court is to achieve justice. Establishing truth, however, can be elusive, and proof in the scientific sense often is not possible in a courtroom. Therefore, the party who argues more convincingly or who presents the preponderance of the evidence in this type of civil suit prevails, and the dispute is settled in a peaceful rather than violent manner. In most lawsuits, the facts are arguable and usually rebuttable. Both disputants are heard carefully by the court, but in the end, only one of them will leave the court a winner.

The party who loses in trial court has recourse to proceed to an appellate court for review of the decision in the court below. The appellate court reviews the record of the trial court and allows both parties to present briefs and arguments about why the decision of the lower court should be overturned or upheld. The appellate court does not examine new evidence or "retry" the case. State court systems have two tiers of appellate review: an intermediate appellate court and the highest court of the state, usually called the state Supreme Court. In the federal court system, decisions of the federal district (trial) court may be appealed to the federal circuit court of appeals. The U.S. Supreme Court has the discretion to review decisions of the highest state courts and of the federal circuit appellate courts, particularly if a constitutional question or right is involved.

This general sketch of the legal system of the United States is intended only as an introductory outline. Both the state and federal court systems have rules of procedure, which at first glance may seem to be mystifying tools of the legal profession. However, a basic familiarity with these rules is well within the comprehension of most health care professionals and will foster a general understanding of what is expected of the litigating parties and how they should proceed from the inception to the conclusion of a lawsuit.

THE CONSTITUTIONAL RIGHT OF PRIVACY IN REPRODUCTIVE DECISIONS

Most legal cases involving genetically defective children derive from claims that parents were deprived of their right to make their own decisions about conceiving and bearing children. Specifically, parents claim that the health care provider was negligent either in performing sterilization surgery or in providing sufficient, accurate information about reproductive risks. The parents claim that this negligence infringed on their rights to privacy and personal autonomy. The right to privacy was first recognized under the Constitution in 1965; before that time, parents had no claim to a constitutionally protected right not to have children.

In 1965, a Connecticut statute banning the use of contraceptives by married couples was held unconstitutional by the U.S. Supreme Court. The Court found the statute to be an impermissible intrusion by the state into the constitutional right to privacy in the marital bedroom (*Griswold v. Connecticut*, 1965). Seven years later, the right to privacy in deciding whether to conceive or bear a child was extended to single persons as well (*Eisenstadt v. Baird*, 1972). Shortly thereafter, the Court extended the constitutional right to privacy to include the right of a woman, in consultation with her physician, to decide to terminate her pregnancy (*Roe v. Wade*, 1973). In this landmark decision, states were proscribed from limiting access to abortions until after the fetus becomes viable, after which a state's interest in the life of the fetus becomes compelling unless the life or the health of the mother is endangered. The strict standards of judicial review and the viability approach of *Roe v. Wade* were somewhat relaxed when the Supreme Court later held that state law could regulate access to abortions as long as the law did not impose an "undue burden" on the woman who seeks to terminate a pregnancy (*Planned Parenthood of Southeastern Pennsylvania v. Casey*, 1992).

This series of Supreme Court decisions has significantly expanded the duty of physicians and genetic counselors to disclose information that could be material, or influential, in a parental decision to conceive and bear children. Parents who are not fully and accurately informed about risks of genetic or other possible defects in their future offspring are now quick to claim that they have been denied their right to privacy in matters of reproductive choice.

THE DOCTRINE OF INFORMED CONSENT IN MEDICAL TREATMENT

The evolution of the common law Doctrine of Informed Consent over the course of the twentieth century has reinforced the right of patients to personal autonomy in making their own decisions about their medical treatment. This right is based on the premise that "every adult of sound mind and body has the right to determine what shall be done with his own body" (*Schloendorf v. Society of New York Hospital*, 1914). Derived from this doctrine is the recognition of tortious conduct of physicians who fail to inform parents about their reproductive risks and options. Parents have successfully claimed that disclosure of these risks and options is necessary for them to make rational, autonomous decisions about family planning. Also relative to these decisions is information about any preconception or prenatal diagnostic tests that could elucidate risks to future offspring. A critical issue in many wrongful birth and wrongful life cases is whether the physician failed to disclose information that was material, or could have been influential, in the patient's decision-making process (Pelias, 1991).

The standard of disclosure used to measure a physician's conduct varies among jurisdictions. Most states adhere to a professional standard of care, the standard of professional conduct that would be expected from a reasonable physician (*Natanson v. Kline*, 1960). Other states, however, look to a standard of care that would be expected by a reasonable patient: the physician's conduct is measured from the viewpoint of the patient, and the physician is expected to disclose any risks and alternatives that may be material for an informed decision by a reasonable person (*Canterbury v. Spence*, 1972). Although the concepts of disclosure and informed consent underlie the allegations in suits for wrongful birth and wrongful life, the fact that these arguments usually are not raised in court strongly supports the view that the parents' right to personal autonomy outweighs the physician's right to exercise his or her professional judgment about how much information to disclose.

EARLY CONCEPTS IN PRECONCEPTION AND PRENATAL TORT LAW

Two additional legal concepts have influenced the development of the torts of wrongful birth and wrongful life. Under a long line of cases in the English common law of property, the right to inherit vests at the moment of conception, so that a child born after the death of a parent may inherit under the testament of that parent (Shaw and Damme, 1976). And in the law of prenatal injury resulting in death shortly after birth, Justice Oliver Wendell Holmes wrote that there is "a conditional prospective liability in tort to one not yet in being" (*Dietrich v. Inhabitants of Northhampton*, 1884). This holding has been the foundation for recovery of damages in cases of injury to the fetus, although some courts have allowed recovery only if the fetus is injured after quickening (*Bonbrest v. Kotz*, 1946) or after the time of viability. The artificial time limits of quickening and viability have been disregarded in later cases, so that all jurisdictions now allow recovery for prenatal injuries, and some courts permit recovery for preconception torts (Shaw, 1980) and for injuries sustained by a fetus that is subsequently stillborn (*Panagopoulos v. Martin*, 1969).

SUITS FOR WRONGFUL BIRTH AND WRONGFUL LIFE

Definitions

When parents claim that they have been wronged by the birth of a child, the courts have distinguished between two causes of action: *wrongful pregnancy* and *wrongful birth*. Suits for *wrongful pregnancy*, occasionally also called wrongful conception, are based on active measures by the parents to avoid any pregnancy, usually by surgical sterilization. When they subsequently have a normal, healthy child, they seek to recover damages from the physician who negligently performed the surgical procedure or whose conduct was otherwise negligent. The damages sought in these cases include general damages for the pain and suffering associated with the first sterilization procedure, the unwanted pregnancy and birth, and for loss of service and consortium. The plaintiff also may seek special damages to cover all medical expenses and the "ordinary" costs of raising the normal child to adulthood. Whether the parents actually do recover damages, and how much they recover, depends on the statutory law, judicial receptivity, precedent, and the litigation climate in the state in which the suit is brought: recovery usually is limited to the damages for the negligent sterilization procedure and prenatal and postnatal care (*C.S. v. Nielson*, 1988; *Hatter v. Landsberg*, 1989; *Simmerer v. Dabbas*, 2000), but occasionally, the parents recover the ordinary costs of rearing a normal child to majority (*Lovelace Medical Center v. Mendez*, 1991).

Parents who sue for *wrongful birth* also may have sought to avoid any pregnancy but eventually had a child with hereditary or environmentally induced defects that require special attention and care over the child's projected lifetime. The parents may have decided not to bear any children because they are or may be at risk of having an abnormal child or not to bear any more children because they already have an abnormal child. Alternatively, they may have been under the mistaken impression that their pregnancy probably was normal, either because their physician told them incorrectly that there was no risk to the fetus or because the physician failed to inform them about available tests or known risks. After the birth of an abnormal child, the parents may sue the physician and any other health care providers involved for misdeeds (malfeasance) or nondeeds (nonfeasance) that occurred either before or after the conception of the abnormal child. Allegations of negligence may include failure to perform a surgical procedure properly, failure to disclose complete information about genetic risks and appropriate tests, or failure to perform appropriate tests accurately. The plaintiff/parents in wrongful birth suits may seek general damages for pain and suffering as well as special damages for all of their expenses, including their own medical expenses, the ordinary costs of rearing the child, and the "extraordinary" costs associated with the child's abnormality, for as long as the child is dependent. Again, whether the parents may recover damages, and how much they may recover, depends on the legal climate in the state where the suit is brought (*Wilson v. Mercy Hospital*, 2003).

Suits for *wrongful life* are brought by or on behalf of a child born with inherited or acquired abnormalities that could have been predicted before conception or during the prenatal period. The plaintiff/child may claim that it would have been better not to be born at all rather than to be born with defects to endure suffering and pain. Alternatively, the child may claim that its damages should be measured by comparing its compromised life with the life of a normal child. The child may seek general damages for its pain and suffering as well as special damages for the costs associated with its defects over its entire lifetime. Another line of cases, now referred to as suits for *dissatisfied life*, has been generated by illegitimate but otherwise normal offspring who sue their parents for the wrongs associated with their illegitimate state. So far, either these cases have been dismissed for want of a cognizable cause of action (e.g., *Lloyd v. Howard*, 1990) or the court has refused to award damages for the wrong committed because the problem is deemed one for legislative rather than judicial solution (e.g., *Zepeda v. Zepeda*, 1963, 1964).

Theories of Recovery in Wrongful Pregnancy and Wrongful Birth

When parents first complained about having unwanted children because of a physician's negligence in a sterilization procedure, the courts stubbornly refused to recognize that the parents had been injured. In these early decisions, the courts applied the "Blessings Theory," which insists that every child is a blessing rather than an injury to its parents (*Christensen v. Thornby*, 1934; *Terrell v. Garcia*, 1973, 1974). These opinions were typified by justifications such as, "Who can put a price tag on a child's smile?" (*Ball v. Mudge*, 1964), and no recovery of damages was allowed. In addition, some state supreme courts have thwarted any recovery in wrongful birth by holding that the court would recognize no cause of action for wrongful birth "absent a clear mandate by the legislature" (*Azzolino v. Dingfelder*, 1985, 1986; *Campbell v. United States*, 1992). Any possibility of recovery also has been precluded in those states that have enacted statutes that proscribe a cause of action for wrongful birth (*Wilson v. Kuenzi*, 1988; *Wood v. University of Utah Medical Center*, 2002).

The notion of children being unqualified blessings gradually gave way to the idea that parents who take active measures to avoid conception could indeed be harmed by the subsequent birth of a child. In suits that fall into the category of wrongful pregnancy, followed by the birth of a normal child, most courts now limit recovery to the costs of the unsuccessful sterilization procedure and prenatal and postnatal expenses and perhaps some recovery for the pain and suffering associated with the sterilization procedure, pregnancy, and birth. However, the ordinary costs of raising a normal child to maturity are disallowed on the theory that the birth of a normal child is not an injury to the parents (*Johnson v. University Hospitals of Cleveland*, 1989).

A third line of reasoning has developed into the so-called benefits rule, which admits that an unwanted child can be both a burden and a benefit to its parents. Under this rule, the court weighs the burdens imposed on the family against the benefits conferred by the child. The monetary value of the burden is then mitigated by the monetary value of the benefits, sometimes in such a manner that the mitigated recovery amounts to nothing. For example, one court concluded that "the benefits of joy, companionship, and affection which a normal, healthy child can provide must be deemed as a matter of law to outweigh the costs of raising that child" (*Butler v. Rolling Hill Hospital*, 1990; see also *Lodato v. Kappy*, 2002). In response to the assertions of several defendants that the parents themselves had a duty to mitigate their damages, a number of courts have clearly stated that plaintiff/parents were under no obligation to mitigate their damages by choosing abortion (*Liddington v. Burns*, 1995) or by placing the unwanted child for adoption (*University of Arizona Health Sciences Center v. Arizona Superior Court*, 1983).

A fourth approach, adopted in some more recent cases, recognizes that the parents are indeed injured by the birth of an unwanted child. In what may be an especially important decision in wrongful pregnancy, the Wisconsin Supreme Court noted that the injury to the parents was not the actual birth of the child but, rather, was injury to their interest in establishing financial security for their family and in providing well for the children they already had (*Marciniak v. Lundborg*, 1990). This court allowed full recovery of ordinary costs of rearing the normal child to adulthood. In cases of wrongful birth of children with abnormalities, the courts are divided about what constitutes full recovery: at least two states still allow recovery only for the costs associated with the sterilization procedure and the unwanted pregnancy (*Pitre v. Opelousas General Hospital*, 1988; *Simmerer v. Dabbas*, 2000); most courts limit recovery to extraordinary costs related to the child's abnormalities (*Fassoulas v. Ramey*, 1984; *Lininger v. Eisenbaum*, 1988; *Arche v. U.S. Department of Army*, 1990), whereas at least two courts have allowed recovery of both the ordinary and extraordinary costs of raising the abnormal child (*Robak v. United States*, 1981; *Naccash v. Burger*, 1982). With regard to the time span of recovery, some courts limit the recoverable amount to the costs generated during the minority of the child (e.g., *Ochs v. Borrelli*, 1982), whereas other courts recognize the ongoing duty of the parents to care for their abnormal child and allow costs over the child's entire lifetime (*Garrison v. Medical Center of Delaware*, 1989; *Lloyd v. North Broward Hospital District*, 1990).

Recent Trends in Wrongful Life Suits Brought by Children

Children are far less successful in their claims for wrongful life than are parents who sue for wrongful birth. Most jurisdictions still deny the child the right to complain for having been born. Some courts have pointed out the logical and legal absurdity of recognizing the child's claim for pain and suffering, because if the negligence had not occurred, the child would not be there to complain; in legal terms, the child "lacks standing" to sue. Most courts state that the reason for denying the child's claim is the impossibility of measuring damages by comparing life compromised by defects to no life at all (*Gleitman v. Cosgrove*, 1967; *Lininger v. Eisenbaum*, 1988; *Hester v. Dwivedi*, 2000). Because of society's regard for the preciousness of all life, some courts argue that it would be against public policy to allow the child to claim that it would have been better not to have been born at all (*Smith v. Cote*, 1986; *Siemieniec v. Lutheran General Hospital*, 1987). Most courts that discuss the issue of public policy insist that the question is one for legislative decision, so that a tort of wrongful life must be recognized by statute before it can be acknowledged by the judiciary (*James G. v. Caserta*, 1985; *Proffitt v. Bartolo*, 1987, 1988).

Nevertheless, despite a general reluctance of the courts to grapple with the issue of public policy, courts in four states have recognized that a wrong has indeed occurred when a child both exists and suffers because of another's negligence. Therefore, the child is granted standing to sue based on a cause of action for wrongful life. The first state to do so was California, in which an intermediate appellate court upheld the claim of a child with Tay–Sachs disease whose parents both were erroneously reported to be noncarriers of the recessive gene (*Curlender v. Bio-Science Laboratories*, 1980). In a second case in California, a child born with hereditary deafness was allowed to recover special damages related to her deafness but was not allowed to collect general damages for being born with defects as opposed to not being born at all (*Turpin v. Sortini*, 1981, 1982). Two children born with fetal hydantoin syndrome were allowed to collect special damages related to their defects over their lifetimes when the Supreme Court of Washington declared that physicians owe a duty to the fetus as well as to the mother (*Harbeson v. Parke-Davis*, 1983). Shortly after the *Harbeson* decision, the Supreme Court of New Jersey allowed a child with congenital rubella syndrome to recover special damages for his extraordinary expenses, both during infancy and adulthood (*Procanik v. Cillo*, 1984). Finally, a child who suffered severe damage as a result of undetected Rh incompatibility was allowed to recover damages in Colorado (*Continental Casualty Co. v. Empire Casualty Co.*, 1985). Although these seminal cases established wrongful life as a tort in four jurisdictions, similar claims in other jurisdictions have been disallowed.

Several arguments on behalf of the child's wrongful life claim have been advanced in trial courts and in appellate hearings. For example, one court has argued that if the parents are compensated for the special medical costs of their abnormal child until majority, then in all fairness, the child should be permitted to recover these costs after majority (e.g., *Simmons v. West Covina Medical Clinic*, 1989). If the parents are dead or are severely impaired themselves, or if the statute of limitations has expired on the parents' claim, allowing the child to recover avoids the injustice that would result if the child had no standing before the court. However, if the child is adopted and the responsibility for its well-being is legally shifted to the adoptive parents, the child's claim for damages extinguishes at the time of adoption. Therefore, the child may claim damages only for the time between birth and adoption (*Cowe v. Forum Group, Inc.*, 1989). Note, also, that a claim for "wrongful adoption," on the basis of later discovered psychologic and physical disorders in the adopted child, has no basis in Constitutional law or under Civil Rights Law, 42 U.S.C. § 1983 (*Collier v. Krane*, 1991).

These and other practical reasons may sway other courts to recognize suits for wrongful life in the future.

Analysis of Alleged Negligent Acts and Outcomes in Wrongful Birth and Wrongful Life Suits

Table 31.1 lists many of the important wrongful birth and wrongful life cases that have been reported in the legal literature since the *Roe v. Wade* abortion decision in 1973. Only

Table 31.1. Selected legal cases involving the birth of abnormal children

Case	Parents' Claim	Child's Claim	Diagnosis
Chromosomal disorders			
Alquijay v. St. Luke's Hospital (1984)	Yes	No	Down syndrome
Atlanta Obstetrics and Gynecology Group v. Abelson (1990)	No	No	Down syndrome
Azzolino v. Dingfelder (1985)	Yes	Yes	Down syndrome
Becker v. Schwartz (1978)	Yes	No	Down syndrome
Berman v. Allen (1981)	Yes	No	Down syndrome
Call v. Kezirian (1982)	Yes	N/A	Down syndrome
Garrison v. Medical Center of Delaware (1989)	Yes	No	Down syndrome
Haymon v. Wilkerson (1987)	Yes	No	Down syndrome
Jenkins v. Hospital of Medical College (1991)	Yes	N/A	Down syndrome
Jorgensen v. Meade Johnson Laboratories, Inc. (1973)	N/A	Yes	Down syndrome
Karlsons v. Guerinot (1977)	Yes	No	Down syndrome
Kassama v. Magat (2002)	No	No	Down syndrome
Phillips v. United States (1980, 1981, 1983)	Yes	No	Familial Down syndrome
Simmons v. West Covina Medical Clinic (1989)	No	No	Down syndrome
Wilson v. Kuenzi (1988)	No	No	Down syndrome
Wood v. University of Utah Medical Center (2002)	No	N/A	Down syndrome
Johnson v. Yeshiva University (1977)	No	No	Cri-du-chat syndrome
Campbell v. United States (1992)	No	N/A	10q chromosome deletion
Davis v. Board of Supervisors (1998)	No	No	Trisomy 9 mosaic
Feigelson v. Ryan (1981)	No	N/A	Chromosomal disorder
Gallagher v. Duke University (1988)	Yes	No	Chromosomal disorder
Lloyd v. North Broward Hospital District (1990)	Yes	No	Chromosomal disorder
Dominant genes			
Brubaker v. Cavanaugh (1982)	No	No	Multiple polyposis of colon
Ellis v. Sherman (1984)	Yes	No	Neurofibromatosis
Speck v. Finegold (1979, 1981)	Yes	No	Neurofibromatosis
Moores v. Lucas (1981)	Yes	N/A	Larsen syndrome
Recessive genes			
Curlender v. Bio-Science Laboratories (1980)	N/A	Yes	Tay–Sachs disease
Didato v. Strehler (2001)	N/A	N/A	Sickle cell β^0-thalassemia
Gildiner v. Thomas Jefferson University Hospital (1978)	Yes	No	Tay–Sachs disease
Goldberg v. Ruskin (1984)	Yes	No	Tay–Sachs disease
Howard v. Lecher (1976, 1977)	Yes	N/A	Tay–Sachs disease
Naccash v. Burger (1982)	Yes	N/A	Tay–Sachs disease
Rubin v. Hamot Medical Center (1984)	N/A	No	Tay–Sachs disease
Dorlin v. Providence Hospital (1982)	Yes	No	Sickle cell anemia
Lininger v. Eisenbaum (1988)	Yes	No	Leber congenital amaurosis
Park v. Chessin (1977, 1978)	Yes	No	Infantile polycystic kidneys
Pitre v. Opelousas General Hospital (1988)	Yes	No	Albinism
Pratt v. University of Minnesota Affiliated Hospitals and Clinics (1987)	Yes	N/A	Oral-facial-digital syndrome
Schroeder v. Perkel (1981)	Yes	N/A	Cystic fibrosis
Turpin v. Sortini (1982)	Yes	Yes	Hereditary deafness
X-linked recessive genes			
Nelson v. Krusen (1984)	Yes	No	Duchenne muscular dystrophy
Payne v. Myers (1987)	Yes	No	Pelizaeus–Merzbacher syndrome
Siemieniec v. Lutheran General Hospital (1987)	Yes	No	Hemophilia B
Wilson v. Mercy Hospital (2003)	No	No	Hemophilia

Table 31.1. Selected legal cases involving the birth of abnormal children (continued)

Case	Parents' Claim	Child's Claim	Diagnosis
Other disorders			
Aquilio v. Nelson (1980)	No	N/A	Rh disease
Continental Casualty Co. v. Empire Casualty Co. (1985)	N/A	Yes	Rh disease
Dyson v. Winfield (2002)	Yes	N/A	Birth defects
Lazevnick v. General Hospital of Monroe County (1980)	Yes	N/A	Rh disease
Renslow v. Mennonite Hospital (1977)	N/A	Yes	Rh disease
Blake v. Cruz (1984)	Yes	No	Rubella
Eisbrenner v. Stanley (1981)	Yes	No	Rubella
Procanik v. Cillo (1984)	N/A	Yes	Rubella
Proffitt v. Bartolo (1987, 1988)	Yes	No	Rubella
Robak v. United States (1980, 1981)	Yes	N/A	Rubella
Strohmaier v. Associates in Obstetrics and Gynecology (1982)	Yes	No	Rubella
Walker v. Mart (1990)	Yes	No	Rubella
Allen v. Colonial Laboratories (1982)	Yes	No	Physical and mental defects
Anderson v. Wiener (1984)	Yes	N/A	Brain damage
Anonymous v. Physician (1980)	Yes	Yes	Physical and mental defects
Comras v. Lewin (1982)	Yes	N/A	"Defective child"
DiNatale v. Lieberman (1982)	Yes	No	Physical and mental defects
Donadio v. Crouse-Irving Memorial Hospital (1980)	No	N/A	Prematurity and blindness
Flickinger v. Wanczyk (1994)	No	No	Hydrocephaly and spina bifida
Arche v. U.S. Department of Army (1990)	Yes	N/A	Severe, permanent handicap
Elliott v. Brown (1978)	N/A	No	Severe deformities
Fassoulas v. Ramey (1984)	Yes	N/A	Severe deformities
Harbeson v. Parke-Davis (1983)	Yes	Yes	Fetal hydantoin syndrome
Ochs v. Borelli (1982)	Yes	N/A	Orthopedic defects
Pines v. Dr. Carlos D. Moreno, Inc. (1990)	Yes	N/A	Cornelia de Lange syndrome
Schreck v. State of New York (1981)	No	N/A	Microcephaly in siblings
Stribling v. DeQuevedo (1980)	Yes	No	Dextrocardia

Note: Brief summaries of these cases are provided in the appendix.

those cases that are appealed to intermediate appellate courts or to the higher supreme court levels are published in the legal literature, and this is only a small fraction of the total number of suits that are filed. Although many cases are decided in trial court, most suits are settled out of court through malpractice insurance or are dismissed on preliminary motions before a trial on the merits actually starts. Recent out-of-court settlements have provided plaintiffs with sums ranging from $450,000 to $2.7 million (*Woodruff v. City and County of San Francisco*, 1995; *Shrader v. Coffineau*, 1996; *Vega v. Del Rosario*, 1996).

The second and third columns of Table 31.1 show that the parents are nearly always successful in their suits for wrongful birth, whereas the child usually is denied his or her claim for wrongful life. Only five cases have recognized a child's cause of action for wrongful life. Of these, three have been decided at the state supreme court level: *Turpin v. Sortini*, in California in 1982; *Harbeson v. Parke-Davis*, in Washington in 1983; and *Procanik v. Cillo*, in New Jersey in 1984. A fourth case, *Curlender v. Bio-Science Laboratories*, was decided at the intermediate appellate level in California in 1980 and was later reinforced by the *Turpin* decision. The fifth case, *Continental Casualty Co. v. Empire Casualty Co.*, was decided at the intermediate appellate level in Colorado.

The appendix at the end of this chapter provides a short summary of each case listed in Table 31.1 and other cases cited in the text. The facts giving rise to allegations of negligence are described briefly, and a summary of the reasoning offered by the court in its published decision is also included.

More complete discussions of these cases and the issues involved are found in the legal literature. The cases themselves are published in the various regional reporters, whereas case reports, or summaries, and commentaries are found in law review journals. Some cases that result in out-of-court settlements are reported in local news journals that circulate in the legal profession. These cases delineate for the physician, genetic counselor, and other health care providers the foundations of legal liability. An understanding of the basic issues in wrongful birth and wrongful life litigation should suggest how health care professionals may reduce or eliminate allegations of negligence in the future.

COMMENTS FROM THE VIEW OF THE CHILD

In a personal injury case in which a fetus was injured in an automobile accident, the Supreme Court of New Jersey announced that "a child has a right to begin life with a sound mind and a sound body" (*Smith v. Brennan*, 1960). This doctrine establishes that the child's right to a healthy life takes precedence over the parents' right to reproduce. The *Curlender* court in California enunciated the concept more clearly:

> One of the fears expressed in the decisional law [about wrongful life suits] is that, once it is determined that such infants have rights cognizable at law, nothing would prevent a plaintiff from bringing suit against its own parents for allowing the plaintiff to be born. In our view, the fear is groundless. The "wrongful-life" cause of action with which we are concerned is based upon negligently caused failure by someone under a duty to do so to inform the prospective parents of facts needed by them to make a conscious choice not to become parents. If a case arose where, despite due care by the medical profession in transmitting the necessary warnings, parents made a choice to proceed with a pregnancy, with full knowledge that a seriously impaired infant would be born, that conscious choice would provide an intervening act of proximate cause to preclude liability insofar as defendants other than the parents were concerned. Under such circumstances, we see no sound public policy which should protect those parents from being answerable for the pain, suffering and misery which they have wrought upon their offspring.

This line of reasoning was quickly criticized by legal commentators, who noted that such reasoning might give rise to a legal duty of the parents to abort a defective fetus. To anyone who believes in the right to life from the moment of conception or who holds fetal life sacred, such a suggestion would be an unreasonable burden. On the other hand, civil libertarians would find it equally distasteful because it violates the concept of parental autonomy in reproductive decision-making.

Soon after the *Curlender* opinion was announced, the California legislature moved quickly to disallow tort actions by children against their parents if the only alternative is not to be born at all. The *California Civil Code* (1982) reads, in part:

> (a) No cause of action arises against a parent of a child based upon the claim that the child should not have been conceived or, if conceived, should not have been allowed to have been born alive.

(b) The failure or refusal of a parent to prevent the livebirth of his or her child shall not be a defense in any action against a third party, nor shall the failure or refusal be considered in awarding damages in any such action.

Part (b) of the act puts physicians on notice that they cannot claim that the parents were intervening parties in the events leading to birth and that the parents might have chosen not to abort if they had been told of the high probability or certainty of defects in the fetus.

A number of cases have established that children may recover for other torts committed before conception, usually physical injury to the fetus (Shaw, 1980). The courts have argued that because the child would have been normal but for the tort, a legal liability accrues at live birth. In response to the suggestion that this is an artificial distinction from wrongful life claims, one might argue that the source of the child's mental and physical abnormalities is irrelevant: the abnormal child both exists and suffers, regardless of whether the abnormalities are caused by external injury, defective genes, an extra chromosome, or a teratogen. If knowledge of increased risks and prenatal diagnostic techniques permits parents to avoid the birth of a child whose life is compromised, then failure to use this expertise results in a compensable wrong to the child. The obligation of the professional is to help future generations be the beneficiaries of increased knowledge and technology.

FUTURE TRENDS

Because of the strongly divisive nature of the continuing controversy about abortion, accurate predictions about the outcome of future litigation are not feasible. If elective abortions become illegal in some states, and if there is no statutory exception for grossly deformed fetuses or fetuses that could be born with grave retardation or serious genetic disease, the courts will be obligated to reconsider their precedential holdings. Undoubtedly, some questions about the negligent acts of physicians will become moot unless new theories of recovery are fashioned. And, tragically, the hard-won constitutional rights of individuals and couples to choose whether to have children will be compromised and, in some cases, denied altogether if no legally compensable injury is identified.

Preconception, but not prenatal, torts could become the only cognizable cause of action, and negligence of the physician in wrongful birth cases could be limited to failure to disclose known risks or failure to disclose availability of tests for parents who could determine their own genetic status before conception. Parents could be advised, for example, to determine whether they both are carriers for a deleterious autosomal recessive gene or whether the woman is a carrier for an X-linked recessive gene. Such an approach would preserve the parents' choice about whether to conceive, but it would not allow them to choose whether to carry a defective fetus to term. The right to be informed about genetic or environmental risks to the fetus and about the right to determine the status of the fetus by prenatal testing will become hollow rights indeed if parents are no longer allowed to act on that knowledge after conception.

APPENDIX: SUMMARIES OF CASES

Allen v. Colonial Laboratories (Florida, 1982). This is a companion case to *DiNatale v. Lieberman* (see below), and the court's opinion applies to both cases.

Alquijay v. St. Luke's Roosevelt Hospital (New York, 1984). Because the woman was 35 years of age when she became pregnant, the physician advised an amniocentesis, which she accepted. The laboratory reported a 46,XY normal karyotype. The child was born with Down syndrome, 47,XX,+21. The trial court dismissed the parents' lawsuit. The intermediate appellate court reinstated the parents' claim of negligence but refused to recognize the child's claim, stating that the recognition of a cause of action for wrongful life would require legislation.

Anderson v. Weiner (New York, 1984). A mother of seven children, three of whom were mildly retarded, had a bilateral tubal ligation. She subsequently gave birth to a child with brain damage and other defects. The child could not sue. The mother's claims for emotional distress and physical pain and suffering during pregnancy and childbirth were recognized, but the court disallowed the parents' claim for lack of informed consent. The parents alleged that the physician failed to inform them that tubal ligations were not always successful, but the court found that the parents had ample time to have an abortion after the pregnancy was discovered. This holding contradicts rulings of most other courts, which state that the parents' decision regarding whether to obtain an abortion is unrelated to the negligent act during surgery.

Anonymous v. Physician (Connecticut, 1980). After a negligently performed tubal ligation, the woman gave birth to a child with both mental and physical defects. The parents' claims were granted by the trial court. The appellate court disallowed claims by the three normal siblings that they had been injured by the birth of the defective sibling, but the court did allow the abnormal child's right to recover under the theory of a preconception tort rather than a "wrongful life" action. The court held that relief can be granted to the injured child directly if competent evidence at trial proves the merits of his claim.

Aquilio v. Nelson (New York, 1980). The parents were Rh-incompatible. Their first child had thrombocytopenia at birth and recovered after treatment. During the second pregnancy, the mother told her physician these facts, and he promised to read the records of her first pregnancy and delivery. The second child was born with severe thrombocytopenia and died 1 day after birth. The parents claimed emotional and physical injury, breach of contract, and fraud for failing to tell the mother that her second child was endangered. The lower court dismissed the suit. The appellate court affirmed, stating that even though the parents were more than bystanders and although the physician did owe them a duty, their emotional distress was too remote from the negligence to be compensable.

Arche v. U.S. Department of Army (Kansas, 1990). In response to questions certified from federal district court, the Supreme Court of Kansas recognized the parents' cause of action for wrongful birth provided that the child was "severely and permanently handicapped," with "such gross deformities, not medically correctable, that the child will never be able to function as a normal human being." Parents would be allowed to recover the extraordinary costs associated with the child's defects, either for the span of the child's life or until the child reached the age of majority, whichever is shorter. A cause of action for wrongful life is not recognized in Kansas.

Atlanta Obstetrics & Gynecology Group v. Abelson (Georgia, 1990). A woman was 37 years old at the time her daughter was born with Down syndrome. The parents alleged wrongful birth resulting from failure of the defendants to counsel the mother about the risks associated with increased maternal age and about the availability of amniocentesis. The child sued for wrongful life. The Supreme Court of Georgia ruled that no causes of action for wrongful birth and wrongful life would be recognized in that state in the absence of legislation to that effect.

Azzolino v. Dingfelder (North Carolina, 1985, 1986). Despite the request of a 36-year-old pregnant woman for an amniocentesis, the procedure was not performed, and her child was born with Down syndrome. The parents sued for wrongful birth, the child sued for wrongful life, and his normal siblings claimed they had suffered because their brother was retarded. The siblings' suit was disallowed, but the intermediate appellate court recognized the claims of both the parents and the child. Noting its departure from the opinions of other courts, the court found that the child's injury was legally cognizable and that the damages of an impaired life could be measured for the child as easily as for the parents. The court argued that the defendant's negligence was the proximate cause of the child's need for special care. The parents' claim for punitive damages, alleging that the defendants had tried to hide their malpractice by altering the dates on the medical records, was inadequate to justify these damages, because the fraud, if any, occurred after the child was born. This holding was later overturned by the North Carolina Supreme Court, which held that neither claims for wrongful birth nor wrongful life were recognized in that state.

Basten v. United States (Alabama, 1994). Parents of a child born with severe neural tube defects sued military physicians under the Federal Tort Claims Act for wrongful birth after they had requested and had been denied access to private, off-base prenatal care. Military medical care included neither maternal serum α-fetoprotein (MSAFP) screening nor ultrasound examinations during pregnancy. Damages to the family included $2.65 million for the care of the child, $900,000 and $700,000 to the mother and father, respectively, for their anguish and mental suffering, $50,000 to each parent for loss of consortium, and $25,000 to the sibling for loss of parental services.

Becker v. Schwartz (New York, 1978). A 38-year-old woman gave birth to a child with Down syndrome. The physician had failed to warn her of increased risk associated with advanced maternal age and had also failed to offer amniocentesis. The court upheld the father's claim for medical expenses but disallowed recovery for the parents' emotional pain and suffering caused by rearing a defective child. Several reasons were given for denying the child's claim: injury not cognizable at law, inability to measure damages, and public policy reasons for protecting the preciousness of life.

Berman v. Allen (New Jersey, 1979, 1981). A child with Down syndrome was born to a 38-year-old woman. The court denied reimbursement for rearing the child, stating that the amounts would be disproportionate to the physician's culpability. However, compensation for emotional anguish was allowed. The child's claims were denied because she had the capacity to love and be loved; one justice dissented, however, and would have allowed the claim for her impaired childhood.

Blair v. Hutzel Hospital (Michigan, 1996). A child with Down syndrome was born to a mother who had not been offered MSAFP testing during pregnancy. The intermediate appellate court agreed that the loss of a 25–30 percent chance of discovering the defect in the fetus was the loss of a "substantial opportunity" to elect to terminate the pregnancy, rather than "mere conjecture," as asserted by the defendants. The court noted that the physician had a duty to ensure that the mother made informed decisions and that failure to inform her fully was a breach of duty.

Blake v. Cruz (Idaho, 1984). The woman suspected that she had rubella during pregnancy, but the physician diagnosed it as roseola and failed to take a blood sample. The child was totally deaf in one ear and had 75 percent hearing loss in the other. The parents were allowed to recover for emotional pain and suffering and for the expenses of maintenance and support of their handicapped child, even beyond the age of majority. The child's claim, however, was disallowed.

Brubaker v. Cavanaugh (Kansas, 1982). A woman whose father had died from multiple polyposis of the colon gave birth to a child. She later developed, the same dominantly inherited disease and died. The widower filed claims for wrongful death of his wife, wrongful birth of his child, and wrongful life on behalf of the child. All causes of action were dismissed because the statute of limitations had expired before the filing of the lawsuit; the court did not rule on the merits of the case.

Call v. Kezirian (California, 1982). A middle-aged woman gave birth to a child with Down syndrome. She alleged failure to warn of increased risks and to offer an amniocentesis test. The parents were awarded special damages for medical costs and for care and training of the retarded child.

Campbell v. United States (Georgia, 1992). A child with 10q⁻ chromosome deletion was born with severe mental and physical retardation. The parents sued the U.S. Army Health Clinic at Fort MacPherson, Georgia. The court noted that a cause of action under the Federal Tort Claims Act must be recognized in the state where the alleged wrongdoing occurred. Because Georgia did not recognize a claim for wrongful birth, the parents at Fort MacPherson had no cognizable claim.

Collier v. Krane (Colorado, 1991). A child was represented by a state adoption agency as being in good health and coming from "good physical and mental stock." After the child was found to have multiple psychologic and physical disorders, the adoptive mother filed suit for "wrongful adoption" and violation of her constitutional rights and civil rights. Federal district court held that no violation of constitutional rights, based on the right of familial association, had occurred, nor was there a violation of civil rights under federal statutes. The court concluded that adoption was a matter of state law, which had no provisions for protecting the "rights" of adoptive parents to obtain a "suitable" child.

Comras v. Lewin (New Jersey, 1982). A woman with diabetes who was of advanced maternal age had a defective child (deformities unspecified). She was not told of her increased risk until the second trimester because the diagnosis of pregnancy was missed by her first physician. She was unable to consent to a late abortion and feared increased risks of an abortion in midpregnancy. She was entitled to recover for wrongful birth.

Continental Casualty Co. v. Empire Casualty Co. (Colorado, 1985). A child who had been severely damaged as a result of Rh incompatibility obtained a favorable jury verdict for wrongful life against the defendant physician. This case affirmed the tort of wrongful life in Colorado and ordered the physician's insurers to honor their professional liability policies with the insured.

Cowe v. Forum Group, Inc. (Indiana, 1989). A profoundly retarded woman requiring complete custodial care gave birth to a son who was conceived while the mother was a resident of an institution for the retarded. The son sued the institution for wrongful life. The intermediate appellate court expanded the cause of action for wrongful life to include the son's unusual situation because his parents were so severely impaired that they were incapable of making decisions about childbearing: except for the negligence of the custodial institution, the child would not have been conceived. The court's decision was "predicated on the needs of the living."

Curlender v. Bio-Science Laboratories (California, 1980). The laboratory wrongfully reported both parents to be noncarriers of the Tay–Sachs gene. Punitive damages for gross negligence were allowed because the laboratory had previously been put on notice that their technical methods were inaccurate. The child's claim for physical pain and suffering and pecuniary loss was unanimously upheld. The court also recognized punitive damages for fraud, oppression, and malice.

Daly v. United States (Washington, 1991). A pre-employment examination by a physician employed by the Veterans Administration revealed lung disease in the prospective employee. This information was not communicated to the prospective employee. Although this case does not involve prenatal or preconception tort, it may be significant because the U.S. Court of Appeals for the 9th Circuit held that an examining physician has a duty to inform persons examined of abnormal test results, even in the absence of a physician–patient relationship.

Davis v. Board of Supervisors of Louisiana State University (Louisiana, 1998). Parents were advised during the twenty-third week of gestation that amniocentesis revealed a chromosome anomaly that could lead to birth defects (trisomy 9 mosaic). The mother refused the option to terminate the pregnancy, claiming that her fetus was viable at 22–23 weeks, while defendants' expert witness placed viability at 26–27 weeks. The parents' claim for wrongful birth was disallowed because the parents failed to support their claim of viability. The child's claim for wrongful life was dismissed because this claim is not recognized in Louisiana.

Didato v. Strehler (Virginia, 2001). Pediatric health care providers failed to inform parents that their second child was a carrier of sickle cell trait. A third child was born with sickle cell β^0 thalassemia. The Supreme Court of Virginia affirmed the defendants' assertion that the plaintiff/parents failed to plead causes of actions that gave rise to a "special relationship" (i.e. a physician–patient relationship) between the plaintiffs and the defendants. However, the parents' assertion that the defendants assumed a duty to convey correct screening results to the parents was remanded for further proceedings on issues of negligence and assumption of duties.

DiNatale v. Lieberman (Florida, 1982). The Florida court of appeals ruled on several issues concerning wrongful birth and wrongful life. The court found that a child with mental or physical defects has no cause of action against anyone for wrongful life. However, the parents can sue for wrongful birth, alleging that a physician or laboratory was negligent in failing to determine the defects prenatally so that they could choose an abortion if they wished. Extraordinary expenses for the care of the defective child could be recovered by the parents. (The child's defects were not specified in the court opinion.)

Donadio v. Crouse-Irving Memorial Hospital (New York, 1980). A child of the mother's twelfth pregnancy was born 10 weeks prematurely and was permanently blinded by oxygen therapy. The parents alleged that her obstetricians failed to evaluate her history of eight previous miscarriages and failed to provide genetic counseling or to refer her to specialists. The appellate court held that there was no cause of action against the obstetricians because their care of the fetus terminated when the infant was born.

Dorlin v. Providence Hospital (Michigan, 1982). A woman was diagnosed as a sickle cell carrier. She was never told the significance of the test result. Four years later, she gave birth to a girl who later developed sickle cell anemia. The trial court dismissed the child's claim for wrongful life, reasoning that the establishment of a new tort claim of such far-reaching significance should be in the province of the legislature. The court barred the mother's claim for wrongful birth under the statute of limitations. The appellate court affirmed, stating that the mother should have discovered the alleged malpractice when she knew that she was a carrier and that her child had the disease.

Dyson v. Winfield (District of Columbia, 2001. The physician prescribed the drug Provera to the plaintiff/patient while she was pregnant. Her child was born with numerous defects and eventually died. In her claim for wrongful birth, the mother sought to recover extraordinary child-rearing expenses and compensation for her emotional distress. The federal district court ruled that the patient could recover extraordinary child-rearing expenses but that she could not recover damages for her emotional distress. The court denied the mother's motion for reconsideration of its holding on emotional distress, noting that the mother had not sustained "physical damage" to herself, as required by law in the District of Columbia.

Eisbrenner v. Stanley (Michigan, 1981). A child was born with congenital rubella syndrome after a physician missed the diagnosis of rubella in the mother. The trial court dismissed the child's claim for wrongful life but refused to grant summary judgment to the physician, who claimed that he did not "cause" the rubella. The appellate court found that the parents had shown a causal connection between the physician's failure to warn the parents and the rubella syndrome in the child, depriving them of the option to choose an abortion. The appellate court affirmed the parents' claims for medical expenses and mental distress.

Elliott v. Brown (Alabama, 1978). A child was born with serious deformities after a failed vasectomy. The parents did not bring suit for themselves but only on behalf of their child. The appellate court unanimously denied the child's claims for wrongful life, citing several reasons. Some judges believed that it was a matter of public policy and should be decided by the legislature; some believed that the injury was not cognizable at law and that it was impossible to measure damages; and two judges believed that they were bound by precedent.

Ellis v. Sherman (Pennsylvania, 1984). After a child was born with a severe form of neurofibromatosis and with mental defects and epilepsy, the father was diagnosed as mildly affected. He had been treated since childhood for recurrent skin problems; several skin tumors had been removed and had been reported to be nonmalignant. Before conception, the child's mother consulted her obstetrician concerning the hereditary nature of her husband's skin problems. She was falsely reassured that his disease would have no affect on her future children. The parents' claims for wrongful birth were recognized, but the child's claim for wrongful life was dismissed. The appellate court held that wrongful life claims are not legally cognizable.

Estate of Doe v. Vanderbilt University, Inc. (Tennessee, 1993). A woman received a transfusion of blood infected with human immunodeficiency virus (HIV) in 1984 and later gave birth to a daughter who subsequently died from acquired immunodeficiency syndrome (AIDS-related disease). The supplier of the blood initiated "look-back" notification procedures in 1986, but only with respect to donors who were known to be HIV-positive in 1986. The court held that the mother had a right to pursue a claim for wrongful birth on the question of negligent failure to notify and as a question of negligence in a medical decision.

Fassoulas v. Ramey (Florida, 1984). After having two children with severe congenital abnormalities, the father had a vasectomy. The couple subsequently had two more children, one normal and one with severe deformities. The parents sued for two wrongful births. The Supreme Court of Florida disallowed the claim for wrongful birth of the normal child, because, as a matter of law and public policy, recovery of damages for the birth of a healthy child are not allowed in that state. The court did, however, recognize the parents' claim for the extraordinary costs of raising the deformed child because there was no valid policy argument against compensating parents for the "financial and emotional drain associated with raising such a child."

Feigelson v. Ryan (New York, 1981). A 36-year-old woman was artificially impregnated with donor sperm. Her child was born with physical abnormalities and mental retardation. At 15 months of age, a chromosomal disorder was found to be the cause of his defects. The mother alleged that if she had been informed of the increased incidence of chromosome abnormalities in births to women older than 35 years of age, she would have had an amniocentesis test and aborted the pregnancy. The trial court granted the physician's motion to dismiss the case, and the mother did not appeal.

Flickinger v. Wanczyk (Pennsylvania, 1994). Parents and a child born with hydrocephalus and spina bifida claimed violation of their civil rights and both wrongful birth and wrongful life. A Pennsylvania statute expressly holds health care professionals immune from liability for negligent provision of fetal screening diagnostic services. The court held that (1) the fact that Pennsylvania specifically refuses to recognize a cause of action for wrongful birth does not encourage negligence on the part of health care providers, and (2) the plaintiffs had no constitutional civil rights action under the wrongful birth statute.

Gallagher v. Duke University (North Carolina, 1988). A first child, who had severe, multiple birth defects and died at 3 weeks of age, was erroneously reported to have a normal karyotype. After a second child was born with similar defects and was found to have an abnormal karyotype, the parents and child sued for wrongful birth and wrongful life. The child's claim was dismissed because wrongful life is not cognizable under North Carolina law. The intermediate appellate court did find, however, that the parents had a claim for "wrongful conception" of a genetically defective child. Parents were allowed to recover damages for the costs of rearing the child, unmitigated by a consideration of the benefits of parenthood, and the mother was allowed a claim for emotional distress. The court limited recovery to extraordinary expenses for the child until the death of the parents, noting that damages are awarded to the parents and that the parents' obligation to support their daughter terminates with their deaths.

Galvez v. Frields (California, 2001). A child born with a neural tube defect sued for wrongful life after his mother's physican had failed to advise her of the availability of the α-fetoprotein test. The child asserted "negligence per se" because the defendant had violated a California regulation that required that such information be conveyed to all pregnant women. After the trial court refused to inform the jury about the doctrine of negligence per se and entered a verdict for the defendant, the child appealed on the question of reversible error. The Court of Appeal remanded the case for trial on all issues.

Garrison v. Medical Center of Delaware (Delaware, 1989). A 39-year-old woman had a timely amniocentesis procedure in the 17th week of pregnancy but was not informed that her fetus had Down syndrome until she was in the third trimester. The child's action for wrongful life was disallowed. The parents were allowed to recover special damages for the extraordinary expenses related to rearing and educating the child. The court noted the parents' statutory obligation to continue to provide for the child as long as she was dependent, through her lifetime, if necessary. In an unusual step, this court also acknowledged the parents' fiduciary relationship to the child and required that the parents account to the court for investments and expenditures of the sums received as damages.

Gildiner v. Thomas Jefferson University Hospital (Pennsylvania, 1978). The parents were known carriers of the Tay–Sachs gene. Amniotic fluid hexosaminidase A was erroneously reported as normal, and the parents were reassured. Their child with Tay–Sachs disease was denied its claim for wrongful life as not cognizable at law, but the court upheld the parents' claim for economic loss, citing its policy in favor of encouraging accurate testing.

Goldberg v. Ruskin (Illinois, 1984). The parents were Jews of Eastern European ancestry. The mother's physician failed to notify the parents that a prenatal diagnostic test was available to determine whether the fetus had Tay–Sachs disease. The court allowed the parents' claim for extraordinary expenses connected with the disease. However, the child's claim for physical pain and suffering was denied because the injury to the child (i.e., being born with defects) was not cognizable at law and because measuring the difference in value between an impaired life and nonexistence was deemed too difficult. One justice dissented, arguing that the child's claim is merely a survival action to recover for the pain and suffering caused by the defendant's negligence and should not be called wrongful life.

Harbeson v. Parke-Davis (Washington, 1983). A woman who was being treated with Dilantin for epilepsy became pregnant. When she asked several physicians who gave her prenatal care if the drug might be dangerous to her fetus, she was told that there might be a slightly increased risk of cleft palate and temporary hirsutism. She had two children with severe fetal hydantoin syndrome. The Washington Supreme Court held that there was a cause of action for both wrongful birth and wrongful life. The court found the doctors negligent for failing to keep up with medical developments and for failing to read the medical literature and to seek consultation. Thus, Washington became the second state to allow recovery for wrongful life. As in the California case (*Turpin v. Sortini*, see below), damages were limited to medical and special education expenses related to the defects.

Haymon v. Wilkerson (District of Columbia, 1987). When a 34-year-old woman asked her physician on several occasions during her pregnancy about having an amniocentesis, she was repeatedly assured that such a test was unnecessary. Her daughter was born with Down syndrome. The child's claim for wrongful life was dismissed by the trial court and was not appealed. The mother's claim for wrongful birth was upheld, and the mother was allowed to seek recovery for extraordinary medical and other expenses related to the child's mental and physical abnormalities. Noting the lack of agreement in other jurisdictions on the question of recovery through only the child's minority or continuing recovery throughout the child's majority, the appeals court left the question for the trial court to decide on remand.

Hester v. Dwivedi (Ohio, 2000). Parents of a child born with birth defects that could have been predicted filed a claim for wrongful birth, noting that their physicians' failure to inform them of prenatal test results deprived them of the opportunity to terminate the pregnancy. Their child sued for wrongful life. The trial court dismissal of the child's claim on the pleadings was the sole question appealed to the Ohio Supreme Court, which affirmed that "the status of being alive simply does not constitute an injury" that is cognizable in tort law. The court further noted that the duty of the defendants extended to the mother, but not to the child.

Howard v. Lecher (New York, 1977). A physician failed to take a genetic and ethnic history of an Ashkenazi Jewish couple, failed to offer heterozygote tests, failed to give genetic counseling, and failed to offer prenatal diagnostic tests. Their child, born with Tay–Sachs disease, did not bring suit. The parents were allowed medical, nursing, hospital, and funeral expenses. The court disallowed the parents' claims for emotional pain and suffering by a 4:3 decision.

Jenkins v. Hospital of Medical College (Pennsylvania, 1991). A woman who had not been advised about the possibility of amniocentesis gave birth to a child with Down syndrome in 1984; she sued for wrongful birth in 1986. In 1988, the Pennsylvania legislature passed an act prohibiting a cause of action for both wrongful birth and wrongful life in that state. The trial court subsequently dismissed the mother's claim, stating that the suit was contrary to Pennsylvania law. On appeal, however, her suit was reinstated when the appellate court ruled that the statute could not be applied retroactively.

Johnson v. Yeshiva University (New York, 1977). After a baby with cri-du-chat syndrome was born in 1969, the parents and their abnormal child brought suit, alleging that the physicians had failed to offer the mother an amniocentesis test, which would have discovered the defect. The highest court in the state of New York upheld the trial court's dismissal of the claims, stating that the doctor owed no duty, under the standard of professional prenatal care as it existed in 1969, to offer the parents a test that was still in the experimental stages of development.

Jorgensen v. Meade Johnson Laboratories, Inc. (Oklahoma, 1973). After using oral contraceptive pills, the mother became pregnant and had twin daughters, both with Down syndrome. One child died before the lawsuit was filed. The father, as administrator of the deceased child's estate, brought a complaint on behalf of both twins, alleging that the contraceptive had caused the nondisjunctional events leading to Down syndrome. The federal appellate court held that if the mother had not been warned of the risks of the medication and if the medication caused the injuries to her ova, then a preconception tort on behalf of the children was allowable. If there is no remedy for defective products on the market before conception, then an infant suffering injuries from a contaminated baby food product or toy manufactured before his or her conception would have no recourse against the manufacturer, with an unjust result. This case is distinguished from wrongful life cases because it is the position of the children/plaintiffs that they would have been born normal except for the manufacturer's negligence, as distinct from not having been born at all.

Karlsons v. Guerinot (New York, 1977). The woman's first child had "unspecified deformities." During her second pregnancy, she was not told that her fetus was at increased risk for Down syndrome. The parents' claims for expenses of care, general support of the child, and emotional anguish were allowed, but the child's claim was denied. The court refused to compare nonexistence to life with defects.

Kassama v. Magat (Maryland, 2002). A mother who gave birth to a child with Down syndrome sued for wrongful birth, and on behalf of her child, for wrongful life. She alleged that her physician had failed to communicate MSAFP test results to her is a timely manner. The physicians alleged contributory negligence on the part of the mother for delaying 4 weeks to have the MSAFP test performed. Results from a subsequent amniocentesis would have been too late for an abortion under Maryland's 24 weeks law. The Court of Appeals affirmed the dismissal of the child's claim, noting that "for purposes of tort law, impaired life is *not* worse than nonlife and, for that reason, is not, and cannot be, an injury." The court affirmed the jury verdict in favor of the defendant/physician, noting that the question of contributory negligence was indeed an appropriate question for the jury, appropriately decided.

Lazevnick v. General Hospital of Monroe County (Pennsylvania, 1980). During her first pregnancy, the mother's blood type was incorrectly listed in her chart as "A-positive" instead of "O-negative." Her second child was born with severe hemolytic anemia and brain damage. The court found that the negligence action was not a case of "wrongful birth" or "wrongful life" but should be labeled as "preconception tort" and allowed the mother's complaints to proceed to trial. The court also found that the hospital, the laboratory supervisor, or the physician may be liable or vicariously liable for the error.

Liddington v. Burns (Oklahoma, 1995). A pregnant woman was informed after an early ultrasound examination that her fetus was "probably" normal. After another ultrasound late in pregnancy revealed that the fetus had severe cerebral and other neurologic deformities, the mother declined a third-trimester abortion. The court negated the defendant physician's argument that ultrasound examinations are "medical procedures which result in abortions" (which doctors in Oklahoma are not required to do). The court also noted that the mother's failure to have a third-trimester abortion did not relieve the physician of liability because such a decision was not a "supervening cause" of the child's abnormalities. This case opened the door in Oklahoma for wrongful birth actions and for recovery of extraordinary medical expenses and other monetary losses proximately caused by the physician's negligence, except for the normal and foreseeable cost of raising a healthy child to majority.

Lininger v. Eisenbaum (Colorado, 1988). A first child born with Leber's congenital amaurosis was misdiagnosed, and the parents were advised that the child's blindness was not hereditary. After their second child was born and both children were diagnosed correctly, the parents and second child sued. The Colorado Supreme Court ruled that the child's claim for wrongful life was not viable in that state, but that the parents stated a viable claim and could recover the extraordinary medical and education expenses related to the second child's hereditary defect. The court noted that if the parents sought to recover expenses beyond the age of majority, they must prove that the child would continue to be dependent on them.

Lloyd v. North Broward Hospital District (Florida, 1990). When a first son was born severely deformed and severely retarded, physicians assured the parents that the child's condition was not hereditary. After the second son was born with abnormalities identical to those of his brother, the parents learned that both boys had the same chromosome abnormality and that it was inherited from their mother. The Florida Court of Appeal ruled that the parents' suit was timely filed because the statute of limitations begins to run when the child is born rather than when the last health advice is given to the parents. The court also ruled that the parents could recover for mental anguish. Because no cause of action for wrongful life is recognized in Florida, the child had no claims for either general or special damages, during either his minority or majority.

Lodato v. Kappy (New Jersey, 2002). Parents and their child with severe birth defects of the central nervous system sued for wrongful birth and wrongful life, respectively. They argued that the physician had failed to note the defects on ultrasound and had failed to offer MSAFP screening. The trial court instructed the jury that if their decision favored the plaintiffs, the physician was entitled to consideration of the joy/benefit rule, so that any monetary damages could be reduced accordingly. Plaintiffs appealed the jury finding and reduction of damages. Appellate court reversed the trial court holding and remanded the case for further proceedings.

Moores v. Lucas (Florida, 1981). A woman who suffered from Larsen syndrome sought genetic counseling concerning its hereditary nature before planning to have children. She was falsely reassured that the condition would not appear in her children. The first child was affected with the dominant form of the disorder. Although the child was not allowed to recover for wrongful life, the parents were entitled to seek past and future medical expenses involved in treating the child's deformities.

Moscatello v. University of Medicine and Dentistry of New Jersey (New Jersey, 2001). Parents and siblings of a child born with disabilities sued for wrongful birth, and the child, who had partial trisomy of chromosome 14 and a partial deletion of chromosome 18, sued for wrongful life. The trial court holding that siblings do not state a cause of action was affirmed on appeal. The trial court finding that the parents' settlement, on advice of their attorney, extinguished the disabled child's wrongful life claim, was reversed on appeal; the appellate court noted that the law does not permit a parent to settle a child's claim without judicial approval and that the child's claim was still viable. The court further noted that the parents could recover extraordinary medical expenses during the child's infancy, while only the child could recover these expenses during majority. The appellate court reinstated the child's claim for extraordinary medical expenses but disallowed his claim for loss of enjoyment of life; this issue was remanded. Finally, on the first question of legal malpractice, the appellate court noted that the original attorney indeed owed a duty to the child, but that this duty was not violated because the child's claim was not extinguished by the settlement with the parents; the dismissal of claims against the attorney was affirmed. The second question of legal malpractice, on the adequacy of the amount of the monetary settlement, was remanded for further proceedings by the mother.

Naccash v. Burger (Virginia, 1982). The father's blood test was wrongly reported to be normal for hexosaminidase A due to the mislabeling of blood samples by a laboratory technician. The child developed Tay–Sachs disease. The physician was found to be vicariously liable, and the parents were allowed to recover for medical expenses and for emotional pain and suffering.

Nelson v. Krusen (Texas, 1984). After her first son developed Duchenne muscular dystrophy, a woman was examined by a leading specialist, who found no abnormalities on neurologic examination, electromyogram, or creatine phosphokinase test. She was negligently reassured that her risk of having another affected child was no greater than that of the general population. A second son showed signs of muscular dystrophy at 3 years of age. The court held that she could maintain a cause of action for negligent genetic counseling and wrongful birth, although the child's claim for wrongful life was denied for reasons of public policy. The court found that the occurrence rule for filing malpractice claims within 2 years of the negligent act was unjust because it would deprive the parents of their day in court; the court adopted the discovery rule in the state of Texas, allowing plaintiffs to file a claim within 2 years after the negligent act was discovered or, by reasonable prudence, should have been discovered.

Ochs v. Borrelli (Connecticut, 1982). After two children were born with congenital skeletal defects, the mother had a tubal ligation, which failed. The third child had even more severe defects. The parents were allowed to recover for the expenses of rearing the third child, which would be offset by the value of "the satisfaction, fun, and joy" of the child's companionship. The court did not find such a determination to be too speculative. The jury awarded $106,360, which included expenses for rearing the child to 18 years of age.

Park v. Chessin (New York, 1977, 1978). The parents' first child died from polycystic kidney disease 5 hours after birth, and an autopsy was performed. The parents were falsely reassured that the condition was not hereditary. Their second child died at 2 years of age of the same condition. The court's findings are the same as those given above in *Becker v. Schwartz* because the two cases were consolidated for judicial review.

Payne v. Myers (Utah, 1987). A first child who had Pelizaeus–Merzbacher syndrome was incorrectly diagnosed by physicians at Handicapped Children's Service in Utah. When the second child was diagnosed as having the same hereditary neurodegenerative disorder, the parents sued for wrongful birth. Shortly before the birth of the second child, the Utah legislature amended a statute to give immunity to state employees for simple negligence. The parents claimed that they had been wronged at the time that they were given incorrect information by the physicians (i.e., before the conception of the second child) and that their claim should therefore not be subject to the immunity granted by the amended statute. The Supreme Court of Utah held that the wrong to the parents accrued at the time of the second child's birth and that their claim was thereby precluded by the amended statute, which was found to be constitutional.

Phillips v. United States (South Carolina, 1983). During her first pregnancy, a 23-year-old woman recorded on her history form that she had a sister with mental retardation. She delivered a healthy child. During her second pregnancy, she recorded the fact that her sister had Down syndrome. She was never given genetic counseling regarding familial Down syndrome and inherited translocations that give rise to Down syndrome children, irrespective of maternal age. She was not karyotyped. She gave birth to a son with translocation Down syndrome and a congenital heart defect, which was not immediately diagnosed. The Federal District Court of South Carolina allowed the parents to recover damages totaling $1,283,765 for all expenses related to their son's condition, including custodial care, calculated on the basis of a 40-year life expectancy.

Pines v. Dr. Carlos D. Moreno, Inc. (Louisiana, 1990). A physician missed a diagnosis of pregnancy and continued to prescribe birth control pills for the mother. When the child was born with Cornelia de Lange syndrome, the mother and child sued, claiming that the mother was denied the opportunity to decide to terminate the pregnancy and that the child's condition was aggravated by the continuing medication. The appellate court reinstated the claims of both plaintiffs, noting that the child was not suing for wrongful life but, rather, for aggravation of her deformities because of negligent prenatal care. The case was remanded for trial on the merits.

Pitre v. Opelousas General Hospital (Louisiana, 1988). Before the birth of their second normal child, a couple decided for financial reasons to limit their family to two children, and the mother had a tubal ligation in conjunction with her second delivery. A third child was subsequently born and was an albino. Both parents and child sued. The Supreme Court of Louisiana held that no cause of action for wrongful life exists in Louisiana and that the parents' claim for wrongful birth was limited to recovering the expenses for the birth of the third child. No damages for rearing the third child were allowed because her albinism was not a reasonably foreseeable consequence of the failed tubal ligation.

Pratt v. University of Minnesota Affiliated Hospital and Clinics (Minnesota, 1987). After having two normal children, a couple had a third child who was born with various defects that were called a "fluke happening" and a "sporadic event" by physicians whom they consulted. A fourth child was born with anomalies similar to those of his older brother, and the children were diagnosed as having oral–facial–digital syndrome type II and/or Dandy–Walker syndrome. The defendants argued that (1) genetic counseling was not medical treatment within the meaning of negligent nondisclosure and (2) depositions of other physicians did not satisfy the requirement of producing expert testimony. Summary judgment in favor of the defendants was reversed on appeal, and the case was remanded for trial.

Procanik v. Cillo (New Jersey, 1984). An infant son was born with severe congenital rubella syndrome, allegedly because the obstetricians caring for the mother failed to discover that she had German measles during her first trimester. The child claimed he would never have been born if the mother had been informed about the risks to the fetus. The New Jersey Supreme Court held that he was entitled to recover damages for his extraordinary medical expenses. His parents had no cause of action for wrongful birth because their statute of limitations had expired. Recovery for the child's emotional distress and "impaired childhood" were considered too speculative for legal recognition. New Jersey became the third state to recognize a cause of action for wrongful life (see *Harbeson v. Parke-Davis*, above, and *Turpin v. Sortini*, below).

Proffitt v. Bartolo (Michigan, 1987). Shortly after becoming pregnant, a woman appeared to have rubella. She was tested, but her physician failed to convey the test results to her. The physician treated the mother for a parasitic infection, after which the mother continued to report chronic headaches, nausea, malaise, and fever. The physician withdrew from caring for the mother. The child, delivered by another physician, was born with severe congenital malformations attributed either to rubella or to other intrauterine infection. The intermediate appellate court upheld the parents' claim for wrongful birth, noting that the parents should be able to recover general damages as well as both their own extraordinary medical expenses and the extraordinary costs of raising the child. However, the court also ruled that the physician owed no duty to the child and that recognition of a claim for wrongful life was a question for either the legislature or the state supreme court to decide.

Provenzano v. Integrated Genetics (New Jersey, 1998). A woman carrying a twin pregnancy had seven ultrasound examinations during the pregnancy and an amniocentesis procedure in the third month. The primary physicians failed to inform the parents that one twin had a subarachnoid cyst and was significantly smaller than the co-twin. The laboratory reported chromosomes to be normal, having missed the finding of trisomy 14 mosaicism. Parents subsequently filed a wrongful birth claim and later a motion to amend their initial allegations to include the second physician who had performed the ultrasound investigations. Defendants moved for a summary judgment. Federal district court denied the plaintiffs' motion to amend on the grounds that the statute of limitations had extinguished the claim against the second physician. The court also denied the defendants' motion for summary judgment on the grounds that the case had significant issues for the trier of fact. These issues included (1) consideration of the defendants' argument that the proximate cause of the parents' injury depended on whether the parents would have aborted the affected twin, and (2) whether inaccurate test results deprived the parents of the right to abort the fetus and "reject a parental relationship." A third issue, whether the second physician could shift culpability to the primary physicians under the "learned intermediary" doctrine, was mooted because the second physician was protected by the statute of limitations.

Reed v. Campagnolo (Maryland, 1993). The mother of a daughter born with spina bifida, hydrocephalus, imperforate anus, ambiguous genitalia, and other urogenital malformations asserted that the physician's failure to inform her about MSAFP testing resulted in valid claims for wrongful birth and lack of informed consent. The district court certified the following questions to the Maryland court of appeals: (1) whether Maryland recognized a cause of action for wrongful birth; and (2) whether continuing a pregnancy is a decision requiring informed consent, so that a physician's failure to inform the patient about tests can give rise to a claim for lack of informed consent.

Renslow v. Mennonite Hospital (Illinois, 1977). A 13-year-old girl who was Rh-negative was wrongly transfused with Rh-positive blood. Eight years later she gave birth to a child with erythroblastosis fetalis, who required an immediate exchange transfusion. The child suffered permanent damage to her brain, nervous system, and other organs. The child's suit was brought against the physician and hospital where the preconception tort had occurred. In a landmark decision, the Illinois Supreme Court held that the infant plaintiff had a cause of action against the physician because the elements of duty, causation, and foreseeability existed even though she was not in existence at the time. It could be reasonably foreseen that the mother would grow up, marry, and have children.

Robak v. United States (Illinois, 1981). The wife of a serviceman had a mild rash during her first month of pregnancy. Physicians at the base clinic told her that the rubella test was negative. Although a second test a few days later was positive, she was never informed, and was not advised of the seriousness of congenital rubella syndrome. Her child was born with a severe body rash and had cataracts, decreased hearing, congenital heart defect, and mental retardation. A trial court awarded the parents $900,000 for the clinic's negligence. The appellate court affirmed.

Rossi v. Somerset Ob-Gyn Assoc. (New Jersey, 1994). When a child born with severe defects sued for wrongful life, the court held that the infant must establish proximate cause by proving that his mother would have chosen abortion if she had been informed about defects in the fetus. Because neither parent would testify that the mother would have aborted the pregnancy, the child's claim would not stand.

Rubin v. Hamot Medical Center (Pennsylvania, 1984). The parents were known heterozygotes for Tay–Sachs but were not warned of the risks of Tay–Sachs disease in their offspring. The child's claim of wrongful life was held to be not legally cognizable; recovery was also precluded on the theory that he was a third-party beneficiary to the physician–parent contract.

Santana v. Zilog, Inc. (Idaho, 1996). A woman who already had three healthy children had six successive miscarriages, all within the first 17 weeks of gestation, while she was employed by Zilog. She later had a fourth healthy child while working in another setting and sued Zilog for wrongful death of the six fetuses caused by her exposure to "dangerous chemicals." The court found no cause of action for the wrongful death of a nonviable fetus because a nonviable fetus was not a "person" in the eyes of the law. The fetus becomes a person only after it is viable and can survive outside the mother's uterus. The court noted that claims for wrongful birth and wrongful life depend on the fetus becoming a "person" at the time of livebirth.

Schreck v. State of New York (New York, 1981). The mother gave birth to a child with microcephaly in 1972. A second child was conceived in 1977, and sonograms of the fetus indicated normal cranial development. On February 2, 1978, a son with microcephaly was born. The trial court permitted the parents to file a late claim in April 1979, alleging negligence in the performance and evaluation of the diagnostic tests and failure to warn them of the possibility of the same genetic defect in a second child. The appellate court ruled that the trial court had erred in allowing the claim to be filed after the statute of limitations had expired and ordered dismissal of the suit.

Schroeder v. Perkel (New Jersey, 1981). The pediatrician failed to diagnose cystic fibrosis in a couple's first child and therefore failed to warn them of the hereditary nature of the disease. A second child was born with cystic fibrosis. The parents were allowed to recover medical expenses for the second child, undiminished by the value of their parenthood.

Sejpal v. Corson (Pennsylvania, 1995). A woman gave birth to a child with Down syndrome and was immediately sterilized, according to prior agreement, before she was informed about her daughter's condition. Noting that the U.S. Supreme Court had refused to hear arguments on the constitutionality of Pennsylvania's ban on a cause of action for wrongful birth, the Superior Court ruled that parents should be allowed to sue for lack of informed consent with respect to her sterilization. The case was remanded for trial with instructions to allow the parents to amend their complaint.

Shrader v. Coffineau (New Jersey, 1996). A child was born with Down syndrome after the physician first reported a MSAFP test to be normal and later failed to correct the error in time to allow the parents a choice about proceeding with the pregnancy. The $1.65 million settlement allotted $1 million for the child's extraordinary expenses related to his disability and $650,000 for the parents' emotional distress.

Siemieniec v. Lutheran General Hospital (Illinois, 1987). A woman who had two cousins with hemophilia sought information about her chances of being a carrier. Her physician informed her about the possibility of prenatal diagnosis but concurred with the opinion of a second physician that the probability of her being a carrier was "very low." After having a son with hemophilia, the parents sued on their own behalf and on behalf of their son. The Supreme Court of Illinois found that the son had "suffered no legally cognizable injury by being brought into existence afflicted with hemophilia" and dismissed his wrongful life claim as contrary to public policy. In allowing the parents' claim for wrongful birth, the court held that the parents' recovery should be limited to the extraordinary medical expenses for their son during his minority. The court disallowed the parents' claim for negligent infliction of emotional distress because they were not in the "zone of physical danger."

Simmerer v. Dabbas (Ohio, 2000). After the mother of two normal children elected a permanent sterilization procedure, she had a third child who was born with a congenital heart defect and died at 15 months. The parents' wrongful pregnancy action was settled for pregnancy-related damages. However, the parents' claim for the third child's medical expenses and emotional stress associated with the child's birth defects was denied. On appeal, the Supreme Court of Ohio affirmed, noting that the physician's negligence in performing the sterilization procedure was not the proximate cause of the medical expenses and emotional stress associated with the child's birth defects: these injuries were "not [a] reasonabl[y] foreseeable" consequence of a failed sterilization procedure.

Simmons v. West Covina Medical Clinic (California, 1989). A woman who had a child with Down syndrome claimed that her physicians were negligent in failing to advise her about a 20 percent chance that a very low serum α-fetoprotein level could be indicative of a fetus with trisomy 21. The intermediate appellate court in California found an insufficient causal connection between the physician's failure to inform the mother and the mother's claim that she would have terminated the pregnancy if she had been adequately informed; both the claims of the mother and the child were disallowed.

Smith v. Saraf (New Jersey, 2001). A woman on active duty in the Air Force became pregnant and subsequently had a son with neural tube defects. The government provided payment for the mother's care by private physicians but required her to obtain medical testing at a military hospital. The private physician twice recommended a triple-screen MSAFP test, which the mother had done twice at the military hospital. The hospital failed to convey the results to the private physician. Parents sued for wrongful birth and, on behalf of their child, for wrongful life, naming both the private physician and the government as defendants. The private physician filed a third-party claim against the government for indemnification and contribution. Under the so-called *Feres* doctrine in federal law, active-duty-service members are barred from recovering from the government under the Federal Tort Claims Act for injuries sustained "incident to service." Federal district court noted (1) the third-party claim for indemnification and contribution against the government, based on either the mother's or father's wrongful birth claim, was barred under the *Feres* doctrine; but (2) that the third-party claim was not barred with respect to the infant's wrongful life claim because the infant's claim was not a derivative of his mother's military status.

Speck v. Finegold (Pennsylvania, 1979, 1981). Two daughters were born with severe neurofibromatosis and mental retardation. Their father had a mild form of the disease. The parents received genetic counseling, and the father had a vasectomy. The wife became pregnant and insisted on an abortion. After the abortion procedure, she realized that she was still pregnant and carried her third child to term. He was born with neurofibromatosis. The parents and child sued for negligent performance of the vasectomy and the abortion. The parents were entitled to recover damages for the child's birth and upbringing and for their own emotional distress, but the child's claim of wrongful life was denied by an equally divided court.

Stribling v. DeQuevedo (Pennsylvania, 1980). After a bilateral tubal ligation, a child was born with dextrocardia. The appellate court recognized the mother's claims for lost earnings and for pain and suffering from surgery. The father was allowed medical expenses for the mother and child, but the parents were denied reimbursement for emotional pain and suffering. The child had no cause of action for wrongful life.

Strohmaier v. Associates in Obstetrics and Gynecology (Michigan, 1982). The facts in this case are nearly identical to those in *Eisbrenner v. Stanley* (see above) and the reasoning is the same. The same appellate court heard both of these cases.

Taylor v. Mercedes (Florida, 2000). After a settlement in a wrongful birth action, a guardian was appointed for monies awarded. When the guardian was subsequently sanctioned by a trial court, with no notice to the guardian, for improper use of the funds from the settlement, he claimed he was entitled to formal notice that he faced sanctions at the subject hearing. The court of appeal noted that surcharging the guardian was an adversarial proceeding that required formal notice and that guardians may waive their right to such notice only in writing.

Turpin v. Sortini (California, 1982). The couple's first child, who was totally deaf, was misdiagnosed in infancy as having normal hearing. Before a second conception, the parents were reassured, but the second child also had hereditary deafness. The Supreme Court of California was the first to recognize a cause of action for wrongful life, which set the precedent throughout the state. Medical expenses and special education expenses for the hearing-impaired children were allowed. By this decision, the court upheld the wrongful life decision in *Curlender v. Bio-Science Laboratories* (1980) and overturned the intermediate appellate court's holding in *Turpin v. Sortini* (1981).

Vega v. Del Rosario (New Jersey, 1996). After a child was born with stumps for arms, a deformed leg on one side, and no leg on the other side, a physician admitted that she had not interpreted a sonogram correctly. The $2.7 million settlement allotted $900,000 for the child's medical expenses and cost of his care, $1.2 million for the mother's claim, and $600,000 for attorney's fees.

Walker v. Mart (Arizona, 1990). When a woman sought obstetrical care, the physician failed to discuss or test for the possibility of rubella during the first trimester. When the child was born with rubella syndrome, the mother sued for herself and on behalf of her daughter, seeking special and general damages for both claims. The Supreme Court of Arizona recognized a cause of action for wrongful birth but denied the child's claim for wrongful life on the ground that any wrong that was done was wrong to the parents rather than to the fetus. The court noted that "bringing a child into the world—even one who is impaired—is not a legally cognizable injury to that child."

Wilson v. Kuenzi (Missouri, 1988). A 36-year-old pregnant woman was neither informed about the availability of amniocentesis nor about the increased risk of birth defects associated with advanced maternal age. A son with Down syndrome was born in 1983. In 1986, the Missouri legislature enacted a law that precludes both wrongful birth and wrongful life actions in that state. The state Supreme Court noted that the statute may not be applied retroactively but nevertheless denied both suits. The court denied the claim for wrongful life because of the difficulty, or impossibility, of calculating damages when comparing the value of an impaired life with the value of nonexistence, "based on considerations of the sanctity of all human life notwithstanding incidental defects." The court justified its denial of the claim for wrongful birth by noting that all courts that have permitted such an action have failed to examine carefully the element of causation: because the physician did not cause the defect, the physician could not be liable.

Wilson v. Mercy Hospital (Michigan, 2003). A mother who had disclosed to her physicians a family history of hemophilia subsequently had an affected child. No tests were carried out while she was pregnant to determine the genetic status of the fetus. In spite of the fact that the tort action for wrongful birth had been abolished in civil litigation in Michigan, she sued for wrongful birth based on gross negligence, claiming that such a cause of action was indeed legally permissible under a subsequently enacted statute. The defendants' motion for summary judgment was affirmed on appeal: the court of appeal noted that a cause of action for wrongful birth was abolished in 1999 and that subsequent legislation on gross negligence would not apply to earlier cases.

Wood v. University of Utah Medical Center (Utah, 2002). Parents of a child born with Down syndrome sued for wrongful birth, alleging that the hospital was negligent in misreading genetic tests and in failing to disclose test results. They further alleged negligent infliction of emotional distress and failure to obtain informed consent, and they challenged the constitutionality of the Utah Wrongful Life Act. The defendants' motion for judgment on the pleadings was granted and later affirmed on appeal. The Utah Wrongful Life Act prohibits lawsuits for wrongful birth. The Supreme Court of Utah noted that the state's Wrongful Life Act did not deprive the plaintiffs of a right that existed at the time the statute was enacted. Further, the Act places no substantial obstacle in the path of the mother who could have aborted her nonviable fetus and therefore did not violate state and federal due process rights or equal protection rights.

Woodruff v. City and County of San Francisco (California, 1995). A mother was an admitted user of crack cocaine and was incarcerated for petty theft when she was 4 months pregnant. She had terminated two previous pregnancies by elective abortion. During her incarceration, three checkup visits at San Francisco General Hospital were canceled. A sonogram during the seventh month of pregnancy revealed a fetus with hydrocephalus, too late for a termination procedure. The city and county settled the case for $405,000.

SUGGESTED READINGS

Allen v. Colonial Laboratories, 409 So.2d 512 (Fla. Dist. Ct. App.), 1982.

Alquijay v. St. Luke's Roosevelt Hospital, 99 A.D.2d 704, 472 N.Y.S.2d 2, 1984.

Anderson v. Wiener, 100 A.D.2d 919, 474 N.Y.S.2d 801, 1984.

Anonymous v. Physician, (Conn. Super. Ct.), 1980.

Aquilio v. Nelson, 78 A.D.2d 195, 434 N.Y.S.2d 520, 1980.

Arche v. U.S. Department of Army, 798 P.2d 477 (Kan.), 1990.

Atlanta Obstetrics & Gynecology Group v. Abelson, 398 S.E.2d 557 (Ga.), 1990.

Azzolino v. Dingfelder, 315 N.C. 103, 337 S.E.2d 528, 1985; cert. denied, 479 U.S. 835, 1986; S.Ct. 131, 93 L.Ed.2d 75, 1986; reh. denied, 319 N.C. 227, 353 S.E.2d 401, 1987.

Ball v. Mudge, 64 Wash.2d 247, 391 P.2d 201, 1964.

Basten v. United States, 848 F.Supp. 962 (M.D. Ala.), 1994.

Becker v. Schwartz, 60 A.D.2d 587, 400 N.Y.S.2d 119, 1977; modified 46 N.Y.2d 401, 386 N.E.2d 807, 413 N.Y.S.2d 895, 1978.

Berman v. Allen, 80 N.J. 421, 404 A.2d 8, 1979; *overruled in part, Schroeder v. Perkel*, 87 N.J. 53, 432 A.2d 834, 1981.

Blair v. Hutzel Hospital, Michigan Lawyers Weekly No. 25336, July 22, 1996.

Blake v. Cruz, 698 P.2d 315 (Idaho), 1984.

Bonbrest v. Kotz, 65 F. Supp. 138 (D.D.C.), 1946.

Brubaker v. Cavanaugh, 542 F. Supp. 944 (D. Kans.), 1982.

Butler v. Rolling Hill Hospital, 582 A.2d 1384 (Pa. Super.), 1990.

California Civil Code, § 43.6 (West), 1982.

Call v. Kezirian, 135 Cal.App.3d 198, 185 Cal.Rptr. 103, 1982.

Campbell v. United States, 962 F.2d 1579 (11th Cir.), 1992.

Canterbury v. Spence, 464 F.2d 772 (D.C. Cir.), 1972.

Christensen v. Thornby, 192 Minn. 123, 255 N.W. 620, 1934.

Collier v. Krane, 763 F.Supp. 473 (D. Colo.), 1991.

Comras v. Lewin, 183 N.J. Super. 42, 443 A.2d 229, 1982.

Continental Casualty Co. v. Empire Casualty Co., 713 P.2d 384 (Colo. App.), 1985.

Cowe v. Forum Group, Inc., 541 N.E.2d 962 (Ind. App. 4 Dist.), 1989.

C.S. v. Nielson, 767 P.2d 504 (Utah), 1988.

Curlender v. Bio-Science Laboratories, 106 Cal.App.3d 811, 165 Cal.Rptr. 477, 1980.

Daly v. United States, 946 F.2d 1467 (9th Cir.), 1991.

Davis v. Board of Supervisors of Louisiana State University Agricultural and Mechanical College, 709 So.2d 1030, 197-0382 (La.App. 4 Cir.), 1998.

Didato v. Strehler, 262 Va. 617,554 S.E.2d 42, 2001.

Dietrich v. Inhabitants of Northhampton, 138 Mass. 14, 52 Am. Rep. 242, 1884.

DiNatale v. Lieberman, 409 So.2d 512 (Fla.), 1982.

Donadio v. Crouse-Irving Memorial Hospital, 75 A.D.2d 715, 427 N.Y.S.2d 118, 1980.

Dorlin v. Providence Hospital, 118 Mich.App. 831, 325 N.W.2d 600, 1982.

Dyson v. Winfield, 129 F.Supp.2d 22 (D.C.), 2001.

Eisbrenner v. Stanley, 106 Mich.App. 351, 308 N.W.2d 209, 1981.

Eisenstadt v. Baird, 405 U.S. 438, 1972.

Elliott v. Brown, 361 So.2d 546 (Ala.), 1978.

Ellis v. Sherman, 330 Pa. Super. 42, 478 A.2d 1339, 1984.

Estate of Doe v. Vanderbilt University, Inc., 824 F. Supp. 746 (M.D. Tenn.), 1993.

Fassoulas v. Ramey, 450 So.2d 822 (Fla.), 1984.

Feigelson v. Ryan, 108 Misc. 2d 192, 437 N.Y.S.2d 229, 1981.

Flickinger v. Wanczyk, 843 F.Supp. 32 (E.D. Pa.), 1994.

Gallagher v. Duke University, 852 F.2d 773 (4th Cir.), 1988.

Garrison v. Medical Center of Delaware, 581 A.2d 288 (Del. Supr.), 1989.

Galvez v. Frields, 88 Cal.App.4th 1410, 107 Cal.Rptr.2d 50, 2001.

Gildiner v. Thomas Jefferson University Hospital, 451 F. Supp. 692 (E.D.Pa.), 1978.

Gleitman v. Cosgrove, 49 N.J. 22, 227 A.2d 689, 1967.

Goldberg v. Ruskin, 128 Ill. App. 3d 1029, 471 N.E.2d 530, 1984.

Griswold v. Connecticut, 381 U.S. 479, 1965.

Harbeson v. Parke-Davis, 98 Wash.2d 460, 656 P.2d 483, 1983.

Hatter v. Landsberg, 563 A.2d 146 (Pa. Super.), 1989.

Haymon v. Wilkerson, 535 A.2d 880 (D.C.App.), 1987.

Hester v. Dwivedi, 89 Ohio St..3d 575, 733 N.E.2d 1161, 2000.

Howard v. Lecher, 52 A.D.2d 420, 386 N.Y.S.2d 460, 1976; affd., 42 N.Y.2d 109, 366 N.E.2d 64, 397 N.Y.S.2d 363, 1977.

James G. v. Caserta, 332 S.E.2d 872 (W.Va.), 1985.

Jenkins v. Hospital of Medical College, 585 A.2d 1091 (Pa. Super.), 1991.

Johnson v. University Hospitals of Cleveland, 540 N.E.2d 1370 (Ohio), 1989.

Johnson v. Yeshiva University, 53 A.D.2d 523, 384 N.Y.S.2d 455, 1976; affd., 42 N.Y.2d 818, 364 N.E.2d 1340, 396 N.Y.S.2d 647, 1977.

Jorgensen v. Meade Johnson Laboratories, Inc., 483 F.2d 237 (10th Cir.), 1973.

Karlsons v. Guerinot, 57 A.D.2d 73, 394 N.Y.S.2d 933, 1977.

Kassama v. Magat, 368 Md. 113, 792 A.2d 1102, 2002.

Keel v. Banach, 624 So.2d 1022 (Ala.), 1993.

Kelly MB. The rightful position in "wrongful life" actions. Hastings Law J 1991;42:505.

Kowitz JF. Not your garden variety tort reform: Statutes barring claims for wrongful life and wrongful birth are unconstitutional under the purpose prong of Planned Parenthood v. Casey. Brooklyn Law Rev 1995;61:235.

Lazevnick v. General Hospital of Monroe County, 499 F. Supp. 146 (M.D.Pa.), 1980.

Liddington v. Burns, 916 F. Supp. 1127 (W.D. Okl.), 1995.

Lininger v. Eisenbaum, 764 P.2d 1202 (Colo.), 1988.

Lloyd v. Howard, 566 So.2d 424 (La.App. 3 Cir.), 1990.

Lloyd v. North Broward Hospital District, 570 So.2d 984 (Fla.App. 3 Dist.), 1990.

Lodato v. Kappy, 353 N.J.Super. 439, 803 A.2d 160, 2002.

Lovelace Medical Center v. Mendez, 805 P.2d 603 (N.M.), 1991.

Marciniak v. Lundborg, 450 N.W.2d 243 (Wis.), 1990.

Moores v. Lucas, 405 So.2d 1022 (Fla. Dist. Ct. App.), 1981.

Morgan v. Christman, Civil Action No. 88-2311-0, D. Kan., 1990 U.S. Dist. LEXIS 15743, October 1, 1990.

Moscatello v. University of Medicine and Dentistry of New Jersey, 342 N.J.Super. 351, 776 A.2d 874, 2001.

Naccash v. Burger, 223 Va. 446, 290 S.E.2d 825, 1982.

Natanson v. Kline, 350 P.2d 1093 (Kan.), 1960.

Nelson v. Krusen, 635 S.W.2d 582 (Tex. Civ. App.), 1982; 678 S.W.2d 918 (Tex.), 1984.

Ochs v. Borrelli, 445 A.2d 883 (Conn.), 1982.

Panagopoulos v. Martin, 295 F. Supp. 220 (S.D.W.V.), 1969.

Park v. Chessin, 60 A.D.2d 80, 400 N.Y.S.2d 110, 1977; *modified sub nom. Becker v. Schwartz*, 46 N.Y.2d 401, 386 N.E.2d 807, 413 N.Y.S.2d 895, 1978.

Payne v. Myers, 743 P.2d 186 (Utah), 1987.

Pelias MZ. Duty to disclose in medical genetics: A legal perspective. Am J Med Genet 1991;39:347.

Phillips v. United States, 508 F. Supp. 537 (D.S.C.), 1980; 508 F. Supp. 544 (D.S.C.), 1981; 566 F. Supp. 1 (D.S.C.), 1981, 575 F. Supp. 1309 (D.S.C.), 1983.

Pines v. Dr. Carlos D. Moreno, Inc., 569 So.2d 203 (La.App. 1 Cir.), 1990.

Pitre v. Opelousas General Hospital, 530 So.2d 1151 (La.), 1988.

Planned Parenthood of Southeastern Pennsylvania v. Casey, 112 S.Ct. 2791, 1992.

Pratt v. University of Minnesota Affiliated Hospital and Clinics, 403 N.W.2d 865 (Minn.App.), 1987.

Procanik v. Cillo, 97 N.J. 339, 478 A.2d 755 (N.J), 1984.

Proffitt v. Bartolo, 412 N.W.2d 232 (Mich.App.), 1987; *lv. denied*, 430 Mich. 860, 1988.

Provenzano v. Integrated Genetics, 22 F.Supp.2d 406 (D.N.J.), 1998.

Reed v. Campagnolo, 810 F.Supp. 167 (D.Md.), 1993.

Renslow v. Mennonite Hospital, 67 Ill.2d 348, 367 N.E.2d 1250, 1977.

Robak v. United States, 503 F. Supp. 982 (N.D.Ill.), 1980; modified, 658 F.2d 471 (7th Cir.), 1981.

Roe v. Wade, 410 U.S. 113, 1973.

Rossi v. Somerset Ob-Gyn Assoc., 879 F. Supp. 411 (D.N.J.), 1994.

Rubin v. Hamot Medical Center, 329 Pa. Super. 439, 478 A.2d 869, 1984.

Santana v. Zilog, Inc., 95 F.3d 780 (9th Cir.), 1996.

Schloendorf v. Society of New York Hospital, 105 N.E. 92 (N.Y.), 1914.

Schreck v. State of New York, 81 A.D.2d 882, 439 N.Y.S.2d 162, 1981.

Schroeder v. Perkel, 87 N.J. 53, 432 A.2d 834, 1981.

Sejpal v. Corson, Pennsylvania Law Weekly, October 23, 1995.

Shaw MW. The potential plaintiff: Preconception and prenatal torts. In: Milunsky A, Annas G, eds. Genetics and the law II. New York: Plenum Press, 1980:225.

Shaw MW, Damme C. Legal status of the fetus. In: Milunsky A, ed. Genetics and the law. New York: Plenum Press, 1976:3.

Shrader v. Coffineau, New Jersey Law Journal 22, May 27, 1996.

Siemieniec v. Lutheran General Hospital, 512 N.E.2d 691 (Ill.), 1987.

Simmerer v. Dabbas, 89 Ohio St.3d 586, 733 N.E.2d 1169, 2000.

Simmons v. West Covina Medical Clinic, 212 Cal. App. 3d 696, 260 Cal. Rptr 772 (Cal.App. 2 Dist.), 1989.

Smith v. Brennan, 31 N.J. 353, 157 A.2d 497, 1960.

Smith v. Cote, 128 N.H. 231, 513 A.2d 341, 1986.

Smith v. Saraf, 148 F.Supp.2d 504 (D.N.J.), 2001.

Speck v. Finegold, 268 Pa. Super. 342, 408 A.2d 496, 1979; affd., 497 Pa. 76, 439 A.2d 110, 1981.

Stribling v. DeQuevedo, 422 A.2d 505 (Pa. Super. Ct.), 1980; 432 A.2d 239 (Pa. Super. Ct.), 1980.

Strohmaier v. Associates in Obstetrics and Gynecology, 122 Mich. App. 116, 332 N.W.2d 432, 1982.

Terrell v. Garcia, 496 S.W.2d 124 (Tex. Civ. App.), 1973; *cert. denied*, 415 U.S. 927, 1974.

Taylor v. Mercedes, 760 So.2d 282 (Fla.App.4 Dist.), 2000.

Turpin v. Sortini, 119 Cal.3d 690, 174 Cal. Rptr. 128, 1981; rev., 31 Cal.3d 220, 643 P.2d 954, 182 Cal. Rptr. 337, 1982.

University of Arizona Health Sciences Center v. Arizona Superior Court, 136 Ariz. 579, 667 P.2d 1294 (Ariz.), 1983.

Vega v. Del Rosario, No. BER-L-7265-91 (N.J. Super. Ct., Bergen Cty., settled April 8, 1996), Medical Malpractice Law & Strategy 4, May, 1996.

Walker v. Mart, 790 P.2d 735 (Ariz.), 1990.

Wilson v. Kuenzi, 751 S.W.2d 741 (Mo. banc), 1988.

Wilson v. Mercy Hospital, 2003 WL 245823 (Mich.App.), 2003.

Wood v. University of Utah Medical Center, 2002 WL 31895671 (Utah), 2002.

Woodruff v. City and County of San Francisco, 932772, The Recorder 1, May 15, 1995.

Zepeda v. Zepeda, 41 Ill. App.2d 240, 190 N.E.2d 849, 1963; cert. denied, 379 U.S. 945, 1964.

Frank A. Chervenak, M.D., and
Laurence B. McCullough, Ph.D.

32

Ethical Issues in the Diagnosis and Management of Genetic Disorders in the Fetus

Ethics is an essential dimension of the clinical management of pregnancies complicated by genetic disorders. Clinicians and patients confront a wide variety of ethical challenges in this context. The purpose of this chapter is to provide clinicians with conceptual and clinical tools to prevent and respond to ethical conflicts among members of the team or between team members, pregnant women, and their partners. To achieve this goal, the chapter begins with an account of an ethical framework that appeals to two main principles of bioethics, beneficence and respect for autonomy.[1,2] On the basis of these two principles, the concept of the fetus as a patient is then elaborated, with particular attention to the implications of this core concept of obstetric ethics for counseling pregnant women whose pregnancies are complicated by genetic disorders. This ethical framework is then used as the basis for a detailed consideration of major ethical issues in the management of such pregnancies: the diagnosis of genetic disorders in the fetus, management of pregnancies complicated by genetic disorders, and research to improve the clinical management of fetal anomalies.

ETHICAL FRAMEWORK

Throughout the history of medical ethics, an important starting point for reflection on ethics in clinical practice has been the clinician's obligation to protect and promote the health-related interests of the patient. This commitment defines what it means to be a health-care professional, but at the same time is quite general in its nature. To make it clinically relevant and applicable, this general guideline needs to be made more clinically specific. To do so, we interpret it from two basic perspectives, that of the clinician and that of the patient.[2]

The Ethical Principle of Beneficence

The ethical principle of beneficence translates into clinical practice medicine's perspective on the health-related interests of the patient. This ethical principle obligates the clinician to seek the greater balance of clinical benefits over clinical harms for the patient as a consequence of clinical management of the patient's condition. On the basis of rigorous clinical judgment, informed by current science, especially evidence-based medicine, and a commitment to excellence in clinical practice, the clinician should identify the clinical strategies that are reliably expected to result in the greater balance of benefits (i.e., the protection and promotion of health-related interests) over clinical harms (i.e., impairments of those interests). The principle of beneficence has a long and illustrious history in the global history of medical ethics. In Western medical ethics, for example, it dates back at least to the time of Hippocrates.[2] Indeed, the Hippocratic Oath enjoins physicians to act in a manner that will "benefit the sick according to my ability and judgment."[3]

The principle of beneficence should not be confused with the principle of nonmaleficence. The latter principle is also known as *Primum non nocere*, or "First, do no harm." It is worth noting that *Primum non nocere* appears neither in the Hippocratic Oath nor in the texts that accompany the Oath. Rather, the principle of beneficence was the primary consideration of the Hippocratic writers. For example, the Hippocratic text, Epidemics, reads, "As to diseases, make a habit of two things—to help or to at least do no harm." [4] Thus, the historical origins of *Primum non nocere* remain obscure. This seemingly arcane historical point is not just historical, but also conceptual and clinical: if *Primum non nocere* were to be made the primary principle of clinical ethics, then virtually all invasive aspects of health care, including many aspects of obstetrics and gynecology, such as invasive prenatal diagnosis, would be unethical because of the risks they involve for patients. If the primary goal is to avoid harm, even drawing blood becomes ethically suspect, especially for patients with a dread of needles.

The Ethical Principle of Respect for Autonomy

A rigorous clinical perspective on the patient's health-related and other interests is not the only legitimate perspective on such interests. The patient's perspective on her own health-related and other interests must also be considered by the clinician.[2] This is because adult patients have developed a set of values and beliefs, according to which they are capable of making judgments about what will and will not protect and promote their health-related and other interests. In particular, all adult pregnant women not in an emergency situation should be assumed to possess the decision-making capacity to determine which clinical strategies for the clinical diagnosis and management of their pregnancies are consistent with their interests and which are not, unless there is reliable evidence of significant clinical deficits in their decision-making processes. In making decisions about their medical care, pregnant women may use values and beliefs that go far beyond health-related interests (e.g., religious beliefs or beliefs about how many children she wants to have). Inasmuch as beneficence-based clinical judgment is limited by the scientific and clinical competencies of medicine, beneficence-based clinical judgment provides the physician no authority to assess the worth or meaning to the pregnant woman of her own non-health-related interests. Such are matters solely for the pregnant woman to determine.

The patient's perspective is translated into clinical practice in the ethical principle of respect for autonomy. This principle obligates the clinician to respect the integrity of the patient's values and beliefs, to respect her perspective on her interests, and to implement only those clinical strategies authorized by her as the result of the informed consent process. The informed consent process is typically understood to have three elements: (1) disclosure by the physician or other relevantly trained and experienced clinician to the patient of adequate information about the patient's condition and its management; (2) understanding of that information by the patient; (3) a voluntary decision by the patient to authorize or refuse proposed treatment.[2,5]

The Ethical Concept of the Fetus as a Patient

The clinician's perspective on the pregnant woman's health-related interests and the commitment to protect and promote her health-related interests create the clinician's beneficence-based obligations to her. At the same time, the woman's own perspective on her interests and the clinician's commitment to respect her values and preferences create the clinician's autonomy-based obligations to her. In contrast, because of its insufficiently developed central nervous system the fetus cannot meaningfully be said to possess values and beliefs. Thus, there is no valid basis for saying that a fetus has a perspective on its interests. It follows that there can be no autonomy-based obligations to any fetus.[2] The clinician nonetheless has a perspective on the fetus's health-related interests and therefore can have beneficence-based obligations to the fetus, but only when the fetus is a patient. Because of its centrality for the ethical management of pregnancies complicated by fetal anomalies, the topic of the fetus as patient requires careful consideration, a task to which we now turn.

One can become a patient without having rights. An important advantage of the concept of the fetus as a patient is that the language of fetal rights or personhood has no meaning and, therefore, no application to the fetus in obstetric ethics, despite its popularity in public and political discourse in many countries. Thus, current controversies about "right to life," especially its possible limited application to patients from non-Western cultures, can be avoided in clinical judgment and decision making about the management of pregnancies complicated by fetal anomalies.

We have argued elsewhere that beneficence-based obligations to the fetus exist when the fetus can later, after birth, become a child and still later achieve independent moral status as a person.[2] The fetus is a patient when two conditions are met: (1) the fetus is presented to the physician or other clinician; and (2) there exist medical and other clinical interventions, whether diagnostic or therapeutic, that can reliably be expected to result in a greater balance of clinical goods over clinical harms for the fetus in its future. The ethical significance of the concept of the fetus as a patient therefore depends on links to its later becoming a child and, later still, achieving independent moral status.

The Viable Fetus as a Patient

One link to becoming a patient is viability, the ability of the fetus to exist ex utero with full technological support. This introduces the first ethical sense of the fetus as a patient. Viability should not be viewed as an exclusively biologic property of the fetus, but in terms of both biologic and technologic factors. Only by virtue of both factors can a viable fetus exist ex utero and subsequently become a child and later achieve independent moral status. Viability is closely correlated with access to technologic capacity. When access to such technology is present, as is the case in the United States and other developed countries, viability occurs at approximately the end of 24 weeks of gestational age.[6,7] This understanding of viability as having a technologic component is not unique to obstetrics, but applies throughout medicine. For example, a patient with massive internal injuries with uncontrolled bleeding but without timely access to rapid transport to surgery is almost certainly nonviable, while the same patient with such access is viable.

The Previable Fetus as a Patient

The only possible link between the previable fetus and the child it can become is the pregnant woman's autonomy. This introduces the second ethical sense of the fetus as patient. This is because technologic factors cannot result in the previable fetus becoming a child: this is simply what *previable* means. When the fetus is previable, the link between a fetus and the child it can later become is established only by the pregnant woman's decision to confer the status of being a patient on her previable fetus in a decision to continue her pregnancy. The previable fetus has no claim to the status of being a patient independently of the pregnant woman's autonomy. The pregnant woman is therefore free to withhold, confer, or, having once conferred, withdraw the status of being a patient on or from her previable fetus according to her own values and beliefs. Having made a decision to continue a previable pregnancy, the woman remains free to revoke that decision. This has direct clinical application to the management of pregnancies complicated by fetal anomalies, as we shall see below. The previable fetus is presented to the clinician solely as a function of the pregnant woman's autonomy.[2]

Prenatal Genetic Counseling

It is usually understood that genetic counseling should be nondirective (see also chapter 1). The concept of the fetus as a patient has considerable clinical significance for genetic counseling because, when the fetus is a patient, directive counseling (i.e., recommending a form of treatment) for fetal benefit is appropriate and, when the fetus is not a patient, nondirective counseling (i.e., offering but not recommending clinical alternatives) is appropriate. Our task now is to explain when each form of counseling is ethically justified.

Counseling Regarding the Viable Fetus

When the viable fetus is a patient, directive counseling for fetal benefit is ethically justified. However, the strength of directive counseling for fetal benefit varies according to the presence and severity of fetal anomalies. As a rule, the more severe the fetal anomaly, the less directive counseling should be for fetal benefit.[8,9] In particular, when there is "(1) a very high probability of a correct diagnosis and (2) either (a) a very high probability of death as an outcome of the anomaly diagnosed or (b) a very high probability of severe irreversible deficit of cognitive developmental capacity as a result of the anomaly diagnosed,"[10] counseling should be nondirective in offering a choice between aggressive and nonaggressive management.[11,12] In contrast, when lethal anomalies can be diagnosed with certainty there are no beneficence-based obligations to provide aggressive treatment.[13–15] Such viable fetuses are appropriately understood to be dying patients. Counseling therefore should be nondirective in offering a choice between nonaggressive management and termination of pregnancy, but directive in recommending against aggressive management for the sake of maternal benefit.[8]

Any directive counseling for fetal benefit must occur in the context of balancing beneficence-based obligations to the viable fetal patient against beneficence-based and autonomy-based obligations to the pregnant woman.[2,15] Any such balancing must recognize that a pregnant woman is obligated only to take reasonable risks of medical interventions that are reliably expected to benefit the viable fetus or child later. On this account, no pregnant woman is obligated to her fetus and to accept the risks to herself of experimental fetal intervention. The unique feature of obstetric ethics is that whether, in a particular case, the viable fetus ought to be regarded as presented to the physician is, in part, a function of the pregnant woman's autonomy.

Any strategy for directive counseling for fetal benefit that takes account of obligations to the pregnant woman must be open to the possibility of conflict between the clinician's recommendation and a pregnant woman's autonomous decision to the contrary. Such conflict should be managed preventively through informed consent as an ongoing dialogue throughout the pregnancy, augmented as necessary by negotiation and respectful persuasion.[2,16]

Counseling Regarding the Previable Fetus

Counseling the pregnant woman regarding the management of fetal anomalies when the fetus is previable should be strictly nondirective in terms of continuing the pregnancy or having an abortion, if she refuses to confer on her fetus the status of being a patient. If she does confer such status in a settled way, at that point beneficence-based obligations to her fetus come into existence, and directive counseling for fetal benefit becomes appropriate for these previable fetuses. Just as for viable fetuses, such counseling must take account of the presence and severity of fetal anomalies, extreme prematurity, and obligations owed to the pregnant woman.

For previable pregnancies in which the woman is uncertain about whether to confer such status, we propose that the fetus be provisionally regarded as a patient.[2] This justifies directive counseling in favor of fetal therapy, when indicated.

In particular, nondirective counseling is appropriate in cases of what we term near-viable fetuses[2] (i.e., those that are 22–23 weeks of gestational age for which there are anecdotal reports of survival).[2,6,7] In the authors' view, aggressive obstetric and neonatal management should be regarded as clinical investigation (i.e., a form of medical experimentation), not the standard of care.[7] There is no ethical obligation on the part of a pregnant woman to confer the status of being a patient on a near-viable fetus, because the efficacy of aggressive obstetric and neonatal management has yet to be proven.

DIAGNOSIS OF GENETIC DISORDERS IN THE FETUS

Competence and Referral in Prenatal Diagnosis

The ethical obligation to provide competent genetic diagnosis derives from both beneficence and respect for autonomy. Either principle alone, and certainly both in combination, require clinicians to provide patients with accurate and reliable clinical information. To meet this ethical obligation, the clinician must address the following ethical considerations.

First, ensuring an appropriate level of competence imposes a rigorous standard of training and continuing education. Two problems result when clinicians do not maintain this baseline level of competence in prenatal diagnosis, including ultrasound and genetics. Clinicians may cause unnecessary harm to the woman or fetal patient (e.g., from mistaken diagnosis of fetal anomalies), thus violating beneficence-based obligations. Incomplete or inaccurate reporting of results by the clinician to the pregnant woman also undermines the informed consent process regarding the management of her pregnancy. This constitutes an unacceptable ethical violation of autonomy-based obligations of the clinician to the pregnant woman.

Second, these obligations have important implications for physicians who employ a genetic counselor. Such physicians are ethically obligated to supervise the genetic counselor's clinical work adequately. To do this adequately the physician should know more than the genetic counselor, especially about the application of sonographic and genetic findings to the diagnosis of anomalies. This more advanced fund of clinical and scientific knowledge is essential for the physician to fulfill his or her additional ethical obligation to regularly review the counselor's work. In addition, physician-employers should provide the opportunity for continuing education for genetic counselors. In medical care, patients properly rely for their protection on the personal and professional integrity of their clinicians. A crucial aspect of that integrity on the part of physicians is willingness to refer to specialists when the limits of their own knowledge are being approached (e.g., detection of a rare genetic anomaly). Like other virtues, such as self-sacrifice and compassion, integrity directs physicians to focus primarily on the patient's interests, as a way to blunt mere self-interest.[2]

Disclosure of Results of Prenatal Diagnosis

Significant clinical ethical issues arise about the disclosure of the results of prenatal diagnosis. The first clinical ethical topic here concerns the phenomenon of the apparent bonding of pregnant women with their fetuses as a result of the pregnant woman seeing the ultrasound images, which experience usually precedes invasive genetic diagnosis.[17] Such bonding can sometimes benefit pregnancies that will be taken to term but at other times can complicate decisions to terminate a pregnancy. We recommend that these matters, like abnormal findings, should be discussed with the pregnant woman.

A second topic is a matter of ongoing debate: the disclosure of the fetus's sex.[2,18] We propose that respect for maternal autonomy dictates responding frankly to requests from the pregnant woman for information about the fetus's sex.

Confidentiality of Findings

Confidentiality concerns the obligation of health care professionals and health care organizations to protect clinical information about patients from unauthorized access.[1,2] These obligations have become especially important with the implementation of the Health Insurance Portability and Accountability Act, or HIPAA.[19] The obligation of confidentiality derives from the principles of beneficence (patients will be more forthcoming) and respect for autonomy (the patient's privacy rights are protected). Others, including the pregnant woman's spouse, sex partner, and family, should be understood to be third parties to the patient–clinician relationship with respect to information about the results of prenatal diagnosis. Diagnostic information about a woman's condition or pregnancy is confidential. It can therefore be justifiably disclosed to third parties only with the pregnant woman's explicit permission. This is because a potentially acceptable condition for releasing confidential information, avoiding grave harm to others, does not apply in this context.[1,2] To avoid awkward situations, clinicians and health care organizations should establish clear policies and procedures that reflect this analysis of the ethics of confidentiality.[20] Doing so will likely meet HIPAA standards. The reader should seek competent legal advice and review of such policies and procedures.

Autonomy-Enhancing Strategies in the Routine Offering of Prenatal Diagnosis

Second-Trimester Ultrasound

To date, the Routine Antenatal Diagnostic Imaging with Ultrasound (RADIUS) trial has been the largest and most expensive prospective study of the routine use of obstetric ultrasound.

RADIUS investigators concluded that screening ultrasound was not found to improve perinatal or maternal outcome significantly, and the investigators concluded that routine obstetric ultrasound is not indicated.[21] The American College of Obstetricians and Gynecologists (ACOG) supported this conclusion in their November 1993 newsletter[22] and in their December 1993 technical bulletin on "Ultrasonography and Pregnancy."[23] The bulletin states that "in the United States the routine use of ultrasonography cannot be supported from a cost-benefit standpoint." The newsletter reports that "the College not recommend routine ultrasound screening." There is, however, no uniform support for this stance. Critics have pointed out scientific shortcomings in both the methods and conclusions of the RADIUS trial.[24,25]

There is, however, another unstated concern about second-trimester ultrasound that we believe needs to be addressed. In our view, ethics is an essential dimension of the routine obstetric ultrasound debate.[2] This is not so much a clinical issue to which there are ethical aspects, but rather, it is a clear example in modern obstetrics in which widespread ignorance of basic ethical concepts can lead to inappropriate clinical judgment and practice.

Respect for autonomy is a central principle of clinical ethics, as noted in the first part of the chapter. This core ethical principle obliges the physician to acknowledge and respect the patient's values, to elicit the patient's preferences, and in the absence of compelling constraints, to implement these preferences. Providing patients with access to information about diagnostic and therapeutic alternatives is an essential component of respect for the patient's autonomy. Failure to provide the patient access to information deprives her of the opportunity to consider alternatives about the management of her pregnancy, some of which may be highly in accord with the patient's values. Nondisclosure of diagnostic alternatives, therefore, seriously impairs the exercise of the patient's autonomy regarding her pregnancy. Routinely offering obstetric ultrasound respects the autonomy of pregnant women, and not routinely offering obstetric ultrasound undermines the autonomy of pregnant women, because the woman's access to the diagnosis of serious anomalies and, therefore, access to abortion for serious fetal anomalies is restricted.[5]

Routinely offering obstetric ultrasound to implement respect for autonomy in clinical practice has important implications. Every pregnant woman should be informed of the availability of this diagnostic method at the physician's initiative.[26] A practice of discussing ultrasound only when women initiate inquiries does not display respect for autonomy because many women are ignorant of this method and the fact that its detection ability is at least three times that of the background detection rate of fetal anomalies.[21,27] Instead, the clinical strategy of prenatal informed consent for sonogram (PICS) should be employed with every pregnant woman.[26]

PICS is best undertaken in several stages. Shortly after the pregnancy has been diagnosed, the pregnant woman's physician should provide her with information about the actual and theoretical benefits and harms of obstetric ultrasound. The pregnant woman should then evaluate this information in terms of her own values, something every autonomous patient can do. It may be helpful to some women to consider, at this point in the process, the physician's scientific evaluation of the clinical data that have been reported in the literature. The pregnant woman should be asked to articulate her preference regarding the use of ultrasound in the management of her pregnancy. The physician should then provide the pregnant woman with the his or her own recommendation, and there should be discussion of any disagreement that may emerge. The woman then can make her decision about whether she wants an ultrasound examination.

PICS establishes an autonomy-based indication for routine obstetric ultrasound.[26] The RADIUS investigators have explicitly objected to this indication,[27] and ACOG, by its si-lence on this matter and its support of the conclusions of the RADIUS study, gives the appearance that it also opposes this indication. As a result, ACOG undercuts the ability of obstetricians to be effective advocates for the autonomy of pregnant women with regard to access to routine obstetric ultrasound. The authors propose that obstetricians act on their autonomy-based obligation to pregnant women and advocate for their autonomy by offering and thereby providing access to routine obstetric ultrasound. There are two possible objections to our proposal: lack of benefit and excessive cost. We will show how each of these objections fails.

Treating the lack of benefit of routine obstetric ultrasound as decisive assumes that clinical considerations always override autonomy-based considerations. However, the ethical framework presented earlier in this chapter calls this assumption into question. The RADIUS trial, which applies to at most 40 percent of women who present for private obstetric care, found that routine ultrasound did not significantly improve outcome in terms of perinatal morbidity or mortality or maternal morbidity.[21] This is only one measure of the efficacy of this diagnostic maneuver. Screening ultrasound accomplished significant improvement in the detection of fetal anomalies, detection of twin pregnancies, diminished usage of tocolysis, and reduction of the occurrence of postdatism.[21,24,25] The RADIUS trial assumed that these possible benefits would be truly clinical benefits only if they showed a documented improvement in perinatal morbidity and mortality.

These are important measures. However, they should not be equated with comprehensive, beneficence-based clinical judgment. Indeed, clinical judgment should not narrow itself only to the measurement of such end points, but should also include the prevention of harm in small but important subsets of patients. The RADIUS study conclusions were slanted by an unjustifiably narrow concept of clinical judgment that is not acceptable in modern obstetrics. The study ignored other clinical realities (prevention of unnecessary tocolysis, early prenatal diagnosis of twin gestations not detected clinically, physician–patient ignorance of the presence of fetal anomalies before delivery, and inappropriate assignment of postdatism) that are also significant in and of themselves in any adequate clinical judgment. Ignorance of clinical realities is not bliss for either the patient or the obstetrician. Lack of available information is not an acceptable standard of care.

In contrast to the narrow view adopted by the RADIUS study, the goal of modern obstetrics should be well-formed clinical judgment. This means that the physician should offer obstetric ultrasound as a matter of prudence to avoid rare adverse outcomes such as unnecessary tocolysis, provided that such benefits outweigh the possibility of harm from erroneous ultrasound diagnoses. Prudential calculations in well-formed clinical judgment consider the seriousness of the outcome rather than just the low incidence of the outcome. With respect to seriousness of outcome, the risks of not performing ultrasound are significant, even though they are of very low incidence. For example, given the seriousness of the outcomes of undetected clinical complications, such as unexpected twins at the time of delivery, it is justifiably risk-averse to attempt to prevent those outcomes when in clinical judgment the risks of not performing the ultrasound outweigh the risks of performing it. In the authors' view, high-quality ultrasound,[26] which is required as a matter of professional integrity, reduces the risk of harm from erroneous ultrasound and, therefore, tips the balance in favor of this prudential judgment. This prudential judgment is not altered by concern for possible bioeffects. This is because there are no documented reproducible ill effects of obstetric ultrasound. Moreover, no credible study has documented a serious bioeffect. Therefore, in prudential clinical judgment, outcomes that remain theoretical have far less weight than serious outcomes that are documented.

An ethical analysis of routine ultrasound based on well-formed clinical judgment supports two important conclusions: (1) end points of overall perinatal morbidity and mortality are not the only measures of clinical judgment, but are only part of it; and (2) prudential clinical judgment supports offering high-quality ultrasound. The first is neutral in the clinical judgment of PICS; the second supports PICS in clinical judgment. Thus, objection to PICS on the ground that it provides no benefit does not succeed. Moreover, given the significance to the pregnant woman of the benefits of PICS, namely to make an informed choice about the management of her pregnancy, central matters of respect for autonomy are at stake. On balance, autonomy-based obligations should clearly be the physician's primary guide in response to objections based on lack of benefit.

Treating the excessive cost of routine obstetric ultrasound as ethically decisive assumes that justice-based considerations or fairness override autonomy-based considerations. However, a central, additional justice-based consideration is cost effectiveness, which concerns identifying the least expensive means to achieve an agreed-upon goal. An important goal of obstetric ultrasound is to detect fetal anomalies. Devore has shown that the cost per detected case of an anomaly in the RADIUS trial was not greatly different from the cost per detected anomaly in the California maternal serum (MSAFP) screening program.[28] Given the improved detection rate in tertiary centers, Devore has shown that the cost per anomaly detected with quality ultrasound is much less.[28] The California MSAFP screening program is a reliable touchstone for cost effectiveness. By this comparison alone, routine obstetric ultrasound is cost effective.

A second justice-based consideration is whether the cost of an intervention in the present saves a greater cost in the future. We interpret Devore's analysis to suggest that routine ultrasound is cost saving because the cost-per-anomaly detected with quality ultrasound is far below the neonatal and lifetime costs of those anomalies, assuming that for many pregnancies in which serious anomalies are detected women will seek a termination.

Suppose for the sake of argument that routine obstetric ultrasound was not cost saving. Should this consideration automatically override respect for autonomy? Those who assume that the answer is "yes" confront a major burden of proof. First, most theories of justice in Western philosophy give paramount consideration to personal autonomy and freedom, including theories of justice based on utilitarianism. It would mark a radical departure from this centuries-long history for the principle of justice to automatically override the principle of respect for autonomy. Justice-based considerations may override autonomy-based considerations when costs are enormous, even when some benefit results. This was not the case before, and is not the case after, the RADIUS study.

Second, in Western democracies, it is already well understood that respect for autonomy can be very costly and that fact, by itself, does not override the importance of autonomy. Matters such as universal suffrage, protection of the rights of citizens accused or convicted of crimes, and the public accountability of government institutions to the electorate are very expensive. No credible argument based on excessive cost has been advanced to override such autonomy-based considerations. Therefore, no credible argument can be advanced against PICS, a far less costly form of respect for autonomy exercised around a central individual and social concern, namely, human reproductive freedom.

First-Trimester Ultrasound and Biochemistry

Recently, first-trimester ultrasound screening for aneuploidy using nuchal translucency determination has become a controversial topic in the ethics of prenatal diagnosis. The term *nuchal translucency* refers to the sonographic measurement of nuchal skin late in the first trimester. A typical feature of newborns with Down syndrome is redundant nuchal skin. This has also been noted with other autosomal trisomies, Turner syndrome, and other disorders.[29] Nuchal edema occurs in the fetus as well, and varying degrees of this are visible sonographically. These range from slight thickening of nuchal skin to cystic hygromas. These are malformations in which dilated lymphatic channels form a soft tissue mass, typically in the posterior neck.

In 1985, Benacerraf et al. reported an association between increased nuchal skin fold thickness in the second trimester and Down syndrome.[30] Although this is a useful second-trimester marker for Down syndrome, only approximately 20–30 percent of fetuses with Down syndrome will have increased nuchal skin fold thickness.[31]

In 1992, Nicolaides et al. described an association with first-trimester nuchal edema and aneuploidy.[31] Numerous studies subsequently described increased nuchal translucency between 10 and 14 weeks in the majority of fetuses with Down syndrome and other forms of aneuploidy. Most early studies defined increased nuchal translucency using a single cutoff, usually 3.0 mm.[32]

Several problems with using a single cutoff in defining abnormal nuchal translucency need to be addressed. One is the fact that nuchal translucency increases with gestational age in normal fetuses.[33] Thus, sensitivity rates for aneuploidy with a single cutoff of 3.0 mm would be lower at earlier gestational ages, and false-positive rates would be higher at later gestational ages. Another problem with ultrasound screening for aneuploidy in the first trimester concerns operator technique in measuring nuchal translucency. Nuchal translucency must be measured with a fetus in the optimal position, with appropriate image magnification and caliper placement.[34] If appropriate techniques are not used, harm may result from both lower detection rates and higher false-positive results.

Finally, maternal age must be an integral part in the estimation of risk in any screening test for aneuploidy. The relative risk of Down syndrome in a fetus with an abnormal nuchal translucency is independent of maternal age. It must be noted, however, that an abnormal nuchal translucency measurement with a maternal-age-related risk of 1 in 100 would reflect a much higher absolute risk of Down syndrome than with an age-related risk of 1 in 1000.[33]

Many studies evaluating nuchal translucency screening for Down syndrome, including those performed in the United States, were performed using single cutoffs, without well-defined techniques, and did not consider maternal age. Not surprisingly, wide ranges of sensitivity and false-positive rates have been described.[35,36]

In 1998, Snijders et al. published the results from the Fetal Medicine Foundation (FMF) multicenter study assessing nuchal translucency screening for Down syndrome. Over 100,000 pregnancies at 22 centers in the United Kingdom were screened from 10 to 14 weeks. All of the participating centers had demonstrated the ability to obtain appropriate nuchal translucency measurements by submitting images to the FMF. The criteria for an appropriate image were magnification such that the fetus occupied at least 75 percent of the image; that the skin could be distinguished from the amnion; and that the maximum thickness of subcutaneous translucency between the skin and soft tissue overlying the cervical spine was measured. Risks for Down syndrome were calculated based on crown- rump length, nuchal translucency, and maternal age.[34]

In 22 centers, 100,311 singleton pregnancies were screened from 10 to 14 weeks. In 96,127 cases, the prenatal or postnatal karyotype was obtained, or a birth of a phenotypically normal child was documented. To determine sensitivity of nuchal translucency, a risk threshold of 1 in 300 was used. There was a risk estimate of 1 in 300, or more in 7,907 normal fetuses (8.3 percent), in 268 of 326 fetuses with Down syndrome (82.2 percent), and 253 of 325 fetuses with other chromosomal abnormalities (77.9 percent).[34]

The FMF has currently accredited numerous international sites. Centers must demonstrate expertise in measuring nuchal translucency, and images from all sonographers must be submitted for review before software for risk estimation is provided. Annual audits of all data and submission of a sample of nuchal translucency images are also required. Investigators outside the United Kingdom have described similar effectiveness of first-trimester ultrasound screening for Down syndrome using software provided by the FMF.[37–41]

In our view, the FMF database demonstrates that nuchal translucency should be regarded as a clearly reliable screen for aneuploidy because of: (1) the universal standard of quality in all FMF testing sites; (2) the large number of patients involved in published reports describing nuchal translucency screening in FMF centers; and (3) the advantages of a large multicenter study, especially in reducing biases when only one center is involved.

First-trimester biochemical screening for aneuploidy has also been described. Using a combination of free β-hCG and pregnancy-associated plasma protein A with maternal age, detection rates of 60–70 percent for Down syndrome have been reported.[42,43] Combining first-trimester serum analytes with nuchal translucency and maternal age, detection rates exceeding 90 percent have been reported and is now considered superior to nuchal translucency alone.[44–46] Sonographic screening for Down syndrome continues to evolve. Absence of the nasal bone[47] and abnormal ductus venosus flow[48] may enhance screening.

In the United States, the FASTER (First And Second Trimester Evaluation of Risk for aneuploidy) trial, sponsored by the National Institutes of Health, is comparing first-trimester nuchal translucency and serum screening with second-trimester serum screening.[36] In this study, patients undergo nuchal translucency screening and first-trimester serum screening, followed by second-trimester serum screening. Results of first-trimester tests are not disclosed to patients until they have undergone second-trimester serum screening.

The investigators of the FASTER trial have stated that "first-trimester methods of screening should be considered investigational" and "patients interested in having first-trimester screening for Down syndrome should be encouraged to do so only in the context of a well-designed clinical trial."[36] We respectfully disagree. Given the scientific rigor and the results of the FMF database, nuchal translucency and biochemical screening should not be considered investigational, but instead is a highly reliable diagnostic screen when performed in expert hands.[49,50]

The ideal combination of tests in aneuploidy screening, and the natural history of the aneuploid fetus with abnormal nuchal translucency are investigational.[36] Nonetheless, investigation in these areas does not negate the established value of first-trimester ultrasound and biochemical screening for aneuploidy, or preclude its use in a noninvestigational setting.

If first-trimester screening for Down syndrome with nuchal translucency and biochemistry is available at specialized centers with expertise and ongoing quality control, patients may benefit in several ways. Some women at high risk based on age or history would prefer to avoid invasive testing because of the associated risk of miscarriage, especially if pregnancy has been achieved after therapy for infertility. These women may choose to undergo invasive testing, however, if there is any evidence of an increased risk based on screening tests. Two studies suggest that the availability of first trimester screening may decrease the rate of invasive testing in high-risk women.[51,52] Undergoing a combination of tests, including first-trimester ultrasound as well as second-trimester serum screening, could increase the likelihood that a fetus with Down syndrome will be identified. Ongoing studies may develop the ability to integrate these and other tests to derive a single estimation of risk in the future.[52]

Other women are determined to undergo invasive testing to exclude the possibility of Down syndrome, but may use nuchal translucency and biochemistry to assist them in choosing between chorionic villus sampling (CVS) and amniocentesis. Although it is not clear that CVS, when performed by an experienced operator, has a significantly higher complication rate than amniocentesis, there is some evidence to suggest slightly higher miscarriage rates with CVS.[53,54] Some women would prefer to avoid CVS and undergo amniocentesis for other reasons. These include the small incidence of placental mosaicism found on CVS, which requires amniocentesis to be performed subsequently, and the ability to screen for neural tube defects by determining amniotic fluid α-fetoprotein (AFP), although the routine determination of amniotic fluid AFP has been questioned.[55] If nuchal translucency and biochemistry were to reveal a substantial risk of Down syndrome, however, some women would be willing to undergo CVS to achieve an earlier diagnosis.

Finally, women considered to be at low risk may be interested in first-trimester screening for Down syndrome. Informed patients are aware that women at any age can give birth to a child with Down syndrome, and they have shown interest in first-trimester screening. If a sensitive first-trimester test with a relatively low false-positive rate is available, this is certainly a reasonable option, as these women could undergo invasive testing if nuchal translucency and biochemistry are abnormal.

Aside from screening for Down syndrome, ultrasound performed to measure nuchal translucency has other benefits. Increased nuchal translucency is associated with other forms of aneuploidy and cardiac anomalies. Many other congenital anomalies have been described in euploid fetuses with increased nuchal translucency as well.[56] Accurate estimation of gestational age, and accurate identification of amnionicity and chorionicity in multifetal gestations are other well-described benefits of first-trimester ultrasound.[57]

The use of nuchal translucency and biochemical screening for Down syndrome also has the potential to harm. Obtaining the ultrasound measurement requires paying meticulous attention to technique; failure to do so could lead to both false-positive and false-negative results. This can lead to higher rates of invasive testing and miscarriage if risks are overestimated, or to women with affected pregnancies not undergoing prenatal diagnosis if the risks are underestimated. Ongoing review of data and follow-up are essential to document the quality of screening in every center providing this service.

It is also important to note that nuchal translucency with biochemistry does not replace second-trimester serum screening, which should be offered if nuchal translucency with biochemistry testing reveals a low risk of Down syndrome. Until different screening tests can be integrated to derive a single estimation of risk, it is important that women be aware that serial screening will result in higher cumulative false-positive rates. This could increase the number of invasive tests performed and lead to a higher rate of loss of normal fetuses.

In summary, it is not reasonable to conclude that the potential harms of first trimester nuchal translucency and biochemical screening outweigh the potential benefits when quality testing is available. Moreover, in our view, the potential benefits do outweigh the potential harms. Beneficence is not the only ethically relevant consideration here. As in second-trimester ultrasound examination, considered alone, respect for autonomy must also be considered. The relevance of respect for autonomy to nuchal translucency and biochemical screening is that first-trimester identification of fetuses at risk provides the option of prenatal testing and the subsequent option of early abortion, which is of considerable value to many women.[58]

Like PICS, discussed above, the counseling process for nuchal translucency and biochemical screening should involve several stages.[26,58] Because nuchal translucency and biochemical screening must be done before 14 weeks of gestation, the physician should discuss these tests with the pregnant woman at the initial prenatal visit. Information should be provided about the actual and theoretic benefits, including potential benefits and harms. The pregnant woman should evaluate this information in terms of her own values and beliefs; this is something every autonomous patient is able to do. The physician should be prepared to discuss his or her scientific evaluation of available data regarding nuchal translucency and biochemical screening for Down syndrome.

After these steps, the pregnant woman should be able to articulate her preference regarding the use of nuchal translucency and biochemistry to screen for Down syndrome in the first trimester. The physician can then make a recommendation to the pregnant woman, if the physician has one. Finally, a thoughtful and sensitive discussion of any disagreement should ensue, after which a woman can make her decision. This process provides a significant role for the judgment of the physician and experience, while maintaining respect for a pregnant woman's autonomy.

It must be noted that the physician should offer the option of first-trimester screening with a pregnant woman only if quality testing is available. It is the responsibility of the physician to ensure that the center to which he or she will refer patients for nuchal translucency screening maintains the highest standards. Without quality testing in experienced centers, the harms of testing may outweigh the benefits.

First-trimester screening when conducted according to accepted standards of quality is a reliable diagnostic screen. There is no beneficence-based argument opposed to offering it, and offering it is an important autonomy-enhancing strategy. Such screening should be offered only in centers where high quality is available. The results of ongoing trials will only enhance this position.[58]

MANAGEMENT OF PREGNANCIES COMPLICATED BY GENETIC DISORDERS

Termination of Pregnancy before Viability

Before viability, the management of a pregnancy complicated by genetic disorders is ethically straightforward. As noted earlier in this chapter, the pregnant woman is free to withhold or withdraw the moral status of being a patient from any previable fetus, including the fetus with anomalies. When an anomaly is detected, counseling by the physician and other clinicians involved in the woman's care should be rigorously nondirective. The clinician should offer medically reasonable alternatives, but not make any recommendations for or against any alternative. Therefore, the woman should be given the choice between abortion and continuing her pregnancy to viability and thus toward term, regardless of any involved clinician's personal views about rearing a child with such an anomaly or about abortion.

If the woman elects to continue her pregnancy, she should be apprised of decisions that will need to be made later, so that she can begin to plan the rearing of her child.[2] If the woman elects an abortion, it should be performed unless her physician has moral objections to abortion, which should be respected by the patient and the physician's colleagues. For this reason, training in performing abortion should not be mandated, although education about abortion and its complications is mandatory. As a matter of professional conscience, a physician unwilling to perform abortions should nonetheless make an appropriate referral.

Respect for autonomy has the important implication that the clinician should not judge the reasons a woman has for aborting a previable pregnancy. Respect for autonomy also means that the clinician should be alert to substantially controlling or even coercive influences on her decisions about the clinical management of a pregnancy, such as from her husband, partner, or potential grandparents, and should advocate for her preferences, whatever they may be, to protect her from such substantial control and coercion.[2]

Fetal Reduction and Selective Termination

An important subset of the option of termination of pregnancies before viability is fetal reduction and selective termination of multiple pregnancies.[59–61] Three ethically justifiable indications for reduction or selective termination of multiple pregnancies have been identified. These are related to three possible goals for a multiple pregnancy: (1) achieving a pregnancy that results in a live birth with one or more infants with minimal neonatal morbidity and mortality, (2) achieving a pregnancy that results in a live birth of one or more infants without anomalies detected antenatally, and (3) achieving a pregnancy that results in a singleton live birth.[62] The ethical justification for these indications is based on the ethical principles of beneficence and respect for the autonomy of the pregnant woman and on the concept of the fetus as a patient as explained above.

First Indication: Achieving a Pregnancy that Results in Live-Birth Infant(s) with Minimal Neonatal Morbidity and Mortality

In cases of multifetal pregnancies being taken to term, the goal of obstetric management is live birth(s) with a minimum of neonatal morbidity and mortality.[62] In triplet or higher-order pregnancies, while this goal is more than remotely possible, there are significant increased risks of fetal morbidity and mortality. In multiple pregnancies of high order, this goal is only remotely possible, or even impossible to achieve, depending on the number of fetuses (four or more). Fetal reduction either makes it possible to achieve, or increases the likelihood of achieving, the goal of the live birth of infant(s) with minimal neonatal morbidity and mortality.[63] The first indication applies to cases in which the woman's goal is to maximize the probability of live birth. In current clinical judgment, this is best achieved by having two fetuses remain after the procedure has been performed.

It may at first appear that this initial indication for fetal reduction is ethically unjustified because it violates beneficence-based obligations to the fetus as a patient. On closer examination, however, this is not the case, because the moral status of being a patient is conferred on the previable fetus only as a function of the pregnant woman's decision to do so, as explained above. The clinical reality is that, for pregnancies in this category, the pregnant woman's decision to confer such status on all of the fetuses will jeopardize all of the fetuses. For some of the fetuses to become patients, the moral status of being a patient must be withheld from others. Thus, fetal reduction does not involve the killing of patients and is, therefore, justified in medical ethics.

An alternative, beneficence-based justification for fetal reduction in this category has been offered in an important pioneering article by Evans et al.[63] These authors apply the ethical principle of proportionality: "Proportionality is the source of the duty, when taking actions involving risks of harm, to balance risks and benefits so that actions have the greatest chance to cause the least harm and the most benefit to persons directly involved." On the basis of this ethical principle they conclude that fetal reduction of multifetal pregnancy is permissible in the clinical ethics of obstetric practice.

Second Indication: Achieving a Pregnancy that Results in Live Birth of Infant(s) without Prenatally Detected Anomalies

In some cases, the goal of obstetric care becomes live birth(s) without antenatally detected fetal anomalies.[62] Given the widespread use of antenatal diagnosis and legal access to abortion in developed countries, this is already an accepted practice. The ethical challenge in this category is the possibility of increased morbidity and mortality to the remaining fetus(es).

When a woman elects to selectively terminate a fetus with a detected anomaly, she, in effect, withholds from that fetus the moral status of becoming a patient and thus cannot reasonably be thought to be violating, in any way, beneficence-based obligations to that fetus; nor can the physician who performs the procedure. Presumably the remaining fetus(es) will be taken to term and thus have conferred on it, or them, by the pregnant woman's decision to do so, the moral status of being a patient. The possible risks of increased morbidity and mortality for remaining fetuses must be evaluated in the particular context of whether the anomaly is of such severity to justify possible compromise of the beneficence-based obligations to the remaining fetus(es). At the present time, risks of the selective termination procedure to the survivor fetus(es) are so infrequent that one cannot justify overriding beneficence-based obligations to remaining fetuses not to perform the procedure.[62]

Third Indication: Achieving a Pregnancy that Results in a Singleton Live Birth

Some cases do not involve fetal reduction as a means to have a successful pregnancy as for the first indication. Nor do they involve selective termination after the antenatal diagnosis of fetal anomalies for the second indication. Instead, they involve the pregnant woman's decision to have a single child rather than more than one child from her pregnancy.[62]

In these cases, the pregnant woman is withholding the moral status of being a patient from one or more of the fetuses, something she is free to do as a matter of exercising her autonomy to set her own goals for her pregnancy, as explained above. The pregnant woman also confers the status of being a patient on the fetus that survives reduction to the singleton (i.e., the one that she intends to take to term). As a consequence, there are beneficence-based obligations on her part and her physician's part to the singleton fetus to avoid significant harm that might result from the reduction. Clinical judgment at this time does not support the contention that harm will occur with high probability.[65] In the case of fetal reduction of twins to a singleton, a randomized clinical trial would be necessary to clearly assess whether the survivor would fare slightly better or slightly worse than twins without intervention. Given that the alternative to reduction of twin gestation is often complete termination, any minor risk of harm becomes moot under beneficence-based judgment when balanced against 100 percent mortality. Therefore, there are no beneficence-based obligations to the surviving singleton fetus not to terminate the pregnancy to a singleton.

Termination of Pregnancy after Viability

After viability, aggressive management is the ethical standard of care in obstetric practice. Aggressive management aims at optimizing perinatal outcome by using effective antepartum and intrapartum diagnostic and therapeutic methods. In addition, there are three other management options, termination of pregnancy, nonaggressive management, and cephalocentesis. We emphasize that these options are ethically challenging and best avoided through early diagnosis.[2]

Termination of pregnancy after fetal viability is ethically permissible when there is (1) certainty of diagnosis, and either (2a) certainty of death as an outcome of the anomaly diagnosed, or (2b) in some cases of short-term survival, certainty of the absence of cognitive developmental capacity as an outcome of the anomaly diagnosed.[2,66] When these criteria are satisfied, recommending a choice between nonaggressive management and termination of pregnancy is justified. Anencephaly is a classic example of a fetal anomaly that satisfies these criteria.[66]

A strong ethical argument can also be made that anomalies such as trisomy 13, trisomy 18, renal agenesis, thanatophoric dysplasia, alobar holoprosencephaly, and hydranencephaly should also count as anomalies that could ethically justify third-trimester abortion.[67] This is because, with these anomalies, either death is already a certain or a near-certain outcome or the certain or near-certain absence of cognitive developmental capacity is tantamount to death, and so in beneficence-based clinical judgment causing death is an acceptable outcome.

For many other anomalies, such as Down syndrome, spina bifida, isolated hydrocephalus, diaphragmatic hernia, achondroplasia, and most cardiac anomalies, neither death nor the absence of cognitive developmental capacity is a certain or near-certain outcome. Although these anomalies do involve incremental risks of mental and physical morbidity and mortality, they do not ethically justify third-trimester abortion. Under no rigorous clinical evaluation can these conditions be regarded as tantamount to death or absence of cognitive developmental capacity. For such anomalies, the beneficence-based prohibition against terminating the life of a viable fetus remains robustly intact. Any clinical judgment that does not address and defeat this beneficence-based prohibition is defective on ethical grounds and therefore is inconsistent with professional integrity.[67,68]

The pregnant woman has the same beneficence-based obligations to the fetal patient as does her physician and she should therefore act on those obligations, provided that the risks to her of doing so are reasonable.[2] The risks of continuing a viable pregnancy to term are in almost all cases reasonable. In the rare instance in which the woman's health necessitates delivery, all efforts should be made to help the child. Thus, the pregnant woman's autonomy should be understood by the woman and her physician to be constrained by the beneficence-based prohibition against killing the third-trimester fetal patient, with the exceptions noted above. Thus, a woman's exercise of autonomy to request a third-trimester abortion for a fetus with an anomaly such as Down syndrome, lacks ethical authority.[2] Therefore, as a matter of professional integrity no physician should carry out such a request.

Many anomalies in children create burdens on patients, parents, society, communities, institutions, and health care professionals. However, although those burdens may often be significant, they are concerns distinct from the doctor's obligation to protect and promote the fetal patient's interest just as they are distinct from what is in any patient's interests. Moreover, in theories of justice that emphasize equality of opportunity for human experience and development, the assumption of such burdens by society would be ethically obligatory.[69] Society has a justice-based obligation to look after its disabled and to maximize their potential so that they can live fulfilling lives. Thus, in addition to violating the beneficence-based prohibition against killing, third-trimester abortion of fetal patients with Down syndrome and the other anomalies listed above enlists medicine to escape from the well-founded, justice-based obligations of parents, institutions, and society to disabled children. We are hard pressed, indeed, to see how this would be consistent with professional integrity and social justice.

Nonaggressive Management

Nonaggressive obstetric management is ethically permissible when there is (1) a very high probability, but sometimes less than complete certainty, about the diagnosis and, either (2a) a very high probability of death as an outcome of the anomaly diagnosed, or (2b) survival with a very high probability of severe and irreversible deficit of cognitive developmental capacity as a result of the anomaly diagnosed.[2,70] When these two criteria apply, a choice between aggressive or nonaggressive management should be offered. Encephalocele is a classic example of a fetal anomaly that satisfies these criteria.

Cephalocentesis

Cephalocentesis involves the drainage of an enlarged fetal head, secondary to hydrocephalus.[71,72] The ethical justification of cephalocentesis varies according to the nature and associated complications of hydrocephalus. Fetal hydrocephalus is caused by the obstruction of cerebrospinal flow and is diagnosed by sonographic signs such as dilatation of the atrium or body of the lateral ventricles.[73] In the third trimester, macrocephaly often accompanies the ventriculomegaly. In addition, sonography can diagnose hydrocephalus in association with gross abnormalities suggestive of poor prognosis, for example, hydranencephaly, microcephaly, encephalocele, alobar holoprosencephaly, or thanatophoric dysplasia with cloverleaf skull.[73] In the absence of defined anatomical abnormalities, however, diagnostic imaging is, at the present time, unable to predict the outcome. Although cortical mantle thickness can be measured with ultrasound, its value as a prognostic index is not established.[73]

Cephalocentesis should be performed under simultaneous ultrasound guidance so that needle placement into the cerebrospinal fluid is facilitated. An 18-gauge needle is used with subsequent collapse of the cranial bones, the end point for this procedure. Enough fluid is drained to permit reduction of the skull diameters so that passage through the birth canal is possible.[74,75] Cephalocentesis is a potentially destructive procedure. Perinatal death following cephalocentesis has been reported in more than 90 percent of cases.[71] The sonographic visualization of intracranial bleeding during cephalocentesis and the demonstration of this hemorrhage at autopsy further emphasize the morbid nature of the procedure. However, if decompression is performed in a controlled manner, the mortality may be reduced.

There is considerable potential for normal, sometimes superior, intellectual function for fetuses with even extreme, isolated hydrocephalus.[76–79] However, as a group, infants with isolated hydrocephalus experience a greater incidence of mental retardation and early death than the general population. In addition, associated anomalies may go undetected, and a fetus may be incorrectly diagnosed as having isolated hydrocephalus.[74,80] One thing is clear in obstetric ethics: A viable at-term fetus with isolated hydrocephalus is a fetal patient, because neither of the two exceptions described above (certainty of diagnosis and certainty of outcome) apply, given the variable outcomes of isolated hydrocephalus.

There are compelling, beneficence-based ethical reasons for concluding that the continuing existence of fetuses with isolated hydrocephalus is in their interest. Beneficence directs the physician to prevent mortality and morbidity for the fetal patient. Beneficence also directs the physician to undertake interventions that ameliorate handicapping conditions such as mental retardation. The probability of mental retardation does not diminish the interests of the fetal patient with isolated hydrocephalus in continuing existence because (1) it is impossible to predict which fetuses with isolated hydrocephalus will have mental retardation, and (2) the degree of mental retardation cannot be predicted in advance.

The beneficence-based obligation of the physician caring for the fetus with macrocephaly is to recommend strongly and to attain the woman's consent to perform a cesarean delivery, because this clinical intervention clearly involves the least risk of mortality, morbidity, and handicap for the fetus compared with cephalocentesis to permit subsequent vaginal delivery. Even when performed under maximal therapeutic conditions (i.e., under sonographic guidance), cephalocentesis cannot reasonably be regarded as protecting or promoting the health-related interests of the fetal patient with isolated hydrocephalus with macrocephaly. This procedure is followed by a high rate of perinatal mortality, fetal heart rate deceleration, and pathologic evidence of intracranial bleeding.[74,80] Cephalocentesis, therefore, cannot reasonably be construed as an ethically justifiable mode of management, insofar as it is inconsistent with beneficence-based obligations to avoid increased mortality and morbidity risks for the fetal patient. Cephalocentesis, employed with a destructive intent, is altogether antithetical to the beneficence-based prohibition against killing.[2]

It is essential in obstetric ethics that beneficence-based obligations to the fetal patient be balanced against beneficence-based and autonomy-based obligations to the pregnant woman. First, the physician has a beneficence-based obligation to avoid performing a cesarean delivery because the possibility of morbidity and mortality for the woman is higher than that associated with vaginal delivery. Respect for autonomy obligates the physician to undertake only those interventions or forms of treatment to which the woman has given voluntary, informed consent. Informed consent is grounded in an autonomy-based right of the pregnant woman to control what happens to her body. In particular, the woman has the right to authorize or refuse operative intervention—those that are, as well as those that are not, consistent with the physician's beneficence-based obligations.[2]

We are now prepared to consider the full complexity of the management of the fetal patient with isolated hydrocephalus with macrocephaly: Beneficence-based and autonomy-based obligations to the pregnant woman, as well as beneficence-based obligations to her fetus, must all be considered for clinical ethical judgment to be complete and therefore reliable. If, with informed consent, the woman authorizes cesarean delivery, there is no conflict among these obligations.

In contrast, her physician faces a significant and challenging ethical conflict if the woman refuses cesarean delivery. This conflict should be resolved in favor of the beneficence-based obligations to the fetal patient, because the harm to the fetal patient is final, namely, death, and will occur with high probability. Moreover, if the fetal patient survives (death is not guaranteed by cephalocentesis), it is likely to be more damaged as a result of intracranial hemorrhage than if cesarean delivery is performed. Morbidity and mortality of the pregnant woman are both minimal and therefore risks that she ought to accept to protect the fetal patient's interest.[2] Such ethical conflict should be prevented by employing the preventive ethics strategies of informed consent as an ongoing dialogue, negotiation, respectful persuasion, and the proper use of ethics committees.[2,16]

If these preventive ethics strategies do not succeed and the pregnant woman continues to refuse cesarean delivery, the physician confronts tragic circumstances. If neither cesarean delivery nor cephalocentesis is performed, the woman is at risk for uterine rupture and death, and the fetal patient is at risk for death. This logic of beneficence-based obligations is to prevent such total and irreversible harm. Therefore, we believe that because of the grave nature of possible consequences for the woman and her fetus, because of the dangers for the woman of performing a surgical procedure on a resistant patient, and because of the pitfalls of attempted legal coercion, the physician should act on beneficence-based obligations to the woman in such an extreme circumstance. The fetal patient is at high risk for death under either alternative. The woman's death, at least, can be avoided. Serious beneficence-based obligations to the fetal patient on the part of both the physician and the pregnant woman will probably be violated and a needless death will most probably result, however, by performing a cephalocentesis. Herein lies the tragedy of these circumstances. To avoid this tragedy, redoubled efforts of preventive ethics should be undertaken. Carefully explaining the fact that cephalocentesis does not guarantee death and may produce a worse outcome is very powerfully persuasive. In the rare cases in which this effort at respectful persuasion fails, cephalocentesis should be performed in the least destructive way possible or an appropriate referral should be made.

Some abnormalities that occur in association with fetal hydrocephalus are severe in nature for the child afflicted with them. We define "severe" abnormalities as those that either are (1) incompatible with continued existence (e.g., bilateral renal agenesis or thanatophoric dysplasia with cloverleaf skull), (2) compatible with survival in some cases but resulting in virtual absence of cognitive function (e.g., trisomy 18 or alobar holoprosencephaly).[81] Because there is no available intervention to prevent postnatal death in the first group, beneficence-based obligations of the physician and the pregnant woman to attempt to prolong the life of the fetal patient are nonexistent. No ethical theory and no version of obstetric ethics based on beneficence and respect for autonomy obligate the physician to attempt the impossible. For the second group, beneficence-based obligations of the physician and the pregnant woman to sustain the life of the fetal patient are minimal because the handicap imposed by the abnormality is severe. In these cases the potential for cognitive development—and therefore the achievement of other "good" for the child (e.g., relationships with others)—are virtually absent. Such fetuses are fetal patients to which there are owed only minimal beneficence-based obligations.

In these circumstances, the woman is therefore released from her beneficence-based obligations to the at-term fetal patient to place herself at risk, because no significant good can be achieved by cesarean delivery for the fetal patient or the child it will become. There remain only the autonomy-based and beneficence-based obligations of the physician to the pregnant woman. After the preceding analysis of these obligations, we conclude that the physician's overriding moral obligations are to the pregnant woman's voluntary and informed decision about the use of cephalocentesis.

Because there are no weighty beneficence-based obligations to the fetus in such clinical and ethical circumstances, the physician may justifiably offer a choice between cesarean delivery and cephalocentesis to enable vaginal delivery. There are obvious advantages to the woman's health by the avoidance of cesarean delivery. However, cesarean delivery permits women who wish to do so to have a live birth and satisfy religious convictions or help with the grieving process. A cesarean delivery performed in this clinical setting is best viewed as an autonomy-based maternal indication. Because the prognosis for infants with hydrocephalus associated with severe anomalies is poor, we believe that intrapartum fetal death resulting from cephalocentesis would not be a tragic outcome in the sense that it would be in the death of a fetal patient with isolated hydrocephalus.

On the continuum between the extreme cases of isolated hydrocephalus and hydrocephalus with severe associated abnormalities, there is a variety of cases of hydrocephalus associated with macrocephaly with other abnormalities with varying degrees of impairment of cognitive physical function. They range from hypoplastic distal phalanges to spina bifida to encephalocele.[74] Because these conditions have varying prognoses, it would be clinically inappropriate, and therefore ethically misleading, to treat this third category as homogeneous. Therefore, we propose a working distinction between different kinds of prognoses. The first we call "probably promising," by which we mean that there is a significant possibility the child will experience cognitive development with learning disabilities and physical handicaps that perhaps can be ameliorated to some extent. The second we call "probably poor." By this phrase, we mean that there is only a limited possibility for cognitive development because of learning disabilities and physical handicaps that cannot be ameliorated to a significant extent. We propose these definitions as tentative, so they are subject to revision as clinical and ethical investigation of such associated anomalies continues. As a consequence, our ethical analysis of these two categories cannot be carried out as extensively as those in the previous two sections. In essence, we propose that the clinical continuum in these cases is paralleled by an ethical continuum or progressively less weighty, beneficence-based obligations to the fetal patient.[81]

When the prognosis is probably promising (e.g., isolated arachnoid cyst), there are serious beneficence-based obligations to the fetal patient. However, they are not necessarily on the same order as those that occur in cases of isolated hydrocephalus. (It has been suggested that any associated anomaly may increase the possibility of a poor outcome.[74]) Therefore, in such cases with a prognosis of probably promising, we propose that the physician recommend cesarean delivery, although perhaps not as vigorously as in cases of isolated hydrocephalus. A pregnant woman's informed refusal of cesarean delivery should therefore be respected.

In cases in which the prognosis, even though uncertain, is probably poor (e.g., encephalocele), beneficence-based obligations to the fetal patient are less weighty than those owed to the fetal patient with a promising prognosis. These cases, then, resemble ethically those of hydrocephalus with severe anomalies, with the proviso that some, albeit limited, benefits can be achieved for the fetal patient by cesarean delivery and aggressive perinatal treatment. Nonetheless, the physician may in these cases justifiably accept an informed voluntary decision by the woman for cephalocentesis followed by vaginal delivery. However, the physician cannot assume an advocacy role for such a decision with the same level of ethical confidence that he or she can in cases of hydrocephalus associated with severe anomalies.

RESEARCH TO IMPROVE CLINICAL MANAGEMENT OF FETAL ANOMALIES

Gene Transfer Research

Sometime in the not-too-distant future, gene transfer technology will be introduced into the clinical setting as human subjects research. Significant ethical challenges regarding the informed consent process for such research will need to be addressed effectively. One of these is known as the therapeutic misconception. Recent studies of the experience of subjects of research have shown that patients are not always aware when they are subjects of research.[82] It has been suggested that the language used during the consent process may contribute to this disturbing lack of understanding.[82] In our judgment, the use of the word *therapy* should be avoided to prevent this lack of understanding. Therefore, phrases such as "innovative therapy," "gene therapy," and "experimental therapy" should not be used in consent forms or in discussions with pregnant women about their participation in gene transfer research. Instead, the consent form and these discussions should be explicit about the fact that the clinical application of gene transfer to the embryo or fetus at this time is research or experimentation.

It is never obligatory for an individual who can consent for himself or herself to consent to become a subject for research. Nor is it obligatory for a surrogate, such as a parent, to consent for a patient not capable of participating in the consent process (e.g., an infant or very young child) to become a subject of research.[5] It therefore follows that no pregnant woman is obligated to consent to gene transfer research on her embryo or fetus, even when the fetus is a patient. This is because no surrogate is obligated to make consent to such a patient becoming a subject of research. It is therefore critical that the consent process make this moral fact very clear to pregnant women and to others who might be involved with them in the consent process for gene transfer research.

Institutional review boards should scrutinize consent forms and procedures to require efforts on the part of investigators to prevent coercion of a woman's decision by internal factors such as unreasoning desperation and external factors such as partners and family members. These recommendations parallel the ethically justified practice of protecting women from subtle coercion in decisions about using assisted reproduction technologies.

Gene transfer research is new, and the informed consent process should be structured with this fact in mind. We recommend, therefore, that the consent process should begin with the research team inviting the pregnant woman to state what she understands about the embryo's or the fetus's diagnosis, available alternatives for managing that diagnosis, and the benefits and risks of those alternatives. If there is no intervention currently available, she should be asked what she understands the prognosis to be. This will be very important for aiding women in understanding the distinction between gene transfer for uniformly lethal conditions and gene transfer for conditions that result in serious morbidity. The research team should be attentive to factual errors and incompleteness in the woman's fund of knowledge. Educating her about the protocol should begin by making sure her initial fund of knowledge is accurate, thus laying a solid intellectual foundation for the rest of the consent process.

That process should continue with an explanation of the embryo's or the fetus's genetic condition and how the gene transfer research is designed to address that condition. She should be given information about the results of animal studies, especially about documented benefits and risks identified in such studies. She should also be informed about the unknown risk that transferred genes could malfunction in unpredictable ways (the law of unintended consequences).

She should then be assisted in identifying her relevant values and beliefs. This can be accomplished in a nondirective fashion by asking what is important to her about this pregnancy, about having children, and about having children with potentially severe health problems. She can then be asked to assess the offered gene transfer research on the basis of her values and beliefs, thus enhancing her autonomy in the consent process.

Throughout the consent process and in the consent form, the options of abortion and nonintervention should be presented as entirely acceptable to the research team. We make this recommendation to reinforce the nondirective character of the informed consent process for gene transfer research.

Current federal regulations continue to require paternal consent.[83] On the account we have given of the fetus as a patient, the father of the fetus does not determine whether the fetus is a patient. There is an obvious moral asymmetry between the father and the pregnant woman during pregnancy, such that his role in decisions about interventions on the fetus should be a function of the pregnant woman's autonomy.

Gene transfer research will be used especially to try to reduce the mortality of uniformly lethal conditions, such as α-thalassemia. The traditional logic of beneficence that drives such research has been that every reduction of mortality from such conditions is worth whatever morbidity that might result for survivors. In the clinical setting, especially in critical care, the traditional logic of beneficence has been appropriately challenged when morbidities eliminate or greatly impair the developmental capacity of survivors. As McCormick put it more than 25 years ago, when critical care results in all of the patient's energies being used in an irreversible struggle to survive, critical care intervention can be stopped.[84] The moral lessons for gene transfer research are twofold. First, if animal studies reduce mortality but survivors are left with devastating morbidity, then human trials should not be started until animal outcomes improve. Second, human trials should include, as a stopping rule, high rates of occurrence of devastating fetal morbidity.

Recall that the previable fetus is a patient solely as a function of the pregnant woman's autonomy. For gene transfer on previable fetuses, the exercise of such autonomy is greatly restricted in the absence of prenatal diagnosis to determine the effectiveness of the gene transfer. In particular, some women may want to terminate a pregnancy before viability, when there is no laboratory evidence of successful transfer. In our view, therefore, offering prenatal diagnosis should be required by institutional review boards for gene therapy interventions with previable fetuses. The consent process should include a careful explanation about the potential for false-negative and false-positive results.

It is an accepted feature of study design in general that clinical trials should be conducted in such a way as to control for the idiosyncratic effects of patients' preferences on results. This, for example, justifies a double-blind study design.

For gene transfer research, this general rule of study design raises significant ethical issues. On the one hand, to get the cleanest results one would not want any pregnancies in which gene transfer occurred to result in elective abortions. On the other hand, it would be desirable to prevent adverse outcomes of gene transfer through abortion in a study population of women who would accept this option.

To address the first problem, one would exclude women who indicated any willingness to consider elective abortion. To address the second problem, one would exclude women who were opposed to abortion. Both solutions share a common and disabling ethical problem: They decide for the woman whether the previable fetus is a patient, thus unjustifiably overriding her autonomy in favor of research considerations, a paternalistic abuse of research subjects.

To avoid this unacceptable ethical problem there should be no exclusion criteria for fetal gene transfer based on willingness to countenance elective abortion. Therefore, study designs would have to include elective abortion and birth of adversely affected infants as hard end points.

Gene transfer research will almost certainly continue to attract a great deal of public concern and attention, especially in print and electronic media. Moreover, institutions that sponsor this research will desire to publicize such research as a way to bring prestige to the institution. These pressures, we fear, could combine to create a very powerful incentive to bypass the rigors of scientific investigation, in particular the intellectual and clinical ethical obligations to report the results of research in the peer-reviewed literature. In accordance with the accepting journals' policies, press conferences are acceptable. This approach prevents the deleterious phenomenon of "science by press conference."

Anecdotal reports by grateful parents of a healthy newborn do not count as evidence for the efficacy and safety of embryo or fetal gene transfer research. It follows that press conferences meeting the stipulations above should not involve parents, and their names should not be released. Parents are free to release private information about themselves to the media. Institutional publicity independent of parents will help maintain the crucial distinction between scientific investigation of experimental intervention and anecdotal reports of benefit or harm.

Fletcher and Richter raised the important ethical concern for germ-line harm that could result from the unknown harms of gene transfer.[85] They propose that somatic cell gene transfer research "ought not be approved unless investigation in animal studies shows that the vector does not convey copies of exogenous genetic material into sex cells of fetuses."[85] This, in our view, is a prudent recommendation designed to prevent unnecessary harm to future generations. As embryo and fetal gene transfer research matures, this position may need to be reconsidered, especially when it is reliably thought that germ-line benefits convincingly outweigh germ-line harms. Any attempt to address this question will be controversial.

Fletcher and Richter also propose that a public body be mandated to "oversee" gene transfer research, at least for the near future.[85] They express confidence that the NIH's Recombinant DNA Advisory Committee (RAC) could effectively play this role. They argue that this public policy response would "continue the tradition of scientific and ethical restraint in the introduction of human gene therapy in medicine."[85] Given the fractious debate about abortion in American society, such public oversight will help increase confidence among the public that gene transfer research, while unavoidably controversial, is accountable to society. The scientific community should welcome such public scrutiny as a way to build and sustain public trust in ethically controversial scientific research. The RAC currently is charged with oversight of gene transfer research.

Fetal Surgery Research

Fetal research is essential for the improvement of clinical management of fetal anomalies.[86] The first stage of such research is innovation, which begins with the design of an intervention and its implementation in animal models, followed by a single case and then a case series. This approach is required to determine the feasibility, safety, and efficacy of innovations. It is a basic tenet of research ethics that potential subjects should be protected from potentially harmful innovation.

Three criteria must be satisfied to conduct such preliminary investigations in an ethically responsible fashion, that is, that takes into account beneficence-based obligations to the fetal patient and beneficence-based obligations to the pregnant woman. The previable fetus is a patient in these cases because the woman has made a decision to continue her pregnancy, to have the opportunity to gain the potential benefits of the innovation. She remains free to withdraw that status before viability.

1. The proposed fetal intervention is reliably expected on the basis of previous animal studies either to be lifesaving or to prevent serious and irreversible disease, injury, or handicap for the fetus;

2. Among possible alternative designs, the intervention is designed in such a way as to involve the least risk of mortality and morbidity to the fetal patient (which is required by beneficence and will satisfy the U.S. research requirement of minimal risk to the fetus)[87]; and

3. On the basis of animal studies and analysis of theoretical risks both for the current and future pregnancies, the mortality risk to the pregnant woman is reliably expected to be low and the risk of disease, injury, or handicap to the pregnant woman is reliably expected to be low or manageable.[86]

The first two criteria appeal to beneficence-based obligations to the fetal patient. Research on animal models should suggest that there would be therapeutic benefit without disproportionate iatrogenic fetal morbidity or mortality. If animal studies result in high rates of mortality or morbidity for the animal fetal subject, then innovation should not be introduced to human subjects until these rates improve in subsequent animal studies.

The third criterion underscores the fact that fetal surgery is also maternal surgery. This criterion is important because it reminds investigators that the willingness of a subject, in this case, the pregnant woman, to consent to risk does not by itself establish whether the risk/benefit ratio is favorable. Investigators have an independent beneficence-based obligation to protect human subjects from unreasonably risky research and should use beneficence-based, not autonomy-based, risk/benefit analyses. Phrases such as "maternal–fetal surgery" are useful if they remind investigators of the need for such comprehensive analysis. If they are used systematically to subordinate fetal interests to maternal interest and rights, and therefore to undermine the concept of the fetus as a patient in favor of the concept that the fetus is merely a part of the pregnant woman, such phrases lack ethical utility.

Preliminary innovation should end and randomized clinical trials begin when there is clinical equipoise, that is, there is "a remaining disagreement in the expert clinical community, despite the available evidence, about the merits of the intervention to be tested."[83] Brody notes that one challenge is identifying how much disagreement can remain for there still to be equipoise.[83] Lilford suggested that when two-thirds of the expert community, measured reliably, no longer disagrees, equipoise is not satisfied.[88] When the experimental intervention is more harmful than nonintervention, equipoise cannot be achieved.

The satisfaction of the previous three criteria, with slight modifications, should count as equipoise in the expert community.

1. The initial case series indicates that the proposed fetal intervention is reliably expected either to be lifesaving or to prevent serious and irreversible disease, injury, or handicap;

2. Among possible alternative designs, the intervention continues to involve the least risk of morbidity and mortality to the fetus; and

3. The case series indicates that the mortality risk to the pregnant woman is reliably expected to be low and the risk of disease, injury, or handicap to the pregnant woman, including for future pregnancies, is reliably expected to be low or manageable.[86]

One good test for the satisfaction of the first and third criteria is significant trends in the data from the case series. When equipoise has been achieved on the basis of these three criteria, randomized clinical trials should commence. They must have relevant and clearly defined primary and secondary end points and a design and sample size adequate to measure these end points.

The above three criteria can also be used to define stopping rules for such a clinical trial. When the data support a rigorous clinical judgment that the first or third criterion is not satisfied, the trial should be stopped.

When the clinical trial is completed, its outcome should be carefully assessed to determine whether the innovative fetal surgery should be regarded as the standard of care. In addition to meeting accepted requirements of scientific rigor, trial results should meet the following three criteria to establish the innovation as a standard of care:

1. The fetal surgery has a significant probability of being lifesaving or of preventing serious or irreversible disease, injury, or handicap for the fetus;
2. The surgery involves low mortality and low or manageable risk of serious and irreversible disease, injury, or handicap to the fetus; and
3. The mortality risk to the pregnant woman is low and the risk of disease, injury or handicap is low or manageable, including for future pregnancies.[86]

Brody underscored the value of data safety and monitoring boards to prevent investigator bias and to protect subjects.[83] Such boards should be used in fetal research, especially to ensure adherence of the above-mentioned ethical criteria as a basis for monitoring such research.

Practicing physicians are ethically justified in informing their patients about relevant clinical investigations, and with the patient's consent, referring them to the investigators. In our view, there is also an obligation to do so in the case of fetal research. The justification for this obligation cannot appeal to benefit to the pregnant woman or fetal patient, because by definition, the existence of clinical investigation does not establish clinical benefit. However, there is an obligation to future patients, pregnant and fetal alike, to establish whether investigative fetal intervention improves the management of pregnancies complicated by fetal anomalies. All physicians should take seriously their obligation to future patients to ensure that innovation has the opportunity to be validated scientifically and ethically, rather than introduced in an unmanaged fashion or simply ignored.

CONCLUSION

Ethics provides clinicians with indispensable conceptual and clinical tools for responsible responses to ethical challenges in the diagnosis and management of genetic disorders in the fetus.[2,89–91] As we have seen in this chapter, these challenges range very widely indeed, from how to counsel pregnant women about prenatal diagnostic screens and tests, to management of both previable and viable pregnancies complicated by fetal anomalies, to gene transfer and procedures performed directly on fetuses and pregnant women in maternal–fetal research. It is a commonplace of the current bioethics literature to start discussion of such topics with a claim that developments in biomedical technology and their clinical application threaten to outstrip our moral concepts and capacities. This chapter is written on the assumption that this is very much not the case. Bioethics has developed very powerful conceptual tools, principally the concept of the fetus as a patient, that are certainly adequate for understanding and responding to the full range of ethical challenges in the diagnosis and management of genetic disorders in the fetus.

The ethical concept of the fetus as a patient guides clinicians in reaching ethically justified balancing of autonomy-based and beneficence-based obligations to the pregnant woman and beneficence-based obligations to the fetus. These obligations can be stratified in a clinically useful fashion into three groups, management of pregnancies before viability, management of pregnancies after viability, and fetal research. For previable pregnancies, respect for the pregnant woman's autonomy is the decisive ethical concern, including the subset of selective termination for multifetal pregnancies. For viable pregnancies, beneficence-based obligations to the fetal patient support aggressive obstetric management with the well-defined exceptions of termination of pregnancy, nonaggressive management, and cephalocentesis. For fetal research, ethically justified criteria for the design, conduct, and evaluation of clinical investigation must take account of obligations to both the pregnant woman and fetal patient.

REFERENCES

1. Beauchamp TL, Childress JF. Principles of biomedical ethics, 5th ed. New York: Oxford University Press, 2000.
2. McCullough LB, Chervenak FA. Ethics in obstetrics and gynecology. New York: Oxford University Press, 1994.
3. Temkin O, Temkin CL, Edelstein L. Ancient medicine. Baltimore: Johns Hopkins University Press, 1967:3.
4. Hippocrates. Epidemics. In: Jones WHS, trans., Hippocrates, vol. 1. Cambridge, MA.: Harvard University Press, 1923:165.
5. Faden RR, Beauchamp TL. A history and theory of informed consent. New York: Oxford University Press, 1986.
6. Hack M, Fanaroff AA. Outcomes of extremely-low-birth-weight infants between 1982 and 1988. N Engl J Med 1989;321:1642.
7. Chervenak FA, McCullough LB. The limits of viability. J Perinat Med 1997;25:418.
8. Chervenak FA, McCullough LB. An ethically justified, clinically comprehensive management strategy for third-trimester pregnancies complicated by fetal anomalies. Obstet Gynecol 1990;75:311.
9. Chervenak FA, McCullough LB. Does obstetric ethics have any role in the obstetrician's response to the abortion controversy? Am J Obstet Gynecol 1990;163:1425.
10. Chervenak FA, McCullough LB. Nonaggressive obstetric management: an option for some fetal anomalies during the third trimester. JAMA 1989;261:3439.
11. Chervenak FA, McCullough LB, Campbell S. Is third trimester abortion justified? Br J Obstet Gynaecol 1995;102:434.
12. Chervenak FA, McCullough LB, Campbell S. Third trimester abortion: is compassion enough? Br J Obstet Gynaecol 1999;106:293.
13. Brett A, McCullough LB. When patients request specific interventions: refining the limits of the physician's obligations. N Engl J Med 1986;315:1347.
14. Chervenak FA, Farley MA, Walters L, et al. When is termination of pregnancy during the third trimester morally justifiable? N Engl J Med 1984;310:501.
15. Chervenak FA, McCullough LB. Perinatal ethics: a practical method of analysis of obligations to mother and fetus. Obstet Gynecol 1985;66:442.
16. Chervenak FA, McCullough LB. Clinical guides to preventing ethical conflicts between pregnant women and their physicians. Am J Obstet Gynecol 1990;162:303.
17. Campbell S, Reading AE, Cox DN, et al. Ultrasound scanning in pregnancy: the short-term psychological effects of early real time scans. J Psychosomat Obstet Gynecol 1986;1:57.
18. Warren MA. Gendercide: the implications of sex selection. Totowa, NJ: Rowman and Littlefield, 1985.
19. Gostin LO. National health information privacy: regulations under the Health Insurance Portability and Accountability Act. JAMA 2001;285:3015.
20. Chervenak FA, McCullough L. Ethics in obstetric ultrasound. J Ultrasound Med 1989;8:493.
21. Ewigman BG, Crane JP, Frigoletto FD, et al. Effect of prenatal ultrasound screening on perinatal outcome. N Engl J Med 1993;329:821.
22. American College of Obstetricians and Gynecologists: Ultrasonography in pregnancy. ACOG Technical Bulletin 187. Washington, DC, ACOG, 1993.
23. American College of Obstetricians and Gynecologists: Newsletter. Washington, DC, ACOG, November 1993.
24. Romero R. Routine obstetric ultrasound. Ultrasound Obstet Gynecol 1993;3:303.
25. Skupski DW, Chervenak FA, McCullough LB. Is routine ultrasound screening for all patients? Clin Perinatol 1994;21:707.
26. Chervenak FA, McCullough LB, Chervenak JL. Prenatal informed consent for sonogram: an indication for obstetric ultrasonography. Am J Obstet Gynecol 1989;161:857.

27. Ewigman BG, Le Fevre M, Bain RP, et al. Ethics and routine ultrasonography in pregnancy. Am J Obstet Gynecol 1990;163:256.

28. Devore G. The routine antenatal diagnostic imaging with ultrasound study: another perspective. Obstet Gynecol 1994;84:622.

29. Jones KL. Smith's recognizable patterns of human malformation, 5th ed. Philadelphia: WB Saunders, 1997.

30. Benacerraf BR, Barss VA, Laboda LA. A sonographic sign for the detection in the second trimester of the fetus with Down's syndrome. Am J Obstet Gynecol 1985;151:1078.

31. Nicolaides KH, Azar G, Byrne D, et al. Fetal nuchal translucency: ultrasound screening for chromosomal defects in first trimester of pregnancy. BMJ 1992;304:867.

32. Pandya PP, Santiago C, Snijders RJ, Nicolaides KH. First trimester fetal nuchal translucency. Curr Opin Obstet Gynecol 1995;7:95.

33. Pandya PP, Snijders RJM, Johnson SJ, et al. Screening for fetal trisomies by maternal age and fetal nuchal translucency thickness at 10 to 14 weeks of gestation. Br J Obstet Gynaecol 1995;102:957.

34. Snijders RJM, Noble P, Sebire N, et al. UK multicentre project on assessment of risk of trisomy 21 by maternal age and fetal nuchal translucency thickness at 10–14 weeks of gestation. Lancet 1998;351:343.

35. American College of Obstetricians and Gynecologists Committee on Genetics. First-trimester screening for fetal anomalies with nuchal translucency. Committee Opinion Number 223. Washington, DC: American College of Obstetricians and Gynecologists, 1999.

36. Malone FD, Berkowitz RL, Canick JA, D'Alton ME. First-trimester screening for aneuploidy: research or standard of care. Am J Obstet Gynecol 2000;182:49.

37. O'Callaghan SP, Giles WB, Raymond SP, et al. First trimester ultrasound with nuchal translucency measurement for Down syndrome risk estimation using software developed by the Fetal Medicine Foundation, United Kingdom—the first 2000 examinations in Newcastle, New South Wales, Australia. Aust NZJ Obstet Gynaecol 2000;40:292.

38. Theodoropoulos P, Lolis D, Papageorgiou C, et al. Evaluation of first-trimester screening by fetal nuchal translucency and maternal age. Prenat Diagn 1998;18:133.

39. Zoppi MA, Ibba RM, Floris M, Monni G. Fetal nuchal translucency screening in 12,495 pregnancies in Sardinia. Ultrasound Obstet Gynecol 2001;18:649.

40. Chasen ST, Sharma G, Kalish RB, Chervenak FA. First-trimester screening for aneuploidy with fetal nuchal translucency in a United States population. Ultrasound Obstet Gynecol 2003;22:149.

41. Wapner RJ, Thorn E, Simpson JL, Pergament E, Silver R, et. al. N Engl J Med 2003; 349:1405–13.

42. Haddow JE, Palomaki GE, Knight GJ, et al.. Screening of maternal serum for fetal Down's syndrome in the first trimester. N Engl J Med 1998;338:955.

43. Krantz DA, Larsen JW, Buchanan PD, Macri JN. First trimester Down syndrome screening; free beta human chorionic gonadotropin and pregnancy-associated plasma protein A. Am J Obstet Gynecol 1996;174:612.

44. Spencer K, Spencer CE, Power M, et al.. One stop clinic for assessment of risk for fetal anomalies: a report of the first year of prospective screening for chromosomal anomalies in the first trimester. BJOG 2000;107:1271.

45. Krantz DA, Hallahan TW, Orlandi F, et al. First-trimester Down syndrome screening using dried blood biochemistry and nuchal translucency. Obstet Gynecol 2000;96:207.

46. Bindra R, Heath V, Liao A, Spencer K, Nicolaides KH. One-stop clinic for assessment of risk for trisomy 21 at 11–14 weeks: a prospective study of 15,030 pregnancies. Ultrasound Obstet Gynecol 2002;20:219.

47. Cicero S, Curcio P, Papageorghiou A, et al. Absence of nasal bone in fetuses with trisomy 21 at 11–14 weeks of gestation: an observational study. Lancet 2001;358:1665.

48. Mavrides E, Sairam S, Hollis B, Thilaganathan B. Screening for aneuploidy in the first trimester by assessment of blood flow in the ductus venosus. Ultrasound Obstet Gynecol 1997;10:381.

49. Nicolaides KH, Sebire NJ, Snijders RJM. The 11–14 week scan. Carnforth, UK: Parthenon Publishing, 1999.

50. Chasen ST, Skupski DW, Chervenak FA, McCullough LB. First-trimester nuchal translucency screening. J Ultrasound Med 2002;21:483.

51. Zoppi MA, Ibba RM, Putzolu M, et al. Nuchal translucency and the acceptance of invasive prenatal chromosomal diagnosis in women aged 35 and older. Obstet Gynecol 2001;97:916.

52. Chasen ST, McCullough LB, Chervenak FA. Is nuchal translucency screening associated with different rates of invasive testing in an older obstetric population? Am J Obstet Gynecol 2004. In press.

53. Wald NJ, Watt HC, Hackshaw AK. Integrated screening for Down's syndrome on the basis of tests performed during the first and second trimesters. N Engl J Med 1999;12:341:461.

54. Alfirevic Z, Gosden CM, Neilson JP. Chorion villus sampling versus amniocentesis for prenatal diagnosis. Cochrane Database Syst Rev 2000;CD000055.

55. Silver RK, Leeth EA, Check IJ. A reappraisal of amniotic fluid alpha-fetoprotein measurement at the time of genetic amniocentesis and midtrimester ultrasonography. J Ultrasound Med 2001;20:631.

56. Souka AP, Snijders RJ, Novakov A, et al. Defects and syndromes in chromosomally normal fetuses with increased nuchal translucency thickness at 10–14 weeks of gestation. Ultrasound Obstet Gynecol 1998;11:391.

57. Kurtz AB, Wapner RJ, Mata J, et al. Twin pregnancies: accuracy of first-trimester abdominal US in predicting chorionicity and amnionicity. Radiology 1992;185:759.

58. Chasen ST, Skupski DW, McCullough LB, Chervenak FA. Prenatal informed consent for sonogram: the time for nuchal translucency has come. J Ultrasound Med 2001;20:1147.

59. Harris LH. Rethinking maternal–fetal conflict: gender and equality in perinatal ethics. Obstet Gynecol 2000;96:786.

60. Steinbock B. Life before birth: the moral and legal status of embryos and fetus. New York: Oxford University Press, 1992.

61. Strong C. Ethics in reproductive and perinatal medicine: a new framework. New Haven: Yale University Press, 1997.

62. Chervenak FA, McCullough LB, Wapner R. Three ethically justified indications for selective termination in multifetal pregnancy: a practical and comprehensive management strategy. J Assist Reprod Genet 1995;12:531.

63. Evans MI, Johnson MP, Quintero RA, Fletcher JC. Ethical issues surrounding multifetal pregnancy reduction and selective termination. Clin Perinatol 1996;23:437.

64. Fletcher JC, Isada NB, Pryde PG, et al. Fetal intracardiac potassium chloride injection to avoid the hopeless resuscitation of an abnormal abortus. II. Ethical issues. Obstet Gynecol 1992;80:310.

65. Evans MI, Goldberg JD, Dommergues M, et al. Efficacy of second trimester selective termination for fetal abnormalities: international collaborative experience among the world's largest centers. Am J Obstet Gynecol 1994;171:90.

66. Chervenak FA, Farley MA, Walters L, et al. When is termination of pregnancy during the third trimester morally justifiable? N Engl J Med 1984;310:501.

67. Chervenak FA, McCullough LB, Campbell S. Is third trimester abortion justified? Br J Obstet Gynaecol 1995;102:434.

68. Chervenak FA, McCullough LB, Campbell S. Third trimester abortion: is compassion enough? Br J Obstet Gynaecol 1999;106:293.

69. Sen A. Inequality reexamined. Cambridge, MA: Harvard University Press, 1992.

70. Chervenak FA, McCullough LB. Nonaggressive obstetric management: an option for some fetal anomalies during the third trimester. JAMA 1989;261:3439.

71. Chervenak FA, Romero R. Is there a role for fetal cephalocentesis in modern obstetrics? Am J Perinatol 1984;1:170.

72. Chasen S, Chervenak FA, McCullough LB. The role of cephalocentesis in modern obstetrics. Am J Obstet Gynecol 2001;185:734.

73. Chervenak FA, Isaacson G, Campbell S. Anomalies of the cranium and its contents: textbook of ultrasound in obstetrics and gynecology. Boston: Little, Brown, 1993:825.

74. Chervenak FA, Berkowitz RL, Tortora M, et al. Management of fetal hydrocephalus. Am J Obstet Gynecol 1985;151:933.

75. Clark SL, DeVore GR, Platt LD. The role of ultrasound in the aggressive management of obstructed labor secondary to fetal malformations. Am J Obstet Gynecol 1985;152:1042.

76. Raimondi AJ, Soare P. Intellectual development in shunted hydrocephalic children. Am J Dis Child 1974;127:664.

77. McCullough DC, Balzer-Martin LA. Current prognosis in overt neonatal hydrocephalus. J Neurosurg 1982;57:378.

78. Sutton LN, Bruce DA, Schut L. Hydranencephaly versus maximal hydrocephalus: an important clinical distinction. Neurosurgery 1980;6:35.

79. Lorber J. The results of early treatment on extreme hydrocephalus. Med Child Neurol (Suppl) 1968;16:21.

80. Nyberg DA, Mack LA, Hirsch J, et al. Fetal hydrocephalus: sonographic detection and clinical significance of associated anomalies. Radiology 1987;163:187.

81. Chervenak FA, McCullough LB. An ethically justified, clinically comprehensive management strategy for third-trimester pregnancies complicated by fetal anomalies. Obstet Gynecol 1990;75:311.

82. Sugarman J, Kass NE, Goodman SN, et al. What patients say about medical research. IRB 1998;20:1.

83. Brody BA. The ethics of research: an international perspective. New York: Oxford University Press, 1998.

84. McCormick RJ. To save or let die: the dilemma of modern medicine. JAMA 1974;229:172.

85. Fletcher JC, Richter G. Human fetal gene therapy: moral and ethical questions. Hum Gene Ther 1996;7:1605.
86. Chervenak FA, McCullough LB. A comprehensive ethical framework for fetal research and its application to fetal surgery for spina bifida. Am J Obstet Gynecol 2002;187:10.
87. Department of Health and Human Services. Regulations for the protection of human subjects. 45 CFR 46.
88. Lilford RJ. The substantive ethics of clinical trials. Clin Obstet Gynecol 1992;35:837.
89. American College of Obstetricians and Gynecologists. Ethics in obstetrics and gynecology. Washington, DC: American College of Obstetricians and Gynecologists, 2002.
90. Association of Professors of Gynecology and Obstetrics. Exploring medical–legal issues in obstetrics and gynecology. Washington, DC: APGO Medical Education Foundation, 1994.
91. FIGO Committee for the Study of Ethical Aspects of Human Reproduction. Recommendations of ethical issues in obstetrics and gynecology. London: International Federation of Gynecology and Obstetrics, 1997.

Aubrey Milunsky, M.B.B.Ch., D.Sc., F.R.C.P.,
F.A.C.M.G., D.C.H.

Appendix: Prenatal Diagnosis of Additional Miscellaneous Genetic Disorders

This appendix briefly mentions a few additional disorders for which prenatal diagnosis either has been achieved or is possible (Table A.1). Careful use of the index will, in all likelihood, reveal some mention of or reference to the overwhelming majority of categorical disorders detectable prenatally. Clearly, the rapid rate of advances in human genetics makes it impossible to deal with every single disorder for which prenatal diagnosis has become possible.

GENETIC SYNDROMIC AND NONSYNDROMIC DEAFNESS/HEARING IMPAIRMENT AND PRENATAL DIAGNOSIS

Hearing loss occurs in between 1 and 2 per 1000 children born, more than 50 percent having a genetic cause. Hundreds of genes are now known to cause deafness/hearing impairment that may be conductive, sensorineural, or mixed. Hearing impairment may be a feature of a genetic syndrome or be nonsyndromic, both with autosomal dominant, recessive, X-linked, or mitochondrial inheritance manifesting before or after language develops.[114]

For the most part, prenatal diagnosis for nonsyndromic hearing impairment appears to have little appeal. Nevertheless, prenatal diagnosis for prelingual deafness based on mutation analysis from amniocyte or chorionic villus sampling (CVS) DNA has been offered.[115]

More than 70 percent of genetic hearing impairment is nonsyndromic. For a number of these disorders, both recessive and dominant as well as X-linked loci are recognized for either the same disorder or an allelic variant. About 80 percent of prelingual nonsyndromic hearing impairment is due to autosomal recessive inheritance, about 20–25 percent is of autosomal dominant origin, and only 1–1.5 percent is X-linked. More than half of those with autosomal recessive nonsyndromic hearing impairment have mutations in the *connexin* (*GJB2*) gene. The common mutation (35delG) in this gene is found in about one in thirty-three Caucasians. A common mutation (167delT) in this gene is found in

Table A.1. Additional selected monogenic disorders for which prenatal diagnosis has been accomplished or is possible

Disorder	MIM No.	Inheritance	Selected Clinical Features	Prenatal Diagnosis	Selected References
Adrenal hypoplasia	300200	X-L	Clinical adrenal insufficiency; possible hypogonadotropic hypogonadism	DNA[a]	1,2
Alagille syndrome	118450	AD	Dysmorphic; neonatal cholestatic jaundice; ocular embryotoxon; pigmentary retinopathy; pulmonary stenosis, peripheral arterial stenosis; skeletal abnormalities	High-resolution chromosome analysis; fluorescence in situ hybridization	3,4
α-1-antitrypsin deficiency	107400	AR	Asthma, emphysema, obstructive lung disease and liver disease	DNA[a]	5
α-thalassemia/mental retardation syndrome	301040	X-L	Severe developmental delay, characteristic facial appearance, genital anomalies, mild thalassemia	DNA[a]	6–8
Amyloidosis, cerebroarterial, Dutch type	104760	AD	Hereditary cerebral hemorrhage with strokes and dementia	DNA[a]	9,10
Amyloidosis, cerebroarterial, Icelandic type	105150	AD	Fatal cerebral hemorrhage in normotensive young adults	DNA[a]	11,12
Amyloidosis, Finnish type	105120	AD	Systemic amyloidosis with corneal lattice dystrophy and peripheral polyneuropathy	DNA[a]	13–15
Aniridia	106210	AD	Variable iris hypoplasia with panocular defects	DNA[a]	16
Aortic aneurysm (familial)	120180	AD	Abdominal aortic aneurysm	DNA[a] and ultrasound	17
Aortic aneurysm, ascending and dissection	134797	AD	Mild aortic root enlargement to aneurysm and/or dissection in the absence of classical signs of Marfan syndrome	DNA[a] and ultrasound	18–21
Bartter syndrome	601678	AR	A salt-losing nephropathy with sensorineural deafness occurring in 1 of 4 variants	DNA[a]	22–25
Bernard-Soulier disease	231200	AR	A bleeding disorder	DNA[a]	26–28
Blomstrand lethal osteochondrodysplasia	215045	AR	Rhizomesomelic short limb skeletal dysplasia, with increased bone density and advance skeletal maturation	By first- or second-trimester ultrasound	29–34
Cardiomyopathy, familial hypertrophic	115195 115196	AD AD	Variable clinical spectrum; heart failure; progressive; sudden death	DNA[a]	35–37
Cardiomyopathy, X-linked dilated	302045	X-L	Heart failure; progressive; arrhythmias	DNA[a]	38–40
Carnitine-acyl-carnitine translocase deficiency	212138	AR	A disorder of long-chain fatty acid oxidation with possible liver failure, and lethal outcome without treatment	DNA[a]	34a

Disease	OMIM	Inheritance	Description	Method	Ref.
Central core disease	130901	AD	Fetal akinesia and death, arthrogryposis, hypotrophy, hypotonia, skeletal abnormalities	DNA[a]	41–43
Cerebro-oculofacio-skeletal syndrome	214150	AR	A nucleotide excision-repair disorder with progressive brain atrophy and calcifications, cataracts, microcornea, optic atrophy, joint contractures, and growth failure	DNA[a]	44
Colon cancer, hereditary nonpolyposis	120435	AD	Nonpolyposis colon cancer	DNA[a]	45,46
Combined hyperlipidemia, familial	238600	AR	Severe hypertriglyceridemia, eruptive xanthomas, hepatosplenomegaly, and (hyperlipidemia type VI) recurrent acute pancreatitis	DNA[a]	47,48
Congenital afibrinogenemia	202400	AR	Bleeding that may be uncontrollable	DNA[a]	49
Congenital insensitivity to pain, anhidrosis	256800	AR	Congenital insensitivity to pain with anhidrosis and recurrent episodes of unexplained fever, self-mutilating behavior, and mental retardation	DNA[a]	50
Conradi-Hunermann-Happle syndrome	302960	X-L	A cholesterol x-linked dominant synthetic disorder resulting in chondrodysplasia punctata primarily in females, mostly lethal in males. Neurocognitive delay. Seizures and congenital anomalies may also be evident.	DNA[a]	51
Diabetes insipidus	125700	AD	Deficient vasopressin synthesis, delayed onset but progressive	DNA[a]	52–54
Diabetes insipidus (nephrogenic)	304800	X-L	Polyuria, polydipsia, and hyposthenuria, resistant to vasopressin. Signs evident within the first week of life. Without diagnosis and treatment, seizures and death will occur.	DNA[a]	55,56
Diastrophic dysplasia, including atelosteogenesis type 2 and achondrogenesis type 1b	222600	AR	Chondrodysplasias of variable severity	DNA[a]	57–60
Dihydropyrimidine dehydrogenase deficiency	274270	AR	Cerebral dysfunction and uraciluria; severe reaction to fluorouracil	DNA[a]	61–63
Elliptocytosis/spherocytosis	182860 182870	AR	Hemolytic anemia	DNA[a]	64–66
Ellis van Creveld syndrome	225500	AR	Dwarfism, polydactyly, and cardiac and multiple other abnormalities	DNA[a]	66a
Factor VII deficiency	227500	AD	A bleeding disorder	DNA[a]	67
Factor X deficiency	227600	AR	Predisposition to prolonged bleeding (e.g., nasal, mucosal, uterine, joints)	DNA[a]	68

(continued)

Table A.1. Additional selected monogenic disorders for which prenatal diagnosis has been accomplished or is possible (*continued*)

Disorder	MIM No.	Inheritance	Selected Clinical Features	Prenatal Diagnosis	Selected References
Foveomacular dystrophy, adult onset with choroidal neovascularization	179605	AD	Macular dystrophy	DNA[a]	69,70
Glanzmann thrombasthenia	273800	AR	A bleeding disorder due to defective platelets	DNA[a]	71
Hereditary nephrolithiasis (Dent disease)	300009	X-L	A renal tubular disorder with proteinuria, hypercalciuria, nephrocalcinosis, renal stones, and renal failure	DNA[a]	72–74
Holoprosencephaly	236100	AD	Developmental abnormality of forebrain and face with wide, intrafamilial variability; marked heterogeneity with at least 6 different genes involved	DNA[a]	75
Hypokalemic periodic paralysis	170400	AD	Episodic paralysis of varying severity	DNA[a]	76–78
Lafora disease	254780	AR	Grand mal seizures and/or myoclonus, rapid mental deterioration and early death	DNA[a]	79,79a
Laron dwarfism	262500	AR	Dwarfism, especially in people of Mediterranean origin	DNA[a]	80,81
Lysinuric protein intolerance	222700	AR	A dibasic amino acid transport disorder	DNA[a]	82
MASA syndrome	303350	X-L	Variable phenotype with hydrocephalus, spastic paraplegia, and agenesis of corpus callosum	DNA[a]	83–84
Molybdenum cofactor deficiency	252150	AR	Mental retardation, dislocated lenses, myoclonic spasms	DNA[a]	86
Muir-Torre syndrome	158320	AD	One or more low-grade visceral malignancies, sebaceous tumors of the skin with or without keratoacanthomas	DNA[a]	87–90
Mullerian duct syndrome, persistent	261550	AR	Otherwise normal 46,XY males who have a uterus, cervix, and fallopian tubes	DNA[a]	91,92
Netherton disease	256500	AR	Severe ichthyosis, frequently lethal	DNA[a]	93
Nijmegen breakage syndrome	251260	AR	An inherited chromosome instability syndrome with microcephaly, dysmorphic facies, immunodeficiency, and predisposition to malignancy	DNA[a]	94

Disorder		Inheritance	Clinical features	Prenatal diagnosis	References
Osteopetrosis, malignant infantile	259700	AR	Macrocephaly, progressive deafness and blindness, anemia, hepatosplenomegaly, dense bones, and other features	DNA[a]	95,96
Pachyonychia congenita type I	177000	AD	Ectodermal dysplasia, severe nail dystrophy, palmoplantar keratoderma and oral lesions	DNA[a]	97,98
Paramyotonia congenita	170500	AD	Cold-induced paradoxical myotonia; possible muscle atrophy; possible episodes of paralysis	DNA[a]	76,99
Protoporphyria, erythropoietic	177000	AD	Photosensitivity; possible acute hepatic failure	DNA[a]	100–103
Retinitis pigmentosa, rhodopsin-related	180380	AD	Vision loss; night blindness	DNA[a]	104
Sorsby fundus dystrophy	136900	AD	Midlife visual impairment leading to blindness	DNA[a]	105–107
Schmid metaphyseal chondrodysplasia	156500	AD	Chondrodysplasia, bow legs, coxa vara	DNA[a]	108
Trichothiodystrophy	601675	AR	Congenital ichthyosis (collodion baby), some with brittle nails and hair and ichthyosiform erythroderma	Fetal hair (eyebrow) biopsy in second trimester for polarized microscopy, electron microscopy, analysis of sulfur content, and staining	109,111
Vitamin D-dependent rickets (type II)	277440	AR	Severe hypocalcemia, growth retardation, and frequent alopecia due to hereditary failure to respond to 1,25-dihydroxyvitamin D^3	Assay to assess binding of 1,25-dihydroxy vitamin D^3	110
Zellweger syndrome	214100	AR	Multiple genes, craniofacial dysmorphism and abnormalities of hands and feet, kidneys, cartilage and brain, inter alia	DNA[a]	112,113

[a]Prenatal diagnosis possible by mutation and/or DNA linkage analysis.

AD = autosomal dominant

AR = autosomal recessive

X-L = sex-linked recessive

Table A.2. Examples of genetic syndromic disorders with deafness/hearing impairment for which prenatal diagnosis might be considered using mutation and/or linkage analysis

Syndrome/Disorder	Genetics	Common Features	Selected References
Alport syndrome	X-L	Progressive nephropathy and ocular lesions	116
Alstrom syndrome	AR	Retinal pigmentary degeneration and blindness, obesity, diabetes mellitus, and chronic nephropathy	117
Bartter syndrome	AR	Renal salt-wasting, hypotension, hypokalemic metabolic alkalosis, hypercalciuria, renal stones	118
Branchio-otorenal syndrome	AD	Preauricular fistula, ear and kidney abnormalities	119
Charcot-Marie-Tooth syndrome	AD	Muscle atrophy, sensory loss and deformities of hands and feet	120
Coffin-Lowry syndrome	X-L	Psychomotor retardation, dysmorphic features, hypotonia, skeletal changes and multiple other variable anomalies	121
Feingold syndrome	AD	Multiple variable anomalies including microcephaly, digital anomalies, esophageal, duodenal or anal atresia, and vertebral, cardiac, and renal abnormalities	122
Focal segmental glomerulosclerosis	AD	Progressive nephropathy	123
Jervell and Lange-Nielsen syndrome	AR	Syncope, cardiac arrhythmias with prolongation of the QT interval, and sudden death	124
Keratitis-ichthyosis deafness syndrome	AD	Visual loss, ichthyosis and palmoplantar keratoderma	125
Norrie disease	X-L	Pseudotumor of the retina and other retinal abnormalities, cataracts, phthisis bulbi, mental retardation	126
Oculodentodigital dysplasia	AD	Craniofacial dysmorphisms (ocular, nasal, and dental) and limb abnormalities, spastic paraplegia and neurodegeneration	127
Oculo-otodental syndrome	AD	Iris and retina colobomas and enlarged teeth	128
Stickler syndrome	AD	Progressive myopia, vitreoretinal degeneration, premature joint degeneration, craniofacial abnormalities, and vertebral irregularities	129
Treacher Collins syndrome	AD	Coloboma of the lower eyelid, micrognathia, microtia, hypoplasia of the zygomatic arches, macrostomia and downward displacement of the lateral canthi	130
Usher type I	AR	Deafness and blindness	131,132
Waardenburg syndrome	AD	Dystopia canthorum (type I), heterochromia irides, hypopigmentation, limb abnormalities (type III), Hirschsprung disease (type IV) (AR)	133–135
Wolfram syndrome type I	AR	Diabetes insipidus, diabetes mellitus, and optic atrophy	136,137
Zellweger syndrome	AR	Liver disease, variable neurodevelopmental delay, retinopathy, mental retardation, short stature, craniofacial dysmorphism, large, soft hands with lax skin and tapering fingers	112

AD = autosomal dominant
AR = autosomal recessive
X-L = sex-linked recessive

about one in twenty-six of those of Ashkenazi Jewish ancestry. Prenatal diagnosis is available only when specific mutations have been recognized in both parents.

Prenatal diagnosis is a more realistic consideration when hearing impairment associated with genetically recognized syndromes is in question. More than 400 genetic syndromes that include hearing impairment have been described, and these account for about 30 percent of cases of prelingual deafness. When prenatal diagnosis is pursued for one of these genetic syndromes, it is invariably the associated features rather than the hearing impairment that provide parents with the greatest concern. A few of these genetic syndromes with associated hearing impairment in which genes have been identified are shown in Table A.2. Generally, prenatal diagnosis would proceed only when a dominant, recessive, or X-linked gene mutation has been predetermined in one or both parents.

PRENATAL DIAGNOSIS OF MITOCHONDRIAL DISORDERS

Primary mitochondrial diseases are due to defects in mitochondrial DNA (mtDNA),[138–140] which are transmitted via maternal inheritance. This means that all mitochondria in the zygote derive from the ovum, thus far with rare exceptions. Hence, an affected mother with a mitochondrial disorder would transmit to all of her children, but subsequently her sons, while affected, would not be transmitters. A characteristic feature of this form of inheritance is that the pathogenic mutations in mtDNA are present in some but not necessarily all mitochondria. This situation, known as heteroplasmy, will be highly variable with greater clinical manifestations reflecting high mutant loads. Moreover, the highly variable distribution of mutations within mtDNA will vary from tissue to tissue. Tissues that are highly dependent on oxidative metabolism, such as the brain, heart, skeletal muscle, retina, renal tubules, and endocrine glands are particularly vulnerable to the effects of mutations in mtDNA. Mitochondrial disorders are more common than originally thought, and current estimates suggest an estimated prevalence of 10–15 cases per 100,000 individuals.[138]

Prenatal diagnosis of mitochondrial disorders is fraught with difficulty. Extremely careful genetic counseling will inform an affected mother of the likely 100 percent transmission of her mutation to all of her offspring. Key to the clinical manifestations is the size of the mutant load transmitted and the tissue distribution of the abnormal mitochondria. Hence, such parents will have to understand that assessment of the mutant load from CVS or amniocyte cells may not necessarily reflect ultimate fetal health and welfare. A low mutant load may not necessarily result in a child with few or no clinical features and, moreover, be uninformative about future health. Notwithstanding the obvious lack of guarantees in these circumstances, a number of cases have been reported for the prenatal diagnosis of Leigh syndrome, more specifically of the T8993G mutation[141–144] and of the T8993C mutation.[145] Although descriptions of "a healthy baby" have followed, much longer follow-up would be necessary for any certainty to attach to such a fortunate result.

In the very difficult circumstances of an affected mother having lost one or more affected children, ovum donation may be a realistic option.

REFERENCES

1. Kinoshita E, Yoshimoto M, Motomura K, et al. DAX-1 gene mutations and deletions in Japanese patients with adrenal hypoplasia congenita and hypogonadotropic hypogonadism. Horm Res 1997;48:29.
2. Peter M, Partsch CJ, Dorr HG, et al. Prenatal diagnosis of congenital adrenal hypoplasia. Horm Res 1996;46:41.

3. Albayram F, Stone K, Nagey D, et al. Alagille syndrome: prenatal diagnosis and pregnancy outcome. Fetal Diagn Ther 2002;17:182.

4. Ropke A, Kujat A, Graber M, et al. Identification of 36 novel Jagged1 (JAG1) mutations in patients with Alagille syndrome. Hum Mutat 2003;21:100.

5. Abbott CM, Lovegrove JU, Whitehouse DB, et al. Prenatal diagnosis of alpha-1 antitrypsin deficiency by PCR of linked polymorphisms: a study of 17 cases. Prenat Diagn 1992;12:235.

6. Gibbons RJ, Brueton L, Buckle VJ, et al. Clinical and hematologic aspects of the X-linked alpha-thalassemia/mental retardation syndrome (ATR-X). Am J Med Genet 1995;55:288.

7. Lamb J, Harris PC, Wilkie AO, et al. De novo truncation of chromosome 16p and healing with (TTAGGG)n in the alpha-thalassemia/mental retardation syndrome (ATR-16). Am J Hum Genet 1993;52:668.

8. Fichera M, Silengo M, Spalletta A, et al. Prenatal diagnosis of ATR-X syndrome in a fetus with a new G>T splicing mutation in the XNP/ATR-X gene. Prenat Diagn 2001;21:747.

9. Bornebroek M, Haan J, Van Duinen SG, et al. Dutch hereditary cerebral amyloid angiopathy: structural lesions an apolipoprotein E genotype. Ann Neurol 1997;41:695.

10. Mann DM, Iwatsubo T, Ihara Y, et al. Predominant deposition of amyloid-beta 42(43) in plaques in cases of Alzheimer's disease and hereditary cerebral hemorrhage associated with mutations in the amyloid precursor protein gene. Am J Pathol 1996;148:1257.

11. Olafsson I, Thorsteinsson L, Jensson O. The molecular pathology of hereditary cystatin C amyloid angiopathy causing brain hemorrhage. Brain Pathol 1996;6:121.

12. Liberski PP, Barcikowska M. Pathology of the vessels in cerebral amyloid angiopathy. Folia Neuropathol 1995;33:207.

13. Kangas H, Paunio T, Kalkkinen N, et al. In vitro expression analysis shows that the secretory form of gelsolin is the sole source of amyloid in gelsolin-related amyloidosis. Hum Mol Genet 1996;5:1237.

14. Paunio T, Sunada Y, Kiuru S, et al. Haplotype analysis in gelsolin-related amyloidosis reveals independent origin of identical mutation (G654A) of gelsolin in Finland and Japan. Hum Mutat 1995;6:60.

15. Carvalho F, Sousa M, Fernandes S, et al. Preimplantation genetic diagnosis for familial amyloidotic polyneuropathy (FAP). Prenat Diagn 2001;21:1093.

16. Churchill AJ, Hanson IM, Markham AF. Prenatal diagnosis of aniridia. Ophthalmology 2000;107:1153.

17. Schrijver I. Liu W, Francke U. The pathogenicity of the Pro1148Ala substitution in the FBN1 gene: causing or predisposing to Marfan syndrome and aortic aneurysm, or clinically innocent? Hum Genet 1997;99:607.

18. Francke U, Berg MA, Tynan K, et al. A Gly1127Ser mutation in an EGF-like domain of the fibrillin-1 gene is a risk factor for ascending aortic aneurysm and dissection. Am J Hum Genet 1995;56:1287.

19. Malee MP, Carr S, Rubin LP, et al. Prenatal ultrasound diagnosis of abdominal aortic aneurysm with fibrotic occlusion in aortic branch vessels. Prenat Diagn 1997;17:479.

20. Kakko S, Raisanen T, Tamminen M, et al. Candidate locus analysis of familial ascending aortic aneurysms and dissections confirms the linkage to the chromosome 5q13-14 in Finnish families. J Thorac Cardiovasc Surg 2003;126:106.

21. Hasham SN, Willing MC, Guo DC, et al. Mapping a locus for familial thoracic aortic aneurysms and dissections (TAAD2) to 3p24-25. Circulation 2003;107:3184.

22. Derst C, Konrad M, Kockerling A, et al. Mutations in the ROMK gene in antenatal Bartter syndrome are associated with impaired K+ channel function. Biochem Biophys Res Commun 1997;230(3):641.

23. International Collaborative Study Group for Bartter-like Syndromes. Mutations in the gene encoding the inwardly-rectifying renal potassium channel, ROMK, cause the antenatal variant of Bartter syndrome: evidence for genetic heterogeneity. Hum Mol Genet 1997;6:17.

24. Shalev H, Ohaly M, Meizner I, et al. Prenatal diagnosis of Bartter syndrome. Prenat Diagn 1994;14:996.

25. Birkenhager R, Otto E, Schurmann MJ, et al. Mutation of BSND causes Bartter syndrome with sensorineural deafness and kidney failure. Nat Genet 2001;29:310.

26. Sachs UJ, Kroll H, Matzdorff AC, et al. Bernard-Soulier syndrome due to the homozygous Asn-45Ser mutation in GPIX: an unexpected, frequent finding in Germany. Br J Haematol 2003;123:127.

27. de la Salle C, Baas MJ, Lanza F, et al. A three-base deletion removing a leucine residue in a leucine-rich repeat of platelet glycoprotein Ib alpha associated with a variant of Bernard–Soulier syndrome (Nancy I). Br J Haematol 1995;89:386.

28. Watanabe R, Ishibashi T, Saitoh Y, et al. Bernard–Soulier syndrome with a homozygous 13 base pair deletion in the signal peptide-coding region of the platelet glycoprotein Ib(beta) gene. Blood Coagul Fibrinolysis 2003;14:387.

29. den Hollander NS, van der harten HJ, Vermeij-Keers C, et al. First-trimester diagnosis of Blomstrand lethal osteochondrodysplasia. Am J Med Genet 1997;73:345.

30. Spranger J, Maroteaux P. The lethal osteochondrodysplasias. In: Harris H, Hirschhorn K, eds. Advances in human genetics, vol. 19. New York: Plenum Press, 1990:1.

31. Young ID, Zuccollo JM, Broderick NJ. A lethal skeletal dysplasia with generalised sclerosis and advanced skeletal maturation: Blomstrand chondrodysplasia? J Med Genet 1993;30:155.

32. Leroy JG, Keersmaeckers G, Coppens M, et al. Blomstrand lethal osteochondrodysplasia. Am J Med Genet 1996;63:84.

33. Galera MF, de Silva Patricio FR, Lederman HM, et al. Blomstrand chondrodysplasia: a lethal sclerosing skeletal dysplasia: case report and review. Pediatr Radiol 1999;29:842.

34. Karperien M, van der Harten HJ, van Schooten R, et al. A frame-shift mutation in the type I parathyroid hormone (PTH)/PTH-related peptide receptor causing Blomstrand lethal osteochondrodysplasia. J Clin Endocrinol Metab 1999;84:3713.

34a. Costa C, Costa JM, Slama A, et al. Mutational spectrum and DNA-based prenatal diagnosis in carnitine-acylcarnitine translocase deficiency. Mol Genet Metab 2003;78:68.

34b. Chalmers RA, Stanley CA, English N, et al. Mitochondrial carnitine-acylcarnitine translocase deficiency presenting as sudden neonatal death. J Pediatr 1997;131:220.

35. Richard P, Charron P, Carrier L, et al. Hypertrophic cardiomyopathy: distribution of disease genes, spectrum of mutations, and implications for a molecular diagnosis strategy. Circulation 2003;107:2227.

36. Havndrup O, Bundgaard H, Andersen PS, et al. Outcome of clinical versus genetic family screening in hypertrophic cardiomyopathy with focus on cardiac beta-myosin gene mutations. Cardiovasc Res 2003;57:347.

37. Takeda N. Cardiomyopathy: molecular and immunological aspects. Int J Mol Med 2003;11:13.

38. Feng J, Yan J, Buzin CH, et al. Mutations in the dystrophin gene are associated with sporadic dilated cardiomyopathy. Mol Genet Metab 2002;77:119.

39. Finsterer J, Stollberger C. The heart in human dystrophinopathies. Cardiology 2003;99:1.

40. Flanigan KM, von Niederhausern A, Dunn DM, et al. Rapid direct sequence analysis of the dystrophin gene. Am J Hum Genet 2003;72:931.

41. Phillips MS, Fujii J, Khanna VK, et al. The structural organization of the human skeletal muscle ryanodine receptor (RYR1) gene. Genomics 1996;34:24.

42. Fletcher JE, Tripolitis L, Hubert M, et al. Genotype and phenotype relationships for mutations in the ryanodine receptor in patients referred for diagnosis of malignant hyperthermia. Br J Anaesth 1995;75:307.

43. Romero NB, Monnier N, Viollet L, et al. Dominant and recessive central core disease associated with RYR1 mutations and fetal akinesia. Brain 2003;126:2341.

44. Graham JM Jr, Anyane-Yeboa K, Raams A, et al. Cerebro-oculo-facio-skeletal syndrome with a nucleotide excision-repair defect and a mutated XPD gene, with prenatal diagnosis in a triplet pregnancy. Am J Hum Genet 2001;69:291.

45. Chung DC, Rustgi AK. The hereditary nonpolyposis colorectal cancer syndrome: genetics and clinical implications. Ann Intern Med 2003;138:560.

46. Robbins DH, Itzkowitz SH. The molecular and genetic basis of colon cancer. Med Clin North Am 2002;86:1467.

47. Pajukanta P, Allayee H, Krass KL, et al. Combined analysis of genome scans of Dutch and Finnish families reveals a susceptibility locus for high-density lipoprotein cholesterol on chromosome 16q. Am J Hum Genet 2003;72:903.

48. Kypreos KE, Li X, van Dijk KW, et al. Molecular mechanisms of type III hyperlipoproteinemia: the contribution of the carboxy-terminal domain of ApoE can account for the dyslipidemia that is associated with the E2/E2 phenotype. Biochemistry 2003;42:9841.

49. Neerman-Arbez M, Vu D, Abu-Libdeh B, et al. Prenatal diagnosis for congenital afibrinogenemia caused by a novel nonsense mutation in the FGB gene in a Palestinian family. Blood 2003;101:3492.

50. Shatzky S, Moses S, Levy J, et al. Congenital insensitivity to pain with anhidrosis (CIPA) in Israeli-Bedouins: genetic heterogeneity, novel mutations in the TRKA/NGF receptor gene, clinical findings, and results of nerve conduction studies. Am J Med Genet 2000;92:353.

51. Milunsky JM, Maher TA, Metzenberg AB. Molecular, biochemical, and phenotypic analysis of a hemizygous male with a severe atypical phenotype for X-linked dominant Conradi–Hunermann–Happle syndrome and a mutation in EBP. Am J Med Genet 2003;116A:249.

52. Christensen JH, Siggaard C, Rittig S. Autosomal dominant familial neurohypophyseal diabetes insipidus. APMIS Suppl 2003;109:92.

53. Wolf MT, Dotsch J, Metzler M, et al. A new missense mutation of the vasopressin-neurophysin II gene in a family with neurohypophyseal diabetes insipidus. Horm Res 2003;60:143.

54. Elias PC, Elias LL, Torres N, et al. Progressive decline of vasopressin secretion in familial autosomal

dominant neurohypophyseal diabetes insipidus presenting a novel mutation in the vasopressin-neuro-physin II gene. Clin Endocrinol 2003;59:511.

55. Asai T, Kuwahara M, Kurihara H, et al. Pathogenesis of nephrogenic diabetes insipidus by aquaporin-2 C-terminus mutations. Kidney Int 2003;64:2.

56. Bichet DG, Turner M, Morin D. Vasopressin receptor mutations causing nephrogenic diabetes insipidus. Proc Assoc Am Physicians 1998;110:387.

57. Rossi A, van der Harten HJ, et al. Phenotypic and genotypic lap between atelosteogenesis type 2 and diastrophic dysplasia. Hum Genet 1996;98:657.

58. Horton WA. Molecular genetic basis of the human chondrodysplasias. Endocrinol Metab Clin North Am 1996;25:683.

59. Superti-Furga A, Rossi A, Steinmann B, et al. Achondrodysplasia family produced by mutations in the diastrophic dysplasia sulfate transporter gene: genotype/phenotype correlations. Am J Med Genet 1996; 63:144.

60. Rossi A, Superti-Furga A. Mutations in the diastrophic dysplasia sulfate transporter (DTDST) gene (SLC26A2): 22 novel mutations, mutation review, associated skeletal phenotypes, and diagnostic relevance. Hum Mutat 2001;17:159.

61. Jakobs C, Stellaard F, Smit LM, et al. The first prenatal diagnosis of dihydropyrimidine dehydrogenase deficiency. Eur J Pediatr 1991;150:291.

62. Wei X, McLeod HL, McMurrough J, et al. Molecular basis of the human dihydropyrimidine dehydrogenase deficiency and 5-fluorouracil toxicity. J Clin Invest 1996;98:610.

63. Gross E, Seck K, Neubauer S, et al. High-throughput genotyping by DHPLC of the dihydropyrimidine dehydrogenase gene implicated in (fluoro) pyrimidine catabolism. Int J Oncol 2003;22:325.

64. Dhermy D, Feo C, Garbarz M, et al. Prenatal diagnosis of hereditary elliptocytosis with molecular defect of spectrin. Prenat Diagn 1987;7:471.

65. Gallagher PG, Romana M, Wong C, et al. Genetic basis of the polymorphisms of the alphaI-domain of spectrin. Am J Hematol 1997;56:107.

66. Delaunay J. Molecular basis of red cell membrane disorders. Acta Haematol 2002;108:210.

66a. Ruiz-Perez VL, Tompson SW, Blair HJ, et al. Mutations in two nonhomologous genes in a head-to-head configuration cause Ellis–van Creveld syndrome. Am J Hum Genet 2003;72:728.

67. Tamary H, Fromovich-Amit Y, Shalmon L, et al. Molecular characterization of four novel mutations causing factor VII deficiency. Hematol J 2000;1:382.

68. Camire R, Ann Denchy R, Day GA 3rd, et al. Prenatal diagnosis of factor X deficiency using a combination of direct mutation detection and linkage analysis with an intragenic single nucleotide polymorphism. Prenat Diagn 2003;23:457.

69. Feist RM, White MF Jr, Skalka H, et al. Choroidal neovascularization in a patient with adult foveomacular dystrophy and a mutation in the retinal degeneration slow gene (Pro 210 Arg). Am J Ophthalmol 1994;118:259.

70. Yang Z, Lin W, Moshfeghi DM, et al. A novel mutation in the RDS/Peripherin gene causes adult-onset foveomacular dystrophy. Am J Ophthalmol 2003;135:213.

71. French DL, Coller BS, Usher S, et al. Prenatal diagnosis of Glanzmann thrombasthenia using the polymorphic markers BRCA1 and THRA1 on chromosome 17. Br J Haematol 1998;102:582.

72. Fisher SE, van Bakel I, Lloyd SE, et al. Cloning and characterization of CLCN5, the human kidney chloride channel gene implicated in Dent disease (an X-linked hereditary nephrolithiasis). Genomics 1995; 29:598.

73. Tanaka K, Fisher SE, Craig IW. Characterization of novel promoter and enhancer elements of the mouse homologue of the Dent disease gene, CLCN5, implicated in X-linked hereditary nephrolithiasis. Genomics 1999;58:281.

74. Thakker RV. Pathogenesis of Dent's disease and related syndromes of X-linked nephrolithiasis. Kidney Int 2000;57:787.

75. Marini M, Cusano R, DeBiasio P, et al. Previously undescribed nonsense mutation in SHH caused autosomal dominant holoprosencephaly with wide intrafamilial variability. Am J Med Genet 2003;117A:112.

76. Ptacek LJ. Channelopathies: Ion channel disorders of muscle as a paradigm for paroxysmal disorders of the nervous system. Neuromuscul Disord 1997;7:250.

77. Sillen A, Sorensen T, Kantola I, et al. Identification of mutations in the CACNL1A3 gene in 13 families of Scandinavian origin having hypokalemic periodic paralysis and evidence of a founder effect in Danish families. Am J Med Genet 1997;69:102.

78. Fouad G, Dalakas M, Servidei S, et al. Genotype–phenotype correlations of DHP receptor alpha 1-subunit gene mutations causing hypokalemic periodic paralysis. Neuromuscul Disord 1997;7:33.

79. Ganesh S, Delgado-Escueta AV, Suzuki T, et al. Genotype-phenotype correlations for EPM2A mutations in Lafora's progressive myoclonus epilepsy: exon 1 mutations associate with an early-onset cognitive deficit subphenotype. Hum Mol Genet 2002;11:1263.

79a. Chan EM, Young EJ, Ianzano L, et al. Mutations in NHLRC1 cause progressive myoclonus epilepsy. Nat Genet 2003;35:125.

80. Wojcik J, Berg MA, Esposito N, et al. Four contiguous amino acid substitutions, identified in patients with Laron syndrome, differently affect the binding affinity and intracellular trafficking of the growth hormone receptor. J Clin Endocrinol Metab 1998;83:4481.

81. Shevah O, Nunez O, Rubinstein M, et al. Intronic mutation in the growth hormone receptor gene in a Peruvian girl with Laron syndrome. J Pediatr Endocrinol Metab 2002;15:1039.

82. Sperandeo MP, Bassi MT, Riboni M, et al. Structure of the SLC7A7 gene and mutational analysis of patients affected by lysinuric protein intolerance. Am J Hum Genet 2000;66:92.

83. Timor-Tritsch IE, Monteagudo A, Haratz-Rubinstein N, et al. Transvaginal sonographic detection of adducted thumbs, hydrocephalus, and agenesis of the corpus callosum at 22 postmenstrual weeks; the masa spectrum or L1 spectrum: a case report and review of the literature. Prenat Diagn 1996;16:543.

84. Pomili G, Venti Donti G, Alunni Carrozza L, et al. MASA syndrome: ultrasonographic evidence in a male fetus. Prenat Diagn 2000;20:1012.

85. Weller S, Gartner J. Genetic and clinical aspects of X-linked hydrocephalus (L1 disease): mutations in the LICAM gene. Hum Mutat 2001;18:1.

86. Johnson JL. Prenatal diagnosis of molybdenum cofactor deficiency and isolated sulfite oxidase deficiency. Prenat Diagn 2003;23:6.

87. Esche C, Kruse R, Lamberti C, et al. Muir-Torre syndrome: clinical features and molecular genetic analysis. Br J Dermatol 1997;136:913.

88. Schwartz RA, Torre DP. The Muir-Torre syndrome: a 25-year retrospect. J Am Acad Dermatol 1995;33:90.

89. Kruse R, Lamberti C, Wang Y, et al. Is the mismatch repair deficient type of Muir–Torre syndrome confined to mutations in the hMSH2 gene? Hum Genet 1996;98:747.

90. Lucci-Cordisco E, Zito I, Gensini F, et al. Hereditary nonpolyposis colorectal cancer and related conditions. Am J Med Genet 2003;122A:325.

91. Lang-Muritano M, Biason-Lauber A, Gitzelmann C, et al. A novel mutation in the anti-mullerian hormone gene as cause of persistent mullerian duct syndrome. Eur J Pediatr 2001;160:652.

92. MacLaughlin DT, Donahoe PK, Mullerian inhibiting substance: an update. Adv Exp Med Biol 2002; 511:25.

93. Bitoun E, Bodemer C, Amiel J, et al. Prenatal diagnosis of a lethal form of Netherton syndrome by SPINK5 mutation analysis. Prenat Diagn 2002;22:121.

94. Kleier S, Herrmann M, Wittwer B, et al. Clinical presentation and mutation identification in the NBS1 gene in a boy with Nijmegen breakage syndrome. Clin Genet 2000;57:384.

95. Sobacchi C, Frattini A, Orchard P, et al. The mutational spectrum of human malignant autosomal recessive osteopetrosis. Hum Mol Genet 2001;10:1767.

96. Bruder E, Stallmach T, Peier K, et al. Osteoclast morphology in autosomal recessive malignant osteopetrosis due to a TC1RG1 gene mutation. Pediatr Pathol Mol Med 2003;22:3.

97. Smith FJ, McKusick VA, Nielsen K, et al. Cloning of multiple keratin 16 genes facilitates prenatal diagnosis of pachyonychia congenita type 1. Prenat Diagn 1999;19:941.

98. Smith F. The molecular genetics of keratin disorders. Am J Clin Dermatol 2003;4:347.

99. Borg K, Ahlberg G, Anvret M. C4342T-mutation in the SCN4A gene on chromosome 17q in a Swedish family with paramyotonia congenita. Neuromuscul Disord 1997;7:231.

100. Cox TM. Erythropoietic protoporphyria. J Inherit Metab Dis 1997;20:258.

101. Imoto S, Tanizawa Y, Sato Y, et al. A novel mutation in the ferrochelatase gene associated with erythropoietic protoporphyria. Br J Haemtol 1996;94:191.

102. Morris SD, Mason NG, Elder GH, et al. Ferrochelatase gene polymorphism analysis for accurate genetic counselling in erythropoietic protoporphyria. Br J Dermatol 2002;147:572.

103. Wiman A, Floderus Y, Harper P. Novel mutations and phenotypic effect of the splice site modulator IVS3-48C in nine Swedish families with erythropoietic protoporphyria. J Hum Genet 2003;48:70.

104. Tessitore A, Toniato E, Gulino A, et al. Prenatal diagnosis of a rhodopsin mutation using chemical cleavage of the mismatch. Prenat Diagn 2002;22:380.

105. Felbor U, Suvanto EA, Forsius HR, et al. Autosomal recessive Sorsby fundus dystrophy revisited: molecular evidence for dominant inheritance. Am J Hum Genet 1997;60:57.

106. Clarke M, Mitchell KW, Goodship J, et al. Clinical features of a novel TIMP-3 mutation causing Sorsby's fundus dystrophy: implications for disease mechanism. Br J Ophthalmol 2001;85:1429.

107. Qi JH, Ebrahem Q, Yeow K, et al. Expression of Sorsby's fundus dystrophy mutations in human retinal pigment epithelial cells reduces matrix metalloproteinase inhibition and may promote angiogenesis. J Biol Chem 2002;277:13394.

108. Milunsky J, Maher T, Lebo R, et al. Prenatal Diagnosis for Schmid metaphyseal chondrodysplasia in twins. Fetal Diagn Ther 1998;13:167.

109. Quintero RA, Morales WJ, Gilbert-Barness E, et al. In utero diagnosis of trichothiodystrophy by endoscopically-guided fetal eyebrow biopsy. Fetal Diagn Ther 2000;15:152.

110. Weisman Y, Jaccard N, Legum C, et al. Prenatal diagnosis of vitamin D-dependent rickets, type II: response to 1,25-dihydroxyvitamin D in amniotic fluid cells and fetal tissues. J Clin Endocrinol Metab 1990;71:937.

111. Botta E, Nardo T, Lehmann AR, et al. Reduced level of the repair/transcription factor TFIIH in trichothiodystrophy. Hum Mol Genet 2002;11:2919.

112. Gootjes J, Schmohl F, Waterham HR, et al. Novel mutations in the PEX12 gene of patients with a peroxisome biogenesis disorder. Eur J Hum Genet 2004;12:115.

113. Matsumoto N, Tamura S, Furuki S, et al. Mutations in novel peroxin gene PEX26 that cause peroxisome-biogenesis disorders of complementation group 8 provide a genotype–phenotype correlation. Am J Hum Genet 2003;73:233.

114. Nance WE. The genetics of deafness. Ment Retard Dev Disabil Res Rev 2003;9:109.

115. Antoniadi T, Pampanos A, Petersen MB. Prenatal diagnosis of prelingual deafness: carrier testing and prenatal diagnosis of the common GJB2 35delG mutation. Prenat Diagn 2001;21:10.

116. Gross O, Netzer KO, Lambrecht R, et al. Meta-analysis of genotype–phenotype correlation in X-linked Alport syndrome: impact on clinical counselling. Nephrol Dial Transplant 2002;17:1218.

117. Benso C, Hadjadj E, Conrath J, et al. Three new cases of Alstrom syndrome. Graefes Arch Clin Exp Ophthalmol 2002;240:622.

118. Hebert SC. Bartter syndrome. Curr Opin Nephrol Hypertens 2003;12:527.

119. Yashima T, Noguchi Y, Ishikawa K, et al. Mutation of the EYA1 gene in patients with branchio-oto syndrome. Acta Otolaryngol 2003;123:279.

120. Kovach MJ, Campbell KC, Herman K, et al. Anticipation in a unique family with Charcot–Marie–Tooth syndrome and deafness: delineation of the clinical features and review of the literature. Am J Med Genet 2002;108:295.

121. Touraine RL, Zeniou M, Hanauer A. A syndromic form of X-linked mental retardation: the Coffin–Lowry syndrome. Eur J Pediatr 2002;161:179.

122. Celli J, Van Bokhoven H, Brunner HG. Feingold syndrome: clinical review and genetic mapping. Am J Med Genet 2003;122A:294.

123. Prakash S, Chung KW, Sinha S, et al. Autosomal dominant progressive nephropathy with deafness: linkage to a new locus on chromosome 11q24. J Am Soc Nephrol 2003;14:1794.

124. Huang L, Bitner-Glindzicz M, Tranebjaerg L, et al. A spectrum of functional effects for disease causing mutations in the Jervell and Lange–Nielsen syndrome. Cardiovasc Res 2001;51:670.

125. Richard G, Rouan F, Willoughby CE, et al. Missense mutations in GJB2 encoding connexin-26 cause the ectodermal dysplasia keratitis-ichthyosis-deafness syndrome. Am J Hum Genet 2002;70:1341.

126. Berger W. Molecular dissection of Norrie disease. Acta Anat (Basel) 1998;162:95.

127. Paznekas WA, Boyadjiev SA, Shapiro RE, et al. Connexin 43 (GJA1) mutations cause the pleiotropic phenotype of oculodentodigital dysplasia. Am J Hum Genet 2003;72:408.

128. Vierra H, Gregory-Evans K, Lim N, et al. First genomic localization of oculo-oto-dental syndrome with linkage to chromosome 20q13.1. Invest Ophthalmol Vis Sci 2002;43:2540.

129. Liberfarb RM, Levy HP, Rose PS, et al. The Stickler syndrome: genotype/phenotype correlation in 10 families with Stickler syndrome resulting from seven mutations in the type II collagen gene locus COL2A1. Genet Med 2003;5:21.

130. Ellis PE, Dawson M, Dixon MJ. Mutation testing in Treacher Collins Syndrome. J Orthod 2002;29:293.

131. Weil D, El-Amraoui A, Masmoudi S, et al. Usher syndrome type I G (USH1G) is caused by mutations in the gene encoding SANS, a protein that associates with the USH1C protein, harmonin. Hum Mol Genet 2003;12:463.

132. Najera C, Beneyto M, Blanca J, et al. Mutations in myosin VIIA (MYO7A) and usherin (USH2A) in Spanish patients with Usher syndrome types I and II, respectively. Hum Mutat 2002;20:76.

133. Baldwin CT, Hoth CF, Amos JA, et al. An exonic mutation in the HuP2 paired domain gene causes Waardenburg syndrome. Nature 1992;355:637.

134. Hoth CF, Milunsky A, Lipsky N, et al. Mutations in the paired domain of the Human PAX3 gene cause

Klein-Waardenburg syndrome (WS-III) as well as Waardenburg syndrome type I (WS-I). Am J Hum Gen 1993;52:455.

135. Read AP. Hereditary deafness: lessons for developmental studies and genetic diagnosis. Eur J Pediatr 2000;159:S232.

136. Lesperance MM, Hall JW 3rd, San Agustin TB, et al. Mutations in the Wolfram syndrome type 1 gene (WFS1) define a clinical entity of dominant low-frequency sensorineural hearing loss. Arch Otolaryngol Head Neck Surg 2003;129:411.

137. Domenech E, Gomez-Zaera M, Nunes V. WFS1 mutations in Spanish patients with diabetes mellitus and deafness. Eur J Hum Genet 2002;10:421.

138. DiMauro S, Schon EA. Mitochondrial respiratory-chain diseases. N Engl J Med 2003:348:2656.

139. DiMauro S, Andreu AL, DeVivo DC. Mitochondrial disorders. J Child Neurol 2002;17 Suppl 3:3535.

140. Sciacco M, Prelle A, Comi GP, et al. Retrospective study of a large population of patients affected with mitochondrial disorders: clinical, morphological and molecular genetic evaluation. J Neurol 2001;248:778.

141. Harding AE, Holt IJ, Sweeney MG, et al. Prenatal diagnosis of mitochondrial DNA 8993T-G disease. Am J Hum Genet 1992;50:629.

142. Ferlin T, Landrieu P, Rambaud C, et al. Segregation of the G8993 mutant mitochondrial DNA through generations and the embryonic tissues in a family at risk of Leigh syndrome. J Pediatr 1997;131:447.

143. White SL, Shanske S, Biros I, et al. Two cases of prenatal analysis for the pathologic T to G substitution at nucleotide 8993 in mitochondrial DNA. Prenat Diagn 1999;19:1165.

144. Bartley J, Senadheera D, Park P, et al. Prenatal diagnosis of T8993G mitochondrial DNA point mutation in amniocytes by heteroplasmy detection. Am J Hum Genet 1996;59:A317.

145. Leshinsky-Silver E, Perach M, Basilevsky E, et al. Prenatal exclusion of Leigh syndrome due to T8993C mutation in the mitochondrial DNA. Prenat Diagn 2003;23:31.

Index

Note: Boldface page numbers indicate main discussion; t denotes tables; and f denotes figures.